Newborn Surgery
Fourth Edition

Newborn Surgery

Fourth Edition

Edited by

Prem Puri
Newman Clinical Research Professor
and
Conway Institute of Biomolecular and Biomedical Research
University College Dublin
and
Beacon Hospital
Dublin, Ireland

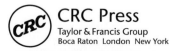
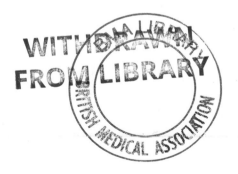

CRC Press
Taylor & Francis Group
Boca Raton London New York

CRC Press is an imprint of the
Taylor & Francis Group, an **informa** business

CRC Press
Taylor & Francis Group
6000 Broken Sound Parkway NW, Suite 300
Boca Raton, FL 33487-2742

© 2018 by Taylor & Francis Group, LLC
CRC Press is an imprint of Taylor & Francis Group, an Informa business

No claim to original U.S. Government works

Printed on acid-free paper

International Standard Book Number-13: 978-1-4822-4770-1 (Pack - Book and eBook)

Visit the Taylor & Francis Web site at
http://www.taylorandfrancis.com

and the CRC Press Web site at
http://www.crcpress.com

To Veena, Abir, Anita, and Niki, for their love and patience.

Contents

Preface to the fourth edition

Newborn surgery has reached a high degree of sophistication and is now recognized as an independent discipline in pediatric surgery. The more comprehensive understanding of the pathophysiology of various neonatal disorders, advances in specialized neonatal anesthesia and intensive care, as well as the introduction of new surgical techniques including minimally invasive surgery have dramatically improved survival in neonatal surgical conditions. Recent advances in the fields of regenerative medicine and tissue engineering offer hope in the future to provide stem cell–based constructs for the reconstruction of some birth defects.

It has been six years since the third edition of the book (published in 2011). The fourth edition of *Newborn Surgery* has been thoroughly revised and updated, and contains 112 chapters by 194 contributors from five continents. This edition contains nine new chapters on key topics, including transition to extrauterine life, specific risks for the preterm infant, access for enteral nutrition, patient safety, tissue engineering and stem cell research, surgical aspects of HIV infection, stridor in infants, stomas of small and large intestine, and spontaneous intestinal perforation. Each chapter has been written by internationally renowned leaders in their respective fields. Several younger surgeons were selected as coauthors, who will become the next generation of leaders in pediatric surgery.

This book is intended for those who have a clinical responsibility for newborn babies. It provides an authoritative, comprehensive, and complete account of the pathophysiology and surgical management of neonatal disorders. The book is specifically designed for pediatric surgeons, trainees in pediatric surgery, pediatric urologists, as well as neonatologists and pediatricians seeking more detailed information on newborn surgical conditions. It is my sincere hope that the readers will find this textbook a useful reference in the management of surgical disorders in the newborn.

I wish to thank most sincerely all the contributors from around the world for their precious time and outstanding work in the preparation of this innovative textbook. I also wish to express my gratitude to Dr. Julia Zimmer and Dr. Hiroki Nakamura for their help with the galley proofs of the book. I wish to thank the editorial staff of CRC Press, particularly Ms. Miranda Bromage, for all their help during the preparation and publication of this book. I am thankful to the National Children's Research Centre, Our Lady's Children's Hospital, Dublin for their support.

Prem Puri
2017

Preface to the third edition

It has been eight years since the second edition of the book was published in 2003. Over the last decade, major advances have occurred in the understanding and treatment of neonatal surgical conditions. Advances in prenatal diagnosis, imaging, intensive care, and minimally invasive surgery have transformed the practice of surgery in the newborn. The third edition of *Newborn Surgery* has been extensively revised and contains 105 chapters by 160 contributors from five continents of the world. This edition contains many new chapters taking account of the recent advances in neonatal surgery. The new chapters include the following: Perinatal Physiology; Clinical Anatomy of the Newborn; Epidemiology of Birth Defects; Fetal Counselling for Surgical Malformations; Neonatal Sepsis; Liver Transplantation; Congenital Pouch Colon; Megacystis Microcolon Intestinal Hypoperistalsis Syndrome; and Urinary Tract Infections. Each chapter has been written by world-class experts in their respective fields, along with their coauthors.

This textbook provides an authoritative, comprehensive, and complete account of the pathophysiology and treatment of various surgical conditions in the newborn. This book should be of interest to all those who have a clinical responsibility for newborn babies. It is particularly intended for trainees in pediatric surgery, established pediatric surgeons, general surgeons with an interest in pediatric surgery, as well as neonatologists and pediatricians seeking more detailed information on newborn surgical conditions.

I wish to thank most sincerely all the contributors for their outstanding work in producing this innovative textbook. I also wish to express my gratitude to Ms. Vanessa Woods and Ms. Lisa Kelly for their skillful secretarial help. I am grateful to Dr. G.P. Seth for reading each and every word of the galley proofs of the entire book. I wish to thank the editorial staff of Hodder Arnold, particularly Mr. Stephen Clausard, for their help during the preparation and publication of this book. I am thankful to the Children's Medical & Research Foundation, Our Lady's Children's Hospital, Dublin for their support.

Prem Puri
2011

Preface to the second edition

The second edition of *Newborn Surgery* has been extensively revised. Many new chapters have been added to take account of the recent developments in the care of the newborn with congenital malformations. This edition, which comprises 97 chapters by 121 contributors from five continents of the world, provides an authoritative, comprehensive, and complete account of the various surgical conditions in the newborn. Each chapter is written by the current leading expert(s) in their respective fields.

Newborn surgery in the twenty-first century demands of its practitioners detailed knowledge and understanding of the complexities of congenital anomalies, as well as the highest standards of operative techniques. In this textbook, great emphasis continues to be placed on providing a comprehensive description of operative techniques of each individual congenital condition in the newborn. The book is intended for trainees in pediatric surgery, established pediatric surgeons, general surgeons with an interest in pediatric surgery, as well as neonatologists and pediatricians seeking more detailed information on newborn surgical conditions.

I wish to thank most sincerely all the contributors for the outstanding work they have done for the production of this innovative textbook. I also wish to express my gratitude to Mrs. Karen Alfred and Ms. Ann Brennan for their secretarial help and to the staff of Hodder Arnold for their help during the preparation and publication of this book. I am grateful to the Children's Medical & Research Foundation, Our Lady's Hospital for Sick Children, Dublin for their support.

Prem Puri
2003

Preface to the first edition

During the last three decades, newborn surgery has developed from an obscure subspecialty to an essential component of every major academic pediatric surgical department throughout both the developed and the developing world. Major advances in perinatal diagnosis, imaging, neonatal resuscitation, intensive care, and operative techniques have radically altered the management of newborns with congenital malformations. Embryological studies have provided new valuable insights into the development of malformations, while improvements in prenatal diagnosis are having a significant impact on approaches to management. Monitoring techniques for the sick neonate pre- and postoperatively have become more sophisticated, and there is now greater emphasis on physiological aspects of the surgical newborn, as well as their nutritional and immune status. This book provides a comprehensive compendium of all these aspects as a prelude to an extensive description of surgical conditions in the newborn. Modern-day newborn surgery demands detailed knowledge of the complexities of newborn problems. Research developments, laboratory diagnosis, imaging, and innovative surgical techniques are all part of the challenge facing surgeons dealing with congenital conditions in the newborn. In this book, a comprehensive description of operative techniques of each individual condition is presented. Each of the contributors was selected to provide an authoritative, comprehensive, and complete account of their respective topics. The book, comprising 90 chapters, is intended primarily for trainees in pediatric surgery, established pediatric surgeons, general surgeons with an interest in pediatric surgery, and neonatologists.

I am most grateful to all contributors for their willingness to contribute chapters at considerable cost of time and effort. I am indebted to Mr. Maurice De Cogan for artwork, Mr. Dave Cullen for photography, and Ms. Ann Brennan and Ms. Deirdre O'Driscoll for skillfull secretarial help. I am grateful to the Children's Research Centre, Our Lady's Hospital for Sick Children, for their support. Finally, I wish to thank the editorial staff, particularly Ms. Susan Devlin, of Butterworth-Heinemann for their help during the preparation and publication of this book.

Prem Puri
1996

Contributors

N. Scott Adzick
Center for Fetal Diagnosis and Treatment
Children's Hospital of Philadelphia
Philadelphia, Pennsylvania

Alessandro de Alarcón
Division of Pediatric Otolaryngology
Cincinnati Children's Hospital Medical Center
Cincinnati, Ohio

Adam C. Alder
Department of Pediatric Surgery
Children's Medical Center
UT Southwestern
Dallas, Texas

Lee W. T. Alkureishi
Division of Plastic Surgery
Northshore University Health System
Chicago, Illinois

Richard G. Azizkhan
Department of Pediatric Thoracic and General Surgery
Hemangioma and Vascular Malformation Center
Cincinnati Children's Hospital Medical Center
Cincinnati, Ohio
and
Omaha Children's Hospital and Medical Center
Omaha, Nebraska

Maria Marcela Bailez
Surgical Department
Garrahans Childrens Hospital
Buenos Aires, Argentina

Bruce S. Bauer
Division of Plastic Surgery
Northshore University Health System
Chicago, Illinois

Spencer W. Beasley
Christchurch School of Medicine
University of Otago
and
Department of Paediatric Surgery
Christchurch Hospital
Canterbury District Health Board
Christchurch, New Zealand

Lorenzo Biassoni
Great Ormond Street Hospital for Children NHS
Foundation Trust
London, United Kingdom

Benjamin O. Bierbach
German Paediatric Heart Center Sankt Augustin
Department of Paediatric Cardiothoracic Surgery
Asklepios Children's Hospital
Sankt Augustin, Germany

Andrea Bischoff
International Center for Colorectal Care
Colorado Children's Hospital
Division of Pediatric Surgery
Department of Surgery
University of Colorado
Aurora, Colorado

Carlos E. Blanco
National Maternity Hospital
Dublin, Ireland

Jose Boix-Ochoa
Autonomous University of Barcelona
Barcelona, Spain

Steven W. Bruch
University of Michigan
Section of Pediatric Surgery
C.S. Mott Children's Hospital
Ann Arbor, Michigan

Christoph Bührer
Department of Neonatology
Charité - Universitätsmedizin Berlin
Berlin, Germany

David M. Burge
Department of Paediatric Surgery and Urology
Southampton Children's Hospital
Southampton, United Kingdom

Paolo Caione
Division of Pediatric Urology
Bambino Gesù Children's Hospital
Rome, Italy

Casey M. Calkins
Department of Pediatric
General and Thoracic Surgery
Children's Hospital of Wisconsin
Milwaukee, Wisconsin

Donna A. Caniano
Department of Surgery
Ohio State University College of Medicine
and
Nationwide Children's Hospital
Columbus, Ohio

Robert Carachi
Department of Surgical Paediatrics
Royal Hospital for Children
Glasgow, United Kingdom

Alonso Carrasco Jr.
Department of Pediatric Urology
Children's Hospital Colorado
Aurora, Colorado

Salvatore Cascio
Department of Paediatric Surgery and Urology
Temple Street Children's University Hospital
Dublin, Ireland

Boris Chertin
Department of Pediatric Urology
Shaare Zedek Medical Center
Hebrew University-Hadassah Medical School
Jerusalem, Israel

Emily R. Christison-Lagay
Yale School of Medicine
and
Yale-New Haven Children's Hospital
New Haven, Connecticut

Joseph Chukwu
Locum Consultant Community Paediatrician
Queen Mary's Hospital
Kent, United Kingdom

Guido Ciprandi
Deparment of Pediatric Surgery
Bambino Gesù Children Hospital
Institute of Scientific Research
Rome, Italy

Paolo de Coppi
Specialist Neonatal and Paediatric Surgery Unit
Great Ormond Street Hospital
and
UCL Great Ormond Street Institute of Child Health
London, United Kingdom

Martin T. Corbally
Department of Surgery
Royal College of Surgeons of Ireland–Medical
University of Bahrain
Adilya, Bahrain
and
King Hamad University Hospital
Al Sayh, Bahrain
and
Children's Hospital Number 2
Ho Chi Minh City, Vietnam
and
Muhimbili National Hospital
Dar es Salaam, Tanzania

Sharon Cox
Division of Paediatric Surgery
University of Cape Town
and
Red Cross War Memorial Children's Hospital
Cape Town, South Africa

Suzanne Crowe
Our Lady's Children's Hospital, Crumlin
Dublin, Ireland

Sam J. Daniel
Department of Pediatric Surgery and Otolaryngology
McGill University
Montreal Children's Hospital
Montreal, Quebec, Canada

Mark Davenport
Department of Paediatric Surgery
King's College Hospital
Denmark Hill, London, United Kingdom

Andrew M. Davidoff
Department of Surgery
St. Jude Children's Research Hospital
and
Departments of Surgery, Pediatrics, and Pathology
and Laboratory Medicine
College of Medicine
University of Tennessee
Memphis, Tennessee

Dawn Deacy
Our Lady's Hospital for Sick Children
Dublin, Ireland

Belinda Hsi Dickie
Department of Pediatric Thoracic and General Surgery
Hemangioma and Vascular Malformation Center
Cincinnati Children's Hospital Medical Center
Cincinnati, Ohio
and
Department of Surgery
Boston Children's Hospital
Boston, Massachusetts

Jens Dingemann
Center of Pediatric Surgery
Hannover Medical School and Bult Children's Hospital
Hannover, Germany

Jonathan Durell
Department of Paediatric Surgery and Urology
Southampton Children's Hospital
Southampton, United Kingdom

Simon Eaton
Department of Paediatric Surgery
UCL Great Ormond Street Institute of Child Health
London, United Kingdom

Yousef El-Gohary
Department of Surgery
Division of Pediatric Surgery
Stony Brook Children's Hospital
and
Stony Brook University Medical Center
Stony Brook, New York

Jack S. Elder
Division of Pediatric Urology
MassGeneral Hospital for Children
Boston, Massachusetts

Brian Eley
Department of Paediatrics and Child Health
University of Cape Town
and
Red Cross War Memorial Children's Hospital
Cape Town, South Africa

Nicholas Eustace
Department of Anaesthesia and Intensive Care Medicine
Temple Street Children's University Hospital
Dublin, Ireland

Mary E. Fallat
Hiram C. Polk Jr. Department of Surgery
Norton Children's Hospital
University of Louisville
Louisville, Kentucky

Benjamin A. Farber
Pediatric Service
Department of Surgery
Memorial Sloan Kettering Cancer Center
New York, New York

Israel Fernandez-Pineda
Department of Surgery
St. Jude Children's Research Hospital
University of Tennessee
Memphis, Tennessee

Steven J. Fishman
Department of Surgery
Boston Children's Hospital
Boston, Massachusetts

David S. Foley
University of Louisville School of Medicine
Louisville, Kentucky

Henri R. Ford
Division of Pediatric Surgery
Children's Hospital Los Angeles
Los Angeles, California

Joseph Fusco
Division of Pediatric Surgery
Department of Surgery
Children's Hospital of Pittsburgh
Pittsburgh, Pennsylvania

Jeffrey W. Gander
Center for Adolescent Bariatric Surgery
Division of Pediatric Surgery
Morgan Stanley Children's Hospital of New York
Presbyterian/Columbia University Medical Center
New York, New York

Michael W. L. Gauderer
University of South Carolina
Columbia, South Carolina
and
School of Medicine Greenville
Greenville, South Carolina

Christopher P. Gayer
Division of Pediatric Surgery
Children's Hospital Los Angeles
Los Angeles, California

John P. Gearhart
Division of Pediatric Urology
Johns Hopkins Brady Urological Institute
Baltimore, Maryland

Keith E. Georgeson
Providence Pediatric Surgery Center
Spokane, Washington, DC

John Gillick
Department of Paediatric Surgery
Temple Street Children's University Hospital
Dublin, Ireland

George K. Gittes
Division of Pediatric Surgery
Department of Surgery
Children's Hospital of Pittsburgh
Pittsburgh, Pennsylvania

Jacqueline J. Glover
Department of Pediatrics
and
Center for Bioethics and Humanities
University of Colorado, Anschutz Medical Campus
Aurora, Colorado

Jamie Golden
Division of Pediatric Surgery
Children's Hospital Los Angeles
Los Angeles, California

Winifred A. Gorman
National Maternity Hospital
Dublin, Ireland

Jan-Hendrik Gosemann
Department of Pediatric Surgery
University of Leipzig
Leipzig, Germany

Andrew Green
Department of Clinical Genetics
Our Lady's Children's Hospital, Crumlin
and
School of Medicine and Medical Science
University College Dublin
Dublin, Ireland

Arin K. Greene
Department of Plastic Surgery
Boston Children's Hospital
Boston, Massachusetts

Tracy C. Grikscheit
Division of Pediatric Surgery
Children's Hospital Los Angeles
Los Angeles, California

Devendra K. Gupta
Department of Pediatric Surgery
All India Institute of Medical Sciences
New Delhi, India

Piotr Hajduk
Department of Paediatric Surgery
Our Lady's Children's Hospital, Crumlin
Dublin, Ireland

Yoshinori Hamada
Department of Surgery
Kansai Medical University
Hirakata, Japan

Philip J. Hammond
Department of Paediatric Surgery
Royal Hospital for Sick Children
Edinburgh, United Kingdom

William J. Hammond
Pediatric Service
Department of Surgery
Memorial Sloan Kettering Cancer Center
New York, New York

Christopher Hart
German Paediatric Heart Center Sankt Augustin
Department of Paediatric Cardiology
Asklepios Children's Hospital
Sankt Augustin, Germany

Roisin Hayes
Department of Radiology
Our Lady's Childrens Hospital, Crumlin
Dublin, Ireland

Melanie Hiorns
Radiology Department
Great Ormond Street Hospital for Children NHS
Foundation Trust
University College London
London, United Kingdom

Michael E. Höllwarth
Department of Paediatric and Adolescent Surgery
Medical University of Graz
Graz, Austria

Mark A. Hughes
Department of Clinical Neurosciences
Little France, Edinburgh, Scotland

Manuela Hunziker
Department of Pediatric Surgery
University Children's Hospital
Zurich, Switzerland

John M. Hutson
Department of Paediatrics
University of Melbourne
and
Department of Urology
The Royal Children's Hospital
and
Douglas Stephens Surgical Research Group
Murdoch Children's Research Institute
Parkville, Victoria, Australia

Aranka Ifert
Department of Dentistry
Goethe University Frankfurt
Frankfurt am Main, Germany

Michele Innocenzi
Division of Pediatric Urology
Bambino Gesù Children's Hospital
Rome, Italy

Vincenzo Jasonni
Giannina Gaslini Institute
and
University of Genoa
Genoa, Italy

Edwin C. Jesudason
NHS Lothian
Astley Ainslie Hospital
Edinburgh, Scotland

Paul R. V. Johnson
Nuffield Department of Surgical Sciences
University of Oxford
and
Department of Paediatric Surgery
Children's Hospital
Oxford, United Kingdom

Jonathan F. Kalisvaart
Providence Sacred Heart Children's Hospital
Spokane, Washington

Jothy Kandasamy
Department of Clinical Neurosciences
Little France, Edinburgh, Scotland

Frederick M. Karrer
University of Colorado School of Medicine
Children's Hospital Colorado
Aurora, Colorado

Richard Keijzer
Division of Pediatric Surgery
Department of Surgery
University of Manitoba
and
Department of Pediatrics and Child Health and Children's
Hospital Research Institute of Manitoba
University of Manitoba
Winnipeg, Manitoba, Canada

J. Kelleher
Department of Radiology
Our Lady's Childrens Hospital, Crumlin
Dublin, Ireland

Emily A. Kieran
Department of Neonatology
National Maternity Hospital
and
National Children's Research Centre
and
School of Medicine and Medical Science
University College Dublin
Dublin, Ireland

Andrew J. Kirsch
Department of Urology
Children's Healthcare of Atlanta
Atlanta, Georgia

Dietrich Kluth
Research Laboratory
Department of Pediatric Surgery
University Hospital Leipzig
Leipzig, Germany

Shannon M. Koehler
Division of Pediatric Surgery
Children's Hospital of Wisconsin
Milwaukee, Wisconsin

Hiroyuki Koga
Department of Pediatric General and Urogenital Surgery
Juntendo University School of Medicine
Tokyo, Japan

Martin Koyle
University of Toronto
and
Women's Auxiliary Chair in Urology & Regenerative
Medicine
The Hospital for Sick Children
Toronto, Ontario, Canada

Jeyanthi Kulasegarah
Department of Otolaryngology
Starship Children's Hospital
Auckland, New Zealand

Balazs Kutasy
Department of Pediatric Surgery
Karolinska University Hospital
Stockholm, Sweden

Kokila Lakhoo
Children's Hospital Oxford
John Radcliffe Hospital
University of Oxford
Oxford, United Kingdom

Ganapathy Lakshmanadass
Department of Paediatric Surgery
National Children's Hospital
Dublin, Ireland

Wolfgang Lambrecht
Department of Pediatric Surgery
University Hospital Hamburg
Hamburg, Germany

Jacob C. Langer
University of Toronto and Pediatric Surgeon
Hospital for Sick Children
Toronto, Ontario, Canada

Hanmin Lee
Department of Surgery
School of Medicine
University of California
San Francisco, California

Maggie K. Lee
Department of Neurosurgery,
The Walton Centre Foundation Trust
Liverpool, United Kingdom

Malcolm A. Lewis
Department of Paediatric Nephrology
Temple Street Children's University Hospital
Dublin, Ireland

Thom Lobe
Beneveda Medical Group
Beverly Hills, California

Paul D. Losty
Division of Child Health
Institute of Translational Medicine
Alder Hey Children's Hospital NHS Foundation Trust
University of Liverpool
Liverpool, United Kingdom

Conor L. Mallucci
Department of Neurosurgery
Alder Hey Childrens NHS Foundation Trust
Liverpool, United Kingdom

Andrea M. Malone
Our Lady's Children's Hospital, Crumlin
Dublin, Ireland

Leopoldo Martinez
Department of Pediatric Surgery
Hospital Universitario La Paz
Universidad Autonoma de Madrid
Madrid, Spain

Praveen Mathur
Department of Pediatric Surgery
SMS Medical College
Jaipur, Rajasthan, India

Girolamo Mattioli
Giannina Gaslini Institute
and
University of Genoa
Genoa, Italy

Judith Meehan
Tallaght Hospital
Trinity College Dublin
Dublin, Ireland

Roman Metzger
Department of Pediatric Surgery
University of Leipzig
Leipzig, Germany
and
Department of Pediatrics and
Adolescent Medicine
Salzburg County Hospital
Salzburg, Austria

William Middlesworth
Department of Surgery
Division of Pediatric Surgery
Morgan Stanley Children's Hospital
of New York-Presbyterian
Columbia University Medical Center
New York, New York

Alastair J. W. Millar
Division of Paediatric Surgery
University of Cape Town
and
Red Cross War Memorial Children's Hospital
Cape Town, South Africa

Robert K. Minkes
Division of Pediatric Surgery
Children's Medical Center Plano
Department of Surgery
UT Southwestern
Plano, Texas

S. Ali Mirjalili
Anatomy and Medical Imaging Department
Faculty of Medical and Health Sciences
University of Auckland
Auckland, New Zealand

Hideshi Miyakita
Department of Urology
Tokai University School of Medicine
Oiso Hospital
Oiso, Japan

Eleanor J. Molloy
Paediatrics and Child Health
Trinity College Dublin
The University of Dublin
Dublin, Ireland

Sam W. Moore
Department of Surgery/Paediatric Surgery
Faculty of Medicine and Health Sciences
University of Stellenbosch
Cape Town, South Africa

Alan E. Mortell
Department of Paediatric Surgery
Our Lady's Children's Hospital, Crumlin
and
Temple Street Children's University Hospital
Dublin, Ireland

Oliver J. Muensterer
Pediatric Surgery
University Medicine Mainz
Johannes Gutenberg University
Mainz, Germany

Azad S. Najmaldin
Leeds Teaching Hospitals
Leeds, United Kingdom

Masaki Nio
Department of Pediatric Surgery
Tohoku University Graduate School of Medicine
Sendai, Japan

Alp Numanoglu
Division of Paediatric Surgery
University of Cape Town
and
Red Cross War Memorial Children's Hospital
Cape Town, South Africa

Kay O'Brien
Department of Anaesthesia and Intensive Care Medicine
Temple Street Children's University Hospital
Dublin, Ireland

Brendan R. O'Connor
Department of Paediatric Surgery
Our Lady's Children's Hospital, Crumlin
Dublin, Ireland

Colm P. F. O'Donnell
Department of Neonatology
National Maternity Hospital
and
National Children's Research Centre
and
School of Medicine and Medical Science
University College Dublin
Dublin, Ireland

Fiona O'Hare
Department of Neonatology
National Maternity Hospital
Dublin, Ireland

Keith T. Oldham
Division of Pediatric Surgery
Medical College of Wisconsin
and
Children's Hospital of Wisconsin
Milwaukee, Wisconsin

Murwan Omer
Coombe Women's and Infants' University Hospital
Discipline of Paediatrics
Trinity College Dublin
Dublin, Ireland

Benjamin Padilla
Department of Surgery
School of Medicine
University of California
San Francisco, California

Konstantinos Papadakis
Harvard Medical School
and
Boston Children's Hospital
Boston, Masachusetts

Stephanie C. Papillon
Division of Pediatric Surgery
Children's Hospital Los Angeles
Los Angeles, California

Dakshesh H. Parikh
Department of Paediatric Surgery
Birmingham Women's and Children's
NHS Foundation Trust
Birmingham, United Kingdom

David A. Partrick
University of Colorado School of Medicine
Children's Hospital Colorado
Aurora, Colorado

Jose L. Peiró
Cincinnati Fetal Center
Pediatric General and Thoracic Surgery Division
Cincinnati Children's Hospital Medical Center (CCHMC)
Cincinnati, Ohio

Alberto Peña
International Center for Colorectal Care
Colorado Children's Hospital
and
Division of Pediatric Surgery
Department of Surgery
University of Colorado
Aurora, Colorado

Agostino Pierro
Division of General and Thoracic Surgery
Hospital for Sick Children
Toronto, Ontario, Canada

Rachael L. Polis
Norton Children's Gynecology
Louisville, Kentucky

Alessio Pini Prato
Department of Paediatric Surgery
Children Hospital
AON SS Antonio e Biagio e Cesare Arrigo
Alessandria, Italy

Kevin C. Pringle
Department of Obstetrics and Gynaecology
University of Otago
Wellington, New Zealand

Prem Puri
Newman Clinical Research Professor
and
Conway Institute of Biomolecular and Biomedical
Research
University College Dublin
and
Beacon Hospital
Dublin, Ireland

Michael P. La Quaglia
Pediatric Service
Department of Surgery
Memorial Sloan Kettering Cancer Center
New York, New York

John Mark Redmond
Our Lady's Children's' Hospital, Crumlin
and
Mater Misericordiae University Hospital
Dublin, Ireland

Denis J. Reen
Conway Institute of Biomolecular and Biomedical
Research
University College Dublin
Dublin, Ireland

Massimo Rivosecchi
Department of Pediatric Surgery
Bambino Gesù Children Hospital
Institute of Scientific Research
Rome, Italy

Jonathan P. Roach
University of Colorado School of Medicine
Children's Hospital Colorado
Aurora, Colorado

Ian H. W. Robinson
Department of Radiology
Temple Street Children's University Hospital
Dublin, Ireland

Udo Rolle
Department of Paediatric Surgery and Paediatric Urology
University Hospital of the Goethe-University Frankfurt
Frankfurt am Main, Germany

John D. Russell
Department of Otolaryngology
Our Lady's Children's Hospital, Crumlin
Dublin, Ireland

Elke Ruttenstock
Department of Pediatric Surgery
The Hospital for Sick Children
Toronto, Ontario, Canada

Frederick C. Ryckman
Cincinnati Children's Hospital
Cincinnati, Ohio

Beth A. Rymeski
Cincinnati Children's Hospital
Cincinnati, Ohio

Mira Sadadcharam
Department of Paediatric Otolaryngology
Royal Manchester Children's Hospital
Manchester, United Kingdom

Robert Sader
Frankfurt Oral Regenerative Medicine (FORM)
Clinic for Maxillofacial and Plastic Surgery
Johann Wolfgang Goethe University

Hideyuki Sasaki
Department of Pediatric Surgery
Tohoku University Graduate School of Medicine
Sendai, Japan

Amulya K. Saxena
Department of Pediatric Surgery
Chelsea and Westminster Hospital NHS Fdn Trust
Imperial College London
London, United Kingdom

Robert C. Shamberger
Harvard Medical School
and
Boston Children's Hospital
Boston, Masachusetts

Shilpa Sharma
Department of Pediatric Surgery
All India Institute of Medical Sciences
New Delhi, India

Stephen J. Shochat
Department of Surgery
St. Jude Children's Research Hospital
Memphis, Tennessee
and
Department of Surgery
Stanford University Medical Center
Standford, California

Scott S. Short
Division of Pediatric Surgery
Children's Hospital Los Angeles
Los Angeles, California

Michael Singh
Department of Paediatric Surgery
Birmingham Women's and Children's
NHS Foundation Trust
Birmingham, United Kingdom

Owen P. Smith
University College Dublin
and
Our Lady's Children's Hospital, Crumlin
Dublin, Ireland

CWN Spearman
University of Cape Town
and
Red Cross War Memorial Children's Hospital
Cape Town, South Africa

Thambipillai Sri Paran
Department of Pediatric Surgery
Our Lady's Children's Hospital
Dublin, Ireland

Charles J. H. Stolar
Columbia University
Division of Pediatric Surgery
College of Physicians and Surgeons
Morgan Stanley Children's Hospital/Columbia University Medical Center
New York, New York

Mark D. Stringer
Departments of Paediatric Surgery and Child Health
Wellington Hospital
University of Otago
Wellington, New Zealand

Peter P. Stuhldreher
Division of Pediatric Urology
Johns Hopkins Brady Urological Institute
Baltimore, Maryland

Yechiel Sweed
Department of Pediatric Surgery
Galilee Medical Center
Nahariya, Israel
and
Faculty of Medicine in the Galilee
Bar Ilan University
Safed, Israel

Tomoaki Taguchi
Department of Pediatric Surgery
Graduate School of Medical Sciences
Kyushu University
Fukuoka, Japan

Yoshiaki Takahashi
Department of Pediatric Surgery
Graduate School of Medical Sciences
Kyushu University
Fukuoka, Japan

Paul K. H. Tam
Department of Surgery
The University of Hong Kong
Queen Mary Hospital
Hong Kong, China

Farhan Tareen
Department of Paediatric Surgery
Our Lady's Children's Hospital, Crumlin
and
Temple Street Children's University Hospital
Dublin, Ireland

David F. M. Thomas
Leeds Teaching Hospitals
and
University of Leeds
Leeds, United Kingdom

Christian Tomuschat
National Children's Research Centre
Our Lady's Children's Hospital
Dublin, Ireland

Juan A. Tovar
Department of Pediatric Surgery
Hospital Universitario La Paz
Universidad Autonoma de Madrid
Madrid, Spain

Benno Ure
Department of Pediatric Surgery
Hannover Medical School
Hannover, Germany

Vijaya M. Vemulakonda
Department of Pediatric Urology
Children's Hospital Colorado
Aurora, Colorado

Rohit Umesh Verma
Department of Otolaryngology
Manchester Royal Infirmary
Manchester, United Kingdom

Eduardo Villamor
Department of Pediatrics
Maastricht University Medical Center (MUMC+)
School for Oncology and Developmental Biology (GROW)
Maastricht, Netherlands

Motoshi Wada
Department of Pediatric Surgery
Tohoku University Graduate School of Medicine
Sendai, Japan

Miho Watanabe
Department of Pediatric Thoracic and General Surgery
Hemangioma and Vascular Malformation Center
Cincinnati Children's Hospital Medical Center
Cincinnati, Ohio

Tomas Wester
Unit of Pediatric Surgery
Karolinska University Hospital
Karolinska Institutet
Stockholm, Sweden

Chad Wiesenauer
Hiram C. Polk Jr. Department of Surgery
Norton Children's Hospital
University of Louisville
Louisville, Kentucky

Duncan T. Wilcox
Department of Pediatric Urology
Children's Hospital Colorado
Aurora, Colorado

Kenneth K. Y. Wong
Department of Surgery
The University of Hong Kong
Queen Mary Hospital
Hong Kong, China

Atsuyuki Yamataka
Department of Pediatric General and Urogenital Surgery
Juntendo University School of Medicine
Tokyo, Japan

Iain Yardley
Evelina London Children's Hospital
London, United Kingdom
and
WHO Service Delivery and Safety
Geneva, Switzerland

George G. Youngson
Department of Paediatric Surgery
Royal Aberdeen Children's Hospital
Aberdeen, Scotland

Alon Yulevich
Department of Pediatric Surgery
Galilee Medical Center
Nahariya, Israel
and
Faculty of Medicine in the Galilee
Bar Ilan University
Safed, Israel

Jessica A. Zagory
Division of Pediatric Surgery
Children's Hospital Los Angeles
Los Angeles, California

Augusto Zani
Division of General and Thoracic Surgery
Hospital for Sick Children
Toronto, Ontario, Canada

Faisal Zawawi
Division of Pediatric Otolaryngology
McGill University
Montreal, Quebec, Canada

Julia Zimmer
National Children's Research Centre
Our Lady's Children's Hospital, Crumlin
Dublin, Ireland
and
Department of Paediatric Surgery
Hannover Medical School
Hannover, Germany

Christoph Zoeller
Department of Pediatric Surgery
Hannover Medical School
Hannover, Germany

PART 1

General

Embryology of malformations

DIETRICH KLUTH, WOLFGANG LAMBRECHT, CHRISTOPH BÜHRER, AND ROMAN METZGER

INTRODUCTION

Approximately 3% of human newborns present with congenital malformations.[1] Without surgical intervention, one-third of these infants would die since their malformations are not compatible with sustained life outside the uterus.[1,2] In figures, this means that in a country such as Germany, nearly 6000 children are born every year with a life-threatening malformation.

Due to the development of prenatal diagnostic procedures, advanced surgical techniques, and intensive postoperative care, most infants with otherwise fatal malformations can be rescued by an operation in the neonatal period. However, morbidity remains high in some of these children[2] with the necessity of repeated operations and hospitalizations despite a successful primary operation. This may also be the fate of many children with non-life-threatening malformations such as hypospadias or cleft palate.

Mortality is still high in newborns with certain malformations such as congenital diaphragmatic hernias (CDHs) or severe combined defects. As a consequence, congenital malformations today are the main cause of death in the neonatal period. In the United States, 21% of neonatal mortality can be related to congenital malformations.[3]

These figures probably do not reflect a real increase in the actual incidence of congenital malformations. The observed mortality shift might rather be due to improved intensive care medicine in today's Western world countries where neonates (even those with birth defects) have a better chance of survival. On the other hand, this statistical shift indicates that knowledge about congenital malformations lags behind the progress clinical research has made in the surrounding fields. Efforts are needed to close the gap and learn more about baby killer no. 1. Identification of teratogens will help to reduce the incidence of malformations when exposure can be avoided, and pathogenetic studies might aid in designing therapeutic measures.

Both treatment and prevention critically depend on basic embryological research.

GENERAL REMARKS ON EMBRYOLOGY AND THE EMBRYOLOGY OF MALFORMATIONS

Despite many efforts, the embryology of numerous congenital anomalies in humans is still a matter of speculation. This is due to the following reasons:

1. A shortage of study material (both normal and abnormal embryos)
2. Various technical problems (difficulties in the interpretation of serial sections, shortage of explanatory three-dimensional reconstructions)
3. Misconceptions and/or outdated theories concerning normal and abnormal embryology

Fortunately, a number of animal models are known today, which allow advanced embryological studies in various embryological fields. Especially for the studies of anorectal malformations, a number of animal models are at hand. In addition, a scanning electron microscopic atlas of human embryos had been published recently, which provides detailed insights into normal human embryology.[4]

Appropriate and illustrative findings in various fields of embryology are still lacking. This explains why today many typical malformations are still not explained satisfactorily. Pediatric surgeons are still confused when they are confronted with the embryological background of normal and abnormal development.

For the described misconceptions and/or outdated theories, Haeckel's "biogenetic law"[5] is one example. According to this theory, a human embryo recapitulates in its individual development (ontogeny) the morphology observed in all life forms (phylogeny). This means that during its development, an advanced species is seen to pass through stages represented by adult organisms of more primitive species.[5]

This theory still has an impact on the nomenclature of embryonic organs and explains why human embryos have "cloacas" like adult birds and "branchial" clefts like adult fish.

Another very popular misconception is the theory that malformations actually represent "frozen" stages of normal embryology ("Hemmungsmißbildung").[6] As a result, our understanding of normal embryology stems more from pathological–anatomic interpretations of observed malformations than from proper embryological studies. The theory of the "rotation of the gut" as a step in normal development is a perfect example for this misconception.

DEFINITION OF THE TERM "MALFORMATION"

After birth, neonates can present with a broad spectrum of deviations from normal morphology. This extends from minor variations of normal morphology without any clinical significance to maximal organ defects with extreme functional deficits of the malformed organs or of the whole organism.

The degree of functional disorder is decisive when dealing with the question of whether a variation of normal morphology has to be viewed as a dangerous malformation requiring surgical correction. This means that functional disturbance is essential when using the term "malformation." Inborn deviations can be detrimental, neutral, or even beneficial; otherwise, evolutionary progress could not take place. An example of a beneficial deviation is the longevity syndrome of people with abnormally low serum cholesterol levels. Abnormalities with little or no functional disturbance might still require surgical correction when patients are in danger of social stigmatization. Coronal or glandular hypospadias might serve as an example for this condition.

ETIOLOGY OF CONGENITAL MALFORMATIONS

In most cases, the etiology of congenital malformations remains unclear. Possible etiological factors are listed in Table 1.1.

In about 20% of cases, genetic factors (gene mutation and chromosomal disorders) can be identified.[1,2,7] In 10%, an environmental origin can be demonstrated.[1,2] In 70%, the factors responsible remain obscure.

Environmental factors

A large number of agents are known that might interfere with the normal development of organ systems during embryogenesis.[1,7] The underlying mechanisms of this interference are poorly understood in most cases. Characteristically, during organogenesis, different organs of the embryo show distinct periods of greatest sensitivity to the action of the teratogen. These phases of greatest sensitivity are called the "teratogenetic period of determination."[8] The typical patterns of some syndromes can be explained by an overlap of these phases during embryological development.

In 1983, Shepard[2] published a catalogue of suspected teratogenic agents. Over 900 agents are known to produce congenital anomalies in experimental animals. In 30 agents, evidence for teratogenic action in humans could be demonstrated. Teratogenic agents can be divided into four groups (Table 1.2).

The teratogenic potential of virus infections,[1] especially rubella and herpes, and that of radiation[1] has been clearly established. Maternal metabolic defects and lack of essential nutritives can be teratogenic. After a vitamin A–free diet[9] and riboflavin-free diet,[10] various congenital malformations were observed in rats and mice. Among these were diaphragmatic hernias, isolated esophageal atresias, and isolated tracheo-esophageal fistulas. Similarly, inappropriate administration of hormones can be associated with intrauterine dysplasias.[11]

Industrial and pharmaceutical chemicals such as tetrachlor-diphenyl-dioxin or thalidomide have inflicted tragedies by their teratogenic action. When thalidomide was prescribed to women in the early 1960s as a "safe" sleeping medication, numerous children were born with dysmelic deformities.[7,12,13] In addition, atresias of the esophagus, the duodenum, and the anus were observed in some children.[12] The data collected suggest that teratogenic agents do not cause new patterns of malformations but rather mimic sporadic birth defects. This had posed problems in identifying thalidomide as the responsible agent. It appears likely that among those 70% congenital malformations with unclear etiology, a considerable percentage might be precipitated by as yet unidentified environmental factors. In a rat model, the herbicide nitrofen (2,4-dichlorophenyl-p-nitrophenyl ether) has been shown to induce CDHs, cardiac abnormalities, and hydronephrosis.[14–18] In 1978, Thompson et al.[19] described the teratogenicity of the anticancer drug Adriamycin in rats and rabbits. More recently, Diez-Pardo et al.[20] re-described

Table 1.1 Etiology of congenital malformations

Genetic disorders	20%
Environmental factors	10%
Unknown etiology	70%

Table 1.2 Teratogenic agents in congenital malformations

Physical agents (radiation, heat, mechanical factors)
Infectious agents (viruses, treponemes, parasites)
Chemicals and drugs (thalidomide, nitrofen)
Environmental agents (hormones, vitamin deficiencies)
Maternal, genetic, and chromosomal disorders
Multifactorial inheritance

Source: Nadler HL. Teratology. In: Welch KJ, Randolph JG, Ravitch MM, O'Neill JA, Rowe MJ (editors). *Pediatric Surgery.* 4th Edition. Chicago: Year Book Medical Publishers, 1986:11–3.

this model with emphasis to its potentials as a model for foregut anomalies. Today, the Adriamycin model is generally described as a model for the VACTERL association (V = vertebral, A = anorectal, C = cardiac, T = tracheal, E = esophageal, R = renal, L = limb).[21,22] Thus, classic malformations such as atresias of the esophagus and the intestinal tract, intestinal duplications, and others can be mimicked by teratogens in animal models.

Genetic factors

Approximately 20% of congenital malformations are of genetic origin. Most surgically correctable malformations are associated with chromosomal disorders, e.g., trisomy 21, 13, or 18, or are of multifactorial inheritance[23] with a small risk of recurrence. The assumption of multifactorial inheritance results from the fact that with nearly all major anomalies familiar occurrences had been observed.[1] In animals, inheritance has also been found for some malformations.[24-27]

EMBRYOLOGY AND ANIMAL MODELS

Over the last two decades, a number of animal models were developed with the potential to gain a better understanding of the morphology of not only malformed but also normal embryos. These animal models can be divided into four subgroups.

Surgical models

In the past, the chicken was an important surgical model to study embryological processes. Due to the easy access to the embryo, its broad availability, and its cheapness, the chicken is an ideal model for experimental studies. It has been widely used by embryologists especially in the field of epithelial/mesenchymal interactions.[28-30] Pediatric surgeons used this model to study morphological processes involved in intestinal atresia formation,[31,32] gastroschisis,[33] and M. Hirschsprung.[34]

The Czech embryologist Lemez[35] used chicken embryos in order to induce tracheal agenesis with tracheo-esophageal fistula.

Apart from these purely embryonic models, a large number of fetal models exist. However, these models were mainly used in order to demonstrate the feasibility of fetal interventions.[36]

Chemical models

A large number of chemicals can have an impact on the normal development of humans and animals alike. The following are the most important chemicals today: (1) Adriamycin,[19,20] (2) etretinate,[37,38] (3) all-trans retinoic acid (ATRA),[39-41] (4) ethylenethiourea,[42-44] and (5) nitrofen.[15,16,18]

While models 1 to 4 are used to study the embryology of atresias of the esophagus, the gut, and the anorectum,

model 5 was developed to study the malformations of the diaphragm, the lungs, the heart, and kidneys (hydronephrosis).

Genetic models

A number of genetic models had been developed that had been used for embryological studies in the past. These animals can be the product of spontaneous mutations or are the result of genetic manipulations, mainly in mice (transgenic mice).

1. Models of spontaneous origin: the SD mouse model[25,27]
2. Inheritance models: the pig model of anal atresia[24,26]
3. "Knockout" models[45-47]

The number of transgenic animal models is growing fast. For pediatric surgeons, those models are of major importance, which result in abnormalities of the fore- and hindgut. Here, interference with the sonic hedgehog pathway has proven to be very effective.[45-47] There are two ways to interfere with that pathway:

1. Targeted deletion of sonic hedgehog (Shh)[45,46]
2. Deletion of one of the three transcription factors Gli1, Gli2, and Gli3[46,47]

In the foregut, targeted deletion of Shh causes esophageal atresia/stenosis, tracheo-esophageal fistulas, and tracheal/lung anomalies in homozygous Shh null mutant mice.[45] In the hindgut, the deletion of Shh caused the formation of "cloacas,"[46] while Gli2 mutant mice demonstrated the "classic" form of anorectal malformations and Gli3 mutants showed minor forms like anal stenosis.[46,47] Interestingly, the morphology of Gli2 mutant mice embryos resembles that of heterozygous SD-mice embryos, while Shh null mutant mice embryos had morphological similarities with homozygous SD-mice embryos. Interestingly, after administration of Adriamycin, changes in the normal pattern of Shh distribution in the developing foregut were demonstrated.[48]

Viral models

Animal models that use virus infections to produce malformations important for pediatric surgeons are very rare. One exception is the murine model of extra hepatic biliary atresia (EHBA). In this model, newborn Balb/c mice are infected with rhesus rotavirus group A.[49] As a result, the full spectrum of EHBA develops as it is seen in newborns with this disease. However, this model is not a model to mimic failed embryology. But it highlights the possibility that malformations are not caused by embryonic disorders but by fetal or even postnatal catastrophes.

This part on embryology and animal models further highlights the importance of the study of normal animal embryos. Today, much information in current textbooks on human embryology stems from studies done in animals of varied species. Many of these are outdated. However, the wide use of transgenic mice in order to mimic congenital malformations makes morphological studies of the various organ systems in normal mice mandatory. Otherwise, the interpretation of the effects of the deletion of genetic information can be very difficult.[50]

EMBRYOLOGY OF MALFORMATIONS

Disturbances of normal embryological processes will result in malformations of organs. This was first shown by Spemann[51] in 1901 by experimentally producing supernumerary organs in the triton embryo after establishing close contact between excised parts of triton eggs and other parts of the same egg. Spemann and Mangold[5] coined the term "induction" to describe this observation. They found that certain parts of the embryo obviously were able to control embryonic development of other parts. These controlling parts were called "organizers."[5] The process of influence itself was called "induction."

It was believed by many scientists in the field that "induction" could serve as the overall principle of hierarchical control of embryonic development. Ensuing investigations, however, made modifications necessary, which finally resulted in a very complex model of organizers and inductors. The nature of inductive substances remained obscure, and attempts to isolate inductive substances, currently called "morphogenes," were unsuccessful.[52] Interestingly, not only live cells could induce development in certain experiments but also dead and denatured materials.[5]

A process essential for the formation of early embryonic organs is the invagination of epithelial sheets. This invagination is preceded by a thickening of the epithelial sheet,[53] a process known as placode formation. The thickening itself is caused by elongation of individual cells of the placode. This process can be studied in detail in epithelial morphogenesis.[54] The same sequence of developmental events has been observed in the formation of the neural plate, in the formation of the optic and lens placode, and in the development of most epitheliomesenchymal organs including the lung, the thyroid gland, and the pancreas. From these observations, it can be concluded that most epithelial cells behave uniformly in the early phase of embryonic development.

Today it is generally accepted that early embryonic organs are especially sensitive for alterations. Therefore, researchers are more and more interested to understand the formation of early embryonic organs.

In 1985, Ettersohn[55] stated that most invaginations are the result of mechanical forces that are local in origin. He focused on three possible mechanisms that might lead to placode formation and subsequent invagination:

1. Change of cell shape by cell adhesion
2. Microfilament-mediated change of cell shape
3. Cell growth and division

In the following part, we will discuss some aspects of these mechanisms.

A teratological method used to determine the function of cell adhesion molecules (CAMs) in vivo during embryogenesis has been reported recently.[56] Mouse hybridoma cells producing monoclonal antibodies against the avian integrin complex were grafted into 2- or 3-day-old chick embryos. Depending on the site of engraftment, local muscle agenesis was observed. This is an example that the immunologic immaturity of the embryo can be exploited to study the contribution of cell attachment molecules to organ development in a functional fashion. A number of monoclonal antibodies directed against cell attachment molecules of various species have become available over the last years, and the structure of the binding molecules has been elucidated biochemically and by cDNA cloning. Functionally, adhesion molecules may be grouped into three families: (1) CAMs, which mediate specific and mostly transient cell recognition of other cells; (2) substrate adhesion molecules (SAMs), necessary for attachment to extracellular matrix proteins; and (3) cell-junctional molecules (CJMs), found in tight and gap junctions. Whereas CJMs apparently play an important role for metabolic signaling within established tissues, CAMs and SAMs are necessary for the formation of histologically distinct structures and directed migration of single cells. Among CAMs and SAMs, at least three families have been identified biochemically: integrins,[57] members of the immunoglobulin superfamily, and LEC-CAMS.[58] Integrins are heterodimeric molecules consisting of a larger α chain, which is associated with a smaller β chain in a calcium-dependent way. Usually, one given α chain might be found in association with various chains, but promiscuity of β chains has been described recently. Functionally, members of the integrin family present as SAMs (adhesion to vitronectin, collagen, fibronectin, complement components, or other intercellular matrix proteins) or CAMs (direct adhesion to other cells via corresponding cell surface target molecules). For example, cells bearing the integrin LFA-1 on their cell surface bind to cells expressing ICAM-1 or ICAM-2, both of which are members of the immunoglobulin superfamily.[59,60] Other members of the immunoglobulin superfamily that are known to be important during morphogenesis include liver CAM[61] (L-CAM) and neural CAM[62,63] (N-CAM). Both show homophilic aggregation; that is, N-CAM serves as a target structure for N-CAM, and L-CAM serves as a target structure for L-CAM, but there is no cross-reactivity. In developing feather placodes in avian embryos, L-CAM and N-CAM are mutually exclusive expressed on epidermal or mesodermal cells, respectively. When the placodes are incubated with antibodies to L-CAM, primarily only epidermal cell-to-cell contact is disturbed.[64] However, the structure of the surrounding mesoderm is altered subsequently, suggesting an inductive signal loop between epidermal and mesodermal cells. A third group of adhesion molecules has been termed LEC-CAMs to indicate that their extracellular part consists of a lectin domain, an epidermal growth factor (EGF)-like domain, and a complement regulatory protein repeat domain. The lectin domain is presumed to contain the active center; binding mediated by the murine homolog to the leukocyte adhesion molecule 1 (LAM-1)[65] can be blocked by mannose-6-phosphate or its polymers.[66] Lectin-dependent organ formation should be accessible experimentally by administration of the respective carbohydrates, but few, if any, data have been reported so far.

Cell shape is mainly maintained by microtubules forming the cellular cytoskeleton. In addition, contractile elements exist such as actin, which are essential for cell movement, the so-called microfilaments. These structures are thought to be essential for the process of placode formation and invagination.[67] Microfilament-mediated change of cell shape is based on the idea that actin filaments could alter the shape of cells by contraction. Most of these filaments are found at the apex of epithelial cells. Contraction of these filaments in each individual cell of a cell layer would result in an increasing infolding of the whole cell layer,[67,68] finally resulting in invagination. It is a disadvantage of this model, however, that there is no apparent reason why apical constriction should proceed by cell elongation.[55]

Cell proliferation is probably an essential factor in the morphogenesis of epitheliomesenchymal organs. During morphogenesis of these organs, repeated invagination can be observed, which might be dependent upon cell proliferation.[69] The way in which epithelial cell growth and proliferation is controlled in the embryo is not clear. However, it is believed that the surrounding mesenchyme might regulate the timing and location of invagination of the epithelial layer. Goldin and Opperman[28] proposed that EGF might be excreted by mesenchymal cells, which would stimulate epithelial cell proliferation and repeated invagination. When agarose pellets impregnated with EGF were cultured alongside 5-day embryonic chick tracheal epithelium, supernumerary buds were induced to form at those sites. EGF and the related peptide transforming growth factor-β (TGFβ) have been shown to lead to precocious eyelid opening when injected into newborn mice.[70] Thus, complex changes of late-stage organ development can be induced by physiological stimuli in the laboratory. Interestingly, EGF is a mitogen for many epithelial cells in vitro without affecting most mesenchymal cells. A large variety of cells have been demonstrated to display the receptor for EGF/TGFβ on their cell surface, which is encoded by the cellular proto-oncogene c-erbB. Structural alterations of this receptor are known to result in uncontrolled proliferation and ultimately malignant transformation. When secreted locally, EGF might provide physically associated cells with appropriate on and off signals required for the formation of complex organs. Other polypeptides, such as platelet-derived growth factor or transforming growth factor-α (TGFα), appear to function in an antagonistic way in that they stimulate rather the proliferation of mesenchymal cells.[71,72] In defined experimental situations, TGFα has been shown to be a mitogen for osteoblasts while being a potent inhibitor of the proliferation of epithelial and endothelial cells at the same time. Embryonic fibroblasts, however, are also inhibited by TGFα.[73] TGFα is a powerful chemotactic agent for fibroblasts and enhances the production of both collagen and fibronectin by these

cells. There are, however, little data available concerning the involvement of these factors during normal and pathologic development of the embryo. Future investigations using such powerful approaches as in situ hybridization with cloned genes, preparation of transgenic animals, and direct administration of the recombinant proteins to various parts of the embryo might shed some light on signaling pathways mediated by soluble cytokines.

The surrounding mesenchyme might limit the expansion of the epithelial bud[74] forcing the epithelial sheet to fold in characteristic patterns. If a growing cell layer is restricted from lateral expansion, "mitotic pressure" by dividing cells will result in elongation of cells and then invagination of the "crowded" cell sheet. This does not necessarily imply that cells divide more rapidly in the region of invagination than in the surrounding areas. The main effect is caused by restriction of lateral expansion.[29,30] In the early anlage of the thymus, cell proliferation counts are actually lower in the thymus anlage than in the surrounding epithelium.[75] Steding[29] and Jacob[30] have shown experimentally that restriction of lateral expansion might be responsible for thickening and subsequent invagination of epithelial sheets. In their experiments, restriction of lateral expansion was caused by a tiny silver ring placed on the epithelium of chick embryos.

EXAMPLES OF PATHOLOGICAL EMBRYOLOGY

The focus of our research has been the embryology of foregut, anorectal, and diaphragmatic malformations. We studied the normal development of all embryonic organs involved by scanning electron microscopy (SEM).[76–82] In addition, we employed two rodent animal models to study malformations of the anorectum and the diaphragm. Pathogenetic concepts concerning these malformations were controversial in the past due to lack of detailed data.

EMBRYOLOGY OF FOREGUT MALFORMATIONS

The differentiation of the primitive foregut into the ventral trachea and dorsal esophagus is thought to be the result of a process of septation.[83] It is guessed that lateral ridges appear in the lateral walls of the foregut, which fuse in midline in a caudocranial direction, thus forming the tracheo-esophageal septum. This theory of septation has been described in detail by Rosenthal[84] and Smith.[85] However, others[86,87] were not able to verify the importance of the tracheo-esophageal septum for the differentiation of the foregut. They instead proposed individually that the respiratory tract develops simply by further growth of the lung bud in a caudal direction.

Using SEM, we studied the development of the foregut in chick embryos.[76,77] In this study, we were unable to demonstrate the formation of a tracheo-esophageal septum (Figure 1.1). A sequence of SEM photographs of staged chick embryos suggests that differentiation of the primitive

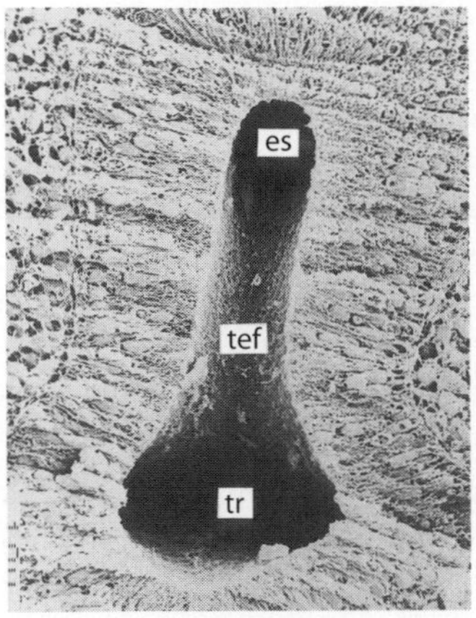

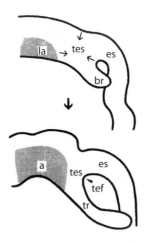

Figure 1.1 SEM photograph of the inner layer of foregut epithelium in a chick embryo (approx. 3.5 days old). View from cranial. Between trachea (tr) on bottom and esophagus (es) on top, the tip of the tracheo-esophageal fold (tef) is recognizable. Lateral ridges or signs of fusion are not found.

foregut is best explained by a process of "reduction of size" of a foregut region called the "tracheo-esophageal space" (Figure 1.2). This reduction is caused by a system of folds that develops in the primitive foregut. They approach each other but do not fuse (Figure 1.2).

Based on these observations, the development of the malformation can be explained by disorders either of the formation of the folds or of their developmental movements:

1. Atresia of the esophagus with fistula (Figure 1.3a): The dorsal fold of the foregut bends too far ventrally. As a result, the descent of the larynx is blocked. Therefore, the tracheo-esophageal space remains partly undivided and lies in a ventral position. Due to this ventral position, it differentiates into trachea.

Figure 1.2 Summarizing sketch of foregut development. The tracheo-esophageal space (tes) is reduced in size by developmental movements of folds (indicated by arrows) (es, esophagus; la, anlage of larynx; br, bronchus; tr, trachea). Short arrow marks tip of tracheo-esophageal fold (tef) (compare Figure 1.1).

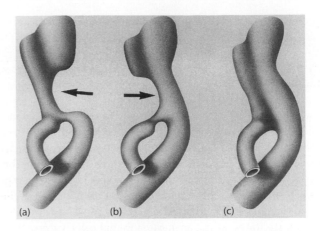

Figure 1.3 Sketch of formal pathogenesis of typical foregut malformations (see text for details): **(a)** atresia of esophagus with fistula; **(b)** atresia of trachea with fistula; **(c)** laryngotracheo-esophageal cleft. Arrows indicate sites of possible deformation of the developing foregut.

2. Atresia of the trachea with fistula (Figure 1.3b): The foregut is deformed on its ventral side. The developmental movements of the folds are disturbed, and the tracheo-esophageal space is dislocated in a dorsal direction. Therefore, it differentiates into esophagus.
3. Laryngotracheo-esophageal clefts (Figure 1.3c): Faulty growth of the folds results in the persistence of the primitive tracheo-esophageal space.

Recently, it has been shown that esophageal atresias and tracheo-esophageal fistulas can be induced by maternal application of Adriamycin into the peritoneal cavity of pregnant rats.[19,20] The dosage may vary between 1.5 and 2.0 mg/kg depending on the number of days it will be given. In most reports, the most promising dosage is 1.75 mg/kg given on days 6–9 of pregnancy. The Adriamycin model has been intensively studied over the last 20 years, resulting in more than 90 reports between 1997 and 2017.[88] It could be demonstrated that, in this model, not only foregut malformations but also atypical patterns of malformation can be observed, which are usually summarized under the term "VATER" or "VACTERL" association.[21,22] Therefore, this model is promising for the studies of not only foregut anomalies but also of anomalies of the hind- and midgut.

DEVELOPMENT OF THE DIAPHRAGM

In the past, several theories were proposed to explain the appearance of posterolateral diaphragmatic defects:

1. Defects caused by improper development of the pleuroperitoneal membrane[89,90]
2. Failure of muscularization of the lumbocostal trigone and pleuroperitoneal canal, resulting in a "weak" part of the diaphragm[89,91]
3. Pushing of intestine through the posterolateral part (foramen of Bochdalek) of the diaphragm[92]

4. Premature return of the intestines into the abdominal cavity with the canal still open[89,91]
5. Abnormal persistence of lung in the pleuroperitoneal canal, preventing proper closure of the canal[93]
6. Abnormal development of the early lung and posthepatic mesenchyme, causing nonclosure of pleuroperitoneal canals[18]

Of these theories, failure of the pleuroperitoneal membrane to meet the transverse septum is the most popular hypothesis to explain diaphragmatic herniation. However, using SEM techniques,[78] we could not demonstrate the importance of the pleuroperitoneal membrane for the closure of the so-called pleuroperitoneal canals (Figure 1.4).

As stated earlier, most authors assume that delayed or inhibited closure of the diaphragm will result in a diaphragmatic defect that is wide enough to allow herniation of gut into the fetal thoracic cavity. However, this assumption is not the result of appropriate embryological observations but rather the result of interpretations of anatomical/pathological findings. In a series of normal staged embryos, we measured the width of the pleuroperitoneal openings and the transverse diameter of gut loops.[82] On the basis of these measurements, we estimated that a single embryonic gut loop requires at least an opening of 450 μm in size to herniate into the fetal pleural cavity. However, in none of our embryos, the observed pleuroperitoneal openings were of appropriate dimensions. This means that delayed or inhibited closure of the pleuroperitoneal canal cannot result in a diaphragmatic defect of sufficient size. Herniation of gut through these openings is therefore impossible. Thus, the proposed theory about the pathogenetic mechanisms of CDH development lacks any embryological evidence. Furthermore, the proposed timing of this process is highly questionable.[79,80]

Recently, an animal model for diaphragmatic hernia has been developed[14–18] using nitrofen as the noxious substance. In these experiments, CDHs were produced in a reasonably high percentage of newborns.[15,16] Most diaphragmatic hernias were associated with lung hypoplasias. Using electron microscopy, our group[79–82] used this model to give a detailed description of the development of the diaphragmatic defect. Our results are as follows.

Timing of diaphragmatic defect appearance

Iritani[18] was the first to notice that nitrofen-induced diaphragmatic hernias in mice are not caused by an improper closure of the pleuroperitoneal openings but rather the result of a defective development of the so-called posthepatic mesenchymal plate (PHMP). In our study in rats, clear evidence of disturbed development of the diaphragmatic anlage was seen on day 13 (left side) and day 14 (right side, Figure 1.5).[79,82] In all embryos affected, the PHMP was too short. This age group is equivalent to 4–5 week old human embryos.[79]

Location of diaphragmatic defect

In our SEM study, the observed defects were localized in the PHMP (Figure 1.5). We identified two distinct types of defects: (1) large "dorsal" defects and (2) small "central" defects.[79] Large defects extended into the region of the pleuroperitoneal openings. In these cases, the closure of the pleuroperitoneal openings was usually impaired by the massive ingrowth of liver (Figures 1.6 and 1.7). If the defects were small, they were consistently isolated from the pleuroperitoneal openings closing normally at the 16th or 17th day of gestation. Thus, in our embryos with CDH, the region of the diaphragmatic defect

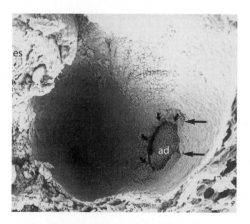

Figure 1.4 SEM photograph of right pleural sac in a rat embryo (approx. 16.5 days old). View from cranial. The so-called pleuroperitoneal canal (PPC) is nearly closed. Small arrows point at the margin of PPC. In the depth of the abdomen, the right adrenals (ad) are seen. Large arrows point at margins of the so-called pleuroperitoneal membrane. Its contribution to the closure of the canal is minimal (es, esophagus).

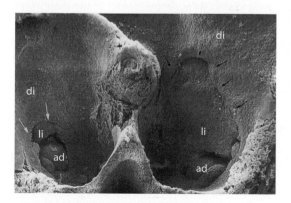

Figure 1.5 Cranial view of the pleural sacs in a rat embryo after exposition to nitrofen on day 11 of pregnancy. The embryo is approx. 15 days old. Note the big defect of the right diaphragmatic primordium. Small black arrows point at margins of the defect, which leaves parts of the liver (li) uncoated. On the left, the diaphragmatic anlage is normal. Note the low position of the cranial border of the pleuroperitoneal opening on this side (white arrows) (ad, adrenals; di, anlage of diaphragm).

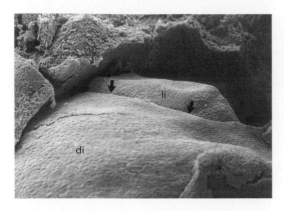

Figure 1.6 Liver (li) protrudes through diaphragmatic defect. Arrows point to the margin of the defect (di, diaphragmatic anlage). Rat embryo (approx. 16 days old), nitrofen exposition on day 11 of pregnancy.

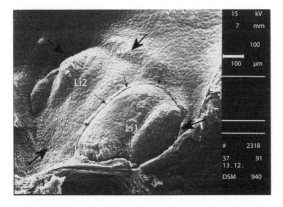

Figure 1.7 SEM photograph of a right pleural sac in a rat embryo after nitrofen exposure on day 11 of pregnancy. The embryo is approximately 15.5 days old. Note the big defect of the right dorsal diaphragm (large arrows). The closure of the pleuroperitoneal canal (PPC) is impaired by the ingrowths of liver (small arrows). Li1 = liver growing through PPC. Li1 + Li2 = liver growing through the defect of the diaphragm.

was a distinct entity and was separated from that part of the diaphragm where the pleuroperitoneal "canals" are localized. We conclude therefore that the pleuroperitoneal openings are not the precursors of the diaphragmatic defect.

Why lungs are hypoplastic

Soon after the onset of the defect in the 14-day-old embryo, liver grows through the diaphragmatic defect into the thoracic cavity (Figure 1.6). This indicates that, from this time on, the available thoracic space is reduced for the lung and further lung growth is hampered. In the following stages, up to two-thirds of the thoracic cavity can be occupied by liver (Figure 1.7). Herniated guts were found in our embryos and fetuses only in late stages of development (21 days and newborns). In all of these, the lungs were already hypoplastic when the bowel entered the thoracic cavity.[79]

Based on these observations, we conclude that the early ingrowth of the liver through the diaphragmatic defect is

the crucial step in the pathogenesis of lung hypoplasia in CDH. This indicates that growth impairment is not the result of lung compression in the fetus but rather the result of growth competition in the embryo: the liver that grows faster than the lung reduces the available thoracic space. If the remaining space is too small, pulmonary hypoplasia will result.

DEVELOPMENT OF THE EMBRYONIC CLOACA (EC)

General remarks on the development of the EC

The terminology of malformations is sometimes confusing. As already mentioned, there is a strong belief that human embryos go through a phase in their development where they have a "cloaca." This belief is based on Haeckel's "biogenetic law."[5] According to this theory, a human embryo recapitulates in its individual development (ontogeny) the morphology observed in all life forms (phylogeny). This means that the development of advanced species passes through stages represented by adult organisms of more primitive species. This theory still has an impact on the nomenclature of embryonic organs.

Literature on "normal cloacal development"

In the literature, several theories have been put forward to explain the differentiation of the "cloaca" into the dorsal anorectum and the ventral sinus urogenitalis. To many authors, this differentiation is caused by a septum that develops cranially to caudally and thus divides the cloaca in a frontal plane. Disorders in this process of differentiation are thought to be the cause of "cloacal" anomalies such as "persistent cloaca" and anorectal malformations.

However, there is no agreement on the mechanisms of septation. While some authors[94,95] believe that the descent of a single fold separates the urogenital part from the rectal part by ingrowth of mesenchyme from cranial, others[96] think that lateral ridges appear in the lumen of the cloaca, which progressively fuse along the midline and thus form the septum. In a recent paper,[97] the process of septation had been questioned altogether.

Own observations

Using SEM techniques, our group studied cloacal development in rat and SD-mice embryos. The SD-mouse is a spontaneous mutation of the house mouse characterized by having a short tail (Figure 1.8). Homozygous or heterozygous offspring of these mice show skeletal, urogenital, and anorectal malformations.[25,28] Therefore, these animals are ideal for the study of the development of anorectal malformations.

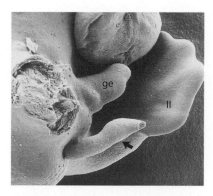

Figure 1.8 Characteristic short tail (arrow) of SD-mouse embryo (approx. 13 days old) (ll, left lower limb; ge, genital tuberculum, abnormal).

Normal "cloacal" embryology (rat)

As in the foregut of chick embryos, signs of median fusion of lateral cloacal parts could not be demonstrated during normal cloacal development in the rat. However, in contradiction to van der Putte,[97] we think that downgrowth of the urorectal fold takes place, although it is probably not responsible for the formation of "cloacal" malformations.

Abnormal "cloacal" embryology (SD-mouse)

"Cloacal" malformations are caused by improper development of the early anlage of the cloacal membrane as demonstrated in SD-mice embryos.[98,99] Our studies of abnormal "cloacal" development in SD-mice had the following results:

1. The basis of the pathogenesis of anorectal malformations is too short a cloacal membrane.
2. The anlage of the cloacal membrane is too short and results in a maldeveloped anlage of the "cloaca," which is missing in its dorsal part (Figure 1.9).
3. The caudal movement of the urorectal fold is impaired in the malformed "cloaca." Thus, the hindgut remains in abnormal contact with the urethral part. This opening is true ectopic and will develop into the recto-urogenital fistula (Figure 1.10).

It is interesting to note that the morphology of the anorectal malformations observed is very similar in all animal models used irrespective of the source of the malformed embryo (spontaneous mutation vs. chemically induced vs. transgenic models).

Critical remarks on the terminology of the "cloaca"

It must be kept in mind that the term "cloaca" is used to describe not only a transitional organ system in human

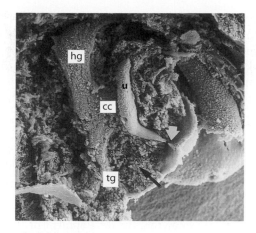

Figure 1.9 Malformed cloaca of SD-mouse embryo (approx. 11 days old). The surrounding mesenchyme is removed by microdissection. View on the basal layer of the cloacal entoderm. The cloaca has lost its contact to the ectoderm of the genitals (white arrow). The dorsal part of the cloaca is missing (black arrow). Tailgut (tg) and hindgut (hg) are hypoplastic. This malformed cloaca developed because the anlage of the cloacal membrane was too short in early embryogenesis (see text for details) (cc, rest of cloaca; u, urachus, rudimentary).

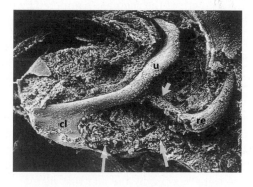

Figure 1.10 Malformed cloaca of SD-mouse embryo (approx. 13 days old). Urachus (u) and rectum (re) nearly normal (cl, ventral part of cloaca with short cloacal membrane). The dorsal part of the cloaca is missing (long white arrows). Short white arrow points to the region of the future fistula.

embryos but also a congenital anomaly in human female newborns and a normal organ in birds.[99]

This may lead to the false conclusion that the morphology of these three entities is similar. This is not the case. Despite the same name, embryonic "cloacas" are morphologically completely different from "cloacas" in female newborns with ARM. And these female "cloacas" are morphologically completely different from cloacas in birds.[100]

The main difference is the presence/absence and position of the anus:

1. In normal embryonic "cloacas," the future anal region is always present.
2. In human "cloacas," the anus is always missing.
3. In birds, the "cloaca" is part of the rectum.

Thus, the anus is always present in birds.

Furthermore, it is obvious that a true definition of the term embryonic "cloaca" is missing. In many papers and textbooks, it is replaced by observations made in female newborns born with the malformation called "cloaca." These are defined as defects "in which the rectum, one or two vaginas and the urinary tract converge into a common channel."[101]

It is believed that they represent malformations that occur in a very early stage of development.[101] Therefore, many authors believe that these malformations are "persistent cloacas."[101]

However, recent observations on the development of the vagina in mice[102] show that the development of the vagina and its downgrowth takes place after the complete separation of urethra and anorectum. As a result, a "cloaca" in the above-mentioned definition does not exist in normal embryos.

How can the female malformation called "cloaca" be explained? In our opinion, this malformation develops in two steps:

1. An anorectal malformation develops as described above.
2. The downgrowth of the vagina is hampered by the abnormal connection between urethra and anorectum (Figure 1.10).

HYPOSPADIAS

Many investigators[103–106] believe that the urethra develops by fusion of the paired urethral folds following the disintegration of the urogenital membrane. Impairment of this process is thought to result in the different forms of hypospadia.[106] However, in our study of normal cloacal development,[107] we were puzzled by the fact that disintegration of the urogenital part of the cloacal membrane could not be observed in rat embryos (Figure 1.11). This finding caused us to call in question the generally assumed concepts of hypospadia formation. Instead we found that

1. The urethra is always present as a hollow organ during embryogenesis of rats, and that it is always in contact with the tip of the genitals.
2. An initially double urethral anlage exists. The differentiation in female and male urethra starts in rats of 18.5 days old. On the other hand, we found no evidence for
   a. The disintegration of the urogenital cloacal membrane
   b. A fusion of lateral portions within the perineum

In our opinion, more than one embryological mechanism is at play in the formation of the hypospadias complex. The moderate degrees, such as the penile and glandular forms, represent a developmental arrest of the genitalia (Figure 1.12). They take their origin from a situation comparable

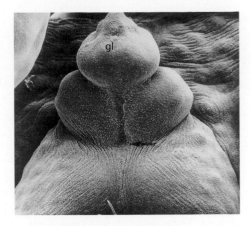

Figure 1.11 Genitals of a normal female rat embryo (approx. 18.5 days old) (gl, glans). Arrow points to future opening of the female urethra. No signs of disintegration of the cloacal membrane.

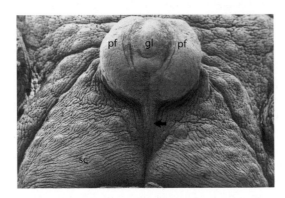

Figure 1.12 Genitals of a normal male rat embryo (approx. 20 days old) (gl, glans; pf, preputial fold; sc, scrotum). Arrow points to the raphe up to this stage; disintegration of the urogenital part of the cloacal membrane was not seen. Note similarity with clinical picture of hypospadia.

to the 20-day-old embryo. Consequently, the penis, not the urethra, is the primary organ of the malformation.

Perineal and scrotal hypospadias are different from the type discussed previously. Pronounced signs of feminization in these forms suggest that we are dealing with a female-type urethra. The origin of this malformation complex is an undifferentiated stage as may be seen in the 18.5-day-old rat embryo.[104]

CONCLUSION

Despite the long history of experimental embryology, we know very little about etiology and pathogenesis of congenital malformations. For decades, hypotheses were abundant while few data existed to support them. The tremendous progress of neighboring biological sciences is now providing powerful tools for researchers in the field, such as recombinant DNA and hybridoma technology. Future investigations will monitor closely how genes are switched on and off during embryogenesis and determine the relation of spatial and temporal disturbances to ensuing malformations. Target structures of chemical or viral teratogens within the embryonic cells await identification. Finally, improved understanding of growth coordination in utero will extend to related areas such as wound healing and proliferation of cancer cells.

REFERENCES

1. Nadler HL. Teratology. In: Welch KJ, Randolph JG, Ravitch MM, O'Neill JA, Rowe MJ (eds). *Pediatric Surgery*, 4th edn. Chicago: Year Book Medical Publishers, 1986: 11–3.

2. Shepard TH. *Catalogue of Teratogenic Agents*, 4th edn. Baltimore: Johns Hopkins Press, 1983.

3. United States National Center for Health Statistics. Monthly Vital Statistics Report, Vol. 31. No. 5. Birth, marriages, divorces, and deaths for May 1982. Hyattsville, MD: Public Health Service, 1982: 1–10.

4. Steding G. *The Anatomy of the Human Embryo. A Scanning Electron-Microscopic Atlas*. Basel: Karger, 2009.

5. Gilbert SF. *Developmental Biology*, 7th edn, Chapter 23. Sunderland, MA: Sinauer Associates, 2003.

6. Schwalbe E. *Die Morphologie der Missbildungen des Menschen und derTiere. 1. Teil Allgemeine Mißbildungslehre (Teratologie)*. Jena, Germany: Gustav Fischer, 1906: 143–4.

7. McCredie J, Loewenthal J. Pathogenesis of congenital malformations. *Am J Surg* 1978; 135: 293–7.

8. Spemann, Mangold, cited by Starck D. *Embryologie*. Stuttgart: Thieme, 1975: 135–63.

9. Warkany J, Roth CB, Wilson JG. Multiple congenital malformations: A consideration of etiological factors. *Pediatrics* 1948; 1: 462–71.

10. Kalter H. Congenital malformations induced by riboflavin deficiency in strains of inbred mice. *Pediatrics* 1959; 23: 222–30.

11. Kalter H. The inheritance of susceptibility to the teratogenic action of cortisone in mice. *Genetics* 1954; 39: 185.

12. Lenz W. Fragen aus der Praxis. *Dtsch Med Wochenschr* 1961; 86: 25–55.

13. Ministry of Health Reports on Public Health and Medical Subjects No. 112. *Deformities Caused by Thalidomide*. London: HMSO, 1964.

14. Ambrose AM, Larson PS, Borcelleca JF, Blackwell Smith Jr R, Hennigar Jr GR. Toxicological studies on 2,4-dichlorophenyl-P-nitrophenyl ether. *Toxicol Appl Pharmacol* 1971; 19: 263–75.

15. Tenbrinck R, Tibboel D, Gaillard JLJ, Kluth D, Bos AP, Lachmann B, Molenaar JC. Experimentally induced congenital diaphragmatic hernia in rats. *J Pediatr Surg* 1990; 25: 426–9.

16. Kluth D, Kangha R, Reich P, Tenbrinck R, Tibboel D, Lambrecht W. Nitrofen-induced diaphragmatic hernia in rats—An animal model. *J Pediatr Surg* 1990; 25: 850–4.

17. Costlow RD, Manson JM. The heart and diaphragm: Target organs in the neonatal death induced by nitrofen (2,4-dichloro-phenyl-P-nitrophenyl ether). *Toxicology* 1981; 20: 209–27.

18. Iritani L. Experimental study on embryogenesis of congenital diaphragmatic hernia. *Anat Embryol* 1984; 169: 133–9.

19. Thompson DJ, Molello JA, Strebing RJ, Dyke IL. Teratogenicity of Adriamycin and daunomycin in the rat and rabbit. *Teratology* 1978; 17: 151–8.

20. Diez-Pardo JA, Baoquan Q, Navarro C, Tovar JA. A new rodent experimental model of esophageal atresia and tracheoesophageal fistula: Preliminary report. *J Pediatr Surg* 1996; 31: 498–502.

21. Beasley SW, Diez-Pardo J, Qi BQ, Tovar JA, Xia HM. The contribution of the Adriamycin-induced rat model of the VATER association to our understanding of congenital abnormalities and their embryogenesis. *Pediatr Surg Int* 2000; 16: 465–72.

22. Orford JE, Cass DT. Dose response relationship between Adriamycin and birth defects in a rat model of VATER association. *J Pediatr Surg* 1999; 34: 392–8.

23. Rosenbaum KN. Genetics and dysmorphology. In: Welch KJ, Randolph MM, Ravitch MM, O'Neill JA, Rowe MJ (eds). *Pediatric Surgery*, 4th edn. Chicago: Year Book Medical Publishers, 1986: 3–11.

24. van der Putte SCJ, Neeteson FA. The pathogenesis of hereditary congenital malformations in the pig. *Acta Morphol Neerl Scand* 1984; 22: 17–40.

25. Kluth D, Lambrecht W, Reich P, Buehrer C. SD mice—An animal model for complex anorectal malformations. *Eur J Pediatr Surg* 1991; 1: 183–8.

26. Lambrecht W, Lierse W. The internal sphincter in anorectal malformations: Morphologic investigations in neonatal pigs. *J Pediatr Surg* 1987; 22: 1160–8.

27. Dunn LC, Gluecksohn-Schoenheimer S, Bryson V. A new mutation in the mouse affecting spinal column and urogenital system. *J Hered* 1940; 31: 343–8.

28. Goldin GV, Opperman LA. Induction of supernumerary tracheal buds and the stimulation of DNA synthesis in the embryonic chick lung and trachea by epidermal growth factor. *J Embryol Exp Morphol* 1980; 60: 235–43.

29. Steding G. Ursachen der embryonalen Epithelverdickung. *Acta Anat* 1967; 68: 37–67.

30. Jacob HJ. Experimente zur Entstehung entodermaler Organanlagen. Untersuchungen an explantierten Hühnerembryonen. *Anat Anzeiger* 1971; 128: 271–8.

31. Molenaar JC, Tibboel D. The pathogenesis of atresias of the small bowel and colon. *S Afr J Surg* 1982; 20: 87–95.

32. Schoenberg RA, Kluth D. Experimental small bowel obstruction in chick embryos: Effects on the developing enteric nervous system. *J Pediatr Surg* 2002; 37: 735–40.

33. Aktuğ T, Hoşgör M, Akgür FM, Olguner M, Kargi A, Tibboel D. End-results of experimental gastroschisis created by abdominal wall versus umbilical cord defect. *Pediatr Surg Int* 1997; 12: 583–6.

34. Meijers JH, van der Sanden MP, Tibboel D, van der Kamp AW, Luider TM, Molenaar JC. Colonization characteristics of enteric neural crest cells: Embryological aspects of Hirschsprung's disease. *J Pediatr Surg* 1992; 27: 811–4.

35. Lemez L. Sites for experimental production of tracheal and/or oesophageal malformations in 4-day-old chick embryos. *Folia Morphol (Praha)* 1980; 28: 52–5.

36. Harrison MR, Jester JA, Ross NA. Correction of congenital diaphragmatic hernia in utero. I. The model: Intrathoracic balloon produces fatal pulmonary hypoplasia. *Surgery* 1980 Jul; 88(1): 174–82.

37. Kubota Y, Shimotake T, Yanagihara J, Iwai N. Development of anorectal malformations using etretinate. *J Pediatr Surg* 1998; 33: 127–9.

38. Liu Y, Sugiyama F, Yagami K, Ohkawa H. Sharing of the same embryogenic pathway in anorectal malformations and anterior sacral myelomeningocele formation. *Pediatr Surg Int* 2003; 19: 152–6.

39. Bitoh Y, Shimotake T, Sasaki Y, Iwai N. Development of the pelvic floor muscles of murine embryos with anorectal malformations. *J Pediatr Surg* 2002; 37: 224–7.

40. Hashimoto R, Nagaya M, Ishiguro Y, Inouye M, Aoyama H, Futaki S, Murata Y. Relationship of the fistulas to the rectum and genitourinary tract in mouse fetuses with high anorectal malformations induced by all-trans retinoic acid. *Pediatr Surg Int* 2002; 18: 723–7.

41. Sasaki Y, Iwai N, Tsuda T, Kimura O. Sonic hedgehog and bone morphogenetic protein 4 expressions in the hindgut region of murine embryos with anorectal malformations. *J Pediatr Surg* 2004; 39: 170–3.

42. Arana J, Villanueva A, Guarch R, Aldazabal P, Barriola M. Anorectal atresia. An experimental model in the rat. *Eur J Pediatr Surg* 2001; 11: 192–5.

43. Qi BQ, Beasley SW, Frizelle FA. Clarification of the processes that lead to anorectal malformations in the ETU-induced rat model of imperforate anus. *J Pediatr Surg* 2002; 37: 1305–12.

44. Yuan ZW, Lui VC, Tam PK. Deficient motor innervation of the sphincter mechanism in fetal rats with anorectal malformation: A quantitative study by fluorogold retrograde tracing. *J Pediatr Surg* 2003; 38: 1383–8.

45. Litingtung Y, Lei L, Westphal H, Chiang C. Sonic hedgehog is essential to foregut development. *Nat Genet* 1998 Sep; 20(1): 58–61.

46. Kim J, Kim P, Hui CC. The VACTERL association: Lessons from the Sonic hedgehog pathway. *Clin Genet* 2001; 59: 306–15.

47. Mo R, Kim JH, Zhang J, Chiang C, Hui CC, Kim PC. Anorectal malformations caused by defects in sonic hedgehog signaling. *Am J Pathol* 2001; 159: 765–74.

48. Arsic D, Cameron V, Ellmers L, Quan QB, Keenan J, Beasley S. Adriamycin disruption of the Shh-Gli pathway is associated with abnormalities of foregut development. *J Pediatr Surg* 2004; 39: 1747–53.

49. Petersen C, Biermanns D, Kuske M, Schäkel K, Meyer-Junghänel L, Mildenberger H. New aspects in a murine model for extrahepatic biliary atresia. *J Pediatr Surg* 1997; 32: 1190–5.

50. Fiegel HC, Rolle U, Metzger R, Geyer C, Till H, Kluth D. The testicular descent in the rat: A scanning electron microscopic study. *Pediatr Surg Int* 2010; 26: 643–7.

51. Spemann H. Entwicklungsphysiologische Studien am Tritonei. ROIIX. *Arch Entw Mech* 1901; 12: 224–64.

52. Murray JD, Maini PK. A new approach to the generation of pattern and form in embryology. *Sri Progr Oxf* 1986; 70: 539–53.

53. Gudernatsch JF. Concerning the mechanisms and direction of embryonic folding. *Anat Rec* 1913; 7: 411–31.

54. Oster G, Alberich P. Evolution and bifurcation of developmental programmes. *Evolution* 1982; 36: 444–59.

55. Ettersohn CA. Mechanisms of epithelial invagination. *Q Rev Biol* 1985; 60: 289–307.

56. Jaffredo T, Horwitz AF, Buck CA, Rong PM, Dieterlen-Lievre F. Myoblast migration specifically inhibited in the chick embryo by grafted CSAT hybridoma cells secreting an anti-integrin antibody. *Development* 1988; 103: 431–46.

57. Ruoslahti E, Pierschbacher MD. 7 New perspectives in cell adhesions: RDG and integrins. *Science* 198; 238: 491–7.

58. Stoolman LM. Adhesion molecules controlling lymphocyte migration. *Cell* 1989; 56: 907–10.

59. Simmons D, Makgoba MW, Seed B. ICAM, an adhesion ligand for LFA-1, is homologous to the neural cell adhesion molecule NCAM. *Nature* 1988; 331: 624–7.

60. Staunton DE, Dustin L, Springer TA. Functional cloning of ICAM-2, a cell adhesion ligand for LFA-1 homologous to ICAM-1. *Nature* 1989; 339: 61–4.

61. Gallin WJ, Sorkin C, Edelman GM, Cunningham BA. Sequence analysis of a cDNA clone encoding the liver cell adhesion molecule, L-CAM. *Proc Natl Acad Sci USA* 1987 May; 84(9): 2808–12.

62. Edelman GM. Morphoregulatory molecules. *Biochemistry* 1988; 27: 3533–43.

63. Rutishauser U, Acheson A, Hall AK, Mann DM, Sunshine J. The neural cell adhesion molecule (NCAM) as a regulator of cell-cell interactions. *Science* 1988; 240: 53–7.

64. Edelman GM. Topobiology. *Sci Amer* 1989; May: 44–52.

65. Tedder TF, Isaacs CM, Ernst TJ, Demetri GD, Adler DA, Disteche CM. Isolation and chromosomal localisation of cDNAs encoding a novel human lymphocyte cell surface molecule, LAM-1. *J Exp Med* 1989; 170: 123–33.

66. Yednock TA, Rosen D. Lymphocyte homing. *Adv Immunol* 1989; 44: 313–78.

67. Spooner BS. Microfilaments, microtubules, and extra-cellular materials in morphogenesis. *BioScience* 1975; 25: 440–51.

68. Baker PC, Schroeder TE. Cytoplasmatic filaments and morphogenetic movement in the amphibian neural tube. *Dev Biol* 1967; 15: 432–50.

69. Alescio T, DiMichele M. Relationship of epithelial growth to mitotic rate in mouse embryonic lung developing in vitro. *Embryol Exp Morphol* 1968; 19: 227–37.

70. Smith JM, Sporn MB, Roberts AB, Derynck R, Winkler ME, Gregory H. Human transforming growth factor-alpha causes precocious eyelid opening in newborn mice. *Nature* 1985; 315: 515–6.

71. Sporn MB, Roberts AB, Wakefield LM, Assoian RK. Transforming growth factor-beta: Biological function and chemical structure. *Science* 1986; 233: 532–4.

72. Sporn MB, Roberts AB, Wakefield LM, de Crombrugghe B. Some recent advances in the chemistry and biology of transforming growth factor-beta. *J Cell Biol* 1987; 105: 1039–45.

73. Anzano MA, Roberts AB, Sporn MB. Anchor-age-independent growth of primary rat embryo cells is induced by platelet-derived growth factor and inhibited by type-beta transforming growth factor. *J Cell Physiol* 1986; 126: 312–8.

74. Nogawa H. Determination of the curvature of epithelial cell mass by mesenchyme in branching morphogenesis of mouse salivary gland. *J Embryol Exp Morphol* 1983; 73: 221–32.

75. Smuts MS, Hilfer SR, Searls RL. Patterns of cellular proliferation during thyroid organogenesis. *J Embryol Exp Morphol* 1978; 48: 269–86.

76. Kluth D, Steding G, Seidl W. The embryology of foregut malformations. *J Pediatr Surg* 1987; 22: 389–93.

77. Kluth D, Habenicht R. The embryology of usual and unusual types of oesophageal atresia. *Pediatr Surg Int* 1987; 1: 223–7.

78. Kluth D, Petersen C, Zimmermann HJ, Mulhaus K. The embryology of congenital diaphragmatic hernia. In: Puri P (ed). *Congenital Diaphragmatic Hernia: Modern Problems in Pediatrics*, Vol. 24. Basel: Karger, 1989: 7–21.

79. Kluth D, Tenbrinck R, v. Ekesparre M, Kangah R, Reich P, Brandsma A, Tibboel D, Lambrecht W. The natural history of congenital diaphragmatic hernia in pulmonary hypoplasia in the embryo. *J Pediatr Surg* 1993; 28: 456–63.

80. Kluth D, Tander B, v. Ekesparre M, Tibboel D, Lambrecht W. Congenital diaphragmatic hernia: The impact of embryological studies. *Pediatr Surg Int* 1995; 10: 16–22.

81. Kluth D, Losty PD, Schnitzer JJ, Lambrecht W, Donahoe PK. Toward understanding the developmental anatomy of congenital diaphragmatic hernia. *Clin Perinatol* 1996; 23: 655–69.

82. Kluth D, Keijzer R, Hertl M, Tibboel D. Embryology of congenital diaphragmatic hernia. *Semin Pediatr Surg* 1996; 5: 224–33.

83. His W. Zur Bildungsgeschichte der Lungen beim menschlichen Embryo. *Arch Anat Entwickl Gesch* 1887; 89–106.

84. Rosenthal AH. Congenital atresia of the esophagus with tracheo esophageal fistula: Report of eight cases. *Arch Pathol* 1931; 12: 756–72.

85. Smith EL. The early development of the trachea and the esophagus in relation to atresia of the esophagus and tracheo-oesophageal fistula. *Contrib Embyol Carneg Inst* 1957; 36:41–57.

86. Zaw Tun HA. The tracheo-esophageal septum—Fact or fantasy? *Acta Anat* 1982; 114: 1–21.

87. O'Rahilly R, Muller F. Chevalier Jackson Lecture. Respiratory and alimentary relations in staged human embryos. New embryological data and congenital anomalies. *Ann Otol Rhinol Laryngol* 1984; 93: 421–9.

88. Medline recherché, http://www.ncbi.nlm.nih.gov /PubMed/.

89. Gray SW, Skandalakis JE. *Embryology for Surgeons*. Philadelphia: Saunders, 1972: 359–85.

90. Grosser O, Ortmann R. *Grundriß der Entwicklungsgeschichte des Menschen*, 7th edn. Berlin: Springer, 1970: 124–7.

91. Holder RM, Ashcraft KW. Congenital diaphragmatic hernia. In: Ravitch MM, Welch KJ, Benson CD, Aberdeen E, Randolph JG (eds). *Pediatric Surgery*, 3rd edn, Vol. 1. Chicago: Year Book Medical Publishers, 1979: 432–45.

92. Bremer JL. The diaphragm and diaphragmatic hernia. *Arch Pathol* 1943; 36: 539–49.

93. Gattone VH II, Morse DE. A scanning electron microscopic study on the pathogenesis of the posterolateral diaphragmatic hernia. *J Submicrosc Cytol* 1982; 14: 483–90.

94. Tourneux F. Sur le premiers developpements du cloaque du tubercle genitale et de l'anus chez l'embryon moutons, avec quelques remarques concernant le developpement des glandes prostatiques. *J Anat Physiol* 1888; 24: 503–17.

95. DeVries P, Friedland GW. The staged sequential development of the anus and rectum in human embryos and fetuses. *J Pediatr Surg* 1974; 9: 755–69.

96. Retterer E. Sur l'origin et de l'evolution de la region ano-génitale des mammiferes. *J Anat Physiol* 1890; 26: 126–216.

97. van der Putte SCJ. Normal and abnormal development of the anorectum. *J Pediatr Surg* 1986; 21: 434–40.
98. Kluth D, Hillen M, Lambrecht W. The principles of normal and abnormal hindgut development. *J Pediatr Surg* 1995; 30: 1143–7.
99. Kluth D, Lambrecht W. Current concepts in the embryology of anorectal malformations. *Semin Pediatr Surg* 1997; 6: 180–6.
100. Salomon FV, Krautwald-Junghanns M. Die Anatomie der Vögel. In: Geyer H, Gille U, Salomon FV (eds). Anatomie für die Tiermedizin, 3rd edn, Chapter 13. Stuttgart: Enke, 2015.
101. Holschneider AM, Scharbatke H. Persistent cloaca—Clinical aspects. In: Holschneider AM, Hutson J (eds). *Anorectal Malformation in Children*, Chapter 10. Heidelberg: Springer, 2006: 2001.
102. Drews U. Helper function of the Wolffian ducts and role of androgens in the development of the vagina. *Sex Dev* 2007: 100–10.
103. Felix W. Die Entwicklung der Harn-und Geschlechtsorgane. In: Keibel F, Mall FP (eds). *Handbuch der Entwicklungsgeschichte des Menschen*, Vol. 2. Leipzig: Hirzel, 1911: 92–5.
104. Spaulding MH. The development of the external genitalia in the human embryo. *Contrib Embryol Carneg* 1921; 13: 67–88.
105. Glenister TW. A correlation of the normal and abnormal development of the penile urethra and of the intraabdominal wall. *J Urol* 1958; 30: 117–26.
106. Gray SW, Skandalakis JE. *Embryology for Surgeons*. Philadelphia: Saunders, 1972: 595–631.
107. Kluth D, Lambrecht W, Reich P. Pathogenesis hypospadias—More questions than answers. *J Pediatr Surg* 1988; 23: 1095–101.

2

Transition to extrauterine life

CARLOS E. BLANCO AND EDUARDO VILLAMOR

INTRODUCTION

In order to succeed in this transition, the respiratory system must be developed enough to assure a sufficient alveolar exchange area, it must have a drive to offer a continuous breathing activity, and the circulatory system should start perfusing the lungs instead of the placenta.

This chapter will discuss the mechanisms preparing the fetus to be born, the transition at birth, and the successful adaptation to the air-breathing world. This chapter will review the respiratory system, the respiratory drive and chemoreceptor role, and the circulatory system including fetal circulation and its changes at birth.

FETAL CIRCULATION AND ITS TRANSITION AT BIRTH

EDUARDO VILLAMOR

The fetal circulation is characterized by high pulmonary vascular resistance (PVR), low systemic vascular resistance (SVR), presence of an additional low resistance vascular bed (i.e., the placental bed), and right-to-left shunting via the foramen ovale and ductus arteriosus (DA).[1] Distribution of blood flow to the lungs, systemic organs, and placenta is determined by local vascularl resistance. The placental vascular bed receives about 40%–50% of the combined ventricular output, whereas the lungs receive less than 10%. In response to fetal hypoxemia, distribution of cardiac output and venous return is altered in an effort to maintain perfusion and O_2 delivery to the vital organs such as the heart, brain, and adrenal glands.[2,3] Thus, during maternofetal hypoxia, the percentage of systemic venous blood not sent to the placenta for oxygenation is decreased, whereas the proportion of umbilical venous blood contributing to fetal cardiac output is increased.[2,3]

The human placenta was widely thought of as a passive organ in which blood flow depends only on the pressure difference between the umbilical arteries and vein connecting it to the fetus.[4,5] However, more recent evidences indicate that the regulation of vasomotor tone in the vessels of the fetoplacental circulation is important to maintain an adequate blood supply that makes possible maternofetal gas and solute exchange.[4-6] As fetoplacental blood vessels lack autonomic innervation, control of vascular tone is mainly influenced by circulating and/or locally released vasoactive agents as well as by physical factors, such as flow or oxygen tension.[7] Accordingly, constriction and relaxation of fetoplacental arteries and veins have been demonstrated in response to a number of agonists and physical stimuli. Moreover, various authors have suggested that the fetoplacental vasculature shows some form of flow matching similar to hypoxic pulmonary vasoconstriction. This mechanism, termed hypoxic fetoplacental vasoconstriction,[6,8,9] would divert blood flow to the placental areas with better maternal perfusion as hypoxic pulmonary vasoconstriction diverts pulmonary blood flow to the better ventilated areas of the lung.[9-11]

Separating the infant from the placenta by clamping the umbilical cord necessitates the rapid switch to pulmonary gas exchange within minutes of birth. This switch not only involves aeration of the airways and gas exchange regions of the lung but also includes a major reorganization of the fetal cardiovascular system.[12] As the lung assumes the respiratory function, the pulmonary circulation undergoes a striking transition characterized by an immediate 8- to 10-fold rise in pulmonary blood flow and a sustained decrease in PVR.[13-16] The postnatal fall in PVR and rise in SVR results in a reversal of the relationships present in the fetus. Moreover, pulmonary blood flow must have the capacity to replace umbilical venous return as the primary source of preload for the left ventricle when the cord is clamped.[12] Increasing blood return to the heart via the pulmonary veins raises the pressure of the left atrium above that of the right, causing a functional closure of the foramen ovale. While the DA is still patent, the flow of blood through it will change to a left-to-right shunt, but the DA normally achieves functional closure within 48 hours after birth. Because the foramen ovale and DA are only functionally closed and the pulmonary circulation is very sensitive to vasoconstrictive stimuli, the neonatal circulatory pattern can readily revert to the fetal pattern. In the following paragraphs, the different circulatory events that take place during the transition between fetal and postnatal life will be analyzed in more detail.

Closure of the ductus venosus

The ductus venosus is a shunt between the umbilical vein and the inferior vena cava, which allows highly oxygenated and nutrient-rich umbilical venous blood to bypass the liver and reach the central circulation rapidly.[1] A large proportion of inferior vena caval return crosses the foramen ovale into the left atrium to the left ventricle, and is thus distributed to the coronary and cerebral circulations. The PO_2 of blood supplying the heart, brain, head, and neck is higher by 4–5 mmHg than that of blood in the descending aorta. Although the ductus venosus has received less attention than the DA, it is now well accepted that it plays a major role in the regulation of fetal circulation. Inlet of the vessel is under active control and a compensatory mechanism, supported by transient dilatation, is supposed to increase oxygenated blood flow through the ductus venosus during hypoxia or reduced umbilical flow.[17] Absence of the ductus venosus is associated with a high incidence of fetal anomalies and adverse outcomes, including associated malformations, chromosomal aberrations, in utero heart failure, and absence of the portal vein.[18] Functional closure of the ductus venosus, which is followed by anatomic closure, is virtually complete within a few weeks of birth. However, the ductus venosus of almost all neonates remains open for a certain period after birth with important variations in the volume of blood flow.[19] Closure of the ductus venosus is more delayed in preterm neonates, and patent ductus venosus appears to be related to alterations in ammonia detoxification, blood coagulation, and regulation of serum total bile acid concentration.[19]

Closure of the foramen ovale

Anatomically, the foramen ovale comprises overlapping portions of septum primum and septum secundum, acting as a one-way flap valve allowing continuous right-to-left flow during fetal life.[20] Immediately after birth, with the acute increase in pulmonary blood flow, left atrium pressure rises to exceed right atrium pressure, pushing septum primum rightward, against septum secundum, shutting the flap of the foramen ovale. Afterward, septum primum fuses to septum secundum, completing septation of the atria. However, in 20% to 25%, incomplete fusion leads to the persistence of the flap valve, leaving a patent foramen ovale.[20] In general, individuals with patent foramen ovale are never identified because they have no symptoms. However, there is increasing interest in the evaluation and treatment of patent foramen ovale, which has been associated with various pathologic conditions, such as cryptogenic stroke,

decompression sickness, platypnea–orthodeoxia syndrome, and migraine.[21]

Fall in PVR

Although the regulation of the pulmonary circulation in the fetus and newborn is under many interacting and redundant signaling pathways, the ability to adapt to changes in the availability of O_2 is probably the most relevant.[22] The fetal lung is continuously exposed to a low O_2 tension, which induces a vigorous hypoxic pulmonary vasoconstriction.[14,23,24] This physiological level of hypoxia maintains the fetal type of circulation and also promotes normal vascular growth. However, an increase in the degree of hypoxia results in abnormal signaling and vascular remodeling.[14,23,24]

At birth, with the onset of breathing, PVR dramatically decreases and pulmonary blood flow increases such that the entire right ventricular output goes to the lung, as they assume the function of gas exchange. The hemodynamic changes in the pulmonary circulation after birth are regulated by various mechanical factors and vasoactive agents in a complicated but coordinated manner. These mechanisms not only are involved in the immediate postnatal fall in PVR but also help maintain the low PVR in the newborn and the adult. Besides the increase in O_2 tension, several other mechanisms contribute to the normal fall in PVR at birth, including the establishment of a gas–liquid interface in the lung, rhythmic distension of the lung, and shear stress.[13,14,25] These physical stimuli act, at least partially, through the production of vasoactive products. An increased release of vasodilators, in particular nitric oxide (NO) and prostaglandin (PG)I_2, and a decreased release of vasoconstrictors such as platelet activating factor (PAF) or endothelin (ET)-1, as well as changes in their signaling pathways, contribute significantly to the fall in PVR.[13,16,26,27] Normally, pulmonary arterial pressure falls to the half of the systemic pressure by 24 hours and then progressively decreases to adult levels within 2–6 weeks.[28] Therefore, the process of pulmonary circulatory transition is not limited to the first moments of extrauterine life, but it extends during the following weeks.[28]

Failure of the pulmonary circulation to undergo a normal transition results in persistent pulmonary hypertension of the newborn (PPHN), a clinical syndrome of various neonatal cardiopulmonary disorders that are characterized by sustained elevation of PVR after birth, leading to right-to-left shunting of blood across the DA or foramen ovale and severe hypoxemia.[14,16] PPHN is a pathophysiological phenomenon occurring in a heterogeneous group of diseases with a wide diversity of etiologies. These range from transient reversible pulmonary hypertension attributable to perinatal insults to irreversible fixed structural malformations of the lung. Diseases associated with the syndrome of PPHN can be classified in three categories[13,15]: (1) maladaptation, in which vessels are presumably of normal structure but have abnormal vasoreactivity; (2) excessive muscularization, in which smooth muscle cell thickness is increased and muscle extends distally to vessels that usually are nonmuscular; and (3) underdevelopment, in which lung hypoplasia is associated with decreased number of pulmonary arteries. Either as a primary condition or secondary to other pulmonary or extrapulmonary diseases, PPHN is an important cause of cardiorespiratory failure and responsible for a relevant percentage of morbidity in the neonatal intensive care units.[13,15] The progress made in our understanding of the regulation of the perinatal pulmonary circulation has helped in the development of new treatments for PPHN, such as NO inhalation, PGI_2 inhalation, inhibition of cGMP degradation by type 5 phosphodiesterase with sildenafil, inhibition of cAMP degradation with milrinone, and inhibition of ET-1 with bosentan.[27]

Closure of the DA

The DA is distinguished from the surrounding vasculature by its embryologic derivation from the left sixth aortic arch, the contribution of migratory neural crest cells, and exquisite sensitivity to oxygen tension.[29] Low O_2 tension, high levels of circulating PGE_2, and locally produced PGE_2 and PGI_2 are the main factors maintaining patency of the DA in utero.[30–32]

Classically, the process of DA is divided into two sequential steps: functional and structural. However, it should be noted that these steps overlap and the causative agents may be shared.[33] Several events promote the constriction of the DA in the full-term newborn: (1) the increase in arterial PO_2, (2) the decrease in blood pressure within the ductus lumen (due to the postnatal decrease in PVR), and (3) the decrease in circulating PGE_2 (due to the loss of placental PG production and the increase in PGs removal by the lung), as well as the decrease in the number of PGE_2 receptors in the ductus wall.[30,31,34] Intertwined with functional closure, structural closure may encompass up to four distinct mechanisms of varying impact depending on the species[33]: (1) development of intimal cushions,[30,33] (2) mechanical solicitation from turbulent blood flow along the narrowing lumen,[33] (3) intramural hypoxia, which inhibits local production of PGE_2 and NO and induces production of growth factors,[30,33] and (4) interaction of platelets with the vessel wall, which adopts a prothrombotic phenotype.[35]

Perspectives

Despite the progress being made in understanding the regulation of the perinatal circulatory transition, much is left unknown. Evidence accumulated during the last two decades demonstrates that alterations in the production and actions of a number of vasoactive agents such as NO, ET-1, prostanoids, PAF, and reactive oxygen species are critically involved in promoting vascular remodeling and augmenting vasoreactivity that lead to PPHN. However, our knowledge about the regulation of the development of the pulmonary circulation at the genetic and molecular levels is scanty.[26] In addition, the cross talk among the multiple signaling pathways involved in the different cell types in the pulmonary vasculature needs to be better understood.[26]

A patient DA (PDA) in the first 3 days of life is a physiologic shunt in healthy term and preterm newborn infants. In contrast, failure of DA closure after birth is a common complication of premature delivery.[32] Even when it does constrict, the premature DA frequently fails to develop profound hypoxia and anatomic remodeling and is, therefore, susceptible to reopening.[34] PDA in preterm infants is associated with significant morbidities including intraventricular hemorrhage, necrotizing enterocolitis, and bronchopulmonary dysplasia. However, there is intense controversy regarding whether PDA is truly causative.[36] Furthermore, it is unknown if prophylactic and/or symptomatic PDA therapy will cause substantive improvements in outcome.[37] Therefore, there is still uncertainty and controversy about the significance, evaluation, and management of PDA in preterm infants, resulting in substantial heterogeneity in clinical practice. A large body of evidence now exists demonstrating that early, routine treatment to induce closure of the ductus in preterm infants, either medically or surgically, in the first 2 weeks after birth does not improve long term. The role of more selective use of medical methods for induction of ductal closure, either for defined high-risk infants in the first 2 postnatal weeks or for older infants with PDA, remains uncertain and requires further study.[38] The hope for future targeted therapies and for the prevention of PDA requires knowledge of the fundamental mechanisms controlling its development and pathogenesis.[36]

The immaturity of the fetal heart and circulatory system, along with pulmonary immaturity, creates many challenges in the care of very preterm infants. Given that premature infants begin extrauterine life before the fetal circulation has finished its maturation, very preterm infants manifest many of the functional and structural characteristics of the fetal cardiovascular system.[39] Therefore, the preterm neonate may not be able to adapt to the sudden increase in SVR because of the immaturity of the myocardium. This may negatively affect preload, afterload, contractility, heart rate, cardiac output, and systemic blood flow, leading to hypotension and possibly shock.[39,40] The immature myocardium has impaired contractility due to a decreased proportion of contractile elements, altered calcium release, altered titin function, decreased β-adrenoceptor number, and decreased sympathetic innervation.[39] When hypoxia associated with perinatal depression occurs at delivery, the myocardium is even more compromised, especially when coupled with acidosis.[39,40] An understanding of the development of the circulatory physiology can assist the practicing clinician with management of circulatory failure in the very preterm infant.[39] Delayed cord clamping, limiting iatrogenic blood loss, judicious use of volume expanders and inotropes for hypotension, and a more conservative approach for PDA are among the current recommendations and standards used in neonatology; but there is still a large amount of research that needs to be done, especially stratifying studies specific to the extremely very low birth weight population.[40]

THE RESPIRATORY SYSTEM

CARLOS E. BLANCO

Fetal breathing movements (FBM)

Periodic non-air intrauterine breathing pattern must change at birth to a continuous air-breathing pattern. This change happens after clamping the umbilical cord, full perfusion of the lungs, changes in temperature, changes in behavioral state, increase in metabolism, increase in afferent input to the central nervous system, changes in levels of prostaglandins, and many other changes associated to the moment of birth.

Breathing-like activity in utero is present from very early in gestation and is the consequence of rhythmic activation of respiratory neurons in the brainstem[41,42]; however, these breathing movements play no part in fetal gas exchange. The efferent activity of these respiratory neurons activates the respiratory motoneurons and hence the muscles, mainly the diaphragm, which generate a negative intrathoracic pressure. In fetal lamb, spasm of the diaphragm at the 38th day of gestation (term 147 days) and rhythmic movements of the diaphragm at the 40th day of gestation have been described.[43] Chronic recordings from fetal lambs in utero performed at approximately 50 days of gestation showed two types of diaphragmatic activity: (1) unpatterned discharge and (2) patterned, bursting discharge.[44] In the human fetus, thoracic movements were observed from the 10–12th week of gestation.[45] At this time in gestation, there is still not a clear pattern and FBM appear to be more "freewheeling."

Later in gestation in the fetal lamb (75–110 days), movements of the diaphragm start to become periodic. At this age, they are often associated with nuchal muscle activity and rapid eye movements.[46,47] A more definitive pattern starts to appear at 108–120 days of gestation when breathing movements become organized into a more complex state, now associated with the presence of rapid eye movements and nuchal muscle activity.[46–49] At this time in gestation, the electroencephalographic activity, commonly known as electrocortical activity (ECoG), still does not show any signs of differentiation. However, by 120–125 days of gestation, the ECoG shows a clear differentiation into low-voltage, high-frequency activity (range 13–30 Hz; low-voltage electrocortigram activity [LVECoG]) and high-voltage, low-frequency activity (3–9 Hz; high-voltage electrocortical activity [HVECoG]).[46,50–52] At this gestational age, breathing movements are rapid and irregular, with a frequency of 0.1–4 Hz and amplitude of 3–5 mmHg, and they produce small movements of tracheal fluid (<1 mL).[53] There are now two clearly defined fetal behavioral states in the fetal lamb: there is no nuchal muscle activity during LVECoG, but rapid eye movements and FBM are present. Polysynaptic spinal reflexes are also relatively inhibited during the LVECoG state.[54] During HVECoG, there are no eye movements or FBM, but nuchal muscle activity is present and polysynaptic reflexes are stronger.[54] The link between ECoG state and FBM implies either that breathing activity is facilitated (or even stimulated) during LVECoG and/or that it is inhibited during HVECoG. During LVECoG, there is more neural activity in cortical and subcortical structures, including the brainstem reticular formation. This facilitatory state could increase the sensitivity for tonic stimuli, such as the level of arterial CO_2, and generate respiratory output. This hypothesis is supported by the observation that there are no breathing movements during fetal hypocapnia even during the LVECoG state.[55] Extending this idea, the absence of FBM during HVECoG could be due to a disfacilitation, as reported during quiet sleep in the adult when slow waves appear in the EEG.[56,57] Other evidence also leads us to believe that during HVECoG, there is an active inhibition of breathing activity because in fetal sheep, FBM and ECoG were dissociated after the brainstem was transected at the level of the colliculi.[58] Furthermore, FBM response to hypercapnia is limited to LVECoG activity in the intact fetus, but hypercapnia can produce continuous breathing in both LVECoG and HVECoG after small bilateral lesions made in the lateral pons.[59] The mechanisms, origin, and location for this inhibition are not clear, but it is known that it is of central origin, and that it can be overridden in utero and at the time of birth when breathing becomes continuous.

Control of fetal breathing movements

The work of Barcroft[60] gave rise to the concept that inhibitory mechanism, which descends from higher centers, is involved in producing apneic periods in the fetus. This inhibitory control develops during the second half of gestation. This work also showed that the inhibition of FBM by hypoxemia is not seen early in gestation, and the descending inhibitory processes develop later. While the inhibition of FBM in HVECoG and in hypoxia involves descending inhibitory processes, they do not necessarily utilize the same neural mechanisms. Barcroft employed similar brainstem transection techniques to those of Lumsden[61] to show that neural structures above the level of the pons do not exert significant control over FBM. These studies were extended by Dawes and coworkers[62] who employed the technique of transection in the chronically instrumented late gestation fetal sheep. They showed that transection at the level of upper midbrain/caudal hypothalamus resulted in FBM, which were episodic but not related to the ECoG. These FBM were still inhibited by hypoxia. This makes it clear that the processes that mediate the inhibition of FBM in HVECoG are different from those that produce the inhibition in hypoxia. Transection through the rostral pons/caudal midbrain produced FBM that occurred almost continuously and were not inhibited by hypoxia. This focused attention on the upper pons in the inhibition of fetal breathing movements in hypoxia. Gluckman and

Johnston[63] pursued this by making lesions in the rostral lateral pons, and compiled a diagram showing areas not needed for the inhibition to be manifest, and the location of an area in the lateral pons that, if lesioned bilaterally, prevented the inhibition.

One of the key questions that emerged from these brainstem studies was whether the descending inhibitory mechanism is capable of inhibiting the input from peripheral chemoreceptors. Once it had been established that the peripheral chemoreceptors are active in utero and respond to natural stimuli such as hypoxia or hypercapnia (see section "Peripheral chemoreceptor function in utero"), it was no longer necessary to view the effect of modest hypoxia in inhibiting FBM as a direct depression of the medulla. The results of transection and lesion studies suggested that stimulation of FBM occurred during hypoxia after the damage to the brainstem, as if a stimulatory effect of the peripheral chemoreceptors had been unmasked. Direct confirmation of this idea came from the study of Johnston and Gluckman[64], who conducted a two-stage procedure: first, lesions were placed as before in the brainstem to prevent the inhibition of FBM in hypoxia or to give an overt stimulation; this was then prevented by chemodenervation at a second operation.

The nature (and indeed the location) of the inhibitory processes is not known. Because the inhibition occurs even in chemodenervated fetuses,[65] it is clear that the neurons involved do not receive an excitatory input from the chemoreceptors. They may therefore be chemoreceptors themselves or receive input from other cells thought to be sensitive to hypoxia, e.g., in the rostral ventrolateral medulla.[66] The neural activity as a whole behaves as a chemoreceptor, because the chemoreceptor stimulant drug almitrine mimics the effects of hypoxia in inhibiting FBM, irrespective of the integrity of the peripheral chemoreceptors.[67] As expected from the discussion above, the stimulatory effect of the drug on the peripheral chemoreceptors only becomes manifest when lesions were placed in the lateral pons,[68] unmasking its peripheral actions.

Peripheral chemoreceptor function in utero

The concept that peripheral chemoreceptors could produce effects on breathing can be traced to experiments conducted over 50 years ago in which breathing was shown to be stimulated in exteriorized midgestation animal fetuses by hypoxia or cyanide.[69] In late gestation, the descending inhibitory effects on breathing arising from the fetal brainstem in hypoxia and with HVECoG (see above) dominate. It was perhaps the increasing interest in these processes that caused the scientific community to lose sight of the implications of the earlier observations. The idea became prevalent that the carotid chemoreceptors were quiescent in utero and were activated at birth, perhaps by the increase in sympathetic nervous activity. In addition, when it became clear that normal fetal arterial PO_2 in late gestation, both in the sheep and the human fetus, was about 3 Kpa (25 mmHg), it was thought that if the chemoreceptors were functional, they would be so intensely stimulated that powerful reflex effects would be induced continuously. This was clearly not the case, although it had been shown that brainstem transection removed inhibitory effects on breathing[60,62] and permitted stimulation of breathing activity during hypoxia. It was therefore essential to readdress the question of arterial chemoreceptor function in utero. It was found that both carotid[70] and aortic[71] chemoreceptors were spontaneously active at the normal arterial PO_2 in fetal sheep, and that they responded with an increase in discharge if PO_2 fell or PCO_2 rose. There were several very important implications of these findings. First, it was clear that the peripheral chemoreceptors would be able to stimulate fetal breathing under some circumstances, but that it was the balance between this stimulatory input and the normally dominant, inhibitory input from higher centers that determined the characteristics of fetal breathing (see above). Second, it redirected attention to the role the carotid chemoreceptors play in initiating cardiovascular reflex responses to hypoxia.[72,73] Last, the observation that the fetal peripheral chemoreceptors discharge spontaneously (at about 5 Hz) at the normal fetal arterial PO_2 made it clear that the rise in PO_2 at birth would silence them. Their sensitivity to PO_2 would then have to reset to the adult range postnatal, and this has generated research into the mechanisms of this resetting.[74,75]

Pharmacological control

Prostaglandins exert a powerful influence on FBM and postnatal breathing. Prostaglandin E2 (PGE2) decreases the incidence of FBM,[76] whereas meclofenamate and indomethacin, inhibitors of PG synthesis, increase FBM.[77-79] The effect of prostaglandins appears to be central, as it is independent of the peripheral chemoreceptors[80] and because central administration of meclofenamate stimulates FBM.[81,82] The same effects can be produced postnatally, with PGE2 decreasing, and meclofenamate and indomethacin increasing, ventilation in lambs.[83,84] However, the change in the concentration of PGE2 that occurs around birth cannot be solely responsible for either the decrease in FBM seen immediately before birth[79,85] or the onset of continuous breathing postnatally.[86] The well-established effects of ethyl alcohol to reduce the incidence of FBM[87] are not mediated by prostaglandin[88] but by adenosine.[89]

Bennet et al.[90] showed that large doses of thyroid releasing hormone (TRH) can induce stimulation of FBM. This effect may be at the level of the respiratory neurons where TRH can be localized, but its physiological significance is not known. This may also be true of the effects of the cholinergic agonist, pilocarpine, and serotonin (5-HT) precursor L-5-hydroxytryptophan (L-5-HTP).[91,92] Both of these agents stimulate FBM, but pilocarpine induces LVECoG and L-5-HTP induces HVECoG. This stresses again the coincidental rather than causal relationship between FBM and LVECoG. 5-HT has been implicated in neural mechanisms controlling adult sheep, but that the site of action in the fetus is not known. A range of opiates has effects on FBM,[93] but the physiological localization of their effects has not been established.

The high rate of progesterone synthesis by the placenta in late gestation exposes the fetus to high concentrations of progesterone and its metabolites. Progesterone can influence fetal behavior, and normal progesterone production tonically suppresses arousal, or wakefulness in the fetus.[94,95]

Last, one of the striking aspects of FBM is that FBM cease 24–48 hours before parturition. The mechanism involved is not known. Kitterman et al.[77] excluded a rise in plasma PGE$_2$, and Parkes et al.[96] showed that it did not occur if the fall in plasma progesterone was prevented.

Lung growth associated to FBM

Fetal breathing movements are necessary for fetal lung growth and maturation. By opposing lung recoil, FBM help to maintain the lung expansion that is now known to be essential for normal growth and structural maturation of the fetal lungs. FBM induce complex and variable changes in thoracic dimensions; these induce small alterations in the shape of the lungs that may act as a stimulus to lung growth. The prolonged absence or impairment of FBM is likely to result in a reduced mean level of lung expansion, which can lead to hypoplasia of the lungs.[97] Moreover, static distension decreases steady-state SP-A and SP-B mRNA levels in whole lung, whereas cyclic stretching increases SP-B and SP-A expression two- to fourfold and enhances 3H-choline incorporation into saturated phosphatidylcholine.[98]

Changes at birth

At birth, breathing activity must become continuous in order to fulfil its gas exchange function. After occlusion of the umbilical cord, the neonatal ECoG still cycles between low- and high-voltage states, which seem to have identical spectral characteristics to the fetal states. LVECoG activity is associated with the absence of nuchal muscle activity, rapid eye movements, and inhibition of polysynaptic reflexes, and HVECoG is associated with presence of nuchal muscle activity, lack of rapid eye movements, and enhanced polysynaptic reflexes.[99] However, despite the fact that after birth the HVECoG state seems to be similar to the equivalent fetal state, breathing activity is present.

Studies of the mechanisms involved in the establishment of continuous breathing at birth have followed two lines: (1) attempts to induce continuous breathing in utero or (2) observation of establishment of continuous breathing during situations aimed at mimicking birth.

It is well established that the inhibition of FBM during HVECoG can be overridden as demonstrated by the presence of continuous breathing during metabolic acidosis,[100,101] administration of prostaglandin synthetase inhibitors,[77,78,82] 5-hydroxytryptophan,[102,103] catecholamines,[103] pilocarpine,[91] thyrotrophin releasing hormone,[104] corticotrophin releasing factor,[90] central or peripheral fetal cooling,[105,106] and by lesions within the CNS (see above). These experiments show that FBM can become continuous through the operation of various mechanisms including disinhibition during HVECoG, changes in the balance between stimulatory and inhibitory neuromodulators, increased arousability, and changes in chemoreceptor sensitivity.[107] Some, but not all, of these mechanisms are likely to play an important role at birth.

Experiments designed to observe changes in breathing activity after cord occlusion have led to two main hypotheses: (1) The exclusion of fetal–placental circulation leads to the disappearance of hormones or neuromodulators, which exert continuous tonic inhibition (through the CNS) during fetal life, and that this allows continuous breathing postnatally.[108–111] There are reports indicating that prostaglandins originating from placental tissue can inhibit fetal breathing activity.[112] Although this is a possible explanation, it is not yet demonstrated that such a substance is responsible for the modulation by ECoG of FBM. It was shown that breathing movements of goat fetuses maintained in an extrauterine incubation system for more than 24 hours were episodic, suggesting that intermittent breathing movements are intrinsic to the fetus, independent of placenta-derived factors.[113] (2) Breathing activity is dependent on the level of PaCO$_2$ in utero and at birth.[55] It is known that during hypocapnia, fetal and neonatal breathing is reduced.[55,106,108] Hypercapnia stimulates breathing activity, but in utero, this is inhibited during quiet sleep. However, this inhibition can be overridden after lesions in the lateral pons[59] or when hypercapnia is combined with cooling.[106] This might be explained by changes in the CO$_2$ sensitivity of central and/or peripheral chemoreceptors or due to changes in the balance between central inhibitory and excitatory mechanisms caused by an increase in afferent input at birth. In this hypothesis, both changes in afferent input from chemoreceptors and thermoreceptors to the CNS, and/or changes in CNS sensitivity to these inputs, are important in the transition from fetal to neonatal breathing. Changes in the plasma level of a placental neuromodulator at birth may then serve to maintain postnatal breathing after its initiation. More insights into these mechanisms may offer an explanation for the occurrence of apneic periods after birth.

Postnatal breathing

Studies to identify brainstem mechanisms that regulate breathing have been conducted in the neonate, in which hypoxia also inhibits breathing but after a transient chemoreceptor-mediated stimulation. Therefore, the reasoning is that similar inhibitory processes to those that operate in the fetus produce the postnatal inhibition of ventilation by hypoxia. Transection of the brainstem through the rostral pons does indeed remove the secondary fall in ventilation[114] as does placement of lesions in the lateral pons[115]. However, these studies did not identify any clear group of neurons involved in mediating the effect. Investigators focused their attention on the red nucleus, located above the pons in the mesencephalon. The transection studies implicate structures in either the rostral pons or caudal mesencephalon, so it is likely that the red nucleus would have been affected. In neonatal rabbits, electrical stimulation of the red nucleus produces a profound inhibition of respiratory output, and bilateral lesions in the red nucleus prevent the inhibition of respiratory output in hypoxia while not affecting the cardiovascular responses. Evidence that neurons in the red nucleus are involved in this effect comes from the observation that chemical stimulation with glutamate also produces an inhibition of respiratory output.[116] Interestingly, the efferent pathway for these cells, rubrospinal tract, runs in precisely the ventrolateral region of the pons lesioned by Gluckman and Johnston[63] in their fetal studies.

The observations on the red nucleus are interesting because in postnatal life, it has been implicated in producing the hypotonia of postural muscles, which occurs in REM sleep. Such hypotonia also occurs in the fetus,[70] but at that time, it is associated with presence, and not absence, of FBM. Once again, behaviorally related and hypoxia-induced inhibition of FBM appears to be distinct. In addition, the brainstem reticular formation and related nuclei associated with sleep and arousal have not been greatly studied in the postnatal period. In one study, Moore et al.[117] reported that cooling the locus coeruleus by a few degrees, sufficient to reduce neuronal activity but not conducted action potentials, prevented the secondary fall in ventilation in hypoxia in neonatal lambs. The locus coeruleus has been implicated in producing arousal at birth.[118] There are also reports that structures as high in the brain as the thalamus are implicated in the descending inhibition of breathing during hypoxia.[119]

While the effects of acute hypoxia on FBM have been widely studied, the effects of prolonged hypoxemia are quite different. Over a period of 6–12 hours, FBM return to their control incidence as does cycling of the ECoG.[120] Studies reveal that the peripheral chemoreceptors are necessary for the return of fetal breathing movements during sustained hypoxia produced by reduced uterine blood flow, but the mechanisms involved are not known.[121]

CONCLUSIONS AND FURTHER DIRECTIONS

Spontaneous breathing movements are present during fetal life, and they are important for normal development of the fetal lungs. Early in gestation, they seem to represent free-running activity of the respiratory centers, not controlled by peripheral mechanisms but probably dependent on a tonic CO_2 drive. Maturation of sleep states brings into play powerful brainstem inhibitory mechanisms that control this activity.

Fetal breathing activity is present during physiological and normal fetal conditions, and it can be monitored non-invasively by ultrasound; therefore, its monitoring could be used to interrogate fetal well-being. A recent Cochrane systematic review did not support its usefulness when included in a biophysical profile to detect high-risk fetuses.[122] However,

the monitoring of fetal breathing activity could be used to predict premature labor.[123] Moreover, there is limited information showing the usefulness of monitoring fetal breathing and body activity during maternal physical activity. More research will be welcomed to assess and determine the intensity of maternal physical activity on the developing fetus.[124]

Birth clearly involves some irreversible processes, the transition to continuous breathing being one. However, breathing remains linked to behavioral and sleep states in the neonate as in the fetus, and clearly there is continuity of some control processes from late gestation to early postnatal life. Some of these processes mature relatively slowly after birth such as resetting of chemoreceptor hypoxia sensitivity and the diminishing influence of descending inhibitory effects on breathing in hypoxia. Understanding these effects will be of vital importance to prevention of SIDS and the care of newborn, especially preterm babies.

REFERENCES

1. Dzialowski EM, Sirsat T, van der Sterren S, Villamor E. Prenatal cardiovascular shunts in amniotic vertebrates. *Respir Physiol Neurobiol* 2011; 178(1): 66–74.
2. Reuss ML, Rudolph AM. Distribution and recirculation of umbilical and systemic venous blood flow in fetal lambs during hypoxia. *J Dev Physiol* 1980; 2(1–2): 71–84.
3. Noori S, Friedlich PS, Seri I. Pathophysiology of shock in the fetus and neonate. In: Polin RA, Fox WW, Abman SH (eds). *Fetal and Neonatal Physiology*. Philadelphia: Saunders, 2004: 772–781.
4. Talbert D, Sebire NJ. The dynamic placenta: I. Hypothetical model of a placental mechanism matching local fetal blood flow to local intervillus oxygen delivery. *Med Hypotheses* 2004; 62(4): 511–9.
5. Sebire NJ, Talbert D. The role of intraplacental vascular smooth muscle in the dynamic placenta: A conceptual framework for understanding uteroplacental disease. *Med Hypotheses* 2002; 58(4): 347–51.
6. Cooper EJ, Wareing M, Greenwood SL, Baker PN. Oxygen tension and normalisation pressure modulate nifedipine-sensitive relaxation of human placental chorionic plate arteries. *Placenta* 2006; 27(4–5): 402–10.
7. Khong TY, Tee JH, Kelly AJ. Absence of innervation of the uteroplacental arteries in normal and abnormal human pregnancies. *Gynecol Obstet Invest* 1997; 43(2): 89–93.
8. Hampl V, Bibova J, Stranak Z, Wu X, Michelakis ED, Hashimoto K, Archer SL. Hypoxic fetoplacental vasoconstriction in humans is mediated by potassium channel inhibition. *Am J Physiol* 2002; 283(6): H2440–9.
9. Weir E, Lopez-Barneo J, Buckler K, SL A. Acute oxygen-sensing mechanisms. *N Engl J Med* 2005; 353(19): 2042–55.

10. Aaronson PI, Robertson TP, Knock GA, Becker S, Lewis TH, Snetkov V, Ward J PT. Hypoxic pulmonary vasoconstriction: Mechanisms and controversies. *J Physiol* 2006; 570(Pt 1): 53–8.

11. Russell MJ, Dombkowski RA, Olson KR. Effects of hypoxia on vertebrate blood vessels. *J Exp Zool Part A Ecol Genet Physiol* 2008; 309A(2): 55–63.

12. Hooper SB, Te Pas AB, Lang J, van Vonderen JJ, Roehr CC, Kluckow M, Gill AW, Wallace EM, Polglase GR. Cardiovascular transition at birth: A physiological sequence. *Pediatr Res* 2015; 77: 608–14.

13. Abman SH. Abnormal vasoreactivity in the pathophysiology of persistent pulmonary hypertension of the newborn. *Pediatr Rev/Am Acad Pediatr* 1999; 20(11): e103–9.

14. Abman SH, Stevens T. Perinatal pulmonary vasoregulation: Implications for the pathophysiology and treatment of neonatal pulmonary hypertension. In: Haddad G, Lister G (eds). *Tissue Oxygen Deprivation: Developmental, Molecular and Integrative Function.* New York: Marcel Dekker, 1996, 367–432.

15. Kinsella JP, Abman SH. Recent developments in the pathophysiology and treatment of persistent pulmonary hypertension of the newborn. *J Pediatr* 1995; 126(6): 853–64.

16. Ziegler JW, Ivy DD, Kinsella JP, Abman SH. The role of nitric oxide, endothelin, and prostaglandins in the transition of the pulmonary circulation. *Clin Perinatol* 1995; 22(2): 387–403.

17. Kiserud T, Ozaki T, Nishina H, Rodeck C, Hanson MA. Effect of NO, phenylephrine, and hypoxemia on ductus venosus diameter in fetal sheep. *Am J Physiol* 2000; 279(3): H1166–71.

18. Contratti G, Banzi C, Ghi T, Perolo A, Pilu G, Visentin A. Absence of the ductus venosus: Report of 10 new cases and review of the literature. *Ultrasound Obstet Gynecol* 2001; 18(6): 605–9.

19. Murayama K, Nagasaka H, Tate K, Ohsone Y, Kanazawa M, Kobayashi K, Kohno Y, Takayanagi M. Significant correlations between the flow volume of patent ductus venosus and early neonatal liver function: Possible involvement of patent ductus venosus in postnatal liver function. *Arch Dis Child Fetal Neonatal Ed* 2006; 91(3): F175–9.

20. Sommer RJ, Hijazi ZM, Rhodes JF, Jr. Pathophysiology of congenital heart disease in the adult: Part I: Shunt lesions. *Circulation* 2008; 117(8): 1090–9.

21. Cruz-Gonzalez I, Solis J, Kiernan TJ, Yan BP, Lam YY, Palacios IF. Clinical manifestation and current management of patent foramen ovale. *Exp Rev Cardiovasc Ther* 2009; 7(8): 1011–22.

22. Ward JP. Oxygen sensors in context. *Biochim Biophys Acta* 2008; 1777(1): 1–14.

23. Abman SH, Accurso FJ, Wilkening RB, Meschia G. Persistent fetal pulmonary hypoperfusion after acute hypoxia. *Am J Physiol* 1987; 253(4 Pt 2): H941–8.

24. Blanco CE, Martin CB, Rankin J, Landauer M, Phernetton T. Changes in fetal organ flow during intrauterine mechanical ventilation with or without oxygen. *J Dev Physiol* 1988; 10(1): 53–62.

25. Abman SH, Chatfield BA, Rodman DM, Hall SL, McMurtry IF. Maturational changes in endothelium-derived relaxing factor activity of ovine pulmonary arteries in vitro. *Am J Physiol* 1991; 260(4 Pt 1): L280–5.

26. Shaul PW. Regulation of vasodilator synthesis during lung development. *Early Hum Dev* 1999; 54(3): 271–94.

27. Gao Y, Raj JU. Regulation of the pulmonary circulation in the fetus and newborn. *Physiol Rev* 2010; 90(4): 1291–335.

28. Haworth SG, Hislop AA. Lung development—The effects of chronic hypoxia. *Semin Neonatol* 2003; 8(1): 1–8.

29. Reese J. Death, dying, and exhaustion in the ductus arteriosus: Prerequisites for permanent closure. *Am J Physiol Regul Integr Comp Physiol* 2006; 290(2): R357–8.

30. Clyman RI. Mechanisms regulating the ductus arteriosus. *Biol Neonate* 2006; 89(4): 330–5.

31. Bouayad A, Hou X, Varma DR, Clyman RI, Fouron J-C, Chemtob S. Cyclooxygenase isoforms and prostaglandin E2 receptors in the ductus arteriosus. *Curr Ther Res* 2002; 63(10): 669–81.

32. Smith GC. The pharmacology of the ductus arteriosus. *Pharmacol Rev* 1998; 50(1): 35–58.

33. Coceani F, Baragatti B. Mechanisms for ductus arteriosus closure. *Semin Perinatol* 2012; 36(2): 92–7.

34. Clyman RI. Mechanisms regulating closure of the ductus arteriosus. In: Polin RA, Fox WW, Abman SH (eds). *Fetal and Neonatal Physiology.* Philadelphia: Saunders, 2004, 743–8.

35. Echtler K, Stark K, Lorenz M, Kerstan S, Walch A, Jennen L et al. Platelets contribute to postnatal occlusion of the ductus arteriosus. *Nat Med* 2010; 16(1): 75–82.

36. Stoller JZ, DeMauro SB, Dagle JM, Reese J. Current perspectives on pathobiology of the ductus arteriosus. *J Clin Exp Cardiolog* 2012; S8: 001.

37. Hamrick SE, Hansmann G. Patent ductus arteriosus of the preterm infant. *Pediatrics* 2010; 125(5): 1020–30.

38. Benitz WE, Committee on Fetus and Newborn. Patent ductus arteriosus in preterm infants. *Pediatrics* 2016; 137(1): 1–6.

39. Finnemore A, Groves A. Physiology of the fetal and transitional circulation. *Semin Fetal Neonatal Med* 2015; 20: 210–6.

40. Evans K. Cardiovascular transition of the extremely premature infant and challenges to maintain hemodynamic stability. *J Perinatal Neonatal Nurs* 2016; 30(1): 68–72.

41. Bystrzycka E, Nail B, Purves MJ. Central and peripheral neural respiratory activity in the mature sheep fetus and newborn lamb. *Respir Physiol* 1975; 25: 199–215.

42. Bahoric A, Chernick V. Electrical activity of phrenic nerve and diaphragm in utero. *J Appl Physiol* 1975; 39: 513–8.

43. Barcroft J. *Researches on Pre-natal Life*. Illinois: Charles C Thomas, 1946: 261–6.

44. Cooke IRC, Berger PH. Precursor of respiratory pattern in the early gestation mammalian fetus. *Brain Res* 1990; 522: 333–6.

45. Vries de JIP, Visser GHA, Prechtl HFR. The emergence of fetal behavior 1. Qualitative aspects. *Early Hum Develop* 1982; 7: 301–22.

46. Clewlow R, Dawes GS, Johnston BM, Walker DW. Changes in breathing, electrocortical and muscle activity in unanaesthetized fetal lambs with age. *J Physiol* 1983; 341: 463–76.

47. Ioffe S, Jansen AH, Chernick V. Maturation of spontaneous fetal diaphragmatic activity and fetal response to hypercapnia and hypoxemia. *J Appl Physiol* 1987; 62: 609–22.

48. Bowes G, Adamson TM, Ritchie BC, Dowling M, Wilkinson MH, Maloney JE. Development of patterns of respiratory activity in unanaesthetized fetal sheep in utero. *J Appl Physiol* 1981; 50: 693–700.

49. Szeto HH, Cheng PY, Decena JA, Wu DL, Cheng Y, Dwyer G. Developmental changes in continuity and stability of breathing in the fetal lamb. *Am J Physiol* 1992; 262: R452–8.

50. Dawes GS, Fox HE, Leduc BM, Liggins GC, Richards RT. Respiratory movements and rapid eye movements sleep in the fetal lamb. *J Physiol Lond* 1972; 220(1): 119–43.

51. Szeto HH, Vo TDH, Dwyer G, Dogramajian ME, Cox MJ, Senger G. The ontogeny of fetal lamb electrocortical activity: A power spectral analysis. *Am J Obstet Gynecol* 1985; 153: 462–6.

52. Szeto HH. Spectral edge frequency as a simple quantitative measure of maturation of electrocortical activity. *Pediatr Res* 1990; 27: 289–92.

53. Harding R, Bocking AD, Sigger JN. Influence of upper respiratory tract on liquid flow to and from fetal lungs. *J Physiol* 1986; 61: 68–71.

54. Blanco CE, Dawes GS, Walker DW. Effects of hypoxia on polysynaptic hind-limb reflexes of unanaesthetized fetal and new-born lambs. *J Physiol* 1983; 39: 453–4.

55. Kuipers IM, Maertzdorf WJ, De Jong DS, Hanson MA, Blanco CE. Effects of mild hypocapnia on fetal breathing and behavior in unanaesthetized normoxic fetal lambs. *J Appl Physiol* 1994; 76: 1476–80.

56. Steriade M, Contreras D, Amzica F. Synchronized sleep oscillations and their paroxysmal developments. *TINS* 1994; 17: 199–208.

57. Phillipson EA, Bowes G, Townsend ER, Duffin J, Cooper JD. Carotid chemoreceptors in ventilatory response to changes in venous CO_2 load. *J Appl Physiol* 1981; 51: 1398–403.

58. Dawes GS, Gardner WN, Johnston BM, Walker DW. Breathing in fetal lambs: The effects of brain stem section. *J Physiol* 1983; 335: 535–53.

59. Johnston BM, Gluckman PD. Lateral pontine lesion affects central chemosensitivity in unanaesthetized fetal lambs. *J Physiol* 1989; 67: 1113–8.

60. Barcroft J. *The Brain and Its Environment*. New Haven: Yale University Press, 1938: 44.

61. Lumsden T. Observations on the respiratory centers. *J Physiol* 1923; 57: 354–67.

62. Dawes GS. The central control of fetal breathing and skeletal muscle movements. *J Physiol* 1984; 346: 1–18.

63. Gluckman PD, Johnston BM. Lesions in the upper lateral pons abolish the hypoxic depression of breathing in unanaesthetized fetal lambs in utero. *J Physiol* 1987; 382: 373–83.

64. Johnston BM, Gluckman PD. Peripheral chemoreceptors respond to hypoxia in pontine-lesioned fetal lambs in utero. *J Appl Physiol* 1993; 75(3): 1027–34.

65. Moore PJ, Parkes MJ, Nijhuis JG, Hanson MA. The incidence of breathing movements in fetal sheep in normoxia and hypoxia after peripheral chemodenervation and brain stem transection. *J Dev Physiol* 1989; 11: 147–51.

66. Nolan PC, Dillon GH, Waldrop TG. Central hypoxic chemoreceptors in the ventrolateral medulla and caudal hypothalamus. *Adv Exp Med Biol* 1995; 393: 261–6.

67. Moore PJ, Hanson MA, Parkes MJ. Almitrine inhibits breathing movements in fetal sheep. *J Dev Physiol* 1989; 11(5): 277–81.

68. Johnston BM, Moore PJ, Bennet L, Hanson MA, Gluckman PD. Almitrine mimics hypoxia in fetal sheep with lateral pontine lesions. *J Appl Physiol* 1990; 69: 1330–5.

69. Hanson MA. Peripheral chemoreceptor function before and after birth. In: Johnston BM, Gluckman P (eds). *Respiratory Control and Lung Development in the Fetus and Newborn*. Perinatology Press, Ithaca, NY, 1986: 311–30.

70. Blanco CE, Dawes GS, Hanson MA, McCooke HB. The response to hypoxia of arterial chemoreceptors in fetal sheep and newborn lambs. *J Physiol* 1984; 351: 25–37.

71. Blanco CE, Dawes GS, Hanson MA, McCooke HB. The arterial chemoreceptors in fetal sheep and newborn lambs. *J Physiol* 1982; 330: 38 pp.

72. Bartelds B, Van Bel F, Teitel DF, Rudolph AM. Carotid, not aortic, chemoreceptors mediate the fetal cardiovascular response to acute hypoxemia in lambs. *Pediatr Res* 1993; 34(1): 51–5.

73. Giussani DA, Spencer JAD, Moore PJ, Bennet L, Hanson MA. Afferent and efferent components of the cardiovascular reflex responses to acute hypoxia in term fetal sheep. *J Physiol* 1993; 461: 431–49.

74. Blanco CE, Hanson MA, McCoocke HB. Effects on carotid chemoreceptor resetting of pulmonary ventilation in the fetal lamb in utero. *J Dev Physiol* 1988; 10: 167–74.

75. Kumar P, Hanson MA. Re-setting of the hypoxic sensitivity of aortic chemoreceptors in the newborn lamb. *J Dev Physiol* 1989; 11: 199–206.

76. Kitterman JA, Liggins GC, Fewell JE, Tooley WH. Inhibition of breathing movements in fetal sheep by Prostaglandins. *J Appl Physiol* 1983 Mar 1; 54: 687–92.

77. Kitterman JA, Liggins GC, Clements JA, Tooley WH. Stimulation of breathing movements in fetal sheep by inhibitors of prostaglandin synthesis. *J Dev Physiol* 1979; 1: 453–66.

78. Wallen LD, Murai DT, Clyman RI, Lee CH, Mauray FE, Kitterman JA. Regulation of breathing movements in fetal sheep by prostaglandin E_2. *J Appl Physiol* 1986; 60: 526–31.

79. Patrick J, Challis JRG, Cross J. Effects of maternal indomethacin administration on fetal breathing movements in sheep. *J Dev Physiol* 1987; 9: 295–300.

80. Murai DT, Wallen LD, Lee CC, Clyman RI, Mauray F, Kitterman JA. Effects of prostaglandins in fetal breathing do not involve peripheral chemoreceptors. *J Appl Physiol* 1987; 62: 271–7.

81. Koos BJ. Central effects on breathing in fetal sheep of sodium meclofenamate. *J Physiol* 1982; 330: 50–1.

82. Koos BJ. Central stimulation of breathing movements in fetal lambs by prostaglandin synthetase inhibitors. *J Physiol* 1985; 362: 455–66.

83. Guerra FA, Savich RD, Clyman RI, Kitterman JA. Meclofenamate increases ventilation in lambs. *J Dev Physiol* 1988;11:1-6.

84. Long WA. Prostaglandins and control of breathing in newborn piglets. *J Appl Physiol* 1988; 64: 409–18.

85. Wallen LD, Murai DT, Clyman RI, Lee CH, Mauray FE, Kitterman JA. Effects of meclofenamate on breathing movements in fetal sheep before delivery. *J Appl Physiol* 1988; 64: 759–66.

86. Lee DS, Choy P, Davi M, Caces R, Gibson D, Hasan SU, Cates D, Rigatto H. Decrease in plasma prostaglandin E_2 is not essential for the establishment of continuous breathing at birth in sheep. *J Dev Physiol* 1989; 12(3): 145–51.

87. Smith GN, Brien JF, Homan J, Carmichael L, Treissman D, Patrick J. Effect of ethanol on ovine fetal and maternal plasma prostaglandin E² concentrations and fetal breathing movements. *J Dev Physiol* 1990; 14: 23–8.

88. Smith GN, Brien JF, Homan J, Carmichael L, Patrick J. Indomethacin reversal of ethanol-induced suppression of ovine fetal breathing movements and relationship to prostaglandin E2. *J Dev Physiol* 1990; 14: 29–35.

89. Watson CS, White SE, Homan JH, Kimura KA, Brien JF, Fraher L, Challis JRG, Bocking AD. Increase cerebral extracellular adenosine and decreased PGE2 during ethanol-induced inhibition of FBM. *J Appl Physiol* 1999; 86: 1410–20.

90. Bennet L, Johnston BM, Vale WW, Gluckman PD. The effects of corticotrophin-releasing factor and two antagonists on breathing movements in fetal sheep. *J Physiol* 1990; 421: 1–11.

91. Hanson MA, Moore PJ, Nijhuis JG, Parkes MJ. Effects of pilocarpine on breathing movements in normal, chemodenervated and brain stem-transected fetal sheep. *J Physiol* 1988; 400: 415–24.

92. Fletcher DJ, Hanson MA, Moore PJ, Nijhuis JG, Parkes MJ. Stimulation of breathing movements by L-5-hydroxytryptophan in fetal sheep during normoxia and hypoxia. *J Physiol* 1988; 404: 575–89.

93. Hasan SU, Lee DS, Gibson DA, Nowaczyk BJ, Cates DB, Sitar DS, Pinsky C, Rigatto H. Effect of morphine on breathing and behavior in fetal sheep. *J Appl Physiol* 1988; 64: 2058–65.

94. Crossley KJ, Nicol MB, Hirst JJ, Walker DW, Thorburn GD. Suppression of arousal by progesterone in fetal sheep. *Reprod Fertil Dev* 1997; 9: 767–73.

95. Nicol MB, Hirst JJ, Walker D, Thorburn GD. Effect of alteration of maternal plasma progesterone concentrations on fetal behavioural state during late gestation. *J Endocrinol* 1997; 152: 379–86.

96. Parkes MJ, Moore PJ, Hanson MA. The effects of inhibition of 3-B hydroxysteroid dehydrogenase activity in sheep fetuses in utero. *Proc Soc Study Fetal Physiol Cairn* 1988; 58.

97. Inanlou MR, Baguma-Nibasheka M, Kablar B. The role of fetal breathing-like movements in lung organogenesis. *Histol Histopathol* 2005 Oct; 20(4): 1261–6.

98. Sanchez-Esteban J, Tsai SW, Sang J, Qin J, Torday JS, Rubin LP. Effects of mechanical forces on lung-specific gene expression. *Am J Med Sci* 1998; 316: 200–4.

99. Blanco CE, Dawes GS, Walker DW. Effects of hypoxia on polysynaptic hind-limb reflexes in new-born lambs before and after carotid denervation. *J Physiol* 1983; 339: 467–74.

100. Molteni RA, Melmed MH, Sheldon RE, Jones MD, Meschia G. Induction of fetal breathing by metabolic acidemia and its effects on blood flow to the respiratory muscles. *Am J Obstet Gynecol* 1980; 136: 609–20.

101. Hohimer AR, Bissonnette JM. Effects of metabolic acidosis on fetal breathing movements in utero. *Respir Physiol* 1981; 43: 99–106.

102. Quilligan EJ, Clewlow F, Johnston BM, Walker DW. Effects of 5-hydroxytryptophan on electrocortical activity and breathing movements of fetal sheep. *Am J Obstet Gynecol* 1981; 141: 271–5.

103. Jansen AH, Ioffe S, Chernick V. Stimulation of fetal breathing activity by beta-adrenergic mechanisms. *J Appl Physiol* 1986; 60: 1938–45.

104. Bennet L, Gluckman PD, Johnston BM. The effects of corticotrophin-releasing hormone on breathing movements and electrocortical activity of the fetal sheep. *J Physiol* 1988; 23: 72–5.

105. Gluckman PD, Gunn TR, Johnston BM. The effect of cooling on breathing and shivering in unanaesthetized fetal lambs in utero. *J Physiol* 1983; 343: 495–506.

106. Kuipers IM, Maertzdorf EJ, De Jong DS, Hanson MA, Blanco CE. Initiation and maintenance of continuous breathing at birth. *Pediatr Res* 1997; 42: 163–8.

107. Lagercrantz H, Pequignot JM, Hertzberg T, Holgert H, Ringstedt T. Birth-related changes of expression and turnover of some neuroactive agents and respiratory control. *Biol Neonate* 1994; 65: 145–8.

108. Adamson SL, Richardson, Homan J. Initiation of pulmonary gas exchange by fetal sheep in utero. *J Appl Physiol* 1987; 62: 989–98.

109. Boddy K, Dawes GS, Fisher R, Pinter S, Robinson JS. Foetal respiratory movements, electrocortical activity and cardiovascular responses to hypoxaemia and hypercapnia in sheep. *J Physiol* 1974; 243: 599–618.

110. Adamson SL, Kuipers IM, Olson DM. Umbilical cord occlusion stimulates breathing independent of blood gases and pH. *J Appl Physiol* 1991; 70: 1796–809.

111. Sawa R, Asakura H, Power G. Changes in plasma adenosine during simulated birth of fetal sheep. *J Appl Physiol* 1991; 70: 1524–28.

112. Alvaro RE, Hasan SU, Chemtob S, Qurashi M, Al-Saif S, Rigatto H. Prostaglandins are responsible for the inhibition of breathing observed with a placental extract in fetal sheep. *Respir Physiol Neurobiol Physiol* 2004 Nov 30; 144(1): 35–44.

113. Kozuma S, Nishina H, Unno N, Kagawa H, Kikuchi A, Fujii T, Baba K, Okai T, Kuwabara Y, Taketani Y. Goat fetuses disconnected from the placenta, but reconnected to an artificial placenta, display intermittent breathing movements. *Biol Neonate* 1999; 75: 388–97.

114. Martin-Body RL. Brain transections demonstrate the central origin of hypoxic ventilatory depression in carotid body-denervated rats. *J Physiol* 1988; 407: 41–52.

115. Martin-Body RL, Johnston BM. Central origin of the hypoxic depression of breathing in the young rabbit. *Respir Physiol* 1988; 71: 25–32.

116. Ackland GL, Noble R, Hanson MA. Red nucleus inhibits breathing during hypoxia in neonates. *Respir Physiol* 1997; 110(2–3): 251–60.

117. Moore PJ, Ackland GL, Hanson MA. Unilateral cooling in the region of locus coeruleus blocks the fall in respiratory output during hypoxia in anaesthetized neonatal sheep. *Exp Physiol* 1996; 81: 983–94.

118. Lagercrantz H. Stress, arousal and gene activation at birth. *Pediatr Res* 1996; 11: 214–8.

119. Chau AF, Matsurura M, Koos B. Glutamate receptors in the thalamus stimulate breathing and modulate sleep state in fetal sheep. *J Soc Gynecol Invest* 1996; 3(2): 252A/388.

120. Bocking AD, Harding R. Effects of reduced uterine blood flow on electrocortical activity, breathing and skeletal muscle activity in fetal sheep. *Am J Obstet Gynecol* 1986; 154: 655–62.

121. Stein P, White SE, Homan J, Blocking AD. Altered fetal cardiovascular responses to prolonged hypoxia after sinoaortic denervation. *Am J Physiol* 1999, 276: R340–46.

122. Lalor JG, Fawole B, Alfirevic Z, Devane D. Biophysical profile for fetal assessment in high risk pregnancies. *Cochrane Database Syst Rev* 2008 Jan 23; (1): CD000038.

123. Honest H, Bachmann LM, Sengupta R, Gupta JK, Kleijnen J, Khan KS. Accuracy of absence of fetal breathing movements in predicting preterm birth: A systematic review. *Ultrasound Obstet Gynecol* 2004 Jul; 24(1): 94–100.

124. Sussman D, Lye SJ, and Wells GD. Impact of maternal physical activity on fetal breathing and body movements. A review. *Early Human Dev* 2016, March; 94: 53–6.

3

Clinical anatomy of the newborn

MARK D. STRINGER AND S. ALI MIRJALILI

INTRODUCTION

A newborn infant more than triples in height and increases in weight some 20-fold before reaching maturity. During the process, structures change in size and position. Some, which are critically important during fetal development, disappear. Most persist but grow at different rates at different ages. It is therefore not surprising that newborn anatomy differs from adults; some of these differences are particularly important for the pediatric surgeon (Table 3.1 and Figure 3.1). This chapter summarizes the applied anatomy of the newborn, emphasizing aspects that are clinically relevant and different to adults.

GROWTH AND PROPORTIONS

Growth can be defined as "the progressive development of a living being or any of its parts from its earliest stage to maturity, including the attendant increase in size."[1] It involves changes in size and mass, and includes processes such as cell division, specialization, and apoptosis. Growth can be proportional but is often differential. For example, the head of a full-term newborn infant accounts for about 25% of its body length and 20% of its body surface area. In adults, these figures are about 13% and 9%, respectively (Figure 3.2). Similarly, the pelvis and lower limbs are proportionately small in the neonate.[2] Body surface area to weight ratio decreases with age: the surface area of a neonate is about 0.25 m² compared to 1.73 m² in an adult. Neonates are consequently more vulnerable to heat loss.

The mean length of the full-term newborn measured from crown to heel is around 48–50 cm and weight 2.7 to 3.8 kg. About 75%–80% of this weight is water and 15%–28% is fat.[3] By 1 year of age, total body water has decreased to adult values of around 60% of body weight.

CARDIOVASCULAR SYSTEM

Circulatory changes after birth

In the fetus, oxygen-rich blood is transported from the placenta via the umbilical vein to the left branch of the portal vein lying within the umbilical recess of the liver (Figure 3.3). The ductus venosus arises from the posterior aspect of the left branch of the portal vein directly opposite the opening of the umbilical vein and passes superiorly and laterally between the left lobe and caudate lobe of the liver to terminate in the left hepatic vein near its entry into the inferior vena cava (IVC). A valve along the anterior margin of the opening of the IVC into the right atrium directs the oxygenated blood through the foramen ovale to the left atrium. Deoxygenated systemic blood returning from the fetal superior vena cava and coronary sinus is directed preferentially to the right ventricle. However, during late gestation, only about 20% of the fetal cardiac output reaches the lungs[4,5] because the ductus arteriosus shunts blood from the pulmonary trunk to the aortic arch, just distal to the origin of the left subclavian artery. At term, the ductus arteriosus is about 8–12 mm long and 4–5 mm wide at its origin from the pulmonary trunk; the thoracic aorta by comparison measures about 5–6 mm in diameter.[3] The walls of the ductus arteriosus are rich in smooth muscle fibers. In the fetus, ductal patency is maintained by locally produced prostaglandins, which inhibit muscle contraction in response to oxygen.

At birth, the lungs inflate and, as a result of mechanical effects and oxygen-induced pulmonary vasodilatation, pulmonary vascular resistance falls. The ductus arteriosus starts to close and pulmonary blood flow increases. Increased venous return to the left atrium causes a rise in left atrial pressure. Right atrial pressure falls as a result of reduced venous return secondary to occlusion of the

Table 3.1 Key anatomical differences between neonates and adults

Cardiovascular System	Recent transition from fetal circulation
	Relatively large heart
	Potential for congenital heart defects
	Prominent thymic shadow on chest x-ray
Respiratory System	Obligate nose breathing
	Short neck with high larynx
	Ability to breathe while suckling
	Subglottis is narrowest part of the airway
	Highly compliant chest wall
	Greater reliance on diaphragm for breathing
Abdomen	Relatively wide abdomen
	Short inguinal canal
	Propensity to inguinal hernias and undescended testes
	Small amount of intra-abdominal fat
	Proportionately large liver
	Poor radiological distinction between small and large bowel
	Small pelvic cavity
	Intra-abdominal bladder and body of uterus
	Proportionately large suprarenal glands
Musculoskeletal System	Proportionately large head, small pelvis, and lower limbs
	Open fontanels
	Relatively underdeveloped face and mandible
	Horizontal auditory tube
	No spinal curvatures (other than shallow sacral curve)
	Absence of most secondary ossification centers
	Shallow acetabulum
	Relatively small gluteal muscles
Nervous System	Relatively large brain with full complement of neurones but incomplete myelination of axons
	Proportionately large cerebral ventricles
	Spinal cord terminates at lower level
Skin	Variable subcutaneous fat (some brown fat)
	Thin skin, immature sweating
	Greater body surface area to weight ratio
	Head accounts for 20% of body surface area

umbilical vein. These changes in atrial pressure force the free lower edge of the primary atrial septum to flatten against and subsequently adhere to the margins of the fossa ovale, resulting in functional closure of the foramen ovale. A permanent seal usually develops during the first year of life.

Cardiovascular adaptation to neonatal life therefore requires the functional closure of three fetal conduits:

- *Foramen ovale.* Incomplete fusion of the primary atrial septum with the limbus of the fossa ovale occurs in up to 25% of individuals,[6] resulting in a small potential atrial communication, a patent foramen ovale (PFO). Typically this has no consequences because of the flap-like arrangement of the opening and differential atrial pressures. However, a PFO may rarely be associated with paradoxical embolism (passage of an embolus from the venous system through an abnormal communication between the chambers of the heart causing a systemic arterial embolus, e.g., an embolic stroke) and an increased risk of decompression sickness in divers.[7] After closure of the foramen ovale, the valve of the IVC that was prominent in the fetus becomes flimsy or disappears.

- *Ductus arteriosus.* In full-term neonates with no congenital heart disease, the ductus arteriosus starts to close immediately after birth. Smooth muscle contraction within the ductus produces an initial functional closure and is probably mediated by several mechanisms: an increased arterial oxygen concentration, suppression of endogenous prostaglandin E2 synthesis, plasma catecholamines, and neural signaling. In addition, ductal blood flow is reversed as a result of increased systemic vascular resistance (due to absence of the placental circulation) and decreased pulmonary vascular resistance. Functional closure is complete within 3 days in more than 90% of term infants.[8]

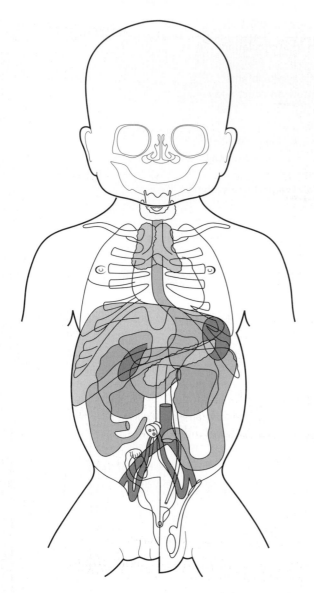

Figure 3.1 Diagram illustrating the relative proportions of viscera in the newborn. (Adapted from Crelin ES. *Functional Anatomy of the Newborn*. New Haven: Yale University Press, 1973, p. 75.)

Structural closure occurs more gradually, leaving the fibrous ligamentum arteriosum connecting the origin of the left pulmonary artery to the underside of the aortic arch. Persistent ductal shunting frequently occurs in preterm infants with respiratory distress.[4]

- *Ductus venosus.* Spontaneous closure of the ductus venosus begins immediately after birth[9] and is usually complete by about 17 days of age.[10,11] Closure may be temporarily delayed in the presence of congenital heart disease, presumably as a result of elevated venous pressure. In the adult, the remnant ligamentum venosum runs within the fissure separating the anatomic left lobe of the liver and the caudate lobe. Persistent patency of the ductus venosus is rare, is more common in boys, and may cause long-term problems such as hepatic encephalopathy.[12]

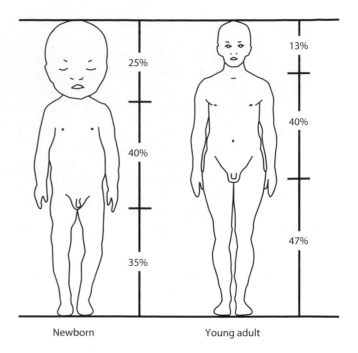

Newborn   Young adult

Figure 3.2 Relative proportions of the head, trunk, and lower limbs in a neonate and adult. (Adapted from Diméglio A. Growth in pediatric orthopaedics. In Morrissy RT, Weinstein SL. *Lovell and Winter's Pediatric Orthopaedics*. 6th edn. Lippincott Williams and Wilkins, 2006, Vol 1, p. 40.)

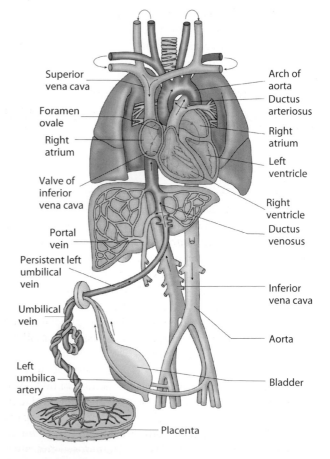

Figure 3.3 Fetal circulation.

The heart

In the full-term neonate, cardiac output measured by Doppler studies is about 250 mL/kg/min, mean systolic blood pressure in the first week is 70–80 mmHg (lower in preterm infants), and heart rate settles within hours of delivery to 120–140 beats/min. As the pulmonary circulation is established, the work of the right side of the heart decreases and the left increases, reflected by changes in ventricular muscle thickness; at birth, the mean wall thickness of both ventricles is about 5 mm, whereas in adults, the left ventricle is about three times as thick as the right.[3] The neonatal heart is relatively large in relation to the thorax and lungs, and consequently, it occupies a larger proportion of the lung fields on a chest radiograph compared to an adult (Figure 3.4[13]).

Congenital cardiac malformations account for up to a quarter of all developmental anomalies (8 per 1000 live births[4]) and include dextrocardia (isolated or part of situs inversus), isomerism, and structural defects (septal defects, abnormal atrioventricular or ventriculoarterial connections, and valvular anomalies). Ventriculoseptal defects are the most frequent, more often affecting the membranous than the muscular part of the interventricular septum. A true atrial septal defect occurs when there is a failure of normal development of the septum primum and/or atrioventricular endocardial cushions. Coarctation of the aorta is often included within the spectrum of congenital heart disease. Typically, there is narrowing or occlusion of the juxtaductal segment of aorta just distal to the origin of the left subclavian artery, although preductal (involving the aortic arch and its branches) and even postductal coarctation can occur.

Neonatal central venous catheters are generally positioned such that the catheter tip lies at the SVC/RA junction on a chest radiograph in order to reduce the small but serious risk of atrial perforation and cardiac tamponade.[14]

Umbilical vessels

The normal umbilical cord contains two thick-walled umbilical arteries and, near the 12 o'clock position, one larger but thin-walled umbilical vein. The presence of a single umbilical artery is associated with an increased risk of other congenital anomalies, particularly renal, vertebral, cardiovascular, and anorectal malformations,[15] and an increased risk of prematurity, growth restriction, and perinatal mortality.[16,17] However, routine karyotyping and renal sonography in an infant with an isolated single umbilical artery is not generally recommended.[16,18]

At birth, the umbilical vessels constrict rapidly in response to a fall in umbilical cord temperature and hemodynamic changes. Occlusion of the umbilical artery is facilitated by the "folds of Hoboken," constriction rings along the length of the umbilical artery produced by oblique or transverse bundles of myofibroblasts.[19] Numerous mediators of umbilical vessel vasoconstriction have been proposed,

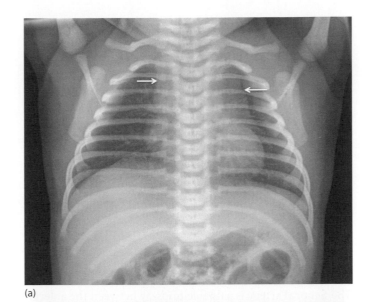

(a)

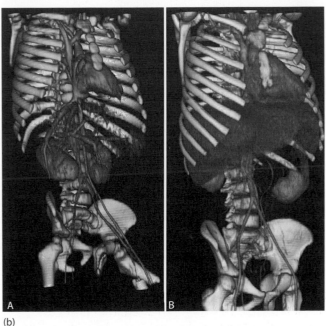

(b)

Figure 3.4 **(a)** Supine anteroposterior neonatal chest radiograph. Note the prominent superior mediastinal thymic shadow (white arrows). Compared to an adult, the hemidiaphragms are relatively flat, the ribs are more horizontal, and the heart size is relatively large (although the transverse cardiothoracic ratio should still be less than 60%). **(b)** 3-D reconstructed CT scan of a neonate (A) and 10-year-old child (B) demonstrating differences in skeletal anatomy including chest shape and rib alignment.

including bradykinin and endothelin-1, some of which are produced locally within the umbilical cord. After birth, the obliterated umbilical arteries become the paired medial umbilical ligaments usually visible under the peritoneum of the anterior abdominal wall below the umbilicus; the proximal parts of each umbilical artery remain patent as the superior vesical artery. The intra-abdominal segment of the umbilical vein becomes the ligamentum teres. The urachus has normally involuted before birth leaving the fibrous median umbilical ligament.

The umbilical artery and vein can be catheterized within 24–48 h of birth to provide vascular access for resuscitation, intravascular monitoring, fluid administration, blood transfusion, and parenteral nutrition.[20] The ideal position for the tip of an umbilical venous catheter is in the IVC, just below the right atrium. The tip of an umbilical artery catheter is usually positioned above the diaphragm but below the ductus arteriosus ("high" position equivalent to T6-9 vertebral level). Sometimes, the catheter tip is sited below the origin of the renal and inferior mesenteric arteries but above the aortic bifurcation ("low" position at L3-4 vertebral level).

Arteries

The femoral artery is palpable midway between the anterior superior iliac spine and pubic tubercle in the neonate[21]; it is therefore more lateral than in an adult where the surface marking is midway between the anterior superior iliac spine and symphysis pubis.[3] The renal arteries have been stated to lie at a higher vertebral level in the neonate than the adult, but recent studies have shown that they are around the level of L1 in both age groups.[22,23] The aortic bifurcation is at the upper rather than the lower border of L4.

Central veins

As in adults, the right and left brachiocephalic veins are formed by the union of the internal jugular and subclavian veins behind the ipsilateral sternoclavicular joint, and the junction between the superior vena cava and right atrium is most commonly behind the right fourth costal cartilage.[24,25] The left brachiocephalic vein lies at a relatively higher level than in adults and is potentially at risk of injury during tracheostomy when the neck is extended.

RESPIRATORY SYSTEM

Upper airway

Relative to an adult, the newborn infant has a large head, short neck, small face and mandible, and large tongue.[26,27] The entire surface of the tongue is within the oral cavity, unlike the adult where the posterior third is in the oropharynx. Neonates are obligate nose breathers and do not begin to breathe orally until about 4 months of age. All these features predispose to upper airway obstruction.

The neonatal nasopharynx curves smoothly backward and downward to join the oropharynx, rather than almost at a right angle as in adults (Figure 3.5).[27] The hyoid bone and larynx are high in the neck. Consequently, the upper margin of the neonate's epiglottis extends to the level of the soft palate, and the nasopharynx is in direct continuity with the larynx. This allows the infant to breathe while suckling. Ingested liquids pass lateral to the epiglottis via the piriform

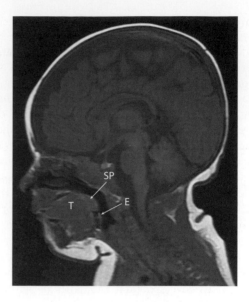

Figure 3.5 Sagittal magnetic resonance image of the upper airway in a newborn. T = tongue, SP = soft palate, E = epiglottis. (Courtesy of Professor Terry Doyle.)

fossae. Despite immature coordination of swallowing and breathing, the risk of aspiration is reduced by the high position of the larynx.

The higher more anterior position of the larynx also means that it is easier to intubate the trachea with a straight-bladed laryngoscope. The narrowest part of the infant's upper airway (about 3.5 mm in a term neonate) is the subglottis at the level of the cricoid cartilage, rather than the vocal cords as in adults. As the infant grows, the larynx descends and the epiglottis loses contact with the soft palate. Gender differences in laryngeal shape and size only begin to appear at about 3 years of age.[26]

Trachea and bronchial tree

The trachea is short, measuring approximately 4–5 cm in length in term neonates[28] and as little as 2–3 cm in premature neonates, making positioning of an endotracheal tube critical. The tip of the tube is usually sited between the clavicles, 1–2 cm above the carina, which corresponds to the vertebral body of T1. As in adults, the trachea starts at the level of the sixth cervical vertebra but bifurcates relatively higher at T3/4 (rather than T4/5 in adults). The trachea is rich in elastic tissue[29] and readily deformable. The right main bronchus is wider and steeper than the left, and the carina is more likely to lie to the left of the midline. Contrary to some reports, an aspirated foreign body is therefore more likely to enter the right lung.[30]

The bronchial tree is developed by the 16th week of intrauterine life; thereafter, conducting airways increase in size but not number.[31] Postnatal lung growth is mostly by alveolar development. Lung volume increases rapidly during infancy. Most alveoli have been formed by 2 years of age and only increase in size thereafter.[32,33] Before the infant takes its first breath, the terminal bronchioles and alveoli are filled with fluid, mostly produced in the lung. There is more fluid in the lungs of a newborn infant delivered by cesarian section than after vaginal delivery. For the alveoli to expand adequately, surface tension must be reduced; this is achieved by the release of surfactant from type II pneumocytes lining the alveoli. Surfactant also prevents alveolar collapse on expiration, which explains why very premature infants with inadequate surfactant production develop respiratory distress. Remodeling of the pulmonary vessels begins immediately after birth to reduce pulmonary vascular resistance.

Thorax and mechanics of breathing

The neonatal thorax has the shape of a truncated cone and is more rounded in circumference (Figure 3.4). Unlike the adult in whom the compliance of the chest wall and lung are similar, the neonate's chest wall is up to five times more compliant than its lungs.[3] Consequently, it is easily deformable, a fact that is readily apparent in the presence of respiratory distress.

The respiratory rate of a newborn at term is about 40–44 breaths/min. The ribs are more horizontal and contribute less to chest expansion. Infants rely mainly on diaphragmatic breathing. The diaphragm is relatively flat at birth (Figure 3.4) and becomes more dome-shaped with growth. Diaphragmatic contraction tends to pull the ribs inward; concomitant outward movement of the abdomen (thoracoabdominal paradox) is a normal finding in newborns. The work of breathing is greater in a neonate than an adult and still greater in a preterm infant.

The neonatal thymus is large (up to 5 cm wide and 1 cm thick) but variable in size at birth. It is a prominent feature on a chest x-ray (Figure 3.4). The gland overlies the trachea, great vessels (especially the left brachiocephalic vein), and the upper anterior surface of the heart. After the first year of life, it becomes progressively less vascular, and the lymphoid tissue is increasingly replaced by fat.

ABDOMINAL WALL AND GASTROINTESTINAL TRACT

Abdominal and pelvic cavities

The neonatal abdomen is relatively wide and protruberant because the diaphragm is flatter and the pelvic cavity smaller. The distance between the costal margin and iliac crest is proportionately greater in the neonate (Figure 3.4). For these reasons, transverse supraumbilical incisions provide good surgical access. The rectus abdominis muscles may be relatively wide apart in the upper abdomen (divarication); this resolves with growth. The inguinal canal in the newborn is short, measuring about 10–15 mm long in boys.[34–36] It subsequently lengthens with growth.

Compared to an adult, the true pelvis in the neonate is small, both relatively and absolutely, is more circular in

cross section, is orientated more horizontally, and has a less pronounced sacral curve. The peritoneal cavity is shallow anteroposteriorly because there is no lumbar lordosis and the paravertebral gutters are poorly developed. The urinary bladder, ovaries, and uterus are all partly intra-abdominal, and the rectum occupies most of the true pelvis (Figure 3.6). The greater omentum is delicate and membranous, rarely extending much below the level of the umbilicus. Indeed, the neonate has altogether less fat in the mesenteries and around the viscera.

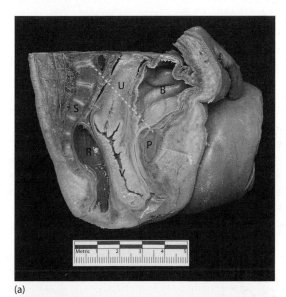

(a)

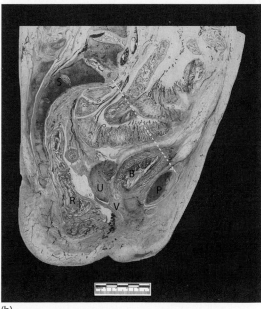

(b)

Figure 3.6 Midline sagittal section of a plastinated neonatal **(a)** and adult **(b)** female pelvis. Note the relative positions of the bladder (B) and uterus (U), the curvature of the sacrum (S), and the angle of the pelvis (dotted line between sacral promontory and pubic bone [P]). V = vagina, R = rectum. (Courtesy of the W.D. Trotter Anatomy Museum, University of Otago.)

Gastrointestinal tract

At term, the newborn esophagus measures about 8–10 cm in length from cricoid to diaphragm[26]; the upper and lower esophageal sphincters each extend over about 1 cm.[37] Lower esophageal sphincter pressure is particularly low during the first month or two of life. The narrowest part of the upper digestive tract is where the cricopharyngeus muscle blends with the upper esophagus, a potential site of esophageal perforation during the passage of a nasogastric tube.[38]

The anterior surface of the stomach is overlapped by the left lobe of the liver, which extends almost to the spleen. The capacity of the neonatal stomach is 30–35 mL at term but reaches 100 mL by the fourth week. Gastric emptying is relatively slow and poorly coordinated in the first few weeks. The small bowel of the newborn is distributed more horizontally because of the shape of the abdominal cavity. The mean length of the small intestine from the duodenojejunal flexure to the ileocecal junction is around 160 cm when measured at term along its antimesenteric border *in vivo*[39] but considerably longer when measured at autopsy.[40] In normal infants, the duodenojejunal flexure lies to the left of the midline, most often at the level of the L1 vertebra, although this level is variable.[41] The superior mesenteric artery typically lies to the left of the superior mesenteric vein. This vascular relationship is often abnormal in patients with intestinal malrotation, although abnormal orientation of these vessels can be seen in some healthy individuals and a normal relationship may sometimes exist in patients with intestinal malrotation.[42]

The mean *in vivo* length of the colon from the ileocecal junction to the upper rectum is 33 cm at term.[39] The cecum and ascending and descending colon are proportionately shorter than in the adult, and the transverse colon, sigmoid colon, and rectum proportionately longer. The cecum tapers to a proportionately large appendix with a relatively wide orifice. The anal canal has well-defined anal columns and prominent anal sinuses[43]; stasis within these sinuses is a putative cause of perianal sepsis, particularly in male infants.[44]

Neonatal small bowel has few circular folds (valvulae conniventes), and the neonatal colon has no haustra. This makes it difficult to distinguish the small and large bowel on plain abdominal radiographs. Their relative position (central versus peripheral) and caliber are a guide, but a contrast study may be required to accurately differentiate small and large bowel pathology.

Liver and spleen

The neonatal liver weighs about 120 g at term and comprises about 4% of body weight (compared to 2% in the adult); it more than doubles in weight during the first year. The relatively large liver fills much of the upper abdomen. Its inferior border extends 1–2 cm below the costal margin. The premature baby's liver is particularly fragile and vulnerable to injury (e.g., from an abdominal retractor). The neonatal

gallbladder is more intrahepatic, and its fundus may not extend below the liver margin.

The tip of the newborn's spleen is often palpable just below the left costal margin. The pancreatic tail is in contact with the spleen, usually at its hilum, in more than 90% of cases, which is a greater proportion than in adults.[45] Accessory spleens are found at autopsy in about 14% of fetuses and neonates as compared to 10% of adults,[46] but it is uncertain whether this is a true increased prevalence.

GENITOURINARY SYSTEM

Genitourinary anomalies are among the commonest congenital malformations, and so it is especially important to understand normal anatomy in the newborn.

Kidneys and suprarenal glands

At birth, the kidneys are about 4–5 cm in length compared to a mean length of 11 cm in adults. Fetal lobulation of the kidneys is still present at birth. Individual nephrons consist of a renal corpuscle with (i) a central glomerulus concerned with plasma filtration and (ii) a renal tubule that produces urine by selective reabsorption of the filtrate. At birth, there are about 1 million renal corpuscles in the cortex of each kidney. Postnatally, cortical nephron mass increases but no new nephrons are made. The glomerular filtration rate (GFR) is low in newborns, particularly in the premature, but in the term infant, the GFR doubles by 2 weeks of age and reaches adult values (120 mL/min per 1.73 m^2) by 1–2 years.[47]

The suprarenal glands are relatively large at birth with a proportionately thick cortex. Their average combined weight is 9 g compared with 7–12 g in the adult. Both glands shrink in the neonatal period.

Bladder and ureter

The bladder is largely intra-abdominal at birth (Figure 3.6) with its apex midway between the pubis and the umbilicus in the unfilled state. Suprapubic aspiration and manual expression of urine are therefore relatively easy. The bladder does not achieve its adult pelvic position until about the sixth year.[3] The intravesical segment of the ureter (intramural and submucosal portions) lengthens from about 0.5 cm in neonates to 1.3 cm (the adult value) by 10–12 years of age. An abnormally short submucosal tunnel predisposes to vesicoureteric reflux (VUR); this type of VUR tends to resolve spontaneously with growth.[48]

Genitalia and reproductive tract

By about the sixth month *in utero*, the testis lies adjacent to the deep inguinal ring connected to the developing scrotum by the gubernaculum. Although the testis originates as a retroperitoneal structure, it is suspended on a short mesentery (mesorchium) within the peritoneal cavity during abdominal "descent."[49] Inguinoscrotal descent of the testis occurs between 25 and 35 weeks postconception; in this phase, it is invaginated into an elongating peritoneal diverticulum, the processus vaginalis, which subsequently becomes obliterated leaving only the tunica vaginalis around the testis. At term, about 4% of boys have an undescended testis(es); the figure is considerably higher in premature infants. By 3 months of age, the prevalence of cryptorchidism has fallen to 1.5%. The timing and process of closure of the processus vaginalis are both uncertain.[50] Surgical studies have shown that a patent processus vaginalis is present in around 60% of contralateral groin explorations *in infants with a unilateral inguinal hernia* in the first 2 months, falling to around 40% after 2 years of age. Autopsy studies have indicated that the processus is patent in about 80% of newborns, decreasing to about 15%–30% in adults. Boys with cryptorchidism have higher patency rates.

The prostate and seminal vesicles are well developed at birth. The penis and scrotum are relatively large, and the scrotum has a broad base and relatively thick walls. The prepuce begins to separate from the glans *in utero* but is usually only partially retractile at birth.

In baby girls, the ovary lies in the lower part of the iliac fossa and only descends into the ovarian fossa within the true pelvis during early childhood as the pelvis deepens. At birth, the ovaries are relatively large and contain the full complement of primary oocytes, each surrounded by a single layer of follicular cells forming primordial follicles. Of the 7 million oocytes estimated to be present in the female fetus, only 1 million remain at birth, and this number decreases further to approximately 40,000 by puberty.

In the term infant, the uterus is about 3–5 cm long and the cervix forms two-thirds or more of its length (Figure 3.6). Female newborns have a relatively prominent clitoris and labia, and the vagina, which is about 3 cm in length, is relatively thick-walled with a fleshy hymen. After withdrawal of maternal hormones, the uterus and the vagina shrink in size.

MUSCULOSKELETAL SYSTEM

Skull and face

The skull vault is formed by intramembranous ossification, the facial skeleton is derived from neural crest membrane bones, and the skull base and some bony pharyngeal arch derivatives (e.g., hyoid bone and ossicles) by endochondral ossification.[3] During birth, the margins of the frontal and parietal bones are able to slide over each other. In the first 2 days of life, palpable overriding of the bones of the vault is common. However, persistent ridging of suture lines may indicate craniosynostosis. Growth at the coronal suture is mostly responsible for fronto-occipital expansion of the skull; premature fusion causes brachycephaly if bilateral and plagiocephaly if unilateral. Growth at the metopic and

sagittal sutures increases skull breadth, the metopic suture fusing at around 18 months of age and the sagittal at puberty. Premature fusion produces the elongated skull of sagittal craniosynostosis, the most common form of craniosynostosis. Premature babies have a tendency to develop a long thin head (dolichocephaly) secondary to postnatal gravitational molding, but this is not due to premature sutural fusion.

Fontanels are formed where several skull vault bones meet. The two most prominent are the anterior fontanel overlying the superior sagittal venous sinus at the junction of the metopic and sagittal sutures (bregma), and the posterior fontanel at the junction of the sagittal and lambdoid sutures (lambda).[51] The size of the anterior fontanel at birth is very variable; if unduly large, it may be an indication of congenital hypothyroidism, raised intracranial pressure or a skeletal disorder.[52] The timing of closure is also variable, but the anterior fontanel is obliterated by 2 years of age in 95% of children[53] and the posterior by 2 months of age.[54]

Postnatal growth of the skull vault is accompanied by disproportionate growth of the facial skeleton and mandible (Figure 3.7). At birth, the bony external ear canal is not developed, and the mastoid process is absent. The facial nerve is therefore more at risk of injury where it emerges from the stylomastoid foramen (e.g., from obstetric forceps). At birth, the two halves of the mandible are united by a fibrous symphysis that fuses in early childhood. The rami are at a more obtuse angle to the body of the mandible. The mandible subsequently changes shape as the teeth erupt and the muscles of mastication and chin develop.

The maxillary and ethmoid sinuses are present at birth, but the sphenoid sinus is poorly developed and the frontal sinuses are absent.[26] The auditory tube is almost horizontal, increasing the risk of middle ear disease; it becomes more vertical during childhood. The hard palate is short, only slightly arched, and ridged by transverse folds, which assist with suckling. The nasolacrimal duct, which drains tear secretions from the conjunctival sac to the inferior meatus of the nasal cavity, is relatively short and wide at birth, but may be obstructed due to incomplete canalization. This can cause excessive tearing, discharge, and infection.

Vertebral column, pelvis, and limbs

The vertebral column in the neonate has no fixed curvatures other than a mild sacral curve. After birth, the thoracic curvature develops first and then, as the infant learns to control its head, sit, stand, and walk, curvatures in the lumbar and cervical spine develop, which help to maintain the center of gravity of the trunk when walking. The sacral promontory "descends" and becomes more prominent. Hemopoiesis occurs in the liver, spleen, and bone marrow in the fetus, but is largely restricted to the bone marrow of the vertebrae, ribs, sternum, proximal long bones, and diploe of the skull after birth.

Of the 800 or so ossification centers in the human skeleton, just over half appear after birth; these include most secondary ossification centers (Figure 3.8). Cartilage is abundant at birth; none of the carpal bones have ossification

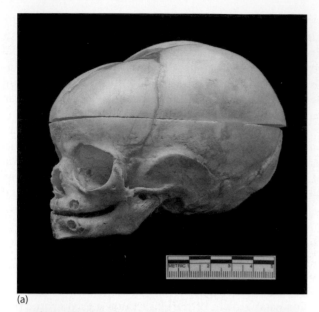

(a)

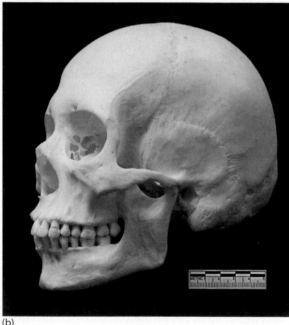

(b)

Figure 3.7 Comparison of a neonatal **(a)** and adult male **(b)** skull. Note the relatively small size of the face and mandible in the neonate, the cranial vault sutures, and the anterior fontanel. The mastoid process has not developed at birth. (Courtesy of the W.D. Trotter Anatomy Museum, University of Otago.)

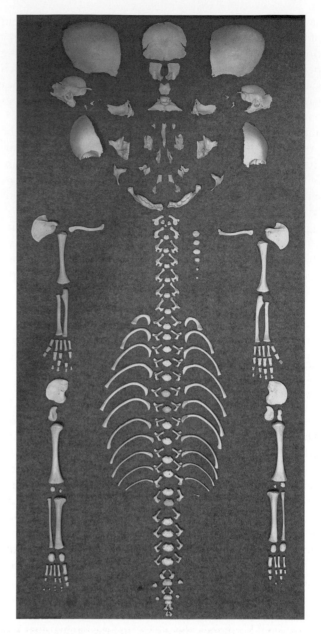

Figure 3.8 Bony skeleton of a newborn baby. There are no carpal bones at birth, there are separate ossification centers for the hip, and secondary centers of ossification in the long bones are absent except for the lower end of the femur and upper end of tibia. Specimen prepared by Professor J.H. Scott in 1895. (Courtesy of the W.D. Trotter Anatomy Museum, University of Otago.)

centers. The only secondary centers of ossification in the long bones at birth are in the femoral and tibial condyles and sometimes in the humeral head.[26] The iliac crest, acetabular floor, and ischial tuberosity are all cartilaginous.

The acetabulum is relatively large and shallow at birth and has a characteristic Y-shaped triradiate cartilaginous epiphyseal plate between the ilium, ischium, and pubis. Nearly one-third of the neonatal femoral head lies outside the acetabulum, making the hip joint easier to dislocate.

Developmental dysplasia of the hip affects about 1 in 100 live births and is more common in girls. The neonatal femoral neck is short, and the femoral shaft is straight. The proximal femoral growth plate in early infancy is intra-articular so that infection in the proximal femoral metaphysis may cause a septic arthritis. The lower limb muscles in the newborn are relatively underdeveloped, and the gluteal muscle mass is small. The thighs tend to be abducted, flexed, and externally rotated, the knees flexed, and the foot dorsiflexed and inverted. In congenital talipes equinovarus (club foot),

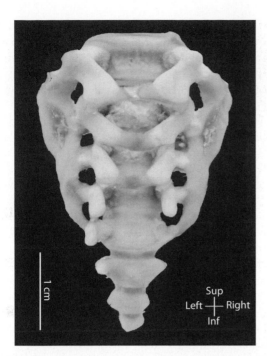

Figure 3.9 Sacrum from a newborn demonstrating the variable development, ossification, and symmetry of the posterior cartilaginous vertebral elements.

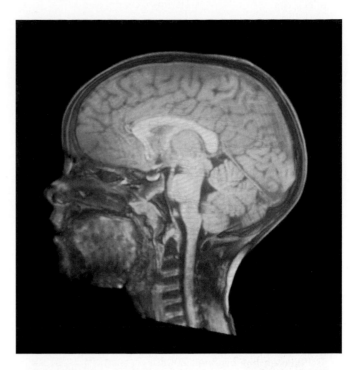

Figure 3.10 3-D volume rendered sagittal MRI scan of the head in an infant.

there is impaired development of the talus causing inversion and supination of the foot and adduction of the forefoot.

Incomplete ossification of the posterior vertebral elements can make palpation of the sacrococcygeal hiatus difficult, increasing the risks of neonatal caudal anesthesia (Figure 3.9).[55] Ultrasound guidance has therefore been recommended when performing this regional block in neonates. Ultrasound has the added advantage of being able to visualize the termination of the dural sac (usually at S2 but at S3 in some), which lies at a variable distance from the sacral cornua.

NERVOUS SYSTEM

At term, the neonatal brain weighs between 300 and 400 g, accounting for about 10% of body weight (compared to 2% in the adult).[26] Brain growth is especially rapid during the first year, when it reaches 75% of its adult volume. The number of neurones is already established at birth, and brain growth is due to an increase in size of nerve cell bodies, further development of neuronal connections, proliferation of neuroglia and blood vessels, and myelination of axons. Myelination is at its peak in the first 6 months of life but continues until maturity.[3] The arrangement of sulci and gyri at birth is similar to the adult, although the central sulcus is slightly further forward and the ventricles are proportionately larger (Figure 3.10). Mean head circumference at term is 34 cm.

The termination of the spinal cord (the conus medullaris) is at a median level of the L2 vertebra in the neonate compared to the lower border of L1 in adults.[56] Variable anatomy means that in some infants, the conus may lie as low

as L3; if the conus is unusually low or immobile on a spinal ultrasound scan, spinal cord tethering should be excluded. The supracristal plane between the tops of the iliac crests is slightly higher (L3/4 rather than L4); a lumbar puncture in the newborn should not be performed above this level.

SKIN AND SUBCUTANEOUS TISSUE

Body fat is laid down in the fetus from about 34 weeks' gestation and, with appropriate intrauterine nutrition, increases until term. Plantar fat pads give the neonate a flat-footed appearance. Brown fat is a modified form of adipose tissue concentrated at the back of the neck, in the interscapular region, and in pararenal areas. It is composed of adipocytes with mitochondria that have large and numerous cristae adapted to heat production. However, the neonate's ability to regulate temperature is poorly developed.

At birth, breast tissue is similarly developed in girls and boys. It may appear prominent due to the influence of maternal hormones, even leading to the secretion of a small amount of fluid (witch's milk). Supernumerary nipple(s) may be found along the mammary ridges (milk lines), which extend from the axilla to the groin.

Neonatal skin is relatively thin, but the ability to see peripheral veins is very dependent on the thickness of the subcutaneous tissues. Common sites for peripheral venous cannulation include the dorsal arch veins of the hands and feet; the cephalic vein at the wrist; the cubital fossa; the great saphenous vein immediately anterior to the medial malleolus or behind the medial aspect of the knee; and the superficial temporal vein anterior to the ear. The saphenous, cephalic and basilic veins are also used for insertion of percutaneous central catheters.

ACKNOWLEDGMENTS

We wish to thank Chris Smith, curator of the W.D. Trotter Anatomy Museum, and Robbie McPhee, medical illustrator and graphic artist, Department of Anatomy, University of Otago, Dunedin, New Zealand.

REFERENCES

1. Sinclair D, Dangerfield P. *Human Growth after Birth*, 6th edn. Oxford: Oxford Medical Publications, 1998.
2. Diméglio A. Growth in pediatric orthopaedics. In: Morrissy RT, Weinstein SL (eds). *Lovell and Winter's Pediatric Orthopaedics*, 6th edn, Vol 1. Philadelphia: Lippincott Williams and Wilkins, 2006: 35–65.
3. Standring S (ed). *Gray's Anatomy*, 40th edn. Philadelphia: Elsevier, 2008.
4. Archer LN. Cardiovascular disease. In: Rennie JM (ed). *Roberton's Textbook of Neonatology*, 4th edn. London: Elsevier Limited, 2005: 619–60.
5. Rasanen J, Wood DC, Weiner S, Ludomirski A, Huhta JC. Role of the pulmonary circulation in the distribution of human fetal cardiac output during the second half of pregnancy. *Circulation* 1996; 94: 1068–73.
6. Hagen PT, Scholz DG, Edwards WD. Incidence and size of patent foramen ovale during the first 10 decades of life: An autopsy study of 965 normal hearts. *Mayo Clin Proc* 1984; 59: 17–20.
7. Holmes DR, Cohen HA, Ruiz C. Patent foramen ovale, systemic embolization, and closure. *Curr Probl Cardiol* 2009; 34: 483–530.
8. Evans NJ, Archer LN. Postnatal circulatory adaptation in healthy term and preterm neonates. *Arch Dis Child* 1990; 65: 24–6.
9. Meyer WW, Lind J. The ductus venosus and the mechanism of its closure. *Arch Dis Child* 1966; 41: 597–605.
10. Loberant N, Barak M, Gaitini D, Herskovits M, Ben-Elisha M, Roguin N. Closure of the ductus venosus in neonates: Findings on real-time gray-scale, color-flow Doppler, and duplex Doppler sonography. *Am J Roentgenol* 1992; 159: 1083–5.
11. Fugelseth D, Lindemann R, Liestol K, Kiserud T, Langslet A. Ultrasonographic study of ductus venosus in healthy neonates. *Arch Dis Child* 1997; 77: F131–4.
12. Stringer MD. The clinical anatomy of congenital portosystemic venous shunts. *Clin Anat* 2008; 21: 147–57.
13. Arthur R. The neonatal chest x-ray. *Paed Resp Rev* 2001; 2: 311–23.
14. Wariyar UK, Hallworth D. *Review of Four Neonatal Deaths due to Cardiac Tamponade Associated with the Presence of a Central Venous Catheter*. London, UK: Department of Health, 2001.
15. Martínez-Frías ML, Bermejo E, Rodríguez-Pinilla E, Prieto D, ECEMC Working Group. Does single umbilical artery (SUA) predict any type of congenital defect? Clinical–epidemiological analysis of a large consecutive series of malformed infants. *Am J Med Genet A* 2008; 146A: 15–25.
16. Mu SC, Lin CH, Chen YL, Sung TC, Bai CH, Jow GM. The perinatal outcomes of asymptomatic isolated single umbilical artery in full-term neonates. *Pediatr Neonatol* 2008; 49: 230–3.
17. Murphy-Kaulbeck L, Dodds L, Joseph KS, Van den Hof M. Single umbilical artery risk factors and pregnancy outcomes. *Obstet Gynecol* 2010; 116: 843–50.
18. Deshpande SA, Jog S, Watson H, Gornall A. Do babies with isolated single umbilical artery need routine postnatal renal ultrasonography? *Arch Dis Child Fetal Neonatal Ed* 2009; 94: F265–7.
19. Röckelein G, Kobras G, Becker V. Physiological and pathological morphology of the umbilical and placental circulation. *Pathol Res Pract* 1990; 186: 187–96.
20. Anderson J, Leonard D, Braner DAV, Lai S, Tegtmeyer K. Umbilical vascular catheterization. *N Engl J Med* 2008; 359: e18.
21. Van Schoor AN, Bosman M, Bosenberg A. Femoral nerve blocks: A comparison of neonatal and adult anatomy. 17th Congress of the International Federation of Associations of Anatomists, Cape Town, South Africa, August 2009.
22. Subramaniam H, Taghavi K, Mirjalili SA. A reappraisal of pediatric abdominal surface anatomy utilizing in vivo cross-sectional imaging. *Clin Anat* 2016; 29: 197–203.
23. Mirjalili SA, McFadden SL, Buckenham T, Stringer MD. A reappraisal of adult abdominal surface anatomy. *Clin Anat* 2012; 25: 844–50.
24. Mirjalili SA, Hale SJ, Buckenham T, Wilson B, Stringer MD. A reappraisal of adult thoracic surface anatomy. *Clin Anat* 2012; 25: 827–34.
25. Tarr GP, Pak N, Taghavi K, Iwan T, Dumble C, Davies-Payne D, Mirjalili SA. Defining the surface anatomy of the central venous system in children. *Clin Anat* 2016; 29: 157–64.
26. Crelin ES. *Functional Anatomy of the Newborn*. New Haven: Yale University Press, 1973.
27. Bosma JF. *Anatomy of the Infant Head,* 1st edn. Baltimore: The Johns Hopkins University Press, 1986: 321–79.
28. Sirisopana M, Saint-Martin C, Wang NN, Manoukian J, Nguyen LH, Brown KA. Novel measurements of the length of the subglottic airway in infants and young children. *Anesth Analg* 2013; 117: 462–70.

29. Kamel KS, Beckert LE, Stringer MD. Novel insights into the elastic and muscular components of the human trachea. *Clin Anat* 2009; 22: 689–97.

30. Tahir N, Ramsden WH, Stringer MD. Tracheobronchial anatomy and the distribution of inhaled foreign bodies in children. *Eur J Pediatr* 2009; 168: 289–95.

31. Jeffery PK. The development of large and small airways. *Am J Respir Crit Care Med* 1998; 157: S174–80.

32. Thurlbeck WM. Postnatal human lung growth. *Thorax* 1982; 37: 564–71.

33. Hislop AA. Airway and blood vessel interaction during lung development. *J Anat* 2002; 201: 325–34.

34. Parnis SJ, Roberts JP, Hutson JM. Anatomical landmarks of the inguinal canal in prepubescent children. *ANZ J Surg* 1997; 67: 335–7.

35. Vergnes P, Midy D, Bondonny JM, Cabanie H. Anatomical basis of inguinal surgery in children. *Anat Clin* 1985; 7: 257–65.

36. Taghavi K, Geneta vP, Mirjalili SA. The pediatric inguinal canal: Systematic review of the embryology and surface anatomy. *Clin Anat* 2016; 29: 204–10.

37. Gupta A, Jadcherla SR. The relationship between somatic growth and in vivo esophageal segmental and sphincteric growth in human neonates. *J Pediatr Gastroenterol Nutr* 2006; 43: 35–41.

38. Gander JW, Berdon WE, Cowles RA. Iatrogenic esophageal perforation in children. *Pediatr Surg Int* 2009; 25: 395–401.

39. Struijs MC, Diamond IR, de Silva N, Wales PW. Establishing norms for intestinal length in children. *J Pediatr Surg* 2009; 44: 933–8.

40. Weaver LT, Austin S, Cole TJ. Small intestinal length: A factor essential for gut adaptation. *Gut* 1991; 32: 1321–3.

41. Koch C, Taghavi K, Hamill J, Mirjalili SA. Redefining the projectional and clinical anatomy of the duodenojejunal flexure in children. *Clin Anat* 2016; 29: 175–82.

42. Dufour D, Delaet MH, Dassonville M, Cadranel S, Perlmutter N. Midgut malrotation, the reliability of sonographic diagnosis. *Pediatr Radiol* 1992; 22: 21–3.

43. Shafik A. A new concept of the anatomy of the anal sphincter mechanism and the physiology of defecation. *Dis Colon Rect* 1980; 23: 170–9.

44. Nix P, Stringer MD. Perianal sepsis in children. *Br J Surg* 1997; 84: 819–21.

45. Üngör B, Malas MA, Sulak O, Albay S. Development of spleen during the fetal period. *Surg Radiol Anat* 2007; 29: 543–50.

46. Cahalane SF, Kiesselbach N. The significance of the accessory spleen. *J Pathol* 1970; 100: 139–44.

47. Lissauer T, Clayden G. *Illustrated Textbook of Paediatrics*, 3rd edn. London: Mosby Elsevier, 2007.

48. Godley ML, Ransley PG. Vesicoureteral reflux: Pathophysiology and experimental studies. In: Gearhart JP, Rink RC, Mouriquand PDE (eds). *Pediatric Urology*, 2nd edn. Philadelphia: Saunders, Elsevier, 2010: 283–300.

49. Lopez-Marambio FA, Hutson JM. The relationship between the testis and tunica vaginalis changes with age. *J Pediatr Surg* 2015; 50: 2075–77.

50. Godbole PP, Stringer MD. Patent processus vaginalis. In: Gearhart JP, Rink RC, Mouriquand PDE (eds). *Pediatric Urology*, 2nd edn. Philadelphia: Saunders, Elsevier, 2010: 577–84.

51. Sundaresan M, Wright M, Price AB. Anatomy and development of the fontanelle. *Arch Dis Child* 1990; 65: 386–7.

52. Davies DP, Ansari BM, Cooke TJ. Anterior fontanelle size in the neonate. *Arch Dis Child* 1975; 50: 81–3.

53. Acheson RM, Jefferson E. Some observations on the closure of the anterior fontanelle. *Arch Dis Child* 1954; 29: 196–8.

54. Bickley LS, Szilagyi PG. *Bates' Guide to Physical Examination and History Taking,* 10th edn, Chapter 18. Philadelphia: Wolters Kluwer Health, 2009: 743–96.

55. Mirjalili SA, Taghavi K, Frawley G, Craw S. Should we abandon landmark-based technique for caudal anesthesia in neonates and infants? *Paediatr Anaesth* 2015; 25: 511–6.

56. Van Schoor AN, Bosman MC, Bosenberg AT. Descriptive study of the differences in the level of the conus medullaris in four different age groups. *Clin Anat* 2015; 28: 638–44.

4

The epidemiology of birth defects

EDWIN C. JESUDASON

BIRTH DEFECTS HELPED DEFINE PEDIATRIC SURGERY

Surgery for birth defects helped create the specialty of pediatric surgery during the middle of the last century. Around this time, pioneering operations were successfully performed to allow the survival of babies with, e.g., esophageal atresia or congenital diaphragmatic hernia (CDH). Indeed, along with innovations such as parenteral nutrition, this concentration of surgical, nursing, and anesthetic expertise now allows high survival rates to be achieved for many previously fatal anomalies. Moreover, for certain conditions that retain high mortality and/or morbidity, fetal surgery represents a promising experimental approach to reduce the harm of birth defects further. Given this progress, it would be tempting to imagine that the problem of birth defects was largely solved.

BIRTH DEFECTS REMAIN POTENT CAUSES OF INFANT MORTALITY AND LONG-TERM DISABILITY

The advances made against infectious disease mean that birth defects represent a leading cause of infant mortality. This holds true in nations with expensive healthcare systems and indeed anywhere that infant mortality has fallen below ~50 per thousand births.[1] Prevention is possible for some of these birth defects: congenital rubella syndrome might be eradicated by an effective program of maternal immunization[2]; a subset of neural tube defects continue to occur due to inadequate implementation of preconceptual folate prophylaxis.[3,4] However, for many defects, prevention is not always possible, feasible, or effective. In these circumstances, the epidemiological challenge extends from new problems like the Zika outbreak to explaining the changed prevalence of familiar defects like gastroschisis (Figure 4.1).[5,6] Hence, birth defects will continue to cause not only infant deaths but also premature birth and chronic disability. Pediatric services have tended to focus on perinatal approaches to birth defects, but it is clear that the needs of long-term survivors have to be considered more fully. For example, the transition toward independent adulthood poses particular challenges. While it is tempting to attribute this to the patients and their families, it is striking how the separate development of pediatric and adult specialists means that there is often a lack of meaningful engagement between the two realms. An upshot is that children and young adults are often "held back" within children's services only then to be ejected belatedly into an adult realm that seems disjointed and unfamiliar. It is likely that pediatric surgeons can do more to address this transition and to cater to the needs of survivors via greater attention to patient-derived outcomes and Engel's biopsychosocial model of health.

BIRTH DEFECT EPIDEMIOLOGY AND TERATOLOGY EMERGED FROM OUTBREAK INVESTIGATION

Like neonatal surgery, teratology and birth defect epidemiology really date from only the mid–twentieth century. Key historical developments include the recognition of congenital rubella syndrome (noted by clinical ophthalmological examination) and the thalidomide disaster (phocomelia and other defects associated with maternal thalidomide administration for morning sickness).[7,8] These chastening episodes illustrated the devastating consequences of prenatal infection and drug exposure respectively. They highlighted the need to formalize birth defect surveillance. Today, this serves a range of important purposes. These include early warning of outbreaks, identification of potential causes, planning neonatal services, informing prenatal counseling, and the comparison of outcomes (as a guide toward best practice).[9]

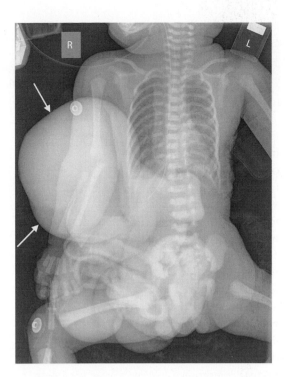

Figure 4.1 Gastroschisis—birth defect prevalences can change. Data from birth defect registries indicate an increase in gastroschisis prevalence. It remains to be seen if the severity of gastroschisis is also increasing: in this severe and unusual example, in addition to the gut, the liver (arrowed) lies outside the neonatal abdomen. Furthermore, the thorax is narrowed; this child needed ventilation immediately from birth. (Image used courtesy of the author.)

CAUSATION OF BIRTH DEFECTS REMAINS OFTEN COMPLEX AND UNCERTAIN

Before considering the methods of birth defect surveillance, it is worth sketching out the developmental biology that underpins birth defects.[10] Causes of birth defects can be considered as parental, fetal, and environmental. In reality, they will often overlap. For example, grandparental behaviors (or exposures) may produce epigenetic modifications that only manifest themselves in the developing fetus.

A familiar example of a parental factor is the impact of maternal age on Down's prevalence.[11] Alternatively, maternal diseases such as diabetes are well-described risk factors for birth defect formation.[12] The role of paternal age and/or exposures is more difficult to quantify.[13] Fetal causes might include genetically determined inborn errors of metabolism such as those causing intersex anomalies in congenital adrenal hyperplasia, chromosomal lesions such as Edwards' etc., and twinning (with its increased risk of birth anomalies). Environmental causes include those related to prenatal drug exposure (alcohol, smoking, illicit drugs, thalidomide, valproate, phenytoin, warfarin, etc.) as well as the impact of intrauterine infections (e.g., toxoplasmosis, rubella, cytomegalovirus, possibly Zika).[14–16] The impact on birth defect prevalence of assisted reproductive technologies such as in vitro fertilization and intracytoplasmic sperm injection is quite difficult to assess.[17] The suggestion that anomaly rates are higher in assisted pregnancies needs to contend with confounding factors, e.g., the increased rates of multiple pregnancy and parental differences that may have created the need for assisted reproduction. Environmental contributors to birth defects may also include *endocrine disruptors*: these estrogenic compounds are conjectured to contribute to anomalies of sexual development in fetal males (e.g., hypospadias) as well as putative impairment of adult male sperm quality.[16] In light of such difficulties in attributing cause, it is simpler to admit that only the minority of birth defects are known to arise from a simple genetic or environmental cause. At present, the remainder appear to have multifactorial origins. In such circumstances, it is helpful to consider birth defect causation as the result of complex interactions between genes and environment. Hence, cases of spina bifida may result from micronutrient deficiency in the context of predisposing enzyme polymorphisms.[18] Similarly, teratogenic drugs may interact with pharmacogenomic predispositions to help explain why only certain pregnancies are affected.[19] Beyond considerations of even complex causation, it remains likely that simple chance has a major role to play (similar to the stochastic effects noted in radiation biology).[20]

BIRTH DEFECTS APPEAR TO ARISE TYPICALLY (BUT NOT EXCLUSIVELY) IN THE FIRST TRIMESTER

Developmental biologists refer to *competence windows* to describe periods in development when particular cells and tissues are capable of responding appropriately to certain growth and transcription factors.[21] In a similar manner, developing organs are contended to have particular temporal windows when an otherwise nonspecific teratogenic stimulus will impact disproportionately on formation of that organ system. During the first trimester, organ morphogenesis predominates, while later trimesters are devoted to organ growth and maturation. Unsurprisingly, therefore, sensitivity to teratogens is held to peak during the first trimester. Hence, pregnant women are advised to avoid medications during this part of gestation in particular. Teleologically, morning sickness, which peaks during the first trimester, is postulated to help reduce ingestion of potential teratogens during this period of maximum vulnerability. While the model of first-trimester teratogenesis appears appropriate for many birth defects, certain anomalies appear to arise later as a result of fetal events, e.g., amniotic band formation, intussusception, or vascular accident. Gastroschisis and intestinal atresiae may be considered in this latter category.[22–24] Indeed, the contrast between exomphalos and gastroschisis in terms of associated anomalies (and hence prognosis) may be explained by the different times they are held to originate in development. Exomphalos is considered an embryonic lesion that is accompanied by contemporaneous lesions of organogenesis in other systems such as the heart. In contrast, gastroschisis is thought to result from a discrete fetal vascular accident (like the associated intestinal atresiae) and to lack extraintestinal manifestations as a consequence. An alternative view, however, is that intestinal atresiae result only rarely from fetal accidents such as intussusception and are in fact better understood as failures of mesenteric vascular development.[25]

A contrast between duodenal atresia and small bowel atresia may likewise be understood as the result of their differing onsets and etiologies. Duodenal atresia was historically explained as an embryonic failure of luminal recanalization; although this "solid core" theory has been contradicted by more recent animal studies, the association between duodenal atresia and other defects (e.g., cardiac lesions, esophageal atresia, and Down's syndrome) supports an embryonic origin of this malformation.[26,27] In contrast, small bowel atresiae are claimed to follow mesenteric vascular occlusion usually in fetal life.[28] Aside from gastroschisis, intestinal atresiae are unlikely to be associated with other structural lesions.

Between these two "extremes" are birth defects where an embryonic lesion has deleterious knock-on effects later in fetal development. Based on experimental models, the neurological sequelae of spina bifida are postulated to result not only from the primary failure of neural tube closure but also from consequent exposure of the neural placode to amniotic fluid.[29] Similarly, lung hypoplasia in CDH may emerge as an embryonic lesion prior to CDH only for compression by the visceral hernia to exacerbate the pulmonary lesion.[30] In circumstances such as these, where the pathology is thought to progress during fetal life, prenatal surgical correction has been a logical proposal to meet the challenge of refractory mortality and morbidity.[31]

CLASSIFICATION OF BIRTH DEFECTS FOR EPIDEMIOLOGICAL PURPOSES

Birth defect epidemiology involves the registration of anomalies by type. At present, birth defect registries such as EUROCAT (European Surveillance of Congenital Anomalies) use a classification scheme based around organ systems (see Table 4.1), specific diagnoses, and International Classification of Diseases codes (see Table 4.2: both tables are derived from data published by EUROCAT at http://www.eurocat-network.eu/access prevalencedata/prevalencetables). Cooperation between registries helps by pooling data and also by building consensus on, e.g., exclusion of minor anomalies without major and/or long-term sequelae (e.g., cryptorchidism or congenital hydrocele) or, e.g., how abnormalities of gut fixation in CDH might be recorded. Although anomalies are currently classified by structural anomaly (e.g., CDH, esophageal atresia) or defined diagnosis (e.g., Down's), it is likely that in the future, anomalies may be classified or at least subgrouped by genotypic differences rather than anatomic details alone. Such distinctions may be

Table 4.1 Birth prevalence of malformations in 2008–2012 grouped by EUROCAT category

Organ system	Live birth + fetal death + termination/10,000 births (to 2 s.f.)
All	260
Congenital heart disease	82
Limb	41
Chromosomal	39
Urinary	34
Nervous system	25
Genital	22
Digestive system	19
Orofacial clefts	14
Abdominal wall defects	6.5
Genetic syndromes + microdeletions	5.0
Respiratory	4.1
Eye	4.2
Ear, face, neck	2.0
Teratogenic syndromes with malformations	1.4

Note: Rates for each category are inclusive of cases with chromosomal lesions and derived from registries with full EUROCAT membership.
Abbreviation: s.f. = significant figures.

prognostically and therapeutically important: e.g., exomphalos in the context of Beckwith–Wiedemann syndrome is associated with the additional hazards of hypoglycemia, macrosomia, and increased tumor risk due to disordered gene imprinting.[32] Hence the anatomic defect (exomphalos) becomes less important than the genetics and its multisystem sequelae. Similarly, it is postulated that subgroups of spina bifida may be folate resistant due to underlying genetic/enzymatic variation.[18,33] The design of preconceptual prophylaxis for birth defects may need to acknowledge pharmacogenomically distinct subgroups to avoid benefits within one subgroup being overlooked due to a surrounding nonresponder cohort.

Having a system of classification is only part of the task. Notification and classification are subject to local variations in practice. When resources exist for expert-mediated classification of birth defects by diagnosis, this approach to birth defect epidemiology appears the best currently available.[34] However, even some North American registries lack clinician input in the classification/assignment of observed birth defects. The impact of this omission on data quality remains to be determined. In the contrasting circumstances of rural China, expert-led assignment of cases has been substituted with simple photographic recording of malformations: this system allows the registry to function but also allows difficult cases to be assigned later after remote assessment of images by experts.[35] In addition, the photographs

Table 4.2 Birth prevalence of malformations of relevance to pediatric surgery (2008–2012) grouped by diagnosis from registries with full EUROCAT membership

Anomaly	Live birth + fetal death + termination/10,000 births
Down's	23
Hypospadias	18
Congenital hydronephrosis	11
Edwards'	5.4
Spina bifida	4.9
Anorectal malformations	3.2
Exomphalos	3.1
Diaphragmatic hernia	2.8
Gastroschisis	2.8
EA/TOF	2.6
Duodenal atresia/stenosis	1.4
Hirschsprung's disease	1.3
Bilateral renal agenesis	1.2
CCAM	1.1
Intestinal atresia/stenosis	0.92
Posterior urethral valves/ prune belly	0.89
Bladder extrophy/epispadias	0.71
Situs inversus	0.68
Indeterminate sex	0.67
Amniotic band	0.51
Biliary atresia	0.31
Conjoined twins	0.18

Note: Rates for each category are inclusive of cases with chromosomal lesions. These are birth prevalences (including fetal death/terminations) and not the prevalences experienced at pediatric surgical units.
Abbreviations: CCAM = congenital cystic adenomatoid malformations, TOF = tracheo-oesophageal fistula.

potentially allow the classifiers to calibrate their judgments against those from other registries.

COUNTING OF BIRTH DEFECTS IS AFFECTED BY THE DEFINITION OF STILLBIRTH

Birth defect epidemiology becomes difficult whenever the classification of defects is not uniform or straightforward. However, an equal challenge remains the counting of birth defects. This task is complicated by practical barriers to case ascertainment (e.g., inadequate resources), the definition of stillbirth, and the effects of prenatal diagnosis and terminations.

Recording of anomaly prevalence lies at the core of birth defect epidemiology. To account for the unknowable incidence of a defect amongst vast numbers of naturally miscarried pregnancies, epidemiologists measure the prevalences of defects within a defined birth cohort: i.e., the number of live and stillborn cases of the defect, as a proportion of all births (live and stillborn). This definition depends on the artificial distinction between miscarriage and stillbirth: EUROCAT's recommendation is that spontaneous pregnancy losses prior to 20 weeks' gestation are counted as miscarriages (and do not contribute to anomaly prevalence), while similar losses at 20 weeks of gestation and beyond are counted as stillbirths (and included in prevalence statistics). Despite these guidelines, several countries have established different demarcations (e.g., 24 or 28 weeks or even 500 g weight). Clearly, some estimate of prenatal birth defects is required to avoid seriously underestimating overall prevalences.[36] However, the demarcation of stillbirths begins to complicate matters. Countries using later gestational cut-offs may underestimate birth defect prevalence compared to registries where 20 weeks is used. Hence, minor changes in convention can lead to large but artificial differences in anomaly prevalence.

While a definition of stillbirths is needed for data collection, the sharp demarcation (whether 20 weeks or later) also appears arbitrary from a biological perspective. Consider, a hypothetical prenatal medical therapy that reduces the prevalence of a specific birth defect. When the anomaly is rare (as most are), it may be difficult to determine whether an observed reduction in prevalence is truly due to fewer malformations or instead due to the promotion of earlier loss of affected pregnancies (i.e., prior to the 20th week or other agreed-upon margin). This latter phenomenon, termed *terathanasia*, has been invoked to explain how folate supplementation might influence the prevalence of neural tube defects.[37]

PRENATAL DIAGNOSIS: THE GREATEST CHALLENGE TO BIRTH DEFECT EPIDEMIOLOGY?

The classification of birth defects and the definition of stillbirth make anomaly surveillance complex. However, the impact of prenatal diagnosis is arguably more important still. Prenatal diagnosis (in particular, nonspecific ultrasound screening) confounds birth defects surveillance in a number of ways:

1. Prenatal diagnosis increases identification of birth defects within the cohort of assessment by diagnosing those who may otherwise have perished prenatally (and were uncounted), or those who may have presented beyond the neonatal period (if at all). Consider prenatal identification of cystic lung lesions. Some would never have been diagnosed (either regressing spontaneously or persisting asymptomatically). Others would have presented later (beyond the scope of the birth defects registry).
2. Prenatal diagnosis alters antenatal management and results in terminations (or fetal intervention), which affects the numbers of birth defects being counted. Most registries try to keep data on terminations for birth

defects, but these data are hard to find when terminations are prohibited by law.

3. Prenatal diagnosis may be inaccurate and unchecked. Pathological verification after termination may be incomplete or absent, yet the presumptive "diagnosis" is included in the birth defect tally.

4. The resources and expertise to perform prenatal sonography vary with location (thereby hampering international comparison of birth defect prevalences).

In summary, the apparently simple task of counting live and stillborn cases for birth defect surveillance is fraught with difficulty once (1) the arbitrary definition of stillbirth is imposed and (2) ubiquitous prenatal imaging prompts both terminations and identification of previously occult "cases."

Given these challenges in data collection, epidemiologists are aided by being able to compare a variety of surveillance databases. Many European registries are incorporated into the EUROCAT initiative. Similarly, several other registries feed into birth defect surveillance data furnished by the World Health Organization (WHO). Their *Birth Defects Atlas* is an interesting publication available in the public domain (http://www.who.int/nutrition/publications /birthdefects_atlas/en/). Most importantly it is instructive to read and consider the caveats that EUROCAT and WHO place upon their data. Their caveats not only highlight the problems discussed in the previous sections but also allude to the ongoing challenge of inadequate resources and expertise for birth defect reporting. This in turn impairs the data accuracy and may help explain insufficient action upon findings. Major studies reinforce the logistical shortcomings of birth defect reporting in the United Kingdom.[38]

PEDIATRIC SURGEONS OFTEN FOCUS ON THEIR INSTITUTIONAL SERIES OF BIRTH DEFECTS

Small institutional series are the staple of pediatric surgeons' reporting. But several studies have shown how institutional series are vulnerable to bias and confounding.[39–41] Indeed, these studies face broader problems than population-based registries. Ascertainment remains a particular issue. For example, prenatal diagnosis, terminations or pretransfer deaths can each foster an impression that the institution is improving its outcomes when, in fact, extramural changes are responsible. Moreover, surgeons try to stratify for disease severity to show that their (good) results are not simply the product of a low-risk caseload (Figure 4.2). But it can be misleading to use the frequency of interventions to stratify for severity in a birth defect cohort. For example, in CDH, the decision to patch and/or use extracorporeal membrane oxygenation (ECMO) and/or nitric oxide may owe more to institutional protocols than differences in pathophysiology between cases.

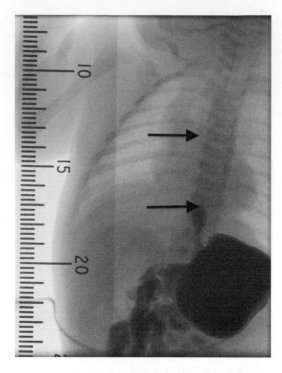

Figure 4.2 Birth defect registries and disease severity. Birth defect registries generally do not distinguish anomaly severity (despite implications for service provision and outcome measures). This gap assessment x-ray for pure esophageal atresia (EA) shows the tip of the oral tube pressed down (upper arrow) and refluxed contrast in the distal pouch (lower arrow). Treated by the author with a single-stage "Bax" jejunal interposition at 7 weeks of age, this anomaly is registered just like the more common EA with distal fistula, despite the very different management and resources required.

A "LIFE-COURSE" APPROACH TO BIRTH DEFECTS

Given the aforementioned caveats, where can pediatric surgery make progress? Advances in prenatal imaging may improve prenatal prognostication and case selection for fetal therapies.[42] But better imaging may also identify more "defects" of questionable significance. To help families balance these developments, pediatric surgeons will need to keep abreast of birth defect epidemiology and to collaborate with other specialties. A larger prize may be realized if pediatric surgery follows epidemiology in widely adopting "life-course" studies to assess the impact over time of correcting birth defects surgically. Embracing a life-course approach means that, like pediatric oncology, further thought and training can be focused on the needs of teenage and young adult (TYA) survivors. Pediatric surgery can also adopt the biopsychosocial model and the creative, problem-solving approach exemplified by, e.g., trauma rehabilitation. These efforts may help the team broach issues well before the hurdles of transitional care. It may also allow such issues to be addressed using the full breadth of nonsurgical, nonpharmacological approaches.

REFERENCES

1. Carmona RH. The global challenges of birth defects and disabilities. *Lancet* 2005; 366(9492): 1142–4.
2. Condon RJ, Bower C. Rubella vaccination and congenital-rubella syndrome in Western-Australia. *Med J Austr* 1993; 158(6): 379–82.
3. Stockley L, Lund V. Use of folic acid supplements, particularly by low-income and young women: A series of systematic reviews to inform public health policy in the UK. *Public Health Nutr* 2008; 11(8): 807–21.
4. Wald N. Prevention of neural-tube defects—Results of the Medical-Research-Council Vitamin Study. *Lancet* 1991; 338(8760): 131–7.
5. Kilby MD. The incidence of gastroschisis—Is increasing in the UK, particularly among babies of young mothers. *Br Med J* 2006; 332(7536): 250–1.
6. Tan KH, Kilby MD, Whittle MJ, Beattie BR, Booth IW, Botting BJ. Congenital anterior abdominal wall defects in England and Wales 1987–93: Retrospective analysis of OPCS data. *Br Med J* 1996; 313(7062): 903–6.
7. Monif GRG, Avery GB, Korones SB, Sever JL. Postmortem isolation of rubella virus from 3 children with rubella-syndrome defects. *Lancet* 1965; 1(7388): 723–4.
8. Taussig HB. Thalidomide and phocomelia. *Pediatrics* 1962; 30(4): 654.
9. Khoury MJ. Epidemiology of birth defects. *Epidemiol Rev* 1989: 244–8.
10. Donnai D, Read AP. How clinicians add to knowledge of development. *Lancet* 2003; 362(9382): 477–84.
11. Hay S, Barbano H. Independent Effects of maternal age and birth-order on incidence of selected congenital malformations. *Teratology* 1972; 6(3): 271.
12. Becerra JE, Khoury MJ, Cordero JF, Erickson JD. Diabetes-mellitus during pregnancy and the risks for specific birth-defects—A population-based case–control study. *Pediatrics* 1990; 85(1): 1–9.
13. Yang Q, Wen SW, Leader A, Chen XK, Lipson J, Walker M. Paternal age and birth defects: How strong is the association? *Hum Reprod* 2007; 22(3): 696–701.
14. Ernhart CB, Sokol RJ, Martier S, Moron P, Nadler D, Ager JW, Wolf A. Alcohol teratogenicity in the human—A detailed assessment of specificity, critical period, and threshold. *Am J Obstet Gynecol* 1987; 156(1): 33–9.
15. Ardinger HH, Atkin JF, Blackston RD, Elsas LJ, Clarren SK, Livingstone S, Flannery DB et al. Verification of the fetal valproate syndrome phenotype. *Am J Med Genet* 1988; 29(1): 171–85.
16. Colborn T, Saal FSV, Soto AM. Developmental effects of endocrine-disrupting chemicals in wildlife and humans. *Environ Health Perspect* 1993; 101(5): 378–84.
17. Hansen M, Kurinczuk JJ, Bower C, Webb S. The risk of major birth defects after intracytoplasmic sperm injection and in vitro fertilization. *N Engl J Med* 2002; 346(10): 725–30.
18. Brody LC, Conley M, Cox C, Kirke PN, McKeever MP, Mills JL, Molloy AM et al. A polymorphism, R653Q, in the trifunctional enzyme methylenetetrahydrofolate dehydrogenase/methenyltetrahydrofolate cyclohydrolase/formyltetrahydrofolate synthetase is a maternal genetic risk factor for neural tube defects: Report of the birth defects research group. *Am J Hum Genet* 2002; 71(5): 1207–15.
19. Leeder JS, Mitchell AA. Application of pharmacogenomic strategies to the study of drug-induced birth defects. *Clin Pharmacol Ther* 2007; 81(4): 595–9.
20. Whitaker SY, Tran HT, Portier CJ. Development of a biologically-based controlled growth and differentiation model for developmental toxicology. *J Math Biol* 2003; 46(1): 1–16.
21. Kim J, Wu HH, Lander AD, Lyons KM, Matzuk MM, Calof AL. GDF11 controls the timing of progenitor cell competence in developing retina. *Science* 2005; 308(5730): 1927–30.
22. Curry JI, McKinney P, Thornton JG, Stringer MD. The aetiology of gastroschisis. *Br J Obstetr Gynaecol* 2000; 107(11): 1339–46.
23. Feldkamp ML, Carey JC, Sadler TW. Development of gastroschisis: Review of hypotheses, a novel hypothesis, and implications for research. *Am J Med Genet A* 2007; 143A(7): 639–52.
24. Byron-Scott R, Haan E, Chan A, Bower C, Scott H, Clark K. A population-based study of abdominal wall defects in South Australia and Western Australia. *Paediatr Perinat Epidemiol* 1998; 12(2): 136–51.
25. Shorter NA, Georges A, Perenyi A, Garrow E. A proposed classification system for familial intestinal atresia and its relevance to the understanding of the etiology of jejunoileal atresia. *J Pediatr Surg* 2006; 41(11): 1822–25.
26. Cheng W, Tam PKH. Murine duodenum does not go through a "solid core" stage in its embryological development. *Eur J Pediatr Surg* 1998; 8(4): 212–5.
27. Meio IB, Siviero I, Ferrante SMR, Carvalho JJ. Morphologic study of embryonic development of rat duodenum through a computerized three-dimensional reconstruction: Critical analysis of solid core theory. *Pediatr Surg Int* 2008; 24(5): 561–5.
28. Koga Y, Hayashida Y, Ikeda K, Inokuchi K, Hashimoto N. Intestinal atresia in fetal dogs produced by localized ligation of mesenteric vessels. *J Pediatr Surg* 1975; 10(6): 949–53.

29. Stiefel D, Meuli M. Scanning electron microscopy of fetal murine myelomeningocele reveals growth and development of the spinal cord in early gestation and neural tissue destruction around birth. *J Pediatr Surg* 2007; 42(9): 1561–5.

30. Jesudason EC. Challenging embryological theories on congenital diaphragmatic hernia: Future therapeutic implications for paediatric surgery. *Ann R Coll Surg Engl* 2002; 84(4): 252–9.

31. Jancelewicz T, Harrison MR. A history of fetal surgery. *Clin Perinatol* 2009; 36(2): 227.

32. Reik W, Walter J. Genomic imprinting: Parental influence on the genome. *Nat Rev Genet* 2001; 2(1): 21–32.

33. Pitkin RM. Folate and neural tube defects. *Am J Clin Nutr* 2007; 85(1): 285S–8S.

34. Lin AE, Forrester MB, Cunniff C, Higgins CA, Anderka M. Clinician reviewers in birth defects surveillance programs: Survey of the National Birth Defects Prevention Network. *Birth Defects Res A Clin Mol Teratol* 2006; 76(11): 781–6.

35. Li S, Moore CA, Li Z, Berry RJ, Gindler J, Hong SX, Liu Y et al. A population-based birth defects surveillance system in the People's Republic of China. *Paediatr Perinat Epidemiol* 2003; 17(3): 287–93.

36. Duke CW, Correa A, Romitti PA, Martin J, Kirby RS. Challenges and priorities for surveillance of stillbirths: A report on two workshops. *Public Health Rep* 2009; 124(5): 652–9.

37. Hook EB, Czeizel AE. Can terathanasia explain the protective effect of folic-acid supplementation on birth defects? *Lancet* 1997; 350(9076): 513–5.

38. Boyd PA, Armstrong B, Dolk H, Botting B, Pattenden S, Abramsky L, Rankin J, Vrijheid M, Wellesley D. Congenital anomaly surveillance in England—Ascertainment deficiencies in the national system. *Br Med J* 2005; 330(7481): 27–29.

39. Mah VK, Zamakhshary M, Mah DY, Cameron B, Bass J, Bohn D, Scott L, Himidan S, Walker M, Kim PC. Absolute vs relative improvements in congenital diaphragmatic hernia survival: What happened to "hidden mortality". *J Pediatr Surg* 2009; 44(5): 877–82.

40. Scott L, Mah D, Cameron B, Grace N, Bass J, Panaeru D, Masiokos P, Bohn D, Wales P, Kim PCW. Apparent truth about congenital diaphragmatic hernia: A population-based database is needed to establish benchmarking for clinical outcomes for CDH. *J Pediatr Surg* 2004; 39(5): 661–5.

41. Harrison MR, Bjordal RI, Langmark F, Knutrud O. Congenital diaphragmatic hernia—Hidden mortality. *J Pediatr Surg* 1978; 13(3): 227–30.

42. Joe BN, Vahidi K, Zektzer A, Chen MH, Clifton MS, Butler T, Keshari K, Kurhanewicz J, Coakley F, Swanson MG. H-1 HR-MAS spectroscopy for quantitative measurement of choline concentration in amniotic fluid as a marker of fetal lung maturity: Inter-and intraobserver reproducibility study. *J Magn Reson Imaging* 2008; 28(6): 1540–5.

5

Prenatal diagnosis of surgical conditions

N. SCOTT ADZICK

INTRODUCTION

Prenatal diagnosis has undergone an explosion of growth in the past two decades. The primary impetus for this rapid expansion has come from the widespread use of prenatal ultrasonography. Most correctable malformations that can be diagnosed in utero are best managed by appropriate medical and surgical therapy after maternal transport and planned delivery at term. Prenatal diagnosis may influence the timing (Table 5.1) or the mode (Table 5.2) of delivery, and in some cases, may lead to elective termination of the pregnancy. In rare cases, various forms of in utero therapy may be possible (Table 5.3).

Prenatal diagnosis has defined a "hidden mortality" for some lesions such as congenital diaphragmatic hernia (CDH), bilateral hydronephrosis (HN), sacrococcygeal teratoma (SCT), and cystic hygroma. These lesions, when first evaluated and treated postnatally, demonstrate a favorable selection bias. The most severely affected fetuses often die in utero or immediately after birth, before an accurate diagnosis has been made. Consequently, such a condition detected prenatally may have a worse prognosis than the same condition diagnosed after delivery.[1] Multidisciplinary care and nondirective counseling are the crux of appropriate prenatal management of most congenital anomalies. The perinatal management of the patients involves many different medical disciplines, including obstetricians, sonographers, neonatologists, geneticists, pediatric surgeons, and pediatricians. It is essential that the affected family be managed using a team approach, and that information and experience be exchanged freely.

In this chapter, we will discuss the prenatal diagnosis of neonatal surgical conditions. First, a brief summary of the diagnostic methods currently available will be given. Then a review of prenatal diagnosis by organ system will be presented.

ULTRASOUND

Ultrasound testing has become a routine part of the prenatal evaluation of almost all pregnancies. It is especially important to perform ultrasound for pregnancies with maternal risk factors (e.g., age over 35 years, diabetes, previous child with anatomic or chromosomal abnormality) and if there is an elevation in maternal serum alphafetoprotein (MSAFP). Most defects can be reliably diagnosed in the late first or early second trimester by a skilled sonographer. Early in gestation, nuchal translucency measurements are an independent marker of chromosomal abnormalities, with a sensitivity of about 60%.[2] This abnormality may be detected on transvaginal ultrasound at 10–15 weeks gestation, thus providing an early test for high-risk pregnancies. Nuchal cord thickening may also be a marker for congenital heart disease[3] and may be a valuable initial screen to detect high-risk fetuses for referral for fetal echocardiography. It is important to remember that sonography is operator-dependent; the scope and reliability of the information obtained are directly proportional to the skill and experience of the sonographer.

MAGNETIC RESONANCE IMAGING

Until recently, the long acquisition times required for magnetic resonance imaging (MRI) were not conducive to fetal imaging because fetal movements resulted in poor quality images. Obtaining adequate images with the traditional spin-echo techniques required fetal sedation or paralysis.[4] With the development of ultrafast scanning techniques, the artifacts caused by fetal motion have almost been eliminated.[5] While fetal MRI is most commonly used to evaluate the fetal central nervous system, the ability to obtain cross-sectional imaging has made this tool a crucial adjunct to ultrasound for many pediatric surgical diseases, including

Table 5.1 Defects that may lead to induced preterm delivery

Obstructive HN
Gastroschisis or ruptured omphalocele
Intestinal ischemia and necrosis secondary to volvulus, meconium ileus, etc.
SCT with hydrops

Table 5.2 Defects that may require caesarian delivery

MMC
Giant omphalocele
Large SCT
Giant neck masses or lung lesions (EXIT procedure)

measurement of lung sizes in CDH and evaluation of airway anatomy in neck masses. This technique is now an important part of prenatal evaluation of fetuses referred to our institution and has greatly enhanced our ability to diagnose and treat fetal malformations.

AMNIOCENTESIS

The first report of the culture and karyotyping of fetal cells from amniocentesis was by Steele and Berg[6] in 1966. Since then, it has become the gold standard for detecting fetal chromosomal abnormalities by karyotyping. It is usually performed at 15–16 weeks gestation and involves a very low risk of fetal injury or loss. Attempts at early amniocentesis (11–12 weeks gestation) have been complicated by a higher pregnancy loss, increased risk of iatrogenic fetal deformities, and increased post-amniocentesis leakage rate.[7] For this reason, the most reliable method for first trimester diagnosis remains chorionic villus sampling (CVS). In addition to screening for the most common chromosomal abnormalities using karyotyping, modern sequence analysis and microarrays have revolutionized our ability to detect small deletions or duplications that are not apparent with karyotyping.[8]

CHORIONIC VILLUS SAMPLING

CVS may be performed at 10–14 weeks gestation and involves the biopsy of the chorion frondosum, the precursor for the placenta. Either a transcervical or transabdominal approach may be used, both under ultrasound guidance. The cells obtained may be subjected to a variety of tests including karyotype, microarray, or enzymatic activity. Due to the high mitotic rate of the chorionic villus cells, results for karyotyping may be obtained in less than 24 hours. Disadvantages include diagnostic errors due to maternal decidual contamination or genetic mosaicism of the trophoblastic layer of the placenta. When performed by experienced operators, the pregnancy loss rate is equivalent to second trimester amniocentesis.[8]

BIOCHEMICAL MARKERS

Maternal blood and amniotic fluid can be screened for the presence of various biochemical markers that indicate fetal disease. About two-thirds of women in the United States currently undergo screening for Down's syndrome and other chromosomal abnormalities with the "triple test," which includes measuring serum alpha-fetoprotein with human chorionic gonadotropin and unconjugated estriol.[9] This screening is performed in the early second trimester, and the detection rate for Down's is 69%, with a 5% false positive test.[10] A positive result on the serum screening test indicates a need for chromosome analysis by amniocentesis.

PERCUTANEOUS UMBILICAL BLOOD SAMPLING

Umbilical venous blood can also be used to determine the karyotype and diagnose various metabolic and hematological disorders. The procedure for obtaining it is performed at around 18 weeks gestation under ultrasound guidance. Karyotype results may be obtained within 24–48 hours. In various large series, the mortality from the procedure has been reported to be 1%–2%, with increasing mortality with long procedure times and multiple punctures.[11–13]

FETAL CELLS IN THE MATERNAL CIRCULATION

Since the advent of fluorescence-activated cell sorting, there has been growing interest and progress in detecting circulating fetal cells or cell-free nucleic acids in maternal blood

Table 5.3 Diseases amenable to fetal surgical intervention in selected cases

Malformation	Effect on development	In utero treatment
Congenital diaphragmatic hernia	Pulmonary hypoplasia, pulmonary hypertension	Tracheal occlusion and release
CCAM or BPS	Pulmonary hypoplasia, hydrops	Thoracoamniotic shunting, lobectomy, maternal steroids
SCT	Massive arteriovenous shunting, placentomegaly, hydrops	Excision
Urethral obstruction	HN, renal dysplasia, lung hypoplasia	V-A shunting, laser ablation of PUV
MMC	Damage to spinal cord, paralysis	Closure of defect

for diagnostic purposes.[14] While the number of intact cells in the circulation is limited, amplification of fetal cell–free nucleic acids using real-time PCR has growing utility in early prenatal diagnosis.[15] Fetal DNA can be detected reliably by 9 weeks and increases with gestational age.[16] This method can be used for gender determination in the first trimester (if Y chromosome sequences are found, the fetus is male and if not, assumed to be female) and can thus be helpful in counseling for X-linked disorders. Rhesus factor determinations are also accurate and can avoid unnecessary treatment of an Rh negative mother if the fetus is also negative. In the future, it may be expanded to detecting paternally inherited single gene mutations. Noninvasive prenatal testing is becoming the routine screening test for prenatal diagnosis of aneuploidies.

PRENATAL DIAGNOSIS OF SPECIFIC SURGICAL LESIONS

Neck masses

Prenatal diagnosis and surgical management can be life-saving for fetuses with airway obstruction. Fetal airway obstruction could be a result of extrinsic compression of the airway by lesions such as cervical teratoma or cystic hygroma, or intrinsic defects in the airway such as congenital high airway obstruction syndrome (CHAOS). Although large congenital neck masses causing airway obstruction previously carried an enormous perinatal mortality,[17] the advent of the ex utero intrapartum treatment (EXIT) procedure[18,19] has improved their outcome by providing a means of controlling the airway during delivery and converting an airway emergency into an elective procedure (Figure 5.1).

Cystic hygroma diagnosed in utero is a severe diffuse lymphatic abnormality, which is frequently associated with hydrops, polyhydramnios, and other abnormalities.[20] Chromosomal abnormalities are very common (62%

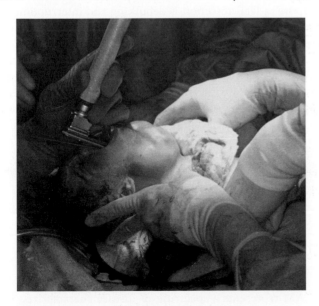

Figure 5.1 EXIT procedure for giant neck mass.

overall), with the most common being Turner's syndrome.[21] There are two groups of prenatally diagnosed cervical lymphangiomas: those diagnosed in the second trimester are usually in the posterior triangle of the neck, have a high incidence of associated abnormalities, and carry a very poor prognosis.[22] Those diagnosed later in gestation are most often isolated lesions and generally do not lead to hydrops. Hydrops is an ominous finding in fetuses with cystic hygroma,[17] as is the presence of aneuploidy and septations in the mass.[23] However, fetuses with normal karyotype, nonseptated masses, and no evidence of hydrops may have a good prognosis.[24] Therefore, it is important to monitor the fetus for development of hydrops by serial evaluations.

Teratomas are asymmetrical lesions that are frequently unilateral, with well-defined margins. They may also be multiloculated, irregular masses with solid and cystic components. Most teratomas contain calcifications. Some fetuses with huge cervical teratomas may also have severe pulmonary hypoplasia with its attendant morbidities, and this possibility should be addressed during prenatal counseling.[25] MRI is a very useful adjunct to ultrasound in evaluating giant neck masses. We have used it successfully for showing the relationship of the mass to the airway in preparation for the EXIT procedure.[26] T1 weighted images may help differentiate teratomas from lymphangiomas.[27]

The EXIT procedure, originally designed for removal of tracheal clips in patients with CDH,[18] has proven lifesaving for many fetuses with giant neck masses.[19,28,29] This procedure involves performing a maternal hysterotomy using the uterine stapling device and obtaining control of the fetal airway while the fetus remains on placental support. In order to prevent uterine contractions during the procedure, the mother is given inhalational anesthetic and tocolytics, warm saline is infused through a level I device, and only the head and shoulders of the fetus are delivered. After attaching a pulse oximeter to the fetal hand to monitor heart rate and oxygen saturation, direct laryngoscopy and, if possible, endotracheal intubation are performed. If the airway cannot be secured in this way, a rigid bronchoscope is inserted to determine the anatomy. If secure airway establishment is still unsuccessful, a tracheostomy can be performed. After securing the airway, surfactant is administered for premature fetuses, the cord is clamped, and the infant is taken to an adjacent operating room for resuscitation and possible immediate resection of the mass. In our most recent review of the EXIT procedure,[28] establishment of a reliable airway was highly successful.

The EXIT procedure has also been useful in the perinatal resuscitation of fetuses with a range of anomalies expected to cause hemodynamic compromise at birth, such as giant lung masses (EXIT to congenital cystic adenomatoid malformation [CCAM] resection),[30] CHAOS,[31] severe congenital heart disease with CDH (EXIT to extracorporeal membrane oxygenation [ECMO]),[32] and even thoracopagus conjoined twins with a single functioning heart.[33] The most critical component of the EXIT procedure is deep inhalational anesthesia, which maximizes uteroplacental blood flow to avoid fetal hypoxia. It is therefore different from a Cesarean section and carries the risk of significant maternal blood loss if there is not careful coordination between the surgical and anesthetic teams.[34]

SACROCOCCYGEAL TERATOMA

SCT is the most common newborn tumor, occurring in 1/35,000 to 40,000 of births.[35] The AAPSS classification[36] defines four types with differing prognoses: Type 1 tumors are external, with at most a small presacral component, and carry the best prognosis. Type 2 tumors are predominantly external with a large intrapelvic portion. Type 3 lesions are predominantly intrapelvic with abdominal extension with only a minor external component. Type 4 lesions are entirely intrapelvic and abdominal. The latter have the worst prognosis since they are difficult to diagnose, sometimes less amenable to surgical resection, and frequently malignant at the time of diagnosis because of the delay in diagnosis. Overall, prenatally diagnosed SCT has a worse prognosis than those diagnosed at time of birth.

On prenatal ultrasound, SCT appears as a mixed solid and cystic lesion arising from the sacrum. The tumor frequently contains calcifications. Since there is acoustic shadowing by the fetal pelvic bones, it is not always possible to determine the most cephalad portion of the tumor by ultrasound. Ultrafast fetal MRI may determine the intrapelvic dimensions of the tumor, spinal canal involvement, and the presence of hemorrhage (Figure 5.2).[37,38] Those fetuses with mainly solid and highly vascular SCT have a higher risk of developing hydrops.[39,40] High output cardiac failure is the result of the hemodynamic effects of the large blood flow to the tumor,[41,42] and anemia from hemorrhage into the tumor may compound this problem. In severe cases, the mother with placentomegaly develops "mirror syndrome," a severe preeclamptic state with vomiting, hypertension, proteinuria, and edema. This phenomenon may be mediated by the release of vasoactive compounds from the edematous placenta. As with other fetal masses, the development of hydrops is a grave sign, with almost 100% mortality without fetal intervention.[43,44]

The prediction of which fetuses with SCT are at highest risk for developing hydrops is therefore the crucial issue in prenatal management. A thorough prenatal evaluation with US, MRI, and fetal echocardiography is important in defining such a group. In a series of 23 cases seen at Children's Hospital of Philadelphia (CHOP) between 2003 and 2006,[45] we observed that rapid tumor growth (>150 cm³/week) identifies a group of fetuses with a higher risk of prenatal mortality. The combined cardiac output correlates with tumor growth, with those fetuses >600 mL/kg/min portending a higher risk of complications. The solid component of the mass is an important prognostic indicator—when the solid tumor volume is normalized to the head volume, fetuses with a ratio <1 all survive, whereas those with a volume >1 have 61% mortality.[46] A similar classification scheme based on size, growth, and vascularity has also been reported.[47]

Prenatal interventions for SCT include cyst aspiration (for those with a dominant cystic component), amnioreduction (for those with severe, symptomatic polyhydramnios with an AFI >35), amnioinfusion (for those with bladder outlet obstruction, to facilitate placement of a vesioamniotic shunt), or open fetal surgery for resection of the mass. The latter option should only be considered for fetuses with impending high-output failure, rapid growth, type I lesion amenable to resection, and gestational age between 20 and 30 weeks. Since our initial report of the first successful case of fetal SCT resection in 1997,[48] we have had seven additional cases, with five survivors.[49] It is important to note that the purpose of fetal resection is debulking and interruption of the "vascular steal," and a complete resection is performed postnatally. Minimally invasive prenatal interventions such as laser vessel ablation, radiofrequency ablation, and alcohol sclerosis have been reported for the management of hydropic fetuses with virtually no success, and thus these approaches should be abandoned.[50] For fetuses older than 28 weeks and impending hydrops, emergent delivery with immediate postnatal resection should be considered. The combined perinatal mortality from both of our published series is 43% (19/44) excluding terminations,[45] illustrating the severity of this disease.

CONGENITAL CHEST LESIONS

CCAM and bronchopulmonary sequestration

CCAM represents a spectrum of disease characterized by cystic lesions of the lung.[51] Macrocystic lesions are larger

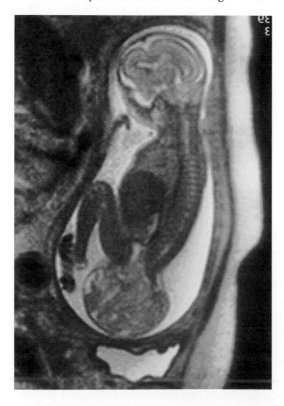

Figure 5.2 MRI of a large SCT.

than 5 mm in diameter and may be solitary cysts that grow to several centimeters (Figure 5.3). Microcystic disease has multiple cystic lesions less than 5 mm in diameter. Prenatal ultrasound can generally distinguish individual cysts in macrocystic disease, while microcystic lesions usually have the appearance of an echogenic, solid lung mass.[52] Bronchopulmonary sequestration (BPS) is an aberrant lung mass that is nonfunctional and usually has a systemic blood supply. The two lesions may be related embryologically, with many reported cases of hybrid lesions that have CCAM-like architecture and a systemic blood supply.[53,54] Some of these lesions may decrease in size during fetal life,[55] but postnatal evaluation is still warranted to detect residual disease for resection[56] because of the risk of pulmonary infections and the development of tumors such as pleuropulmonary blastoma.

MRI is useful in delineating normal lung from abnormal.[57] In CCAM, the number and size of cysts contribute to the signal intensity on T2-weighted images.[5] MRI can also define BPS from surrounding lung due to its high signal intensity and homogeneous appearance.[57] Ultrasound with color flow Doppler is more accurate in demonstrating systemic feeding vessels. MRI may also be helpful in making the correct diagnosis in cases where ultrasound is ambiguous. In a series of 18 lung lesions that were viewed with both ultrasound and MRI, multiple chest abnormalities were misdiagnosed as CCAM on the ultrasound, including CDH, tracheal atresia, pulmonary agenesis, neurenteric cyst, bronchial stenosis, and BPS.[57] MRI helped establish the correct diagnosis in these cases and was thus crucial for perinatal management.

Polyhydramnios is a frequent accompanying finding in fetuses with large chest masses. This is likely due to esophageal compression caused by the large thoracic mass, decreasing the fetal ability to swallow amniotic fluid.[58] The most important prognostic indicator in fetuses with CCAM is the development of hydrops. Hydrops is secondary to obstruction of the vena cava or cardiac compression from extreme mediastinal shift.[59] Historically, the development

of hydrops has indicated a grave prognosis with 100% mortality,[58] and it is important to predict which fetuses are at high risk for this complication. The volume of the CCAM compared to the head circumference (CCAM volume ratio [CVR]) is an important prognostic indicator: fetuses with a CVR greater than 1.6 are more likely to develop hydrops.[60] It is also important to recognize that there is an expected period of lesion growth during the second trimester, after which the mass usually gets smaller with respect to the fetus. Therefore, CVR should be measured at multiple consecutive visits. Fetuses with extralobar BPS can also develop pleural effusions.

For fetuses with large macrocystic CCAMs with a dominant cyst, or large pleural effusion causing pulmonary hypoplasia, thoracoamniotic shunting may be lifesaving: In our series of 19 high-risk fetuses who underwent prenatal shunt placement,[61] survival was 67% (6/9) in the pleural effusion group and 70% (7/10) for the CCAM group, with an average age of delivery at 33+ weeks. However, we have reported an increased risk of chest wall anomalies if shunts are placed prior to 20 weeks gestation.[62]

Fetuses with large microcystic CCAMs (thus not amenable for shunting) and signs of hydrops are more problematic. After 32 weeks gestation, delivery with immediate resection is the optimum management. In fact, given the high risk of perinatal circulatory collapse secondary to mediastinal shift and inability to ventilate, we currently perform an EXIT procedure with resection of the mass on placental support.[30] EXIT to ECMO strategy for severe masses has also been described.[63] For those fetuses <32 weeks with hydrops, open fetal surgery with thoracotomy and resection of the mass may be offered at select centers. At CHOP, we have performed 27 cases of in utero resection of fetal lung lesions for hydrops between 21 and 31 weeks gestation.[52] There were 18 healthy survivors, all of whom at resolution of hydrops at 1–2 weeks after the operation. Nine fetuses had in utero demise, with six intraoperative deaths. Intraoperative hemodynamic compromise secondary to acute changes in cardiac output upon delivery of the mass has led us to adopt a method of continuous intraoperative cardiac monitoring, with volume resuscitation of the fetus and administration of atropine prior to thoracotomy.[64] Grethel et al.[65] have reported a similar experience at University of California, San Francisco (UCSF), in which open resection of the mass in fetuses with hydrops led to the survival of 15 of 30 fetuses. While minimally invasive methods such as intrathoracic YAG laser therapy have been described,[66] technical limitations leading to damage to adjacent normal lung and ribs should prohibit offering such treatments until proven in animal models.

The recognition that maternal administration of steroids can reverse hydrops has been an exciting new development in the antenatal management of CCAM, with survival of all three hydropic fetuses in the initial report.[67] The experience at CHOP has also been favorable[68]: 11 fetuses (10 microcystic, 1 macrocystic) were given maternal betamethasone, with survival of all 5 hydropic fetuses and all 7 fetuses with CVR > 1.6 (compared to a mortality of 100% and 56%,

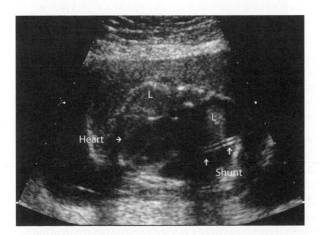

Figure 5.3 Ultrasound image of large CCAM following the placement of a thoracoamniotic shunt. L = lung.

respectively, in historical controls). Only one patient still needed fetal intervention, while one needed resection on EXIT due to the large size of the mass; the remaining nine fetuses underwent vaginal delivery with postnatal resection without complication. The salutary effects of steroids cannot simply be ascribed to reductions in the size or rate of growth of the CCAM as there was variable growth in these patients and a natural growth plateau is well described.[56,69-71] Further studies into the basic biology of CCAM to understand how steroids may influence alveolar maturation or hydrops are areas of active research interests in several laboratories. Our current algorithm for the management of hydropic fetuses with microcystic CCAM prior to 32 weeks is to administer steroids with close observation and open lobectomy if hydrops fails to resolve.

Congenital diaphragmatic hernia

Herniation of abdominal viscera into the chest in utero occurs most commonly due to failure of the pleuroperitoneal folds to fuse normally. The left side is affected five times more commonly than the right. The ultrasonographic diagnostic criteria include herniated abdominal viscera, abnormal upper abdominal anatomy, mediastinal shift away from the side of herniation, and, in severe cases, polyhydramnios. The extent of pulmonary hypoplasia is proportional to the timing of herniation, the size of the diaphragmatic defect, and the amount of viscera herniated. Despite earlier impressions that CDH was infrequently associated with other serious congenital lung lesions, recent reports state that other major anomalies occur in 10%–50% of cases, including a high proportion of chromosomal abnormalities and cardiac anomalies.

The presence of abdominal contents intrathoracically on a transverse sonographic scan at the level of a four-chamber view of the heart is required for diagnosis. In the case of a right-sided defect, the presence of liver and especially gallbladder in the chest makes the diagnosis more clear-cut. MRI is superior in defining the position of the liver in CDH (above or below the diaphragm), which carries important prognostic significance (Figure 5.4).[72,73] Since the extent of pulmonary hypoplasia is an important prognostic indicator, MRI has the potential to become a very useful tool for more accurate measurement of hypoplastic and contralateral lung volumes as well as the extent of liver herniation.[74-76]

The best predictor of outcome in left CDH has been the right lung to head circumference ratio (LHR), defined as right lung area (measured at the level of the transverse four-chamber cardiac view) divided by head circumference (Figure 5.5).[77] The utility of LHR in predicting survival has been validated prospectively[78] and in a multicenter trial.[79] The position of the liver is an independent prognostic indicator. For example, in our experience, fetuses who have an intrathoracic liver ("liver up") need ECMO more frequently than those with the liver down (80% vs. 25%) and have a higher mortality (45% vs. 93%).[80] Given the age-related changes in normal lung area compared to

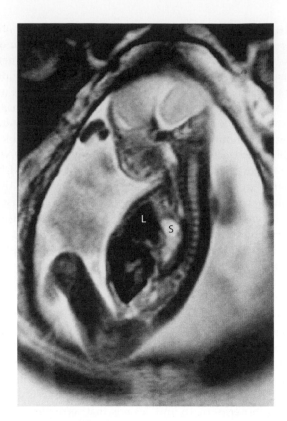

Figure 5.4 MRI of a CDH showing liver (L) and stomach (S) in the chest.

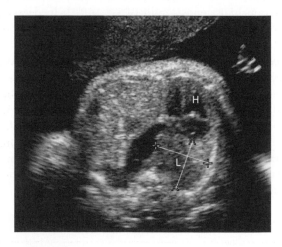

Figure 5.5 Ultrasound of CDH at the level of the transverse four-chamber view of the heart (H) showing measurements used for LHR calculation on the right lung (L).

head circumference through gestation, another commonly used approach is to normalize the LHR to the expected mean LHR for that gestational age, thus obtaining an "observed to expected" (O:E) ratio. CDH fetuses with an LHR O:E <25% have survival of 15%, whereas those with an LHR O:E of >45% have an excellent survival.[81] Right-sided CDH has a higher rate of prenatal complications such as polyhydramnios, premature rupture of membranes, and preterm labor.[82]

The realization that infants with severe CDH succumb to pulmonary hypertension (more so than pulmonary hypoplasia) has fueled interest in measuring prenatal surrogates of this parameter to guide counseling and management. Fetal echocardiography may be used to measure pulmonary artery diameter,[83,84] peak early diastolic reversed flow velocity,[85] as well as pulmonary artery reactivity to maternal hyperoxygenation.[86]

The strategy for in utero treatment of CDH has undergone many permutations in the last two decades, with the current approach involving tracheal occlusion using a percutaneous, fetoscopically placed balloon (FETO) and subsequent reversal of occlusion prior to delivery (reviewed in Refs. 87 and 88). The basis for this approach is the recognition that fetal tracheal occlusion leads to compensatory lung growth due to decrease in lung liquid egress, as confirmed in lamb models of CDH.[89] Given the embryology of lung growth, occlusion earlier in gestation, prior to the pseudoglandular stage of lung development, may lead to more reliable lung growth. The outcome in fetuses after tracheal occlusion has been favorable in both the lamb model[90] and in initial clinical reports.[91,92] Although a subsequent randomized clinical trial comparing prenatal tracheal occlusion (using a clip or balloon, but without reversal) did not show a treatment benefit,[93] this may have been secondary to a generous inclusion criterion (LHR < 1.4) as well as preterm labor—still the Achilles' heel of fetal surgery. Furthermore, reversal of occlusion may confer more benefit. The European experience with fetal occlusion and reversal has been quite favorable. Jani et al.[94] reported on 24 fetuses (LHR <1, liver up) that underwent FETO between 26 and 28 weeks, with 12 undergoing reversal at 34 weeks and 12 undergoing delivery via EXIT. Survival to discharge was 50% overall (83% in the in utero reversal group; 33% in the EXIT group) compared to 9% in historical controls with the same disease severity. The mean gestational age at delivery was 33.5 weeks, although preterm premature rupture of membranes (PPROM) was still seen in 17% of patients at 28 weeks and 33% at 32 weeks. A prospective randomized trial (the TOTAL trial) is in process in Europe.

GASTROINTESTINAL LESIONS

Esophageal and bowel atresias

Esophageal atresia is typically diagnosed on prenatal ultrasound by the presence of a small or absent stomach bubble and polyhydramnios, but no ultrasound finding is sensitive or specific for esophageal atresia.[95] Esophageal atresia is associated with anatomic and chromosomal abnormalities in 63% of cases,[96] most notably trisomy 18 and VACTERL (vertebral anomalies, anal atresia, cardiac anomalies, tracheoesophageal fistula, renal agenesis, and limb defects). Duodenal atresia has a characteristic "double bubble" appearance on prenatal ultrasound, resulting from dilatation of the stomach and proximal duodenum. The incidence of associated malformations is high (57% in one recent series[97]—classically with Down's syndrome and endocardial cushion defects), and those who are prenatally diagnosed are more likely to have associated anomalies.[97] In a recent review of all small intestinal atresias, Hemming and Rankin[98] reported that 25% have chromosomal anomalies and 25% have other structural anomalies.

There are many bowel abnormalities that may be noted on prenatal ultrasound (dilated bowel, ascites, cystic masses, hyperperistalsis, polyhydramnios); however, none is absolutely predictive of postnatal outcome. Patients with obstruction frequently have findings of increased bowel diameter (especially in the third trimester), hyperperistalsis, or polyhydramnios, but ultrasound is much less sensitive in diagnosing large bowel anomalies than those in small bowel.[99] Since the large bowel is mostly a reservoir, with no physiologic function in utero, defects in this region such as anal atresia or Hirschsprung's disease are difficult to detect, although low MSAFP may be a marker for anal atresia.[100] Small bowel obstruction may be associated with cystic fibrosis; therefore, all such fetuses should undergo perinatal evaluation for this disease.[99]

ABDOMINAL WALL DEFECTS

Omphalocele is thought to be secondary to failure of the abdominal viscera to return to the abdomen in the 10th week of gestation.[101] It characteristically has a viable sac composed of amnion and peritoneum containing herniated abdominal contents. The defect is in the midline, usually near the insertion point of the umbilical cord. Ultrasound may demonstrate the internal viscera and sometimes the liver within the sac. Ascites may also be present. Since chromosomal and structural abnormalities are very common in omphalocele (cardiac and renal anomalies, chromosomal anomalies including Beckwith–Wiedemann syndromes and Pentalogy of Cantrell), fetuses with this defect should be screened by karyotype in addition to a detailed sonographic review and echocardiogram.[102] Omphalocele is rarely seen as part of the OEIS sequence (omphalocele, exstrophy of the bladder, imperforate anus, and spinal anomalies),[103] requiring multiple operations with considerable morbidity. Patients with giant omphaloceles (containing predominantly liver, with a defect >5 cm) can have a prolonged course with high long-term morbidity, especially with respiratory and feeding difficulties.[104]

Gastroschisis is more often an isolated lesion with a right para-umbilical defect.[102] There is no membrane covering the exposed bowel. On ultrasound, the bowel appears free-floating, and the loops may appear thickened due to peel formation from exposure to amniotic fluid (Figure 5.6). Dilated loops of bowel may be seen from obstruction secondary to protrusion from a small defect or from the presence of an atresia, seen in 8–10% in most series. The pathophysiology of bowel damage is likely due to amniotic fluid exposure and bowel constriction, the latter leading to ischemia and venous obstruction.[105,106] There is a rate of third trimester fetal demise in about

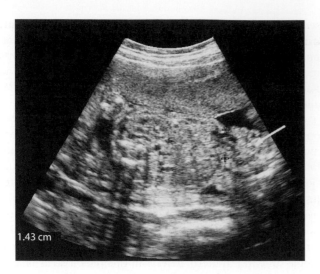

Figure 5.6 Ultrasound of a fetus with gastroschisis with crossmarks showing the abdominal wall defect and arrow indicating extra-abdominal bowel.

5%,[107] highlighting the need for careful, serial monitoring once the diagnosis is made. Many infants have intrauterine growth retardation: 70% are below the 50th percentile at birth (this number may be overestimated on prenatal measurements, since the abdominal cavity is small because of the defect).[102]

Predicting outcome in fetuses with gastroschisis based on prenatal ultrasound findings remains a challenge. Analysis of infants with gastroschisis has led to the definition of two groups of patients: simple (isolated gastroschisis, very low mortality) vs. complex (those who also have bowel atresias, perforation, volvulus, or bowel necrosis and a higher mortality [28% in Ref. 108; 8.7% in Ref. 109]). It is therefore crucial to develop prenatal diagnostic criteria for prediction of postnatal outcome. In addition, the timing of delivery has been an unanswered question: the urgency to prevent in utero bowel damage must be tempered with the risks of prematurity in these infants, many of whom are small for gestational age. Both ultrasound and biochemical characteristics have been examined to address this issue. Examination of amniotic fluid for markers of fetal distress such as meconium[110] and β-endorphin[111] may carry prognostic significance but is not currently used in clinical practice. Ultrasound characteristics such as bowel dilatation, bowel wall thickening, and mesenteric flow have been studied by many groups as possible prognostic indicators. We recently reviewed our experience with 64 cases of gastroschisis seen at CHOP between 2000 and 2007[112]; 53 were simple and 11 were complex (17%). There were three in utero mortalities (two fetal demises and one termination) with an overall perinatal mortality of 9%. Interestingly, prenatal ultrasound findings were not predictive of the postnatal course for any of the parameters examined (simple vs. complex, primary vs. silo, hospital length, time to enteral feedings, etc.).

The question of whether Caesarian section delivery would protect the exposed bowel from further damage during delivery has been considered but does not appear to confer any outcome benefit.[113,114] Thus, the mode of delivery for abdominal wall defects can be vaginal except in cases of giant omphalocele, in whom the risk of liver rupture and dystocia mandates a Caesarian section. The issue of whether transport prior to delivery impacts outcome (secondary to ongoing ischemia and damage to the exposed intestines during transport) has also been studied and, interestingly, did not appear to make a difference in one series.[115] Our current strategy for management is serial ultrasounds to monitor for signs of fetal distress, with planned delivery at term and either primary or silo closure.

PRENATAL DIAGNOSIS OF RENAL ANOMALIES

Prenatally diagnosed HN represents a broad spectrum of diseases with widely disparate prognoses (reviewed in Ref. 116). The ultrasound findings of HN include dilated renal pelvis and calyces, with or without dilatation of the bladder and ureter, depending on the cause of HN (Figure 5.7). The Society for Fetal Urology defines four grades with increasing severity, with grade 1 being split pelvis only and grade 4 being dilated pelvis with distended calyces and thinned parenchyma.[117] In addition, an anterior–posterior diameter >10 mm has been suggested as being predictive of fetuses who will need some postnatal intervention.[118] The differential diagnosis of prenatal HN includes ureteropelvic junction (UPJ) obstruction, multicystic kidney, primary obstructive megaureter, ureterocele, ectopic ureter, and posterior urethral valves (PUV).[119] Severe, bilateral HN leads to oligohydramnios with a fetus small for gestational age. Because of the lack of amniotic fluid, ultrasound diagnosis may be difficult and MRI may help define the cause of HN.[5]

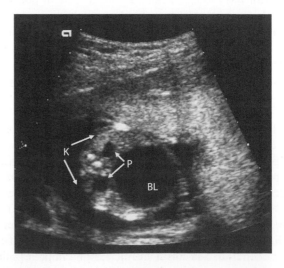

Figure 5.7 Ultrasound of HN showing enlarged bladder (BL), compressed renal parenchyma (K), and dilated renal pelvises (P).

UPPER URINARY TRACT OBSTRUCTION

The most common cause of prenatal HN is UPJ obstruction. The prognosis of prenatally diagnosed HN is excellent, if there is unilateral disease[120] and if the renal pelvic diameter is less than 10 mm.[121] In one large series, 80% were normal at 3 years and 17% were normal at birth, suggesting spontaneous resolution of the problem.[122] Only 17% needed surgical intervention. Prenatally diagnosed HN requires follow-up with ultrasound at birth and at 1 month. If there is any evidence of abnormality, a voiding cystourethrogram and diuretic renal scintigram should be performed.[123]

LOWER URINARY TRACT OBSTRUCTION

The most common cause of lower urinary tract obstruction (LUTO) is PUV; it is also seen in prune belly syndrome and urethral atresia.[124] The most important factor in the morbidity and mortality from fetal urethral obstruction is pulmonary hypoplasia secondary to oligohydramnios.[125] For patients with PUV, prenatal diagnosis defines a subgroup of patients with very poor prognosis, with 64% incidence of renal failure and transient pulmonary failure, compared to 33% in the postnatally diagnosed group.[126] Serial fetal urine analysis may provide prognostic information in this group of fetuses. Drainage of the bladder three times at 48–72 hour intervals with measurement of sodium, chloride, osmolality, calcium, β-2 microglobulin, and total protein should be performed to determine renal function. In this strategy, the later taps indicate the characteristics of recently produced urine, and a decrease in the electrolytes, proteins, and tonicity correlates with a favorable outcome.[124]

The rationale for prenatal intervention originates from sheep models of the disease, in which bladder outlet obstruction in fetal lambs reproduced the pulmonary hypoplasia and renal dysplasia seen in patients with bilateral obstructive uropathy.[127] Correction of the obstruction led to normal lung growth.[128] Fetal intervention in prenatal obstructive uropathy is only warranted in male fetuses with oligohydramnios, bladder distention, and bilateral HN (with no other abnormalities), who have improving urine profiles with serial bladder drainage.[129] In female fetuses, LUTO is generally part of a complex cloacal anomaly, and fetal intervention has not been beneficial. Male fetuses may be considered for vesicoamniotic (V-A) shunting,[130] and fetal microcystoscopy and mechanical valve disruption have been reported.[131]

Although V-A shunting in a fetus with oligohydramnios can be technically challenging, the survival benefit of prenatal shunting in carefully selected populations of fetuses has been reported, with 43% of patients having normal renal function 2 years after birth.[132] We reported our series of 18 patients who had V-A shunts for PUV (7), prune belly syndrome (7), and urethral atresia (4).[133] Eight patients have good renal function, four have mild renal insufficiency, and six required hemodialysis with subsequent transplantation. Respiratory problems and frequent urinary tract infections were seen in eight and nine patients, respectively. While short-term outcomes are variable in different reports,[120] a recent meta-analysis[134] determined that in utero drainage improved survival compared to postnatal management alone in the group of fetuses with poor prognosis. Patients who have been shunted can still die from pulmonary hypoplasia as well as renal failure. A prospective randomized trial (PLUTO) in Europe showed difficulties in patient recruitment, a higher survival with V-A shunting, but less than optimal renal function in some survivors.[135]

MYELOMENINGOCELE

Myelomeningocele (MMC) is a neural tube defect characterized by the protrusion of the spinal cord and meninges through open vertebral arches. It is the most common form of spina bifida, which affects 1 in 2000 births per year. Maternal serum testing identifies 75%–80% of pregnancies with MMC by 16 weeks of age.[136] If an increase in serum AFP is noted, amniocentesis is performed to assess amniotic fluid AFP and acetylcholinesterase to confirm the diagnosis.[137] The ultrasound characteristics include the "lemon" and "banana" signs, which are scalloping of the frontal bone and abnormal anterior curvature of the cerebellar hemispheres, respectively.[138] Most fetuses have an associated Arnold–Chiari malformation, characterized on fetal MRI by the caudal displacement of the vermis and cerebellum with midbrain herniation through the foramen magnum. Ultrasound confirmation can be made as early as 18 weeks, which allows localization of the defect as well as assessment of limb function, and the presence of clubbing or of the Arnold–Chiari malformation (Figure 5.8).

Analysis of the potential benefits of fetal repair of MMC has been accomplished in sheep models of the defect,[139–141] thus providing a compelling reason for in utero repair, the first nonlethal disease to be considered for this treatment. The goals of fetal repair are to prevent the chemical and mechanical trauma to the exposed spinal cord, to resolve

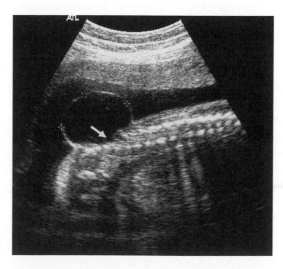

Figure 5.8 Ultrasound of a fetus with MMC showing the sac (crossmarks) over the spinal defect (arrow).

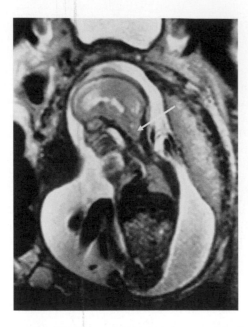

Figure 5.9 MRI of a fetus with MMC showing hindbrain herniation (arrow).

the hindbrain herniation frequently seen with this defect, to decrease the need for postnatal ventriculoperitoneal shunt, and to allow time for possible neural regeneration after repair. We reported the first open repair of fetal MMC, which led to improved neurological outcome[142] and resolution of the Arnold–Chiari malformation (Figure 5.9). Long-term analysis of patients who underwent in utero repair has indicated that this may lead to a decreased need for ventriculoperitoneal shunting[143,144] as well as improved brainstem function[145] and neurodevelopmental outcomes.[146] The multicenter Management of Myelomeningocele Study (MOMS trial) demonstrated benefits of prenatal repair such as a decreased rate of ventricular shunting and improved motor function including the ability to walk.[147]

CONCLUSIONS

Prenatal ultrasound has led to a rapid increase in the number of pediatric surgical conditions diagnosed in utero. Prenatal detection and serial sonographic study of fetuses with anatomic lesions now make it possible to define the natural history of these abnormalities, determine the pathophysiologic causes that affect outcome, and formulate management based on prognosis. Since many congenital anomalies are associated with others, it is important to perform a careful ultrasound evaluation and karyotype analysis when one abnormality is discovered.

Careful evaluation of patients followed prenatally and postnatally, as well as studies of congenital defects in animal models, has defined select populations of fetuses who may benefit from prenatal intervention. In most cases, these are fetuses who would not be expected to survive the prenatal period given the natural history of their disease. Further progress in prenatal diagnosis and monitoring as well as continued

reevaluation of outcomes will undoubtedly tune our current algorithms regarding the management of these congenital anomalies. Pediatric surgeons have a unique opportunity to continue to shape this exciting field in the new millennium.

REFERENCES

1. Harrison MR, Bjordal RI, Langmark F, Knutrud O. Congenital diaphragmatic hernia: The hidden mortality. *J Pediatr Surg* 1978; 13: 227–30.
2. Taipale P, Hiilesmaa V, Salonen R, Ylostalo P. Increased nuchal translucency as a marker for fetal chromosomal defects [see comments]. *N Engl J Med* 1997; 337: 1654–8.
3. Hyett J, Perdu M, Sharland G, Snijders R, Nicolaides KH. Using fetal nuchal translucency to screen for major congenital cardiac defects at 10–14 weeks of gestation: Population based cohort study [see comments]. *BMJ* 1999; 318: 81–5.
4. Daffos F, Forestier F, Mac Aleese J, Aufrant C, Mandelbrot L, Cabanis EA, Iba-Zizen MT, Alfonso JM, Tamraz J. Fetal curarization for prenatal magnetic resonance imaging. *Prenat Diagn* 1988; 8: 312–4.
5. Hubbard AM, Harty MP, States LJ. A new tool for prenatal diagnosis: Ultrafast fetal MRI. *Semin Perinatol* 1999; 23: 437–47.
6. Steele MW, Breg WR, Jr. Chromosome analysis of human amniotic-fluid cells. *Lancet* 1966; 1: 383–5.
7. Delisle MF, Wilson RD. First trimester prenatal diagnosis: Amniocentesis. *Semin Perinatol* 1999; 23: 414–23.
8. Wapner RJ, Martin CL, Levy B, Ballif BC, Eng CM, Zachary JM, Savage M et al. Chromosomal microarray versus karyotyping for prenatal diagnosis. *N Engl J Med* 2012; 367: 2175–84.
9. Canick JA, Kellner LH. First trimester screening for aneuploidy: Serum biochemical markers. *Semin Perinatol* 1999; 23: 359–68.
10. Wald NJ, Kennard A, Hackshaw A, McGuire A. Antenatal screening for Down's syndrome [published erratum appears in J Med Screen 1998;5(2):110 and 1998;5(3):166]. *J Med Screen* 1997; 4: 181–246.
11. Duchatel F, Oury JF, Mennesson B, Muray JM. Complications of diagnostic ultrasound-guided percutaneous umbilical blood sampling: Analysis of a series of 341 cases and review of the literature. *Eur J Obstet Gynecol Reprod Biol* 1993; 52: 95–104.
12. Hickok DE, Mills M. Percutaneous umbilical blood sampling: Results from a multicenter collaborative registry. The Western Collaborative Perinatal Group. *Am J Obstet Gynecol* 1992; 166: 1614–7; discussion 7–8.
13. Boulot P, Deschamps F, Lefort G, Sarda P, Mares P, Hedon B, Laffargue F, Viala JL. Pure fetal blood samples obtained by cordocentesis: Technical aspects of 322 cases. *Prenat Diagn* 1990; 10: 93–100.

14. Herzenberg LA, Bianchi DW, Schroder J, Cann HM, Iverson GM. Fetal cells in the blood of pregnant women: Detection and enrichment by fluorescence-activated cell sorting. *Proc Natl Acad Sci USA* 1979; 76: 1453–5.

15. Maron JL, Bianchi DW. Prenatal diagnosis using cell-free nucleic acids in maternal body fluids: A decade of progress. *Am J Med Genet C Semin Med Genet* 2007; 145C: 5–17.

16. Guibert J, Benachi A, Grebille AG, Ernault P, Zorn JR, Costa JM. Kinetics of SRY gene appearance in maternal serum: Detection by real time PCR in early pregnancy after assisted reproductive technique. *Hum Reprod* 2003; 18: 1733–6.

17. Langer JC, Fitzgerald PG, Desa D, Filly RA, Golbus MS, Adzick NS, Harrison MR. Cervical cystic hygroma in the fetus: Clinical spectrum and outcome. *J Pediatr Surg* 1990; 25: 58–61; discussion 61–2.

18. Mychaliska GB, Bealer JF, Graf JL, Rosen MA, Adzick NS, Harrison MR. Operating on placental support: The ex utero intrapartum treatment procedure. *J Pediatr Surg* 1997; 32: 227–30; discussion 30–1.

19. Liechty KW, Crombleholme TM, Flake AW, Morgan MA, Kurth CD, Hubbard AM, Adzick NS. Intrapartum airway management for giant fetal neck masses: The EXIT (ex utero intrapartum treatment) procedure. *Am J Obstet Gynecol* 1997; 177: 870–4.

20. Liechty KW, Crombleholme TM. Management of fetal airway obstruction. *Semin Perinatol* 1999; 23: 496–506.

21. Descamps P, Jourdain O, Paillet C, Toutain A, Guichet A, Pourcelot D, Gold F, Castiel M, Body G. Etiology, prognosis and management of nuchal cystic hygroma: 25 new cases and literature review. *Eur J Obstet Gynecol Reprod Biol* 1997; 71: 3–10.

22. Gallagher PG, Mahoney MJ, Gosche JR. Cystic hygroma in the fetus and newborn. *Semin Perinatol* 1999; 23: 341–56.

23. Brumfield CG, Wenstrom KD, Davis RO, Owen J, Cosper P. Second-trimester cystic hygroma: Prognosis of septated and nonseptated lesions. *Obstet Gynecol* 1996; 88: 979–82.

24. Nadel A, Bromley B, Benacerraf BR. Nuchal thickening or cystic hygromas in first- and early second-trimester fetuses: Prognosis and outcome. *Obstet Gynecol* 1993; 82: 43–8.

25. Liechty KW, Hedrick HL, Hubbard AM, Johnson MP, Wilson RD, Ruchelli ED, Howell LJ, Crombleholme TM, Flake AW, Adzick NS. Severe pulmonary hypoplasia associated with giant cervical teratomas. *J Pediatr Surg* 2006; 41: 230–3.

26. Hubbard AM, Crombleholme TM, Adzick NS. Prenatal MRI evaluation of giant neck masses in preparation for the fetal EXIT procedure. *Am J Perinatol* 1998; 15: 253–7.

27. Hubbard AM, Harty P. Prenatal magnetic resonance imaging of fetal anomalies. *Semin Roentgenol* 1999; 34: 41–7.

28. Laje P, Johnson MP, Howell LJ, Bebbington MW, Hedrick HL, Flake AW, Adzick NS. Ex utero intrapartum treatment (EXIT) in the management of giant cervical teratomas. *J Pediatr Surg* 2012; 47: 1208–16.

29. Hirose S, Farmer DL, Lee H, Nobuhara KK, Harrison MR. The ex utero intrapartum treatment procedure: Looking back at the EXIT. *J Pediatr Surg* 2004; 39: 375–80; discussion 380.

30. Hedrick HL, Flake AW, Crombleholme TM, Howell LJ, Johnson MP, Wilson RD, Adzick NS. The ex utero intrapartum therapy procedure for high-risk fetal lung lesions. *J Pediatr Surg* 2005; 40: 1038–43; discussion 1044.

31. Crombleholme TM, Sylvester K, Flake AW, Adzick NS. Salvage of a fetus with congenital high airway obstruction syndrome by ex utero intrapartum treatment (EXIT) procedure. *Fetal Diagn Ther* 2000; 15: 280–2.

32. Kunisaki SM, Barnewolt CE, Estroff JA, Myers LB, Fauza DO, Wilkins-Haug LE, Grable IA et al. Ex utero intrapartum treatment with extracorporeal membrane oxygenation for severe congenital diaphragmatic hernia. *J Pediatr Surg* 2007; 42: 98–104; discussion 104–6.

33. Mackenzie TC, Crombleholme TM, Johnson MP, Schnaufer L, Flake AW, Hedrick HL, Howell LJ, Adzick NS. The natural history of prenatally diagnosed conjoined twins. *J Pediatr Surg* 2002; 37: 303–9.

34. Butwick A, Aleshi P, Yamout I. Obstetric hemorrhage during an EXIT procedure for severe fetal airway obstruction. *Can J Anaesth* 2009; 56: 437–42.

35. Flake AW. Fetal sacrococcygeal teratoma. *Semin Pediatr Surg* 1993; 2: 113–20.

36. Altman RP, Randolph JG, Lilly JR. Sacrococcygeal teratoma: American Academy of Pediatrics Surgical Section Survey—1973. *J Pediatr Surg* 1974; 9: 389–98.

37. Danzer E, Hubbard AM, Hedrick HL, Johnson MP, Wilson RD, Howell LJ, Flake AW, Adzick NS. Diagnosis and characterization of fetal sacrococcygeal teratoma with prenatal MRI. *AJR Am J Roentgenol* 2006; 187: W350–6.

38. Kirkinen P, Partanen K, Merikanto J, Ryynanen M, Haring P, Heinonen K. Ultrasonic and magnetic resonance imaging of fetal sacrococcygeal teratoma. *Acta Obstet Gynecol Scand* 1997; 76: 917–22.

39. Westerburg B, Feldstein VA, Sandberg PL, Lopoo JB, Harrison MR, Albanese CT. Sonographic prognostic factors in fetuses with sacrococcygeal teratoma. *J Pediatr Surg* 2000; 35: 322–5; discussion 325–6.

40. Holterman AX, Filiatrault D, Lallier M, Youssef S. The natural history of sacrococcygeal teratomas diagnosed through routine obstetric sonogram: A single institution experience. *J Pediatr Surg* 1998; 33: 899–903.

41. Bond SJ, Harrison MR, Schmidt KG, Silverman NH, Flake AW, Slotnick RN, Anderson RL, Warsof SL, Dyson DC. Death due to high-output cardiac failure in fetal sacrococcygeal teratoma. *J Pediatr Surg* 1990; 25: 1287–91.

42. Schmidt KG, Silverman NH, Harison MR, Callen PW. High-output cardiac failure in fetuses with large sacro-coccygeal teratoma: Diagnosis by echocardiography and Doppler ultrasound. *J Pediatr* 1989; 114: 1023–8.

43. Chisholm CA, Heider AL, Kuller JA, von Allmen D, McMahon MJ, Chescheir NC. Prenatal diagnosis and perinatal management of fetal sacrococcygeal teratoma. *Am J Perinatol* 1999; 16: 47–50.

44. Bullard KM, Harrison MR. Before the horse is out of the barn: Fetal surgery for hydrops. *Semin Perinatol* 1995; 19: 462–73.

45. Wilson RD, Hedrick H, Flake AW, Johnson MP, Bebbington MW, Mann S, Rychik J, Liechty K, Adzick NS. Sacrococcygeal teratomas: Prenatal surveillance, growth and pregnancy outcome. *Fetal Diagn Ther* 2009; 25: 15–20.

46. Sy ED, Filly RA, Cheong ML, Clifton MS, Cortes RA, Ohashi S, Takifuji K et al. Prognostic role of tumor-head volume ratio in fetal sacrococcygeal teratoma. *Fetal Diagn Ther* 2009; 26: 75–80.

47. Benachi A, Durin L, Maurer SV, Aubry MC, Parat S, Herlicoviez M, Nihoul-Fekete C, Dumez Y, Dommergues M. Prenatally diagnosed sacrococcy-geal teratoma: A prognostic classification. *J Pediatr Surg* 2006; 41: 1517–21.

48. Adzick NS, Crombleholme TM, Morgan MA, Quinn TM. A rapidly growing fetal teratoma. *Lancet* 1997; 349: 538.

49. Hedrick HL, Flake AW, Crombleholme TM, Howell LJ, Johnson MP, Wilson RD, Adzick NS. Sacrococcygeal teratoma: Prenatal assessment, fetal intervention, and outcome. *J Pediatr Surg* 2004; 39: 430–8; discussion 430–8.

50. Makin EC, Hyett J, Ade-Ajayi N, Patel S, Nicolaides K, Davenport M. Outcome of antenatally diagnosed sacrococcygeal teratomas: Single-center experience (1993–2004). *J Pediatr Surg* 2006; 41: 388–93.

51. Stocker JT, Madewell JE, Drake RM. Congenital cystic adenomatoid malformation of the lung. Classification and morphologic spectrum. *Hum Pathol* 1977; 8: 155–71.

52. Adzick NS. Management of fetal lung lesions. *Clin Perinatol* 2009; 36: 363–76, x.

53. Cass DL, Crombleholme TM, Howell LJ, Stafford PW, Ruchelli ED, Adzick NS. Cystic lung lesions with systemic arterial blood supply: A hybrid of congenital cystic adenomatoid malformation and bronchopulmo-nary sequestration. *J Pediatr Surg* 1997; 32: 986–90.

54. Conran RM, Stocker JT. Extralobar sequestration with frequently associated congenital cystic adeno-matoid malformation, type 2: Report of 50 cases. *Pediatr Dev Pathol* 1999; 2: 454–63.

55. Hedrick MH, Jennings RW, MacGillivray TE, Rice HE, Flake AW, Adzick NS, Harrison MR. Chronic fetal vascular access. *Lancet* 1993; 342: 1086–7.

56. Winters WD, Effmann EL, Nghiem HV, Nyberg DA. Disappearing fetal lung masses: Importance of postnatal imaging studies. *Pediatr Radiol* 1997; 27: 535–9.

57. Hubbard AM, Adzick NS, Crombleholme TM, Coleman BG, Howell LJ, Haselgrove JC, Mahboubi S. Congenital chest lesions: Diagnosis and characterization with prenatal MR imaging. *Radiology* 1999; 212: 43–8.

58. Adzick NS, Harrison MR, Crombleholme TM, Flake AW, Howell LJ. Fetal lung lesions: Management and outcome. *Am J Obstet Gynecol* 1998; 179: 884–9.

59. Rice HE, Estes JM, Hedrick MH, Bealer JF, Harrison MR, Adzick NS. Congenital cystic adenomatoid mal-formation: A sheep model of fetal hydrops. *J Pediatr Surg* 1994; 29: 692–6.

60. Crombleholme TM, Coleman B, Hedrick H, Liechty K, Howell L, Flake AW, Johnson M, Adzick NS. Cystic adenomatoid malformation volume ratio predicts outcome in prenatally diagnosed cystic adenoma-toid malformation of the lung. *J Pediatr Surg* 2002; 37: 331–8.

61. Wilson RD, Baxter JK, Johnson MP, King M, Kasperski S, Crombleholme TM, Flake AW, Hedrick HL, Howell LJ, Adzick NS. Thoracoamniotic shunts: Fetal treatment of pleural effusions and congenital cystic adenomatoid malformations. *Fetal Diagn Ther* 2004; 19: 413–20.

62. Merchant AM, Peranteau W, Wilson RD, Johnson MP, Bebbington MW, Hedrick HL, Flake AW, Adzick NS. Postnatal chest wall deformities after fetal tho-racoamniotic shunting for congenital cystic adeno-matoid malformation. *Fetal Diagn Ther* 2007; 22: 435–9.

63. Kunisaki SM, Fauza DO, Barnewolt CE, Estroff JA, Myers LB, Bulich LA, Wong G et al. Ex utero intra-partum treatment with placement on extracorporeal membrane oxygenation for fetal thoracic masses. *J Pediatr Surg* 2007; 42: 420–5.

64. Keswani SG, Crombleholme TM, Rychik J, Tian Z, Mackenzie TC, Johnson MP, Wilson RD et al. Impact of continuous intraoperative monitoring on out-comes in open fetal surgery. *Fetal Diagn Ther* 2005; 20: 316–20.

65. Grethel EJ, Wagner AJ, Clifton MS, Cortes RA, Farmer DL, Harrison MR, Nobuhara KK, Lee H. Fetal intervention for mass lesions and hydrops improves outcome: A 15-year experience. *J Pediatr Surg* 2007; 42: 117–23.

66. Bruner JP, Jarnagin BK, Reinisch L. Percutaneous laser ablation of fetal congenital cystic adenomatoid malformation: Too little, too late? *Fetal Diagn Ther* 2000; 15: 359–63.

67. Tsao K, Hawgood S, Vu L, Hirose S, Sydorak R, Albanese CT, Farmer DL, Harrison MR, Lee H. Resolution of hydrops fetalis in congenital cystic adenomatoid malformation after prenatal steroid therapy. *J Pediatr Surg* 2003; 38: 508–10.

68. Peranteau WH, Wilson RD, Liechty KW, Johnson MP, Bebbington MW, Hedrick HL, Flake AW, Adzick NS. Effect of maternal betamethasone administration on prenatal congenital cystic adenomatoid malformation growth and fetal survival. *Fetal Diagn Ther* 2007; 22: 365–71.

69. Kunisaki SM, Barnewolt CE, Estroff JA, Ward VL, Nemes LP, Fauza DO, Jennings RW. Large fetal congenital cystic adenomatoid malformations: Growth trends and patient survival. *J Pediatr Surg* 2007; 42: 404–10.

70. MacGillivray TE, Harrison MR, Goldstein RB, Adzick NS. Disappearing fetal lung lesions. *J Pediatr Surg* 1993; 28: 1321–4; discussion 1324–5.

71. Morris LM, Lim FY, Livingston JC, Polzin WJ, Crombleholme TM. High-risk fetal congenital pulmonary airway malformations have a variable response to steroids. *J Pediatr Surg* 2009; 44: 60–5.

72. Hubbard AM, Crombleholme TM, Adzick NS, Coleman BG, Howell LJ, Meyer JS, Flake AW. Prenatal MRI evaluation of congenital diaphragmatic hernia. *Am J Perinatol* 1999; 16: 407–13.

73. Hubbard AM, Adzick NS, Crombleholme TM, Haselgrove JC. Left-sided congenital diaphragmatic hernia: Value of prenatal MR imaging in preparation for fetal surgery. *Radiology* 1997; 203: 636–40.

74. Jani J, Cannie M, Sonigo P, Robert Y, Moreno O, Benachi A, Vaast P, Gratacos E, Nicolaides KH, Deprest J. Value of prenatal magnetic resonance imaging in the prediction of postnatal outcome in fetuses with diaphragmatic hernia. *Ultrasound Obstet Gynecol* 2008; 32: 793–9.

75. Walsh DS, Hubbard AM, Olutoye OO, Howell LJ, Crombleholme TM, Flake AW, Johnson MP, Adzick NS. Assessment of fetal lung volumes and liver herniation with magnetic resonance imaging in congenital diaphragmatic hernia. *Am J Obstet Gynecol* 2000; 183: 1067–9.

76. Williams G, Coakley FV, Qayyum A, Farmer DL, Joe BN, Filly RA. Fetal relative lung volume: Quantification by using prenatal MR imaging lung volumetry. *Radiology* 2004; 233: 457–62.

77. Metkus AP, Filly RA, Stringer MD, Harrison MR, Adzick NS. Sonographic predictors of survival in fetal diaphragmatic hernia. *J Pediatr Surg* 1996; 31: 148–51; discussion 51–2.

78. Lipshutz GS, Albanese CT, Feldstein VA, Jennings RW, Housley HT, Beech R, Farrell JA, Harrison MR. Prospective analysis of lung-to-head ratio predicts survival for patients with prenatally diagnosed congenital diaphragmatic hernia. *J Pediatr Surg* 1997; 32: 1634–6.

79. Jani J, Keller RL, Benachi A, Nicolaides KH, Favre R, Gratacos E, Laudy J et al. Prenatal prediction of survival in isolated left-sided diaphragmatic hernia. *Ultrasound Obstet Gynecol* 2006; 27: 18–22.

80. Hedrick HL, Danzer E, Merchant A, Bebbington MW, Zhao H, Flake AW, Johnson MP et al. Liver position and lung-to-head ratio for prediction of extracorporeal membrane oxygenation and survival in isolated left congenital diaphragmatic hernia. *Am J Obstet Gynecol* 2007; 197: 422.e1–4.

81. Jani JC, Peralta CF, Ruano R, Benachi A, Done E, Nicolaides KH, Deprest JA. Comparison of fetal lung area to head circumference ratio with lung volume in the prediction of postnatal outcome in diaphragmatic hernia. *Ultrasound Obstet Gynecol* 2007; 30: 850–4.

82. Hedrick HL, Crombleholme TM, Flake AW, Nance ML, von Allmen D, Howell LJ, Johnson MP, Wilson RD, Adzick NS. Right congenital diaphragmatic hernia: Prenatal assessment and outcome. *J Pediatr Surg* 2004; 39: 319–23; discussion 319–23.

83. Sokol J, Bohn D, Lacro RV, Ryan G, Stephens D, Rabinovitch M, Smallhorn J, Hornberger LK. Fetal pulmonary artery diameters and their association with lung hypoplasia and postnatal outcome in congenital diaphragmatic hernia. *Am J Obstet Gynecol* 2002; 186: 1085–90.

84. Sokol J, Shimizu N, Bohn D, Doherty D, Ryan G, Hornberger LK. Fetal pulmonary artery diameter measurements as a predictor of morbidity in antenatally diagnosed congenital diaphragmatic hernia: A prospective study. *Am J Obstet Gynecol* 2006; 195: 470–7.

85. Moreno-Alvarez O, Hernandez-Andrade E, Oros D, Jani J, Deprest J, Gratacos E. Association between intrapulmonary arterial Doppler parameters and degree of lung growth as measured by lung-to-head ratio in fetuses with congenital diaphragmatic hernia. *Ultrasound Obstet Gynecol* 2008; 31: 164–70.

86. Broth RE, Wood DC, Rasanen J, Sabogal JC, Komwilaisak R, Weiner S, Berghella V. Prenatal prediction of lethal pulmonary hypoplasia: The hyperoxygenation test for pulmonary artery reactivity. *Am J Obstet Gynecol* 2002; 187: 940–5.

87. Deprest JA, Gratacos E, Nicolaides K, Done E, Van Mieghem T, Gucciardo L, Claus F et al. Changing perspectives on the perinatal management of isolated congenital diaphragmatic hernia in Europe. *Clin Perinatol* 2009; 36: 329–47, ix.

88. Jelin E, Lee H. Tracheal occlusion for fetal congenital diaphragmatic hernia: The US experience. *Clin Perinatol* 2009; 36: 349–61, ix.

89. DiFiore JW, Fauza DO, Slavin R, Peters CA, Fackler JC, Wilson JM. Experimental fetal tracheal ligation reverses the structural and physiological effects of pulmonary hypoplasia in congenital diaphragmatic hernia. *J Pediatr Surg* 1994; 29: 248–56; discussion 256–7.

90. Davey MG, Hooper SB, Tester ML, Johns DP, Harding R. Respiratory function in lambs after in utero treatment of lung hypoplasia by tracheal obstruction. *J Appl Physiol* 1999; 87: 2296–304.

91. Flake AW, Crombleholme TM, Johnson MP, Howell LJ, Adzick NS. Treatment of severe congenital diaphragmatic hernia by fetal tracheal occlusion: Clinical experience with fifteen cases. *Am J Obstet Gynecol* 2000; 183: 1059–66.

92. Harrison MR, Mychaliska GB, Albanese CT, Jennings RW, Farrell JA, Hawgood S, Sandberg P, Levine AH, Lobo E, Filly RA. Correction of congenital diaphragmatic hernia in utero IX: Fetuses with poor prognosis (liver herniation and low lung-to-head ratio) can be saved by fetoscopic temporary tracheal occlusion. *J Pediatr Surg* 1998; 33: 1017–22; discussion 1022–3.

93. Harrison MR, Keller RL, Hawgood SB, Kitterman JA, Sandberg PL, Farmer DL, Lee H, Filly RA, Farrell JA, Albanese CT. A randomized trial of fetal endoscopic tracheal occlusion for severe fetal congenital diaphragmatic hernia. *N Engl J Med* 2003; 349: 1916–24.

94. Jani J, Gratacos E, Greenough A, Pieró JL, Benachi A, Harrison M, Nicolaïdes K, Deprest J; FETO Task Group. Percutaneous fetal endoscopic tracheal occlusion (FETO) for severe left-sided congenital diaphragmatic hernia. *Clin Obstet Gynecol* 2005; 48: 910–22.

95. Stringer MD, McKenna KM, Goldstein RB, Filly RA, Adzick NS, Harrison MR. Prenatal diagnosis of esophageal atresia. *J Pediatr Surg* 1995; 30: 1258–63.

96. Sparey C, Jawaheer G, Barrett AM, Robson SC. Esophageal atresia in the Northern Region Congenital Anomaly Survey, 1985–1997: Prenatal diagnosis and outcome. *Am J Obstet Gynecol* 2000; 182: 427–31.

97. Choudhry MS, Rahman N, Boyd P, Lakhoo K. Duodenal atresia: Associated anomalies, prenatal diagnosis and outcome. *Pediatr Surg Int* 2009; 25: 727–30.

98. Hemming V, Rankin J. Small intestinal atresia in a defined population: Occurrence, prenatal diagnosis and survival. *Prenat Diagn* 2007; 27: 1205–11.

99. Corteville JE, Gray DL, Langer JC. Bowel abnormalities in the fetus—Correlation of prenatal ultrasonographic findings with outcome. *Am J Obstet Gynecol* 1996; 175: 724–9.

100. Van Rijn M, Christaens GC, Hagenaars AM, Visser GH. Maternal serum alpha-fetoprotein in fetal anal atresia and other gastro-intestinal obstructions [see comments]. *Prenat Diagn* 1998; 18: 914–21.

101. Langer JC. Gastroschisis and omphalocele. *Semin Pediatr Surg* 1996; 5: 124–8.

102. Wilson RD, Johnson MP. Congenital abdominal wall defects: An update. *Fetal Diagn Ther* 2004; 19: 385–98.

103. Tiblad E, Wilson RD, Carr M, Flake AW, Hedrick H, Johnson MP, Bebbington MW, Mann S, Adzick NS. OEIS sequence—A rare congenital anomaly with prenatal evaluation and postnatal outcome in six cases. *Prenat Diagn* 2008; 28: 141–7.

104. Biard JM, Wilson RD, Johnson MP, Hedrick HL, Schwarz U, Flake AW, Crombleholme TM, Adzick NS. Prenatally diagnosed giant omphaloceles: Short- and long-term outcomes. *Prenat Diagn* 2004; 24: 434–9.

105. Langer JC, Adzick NS, Filly RA, Golbus MS, deLorimier AA, Harrison MR. Gastrointestinal tract obstruction in the fetus. *Arch Surg* 1989; 124: 1183–6; discussion 1187.

106. Crombleholme TM, Harrison MR, Golbus MS, Longaker MT, Langer JC, Callen PW, Anderson RL, Goldstein RB, Filly RA. Fetal intervention in obstructive uropathy: Prognostic indicators and efficacy of intervention. *Am J Obstet Gynecol* 1990; 162: 1239–44.

107. Crawford RA, Ryan G, Wright VM, Rodeck CH. The importance of serial biophysical assessment of fetal wellbeing in gastroschisis. *Br J Obstet Gynaecol* 1992; 99: 899–902.

108. Molik KA, Gingalewski CA, West KW, Rescorla FJ, Scherer LR, Engum SA, Grosfeld JL. Gastroschisis: A plea for risk categorization. *J Pediatr Surg* 2001; 36: 51–5.

109. Abdullah F, Arnold MA, Nabaweesi R, Fischer AC, Colombani PM, Anderson KD, Lau H, Chang DC. Gastroschisis in the United States 1988–2003: Analysis and risk categorization of 4344 patients. *J Perinatol* 2007; 27: 50–5.

110. Api A, Olguner M, Hakguder G, Ates O, Ozer E, Akgur FM. Intestinal damage in gastroschisis correlates with the concentration of intraamniotic meconium. *J Pediatr Surg* 2001; 36: 1811–5.

111. Mahieu-Caputo D, Muller F, Jouvet P, Thalabard JC, Jouannic JM, Nihoul-Fékété C, Dumez Y, Dommergues M. Amniotic fluid beta-endorphin: A prognostic marker for gastroschisis? *J Pediatr Surg* 2002; 37: 1602–6.

112. Badillo AT, Hedrick HL, Wilson RD, Danzer E, Bebbington MW, Johnson MP, Liechty KW, Flake AW, Adzick NS. Prenatal ultrasonographic gastrointestinal abnormalities in fetuses with gastroschisis do not correlate with postnatal outcomes. *J Pediatr Surg* 2008; 43: 647–53.

113. How HY, Harris BJ, Pietrantoni M, Evans JC, Dutton S, Khoury J, Siddiqi TA. Is vaginal delivery preferable to elective cesarean delivery in fetuses with a known ventral wall defect? *Am J Obstet Gynecol* 2000; 182: 1527–34.

114. Segel SY, Marder SJ, Parry S, Macones GA. Fetal abdominal wall defects and mode of delivery: A systematic review. *Obstet Gynecol* 2001; 98: 867–73.

115. Murphy FL, Mazlan TA, Tarheen F, Corbally MT, Puri P. Gastroschisis and exomphalos in Ireland 1998–2004. Does antenatal diagnosis impact on outcome? *Pediatr Surg Int* 2007; 23: 1059–63.

116. Yiee J, Wilcox D. Management of fetal hydronephrosis. *Pediatr Nephrol* 2008; 23: 347–53.

117. Fernbach SK, Maizels M, Conway JJ. Ultrasound grading of hydronephrosis: Introduction to the system used by the Society for Fetal Urology. *Pediatr Radiol* 1993; 23: 478–80.

118. Wollenberg A, Neuhaus TJ, Willi UV, Wisser J. Outcome of fetal renal pelvic dilatation diagnosed during the third trimester. *Ultrasound Obstet Gynecol* 2005; 25: 483–8.

119. Elder JS. Antenatal hydronephrosis. Fetal and neonatal management. *Pediatr Clin North Am* 1997; 44: 1299–321.

120. Coplen DE. Prenatal intervention for hydronephrosis. *J Urol* 1997; 157: 2270–7.

121. Fasolato V, Poloniato A, Bianchi C, Spagnolo D, Valsecchi L, Ferrari A, Paesano P, Del Maschio A. Feto-neonatal ultrasonography to detect renal abnormalities: Evaluation of 1-year screening program. *Am J Perinatol* 1998; 15: 161–4.

122. Kitagawa H, Pringle KC, Stone P, Flower J, Murakami N, Robinson R. Postnatal follow-up of hydronephrosis detected by prenatal ultrasound: The natural history. *Fetal Diagn Ther* 1998; 13: 19–25.

123. Johnson MP, Freedman AL. Fetal uropathy. *Curr Opin Obstet Gynecol* 1999; 11: 185–94.

124. Wu S, Johnson MP. Fetal lower urinary tract obstruction. *Clin Perinatol* 2009; 36: 377–90, x.

125. Nakayama DK, Harrison MR, de Lorimier AA. Prognosis of posterior urethral valves presenting at birth. *J Pediatr Surg* 1986; 21: 43–5.

126. Reinberg Y, de Castano I, Gonzalez R. Prognosis for patients with prenatally diagnosed posterior urethral valves. *J Urol* 1992; 148: 125–6.

127. Harrison MR, Ross N, Noall R, de Lorimier AA. Correction of congenital hydronephrosis in utero. I. The model: Fetal urethral obstruction produces hydronephrosis and pulmonary hypoplasia in fetal lambs. *J Pediatr Surg* 1983; 18: 247–56.

128. Harrison MR, Golbus MS, Filly RA, Callen PW, Katz M, de Lorimier AA, Rosen M, Jonsen AR. Fetal surgery for congenital hydronephrosis. *N Engl J Med* 1982; 306: 591–3.

129. Walsh DS, Johnson MP. Fetal interventions for obstructive uropathy. *Semin Perinatol* 1999; 23: 484–95.

130. Quintero RA, Johnson MP, Romero R, Smith C, Arias F, Guevara-Zuloaga F, Cotton DB, Evans MI. In-utero percutaneous cystoscopy in the management of fetal lower obstructive uropathy. *Lancet* 1995; 346: 537–40.

131. Clifton MS, Harrison MR, Ball R, Lee H. Fetoscopic transuterine release of posterior urethral valves: A new technique. *Fetal Diagn Ther* 2008; 23: 89–94.

132. Freedman AL, Johnson MP, Smith CA, Gonzalez R, Evans MI. Long-term outcome in children after antenatal intervention for obstructive uropathies [see comments]. *Lancet* 1999; 354: 374–7.

133. Biard JM, Johnson MP, Carr MC, Wilson RD, Hedrick HL, Pavlock C, Adzick NS. Long-term outcomes in children treated by prenatal vesicoamniotic shunting for lower urinary tract obstruction. *Obstet Gynecol* 2005; 106: 503–8.

134. Clark TJ, Martin WL, Divakaran TG, Whittle MJ, Kilby MD, Khan KS. Prenatal bladder drainage in the management of fetal lower urinary tract obstruction: A systematic review and meta-analysis. *Obstet Gynecol* 2003; 102: 367–82.

135. Morris RK, Malin GL, Quinlan-Jones E, Middleton LJ, Hemming K, Burke D, Daniels JP et al. Percutaneous vesicoamniotic shunting versus conservative management for fetal lower urinary tract obstruction (PLUTO): A randomized trial. *Lancet* 2013; 382: 1496–506.

136. Platt LD, Feuchtbaum L, Filly R, Lustig L, Simon M, Cunningham GC. The California Maternal Serum alpha-Fetoprotein Screening Program: The role of ultrasonography in the detection of spina bifida. *Am J Obstet Gynecol* 1992; 166: 1328–9.

137. Olutoye OO, Adzick NS. Fetal surgery for myelomeningocele. *Semin Perinatol* 1999; 23: 462–73.

138. Van den Hof MC, Nicolaides KH, Campbell J, Campbell S. Evaluation of the lemon and banana signs in one hundred thirty fetuses with open spina bifida. *Am J Obstet Gynecol* 1990; 162: 322–7.

139. Bouchard S, Davey MG, Rintoul NE, Walsh DS, Rorke LB, Adzick NS. Correction of hindbrain herniation and anatomy of the vermis after in utero repair of myelomeningocele in sheep. *J Pediatr Surg* 2003; 38: 451–8; discussion 451–8.

140. Meuli M, Meuli-Simmen C, Hutchins GM, Yingling CD, Hoffman KM, Harrison MR, Adzick NS. In utero surgery rescues neurological function at birth in sheep with spina bifida. *Nat Med* 1995; 1: 342–7.

141. Yoshizawa J, Sbragia L, Paek BW, Sydorak RM, Yamazaki Y, Harrison MR, Farmer DL. Fetal surgery for repair of myelomeningocele allows normal development of anal sphincter muscles in sheep. *Pediatr Surg Int* 2004; 20: 14–8.

142. Adzick NS, Sutton LN, Crombleholme TM, Flake AW. Successful fetal surgery for spina bifida [letter] [see comments]. *Lancet* 1998; 352: 1675–6.

143. Farmer DL, von Koch CS, Peacock WJ, Danielpour M, Gupta N, Lee H, Harrison MR. In utero repair of myelomeningocele: Experimental pathophysiology, initial clinical experience, and outcomes. *Arch Surg* 2003; 138: 872–8.

144. Tulipan N, Sutton LN, Bruner JP, Cohen BM, Johnson M, Adzick NS. The effect of intrauterine myelomeningocele repair on the incidence of shunt-dependent hydrocephalus. *Pediatr Neurosurg* 2003; 38: 27–33.

145. Danzer E, Finkel RS, Rintoul NE, Bebbington MW, Schwartz ES, Zarnow DM, Adzick NS, Johnson MP. Reversal of hindbrain herniation after maternal–fetal surgery for myelomeningocele subsequently impacts on brain stem function. *Neuropediatrics* 2008; 39: 359–62.

146. Johnson MP, Gerdes M, Rintoul N, Pasquariello P, Melchionni J, Sutton LN, Adzick NS. Maternal–fetal surgery for myelomeningocele: Neurodevelopmental outcomes at 2 years of age. *Am J Obstet Gynecol* 2006; 194: 1145–50; discussion 1150–2.

147. Adzick NS, Thom EA, Spong CY, Brock JW 3rd, Burrows PK, Johnson MP, Howell LJ et al. A randomized trial of prenatal versus postnatal repair of myelomeningocele. *N Engl J Med* 2011; 364: 993–1004.

6

Fetal counseling for surgical malformations

KOKILA LAKHOO

INTRODUCTION

Pediatric surgeons are often called to counsel parents once a surgical abnormality is diagnosed on a prenatal scan. The referral base for a pediatric surgeon now includes the perinatal period. Expertise in surgical correction of congenital malformations may favorably influence the perinatal management of prenatally diagnosed anomalies by changing the site of delivery for immediate postnatal treatment; altering the mode of delivery to prevent obstructed labor or hemorrhage: early delivery to prevent ongoing fetal organ damage; or treatment in utero to prevent, minimize, or reverse fetal organ injury as a result of a structural defect. Recent literature has confirmed the favorable impact of prenatal surgical consultation in influencing the site of delivery in 37% of cases, changing the mode of delivery in 6.8%, reversing the decision to terminate a pregnancy in 3.6%, and influencing the early delivery of babies in 4.5%.

The pediatric surgeon performing prenatal consultations must be aware of differences between the prenatal and postnatal natural history of the anomaly. There is often a lack of understanding of the natural history and prognosis of a condition presenting in the newborn and the same condition diagnosed prenatally.

The diagnosis and management of complex fetal anomalies require a multidisciplinary team encompassing obstetricians, neonatologists, geneticists, pediatricians, pediatric surgeons, and occasional other specialists with expertise to deal with all the maternal and fetal complexities of a diagnosis of a structural defect. This team should be able to provide information to prospective parents on fetal outcomes, possible interventions, appropriate setting, time and route of delivery, and expected postnatal outcomes. The role of the surgical consultant in this team is to present information regarding the prenatal and postnatal natural history of an anomaly, its surgical management, and the long-term outcome.

CONGENITAL MALFORMATION

Congenital malformations account for one of the major causes of perinatal mortality and morbidity. Single major birth defects affect 3% of newborns, and 0.7% of babies have multiple defects. The prenatal hidden mortality is higher since the majority abort spontaneously. Despite improvements in perinatal care, serious birth defects still account for 20% of all deaths in the newborn period and an even greater percentage of serious morbidity later in infancy and childhood. The major causes of congenital malformation are chromosomal abnormalities, mutant genes, multifactorial disorders, and teratogenic agents.

PRENATAL DIAGNOSIS

Prenatal diagnosis has remarkably improved our understanding of surgically correctable congenital malformations. It has allowed us to influence the delivery of the baby, offer prenatal surgical management, and discuss the options of termination of pregnancy for seriously handicapping or lethal conditions. Antenatal diagnosis has also defined an in utero mortality for some lesions such as diaphragmatic hernia and sacrococcygeal teratoma (SCT) so that true outcomes can be measured. Prenatal ultrasound (US) scanning has improved since its first use 30 years ago, thus providing better screening programs and more accurate assessment of fetal anomaly. Screening for Down syndrome may now be offered in the first trimester (e.g., nuchal scan combined test) (Figure 6.1) or second trimester (e.g., quadruple blood test). Better resolution and increased experience with US scans has led to the recognition of US soft markers, which have increased the detection rate of fetal anomalies but at the expense of higher false-positive rates.

Routine US screening identifies anomalies and places these pregnancies in the high-risk categories with maternal diabetes, hypertension, genetic disorders, raised alpha-fetoprotein (AFP), etc. High-risk pregnancies may be offered further invasive diagnostic investigations such as amniocentesis or chorionic villous sampling (CVS). Structural abnormalities difficult to define on US such as hindbrain lesions or the presence of oligohydramnios are better imaged on ultrafast magnetic resonance imaging (MRI). With the increasing range of options and sophistication of diagnostic methods, parents today are faced with more information, choice, and decisions than ever before, which can create as well as help to solve dilemmas. The different tests and screening procedures commonly in use are outlined here.

US examination

US scans are routinely performed at 18–20 weeks gestation as part of the prenatal screening for all pregnancies in England and Wales. Older mothers are routinely screened but in addition are offered invasive testing. Pregnancies with maternal risk factors such as raised AFP levels, genetic disorders, and family history of chromosomal abnormalities or monochorionic twins that carry a high risk for chromosomal anomalies are offered earlier scans in the first trimester. Abnormalities such as diaphragmatic hernia may be detected as early as 11 weeks gestation. First-trimester scans are also useful for accurately dating pregnancies and defining chorionicity in multiple pregnancies.

Recently, nuchal translucency (NT) measurements have emerged as an independent marker of chromosomal abnormalities (with a sensitivity of 60%), structural anomalies (particularly cardiac defects), and some rare genetic syndromes. It involves measuring the area at the back of the fetal neck at 11–14 weeks gestation (Figure 6.1). The mechanisms by which some abnormalities give rise to this transient anatomical change of NT are poorly understood. Although some abnormalities can be seen at the time of the nuchal scan (11–14 weeks), most are detected at the 18th- to 20th-week anomaly scan. Some abnormalities such as gastroschisis have a higher detection rate on a scan than others, e.g., cardiac abnormalities.

If the NT measurement is increased and the karyotype is normal, there is a higher risk for a cardiac anomaly, and these high-risk fetuses may be referred for fetal echocardiography, which provides better prenatal cardiac assessment than the routine screening scan. US surveillance is essential during the performance of invasive techniques such as amniocentesis, CVS, and shunting procedures. It is also useful for assessing fetal viability before and after such procedures. Some abnormalities such as tracheoesophageal fistula (TOF), bowel atresia, diaphragmatic hernia, and hydrocephaly may present later in pregnancy and are thereby not detected on the routine 18th-week scan.

Overall, around 60% of structural birth defects are detected prenatally, but the detection rate varies from 0% (isolated cleft palate) to close to 100% (gastroschisis) depending on the defect. True wrong diagnoses are rare, but false-positive diagnoses do occur; some are due to natural prenatal regression, but most are due to US soft markers.

US soft markers are changes noted on prenatal scan that are difficult to define. Examples are echogenic bowel,[1] hydronephrosis, and nuchal thickening. Their presence creates anxiety amongst sonographers since the finding may be transient with no pathological relevance or may be an indicator of significant anomalies such as chromosomal abnormalities, cystic fibrosis (echogenic bowel), Down syndrome (nuchal thickening), or renal abnormalities (hydronephrosis). Once soft markers are detected, whether they should be reported or further invasive tests offered is a dilemma faced by obstetricians. Reporting these markers has increased detection rates at the expense of high false-positive rates.

US is routinely performed as a prenatal screening test. The reliability of the information obtained is dependent on the expertise and experience of the person performing the scan. In a recent study, congenital anomalies noted at birth were diagnosed on prenatal scan in 64% of cases, with 0.5% opting for termination.

Minimally invasive techniques

CELL-FREE FETAL DNA

The identification of cell-free fetal DNA (cffDNA) in the maternal circulation triggered an increase in research with the aim of developing safer, minimally invasive prenatal diagnosis. It is placental based and detectable from 4 weeks gestation and is rapidly cleared after delivery. The majority of cffDNA is maternal, with only 3%–6% originating from the fetus. Difficulties with separating these means that applications have focused on detection of genetic material that should not be present in the mother, such as Y chromosome sequences. Fetal Rh-D typing using cffDNA has now almost completely replaced invasive testing for determination of fetal blood group in the United Kingdom.

PREIMPLANTATION GENETIC DIAGNOSIS

For couples known to be carrying a genetic disorder, the process of invasive prenatal diagnosis and potential termination of pregnancy can be distressing. Preimplantation genetic diagnosis (PGD) involves generation of embryos by in vitro fertilization (IVF) and then sampling at the eight-cell stage. The genetic analysis is carried out the same day and only unaffected embryos are transferred into the uterus.

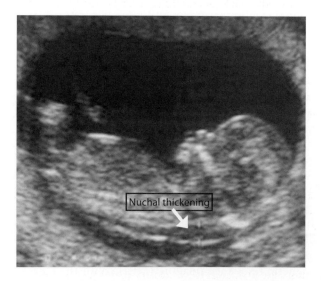

Figure 6.1 Nuchal thickening.

PGD is extremely promising for families affected by genetic disorders but has also given rise to many legal and ethical challenges such as its use to produce an unaffected, human leukocyte antigen (HLA)-compatible "savior sibling."

Invasive diagnostic tests

Amniocentesis and CVS are the two most commonly performed invasive diagnostic tests.

AMNIOCENTESIS

Amniocentesis is commonly used for detecting chromosomal abnormalities and less often for molecular studies, metabolic studies, and fetal infection. It is performed after 15 weeks gestation and carries a low risk of fetal injury or loss (0.5%–1%). Full karyotype analysis takes approximately 2 weeks, but newer rapid techniques using fluorescent in situ hybridization (FISH) or polymerase chain reaction (PCR) can give limited (usually for trisomies 21, 18, and 13) results within 2–3 days.

CHORIONIC VILLOUS SAMPLING

CVS is the most reliable method for first-trimester diagnosis and may be performed at 10–14 weeks gestation. The test involves US-guided biopsy of the chorionic villi. The added risk of fetal loss is approximately 1%–2%. The samples obtained may be subjected to a variety of tests including full karyotype, rapid karyotyping (FISH–PCR), enzyme analysis, or molecular studies. Approximate timing of chromosomal results is 1–2 weeks for karyotyping and 2–3 days for FISH and PCR.

PRENATAL MATERNAL SERUM SCREENING

Interest in detecting circulating fetal cells in maternal blood for diagnostic purposes has grown since the advent of fluorescence-activated cell sorting (FACS). The observation of high levels of AFP in amniotic fluid of pregnancies complicated by open neural tube defects (NTDs) popularized this test.[1] However, with increasing accuracy of US diagnosis, maternal serum screening of AFP solely for identification of NTDs cannot be justified. The more popular maternal serum screening test is the triple test (human chorionic gonadotrophin [HCG], AFP, estrogen) used in combination with the nuchal scan.

FETAL BLOOD SAMPLING

Rapid karyotyping of CVS and FISH and PCR of amniotic fluid samples have replaced fetal blood sampling (FBS) for many conditions. However, FBS is still required for the diagnosis and treatment of hematological conditions and some viral infections. When required, it is best performed by US-guided needle sampling after 18 weeks gestation rather than the more invasive fetoscopic technique. Mortality from this procedure is reported to be 1%–2%.

FETAL SURGERY

Fetal intervention encompasses a range of procedures on the fetus with congenital structural anomalies, while still on the placental circulation. There is a spectrum of interventions ranging from simple aspiration of cysts to open fetal surgery. The concept of fetal surgery was conceived in order to prevent fetal or early postnatal death, or to prevent permanent irreversible organ damage. The benefit of these procedures has to be balanced with risks to both the mother and the fetus. Open fetal surgery, more commonly conducted in North American centers, involves open surgery to the uterus in order to operate on the fetus. Fetal intervention centers in Europe more commonly use minimally invasive fetoscopic surgery. Minimally invasive techniques such as ablation of vessels in SCT, fetoscopic ablation of posterior urethral valves (PUVs), tracheal occlusion for congenital diaphragmatic hernia (CDH), etc. are currently under trial. However, laser ablation in twin-to-twin transfusion is now well established.

GENETIC DIAGNOSES

Antenatal detection of genetic abnormalities is increasing especially in high-risk pregnancies. Previously undiagnosed conditions such as cystic fibrosis, Beckwith–Wiedemann syndrome, Hirschsprung disease, sickle cell disease, etc. may be detected prenatally following invasive testing and genetic counseling and assessment offered early in pregnancy.

Future developments

The aim of prenatal diagnosis and testing is to have 100% accuracy without fetal loss or injury and no maternal risk. National plans to improve Down screening using US and biochemical combination tests are now in place in the United Kingdom. Research into new markers for chromosomal abnormalities is ongoing. The fetal nasal bone is one such example, which may assist in detecting babies with chromosomal abnormalities.

Management of Rhesus disease is showing promise whereby fetal blood groups may be determined from maternal blood samples through detection of free fetal DNA. The search for fetal components in maternal blood is an exciting and expanding field of research since past and present efforts to isolate and use them for diagnosis have met with little success. Rapid detection techniques versus traditional cultures for karyotyping are currently under debate at present.

Three-dimensional images from new US machines may have a useful role in diagnosis and assessment of facial deformities such as cleft lip and palate. MRI may assist in better defining some lesions difficult to view on conventional prenatal scanning, such as presacral teratoma, PUVs in the presence of oligohydramnios, and hindbrain lesions.

SPECIFIC SURGICAL CONDITIONS

Congenital diaphragmatic hernia

CDH accounts for 1 in 3000 live births and challenges the neonatologist and pediatric surgeons in the management of this high-risk condition (Figure 6.2). Mortality remains high (more than 60%) when the hidden mortality of in utero

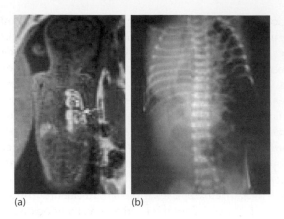

Figure 6.2 Congenital left diaphragmatic hernia shown on **(a)** prenatal MRI and **(b)** postnatal radiograph.

death and termination of pregnancy are taken into account. Lung hypoplasia and pulmonary hypertension account for most deaths in isolated CDH newborns. Associated anomalies (30%–40%) signify a grave prognosis with a survival rate of less than 10%.

In the United Kingdom, most CDHs are diagnosed at the 20th-week anomaly scan with a detection rate approaching 60%, although as early as 11 weeks gestation has been reported. MRI has a useful role in accurately differentiating CDH from cystic lung lesions and may be useful in measuring fetal lung volumes as a predictor of outcome. Cardiac anomalies (20%), chromosomal anomalies of trisomy 13 and 18 (20%), and urinary, gastrointestinal, and neurological anomalies (33%) can coexist with CDH and should be ruled out by offering the patient a fetal echocardiogram, amniocentesis, and detailed anomaly scan. For these associated anomalies and in isolated lesions, early detection, liver in the chest, polyhydramnios, and fetal lung-to-head ratio (LHR) of less than 1 are implicated as poor predictors of outcome.

Greater consistency and accuracy in predictive value can be obtained by using the observed-to-expected LHR (O/E LHR). The O/E LHR was developed in response to the observation that lung growth is four times that of head growth in the third trimester. The O/E LHR (by taking a transverse section of the fetal chest demonstrating the four-chamber view of the heart and multiplying the contralateral lung area's longest diameter by the longest perpendicular to it) is said to eliminate miscalculation. The O/E LHR is lower in fetuses with CDH compared to normal fetuses, and lower still in babies who die with CDH than those who survive.

In these patients with poor prognostic signs, fetal surgery for CDH over the last two decades has been disappointing; however, benefit from fetal intervention with tracheal occlusion (FETO) awaits randomized studies. One ongoing trial in Europe aims to enroll patients with severe hypoplasia (O/E LHR <25%) and randomize half to FETO. The acronym for the trial is TOTAL (Tracheal Occlusion to Accelerate Lung Growth, www.totaltrial.eu).

Favorable outcomes in CDH with the use of antenatal steroids has not been resolved in the clinical setting. Elective delivery at a specialized center is recommended with no benefit from caesarean section.

Postnatal management is aimed at reducing barotrauma to the hypoplastic lung by introducing high-frequency oscillatory ventilation (HFOV) or permissive hypercapnea, and treating the severe pulmonary hypertension with nitric oxide. No clear benefits for CDH with extracorporeal membrane oxygenation (ECMO) have been concluded in a 2002 Cochrane ECMO study.

Surgery for CDH is no longer an emergency procedure. Delayed repair following stabilization is employed in most pediatric surgical centers. Primary repair using the transabdominal route is achieved in 60%–70% of patients, with the rest requiring a prosthetic patch. Complications of sepsis or reherniation with prosthetic patch requiring revision are recorded in 50% of survivors.

Cystic lung lesions

Congenital cystic adenomatoid malformations (CCAMs), bronchopulmonary sequestrations (BPSs), or "hybrid" lesions containing features of both are common cystic lung lesions noted on prenatal scan (Figures 6.3 and 6.4). Less common lung anomalies include bronchogenic cysts, congenital lobar emphysema, and bronchial atresia. Congenital cystic lung lesions are rare anomalies, with an incidence of 1 in 10,000 to 1 in 35,000.

Prenatal detection rate of lung cysts at the routine 18th- to 20th-week scan is almost 100% and may be the most common mode of actual presentation. Most of these lesions are easily distinguished from CDH; however, sonographic

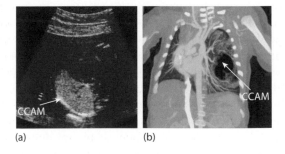

Figure 6.3 **(a)** Prenatal diagnosis of CCAM and **(b)** reconstruction CT scan of a large CCAM of the left upper lobe.

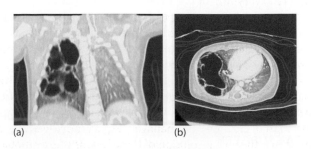

Figure 6.4 **(a)** Chest radiograph and **(b)** CCAM of right upper lobe.

features of CCAM or BPS are not sufficiently accurate and correlate poorly with histology. MRI, though not routinely used, may provide better definition for this condition; however, inaccuracies were reported in 11% of cases.

Bilateral disease and hydrops fetalis (5%) are indicators of poor outcome, whereas mediastinal shift, polyhydramnios, and early detection are not poor prognostic signs. In the absence of termination, the natural fetal demise of antenatally diagnosed cystic lung disease is 28%. Spontaneous involution of cystic lung lesions can occur, but complete postnatal resolution is rare, and apparent spontaneous "disappearance" of antenatally diagnosed lesions should be interpreted with care, as nearly half of these cases subsequently require surgery.

Close monitoring of the antenatally detected lesion with serial USs to detect the size of the lesion, location, volume, blood supply, and compromise to the fetus is performed. The cystic adenomatous malformation volume ratio predicts an 80% increased risk of hydrops fetalis if more than 1.6; a ratio less than 1.6 is associated with a survival rate of 94% and less than 3% risk of hydrops fetalis.

In only 10% of cases, the need for fetal intervention arises. The spectrum of intervention include simple centesis of amniotic fluid, thoracoamniotic shunt placement, percutaneous laser ablation, and open fetal surgical resection. Maternal steroid administration has also been reported to have a beneficial effect on some CCAMs, although the mechanism is unclear. A large cystic mass and hydrops in isolated cystic lung lesions are the only real indication for fetal intervention.

Normal vaginal delivery in recommended unless maternal condition indicates otherwise. Large lesions are predicted to become symptomatic shortly after birth (as high as 45% in some series); thus, delivery at a specialized center would be appropriate. However, smaller lesions are less likely to be symptomatic at birth, and delivery could be done at the referring institution with follow-up in a pediatric surgery clinic.

Postnatal management is dictated by clinical status at birth. Symptomatic lesions require urgent radiological evaluation with chest radiograph and, ideally, computed tomography (CT) scan (Figure 6.2) followed by surgical excision. In asymptomatic cases, postnatal investigation consists of chest CT scan within 1 month of birth, even if regression or resolution is noted on prenatal scanning. Plain radiography should not be relied upon since it will miss and underestimate many lesions.

Surgical excision of postnatal asymptomatic lesions remains controversial, with some centers opting for conservative management. The approach to treating this asymptomatic group has evolved in some centers, whereby a CT scan is performed within 1 month postbirth, followed by surgery before 6 months of age due to the inherent risk of infection and malignant transformation. Small lesions, less than 1 cm, may be managed expectantly, bearing in mind that the true resolution of these lesions is exceptional. Successful outcome of greater than 95% has been reported for these surgically managed asymptomatic lung lesions.

Congenital high airway obstruction syndrome (CHAOS) is usually caused by laryngeal atresia or tracheal obstruction and can be detected from about 17 weeks. Due to lack of communication, fluid is accumulated in the tracheobronchial tree. Sonographic appearance of CHAOS has distinctive features of bilaterally massively enlarged, uniformly hyperechogenic lungs, with eversion of the diaphragm and compression of the heart. It results in a picture suggestive of a small heart surrounded by massive lungs. In some, the absence of tracheal flow in color Doppler can be visualized during fetal breathing movements. CHAOS is usually isolated but may be a feature of Fraser syndrome. The antenatal history of CHAOS depends on the severity of obstruction; however, in the vast majority of cases, this condition is fatal.

Abdominal wall defects

Abdominal wall defects in fetuses include gastroschisis, exomphalos, bladder exstrophy complex, cloacal exstrophy, and body stalk syndrome. The defects that occur more commonly are gastroschisis and exomphalos, but these are distinct abdominal wall defects with an unclear etiology and a controversial prognosis. Attention may be drawn to their presence during the second trimester because of raised maternal serum APF level or abnormal US scan.

EXOMPHALOS

Exomphalos is characteristically a midline defect, at the insertion point of the umbilical cord, with a viable sac composed of amnion and peritoneum containing herniated abdominal contents (Figure 6.5). Incidence is known to be 1 in 4000 live births. Associated major abnormalities—which include trisomy 13, 18, and 21; Beckwith–Wiedemann syndrome (macroglossia, gigantism, exomphalos); pentology of Cantrell (sternal, pericardial, cardiac, abdominal wall, and diaphragmatic defect); and cardiac, gastrointestinal, and renal abnormalities—are noted in 60%–70% of cases. Thus karyotyping, in addition to detailed sonographic review and fetal echocardiogram, is essential for complete prenatal screening. Fetal intervention is unlikely in this condition. If termination is not considered, normal vaginal delivery at a center with neonatal surgical expertise is recommended and delivery by caesarean section only reserved for large exomphalos with exteriorized liver to prevent damage.

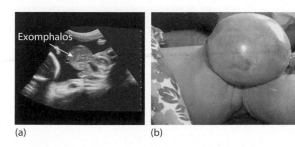

(a) (b)

Figure 6.5 **(a)** Prenatal and **(b)** postnatal images of exomphalos.

Surgical repair includes primary closure or a staged repair with a silo for giant defects. Occasionally, in vulnerable infants with severe pulmonary hypoplasia or complex cardiac abnormalities, the exomphalos may be left intact and allowed to slowly granulate and epithelialize by application of antiseptic solution. Postnatal morbidity occurs in 5%–10% of cases. Malrotation and adhesive bowel obstruction does contribute to mortality in isolated exomphalos; however, the majority of these children survive to live normal lives.

GASTROSCHISIS

Gastroschisis is an isolated lesion that usually occurs on the right side of the umbilical defect with evisceration of the abdominal contents directly into the amniotic cavity (Figure 6.6). The incidence has increased from 1.66 per 10,000 births to 4.6 per 10,000 births, affecting mainly young mothers typically less than 20 years old. Associated anomalies are noted in only 5%–24% of cases with bowel atresia, the most common coexisting abnormality. On prenatal scan with a detection rate of 100%, the bowel appears to be free-floating, and the loops may appear to be thickened due to damage by amniotic fluid exposure causing a "peel" formation. Dilated loops of bowel (Figure 6.3) may be seen from obstruction secondary to protrusion from a defect or atresia due to intestinal ischemia.

Predicting outcome in fetuses with gastroschisis based on prenatal US findings remains a challenge. There is some evidence that US monitoring of growth, umbilical artery Doppler, and bowel diameter measurements lead to early detection of complications and can help improve mortality. However, a recent systematic review looking at the outcome of antenatal bowel dilatation showed no difference in mortality, length of bowel resection, time to feeding, or length of hospital stay. To reduce the rate of third-trimester fetal loss, serial USs are performed to monitor the development of bowel obstruction, and delivery at around 37 weeks is recommended at a center with neonatal surgical expertise.

A recent study[5] has challenged elective preterm delivery with a randomized control trial. Delivery by caesarean section has no advantage over normal vaginal route. Despite efforts to plan elective delivery, 50% of cases will require emergency caesarean section due to development of fetal distress.

Various methods of postnatal surgical repair include the traditional primary closure, reduction of bowel without anesthesia, reduction by preformed silo, or reduction by means of a traditional silo. Coexisting intestinal atresia could be repaired by primary anastomosis or staged with stoma formation. Variation in achieving full enteral feeding due to prolonged gut dysmotility is expected in all cases.

The long-term outcome in gastroschisis is dependent on the condition of the bowel. In uncomplicated cases, the outcome is excellent in more than 90%. The mortality of live-born infants is 5%, with a further 5% suffering short bowel syndrome and 10% requiring surgery for adhesive bowel obstruction. Late third-trimester fetal loss should always be mentioned during fetal counseling.

Tracheoesophageal fistula and esophageal atresia

Repair of TOF)/esophageal atresia (EA) is a condition that measures the skill of pediatric surgeons from trainee to independent surgeon (Figure 6.7). The incidence is estimated at 1 in 3000 births. Prenatally, the condition may be suspected from maternal polyhydramnios and absence of a fetal stomach bubble at the 20th-week anomaly scan. Prenatal scan diagnosis of TOF/OA is estimated to be less than 42%

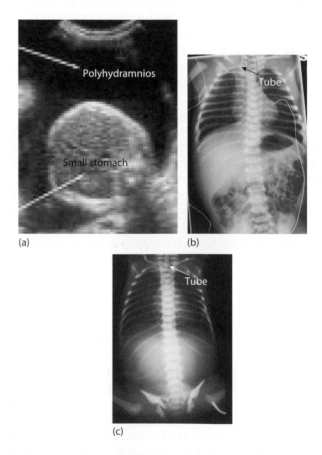

(a)   (b)

(c)

Figure 6.7 **(a)** Prenatal imaging of suspected TOF with polyhydramnios and small stomach. **(b)** Plain radiograph showing esophageal pouch tube and distal gas confirming tracheoesophageal fistula with esophageal atresia. **(c)** Plain radiograph showing esophageal pouch tube and no abdominal gas, confirming isolated esophageal atresia.

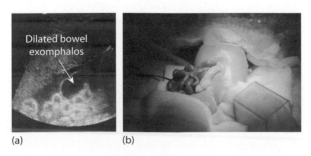

(a)   (b)

Figure 6.6 **(a)** Prenatal and **(b)** postnatal images of gastroschisis.

sensitive, with a positive predictive value of 56%. Additional diagnostic clues are provided by associated anomalies such as trisomy (13, 18, and 21), VACTERAL sequence (vertebral, anorectal, cardiac, tracheoesophageal, renal, limbs), and CHARGE association (coloboma, heart defects, atresia choanae, retarded development, genital hypoplasia, ear abnormality). These associated anomalies are present in more than 50% of cases and worsen the prognosis; thus, prenatal karyotyping is essential. Duodenal atresia may coexist with TOF/OA. The risk of recurrence in subsequent pregnancies for isolated TOF/OA is less than 1%. Delivery is advised to be at a specialized center with neonatal surgical input.

Postnatal surgical management is dependent on the size and condition of the baby, length of esophageal gap, and associated anomalies. Primary repair of the esophagus is the treatment of choice; however, if not achieved, staged repair with upper esophageal pouch care and gastrostomy or organ replacement with stomach or large bowel are other options. Associated anomalies require evaluation and treatment.

Long-term outcomes are indicated by improved perinatal management and inherent structural and functional defects in the trachea and esophagus. In early life, growth of the child is reported to be below the 25th centile in 50% of cases, respiratory symptoms are reported in two-thirds of TOF/OA, and gastroesophageal reflux is recorded in 50% of patients. Quality of life is better in the isolated group with successful primary repair as compared to those with associated anomalies and delayed repair.

Gastrointestinal lesions

The presence of dilated loops of bowel (>15 mm in length and 7 mm in diameter) on prenatal US scan is indicative of bowel obstruction.

Duodenal atresia has a characteristic "double-bubble" appearance on prenatal scan, resulting from the simultaneous dilatation of the stomach and proximal duodenum. Detection rate on second-trimester anomaly scan is almost 100% in the presence of polyhydramnios and the double-bubble sign. However, a late trimester event may only be detected due to polyhydramnios or not detected at all. Associated anomalies are present in approximately 50% of cases, most notably trisomy 21 in 30% of cases, cardiac anomalies in 20%, and the VACTERL association (vertebral, anorectal, cardiac, tracheoesophageal, renal, and limbs).

The incidence of duodenal atresia is 1 in 5000 live births. The postnatal survival rate is >95%, with associated anomalies, low birth weight, and prematurity contributing to the <5% mortality. Temporary delay in enteral feeding occurs due to the dysmotility in the dilated stomach and duodenum.

There are many bowel abnormalities that may be noted on prenatal scanning (dilated bowel, ascites, cystic masses, hyperperistalsis, poyhydramnios, and echogenic bowel); however, none is absolutely predictive of postnatal outcome. Patients with obstruction frequently have findings (especially in the third trimester) of bowel dilatation (Figure 6.8),

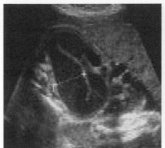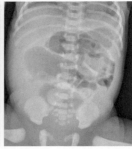

Figure 6.8 **(a)** Prenatal and **(b)** postnatal imaging of intestinal atresia.

polyhydramnios, and hyperperistalsis, but US is much less sensitive in diagnosing large bowel anomalies than those in small bowel. Since the large bowel is mostly a reservoir, with no physiologic function in utero, defects in this region such as anorectal malformations or Hirschsprung disease are very difficult to detect. Bowel dilatation and echogenic bowel may be associated with cystic fibrosis; therefore, all such fetuses should undergo postnatal evaluation for this disease. Prenatally diagnosed small bowel atresia does not select for a group with a worse prognosis, and survival rates are 95%–100%.

Abdominal cysts

Abdominal cystic lesions are not an uncommon diagnosis at antenatal US examination. A cystic mass identified in this way may represent a normal structural variant or a pathological entity requiring surgical intervention postnatally. Despite increasingly sophisticated equipment, some congenital anomalies have significant false-positive rates on US, and fetal cystic abdominal masses in particular can be difficult to diagnose accurately. Excluding cysts of renal origin, the differential diagnosis includes ovarian cysts, enteric duplication cysts, meconium pseudocysts, mesenteric cysts and choledochal cysts. Less common diagnoses include extralobar pulmonary sequestration and pancreatic, splenic, urachal, and adrenal cysts. Almost all cysts are benign, and many are self-limiting; however, these cysts create a high level of anxiety for the prospective parents, especially suspected adrenal cysts. Regular antenatal consultation and fetal counseling by the appropriate team may reduce parental anxiety levels. There is a very small role for fetal intervention. Diagnostic accuracy is greater than 90%. Resolution of these cysts was reported in 30% of cases, and of all the antenatally diagnosed cysts, 40% will come to surgical intervention. Postnatal imaging is essential (Figure 6.9).

Sacrococcygeal teratoma

SCT is the most common neonatal tumor, accounting for 1 in 35,000–40,000 births (Figure 6.10). Four types have been defined:

- Type 1—external tumor with a small presacral component
- Type 2—external tumor with a large presacral component

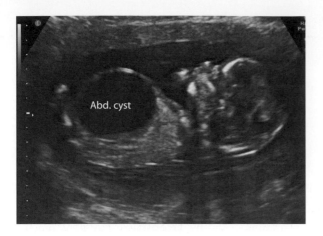

Figure 6.9 Nonspecific prenatal cyst showed complete resolution on postnatal Imaging.

- Type 3—predominantly presacral with a small external component
- Type 4—entirely presacral

The latter carries the worst prognosis due to delay in diagnosis and malignant presentation. Doppler US is the diagnostic tool; however, fetal MRI provides better definition of the intrapelvic component. SCT is a highly vascular tumor, and the fetus may develop high cardiac output failure, anemia, and ultimately hydrops, with a mortality of almost 100%. Fetal treatment of tumor resection or ablation of feeding vessel has been attempted in hydropic patients. Caesarean section may be offered to patients with large tumors to avoid the risk of bleeding during delivery. Postnatal outcomes following surgery in type 1 and 2 lesions are favorable; however, type 3 and 4 tumors may present with urological and bowel problems, with less favorable outcomes. Long-term follow-up with AFP and serial pelvic US is mandatory to exclude recurrence of the disease.

Renal anomalies

Urogenital abnormalities are among the most common disorders seen in the perinatal period and account for almost

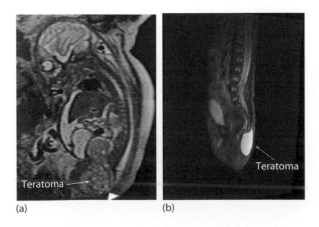

(a)   (b)

Figure 6.10 **(a)** Prenatal MRI and **(b)** postnatal image of sacrococcygeal teratoma.

20% of all prenatally diagnosed anomalies. The routine use of antenatal US scans has resulted in the early detection of these conditions and, in selected cases, has led to the development of management strategies including fetal intervention aimed at preservation of renal function. Two major issues are the indications for intervention in bladder outlet obstruction and early pyeloplasty in infancy in cases with hydronephrosis.

Prenatal evaluation of a dilated urinary tract is based on serial US scans as well as measurement of urinary electrolytes. Ultrasonography provides measurements of the renal pelvis, assessment of the renal parenchyma, as well as detection of cysts in the cortex. In severe disease, lack of amniotic fluid may make US assessment of the renal tract difficult, and MRI may be helpful. Oligohydramnios is indicative of poor renal function and poor prognosis owing to the associated pulmonary hypoplasia. Urogenital anomalies coexist with many other congenital abnormalities, and amniocentesis should be offered in appropriate cases. It is estimated that 3% of infants will have an abnormality of the urogenital system, and half of these will require some form of surgical intervention.

UPPER URINARY TRACT OBSTRUCTION

Antenatal hydronephrosis accounts for 0.6%–0.65% pregnancies. The most common cause of prenatal hydronephrosis is pelviureteric junction (PUJ) obstruction, others being transient hydronephrosis, physiological hydronephrosis, multicystic kidney, PUVs, ureterocele, ectopic ureter, etc. The prognosis of antenatally diagnosed hydronephrosis in unilateral disease with renal pelvic diameter of <10 mm is excellent. Spontaneous resolution is noted in 20% of patients at birth and 80% at 3 years of age. Only 17% of prenatally diagnosed hydronephroses need surgical intervention. Postnatal management of hydronephrosis requires US at birth and at 1 month of age, and further evaluation with radiology and scintigraphy if an abnormality is suspected.

LOWER URINARY TRACT OBSTRUCTION

PUVs are the most common cause for lower urinary tract obstruction in boys, with an incidence of 1 in 2000–4000 live male births (Figure 6.11). The diagnosis of PUV is suspected on the prenatal US finding of bilateral hydronephrosis associated with a thickened bladder and decreased amniotic fluid volume. Serial fetal urine analysis may provide prognostic information on renal function. Prenatal diagnosis for patients with PUV is a poor prognostic sign, with 64% incidence of renal failure and transient pulmonary failure, compared to 33% in postnatally diagnosed patients. Pulmonary hypoplasia secondary to oligohydramnios largely contributes to the morbidity and mortality from fetal urethral obstruction. Outcomes of fetal intervention with vesicoamniotic shunting or fetal cystoscopic ablation of the urethral valve are still under review and await a multicenter trial.

Postnatal management includes US confirmation of the diagnosis, bladder drainage via a suprapubic or urethral route, and contrast imaging of the urethra. Primary PUV ablation, vesicostomy, and ureterostomy are postnatal

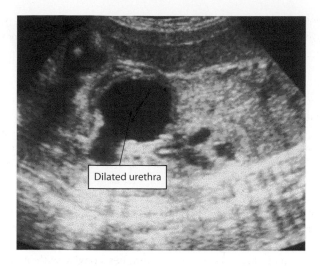

Figure 6.11 Keyhole sign of posterior urethral valves.

surgical options. The overall outcome from this disease is unfavorable.

CONCLUSION

The boundaries of pediatric surgical practice have been extended by prenatal diagnosis. The care of patients with surgically correctable defects can now be planned prenatally with the collaborative effort of obstetricians, geneticists, neonatologists, and pediatric surgeons. Essential to prenatal counseling is the understanding of the specific surgical condition's prenatal natural history, the limitations of prenatal diagnosis, the detection of associated anomalies, the risks and indications of fetal intervention programs, and postnatal outcomes. Prenatal counseling is an essential component of pediatric surgical practice and should be ensured in the training program for future pediatric surgeons.

REFERENCES

1. Collins S, Impey L. Prenatal diagnosis: Types and techniques. EHD 2012; 88(1): 3–8.
2. Brock DJH, Sutcliffe RG. Alpha-fetoprotein in the antenatal diagnosis of anencephaly and spina bifida. Lancet 1972; 2:197–9.
3. Lakhoo K (Guest ed). Neonatal surgical conditions. In: Mallouf E (ed). Best Practice Guidelines (EHD), 2014; 90: 917–50.

FURTHER READING

1. Chevalier RL. Perinatal obstructive nephropathy. *Semin Perinatol* 2004; 28: 124–31.
2. Gajewska-Knapik K, Impey L. Congenital lung lesions: Prenatal diagnosis and intervention. *Semin Paediatr Surg* 2015; 24(4): 156–9.
3. Holmes N. Management of Posterior Urethral Valves. Up to Date December 2015.
4. Puri A, Grover VP, Agarwala S, Mitra DK, Bhatnagar V. Initial surgical treatment as a determinant of bladder dysfunction in posterior urethral valves. *Pediatr Surg Int* 2002; 18: 438–43.
5. Sudhakaran N, Sothinathan U, Patel S. Fetal surgery. *EHD* 2012; 88(1): 15–9.
6. Tailor J, Roy PG, Hitchcock R, Grant H, Johnson P, Joseph VT, Lakhoo K. Long term functional outcome of sacrococcygeal teratoma in a UK regional centre (1993–2006). *Pediatr Hematol Oncol* 2009 Mar; 31(3): 183–6.
7. Thakkar HS, Bradshaw C, Impey L, Lakhoo K. Postnatal outcomes of antenatally diagnosed intraabdominal cysts: A 22-year single-institution series. *Pediatr Surg Int* 2015; 31(2) :187–90.

7

Fetal and birth trauma

PREM PURI AND PIOTR HAJDUK

FETAL TRAUMA

Traumatic injuries in pregnancy are a major cause of non-obsterics maternal and neonatal morbidity and mortality.[1-4] About 40 years ago, it was estimated that 6%–8% of pregnant women were affected by accidental injury.[5] This number is likely to be greater now because more active lifestyles led by pregnant women in today's society may put them at increased risk of injury. When a pregnant woman presents with a major trauma, two lives are at risk. The survival of the fetus depends primarily on maternal survival,[5] but occasionally, the extent of maternal injury does not correlate with the degree of fetal injury.[1,6,7]

Treatment priorities for traumatic pregnant women remain the same as in patients who are not pregnant, although resuscitation and stabilization should be modified to account for the anatomical and physiological changes of the pregnancy.[8] The first consideration in the management of maternal trauma in an accident is to ensure the survival of the mother, as is recommended by the Advanced Trauma Life Support Program.

Assessment of the fetus forms part of the secondary survey of the mother and should be performed in conjunction with an obstetrician, because beyond 24 weeks gestational age, the fetus is potentially viable if urgent delivery is required.

Assessment of the fetus includes the following: the date of the last menstrual period, measuring the fundal height, examination for uterine contractions and tenderness, fetal movements, and fetal heart rate. An important part is the vaginal examination for amniotic fluid or blood.

Fetal distress can occur at any time and without warning. The fetus should be continually monitored to ensure early recognition of fetal distress by using the ultrasonic Doppler cardioscope. Signs of fetal distress include the following: bradycardia (<110 b.p.m.), inadequate accelerations in fetal heart rate in response to uterine contraction, and late decelerations in fetal heart rate in response to uterine relaxation.

In blunt maternal–fetal trauma, placental abruption is the leading cause of death with maternal survival.[9,10] Occasionally, minor maternal trauma may disrupt the placenta "lifeline" by shearing the relatively rigid placenta from the more elastic uterine wall, thereby leading to fetal distress and subsequent fetal death.[6] The clinical signs of placental abruption include the following: vaginal bleeding, uterine irritability, abdominal tenderness, increasing fundal height, maternal hypovolemic shock, and fetal distress. Although the common classical presentation of placental abruption involves vaginal bleeding and abdominal pain, some cases of traumatic abruption occur without these symptoms, and fetal distress may not develop for several hours.

The fetus should be considered salvageable in the face of severe or even mortal maternal injury, and more than 150 cases of successful postmortem cesarean section delivery and numerous deliveries of normal neonates just before maternal death have been described.[11,12] Fetal injuries after trauma may be treatable, but only if they are recognized. Penetrating trauma by gunshot or stab wounds, although rare,[6] is usually obvious, and thus, appropriate surgical intervention has to be undertaken (Figure 7.1a,b). Although most cases of penetrating fetal trauma are fatal to the fetus, some cases of fetal salvage have been reported.[13] In contrast, surgically treatable fetal injury may go unrecognized after blunt maternal trauma, while these injuries are much more frequent. Thus, one can recognize that after 24 weeks' gestation, cesarean section for fetal salvage is indicated in the presence of placental abruption with fetal distress or treatable life-threatening fetal injury, or if there is obvious impending or recent maternal death.

A pediatric surgeon should participate in the evaluation and management of both the pregnant patient and the neonate delivered after maternal trauma, together with the obstetrician and the neonatologist. Pregnant women should be hospitalized after trauma for appropriate evaluation and fetal monitoring, in the hope of decreasing trauma-related fetal deaths. In recent years, it is expected that every

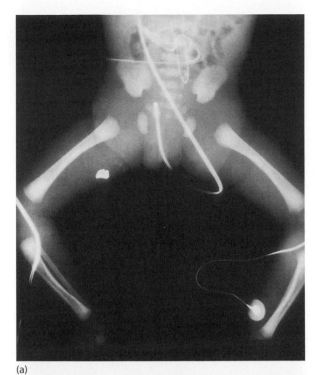

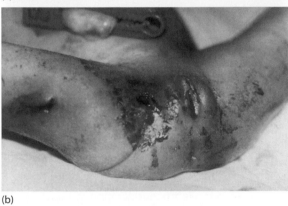

(a)

(b)

Figure 7.1 (a) X-ray of a neonate born to a mother who sustained accidental gunshot wounds to her abdomen. Note metallic pellet in the right thigh. (b) Clinical photograph of the same infant showing entry wound in the right thigh.

pediatric surgeon must be familiar with the treatment of pediatric trauma. The treatment of the traumatic pregnant woman and the fetus must be part of this skill, especially if the fetus is to be considered a patient.

BIRTH TRAUMA

Birth injuries are defined as injuries associated with mechanical forces producing hemorrhage, edema, tissue disruption, or alteration of organ function occurring during the intrapartum period.[14] With the improvement in obstetric techniques, increased frequency of cesarean section in potentially difficult deliveries, decreased use of difficult forceps, and utilization of fetal heart rate and determination of acid–base status to monitor the fetus during labor, the incidence of birth injuries has decreased in recent years.[15] Furthermore, use of prenatal ultrasonography (US) has allowed early identification of the risk factors for possible birth trauma, including fetal size and position and enlarged fetal organs or masses. Nevertheless, birth injuries still occur and represent an important problem for the clinician; the incidence of birth trauma is reported to be 2–8 per 1000 live births.[16,17]

Birth injury is usually associated with unusual compressive or traction forces in association with abnormal presentation of the fetus. Factors that predispose to birth injury include primiparity, cephalopelvic disproportion, dystocia, prematurity, prolonged labor, macrosomia, abnormal presentation, forceps application, version, and extraction.[14,16,17] The newborn at greatest risk for birth injury is the one in breech presentation.

Types of birth trauma

HEAD INJURIES

Caput succedaneum

Caput succedaneum is a diffuse edematous, occasionally hemorrhagic swelling of the scalp, superficial to the periosteum, occurring secondary to compression of the presenting part during prolonged labor. Usually, caput succedaneum requires no treatment, and the swelling disappears spontaneously in a week or so. Rarely, hemorrhage into soft tissue may cause anemia that requires blood transfusion or may lead to hyperbilirubinemia, or both.[18]

Cephalhematoma

Cephalhematoma is a subperiosteal collection of blood most often found in the parietal region and sharply delineated by the surrounding suture lines (Figure 7.2). In 10%–25% of cephalhematomas there is an underlying skull fracture, which is usually of linear type and clinically unimportant.[19] The precise mechanism of production of cephalhematoma is not well established. Repeated buffeting of the fetal skull against the maternal pelvis during a prolonged labor and mechanical trauma caused by the use of forceps and vacuum extractor in delivery have been implicated as important factors. Cephalhematomas have been reported to originate in utero, antipartum. Petrikovsky et al.[20] found seven cases of cephalhematomas identified prenatally in 16,292 fetuses during comprehensive US examinations. Premature rupture of the membranes was seen and was suggested as an associated factor.

Most cephalhematomas resolve spontaneously within a few weeks. Aspiration of the hematoma is contraindicated because of the risk of introducing infection. Drainage and antibiotic therapy are only indicated in the rare case of superinfection of the cephalhematoma.[17] Occasionally, serious complications such as anemia, jaundice, abscess, septicemia, meningitis, osteomyelitis, disseminated intravascular coagulation, shock with acute hemorrhage, and depressed skull fractures have been reported in association with cephalhematomas.[14,21,22] Management involves careful observation for these complications.

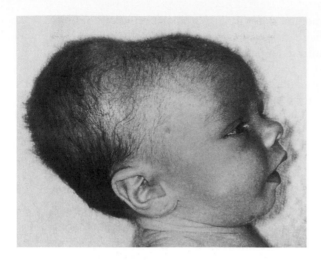

Figure 7.2 Large cephalhematoma.

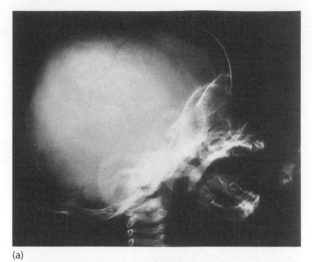

(a)

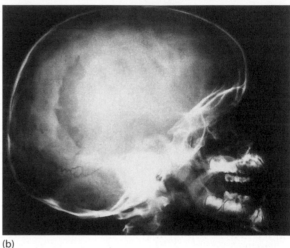

(b)

Figure 7.3 **(a)** Linear fracture of left parietal bone at birth. **(b)** Three years later, the patient presented with a pulsatile swelling in the left parietal region. X-ray shows an extensive bone defect due to leptomeningeal cyst.

Skull fractures

Most of the skull fractures are linear, occurring in association with cephalhematomas and usually involving the parietal bones (Figure 7.3a). No specific treatment is required for linear fractures, but skull x-rays should be repeated when the infant reaches 2–4 months of age to rule out "growing fracture of the skull" associated with a leptomeningeal cyst (Figure 7.3b). A leptomeningeal cyst can occur rarely if the trauma causing the linear fracture tears the underlying dura, thereby permitting herniation of the meninges and brain. This requires surgical intervention to avoid progressive brain damage.[23]

Depressed skull fractures are most often caused by pressure of the fetal head against the maternal pelvis or in association with forceps delivery (Figure 7.4). In babies with no abnormal neurological signs, expectant treatment has been associated with spontaneous resolution.[24] Several nonsurgical techniques for elevation of depressed skull fracture in the newborn have been described, including suction with a breast pump or vacuum extractor, and by digital manipulation. Fracture reduction by neurosurgical elevation should be considered when the depth is more than 2 cm.[25] Indications for surgical elevation of depressed skull fracture include the following[24]:

1. Radiographic evidence of bone fragments within the brain
2. Neurological deficit
3. Signs of increased intracranial pressure
4. Failure to elevate the fracture by closed manipulation

Intracranial hemorrhage

Intracranial hemorrhage following birth trauma may occur in the epidural space, the subarachnoid space, or the subdural space, or within the brain.

Epidural hemorrhage in newborns is rare, typically associated with an instrument-assisted vaginal delivery. A linear skull fracture accompanies neonatal epidural

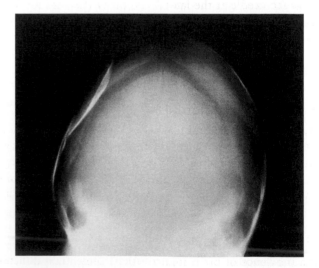

Figure 7.4 Depressed fracture of right parietal bone following forceps delivery.

hemorrhage in the majority of cases and may be associated with a cephalhematoma. As in adults, there may be a delay in the onset of symptoms. The classically described middle meningeal artery laceration from the temporal bone fracture does occur, but neonatal epidural hemorrhage may also be caused by a sinus or vein injury. Treatment of the neonatal epidural hemorrhage is dependent on prompt recognition and typically requires surgical intervention.[26]

Subarachnoid hemorrhage is the most common form of birth-related traumatic intracranial hemorrhage in the newborn.[19] Blood in the subarachnoid space can be documented by lumbar puncture and the diagnosis confirmed by computerized tomography (CT) scan. In the vast majority of cases, traumatic subarachnoid hemorrhage is benign and does not require any treatment. Occasionally, it may result in a communicating hydrocephalus. Subdural hemorrhage is caused by rupture of the cerebral veins bridging the subdural space, occurring as a result of excessive molding of the baby's head during labor or delivery. Most subdural hematomas are infratentorial and bilateral, but occasionally, they have been described in the posterior fossa. Principal factors that predispose to the occurrence of subdural hematoma include large-size infants,[19] breech delivery,[27] and forceps extraction in primiparous women.[28] Clinical features of neonatal subdural hemorrhage may include pallor, vomiting, irritability, seizures, unequal pupils, drowsiness, hypotonia, high-pitched cry, tense fontanelle, and retinal hemorrhages. The diagnosis is confirmed by a subdural tap, CT scan (Figure 7.5), or magnetic resonance imaging (MRI).[29] Although US is a standard practice for detecting germinal matrix hemorrhage in the preterm neonate,[30] it is unlikely to be as accurate as a CT scan in diagnosing peripheral lesions in subarachnoid or subdural space.[31] MRI imaging in general has high sensitivity for intracranial hemorrhage and, with its lack of ionizing radiation, is a favorable technique for the further evaluation of birth trauma over CT, especially for a neonate.[32,33] The treatment consists of repeated tapping of the subdural space using a 20-gauge needle at the lateral margin of the anterior fontanelle. In most cases, subdural collections can be treated successfully with repeated taps. Rarely, membrane stripping or subdural space shunting may be required to deal with persistent subdural collections.

Intracerebral hemorrhage

Traumatic intracerebral hemorrhage is the least common intracranial hemorrhage in the newborn.[19] The clinical features are those of increased intracranial pressure. The diagnosis can be made with cerebral US, CT scan, or MRI, and regression or complications can be monitored with serial studies.[29]

SPINAL CORD INJURIES

The incidence of birth injury to the spinal cord is difficult to determine because most neonatal postmortem examinations do not include complete examination of the

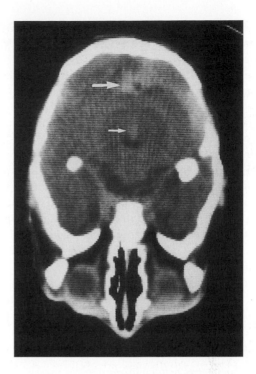

Figure 7.5 CT brain scan without intravenous contrast medium in a newborn, showing blood in the subarachnoid space (large white arrow) and blood in the floor of the fourth ventricle (small white arrow).

spinal cord.[34] The leading cause of neonatal spinal cord injury is delivery of the fetus with marked hyperextension of the neck in a breech presentation. Approximately 75% of reported spinal cord injuries occurred in infants delivered vaginally in breech presentation.[35] Other predisposing factors are prematurity, shoulder dystocia, intrauterine hypoxia, and precipitous delivery.[36] The application of compressive forceps to the fetal spine during fundal pressure to relieve shoulder dystocia has been reported to result in lower thoracic spinal cord injury in the newborn.[37] The site of spinal cord injury following breech delivery is usually in the lower cervical and upper thoracic region, while injury following vertex presentation is usually located in the upper or midcervical level.[19] The injury is usually caused by stretching of the cord and not by compression. The most common mechanism responsible for spinal cord injury is the use of excessive longitudinal traction on the trunk while the head is still engaged in the pelvis.[38] The spinal cord is relatively inelastic compared with the vertebral fracture or dislocation, or both, and cord transection.

The clinical manifestations of spinal cord injury may fit into one of the following four recognized groups, depending on the severity of the damage incurred[21,39]:

1. Babies who are stillborn or die immediately after birth due to a high cervical or brainstem lesion
2. Neonates who die shortly after birth due to respiratory depression and complications and who generally have upper cervical and midcervical lesions

3. Long-term survivors who have flaccid paralysis in the neonatal period and proceed to develop spasticity and hyperreflexia in the ensuing months

4. Those with minimal neurological signs or spasticity who are often classified as having cerebral palsy[40]

The symptoms in these patients result from partial spinal cord injury or cerebral hypoxia.

When spinal cord injury is suspected, definition of the underlying pathology can be difficult using standard diagnostic procedures, including plain x-ray and CT, with or without myelography. MRI, with its excellent definition and low risk of complication, is the best diagnostic tool available to evaluate clinically suspected spinal cord pathology.[41] Spinal US is a good imaging method for guiding diagnosis of traumatic spinal cord lesions.[42]

Treatment of spinal cord injuries is supportive and includes physiotherapy, braces, and urological, orthopedic and psychological care. Surgery has little to offer to patients with these types of injuries. Great emphasis should be placed on prevention of spinal cord injury in the newborn.

PERIPHERAL NERVE INJURIES

Injury to the peripheral nerves in the newborn is usually caused by excessive traction or direct compression of nerves during delivery. The nerves most commonly involved are the brachial plexus, facial nerve, and phrenic nerve.

Brachial plexus injury

With the improvement in obstetric techniques, the incidence of birth-related brachial plexus injuries has decreased considerably in recent years. The incidence of brachial plexus birth palsy is estimated to be between 0.4 and 4 per 1000 live births.[43] The injury is usually caused by traction and stretching of the plexus. All lesions occur in the plexus above the level of the clavicle and range from simple neuropraxia, classified by Sunderland[44] as grade I, to full neurotemesis when associated with root avulsion, classified as grade V. Perinatal risk factors include large-for-gestational-age infants (macrosomia), multiparous pregnancies, previous deliveries resulting in brachial plexus birth palsy, prolonged labor, breech delivery, assisted (vacuum or forceps) difficult deliveries, shoulder dystocia, and/or asphyxiated infant.[45–47] Whereas a mechanical basis for brachial plexus injury is well accepted, delivery by cesarean does not exclude the possibility of birth palsy.[43]

Brachial plexus injury has been divided into three main types depending on the site of the injury:

1. Erb's palsy, which results from injury of the fifth and sixth cervical nerve roots, is by far the most common type of injury. The affected arm hangs limply adducted and internally rotated at the shoulder, and extended and pronated at the elbow with a flexed wrist in the typical "waiter's tip" posture (Figure 7.6). The Moro, biceps, and redial reflexes are absent on the affected side. The grasp reflex is intact. These clinical findings are the result of paralysis of the deltoid, supraspinatus, infraspinatus, brachioradialis, and supinator brevis muscles.

2. Klumpke's paralysis results from injury of the eighth cervical and first thoracic nerve roots and is extremely rare as an isolated entity. The intrinsic muscles of the hand and flexors of the wrist and fingers are affected. The grasp reflex is absent. Injury involving the cervical sympathetic fibers of the first thoracic root may result in ipsilateral Horner's syndrome.

3. Injury to the entire brachial plexus results in a flaccid arm with absence of sweating, sensation, and deep tendon reflexes.

The differential diagnosis includes the following: fracture of the clavicle or humerus, traumatic epiphysiolysis of the proximal epiphysis of the humerus, and shoulder dislocation. These injuries can occur in addition to the plexus paralysis or a phrenic nerve palsy. A radiograph of the chest, shoulder, upper arm, and clavicle should be obtained. Electromyography, an exam that is difficult to perform and interpret in the newborn or the infant, currently plays a limited role in the diagnosis of brachial plexus injury. However, it may be useful in the preoperative workup, determining the extent and site of injury, and evaluating the prognosis. MRI or CT myelography of the cervical spine is a very useful exam in preoperative planning.[48–50]

Serial physical examination of children with brachial plexus injury is recommended, because it is essential to predict recovery and determine the need for additional therapeutic or surgical intervention. Passive range of motion and active muscle strength should be assessed. Assessing infants

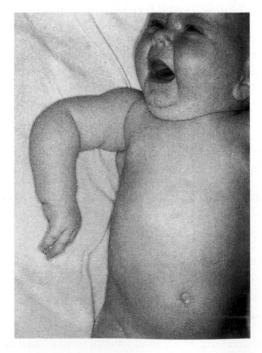

Figure 7.6 Erb's palsy. Characteristic deformity of right arm.

often requires approximation of function by observing spontaneous activity and assessing reflexes (Moro reflex, asymmetric tonic neck, and symmetric tonic neck). Most authors agree that brachial plexus lesions are most often transitory, with 75%–95% of cases advancing to complete recuperation.[51–53] The most recent studies report a lower rate of 66%, with a residual deficit in 20%–30% and considerable alteration of function in 10%–15% of cases.[45,52,54] Total paralysis and the presence of Horner's syndrome are the main factors announcing a poor prognosis.[50] The main principle of management is to maintain the range of "motion" in the affected joints. Treatment should be delayed for a period of 2 weeks after the trauma, in which immobilization of the hand and stretched nerve fibers will allow a spontaneous cure. During the first 2 weeks, the arm has to be adducted to the thorax. Abduction and external rotation position of the shoulder must be prevented due to considerable tension on the brachial plexus in that position. In the other joints, careful passive physiotherapy should be carried out. Thereafter, gentle range-of-motion exercises to shoulder, elbow, wrist, and small joints of the hand may have to be started.

The prognosis of brachial plexus paralysis is better in the Erb's patient than in the patient with Klumpke's variety and, in both of these groups, is better than in total paralysis. In the majority of Erb's palsy cases, a partial or complete recovery can be achieved.[55] Surgical exploration and repair of brachial plexus birth injuries are recommended only when there is no recovery of the biceps by 3 months of age. An electromyography and MRI or myelogram with CT scanning are performed preoperatively.[48,50] Advances in microsurgical techniques and reconstruction of the injured plexus by grafting from the sural nerve can significantly improve the functional result.[48,56,57] Recent use of synthetic collagen nerve conduits has shown very good results in select short-segment brachial plexus repairs.[58] The advantages of synthetic grafts over conventional autologous grafts include eliminating donor site morbidity, increasing the amount of graft material available, and providing direct conduits for neural growth factors produced by the proximal segment to reach the distal segment.

Facial nerve injury

Facial palsy secondary to birth trauma is usually unilateral and most commonly follows compression of the peripheral portion of the nerve, either near its emergence from the stylomastoid foramen or where the nerve transverses the ramus of the mandible. The mechanism of injury is usually either direct trauma from forceps or compression of the side of the face and nerve against the sacral promontory. The affected infant has absent or decreased forehead wrinkling, a persistently open eye, a decreased nasolabial fold, and flattening of the corner of the mouth on the affected side (Figure 7.7). Treatment is conservative, since spontaneous recovery occurs within 1 month in most cases of birth-related facial palsy.[17,47] Initial treatment should be directed at protecting the corneal epithelium from drying with the use of methylcellulose drops instilled every 4 hours. Rarely,

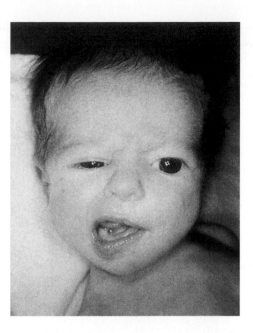

Figure 7.7 Left facial nerve palsy following difficult forceps. Note obliteration of left nasolabial fold with typical deformity of mouth and wide-open left eye.

there is a need for surgical intervention and neurolysis or a nerve cable transplant for the injured or degenerative facial nerve, after confirming the diagnosis by electromyographic and electroneurographic tests.[59]

Phrenic nerve injury

Diaphragmatic paralysis in the neonate results from stretching or avulsion of the fourth and fifth cervical roots, which form the phrenic nerve. The most common cause of phrenic nerve injury is a difficult breech delivery. The majority of injuries are unilateral with right-side dominancy (80%). Bilateral diaphragmatic paralysis is rare. Approximately 78% of cases of birth-related phrenic nerve injury have an associated brachial plexus injury.[60–63]

The clinical features of diaphragmatic paralysis are nonspecific and include respiratory distress with tachypnea, cyanosis, and recurrent atelectasis or pneumonia. Chest x-ray demonstrates an elevated hemidiaphragm about two intercostal spaces higher than the adjacent diaphragm (Figure 7.8a). Diagnosis is confirmed on fluoroscopy, which shows an immobile diaphragm or an abnormal elevation of the diaphragm during inspiration constituting paradoxical movement. Real-time US can also be employed to diagnose phrenic nerve paralysis and can be performed in the intensive care unit in very young babies (Figure 7.8b).

Initial supportive management usually includes mechanical ventilation, oxygen, chest physiotherapy, antibiotics, and nasogastric tube feedings to avoid failure to thrive and to ensure weight gain. Some patients who have severe or increasing respiratory distress may be managed by continuous positive airway pressure (CPAP).[61,62]

Most infants with diaphragmatic paralysis make a complete recovery after conservative treatment (Figure 7.8c).

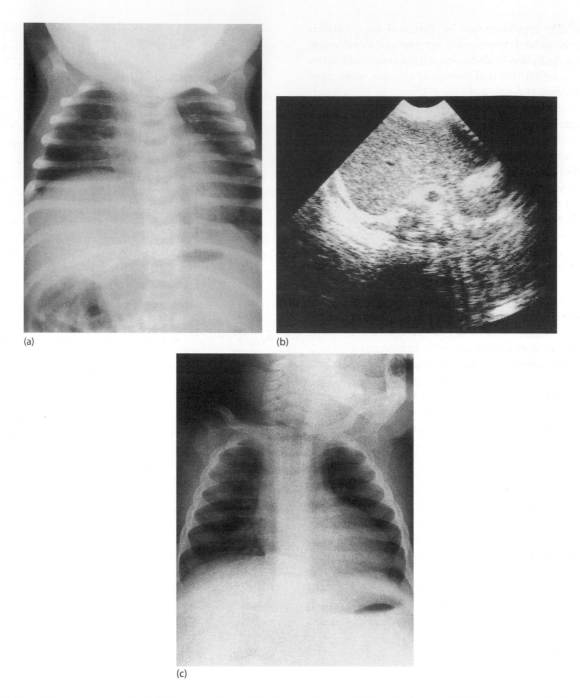

Figure 7.8 Phrenic nerve paralysis. **(a)** Chest radiography shows elevated right diaphragm. **(b)** Transverse real-time sonogram showing blurring in the region of left diaphragm due to respiratory movement. Right diaphragm did not move and is sharply outlined along the liver. **(c)** Chest x-ray 3 months later shows normal right diaphragm after conservative treatment.

Surgery may be required if there is persistent paralysis after 2 weeks of mechanical ventilation or 3 months of medical treatment. However, a recent finding showed that spontaneous recovery was limited after 1–2 months of age, suggesting that early surgical intervention is necessary to obtain a complete resolution of respiratory failure and to gain enough space for subsequent lung development.[61–63] The procedures employed include plication of the diaphragm via thoracoscopy or thoracostomy[61] or incision and replacement of the diaphragm.[64]

INTRA-ABDOMINAL INJURIES

Birth trauma involving intra-abdominal organs is relatively uncommon. The organs most commonly involved are the liver, spleen, adrenal, and kidney.

Liver

The liver is the most commonly injured abdominal organ during the birth process. Factors that predispose to liver trauma include breech presentation, infants with hepatomegaly, large infants, prematurity, and coagulation disorders.[17] The mechanism of birth-related liver injury is thought to be either (1) thoracic compression and pulling of the hepatic ligaments with consequent tearing of the liver parenchyma or (2) direct pressure on the liver leading to subcapsular hemorrhage or rupture.[17]

Hepatic trauma more commonly results in subcapsular hemorrhage than actual rupture of the liver. The infant with subcapsular hemorrhage usually appears to be normal for the first 3 days of life, when the capsule ruptures and there is extravasation of blood into the peritoneal cavity. This is followed by sudden circulatory collapse, abdominal distension and a rapid drop in the hematocrit value. If the processus vaginalis is patent, blood may be seen in the scrotum, suggesting hemoperitoneum. In patients with primary rupture of the liver, major intraperitoneal bleeding occurs immediately, resulting in severe shock and abdominal distension. Abdominal radiographs are not usually very helpful but may show uniform opacity of the abdomen, indicating free intraperitoneal fluid. Abdominal US may confirm the diagnosis and is also useful in differentiating a solid liver tumor from an unruptured subcapsular hemorrhage. A CT scan is recommended, only if the patient is hemodynamically stable (Figure 7.9a–d). Immediate management consists of blood transfusion to restore the blood volume and recognition and correction of any coagulation disorder. This is followed by an immediate laparotomy, with evacuation of the hematoma and repair of any laceration by sutures or by fibrin glue.[65]

Spleen

Rupture of the spleen in the newborn occurs much less often than does rupture of the liver. The predisposing factors and mechanism of injury are quite similar to those of rupture of the liver. Although splenomegaly increases the risk, the vast majority of splenic injuries occur in a spleen of normal size.[66] The presenting features are cardiovascular collapse and abdominal distension. Abdominal radiographs may indicate free fluid in the peritoneal cavity. US scan and abdominal and pelvic CT are recommended to confirm diagnosis.

Nonoperative management of pediatric splenic injuries is now recognized as the treatment of choice in most of the cases. This typically involves following vital signs, serial hematocrits, and physical examination. Blood transfusions are administered as required. Hemodynamically unstable newborns usually with immediate massive hemorrhage may require exploratory laparotomy. In recent years, repair of the spleen has been advocated because of the risk of subsequent serious infections following splenectomy. Since there is a critical mass of the spleen, which prevents overwhelming postsplenectomy infection (OPSI),[67,68] every surgeon should do the utmost to preserve as much of the injured spleen as possible. Fibrin glue, splenorrhaphy, and partial splenectomy are the preferred surgical procedures.[17,69–71] This conservative surgical approach is advocated not only because of the OPSI but also because of the absence of regeneration of the injured spleen after partial splenectomy, which has been proven in animals.[72]

Adrenal

Neonatal adrenal hemorrhage occurs most commonly following a prolonged and difficult labor, culminating in a traumatic delivery. Other contributing factors include asphyxia, prematurity, placental hemorrhage, hemorrhagic disease of the newborn, septicemia, renal vein thrombosis, increased vascularity, and congenital syphilis.[73–78] The right adrenal is involved in over 70% of cases, with bilateral involvement in 5%–10%.[79,80] The presenting features vary with the degree of bleeding. The classical adrenal hemorrhage usually presents between birth and the fourth day of life as an abdominal mass with fever and jaundice or anemia.[78] The differential diagnosis may include adrenal cyst, neuroblastoma, and Wilms' tumor. Diagnosis of neonatal adrenal hemorrhage may be confirmed with a combination of US and CT. Sonography would reveal a suprarenal mass that initially is echogenic and subsequent changes to a cyst-like structure probably indicating fragmentation of the clot (Figure 7.10a,b). A "rim" suprarenal calcification may be seen on abdominal radiographs 2–4 weeks after hemorrhage.[73,81]

In patients with retroperitoneal hemorrhage, treatment consists of blood transfusion, close observation, and follow-up US studies. In infants with massive intraperitoneal hemorrhage, surgical intervention consists of laparotomy, evacuation of hematoma, ligation of bleeders, or adrenalectomy if indicated. It must be remembered that the underlying pathology may be a neuroblastoma,[82,83] and a biopsy should always be taken. Infrequently, a suspicion of an adrenal abscess ensues. In such a situation, a drainage procedure must be performed either percutaneously with US guidance or by operative exploration.

Kidney

Birth-related trauma is rare. Rupture of the kidney in the newborn is usually associated with an underlying congenital anomaly.[84] The presenting signs are hematuria and renal mass. CT is the modality of choice in the evaluation of renal injuries. Renal US may demonstrate renal rupture (Figure 7.11) or ascites. It plays an important role during the follow-up period. Treatment consists of conservative management if possible. Only in cases of severe bleeding or a total rupture of parenchyma or pelvis is a laparotomy indicated, with the correction of underlying congenital anomaly whenever it is necessary.

BONY INJURIES

Fractures due to birth trauma almost always involve the clavicle, humerus, or femur. Epiphyseal separations usually involve upper and lower humeral and upper femoral epiphyses. Dislocations caused by birth trauma are rare.

Fracture of the clavicle

Fracture of the clavicle is the most common fracture in the newborn, usually occurring during a difficult delivery associated with large infants, breech presentation, and shoulder

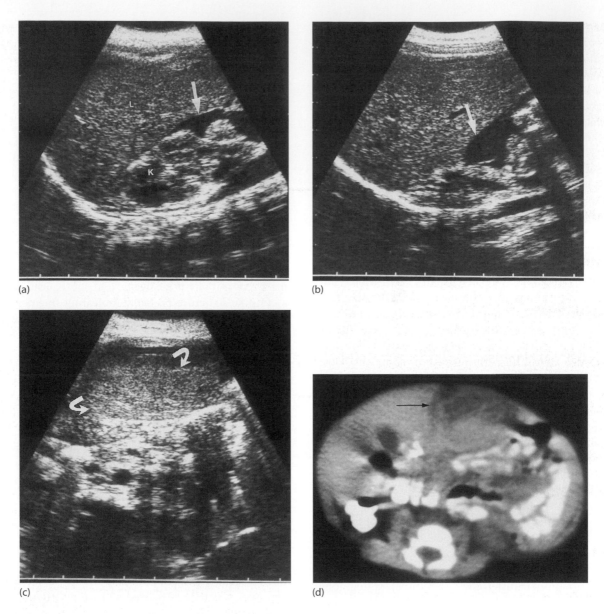

Figure 7.9 Newborn who developed a distended abdomen postdelivery. **(a,b)** Sonographic scan at 36 hours shows echo-poor material due to fresh hemorrhage (white arrow) between the anterior aspect of the right kidney (K) and the inferior aspect of the right lobe of the liver (L). **(c)** Scan through left lobe of liver demonstrating an area of increased echogenicity in keeping with hemorrhage at site of laceration (curved arrows). **(d)** Laceration in left lobe confirmed on CT scan (black arrow).

dystocia.[85] Most fractures are of the greenstick type, occurring in the middle third of the clavicle, but occasionally, the fracture is complete (Figure 7.12). Undisplaced fractures require no treatment. Fractures with marked displacement should be immobilized with a figure-of-eight bandage. Recovery is usually excellent.

Fracture of the humerus

Fractures of the humerus usually occur in the middle third of the shaft and are either transverse or spiral. They are usually greenstick fractures, but occasionally, complete fracture with overriding of fragments may occur. The most common mechanisms responsible for fracture are believed to be traction on the extended arm in the breech presentations and axillary traction to disengage an impacted shoulder in vertex presentations. Treatment consists of strapping the arm to the chest. Complete healing of the fracture fragments usually occurs by 3 weeks.

Fracture of the femur

Femoral shaft fractures usually occur in the middle third and are transverse. The injury usually follows a breech delivery. X-ray invariably shows overriding of the fracture fragments. Treatment consists of Bryant's traction for 3–4 weeks. The prognosis in femoral fractures is usually excellent.

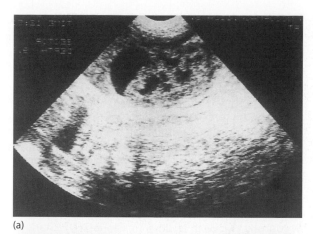

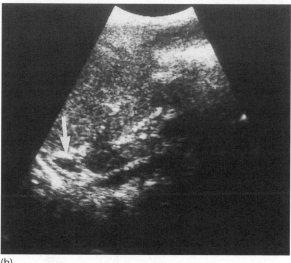

Figure 7.10 **(a)** Right suprarenal echo-poor mass representing a right adrenal hemorrhage (between cursors) in an infant who suffered birth asphyxia. **(b)** Scan performed 1 month later, showing that hemorrhage has almost cleared. Small residual echo-poor area persists (white arrow).

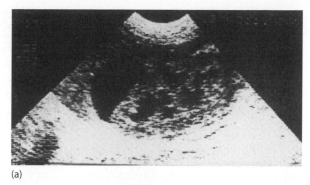

(a)

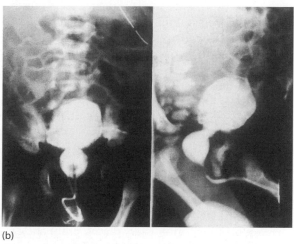

(b)

Figure 7.11 **(a)** Longitudinal sonogram showing an echolucent area in upper pole of right kidney consistent with an intracapsular rupture. Both ureters were hydronephrotic with dilated bladder on sonography. **(b)** Voiding cystogram in the same patient confirmed posterior urethral valves.

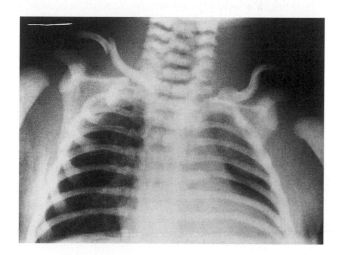

Figure 7.12 Fracture of right clavicle. Typical fracture of middle third of clavicle following forceps delivery.

Epiphyseal separations

The epiphyseal separation or fracture occurs through the hypertrophied layer of cartilage cells in the epiphysis. The most common cause is a difficult breech delivery.[86] A fracture through the proximal epiphyseal plate of the humerus is the most common epiphyseal cartilage injury. Fractures entirely confined to the epiphyseal cartilage cannot be demonstrated radiologically. However, in many cases, the fracture extends through a part of the metaphysis, separating a tiny bony fragment. This fragment is attached to the epiphysis, and if no displacement of the epiphysis has occurred, the fragment may be the only radiographic evidence of fracture. An increased distance of the metaphysis from the joint compared with the opposite side can also indicate fracture through the epiphyseal plate. After 1–2 weeks, a callus becomes visible, confirming the nature of the injury. Diagnosis at the initial stage has to be made primarily on clinical findings of pain on passive motion, swelling, and impaired movement around the joint. Recent reports suggest that epiphyseal separation can be studied by sonography and without the common use of arthrography.[86,87] Treatment of a fracture of the proximal epiphysis of the humerus consists of immobilization of the arm by the side with a sling in 90° flexion.

Epiphysiolysis of the proximal femur is sometimes confused with congenital dislocation of the hip and septic arthritis, and can occur not only after normal delivery but also after delivery by cesarean section.[88] Treatment for a fracture of the proximal epiphysis of the femur is by traction and spica cast for 2 months.

TRAUMA TO THE GENITALIA

Breech delivery is the most common cause of tissue injuries involving the external genitalia. Edema, ecchymoses, and hematomas of the scrotum or the labia majora can occur. No treatment is needed. Spontaneous resolution of edema occurs within 24–48 hours and of discoloration within 4–5 days.

If the tunica vaginalis is injured and blood fills its cavity, a hematocele is formed. The differential diagnosis should include neonatal torsion and patent processus vaginalis.[89,90] An iatrogenic injury to the scrotum with resultant castration during breech extraction has been reported.[91]

REFERENCES

1. Schiff MA, Holt VL, Daling JR. Maternal and infant outcomes after injury during pregnancy in Washington State from 1989 to 1997. *J Trauma* 2002; 53(5): 939–45.
2. Shah KH et al. Trauma in pregnancy: Maternal and fetal outcomes. *J Trauma* 1998; 45(1): 83–6.
3. Weiss HB, Songer TJ, Fabio A. Fetal deaths related to maternal injury. *JAMA* 2001; 286(15): 1863–8.
4. Murphy DJ et al. A cohort study of maternal and neonatal morbidity in relation to use of sequential instruments at operative vaginal delivery. *Eur J Obstet Gynecol Reprod Biol*, 2011; 28: 41–5.
5. Hoff WS et al. Maternal predictors of fetal demise in trauma during pregnancy. *Surg Gynecol Obstet* 1991; 172(3): 175–80.
6. Farmer DL et al. Fetal trauma: Relation to maternal injury. *J Pediatr Surg* 1990; 25(7): 711–4.
7. El Kady D et al. Trauma during pregnancy: An analysis of maternal and fetal outcomes in a large population. *Am J Obstetr Gynecol* 2004; 190(6): 1661–8.
8. Nash P, Driscoll P. ABC of major trauma. Trauma in pregnancy. *BMJ* 1990; 301(6758): 974–6.
9. Oxford CM, Ludmir J. Trauma in pregnancy. *Clin Obstetr Gynecol* 2009; 52(4): 611–29.
10. Curet MJ et al. Predictors of outcome in trauma during pregnancy: Identification of patients who can be monitored for less than 6 hours. *J Trauma* 2000; 49(1): 18–25.
11. Ciuil ID, Talucci RC, Schwab CW. Abdominal trauma. *J Trauma* 1988; 28: 708–10.
12. Arthur RK. Postmortem cesarean section. *Am J Obstet Gynecol* 1978; 132(2): 175–9.
13. Buchsbaum HJ, Staples Jr PP. Self-inflicted gunshot wound to the pregnant uterus: Report of two cases. *Obstet Gynecol* 1985; 65(3): 32–5.
14. Curran JS. Birth-associated injury. *Clin Perinatol* 1981; 8(1): 111–29.
15. Levine MG et al. Birth trauma: Incidence and predisposing factors. *Obstet Gynecol* 1984; 63(6): 792–5.
16. Berle P. Incidence of birth injuries to newborn infants in relation to birth weight. An analysis of the Hessen perinatal study. *Geburtshilfe Frauenheilkd* 1995; 55(1): 23–7.
17. Schullinger JN. Birth trauma. *Pediatr Clin North Am* 1993; 40(6): 1351–8.
18. Murphy WJ. Birth trauma. In: Cloherty JP, Stark A (eds). *Manual of Neonatal Care*, 2nd edn. Boston: Little, Brown, 1985: 251–5.
19. Painter MJ, Bergman I. Obstetrical trauma to the neonatal central and peripheral nervous system. *Semin Perinatol* 1982; 6(1): 89–104.
20. Petrikovsky BM et al. Cephalhematoma and caput succedaneum: Do they always occur in labor? *Am J Obstet Gynecol* 1998; 179(4): 906–8.
21. Zelson C, Lee SJ, Pearl M. The incidence of skull fractures underlying cephalhaematomas in newborn infants. *J Pediatr* 1974; 85: 371–3.
22. Raffensperger JG (ed). Trauma in neonate. In: *Swenson's Pedriatic Surgery*, 5th edn. Norwalk: Appleton and Lange, 1990: 339–42.
23. Kingsley D, Till K, Hoare R. Growing fractures of the skull. *J Neurol Neurosurg Psychiatr* 1978; 41(4): 312–8.
24. Loeser JD, Kilburn HL, Jolley T. Management of depressed skull fracture in the newborn. *J Neurosurg* 1976; 44(1): 62–4.
25. Hung K-L, Liao H-T, Huang J-S. Rational management of simple depressed skull fractures in infants. *J Neurosurg Pediatr* 2005; 103(1): 69–72.
26. Reichard R. Birth injury of the cranium and central nervous system. *Brain Pathol* 2008; 18(4): 565–70.
27. Abroms IF et al. Cervical cord injuries secondary to hyperextension of the head in breech presentations. *Obstet Gynecol* 1973; 41(3): 369–78.
28. O'Driscoll K et al. Traumatic intracranial haemorrhage in firstborn infants and delivery with obstetric forceps. *Br J Obstet Gynaecol* 1981; 88(6): 577–81.
29. Barnes PD. Neuroimaging and the timing of fetal and neonatal brain injury. *J Perinatol* 2001; 21(1): 44–60.
30. Huang C-C, Shen E-Y. Tentorial subdural hemorrhage in term newborns: Ultrasonographic diagnosis and clinical correlates. *Pediatr Neurol* 1991; 7(3): 171–7.
31. Gupta SN, Kechli AM, Kanamalla US. Intracranial hemorrhage in term newborns: Management and outcomes. *Pediatr Neurol* 2009; 40(1): 1–12.
32. Rooks VJ et al. Prevalence and evolution of intracranial hemorrhage in asymptomatic term infants. *AJNR Am J Neuroradiol* 2008; 29(6): 1082–9.

33. Looney CB et al. Intracranial hemorrhage in asymptomatic neonates: Prevalence on mr images and relationship to obstetric and neonatal risk factors 1. *Radiology* 2007; 242(2): 535–41.
34. Bucher HU et al. Birth injury to the spinal cord. *Helv Paediatr Acta* 1979; 34(6): 517–27.
35. Byers RK. Spinal-cord injuries during birth. *Dev Med Child Neurol* 1975; 17(1): 103–10.
36. De Sousa SW, Davis JA. Spinal cord damage in a newborn infant. *Arch Dis Child* 1974; 49: 70–1.
37. Hankins GDV. Lower thoracic spinal cord injury— A severe complication of shoulder dystocia. *Am J Perinatol* 1998; 15(07): 443–4.
38. Tan KL. Elevation of congenital depressed fractures of the skull by the vacuum extractor. *Acta Paediatr Scand* 1974; 63(4): 562–4.
39. Koch BM, Eng GM. Neonatal spinal cord injury. *Arch Phys Med Rehabil* 1979; 60(8): 378–81.
40. Nelson KB, Ellenberg JH. Obstetric complications as risk factors for cerebral palsy or seizure disorders. *J Am Med Assoc* 1984; 251: 1843–8.
41. Mills JF et al. Upper cervical spinal cord injury in neonates: The use of magnetic resonance imaging. *J Pediatr* 2001; 138(1): 105–8.
42. Filippigh P et al. Sonographic evaluation of traumatic spinal cord lesions in the newborn infant. *Pediatr Radiol* 1994; 24(4): 245–7.
43. Foad SL, Mehlman CT, Ying J. The epidemiology of neonatal brachial plexus palsy in the United States. *J Bone Joint Surg Am* 2008; 90(6): 1258–64.
44. Sunderland, S (ed). *Nerves and Nerve Injuries*, vol. 133. Edinburgh: Churchill Livingstone, 1978.
45. Hoeksma AF et al. Neurological recovery in obstetric brachial plexus injuries: An historical cohort study. *Dev Med Child Neurol* 2004; 46(2): 76–83.
46. Water PM. Obstetric brachial plexus injuries: Evaluation and management. *Am Acad Orthop Surg* 1997; 5: 205–14.
47. Eng GM. Neuromuscular diseases., In: Avery GB (ed). *Neonatalogy*. Philadelphia: JB Lippincott, 1980: 987–92.
48. Hunt D. Surgical management of brachial plexus birth injuries. *Dev Med Child Neurol* 1988; 30(6): 824–8.
49. Kwast O. Electrophysiological assessment of maturation of regenerating motor nerve fibres in infants with brachial plexus palsy. *Dev Med Child Neurol* 1989; 31(1): 56–65.
50. Abid A. Brachial plexus birth palsy: Management during the first year of life. *Orthop Traumatol Surg Res* 2016; 102(1 Suppl): S125–32.
51. Greenwald AG, Schute PC, Shiveley JL. Brachial plexus birth palsy: A 10-year report on the incidence and prognosis. *J Pediatr Orthop* 1984; 4(6): 689–92.
52. Pondaag W et al. Natural history of obstetric brachial plexus palsy: A systematic review. *Dev Med Child Neurol* 2004; 46(2): 138–44.
53. Michelow BJ et al. The natural history of obstetrical brachil plexus palsy. *Plast Reconstruct Surg* 1994; 93(4): 675–80.
54. Jackson ST, Hoffer MM, Parrish N. Brachial-plexus palsy in the newborn. *J Bone Joint Surg* 1988; 70(8): 1217–20.
55. Donn SM, Faix RG. Long-term prognosis for the infant with severe birth trauma. *Clin Perinatol* 1983; 10(2): 507–20.
56. Laurent JP, Lee RT. Topical review: Birth-related upper brachial plexus injuries in infants: Operative and nonoperative approaches. *J Child Neurol* 1994; 9(2): 111–7.
57. Piatt Jr JH. Neurosurgical management of birth injuries of the brachial plexus. *Neurosurg Clin N Am* 1991; 2(1): 175–85.
58. Ashley WW, Weatherly T, Park TS. Collagen nerve guides for surgical repair of brachial plexus birth injury. *J Neurosurg Pediatr* 2006; 105(6): 452–6.
59. Kornblut AD. Facial nerve injuries in children. *Ear Nose Throat J* 1977; 56(9): 369–76.
60. Shiohama T et al. Phrenic nerve palsy associated with birth trauma—Case reports and a literature review. *Brain Dev* 2013; 35(4): 363–6.
61. Bowerson M, Nelson VS, Yang LJS. Diaphragmatic paralysis associated with neonatal brachial plexus palsy. *Pediatr Neurol* 2010; 42(3): 234–6.
62. Stramrood Claire AI et al. Neonatal phrenic nerve injury due to traumatic delivery. *J Perinat Med* 2009; 37(3): 293–6.
63. de Vries TS, Koens BL, Vos A. Surgical treatment of diaphragmatic eventration caused by phrenic nerve injury in the newborn. *J Pediatr Surg* 1998; 33(4): 602–5.
64. Bowen TE, Zajtchuk R, Albus RA. Diaphragmatic paralysis managed by diaphragmatic replacement. *Ann Thorac Surg* 1982; 33(2): 184–8.
65. Blocker SH, Ternberg JL. Traumatic liver laceration in the newborn: Repair with fibrin glue. *J Pediatr Surg* 1986; 21(4): 369–71.
66. Gresham EL. Birth trauma. *Pediatr Clin North Am* 1975; 22(2): 317–28.
67. Van Wyck DB et al. Critical splenic mass for survival from experimental pneumococcemia. *J Surg Res* 1980; 28(1): 14–7.
68. Coil Jr JA et al. Pulmonary infection in splenectomized mice: Protection by splenic remnant. *J Surg Res* 1980; 28(1): 18–22.
69. Matsuyama S, Suzuki N, Nagamachi Y. Rupture of the spleen in the newborn: Treatment without splenectomy. *J Pediatr Surg* 1976; 11(1): 115–6.
70. Chryss C, Aaron WS. Successful treatment of rupture of normal spleen in newborn. *Am J Dis Child* 1980; 134(4): 418–9.
71. Bickler S et al. Nonoperative management of newborn splenic injury: A case report. *J Pediatr Surg* 2000; 35(3): 500–1.

72. Bar-Maor JA, Sweed Y, Shoshany G. Does the spleen regenerate after partial splenectomy in the dog? *J Pediatr Surg* 1988; 23(2): 128–9.
73. Mittelstaedt CA et al. The sonographic diagnosis of neonatal adrenal hemorrhage. *Radiology* 1979; 131(2): 453–7.
74. Eklöf O et al. Perinatal haemorrhagic necrosis of the adrenal gland. A clinical and radiological evaluation of 24 consecutive cases. *Pediatr Radiol* 1975; 24(4): 31–6.
75. Khuri FJ et al. Adrenal hemorrhage in neonates: Report of 5 cases and review of the literature. *J Urol* 1980; 124(5): 684–7.
76. Pery M, Kaftori JK, Bar-Maor JA. Sonography for diagnosis and follow-up of neonatal adrenal hemorrhage. *J Clin Ultrasound* 1981; 9(7): 397–401.
77. Lebowitz JM, Belman AB. Simultaneous idiopathic adrenal hemorrhage and renal vein thrombosis in the newborn. *J Urol* 1983; 129(3): 574–6.
78. Cheves H et al. Adrenal hemorrhage with incomplete rotation of the colon leading to early duodenal obstruction: Case report and review of the literature. *J Pediatr Surg* 1989; 24(3): 300–2.
79. Gross M, Kottmeier PK, Waterhouse K. Diagnosis and treatment of neonatal adrenal hemorrhage. *J Pediatr Surg* 1967; 2(4): 308–12.
80. Pond GD, Haber K. Echography: A new approach to the diagnosis of adrenal hemorrhage of the newborn. *J Can Assoc Radiol* 1976; 27(1): 40–4.
81. Brill P, Krasna I, Aaron H. An early rim sign in neonatal adrenal hemorrhage. *Am J Roentgenol* 1976; 127(2): 289–91.
82. Murthy TV, Irving IM, Lister J. Massive adrenal hemorrhage in neonatal neuroblastoma. *J Pediatr Surg* 1978; 13(1): 31–4.
83. Croitoru DP, Sinsky AB, Laberge JM. Cystic neuroblastoma. *J Pediatr Surg* 1992; 27(10): 1320–1.
84. Cromie WJ. Genitourinary injuries in the neonate. Perinatal care. *Clin Pediatr (Phila)* 1979; 18(5): 292–3, 295.
85. Hsu T-Y et al. Neonatal clavicular fracture: Clinical analysis of incidence, predisposing factors, diagnosis, and outcome. *Am J Perinatol* 2002; 19(01): 017, 022.
86. Zeiger M, Dorr U, Schulz RD. Sonography of slipped humeral epiphysis due to birth injury. *Pediatr Radiol* 1987; 17: 425–6.
87. Broker FH, Burbach T. Ultrasonic diagnosis of separation of the proximal humeral epiphysis in the newborn. *J Bone Joint Surg* 1990; 72A: 187–91.
88. Prevot J, Lascombes P, Blanquart D. Geburtstraumatische epiphysenlosung des proximalen femurs 4 falle. *Z Kinerchir* 1989; 44: 289–92.
89. Finan BF, Redman JF. Neonatal genital trauma. *Urology* 1985; 25(5): 532–3.
90. Diamond DA et al. Neonatal scrotal haematoma: Mimicker of neonatal testicular torsion. *BJU Int* 2003; 91(7): 675–7.
91. Samuel G. Castration at birth. *Br Med J* 1988; 297: 1313–4.

8

Transport of the surgical neonate

PREM PURI AND JULIA ZIMMER

INTRODUCTION

The successful outcome of an operation performed on a newborn with congenital anomalies depends not only on the skill of the pediatric surgeon, but also on that of a large interdisciplinary team consisting of neonatologist/pediatrician, anesthetist, radiologist, pathologist, biochemist, nurses, and others necessary for dealing satisfactorily with the newborn subjected to surgery.

The pediatric transport team is a natural physical extension of the neonatal or pediatric intensive care unit and should be able to provide advanced critical care management for children at remote sites and during transport to a tertiary center.[1] Advances in neonatal intensive care dictate that effective and efficient treatment of the sickest neonates can only be available by concentrating resources such as equipment and skilled staff in a few specialist pediatric centers that have responsibilities to a particular region.[2] There has been a marked change in the last two decades with regard to the knowledge, capabilities, and delivery of neonatal transport.[3,4] Neonates with congenital malformations will therefore have to be transported safely to these centers, sometimes over considerable distances.

PRENATAL TRANSFER

Nowadays, it is general consensus that the best and safest way to care for both the mother and the newborn is the transfer of the pregnant woman before delivery to a high-risk perinatal center.[2] Several studies support this *in utero* transportation of the high-risk fetus, particularly for extremely preterm and very-low-birth-weight (VLBW) babies and those with life-threatening neonatal surgical problems.[5–9]

Hypothermia remains a main problem in these babies as it adversely affects neonatal outcome, and poor posttransfer temperature seems to be an independent predictor of mortality.[10,11]

PRETRANSFER MANAGEMENT

Transferring a newborn without proper stabilization is associated with increased morbidity and mortality. The golden rule is still that no neonate should be transported unless his/her condition has been sufficiently stabilized to survive the expected duration of the journey.[8] Nevertheless, studies have shown show that, regardless of their clinical status, a high percentage of referred neonates suffer deterioration during transport, resulting in a higher risk of early neonatal mortality.[10] Therefore, precaution and careful attention to pretransfer management will provide a higher margin of safety during the journey, especially as the transport environment is usually noisy and the access to the patient is restricted, leading to potential difficulties in providing adequate treatment should problems arise.[12] All babies must be properly resuscitated before the journey is undertaken.[2,8] All drugs, fluids, and equipment that are necessary for transfer should be carried by the transport team (Table 8.1).[13]

Airway management

It should be ensured that the airway is clear, that the baby is well oxygenated, and that ventilation can be maintained during transport. If any risk for deterioration of spontaneous breathing is present, the child should be intubated before departure,[12] as emergency intubation while travelling is often difficult or hazardous. Except in patients with a fractured base of the skull, nasal obstruction, or significant coagulopathy, every child should be intubated nasotracheally.[13] All intubated patients need to be suctioned regularly.

Temperature regulation

Thermoregulation requires critical attention. Hypothermia causes an increase in the neonate's metabolic rate with a subsequent increase in glucose and oxygen use ensuing

Table 8.1 Transfer equipment for neonatal transports

Transport incubator/warm environment
Monitors—ECG, BP, pulse oximeter, temperature
Infusion pumps
Resuscitation drugs and equipment
Supply for respiratory support: bags and masks, portable oxygen supply, ventilator, oropharyngeal airways, endotracheal tubes
Portable nitric oxide supply
Thorax drainage sets
Document folder with all relevant information of patient and parents
Maps/navigation system
Mobile telephone

acidosis and if not reversed, persistent pulmonary hypertension of the neonate develops.[7] Neonates are unable to maintain thermogenesis through shivering, and their heat-producing mechanism is limited to metabolism of brown fat and peripheral vasoconstriction.[11,14] Hypothermia with a core body temperature below 36.4°C (97.5°F) in neonates has been correlated with increased mortality.[11] This can all be avoided by warming the baby to a core temperature of at least 36.5°C and using a prewarmed transport incubator in a prewarmed ambulance.[11] Hypothermia can also occur as a sign of infection and should implicate diagnostic evaluation and antibiotic treatment if required.[14] Hyperthermia above 37°C (98.6°F) should be avoided as it is associated with perinatal depression and hypoxic brain injury.[14]

Circulation

Two reliable and secure routes of venous access should be in place. Many surgical newborns have abnormal losses of water, electrolytes, and proteins, which must be replaced to prevent hypovolemia and shock. Intravenous (IV) fluids must be initiated immediately, and sometimes, initiation of inotropic catecholamines may be warranted.[5,7,12] A urinary catheter should be inserted in any patient to closely monitor urinary output in any patient in whom there will be excessive fluid losses.

Every neonate requiring transport must have an adequately sized functioning nasogastric tube to prevent vomiting and aspiration. It should be taped securely in position and kept on open drainage or attached to a low-pressure suction pump, which should be aspirated frequently to prevent occlusion.[12] Glucose blood levels should be monitored regularly and corrected if necessary.[7]

Documentation

Furthermore, some essential data should be transferred with the infant. A copy of the infant's chart with completed medical notes, all x-rays/ultrasound scans, laboratory reports, and nursing documentation (urine output, passage of stools, eye prophylaxis, hepatitis vaccine, blood type, other medication administration) should accompany the patient. It should be clearly documented whether vitamin K was given. Prophylactic broad-spectrum antibiotics should be started if there is a risk of infection. A parental consent for operation, signed by the mother if the parents are not married, should be sent together with a contactable phone number to be able to explain to the parents the surgical condition of their child and the operative procedure. A sample of maternal blood should be sent for cross-matching, along with a cord blood specimen and a copy of maternal records (including complete maternal history and labor and delivery records).

TRANSPORT TEAM

It widely accepted that specific transport training is required by staff who will be called upon to transfer neonatal patients.[15,16] Local and individual circumstances will determine whether the referring or specialist center will send a transport team. The composition of the team may also vary from institution to institution. Ideally, the transport team consists of a transport neonatologist/pediatrician and a trained neonatal nurse familiar with and able to anticipate potential problems associated with specific lesions.[7] They should be familiar with all equipment and its function and should be experienced in stabilizing an infant in suboptimal conditions. A further option is the use of advanced neonatal nurse practitioners (ANNPs), who have been shown to provide comparable care to trainee pediatricians.[16] Some institutions have formed a nursing transport team trained and experienced in the transfer of sick neonates, guiding the doctors, and operating the equipment.[17] However, a recent Cochrane analysis has shown that there is no credible evidence from literature-based randomized trials to support or confute the benefits of specialist neonatal transport staff for neonatal outcome of morbidity and mortality.[18]

TRANSPORT VEHICLES

Selection of a transport vehicle is dependent on the distance travelled, geography, weather conditions, ground traffic, vehicle availability, size of the transport team, the nature of the infant's problem, and the need for speed.[2] Deterioration of the medical condition can be influenced by transport-related factors such as response and stabilization time or the mode of transport.[19-23]

A variety of conveyances are in popular use, including ground ambulances, helicopters, and fixed-wing aircraft. Air transport has several disadvantages. A major disadvantage is that separate ground transport must be arranged at both ends to move the baby between the airport and the hospital. The exception arises in those circumstances in which helicopter landing sites are available at both receiving and referring institutions. Vibration is not usually detrimental to the infant, but can dislodge lines and tubes and adversely affect monitoring equipment.[24] Noise, vibration, and poor lighting make in-flight monitoring of the infant difficult in a rotary-wing aircraft (helicopter).[7,8] This problem is not experienced to such a significant degree in a fixed-wing aircraft. Overall, the noise and vibrations may cause distress and discomfort to the infant, leading to a deteriorating clinical condition, and thus, it is logical to minimize these as much as possible.[24] The transport incubator as well as the infant in the incubator himself/herself should be securely strapped in case of turbulence of the plane. Moreover, the space in a plane is limited and can cause difficulties in manipulating the airway.[7,8]

The negative effects of altitude on the neonate's body can be detrimental.[25] With increasing altitude, the partial pressure of oxygen decreases; therefore, diffusion of oxygen across the alveolar membranes becomes more difficult, resulting in decreasing oxygen saturation in the infant. To maintain the same level of oxygenation, a higher percentage of oxygen may be required. Moreover, the barometric pressure will also decrease with increasing altitude, the volume of gas will increase, and any air trapped in a body cavity will expand. This could have a dramatic effect on pulmonary function,[7] and small insignificant air leaks can become dangerous. This is particularly important in the setting of pneumothoraces, pneumoperitoneum, or intramural gas.[24] It is therefore important to ensure that all air leaks are drained if possible.

Monitoring is essential during transfer because clinical assessment can be limited due to suboptimal lighting, noise, vibration, and lack of space. Invasive and noninvasive measures of arterial pressure, pulse oximetry, electrocardiograph (ECG), core temperature measurement, and pressure transducers for central venous and intracranial pressure readouts must be present. All monitors and syringe pumps should be battery operated.[5] An appropriate stock of airway and ventilatory equipment (self-inflating resuscitation bags, masks, airways, laryngoscopes, uncuffed neonatal endotracheal tubes of various sizes, humidifiers, portable suction apparatus, oxygen supplies, etc.) as well as IV supplies, intraosseous needles, chest tubes, umbilical catheter kits, and emergency drugs should be present at any time.[7]

Because of the very different nature of air travel compared to ground travel, it is imperative that staff receive training specifically directed at both the environment and specific problems that they may encounter in each situation, including logistics (landing sites), airborne environment, and safety issues.[16]

TRANSPORT INCUBATORS

Standard requirements for transport incubators are established in an international standard.[26,27] Currently available portable incubators (Figure 8.1) are designed and equipped for transporting sick newborns.[28] The incubator is a central piece of equipment that has to provide warmth, visibility, and access. It should be able to maintain a specific

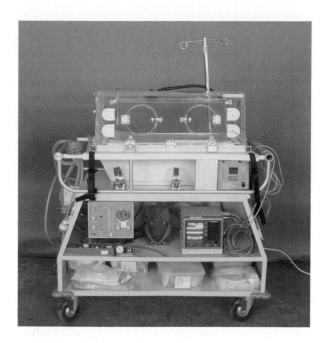

Figure 8.1 A portable incubator.

temperature under a variety of different ambient conditions (e.g., −15°C/5°F to 28°C/82°F).[26] The patient compartment of the transport incubator must be equipped with a front flap for loading and so that there is good access to the neonate in the event of an emergency.[26] It should also be able to run on batteries and must be equipped with its recharger. Guidelines state that the energy of the battery should be sufficient for a minimum of 90 minutes at an ambient temperature of 15°C/59°F.[26] It should be equipped with a cardiorespiratory monitor, pulse oximeter, infusion pump, oxygen analyzer, oxygen and air cylinders, double Plexiglas walls, and shock-absorbing wheels.[7] In the case of transporting very sick neonates and preterm babies, ventilation may be required. In these cases, the incubator should be equipped with a mechanical ventilator which is time-cycled, pressure-limited and capable of delivering conventional ventilations and constant positive airway pressure (CPAP).[26] When securing the neonate in the incubator, one must bear in mind the size of the infant, extreme sensitivity of preterm skin, reduced muscle tone, low body profile, and body weight distribution.[29]

TRANSPORT PROCEDURE

The perfect transfer does not exist yet. It involves early and effective communication between the referring and specialist center, stabilization of the baby pretransfer, and provision of special needs and care during transport.[12] All too often, transport is hastily arranged and conducted in a vacuum of communication, resulting in preventable catastrophes such as vomiting and aspiration, hypothermia, hypovolemia, and airway obstruction,[6] and in the majority of cases, most adverse events arise from poor planning and preparation. Ideally, transfer is arranged at a senior level, i.e., a telephone conversation between a specialist pediatric registrar or consultant pediatrician in the referring center and specialist surgical registrar or consultant pediatric surgeon in the receiving center.[30]

Of increasing relevance is the so-called family-centered care during the transport procedure[31,32] as parental accompaniment has been found to be emotionally beneficial to the child and to reduce parental anxiety.[32]

RECEIVING CENTER

Continuation of care is essential to improving neonatal outcome. On arrival at the tertiary center, a brief report of prenatal, labor, and delivery history should be given by the transport team to the intensive care unit staff, together with details of the newborn's resuscitation and any problems experienced during transfer.[7] The accompanying pediatrician should review the baby and all documents together with the accepting surgeon and neonatologist/pediatrician or anesthetist, if necessary. The parents should be introduced to all staff who will be involved in the care of their baby. Every procedure should be explained in a clear and comprehensive language to avoid confusion and parental fear. The consent form should be updated if necessary. Blood tests and radiological examinations can be ordered subsequently.

SPECIAL CONSIDERATIONS

Gastroschisis

The baby with gastroschisis is at a higher risk for hypothermia, excessive fluid loss, shock, and infection due to lack of a covering peritoneal/amniotic membrane, which gives rise to exposed viscera and peritoneal surfaces. Therefore, radiant heating should be available in the room, and the baby should be kept in a warmed incubator. Intestinal strangulation, necrosis, and obstruction may also occur due to the small size of the paraumbilical defect. Treatment starts immediately after delivery in order to prevent fluid loss and hypothermia (Table 8.2). Intubation and ventilation is carried out if required, and immediate resuscitation with adequate IV fluids (minimum 120 mL/kg per 24 hours)

Table 8.2 Stabilization of a newborn with anterior abdominal wall defect prior to transfer to a referral center

Warm environment
Evaluate respiratory status
Nasogastric tube
Gastroschisis: wrap cling film around defect
Omphalocele: wrap dry gauze around sac
IV fluids, correct deficits
Antibiotics
Vitamin K
Urinary catheter

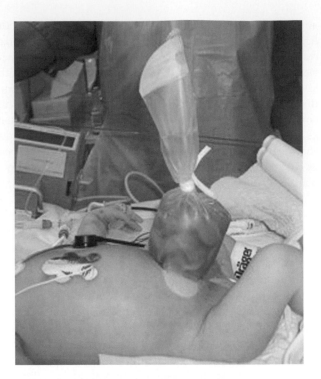

Figure 8.2 Gastroschisis with silo placement.

to overcome substantial water, electrolyte, and protein loss is started. Pulse rate, mean arterial pressure, and glucose level should be observed. Ensure that vitamin K is given and broad-spectrum antibiotics (ampicillin, gentamicin and metronidazole) are commenced to reduce contamination of the exposed intestinal loops. A nasogastric tube is passed for intestinal decompression and prevention of pulmonary aspiration. A urinary catheter is passed to decompress the bladder and to monitor urinary output. In many instances, the viscera are wrapped in sterile gauze that has been soaked in warm sterile saline, and then the abdomen, along with the covered defect, is wrapped in dry sterile gauze. This may, however, induce hypothermia as the gauze cools. If the gauze is allowed to dry, this may stick to the intestinal surface and cause serosal injury when trying remove it.[33] Ideally, the bowel should be placed in sterile clear plastic bag or silo (Figure 8.2). If this is not available, the bowel is localized in the center of the abdomen, and cling film is used to encircle the exposed intestine and is wrapped around the infant.[34] These measures minimize heat loss and trauma to the exposed viscera. The positioning of the infant is very important for preventing bowel ischemia. If the infant is supine and the bowel lies on one side, there is a risk of ischemia to the bowel if the superior mesenteric artery becomes kinked. Hence, the best position is a right lateral position so that the superior mesenteric artery exits straight from the defect.

Omphalocele

As with any abdominal wall defect, the care of the neonate begins with resuscitation. Initially, the respiratory situation needs to be stabilized and the sac protected from rupture and infection, and to minimize heat loss.[34] A nasogastric tube is passed immediately to decompress the stomach and bowel. IV fluids, broad-spectrum antibiotics, and vitamin K should be started. The defect must be inspected to ensure that the sac is intact.[35] The sac should be stabilized in the middle of the abdomen to prevent kinking of the vessels and covered with a sterile, dry, nonadherent dressing to prevent trauma and heat loss. If the sac is ruptured, then the exposed bowel is treated as it is for gastroschisis.[35]

Pierre Robin syndrome

Babies with Pierre Robin syndrome carry a high risk of tongue swallowing and asphyxiation. The baby should be nursed prone to prevent the tongue from falling back into the airway and an oropharyngeal airway inserted.[6]

Choanal atresia

Neonates with choanal atresia suffer from intermittent hypoxia. The baby should be nursed with an appropriately sized and secured oropharyngeal airway with the end or teeth cut off to keep the mouth open.[12] One must ensure that the airway does not go too far into the pharynx as it may enter the esophagus and occlude the airway. In emergencies, the successful usage of larynx masks has been reported.[36]

Myelomeningocele

Infants with myelomeningocele (MMC) should be nursed prone in order to prevent trauma and pressure on the spinal area. A warm, sterile, saline-soaked dressing is placed over the lesion and cling film wrapped around the baby to prevent drying and dehiscence. If the sac is ruptured and cerebrospinal fluid is leaking, or if the MMC is open, it should be covered with Betadine- or chlorhexidine-soaked gauze and IV broad-spectrum antibiotics started. Care must be taken to prevent fecal contamination in sacral lesions.[7] Careful observation and documentation of neurological function is essential before, during, and after transport, including evaluation of the sensorimotor level and assessment of the degree of hydrocephalus.[7]

Bladder exstrophy

At birth, the umbilical cord should be ligated close to the abdominal wall and the umbilical clamp removed to prevent mechanical damage to the bladder mucosa and excoriation of the bladder surface.[5,37] Trauma and damage to the exposed bladder mucosa and plate should be avoided by covering the defect with cling film wrapped around the baby to prevent the mucosa from sticking to clothing or diapers. This will allow urine to escape while establishing a barrier between the environment and the fragile bladder mucosa. Old urine, mucus, and any detritus should be washed from the surface of the bladder with warmed sterile saline at each diaper change.[37] Prophylactic antibiotics should be started immediately.

Cloacal exstrophy

The same measurements to protect the omphalocele sac as discussed under the section "Omphalocele" are applicable.

Esophageal atresia with tracheoesophageal fistula

Most babies with esophageal atresia (EA) become symptomatic soon after birth. Symptoms include excessive drooling, coughing, or choking with the first feed. Once the diagnosis of EA is suspected, the baby should be transferred to a tertiary referral center for further investigation and surgery. Some babies will require endotracheal intubation and ventilation. These infants are particularly at risk because mechanical ventilation is relatively ineffective due to the presence of a fistula. Therefore, the tip of the endotracheal tube should be placed proximal to the carina but distal to the fistula. If the fistula is next to the carina, the fistula can be temporarily occluded with a Fogarty catheter.[38] However, urgent transfer and ligation of the fistula are essential.

Generally, the infant should be handled with care and crying avoided to reduce the risk of aspiration and abdominal distension, and thereby, respiratory distress.[5] Moreover, the baby should be well oxygenated at all times and kept in a warm environment. Regurgitation of gastric contents through the fistula during transport can be prevented by keeping the head of the baby in a slightly elevated position (30°) or nursing the baby prone or in a right lateral position and thereby decreasing the work of breathing and improving oxygenation.[5] The blind upper esophageal pouch should be kept empty. A Replogle sump catheter should be placed in the pouch and connected to low-intermittent or low-continuous suction in order to prevent accumulation of saliva. As these double-lumen esophageal tubes have a tendency to become blocked with mucus, they should be irrigated frequently during transport. IV fluids should be started to provide maintenance and supplemental fluids and electrolytes to compensate for esophageal secretion losses. Infection should be prevented and any existing pneumonitis treated by broad-spectrum antibiotics. Vitamin K should be administered prior to transfer.

Congenital diaphragmatic hernia

The initial objective for the neonatologist and anesthetist is to stabilize the critically ill neonate before transport to the referral center (Table 8.3). A nasogastric tube should be passed immediately on diagnosis to decompress the gastrointestinal tract and to prevent further compression of the lung. If congenital diaphragmatic hernia (CDH) is diagnosed

Table 8.3 Stabilization of a neonate with congenital diaphragmatic hernia prior to transport

Maintain warm environment
Nasogastric tube
Intubation and ventilation
IV fluids
Arterial blood gases
Antibiotics
Vitamin K

prenatally, most centers perform endotracheal intubation and mechanical ventilation directly after birth, which helps to maintain cardiopulmonary stability and impede the natural descent into hypoxemia and hypercapnia.[39]

Full sedation and paralysis and gentle ventilation will reduce the risk of barotraumas in the setting of hypoplastic, delicate lungs. Mask ventilation should be avoided because it will distend the stomach and further compromise the respiratory status. Hyperventilation, using low pressures and high oxygen content, correction of acidosis, and prevention of thermal and metabolic stress are recommended to prevent pulmonary hypertension.[7] Some infants need high-frequency oscillatory ventilation (HFOV) when conventional ventilation proves ineffective. The rationale is that small tidal volumes and gas transport by augmented diffusion result in a lower shear stress and fewer barotraumas.[40] As there is frequently no oscillatory ventilation option available on transport ventilators, clinical teams will usually have to convert to standard ventilation for transfer.[41]

$PaCO_2$ levels and the oxygenation index can be used as a biomarker of effective CDH management,[39,42,43] and the simplified formula of blood gas (PaO_2–$PaCO_2$) in the post-delivery period can predict the need for extracorporeal membrane oxygenation (ECMO) or death.[44]

Careful attention to fluid balance with IV fluids, fresh-frozen plasma (FFP), and catecholamines, if necessary, should be started to maintain adequate peripheral perfusion without causing pulmonary overload.[40] Prophylactic antibiotics should be started and vitamin K administered. Venous access through the umbilicus is useful for obtaining mixed venous blood gas specimens and monitoring central venous pressures if passed across the liver into the right atrium. Arterial access with an umbilical artery catheter will allow monitoring of systemic blood pressure and blood gas measurements at the postductal level. The baby will also need a right radial arterial line to measure preductal blood gases, and a preductal pH ≥ 7.2 with an oxygen saturation of 85%–90% is acceptable.[39] This can be inserted on arrival at the referral center. Acute deterioration of the infant's condition can occur during transfer due to a pneumothorax. Equipment for intercostal drainage must be available since it can be a lifesaving maneuver.[7]

There has been tremendous growth in the use of extracorporeal life support for neonatal cardiopulmonary

failure in the last decades. ECMO has been used as a salvage procedure in high-risk neonates with CHD who fail to respond to mechanical ventilation and meet entry criteria. ECMO is able to partly take over oxygenation and carbon dioxide removal, and thereby may allow respiratory settings to be adjusted to the mechanical and gas exchange properties of the diseased lung.[45] Despite the common use of ECMO for high-risk neonates with CDH, a Cochrane review found that its benefit is unclear.[46] Other studies were also unable to show a survival benefit of ECMO usage in CDH patients.[47,48]

The number of centers providing ECMO is still limited, so special services are needed to transport critically ill neonates to these clinics. Transportable ECMO systems can effectively stabilize and transport high-risk neonates to an ECMO-competent center.[49] The use of inhaled nitric oxide (NO) leads to a reduction in endogenous production of NO, but its value in patients with CDH is still controversial.[40,50] Studies have shown that there is an immediate short-term improvement in oxygenation seen in some treated infants, and this may be of benefit in stabilizing infants for transport and initiation of ECMO. However, inhaled NO did not reduce the need for ECMO.[39,51]

Intestinal obstruction

Intestinal obstruction can occur as a result of a number of conditions, e.g., malrotation, duplication of the alimentary tract, intestinal atresias, necrotizing enterocolitis (NEC), Hirschsprung disease, meconium ileus, and anorectal anomalies. The main objectives are to decompress the bowel and prevent aspiration, accurately estimate and correct fluid losses, and minimize heat loss. A nasogastric tube should be passed to minimize distension and suction carried out regularly and left on free drainage between aspirations. Serum electrolytes and proteins are sequestered in the intestinal wall and lumen, and isotonic IV fluids and colloids should be started to correct acid–base and volume deficits.[33] These must be reviewed and adjusted every 6–8 hours according to the needs of the infant. Broad-spectrum antibiotics should be started prophylactically.

Necrotizing enterocolitis

Neonates with NEC usually are transferred only if surgery is required in case of perforation of gangrenous bowel resulting in pneumoperitoneum or progressive clinical deterioration with evidence of peritonitis.[12] Usually, they are critically ill with sepsis and shock. Prompt resuscitation with crystalloids, colloids, or blood to correct acidosis is started prior to departure. Ventilation with intermittent positive pressure and inotropic support is often required.[5] Blood pressure and blood glucose must be monitored closely. A sump nasogastric tube on continuous suction is passed and suctioned regularly prior to and during transport. Broad-spectrum antibiotics to cover for gram-positive, gram-negative, and anaerobic coverage are started.[33]

CONCLUSION

The approach to the care of the high-risk newborn has changed dramatically in the last two decades. The newborn with a serious congenital malformation requires assessment and stabilization by experienced staff prior to and during transport to the regional center. Stabilization of high-risk newborns before transport is associated with a reduction in perinatal morbidity and mortality. The pediatric transport team plays a vital role in the transport of these patients to tertiary pediatric facilities. The overall aim of transport of the surgical neonate should be to bring the services of the intensive care unit to the patient's bedside during transport to a specialist center.

REFERENCES

1. Ajizian SJ, Nakagawa TA. Interfacility transport of the critically ill pediatric patient. *Chest* 2007; 132: 1361–67.
2. Messner H. Neonatal transport: A review of the current evidence. *Early Hum Dev* 2011; 87 Suppl 1: S77.
3. Ratnavel N. Safety and governance issues for neonatal transport services. *Early Hum Dev* 2009; 85: 483–6.
4. Moss SJ, Embleton ND, Fenton AC. Towards safer neonatal transfer: The importance of critical incident review. *Arch Dis Child* 2005; 90: 729–32.
5. McHugh P SM. Transport of sick infants and children. In: Atwell JD (ed). *Paediatric Surgery*. London, New York: Arnold; Oxford University Press, 1998: 73–89.
6. Harris BA, JR, Wirtschafter DD, Huddleston JF, Perlis HW. In utero versus neonatal transportation of high-risk perinates: A comparison. *Obstet Gynecol* 1981; 57: 496–9.
7. Paxton JM. Transport of the surgical neonate. *J Perinat Neonatal Nurs* 1990; 3: 43–9.
8. Pieper CH, Smith J, Kirsten GF, Malan P. The transport of neonates to an intensive care unit. *S Afr Med J* 1994; 84: 801–3.
9. Chien LY, Whyte R, Aziz K, Thiessen P, Matthew D, Lee SK. Improved outcome of preterm infants when delivered in tertiary care centers. *Obstet Gynecol* 2001; 98: 247–52.
10. Goldsmit G, Rabasa C, Rodriguez S, Aguirre Y, Valdes M, Pretz D et al. Risk factors associated to clinical deterioration during the transport of sick newborn infants. *Arch Argent Pediatr* 2012; 110: 304–9.
11. McCall EM, Alderdice FA, Halliday HL, Jenkins JG, Vohra S. Interventions to prevent hypothermia at birth in preterm and/or low birthweight infants. *Cochrane Database Syst Rev* 2008:CD004210.
12. Lloyd DA. Transfer of the surgical newborn infant. *Semin Neonatol* 1996; 1: 241–8.
13. Macrae DJ. Paediatric intensive care transport. *Arch Dis Child* 1994; 71: 175–8.
14. Gillick J, Puri P. Pre-operative management and vascular access. In: Puri P, Höllwarth ME (eds). *Pediatric Surgery: Diagnosis and Management*. Berlin, Heidelberg: Springer, 2009: 27–38.
15. Orr RA, Felmet KA, Han Y, McCloskey KA, Dragotta MA, Bills DM et al. Pediatric specialized transport teams are associated with improved outcomes. *Pediatrics* 2009; 124: 40–8.
16. Fenton AC, Leslie A. Who should staff neonatal transport teams? *Early Hum Dev* 2009; 85: 487–90.
17. Leslie AJ, Stephenson TJ. Audit of neonatal intensive care transport—Closing the loop. *Acta Paediatr* 1997; 86: 1253–6.
18. Chang ASM, Berry A, Jones LJ, Sivasangari S. Specialist teams for neonatal transport to neonatal intensive care units for prevention of morbidity and mortality. *Cochrane Database Syst Rev* 2015; 10: CD007485.
19. Qiu J, Wu X, Xiao Z, Hu X, Quan X, Zhu Y. Investigation of the status of interhospital transport of critically ill pediatric patients. *World J Pediatr* 2015; 11: 67–73.
20. Borrows EL, Lutman DH, Montgomery MA, Petros AJ, Ramnarayan P. Effect of patient- and team-related factors on stabilization time during pediatric intensive care transport. *Pediatr Crit Care Med* 2010; 11: 451–6.
21. Abdel-Latif ME, Berry A. Analysis of the retrieval times of a centralised transport service, New South Wales, Australia. *Arch Dis Child* 2009; 94: 282–6.
22. Ramnarayan P, Thiru K, Parslow RC, Harrison DA, Draper ES, Rowan KM. Effect of specialist retrieval teams on outcomes in children admitted to paediatric intensive care units in England and Wales: A retrospective cohort study. *Lancet* 2010; 376: 698–704.
23. Ramnarayan P. Measuring the performance of an inter-hospital transport service. *Arch Dis Child* 2009; 94: 414–6.
24. Gajendragadkar G, Boyd JA, Potter DW, Mellen BG, Hahn GD, Shenai JP. Mechanical vibration in neonatal transport: A randomized study of different mattresses. *J Perinatol* 2000; 20: 307–10.
25. Jackson L, Skeoch CH. Setting up a neonatal transport service: Air transport. *Early Hum Dev* 2009; 85: 477–81.
26. Koch J. Transport incubator equipment. *Semin Neonatol* 1999; 4:241–5.
27. International Electrotechnical Commission (IEC). IEC 60601-2-19, IEC 60601-2-20. *Particular Requirements for the Basic Safety and Essential Performance of Infant Incubators*, 2nd edn. 2009, accessible via https://webstore.iec.ch/publication/2622 and https://webstore.iec.ch/publication/2626.
28. Donn SM, Faix RG, Gates MR. Neonatal transport. *Curr Probl Pediatr* 1985; 15: 1–65.
29. Kempley ST, Ratnavel N, Fellows T. Vehicles and equipment for land-based neonatal transport. *Early Hum Dev* 2009; 85: 491–5.

30. Driver C, Robinson C, De Caluwe D et al. The quality of inter-hospital transfer of the surgical neonate. *Today's Emerg* 2000; 6: 102–5.

31. Mullaney DM, Edwards WH, DeGrazia M. Family-centered care during acute neonatal transport. *Adv Neonatal Care* 2014; 14 Suppl 5: S16–23.

32. Joyce CN, Libertin R, Bigham MT. Family-centered care in pediatric critical care transport. *Air Med J* 2015; 34: 32–6.

33. Das UG, Leuthner SR. Preparing the neonate for transport. *Pediatr Clin North Am* 2004; 51: 581–98, vii.

34. Gamba P, Midrio P. Abdominal wall defects: Prenatal diagnosis, newborn management, and long-term outcomes. *Semin Pediatr Surg* 2014; 23: 283–90.

35. Ledbetter DJ. Gastroschisis and omphalocele. *Surg Clin North Am* 2006; 86: 249–60, vii.

36. Trevisanuto D, Verghese C, Doglioni N, Ferrarese P, Zanardo V. Laryngeal mask airway for the inter-hospital transport of neonates. *Pediatrics* 2005; 115: e109–11.

37. Metcalfe PD, Schwarz RD. Bladder exstrophy: Neonatal care and surgical approaches. *J Wound Ostomy Continence Nurs* 2004; 31: 284–92.

38. Alberti D, Boroni G, Corasaniti L, Torri F. Esophageal atresia: Pre and post-operative management. *J Matern Fetal Neonatal Med* 2011; 24 Suppl 1: 4–6.

39. McHoney M. Congenital diaphragmatic hernia, management in the newborn. *Pediatr Surg Int* 2015; 31: 1005–13.

40. Davis CF, Sabharwal AJ. Management of congenital diaphragmatic hernia. *Arch Dis Child Fetal Neonatal Ed* 1998; 79: F1–3.

41. Fenton AC, Leslie A, Skeoch CH. Optimising neonatal transfer. *Arch Dis Child Fetal Neonatal Ed* 2004; 89: F215–9.

42. Salas AA, Bhat R, Dabrowska K, Leadford A, Anderson S, Harmon CM et al. The value of $Pa(CO_2)$ in relation to outcome in congenital diaphragmatic hernia. *Am J Perinatol* 2014; 31: 939–46.

43. Ruttenstock E, Wright N, Barrena S, Krickhahn A, Castellani C, Desai AP et al. Best oxygenation index on day 1: A reliable marker for outcome and survival in infants with congenital diaphragmatic hernia. *Eur J Pediatr Surg* 2015; 25:3–8.

44. Park HW, Lee BS, Lim G, Choi Y, Kim EA, Kim K. A simplified formula using early blood gas analysis can predict survival outcomes and the requirements for extracorporeal membrane oxygenation in congenital diaphragmatic hernia. *J Korean Med Sci* 2013; 28: 924–8.

45. Lewandowski K. Extracorporeal membrane oxygenation for severe acute respiratory failure. *Crit Care* 2000; 4: 156–68.

46. Mugford M, Elbourne D, Field D. Extracorporeal membrane oxygenation for severe respiratory failure in newborn infants. *Cochrane Database Syst Rev* 2008: CD001340.

47. Davis PJ, Firmin RK, Manktelow B, Goldman AP, Davis CF, Smith JH et al. Long-term outcome following extracorporeal membrane oxygenation for congenital diaphragmatic hernia: The UK experience. *J Pediatr* 2004; 144: 309–15.

48. Morini F, Goldman A, Pierro A. Extracorporeal membrane oxygenation in infants with congenital diaphragmatic hernia: A systematic review of the evidence. *Eur J Pediatr Surg* 2006; 16: 385–91.

49. Cornish JD, Carter JM, Gerstmann DR, Null DM, JR. Extracorporeal membrane oxygenation as a means of stabilizing and transporting high risk neonates. *ASAIO Trans* 1991; 37: 564–8.

50. Tiryaki S, Ozcan C, Erdener A. Initial oxygenation response to inhaled nitric oxide predicts improved outcome in congenital diaphragmatic hernia. *Drugs R D* 2014; 14: 215–9.

51. Oliveira CA, Troster EJ, Pereira CR. Inhaled nitric oxide in the management of persistent pulmonary hypertension of the newborn: A meta-analysis. *Rev Hosp Clin Fac Med Sao Paulo* 2000; 55: 145–54.

9

Specific risks for the preterm infant

EMILY A. KIERAN AND COLM P. F. O'DONNELL

INTRODUCTION

Approximately 5%–18% of babies are born preterm (i.e., before 37 weeks of completed gestation) worldwide. Prematurity affects about 7%–12% of births in developed countries.[1,2] In the United Kingdom, an estimated 10% of infants are delivered prematurely and 12% in the United States.[2] The World Health Organization divides preterm infants into three subcategories based on gestational age: extremely preterm infants born at <28 weeks; very preterm infants born at 28–31 weeks and 6 days gestation; and moderate to late preterm infants born at 32–37 weeks.[1] In developed countries, prematurity is the leading cause of neonatal mortality, and preterm babies are at a greater overall risk of morbidity and long-term adverse outcomes than infants born at term.[3,4] Extremely preterm infants are at highest risk; and the chances of survival without long-term sequelae increases with increasing gestation at birth.[5] Advances in the care of extremely preterm infants over the last decades have increased rates of survival, and published data show improved outcomes for these infants. However, with medical advances, infants are surviving from much earlier gestations, and therefore, we still see poor outcomes with a high rate of long-term neurodevelopmental problems.[5–7] The reasons why infants are born preterm vary. Some preterm infants are delivered spontaneously, while others are delivered early because obstetricians identify conditions that pose risks to the mother (e.g., preeclampsia) or fetus (e.g., growth restriction due to placental insufficiency). The proportion of preterm infants whose delivery is planned is greater in developed than in developing countries and has increased in developed countries over time. This is likely due to improved antenatal care identifying risks to the mother and the fetus, and also because the improved outcomes for preterm infants mean that early delivery is not now the "death sentence" that it once may have been.

Preterm infants differ from term infants in size and appearance as the major period of in utero growth is in the third trimester of pregnancy (weeks 28–37). Birth weight is the measure most commonly used to express the size of an infant and to record growth over time. It is also used to describe categories of infants born prematurely (low birth weight [LBW] <2500 grams; very low birth weight [VLBW] <1500 grams; extremely low birth weight [ELBW] <1000 grams).[8]

When infants are born prematurely, their various organs and body systems have had less time to develop in utero. After birth, the preterm infant has to adapt to extrauterine life while also ensuring the ongoing development and maturation of the organs that should have continued in utero during the third trimester of pregnancy. Preterm infants can experience difficulties affecting all body systems at various stages during their stay in the neonatal intensive care unit (NICU).

GENERAL

Preterm infants often need support immediately after birth. A pediatric team should be present in the delivery room for every anticipated preterm delivery. The number of staff and experience required depend on the gestational age, birth weight, and number of infants, with more and more experienced staff needed for more immature babies, smaller babies, and multiple births.

Due to a combination of their low birth weight, large ratio of body surface area to mass, thin fragile skin, and relatively low percentage of insulating brown fat, preterm infants are at risk of heat loss and hypothermia. Newborn infants' total body water content is much higher than that of older children and adults. Preterm infants, with their thin fragile skin, lose water by evaporation through the skin. Immediately after birth, extremely preterm infants are often placed under a radiant heat source and in a polyethylene (food-grade clear plastic) bag or wrap to minimize evaporative heat losses. On admission to the NICU, they should be cared for in a neutral thermal environment, ideally in a prewarmed, closed incubator, until they are mature enough to maintain their own temperature in ambient room temperature in an open cot. Extremely preterm infants are most at risk of water loss and should be cared for in humidified incubators to minimize water loss by evaporation. Preterm infants should only be cared for on an open exposed surface under radiant heat if easy access is required e.g., for procedures such as central vascular catheter (CVC) insertion.

Preterm infants, in particular ELBW infants with intrauterine growth restriction (IUGR), are at increased risk of developing hypoglycemia compared to term infants. They should have their blood sugar level (BSL) checked on admission to the NICU and should be commenced on a dextrose containing intravenous solution as soon as possible to maintain BSL in an acceptable range, ideally >2.6 mmol. Prolonged symptomatic hypoglycemia may lead to long-term neurodevelopmental consequences.

RESPIRATORY

Respiratory distress syndrome

The most common respiratory disorder that preterm infants experience is respiratory distress syndrome (RDS). RDS was originally called hyaline membrane disease (HMD) due to the characteristic appearance of inflammatory exudates (*hyaline membranes*) seen on histopathological examination of postmortem lung specimens of preterm infants who died from hypoxic respiratory failure. RDS is caused by the combination of structural lung immaturity and a deficiency in the production and function of surfactant in the preterm lung. Alveolar development and native surfactant production in the lungs occur from 23 weeks gestation and continue into early childhood. The more premature an infant is born, the higher his/her risk of developing RDS, and the more severe the course may be.

Clinical signs of RDS develop within the first few hours and worsen over the first 48–72 hours of life. Babies may die from their lung immaturity within this time, or their signs may gradually improve thereafter. The typical clinical features of RDS are tachypnea (>60 breaths per minute); expiratory grunting; intercostal, subcostal, and sternal recessions; nasal flaring; and cyanosis and low oxygen saturations. These may be further complicated by apnea and bradycardia. The structural and functional immaturity of the preterm lung makes it difficult for babies to clear the lung of fluid, recruit lung volume, and maintain a functional residual capacity of gas in the lung at end-expiration to facilitate gas exchange. This leads to widespread atelectasis and characteristic changes on chest radiographs (low-volume lungs that have diffuse *ground-glass* opacification with *air bronchograms* visible in the lung fields).

Significant advances in the prevention and management of RDS have occurred over the last 40 years. Administration of intramuscular corticosteroids to women who are at risk of delivering preterm reduces the risk of death from and severity of respiratory disease in preterm infants.[9–11] Respiratory support—supplemental oxygen, continuous positive airway pressure (CPAP), and mechanical ventilation—was widely used from the 1980s. Exogenous surfactant therapy was a tremendous advance for preterm infants as it reduced mortality and respiratory morbidity in babies with RDS.[18–23] Improvements in knowledge and methods of invasive and noninvasive ventilation in preterm infants has have also improved their outcome.[12–17]

Pneumothorax

Pneumothoraces in preterm infants are associated with increased mortality and severity of lung disease along with other long-term morbidities. The main precipitator of pneumothoraces is RDS, and similar to RDS, the risk of pneumothorax is higher in more preterm infants, with approximately 7% of infants born at <29 weeks gestation affected.[16,17,24] Signs of pneumothorax include a marked deterioration in respiratory status with increased clinical signs of respiratory distress and increased oxygen requirements; blood gas analysis may show hypoxia, hypercapnia, and respiratory acidosis. Breath sounds may be decreased on the affected side, and there may be asymmetry of chest wall movement on examination. Diagnosis is confirmed by chest x-ray or, in emergencies, chest transillumination with a cold light source. Small pneumothoraces in a stable infant may resolve spontaneously; however, the majority of large pneumothoraces, especially those under tension with midline shift, are treated with chest drain insertion or needle aspiration with or without chest drain insertion.

Pulmonary hemorrhage

Pulmonary hemorrhage—bleeding directly into the lung parenchyma—is reported in 3%–7% of preterm infants with RDS and is associated with significant mortality and morbidity.[22,24] It is characterized by fresh blood seen coming up the trachea and into the mouth or out the endotracheal tube if the infant is receiving mechanical ventilation. The causes of pulmonary hemorrhage are poorly understood. It is thought to be associated with abnormal and rapidly changing blood flow in the vessels in the lungs over the first few days of life.[23,25] Associated factors include RDS, invasive mechanical ventilation, patent ductus arteriosus (PDA), and coagulopathy. There is a statistically significant increased incidence in preterm infants who receive prophylactic surfactant, but not in infants who receive surfactant as a rescue therapy for RDS.[26,27] There are few proven treatments for pulmonary hemorrhage. Strategies commonly used include measures to increase the mean airway pressure during mechanical ventilation (e.g., relatively higher positive end-expiratory pressure, high-frequency oscillation) and to close a PDA.

Bronchopulmonary dysplasia and chronic lung disease

Chronic respiratory insufficiency is a leading cause of death in preterm infants and is associated with poor neurodevelopmental outcome in survivors. The term *bronchopulmonary dysplasia* (BPD) was originally used to describe the findings on histological examination of samples of lung tissue taken from preterm infants who had died from respiratory failure. As more preterm infants survived, the term *BPD* was applied to infants who had characteristic changes on chest x-ray and were oxygen dependent at 28 days of life. As greater numbers of infants born at earlier gestations survived, it became apparent that 28 days of life was quite a different stage of development for infants born at 24 weeks compared to infants born at 34 weeks of gestation. Chronic lung disease (CLD) of prematurity was thus diagnosed in infants who still had an oxygen requirement at 36 weeks corrected gestational age (CGA). The risk of BPD is highest in infants born extremely preterm and VLBW, with 25%–30% of VLBW infants requiring supplemental oxygen at 36 weeks CGA.[22] BPD is caused by a combination of factors and is most frequently seen, but not specific to, infants who had severe RDS requiring prolonged mechanical ventilation and with high oxygen requirements. Consequences of BPD include long-term oxygen therapy including the potential need for home therapy; feeding difficulties necessitating long-term nasogastric/gastrostomy feeding; increased energy expenditure and subsequent poor growth and nutritional deficiencies; and increased susceptibility to respiratory infections, in particular, bronchiolitis caused by respiratory syncytial virus (RSV).

Apnea of prematurity

Apnea of prematurity is an exaggeration of the periodic breathing pattern seen in newborns and is characterized by pauses in breathing (often for more than 10–20 seconds) and accompanied by episodes of bradycardia and falls in oxygen saturation. It typically affects infants born at <32 weeks gestation. Most episodes of apnea are brief; however, prolonged episodes that are associated with bradycardia and low oxygen saturations should be prevented as both factors have been associated with an increased risk of long-term neurodevelopmental problems. Treatment options include gentle tactile stimulation, nasal CPAP with or without supplemental inflating pressure, and the use of methylxanthines, caffeine or theophylline. Caffeine has been proven to lower the incidence of BPD.[28]

CARDIOVASCULAR

Blood pressure

There is little consensus on either the normal range of systemic blood pressure in preterm infants or the optimal method of treatment for infants whose blood pressure is considered low.[29,30] An ELBW infant's blood pressure generally spontaneously increases over the first 24 hours of life. A commonly used definition for *normal* blood pressure in preterm newborns is that the mean arterial pressure reading, taken from an invasive arterial catheter, should be equal to or above the gestational age in weeks. Clinicians looking after preterm infants should take into account other clinical signs of organ and tissue perfusion such as capillary refill time, urine output, and laboratory markers such as blood lactate. Infants who are determined to have low blood pressure are often treated with volume expanders (e.g., normal saline) and vasoactive medications (e.g., dopamine, dobutamine, adrenaline), and sometimes with steroids (e.g., hydrocortisone). The rates of treatment for hypotension vary widely between centers.

Patent ductus arteriosus

The ductus arteriosus is a vessel that connects the pulmonary artery and descending aorta in the fetus. In the days after birth, the ductus closes as the infant adapts to extrauterine life. If it fails to close, the PDA provides a persistent connection between the pulmonary artery and aorta. Extremely preterm infants are at greatest risk of developing a PDA. The clinical significance depends on the amount and direction of blood flow across the open duct. Over the first few days of life, when the pulmonary blood pressures decrease and systemic blood pressure increases, blood flows in a left-to-right (systemic to pulmonary) direction across the duct. Clinical signs of a PDA include a pan-systolic murmur on auscultation, bounding peripheral pulses on palpation, and a wide pulse pressure (large difference between systolic and diastolic blood pressure measurements). Diagnosis of a PDA is made on echocardiography. Concerns may arise if the left-to-right-side flow of blood causes increased pulmonary blood flow, which can result in pulmonary overload and pulmonary hypertension, and decreased systemic blood flow, leading to hypoperfusion of other organs including the brain. The majority of PDAs close spontaneously over time. However, there are treatment options available if the duct is thought to be causing significant compromise. The prostaglandin synthase inhibitors indomethacin and ibuprofen can be used to treat a known PDA or *prophylactically* to prevent PDA.[31–34] Surgical ligation of PDA, via left lateral thoracotomy, can be carried out in some preterm infants in whom the PDA is thought to be causing significant problems such as dependence on mechanical ventilation.

Congenital heart disease

Similar to infants born at term, preterm infants are at risk of congenital structural cardiac defects. Preterm infants born with defects that require surgical intervention have a significantly poorer prognosis than term infants with similar lesions due to their smaller size and technical difficulty in carrying out surgical repair. Frequently, these infants have to grow before surgical correction can be attempted, and the mortality and morbidity of preterm infants who do reach surgery is higher than term infants undergoing similar operations.

CENTRAL NERVOUS SYSTEM

Intraventricular hemorrhage

Intraventricular hemorrhage (IVH) is the most common neurological complication of preterm delivery and is associated with an increased risk of adverse long-term neurological outcome. IVH is diagnosed and monitored on cranial ultrasound carried out sequentially over the first few days of life and throughout admission to the NICU. IVH are caused by bleeding from the germinal matrix, the small network of capillaries around the caudate nucleus of the immature brain, into the surrounding ventricular system. The germinal matrix disappears by 32 weeks gestation,[2] and therefore, the infants most at risk of developing an IVH and in particular severe IVH are the most premature infants. Typically, IVH develops within the first 72 hours of birth. IVHs are traditionally graded from I to IV.[35] The term *grade I–II* IVH usually describes a small amount blood that is visible within the ventricles. *Grade III* IVH usually means that the intraventricular blood has caused ventricular dilatation, and *grade IV* means that blood is visible in the brain parenchyma, with 10%–20% of infants born before 30 weeks gestation being affected.[36] The most severe complications of IVH are typically seen in grade III–IV bleeds and include posthemorrhagic ventricular dilatation (PHVD) with subsequent hydrocephalus, which may necessitate ventricular access device or ventricular–peritoneal shunt insertion, and porencephalic cyst formation. The rate of grade III and IV IVH[35] in babies born at 501–1500 grams has been reported as 6.4%.[5] The presence of these complications, particularly if bilateral, is associated with a poorer prognosis, with a high risk of mortality and cerebral palsy and significant learning difficulties in survivors.[6,7,36] However, prognosis varies with gestational age, and grade I–II IVH is not predictive of poor outcome.

Cystic periventricular leukomalacia

Cystic periventricular leukomalacia (PVL) describes a pattern of brain injury—holes (cysts) visible in the periventricular white matter—seen on ultrasound. The cause of PVL is thought to be a combination of factors including in utero stress, decreased cerebral blood flow, hypoxia, acidosis, inflammation, and infection. The infants most at risk are the smallest and sickest of infants in the NICU. Unlike IVH, PVL typically only appears on ultrasound 3 or more weeks after the causative event. Over time, single or multiple cystic areas can develop in the periventricular lesions, cystic PVL. Similar to IVH, infants with PVL are at a significant risk of morbidity and long-term neurodevelopmental complications,[6,7,37] with extensive bilateral cystic PVL being strongly predictive of severe motor impairment.

RETINOPATHY OF PREMATURITY

Blood vessels start to proliferate in the retina of the fetus after 30–32 weeks of gestation. Infants, particularly those born before 30 weeks gestation, are at increased risk of disorganized proliferation of blood vessels after 32 weeks postmenstrual age. Unchecked, this can lead to retinal scarring, sight loss, and eventual retinal detachment, and was responsible for an epidemic of blindness in preterm survivors in the 1950s and 1960s. Extreme preterm birth and prolonged exposure to high concentrations of supplemental oxygen increase the risk of retinopathy of prematurity (ROP). However, blindness is now an unusual outcome amongst preterm survivors, thanks largely to effective treatments (laser photocoagulation and intravitreal injection of anti–vascular endothelial growth factors) that are given to infants identified following the regular and routine ophthalmological screening.

GASTROINTESTINAL TRACT

Feeding and nutrition

Like all newborn infants, preterm infants lose weight over the first few days of life. In the third trimester, the fetus gains approximately 100–150 grams per week in utero. Preterm infants have a much higher rate of energy expenditure than if they remained in the uterus; for this reason, they in general take longer than term infants to regain their birth weight. As they are growing rapidly and have high energy requirements, it is important to give preterm infants sufficient energy and nutrients to meet their needs. The optimum way to feed a newborn infant is enterally. However, preterm infants may only tolerate small volumes of feed in the first few days of life, and this volume may only increase gradually over the first week or two of life. To ensure they receive adequate fluid and nutrients, extremely preterm infants often receive parenteral nutrition (PN) while enteral feeding is established. Preterm infants are often unable to coordinate the combination of the suck and swallow reflexes, and when they can, they often tire before they take a volume of oral feeds sufficient for their needs. As a result, preterm infants are fed wholly or partially through a naso/orogastric tube until approximately 33–35 weeks corrected gestation.

Necrotizing enterocolitis

Necrotizing enterocolitis (NEC) is the most common severe gastrointestinal problem that affects preterm infants, and it significantly increases their rates of mortality and morbidity.[2,38–41] NEC is primarily a disease of prematurity; however, term infants with specific risk factors, including perinatal asphyxia, congenital cardiac disease requiring surgery, and structural gastrointestinal conditions such as Hirschsprung's disease, may be affected.[8] Reported rates of NEC among VLBW infants range from 5% to 11%, and, as with other complications of prematurity, the more immature the infant, the greater risk (14% of infants <26 weeks, decreasing to 1% of infants born at >32 weeks).[2,5,8,24,42,43]

Typically, NEC develops in the second to third week of life; however, it is not uncommon for extremely preterm infants who develop NEC to acutely deteriorate after the first month of life after a period of relative stability. Signs associated with the onset of NEC include abdominal distension and tenderness with or without discoloration, bilious vomits or aspirates from the naso/orogastric tube, and fresh blood in the stool. Other clinical signs include those associated with sepsis such as apnea and bradycardia, tachycardia, hypotension, temperature instability, poor perfusion, and shock.

The exact cause of NEC remains unknown. However, multiple risk factors are thought to play a contributing role; these include fetal growth restriction and decreased blood supply to the GIT either in utero or postnatally. The risk of NEC is increased in preterm infants who receive formula feed, with maternal breast milk known to be of benefit in preventing the development of NEC. The disease process starts as inflammation in the bowel wall, which progresses to tissue necrosis and eventually bowel perforation. It may be localized to one area of the bowel wall but in more severe cases is generalized and extensive. Any part of the gastrointestinal tract (GIT) can be affected; however, the terminal ileum, cecum, and ascending colon are the common sites. Diagnosis is made from clinical signs and symptoms and radiological characteristic findings on plain film of the abdomen (PFA). Abnormalities on PFA include dilated bowel loops, thickening of bowel wall, and intramural air (pneumatosis intestinalis). Air may be visible in the portal venous system, and free air may be seen if perforation occurs.

Initial management of NEC is to withhold enteral feeds and commence broad-spectrum antibiotics, which provide cover against both Gram-positive and Gram-negative organisms. If bowel perforation occurs, surgical intervention should be considered.[38,44,45] One small randomized trial showed no difference in the rates of short-term outcomes among preterm infants with perforated NEC who had either primary peritoneal drainage or a laparotomy.[45] Long-term complications of NEC include poor growth and weight gain and poorer neurodevelopmental outcome.[40,41] Stricture formation, and the possibility of associated intestinal obstruction, is a risk in infants who have recovered from NEC.

Spontaneous bowel perforation

Spontaneous bowel perforation affects extremely preterm infants. Typically, it has an earlier onset than bowel perforation associated with NEC and occurs in the first week of life before the infant is established on enteral feeds. The management is similar to that of perforated NEC.

Inguinal hernia

Inguinal hernias are commonly seen in preterm infants, with a reported incidence of 9% in all infants ≤32 weeks, 11% in infants born <1500 grams, and 17% in infants born <1000 grams.[8,46] They are seen in boys much more frequently than girls and can be unilateral or bilateral. The high incidence in convalescing preterm infants is thought to be due to a combination of weak abdominal muscles and a long period

of relatively high intra-abdominal pressure associated with BPD and respiratory support. There is a high risk of strangulation, and therefore, inguinal hernias should be repaired as soon as the infant is stable and suitable for anesthetic. Inguinal hernias should be monitored closely for signs of strangulation, and parents should be educated on the signs and symptoms of hernia strangulation and be aware of the need for urgent presentation to a pediatric surgical center if strangulation occurs.

Umbilical hernia

Preterm infants are more at risk than term infants for developing umbilical hernias. Similar to inguinal hernia, they are more common in extremely preterm infants and infants with BPD. Incarceration of an umbilical hernia is rare, and in general, they resolve over time during the first year of life.

INFECTION

Preterm infants are at an increased risk of sepsis compared to their term counterparts. Infants who develop early-onset sepsis (EOS, <72 hours of life) or late-onset sepsis (LOS, onset at ≥72 hours of life) have increased risk of mortality and morbidity. Group B streptococcus and coliforms such as *Escherichia coli* are the most common organisms to cause EOS, while LOS is mainly caused by organisms that are skin commensals, such as coagulase-negative staphylococcus. Indwelling devices such as central venous catheters, peripheral venous or arterial lines, endotracheal tubes, and chest drains increase the risk of infection and act as a focus for infection. They should therefore only be inserted if absolutely necessary and should be removed as soon as possible. Strict antiseptic techniques should be followed when carrying out any invasive procedure in a preterm infant, and the skin should be monitored closely for signs of breakdown.

OTHER

Hyperbilirubinemia

Unconjugated hyperbilirubinemia is extremely common in preterm infants in the first week of life and should be treated with phototherapy, as prolonged high levels of bilirubin can be neurotoxic. Threshold levels for treatment vary depending on the gestational age of the infant, with treatment being required earlier for the more premature infants. Reference graphs for treatment levels for each gestational age are available.[47]

Electrolytes

Extremely preterm infants, especially infants born at less than 27 weeks gestation, are at risk of developing life-threatening electrolyte imbalances over the first few days of life. Of particular concern is the serum potassium level in ELBW infants, as hyperkalemia can cause disturbances of cardiac rhythm, particularly in the setting of hypocalcemia.

Anemia

A newborn infant's blood volume is approximately 80 mL/kg. Preterm infants may require transfusion for acute blood loss (e.g., due to pulmonary hemorrhage), but more commonly, they are transfused for iatrogenic anemia caused by repeated blood sampling. Typical anemia of prematurity occurs from a few weeks to months of life. It is caused by a combination of decreased red cell production and shortened red cell life span along with increased red blood cell requirements due to rapid body growth.

REFERENCES

1. World Health Organization; Preterm birth. Fact sheet N° 363, November 2012. http://www.who.int /mediacentre/factsheets/fs363/en/.
2. Lissauer T, Fanaroff AA. *Neonatology at a Glance*, 2nd edn. Wiley-Blackwell Press, Hoboken, NJ, 2011.
3. Bhutta AT, Cleves MA, Casey PH, Cradock MM, Anand KJ. Cognitive and behavioural outcomes of school aged children who were born preterm: A meta-analysis. *JAMA* 2002; 288: 728–37.
4. Marlow N, Wolke D, Bracewell MA, Samara M. Neurologic and developmental disability at six years of age after extremely preterm birth. *N Engl J Med* 2005; 352: 9–19.
5. Horbar JD, Carpenter JH, Badger GJ, Kenny MJ, Soll RF, Morrow KA, Buzas JS. Mortality and neonatal morbidity among infants 501–1500 grams from 2000 to 2009. *Pediatrics* 2012; 129: 1019–26.
6. Costeloe KL, Hennessy EM, Haider S, Stacey F, Marlow N, Draper ES. Short term outcomes after extreme preterm birth in England: Comparison of two birth cohorts in 1995 and 2006 (the EPICure studies). *BMJ* 2012; 345: e7976.
7. Moore T, Hennessy EM, Myles J, Johnson SJ, Draper ES, Costeloe KL, Marlow N. Neurological and developmental outcome in extremely preterm children born in England in 1995 and 2006: The EPICure studies. *BMJ* 2012; 345: e7961
8. Rennie JM. *Rennie and Roberton's Textbook of Neonatology*, 5th edn. Churchill Livingstone Elsevier, London, 2012.
9. Liggins GC, Howie RN. A controlled trial of antepartum glucocorticoid treatment for prevention of the respiratory distress syndrome in premature infants. *Pediatrics* 1972; 50: 515–25.
10. Papageorglou AN, Desgranges MF, Masson M, Colle E, Shatz R, Gelfand MN. The antenatal use of betamethasone in the prevention of respiratory distress syndrome: A controlled double-blind study. *Pediatrics* 1979; 63: 73–9.
11. Gamsu HR, Mullinger BM, Donnai P, Dash CH. Antenatal administration of betamethasone to prevent respiratory distress syndrome in preterm infants: Report of a UK multicentre trial. *Br J Obstet Gynaecol* 1989; 96: 401–10.
12. Chernick V. Continuous distending pressure in hyaline membrane disease: Of devices, disadvantages, and a daring study. *Pediatrics* 1973; 52: 114–5.
13. Cox JMR, Boehm JJ, Millare EA. Individual nasal masks and intranasal tubes: A non-invasive neonatal technique for the delivery of continuous positive airway pressure (CPAP). *Anaesthesia* 1974; 29: 597–600.
14. Kattwinkel J, Fleming D, Cha CC, Fanaroff AA, Klaus MH. A device for administration of continuous positive airway pressure by the nasal route. *Pediatrics* 1973; 52: 131–4.
15. Rhodes PG, Hall RT. Continuous positive airway pressure delivered by face mask in infants with the idiopathic respiratory distress syndrome: A controlled study. *Pediatrics* 1973; 52: 1–5.
16. Morley CJ, Davis PG, Doyle LW, Brion LP, Hascoet JM, Carlin JB; COIN Trial Investigators. Nasal CPAP or intubation at birth for very preterm infants. *N Engl J Med* 2008; 358: 700–8.
17. SUPPORT Study Group. Early CPAP versus surfactant in extremely preterm infants. *N Engl J Med* 2010; 362: 1970–9.
18. Fujiwara T, Maeta H, Chida S, Morita T, Watabe Y, Abe T. Artificial surfactant therapy in hyaline-membrane disease. *Lancet* 1980; 1: 55–9.
19. Hallman M, Merritt TA, Jarvenpaa A-L et al. Exogenous human surfactant for treatment of severe respiratory distress syndrome: A randomized prospective clinical trial. *J Pediatr* 1985; 106: 963–9.
20. Enhorring G, Shennan A, Possmayer F, Dunn M, Chen CP, Milligan J. Prevention of neonatal respiratory distress syndrome by tracheal instillation of surfactant: A randomized clinical trial. *Pediatrics* 1985; 76: 145–53.
21. Shapiro DL, Notter RH, Morin FC III et al. Double-blind, randomised trial of a calf lung surfactant extract administered at birth to very premature infants for prevention of RDS. *Pediatrics* 1985; 76: 593–9.
22. Jobe AH. Pulmonary surfactant therapy. *N Engl J Med* 1993; 328: 861–8.
23. Wiswell TE. Expanded uses of surfactant therapy. *Clin Perinatol* 2001; 28: 695–711.
24. Stoll BJ, Hansen NI, Bell EF et al. Neonatal outcomes of extremely preterm infants from the NICHD Neonatal Research Network. *Pediatrics* 2010; 126: 443–56.
25. Papworth S, Cartlidge PHT. Pulmonary haemorrhage. *Curr Paediatr* 2001; 11: 167–71.
26. Aziz A, Ohlsson A. Surfactant for pulmonary haemorrhage in Neonates. *Cochrane Database Syst Rev* 2012; 7: CD005254.

27. Soll R, Ozek E. Multiple versus single doses of exogenous surfactant for the prevention or treatment of neonatal respiratory distress syndrome. *Cochrane Database Syst Rev* 2009; 1: CD000141.

28. Schmidt B, Roberts R, Davis P et al. Caffeine therapy for apnea of prematurity. *N Engl J Med* 2006; 354:2112–20.

29. Dempsey EM, Barrington KJ. Treating hypotension in the preterm infant: When and with what: A critical and systematic review. *J Perinatol* 2007; 27: 469–78.

30. Dempsey EM, Barrington KJ. Diagnostic criteria and therapeutic interventions for the hypotensive very low birth weight infant. *J Perinatol* 2006; 26: 677–81.

31. Ohlsson A, Walia R, Shah SS. Ibuprofen for the treatment of patient ductus arteriosus in preterm and/or low birth weight infants. *Cochrane Database Syst Rev* 2013; CD003481.

32. Van Overmeire B, Follens I, Hartmann S, Cretan WL, Van Acker KJ. Treatment of patient ductus arteriosus with ibuprofen. *Arch Dis Child Fetal Neonatal ED* 1997; 76: 179–84.

33. Ment LR, Ehrenkranz RA, Duncan CC et al. Low-dose indomethacin and prevention of intraventricular hemorrhage: A multicenter randomised controlled trial. *Pediatrics* 1994; 93: 543–50.

34. Schmidt B, Davis P, Moddemann D et al. Long-term effects of indomethacin prophylaxis in extremely-low-birth-weight infants. *N Engl J Med* 2001; 344: 1966–72.

35. Papile LA, Burstein J, Burstein R, Koffler H. Incidence and evolution of subependymal and intraventricular haemorrhage: A study of infants with birthweights less than 1500 gm. *J Pediatrics* 1978; 92: 529–34.

36. Adams Chapman I, Hansen NI, Stoll BJ et al. Neurodevelopmental outcome of ELBW infants with posthemorrhagic hydrocephalus requiring shunt insertion. *Pediatrics* 2008; 121: e1167–77.

37. Dyet LE, Kennea N, Counsell SJ et al. Natural history of brain lesions in extremely preterm infants studied with serial magnetic resonance imaging from birth and neurodevelopmental assessment. *Pediatrics* 2006; 118: 536–48.

38. Neu J, Walker WA. Necrotizing enterocolitis. *N Engl J Med* 2011; 364: 255–64.

39. Fitzgibbons SC, Ching Y, Yu D et al. Mortality of necrotizing enterocolitis expressed by birth weight categories. *J Pediatr Surg* 2009; 44: 1072–5.

40. Rees CM, Pierro A, Eaton S. Neurodevelopmental outcomes of neonates with medically and surgically treated necrotising enterocolitis. *Arch DIs Child Fetal Neonatal Ed* 2007; 92: F193–8.

41. Hintz SR, Kendrick DE, Stoll BJ et al. Neurodevelopmental and growth outcomes of extremely low birth weight infants after necrotising enterocolitis. *Pediatrics* 2005; 115: 696–703.

42. Rees CM, Eaton S, Pierro A. National prospective surveillance study of necrotizing enterocolitis in neonatal intensive care units. *J Pediatr Surg* 2010; 45: 1391–7.

43. Yee WH, Soraisham AS, Shah VS, Aziz K, Yoon W, Lee SK; the Canadian Neonatal Network. Incidence and timing of presentation of necrotizing enterocolitis in preterm infants. *Pediatrics* 2012; 129: e298–304.

44. Rees CM, Hall NJ, Eaton S, Pierro A. Surgical strategies for necrotising enterocolitis: A survey of practice in the United Kingdom. *Arch DIs Child Fetal Neonatal Ed* 2005; 90: F152–5.

45. Moss RL, Dimmitt RA, Barnhart DC et al. Laparotomy versus peritoneal drainage for necrotizing enterocolitis and perforation. *N Engl J Med* 2006; 354: 2225–34.

46. Kumar VH, Clive J, Rosenkrantz TS, Bourque MD, Hussain N. Inguinal hernia in preterm infants (≤32 weeks gestation). *Pediatr Surg Int* 2002; 18: 147–52.

47. National Institute for Health and Clinical Excellence, 2010. Neonatal Jaundice. Clinical Guideline 98. http://www.nice.org.uk/CG98.

10

Preoperative assessment

JOHN GILLICK, DAWN DEACY, AND PREM PURI

INTRODUCTION

Many congenital defects that are of interest to the pediatric surgeon can now be detected before birth; thus, the preoperative assessment of the newborn with a possible congenital anomaly starts in utero. When serious malformations incompatible with postnatal life are diagnosed early enough, the family may have the option of terminating the pregnancy in some countries. It is extremely beneficial for parents if the pediatric surgeon who is likely to manage the infant postnatally is available antenatally to provide information, be involved in management decisions, and counsel the family before birth.[1] The main goal of prenatal diagnosis is to improve the prenatal care by maternal transport to an appropriate center and delivering the baby in a timing and mode that are appropriate for the specific fetal malformation. Multidisciplinary meetings in which obstetric, neonatal, and pediatric surgical expertise is present are commonplace in most large pediatric institutions. They undoubtedly improve postnatal outcome, but as always, effective communication between all disciplines is vital. Prenatal intervention for certain congenital anomalies has been reported extensively in recent years. The success of fetal surgery has varied from condition to condition; for instance, antenatal closure of myelomeningocele is associated with a lesser requirement for subsequent ventricular shunting and improved motor outcomes at 30 months.[2] However, vesicoamniotic shunting for posterior urethral valves has not proved to be the cure-all it was once hoped to be.[3] But it seems clear that fetal surgical intervention is here to stay and is likely to continue to expand its repertoire.[4,5] At present, however, almost all congenital malformations can be successfully managed after birth.

During the past two decades, there have been significant advances in modes and techniques for prenatal diagnosis. These modes include amniocentesis, amniography, fetoscopy, fetal sampling, and ultrasonography. The latter, enabling direct imaging of fetal anatomy, is a noninvasive technique, safe for both the fetus and the mother.[6] With further advances in screening techniques, and combining various antenatal screening modalities, such as the Serum, Urine and Ultrasound Screening Study (SURUSS) for Down syndrome,[7] the efficacy and safety of antenatal screening has improved. However, it is important to remember that sonography is operator dependent and the reliability of the information obtained is directly proportional to the skill and experience of the sonographer. For example, it is important to distinguish duodenal from jejunal obstruction in a fetus with polyhydramnios, because duodenal obstruction is associated with Down syndrome and requires further genetic evaluation, while jejunal obstruction does not.

The real-time sonography may yield important information on fetal malformation, fetal movement, and fetal vital functions such as breathing movements and heart rate variability. Again, this information may guide postnatal intervention.[8,9] Serial sonographic evaluations are particularly useful in following the progression or regression of any fetal disease. All this important information is an integral part of the preoperative assessment of a newborn with any kind of congenital malformation (Figures 10.1 and 10.2).

Neonates born with congenital malformations are usually in urgent need of surgery and, in addition to their surgical problem, may suffer from a multitude of medical problems. Furthermore, they are at a period when significant physiological and maturational changes, involving transition from fetal to extrauterine life, are occurring. The surgical and anesthetic intervention at this time may affect this transition by interfering with normal homeostatic controls of circulation, ventilation, temperature, fluid, and metabolic balance. To facilitate a smooth preoperative course, close cooperation among the neonatologist, pediatric surgeon, and pediatric anesthesiologist is necessary.

All neonates undergoing surgery must be carefully assessed preoperatively, giving particular attention to the following:

- History and physical examination
- Maintenance of body temperature

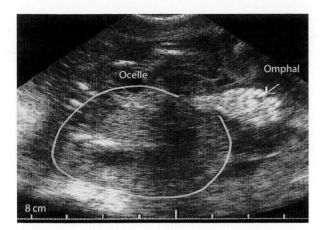

Figure 10.1 Transvaginal ultrasonogram showing a 15-week-old fetus with omphalocele (arrow). Bowel loops protrude through the abdominal wall defect.

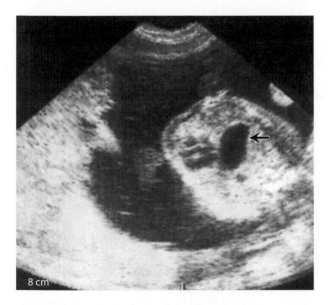

Figure 10.2 Transvaginal ultrasonogram showing a 16-week-old fetus with diaphragmatic hernia. The dilated stomach (arrow) appears in the left hemithorax adjacent to the heart.

- Respiratory function
- Cardiovascular status
- Metabolic status
- Coagulation abnormalities
- Laboratory investigations
- Vascular access
- Fluid and electrolytes, and metabolic responses

HISTORY AND PHYSICAL EXAMINATION

The history of a newborn starts months before delivery, as many of the congenital malformations (e.g., Bochdalek hernia, omphalocele, gastroschisis, sacrococcygeal teratoma and others) nowadays are known to the pediatric surgeon prenatally. The increasing importance of antenatal

pediatric surgical input in counseling parents has been recently reported.[10,11] Not only are the anatomical and structural anomalies important, but even more so are metabolic abnormalities or chromosomal aberrations, which must be diagnosed prenatally or immediately after birth.

Anticipation of a problem in the delivery room is often based on prenatal diagnosis. For example, identification of trisomy 21 in the fetus will increase the neonatologist's awareness in evaluating the infant for those abnormalities closely associated with this chromosomal defect, e.g., evaluation for duodenal atresia and congenital heart disease. Conversely, prenatal identification of specific fetal anomalies should signal the pediatrician to evaluate the infant for a chromosomal abnormality.[7]

The most important recent advance in prenatal detection of anatomical problems has been the development of fetal ultrasonography. In experienced hands, this mode of imaging can be used to detect a wide range of fetal problems and guide postnatal prognosis,[12] ranging from relatively minor abnormalities to major structural defects. However, this anatomical prenatal diagnosis is only one of the tools that aid in planning care management. An accurate and well-documented family history may increase the suspicion that an infant is at risk for an anatomical defect linked to an inherited disorder. In other cases, only the evidence of polyhydramnios should significantly increase suspicion of congenital anomalies.

Most problems are best managed expectantly by natural labor and vaginal delivery. Opinion remains divided on the benefits of elective cesarean section or preterm delivery for abdominal wall defects, with some authorities finding only limited usefulness,[13] and others suggesting that it results in an improved surgical outcome.[14] Certain malformations, however, such as conjoined twins,[15] giant omphalocele, sacrococcygeal teratoma, or large cystic hygroma, often require cesarean section for delivery.

After birth, the assessment of the degree of prematurity, which is an integral part of the physical examination, and the specific type of congenital anomaly must be identified and recorded because of the profound anesthetic and postoperative implications that are involved. The normal full-term infant has a gestational age of 37 weeks or more and a body weight greater than 2500 g. Infants born with a birth weight of less than 2500 g are defined as being of low birth weight (LBW). Babies may be of LBW because they have been born too early (preterm—earlier than 37 weeks' gestational age) or because of intrauterine abnormalities affecting growth (growth retardation). *Small-for-gestational-age* (SGA) infants are those whose birth weight is less than the 10th percentile for their age. Infants may, of course, be both growth retarded and born preterm.

The principle features of prematurity are as follows:

- A head circumference below the 50th percentile
- A thin, semitransparent skin
- Soft, malleable ears
- Absence of breast tissue

- Absence of plantar creases
- Undescended testicles with flat scrotum and, in females, relatively enlarged labia minora

The physiological and clinical characteristics of these babies are as follows:

- Apneic spells
- Bradycardia
- Hypothermia
- Sepsis
- Hyaline membrane disease
- Blindness and lung injury due to use of high levels of oxygen
- Patent ductus arteriosus

In the SGA infant, although the body weight is low, the body length and head circumference approach those of an infant of normal weight for age. These babies are older and more mature. Their clinical and physiological characteristics are as follows:

- Higher metabolic rate
- Hypoglycemia
- Thermal instability
- Polycythemia
- Increased risk of meconium aspiration syndrome (MAS)

In relation to these differences, three important observations have been reported:

1. LBW infants have a mortality 10 times that of full-sized infants.
2. More than 75% of overall perinatal mortality is related to clinical problems of LBW infants.
3. The rate of anatomical malformation in LBW infants is higher than for infants at term.[16]

MAINTENANCE OF BODY TEMPERATURE

The mean and range of temperature for newborns are lower than previously described, and most temperatures ≤ 36.3°C are, in fact, within the normal range.[17] Newborn infants, particularly premature infants, have a poor thermal stability because of a higher surface area/weight ratio, a thin layer of insulating subcutaneous fat, and a high thermoneutral temperature zone. The newborn readily loses heat by conduction, convection, radiation, and evaporation, with the major mechanism being radiation. Shivering thermogenesis is absent in the neonate, and the heat-producing mechanism is limited to nonshivering thermogenesis through the metabolism of brown fat.[18] Cold stress in these neonates leads to an increase in metabolic rate and oxygen consumption, and calories are consumed to maintain body temperature. If prolonged, this leads to depletion of the limited energy reserve and predisposes to hypothermia and increased mortality. Hypothermia can also suggest infection and should trigger diagnostic evaluation and antibiotic treatment if required.[19]

Illness in the newborn, particularly when associated with prematurity, further compounds the problems in the maintenance of body temperature. The classic example for such an illness is the newborn with omphalocele or gastroschisis. In their group of 23 neonates with gastroschisis, Muraji et al.[20] found that hypothermia (31°C–35.4°C), which was found in seven patients upon arrival at the hospital, was the most serious preoperative problem. To minimize heat losses, it is desirable that most sick neonates be nursed in incubators within a controlled temperature. These incubators are efficient for maintaining the baby's temperature but do not allow adequate access to the sick baby for active resuscitation and observation. Overhead radiant heaters, servo-controlled by a temperature probe on the baby's skin, are preferred and effective in maintaining the baby's temperature; they also provide visual and electronic monitoring and access for nursing and medical procedures. Recent studies are investigating the value of plastic coverings, hats, and heated humidified gas in maintaining euthermia.[21] In addition, hyperthermia should be avoided, because it is associated with perinatal respiratory depression and detrimental outcomes in the short-term period postdelivery.

The environmental temperature must be maintained near the appropriate thermoneutral zone for each individual patient because the increase in oxygen consumption is proportional to the gradient between the skin and the environmental temperature.[22] This is 34°C–35°C for LBW infants up to 12 days of age and 31°C–32°C at 6 weeks of age. Infants weighing 2000–3000 g have a thermoneutral zone of 31°C–34°C at birth and 29°C–31°C at 12 days. In an incubator, either the ambient temperature of the incubator can be monitored and maintained at thermoneutrality, or a servo system can be used. The latter regulates the incubator temperature according to the patient's skin temperature, which is monitored by means of a skin probe on the infant. The normal skin temperature for a full-term infant is 36.2°C, but because of many benign factors such as excessive bundling, ambient temperature may affect body temperature. Diurnal and seasonal variations in body temperature have also been described.[17] Thus, the control of the thermal environment of the newborn, and especially the ill baby with congenital malformations, is of the utmost importance to the outcome.

RESPIRATORY FUNCTION

Assessment of respiratory function is essential in all neonates undergoing surgery. The main clinical features of respiratory distress are restlessness, tachypnea, grunting, nasal flaring, sternal recession, retractions, and cyanosis. These symptoms are occasionally present in the delivery room due to anatomical abnormalities involving the airway and lungs and require the most urgent therapy.[23] Table 10.1 lists some common conditions that may be present with

Table 10.1 Approach to respiratory distress postdelivery

Condition	Prenatal and perinatal associations	Clinical features	Chest radiographic findings[a]	Initial therapy
Respiratory distress syndrome (RDS)	Prematurity, lung immaturity, asphyxia, maternal diabetes, male sex	Increasing respiratory distress after birth, tachypnea, grunting, rib retractions or nasal flaring	Diffuse reticulogranular pattern, air bronchograms	Oxygen, assisted ventilation
Air Leak Syndromes				
Pneumothorax	RDS, meconium aspiration, endotracheal resuscitation, diaphragmatic hernia, assisted ventilation	Acute onset of sternal recession, tachypnea, cyanosis, shift in apex beat position	Intrapleural air, mediastinal shift; varying degrees of lung collapse which is always symmetrical toward the hilum	Oxygen, needle aspiration, chest drain; additional tubes may be needed when large leaks from the lung tissue are present
Diaphragmatic hernia (Bochdalek)	Polyhydramnios	Sudden respiratory distress usually soon after birth, dyspnea, cyanosis, scaphoid abdomen, shift in heart sounds, decreased breaths sounds in one hemithorax (usually left)	Bowel pattern in one hemithorax, mediastinal shift with compression of the contralateral lung. Abdominal bowel gas is sparse or absent.	Nasogastric decompression; intubation and ventilation
Lung Abnormalities				
Lobar emphysema	Occasionally associated with congenital malformations of the heart and great vessels	Rapidly progressive respiratory distress with dyspnea and cyanosis, absent or diminished breath sounds over the affected side and displacement of the mediastinum	Hyperinflation of the affected side—usually left upper (increased translucency). Mediastinum may be shifted.	Thoracotomy and lobectomy required. During induction of anesthesia, the ventilator pressures must be kept as low as possible until the chest is open.
Congenital cystic adenomatoid malformation (CCAM)	Fetal hydrops, polyhydramnios, pulmonary hypoplasia, mediastinal shift, type II—associated anomalies including prune belly syndrome and pectus excavatum. 25% of infants are stillborn.	Severe respiratory distress as above, often within hours of birth	Homogeneous mass or multicystic lesion on chest x-ray, mediastinal shift. The normal location of the stomach is of help in differentiating between CCAM and diaphragmatic hernia.	Thoracotomy and lobectomy

(Continued)

Table 10.1 (Continued) Approach to respiratory distress postdelivery

Condition	Prenatal and perinatal associations	Clinical features	Chest radiographic findings[a]	Initial therapy
Esophageal atresia with tracheoesophageal fistula	Polyhydramnios, associated malformations (vertebral, anal, cardiac, tracheo-esophageal, renal, limb [VACTERL]), excessive nasopharyngeal saliva	Mild respiratory distress. Early chest auscultation is normal. The abdomen may show progressive distension (in the common case of atresia and fistula).	Wide, air-filled pouch in the neck or upper mediastinum. Aspiration may be noted, usually in the right upper lobe. Radioopaque nasogastric tube will be seen to stop and coiled in the blind pouch. The abdomen frequently shows hyperaeration of the intestines.	Position of the infant with head elevated 45° or prone position. Place Replogle tube in the blind proximal pouch and connect it to continuous suction. Antibiotics. Evaluate associated congenital malformations.
Airway Abnormalities				
Choanal atresia and supralaryngeal lesions	None	Cyanosis at rest, pink when crying; inability to pass catheter through nares; noisy upper airway	None	Placement or oral airway

[a] Combined chest and abdominal film is recommended in every newborn baby presenting with respiratory distress. An opaque nasogastric tube in the stomach has an important role in both diagnosis and treatment.

respiratory distress at birth. These conditions include the following: diaphragmatic hernia (Bochdalek), lobar emphysema, pneumothorax, esophageal atresia with or without tracheoesophageal fistula, congenital airway obstruction, congenital cystic adenomatoid malformation of the lung, MAS, and aspiration pneumonia. It is important to recognize that more than one condition may be present in the same patient.

If there is any clinical suspicion or sign of respiratory insufficiency, a chest x-ray should be obtained immediately after the resuscitation to determine the cause of respiratory distress. All babies with respiratory distress should have a radiopaque nasogastric tube passed and a radiograph taken that includes the chest and abdomen in order to localize the esophagus, stomach, and bowel gas, and to avoid misdiagnosis, for example, a diaphragmatic hernia that can be mistaken for a cystic adenomatoid malformation of the lung.[24] Blood gas studies are essential in the diagnosis and management of respiratory distress. Arterial pO_2 and pCO_2 indicate the state of oxygenation and ventilation, respectively. In the newborn,[25] repeated arterial blood samples may be obtained either by catheterization of an umbilical artery or by cannulation of radial, brachial, or posterior tibial arteries. An important alternative is noninvasive monitoring techniques with transcutaneous pO_2 monitors or pulse oximeters.[26] Monitoring of arterial pH is also essential in patients with respiratory distress. Acidosis in the neonate produces pulmonary arterial vasoconstriction and myocardial depression. Respiratory alkalosis causes decreased cardiac output,

decreased cerebral blood flow, diminished oxyhemoglobin dissociation, and increased airway resistance with diminished pulmonary compliance.[27]

Respiratory failure is the leading cause of death in the neonate. High-frequency ventilation, use of surfactant, use of inhaled nitric oxide (iNO), and extracorporeal membrane oxygenation (ECMO) have been shown to improve survival in select neonates.[28-31] ECMO provides long-term cardiopulmonary support for patients with reversible pulmonary and/or cardiac insufficiency. It is well accepted as a standard of treatment for neonatal respiratory failure refractory to conventional techniques of pulmonary support.[29] Typically, patients considered for ECMO are 34 gestational weeks or older or weigh more than 2000 g, have intracranial hemorrhages less than grade 2, have no significant coagulopathies, and have had mechanical ventilation for fewer than 7–10 days. Our knowledge of the benefits and associated risks of neonatal ECMO continue to evolve.[32]

Improvements in other support modalities, such as iNO, have tempered the use of ECMO in recent years.[32] More recently, a respiratory strategy based on permissive hypercapnia has been implemented, but its long term benefits have yet to be confirmed.[33] This strategy focuses on avoiding volutrauma/barotraumas/oxygen toxicity while using preductal oximetry to guide therapeutic interventions. Oxygen is administered to maintain the preductal $SaO_2 >$ 90% ($pO_2 > 60$ mmHg), with a corresponding pCO_2 of less than 60 mmHg and pH of more than 7.2. An important feature of this strategy is the minimal use of a muscle relaxant.

Muscle paralysis not only eliminates the infant's inherent respiratory effort but also predisposes the infant to develop tissue edema, while also accelerating lung injury.[34]

Surfactant replacement is commonly used in the clinical management of neonates with respiratory distress syndrome (RDS). It may also be effective in other forms of lung disease, such as MAS, neonatal pneumonia, the "adult" form of acute respiratory distress syndrome (ARDS), and congenital diaphragmatic hernia (CDH). It ensures that alveolar stability is promoted, atelectasis is reduced, edema formation is decreased, and the overall work of respiration is minimized.[31]

Nitric oxide (iNO) is available for treatment of persistent pulmonary hypertension of the neonate (PPHN). It decreases pulmonary vascular resistance, leading to diminished extrapulmonary shunt, and has a microselective effect, which improves ventilation/perfusion matching. Unfortunately the beneficial effects of iNO in premature infants are less clear cut, and its use in these patients has been cautioned.[30,35] In newborns with severe lung disease, high-frequency oscillatory ventilation (HFOV) is frequently used to optimize lung inflation and minimize lung injury. Further studies are needed in order to elucidate the benefits of HFOV compared to conventional ventilation in neonates, particularly those who are extremely preterm.[36]

In summary, the type of respiratory care in particular neonates will always depend upon clinical and radiological findings supported by blood gas estimations.

CARDIOVASCULAR STATUS

At birth, the circulation undergoes a rapid transition from fetal to neonatal pattern. The ductus arteriosus normally closes functionally within a few hours after birth, while anatomical closure occurs 2–3 weeks later.[37] Prior to birth, the pulmonary arterioles are relatively muscular and constricted. With the first breath, total pulmonary resistance falls rapidly because of the unkinking of the vessels with expansion of the lungs and also because of the vasodilatory effect of inspired oxygen. However, during the first few weeks of life, the muscular pulmonary arterioles retain a significant capacity for constriction, and any constricting influences such as hypoxia may result in rapid return of pulmonary hypertension.[23]

The management of neonates with congenital malformation is frequently complicated by the presence of congenital heart disease. At this time of life, recognition of heart disease is particularly difficult. There may be no murmur audible on first examination, but a loud murmur can be audible a few hours, days, or a week later.[38] A newborn undergoing surgery should have a full cardiovascular examination and a chest x-ray. The presence of cyanosis, respiratory distress, cardiac murmurs, abnormal peripheral pulses, or congestive heart failure should be recorded. If there is suspicion of a cardiac anomaly, the baby should be examined by a pediatric cardiologist. In recent years, the use of the noninvasive technique of echocardiography allows accurate anatomical diagnosis of cardiac anomalies, in many cases prenatally.[8]

METABOLIC STATUS

Acid–base balance

The buffer system, renal function, and respiratory function are the three major mechanisms responsible for the maintenance of normal acid–base balance in body fluids. Most newborn infants can adapt competently to the physiological stresses of extrauterine life and have a normal acid–base balance. However, clinical conditions such as RDS, sepsis, congenital renal disorders, and gastrointestinal disorders may result in gross acid–base disturbances in the newborn. Four basic disturbances of acid–base physiology are metabolic acidosis, metabolic alkalosis, respiratory acidosis, and respiratory alkalosis. In a newborn undergoing surgery, identification of the type of disorder, whether metabolic or respiratory, simple or mixed, is of great practical importance to permit the most suitable choice of therapy, and for it to be initiated in a timely fashion.[39] The acid–base state should be determined by arterial blood gas and pH estimation, and must be corrected by appropriate metabolic or respiratory measures prior to operation.

Hypoglycemia

The mechanisms of glucose homeostasis are not well developed in the early postnatal period; this predisposes the neonate, especially the premature neonate, to the risk of both hypoglycemia and hyperglycemia. Prenatally, the glucose requirements of the fetus are obtained almost entirely from the mother, with very little derived from fetal gluconeogenesis. Following delivery, the limited liver glycogen stores are rapidly depleted, and the blood glucose level then depends on the infant's capacity for gluconeogenesis, the adequacy of substitute stores, and energy requirements. From a glucose metabolism point of view, the neonate is considered to be in transition between the complete dependence of the fetus and the complete independence of the adult.[40] Table 10.2 identifies infants who are at risk for developing

Table 10.2 Categories of hypoglycemia

Limited glycogen stores
    Prematurity
    Prenatal stress
    Glycogen storage disease
Hyperinsulinism
    IDM (infant of diabetic mother)
    Nesidioblastosis/pancreatic islet adenoma
    Beckwith–Wiedemann syndrome
    Erythroblastosis fetalis/exchange transfusion
    Maternal drugs
Diminished glucose production
    SGA
    Rare inborn errors

Source: Ogata ES, Carbohydrate metabolism in the fetus and neonate and altered glucoregulation, *Pediatr Clin North Am* 1986;33:25–45.

hypoglycemia according to three mechanisms: (1) those with limited glycogen stores, (2) hyperinsulinism, and (3) diminished glucose production.[41] Premature and LBW infants (especially SGA infants) are at increased risk of both hypoglycemia and hyperglycemia due to immature postnatal metabolic and hormonal adaptation.[40,42] Surgical stress and concomitant feeding practices may further exacerbate matters. Interestingly, operative stress in neonates causes significantly less energy expenditure than comparable procedures in adult practice.[43]

Hypoglycemia is usually defined as a serum glucose level <1.6 mmol/L in the full-term neonate and <1.1 mmol/L in the LBW infant during the first 3 days of life. After 72 hours, serum glucose concentration should always be above 2.2 mmol/L.

Hypoglycemia may be asymptomatic or associated with a number of nonspecific signs such as apathy, apnea, a weak or high-pitched cry, cyanosis, hypotonia, hypothermia, tremors, and convulsions. The differential diagnosis includes other metabolic disturbances or sepsis. The possibility of hypoglycemia must be anticipated to prevent avoidable brain damage.

All neonates undergoing surgery should have an infusion of 10% glucose at a rate of 75–100 mg/kg body weight per 24 hours, and blood glucose levels should be monitored every 4–6 hours by Dextrostix estimation and/or by blood sugar determinations. Blood glucose level should be maintained above 2.5 mmol/L at all times. The symptomatic infant should be treated urgently with 50% dextrose, 1–2 mL/kg intravenously, and maintenance i.v. dextrose 10%–15% at 80–100 mL/kg per 24 hours.

Hypocalcemia

Hypocalcemia is usually defined as a serum calcium value <1.8 mmol/L. However, occasionally, the ionized fraction of the serum calcium may be low, but without a great reduction of the total serum calcium level concomitantly and with the end result of clinical hypocalcemia. This may occur in newborns undergoing exchange transfusion, or in any surgical baby receiving bicarbonate.

Hypocalcemia occurs usually during the first few days of life, with the lowest levels of serum calcium seen during the first 48 hours. The most common causes of neonatal hypocalcemia include decreased calcium stores and decreased renal phosphate excretion. The LBW infants are at greater risk, particularly if they are premature or associated with a complicated pregnancy or delivery. Hypocalcemia may be asymptomatic or associated with nonspecific signs such as jitteriness, muscle twitching, vomiting, cyanosis, and convulsions. Asymptomatic hypocalcemia can be effectively treated by a continuous infusion of 10% calcium gluconate 75 mg kg^{-1} day^{-1} and can be prevented by adding calcium gluconate to daily maintenance therapy. The symptomatic patients should be treated by slow i.v. administration of 10% calcium gluconate, 6 mL in a LBW infant and 10 mL in a full-term infant, with monitoring of heart rate to prevent too rapid an injection. Serum calcium levels should be maintained within the 2.0–2.63 mmol/L (8–10.5 mg%) range.

Hypomagnesemia

Hypomagnesemia may occur in association with hypocalcemia in SGA infants and neonates with increased intestinal losses. If there is no response to correction of calcium deficiency, a serum magnesium level should be obtained. The treatment of hypomagnesemia is by i.v. infusion of 50% magnesium sulfate 0.2 mL/kg every 4 hours until the serum magnesium level is normal (0.7–1.0 mmol/L).

Hyperbilirubinemia

Jaundice in the newborn is a common physiological problem seen in 60% of term neonates and 80% of premature infants.[44] It is the result of a combination of shortened red cell survival, with a consequent increase in bilirubin load, and an immature glucuronyl transferase enzyme system with a limited capacity for conjugating bilirubin. This results in transient physiological jaundice, which reaches a maximum at the age of 3–4 days but returns to normal levels at the end of the first week, and the bilirubin level does not exceed 170 mmol/L.

Hyperbilirubinemia in the newborn may have a pathological basis such as severe sepsis, Rh and ABO incompatibilities, and congenital hemolytic anemias. Neonatal hemolytic jaundice usually appears during the first 24 hours of life, whereas physiological jaundice, as mentioned before, reaches a peak between 2 and 5 days of life. Other causes for prolonged hyperbilirubinemia, including those often associated with surgical conditions, are as follows: biliary obstruction, hepatocellular dysfunction, and upper intestinal tract obstruction. The diagnosis of extrahepatic biliary obstruction should be done as early as possible, because early operations for biliary atresia are essential to obtain good short-term as well as long-term results.[45] The major concern in neonatal hyperbilirubinemia (high levels of unconjugated bilirubin) is the risk of kernicterus (bilirubin deposition in the brain), which can result in brain damage.

Predisposing factors for jaundice include the following: hypoalbuminemia (circulating bilirubin is bound to albumin), hypothermia, acidosis, hypoglycemia, hypoxia, caloric deprivation, and the use of drugs (e.g., gentamicin, digoxin, furosemide). When the serum bilirubin concentration approaches a level at which kernicterus is likely to occur, hyperbilirubinemia must be treated. The infant's gestational age must be taken into account, as kernicterus can occur in the absence of profound hyperbilirubinemia in premature infants. In most patients, other than those with severe hemolysis, phototherapy is a safe and effective method of treating hyperbilirubinemia. When the serum indirect bilirubin level rises early and rapidly and exceeds 340 mmol/L, hemolysis is usually the reason, and exchange transfusion is indicated.

COAGULATION ABNORMALITIES

Coagulation abnormalities in the neonate should be sought preoperatively and treated. The newborn is deficient in vitamin K, and this should be given as 1 mg prior to surgery in order to prevent hypoprothrombinemia and hemorrhagic disease of the newborn. Thus, 1 mg vitamin K should be administered by i.m. or i.v. injection to every newborn undergoing surgery. Neonates with severe sepsis, such as those with necrotizing enterocolitis, may develop disseminated intravascular coagulopathy with a secondary platelet deficiency. Such patients should be given fresh-frozen plasma, fresh blood, or platelet concentrate preoperatively.

Bleeding has been one of the major risks associated with neonatal ECMO.[46] Hemostatic adjuncts and antiplatelet agents are used sparingly and with caution while on ECMO due to the concern of severe thrombotic events and the lack of supporting evidence.[47] Heparin-bonded circuits are becoming more widely used and may assist in minimizing systemic heparinization in select patients, such as those who develop an intracerebral bleed or CDH patients needing to be repaired on ECMO.[48]

The potential for an increased rate of intraventricular hemorrhage (IVH) has also been reported in preterm neonates following iNO therapy. iNO leads to a prolonged bleeding time and an inhibition of platelet aggregation.

LABORATORY INVESTIGATIONS

A newborn undergoing surgery should have blood drawn on admission for the various investigations, including full blood count, serum sodium, potassium and chloride, urea, calcium, magnesium, glucose, bilirubin, and group and cross-match. Blood gas and pH estimation should also be obtained to assess acid–base state and the status of gas exchange. The availability of micro methods in the laboratory has minimized the amount of blood required to do the aforementioned blood tests. The coagulation status of infants who have been asphyxiated may be abnormal and should be evaluated.[49] Neonatal sepsis can result in disseminated intravascular clotting and severe thrombocytopenia. A platelet count <50,000/mm^3 in the neonate is an indication for preoperative platelet transfusion. Blood cultures should be obtained wherever there is a suspicion of sepsis.

VASCULAR ACCESS

Most newborns with surgical conditions cannot be fed in the operative and early postoperative periods. It is essential, therefore, to administer fluids in these patients by the i.v. route. With the availability of 22- to 24-gauge plastic cannulas, percutaneous cannulation of veins has become possible even in small premature infants. Scalp veins and veins of the dorsum of the hand and palmar surface of the wrist are the most common sites used for starting i.v. infusion. With the improvements of techniques and equipment, it is now rarely necessary to perform a "cut-down" in order to administer i.v. fluids.

Longer-term venous access can be obtained with fine percutaneous intravascular central catheters inserted at the bedside without general anesthesia: so-called PICC lines (peripherally inserted central venous catheters [CVCs]). Theses catheters can be successfully inserted by dedicated nursing personnel[50] and provide long-term venous access with a reduced incidence of thromboembolic complications. To minimize complications, it is important to ensure that the catheter tip resides in a central vein.[51]

Adequacy of the intravascular volume and the function of the heart can be assessed by a CVC, which can be inserted through the umbilical vein, internal jugular vein, subclavian vein, and femoral vein. Usually, catheters are placed using the Seldinger technique. This central line is often mandatory and a basic monitoring device for the anesthetist at the time of operation, and sometimes can be performed in the theatre immediately before starting the operation. It is a useful instrument for fluid resuscitation, administration of medication, and central venous pressure monitoring. The next step in the venous access hierarchy is the tunneled central line (commonly Hickman or Broviac). These are typically placed in either a neck or groin vein in neonates. PICC and tunneled central lines are relatively comparable in terms of efficacy and complications; however, if access is required for longer than 2 weeks, a tunneled central line is more suitable.[52] However, CVC lines are not free from risks. Incidence of sepsis in neonates with central lines has been reported at 28%.[53] Most catheter-related bloodstream infections respond to appropriate antibiotic treatment and/or catheter removal.[54]

Critically ill neonates will require an arterial line especially at the time of operation, either because of the surgery, when it is expected to result in significant fluid shift and hemodynamic instability, or because of significant underlying cardiopulmonary disease of the newborn. This arterial line is for monitoring the hemodynamic and biochemical status, especially throughout the operative procedure. Right radial artery percutaneous catheterization is preferred because it allows sampling of preductal blood for measurement of oxygen tension. If the neonate has already had an umbilical artery catheter, it is safer to use it strictly for the purpose of blood pressure monitoring and blood sampling and not for the administration of drugs.

A good fixation of all these venous and arterial lines is essential as these newborns have to be transported frequently, and reinsertion of these vascular lines can be very difficult.

In an emergency, temporary vascular access can also be obtained by the intraosseous route.[55]

FLUID AND ELECTROLYTES, AND METABOLIC RESPONSES

Estimation of the parental fluid and electrolyte requirements is an essential part of management of newborn infants with surgical conditions. Inaccurate assessment of fluid requirements, especially in premature babies and LBW infants, may result in a number of serious complications.[56] Inadequate fluid intake may lead to dehydration, hypotension, poor perfusion with acidosis, hypernatremia, and cardiovascular collapse. Administration of excessive fluid may result in pulmonary edema, congestive heart failure, opening of ductal shunts, bronchopulmonary dysplasia, and cerebral IVH.

In order to plan accurate fluid and electrolyte therapy for the newborn, it is essential to understand the normal body "water" consumption and the routes through which water and solute are lost from the baby. In fetal life around 16 weeks' gestation, total body water (TBW) represents approximately 90% of total body weight, and the proportions of extracellular and intracellular water components are 65% and 25%, respectively.[57] At term, these two compartments constitute about 45% and 30%, respectively, of total body weight, indicating that (1) a shift from extracellular water to intracellular water occurs during development from fetal to neonatal life and (2) relative TBW and extracellular fluid volume both decrease with increasing gestational age.[57] SGA infants have greater TBW than appropriate for gestational-age infants.[58]

In very small premature infants, water constitutes as much as 85% of total body weight, and in the term infant, it represents 75% of body weight. The TBW decreases progressively during the first few months of life, falling to 65% of body weight at the age of 12 months, after which it remains fairly constant.[59] The extracellular and intracellular fluid volumes also change with growth. These changes are shown in Table 10.3.

The objectives of parenteral fluid therapy are to provide the following:

- Maintenance fluid requirements needed by the body to maintain vital functions
- Replacement of preexisting deficits and abnormal losses
- Basic maintenance requirement of water for growth

Maintenance fluid requirement consists of water and electrolytes that are normally lost through insensible loss, sweat, urine, and stools. The amount lost through various sources must be calculated to determine the volume of fluid to be administered. Insensible loss is the loss of water from the pulmonary system and evaporative loss from the skin. Approximately 30% of the insensible water loss occurs through the pulmonary system as moisture in the expired gas; the remainder (about 70%) is lost through the skin.[59]

Numerous factors are known to influence the magnitude of insensible water loss. These include the infant's environment (ambient humidity and ambient temperature[22]), metabolic rate,[60] respiratory rate, gestational maturity, body size, surface area, fever, and the use of radiant warmers and phototherapy.[61] In babies weighing less than 1500 g at birth, insensible loss may be up to three times greater than that estimated for term infants.[62] Faranhoff and colleagues found insensible water loss in infants weighing less than 1250 g to be 60–120 mL kg^{-1} day^{-1}.[63] Chief among the factors that affect insensible water loss are the gestational age of the infant and the relative humidity of the environment.[64] Recently, it has been reported that the application of a semipermeable polyurethane membrane (Tegaderm) to skin of extremely-low-birth-weight (ELBW) infants shortly after birth decreased postnatal fluid and electrolyte disturbances and significantly improved their outcome by reducing severity of lung disease and decreasing mortality.[65]

Respiratory water loss is approximately 5 mL/kg per 24 hours and is negligible when infants are intubated and on a ventilator. Water loss through sweat is generally negligible in the newborn except in patients with cystic fibrosis or severe congestive heart failure, or at high environmental temperature. Fecal water losses are 5–20 mL kg^{-1} day^{-1}.

RENAL FUNCTION, URINE VOLUME, AND URINE CONCENTRATION IN THE NEWBORN

The kidneys are the final pathway regulating fluid and electrolyte balance of the body. The urine volume is dependent on water intake, the quantity of solute for excretion, and the maximal concentrating and diluting abilities of the kidney. Renal function in the newborn infant varies with gestational age and should be evaluated in this context. Very preterm infants younger than 34 weeks' gestational age have reduced glomerular filtration rate (GFR) and tubular immaturity in the handling of the filtered solutes when compared to term infants. Premature infants between 34 and 37 weeks' gestational age undergo rapid maturation of renal

Table 10.3 Changes in total body water (TBW) and body compartments during development

Age	TBW (% body weight)	Extracellular fluid (% body weight)	Intracellular fluid (% body weight)
Premature	75–80	–	–
Newborn	70–75	45	35
3 months	70	35	35
1 year	60	27	40–45
Adolescence			
Male	60	20	40–45
Female	55	18	40

Table 10.4 Metabolic and electrolyte changes of the healthy newborn[a]

Variable	Phase I	Phase II	Phase III
Age	1–3 days	3–6 days	6–7 days
Intake	Low consumption of breast milk	Intake of breast milk rose progressively	Intake of breast milk stable
Body weight	Decreases	Begins to rise	Increases
K+ metabolism	Negative balance	Positive balance[b]	Positive balance
Na+ metabolism	Negative balance	Positive balance	Positive balance
Cl- metabolism	Negative balance	Positive balance	Positive balance
H$_2$O metabolism	Negative balance	Negative balance	± Balance[c]
Urine volume	Small output	Increased	Stable
N metabolism	Negative balance	Positive balance	Positive balance
Caloric metabolism	Negative balance	Positive[d]	Positive balance

Source: From Wilkinson et al., Metabolic changes in the newborn, Lancet 1962;1(7237):983–7, with permission.

[a] This group of 10 male newborn babies includes 5 who were healthy and 5 who suffered degrees of fetal distress.

[b] Potassium probably gives the most sensitive indication of metabolic changes at this time of life. The day on which potassium balance first became positive varied a good deal.

[c] Balance may be slightly positive or slightly negative.

[d] Transition to positive balance. In preterm, infants all three phases can last longer and have more profound changes.

function similar to term infants with rapid establishment of glomerulotubular balance early in the postnatal period.[66] Extremely premature infants followed to school age, however, demonstrate a reduced GFR compared to term infants, presumably due to impaired postnatal nephrogenesis.[67]

The full-term newborn infant can dilute urine to osmolarities of 30–50 mmol/L and can concentrate it to 550 mmol/L by approximately 1 month of age. The solute for urinary excretion in infants varies from 10 to 20 mmol per 100 cal metabolized, which is derived from endogenous tissue catabolism and exogenous protein and electrolyte intake. In this range of renal solute load, a urine volume of 50–80 mL/100 cal would provide a urine concentration of between 125 and 400 mmol/L. If the volume of fluid administered is inadequate, urine volume falls, and concentration increases. With excess fluid administration, the opposite occurs. We aim to achieve a urine output of 2 mL/kg/hour, which will maintain a urine osmolarity of 250–290 mmol/kg (specific gravity, 1009–1012) in newborn infants. For older infants and children, hydration is adequate if the urine output is 1–2 mL/kg/hour, with an osmolarity between 280 and 300 mmol/kg.

Accurate measurements of urine flow and concentration are fundamental to the management of critically ill infants and children, especially those with surgical conditions and extensive tissue destruction or with infusion of high osmolar solutions. In these situations, it is recommended that urine volume be collected and measured accurately.

SERUM ELECTROLYTES AND METABOLIC RESPONSES IN NEONATAL SURGICAL PATIENTS

Electrolyte and metabolic responses to surgical trauma in neonates must be assessed against the background of the normal metabolic responses of an infant to extrauterine life. Table 10.4 represents a reasonable composite of some of the changes occurring in the metabolism of electrolytes, nitrogen, water, and calories in healthy newborn infants.[68] After birth, the neonate must make a transition from the assured continuous transplacental supply of glucose to a variable fat-based fuel economy. The normal infant born at term accomplishes this transition through a series of well-coordinated metabolic and hormonal adaptive changes. In premature and growth-retarded infants, there is impaired ketogenesis, in addition to imprecise neonatal insulin secretion in response to blood glucose.[42] In response to sepsis or surgical trauma, it seems that neonates divert the products of protein synthesis/breakdown from growth to tissue repair. Following surgical stress, oxygen consumption and energy expenditure in neonates return to baseline figures after 12–24 hours.[43] This is greatly different from the situation in adult surgical practice.

Table 10.5 shows fluid and electrolyte disturbances, their mechanisms, and treatment of common neonatal surgical conditions.

PREOPERATIVE MANAGEMENT OF VARIOUS SURGICAL NEONATAL CONDITIONS

Preoperative management is critical to the success of surgical intervention and the postoperative restoration of normal function. It has been observed that patients who have operations conserve sodium postoperatively.[69] In fact, this sodium concentration is usually caused by hypovolemia, which has its genesis in preoperative dehydration, because of various surgical conditions. The remedy is to provide parenteral maintenance fluid preoperatively when oral restriction of

Table 10.5 Fluid and electrolyte disturbances in common neonatal surgical conditions

Neonatal condition	Fluid and electrolyte disturbances	Mechanism	Treatment
Tracheoesophageal fistula	Mild dehydration	External loss of salivary secretions, lack of intake	Volume replacement with dextrose–saline
	Hyponatremia		
Pyloric stenosis	Dehydration, hypokalemia, hypochloremia, metabolic alkalosis	Loss of gastric secretions, hydrogen ions, potassium, and chloride	Volume replacement with dextrose–saline and potassium chloride
Pyloric atresia			
Peritonitis			
Necrotizing enterocolitis	Severe dehydration	Shift of fluids into third space, loss of sodium in stool or emesis, low blood pressure with poor peripheral perfusion	Fast volume replacement
Perforated viscus	Hyponatremia		Blood or blood products
	Metabolic acidosis, hyperkalemia, high levels of BUN		Dextrose–saline
Upper intestinal obstruction			
Duodenal atresia	Mild to severe dehydration	Loss of gastric and duodenal fluids: hydrogen ions, chloride, and bicarbonate	Volume replacement with dextrose–saline and potassium chloride
Malrotation (Ladd bands)	Hypothermia, hypochloremia, hypocalcemia		
Midgut volvulus			
Low intestinal obstruction			
Ileal atresia	Dehydration, hyponatremia, metabolic acidosis, hypokalemia	Loss of fluids into the intestine; enterocolitis	Fluid replacement by dextrose–saline, plasma, and blood as needed
Hirschsprung disease			
Imperforate anus			
Abdominal wall defects			
Omphalocele	Severe dehydration, metabolic acidosis, hyponatremia	Loss of serum from the intestinal wall in gastroschisis; aspiration of large volume of bile by nasogastric catheter; low perfusion	Urgent fluid replacement by plasma, albumin, Ringer's lactate
Gastroschisis			

fluid is required. Some patients may need fluid resuscitation preoperatively, and their extracellular fluid volume must be restored. Assessment of adequacy of the intravascular space can be done by measurement of pulse, blood pressure, capillary filling in the skin, core temperature, temperature of the skin, urine output, specific gravity, and urinary sodium level. In addition to vital signs, an accurate weight, and especially changes in weight, electrolyte levels and calcium and blood gas analyses should be obtained. Attempts should be made to correct any abnormalities encountered during this assessment.

Newborn surgical patients shift large amounts of protein and water into tissues or into potential spaces such as the peritoneal or pleural cavity. These so-called third-space losses are hard to quantify. Inadequate replacement of these losses can cause hypovolemia and shock. This is commonly seen in peritonitis (e.g., necrotizing enterocolitis, perforated viscus) and other congenital abnormalities such as gastroschisis and omphalocele. Infusion of colloid in the form of fresh-frozen plasma, 5% albumin, packed red cells, whole blood, or plasma-like product is required to maintain intravascular integrity in the face of protein and fluid losses.

Table 10.6 Electrolyte content of bodily fluids[a]

Fluid	Na$^+$	K$^+$	Cl$^-$	HCO$_3^-$
Gastric	20–80	5–30	100–140	0
Pancreatic	120–140	5–15	90–120	110
Bile	130–160	5–15	80–120	40
Small intestine	100–140	5–25	90–135	30
Ileostomy	45–135	3–15	20–115	13–100
Diarrhea	10–90	10–80	10–110	15–50
Sweat				
Normal	10–30	3–10	10–35	0
Cystic fibrosis	50–130	5–25	50–110	0

Source: Reproduced with permission from Chesney RW and Zelikovic I, Pre- and post-operative fluid management in infancy, Pediatr Rev 1989;11:153–8.

[a] Values are in mEq/L.

Enterocolitis complicating Hirschsprung disease or other intestinal obstructive lesions can cause massive losses of fluid and electrolytes and result in hypovolemia, hyponatremia, metabolic acidosis, and hypokalemia. In the presence of severe enterocolitis secondary to obstruction, with accompanying large fluid losses into the intestine, adequate preoperative fluid replacement is mandatory to ensure a reasonable outcome. Intraoperative homeostasis should be maintained through administration of appropriate volumes of isotonic crystalloid and colloid.[70] The benefits of colloid over crystalloid solutions in pediatric practice are as of yet unproven and based on results extrapolated from adult practice.

Vomiting of gastric contents as a result of gastric outlet obstruction caused by a duodenal obstruction, pyloric stenosis, intestinal bands, or malrotation results in a chronic loss of gastric contents and primary hydrogen and chloride ions, in turn resulting in hypochloremic alkalosis. Chronic hypochloremic alkalosis results in hypokalemia. In renal compensation, hydrogen ions are conserved at the expense of potassium loss. Preoperative management of patients with gastric outlet obstruction includes fluid replacement and at least potential correction of the hypochloremic alkalosis by infusion of chloride and potassium chloride (Table 10.5). This preoperative metabolic correction greatly enhances surgical outcome. Table 10.6 represents the electrolyte content of bodily fluids, which are lost by various routes and must be corrected with the appropriate balance to be replaced accurately.

Bilateral obstruction uropathy exhibits a number of important and sometimes complex abnormalities of electrolyte metabolism and acid–base regulation. Depending on the severity of a lesion, patients can have dehydration, fluid overload, hypernatremia, hyponatremia, hyperkalemia, renal tubular acidosis, and azotemia with variable degrees of renal failure. Patients with water and salt-losing nephropathy need additional salt and water supplements. Patients with defective dilutional capacity and renal failure require fluid restriction. Patients with renal tubular acidosis require bicarbonate supplementation with or without potassium exchange resins.

FLUID MANAGEMENT PROGRAM

Based on a consideration of the sources of water loss, an average parenteral fluid design for an infant receiving no oral feeding should provide about 40 mL of water per 100 cal metabolized for insensible loss and 50–80 mL/100 cal for urine, with about 5 mL/100 cal for stool water, resulting in a total volume of 100–125 mL/100 cal for the maintenance fluid losses under baseline conditions per 24 hours. LBW infants will require considerably more fluid because of an increasing insensible loss. Neonates weighing less than 1000 g may need 160 mL/kg per 24 hours, and those over 1000 g may require 110–130 mL/kg per 24 hours. With premature infants, a fluid intake >170 mL/kg per 24 hours is associated with an increased risk of congestive cardiac failure, patent ductus arteriosus, and necrotizing enterocolitis.

Serial measurements of body weight are a useful guide to TBW in infants. Fluctuations over a 24-hour period are primarily related to loss or gain of fluid, 1 g body weight being approximately equal to 1 mL water. Errors will occur if changes in clothing, dressings, and tubes are not accounted for and if scales are not regularly calibrated.

The assessment of hydration status in every newborn surgical patient is essential for the infant's outcome. This can best be obtained by changes in body weight, measurement of urine flow rate, concentration of urine, hematocrit, and total serum protein. Estimation of serum electrolytes, urea, sugar, and serum osmolarity gives a good indication of the hydration status.

REFERENCES

1. Benachi A, Sarnacki S. Prenatal counselling and the role of the paediatric surgeon. Semin Pediatr Surg 2014; 23(5): 240–3.
2. Adzick NS, Thom EA, Spong CY, Brock JW, 3rd, Burrows PK, Johnson MP et al. A randomized trial of prenatal versus postnatal repair of myelomeningocele. N Engl J Med 2011; 364(11): 993–1004.

3. Morris RK, Malin GL, Quinlan-Jones E, Middleton LJ, Diwakar L, Hemming K et al. The percutaneous shunting in lower urinary tract obstruction (PLUTO) study and randomised controlled trial: Evaluation of the effectiveness, cost-effectiveness and acceptability of percutaneous vesicoamniotic shunting for lower urinary tract obstruction. *Health Technol Assess* (Winchester, England) 2013; 17(59): 1–232.

4. Vrecenak JD, Flake AW. Fetal surgical intervention: Progress and perspectives. *Pediatr Surg Int* 2013; 29(5):407–17.

5. Wenstrom KD, Carr SR. Fetal surgery: Principles, indications, and evidence. *Obstetr Gynecol* 2014; 124(4): 817–35.

6. Torloni MR, Vedmedovska N, Merialdi M, Betran AP, Allen T, Gonzalez R et al. Safety of ultrasonography in pregnancy: WHO systematic review of the literature and meta-analysis. *Ultrasound Obstetr Gynecol* 2009; 33(5): 599–608.

7. Wald NJ, Rodeck C, Hackshaw AK, Rudnicka A. SURUSS in perspective. *Semin Perinatol* 2005; 29(4): 225–35.

8. Donofrio MT, Skurow-Todd K, Berger JT, McCarter R, Fulgium A, Krishnan A et al. Risk-stratified postnatal care of newborns with congenital heart disease determined by fetal echocardiography. *J Am Soc Echocardiogr* 2015; 28(11): 1339–49.

9. Holland BJ, Myers JA, Woods CR, Jr. Prenatal diagnosis of critical congenital heart disease reduces risk of death from cardiovascular compromise prior to planned neonatal cardiac surgery: A meta-analysis. *Ultrasound Obstetr Gynecol* 2015; 45(6): 631–8.

10. Lakhoo K. Fetal counselling for surgical conditions. *Early Hum Dev* 2012; 88(1): 9–13.

11. Patel P, Farley J, Impey L, Lakhoo K. Evaluation of a fetomaternal–surgical clinic for prenatal counselling of surgical anomalies. *Pediatr Surg Int* 2008; 24(4): 391–4.

12. Policiano C, Djokovic D, Carvalho R, Monteiro C, Melo MA, Graca LM. Ultrasound antenatal detection of urinary tract anomalies in the last decade: Outcome and prognosis. *J Matern Fetal Neonatal Med* 2015; 28(8): 959–63.

13. Al-Kaff A, MacDonald SC, Kent N, Burrows J, Skarsgard ED, Hutcheon JA. Delivery planning for pregnancies with gastroschisis: Findings from a prospective national registry. *Am J Obstetr Gynecol* 2015; 213(4): 557.e1–8.

14. Baud D, Lausman A, Alfaraj MA, Seaward G, Kingdom J, Windrim R et al. Expectant management compared with elective delivery at 37 weeks for gastroschisis. *Obstetr Gynecol* 2013; 121(5): 990–8.

15. O'Brien P, Nugent M, Khalil A. Prenatal diagnosis and obstetric management. *Semin Pediatr Surg* 2015; 24(5): 203–6.

16. Cook R. The low birth weight baby In: Lister J, Irving I (eds). *Neonatal Surgery*, 3rd edn. London: Butterworths, 1990: 77–88.

17. Takayama JI, Teng W, Uyemoto J, Newman TB, Pantell RH. Body temperature of newborns: What is normal? *Clin Pediatr* 2000; 39(9): 503–10.

18. Power G, Blood A. Thermoregulation. In: Polin R, Fox W, Abman S (eds). *Fetal and Neonatal Physiology*. 1, 4th edn. Philadelphia: Elsevier, 2011: 615–24.

19. Laptook AR, Salhab W, Bhaskar B. Admission temperature of low birth weight infants: Predictors and associated morbidities. *Pediatrics* 2007; 119(3): e643–9.

20. Muraji T, Tsugawa C, Nishijima E, Tanano H, Matsumoto Y, Kimura K. Gastroschisis: A 17-year experience. *J Pediatr Surg* 1989; 24(4): 343–5.

21. Chitty H, Wyllie J. Importance of maintaining the newly born temperature in the normal range from delivery to admission. *Semin Fetal Neonatal Med* 2013; 18(6): 362–8.

22. Hey EN. The relation between environmental temperature and oxygen consumption in the new-born baby. *J Physiol* 1969; 200(3): 589–603.

23. Avery GB, MacDonald MG, Seshia MMK, Mullett MD (eds). *Avery's Neonatology: Pathophysiology & Management of the Newborn*, 7th edn. Philadelphia: Lippincott Williams & Wilkins, 2015.

24. Walker J, Cudmore RE. Respiratory problems and cystic adenomatoid malformation of lung. *Arch Dis Child* 1990; 65(7 Spec No): 649–50.

25. Askin DF. Interpretation of neonatal blood gases, Part I: Physiology and acid–base homeostasis. *Neonatal Netw* 1997; 16(5): 17–21.

26. Perlman JM, Wyllie J, Kattwinkel J, Atkins DL, Chameides L, Goldsmith JP et al. Neonatal resuscitation: 2010 International Consensus on Cardiopulmonary Resuscitation and Emergency Cardiovascular Care Science with Treatment Recommendations. *Pediatrics* 2010; 126(5): e1319–44.

27. Philippart AI, Sarnaik AP, Belenky WM. Respiratory support in pediatric surgery. *Surg Clin North Am* 1980; 60(6): 1519–32.

28. Shetty S, Greenough A. Neonatal ventilation strategies and long-term respiratory outcomes. *Early Hum Dev* 2014; 90(11): 735–9.

29. Mugford M, Elbourne D, Field D. Extracorporeal membrane oxygenation for severe respiratory failure in newborn infants. *Cochrane Database Syst Rev* 2008(3): Cd001340.

30. Cole FS, Alleyne C, Barks JD, Boyle RJ, Carroll JL, Dokken D et al. NIH Consensus Development Conference statement: Inhaled nitric-oxide therapy for premature infants. *Pediatrics* 2011; 127(2): 363–9.

31. McCabe AJ, Wilcox DT, Holm BA, Glick PL. Surfactant—A review for pediatric surgeons. *J Pediatr Surg* 2000; 35(12): 1687–700.

32. Gray BW, Shaffer AW, Mychaliska GB. Advances in neonatal extracorporeal support: The role of extracorporeal membrane oxygenation and the artificial placenta. *Clin Perinatol* 2012; 39(2): 311–29.

33. Ryu J, Haddad G, Carlo WA. Clinical effectiveness and safety of permissive hypercapnia. *Clin Perinatol* 2012; 39(3): 603–12.

34. Taguchi T. Current progress in neonatal surgery. *Surg Today* 2008; 38(5): 379–89.

35. Askie LM, Ballard RA, Cutter GR, Dani C, Elbourne D, Field D et al. Inhaled nitric oxide in preterm infants: An individual-patient data meta-analysis of randomized trials. *Pediatrics* 2011; 128(4): 729–39.

36. Cools F, Offringa M, Askie LM. Elective high frequency oscillatory ventilation versus conventional ventilation for acute pulmonary dysfunction in preterm infants. *Cochrane Database Syst Rev* 2015; 3: Cd000104.

37. Heymann MA, Rudolph AM. Control of the ductus arteriosus. *Physiol Rev* 1975; 55(1): 62–78.

38. McNamara DG. Value and limitations of auscultation in the management of congenital heart disease. *Pediatr Clin North Am* 1990; 37(1): 93–113.

39. Askin DF. Interpretation of neonatal blood gases, Part II: Disorders of acid–base balance. *Neonatal Netw* 1997; 16(6): 23–9.

40. Cowett RM, Farrag HM. Selected principles of perinatal–neonatal glucose metabolism. *Semin Neonatol* 2004; 9(1): 37–47.

41. Ogata ES. Carbohydrate metabolism in the fetus and neonate and altered glucoregulation. Pediatr Clin North Am 1986; 33: 25–45.

42. Ogilvy-Stuart AL, Beardsall K. Management of hyperglycaemia in the preterm infant. *Arch Dis Child Fetal Neonatal Ed* 2010; 95(2): F126–31.

43. Pierro A, Eaton S. Metabolism and nutrition in the surgical neonate. *Semin Pediatr Surg* 2008; 17(4): 276–84.

44. Namasivayam A, Carlo W. Jaundice and hyperbilirubinemia in the newborn. In: Kliegman R, Stanton B, St. Geme J, Schor F, Behrman R (eds). *Nelson Textbook of Pediatrics*, 19th edn. Philadelphia: Saunders, 2011: 603–12.

45. Lin JS, Chen SC, Lu CL, Lee HC, Yeung CY, Chan WT. Reduction of the ages at diagnosis and operation of biliary atresia in Taiwan: A 15-year population-based cohort study. *World J Gastroenterol* 2015; 21(46): 13080–6.

46. Sell LL, Cullen ML, Whittlesey GC, Yedlin ST, Philippart AI, Bedard MP et al. Hemorrhagic complications during extracorporeal membrane oxygenation: Prevention and treatment. *J Pediatr Surg* 1986; 21(12): 1087–91.

47. Saini A, Spinella PC. Management of anticoagulation and hemostasis for pediatric extracorporeal membrane oxygenation. *Clin Lab Med* 2014; 34(3): 655–73.

48. Lawson DS, Lawson AF, Walczak R, McRobb C, McDermott P, Shearer IR et al. North American neonatal extracorporeal membrane oxygenation (ECMO) devices and team roles: 2008 survey results of Extracorporeal Life Support Organization (ELSO) centers. *J Extra-corp Technol* 2008; 40(3): 166–74.

49. Del Vecchio A. Evaluation and management of thrombocytopenic neonates in the intensive care unit. *Early Hum Dev* 2014; 90 Suppl 2: S51–5.

50. Sharpe E, Pettit J, Ellsbury DL. A national survey of neonatal peripherally inserted central catheter (PICC) practices. *Adv Neonatal Care* 2013; 13(1): 55–74.

51. Jumani K, Advani S, Reich NG, Gosey L, Milstone AM. Risk factors for peripherally inserted central venous catheter complications in children. *JAMA Pediatr* 2013; 167(5): 429–35.

52. Milstone AM, Reich NG, Advani S, Yuan G, Bryant K, Coffin SE et al. Catheter dwell time and CLABSIs in neonates with PICCs: A multicenter cohort study. *Pediatrics* 2013; 132(6): e1609–15.

53. Freeman JJ, Gadepalli SK, Siddiqui SM, Jarboe MD, Hirschl RB. Improving central line infection rates in the neonatal intensive care unit: Effect of hospital location, site of insertion, and implementation of catheter-associated bloodstream infection protocols. *J Pediatr Surg* 2015; 50(5): 860–3.

54. Benjamin DK, Jr., Miller W, Garges H, Benjamin DK, McKinney RE, Jr., Cotton M et al. Bacteremia, central catheters, and neonates: When to pull the line. *Pediatrics* 2001; 107(6): 1272–6.

55. Kissoon N, Orr RA, Carcillo JA. Updated American College of Critical Care Medicine—Pediatric advanced life support guidelines for management of pediatric and neonatal septic shock: Relevance to the emergency care clinician. *Pediatr Emerg Care* 2010; 26(11): 867–9.

56. Oh W. Fluid and electrolyte management of very low birth weight infants. *Pediatr Neonatol* 2012; 53(6): 329–33.

57. Friis-Hansen B. Water distribution in the foetus and newborn infant. *Acta Paediatr Scand* 1983; 305: 7–11.

58. Meio MD, Sichieri R, Soares FV, Moreira ME. Total body water in small- and appropriate-for-gestational age newborns. *J Perinat Med* 2008; 36(4): 354–8.

59. Statter MB. Fluids and electrolytes in infants and children. *Semin Pediatr Surg* 1992; 1(3): 208–11.

60. Roy RN, Sinclair JC. Hydration of the low birthweight infant. *Clin Perinatol* 1975; 2(2): 393–417.

61. Engle WD, Baumgart S, Schwartz JG, Fox WW, Polin RA. Insensible water loss in the critically III neonate. Combined effect of radiant-warmer power and phototherapy. *Am J Dis Child* 1981; 135(6): 516–20.

62. Bell EF, Gray JC, Weinstein MR, Oh W. The effects of thermal environment on heat balance and insensible water loss in low-birth-weight infants. *J Pediatr* 1980; 96(3 Pt 1): 452–9.

64. Fanaroff AA, Wald M, Gruber HS, Klaus MH. Insensible water loss in low birth weight infants. *Pediatrics* 1972; 50(2): 236–45.
65. Hammarlund K, Sedin G, Stromberg B. Transepidermal water loss in newborn infants. VIII. Relation to gestational age and post-natal age in appropriate and small for gestational age infants. *Acta Paediatr Scand* 1983; 72(5): 721–8.
66. Bhandari V, Brodsky N, Porat R. Improved outcome of extremely low birth weight infants with Tegaderm application to skin. *J Perinatol* 2005; 25(4): 276–81.
67. Shaffer SE, Norman ME. Renal function and renal failure in the newborn. *Clin Perinatol* 1989; 16(1): 199–218.
67. Rodriguez-Soriano J, Aguirre M, Oliveros R, Vallo A. Long-term renal follow-up of extremely low birth weight infants. *Pediatr Nephrol* 2005; 20(5): 579–84.
68. Wilkinson AW, Stevens LH, Hughes EA. Metabolic changes in the newborn. *Lancet* 1962; 1(7237): 983–7.
69. Winters RW. *The Body Fluids in Pediatrics: Medical, Surgical, and Neonatal Disorders of Acid–Base Status, Hydration, and Oxygenation*, 1st edn. Boston: Little, 1973.
70. National Clinical Guideline Centre. *IV Fluids in Children: Intravenous Fluid Therapy in Children and Young People in Hospital*. London: National Institute for Health and Care Excellence (UK), December 2015.

11

Anesthesia

NICHOLAS EUSTACE AND KAY O'BRIEN

Over the past 80 years or so, provision of anesthesia for the neonate requiring surgery has developed from being a relatively haphazard affair to achieving the status of a recognized subspecialty. The improved survival rates seen following surgery, where even the smallest and sickest infants are concerned, have been due in no small part to advances in anesthetic management. Equally important has been an increased appreciation of the need for an efficient smooth-working team. The success of neonatal surgery depends on maximum cooperation between surgeon, anesthetist, neonatologist, and nursing and paramedical personnel. It is appropriate, therefore, that everyone involved in the care of neonates, whether working inside or outside the operating theater, should be familiar with the basic techniques used in maintaining a favorable physiologic milieu in the face of surgical intrusion, while at the same time ensuring adequate anesthesia. This chapter will consider the preoperative evaluation and preparation of the surgical neonate, anesthetic equipment, choice of anesthetic agent and technique (with reference to the pharmacology of the newborn), induction of anesthesia and endotracheal intubation, maintenance and reversal of anesthesia, perioperative monitoring and fluid therapy, the anesthetic implications of congenital anomalies, and finally, specific considerations for the premature infant undergoing surgery.

PREOPERATIVE PREPARATION AND EVALUATION

Much neonatal surgery is performed on an emergency basis. However, operation is rarely so urgent as not to allow for adequate evaluation and stabilization beforehand. The cornerstone of preoperative anesthetic management is a detailed knowledge of the infant's history combined with a thorough physical examination. Consideration must also be given to the specific surgical procedure to be undertaken and its implications in terms of potential blood loss, monitoring requirements, and postoperative care.

History

Although many neonates requiring surgery are aged only a few hours, considerable information that is useful as regards anesthetic management will have been accumulated by the time of the anesthetist's visit. This information should be obtained from the parent(s) (if available) and medical and nursing colleagues. Of profound importance is an accurate estimation of gestational age, as prematurity has profound implications for the anesthetist (see later). Trends in blood pressure and heart rate, including bradycardias, body weight, fluid intake and output, laboratory measurements, x-ray appearances, and the extent of any respiratory support required or apneas, are very helpful in planning anesthetic technique, anticipating problems, and planning postoperative management. A knowledge of recent and current drug therapy is essential.

Physical examination

The anesthetist should make a brief appraisal of the infant's overall condition and follow this with a careful assessment of individual body systems. The neonate's weight should be recorded accurately. Overhydration or hypovolemia can be detected by assessment of skin turgor, the anterior fontanelle, and liver size. Peripheral vasoconstriction may indicate either hypovolemia or acidosis. Signs of respiratory failure include nasal flaring, tachypnea, chest wall recession, grunting respiration, or apneic spells. Airway anatomy should be carefully assessed in order that potential difficulties with endotracheal intubation can be anticipated. One should look for *other* associated congenital anomalies in the surgical neonate. This is particularly so when examining the cardiovascular system (e.g., one-third of infants with esophageal atresia also have some form of congenital heart disease). Accurate preoperative neurological assessment is mandatory in infants presenting for anesthesia for neurosurgery. Finally, potential difficult intravenous (i.v.) access and the possible need for central access for inotropes or postoperative total parenteral nutrition should be evaluated.

Laboratory investigations

Minimum laboratory data required include full blood count, blood urea and serum electrolytes, blood glucose and calcium, and coagulation profile. Arterial blood gas analysis for pH, oxygen and carbon dioxide partial pressure (pO_2 and pCO_2), and bicarbonate levels is also frequently indicated. The preoperative hemoglobin level should be at least 12 g/dL—if lower, consideration should be given to transfusion with packed red blood cells prior to anesthesia and surgery. Any dehydration, hypovolemia, hypoglycemia, hypocalcemia, or hypokalemia or hyperkalemia should be corrected. pH, pO_2, pCO_2, and body temperature should be normalized.

Premedication

Sedative premedication is not used in neonates. However many pediatric anesthetists consider it advisable to administer an anticholinergic drug in order to reduce secretions and to protect against bradycardia. Atropine is the most widely used drug, usually in a dose of 0.02 mg/kg by i.v. injection immediately prior to induction of anesthesia.

Prior to transfer to the operating theater, the anesthetist should confirm the following:

- The infant has been fasting for at least 2 hours (but not for much longer unless an i.v. fluid infusion is in progress)
- Blood has been crossmatched (if indicated)
- Vitamin K, 0.5–1 mg intramuscular (i.m.), has been administered (to allow for possible deficiency in vitamin K–dependent clotting factors)
- The stomach has been decompressed (especially in cases of intestinal obstruction)

Estimated blood volume, allowable blood loss, and maintenance fluid requirements should be calculated. Where it is anticipated that multiple vascular access routes will be required (e.g., for central venous pressure or direct arterial pressure monitoring), it may be advisable to establish these in the intensive care unit (ICU) before transfer to the operating theater, as it is usually easier to maintain an infant's body temperature in the ICU environment. Importantly, overall fitness must be assessed in light of the urgency of surgery. This may require consultation between anesthetist, surgeon, and other interested personnel. If transfer to the operating theater is considered to be unacceptably hazardous, for example, in the case of some extremely ill and low-birth-weight infants, it may be advantageous to undertake surgery in the ICU itself.[1,2]

TRANSFER TO THE OPERATING THEATER

The time during which the neonate is transferred to the operating theater is one that is not without hazard. Risks are minimized if he or she is accompanied by experienced medical and nursing personnel and if the theater is close at hand. Transfer should be in either an incubator or an isolette with overhead heater to reduce heat loss. Any treatment in progress (e.g., i.v. fluid or drug infusion, respiratory support) should be continued by the use of battery-operated infusion pumps and portable respiratory equipment. Monitoring should not be interrupted during this hazardous phase.

OPERATING THEATER AND ANESTHETIC EQUIPMENT

The prime objectives of neonatal anesthesia are the provision of sleep, analgesia, life support, intensive surveillance, and appropriate operating conditions for the infant requiring surgery. In order for these to be achieved, it is imperative that both operating theater environmental conditions and anesthetic equipment be appropriate. It has been shown that maximum heat loss occurs between the time of arrival of the neonate in theater and the skin incision. Measures should be taken to minimize the risk and extent of this occurrence. Before the infant arrives, the theater, which should be draught free, should be warmed to a temperature of 24°C or 25°C. Once the baby is removed from the incubator or isolette, he or she should be placed on a water or air mattress that has been heated to 40°C and kept covered as much as possible—plastic drapes and blankets are particularly useful in this regard. If an overhead radiant heater is available, it should be set to maintain skin temperature at 36°C. Other measures that assist in maintaining body temperature during this critical period include warming and humidifying inspired anesthetic gases and warming i.v. and skin preparation fluids.

Breathing systems

An appropriate anesthetic circuit for use in infants needs to be light, have minimal resistance and dead space, allow for warming and humidifying of inspired gases, and be adaptable to spontaneous, assisted, or controlled ventilation. While the T-piece system originally designed by Philip Ayre[3] and later modified by Rees[4] is still used by some, circle systems are currently more popular. Connectors and tubes should also offer minimal flow resistance and dead space.

Most endotracheal tubes used during neonatal anesthesia are manufactured out of polyvinyl chloride. A knowledge of the probable diameter and length of tube appropriate for any given infant is essential but must always be confirmed clinically. The optimal diameter is the largest that will pass easily through the glottis and subglottic region and will produce a slight leak when positive pressure is applied. A convenient guideline for length of orotracheal tube from gum to midtrachea is 7 cm for an infant weighing 1 kg, with an additional centimeter for each kilogram increase in weight.[5] Use of an endotracheal tube of too large a diameter may result in tracheal wall damage, while excess length leads to endobronchial intubation. Newer cuffed pediatric endotracheal tubes are available, (Microcuff by Kimberly-Clarke), but the recommended size must be used.[6] Once satisfactory positioning has been confirmed visually and by auscultation of both lungs, the tube should be taped securely to prevent accidental extubation. Consideration should be given to secondary fixation to the forehead to prevent rotational movement. Face masks are generally used for only brief periods in neonates but should provide a good fit and have a low dead space. Oral airways are not generally necessary except in cases of choanal atresia but have the advantage of splinting the endotracheal tube and preventing lateral movement.

The incidence of airway complications associated with the laryngeal mask airway (LMA) in infants is high.[7] However, the device can occasionally prove useful, especially when endotracheal intubation is difficult.[8,9]

Laryngoscopes

Because of the anatomical peculiarities of the infant's airway, most anesthetists prefer to use a laryngoscope with a straight blade, lifting the epiglottis forward from behind to facilitate intubation. The Miller number 0 and 1 blades are suitable in most cases. A recent advance has been the development of videolaryngoscopes such as the GlideScope, for use in neonates.[10]

Ventilators

Most infants and children can be ventilated using standard adult ventilators provided the ventilator is of low internal compliance and equipped with pediatric breathing tubes. The ventilator should be capable of delivering small tidal volumes and rapid respiratory rates, and have an adjustable inspiratory flow rate and inspiratory–expiratory ratio so that peak airway pressure is kept as low as possible.[11] Pressure-controlled ventilation is widely used in order to minimize the risk of pulmonary barotrauma. A suitable temperature-controlled humidifier should be incorporated in the inspiratory side of the ventilator circuit. The ability to deliver air–oxygen mixtures through the ventilator or anesthetic circuit should be available.

Monitoring equipment

A complete range of monitoring equipment suitable for infant use is required.

CHOICE OF ANESTHETIC AGENT AND TECHNIQUE

Neonates perceive pain, while even babies born at 28 weeks gestation mount a substantial and potentially harmful response to surgically induced stress.[12] Thus, few would argue with the contention that adequate anesthesia must be provided for all infants undergoing surgery. The anesthetic agents employed are similar to those used for older children and adults. However, the responses of the neonate to these potent drugs differ in a number of respects from those seen in older patients. An understanding of these differences is essential for the safe conduct of neonatal anesthesia and also influences choice of anesthetic agent and technique. The issue of possible neurotoxic effects of general anesthetics on the developing brain has received considerable attention in recent years, and there seems little doubt that until there is more clarity as regards the actual degree of risk, any surgery that is truly elective should be deferred until the infant attains an as-yet undefined older age.[13,14]

Inhalation agents

Inhalation induction of anesthesia with either air or nitrous oxide, oxygen, and a volatile agent remains popular. Provided that respiration is not depressed, both induction of and emergence from anesthesia are rapid in infants. The reasons for this are multiple but include the relatively higher cardiac output, greater alveolar ventilation, smaller functional residual capacity, and larger proportion of vessel-rich tissues relative to body mass seen in the newborn infant.[15,16] All potent inhalation agents lead to a dose-related depression of spontaneous respiration.[17] This is particularly important in the neonate, in whom the ventilatory response to hypoxia is one of hypoventilation. An additional consideration is that the minimal alveolar concentration (MAC) of inhaled agents required to prevent reflex responses to surgical stimulation varies with age.

HALOTHANE

Halothane was, for many years, the most widely used volatile anesthetic for inhalation induction in infants and young children. This is largely because it is usually associated with a smooth induction without irritant effects on the airway. It has been superseded in patients of all ages by agents that offer greater hemodynamic stability to the extent that it is currently unavailable in many parts of the world.

ISOFLURANE

Despite its lower blood gas solubility coefficient, inhalation induction with isoflurane is generally not as rapid or as smooth as with halothane. Indeed, this agent has been shown to be associated with a significant incidence of hypoxic episodes during inhalation induction of anesthesia in older children. Sedative premedication and use of a high inspired isoflurane concentration from the outset[18] both reduce the incidence of these adverse occurrences but are relatively contraindicated in the surgical neonate. Isoflurane has been shown to maintain systolic arterial pressure in the normal range even in preterm neonates and, unlike halothane, does not sensitize the myocardium to the effects of circulating catecholamines. It has considerable potentiating effects on nondepolarizing muscle relaxants, so that lower doses of the latter can be used. Metabolic degradation of the agent is minimal and recovery rapid. In summary, isoflurane is an excellent agent for maintenance of anesthesia but has limited use for inhalation induction.

ENFLURANE

This agent is rarely used in neonatal and pediatric anesthesia because its irritant effects render it relatively unsatisfactory for inhalation induction.

DESFLURANE

Airway irritant effects also render desflurane unsuitable for inhalation induction in pediatric practice. However, recovery times in infants are shorter than those following other volatile anesthetics. The agent has been recommended for maintenance of anesthesia in the ex-premature infant prone to apnea and ventilatory depression.[19]

SEVOFLURANE

Sevoflurane has replaced halothane for the induction of anesthesia in neonates and children. It lacks the airway irritation associated with other newer inhalation agents and provides cardiovascular stability. Induction time is similar to halothane.[20] Infants undergoing inguinal herniotomy with sevoflurane have a slower recovery than those with desflurane but no difference in postoperative respiratory events.[21] Higher concentrations of sevoflurane, commonly used for induction of anesthesia, can be associated with epileptiform electroencephalogram (EEG) changes.[22] In older children, the agent is associated with emergence delirium.[23]

NITROUS OXIDE

This gas does not provide adequate anesthesia when used alone with oxygen. It is most often employed as a carrier that supplements potent volatile anesthetics, thereby reducing the concentration required and minimizing cardiovascular depressant effects. Animal work indicated that it might induce pulmonary vasoconstriction, with resultant increased right-to-left shunting in the newborn, but this does not appear to be so.[24] It does cause moderate respiratory and cardiovascular depression. One limitation to the use of nitrous oxide in neonatal anesthesia is the fact that it is many times more soluble in blood than is nitrogen. As a result, the inhalation and subsequent diffusion of the gas cause an increase in the volume of compliant spaces. It follows that the agent should not be used in infants with congenital diaphragmatic hernia, lobar emphysema, or bowel obstruction.

Intravenous agents

THIOPENTONE

Despite the fact that it was introduced to anesthetic practice over 70 years ago and that many supposedly superior agents have since been developed, many still consider this drug to be the preferred agent for i.v. induction in infants. The induction dose [ED]$_{50}$ (effective dose, 3.4 mg/kg) is lower in neonates less than 14 days of age than in older infants.

PROPOFOL

Propofol is a highly lipophilic short-acting anesthetic agent. It has a rapid onset and short duration of action. It is currently unlicensed for use in neonates in many countries. Despite this, it is increasingly used for the induction of anesthesia in the newborn. The clearance of propofol in neonates is slower than in older pediatric patients to the extent that they are at risk of longer recovery.[25] A randomized study in infants found it to be more effective at facilitating intubation than a morphine, atropine, and succinylcholine combination.[26] It has been used successfully in the management of pyloric stenosis.[27]

KETAMINE

This agent is associated with greater cardiovascular stability than many other anesthetic drugs.[28] However, its metabolism is considerably delayed in infants below 1 year of age. It has the advantages of having a profound analgesic effect and of being capable of being given by i.m. injection.

Neuromuscular blocking agents

SUCCINYLCHOLINE

Succinylcholine has the advantage of having both a rapid onset (30 seconds) and short duration of action. Relatively higher doses (2 mg/kg) of this drug are required to produce full relaxation in infants than in adults (1 mg/kg). This is because of the neonate's larger extracellular fluid space, throughout which the drug is distributed. Succinylcholine is metabolized by plasma pseudocholinesterase. Although plasma levels of this enzyme are low in the first 6 months of life, activity is adequate to metabolize the drug, and recovery occurs after a similar time to that seen in adults (approximately 4 minutes).

Because of the number of side effects, including bradycardia, hyperkalemia, and triggering of malignant hyperpyrexia reactions associated with this agent, it has been suggested that its use in young infants should be reevaluated. However, it remains widely used in neonates.[29]

Nondepolarizing muscle relaxants

For many years, it was generally agreed that newborn infants exhibited an increased sensitivity to these agents, but recent studies have demonstrated that full relaxation demands doses similar to those used in adults. A lower plasma concentration is required (presumably because of immaturity of the neuromuscular junction), but this is produced in any event by distribution of injected drug throughout the relatively larger extracellular fluid compartment. Alterations in plasma protein binding may also play a role in determining dose requirements, which are much more variable than in adults. It follows that careful titration of dose against response is advisable and that these drugs should be administered slowly to neonates. Use of a peripheral nerve stimulator as a guide to degree of relaxation is strongly recommended.[30]

ATRACURIUM AND VECURONIUM

These two agents were introduced because their duration of action was intermediate between that of succinylcholine and older nondepolarizing muscle relaxants such as pancuronium and because they offered increased cardiovascular stability. In addition, atracurium is attractive in that its metabolism is independent of hepatic and renal function, although it is dependent on pH and temperature. Recommended initial doses are 0.3–0.5 mg/kg for atracurium and 0.05–0.1 mg/kg for vecuronium. Because of their pharmacokinetic profiles, both drugs are suitable for use by continuous i.v. infusion, although atracurium infusion requirements show marked individual variation.

Nightingale found the duration of effect of atracurium to be longer in infants less than 3 days of age.[31] Other studies have shown the dose–response curves of this agent to be parallel in infants, older children, and adults, and in fact demonstrate recovery times to be shorter in infants.[32] Histamine release, an occasional problem with the drug in adults, is rarely seen in pediatric practice.

Vecuronium, on the other hand, has been found to have a longer recovery time in infants compared to older children and adults and should be regarded as a long-acting muscle relaxant in this age group.[33]

MIVACURIUM

Mivacurium is a short-acting nondepolarizing neuromuscular agent that is rapidly hydrolyzed by plasma pseudocholinesterase. The time course of block produced by the drug is more rapid in younger pediatric patients.[34] Satisfactory intubating conditions are not achieved as quickly as with succinylcholine, but serious side effects occur less frequently.

ROCURONIUM AND SUGAMMADEX

Rocuronium is a member of the aminosteroid family of neuromuscular blocking drugs similar to vecuronium. It has the advantage of providing a rapid onset of action similar to that of suxamethonium without the side effects associated with it. Its duration of action is similar to vecuronium. The recommended doses to provide optimal intubation conditions are 0.3–1 mg/kg.[35] It is felt that the duration of action of rocuronium in neonates is longer than in older children.[36]

Sugammadex is a selective muscle relaxant binding agent that was designed to specifically reverse the effects of aminosteroid muscle relaxants. It encapsulates rocuronium, forming a tightly bound complex that prevents the muscle relaxant from acting at the receptors. Doses prescribed are 2–4 mg/kg when reversing rocuronium-induced muscle relaxation.[37] Data for neonates is currently unavailable.

ANALGESIA

There is no doubt whatsoever that neonates perceive and respond to pain. Effective management of intraoperative and postoperative pain is required to minimize acute physiological and behavioral distress and may also improve acute and long-term outcomes.[38] Opioids, most commonly morphine, remain the gold standard in treating severe postoperative pain in neonates and infants despite concerns about adverse effects, such as respiratory depression. Care must be taken as the neonate has decreased opioid requirements compared to older children.[39] The reasons for this include immaturity of hepatic enzyme systems leading to impaired conjugation and glucuronide excretion and the greater permeability of the infant blood–brain barrier to these drugs.

It follows that where narcotics are administered to neonates intraoperatively, dosage regimens should be modified so that patient safety is not compromised. Morphine (0.05–0.1 mg/kg) and fentanyl (0.005–0.02 mg/kg) given intravenously are the two most widely used drugs, with the latter being particularly well tolerated hemodynamically. Intraoperative infusions of ultra-short-acting opioids have been used successfully, but there are limited specific data to guide remifentanil dosing in neonates.

Intravenous morphine remains popular for provision of postoperative analgesia in ventilated infants and those nursed in high-dependency areas. Morphine administration protocols vary and include continuous infusions, intermittent bolus doses, and nurse-controlled analgesia (NCA). Continuous infusion rates of 0.01–0.03 mg/kg per hour are common, but the lowest effective dose must always be used. NCA is delivered via the same type of pump as patient-controlled analgesia (PCA) with a prescribed bolus and dose interval. Occasionally, background infusions are utilized, but they may increase the risk of respiratory depression in nonventilated patients.[40] Respiratory monitoring should be continued for 24 hours after the last dose of opioid. The situation with regard to other infants is more difficult. It should be recognized that while failure to treat discomfort or pain effectively may have significant long-term effects, overaggressive treatment has its own morbidity.

The use of combined analgesic regimens, leading to adequate analgesia with lower doses of opioids and reduced side effects, has shown some promise. Opioid sparing has been demonstrated in some studies with paracetamol.[41] Nonsteroidal anti-inflammatory drugs are not widely used for analgesia in infants.[42] Currently, there is little evidence to support the use of newer opioids, e.g., tramadol, as an adjunctive therapy.[43] Codeine was used in the past for mild to moderate pain, but its use has been largely discontinued due to risks of respiratory depression, and its use is no longer recommended.

Paracetamol has become commonly used to treat mild to moderate pain. Its pharmacokinetic profile has been well documented following administration via both the rectal and i.v. routes.[44,45] Due to the risk of accidental overdosage, dosage schedules should be frequently reviewed.

Regional anesthesia

It should not be forgotten that local or regional anesthetic techniques (e.g., epidural block, intrathecal block, peripheral nerve block, transversus abdominis plane [TAP] block, wound infiltration, etc.) may be used as alternative methods of providing analgesia for infants during and after surgery. These methods may be particularly valuable, especially in the high-risk ex-premature infant.[46,47] The availability of ultrasound has provided a useful adjunct in identification of anatomical structures, thereby enabling better placement of local anesthetic.[48]

Induction of anesthesia and endotracheal intubation

Most pediatric anesthetists advocate that infants should have anesthesia induced and a muscle relaxant administered prior to attempts at endotracheal intubation. Induction technique depends on (1) the age, size, and physical status of the infant; (2) the relative hazard of regurgitation; and (3) the personal preference of the anesthetist. In most instances, i.v. induction followed by administration of a muscle relaxant is satisfactory. Inhalation induction is an acceptable alternative. In either case, i.v. access should be established beforehand, and the induction itself should be preceded by a short period of preoxygenation.

Intubation is best accomplished with the infant's head extended at the atlanto-occipital joint. The laryngoscope blade is inserted into the right side of the mouth, displacing the tongue to the left. As the blade is advanced the epiglottis, comes into view. In the neonate, this structure is long and floppy, and it should be displaced anteriorly from behind to aid visualization of the larynx. If difficulty is encountered, the little finger of the left hand can be used to press gently on the larynx to improve visualization. The use of an atraumatic but rigid bougie can also be extremely valuable in these cases. Once intubation has been achieved, one should carefully auscultate both lungs to check for equal air entry, and the endotracheal tube should be securely fixed.

If it is considered at the time of induction of anesthesia that postoperative mechanical ventilation will be required, the tube should be inserted by the nasal rather than the oral route. It is difficult to manipulate Magill's forceps in the mouth of a small infant, but flexing the neck usually facilitates passage of nasotracheal tubes.

MAINTENANCE OF ANESTHESIA

Because of the vulnerability of the infant's respiratory system, spontaneous respiration is not used for long periods in the anesthetized neonate. Mechanical ventilation helps ensure adequate gas exchange and also leaves the hands of the anesthetist free to perform other tasks. Suitable ventilators have already been discussed and, depending on the particular machine available, may be set in either pressure or volume control modes, with a ventilatory rate of 30–40 per minute with an inspiratory time of approximately 0.6 second. With the latter, a delivered tidal volume of approximately 8–10 mL/kg is appropriate. Inspired gases should be warmed and humidified to prevent damage to the mucosal lining of the respiratory tract and to minimize heat loss. Manual ventilation allows rapid detection of airway obstruction or disconnection, and is particularly useful during thoracic surgery.

The most widely used agents for maintenance of anesthesia in the neonatal population are isoflurane and sevoflurane, usually combined with 50% oxygen with air, along with a small dose of relaxant.

Consideration should be given to using the lowest inspired concentration of oxygen where possible.

REVERSAL AND EXTUBATION

If a volatile agent has been used for maintenance of anesthesia, it should be discontinued shortly prior to the end of surgery. Once surgery has been completed, residual muscle relaxation is reversed by either neostigmine (0.06 mg/kg) or edrophonium (1 mg/kg) combined with either atropine (0.02–0.03 mg/kg) or glycopyrrolate (0.01 mg/kg). Sugammadex may also be used if rocuronium was the muscle relaxant used during surgery. Controlled ventilation is continued with 100% oxygen or with oxygen in air until spontaneous respiration has returned. Suctioning through the endotracheal tube is carried out if secretions are obviously present. The nostrils should be gently suctioned as a routine. The infant should not be extubated until fully awake and breathing adequately. In most cases, reversal of neuromuscular blockade and resumption of spontaneous respiration occur rapidly. Care is taken to correct hypothermia, acidosis, or hypoglycemia.

MONITORING

The clinical condition of the anesthetized neonate can deteriorate more rapidly and with less warning than that of patients in any other age group. It follows that careful and continuous monitoring is essential. While no piece of machinery will adequately replace the careful anesthetist, there are a number of devices available that provide helpful information that cannot be gleaned by clinical means alone. The monitoring employed in any particular case depends upon the physical status of the infant and the surgical procedure to be undertaken.

The following should be positioned prior to induction (and, indeed, regarded as the minimum equipment required for monitoring anesthetized neonates):

- Electrocardiogram (ECG)
- Blood pressure cuff
- Core temperature probe
- Pulse oximeter probes (preductal and postductal)
- End-tidal carbon dioxide monitor

Most neonates undergoing anesthesia and surgery require additional monitoring. The various options available will be discussed in relation to the particular body system being monitored.

Respiration

Chest wall movement should be observed continuously if at all possible. When mechanical ventilation is employed, airway pressure and minute volume alarms are mandatory. Oxygenation and adequacy of gas exchange are monitored continuously by pulse oximetry and breath-by-breath end-tidal anesthetic agent and carbon dioxide measurement. Serial arterial blood gas analysis is mandatory in critically ill infants undergoing major surgery.

Cardiovascular function

Blood pressure monitoring is essential because of the reduced cardiovascular reserve of the neonate and the risk of hypotension if high concentrations of inhaled anesthetics are used. Automated oscillotonometry is employed in most instances, but concern has been expressed about the accuracy of the devices used when blood pressure is low. The cuff should be of appropriate width (approximately 4 cm).

If either the infant's physical status or the type of surgery to be performed necessitates continuous monitoring of blood pressure, an arterial line is inserted in a suitable vessel, the cannula being connected to a pressure transducer by narrow-bore tubing.

Central venous pressure monitoring is useful in infants with congenital heart disease, and also if significant blood loss (and replacement) is anticipated. The right internal jugular vein is usually the simplest to cannulate. Ultrasound is increasingly used to guide placement of central lines in neonates.

Fluid balance

The goal of intraoperative fluid management is to sustain homeostasis by providing the appropriate amount of parenteral fluid to maintain adequate intravascular volume, cardiac output, and, ultimately, oxygen delivery to tissues at a time when normal physiological functions are altered by surgical stress and anesthetic agents.[48] Maintenance fluid requirements vary considerably within the neonatal period itself but may be taken as being approximately 4 mL/kg per hour for infants older than 5 days of age. Assuming there is no preoperative fluid deficit, an i.v. infusion set at the usual maintenance rate should be commenced prior to induction of anesthesia. The composition of the administered fluid will vary according to the maturity of the baby and preoperative electrolyte and glucose levels. Because of the problems associated with hyperglycemic states in infancy and hyponatremia, care should be taken with the use of 10% dextrose infusions.[49] It is important to take into account the volume of drug diluents administered during anesthesia and surgery when calculating fluid balance.

Blood and fluid loss can be extensive and very difficult to measure during neonatal surgery. The former is best estimated by the use of small volume suction traps, by weighing small numbers of surgical swabs before they dry out, and by serial hemoglobin measurements. During lengthy surgery, serum electrolytes and blood glucose should be measured at regular intervals. Urine output may be monitored by the use of bladder catheterization. Estimated third-space loss may be replaced by continuous administration of lactated Ringer's solution at 3–5 mL/kg per hour.

Volume replacement should be undertaken when blood loss is expected to exceed 5%–10% of circulating blood volume using either 5% albumen or an isotonic crystalloid. Because of the high hematocrit at birth, red-cell replacement is seldom required during most routine neonatal surgical procedures. When required, the blood used should be as fresh as possible. Adequacy of volume replacement can be assessed by monitoring of blood pressure, heart rate, central venous pressure, acidosis on arterial blood samples, and urine output.

ANESTHESIA FOR SPECIFIC SURGICAL CONDITIONS

Esophageal atresia

Once a diagnosis of esophageal atresia (with or without fistula) has been made, the blind upper pouch should be continuously aspirated using a Replogle or similar tube. In general, operation may be safely delayed pending improvement of any aspiration pneumonia that has developed.[50]

Because of the high incidence of associated congenital heart disease, preoperative cardiology assessment, including echocardiography, is essential. Prethoracotomy bronchoscopy is practiced in some centers and may influence subsequent management.[51] Anesthesia is similar to that for other neonatal procedures, but special care must be taken with positioning of the endotracheal tube, the tip of which should be located above the carina but below any fistula present. Surgical retraction during the operation may compromise either respiratory or cardiac function, so that close monitoring is essential. Extubation may occasionally be possible at the end of the procedure.

Congenital diaphragmatic hernia

This condition was formerly regarded as one of the great emergencies of pediatric surgical practice, but it is now agreed that operation should be postponed until adequate gas exchange has been obtained and the infant is hemodynamically stable.[52]

Positive-pressure ventilation using bag and mask should be avoided prior to endotracheal intubation, as expansion of the viscera contained within the hernia will cause further lung compression. Nitrous oxide should be avoided for the same reason. A reasonable anesthetic technique includes controlled ventilation with fentanyl 0.01–0.02 mg/kg, intermediate-acting muscle relaxant, and 100% oxygen or oxygen in air as required. Great caution should be exercised in the use of volatile anesthetic agents. Airway pressures should be kept as low as possible. Should advanced ventilatory techniques such as high-frequency oscillation or nitric oxide be required in order to achieve preoperative stabilization, these may be safely continued during surgery.[53]

Most infants will require mechanical ventilation, sedation and muscle relaxation, and the management of pulmonary hypertension in the postoperative period.

Intestinal obstruction

The various forms of neonatal intestinal obstruction account for approximately 35% of all surgical procedures in the newborn. The major anesthetic problems are those of fluid and electrolyte imbalance (which must be corrected preoperatively), abdominal distension (causing respiratory embarrassment), and the risk of regurgitation and aspiration of gastric contents into the lungs. Following decompression of the stomach, a rapid-sequence induction incorporating preoxygenation, thiopentone or propofol, and succinylcholine with gentle cricoid pressure is advised. Anesthesia is then continued in the usual way.

Exomphalos and gastroschisis

Exomphalos is associated with other midline defects, especially cardiac anomalies, so that preoperative echocardiography is required. This is not true of neonates with gastroschisis. Anesthetic concerns include heat and fluid loss from the exposed bowel and the fact that closure of the abdominal wall defect may push the diaphragm cephalad, thus compromising respiratory function. Special care must be taken to keep heat loss to a minimum. Fluid requirements are much greater than in normal neonates. To maintain plasma oncotic pressure, at least 25% of fluid intake should be given as a colloid. Often, gastroschisis is closed following staged procedures using a silastic silo. The extent of respiratory compromise can assist the anesthetist in advising the surgeon on whether or not primary closure is feasible. A proportion of infants, especially after repair of gastroschisis, require postoperative mechanical ventilation. Increasingly, neonates born with a large exomphalos have the defect closed in stages over a prolonged period, requiring a tracheostomy and long-term ventilation.

Congenital lobar emphysema

This condition may cause severe respiratory distress in the neonatal period. Induction of anesthesia for lobectomy should be as smooth as possible—struggling may trap large amounts of air in the affected lobe during violent inspiratory efforts.[54] Nitrous oxide can also increase the volume of trapped air considerably and is contraindicated. Great care should be taken with controlled ventilation because of the risk of pneumothorax.

Myelomeningocele

If the defect is large, heat and fluid loss during surgery can pose problems and should be monitored as closely as possible. Surgery is carried out with the infant in the prone position, and the chest and pelvis should be supported with pads so that the abdomen remains free from external pressure. Precautions should be taken to limit the patient's exposure to latex in theater. Postoperatively, the neonate should be monitored for apnea and increasing intracranial pressure.

SPECIAL CONSIDERATIONS FOR THE PREMATURE INFANT

Congenital defects occur more commonly in preterm infants, so that surgery is frequently required. Organs and enzyme systems are very immature, and meticulous attention to detail during anesthetic and surgical management is imperative if survival rates are to be high. The large body surface area and lack of subcutaneous fat make maintenance of body temperature even more difficult than in term infants, so that a high neutral thermal environment is essential. Respiratory fatigue occurs very easily and may be exacerbated by residual lung damage following mechanical ventilation, persistent fetal circulation, and oxygen dependency. The response to exogenous vitamin K is less satisfactory than in term infants, and there is an increased risk of bleeding. In addition, anemia is common because of reduced erythropoiesis, a short erythrocyte life span, and iatrogenic causes such as frequent blood sampling. Fluid and electrolyte management can be difficult—insensitive losses are high and hypoglycemia and hypocalcemia occur easily, while renal function and the ability of the cardiovascular system to tolerate fluid loads are reduced.

Premature infants with a history of idopathic apneic episodes preoperatively are more prone than other infants to develop life-threatening apnea during recovery from anesthesia. It is recommended that infants born prematurely who undergo anesthesia and surgery while less than 60 postconceptual weeks of age should have respiratory monitoring for at least 12 hours postoperatively in order to prevent apnea-related complications.[55]

REFERENCES

1. Besag FMC, Singh MP, Whitelaw AGL. Surgery of the ill, extremely low birth weight infant: Should transfer to the operating theatre be avoided? *Acta Paediatr Scand* 1998; 73: 594–5.
2. Frawley G, Bayley G, Chondros P. Laparotomy for necrotizing enterocolitis: Intensive care nursery compared with operating theatre. *J Paediatr Child Health* 1999; 35: 291–5.
3. Ayre P. Endotracheal anaesthesia for babies with special reference to hare-lip and cleft palate operations. *Anesth Analg* 1937; 16: 330–3.
4. Rees GJ. Neonatal anaesthesia. *Br Med Bull* 1958; 14: 38–41.

5. Tochen ML. Orotracheal intubation in the newborn infant: A method for determining depth of tube insertion. *J Pediatr* 1979; 95: 1050–1.

6. Litman RS, Maxwell LG. Cuffed versus uncuffed endotracheal tubes in pediatric anaesthesia: The debate should finally end. *Anaesthesiology* 2013; 118: 500–1.

7. Harnett M, Kinirons B, Heffernan A et al. Airway complications in infants: Comparison of laryngeal mask airway and the facemask–oral airway. *Can J Anaesth* 2000; 47: 315–8.

8. Bahk J-H, Choi I-H. Tracheal tube insertion through laryngeal mask airway in paediatric patients. *Paediatr Anaesth* 1999; 9: 95–6.

9. Ellis DS, Potluri PK, O'Flaherty JE, Baum VC. Difficult airway management in the neonate: A simple method of intubating through a laryngeal mask airway. *Paediatr Anaesth* 1999; 9: 460–2.

10. Fiadjoe JE, Gurnaney H, Dalesio N et al. A prospective randomized equivalence trial of the GlideScope Cobalt® video laryngoscope to traditional direct laryngoscopy in neonates and infants. *Anesthesiology* 2012; 116: 622–8.

11. Walker I, Lockie J. In Sumner E, Hatch DJ (eds). *Paediatric Anaesthesia*. London: Arnold, 2000: 174.

12. Anand KJS, Hickey PR.Pain and its effects in the human neonate and fetus. *N Engl J Med* 1987; 317: 1321–9.

13. Sinner B, Becke K, Engelhard K. General anaesthetics and the developing brain: An overview. *Anaesthesia* 2014; 69: 1009–22.

14. Sanders RD, Davidson A. Anesthetic-induced neurotoxicity of the neonate: Time for clinical guidelines? *Pediatr Anesth* 2009; 19: 1141–6.

15. Salanitre E, Rackow H. The pulmonary exchange of nitrous oxide and halothane in infants. *Anesthesiology* 1969; 30: 388–94.

16. Steward DJ, Creighton RE. The uptake and excretion of nitrous oxide in the newborn. *Can Anaesth Soc J* 1978; 25: 215–7.

17. Hatch D, Fletcher M. Anaesthesia and the ventilatory system in infants and young children. *Br J Anaesth* 1992; 68: 398–410.

18. Warde D, Nagi H, Raftery S. Respiratory complications and hypoxic episodes during inhalation induction with isoflurance in children. *Br J Anaesth* 1991; 66: 327–30.

19. Wolf AR, Lawson RA, Dryden CM, Davies FW. Recovery after desflurane anaesthesia in the infant: Comparison with isoflurane. *Br J Anaesth* 1996; 76: 362–4.

20. O'Brien K, Robinson DN, Morton NS. Induction and emergence in infants less than 60 weeks postconceptual age: Comparison of thiopental, halothane, sevoflurane and desflurane. *Br J Anaesth* 1998; 80: 456–9.

21. Sale SM, Read JA, Stoddart PA, Wolf AR. Prospective comparison of sevoflurane and desflurane in formerly premature infants undergoing inguinal herniotomy. *Br J Anaesth* 2006; 96: 774–8.

22. Constant I, Seeman R, Murat I. Sevoflurane and epileptiform EEG changes. *Pediatr Anesth* 2005; 15: 266–74.

23. Gordana P, Vlajkovic MD, Sindjelic RP. Emergence delirium in children: Many questions, few answers. *Anesth Analg* 2007; 104: 84–91.

24. Hickey PR, Hansen DD, Stafford M et al. Pulmonary and systemic haemodynamic effects of nitrous oxide in infants with normal and raised pulmonary vascular resistance. *Anesthesiology* 1986; 65: 374–8.

25. Allegaert K. Is Propofol the perfect hypnotic agent for procedural sedation in neonates? *Curr Clin Pharmacol* 2009; 4: 84–6.

26. Ghanta S, Abdel-Latif ME, Lui K et al. Propofol compared with morphine, atropine, and suxamethonium regimen as induction agents for neonatal endotracheal intubation: A randomized trial. *Pediatrics* 2007; 119: 1248–55.

27. Dubois MC, Troje C, Martin C et al. Anesthesia in the management of pyloric stenosis. Evaluation of the combination of propofol-halogenated anesthetics. *Ann Fr Anesth Réanim* 1993; 12: 566–70.

28. Friesen RH, Henry DB. Cardiovascular changes in preterm neonates receiving isoflurane, halothane, fentanyl and ketamine. *Anesthesiology* 1986; 64: 238–42.

29. Rawicz M, Brandom BW, Wolf A. The place of suxamethonium in pediatric anesthesia. *Pediatr Anesth* 2009; 19: 561–70.

30. Driessen JJ, Robertson EN, Booij LH. Acceleromyography in neonates and small infants: Baseline calibration and recovery of the responses after neuromuscular blockade with rocuronium. *Eur J Anaesthesiol* 2005; 22: 11–5.

31. Nightingale DA Use of atracurium in neonatal anaesthesia. *Br J Anaesth* 1986; 58 (Suppl 1): 32–36S.

32. Brandom BW, Woelfel SK, Cook DR et al. Clinical pharmacology atracurium in infants. *Anesth Analg* 1984; 63: 309–12.

33. Fisher DM, Miller RD. Neuromuscular effects of vecuronium (ORG NC45) in infants and children during N_2O, halothane anesthesia. *Anesthesiology* 1983; 58: 519–25.

34. Brandom BW, Meretoja OA, Simhi E et al. Age related variability in the effects of mivacurium in paediatric surgical patients. *Can J Anaesth* 1998; 45: 410–6.

35. Cheng CA, Aun CS, Gin T. Comparison of rocuronium and suxamethonium for rapid tracheal intubation in children. *Paediatr Anaesth* 2002; 12: 140–5.

36. Driessen JJ, Robertson EN, Van Egmond J, Booij LH. The time-course of action and recovery of rocuronium 0.3 mg × kg(−1) in infants and children

during halothane anaesthesia measured with acceleromyography. *Paediatr Anaesth* 2000; 10: 493–7.

37. Walker Suellen M. Neonatal pain. *Pediatr Anesth* 2014; 24(1): 39–48.

38. Taylor J, Liley A, Anderson BJ. The relationship between age and morphine infusion rate in children. *Pediatr Anesth* 2013; 23(1): 40–4.

39. Howard RF, Lloyd-Thomas A, Thomas M et al. Nurse-controlled analgesia (NCA) following major surgery in 10,000 patients in a children's hospital. *Pediatr Anesth* 2010; 20(2): 126–34.

40. Ceelie I, de Wildt SN, van Dijk M et al. Effects of intravenous paracetamol on postoperative morphine requirements in neonates and infants undergoing major noncardiac surgery: A randomized controlled trial. *JAMA* 2013; 309(2): 149–54.

41. Use of nonsteroidal anti-inflammatory drugs in infants. A survey of members of the Association of Paediatric Anaesthetists of Great Britain and Ireland. *Pediatr Anesth* 2007; 17: 183–94.

42. Olischar M, Palmer GM, Orsini F et al. The addition of tramadol to the standard iv acetaminophen and morphine infusion for postoperative analgesia in neonates offers no clinical benefit: A randomized controlled trial. *Pediatr Anesth* 2014; 24(11): 1149–57.

43. Hansen TG, O'Brien K, Morton NS, Rasmussen SN. Plasma paracetamol concentrations and pharmacokinetics following rectal administration in neonates and young infants. *Acta Anaesthesiol Scand* 1999; 43(8): 855–9.

44. Allegaert K, Palmer GM, Anderson BJ. The pharmacokinetics of intravenous paracetamol in neonates: Size matters most. *Arch Dis Chil* 2011; 96(6): 575–80.

45. Davidson AJ, Morton NS, Arnup SJ et al. Apnoea after awake regional and general anesthesia in infants: The general anesthesia compared to spinal anesthesia study—Comparing apnoea and neurodevelopmental outcomes, a randomized control trial. *Anesthesiology* 2015; 123(1): 38–54.

46. Jones LT, Craven PD, Lakkundi A, Foster JP et al. Regional (spinal, epidural, caudal) versus general anaesthesia in preterm infants undergoing inguinal herniorrhaphy in early infancy. *Cochrane Database Syst Rev* 2015; 6: CD003669.

47. Tirmizi H. Spinal anesthesia in infants: Recent developments. *Curr Opin Anaesthesiol* 2015; 28(3): 333–8.

48. Leelanukrom R, Cunliffe M. Intraoperative fluid and glucose management in children. *Paediatr Anaesth* 2000; 10: 353–9.

49. Bush GH, Steward DJ. Can persistent cerebral damage be caused by hyperglycaemia? *Paediatr Anaesth* 1995; 5: 385–7.

50. Spitz L, Kiely E, Brereton RJ. Esophageal atresia: Five year experience with 148 cases. *J Pediatr Surg* 1987; 22: 103–8.

51. Kosloske AN, Jewell PF, Cartwright KC. Crucial bronchoscopic findings in esophageal atresia and tracheoesophageal fistula. *J Pediatr Surg* 1988; 23: 466–70.

52. Langer JC, Filler RM, Bohn DJ et al. Timing of surgery for congenital diaphragmatic hernia: Is emergency operation necessary? *J Pediatr Surg* 1988; 23: 731–4.

53. Bouchut J-C, Dubois R, Moussa M et al. High frequency oscillatory ventilation during repair of neonatal congenital diaphragmatic hernia. *Paediatr Anaesth* 2000; 10: 377–9.

54. Cote CJ. The anesthetic management of congenital lobar emphysema. *Anesthesiology* 1978; 49: 296–8.

55. Kurth CD, Spritzer AR, Broennle AM, Downes JJ. Postoperative apnea in preterm infants. *Anesthesiology* 1987: 66: 486–8.

12

Postoperative management of the surgical neonate

SUZANNE CROWE

INTRODUCTION

As each year passes, there are advances in the perioperative management of critically ill newborns who require surgery. Developments in surgical techniques and equipment available have facilitated challenging surgical repairs in smaller infants.[1,2] This has been coupled with new anesthesia modalities, in particular with regard to regional anesthesia, and rapidly metabolized medications such as desflurane and remifentanil.[3–5] Increased operative intervention in preterm and low-birth-weight infants has increased the demand for postoperative high-dependency and intensive care.[6] Alternative respiratory and cardiovascular support in the form of extracorporeal life support, inhaled nitric oxide (NO), and high-frequency oscillation have expanded the potential to support these severely compromised infants.

Differences in physiology and pharmacology in the preterm and term neonate have a direct impact on their capacity to adapt to surgical intervention and to recover in the postoperative period. Pulmonary vascular resistance (PVR) is elevated in the first 10 days of life, which increases the potential to develop right-to-left shunt through the ductus arteriosus. This response occurs particularly in response to hypoxia or metabolic acidosis. There are distinct differences in the coagulation system as plasma levels and activities are low at the time of birth and then increase in the first few months of life. Total body water is higher in the newborn, especially the premature infant, and glomerular filtration rate (GFR) is low in the first few days of life. Thermoregulation mechanisms are poorly developed and require support. The newborn increases cardiac output by increasing heart rate because stroke volume is relatively fixed due to the thin-walled myocardium at birth. The usual stress response to surgery through hormone release and metabolic modulation is altered in the newborn, which has implications for cardiovascular monitoring, support, and sedation and analgesia. This chapter focuses on the physiological features of the surgical neonate in the postoperative period.

RESPIRATORY MANAGEMENT

Neonates have little functional respiratory reserve, which means they have a limited capacity to compensate for changes in respiratory demand. All other systems have a direct impact on respiratory function: cardiac, renal, neurological, immunological, and hematological. Changes that occur in these systems quickly alter respiratory demand and function, which the sick newborn infant may struggle to compensate for. Respiratory muscle fatigue occurs rapidly, due to reduced lung compliance, relative immaturity of the bronchioles and alveoli, and a compliant chest wall. Combined with the neonatal immature respiratory center, apnea develops early when the infant becomes ill. Major abdominal or thoracic surgical procedures that adversely affect the mechanics of the respiratory system make the neonate vulnerable to respiratory failure in the postoperative period. Particular abnormalities such as gastroschisis and congenital diaphragmatic hernia repair cause an increase in intra-abdominal pressure, with upward displacement of the diaphragm and a reduction in lung compliance. Normal tidal ventilation is just above the closing volume for the neonate, so that a reduction in tidal volumes due to abdominal splinting may lead to collapse of alveoli and loss of surface area available for gas exchange. Atelectasis leads to hypoxemia, hypercarbia, and respiratory acidosis. As the pulmonary vasculature bed remains sensitive to changes in pH, the resistance of the pulmonary circulation increases in response to respiratory acidosis, compromising the function of the right side of the heart. To prevent this physiological deterioration, neonates benefit from postoperative respiratory support.[7] The more complex the surgery, with longer duration and requirement for blood transfusion, the more likely that the infant will require a period of ventilation. This is especially the case in premature infants and those with other congenital anomalies. Advances in regional anesthesia have allowed earlier separation from ventilation as the placement of effective local anesthetic blocks reduces the use of opiates in the early postoperative period.

VENTILATORY SUPPORT

Positive-pressure ventilation

Modern ventilators in the neonatal intensive care unit (NICU) and pediatric intensive care unit (PICU) have been designed to meet the needs of children recovering from major surgery. Oxygen and air are mixed from a pipeline supply at 50 psi. Microprocessors control the inspiratory and expiratory valves, and the gas is humidified and warmed before being delivered to the patient. The expiratory valves control the level of positive end-expiratory pressure (PEEP) applied to each cycle of respiration. Various modes of ventilation are available, ranging from complete mandatory ventilation to synchronized support ventilation and spontaneous pressure support. The range of modes allow the infant to be weaned gently from breathing support, with less lung damage than was previously associated with ventilation in children.[8]

The surgical neonate is generally commenced on time-cycled pressure-limited ventilation. A preselected pressure is set, defined as the peak inspiratory pressure (PIP), and is chosen to deliver an adequate tidal volume, taking into account the compliance of the lung and the airway resistance. In uncomplicated postoperative ventilation, PIP is usually 15–20 cm H_2O. This pressure may need to be increased significantly if there is reduced lung compliance due to pulmonary edema or increased airway resistance due to decreased thoracic compliance. The airway pressure at the end of expiration (normally zero during spontaneous respiration) may need to be increased to 5–10 cm H_2O to prevent alveolar collapse at the end of each breath. The rate of the inflations delivered by the ventilator is related to the need to excrete carbon dioxide and is usually 28–36 breaths per minute (bpm).

Patient-triggered ventilation and synchronized ventilation

Synchronized patient-triggered ventilation has many advantages in the neonate. It reduces the requirement for sedation and neuromuscular medications as the infant coordinates his/her breathing with pressure assist. Neuromuscular medications can have a prolonged duration of effect due to immature drug metabolism and renal excretion. The ventilator uses an inspiratory flow-generated trigger, which senses the commencement of inspiration and provides a set-pressure or set-volume assist. The sensitivity of the trigger may be varied by the operator, to allow earlier opening of the inspiratory valve and initiation of respiratory effort. This can either be triggered in the pressure or volume control modes as pressure support ventilation (PSV) or synchronous intermittent mandatory ventilation (SIMV), or be completely independent of

the machine in the continuous positive airway pressure (CPAP) mode. Patient-generated triggering maintains muscle function during ventilation and facilitates weaning and separation from the ventilator. Different modes of ventilation have been compared in neonates with respiratory failure, most commonly in lung disease of prematurity.[9,10] There is some evidence from these randomized controlled trials (RCTs) that synchronized modes of patient-triggered ventilation may reduce air leak and reduce the duration of ventilation required.[11,12] The terminology and most common modes of ventilatory support are summarized in Table 12.1.

High-frequency oscillatory ventilation

Increased understanding of the importance of limiting peak pressures when inflating the lungs has led to the widespread use of high-frequency oscillatory ventilation (HFOV).[13,14] This mode of ventilation recruits alveoli to participate in gas exchange, keeping the lung open with a constant distending pressure. This is sometimes referred to as the "open lung" approach. Excretion of carbon dioxide is managed by adjustments to the frequency and magnitude of oscillation, and oxygenation is achieved by adjusting the mean airway pressure and the inspired content of oxygen.[15] Recruitment and stabilization of lung volumes is both pressure and time dependent.[16] In 1996, the prospective randomized trial of high frequency oscillatory ventilation versus conventional ventilation (PROVO) trial used a clearly defined lung recruitment protocol with all patients receiving surfactant and demonstrated a reduction in hospital length of stay and the incidence of chronic lung disease.[17] Commencing HFOV early rather than after lung damage has been sustained appears to improve outcome, especially in premature infants.[14,17] Some relevant features of HFOV and high-frequency jet ventilation (HFJV) are summarized in Table 12.2.

Lung-protective ventilation

The intervention of tracheal intubation and ventilation generally aims to restore blood gas analysis to within normal limits for oxygen, carbon dioxide exchange, and pH. However, achieving blood gas values within the normal range comes at a cost due to adverse consequences of PPV. High inflation pressures used to reduce carbon dioxide can result in ventilator-associated lung injury.[18] This may impact on both the lung parenchyma and the vasculature. Animal models of ventilator-induced lung injury demonstrate pulmonary edema, hyaline membrane formation, and pulmonary epithelial cell injury, which can be produced with lung inflation pressures of just 30 cm H_2O. Limiting the pressure within the lung and accepting relative hypercarbia has become known as lung-protective ventilation and is used especially in the context of premature lungs and dysplastic lungs.[19] There is also increasing evidence that hypocarbia may be injurious to the developing neonatal brain, as

Table 12.1 Commonly used forms of positive-pressure ventilation and terminology

Terminology	Descriptor	Comments
Volume ventilation or volume control ventilation	Preset TV. Patient cannot trigger the ventilator. Tidal volume is constant, while PIP may vary.	Most commonly used mode in adults and older children. Also effective in smaller children with minimal ETT leaks.
Pressure ventilation or pressure control ventilation	Preset pressure. Patient cannot trigger the ventilator. PIP is constant, but tidal volume may vary.	Commonly used in neonates. Increasing use in adults to prevent ventilator-induced lung injury in patients with ARDS.
Continuous positive airway pressure (CPAP)	Spontaneous breathing mode with no mechanically delivered breaths and positive end-expiratory pressure. High gas flow delivered by a demand valve.	First introduced to treat preterm infants with lung disease of prematurity. Now commonly used as a pre-extubation mode of respiratory support.
Assist-control ventilation	Minimum rate and TV (or pressure) set. Patient may trigger inspiration at a more rapid rate.	Common form of weaning from mechanical ventilation.
Assisted ventilation	All breaths are patient triggered at the ventilator's set volume or pressure.	Most commonly used as *pressure support* ventilation.
Mandatory ventilation, intermittent mandatory ventilation (IMV), or synchronized intermittent mandatory ventilation (SIMV)	Machine-generated breath that is triggered, limited, and cycled by the ventilator.	Not commonly used.
High-frequency positive-pressure ventilation (HFPPV)	Positive pressure delivered at rates >60/min by a conventional ventilator.	Commonly used in neonates with severe hypoxic respiratory failure.
Noninvasive ventilation (NIV), commonly known as bilevel positive airway pressure (BiPAP)	Positive pressure delivered by either nasal or face mask. Commonly used as a bilevel device with preselected inspiratory airway pressure (IPAP) and expiratory airway pressure (EPAP).	Increasingly used in patients with less severe lung disease and in premature infants. Avoids the need for intubation and risk of ventilator-associated pneumonia (VAP).
Neurally adjusted ventilator assist (NAVA)	Positive pressure initiated by detection of electrical activity in the diaphragm. May be delivered via endotracheal tube or noninvasive mask.	Comfortable weaning mode, which improves synchrony with the ventilator and allows reduction in sedation.

Note: ARDS: acute respiratory distress syndrome; TV: tidal volume.

Table 12.2 Characteristics of high-frequency ventilators

	HFOV	HFJV
Rate	180–900/min	100–600/min
VT	At high rates (>10 Hz), minimal TV. TV increases as rates decreases.	TV 2–5 mL/kg
Expiration	Active	Passive
Gas movement	Diffusion	Diffusion plus bulk flow
Indications	Used in lung disease associated with low lung compliance (MAS, IRDS) as part of an open lung strategy. Also has been extensively used in CDH.	IRDS, MAS, and bronchopleural fistula

Note: Hz: cycles per second; IRDS: infant respiratory distress syndrome; MAS: meconium aspiration syndrome; VT: tidal volume.

it impairs blood flow within the brain. Hyperventilation as a strategy to close the ductus arteriosus is no longer carried out as a result of these concerns. Earlier application of surfactant and nasal CPAP in the neonates has improved the outcome in premature infants with moderately severe forms of respiratory distress syndrome (RDS).[20,21]

Setting ventilator parameters

The choice of ventilation mode in each newborn is dependent on the condition of the infant on arrival in the PICU/NICU, and the expected course for any known pathology, e.g., giant exomphalos or tracheoesophageal fistula. The objective is to maintain gas exchange within a physiological range (PaO$_2$ 8–12 kPa, PCO$_2$ 5–6.5 kPa), using the lowest inspired concentration of oxygen and airway pressures compatible with that aim. This is straightforward when the lungs are normal but may require advanced ventilatory strategies in the presence of congenital or acquired abnormalities of the thorax and/or abdomen. An infant with normal lung compliance and airway resistance placed on a preset pressure ventilator would require a PIP of 10–20 cm H$_2$O, a rate of 25–35 bpm, a FiO$_2$ of 0.21–0.35, and a PEEP of 3–5 cm H$_2$O. Within an hour of commencement, a chest radiograph should be carried out to ensure optimum lung field expansion, and blood gas analysis performed to ensure hyperventilation is avoided.

Respiratory monitoring

Blood gas monitoring: Monitoring of respiratory function in the postoperative period requires measurement of gas exchange. The most reliable and accurate method is to measure PaO$_2$, PaCO$_2$, and pH from an arterial sample. The most common sites for invasive monitoring are the umbilical artery in newborns and radial or dorsalis pedis arteries in older infants. Samples drawn from the right radial artery in the newborn will measure preductal values, whereas the other sites will be postductal. On some occasions, the left subclavian artery is beside the origin of the duct and will therefore measure similarly to the right radial. Automated blood gas machines now require less than 0.2 mL of blood for analysis, which reduces the need for blood transfusions due to frequent sampling in the sick neonate. Capillary blood from a well-perfused area of skin is used to provide samples for blood gas analysis, particularly if there is no direct arterial access.

Noninvasive oxygenation and CO$_2$ monitoring: Pulse oximetry measures arterial saturation and heart rate on a beat-to-beat basis in a reliable and accurate fashion. The absolute values do not correlate well with measured values at arterial saturations less than 70% and in low cardiac output states where there is peripheral hypoperfusion. Careful sensor placement is important as the probe is sensitive to light artifact. It is a useful monitor in the critical care and operating theatre environment as it rapidly reflects response to intervention such as suctioning and changes in ventilation. Due to the shape of the oxygen dissociation curve, high PaO$_2$ levels (>95 mm Hg, 12.6 kPa) will

not be accurately reflected by saturation measurements. Transcutaneous probes for both oxygen and carbon dioxide are also used, especially in premature infants. Both probes heat the skin to 41°C–44°C, augmenting cutaneous blood flow. Indirect monitors of gas exchange should be confirmed occasionally using an arterial sample. Greater accuracy is obtained by careful maintenance of the probes and care in calibration and application to the skin. Due to the risk of skin damage from the heating element, the probe site must be rotated every 4–6 hours. End-tidal CO$_2$ monitoring or capnography uses infrared measurement of CO$_2$ and provides a continuous indirect assessment of the CO$_2$ with each expired breath. It is a standard monitor available in most critical care units. In the presence of lung disease, the difference between the end-tidal CO$_2$ measurement and the PCO$_2$ in blood increases, and the validity of end-tidal CO$_2$ as a monitor declines. Because the connector is still quite cumbersome, it increases the dead space volume and may make spontaneous respiration more difficult in smaller patients.

CARE OF THE INTUBATED PATIENT IN THE PICU

Endotracheal tube (ETT) size and positioning: Newborns are commonly managed with nasotracheal tubes rather than oral tubes unless there is a congenital abnormality of or injury to the nasal area that precludes use. Nasal ETTs provide greater patient comfort and security, require less sedation to tolerate, and allow better oral care. The tube may be securely fastened to the face and nose, reducing the possibility of accidental extubation. In older children, oral tubes are satisfactory for brief periods of ventilation, but nasal tubes are frequently preferred. The ETT size is selected on the basis of weight and age (Table 12.3). In terms of length, the tip of the ETT should be between the heads of the clavicles on a plain radiograph of the chest. If a tube tip is lower than this, it may enter the right main bronchus, causing right upper lobe collapse and/or left lung collapse. This can be a cause of substantial and avoidable morbidity. A plain film of the chest should be obtained after endotracheal intubation or repositioning of the ETT to verify correct position. The proximal end of the ETT should protrude sufficiently far from the nose so that the tube connector does not compress the external nares and result in a pressure-related erosion of the skin or cartilage.

Table 12.3 Endotracheal tube size selection

Age	Endotracheal tube diameter (mm)
Preterm	2.0–2.5
Term newborn	3.0–3.5
1 month	3.5
1–6 months	3.5–4.0
1 year	4.5

Cuffed low-pressure ETTs are being used increasingly in infants, as they facilitate easier management of leak around the ETT and may reduce the incidence of ventilator-associated pneumonia, as secretions do not pass freely around the ETT and into the bronchial tree. When using an uncuffed ETT, a large leak can make ventilation extremely difficult. This is especially relevant in the postoperative period when high-pressure ventilation may initially be required. Very small tubes such as the 2.5 and 3.0 are prone to blocking with retained secretions, and routine suctioning is key in maintaining the patency and efficiency of the ETT. Suctioning may be hazardous, particularly in small infants and the premature infant, leading to hypoxia and bradycardia even when carried out with meticulous care. Suction support with preoxygenation is a feature offered on ventilators, which provides assistance in managing this complication.

Endotracheal suctioning may be used to perform a modified bronchoalveolar lavage and extract samples of alveolar secretions to be examined microbiologically. Information gained about organisms cultured may direct further treatment if infection is suspected clinically.

All ventilators combine ventilation with humidification. Humidification is important in the management of the infant's temperature and in prevention of ventilator-associated pneumonia. Loose secretions are easier to suction out of the bronchial tree; thick dry secretions risk being retained to cause plugging and atelectasis. The goal of the humidifier is to deliver fully saturated gases at a temperature of 37°C to the ETT. When infants wean from ventilation and extubate, they may continue to need supplemental oxygen and/or noninvasive ventilation—these support modalities require humidification also.

MANAGEMENT OF THE NEWBORN WITH HYPOXIC RESPIRATORY FAILURE

Neonates may present shortly after delivery with hypoxic respiratory failure. Cardiac causes must be excluded quickly. The most common cause is persistent pulmonary hypertension of the newborn (PPHN). PPHN may develop rapidly if the reactive pulmonary vascular bed is exposed to acidosis or hypoxia. This may occur in the context of meconium aspiration, airway obstruction, or sepsis. Support of the hypoxic newborn requires neonatal or pediatric intensive care admission, with commencement of HFOV.[22] Inotropic infusions are frequently needed to provide an adequate perfusion pressure as the right side of the heart struggles to pump against the high resistance of the pulmonary bed. If the right ventricle begins to fail, the left ventricular function becomes impaired, and extreme systemic hypotension and organ hypoperfusion may follow.

Nitric oxide

Inhaled NO is generally employed with HFOV in the management of these critically unwell infants.[23] NO induces relaxation of the muscular endothelium in the pulmonary vessels, which may reverse the pulmonary hypertension. When administered by the inhaled route, NO diffuses rapidly from the alveolus into the endothelial cell and the vascular smooth muscle, where it stimulates guanylate cyclase to produce cyclic guanosine monophosphate (cGMP). A series of RCTs have shown that inhaled NO improves oxygenation and reduces the need for extracorporeal membrane oxygenation (ECMO) in term neonates with PPHN.[24-26] Although the response may be dramatic, not all infants respond. Infants with right-to-left shunt without extensive parenchymal lung disease generally respond better. If there is extensive lung disease secondary to meconium aspiration or hypoplasia, reversal may not occur to the same extent.

Two phosphodiesterase inhibitors, dipyridamole and sildenafil, have been successfully used to treat the rebound pulmonary hypertension associated with the withdrawal of inhaled NO.[27] Sildenafil by continuous infusion has also been shown to be effective in infants with PPHN who have not been responsive to inhaled NO.[28] Both inhibitors may be used in combination for severe hypoxia, e.g., infants with congenital diaphragmatic hernia.

Surfactant replacement therapy

An important advance in neonatal medicine was the synthesis and introduction of surfactant replacement therapy for the treatment of lung disease of prematurity. It is administered prophylactically in patients at risk for or with established lung disease of prematurity.[29] When combined with lung-protective ventilation, it reduces the incidence of air leak and mortality.[30,31] Natural surfactant may contain additional proteins that have anti-inflammatory properties. It has been trialed in other diagnostic groups but without the same positive results. Human studies have shown that the use of surfactant replacement therapy in infants with meconium aspiration is associated with decreased need for ECMO.[32]

WEANING FROM VENTILATION

Reducing reliance on ventilatory support as quickly as possible is key to the avoidance of complications of ventilation. Cessation of medications that interfere with respiratory muscle function, i.e., muscle relaxants and, to a lesser extent, opiates, is vital in maintaining the function of the diaphragm and intercostal muscles. Gradual reduction in ventilator support may be achieved in a number of different ways, but they generally incorporate a reduction in pressure support to each breath and a reduction in the number of mandatory breaths delivered by the ventilator. As the strength and efficiency of spontaneous ventilation increases, the patient is moved to a completely spontaneous mode in the form of pressure support (PS)/CPAP. When the pressure support approaches physiological level, i.e., 5–7 cm H_2O, and the PEEP required is 3–5 cm H_2O, in <40% oxygen, extubation may be considered. However, the overall condition of the patient must be included in this decision. If using a cuffed ETT, the cuff is deflated, and the presence of a leak around the ETT is verified. More recently, neurally adjusted ventilation assist (NAVA) is employed as a weaning mode of ventilation. It allows the patient to be awake and comfortable when triggering assisted breaths, as the electrical activity of the diaphragm is sensed early in the respiratory cycle and assistance is delivered proportional to the activity of the diaphragm. This allows the infant to vary the size and frequency of each breath while being assisted.

POSTOPERATIVE SEDATION AND ANALGESIA

It is now widely understood and accepted that neonates require sedation and analgesia to facilitate safe and humane surgical management. Effective pain relief reduces the hormonal stress response to surgery and reduces hypertension and intraventricular hemorrhage in the preterm infant.[33] Analgesia improves glucose homeostasis, reduces airway pressures, and reduces circulating endogenous catecholamines.[34] The most common opiates used in neonatal critical care are fentanyl, morphine, and remifentanil.[35] Benzodiazepines are used as an adjunct, to produce sedation, usually in the form of midazolam or lorazepam. A summary of agents employed is in Table 12.4. The proliferation of catheter-based regional anesthetic techniques in recent years has reduced the requirement for opiate analgesia.[36] Local anesthetic blocks are sited in the operating room using ultrasound guidance and are continued using continuous infusion of levobupivicaine through indwelling catheters.

HEMODYNAMIC SUPPORT IN THE NEWBORN

Cardiac output is a the product of heart rate times the stroke volume, with increase in output dependent on the ability to increase heart rate or vary stroke volume. Stroke volume is influenced by venous return (preload), impedance (afterload) to left or right ventricular output, and contractility of the myocardial muscle. The newborn myocardium is relatively immature, with little capacity to increase stroke volume. Therefore, cardiac output is largely dependent on heart rate. Compensation for falling stroke volume occurs by increasing heart rate. Blood pressure does not reflect compensation through heart rate increase and vasoconstriction, so that decompensation appears to occur suddenly, with hypotension as a late sign. Cardiac output may be estimated from the clinical parameters of heart rate, blood pressure, urine output, and skin/core temperature gradient. These parameters are combined with blood gas analysis to examine the base deficit, serum lactate, and mixed venous saturation if the blood sample is taken from a central venous line. Measurement of central venous pressure (CVP) allows optimization of right atrial filling pressure and preload.

Central venous access may be established through the internal jugular, subclavian, or femoral vein in the neonate. Ultrasonography is now part of standard practice to guide placement of central access, which is technically challenging in very small infants. The cannulation of the

Table 12.4 Commonly used agents for anesthesia and analgesia in newborns

Drug	Classification	Comments	Commonly used dosages
Morphine	Narcotic	Good analgesic effect with sedation. Cumulative effect in newborns. Withdrawal effects with sustained usage.	20–30 µg kg^{-1} hour^{-1} in ventilated patients
Fentanyl	Short-acting narcotic	Potent, short-acting narcotic. Commonly used for procedural sedation in ventilated patients.	1–2 µg kg^{1} hour^{-1} as a stat dose; 0.5–2 µg kg^{-1} hour^{-1} as an infusion
Midazolam	Short-acting benzodiazepine	Used as sedation either as a stat dose or by continuous infusion.	1–4 µg kg^{-1} min^{-1} by continuous iv infusion; stat dose 0.1–0.2 mg/kg
Lorazepam	Benzodiazepine	More prolonged effect than midazolam. Potent anticonvulsant.	For seizures, 0.05 mg/kg iv
Ketamine	Dissociative anesthetic agent. Can be given by im or iv injection.	Good analgesic properties. Used for procedural sedation/anesthesia. Sympathomimetic effect increases blood pressure.	Stat dose for induction of anesthesia 1–2 mg/kg iv
Acetaminophen	COX inhibitor. Available as oral or rectal preparation.	Useful for mild procedural pain and as an antipyretic.	10–15 mg/kg per dose
Sucrose	Stimulates endogenous opioids	Useful for procedural analgesia.	2 mL po for term infants

Note: im: intramuscular; iv: intravenous; po: oral.

radial, posterior tibial, dorsalis pedis, or femoral artery with a 22- or 24-gauge cannula facilitates direct arterial pressure measurement and access for sampling for blood gas analysis, and electrolyte and acid/base measurement. Umbilical venous and arterial lines may be sited shortly after delivery of the infant and may be used for a short time. They can cause renal or gut ischemia if not positioned correctly.

Management of the infant with clinical signs of shock is focused on increasing preload by volume expansion with 1–20 mL/kg crystalloid or colloid boluses, followed by reassessment of the clinical picture. Further fluid boluses are frequently necessary. If increasing preload does not improve systemic perfusion, vasoactive medications may be required to support organ perfusion.

VASOACTIVE MEDICATION THERAPY IN NEONATES

Vasoactive medications produce vasodilation or vasoconstriction. Some medications also produce an increase in contractility due to direct action on the cardiac myocyte. By altering tissue oxygen delivery, heart rate, filling pressures, afterload, and contractility, these medications affect myocardial work and increase oxygen consumption. Figure 12.1 illustrates the effects of fluid administration and inotropes on the neonatal cardiac output. An ideal agent would have a balanced effect, increasing contractility and decreasing afterload, with minimal heart rate change. This medication currently does not exist, so combinations of drugs are used

to maximize systemic perfusion and reduce side effects. There are a limited number of studies looking at inotropes and their effects in the neonate, with most concentrating on the infant post–cardiac surgery.[37,38]

The available vasoactive medications and their effects are summarized in Table 12.5. Generally, a beta or alpha receptor agonist such as noradrenaline or adrenaline is combined with a phosphodiesterase inhibitor such as milrinone or enoximone.[39–41] Vasopressin is a potent medication, which produces vasoconstriction independent of the beta and alpha receptors, and is used in inotrope-resistant shock, e.g., gram-negative sepsis.[42] Vasodilators in the form of sodium nitroprusside are occasionally used to reduce systemic vascular resistance (afterload). Steroids are used in inotrope-resistant shock, producing an increased perfusion pressure secondary to the effects of aldosterone.[43,44]

Fluid management and renal function

Maintenance of normal fluid and electrolyte homeostasis is challenging in the neonate as the kidneys are functionally immature. GFR is lower in the preterm infant than the term neonate, with the term neonate capable of producing dilute urine (30–50 mOsm/L), retaining adequate sodium with normal sodium intake. The kidney in the preterm infant is inefficient at conserving sodium and yet is relatively insensitive to the effects of circulating antidiuretic hormone (ADH). This reduces the capacity of the infant to produce a concentrated urine if necessary, e.g., in dehydration. The newborn has a higher proportion of extracellular water,

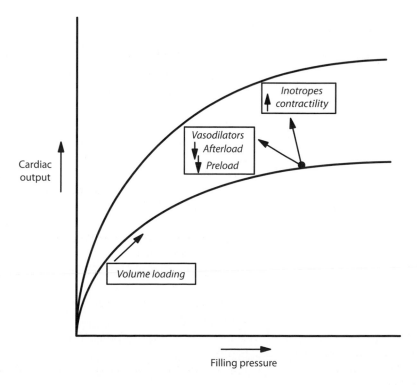

Figure 12.1 Effect of increasing right atrial filling pressures, vasodilator drugs, and inotropes on cardiac output (Frank–Starling curve).

Table 12.5 Vasoactive drugs used for hemodynamic support

	Effect of vasoactive drugs	
Drug	Site of action	Dose
Dopamine	β1 effects on myocardium; peripheral α effects at high doses; indirect release of noradrenaline; renal vasodilation through dopaminergic receptors in kidney	1–10 µg kg^{-1} min^{-1} β effects 10–20 µg kg^{-1} min^{-1} α and β effects >20 µg kg^{-1} min^{-1} α effects
Dobutamine	β1 effects on myocardium; weak α and β2 effects at periphery	5–15 µg kg^{-1} min^{-1}
Epinephrine	β1 effects on myocardium; β2 effects at periphery; peripheral α effects	0.01–0.1 µg kg^{-1} min^{-1}
Norepinephrine	Predominantly α effects; potent vasoconstrictor; pressor with only minimal inotropic properties	0.01–0.1 µg kg^{-1} min^{-1}
Milrinone	Phosphodiesterase inhibitor; acts by increasing cGMP; vasodilator and inotropic effects	0.33–1 µg kg^{-1} min^{-1}
Vasopressin	Acts on V1 receptors in the vascular	0.002–0.0004 µg kg^{-1} min^{-1}	Bed via cAMP; no effect on heart rate

Note: cAMP: cyclic adenosine monophosphate.

which alters the pharmokinetics of medications administered. Fluid balance in the newborn depends on a balance between fluid loss (evaporative, renal, gastrointestinal tract [GIT]) and the intake required for maintaining organ perfusion and growth. Full maintenance fluid requirements for the nonventilated term newborn commence at 60 mL/kg per 24 hours on the first day of life and increase to 100–150 mL/kg per 24 hours by day 7. Fluids are administered as saline 0.9% or 0.45%, with dextrose 5%–10%. Losses from the gastrointestinal (GI) tract due to nasogastric suction, enterocolic fistulas, or high-output stomas can be underestimated and should be measured and replaced.

The hormonal stress response to surgery includes increased release of ADH and cortisol. Anesthetic medications, opiates, and PPV also increase ADH release, causing the infant to retain free water and excrete more concentrated urine. Using hypotonic intravenous solutions as maintenance fluids results in further accumulation of electrolyte free water and can cause hyponatremia.[45,46] All infants on intravenous fluids should have daily assessment of fluid requirements and serum electrolyte levels. When a newborn is on ventilatory support, his/her fluid intake is reduced to 70% of normal requirements as humidification of the ventilator gases reduces insensible fluid loss from the lungs.

A urine output of >1 mL/kg per hour is accepted as adequate and reflects sufficient volume preload and organ perfusion. Short periods of oliguria may follow surgery due to increased ADH levels, but persistent oliguria or anuria needs further management as it may indicate prerenal, postrenal, or intrinsic renal impairment. Prerenal failure is generally due to decreased renal blood flow associated with fluid loss or inadequate fluid resuscitation in a sick infant.

A fluid bolus of 20 mL/kg crystalloid or colloid may restore circulating blood volume and renal perfusion. If there is no urine produced following an initial fluid bolus, further fluid administration may be required. Intrinsic renal failure is an infrequent but more serious complication. It is also more difficult to manage. Causes include congenitally abnormal kidneys (cystic or dysplastic), prolonged intraoperative renal ischemia, or vascular abnormalities of the kidney. Drugs such as indomethacin, nonsteroidal antiinflammatories, and aminoglycosides can cause intrinsic renal damage. If red cells, casts, or protein is found on urinalysis, in association with high urinary sodium losses, it is more likely to be intrinsic renal disease rather than prerenal failure. Management of renal failure focuses on elimination of causes, fluid restriction, and treatment of hyperkalemia. Peritoneal dialysis may be used to support renal recovery.[47] Renal replacement therapy in the form of continuous hemofiltration is not generally performed in newborns, due to availability of suitable equipment and the risks of systemic heparinization.

Temperature regulation and metabolism

Temperature: To maintain a normal body temperature, the neonate has to balance heat loss with heat production. With a large surface area–to–body ratio, the neonate tends to lose heat rapidly by conduction, convection, evaporation, and radiation. The newborn has a limited ability to raise its body temperature through heat production from metabolism of brown fat stores and glucose. This is inability is exaggerated in the premature infant, who is poikilothermic and vulnerable to cold-induced metabolic acidosis, hypoglycemia, increased oxygen consumption, and weight loss. Critically ill neonates need to be nursed in a warm environment to protect them from the effects of cold stress. If hemodynamically stable, the infant is nursed in an incubator with an internal temperature regulated at 32°C–36°C, which will eliminate conductive and convective heat losses. If the infant needs to be nursed outside the incubator, a radiant warmer bed or platform may be used.

Metabolism—Glucose metabolism is immature in the newborn period, and the sick infant may develop hypoglycemia rapidly. This is as a result of diminished glycogen stores (inadequate hepatic stores in the premature infant or depletion from catecholamine-stimulated breakdown in stress) or due to hyperinsulinism in diabetic mothers. Infants born with intrauterine growth retardation are also vulnerable to development of hypoglycemia due to reduced hepatic gluconeogenesis. Failure to recognize and treat neonatal hypoglycemia results in seizures and cerebral injury. Neonates who are not feeding require maintenance fluid containing dextrose, usually 10%. Blood glucose measurement should be performed regularly as part of normal nursing care. Glucagon and steroid administration is occasionally required to bring the blood sugar level into the normal range (2–6 mmol). Infants receiving intravenous dextrose or total parenteral nutrition may experience rebound hypoglycemia if the infusion is stopped abruptly due to increased blood insulin levels.

Hypocalcemia is common in the newborn period, especially in critically ill newborns, infants of diabetic mothers, and infants who have received large volume blood transfusion. Measurements of total serum calcium do not accurately reflect the level of ionized calcium in the blood. Reduced circulating calcium levels can cause seizures, apnea, and low cardiac output as the neonatal myocardium is very sensitive to changes in calcium serum levels. Replacement using intravenous calcium infusion must be carried out using central venous access as calcium is extremely irritant to small peripheral veins and tissues.

REFERENCES

1. Smithers CJ, Hamilton TE, Manfredi MA, Rhein L, Ngo P, Gallagher D et al. Categorization and repair of recurrent and acquired tracheoesophageal fistulae occurring after esophageal atresia repair. *J Pediatr Surg* 2016 Aug 31 pii; S0022-3468(16)30288-3.
2. Nose S, Sasaki T, Saka R, Minagawa K, Okuyama H. A sutureless technique using cyanoacrylate adhesives when creating a stoma for extremely low birth weight infants. *Springer Plus* 2016 Feb 27;5:189 eCollection 2016-10-3.
3. Davidson AJ, Morton NS, Arnup SJ, de Graaff JC, Disma N, Withington DE et al. Apnoea after awake regional and general anesthesia in infants: The general anesthesia compared to spinal anaesthesia study—Comparing apnoea and neurodevelopmental outcomes, a randomized controlled trial. *Anesthesiology* 2015 Jul; 123(1):38–54.
4. Sale SM, Read JA, Stoddart PA, Wolf AR. Prospective comparison of sevoflurane and desflurane in formerly premature infants undergoing inguinal herniotomy. *Br J Anaesth* 2006 Jun; 96(6): 774–8.
5. Sammartino M, Garra R, Sbaraglia F, De Riso M, Continolo N, Papacci P. Experience of remifentanil in extremely low-birth-weight babies undergoing laparotomy. *Pediatr Neonatol* 2011 Jun; 52(3): 176–9.
6. Eicher C, Seitz G, Bevot A, Moll M, Goelz R, Arand J et al. Surgical management of extremely low birth weight infants with neonatal bowel perforation: A single-centre experience and a review of the literature. *Neonatology* 2012; 101(4): 285–92.
7. Greenough A, Dimitriou G, Prendergast M, Milner AD. Synchronised mechanical ventilation for respiratory support in newborn infants. *Cochrane Database Syst Rev* 2008(1): CD000456.
8. Dassieu G, Brochard L, Benani M, Avenel S, Danan C. Continuous gas insufflation in preterm infants with hyaline membrane disease. A prospective randomised trial. *Am J Respir Crit Care Med* 2000; 162(3 Pt 1): 826–31.
9. Davis P, Henderson-Smart D. Post-extubation prophylactic nasal continuous positive airway pressure in preterm infants: A systematic review and meta-analysis. *J Paediatr Child Health* 1999; 35(4): 367–71.
10. Kamper J, Wulff K, Larsen C, Lindequist S. Early treatment with nasal continuous positive airway pressure in very low birth weight infants. *Acta Paediatr* 1993; 82(2): 193–7.
11. Courtney SE, Barrington KJ. Continuous positive airway pressure and non-invasive ventilation. *Clin Perinatol* 2007 Mar; 34(1): 73–92.
12. Robertson NJ, Hamilton PA. Randomised trial of elective continuous positive airway pressure (CPAP) compared with rescue CPAP after extubation. *Arch Dis Child Fetal Neonatal Ed* 1998; 79(1): F58–60.
13. Clark RH, Yoder BA, Sell MS. Prospective randomised comparison of high request oscillation and conventional ventilation in candidates for extracorporeal membrane oxygenation. *J Pediatr* 1994; 124(3): 447–54.
14. Thome U, Kossel H, Lipowsky G, Porz F, Furste HO, Genzel-Boroviczeny O et al. Randomised comparison of high frequency ventilation with high rate intermittent positive pressure ventilation in preterm infants with respiratory failure. *J Pediatr* 1999; 135(1): 39–46.
15. Courtney SE, Durand DJ, Asselin JM, Hudak ML, Aschner JL, Shoemaker CT. High frequency oscillatory ventilation vs. conventional mechanical ventilation former low birth weight infants. *N Engl J Med* 2002 Aug 29; 347(9): 643–52.

16. Johnson AH, Peacock JL, Greenough A, Marlow N, Limb ES, Marston L et al. High frequency oscillatory ventilation for the prevention of chronic lung disease of prematurity. *N Engl J Med* 2002 Aug 29; 347(9): 633–42.

17. Gerstmann DR, Minton SD, Stoddard RA, Meredith KS, Monaco F, Bertrand JM et al. The Provo Multicenter early high frequency oscillatory ventilation trial: Improved pulmonary and clinical outcome in respiratory distress syndrome. *Pediatrics* 1996; 98: 1044–57.

18. Miguet D, Claris O, Lapillonne A, Bakr A, Chappuis JP, Salle BL. Preoperative stabilisation using high frequency oscillatory ventilation in the management of congenital diaphragmatic hernia. *Crit Care Med* 1994; 22(9 Suppl): S77–82.

19. Rimensberger PC, Pache JC, McKerlie C, Frndova H, Cox PN. Lung recruitment and lung volume maintenance: A strategy for improving oxygenation and preventing lung injury during both conventional mechanical ventilation and high frequency oscillation. *Intensive Care Med* 2000; 26(6): 745–55.

20. Verder H, Albertsen P, Ebbesen F, Greisen G, Robertson B, Bertelsen A et al. Nasal continuous positive airway pressure and early surfactant therapy for respiratory distress syndrome in newborns of less than 30 weeks gestation. *Pediatrics* 1999; 103(2): E24.

21. Verder H, Robertson B, Greisen G, Ebbesen F, Albertsen P, Lundstrom K, Jacobsen T. Surfactant therapy and nasal continuous positive airway pressure for newborns with respiratory distress syndrome. Danish-Swedish Multicenter Study Group. *N Engl J Med* 1994; 331(16): 1051–5.

22. Carter JM, Gerstmann DR, Clark RH. High frequency oscillatory ventilation and extra corporeal membrane oxygenation for the treatment of acute neonatal respiratory failure. *Pediatrics* 1990; 85: 159–64.

23. Davidson D, Barefield ES, Kattwinkel J, Dudell G, Damask M, Straube R et al. Inhaled nitric oxide for the early treatment of persistent pulmonary hypertension of the term newborn: A randomised, double-masked, placebo-controlled, dose-response, multi-centre study. *Paediatrics* 1998; 101(3): 325–34.

24. Kinsella JP, Walsh WF, Bose CL, Gerstmann DR, Labella JJ, Sardesai S et al. Inhaled nitric oxide in premature neonates with severe hypoxaemic respiratory failure: A randomised controlled trial. *Lancet* 1999; 354(9184): 1061–5.

25. The Neonatal Inhaled Nitric Oxide Study Group. Inhaled nitric oxide in full-term and nearly full-term infants with hypoxic respiratory failure. *N Engl J Med* 1997 Feb 27; 336(9): 597–604.

26. Christou H, Van Marter LJ, Wessel DL, Allred EN, Kane JW, Thompson JE et al. Inhaled nitric oxide reduces the need for extracorporeal membrane oxygenation in infants with persistent pulmonary hypertension of the newborn. *Crit Care Med* 2000; 28(11): 3722–7.

27. Atz AM, Wessel DL. Sildenafil ameliorates effects of inhaled nitric oxide withdrawal. *Anesthesiology* 1999; 91(1): 307–10.

28. Steinhorn PH, Kinsella JP, Pierce C, Butrous G, Dilleen M, Oakes M, Wessel DL. Intravenous sildenafil in the treatment of neonates with persistent pulmonary hypertension. *J Pediatr* 2009 Dec; 155(6): 841–7.

29. Engle WA. Surfactant replacement therapy for respiratory distress in the preterm and term neonate. *Pediatrics* 2008 Feb; 121(2): 419–32.

30. Lotze A, Mitchell BR, Bulas DI, Zola EM, Shalwitz RA, Gunkel JH. Multicenter study of surfactant (beractant) use in the treatment of term infants with severe respiratory failure. Survanta in Term Infants Study Group. *J Pediatr* 1998; 132(1): 40–7.

31. Boloker J, Bateman DA, Wung JT, Stolar CJ. Congenital diaphragmatic hernia in 120 infants treated consecutively with permissive hyper apnoea/ spontaneous respiration/elective repair. *J Pediatr Surg* 2002 Mar; 37(3): 357–66.

32. El Shahed AI, Dargaville P, Ohlsson A, Soll RF. Surfactant for meconium aspiration syndrome in full term/near term infants. *Cochrane Database Syst Rev* 2007(3): CD002054.

33. Anand KJ, Hansen DD, Hickey PR. Hormonal-metabolic stress responses in neonates undergoing cardiac surgery. *Anaesthesiology* 1990; 73(4): 661–70.

34. Anand KJ, Hall RW. Pharmacological therapy for analgesia and sedation in the newborn. *Arch Dis Child Fetal Neonatal Ed* 2006 Nov; 91(6): F448–53.

35. Hall RW, Anand KJS. Pain management in newborns. *Clin Perinatol* 2014 Dec; 41(4): 895–924.

36. Walker SM. Neonatal pain. *Paediatr Anaesth* 2014 Jan; 24(1): 39–48.

37. Subhedar NV, Shaw NJ. Dopamine versus dobutamine for hypotensive preterm infants. *Cochrane Database Syst Rev* 2003(3): CD001242.

38. Valverde E, Pellicer A, Madero R, Elorza D, Quero J, Cabanas F. Dopamine versus epinephrine for cardiovascular support in low birth weight infants: Analysis of systemic effects and neonatal clinical outcomes. *Pediatrics* 2006 Jun; 117(6): e1213–22.

39. Brierley J, Carcillo JA, Choong K, Cornell T, DeCaen A, Deymann A et al. Clinical practice parameters for hemodynamic support of pediatric and neonatal septic shock: 2007 update from American College of Critical Care Medicine. *Crit Care Med* 2009 Feb; 37(2): 666–88.

40. Chang AC, Atz AM, Wernovsky G, Burke RP, Wessel DL. Milrinone: Systemic and pulmonary hemodynamic effects in neonates after cardiac surgery. *Crit Care Med* 1995 Nov; 23(11): 1907–14.

41. Hoffman TM, Wernovsky G, Atz AM, Kulik TJ, Nelson DP, Chang AC et al. Efficacy and safety of milrinone in preventing low cardiac output syndrome in infants and children after corrective surgery for congenital heart disease. *Circulation* 2003 Feb 25; 107(7): 996–1002.

42. Choong K, Bohn D, Fraser DD, Gaboury I, Hutchison JS, Joffe AR et al. Vasopressin in Pediatrics vasodilatory shock: A multicenter randomised controlled trial. *Am J Respir Crit Care Med* 2009 Oct 1; 180(7): 632–9.

43. Higgins S, Friedlich P, Seri I. Hydrocortisone for hypotension and vasopressin dependence in preterm neonates: A meta-analysis. *J Perinatol* 2010 Jun; 30(6): 373–8.

44. Subhedar NV, Duffy K, Ibrahim H. Corticosteroids for treating hypotension in preterm infants. *Cochrane Database Syst Rev* 2007(1): CD003662.

45. Choong K, Kho ME, Menon K, Bohn D. Hypotonic versus isotonic saline in hospitalised children: A systematic review. *Arch Dis Child* 2006 Oct; 91(10): 828–35.

46. Montanana PA, Modesto i Alapont V, Ocon AP, Lopez PO, Lopez Prats JL, Toledo Parreno JD. The use of isotonic fluid as maintenance therapy prevents iatrogenic hyponatraemia in pediatrics: A randomised, controlled open study. *Pediatr Crit Care Med* 2008 Nov; 9(6): 589–97.

47. Gouyon JB, Guignard JP. Management of acute renal failure in newborns. *Pediatr Nephrol* 2000; 14(10–11): 1037–44.

13

Fluid and electrolyte balance in the newborn

JUDITH MEEHAN, JOSEPH CHUKWU, WINIFRED A. GORMAN, AND ELEANOR J. MOLLOY

INTRODUCTION

Infants are born into a low-humidity, gaseous environment from the liquid intrauterine world. Term and preterm neonates have different fluid requirements and electrolyte changes to older children and adults especially at this time of rapid postnatal transition.

WATER DISTRIBUTION IN THE FETUS AND THE NEWBORN INFANT

Fetal body composition alters progressively throughout pregnancy. Throughout pregnancy, the amount of protein and fat in the fetus increases. Preterm neonates have more water, and they may lose 10%–15% of their weight in the first week of life. At 1 kg birth weight (approximately 28 weeks gestation), the fetus comprises about 80% of its weight as water; by full term, water content is 75% and by 3 months of age (~5 kg) 60%.[1-3] Small for gestational age (SGA) preterm infants may have a higher proportional body water content: 90% for SGA infants versus 84% for appropriate for gestational age (AGA) infants at 25–30 weeks gestation.[4] At 23 weeks gestation, infants are composed of 90% water comprising 60% extracellular fluid (ECF) and 30% intracellular fluid (ICF; Figure 13.1).

The total intracellular water content of the fetus and the newborn infant's body increases directly in proportion to cell mass. Twenty-five percent of the weight of the very immature fetus early in pregnancy is intracellular water, and this increases to 35% at birth and 40% by 3 months of age. Body fat content increases from about 1% in the very early fetus to 15% at birth and 30% at 3 months of age.[1] Fat has a low water content.[1] The SGA infant with a low body fat content has a greater proportion of body weight as water than the AGA infant.

FUNCTIONAL ADJUSTMENTS TO POSTNATAL LIFE

Renal blood flow

Functional nephrons are first present in the fetus at approximately 8 weeks gestation. Nephrons develop in a centrifugal pattern with juxtamedullary nephrons developing first. The full complement of glomeruli is present by 34 weeks gestation. Renal blood supply arises from the aorta between T12 and L2, a relationship that remains constant between 24 and 44 weeks gestation. As the renal arteries divide into segmental end arteries, the renal tissue in their area of distribution is very vulnerable to ischemia, thus follows the recommendation that umbilical artery catheters should not be positioned between T12 and L3.[5,6]

Renal blood flow and glomerular filtration rate (GFR) *in utero* increase gradually with gestational age. Growth of nephrons accounts for the increases in GFR in the fetus. Vascular resistance is high in the fetal kidney and restricts renal blood flow and glomerular filtration *in utero*. The proportion of cardiac output that is distributed to the kidneys during fetal life is about 2%–3%.[5-7] It increases to about 6% during the first week of life and approximates 15%–18% during the first month of life. In adults, the kidneys receive 20%–25% of the cardiac output. The low renal blood flow during fetal life results from a high renal vascular resistance. Factors that may contribute to renal dysfunction in neonates include prematurity, medication (gentamicin, cephalosporin, NSAIDs, Frusemide), hypoxia, congenital renal tract anomalies, and excessive fluid loss.

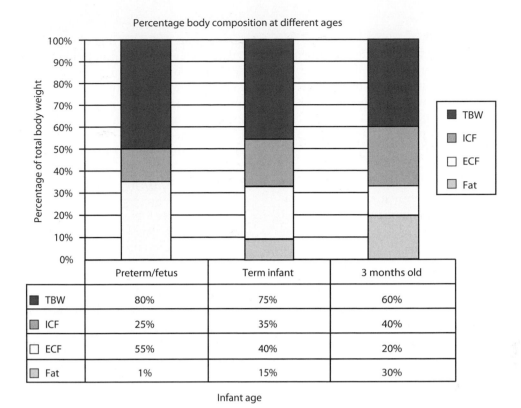

Figure 13.1 Body fluid/fat composition at different ages. TBW: total body water; ICF: intracellular fluid; ECF: extracellular fluid.

The chart is titled "Percentage body composition at different ages" with the y-axis labeled "Percentage of total body weight" and the x-axis labeled "Infant age".

	Preterm/fetus	Term infant	3 months old
■ TBW	80%	75%	60%
▨ ICF	25%	35%	40%
☐ ECF	55%	40%	20%
▥ Fat	1%	15%	30%

Glomerular filtration rate

Glomerular filtration begins between 9 and 12 weeks gestation in the human fetus and contributes to amniotic fluid. In fetal sheep, GFR increases by 2.5 times during the last trimester and parallels the rise in fetal body weight and kidney weight.[8–10] At delivery, there is a positive correlation between GFR and gestational age in newborn infants delivered between 27 and 43 weeks gestation.[11]

In the first 24 hours after delivery, there is a threefold increase in GFR in the term but not preterm infant, although there is no increase in total renal blood flow or in systemic blood pressure. Changes in GFR at birth may be influenced by plasma adrenaline and noradrenaline,[12,13] renin–angiotensin, prostaglandin, arginine vasopressin,[14–16] and plasma cortisol.[17] Indomethacin use in the preterm neonates has been shown to increase the resistance of the renal vascular bed thereby decreasing renal perfusion.[18] Each of these or a combination of these hormones may influence glomerular filtration by decreasing glomerular vascular resistance and recruiting superficial cortical nephrons.

WATER HOMEOSTASIS

The diluting segment of the distal tubule and ascending limb of the loop of Henle develops relatively early in nephrogenesis. When challenged with a water load, both the term and the preterm infants can dilute their urine to osmolalities to 50 and 70 mOsm/kg water, respectively. Glomerular filtration, however, is low, and this limits the quantity of urine that can be excreted even in the presence of a potent dilutional capacity. The newborn kidney of both the term and preterm infants has relatively low osmolality in the renal medulla, and this limits the effectiveness of the countercurrent concentrating mechanism in the loop of Henle.[19,20] In the term infant, urine can be concentrated to a maximum of 600–700 mOsm/L, considerably less than that of 1200 mOsm/L in the older child or adult. Thus, both the preterm and full-term neonates are unable to handle either fluid deprivation or overload, underlining the need for accurate assessment of fluid requirements.[21]

Immediately after birth, a physiological acute isotonic volume contraction occurs predominantly in the extracellular water with the corresponding postnatal weight loss. Weight loss is greater and lasts longer in infants with less advanced gestational age.

Insensible water loss

Insensible water loss is the continuous invisible loss of water by evaporation that occurs from the skin and lung surface. Insensible water loss needs inclusion in the estimation of total fluid requirements.[22] Transepidermal water loss (TEWL) accounts for about two thirds of insensible water loss, while respiratory water loss accounts for one third. Insensible water loss is greater in less mature infants.[23]

Sweating

Sweating occurs to only a very limited extent in response to a thermal stimulus in the term infant, despite the fact that the full complement of sweat glands is present at birth. Although even the most immature infant soon develops the ability to sweat in response to heat stress, the efficiency of sweating as a thermoregulatory process is poor.[24]

Transepidermal water loss

Evaporation of water from the skin surface occurs continuously by diffusion.[25,26] The quantity of water lost is determined by the relative humidity of the infant's surrounding atmosphere particularly in the preterm infant: skin maturation - immature skin keratinization.

TEWL is closely related to thermal balance—there is heat loss whenever water evaporates from a surface (1 g water = 0.58 kcal of heat loss). In a term baby under stable environmental conditions, TEWL can be elevated, accounting for as much as 70 cal/kg/day heat loss (more than half of the caloric intake of the preterm infant). Preterm infant TEWL is greatly increased as gestational age decreases due to the large ratio of surface area to weight and the immature epidermal barrier to water. TEWL from the skin is exaggerated by postnatal trauma to the skin, for example, from adhesive tape applied to the skin for attachment of monitors. Incidentally, neonatal skin barrier dysfunction using TEWL predicts food allergy at 2 years of age, supporting the concept of transcutaneous allergen sensitization.[27]

In addition, placing impermeable plastic sheets over and under the baby or the use of plastic bags can significantly reduce TEWL of the infant surgical patient.[28] After birth regardless of gestation, the skin matures and skin permeability to water falls. However, in the extremely preterm infant, this maturation may be extremely slow and extracellular water loss has been shown to be higher than normal at 28 days postnatal age.[29,30] TEWL gradually decreases over the first 7 days of life and is significantly lower in infants whose mothers had received prenatal steroids. However, Jain et al. failed to demonstrate any maturational effect of antenatal steroids on transepidermal loss in preterm infants.[31–33] Maximizing incubator humidity can reduce TEWL.[34] Insensible water loss in infants weighing <1 kg is reduced to <40 mL/kg/day if ambient humidity is above 90%.[35]

Respiratory water loss

Respiratory loss represents 39% of insensible water loss in term infants. Inspired air becomes fully saturated with water in the upper respiratory tract, and some water is lost as this air is expired. Similarly, tachypnea increases water loss. The relative humidity of the air before inspiration also has an influence; the higher the humidity, the less water needs to be added and the less lost. Ventilated infants inspire humidified air delivered, reducing respiratory water loss by a third.[36]

FLUID AND ELECTROLYTE MANAGEMENT

Infants admitted to a neonatal intensive care unit who are unable to exclusively feed orally require careful management of fluid and electrolyte balance. Additional difficulties may occur if the infant is preterm and if, as frequently happens in babies requiring surgery, there are additional losses from the intestine or the kidneys as a result of a complex surgical problem. When planning maintenance fluid therapy for an infant, all the variables that have already been discussed that may influence fluid requirements must be taken into account. Any guidelines for fluid and electrolyte therapy must be modified to suit an individual infant's requirements. Tables 13.1 and 13.2 give some guidelines that may be used and modified appropriately.[37] Preterm infants

Table 13.1 Fluid requirement in the newborn

	Fluid volume (mL/kg)	Fluid type
Baby Nursed in Incubator		
Day 1	60	10% dextrose/TPN
Day 2	80	Plasmalyte in 10% dextrose/TPN
Day 3	100	Plasmalyte/10% dextrose/TPN
Day 4	120	Plasmalyte/10% dextrose/TPN
Day 5	150	Plasmalyte/10% dextrose/TPN
Baby Nursed under Radiant Warmer		
Day 1	80	10% dextrose/TPN (5% dextrose if Bwt < 1500 g)
Day 2	100	Plasmalyte in 10% dextrose/TPN
Day 3	120	Plasmalyte/10% dextrose/TPN
Day 4	140	Plasmalyte/10% dextrose/TPN
Day 5	150	Plasmalyte/10% dextrose/TPN

Note: Restricted fluids—two thirds of normal maintenance fluids. Very low birth weight infants frequently require even higher initial rates of fluid administration and frequent reassessment of serum electrolytes, urine output, and body weight.

Table 13.2 Maintenance electrolyte therapy

	Per kg/day
Sodium	2–4 mmol
Potassium	1–3 mmol
Calcium	5–10 mL of 10% calcium gluconate (1.125–2.25 mmol calcium)

<1.5 kg should be commenced on total parenteral nutrition in the first few hours of life to optimize their nutrition and then, expressed breast milk once available. Further discussion of neonatal enteral and parenteral nutrition is beyond the scope of this chapter.

Increased fluid requirements may occur in the following circumstances:

- *Low birth weight infants <1.5 kg.* The very low birth weight infant has a very high insensible loss of fluid and thus increased requirements for free water.
- *Phototherapy.* Phototherapy increases insensible water loss by evaporation; thus, fluid intake should be increased by 10 mL/kg/day per number of phototherapy unit light used in the infant >1.5 kg and 20 mL/kg/day per number of lights used with birth weights <1.5 kg.[38,39]
- *Radiant warmer.* Nursing on a radiant warmer increases insensible fluid loss by a mean of 0.94 mL/kg/h[40] when compared with incubators. This increased water loss is not prevented by using a heat shield but may be prevented by using a plastic blanket.[40–42] Use of a humidified incubator is preferable especially in preterm babies.
- *Polyuric renal failure (especially in infants <26 weeks gestation).* Maintenance fluids will require very frequent readjustment guided by regular monitoring of the weight and the serum electrolytes.

Maintenance fluid therapy may need to be decreased in the following circumstances:

- Inappropriate ADH secretion
- Congestive heart failure
- Oliguric renal failure
- Patent ductus arteriosus

Conservative patent ductus arteriosus (PDA) management involves fluid restriction to a total fluid intake of 120 mL/kg/day.[43] A high PDA closure rate (up to 100%) in preterm infants with PDA managed conservatively with fluid restriction (130 m/kg/day) and adjustment of ventilation (reducing inspiration time and increasing the peak end expiratory pressure) may be achieved.[44] The detailed management of PDA with pharmacotherapy and surgery is beyond the scope of this chapter.

In assessing the infant's water requirements, one needs to evaluate weight change, urine output, specific gravity and osmolality, serum sodium and creatinine, and blood urea and osmolality. Normal urine output is 2–4 mL/kg/h. In the first 24 hours of life, urinary output may be very low or even absent. During recovery from a severe illness associated with fluid retention or edema, polyuria may occur. A physiological diuresis (water loss) of up to 10% of body weight occurs over the first 4–5 days of life. This diuresis has the effect of decreasing total body water content by contracting the ECF volume. It is greater in the preterm infant whose total body water content is higher than that of the term infant. This water loss occurs despite usual fluid intakes and is typically accompanied by a negative sodium balance even when sodium is provided.

High fluid intake (>170 mL/kg/day) increases the likelihood of symptomatic patent ductus arteriosus.[45] High fluid intake and or high sodium intake may also increase the likelihood of respiratory complications both in the short term and in the longer term by increasing the frequency of chronic lung disease (CLD).[46,47]

Sodium regulation

Maintenance of normal serum sodium (135–140 mmol/L) is principally controlled by the kidneys. The amount of sodium that can be excreted is limited by the GFR, and the ability of the kidney to excrete a sodium load is diminished as compared with adults and falls progressively with decreasing gestational age.[48–50] Preterm infants have a higher fractional sodium excretion than full-term infants.[48] Extrauterine existence accelerates tubular sodium reabsorption but not GFR, whose maturation is related to postconceptual age. Al-Danhan et al.[48,49] demonstrated that preterm infants of <30 weeks gestation require a minimum of 5 mmol/kg/day of sodium and those of 30–35 weeks gestation require 4 mmol/kg/day to achieve a positive sodium balance and maintain normal serum sodium.

Intestinal absorption of sodium in the very preterm infant is low and improves progressively with increasing gestational age.[49] Neonates undergoing intensive care may gain significant amounts of fluid and sodium from drugs, bronchial lavage, and flushing of catheters, sources that are often overlooked. Hypernatremia may occur, especially in the very low birth weight infant, and may have adverse effects.[51]

Antenatal steroids induce maturation of renal tubular function. Infants who have been exposed to prenatal steroids have an earlier diuresis and natriuresis.[31] Randomized controlled trials have shown that early sodium administration increases the risks of hypernatremia, particularly if TEWL is high and water intake is limited, and increases the risks of respiratory morbidity by impeding the normal, physiological loss of ECF. Subsequently, once nutritional intake is sufficient to support growth, the extremely preterm infant is at risk of chronic sodium depletion. At this stage, an intake of at least 4 mmol/kg/day is required, or more particularly in the absence of antenatal steroid exposure.[52–56]

Renal response to antidiuretic hormone

The human fetal pituitary secretes antidiuretic hormone (ADH) from 12 weeks gestation onward. Labor and delivery are associated with a surge in ADH secretion in cord blood. Both term and preterm infants are capable of an appropriate ADH response to stimuli. Although ADH levels in newborn infants are similar to adults, the antidiuretic response to ADH is blunted because a lower concentration gradient in the renal medulla lessens its effectiveness and low numbers of ADH receptors. Excess ADH can cause a drop in urine output and hyponatremia.[14,57]

Factors that result in excess or inappropriate secretion of ADH (SIADH) in the newborn include birth asphyxia, surgery, hypoxia, severe lung disease, positive pressure ventilation, intracranial hemorrhage, and pneumothorax. SIADH results in weight gain, hyponatremia, and oliguria. SIADH is diagnosed by documenting hyponatremia in association with low serum osmolality and high or normal urine osmolality and high urinary sodium due to continued excretion of sodium in urine despite low serum sodium. There is usually no evidence of fluid depletion. It is also important to note that the renal, adrenal, and thyroid functions are usually normal in SIADH. Management is by fluid restriction in addition to alleviating the primary cause.[58]

Sodium balance

Sodium is not required during the first 24 hours of life, during which time urine and sodium output are low. Sodium supplementation of 2–4 mmol/kg/day should be given when weight loss of approximately 5%–10% of birth weight and postnatal diuresis have occurred.

Hyponatremia, defined as Na+ <130 mmol/L, may occur in the following circumstances:

- Laboratory error.
- Excess antidiuretic hormone secretion, where low urinary loss of water results in dilutional hyponatremia.
- Large renal tubular losses of sodium as occurs in extreme prematurity or polyuric renal failure.
- Congestive heart failure with dilutional hyponatremia.
- Diuretic therapy with loss of sodium via the renal tubules.
- Hypoadrenalism: congenital Addison's disease, septic shock with adrenal failure, salt-wasting adrenogenital syndrome.
- Maternal hyponatremia.[59]
- Factitious hyponatremia as a result of hyperglycemia or hyperlipidemia.
- Inadequate sodium intake in preterm infants with excessive renal sodium loses.
- Excessive large intakes of free water or electrolyte-free solutions like dextrose water.
- Congenital syndromes such as Bartter syndrome, which is a genetic defect caused by a defect in the kidneys'

ability to reabsorb sodium. This results in a rise in rennin and aldosterone, and potassium wasting in addition to excess sodium loss through the urine.

Hypernatremia, serum sodium >145 mmol/L, may occur in the following circumstances:

- Laboratory error
- High insensible water loss, which is incompletely replaced
- High urinary water losses, which are not replaced
- Maternal hypernatremia
- Deficiency of antidiuretic hormone
- Rarely, excessive administration of Na+ in intravenous fluid flushes
- Excessive sodium bicarbonate administration in infants with metabolic acidosis

Hypernatremia and fluctuations of sodium seem to be related to early severe intraventricular hemorrhage (IVH) among preterm infants,[60,61] and increasing intake of sodium appears to be a modifiable risk factor for IVH in very low birth weight infants. The association of high sodium intake with IVH was of similar magnitude to traditionally recognized risk factors such as pneumothorax.

Potassium balance

Potassium is predominantly an intracellular ion. No potassium is required on the first day of life. After this, intakes of 1–3 mmol/kg/day should replace losses and maintain a normal serum potassium of 3.5–5.8 mmol/L (Table 13.2). Potassium should be cautiously administered in infants with renal dysfunction and the very low birth weight infant whose ability to excrete potassium may be limited. Early non oliguric hyperkalemia may occur in 30%–50% of infants with birth weight <1 kg as a result of a potassium shift from intracellular to extracellular space. Hyperkalemia will be exaggerated by hypoxia, metabolic acidosis, catabolic stress, and oliguria. The hyperkalemia may be severe enough to cause life-threatening arrhythmias.[8,62–65]

Hyperkalemia, serum K+ >6 mmol/L in a sample that is not hemolyzed, becomes concerning when >6.5 mmol/L or if ECG changes occur. ECG changes in hyperkalemia vary from peaked T waves, as the earliest sign, to a widened QRS complex, bradycardia, tachycardia, supraventricular tachycardia, ventricular tachycardia, and ventricular fibrillation

Hyperkalemia may occur in the following circumstances:

- Laboratory error or hemolysis of blood sample
- Severe metabolic acidosis: with each 0.1 pH drop, serum potassium increases by 0.6 mmol/L
- Tissue cell death with release of intracellular potassium, e.g., release of K+ from neuronal cells and RBCs post IVH, trauma, or surgery
- Acute renal failure
- Very low birth weight in the absence of renal failure

- Very low birth weight in the absence of antenatal steroids
- Adrenal insufficiency secondary to acute adrenal failure as in sepsis/shock or congenital adrenal hyperplasia
- Severe hemolytic anemia

Management of Hyperkalemia (Figure 13.2)

- Avoid potassium in all infusions in the first day of life.
- Infants born <28 weeks gestation should have serum potassium levels recorded from 12–48 hours of age. Blood gas analysis will identify the neonate with rising potassium levels. Laboratory measurement of serum potassium should be performed 12 hourly for the first 48–72 hours of life.
- Only blood from umbilical arterial line, peripheral arterial line, arterial stab, or free-flowing venous sample should be used.
- Treatment of hyperkalemia should commence if serum K+ ≥7 mmol/L confirmed on a nonhemolyzed arterial/venous sample and/or ECG changes are present and serum K+ ≤7 mmol/L.
- ECG changes include tall peaked T waves, prolonged PR interval, small/absent P waves, widening of the QRS complex, and asystole.

Treatments used in premature infants with non-oliguric hyperkalemia aim to decrease the arrhythmogenicity of hyperkalemia, redistribute potassium into the intracellular space, or remove potassium from the body.[66]

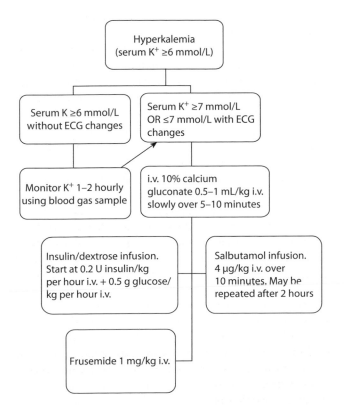

Figure 13.2 Management of hyperkalemia.

Sodium bicarbonate is not recommended. If acidosis is present, the underlying cause should be treated. Ion exchange resins are also not recommended. They have been shown to cause intestinal obstruction and perforation. Also gastric masses found at autopsy were devoid of potassium, indicating that no exchange had occurred. A recent Cochrane study of interventions for neonatal non-oliguric hyperkalemia found limited information from small studies of uncertain quality and made no firm recommendations for clinical practice. The combination of insulin and glucose is preferred over treatment with rectal cation–resin for hyperkalemia in preterm infants. Both the combination of insulin and glucose and salbutamol (albuterol) inhalation deserve further study. Other potentially effective interventions for non-oliguric hyperkalemia (diuretics, exchange transfusion, peritoneal dialysis, and calcium) have not been tested in randomized controlled trials.[67]

CAUSES OF HYPOKALEMIA

Hypokalemia, serum potassium <3.5 mmol/L, may occur in the following circumstances:

- Laboratory error.
- Alkalosis lowers serum potassium by shifting the potassium load intracellularly, but does not lower total body potassium.
- Polyuric renal failure.
- Gastrointestinal losses through vomiting or diarrhea or pooling of fluid in a "third space," such as dilated loops with intestinal obstruction.
- Diuretic therapy.
- Inadequate intake.
- NG aspirate losses not replaced with appropriate fluids.
- Bartter syndrome as mentioned previously, which results in potassium wasting.

Hypokalemia predisposes to cardiac arrhythmias, paralytic ileus, urinary retention and respiratory muscle paralysis. Thus potassium balance must be carefully monitored, taking into account the influence that pH may have on the serum potassium, in that alkalosis shifts potassium which is predominantly an intracellular ion into the cells and acidosis has the reverse effect and that both hyper- and hypokalemia will have adverse effects.

Acid–base balance

Normal values for pH are similar to those in the adult; however, pCO_2 and serum bicarbonate are both slightly lower in the newborn infant than in the adult.[58,59] The lungs and the kidney both have important roles in the maintenance of acid–base balance. The lung excretes volatile acid formed during metabolism as CO_2. Respiratory failure will cause accumulation of CO_2 and respiratory acidosis.

METABOLIC ACIDOSIS

The normal kidney has a vital role in regulation of serum bicarbonate. In mature subjects, serum bicarbonate is maintained at approximately 25 mmol/L, but preterm infants have a lower threshold.[68] The kidney also has an important role in the excretion of nonvolatile acid (mainly sulfur-containing amino acids) produced by metabolism.

Causes of metabolic acidosis

1. Perinatal asphyxia
2. Severe hypotension with impaired tissue perfusion
3. Acute renal failure
4. Acute diarrhea and dehydration
5. Excess ileal loss
6. Excess protein administration, e.g., excess amino acid in parenteral nutrition
7. Inborn errors of metabolism (e.g., organic acidemia)
8. Sepsis

Acute metabolic acidosis is common in the critically ill newborn. Treatment requires management of the underlying cause. Sodium bicarbonate may be used for severe acidosis by giving a dose of 1–2 mmol/kg of 4.2% sodium bicarbonate diluted in equal volume of water. There is currently no evidence from randomized controlled trials to support its routine use in neonatal resuscitation.[69] Its effect on morbidity and mortality has not been well demonstrated. There is controversy about the value of intravenous sodium bicarbonate for correction of metabolic acidosis.[70] It is no longer recommended for resuscitation in newborn infants, and although it may correct acidosis in hypotensive shocked infants, this has not been shown to result in improvement in blood pressure or perfusion.[71] Sodium bicarbonate infusion has potential side effects. Myocardial function may be depressed from the osmolar load with severe acidosis. Paradoxical intracellular acidosis may occur as well as a reduction in cerebral blood flow and increased risk of IVH. Use of sodium bicarbonate is therefore discouraged unless the infant has prolonged acidosis not responsive to other therapies including adequate ventilation.

Causes of metabolic alkalosis

Persistent vomiting causes hypochloremic alkalosis and body potassium depletion. This may occur with untreated pyloric stenosis or upper intestinal obstruction. Correction is by replacement of fluid, sodium chloride, and potassium. Rehydration and correction of depleted electrolytes will be followed by correction of the metabolic alkalosis. Chronic respiratory acidosis as in CLD may cause renal re-regulation of the sodium bicarbonate level at a higher threshold until pH is normal. Infants with chronic hypercapnia regularly have a serum bicarbonate of greater than 30 mmol/L. Permissive hypercapnia or controlled ventilation is a strategy adopted to limit the damage done by excessive mechanical ventilation pressures or volumes to the lungs in order to decrease the incidence of CLD.[72]

Glucose homeostasis

Glucose is the most important substrate for brain metabolism and whereas ketones, glycerol and lactate can be used, a continuous supply of glucose is essential for normal neurological function.[73,74] Fetal blood glucose is identical to that of maternal blood glucose since passive transfer of glucose occurs across the placenta.

HYPOGLYCEMIA

Immediately after delivery, blood glucose falls to ~2.5 mmol/L (45 mg/dL) in the term infant. Following delivery a combination of hormonal responses (glucagon, growth hormone, thyroxine) and oral feeds or in their absence intravenous fluids, serve to maintain blood glucose within a normal range. There is no consensus regarding the definition of hypoglycemia in the neonate.[73,74] Blood glucose levels between 2.5 mmol/L (45 mg/dL) and 7.2 mmol/L (130 mg/dL) are accepted as being safe. Symptomatic hypoglycemia results in cyanosis, apnea, lethargy, seizures, or coma. Blood sugar values represent a continuum, and there is no specific value at which brain-damaging hypoglycemia will always occur.[71,75] However, brain MRI scans after symptomatic neonatal hypoglycemia (median glucose level 1 mmol/L) without evidence of hypoxic–ischemic encephalopathy reveal white matter injury in 94% and neurodevelopmental impairment in 64% at 18 months.[76]

In the newborn infant requiring surgery, hypoglycemia is most commonly caused by vomiting or inadequate intake of fluids. Other contributing factors may include prematurity, septicemia, hypothermia, or hyperinsulinism as may occur in an infant of a diabetic mother. Infants with Beckwith–Wiedemann syndrome, who frequently may have omphalocele, commonly have elevated blood insulin levels and severe hypoglycemia.

Blood sugar in the infant at risk should be monitored at the bedside using a bedside screening glucose analyzer. Blood sugars below 2–2.5 mmol/L should be acted upon by giving a feed or a bolus of intravenous 10% dextrose as appropriate for the individual infant. Significant hypoglycemia should be confirmed by laboratory blood sugar before definitive action, such as intravenous glucose being given. This is because all screening methods are not completely accurate at low blood sugar levels.

HYPERGLYCEMIA

A blood glucose >14 mmol/L (250 mg/dL) may cause a hyperosmolar state with glucosuria, osmotic diuresis, and dehydration. This elevated plasma osmolality increases the risk of intracranial hemorrhage at least in the infant of less than 32 weeks gestation. Hyperglycemia most commonly occurs in the very low birth weight infant who is receiving large amounts of fluids to counteract insensible loss and whose ability to metabolize dextrose or glucose is limited. Hyperglycemia may also be due to defective islet cell processing of proinsulin, insulin resistance nonsuppression of endogenous glucose production during continuous exogenous glucose infusion.[77,78] Infusion of small doses of insulin may be required to counteract intractable hyperglycemia.[77] Extremely low birth weight babies require a higher total dose of insulin for longer periods than low birth weight preterms. Hyperglycemia is related to defective islet beta-cell processing of proinsulin, partial insulin resistance, and failure to suppress hepatic glucose production during parenteral glucose infusion. Exogenous insulin infusion partially reduces endogenous glucose production in preterm newborn infants. This treatment is efficient and safe when used with caution.[77]

After initial hypoglycemia, due to limited glycogen and fat stores, preterm babies often become hyperglycemic because of a combination of insulin resistance and relative insulin deficiency. Hyperglycemia is associated with increased morbidity and mortality in preterm infants, but what should be considered optimal glucose control, and how best to achieve it, has yet to be defined in these infants. In the first week of life, 80% of infants have glucose levels >8 mmol/L, and 32% have glucose levels >10 mmol/L >10% of the time. Independent risk factors for hyperglycemia include increasing prematurity, small size at birth, use of inotropes, lipid infusions, and sepsis. There was a lack of association between the rate of dextrose infused and risk of hyperglycemia in the Neonatal Insulin Therapy in Europe (NIRTURE) Trial.[79] This study included 195 very low birthweight (VLBW) infants randomized in a multicenter study to continuous infusion of insulin at a dose of 0.05 U per kilogram of body weight per hour with 20% dextrose support and 194 to standard neonatal care on days 1 to 7. Early insulin therapy offered little clinical benefit in very low birth weight infants and reduced hyperglycemia but increased hypoglycemia.[80] The use of insulin in preterm infants and prevention of hyperglycemia could also affect immune function, lipid metabolism, growth, and IGF-I generation leading to improved short-term clinical outcomes such as retinopathy of prematurity.[78]

Calcium homeostasis

Calcium has a key role in many physiological processes, including activation and inhibition of enzymes, intracellular regulation of metabolic sequences, secretion and action of hormones, blood coagulation, muscle contraction, and nerve transmission. Ninety-nine percent of total body calcium is in the bones, to which it gives structural support. Only about 1% is in the ECF and soft tissues.[81] Calcium is present in the ECF in three fractions: 30%–50% is bound to protein, principally albumin; 5%–15% is complexed with citrate, lactate, bicarbonate, and inorganic ions; and 5%–15% is ionized—this is the metabolically active fraction of calcium. Calcium concentration reported as mg/dL can be converted to molar units by

dividing by 4 (e.g., 10 mg/dL converts to 2.5 mmol/L).[37,82–84] If serum albumin is low, total serum calcium falls, but the serum level of ionized calcium is unchanged. Serum calcium could be corrected for the level of serum albumin using the formula

$$\text{corrected calcium} = (0.8 \times [\text{normal albumin} - \text{neonatal albumin}]) + \text{serum Ca}$$

Hydrogen ions compete with calcium for albumin binding sites. Thus, acidosis increases serum ionized calcium levels without influencing total serum calcium levels. Prenatally, calcium is actively transported across the placenta from mother to fetus against a concentration gradient, which results in fetal hypercalcemia at the end of the last trimester and immediately after birth. Cord serum calcium in the full-term infant is approximately 2.75 mmol/L.[83] In healthy full-term infants, calcium concentrations decrease for the first 24–48 hours and reach a nadir of 1.8–2.1 mmol/L. Thereafter, calcium concentrations progressively rise to the mean values observed in older children. This transient drop in serum calcium is exaggerated in the preterm infant. Metabolic bone disease is a common feature especially in extreme preterm infants less than 28 weeks gestation and results from inadequate supply of nutrients (vitamin D, calcium, and phosphate), prolonged period of total parenteral nutrition, and prolonged period of immobilization. The main features that manifest between the 10th and 16th week of life include decreased bone mineral density, osteopenia with or without other features of rickets.

HYPOCALCEMIA

This is defined as a total serum calcium concentration <2.0 mmol/L in the term infant and <1.7 mmol/L in the preterm infant.[82] Normal serum ionized calcium in the newborn infant is 1–1.5 mmol/L.[83–85]

Causes of hypocalcemia

1. Infants of diabetic mothers
2. Asphyxia
3. Sepsis
4. Di George's syndrome/22q deletion syndrome
5. Diuretics especially frusemide
6. Hypomagnesemia
7. Maternal hyperparathyroidism
8. Prematurity
9. Vitamin D deficiency

Clinical manifestations

The majority of hypocalcemia is asymptomatic. The symptoms when they occur include jitteriness and seizures. An electrocardiographic $Q–T_c$ interval longer than 0.4 seconds may occur.

Management

Early asymptomatic mild neonatal hypocalcemia does not require treatment. Infants receiving intravenous fluids should be provided with calcium gluconate as maintenance. Brown et al.[86] have shown that aggressive attempts at normalizing serum calcium in sick preterm infants may be ineffective and even hazardous; thus, at the least, in the first week of life, maintenance of serum calcium at a level of 2.0 mmol/L is adequate.

Symptomatic hypocalcemia should be treated with a slow infusion of intravenous calcium gluconate (5 mL 10% calcium gluconate = 1.1 mmol = 45 mg elemental calcium). Extreme care should always be taken when infusing calcium as extravasation can cause severe burns to the surrounding skin and subcutaneous tissue. Emergency treatment of hypocalcemia is only required if the infant is symptomatic. Symptoms include jitteriness, seizures, lethargy, poor feeding, and vomiting [bolus 1–2 mL 10% calcium gluconate IV (0.45 mmol = 18 mg elemental calcium) IV slowly]. Symptoms are uncommon at serum calcium above 1.8 mmol/L and become common at serum calcium <1.5 mmol/L. Oral calcium supplements in the form of Calcium Sandoz provides 2.7 mmol (110 mg) elemental calcium 2.5 mL (50 mg) per kg per day may be given with feeds if the infant on feeds has asymptomatic hypocalcemia, requiring treatment. Symptomatic hypocalcemia unresponsive to calcium therapy may be due to hypomagnesemia. This can be treated with 50% magnesium sulfate either intravenously or intramuscularly.[87]

PERIOPERATIVE MANAGEMENT

Preoperative fluid and electrolyte problems in the neonate

Heird and Winters[88] have summarized the metabolic responses of the normal neonate in the first weeks of life. Preoperatively, infants with abnormalities requiring surgery, especially those of the gastrointestinal tract, may have a variety of electrolyte abnormalities.[88–90] If there has been a delay in recognition of gastrointestinal obstruction and the infant has been vomiting for a period of time, he or she will be dehydrated (Table 13.3).

Upper intestinal obstruction, for example, pyloric stenosis, results in loss of hydrochloric acid from the stomach, and small amounts of sodium and potassium. The kidney then conserves hydrogen ions at the expense of potassium and sodium. Bicarbonate is excreted by the kidney along with sodium and potassium, and the urine pH is alkaline.

Potassium and sodium depletion occurs. As loss of potassium and sodium progresses, and the body stores are diminished, the kidney ceases to excrete these ions with bicarbonate. Sodium and potassium are now conserved by the kidney, and hydrogen ion is lost instead causing a severe hypochloremic metabolic alkalosis. Correction must be with adequate fluid-containing sodium chloride and potassium chloride, as body stores of all these ions are depleted. Infants with lower intestinal obstruction, such as Hirschsprung's disease or other intestinal obstructive lesions, may pool large amounts of fluid and electrolytes in dilated intestinal loops; this may result in intravascular dehydration with hyponatremia, hypokalemia, and metabolic acidosis.

Neonates with necrotizing enterocolitis, peritonitis, or septic shock may have "third space" loss of fluid into the peritoneum, pleural fluid, or interstitial tissues with resultant hypoproteinemia and marked interstitial edema. Additionally, many of these infants are ventilated, sedated, and paralyzed. Immobility resulting from paralysis will accentuate peripheral pooling of interstitial fluid. Intravascular dehydration and hypoproteinemia and hyponatremia will result.

Preoperatively, the infant's hydration should be assessed on the basis of weight, pulse, blood pressure, capillary filling time, blood urea, electrolytes, urine output, specific gravity, and electrolyte content.

Intraoperative management

Careful attention to fluid and electrolyte balance intraoperatively is essential, including blood pressure, pulse, and temperature. During major procedures, intravascular lines allow blood pressure and central venous pressure

Table 13.3 Electrolyte composition of body fluids

Body fluid	Electrolytes (mEq/L)				
	Na+	K+	Cl–	HCO₃	pH
Gastric	70	5–15	120	0	1
Pancreas	140	5	50–100	100	9
Bile	130	5	100	40	8
Ileostomy	130	15–20	120	25–30	8
Diarrhea	50	35	40	50	>7

Sources: Adapted from Wait RB, Kahng KU: Fluids and electrolytes and acid–base balance. In Greenfield LJ, Mulholland MW, Oldham KKT et al. (eds): *Surgery, Scientific Principles and Practice.* Philadelphia, JB Lippincott Co., 1993, p. 223; Pitkin RM, *Clin. Perinatol* 1983 Oct;10(3):575–92; Namgun GR et al. Disorders of calcium and phosphorous metabolism in infants and children 1988:253–271.

monitoring. Urine output should also be measured and oxygenation and ventilation with blood gases and pulse oximetry.

Loss of fluid and heat from exposed peritoneal surfaces should be taken into account and minimized by keeping the operating room sufficiently warm. Acute blood loss should be replaced.[89]

Postoperative management

Patients who have been adequately managed pre- and intraoperatively may be well hydrated, immediately, postoperatively. If the infant had hypotension, transient renal failure with oliguria may occur and may be managed with fluid restriction and correction of electrolyte abnormalities. Inappropriate secretion of antidiuretic hormone is common and results from pain and/or ventilation, resulting in fluid retention and hyponatremia; thus, care must be taken to avoid overhydration, which will encourage both of these. Respiratory acidosis should be corrected by appropriate ventilation. Metabolic acidosis may occur postoperatively in the infant who is persistently hypotensive or hypoxic or who has ongoing tissue necrosis (i.e., severe necrotizing enterocolitis). This must be addressed by correcting the underlying cause of acidosis and by giving sodium bicarbonate. Fluids lost through nasogastric suctioning or drainage must be replaced at regular intervals by normal saline with maintenance potassium added; if losses are from the small intestine, it has been recommended that a small amount of bicarbonate be also added. Where large fluid losses occur from aspiration, calculation of the electrolyte content of these fluids may help plan replacement (Table 13.3).[87,88]

Nitrogen excretion occurs in neonates postoperatively. Thus, early attention must be given to beginning parenteral nutrition in infants in whom early feeding is not foreseen.

FLUID AND ELECTROLYTE BALANCE IN SEPTIC SHOCK

Many surgical conditions predispose to sepsis and shock, including necrotizing enterocolitis, Hirschsprung's disease with enterocolitis, and volvulus. The risk of septicemia with hypotension is even higher if the infant is also preterm. Shock is a stage of acute cardiovascular dysfunction in which the delivery of oxygen and nutrients is insufficient to meet metabolic demands of the tissues. Endotoxin appears to be the common etiological factor in septic shock.[91,92]

Metabolic substrates, i.e., oxygen, glucose, and fatty acid, are available, but their utilization is impaired causing multiple organ failure. Capillary permeability increases, and fluid and protein leak into the interstitial fluid resulting in tissue edema, hypoproteinemia, and a fall in the intravascular fluid volume. Pulmonary hypertension, followed by marked pulmonary edema, occurs with severe respiratory distress. Myocardial depression results in decreased cardiac output.

Clinical manifestations

Neonatal bacterial septicemia may be fulminant and fatal. A high index of suspicion by the nursing and medical staff is essential. Presenting features are subtle and may be recognized only by an experienced nurse or doctor. The infant may merely appear "off color." Early signs of sepsis include lethargy, irritability, apnea and temperature instability, elevated C-reactive protein, and increased immature to total neutrophil ratio.

Management

Shock must be reversed with rapid infusion of fluid and colloid to replete the intravascular space. Normal saline at a volume of 10–20 mL/kg can be infused over 20–60 minutes.[88] Inotropic agents may be needed to increase cardiac output—dopamine improves cardiac contractility (5–20 μg/kg per minute) and in a low dose (<5 μg/kg per minute) also increases blood flow to the kidneys and the intestine; high doses have the opposite effect. Alternative drugs are dobutamine, milrinone, or isoproterenol. Patients with profound hypotension and myocardial depression may respond only to infusion of epinephrine or norepinephrine. Hydrocortisone at stress doses could be used to treat recalcitrant hypotension not responsive to full doses of inotropes and intravascular volume repletion. Administration of corticosteroids leads to rapid resolution of the hypotension without increasing the risk of spontaneous intestinal perforation, grade III–IV IVH, periventricular leukomalacia, and sepsis (bacterial or fungal). Hyperkalemia results from oliguria and tissue catabolism, and hyponatremia results from increased total body water and inappropriate ADH secretion.

In the Fluid Expansion as Supportive Therapy (FEAST) trial, Maitland et al. randomized 3,141 children over 60 days old with severe febrile illness and impaired perfusion to one of three arms: 20 to 40 mL/kg of 5% albumin, 0.9% saline boluses, or no bolus at all, at hospital admission in six sites located in Uganda, Kenya, or Tanzania. All children received maintenance fluids and the standard of care recommended by guidelines. The primary endpoint was 48-h mortality. Forty-eight-hour mortality was 10.6% and 10.5% in the albumin-bolus and saline-bolus groups, respectively, and 7.3% in the control group. Four-week mortality rates were 12.2%, 12.0%, and 8.7%, respectively. Most deaths (87%) occurred before 24 hours. At a scheduled interim data review in January 2011, with data available from 2,995 children, a data and safety monitoring committee recommended stopping enrollment because it was unlikely that the bolus arms would prove to be superior. The authors could not identify any subgroup in which fluid resuscitation was beneficial, which was remarkable given that many of the baseline characteristics of the children in this study are considered to be important criteria for bolus-fluid therapy.[93] These results may not be directly applicable to a developed world setting but suggests that future therapy should be directed at a more cautious approach to fluid resuscitation.

ACUTE RENAL FAILURE

Acute renal failure is common in the seriously ill neonate requiring surgery. It may be prerenal as a result of severe dehydration, hypotension, abdominal distension, or sepsis. It may result from congenital severe intrinsic renal disease. It may be obstructive and result from severe obstruction in the urinary collecting system, e.g., urethral valves.[92,94]

Prerenal failure is the most common form of acute renal failure in the surgical neonate, and results from a severe decrease in renal perfusion usually as a result of profound hypotension from blood loss, sepsis, severe necrotizing enterocolitis, or intestinal obstruction with loss of fluid into dilated intestinal loops.

Primary fascial closure of omphalocele or gastroschisis carries the risk of placing the abdominal contents under pressure, which may cause a reduction in cardiac output, hypotension, bowel ischemia, venostasis, and postoperative renal failure. Limited data suggest that an intragastric pressure >20 mmHg or an increase in central venous pressure of 4 mmHg or more indicates the need of a staged repair using a pouch.[95] Additionally, newborn infants with abdominal wall defects have significantly increased fluid requirements preoperatively as major insensible water losses occur when eviscerated bowel is exposed to air, and a perioperative third space is frequently associated. These conditions also favor hypovolemia, hypoperfusion of the kidney, and postoperative renal failure.

Renal vein or renal artery thrombosis, if bilateral, may be associated with acute renal failure. Treatment is by early aggressive fluid replacement until blood pressure normalizes, and then by meticulous adjustment of fluid and electrolyte balance until recovery of renal function occurs. Peritoneal dialysis may be required until renal function recovers. Recovery is associated with a polyuric phase, which also requires ongoing care with replacement of large amounts of water, potassium, and sodium via the kidneys.

Renal failure due to obstruction and due to congenital malformations is often associated with severe irreversible renal diseases not compatible with normal extrauterine life. The focus of care must initially be to decide on the appropriateness of active management. Further discussion of renal failure management is outside the scope of this chapter.

CONCLUSION

Major changes in body composition and in fluid and electrolyte balance occur during the transition to extrauterine life. These changes are even more marked in the preterm infant. The newborn infant who has a disorder requiring surgery has additional possible disorders of fluid and electrolyte balance. Future research and audit of fluid management strategies are vital to prevent hypernatremia, hyperglycemia, and hyponatremia, and adverse neurodevelopmental sequelae.

REFERENCES

1. Friis-Hansen B. Water distribution in the foetus and newborn infant. *Acta Paediatr Scand Suppl* 1983; 305:7–11.
2. Costarino A, Baumgart S. (1986) Modern fluid and electrolyte management of the critically ill premature infant. *Pediatr Clin North Am* 1986 Feb; 33(1):153–78.
3. Ziegler EE, O'Donnell AM, Nelson SE, Fomon SJ. Body composition of the reference fetus. *Growth* 1976 Dec; 40(4):329–41.
4. Hartnoll G, Betremieux P, Modi N. Body water content of extremely preterm infants at birth. *Arch Dis Child Fetal Neonatal Ed* Jul 2000; 83(1):F56–9.
5. Robillard JE, Namamura KT, Matherne GP, Jose PA. Renal hemodynamics and functional adjustments to postnatal life. *Semi Perinatol* 1988 Apr; 12(2):143–50.
6. Fletcher M, Mhaira G, McDonald MG, Avery GB (eds). *Atlas of Procedures in Neonatology.* Philadelphia: Lippincott, 1983.
7. Rudolph AM, Heymann MA. Circulatory changes during growth in the fetal lamb. *Circ Res* 1970 Mar; 26(3):289–99.
8. Robillard JE. Renal function during fetal life. In: Barrett TM, Ellis ED, Harmon WE (eds). *Pediatric Nephrology*, 4th edn. Baltimore: Lippincott and Williams and Wilkins, 1999:Chapter 1, 23.
9. Robillard JE, Kulvinskas C, Sessions C, Burmeister L, Smith FG Jr. Maturational changes in the fetal glomerular filtration rate. *Am J Obstet Gynecol* 1975 Jul1; 122(5):601–6.
10. Nakamura KT, Matherne GP, McWeeney OJ, Smith BA, Robillard JE. Renal Haemodynamics and functional changes during the transition from fetal to newborn life in sheep. *Pediatr Res* 1987 Mar; 2(3):229–34.
11. Coulthard MG. Maturation of glomerular filtration in preterm and mature babies. *Early Hum Dev* 1985 Sep; 11(3–4):281–92.
12. Wilkins BH. Renal function in sick very low birth weight infants: 1. Glomerular filtration rate. *Arch Dis Child* 1992 Oct; 67(10 spec No):1140–5.
13. Siegal SR. Hormonal and renal interaction in body fluid regulation in the newborn infant. *Clin Perinatol* 1982 Oct; 9(3):535–7.
14. Ervin MG. Perinatal fluid and electrolyte regulation: Role of arginine vasopressin. *Semin Perinatol* 1988 Apr; 12(2):134–42.
15. Stegner HRH, Commetz JC. The role of arginine vasopressin in the regulation of water metabolism in premature infants in the first days of life. *Horm Res* 1987; 28(1):30–6.

16. Aperia A, Broberger O, Elinder G. Herin P, Zetterstrom R. Postnatal development of renal function in preterm and full term infants. *Acta Paediatr Scand* 1981 Mar; 70(2):183–7.

17. Hill KJ, Lumbers ER. The effect of cortisol on fetal renal function. *J Austral, Perinatal Soc Proc, 3rd Congress* 1985:137.

18. van Bel F, Guit GL, Schipper J, van de Bor M, Baan J. Indomethacin-induced changes in renal blood flow velocity waveform in premature infants investigated with color Doppler imaging. *J Pediatr* 1991 Apr; 118(4(pt 1)):621–6.

19. Apeira A, Broberger O, Herin, P, Thodenius K, Zetterstrom R. Postnatal control of water and electrolyte homeostasis in preterm and full term infants. *Acta Paediatr Scand Suppl* 1983; 305:61–5.

20. Gallini F, Maggio L, Romagnoli C, Marrocco G, Tortorolo G. Progression of renal function in preterm neonates with gestational age less than or equal to 32 weeks. *Pediatr Nephrol* 2000 Nov; 15(1–2):119–24.

21. Kavvadia V, Greenough A, Dimitriou G, Forsling ML. Randomized trial of two levels of fluid input in the perinatal period—Effect on fluid balance, electrolyte and metabolic disturbances in ventilated VLBW infants. *Acta Paediatr* 2000 Feb; 89(2):237–41.

22. Hey EN, Katz G. Evaporative water loss in the newborn baby. *J Physiol* 1969 Feb; 200(3):605–19.

23. Chiou YB, Blume-Peytavi U. Stratum corneum maturation. A review of neonatal skin function. *Skin Pharmacol Physiol* Mar–Apr 2004;17(2):57–66.

24. Harpin VA, Rutter N. Sweating in preterm babies. *J Peds* 1982 Apr; 100(4):614–9.

25. Fanaroff AA, Wald M, Gruber HS, Kalus MH. Insensible water loss in low birth weight infants. *Pedriatics* 1972 Aug; 50(2):236–45.

26. Harpin VA, Rutter N. Barrier properties of the newborn infant's skin. *J Pediatr* 1983 Mar; 102(3):419–25.

27. Kelleher MM, Dunn-Galvin A, Gray C1, Murray DM, Kiely M, Kenny L, McLean WH, Irvine AD, Hourihane JO. Skin barrier impairment at birth predicts food allergy at 2 years of age. *J Allergy Clin Immunol* 2016 Feb 25; pii:S0091–6749(16)00113–5.

28. Marc I, Rowe MI, Taylor M. Transepidermal water loss in the infant surgical patient. *J Pediatr Surg* 1981 Dec; 16(6):878–81.

29. Rutter N, Hull D. Water loss from the skin of term and pre term babies. *Arch Dis Child* 1979 Nov; 54(11):858–68.

30. Agren J, Sjors G, Sedin G. Transepidermal water loss in infants born at 24 and 25 weeks of gestation. *Acta Paediatr* 1998 Nov; 87(11):85–90.

31. Omar SA, DeCristofaro JD, Agarwal BI, La Gamma EF. Effects of prenatal steroids on water and sodium homeostasis in extremely low birth weight neonates, *Pediatrics* 1999 Sep; 104(3 pt 1):482–8.

32. Jain A, Rutter N. Cartlidge PH. Influence of antenatal steroids and sex on maturation of the epidermal barrier in the preterm infant. *Arch Dis Child Fetal Neonatal Ed* 2000 Sep; 83(2):F112–6.

33. Hammarlund K, Sedin G. Transepidermal water loss in newborn infants: III. Relation to gestational age. *Acta Paediatr Scand* 1979 Nov; 68(6):795–801.

34. Hartnoll G. (2003) Basic principles and practical steps in the management of fluid balance in the newborn. *Semin Neonatol* 2003 Aug; 8(4):307–13.

35. Takahashi N, Hoshi J, Nishida H. Water balance, electrolyte and acid base balance in extremely premature infants. *Acta Paediatr Jpn* 1994 Jun; 36(3):250–5.

36. Sosulski R, Polin RA, Baumgart S. Respiratory water loss and heat balance in intubated infants receiving humidified air. *J Pediatr* 1983 Aug; 103(2):307–10.

37. Simmons, CF Jr. Fluid and electrolyte management. In: Cloherty JP, Stark AR (eds). *Manual of Neonatal Care*. Philadelphia: Lippincott-Raven, 1988:Chapter 9, 87–100.

38. William OH, Karecki H. Phototherapy and insensible water loss in the newborn infant. *Am J Dis Child* 1972; 124:230–2.

39. Bell EF, Neidich GA, Cashore WJ, Oh W. Combined effect of radiant warmer and phototherapy on insensible water loss in low birth weight infants. *J Pediatr* 1979 May; 94(5):810–3.

40. Flenady VJ, Woodgate PG. Radiant warmers versus incubators for regulating body temperature in newborn infants. *Cochrane Database Syst Rev* 2003; (4):CD000435.

41. Meyer MP, Payton MJ, Salmon A, Hitchinson C, de Klerk A. A clinical comparison of radiant warmer and incubator care for preterm infants from birth to 1800 grams. *Pediatrics* 2001 Aug; 108(2):395–401.

42. Baumgart S. Reduction of oxygen consumption, insensible water loss, and radiant heat demand with use of a plastic blanket for low birth weight infants under radiant warmers. *Pediatrics* 1984 Dec; 74(6):1022–8.

43. Yu VYH. Patent ductus arteriosus in the preterm infant. *Early Hum Dev* 1993 Nov 1; 35(1):I–14.

44. Vanhaesebrouck S, Zonnenberg I, Vandervoort P, Bruneel E, Van Hoestenberghe M, Theyskens C. Conservative treatment for patent ductus arteriosus in the preterm. *Arch Dis Child Fetal Neonatal Ed* 2007 Jul; 92(4):F244–7. Epub 2007 Jan 9.

45. Bell EF, Warburton D, Stonestreet BS, Oh W. Effect of fluid administration on the development of symptomatic patent ductus arteriosus and congestive heart failure in premature infants. *N Engl J Med* 1980 Mar 13; 302(11):598–604.

46. Brown E, Start A, Sosenko I, Lawson EE, Avery ME. Bronchopulmonary dysplasia: Possible relationships to pulmonary edema. *J Pediatr* 1978 Jun; 92(6):982–4.

47. Stephens BE, Gargus RA, Walden RV, Mance M, Nye J, McKinley L, Tucker R, Vohr BR. Fluid regimens in the first week of life may increase risk of patent ductus arteriosus in extremely low birth weight infants. *J Perinatol* 2008 Feb; 28(2):123–8. Epub 2007 Nov 29.

48. Al-Danhan J, Haycock GB, Chantler C, Stimmler L. Sodium homeostasis in term and preterm neonates: I. Renal aspects. *Arch Dis Child* 1983 May; 58(5):335–42.

49. Al-Danhan J, Haycock GB, Chantler C, Stimmler L. Sodium homeostasis in term and preterm neonates: III. Effects of salt supplementation. *Arch Dis Child* 1984 Oct; 59(10):945–50.

50. Tulassay T, Rascher W, Seyberth H, Lang R, Toth M, Sulyok E. Role of atrial natriuretic peptide and sodium homeostasis in premature infants. *J Paediatr* 1986 Dec; 109(6):1023–7.

51. Noble-Jamieson CM, Kuzmin P, Airede KI. Hidden sources of fluid and sodium intake in ill newborns. *Arch Dis Child* 1986 July; 61(7):695–6.

52. Haycock GB. The influence of sodium on growth in infancy. *Pediatr Nephrol* 1993 Dec; 7(6):871–5.

53. Schaffer SG, Meade VM. Sodium balance and extracellular volume regulation in very low birth weight infants. *J Pediatr* 1989 Aug; 115(2):285–90.

54. Hartnoll G, Betremieux P, Modi N. Randomised controlled trial of postnatal sodium supplementation on body composition in 25–30 week gestation infants. *Arch Dis Child Fetal Neonatal Ed* 2000 Jan; 82(1):F24–8.

55. Costarino AT, Gruskay JA, Corcoran L, Polin RA, Baumgart S. Sodium restriction versus daily maintenance replacement in very low birth weight premature neonates: A randomised, blind therapeutic trial. *J Pediatr* 1992 Jan; 120(1):99–106.

56. Modi N. Hyponatraemia in the newborn. *Arch Dis Child Fetal Neonatal Ed* 1998 Mar; 78(2):F81–4.

57. Rees L, Brook CG, Shaw JC, Forsling ML. Hyponatraemia in the first week of life in preterm infants. Part I Arginine vasopressin secretion. *Arch Dis Child* 1984 May: 59(5):414–22.

58. Weinberg JA, Weitzman RE, Zakauddin S, Leake RD. Inappropriate secretion of antidiuretic hormone in a premature infant. *J Pediatr* 1977 Jan; 90(1):111–4.

59. Singhi S, Chookang E, Kalghatgi S. Iatrogenic neonatal and maternal hyponatraemia following oxytocin and aqueous glucose infusion during labour. *Br J Obstet Gynaecol* 1985 Apr; 92(4):356–63.

60. Lim WH, Lien R, Chiang MC, Fu RH, Lin JJ, Chu SM, Hsu JF, Yang PH. Hypernatremia and grade III/IV intraventricular hemorrhage among extremely low birth weight infants. *J Perinatol* 2011 Mar; 31(3):193–8.

61. Barnette AR, Myers BJ, Berg CS, Inder TE. Sodium intake and intraventricular hemorrhage in the preterm infant. *Ann Neurol* 2010 Jun; 67(6):817–23.

62. Lorenz JM, Kleinman A, Markarian K. Potassium metabolism in extremely low birth weight infants in the first week of life. *J Pediatr* 1997 Jul; 131(1 pt 1):81–6.

63. Sato K, Kondo T, Iwao H, Honda S, Ueda K. Internal potassium shift in premature infant: Cause of nonoliguric hyperkalaemia. *J Pediatr* 1995 Jan; 126(1):109–13.

64. Stefano JL, Norman ME, Morales MC, Goplerud JM, Ishra OP, Deliviria-Papadopoulos M. Decreased erythrocyte Na+, K+—ATPase activity associated with cellular potassium loss in extremely low birth weight infants with nonologuric hyperkalemia. *J Pediatr* 1993 Feb; 122(2):277–81.

65. Kluckow M, Evans N. Low systemic blood flow and hyperkalemia in preterm infants. *J Pediatr* 2001 Apr; 139(2):227–32.

66. O'Hare FM, Molloy EJ. What is the best treatment for hyperkalaemia in a preterm infant? *Arch Dis Child* 2008 Feb; 93(2):174–6.

67. Vemgal P, Ohlsson A. Interventions for non-oliguric hyperkalaemia in preterm neonates. *Cochrane Database Syst Rev* 2012 May 16; 5:CD005257.

68. Ramiro-Tolentino SB, Markarian K, Kleinman LI. Renal bicarbonate excretion in extremely low birth weight infants. *Pediatrics* 1996 Aug; 98(2):256–61.

69. Kapadia VS, Wyckoff MH. Drugs during delivery room resuscitation—What, when and why? *Semin Fetal Neonatal Med* 2013 Dec; 18(6):357–61.

70. Berg CS, Barnette AR, Myers BJ, Shimony MK, Barton AW, Inder TE. Sodium bicarbonate administration and outcome in preterm infants. *J Pediatr* 2010 Oct; 157(4):684–7.

71. Burchfield DJ. Medication use in neonatal resuscitation. *Clin Perinatol* 1999 Sep; 26(3):683–91.

72. Varughese M, Patole S, Shama A, Whithall J. Permissive hypercapnia in neonates: The case of the good, the bad, and the ugly. *Pediatr Pulmonol* 2002 Jan; 33(1):56–64.

73. Koh TH, Eyre JA, Aynsley-Green A. Neonatal hypoglycaemia—The controversy regarding definition. *Arch Dis Child* 1988 Nov; 63(11):1386–8.

74. Cornblath M, Hawdon J, William A, Aynsley-Green A, Ward-Platt M, Schwartz R, Kalhan S. Controversies regarding definition of neonatal hypoglycemia: Suggested operational thresholds. *Pediatrics* 2000; 105(5):1141–114.

75. Koh TH, Aynsley-Green A, Tarbit M, Eyre JA. Neural dysfunction during hypoglycaemia. *Arch Dis Child* 1988 Nov; 63(11):1353–8.

76. Burns CM, Rutherford MA, Boardman JP, Cowan FM. Patterns of cerebral injury and neurodevelopmental outcomes after symptomatic neonatal hypoglycaemia. *Pediatrics* 2008 Jul; 122(1):65–74.

77. Mitanchez D. Glucose regulation in preterm newborn infants. *Horm. Res.* 2007; 68(6):265–71. Epub 2007 Jun 20.

78. Beardsall K, Dunger D. Insulin therapy in preterm newborns. *Early Hum Dev* 2008 Dec; 84(12):839–42. Epub 2008 Oct 10.

79. Beardsall K, Vanhaesebrouck S, Ogilvy-Stuart AL, Vanhole C, Palmer CR, Ong K, van Weissenbruch M, Midgley P, Thompson M, Thio M, Cornette L, Ossuetta I, Iglesias I, Theyskens C, de Jong M, Gill B, Ahluwalia JS, de Zegher F, Dunger DB. Prevalence and determinants of hyperglycemia in very low birth weight infants: Cohort analyses of the NIRTURE study. *J Pediatr* 2010 Nov; 157(5):715–9.e1–3.

80. Beardsall K, Vanhaesebrouck S, Ogilvy-Stuart AL, Vanhole C, Palmer CR, van Weissenbruch M, Midgley P, Thompson M, Thio M, Cornette L, Ossuetta I, Iglesias I, Theyskens C, de Jong M, Ahluwalia JS, de Zegher F, Dunger DB. Early insulin therapy in very-low-birth-weight infants. *N Engl J Med* 2008 Oct 30; 359(18):1873–84.

81. Bozzetti V, Tagliabue P. Metabolic bone disease in preterm newborn: An update on nutritional issues. *Ital J Pediatr* 2009 Jul 14; 35(1):20.

82. Scott SM, Ladenson JH, Aguanna JJ, Walgate J, Hillmann LS. Effect of calcium therapy in the sick premature infant with early neonatal hypocalcemia. *J Pediatr* 1984 May; 104(5):747–51.

83. Pitkin RM. Endocrine regulation of calcium homeostatis during pregnancy. *Clin Perinatol* 1983 Oct; 10(3):575–92.

84. Namgun GR, Bainbridge R, Cruz MR, Tsang RC. Disorders of calcium and phosphorus metabolism in infants and children. 1988; 12:253–71.

85. Solden SJ, Hicks JM. *Pediatric Reference Ranges.* Washington: AA Press, 1995:39.

86. Brown DR, Steranka BH, Taylor FH. Treatment of early-onset neonatal hypocalcemia. Effects on serum calcium and ionized calcium. *Am J Dis Child* 1981 Jan; 135(1):24–8.

87. Tsang RC. Calcium, phosphorous and magnesium metabolism. In: Polin RA, Fox WA (eds). *Fetal and Neonatal Physiology.* Philadelphia: Saunders, 1992.

88. Heird WC, Winters R. The body fluids in paediatrics. In: Winters R (ed). *Fluid Therapy for the Pediatric Surgical Patient.* Boston: Little Brown, 1973.

89. Rice HE, Caty MG, Glick PL. Fluid therapy for the pediatric surgical patient. *Pediatr Clin North Am* 1998 Aug; 45(4):719–27.

90. Wait RB, Kahng KU. Fluids and electrolytes and acid-base balance. In: Greenfield LJ, Mulholland MW, Oldham KT. et al (eds). *Surgery Scientific Principles and Practice.* Philadelphia: JB Lippincott Co., 1993:23.

91. Butt W. Septic shock. *Pediatr. Clin North Am* 2001 Jun; 48(3):601–19, viii.

92. Toth-Heyn P, Drukker A, Guignard JP. The stressed neonatal kidney: From pathophysiology to clinical management of neonatal vasomotor nephropathy. *Pediatr Nephrol* 2000 Mar; 14(3):227–39.

93. Maitland K, Kiguli S, Opoka R, Engoru C, Olupot-Olupot P, Akech S, Nyeko R, Mtove G, Reyburn H, Lang T, Brent B, Evans JA, Tibenderana JK, Crawley J, Russell EC, Levin M, Babiker AG, Gibb DM. FEAST Trial Group. Mortality after fluid bolus in African children with shock. *N Engl J Med* 2011; 364:2483–95. doi: 10.1056/NEJMoa1101549.

94. Gouyon JB, Guignard JP. Management of acute renal failure in newborns. *Pediatr Nephrol* 2000 Sep; 14(10–11):1037–44.

95. Yaster M, Scherer TL, Stone MM, Maxwell LG, Schleien CL, Wetzel R, Buck JR, Nichols D, Colombani P, Dudgeon DL et al. Prediction of successful primary closure of congenital abdominal wall defects using intraoperative measurements. *J Pediatr Surg* 1989 Dec; 24(12):1217–20.

14

Nutrition

SIMON EATON AND AGOSTINO PIERRO

INTRODUCTION

The newborn infant requires nutrition not only for tissue maintenance and normal metabolism but also for growth—a term newborn grows at a rate of 25–30 g per day over the first 6 months of life, so that weight has doubled by the age of 5 months. The newborn infant is in a "critical epoch" of development not only for the organism as a whole but also for the individual organs and most significantly for the brain, so a significant period of inadequate nutrition may not only affect short-term outcomes but may also be a risk factor for the long-term menace of stunted mental and physical development. As well as providing the components necessary for increase in tissue mass, adequate provision of the nutrients required to mount an appropriate immune response is extremely important, as infection and sepsis may impair growth and neurodevelopmental outcome.[1] Hence, where indicated, early intervention with appropriate artificial nutritional support is of paramount importance.

The optimum nutritional route is oral enteral feeding; however, artificial enteral feeding or parenteral nutrition (PN) may be required if adequate oral feeds cannot be tolerated. The basic principle underlying choice of feeding routes is that the most physiological route safely possible should be used: gastric feeds are preferred over jejunal feeds, enteral feeds are preferred over parenteral feeds, etc. Various investigators have highlighted the importance of introducing enteral nutrition as soon as possible in surgical neonates. The beneficial effects of minimal enteral feeding on the immune system, infection rate, and liver function have been elucidated.

Growth monitoring

Artificial enteral nutrition and PN are both nutritional interventions, and nutritional outcomes should be assessed in order to determine the effectiveness of these interventions. Growth of all pediatric surgical patients, especially those receiving artificial nutritional support, should be monitored longitudinally using appropriate national charts (e.g., those available from the Royal College of Paediatrics and Child Health in the United Kingdom and Centers for Disease Control and Prevention in the United States). In the absence of national charts, those available from the World Health Organization should be used.

BODY COMPOSITION AND ENERGY REQUIREMENTS OF THE NEONATE

Newborn infants grow very rapidly and have higher energy expenditure and lower caloric reserves than adults, and therefore do not tolerate prolonged periods of starvation. The body composition of newborn infants is markedly different from that of adults: total body water varies from 87% of body weight at 24–25 weeks gestation to 71% at term and 50% in adulthood (Figure 14.1).[2] This decline in body water reflects also an increase in energy content of the body. The ratio between resting energy expenditure (REE, in kcal kg^{-1} day^{-1}) to nonprotein energy reserve (in kcal/kg) gives an approximate estimate of the energy reserve of the infants. This is only ~2 days at 24–25 weeks gestation, increases to ~20 days at term as glycogen and fat stores increase (Figure 14.1),[2] and is in excess of 50 days in the adult, hence the urgent need for adequate caloric intake in very-low-birth-weight (VLBW) and/or extremely-low-birth-weight (ELBW) infants after birth. Early PN in VLBW infants has been shown to be beneficial,[3] although there is controversy on how "aggressive" nutritional intervention should be in preterm infants. Full-term neonates have a higher content of endogenous fat (approximately 600 g) and therefore can tolerate a few days of undernutrition. Nevertheless, adequate nutrition in excess of basic requirements, i.e., enough to support growth, should be instituted as soon as practicable. Although adults following surgery or trauma have increased energy requirements, there is no strong evidence that increased energy should be provided to septic or surgical neonates.[4] The total energy requirement for an ELBW (i.e., <1000 g) preterm infant fed enterally is 130–150 kcal kg^{-1} day^{-1},[5] and that of a term infant is 100–120 kcal kg^{-1} day^{-1},

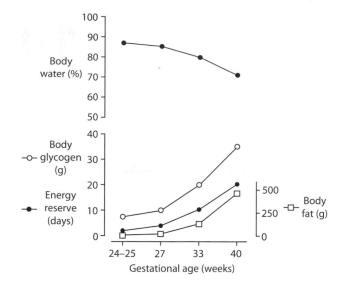

Figure 14.1 Body water and energy stores according to gestational age.

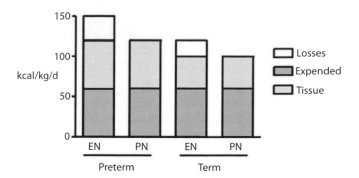

Figure 14.2 Partition of energy metabolism in preterm and term infants receiving nutrition enterally (EN) or parenterally (PN). "Expended" includes basal metabolic rate, activity, the energy expended in laying down new tissue, and thermoregulation. "Tissue" is the amount of energy actually stored in new tissue. "Losses" include losses in stool etc. (Data from Koletzko B et al., Guidelines on Paediatric Parenteral Nutrition of the European Society of Paediatric Gastroenterology, Hepatology and Nutrition (ESPGHAN) and the European Society for Clinical Nutrition and Metabolism (ESPEN), supported by the European Society of Paediatric Research (ESPR), *J Pediatr Gastroenterol Nutr*, 2005, 41 Suppl 2, S1–S87. Tsang RC et al., *Nutrition of the Preterm Infant: Scientific Basis and Practical Guidelines*, 2nd ed., 2005.)

compared to 60–80 kcal kg^{-1} day^{-1} for a 10-year old and 30–40 kcal kg^{-1} day^{-1} for a 20-year old individual.[6] Of the 100–120 kcal kg^{-1} day^{-1} required by the term infant, approximately 40–70 kcal kg^{-1} day^{-1} is needed for maintenance metabolism, 50–70 kcal kg^{-1} day^{-1} for growth (tissue synthesis and energy stored), and up to 20 kcal kg^{-1} day^{-1} to cover energy losses in excreta. Newborn infants receiving total parenteral nutrition (TPN) require fewer calories (110–120 kcal kg^{-1} day^{-1} for a preterm infant and 90–100 kcal kg^{-1} day^{-1} for a term infant),[4] due to the absence of energy losses in excreta and to the fact that energy is not required for thermoregulation when the infant is in an incubator. These data are shown diagrammatically in Figure 14.2, but it should be stressed that energy requirements vary greatly. Several equations have been used to estimate the REE, and therefore the energy requirements, of infants and children. The most frequently used are those of the World Health Organization (WHO),[6] Schofield,[7] and Harris and Benedict.[8] These are based on weight, height, and/or age; are based on measurements of orally fed, healthy individuals; and thus take no account of the abnormal physiology and/or pathology of infants requiring artificial nutritional support. Although adults show large increases in REE following trauma, surgery, or burns or during severe infection, this does not appear to be true for infants, although there are few studies in this area. Critically ill, postsurgical ventilated premature neonates,[9] neonates with necrotizing enterocolitis,[10] and surgical infants (with or without extracorporeal membrane oxygenation [ECMO])[11] were shown to have similar REE values to healthy neonates, whereas others have suggested that REE is increased during neonatal sepsis[12] and that REE correlates with severity of illness during sepsis in neonates.[13] Another study, examining the immediate postoperative response to neonatal surgery, found that there is a peak in REE 4 hours after surgery, which was short-lived, returning to baseline within 12–24 hours after

surgery.[14] Thus, there is no clear indication that increased energy should be provided to septic or surgical neonates,[4] although there are scant data on either postsurgical energy metabolism or growth of surgical infants.

REE is directly proportional to growth rate in healthy infants, and growth is retarded during acute metabolic stress. Studies in adult surgical patients have shown that operative stress causes marked changes in protein metabolism characterized by a postoperative increase in protein degradation, negative nitrogen balance, and a decrease in muscle protein synthesis. However, changes in whole-body protein flux, protein synthesis, amino acid oxidation, or protein degradation do not seem to occur in infants and young children undergoing major operations,[15] which led us to speculate that infants and children divert protein and energy from growth to tissue repair, thereby avoiding the overall increase in energy expenditure and catabolism seen in the adult.[10,15]

Nutritional problems in infants and children requiring surgery are not unusual. The real nutritional challenge is not represented by the operation per se but by the clinical condition of the patient. Examples include intrauterine growth retardation in small-for-gestational-age preterm infants, infants who have suffered massive intestinal resection for necrotizing enterocolitis, and infants with motility disorders of the intestine following surgery for atresia, malrotation and midgut volvulus, meconium ileus, or gastroschisis.

Nutritional integrity particularly in the neonatal period should be maintained regardless of the severity of the illness or organ failure due to the limited energy and protein

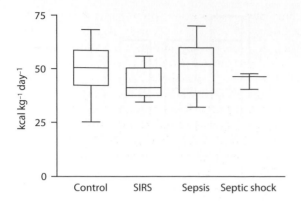

Figure 14.3 Resting energy expenditure in critically ill infants and controls. Indirect calorimetry was performed on infants and children with systemic inflammatory response syndrome (SIRS), sepsis, septic shock, and controls. Results are expressed as median, range, and interquartile range. There were no significant differences between the groups. See Ref. 50.

stores in neonates. Infants and children require nutrition for maintenance of protein status as well as for growth and wound healing. One considerable challenge in pediatrics is represented by nutrition support during critical illness and sepsis. Keshen et al.[16] have shown that parenterally fed neonates on extracorporeal life support are in hypermetabolic and protein catabolic states. These authors recommend the provision of additional protein and nonprotein calories to attenuate the net protein losses.

The existing knowledge on the metabolic response to sepsis in infants is limited. There are conflicting reports on whether critically ill infants are hypermetabolic.[11,17,18] However, most studies suggest that infants with sepsis do not become hypermetabolic[19,20] (Figure 14.3) and that septic neonates with necrotizing enterocolitis do not show any increase in whole-body protein turnover, synthesis, and catabolism.[10] However, the conflicting data may reflect measurements taken at different times in infants with differing degrees of sepsis.[21]

From these studies, it is clear that the metabolic rate and hormonal response to surgery, stress, and sepsis in infants may well be different from that of adults, and therefore, it is not possible to adapt nutritional recommendations made for adults to the neonatal population. It is possible that neonates divert the products of protein synthesis and breakdown from growth into tissue repair. This may explain the lack of growth commonly observed in infants with critical illness or sepsis. Further studies are needed in this field to delineate the metabolic response of neonates and children to trauma and sepsis, explore the relationship between nutrition and immunity, and design the most appropriate diet.

PARENTERAL NUTRITION

Indications

PN should be utilized when enteral feeding is impossible, inadequate, or hazardous, but should be given for the shortest period of time possible and the proportion of nutrition given enterally increased as tolerated. Energy reserves are such that stable term infants can tolerate 3–4 days without enteral feeds before starting PN, if it is anticipated that enteral nutrition may be resumed within this time. Premature neonates have smaller energy reserves, and the time before introducing PN is much shorter.

The most frequent indications in pediatric surgery are intestinal obstruction due to congenital anomalies, although acquired conditions may require PN for variable lengths of time. Although infants with some neonatal surgical conditions, such as gastroschisis, are all likely to receive PN, there are some other congenital anomalies where the use of PN is more controversial, for example, duodenal atresia, in which many surgeons would routinely initiate PN, whereas some surgeons preferentially manage patients without PN by the use of transanastomotic tubes.[22] In addition to congenital bowel obstruction, PN may also be used in cases of postoperative ileus, necrotizing enterocolitis, short-bowel syndrome, gastroenterological indications, and respiratory comorbidity.

Route of administration

As phlebitis may develop with the use of peripheral veins with solutions exceeding 600 mOsm, it is not possible to administer adequate calories peripherally for the growth of ELBW infants, and peripheral veins are only used for short-term, partial, nutritional supplementation. In neonates, the umbilical vessels can be used for provision of PN centrally, although the risk of complications increases if umbilical catheters are used for more than 5 days (arterial) or 14 days (venous).[4] Central venous catheters can either be placed percutaneously directly in a deep vein, with subcutaneous tunneling of the extravascular part of the line, or be a peripherally inserted central catheter (PICC). Although there has been a systematic review comparing outcomes in neonates administered PN through percutaneous central venous catheters versus peripheral cannulae, the authors concluded that there was insufficient evidence to make formal recommendations.[23] For consideration of technical aspects of placement and management, the reader is directed to the European Society for Paediatric Gastroenterology Hepatology and Nutrition (ESPGHAN)/ European Society of Parenteral and Enteral Nutrition (ESPEN) guidelines.[4]

Components of PN

The PN formulation includes carbohydrate, fat, protein, electrolytes, vitamins, trace elements, and water. The caloric needs for TPN are provided by carbohydrate and lipid. Protein is not used as a source of calories, since the catabolism of protein to produce energy is an uneconomic metabolic process compared to the oxidation of carbohydrate and fat, which produces more energy at a lower metabolic cost. The ideal TPN regimen therefore should provide enough amino acids for protein turnover and tissue growth, and sufficient calories to minimize protein oxidation for energy.

FLUID REQUIREMENTS

As noted previously, the proportion of body weight as water decreases with postnatal age (Figure 14.1). In addition, the proportion of total body water that is extracellular also decreases, from 65% at 26 weeks gestation to 40% at term and 20% in childhood.[24] This contributes to an expected weight loss in the first days of life. Any newborn infant deprived of oral fluids will lose body fluids and electrolytes in urine, stools, sweat, and evaporative losses from the lungs and the skin. The insensible water losses from the skin are particularly high (up to 80–100 mL kg^{-1} day^{-1}) in very-low-birth-weight or extremely premature infants.[24] This is due to the very large surface area relative to body weight, to the very thin and permeable epidermis, to reduced subcutaneous fat, and to the large proportion of total body water and extracellular water.[24] The preterm infant requires larger amounts of fluid to replace the high obligatory renal water excretion due to the limited ability to concentrate urine. In surgical newborns, it is not unusual to have significant water losses from gastric drainage and gastrointestinal stoma. Phototherapy may also increase losses. In order to reduce the water losses, it is important to use double-walled incubators, to place the infant in relatively high humidity, to use warm humidified air via the endotracheal tube, and in premature babies, to cover the body surface with an impermeable sheet. However, overhydration is potentially a problem, leading to complications such as pulmonary edema, and fluid restriction may be necessary for treatment of patent ductus arteriosus, renal insufficiency, and chronic lung disease. A recent report highlighted the poor fluid management of many neonates receiving PN.[25] Fluid restriction, or a requirement to administer other fluids in significant volume, can result in the delivery of macronutrients being less than current recommendations. A meta-analysis showed that although a liberal fluid regime decreased weight loss in premature infants on the first days of life, it significantly increased the risk of mortality and the incidence of patent ductus arteriosus and necrotizing enterocolitis (NEC).[26] Thus the recommended fluid intakes of neonates fall between 60 and 80 mL kg^{-1} day^{-1} (for premature infants on the first day of life) and 140 and 170 mL kg^{-1} day^{-1} (for neonates during the stable growth phase).[4] Hence, a one-size-fits-all prescription is inappropriate, and frequent monitoring of weight, urine output, and urea and electrolytes, with reassessment of fluid prescription, should be mandatory in the first weeks of life.

ENERGY SOURCES

Carbohydrates and fat provide the main energy sources in the diet, and this is reflected by their importance as a source of calories in PN. Glucose is a main energy source for body cells and should be the primary energy substrate in PN, covering 60%–70% of nonprotein calories.[4] The amount of glucose that can be infused safely depends on the clinical condition and maturity of the infant, as the ability of neonates to metabolize glucose may be impaired by prematurity and low birth weight. Since (1) pancreatic islet cell function is relatively unresponsive for the first 2 weeks of neonatal life, (2) glycogen stores are limited (Figure 14.1); (3) gluconeogenesis may be impaired; and (4) liver and peripheral tissues are relatively insensitive to insulin, so premature neonates are at risk from both hypoglycemia and hyperglycemia. Glucose infusion should be at least at a rate capable of maintaining blood glucose above 2.6 mmol/L, the current consensus definition of neonatal hypoglycemia.[27] As the rate of endogenous glucose metabolism in neonates is of the order of 5 mg kg^{-1} min^{-1}, this should be considered the lowest infusion rate likely to avoid hypoglycemia.[4] As glucose tolerance increases, the rate of glucose infusion can be increased. However, carbohydrate conversion to fat (lipogenesis) occurs when glucose intake exceeds metabolic needs. The potential risks associated with this process are twofold: accumulation of the newly synthesized fat in the liver and aggravation of respiratory acidosis resulting from increased CO_2 production, although whether these are clinically relevant in PN-fed infants is uncertain. In addition, hyperglycemia in ELBW infants is a risk factor for late-onset sepsis, mortality, and the risk of developing advanced NEC. Hyperglycemia occurs frequently during the course of PN, particularly while the glucose concentration of the infusate is being increased, but most patients will produce adequate endogenous insulin to metabolize the carbohydrate load within hours. Hyperglycemia can also be a sign of impending infection and has also been associated with development of NEC. The treatment of symptomatic hyperglycemia is usually reduction of the infusion rate, but exogenous insulin is sometimes given to ELBW infants with glucose intolerance. A rapid increase in plasma glucose concentration precedes development of NEC, and infants with established NEC have both a high prevalence of hyperglycemia and a worse outcome if hyperglycemic.[28] Hypoglycemia usually results from sudden interruption of an infusion containing a high glucose concentration.

Lipids provide an energy-dense (9 kcal/g of fat), isotonic alternative to glucose as an energy source for PN, which also prevents essential fatty acid deficiency and facilitates provision of fat-soluble vitamins. Combined infusion of glucose and lipids confers metabolic advantages over glucose, because it lowers the metabolic rate and increases the efficiency of energy utilization.[4] There is a close interdependence of carbohydrate and lipid infusion rates on the one hand, and net fat deposition or oxidation on the other (Figure 14.4). When the intake of glucose calories exceeds 18 g kg^{-1} day^{-1} (i.e., REE), net fat oxidation is minimal regardless of fat intake, and net fat synthesis takes place.[29] However, lipid utilization is often low and unpredictable in neonates, and consequently, lipids are usually introduced slowly, especially in premature neonates.[4]

Historically, the first and most commonly used fat emulsions for PN in pediatrics are based on soybean oil, in which the lipid is present as long-chain triglycerides (LCTs). Medium-chain triglycerides (MCTs) can increase

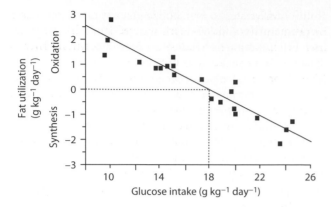

Figure 14.4 Linear relationship between glucose intake and fat utilization ($r = -0.9$; $p < .0001$). Lipogenesis is significant when glucose intake exceeds 18 g kg^{-1} day^{-1}. (From Pierro A et al., Utilisation of intravenous fat in the surgical newborn infant, *Proc Nutr Soc*, 1993, 52, 237A. With permission.)

net fat oxidation without increasing metabolic rate when used to partially replace LCT.[30] MCT/LCT mixtures may improve essential fatty acid status (by protecting essential fatty acids from oxidation). In the last 10 years, several other lipid emulsions have been introduced, based on varying proportions of MCTs, monounsaturated triglycerides (i.e., olive oil), or Ω-3 polyunsaturated triglycerides (i.e., fish oil). These have been utilized in several small-scale studies, in both premature infants and surgical infants. The potential routine use of these novel lipids is complicated by differences in licensing between different geographical areas and by the maximal rate of administration within the license. The main aim of the use of novel lipids, however, is to prevent or treat cholestasis; this will be considered in Section "Hepatic Complications."

High doses of lipid or an accidental rapid infusion of lipid may lead to fat overload syndrome, characterized by an acute febrile illness with jaundice and abnormal coagulation and respiratory problems, so lipids are usually advanced slowly, with close monitoring of triglyceride levels.[4] Peroxidation in stored fat emulsions and the generation of free radicals during intravenous infusion of fat in premature infants have been reported.[31] However, the degree of free radical production is linked to the rate of lipid oxidation, as it has been shown that a reduction in the carbohydrate-to-fat ratio in a PN diet will result in increased oxidation of administered fat and a decrease in free radical–mediated lipid peroxide formation.[32]

AMINO ACIDS

In contrast to healthy adults, who exist in a state of neutral nitrogen balance, infants and children need to be in positive nitrogen balance in order to achieve satisfactory growth and development. Preterm infants who are receiving glucose alone lose protein quickly (at the rate of 1%–2% body protein per day), so they should start to receive at least 1–1.5 g kg^{-1} day^{-1} amino acids parenterally if not receiving enteral

nutrition.[33] Infants are efficient at retaining nitrogen and can retain up to 80% of the metabolizable protein intake on both oral and intravenous diets.[33] Protein metabolism, and deposition of body protein for growth, is dependent upon both protein and energy intake, so that above an energy intake of 70 kcal kg^{-1} day^{-1}, the major determinant of nitrogen retention in preterm infants is the amino acid intake.[33] The PN amino acid requirement of term newborn infants is between 2.5 and 3.0 g kg^{-1} day^{-1}, which allows for accretion of body protein.[33] Complications like azotemia, hyperammonemia, and metabolic acidosis have been described in patients receiving high levels of intravenous amino acids[33] but rarely seen with amino acid intake of 2–3 g kg^{-1} day^{-1}.[33] In patients with severe malnutrition or with additional losses (i.e., jejunostomy, ileostomy), protein requirements are higher. The nitrogen source of PN is provided as a mixture of amino acids, and mixtures specifically formulated for neonates are available. However, the ideal amino acid composition for term and preterm infants is uncertain. As well as the amino acids usually considered essential for adult humans, histidine is considered essential for infants, and the following amino acids have all been considered "conditionally essential" for neonates: arginine, cysteine, glutamine, taurine, and tyrosine.

Glutamine is excluded from PN amino acid mixtures because of poor stability, although it can now be added as a dipeptide. Glutamine is important for the immune system and the intestine, as well as being essential as a nitrogen carrier between organs. It has been hypothesized that glutamine supplementation to parenterally fed neonates would decrease the incidence of infection and decrease time to full enteral feeding. One randomized controlled trial (RCT)[34] in surgical infants found that parenteral glutamine supplementation had no significant effect on intestinal permeability or nitrogen balance, although this study was not powered to detect differences in clinical end points such as incidence of sepsis or duration of PN. A large multicenter RCT of glutamine-supplemented PN showed that although glutamine did not decrease the time to full enteral feeds, or the incidence of sepsis over the full period of PN, it did significantly decrease the incidence of sepsis during the period of exclusive parenteral feeding, i.e., before any enteral nutrition was introduced.[35]

MINERALS, VITAMINS, AND TRACE ELEMENTS

Minerals, vitamins, and trace elements are important structurally, as cofactors, or as components of enzymes, and provision of adequate supplies is important for the growing neonate. Fe, Ca, P, and Mg should all be provided in adequate amounts for growth and development but, conversely, can cause problems if provided in excess of needs or if their metabolism is impaired. In addition, administration of adequate amounts can be problematic because of lack of stability in solution or lack of compatibility with other components. Consequently, iron is often only supplemented in longer-term PN,[4] whereas calcium and phosphate supply depends on solubility in PN mixtures.[4] Vitamins and trace elements are particularly important in maintenance of the body's antioxidant defenses: vitamins C and E; selenium (for glutathione peroxidase); copper, zinc, and manganese (all for superoxide dismutases); chromium; iodine; and molybdenum can all be added to PN. However, for many of these, the precise requirements are not known. Although there is evidence that selenium supplementation may be beneficial, selenium status varies widely geographically, so global recommendations are difficult.[36] It is suggested that if the duration of PN is less than 4 weeks, of the trace elements, only zinc needs to be added.[4] There is little specific evidence for individual vitamin requirements, and the current recommendations are to continue with the available vitamin mixtures, which do not appear to cause toxicity or deficiency in the majority of children.[4]

Complications of PN

INFECTIOUS COMPLICATIONS

In spite of significant improvement in the management of PN, including the introduction of nutrition support teams, infection is still a major problem. More than 50% of surgical infants on PN have at least one suspected episode of sepsis, and around 30% of surgical neonates have at least one positive blood culture.[35] Repeated episodes of sepsis may lead to impaired liver function, critical illness, and removal of central venous catheters. Although catheter-borne infections, which can be reduced by rigorous precautions, such chlorhexidine antisepsis,[37] are important, microbial translocation from the intestine is also a significant source of infection in surgical infants on PN.[38] Infection with enteric microorganisms occurs significantly later than presumed catheter-related infection,[39] supporting the hypothesis that a progressive impairment of host defenses[40] and/or increased intestinal permeability may allow translocation of enteric organisms after an extended period of PN.

MECHANICAL COMPLICATIONS

Mechanical complications related to the intravenous infusion of nutrients are not uncommon. Table 14.1 lists the mechanical complications reported in the literature. Extravasation of PN solution is a common complication of peripheral PN. Unfortunately, even a low osmolarity solution is detrimental for peripheral veins leading to inflammation and extravasation of the solution, which can cause tissue necrosis and infection. Extravasation injury is treated with occlusive dressings or hyaluronidase irrigation, but there

Table 14.1 Mechanical complications of parenteral nutrition

Extravasation of parenteral nutrition solution
Blockage of the central venous line
Migration of the central venous line
Breakage of the infusion line
Right atrium thrombosis
Cardiac tamponade (perforation of right atrium or vena cava)

is little evidence base for the best treatment in neonates.[41] Intravenous lines may become clogged from thrombus formation, calcium precipitates, or lipid deposition. There is disagreement on the ideal position of central venous lines (CVLs) for PN in infants. Some authors advocate the atrium as the ideal position because this would give less chance of catheter dysfunction, whereas others believe that placement in the superior vena cava would reduce the risk of perforation. The current ESPGHAN/ESPEN recommendations are that the catheter tip should lie outside the atrium,[4] but because complications of either approach are very rare (albeit potentially life threatening), there is a paucity of evidence from RCTs.

HEPATIC COMPLICATIONS

The hepatobiliary complications related to PN remain serious and often life threatening. The commonest hepatobiliary complication of PN in neonates is cholestasis. The clinical significance of this cholestasis itself is unknown, but if untreated, intestinal failure–associated liver disease (IFALD) may occur, which can result in the need for liver transplantation or can result in death. IFALD has been defined by the British Society of Paediatric Gastroenterology, Hepatology and Nutrition as follows:

- Type 1 early IFALD—persistent elevation of alkaline phosphatase (ALP) and γ-glutamyl transferase (γGT) greater than 1.5 times the upper limit of reference range for at least 6 weeks
- Type 2 established IFALD—elevation of ALP and γGT as in type 1, together with elevation of total bilirubin (>50 μmol/L), with a conjugated fraction of at least 50%
- Type 3 late IFALD—elevated ALP, total bilirubin, and clinical signs of end-stage liver disease

Type 1 is thought to be reversible; type 2 is potentially reversible if enteral feeding is increased, PN reduced, and repeated episodes of catheter-related sepsis are prevented. The incidence of IFALD depends on the length of time on PN, and occurs in up to 50% of infants receiving long-term PN.[42] Although the frequency of this complication seems to be diminishing, this is probably related to the more aggressive transition to enteral feeding rather than to an improvement in the intravenous diet. Various clinical factors are thought to contribute to the development of PN-related cholestasis. These include prematurity, low birth weight, duration of PN, immature enterohepatic circulation, intestinal microflora, septicemia, failure to implement enteral nutrition, short-bowel syndrome due to resection, and number of laparotomies. In addition to the effects of ELBW, and length of time on PN, infants receiving PN for either gastroschisis or jejunal atresia seem to be at particular risk. PN-related cholestasis has a higher incidence in premature infants than in children and adults. This may be due to the immaturity of the biliary secretory system since bile salt pool size, synthesis, and intestinal concentration are low in premature infants in comparison with full-term infants. PN-related cholestasis and IFALD are diagnoses of exclusion without any specific marker yet available. Therefore, infants with cholestasis (conjugated bilirubin >2.0 mg/dL) who are receiving or have received PN must have an appropriate diagnostic evaluation to exclude other causes of cholestasis, such as bacterial and viral infections, metabolic diseases (e.g., alpha-1-antitrypsin deficiency, tyrosinemia), and congenital anomalies (e.g., Alagille syndrome, biliary atresia, choledocal cyst).

The etiology of PN-related cholestasis remains unclear. Possible causes include the toxicity of components of PN, lack of enteral feeding, continuous nonpulsatile delivery of nutrients and host factors, infection, and sepsis. In particular, the lipid component of PN has been particularly implicated, and many units now use alternative lipid management strategies (see Section "Hepatic Complications"). In addition to lipid management, careful management of these patients under a multidisciplinary team seems to be beneficial.[43] Bowel lengthening procedures, such as the Serial Transverse Enteroplasty (STEP) procedure or longitudinal intestinal lengthening, may help transition to enteral nutrition,[44] whereas in those with advanced liver disease and no prospect of enteral autonomy, transplantation may be considered.

Parenteral nutrition-associated cholestasis (PNAC) and IFALD have been linked to the use of soybean oil, although other factors are thought to be involved. Soybean oil contains mostly Ω-6 fatty acids, which are thought to be pro-inflammatory compared with Ω-3 fatty acids. In addition, the amount of phytosterols delivered in soybean-based lipid emulsions is relatively high, and phytosterol accumulation has been postulated to cause PNAC/IFALD.[45] Hence, in recent years, there has been great interest in adopting hepatoprotective lipid management strategies in PN of surgical infants and children to either prevent or reverse cholestasis. Several different approaches have been adopted:

1. Decreasing the amount of lipid administered. This can also be achieved by limiting the time on lipid, by lipid-free hours or days. This could potentially result in poor growth due to inadequate calories.
2. Use of Omegaven, a lipid emulsion of 10% fish oil. Fish oil is high in Ω-3 fatty acids and low in phytosterols, so it has been suggested to reverse cholestasis in surgical infants on long-term PN.[46] Use of Omegaven as the only lipid source could, however, potentially result in essential fatty acid deficiency, due to lack of Ω-6 fatty acids, and could also result in poor growth, as the dose of Omegaven is limited to 1.0 g kg^{-1} day^{-1} (compared with 3 g kg^{-1} day^{-1} for soybean-based lipid emulsions).
3. Use of lipid emulsions containing a mixture of LCTs and MCT triglycerides. This has the advantage of increasing fat utilization,[30] ability to use at up to 3 g kg^{-1} day^{-1}, and decreasing the phytosterols and Ω-6 fatty acids administered while ensuring adequate delivery of essential fatty acids.

4. Use of mixed lipid emulsions such as SMOF, which is a mixture of soybean, medium-chain, olive, and fish triglycerides.[47] This has the advantages of lowered amounts of phytosterols and Ω-6 fatty acids, increased fat utilization, delivery of Ω-3 fatty acids, and ability to use at up to 3 g kg^{-1} day^{-1}.

Despite these different approaches, the evidence base supporting any lipid management strategy is lacking due to the paucity of RCTs in this area. It is difficult to design and implement good-quality RCTs, as units already use a variety of alternate lipid management strategies. It is also questionable whether maintaining an infant on a high dose of soybean-based lipid emulsion after the onset of PNAC/IFALD is ethical, so that it is difficult to decide on an appropriate comparison group.

Enteral nutrition

The energy requirement of an infant fed enterally is greater than the intravenous requirement because of the energetic cost of absorption from the gastrointestinal tract and energy lost in the stools (Figure 14.2).

FEEDING ROUTES

Alternative feeding routes where neonates are unable to feed orally include nasogastric or orogastric tubes, nasojejunal tubes, gastrostomy tubes, or jejunostomy tubes. Gastric feeding is generally preferable to intestinal feeding because it allows for a more natural digestive process, i.e., it allows action of salivary and gastric enzymes and the antibacterial action of stomach acid. In addition, gastric feeding is associated with a larger osmotic and volume tolerance and a lower frequency of diarrhea and dumping syndrome. Thus, transpyloric feeds are usually restricted to infants (1) unable to tolerate nasogastric or orogastric feeds; (2) at increased risk of aspiration; or (3) with anatomical contraindications to gastric feeds, such as microgastria. Neonates are obligatory nose breathers, and therefore orogastric feeding may be preferable over nasogastric feeding in preterm infants to avoid upper airway obstruction. However, nasogastric tubes are easier to secure and may involve a lower risk of displacement. In infants requiring gastric tube feeding for extended periods (e.g., more than 6–8 weeks), it is advisable to insert a gastrostomy, to decrease the negative oral stimulation of repeated insertion of nasal or oral tubes. The tube can be inserted using an open, endoscopic, or laparoscopic approach. In infants with significant gastroesophageal reflux, fundoplication with gastrostomy tube or enterostomy tube placement is indicated. In preterm infants with gastroesophageal reflux, enteral feeding can be established via a nasojejunal tube inserted under fluoroscopy. Nasojejunal feeding usually minimizes the episodes of gastroesophageal reflux and its consequences. However, it is common for these tubes to dislocate back in the stomach. Regular analysis of the pH in the aspirate is essential to monitor the correct position of the tube. Feeding jejunostomy tubes can be inserted through existing gastrostomy or directly into the jejunum via laparotomy or laparoscopy.

SELECTION OF ENTERAL FEEDS

Breast milk is the ideal feed for infants because it has specific anti-infectious activities and aids gastrointestinal maturation and neurological development. When breast milk is not available, chemically defined formulae can be used, which are designed either for term infants or specifically for preterm infants. If malabsorption is present and persists, an appropriate specific formula should be introduced. A soy-based disaccharide-free feed is used when there is disaccharide intolerance resulting in loose stools containing disaccharides. For fat malabsorption, a formula containing MCTs should be used. An elemental (free amino acids) or semielemental (protein hydrolysate containing dipeptides and tripeptides) formula may be indicated when there is severe malabsorption due to short-bowel syndrome or severe mucosal damage as in NEC. Semielemental preparations have the advantage of a lower osmolality, are well absorbed, and have a more palatable taste. Infants recovering from NEC pose a particular problem, as malabsorption may be severe and prolonged. These infants may have had their small bowel resected, in addition to which the remaining bowel may not have healed completely by the time feeds are begun. Feeding may provoke a relapse of the necrotizing enterocolitis, and feeding should therefore be introduced cautiously. However, there is no strong evidence for the time to reintroduce enteral feeds in infants who have had NEC.[48] For persistent severe malabsorption, a modular diet may be necessary. Glucose, amino acid, and MCT preparations are provided separately, beginning with the amino acid solution and adding the glucose and then the fats as tolerated. Minerals, trace elements, and vitamins are also added. These solutions have a high osmolality and, if given too quickly, may precipitate dumping syndrome, with diarrhea, abdominal cramps, and hypoglycemia. It is important, therefore, to start with a dilute solution and increase slowly the concentration and volume of each component. This may take several weeks, and infants will need PN support during this period.

ADMINISTRATION OF ENTERAL FEEDS

Enteral feeds can be administered as boluses, continuous feeds or combination of the two. Bolus feeds are more physiological and are known to stimulate intestinal motility, enterohepatic circulation of bile acids, and gallbladder contraction[49] continuous enteral feeding leads to an enlarged, noncontractile gallbladder in infants. Contraction is observed immediately after resuming bolus enteral feeds, and gallbladder volume returns to baseline after 4 days. Therefore, the mode of feeding has important bearings on the motility of the extrahepatic biliary tree. Bolus feeds mimic or supplement meals and are easier to administer than continuous feeds since a feeding pump is not required. Bolus feeds are usually given over 15–20 minutes and usually every 3 hours; term infants can tolerate a period of 4 hours without feeds before hypoglycemia occurs. In preterm neonates or in neonates soon after surgery, feeds every 2 hours are occasionally given. Where bolus feeds are not tolerated, for example, in the presence of gastroesophageal reflux, continuous feeds should be administered via an infusion pump over 24 hours. This modality of feeding is used in infants with gastroesophageal reflux, delayed gastric emptying, or intestinal malabsorption. Infants with jejunal tubes should receive continuous feeds and not bolus feeds, as the stomach is no longer providing a reservoir.

COMPLICATIONS OF ENTERAL TUBE FEEDING

Enteral tube feeding is associated with fewer complications than parenteral feeding. The complications can be mechanical, including tube blockage, tube displacement or migration, and intestinal perforation. Although infection is less of a risk than with PN, the risk of infected enteral feeds should not be ignored. Other complications involve the gastrointestinal tract. These include gastroesophageal reflux with aspiration pneumonia, dumping syndrome, and diarrhea. Jejunostomy tubes inserted at laparotomy can be also associated with intestinal obstruction. The use of hyperosmolar feeds has been associated with development of necrotizing enterocolitis, dehydration, and rarely, intestinal obstruction due to milk curds.

In surgical infants, enteral feeding often results in vomiting, interruption of feeding, inadequate calorie intake and rarely in necrotizing enterocolitis. In infants with congenital gastrointestinal anomalies, exclusive enteral feeding is commonly precluded for some time after surgery due to large gastric aspirate and intestinal dysmotility. Therefore, appropriate calorie intake is established initially by TPN. Supplementary enteral feeding is introduced when intestinal motility and absorption improve. The percentage of calories given enterally is gradually increased at the expense of intravenous calorie intake. This transition time from TPN to total enteral feeding could be quite long. The presence of significant gastric aspirate often induces clinicians and surgeons not to use the gut for nutrition. However, minimal enteral feeding can be implemented early in these patients even if its nutritional value is questionable. Minimal enteral feeding may be all that is required to enhance some immunological function. Okada et al.[50] have shown that the introduction of small volumes of enteral feed improved the impaired host bactericidal activity against coagulase-negative staphylococci and the abnormal cytokine response observed during TPN. The increase in bactericidal activity against coagulase-negative staphylococci after the addition of small enteral feeds in patients on PN was significantly correlated with the duration of enteral feeding. This implies that stimulation of the gastrointestinal tract may modulate immune function in neonates and prevent bacterial infection.

CONCLUSION AND FUTURE DIRECTIONS

Nutrition of surgical infants and children is complicated by the requirement for growth. Inadequate or unbalanced nutrition may lead to future problems for these children, and we are now able to start to improve nutrition delivery in order to optimize outcomes as well as survival. Despite advances in nutritional care, such as the multidisciplinary approach, complications such as sepsis and cholestasis remain relatively frequent. Future research should be aimed toward the prevention and treatment of these complications of artificial nutritional support.

REFERENCES

1. Stoll BJ, Hansen NI, Adams-Chapman I et al. Neurodevelopmental and growth impairment among extremely low-birth-weight infants with neonatal infection. *JAMA* 2004; 292: 2357–65.

2. Denne SC, Poindexter BB, Leitch CA, Ernst JA, Lemons PK, Lemons JA. Nutrition and metabolism in the high-risk neonate. In: Martin RJ, Fanarof AA, Walsh MC (eds). *Fanaroff and Martin's Neonatal–Perinatal Medicine*, 8th edn. Philadeplhia, PA: Mosby-Elsevier, 2006: 661–93.

3. Wilson DC, Cairns P, Halliday HL et al. Randomised controlled trial of an aggressive nutritional regimen in sick very low birthweight infants. *Arch DisChild Fetal Neonatal Ed* 1997; 77: F4–11.

4. Koletzko B, Goulet O, Hunt J et al. Guidelines on paediatric parenteral nutrition of the European Society of Paediatric Gastroenterology, Hepatology and Nutrition (ESPGHAN) and the European Society for Clinical Nutrition and Metabolism (ESPEN), supported by the European Society of Paediatric Research (ESPR). *J Pediatr Gastroenterol Nutr* 2005; 41 Suppl 2: S1–87.

5. Tsang RC, Uauy R, Koletzko B, Zlotkin SH. *Nutrition of the Preterm Infant: Scientific Basis and Practical Guidelines*, 2nd edn. Cincinnati, OH: Digital Educational Publishing, Inc. 2005.

6. FAO/WHO/UNU. *Human Energy Requirements: Report of a Joint FAO/WHO/UNU Expert Consultation*, Rome, Italy: FAO, 2004: 1–96.

7. Schofield WN. Predicting basal metabolic rate, new standards and review of previous work. *Hum Nutr Clin Nutr* 1985; 39 Suppl 1: 5–41.

8. Harris JA, Benedict FG. *A Biometric Study of Basal Metabolism in Man*. Washington, DC: Carnegie Institute of Washington. 1919.

9. Garza JJ, Shew SB, Keshen TH et al. Energy expenditure in ill premature neonates. *J Pediatr Surg* 2002; 37: 289–93.

10. Powis MR, Smith K, Rennie M et al. Characteristics of protein and energy metabolism in neonates with necrotizing enterocolitis—A pilot study. *J Pediatr Surg* 1999; 34: 5–10.

11. Jaksic T, Shew SB, Keshen TH et al. Do critically ill surgical neonates have increased energy expenditure? *J Pediatr Surg* 2001; 36: 63–7.

12. Bauer J, Hentschel R, Linderkamp O. Effect of sepsis syndrome on neonatal oxygen consumption and energy expenditure. *Pediatrics* 2002; 110: art-e69.

13. Mrozek JD, Georgieff MK, Blazar BR et al. Effect of sepsis syndrome on neonatal protein and energy metabolism. *J Perinatol* 2000; 20: 96–100.

14. Jones MO, Pierro A, Hammond P et al. The metabolic response to operative stress in infants. *J Pediatr Surg* 1993; 28: 1258–62.

15. Powis MR, Smith K, Rennie M et al. Effect of major abdominal operations on energy and protein metabolism in infants and children. *J Pediatr Surg* 1998; 33: 49–53.

16. Keshen TH, Miller RG, Jahoor F et al. Stable isotopic quantitation of protein metabolism and energy expenditure in neonates on- and post-extracorporeal life support. *J Pediatr Surg* 1997; 32: 958–62.

17. Chwals WJ, Lally KP, Woolley MM et al. Measured energy expenditure in critically ill infants and young children. *J Surg Res* 1988; 44: 467–72.

18. Coss-Bu JA, Klish WJ, Walding D et al. Energy metabolism, nitrogen balance, and substrate utilization in critically ill children. *Am J Clin Nutr* 2001; 74: 664–9.

19. Turi RA, Petros A, Eaton S et al. Energy metabolism of infants and children with systemic inflammatory response syndrome and sepsis. *Ann Surg* 2001; 233: 581–7.

20. Taylor RM, Cheeseman P, Preedy VR et al. Can energy expenditure be predicted in critically ill children? *Pediatr Crit Care Med* 2003; 4: 176–80.

21. Skillman HE, Wischmeyer PE. Nutrition therapy in critically ill infants and children. *J Parent Enteral Nutr* 2008; 32: 520–34.

22. Bishay M, Lakshminarayanan B, Arnaud A et al. The role of parenteral nutrition following surgery for duodenal atresia or stenosis. *Pediatr Surg Int* 2013; 29: 191–5.

23. Ainsworth SB, Clerihew L, McGuire W. Percutaneous central venous catheters versus peripheral cannulae for delivery of parenteral nutrition in neonates. *Cochrane Database Syst Rev* 2007: CD004219.

24. Modi N. Fluid and electrolyte balance. In: Rennie JM (ed). *Roberton's Textbook of Neonatology*, 4th edn. London, United Kingdom: Elsevier Churchill Livingstone, 2005: 335–54.

25. NCEPOD. A mixed bag: An enquiry into the care of hospital patients receiving parenteral nutrition. In: Stewart JAD et al. (eds). London: National Confidential Enquiry into Patient Outcome and Death, 2010.

26. Bell EF, Acarregui MJ. Restricted versus liberal water intake for preventing morbidity and mortality in preterm infants. *Cochrane Database Syst Rev* 2001: CD000503.

27. Cornblath M, Hawdon JM, Williams AF et al. Controversies regarding definition of neonatal hypoglycemia: suggested operational thresholds. *Pediatrics* 2000; 105: 1141–5.

28. Hall NJ, Peters M, Eaton S et al. Hyperglycemia is associated with increased morbidity and mortality rates in neonates with necrotizing enterocolitis. *J Pediatr Surg* 2004; 39: 898–901.

29. Pierro A, Jones MO, Hammond P, Nunn A, Lloyd DA. Utilisation of intravenous fat in the surgical newborn infant. *Proc Nutr Soc* 1993; 52: 237A.

30. Donnell SC, Lloyd DA, Eaton S et al. The metabolic response to intravenous medium-chain triglycerides in infants after surgery. *J Pediatr* 2002; 141: 689–94.

31. Pitkanen O, Hallman M, Andersson S. Generation of free-radicals in lipid emulsion used in parenteral-nutrition. *Pediatr Res* 1991; 29: 56–9.

32. Basu R, Muller DPR, Eaton S et al. Lipid peroxidation can be reduced in infants on total parenteral nutrition by promoting fat utilisation. *J Pediatr Surg* 1999; 34: 255–9.

33. Zlotkin SH, Bryan MH, Anderson GH. Intravenous nitrogen and energy intakes required to duplicate in utero nitrogen accretion in prematurely born human infants. *J Pediatr* 1981; 99: 115–20.

34. Albers MJ, Steyerberg EW, Hazebroek FW et al. Glutamine supplementation of parenteral nutrition does not improve intestinal permeability, nitrogen balance, or outcome in newborns and infants undergoing digestive-tract surgery: Results from a double-blind, randomized, controlled trial. *Ann Surg* 2005; 241: 599–606.

35. Ong EGP, Eaton S, Wade AM et al. Randomized clinical trial of glutamine-supplemented versus standard parenteral nutrition in infants with surgical gastrointestinal disease. *Br J Surg* 2012; 99: 929–38.

36. Darlow BA, Austin NC. Selenium supplementation to prevent short-term morbidity in preterm neonates. *Cochrane Database Syst Rev* 2003: CD003312.

37. Bishay M, Retrosi G, Horn V et al. Chlorhexidine antisepsis significantly reduces the incidence of sepsis and septicemia during parenteral nutrition in surgical infants. *J Pediatr Surg* 2011; 46: 1064–9.

38. Pierro A, van Saene HKF, Donnell SC et al. Microbial translocation in neonates and infants receiving long-term parenteral-nutrition. *Arch Surg* 1996; 131: 176–9.

39. Bishay M, Retrosi G, Horn V et al. Septicaemia due to enteric organisms is a later event in surgical infants requiring parenteral nutrition. *Eur J Pediatr Surg* 2012; 22: 50–3.

40. Okada Y, Klein NJ, van Saene HK et al. Bactericidal activity against coagulase-negative staphylococci is impaired in infants receiving long-term parenteral nutrition. *Ann Surg* 2000; 231: 276–81.

41. Wilkins CE, Emmerson AJB. Extravasation injuries on regional neonatal units. *Arch Dis Child* 2004; 89: F274–5.

42. Lauriti G, Zani A, Aufieri R et al. Incidence, prevention, and treatment of parenteral nutrition–associated cholestasis and intestinal failure–associated liver disease in infants and children: A systematic review. *J Parenter Enteral Nutr* 2014; 38: 70–85.

43. Bishay M, Pichler J, Horn V et al. Intestinal failure–associated liver disease in surgical infants requiring long-term parenteral nutrition. *J Pediatr Surg* 2012; 47: 359–62.

44. Sudan D, Thompson J, Botha J et al. Comparison of intestinal lengthening procedures for patients with short bowel syndrome. *Ann Surg* 2007; 246: 593–601.

45. Clayton PT, Bowron A, Mills KA et al. Phytosterolemia in children with parenteral nutrition-associated cholestatic liver disease. *Gastroenterology* 1993; 105: 1806–13.

46. Puder M, Valim C, Meisel JA et al. Parenteral fish oil improves outcomes in patients with parenteral nutrition–associated liver injury. *Ann Surg* 2009; 250: 395–402.

47. Goulet O, Antebi H, Wolf C et al. A new intravenous fat emulsion containing soybean oil, medium-chain triglycerides, olive oil, and fish oil: A single-center, double-blind randomized study on efficacy and safety in pediatric patients receiving home parenteral nutrition. *J Parenter Enteral Nutr* 2010; 34: 485–95.

48. Bohnhorst B, Muller S, Dordelmann M et al. Early feeding after necrotizing enterocolitis in preterm infants. *J Pediatr* 2003; 143: 484–7.

49. Jawaheer G, Pierro A, Lloyd D et al. Gall-bladder contractility in neonates—Effects of parenteral and enteral feeding. *Arch Dis Child* 1995; 72: F200–2.

50. Okada Y, Klein N, van Saene HK et al. Small volumes of enteral feedings normalise immune function in infants receiving parenteral nutrition. *J Pediatr Surg* 1998; 33: 16–9.

15

Access for enteral nutrition

MICHAEL W. L. GAUDERER AND JULIA ZIMMER

INTRODUCTION

Adequate nutrition in neonates and infants is of major importance to assure optimal health, growth, and development and to support recovery during illness or after surgery. Both enteral and parenteral application routes may be used to provide a patient's caloric requirements. Enteral nutrition can be delivered via an enteral feeding tube (nasogastric/nasoduodenal/nasojejunal, orogastric/oroenteric), a gastrostomy, or a jejunostomy.

Gastrostomy is one of the oldest abdominal operations in continuous use[1] and has played an important role in the management of various surgical conditions of the neonate.[1-6] The procedure was frequently employed for feeding as well as intestinal decompression. In the past decades, there has been remarkable improvement in surgical techniques for gastrostomy placement. Contemporary approaches include techniques with laparotomy (or "open"), such as the Stamm procedure, or minimally invasive techniques, including the percutaneous endoscopic gastrostomy (PEG), the interventional-radiologic guided gastrostomy (IRG), the laparoscopically assisted gastrostomy (LAP), and the laparoscopically assisted percutaneous endoscopic gastrostomy (LA-PEG).[7] Delivery of enteral nutrition may also be post-pyloric (duodenal or jejunal) or gastrojejunal.[8] The optimal method of enterostomy must be carefully chosen according to patients' comorbidities and habitus, and caretakers' experience. New techniques such as fluoroscopic guidance or electromagnets permit tube placement in the small bowel without radiographic confirmation.

Depending on the clinical circumstances and the provider's level of comfort, there is a broad array of enterostomy devices available, either traditional (long) tubes or skin-level devices (buttons or balloon type).

Gastrostomies are these days used not only in patients with major congenital anomalies of the gastrointestinal tract and abdominal wall but in an increased number of infants and children without surgical pathology. In most of these, the indication is an inability to swallow, usually secondary to central nervous system impairment. Ironically, often these are patients who have survived because of aggressive neonatal resuscitation and technological advances.

INDICATIONS

In infants, the three main indications are long-term feeding, decompression, or a combination of both modalities. Additional indications include gastric access for esophageal bougienage and administration of medications.

Nasogastric feeding tube versus gastrostomy

Because the newer 5F and 8F infant feeding tubes are highly biocompatible and remain smooth and soft for prolonged periods of time, they are usually well tolerated, even by the smallest premature infants. In general, feeding tubes should be preferred if the expected length of enteral access is up to 1–2 months. Beyond this arbitrary time frame, complications such as naso-otopharyngeal infections and gastro-esophageal reflux tend to increase. Gastrostomies should be considered when direct gastric access for feeding or the administration of medication is expected to last more than several months.

Nasogastric decompression tube versus gastrostomy

With careful attention to appropriate intragastric position and regular flushing, nasogastric or orogastric tubes generally decompress more effectively than do gastrostomy tubes. The newer 8F or 10F tubes are well tolerated for up to several weeks. The author's preference when performing gastric decompression lasting up to 3–4 weeks in newborns is a 10- to 20-inch-long (38–51 cm), 8F single-lumen tube. Longer tubes are prone to plugging, thus becoming ineffective. It should be remembered that most commercially available 8F tubes are designed for feeding and have only two holes. Additional holes of appropriate size should therefore be added. However, care must be taken not to make the holes too big in order to avoid kinking. These 8F tubes should be attached directly or via a short connecting tube to a spill-resistant open container and irrigated regularly. No suction should be applied to single-lumen tubes. Double-lumen (vented) catheters, such as the 10F Replogle tube, originally designed for the aspiration of saliva in patients with esophageal atresia, tend to be much stiffer and are therefore more likely to cause problems. Additionally, if the venting lumen is obstructed and suction is applied, mucosa is sucked into the holes, leading to trauma and rendering the tube ineffective.

Before performing an enteral access in a neonate, several essential issues need to be addressed and clarified to identify the optimal method for enteral nutrition: (1) medical cause for the child's underlying condition/chance of recovery, (2) length of the anticipated need, (3) anatomical or physiological abnormalities, and (4) what the most efficient workup is and why.

In the author's experience, nasogastric/nasojejunal tubes are mostly only suitable for short-term use (±1–3 months). In case of long-term usage (over ±3 months), gastrostomies are recommendable. If additionally, a stomach bypass is required, a gastrostomy with a jejunal extension tube should be placed or a jejunostomy created.

GASTROSTOMY IN SELECT NEONATAL SURGICAL PATHOLOGY

Esophageal abnormalities

Once considered essential in the management of patients with esophageal atresia, gastrostomies are no longer employed routinely. The analysis of large series demonstrates that esophago-esophagostomy without the use of a gastrostomy is safe[9] and may in fact be beneficial for decreasing the incidence of gastroesophageal reflux.[10] A gastrostomy is indicated in esophageal atresia without fistula, when a difficult repair or a stormy course is anticipated, in staging procedures, and when the child has associated anomalies that may interfere with feeding. The stoma, employed for the decompression or feeding, can also be used to provide access for the management of anastomotic complications such as leakage or strictures.

Duodenal obstruction

Congenital duodenal obstruction is usually associated with proximal duodenal dilatation and atony as well as gastric dilatation. Total parenteral nutrition and nasogastric decompression are generally effective in postoperative management. However, if the need for prolonged gastric decompression is anticipated, a valuable alternative in this setting is the placement of a fine silicone rubber catheter alongside a gastrostomy catheter, across the anastomosis and into the proximal jejunum[1,11] (Figure 15.1). Although these tubes are at times difficult to place and maintain, this simple and

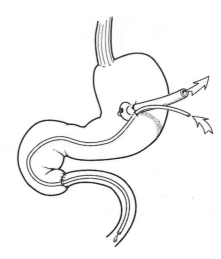

Figure 15.1 Traditional combination gastric decompression and intrajejunal feeding, demonstrated diagrammatically in a newborn with repaired duodenal atresia.

time-honored technique can decrease or eliminate the need for parenteral nutrition.

Major abdominal wall defects

Prolonged ileus typically follows the repair of gastroschisis and, occasionally, other major wall defects. Although decompressive gastrostomies are not routinely employed, they can be helpful in patients with gastroschisis and associated atresia, particularly those requiring long-term continuous feeding.

Short-gut syndrome

Infants who have lost over 50% of their small bowel have profound alteration of gastrointestinal physiology. Initial gastric hypersecretion may require prolonged drainage. As the remaining intestine undergoes adaptive changes, continuous enteral feedings become necessary. As this latter process can be fairly lengthy, direct gastric access via gastrostomy is desirable.

Other surgical pathology

In any neonatal or infant condition in which a prolonged ileus or partial luminal occlusion (e.g., recurrent adhesive bowel obstruction, complicated meconium ileus, small bowel Hirschsprung disease) is anticipated or in whom a complex feeding regimen is likely (e.g., those with intestinal lymphangiectasia), a gastrostomy can facilitate management. Gastrostomies are also helpful in some children with extra-abdominal surgical pathologies (Figure 15.2).

"Nonsurgical" pathology

The number of pediatric patients with an inability to swallow referred to a surgeon for the placement of a gastrostomy

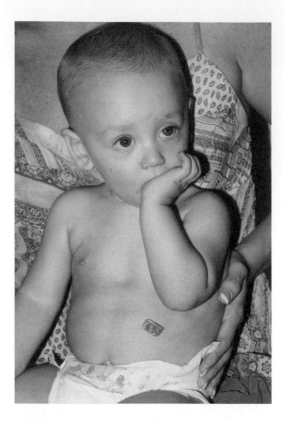

Figure 15.2 Ten-month-old child who presented with respiratory distress shortly after birth because of a large left cervical neuroblastoma. The lesion was fully resected on the second day of life. However, the extensive dissection resulted in difficulty swallowing. A PEG was placed at age 4 weeks and swallowing therapy initiated. Normal feeding gradually returned, and a few weeks after this picture was taken, the gastrostomy could be removed. The only residual side effect is a left-sided Horner syndrome.

continues to increase. The main indications in infants are swallowing difficulty secondary to central nervous system lesions as well as other abnormalities of deglutition, feeding supplementation, large-volume medications, and chronic malabsorption syndromes. Because the neurologically impaired children frequently have foregut dysmotility and gastroesophageal reflux in addition to swallowing difficulties, antireflux procedures are at times added to gastrostomies. There are conflicting results about an increased risk of pathologic gastroesophageal reflux after gastrostomy tube placement in neurologically impaired children, resulting in divergent recommendations of simultaneous antireflux surgery.[12,13] A recent Cochrane analysis found that the question of whether to use gastrostomy only or gastrostomy plus fundoplication remains debatable as there are currently no sufficient trials available for comparison.[14]

In general, gastrostomy and gastrojejunostomy procedures in neurologically impaired and chronically ventilator-dependent infants and children have a significant risk of postoperative complications, morbidity, and mortality.[15,16]

ADVANTAGES AND DISADVANTAGES OF GASTROSTOMIES

Direct access to the stomach provides the surgeon with valuable perioperative access for drainage of air or fluids, a reliable long-term source of intermittent or continuous administration of nutrients, or a combination of both. As stated, nasogastric tubes tend to drain better than gastrostomies in the immediate postoperative period. However, a gastrostomy can eliminate the need for long-term nasogastric or orogastric intubation and the complications associated with placement and maintenance of these tubes. Gastrostomies interfere less with oral feedings than do nasogastric tubes, although the newer, smaller catheters are better tolerated. Gastrostomies are preferred over jejunostomies because the latter are less physiological and more prone to mechanical complications.[1]

The disadvantages of gastrostomies in the neonatal period include the need for an operative intervention with or without laparotomy; the observation that the procedure is not always simple, particularly if the child has associated anomalies; and the observation that gastrostomy placement may interfere with gastric emptying and increase the incidence of gastroesophageal reflux.[1,10] It has also been recognized that both nasogastric tubes and gastrostomies may promote gastric colonization with bacteria. Gastrostomies, as well as any other enteral tubes placed in infants, are associated with a long list of potential early and late complications.[1,7,17–21]

The obvious advantage of jejunostomies is the gastric bypass. Gastrojejunal tubes may eliminate the need for antireflux surgery in patients with gastroesophageal reflux.[22]

On the contrary, gastrojejunal tubes are difficult to place and to maintain and need frequent exchanges, usually every 3 months.[8] They provide a less physiologic nutrition as the feedings are usually continuous administered rather than in bolus feedings. Jejunostomies have been found to provide more complications, such as internal hernia and volvulus (the latter particularly in the Roux-en-Y jejunostomies or the "dissociation" technique bypassing the stomach as described by Bianchi). A notable morbidity after gastrojejunal tube placement has been described ranging from persistent reflux to dislodgement and intestinal perforation.[21]

Gastrojejunal and jejunal buttons have the same design as gastrostomy buttons but, additionally, a long distal jejunal tube component.[8] Nowadays, the smallest gastrojejunal button is a 14F button, which is useful in smaller children needing both jejunal access for feedings and gastric decompression.[8] Jejunal buttons (which do not have a gastric lumen) are used in children requiring only jejunal feeding without the need for gastric venting or intragastric access.[8]

TECHNIQUE

There are multiple approaches to construct a gastrostomy. These techniques and their many variations are based on three fundamental principles:

1. Formation of a serosa-lined channel from the anterior gastric wall around a catheter. This catheter is placed in the stomach and exits either parallel to the serosa, as in the Witzel technique, or vertically, as in the Stamm or Kader approaches.[1,23]

2. Construction of a tube or conduit from a full-thickness gastric wall flap, leading to the skin surface. A catheter is then introduced intermittently for feeding. Several different configurations of the gastric wall flap have been described.[1,23]

3. Percutaneous techniques, i.e., without laparotomy, in which the introduced catheter holds the gastric and abdominal walls in apposition, with or without the aid of special fasteners.[1,23]

The Stamm technique, illustrated in this section, is the most widely employed gastrostomy with laparotomy in the neonatal setting, either as an isolated intervention or when employed in conjunction with another intra-abdominal procedure. It can be used in children of any size and even on the smallest stomach (e.g., in newborns with esophageal atresia without fistula). A standard gastrostomy tube or a skin-level device can be placed under local anesthesia, although general anesthesia is preferred because abdominal wall relaxation is required. The procedure is usually short. After the tract is well healed, this stoma is suitable for the passage of dilators or guide wires.

The construction of a gastric wall tube is difficult in very young children. For a variety of reasons, this approach is not appropriate for newborns.

The first of the gastrostomies without laparotomy was PEG, initially developed for high-risk pediatric patients. The diagrams (Figures 15.9 through 15.12) represented follow the initial description of the "pull" PEG.[24] It has been employed in neonates weighing as little as 2.5 kg, usually for the purpose of long-term enteral feeding.[4,25–27] Although there is no need for abdominal wall relaxation, general endotracheal anesthesia is employed in this age group so that the airway is protected from compression during endoscopy. The procedure is very short, and there is no postoperative ileus, no potential for bleeding or wound disruption, and only minimal interference with subsequent interventions on the stomach, such as a fundoplication. The main disadvantage of this and other pure endoscopic techniques is that the virtual space between the stomach and the abdominal wall cannot be visualized. This shortcoming can be overcome by the addition of laparoscopic control.[28,29] Although in the typical PEG, a long tube is initially employed, a primary insertion of a skin-level device is also possible.[30,31]

Several other methods of gastrostomy without laparotomy have been introduced, and most are suitable for newborns. One of these is the percutaneous endoscopic "push" technique, which is performed with the aid of needle-deployed gastric anchors or T-fasteners, and the Seldinger method of guide-wire introduction followed by progressive tract dilatations. A long tube or skin-level gastrostomy device is then inserted.[32] A similar approach is used by interventional radiologists and found to be suitable for even very small stomachs.[33–35]

In the last couple of decades, minimally invasive, laparoscopically aided approaches have been introduced. These are essentially expansions of the aforementioned methods, significantly increasing the choices of gastric access techniques available to surgeons managing infants.[36–38]

Comparative studies regarding efficacy, outcome, and complications of the different techniques are constantly published identifying the LAP procedure as the currently favorable approach.[7,16,17,39–42]

One of the most widely employed laparoscopically aided gastrostomies is illustrated in this section (Figures 15.13 through 15.15). For infants with an abnormal epigastric anatomy, in whom the aforementioned techniques are difficult or impossible to perform, a hybrid procedure employing a mini-laparotomy and the PEG principle was developed.[43]

STAMM GASTROSTOMY

The child is placed on the table with a small roll behind the back. When possible, a nasogastric tube is inserted for decompression and to help identify the stomach, if necessary. A small transverse incision is made over the left upper rectus abdominis muscle (Figure 15.3). This incision should be neither too high, because it would bring the catheter too close to the costal margin, nor too low, avoiding the colon and the small bowel. A short vertical incision is an alternative. However, this approach is less desirable because the linea alba is the thinnest area of the abdominal wall. Bleeders are simply clamped. Fascial layers are incised transversely and the rectus muscle retracted or transected. When identification of the stomach is not immediate, downward traction of the flimsy greater omentum readily allows visualization of the transverse colon and stomach.

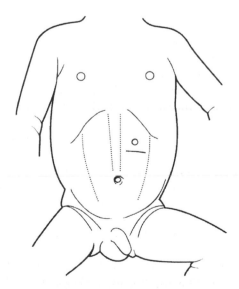

Figure 15.3 Gastrostomy incision and catheter exit site. An alternative is a short vertical midline incision.

The site of gastrotomy placement on the anterior gastric wall is critical in infants. A position midway between the pylorus and the esophagus is chosen (Figure 15.4). The site should be neither too high, because this would interfere with a fundoplication should one be needed in the future, nor too low, because stomas at the level of the antrum are prone to leakage and pyloric obstruction by the catheter. The surgeon must not place the catheter too close to the greater curvature, to avoid the so-called gastric pacemaker and to minimize the potential for gastrocolic fistula.[1]

The anterior gastric wall is lifted with two guy sutures (4-0 silk) at the site of the stoma, ensuring that the posterior wall is not included (Figures 15.4 through 15.7). A concentric purse-string suture (4-0 synthetic, absorbable material) is placed (Figures 15.4 through 15.6). The gastrotomy, at the center of the purse string, is made sharply through the serosa and muscular wall of the stomach.

A small hemostat is introduced to confirm access into the gastric lumen. We prefer a mushroom-type catheter (de Pezzer), sizes 12–14F gauge, for neonates. The mushroom head of the catheter is stretched with a short stylet to allow atraumatic introduction into the stomach (Figure 15.5). The purse string is tied to invert the seromuscular gastric wall around the tube (Figure 15.6). Other suitable catheters are the Malecot or the T-tube, but both have the disadvantage of becoming more easily dislodged. However, a short T-tube is useful if the stomach is very small. It is also our preferred tube for infant jejunostomies. We avoid the Foley or balloon-type catheters because the main lumen is proportionately smaller and the balloon occupies more intragastric space. Long balloon-type catheters, which may rupture, also have a greater propensity for distal migration into the small bowel. Skin-level devices (buttons or balloon type) may be inserted during the operation, instead of the

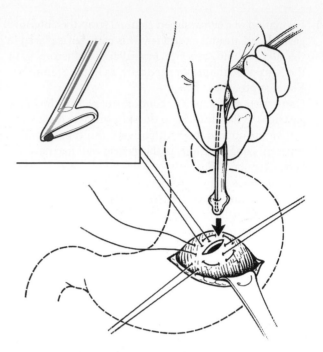

Figure 15.5 Introduction of a de Pezzer catheter using a simple stylet. The inset shows insertion of a PEG-type catheter.[23]

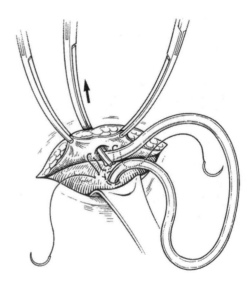

Figure 15.6 The purse-string suture is tied. The continuous monofilament suture, used to anchor the stomach to the anterior abdominal wall, has been partially placed. The catheter is brought out through the counterincision.[23]

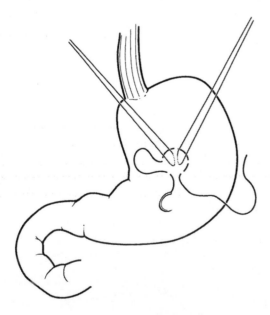

Figure 15.4 Gastrotomy site on the anterior gastric wall. The traction guy sutures and the purse-string suture are depicted.

traditional long tubes.[23] The exit site for the catheter should be through the midportion of the rectus muscle about 1–2 cm above or below the laparotomy incision (Figures 15.3 and 15.6 through 15.8). Although some surgeons bring the catheter out by way of the primary abdominal incision, wound complications that may occur in this setting tend to be more complex.[1] Once the exit site is chosen, the anterior gastric wall is secured to the posterior aspect of the anterior abdominal wall with four equidistant sutures or, as illustrated, with a continuous suture of double-ended

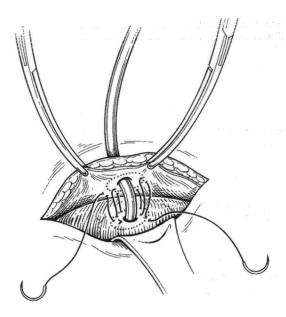

Figure 15.7 The continuous monofilament suture placement is continued anteriorly and then tied. This provides a 360° fixation of the stomach to the anterior abdominal wall with a watertight seal.[23]

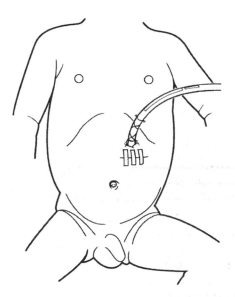

Figure 15.8 Completed procedure. The subcuticular closure, adhesive strips, and secured gastrostomy catheter are depicted. The immobilizing sutures are removed after several days, and a small crossbar is placed to prevent distal catheter migration. An alternative is the placement of a "button" or a balloon-type skin-level device, instead of a long tube, at the initial procedure.[23]

4-0 synthetic monofilament thread[27] (Figures 15.6 and 15.7). The catheter position is tested by injecting and aspirating saline. Gentle traction on the catheter assures that its intragastric position is maintained.

The posterior rectus sheath is closed with a running suture of 4-0 absorbable, synthetic material. The anterior rectus sheath is approximated with interrupted sutures of the same material.

The subcutaneous layer is closed with a couple of 5-0 or 6-0 synthetic, absorbable sutures. The skin can be approximated with either interrupted or continuous 5-0 or 6-0 subcuticular sutures. Adhesive strips cover the incision (Figure 15.8). The catheter is firmly secured with two sutures of 3-0 or 4-0 synthetic monofilament thread. These sutures are removed after 1 week, and a small crossbar is placed loosely to prevent distal catheter migration. Occlusive dressings are not used after the first couple of postoperative days. Conversion of a long tube to a button can be performed after a firm adherence between gastric and abdominal wall is established.

Percutaneous endoscopic gastrostomy

The PEG technique, as initially described,[24] is applicable to neonates and small infants.[27] The procedure must, however, be done with great precision and endoscopic skill. PEG incorporates four basic elements:

1. Gastroscopic insufflation brings the stomach into apposition to the anterior abdominal wall (Figure 15.9).
2. With the stomach apposed to the abdominal wall, a cannula is introduced percutaneously into the gastric lumen under direct endoscopic guidance (Figure 15.10).
3. This cannula serves as access to introduce a guide wire, which is then withdrawn out of the patient's mouth with the gastroscope (Figure 15.11). A tract is thus established.
4. A PEG catheter with a tapered end is attached to the oral end of the guide wire and pulled in a retrograde fashion until it assumes its final position, keeping the stomach firmly apposed to the abdominal wall (Figure 15.12).

Although there are multiple variations of the original PEG technique[1,24,28–32] and several types of catheters, one must be cautious, because most of these are not suitable for use in infants. We employ a 16F-gauge (or smaller) commercially available silicone rubber pediatric PEG catheter. Larger, stiffer catheters, or those with a stiff, noncollapsible inner retainer, can easily tear the infant's esophagus.

A single dose of an intravenous (i.v.) broad-spectrum antibiotic is administered at the outset. The child remains in the supine position throughout the procedure. The abdomen is cleansed and sterilely draped. Gastroscopy is performed with the smallest pediatric gastroscope available. The scope is inserted and advanced slowly into the stomach, at which point the light is seen through the left-upper-quadrant abdominal wall. With the gastroscope in place, insufflation distends the stomach, apposes it against the anterior abdominal wall, and displaces the colon downward. When the room lights are dimmed, the gastric contour is clearly visible, particularly in small children.

The preferred gastrostomy site is over the midportion of the left rectus muscle, as depicted in the inset of Figure 15.9. Digital pressure is exerted at this site, and this is seen by the endoscopist as a *polypoid lesion* or *mound* on the anterior gastric wall (gastric transillumination and endoscopically

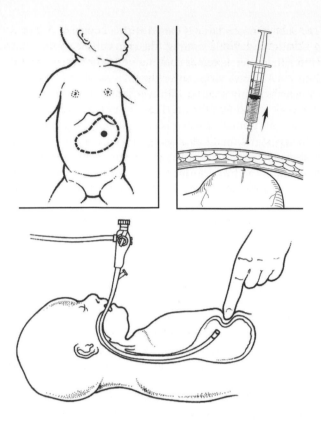

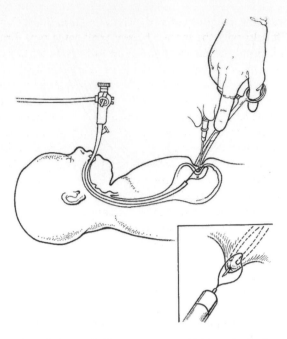

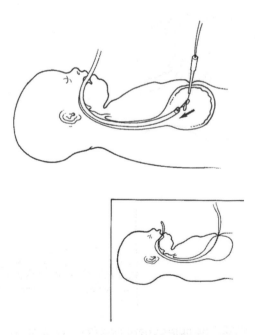

Figure 15.9 Percutaneous endoscopic gastrostomy (PEG). The air insufflated through the endoscope approximates the stomach to the abdominal wall and displaces the colon caudally. Digital pressure is applied to the proposed gastrostomy site, which usually corresponds to the area where transillumination is brightest. Transillumination and clear visualization of an anterior gastric wall indentation are key points. Without these, an open or laparoscopic technique should be employed. Long-lasting local anesthetic is drawn into a syringe and the proposed PEG site injected. The needle is advanced further, and continuous aspirating pressure is applied to the plunger. Air aspiration should only occur when the tip of the needle enters the gastric lumen. (From Gauderer M, Gastrostomy, in Spitz L and Coran AG, editors, *Operative Pediatric Surgery*, 6th ed., London: Hodder Arnold, 2006, 330–55.)

Figure 15.10 A small skin incision is made and a Kelly-type hemostat applied to maintain the intragastric indentation. The endoscopist places the polypectomy snare around the "mound"; the cannula is introduced between the slightly spread prongs of the hemostat and then thrust through the abdominal and gastric walls into the open snare. The snare is partially closed but not tightened around the cannula. (From Gauderer M, Gastrostomy, in Spitz L and Coran AG, editors, *Operative Pediatric Surgery*, 6th ed., London: Hodder Arnold, 2006, 330–55.)

Figure 15.11 The needle is removed and the guide wire inserted. The polypectomy snare grasps the guide and exits it through the mouth. An alternative to the polypectomy snare is an alligator or biopsy forceps. (From Gauderer M, Gastrostomy, in Spitz L and Coran AG, editors, *Operative Pediatric Surgery*, 6th ed., London: Hodder Arnold, 2006, 330–55.)

visualized digital indentation of the stomach are the most important factors in safe PEG placement). The endoscopist then places an endoscopic polypectomy snare around this invagination of the anterior gastric wall. Digital pressure is released, and a 0.5–0.7 cm skin incision is made. A hemostat with slightly opened prongs is placed in the incision, recreating and maintaining the intragastric mound (Figure 15.10). Through this incision and through the prongs of the hemostat, a 16-gauge, smoothly tapered, i.v. cannula and needle are thrust through abdominal and gastric walls under endoscopic visualization. This should be performed quickly to avoid displacing the stomach from the abdominal wall. The snare, if properly positioned initially, will be around the advancing cannula. If not, it can be maneuvered to encircle the cannula. A long, monofilament synthetic suture or a plastic-covered steel guide wire is then advanced through the cannula and grasped by the snare (Figure 15.11). If there is difficulty with the snare, a biopsy or alligator-type forceps may be used. As the gastroscope and snare are withdrawn, the suture is brought out of the patient's mouth (Figure 15.11, inset). The previously selected PEG catheter is then connected to the suture outside the patient's mouth, and both suture and catheter are coated with a water-soluble lubricant. Traction on the abdominal portion of the suture or guide wire pulls the catheter in a retrograde fashion, through the mouth, esophagus, and stomach, and across the abdominal wall (Figure 15.12). The gastroscope is reintroduced to verify the catheter position under direct vision. While re-endoscopy might theoretically be unnecessary, we believe it adds safety to the procedure.

Traction on the catheter is continued until the inner catheter retainer or "dome" loosely touches the gastric mucosa (Figure 15.12). Markings on the commercially available catheters, or markings added to tubes without marks, are helpful in indicating the final position of the tube. The external crossbar is then placed (Figure 15.12). Excessive pressure by the external crossbar on the abdominal wall will produce pressure necrosis and eventual catheter extrusion, and should be avoided. The tapered catheter end is cut off and a connector attached. Tape is used for temporary catheter immobilization. Although the tube can be used immediately, we have arbitrarily placed it to gravity drainage for the first 24 hours and instituted tube feedings the

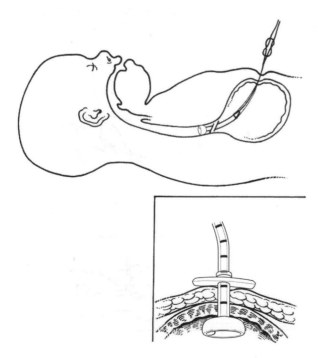

Figure 15.12 The appropriate-size PEG catheter is attached to the oral end of the guide wire and pulled in a retrograde manner through the infant's esophagus and stomach, and then across gastric and abdominal walls. The inset shows the position of the catheter at the end of the procedure. (From Gauderer M, Gastrostomy, in Spitz L and Coran AG, editors, *Operative Pediatric Surgery*, 6th ed., London: Hodder Arnold, 2006, 330–55.)

day after the procedure. The catheter may be converted to a skin-level device by using the external port valve at any time. To replace the PEG catheter with a button or balloon-type skin-level device, we find that it is prudent to wait until firm adhesions between the stomach and abdominal wall are established. This may take 1–3 months or longer.

Minimally invasive gastrostomies

The most recent development in pediatric gastrostomy technique was the introduction of pediatric LAP gastrostomy in the 1990s, combining the advantages of minimally invasive PEG placement with the safety of the open procedure.[7] Hereby, two variations have been reported, a LAP and a LA-PEG.[7,28,44–51]

Laparoscopically assisted gastrostomies

Direct visualization by a laparoscope expands the options for constructing a gastrostomy.[31–36,52] Several approaches have been described. In addition to the videoscopically controlled PEG, the two most common methods are adaptations of the Stamm technique and modifications of the push PEG.[49,51] Our preference is for the latter because in order to place a purse-string suture through the exposed segment of the anterior gastric wall, the trocar site must be sufficiently enlarged. This may predispose the site to leakage. To temporarily anchor the stomach to the abdominal wall, different approaches may be employed, notably T-fasteners and U-stitches. The most suitable site for the gastrostomy is selected in the left upper quadrant and marked. A nasogastric tube is inserted. Pneumoperitoneum is established in the child's size-appropriate manner, a trocar is placed at the umbilicus, and the laparoscope is introduced. A needle is pushed through the previously marked abdominal wall site, and the appropriate relation between the anterior gastric wall and the stoma site established. A small skin incision is made and a 5 mm trocar inserted. A grasper is introduced, and the gastrotomy site on the anterior gastric wall is lifted toward the parietal peritoneum (Figure 15.13). A U-stitch is passed through the abdominal wall, through the anterior gastric wall, and back out through the abdominal wall. A second U-stitch is passed parallel to the first one, 1–2 cm apart (Figure 15.13). The sutures are lifted, maintaining the stomach in contact with the abdominal wall. The grasper and the trocar are removed. The stomach is insufflated with air through the nasogastric tube, and a needle is inserted through the trocar site into the gastric lumen, between the two U-stitches. A Seldinger-type guide wire is passed through the needle into the stomach (Figure 15.14). The tract is dilated over the guide wire to the size required to insert either a Foley-type catheter or a balloon-type skin-level device. These are placed over the same guide wire. Stiffening of the catheter shaft with a thin metallic dilator is helpful. The previously placed U-stitches are tied over the wings of the button (Figure 15.15). If a long tube is placed, a pair of bolsters is employed. Care must be taken to avoid excessive tension.

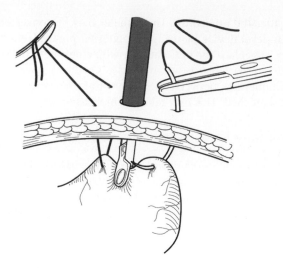

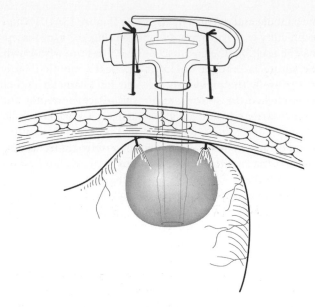

Figure 15.13 Laparoscopically assisted gastrostomy. Following the establishment of pneumoperitoneum and insertion of a trocar at the gastrostomy site, a grasper is introduced, and the appropriate portion of the anterior gastric wall is lifted. Two sutures are placed in the depicted manner. (From Gauderer M, Gastrostomy, in Spitz L and Coran AG, editors, *Operative Pediatric Surgery*, 6th ed., London: Hodder Arnold, 2006, 330–55.)

Figure 15.15 A balloon-type "button" has been placed. The previously placed U-stitches are tied over the "wings" of the skin-level device. (From Gauderer M, Gastrostomy, in Spitz L and Coran AG, editors, *Operative Pediatric Surgery*, 6th ed., London: Hodder Arnold, 2006, 330–55.)

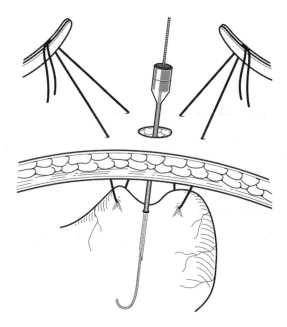

Figure 15.14 The stomach is insufflated with air through the nasogastric tube, and a needle is inserted through the trocar site into the gastric lumen, between the two U-stitches. A Seldinger-type guide wire is passed through the needle into the stomach. The tract is dilated over the guide wire to the size required to insert either a Foley-type catheter, a balloon-type skin-level device, or another low-profile access device. These are placed over the same guide wire. (From Gauderer M, Gastrostomy, in Spitz L and Coran AG, editors, *Operative Pediatric Surgery*, 6th ed., London: Hodder Arnold, 2006, 330–55.)

In the past decades, various working groups have variated and improved the LAP procedure, such as one- or two-trocar techniques or microinvasive strategies[42,44,45,50,53]: One-trocar aided gastrostomy has been shown to be feasible by Kawahara et al.[53] Patel and colleagues[45] developed a modified two-port LAP approach using the Seldinger technique with serial dilatation and tube insertion through a peel-away sheath for children with epidermolysis bullosa.

Turial et al.[50] introduced microlaparoscopic-assisted gastrostomy where a 1.7 or 1.9 mm 0-degree camera is inserted through the umbilicus and a 5 mm port is placed over the stomach at the designated site for the tube placement. The stomach is grasped and exteriorized and a gastrostomy opened, followed by a balloon gastrostomy tube placement.

Stitch technique has also been modified by several authors, e.g., replacement of single U-stitches with a continuous double U-stitch suture,[54] subcutaneous placement of absorbable stay sutures,[55] or laparoscopically placed sutures to secure the stomach to the abdominal wall.[56]

Laparoscopic-assisted percutaneous endoscopic approach

To achieve optimal visualization of the operation sites, LAP gastrostomy placement has been combined with the traditional PEG technique. Here as well, various working groups developed and adapted different operating strategies during the course of time.[49,57–60]

The gastroscope is placed within the stomach, and a port is introduced trough the umbilicus. Pneumoperitoneum is achieved depending on the patient's age. A camera is introduced into the peritoneal cavity, the ideal gastrostomy site, and a skin incision is made for the abdominal wall exit site. Under direct visualization by both gastroscope and laparoscope, T-fastener pexy sutures can be placed from the proposed gastrostomy site on the abdominal wall into the insufflated stomach. The next step is a needle placement at the center of the sutures from the abdominal incision into the stomach through which a guide wire is passed. Under visualization, an appropriate-size dilator–peel-away sheath is passed over this guide wire into the stomach followed by removal of both guide wire and dilator (Seldinger technique). Then an appropriate-size button is introduced through the peel-away sheath. The latter is removed, and the balloon is inflated with water (usually 3–5 mL). The pexy sutures are pulled outside and tied subcutaneously, leaving the gastrostomy button in the center of the sutures at the proposed gastrostomy button site. Inspection with both gastroscope and laparoscope ensures a proper gastrostomy tube placement. Gastroscope, camera, and port are removed, and the port site is closed with a dissolvable stitch after removal of the port and desufflation of the peritoneal cavity (technique adapted from Livingston et al.[49] and Hassan and Pimpalwar[59]).

In variation, two transabdominal incisions can be made for laparoscopic working instruments besides the umbilical port, and only three sutures may be placed around a proposed gastrostomy site.[60]

Other authors suggest to insert two U-stitches on a large needle through skin and abdominal wall into the gastric lumen and lead them back out again under endoscopic vision.[57] The needle and guide wire are placed between these two stitches, and subsequently, a dilatator and button are introduced. The U-sutures are then tied down over cotton bolsters to appose the stomach to the abdominal wall.[57]

SELECT COMPLICATIONS OF GASTROSTOMIES

Although frequently considered a "simple" procedure and often delegated to a junior member of the surgical team, a gastrostomy has considerable potential for early and late morbidity, particularly among neonates.

Complications related to operative technique

SEPARATION OF STOMACH FROM ABDOMINAL WALL

This serious mishap most commonly occurs after early gastrostomy tube reinsertion, before a firm adhesion between gastric and abdominal walls has occurred. However, it can also occur at any time thereafter. During the attempt to replace a dislodged catheter, the stomach is pushed away from the abdominal wall; that displacement leads to a partial or complete separation of the stoma. If recognition of the problem is delayed, severe peritonitis and death may result.[1–3,6,20,26] To avoid this and other mechanical problems, the stomach must be firmly anchored to the anterior abdominal wall and the catheter well secured to the skin, particularly with the open, Stamm-type techniques. In the event of early removal or dislodgement of the tube, the tract can be gently probed and a thin Foley catheter inserted. This must be followed by injection of a radio-opaque contrast material under fluoroscopy to assure an intragastric position of the tube and absence of intraperitoneal leakage. If there is any question about the position of the catheter, prompt exploration is necessary.

WOUND SEPARATION, DEHISCENCE, AND VENTRAL HERNIA

The aforementioned are usually the result of technical problems and carry high morbidity and mortality rates.[1,3,6] Leakage from an enlarged incision can be life threatening.[6] Such mishaps can be minimized by the use of appropriate, small incisions and by bringing the tube out through a counterincision. These complications will not occur after a PEG, or a LAP gastrostomy, because there is no laparotomy.

HEMORRHAGE

Major bleeding is described in pediatric series[3,5] and is usually related to inadequate hemostasis at the time of catheter insertion. Gentle traction on the catheter can control the bleeding, but reoperation may become necessary.[20]

INFECTION

This complication can occur with any type of gastrostomy.[1,5,6,20,26,61] Although usually limited to the skin and subcutaneous tissue, it can lead to full-thickness abdominal wall loss. Infections are less common following PEG placement or LAP gastrostomy and can usually be avoided through the use of prophylactic antibiotic administration and a skin incision only slightly larger than the diameter of the tube.

INJURY TO THE POSTERIOR WALL OF THE STOMACH

The posterior gastric wall can be damaged or perforated not only during the initial procedure[62] but also later during catheter change.[1] Once the tube is introduced, air or saline should be injected to test the tube's position and function.

INJURY TO OTHER ORGANS

During open procedures, damage to the liver and spleen can occur through the improper use of retractors or other instruments. The distended colon may be mistaken for the stomach, particularly in patients with intra-abdominal adhesions in whom mobility of intestinal loops is limited.

GASTROCOLIC FISTULA

Although it can occur with any gastrostomy, this complication is more likely with the percutaneous endoscopic techniques.[1] With proper technique, however, this problem should be rare. During the PEG procedure, the importance of appropriate gastric insufflation with downward colonic displacement, transillumination, and the indentation on the anterior abdominal wall cannot be overemphasized. On the other hand, overinflation must be avoided because it can distort the local anatomy, including the position of the colon. Additionally, air-filled small bowel loops will displace the colon cranially and move it between the stomach and the abdominal wall.

Complications related to care of stoma

SKIN IRRITATION AND MONILIASIS

Next to granulation tissue, these are the most frequent problems encountered. Usually related to leakage, and compounded by occlusive dressings, irritation is best prevented by avoiding any occlusive devices, including nipples, tape, or gauze pads.[1] The site should be kept open and dry at all times. Ointments and other solutions, except for the treatment of moniliasis, should be avoided. Catheters, if kept long, can be immobilized with a small external crossbar.

TUBE PLUGGING

Catheters must be flushed with water after each feeding to prevent blockage. In neonates the amount should be small and added to the fluid intake.

ADMINISTRATION OF IMPROPER FEEDINGS

Careful and slow administration of the appropriate nutrient prevents metabolic abnormalities as well as diarrhea and excessive reflux.

DELAY IN THE REINTRODUCTION OF A DISLODGED CATHETER

Accidental dislodgement of long gastrostomy catheter is fairly common. The catheter must be replaced before the tract closes, which can be in a few hours unless it is well matured and epithelium lined. Careful dilation of the tract is usually successful.

In gastrostomy skin-level devices with jejunal extension, dislodgment of the tube from the jejunum back into the stomach can occur, which usually requires radiologic (fluoroscopy) or endoscopic guided repositioning.

TRAUMA DURING REINSERTION OF CATHETER

Improper catheter reintroduction can lead to damage to the pancreas, liver, or spleen, particularly if long stylets or other traumatic instruments are used to elongate a mushroom-type tip. Small children are more prone to this complication, given the short distance of these organs from the abdominal wall. Gentle insertion and aiming toward the gastric cardia or fundus is the method least likely to project injury.

Complications related to catheters

GRANULATION TISSUE

This is by far the most frequent problem associated with gastrostomies. Usually, granulation tissue formation is mild, and a few applications of silver nitrate are curative. If this condition is neglected, however, granulation tissue will predispose to leakage, bleeding, and chronic discharge. With excessive growth, excision and cauterization become necessary. Granulation tissue formation will cease once epithelialization of the tract has occurred. We have found that a cream combining an antifungal and a steroid preparation helps to minimize the formation of this abnormal tissue.

LEAKAGE

Severe continuous leakage is uncommon in properly constructed gastrostomies.[1,6] However, severe widening of the stoma can lead to skin excoriation, dislodgment of the tube, metabolic imbalance, and even death.[1,6] the main cause of leakage in most children is enlargement of the stoma by the pivoting motion of the gastrostomy tube, which is often too large or too stiff.[1] Catheters brought through the incision or the thinner midline are more prone to this problem. Management of leakage begins with control of granulation tissue and placement of a smaller, softer catheter to avoid pivoting motion. A variety of other methods have been tried with varying degrees of success.[1] In extreme cases, reoperation or stoma relocation becomes necessary.

INTERNAL MIGRATION

Distal migration of a long catheter producing high intestinal obstruction is a well-known problem.[1,6] It can occur with any gastric tube but is particularly common with long, balloon-type catheters.

EXTERNAL MIGRATION

Overzealous approximation of external immobilizing devices, such as the bumper, can lead to embedding of the inner crossbar of the PEG catheter, mushroom tip, or balloon in the gastric and abdominal wall.[1] The resulting so-called buried bumper syndrome (BBS) is defined as the migration of the internal fixation device (bumper) of the PEG tube alongside the stoma tract out of the stomach over a variable distance with complete or partial loss of tract patency between the stomach and the PEG tube tip.[16,63] The bumper can end up anywhere between the stomach mucosa and the skin surface, which is typical for rigid or semirigid internal immobilization devices.[63]

The usual presentations are malfunction with limited flow, leakage, lack of to-and-fro motion of the catheter, and the formation of an abscess. The catheter should be removed and replaced. This problem can be avoided by giving the catheter enough "play," i.e., a little to-and-fro motion.

However, BBS is quite rare in neonates due to their thin abdominal wall. Since the development of skin-level devices such as buttons, problems with BBS decreased markedly.

PERFORATION OF ESOPHAGUS AND SMALL BOWEL

The balloon of a Foley-type catheter can be accidentally inflated in the esophagus[64] or small bowel,[65] leading to wall disruption.

PERSISTENT GASTROCUTANEOUS FISTULA

In the longstanding gastrostomy, an epithelium-lined channel will form. Although most stomas close spontaneously after a few days, excision of the tract with simple closure is indicated if drainage persists after several weeks.[1]

Prevention

As outlined in the previous segment, a long list of complications is recorded, which can be particularly dangerous in the newborn age group. Most of the common gastrostomy care–related problems can be prevented with meticulous attention to detail during placement and subsequent follow-up.[26] The use of skin-level devices such as the original gastrostomy button,[1] the balloon-type versions, or the externally placed port valve has dramatically decreased the most common problems associated with older, long tubes. Many techniques, whether open, endoscopic, or laparoscopically aided, now permit the initial placement of one of these well-tolerated skin-level devices (Figures 15.16 and 15.17). Jejunostomy and gastrojejunal tubes are even more prone to complications, as outlined in the previous

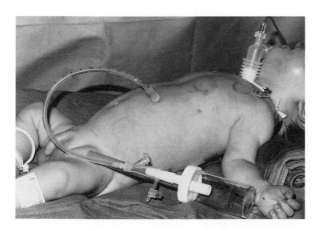

Figure 15.16 Completed percutaneous endoscopic gastrostomy and tracheostomy in a 4-month-old child, weighing 3.5 kg, with poor swallowing and severe bronchopulmonary dysplasia. The child was born prematurely at 29 weeks' gestation and was hospitalized following an eventful neonatal course. Sutures are not used after the PEG, and the catheter is connected to a small clear plastic trap. After 24 hours, the external crossbar is checked and loosened, if necessary, to accommodate for wound edema. Feedings are then started. Notice the tracheal traction sutures used as safety measures with the child's tracheostomy and the scar of a previously repaired inguinal hernia. (From Ferguson DR et al., Placement of a feeding button ("one-step button") as the initial procedure, *Am J Gastroenterol*, 1993;88:501–04.)

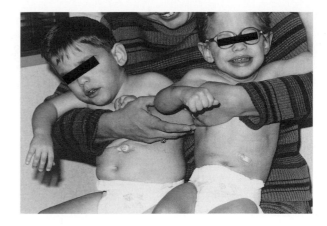

Figure 15.17 Two former premature infants with complex neonatal courses. Both receive supplemental feedings and medication via the gastrostomy. The child on the left has a balloon-type skin-level device, and the one on the right has an original, low-profile gastrostomy button.

segment. A gastrojejunal button that is too big may cause pyloric obstruction in smaller children.[8]

CONCLUSION

Although gastrostomy is a basic and fairly simple procedure, the surgeon must carefully consider the advantages versus disadvantages when using it in conjunction with another major intervention in the newborn. So far, jejunostomies play only a minor role for nutritional access in neonates and infants. If the gastrostomy is used for long-term enteral feeding, careful consideration must be given not only to the often difficult ethical problems encountered in some neonatal patients, but also to the duration of these enteral feedings, potential complications, and the problem of gastroesophageal reflux. These children benefit from a team approach, including the neonatologist, pediatric surgeon, pediatric gastroenterologist, primary nurse, and nutritionist. It is also paramount that the parents or caregivers be an integral part of the decision-making process at the different stages of management. Long-term follow-up is essential, and its importance cannot be overemphasized. Whether the gastrostomy is placed as an adjunct or for the prime purpose of feeding, every effort should be directed toward resuming oral feeding whenever possible.

REFERENCES

1. Gauderer MW, Stellato TA. Gastrostomies: Evolution, techniques, indications, and complications. *Curr Probl Surg* 1986; 23: 657–719.
2. Meeker IA, Snyder WH. Gastrostomy for the newborn surgical patient: A report of 140 cases. *Arch Dis Child* 1962; 37: 159–66.
3. Meier H, Willital GH. Gastrostomy in the newborn—Indication, technique, complications (author's transl). *Z Kinderchir* 1981; 34: 82–6.

4. Srinivasan R, Irvine T, Dalzell M. Indications for percutaneous endoscopic gastrostomy and procedure-related outcome. *J Pediatr Gastroenterol Nutr* 2009; 49: 584–8.

5. Vengusamy S, Pildes RS, Raffensperger JF, Levine HD, Cornblath M. A controlled study of feeding gastrostomy in low birth weight infants. *Pediatrics* 1969; 43: 815–20.

6. Haws EB, Sieber WK, Kiesewetter WB. Complications of tube gastrostomy in infants and children. 15-year review of 240 cases. *Ann Surg* 1966; 164:284–90.

7. Baker L, Beres AL, Baird R. A systematic review and meta-analysis of gastrostomy insertion techniques in children. *J Pediatr Surg* 2015; 50: 718–25.

8. Vermilyea S, Goh VL. Enteral feedings in children: Sorting out tubes, buttons, and formulas. *Nutr Clin Pract* 2016; 31: 59–67.

9. Louhimo I, Lindahl H. Esophageal atresia: Primary results of 500 consecutively treated patients. *J Pediatr Surg* 1983; 18: 217–29.

10. Spitz L, Kiely E, Brereton RJ. Esophageal atresia: Five year experience with 148 cases. *J Pediatr Surg* 1987; 22: 103–8.

11. Coln D. Simultaneous drainage gastrostomy and feeding jejunostomy in the newborn. *Surg Gynecol Obstet* 1977; 145: 594–95.

12. Barnhart DC. Gastroesophageal reflux disease in children. *Semin Pediatr Surg* 2016; 25: 212–18.

13. Kakade M, Coyle D, McDowell DT, Gillick J. Percutaneous endoscopic gastrostomy (PEG) does not worsen vomiting in children. *Pediatr Surg Int* 2015; 31: 557–62.

14. Gantasala S, Sullivan PB, Thomas AG. Gastrostomy feeding versus oral feeding alone for children with cerebral palsy. *Cochrane Database Syst Rev* 2013: CD003943.

15. Chatwin M, Bush A, Macrae DJ, Clarke SA, Simonds AK. Risk management protocol for gastrostomy and jejunostomy insertion in ventilator dependent infants. *Neuromuscul Disord* 2013; 23: 289–97.

16. Liu R, Jiwane A, Varjavandi A, Kennedy A, Henry G, Dilley A et al. Comparison of percutaneous endoscopic, laparoscopic and open gastrostomy insertion in children. *Pediatr Surg Int* 2013; 29: 613–21.

17. Landisch RM, Colwell RC, Densmore JC. Infant gastrostomy outcomes: The cost of complications. *J Pediatr Surg* 2016; 51: 1976–82

18. Adams SD, Baker D, Takhar A, Beattie RM, Stanton MP. Complication of percutaneous endoscopic gastrostomy. *Arch Dis Child* 2014; 99: 788.

19. Naiditch JA, Lautz T, Barsness KA. Postoperative complications in children undergoing gastrostomy tube placement. *J Laparoendosc Adv Surg Tech A* 2010; 20: 781–5.

20. Friedman JN, Ahmed S, Connolly B, Chait P, Mahant S. Complications associated with image-guided gastrostomy and gastrojejunostomy tubes in children. *Pediatrics* 2004; 114: 458–61.

21. Campwala I, Perrone E, Yanni G, Shah M, Gollin G. Complications of gastrojejunal feeding tubes in children. *J Surg Res* 2015; 199: 67–71.

22. Axelrod D, Kazmerski K, Iyer K. Pediatric enteral nutrition. *JPEN J Parenter Enteral Nutr* 2006; 30: S21–6.

23. Gauderer M. Gastrostomy. In: Spitz L, Coran AG, (eds). *Operative Pediatric Surgery*, 6th edn. London: Hodder Arnold, 2006: 330–55.

24. Gauderer MW, Ponsky JL, Izant RJ, JR. Gastrostomy without laparotomy: A percutaneous endoscopic technique. *J Pediatr Surg* 1980; 15: 872–5.

25. Lalanne A, Gottrand F, Salleron J, Puybasset-Jonquez AL, Guimber D, Turck D et al. Long-term outcome of children receiving percutaneous endoscopic gastrostomy feeding. *J Pediatr Gastroenterol Nutr* 2014; 59: 172–6.

26. Beres A, Bratu I, Laberge J-M. Attention to small details: Big deal for gastrostomies. *Semin Pediatr Surg* 2009; 18: 87–92.

27. Wilson L, Oliva-Hemker M. Percutaneous endoscopic gastrostomy in small medically complex infants. *Endoscopy* 2001; 33: 433–6.

28. Stringel G, Geller ER, Lowenheim MS. Laparoscopic-assisted percutaneous endoscopic gastrostomy. *J Pediatr Surg* 1995; 30: 1209–10.

29. Croaker GD, Najmaldin AS. Laparoscopically assisted percutaneous endoscopic gastrostomy. *Pediatr Surg Int* 1997; 12: 130–1.

30. Ferguson DR, Harig JM, Kozarek RA, Kelsey PB, Picha GJ. Placement of a feeding button ("one-step button") as the initial procedure. *Am J Gastroenterol* 1993; 88: 501–4.

31. Novotny NM, Vegeler RC, Breckler FD, Rescorla FJ. Percutaneous endoscopic gastrostomy buttons in children: Superior to tubes. *J Pediatr Surg* 2009; 44: 1193–6.

32. Robertson FM, Crombleholme TM, La Latchaw, Jacir NN. Modification of the "push" technique for percutaneous endoscopic gastrostomy in infants and children. *J Am Coll Surg* 1996; 182: 215–8.

33. Am Cahill, Kaye RD, Fitz CR, Towbin RB. "Push–pull" gastrostomy: A new technique for percutaneous gastrostomy tube insertion in the neonate and young infant. *Pediatr Radiol* 2001; 31: 550–4.

34. Aziz D, Chait P, Kreichman F, Langer JC. Image-guided percutaneous gastrostomy in neonates with esophageal atresia. *J Pediatr Surg* 2004; 39: 1648–50.

35. Chait PG, Weinberg J, Connolly BL, Pencharz P, Richards H, Clift JE et al. Retrograde percutaneous gastrostomy and gastrojejunostomy in 505 children: A 4 1/2-year experience. *Radiology* 1996; 201: 691–5.

36. Humphrey GM, Najmaldin A. Laparoscopic gastrostomy in children. *Pediatr Surg Int* 1997; 12: 501–4.

37. Jones VS, La Hei ER, Shun A. Laparoscopic gastrostomy: The preferred method of gastrostomy in children. *Pediatr Surg Int* 2007; 23: 1085–9.

38. Rothenberg SS, Bealer JF, Chang JH. Primary laparoscopic placement of gastrostomy buttons for feeding tubes. A safer and simpler technique. *Surg Endosc* 1999; 13: 995–7.

39. Merli L, Marco EA de, Fedele C, Mason EJ, Taddei A, Paradiso FV et al. Gastrostomy placement in children: Percutaneous endoscopic gastrostomy or laparoscopic gastrostomy? *Surg Laparosc Endosc Percutan Tech* 2016; 26: 381–4.

40. Franken J, Mauritz FA, Suksamanapun N, Hulsker CCC, van der Zee DC, van Herwaarden-Lindeboom MYA. Efficacy and adverse events of laparoscopic gastrostomy placement in children: Results of a large cohort study. *Surg Endosc* 2015; 29: 1545–52.

41. Petrosyan M, Am Khalafallah, Franklin AL, Doan T, Kane TD. Laparoscopic gastrostomy is superior to percutaneous endoscopic gastrostomy tube placement in children less than 5 years of age. *J Laparoendosc Adv Surg Tech A* 2016; 26: 570–3.

42. Akay B, Capizzani TR, Am Lee, Drongowski RA, Geiger JD, Hirschl RB et al. Gastrostomy tube placement in infants and children: Is there a preferred technique? *J Pediatr Surg* 2010; 45: 1147–52.

43. Gauderer MW. Experience with a hybrid, minimally invasive gastrostomy for children with abnormal epigastric anatomy. *J Pediatr Surg* 2008; 43: 2178–81.

44. Baker L, Emil S, Baird R. A comparison of techniques for laparoscopic gastrostomy placement in children. *J Surg Res* 2013; 184: 392–6.

45. Patel K, Wells J, Jones R, Browne F, Moss C, Parikh D. Use of a novel laparoscopic gastrostomy technique in children with severe epidermolysis bullosa. *J Pediatr Gastroenterol Nutr* 2014; 58: 621–3.

46. Am Thaker, Sedarat A. Laparoscopic-assisted percutaneous endoscopic gastrostomy. *Curr Gastroenterol Rep* 2016; 18: 46.

47. Zamakhshary M, Jamal M, Blair GK, Murphy JJ, Webber EM, Skarsgard ED. Laparoscopic vs percutaneous endoscopic gastrostomy tube insertion: A new pediatric gold standard? *J Pediatr Surg* 2005; 40: 859–62.

48. Georgeson KE. Laparoscopic fundoplication and gastrostomy. *Semin Laparosc Surg* 1998; 5: 25–30.

49. Livingston MH, Pepe D, Jones S, Butter A, Merritt NH. Laparoscopic-assisted percutaneous endoscopic gastrostomy: Insertion of a skin-level device using a tear-away sheath. *Can J Surg* 2015; 58: 264–68.

50. Turial S, Schwind M, Engel V, Kohl M, Goldinger B, Schier F. Microlaparoscopic-assisted gastrostomy in children: Early experiences with our technique. *J Laparoendosc Adv Surg Tech A* 2009; 19 Suppl 1: S229–31.

51. Vasseur MS, Reinberg O. Laparoscopic technique to perform a true Stamm gastrostomy in children. *J Pediatr Surg* 2015; 50: 1797–800.

52. Georgeson KE. Laparoscopic gastrostomy and fundoplication. *Pediatr Ann* 1993; 22: 675–7.

53. Kawahara H, Kubota A, Okuyama H, Shimizu Y, Watanabe T, Tani G et al. One-trocar laparoscopy-aided gastrostomy in handicapped children. *J Pediatr Surg* 2006; 41: 2076–80.

54. Backman T, Sjovie H, Kullendorff C-M, Arnbjornsson E. Continuous double U-stitch gastrostomy in children. *Eur J Pediatr Surg* 2010; 20: 14–7.

55. Antonoff MB, Hess DJ, Saltzman DA, Acton RD. Modified approach to laparoscopic gastrostomy tube placement minimizes complications. *Pediatr Surg Int* 2009; 25: 349–53.

56. Villalona GA, Mckee MA, Diefenbach KA. Modified laparoscopic gastrostomy technique reduces gastrostomy tract dehiscence. *J Laparoendosc Adv Surg Tech A* 2011; 21: 355–9.

57. Nixdorff N, Diluciano J, Ponsky T, Chwals W, Parry R, Boulanger S. The endoscopic U-stitch technique for primary button placement: An institution's experience. *Surg Endosc* 2010; 24: 1200–3.

58. Idowu O, Driggs XA, Kim S. Laparoscopically assisted antegrade percutaneous endoscopic gastrostomy. *J Pediatr Surg* 2010; 45: 277–9.

59. Hassan SF, Pimpalwar AP. Modified laparoendoscopic gastrostomy tube (LEGT) placement. *Pediatr Surg Int* 2011; 27: 1249–54.

60. Smitherman S, Pimpalwar A. Laparoendoscopic gastrostomy tube placement: Our all-in-one technique. *J Laparoendosc Adv Surg Tech A* 2009; 19: 119–23.

61. Goldin AB, Heiss KF, Hall M, Rothstein DH, Minneci PC, Blakely ML et al. Emergency department visits and readmissions among children after gastrostomy tube placement. *J Pediatr* 2016; 174: 139–145.e2.

62. Tomicic JT, Luks FI, Shalon L, Tracy TF. Laparoscopic gastrostomy in infants and children. *Eur J Pediatr Surg* 2002; 12: 107–10.

63. Cyrany J, Rejchrt S, Kopacova M, Bures J. Buried bumper syndrome: A complication of percutaneous endoscopic gastrostomy. *World J Gastroenterol* 2016; 22: 618–27.

64. Abrams LD, Kiely EM. Oesophageal rupture due to gastrostomy catheter. *Z Kinderchir* 1981; 33: 274–5.

65. Ballinger W2, McLaughlin ED, Baranski EJ. Jejunal overlay closure of duodenum in the newborn: Lateral duodenal tear caused by gastrostomy tube. *Surgery* 1966; 59: 450–4.

16

Stomas of small and large intestine

ANDREA BISCHOFF AND ALBERTO PEÑA

INTRODUCTION

The creation of an intestinal stoma is an operation frequently performed in pediatric surgery, especially for cases of anorectal malformations and necrotizing enterocolitis, and frequently indicated for Hirschsprung disease. Its purpose is to divert the fecal stream for different reasons. The diversion can be total (separated stomas) or partial (loop colostomies).

In the management of anorectal malformations, the goal of a colostomy is slightly different. The colostomy must decompress the gastrointestinal tract but must be totally diverting to avoid fecal contamination of the urinary tract, since over 85% of the patients with an anorectal malformation have a distal communication with the urogenital tract. In order to achieve these goals, we recommend a colostomy located in the left lower quadrant of the abdominal wall, with separated stomas (Figure 16.1). The proximal stoma is created using the lowest portion of the descending colon, taking advantage of its attachments to the posterior and lateral abdominal wall, which helps to avoid prolapse. The colostomy must be created leaving enough distal colon (sigmoid) for the future pull-through. The proximal stoma should be matured and located in the center of a triangle formed by the last left rib, the umbilicus, and the iliac crest, in order to allow a colostomy bag to be adapted to a flat surface of the abdomen. The distal stoma must be separated enough from the proximal one to be sure that it is possible to adapt a stoma bag onto it, without overlying the mucous fistula. In addition, the mucous fistula should be made very small and flat (Figures 16.1 and 16.2), since it is only used for irrigation and injection of contrast material to define the anatomy of the malformation prior to the main repair.[1] This maneuver helps to avoid prolapse of this distal mobile segment of the sigmoid.

An important step during the creation of a colostomy consists in irrigating, with saline solution, the distal portion of the bowel until it is completely clean of meconium.

Leaving meconium distally can result in infection and contamination of the urinary tract.

Due to the fact that we work at a pediatric colorectal referral center, we frequently receive patients born with an anorectal malformation who had a colostomy done elsewhere, at birth, and were referred to us thereafter for definitive reconstruction.[2] Because of this, we have been exposed to a great variety of colostomies. This has allowed us to learn about the advantages and disadvantages of the different types, the most common complications, and how to deal with them, and to describe strategies to avoid them.

MOST COMMON ERRORS

Stoma mislocation

This type of error may occur in different ways:

1. *Proximal and distal stomas placed too close to each other.* When this happens, the colostomy bag covers both stomas and allows for passage of stool from the proximal to the distal colon. As a consequence, some patients suffer from recurrent urinary tract infections. Also, the stoma bag may be difficult to adapt to the skin. The management of this problem can include (1) performing the main repair earlier than anticipated and (2) revising the stomas by separating them.

   The decision will depend on the specific clinical circumstances. If the surgeon decides to perform the main repair earlier than anticipated, he/she must keep in mind that there is a possibility that the patient may pass stool through a reconstructed area, which may increase the risk of infection. To avoid that, the surgeon may (a) clean the entire gastrointestinal tract preoperatively and then keep the patient fasting for a period of time (about a week) receiving parenteral nutrition or (b) use a purse-string, long-term absorbable suture in the distal

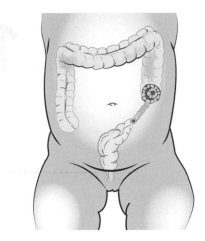

Figure 16.1 Descending colostomy, with mucous fistula.

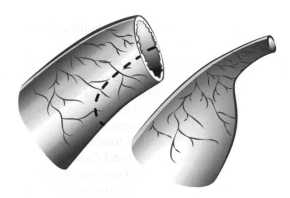

Figure 16.2 Distal stoma made tiny and flat to help avoid prolapse.

stoma to occlude its lumen temporarily and avoid the distal passage of fecal material postoperatively.

2. *Colostomy created too distal in the sigmoid, not allowing enough distal length for the rectal pull-through* (Figure 16.3). In this case the surgeon has several options. The first is to perform the pull-through, taking

down the distal stoma (mucous fistula) and closing it as a Hartman pouch. Sometimes the piece of bowel is so short that it will make a very difficult future colostomy closure, since the anastomosis will have to be done deep down in the pelvis, behind the bladder. The second option is to close the colostomy at the time of the main repair and then pull down the rectum, leaving the patient without the benefit of a protective colostomy. For that, we recommend cleaning the entire gastrointestinal tract preoperatively and leaving the patient fasting 7–10 days, receiving parenteral nutrition. The third option is to close the colostomy, pull the rectum down, and create a proximal new colostomy to divert the stool and protect the perineum.

It is vital to try to save the distal rectum, and avoid discarding it and pulling through the proximal stoma. This is particularly important in patients with anorectal malformation. The resection of the rectum means the removal of the natural human fecal reservoir; this results in having frequent bowel movements and sometimes, tendency to diarrhea. All this seriously interferes with the toilet training process; patients with potential for bowel control will suffer from fecal incontinence.

3. *Inverted stomas* (Figure 16.4). The functional (proximal stoma) is inadvertently placed in the location of the mucous fistula and vice versa. An additional problem occurs because the surgeon mistakenly tapers the proximal bowel, assuming that it is the mucous fistula, which may provoke an obstruction. This complication may require a reoperation. Furthermore, since the stomas are inverted, the mucous fistula (distal stoma) is erroneously placed in the location of the proximal stoma, (high in the abdomen), which will interfere with the pull-through.

4. *Sigmoid colostomy in the upper abdomen* (Figure 16.5). In this case the surgeon planned to do a transverse colostomy. Consequently, he/she made an incision in the upper abdomen, found a piece of colon and brought it out as a colostomy believing it was the transverse colon. Instead a sigmoidostomy was inadvertently opened in

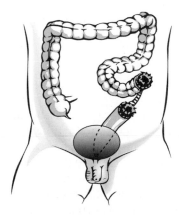

Figure 16.3 Colostomy placed too distal with not enough distal bowel for the pull-through.

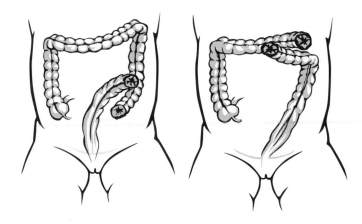

Figure 16.4 Inverted stomas.

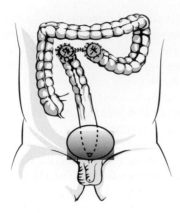

Figure 16.5 Right upper sigmoidostomy instead of a right transverse colostomy.

the upper abdomen, which then can interfere with the pull-through. When opening a transverse colostomy, the surgeon must remember that newborns have a very dilated and mobile sigmoid colon that can reach the diaphragm. When this error is detected, prior to the pull-through, the colostomy must be moved to the lower abdomen.

The diagnosis of a mislocated colostomy is best determined by a distal colostogram, which is a routine study done prior to the main repair of an anorectal malformation.

Prolapse

The second most common complication observed in colostomies is prolapse. This can be a serious complication that can result in intestinal loss due to ischemia. We believe that most prolapses can be avoided by creating the colostomy adjacent to a fixed portion of the colon. If the colostomy has to be created in a mobile portion of the bowel, we recommend that it be fixed to the anterior abdominal wall, approximately 6–7 cm proximal to the stoma. In Figure 16.6, one can identify the mobile and fixed portions of a normally rotated colon, and understand the segments

that are prone to prolapse and will need fixation to the abdominal wall.

When a patient presents to us with significant prolapse, we recommend a surgical repair. Our technique consists in inserting a large amount of packing gauze soaked in povidone–iodine in the prolapsed bowel, gently reducing the prolapse. Then the abdomen is palpated, feeling for the mass that corresponds to the packing gauze inside the bowel, naturally oriented inside the abdomen. A transverse incision is then made on top of the palpated mass, usually about 5 cm away from the stoma, opening skin, subcutaneous tissue, muscle, aponeurosis, and peritoneum. The bowel full of gauze is easily identified. The peritoneum and aponeurosis are closed with interrupted long-term absorbable stitches, including in each stitch a bite of the bowel wall (without taking the packing gauze), securing it to the abdominal wall, which helps to avoid future prolapse. When using this technique, the stoma does not need to be touched.

Stenosis

This happens more often than doctors suspect, and patients may suffer from obstructive symptoms. When opening a stoma, we specifically recommend creating an adequate space to pass through the functional bowel, without being compressed by the fascia. In other words, we specifically avoid creating stomas through a simple stab wound. We resect a circle of skin, as well as a circle of aponeurosis, muscle, and peritoneum. Most cases of stoma stenosis do not respond to dilations and need reoperation.

Retraction

This complication is a result of a technical mistake and therefore a preventable problem. An acute, early retraction can be a surgical emergency. A late retraction may represent a serious difficulty in managing the stoma, since it will be hard to adapt the stoma bag. Reoperation with mobilization of the stoma higher above the skin surface is required.

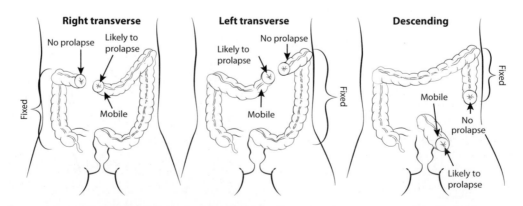

Figure 16.6 Right transverse colostomy (distal stoma likely to prolapse), left transverse colostomy (proximal stoma likely to prolapse), descending colostomy (distal stoma likely to prolapse).

STOMAS IN CLOACAL EXSTROPHY

A special comment should be made about stomas in patients born with cloacal exstrophy.[3,4] A common misconception is that these patients have a short and therefore useless colon. As a consequence, many surgeons perform an ileostomy at birth, leaving the colon distally attached to the urinary tract or simply discarding it. However, the colon is extremely valuable for these patients, allowing them to form solid stool and making them future candidates for a colonic pull-through.[4] It is very important to incorporate every single piece of colon into the fecal stream, regardless of how small it is. In other words, these patients must receive a real end colostomy. Over time, those small pieces of bowel grow considerably. Another advantage of incorporating colon in the fecal stream is that those patients become easier to manage than a patient having an ileostomy. We have reoperated on patients initially managed in other institutions, in order to incorporate a piece of colon that was left distally defunctionalized. We call that procedure "rescue operation," and it consists in closing the ileostomy, separating the colon from the urinary tract, and creating a real end colostomy.[5]

Leaving a piece of colon distally attached to the urinary tract may produce severe hyperchloremic acidosis as a consequence of absorption of urine.

ILEOSTOMIES

Another special comment should be made about ileostomies, a common procedure done for total colonic aganglionosis[6] and necrotizing enterocolitis. Since by definition, the ileostomy will always be made in a mobile portion of the intestine, the risk of prolapse is very high; therefore, we recommend fixing the bowel to the anterior abdominal wall, approximately 6–7 cm proximal to the stoma. All the other complications described for colostomy apply for ileostomies. Other particular issues associated with ileostomy include managing the possible electrolyte disturbances. Patients need to maintain good hydration, and parents need to be keen observers of stoma output. These patients tend to have significant sodium losses and may need oral sodium supplementation.

COLOSTOMY CLOSURE

Colostomy closure in the pediatric population is also associated with a high morbidity rate due to potential avoidable complications such as anastomotic dehiscence, stricture, wound infection, bleeding, and death.[7–23]

Our perioperative protocol for colostomy closure[23] consists in (1) admission on the day before surgery; (2) clear liquids by mouth; (3) repeat proximal stoma irrigations with saline solution 24 hours prior to the operation; (4) administration of intravenous (IV) antibiotics during anesthesia induction and continued for 48 hours; and (5) meticulous surgical technique that includes the following:

1. Packing of the proximal stoma
2. Plastic drape to immobilize the surgical field
3. Multiple silk sutures in the mucocutaneous junction of the stomas to provide uniform traction that allows the surgeon to identify the correct dissection plane, remaining as close as possible to the bowel wall (Figure 16.7)
4. Careful hemostasis
5. Emphasis in avoiding contamination
6. Cleaning the edge of the stomas to allow a precise anastomosis (Figure 16.8)
7. A two-layer, end-to-end anastomosis with separated long-term 6-0 absorbable sutures (Figure 16.9)
8. Generous irrigation of the peritoneal cavity and subsequent layers of the abdominal wall, with saline solution
9. Closure by layers to avoid dead spaces and hematomas
10. Wound coverage with Dermabond (Figure 16.10)

In postoperative care, no nasogastric tubes are used, and the patients receive clear fluids on the first postoperative day, if they are not distended or nauseated. Most of the patients can be discharged home on the second or third day following the operation.

When the size discrepancy between proximal and distal stoma is more than 5:1, with the distal stoma diameter being less than 1 cm, the colostomy closure can present a serious

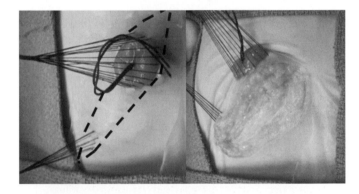

Figure 16.7 Multiple silk sutures in the mucocutaneous junction, which allow for a uniform traction. The dotted line shows the elliptical incision. The opening is performed layer by layer.

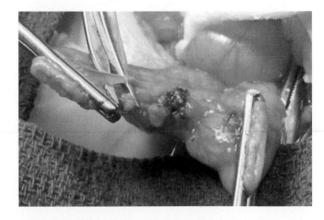

Figure 16.8 Cleaning the edges of the stomas, preparing for the anastomosis.

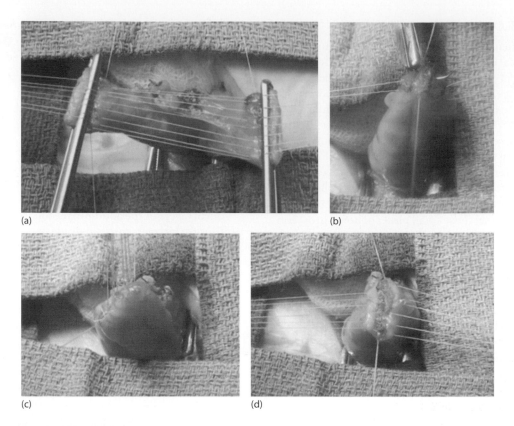

(a)

(b)

(c)

(d)

Figure 16.9 Two-layer anastomosis: **(a)** external layer of posterior wall, **(b)** internal layer of posterior wall **(c)** internal layer of anterior wall, and **(d)** external layer of anterior wall.

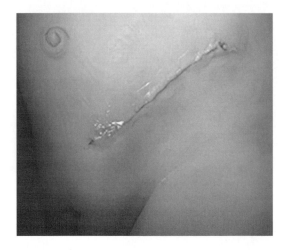

Figure 16.10 Closed wound, covered with Dermabond.

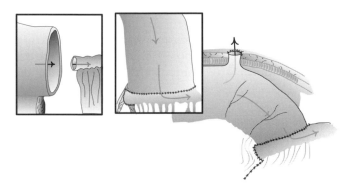

Figure 16.11 End-to-side anastomosis for size discrepancy greater than 5:1. Window-type stoma created about 5–10 cm proximal to the anastomosis.

technical challenge; for that, we use the same technique that we have used for cases of colonic atresia. The technique consists in performing an end-to-side anastomosis plus a window-type stoma created about 5–10 cm proximal to the anastomosis (Figure 16.11). During the first few postoperative days, one can see a large fecal output through the window; eventually, the output decreases, and the amount of stool passing through the downstream bowel increases, until the window closes up, the anastomosis is efficient, and the microcolon gradually grows.

REFERENCES

1. Gross GW, Woflson PJ, Peña A. Augmented-pressure colostogram in imperforate anus with fistula. *Pediatr Radiol* 1991; 21(8): 560–2.
2. Peña A, Migotto-Krieger M, Levitt MA. Colostomy in anorectal malformations: A procedure with serious but preventable complications. *J Pediatr Surg* 2006; 41: 748–56.
3. Soffer SZ, Rosen NG, Hong AR et al. Cloacal exstrophy: A unified management plan. *J Pediatr Surg* 2000; 35(6): 932–7.

4. Levitt MA, Mak GA, Falcone RA, Peña A: Cloacal exstrophy—Pull through or permanent stoma? A review of 53 patients. *J Pediatr Surg* 2008; 43(1): 164–70.

5. Bischoff A, Brisighelli G, Levitt MA, Pema A. The "rescue operation" for patients with cleacal exstrophy and its variants. *Pediatr Sung Imt* 2014; 30: 723–7.

6. Bischoff A, Levitt MA, Peña A. Total colonic aganglionosis: A surgical challenge. How to avoid complications? *Pediatr Surg Int* 2011; 27(10): 1047–52.

7. Kiely EM, Sparnon AL. Stoma closure in infants and children. *Pediatr Surg Int* 1987; 2: 95–7.

8. Millar AJK, Lakhoo K, Rode H et al. Bowel stomas in infants and children. A 5 year audit of 203 patients. *S Afr J Chir* 1993; 3: 110–3.

9. Rees BI, Thomas DFM, Negam M. Colostomies in infancy and childhood. *Z Kinderchir* 1982; 36: 100–2.

10. Ekenze SO, Agugua-Obianyo NEN, Amah CC. Colostomy for large bowel anomalies in children: A case controlled study. *Int J Surg* 2007; 5: 273–7.

11. Mollitt DL, Malangoni MA, Ballantine TVN et al. Colostomy complications in children. An analysis of 146 cases. *Arch Surg* 1980; 115: 445–58.

12. Uba AF, Chirdan LB. Colostomy complications in children. *Ann Afr Med* 2003; 2: 9–12.

13. Steinau G, Ruhl KM, Hornchen H et al. Enterostomy complications in infancy and childhood. *Langenbeck's Arch Surg* 2001; 386: 346–9.

14. Das S. Extraperitoneal closure of colostomy in children. *J Indian Med Assoc* 1991; 89: 253–5.

15. Chandramouli B, Srinivasan K, Jagdish S et al. Morbidity and mortality of colostomy and its closure in children. *J Pediatr Surg* 2004; 39: 596–9.

16. Miyano G, Yanai T, Okazaki T et al. Laparoscopy-assisted stoma closure. *J Laparoendosc Adv Surg Tech A* 2007; 17: 395–8.

17. Figueroa M, Bailez M, Solana J. Morbilidad de la colostomia en ninos con malformaciones anorrectales (MAR). *Cir Pediatr* 2007; 20: 79–82.

18. Nour S, Beck J, Stringer MD. Colostomy complications in infants and children. *Ann R Coll Surg Engl* 1996; 78: 526–30.

19. Dobe CO, Gbobo LI. Childhood colostomy and its complications in Lagos. *East Central Afr J Surg* 2001; 6: 25–9.

20. Macmahon RA, Cohen SJ, Eckstein HB. Colostomies in infancy and childhood. *Arch Dis Childh* 1963; 38: 114–7.

21. Rickwood AMK, Hemlatha V, Brooman P. Closure of colostomy in infants and children. *Br J Surg* 1979; 66: 273–4.

22. Brenner RW, Swenson O. Colostomy in infants and children. *Surg Gynecol Obstet* 1967; 124: 1239–44.

23. Bischoff A, Levitt MA, Lawal TA et al. Colostomy closure: How to avoid complications. *Pediatr Surg Int* 2010; 26: 1087–92.

17

Vascular access in the newborn

BETH A. RYMESKI AND FREDERICK C. RYCKMAN

INTRODUCTION

Although only a small fraction of all neonates require extensive resuscitation, the large number of births throughout the world ensures that adequate neonatal intensive care facilities remain on the cutting edge of technology. Advancements in monitoring, ventilatory support, vascular access, and maintenance of core body temperature have been paramount in the vast increase in the survival rates of newborns.[1] New innovations in size and materials coupled with new routes of vascular access have been paramount for neonatologists with regard to invasive monitoring, ionotropic support, and total parental nutrition. Invasive monitoring includes both continuous blood pressure measurements and the ability to obtain arterial blood for up-to-the-minute blood gas measurements for ventilatory support. Smaller catheter size and peripheral central routes have enabled the neonatologist to maximize the use of blood products, electrolytes, drug delivery, and nutrition, especially in those neonates who are unable to tolerate enteral nutrition for long periods of time. Advances in medical devices and refinement of techniques now allow for smaller and sicker neonates to gain the same advantage that was once only available to larger infants within the intensive care unit.

ARTERIAL CANNULATION

Invasive access to the arterial system has been a mainstay in the monitoring of the critically ill patient for decades. Short-term arterial access has circumvented the need for numerous heel sticks or difficult arterial punctures for blood gas analysis utilized for ventilatory changes. Continuous blood pressure monitoring allows for up-to-the-minute decision making when using supportive vasoactive medications and can also be used to draw needed blood studies, obviating frequent venipunctures. The majority of these cannulas can be placed by percutaneous insertion techniques at the bedside.

Maintenance

Catheters within the arterial system are particularly prone to thrombosis, which guides their general care. Continuous infusion of a balanced saline solution with heparin (1 unit/mL) at a minimum of 0.5 mL/hour for all arterial lines helps to ensure patency. The type of fluid can be altered, dictated by the clinical situation. Arterial catheters are flushed with 0.5 mL of normal saline over 5 seconds after each blood draw to clear the system.

Blood pressure monitoring devices are connected by three-way stopcocks for ease of blood draws and to ensure sterility. Transducers are leveled to the phlebostatic axis (located at the fourth intercostal space and one-half the anterior–posterior [AP] diameter of the chest). The system is zeroed with the transducer in this position at the initial setup, at each shift change, and with position change of the transducer. The waveform can become dampened due to microthrombi or positioning, or from mechanical disturbances within the system. Once a waveform appears dampened, all connections are checked and secured, the tubing is evaluated for air within the system (this tends to blunt the actual pressure reading), and the catheter is then irrigated. The infant or catheter can be repositioned and the limb immobilized if necessary.

Consideration should be made of suturing the catheter in place to provide stability and promote safety. Transparent dressings (such as Tegaderm or Opsite) are utilized to facilitate inspection of the insertion site while maintaining sterility. The connections, catheter, stitches, and tubing are examined and their status documented routinely to ensure that they are intact. Intravenous (IV) fluids are changed every 24 hours, and the tubing is changed every 72 hours utilizing sterile technique. Transducers are changed every 72 hours as well. Nursing assessment of color, pulses, capillary refill, and temperature is documented every 2 hours, and the position of deeper indwelling catheters (i.e., umbilical arterial catheters) is documented with radiographs following placement and as indicated.

Complications

Most complications with peripherally inserted arterial catheters arise due to thromboembolic events or vasospasm.[2,3] Treatment is prompt removal at the first sign of blanching of the distal extremities. Further treatment includes the use of heparin or tissue plasminogen activator (tPA) and, in rare circumstances, surgical removal of clot if extremity tissue viability is compromised. Infectious complications are rare with arterial catheters as long as appropriate measures as described previously are followed.

Umbilical artery catheters (UACs) have a higher risk of thromboembolism, especially when they are placed in the low-lying position (L3–L5).[4] The infectious rates are similar to central venous catheter (CVC) rates.[3] We tend to remove these catheters within 5 days of being placed to help prevent these issues. Studies have also shown that there in no evidence that prophylactic antibiotics are useful with these catheters.[5]

UMBILICAL ARTERY CATHETERIZATION

Frequently, neonates transferred to a neonatal intensive care unit (NICU) with surgical capability have already had umbilical catheters placed at the referral hospital. Although this is not a common procedure performed by most pediatric surgeons, the ability to place these catheters is a valuable tool in the invasive monitoring of the critically ill neonate.

One or both umbilical arteries may be cannulated for continuous blood pressure monitoring or for frequent arterial blood gas measurements for ventilator management. Resuscitation fluids and medications can be delivered via these cannulas in urgent situations but are best infused using venous access sites, discussed later in this chapter. UAC placement is contraindicated in infants with omphalocele, omphalitis, umbilical cord anomalies, necrotizing enterocolitis, or signs of peritonitis or lower extremity vascular compromise.

Access technique

Catheter length should be established prior to initiating the procedure using standardized graphs, which utilize the length of the shoulder to the umbilical cord in centimeters to estimate the position of the catheter.[6] Calculations can also be performed using birth weight (BW) to estimate the desired position of the catheter (high T6–T9, low L3–L5), such as those described by Shukla and Ferrara[7]:

Low catheter position umbilical artery (UA)

length (cm) = BW(kg) + 7

High catheter position UA length (cm) = (3 × BW(kg)) + 9

Since this may not be accurate in very-low-BW infants, Wright et al.[8] suggest using the formula UA length (cm) = (4 × BW (kg)) + 7 for those infants less than 1500 g for a high-lying position. We generally attempt to place UACs in the high-lying position to theoretically decrease the rates of

thrombosis and intestinal ischemia given previous studies.[4] In all cases, an abdominal radiograph is used to check the catheter position prior to the completion of the procedure (Figure 17.1).

Standard umbilical catheters measure 3.5 Fr (premature) to 5 Fr (full term) and can be purchased from various manufacturers. The infant is generally placed under a radiant warmer with the surgeon donning standard sterile equipment. The umbilical stump and surrounding abdominal skin is prepped with a surgical prep solution and the field draped. A minor instrument set including forceps, hemostats, and needle drivers is all that is needed for catheter placement. Appropriate fluids should be available to infuse into the catheter upon gaining access. We prefer to use ¼ normal saline with heparin (1 unit/mL) to keep the line patent. The catheter should be flushed with sterile saline prior to insertion. The umbilical stump is grasped, and umbilical tape is used to encircle the stump below skin level to prevent bleeding. The stump is cut with care to leave adequate length for ease of manipulation during placement. One umbilical artery is identified—the vein is normally larger and thin walled, and the arteries are small, thick walled, and normally two in number—and gently dilated with either a hemostat or forceps. Either a 3.5 Fr (infants less than 2 kg) or 5 Fr (those greater than 2 kg) previously flushed catheter is then passed into the lumen with gentle traction applied to

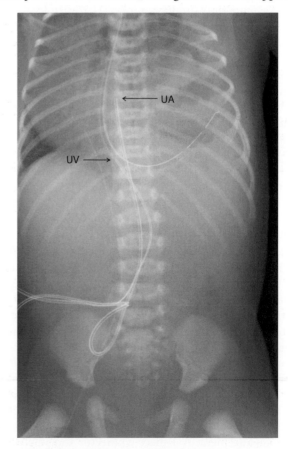

Figure 17.1 Radiograph of high-lying umbilical artery catheter (UA) and umbilical vein catheter (UV) in desired position.

the umbilical stump. Blood return is usually encountered when the catheter enters the iliac artery. The catheter is then advanced to the desired position and secured with suture through the substance of the cord. Radiographs can be used to confirm position prior to breaking sterile conditions to allow for manipulation. The desired fluids and measurement devices are then secured to the catheter by way of a three-way stopcock mechanism or manifold.

ALTERNATIVE METHOD FOR UMBILICAL ARTERY CANNULATION

At times, the umbilical cord is too short or dry to allow for easy cannulation. Access to both umbilical arteries can be achieved through an infraumbilical incision and blunt dissection through the subcutaneous tissues. Once the umbilical arteries are encountered, proximal and distal control can be gained by silk or long-term absorbable sutures. The artery can be accessed by making a transverse arteriotomy through the anterior one-half of the artery, allowing direct catheter passage. The distal control suture is tied to secure the artery and the catheter. The incision can be closed with interrupted suture and a sterile dressing applied.

RADIAL ARTERY CANNULATION

The most common site for peripheral arterial access is the radial artery. It provides a site that is ideal to access due to its consistent anatomical relationships, collateral blood flow, and easy access for nursing maintenance. Most radial arterial lines can be placed percutaneously, which helps to maintain sterility and allows for potential recannulation in the future. In rare instances, a cut-down technique is required for direct access to the artery.

Access technique

Collateral circulation of the hand should always be assessed (Allen test) and documented prior to radial or ulnar artery access attempts. Blanching or cyanosis of the fingers or hand should preclude placement. The radial artery can be palpated medial to the styloid process of the radius along the proximal wrist crease. The infant's forearm is placed on an arm board with the wrist dorsiflexed approximately 30–45 degrees (Figure 17.2). The wrist is then prepped (Betadine solution) and draped in a sterile fashion. Local anesthetic can be used but will sometimes obscure the radial pulse and is generally avoided. A 22 or 24 Fr needle catheter is inserted at approximately a 20-degree angle until blood can be seen within its hub. The catheter tip is then gently advanced into the vessel while removing the needle. If resistance is met, a small guidewire (Cook 0.015" fixed-core guidewire) can be passed into the catheter to aid in manipulation and to allow easier advancement. A T-piece connector and stopcock are then attached to the catheter, and it is flushed to ensure patency. The arterial line is then stitched into place and dressed with a transparent dressing. Ultrasound guidance

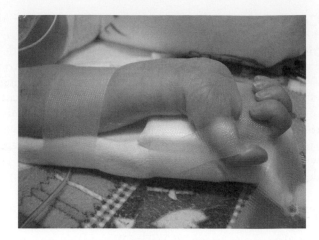

Figure 17.2 Positioning for radial arterial catheter.

to identify the radial artery and visualize the needle in the center of the artery can be helpful when utilized by providers who are trained to use ultrasound for vascular access.

If a cut-down approach is necessary, a small transverse incision can be made proximal to the joint over the point of maximal impulse. Blunt dissection is usually all that is necessary parallel to the vessel course for adequate exposure. Once exposure is obtained, proximal and distal control is secured with silk or long-term absorbable suture ties. Once again, a 22 or 24 Fr catheter is used to gain percutaneous access with gentle traction on the distal control suture. A guidewire (Cook 0.015" fixed-core guidewire) can also be useful in this setting to guide the catheter into place once blood is obtained within the hub. Backflow of arterial blood ensures successful placement. Distal vascular occlusion to prevent back-bleeding is generally not necessary, and the control sutures can be removed following the procedure. The skin site is then closed with interrupted sutures, and the catheter is sutured into place at the skin level. The catheter is then dressed and accessed in a similar manner as earlier described.

PEDAL ARTERIAL CANNULATION

The next most commonly used sites for arterial cannulation are the posterior tibial and dorsalis pedis arteries. Once again, these sites allow for collateral blood flow and easy maintenance. Access can be obtained percutaneously or by cut-down. The anatomical relationship of the posterior tibial artery posterior to the medial malleolus provides an easy site for surgical access. Insertion techniques are similar to those described for the radial artery. The line is then immobilized in a similar manner.

AXILLARY AND FEMORAL ARTERIAL CANNULATION

These sites are generally reserved for emergent situations where peripheral arterial pulses are weak and access is unobtainable. The high risk of vasospasm and embolization to the extremities and minimal collateral blood flow preclude their everyday use. In the urgent situation that these lines are required, they should be removed as soon as clinically possible.

Percutaneous access can be obtained via the axillary artery with the arm extended beyond the horizontal and midway through its course. A guidewire is generally not needed for this catheter placement. Access to the femoral artery can be gained below the inguinal ligament also by percutaneous methods. Guidewires are generally used to ensure correct position within the iliac artery. They are secured in a similar manner to the peripherally placed lines.

VENOUS CANNULATION

The ability to gain venous access in newborns has been available for decades and allows neonatologists and surgeons the ability to provide consistent vascular access to deliver critical care. New catheter materials including plastic and silicone allow for small-bore devices and the cannulation of the smallest of veins. Temporary peripheral access can be easily obtained in the newborn at the bedside with 24 Fr angiocatheters or by umbilical vein catheterization. This access, however, is temporary, and often, central IV access is needed for long-term parental nutrition or vasoactive medication drips.

Newer access methods including peripheral intervenous central catheters (PICCs) are now the mainstay for central venous access in the neonatal intensive care setting. The ability to insert these catheters at the bedside, coupled with decreased expense and rapid insertion times, has significantly decreased the need for both cut-down and umbilical catheter access in these babies. Occasions still arise when a PICC line is unable to be placed, is of insufficient size to accommodate all of the needs of the patient, or emergency resuscitation dictates the need for expedited central venous access. It is imperative for the pediatric surgeon to be skilled in all these access modalities.

Maintenance

Many hospitals have established designated central line teams to manage the everyday care of CVCs. Dedicated care teams in combination with nursing staff familiar with the care protocols and requirements are central to providing consistent daily care for CVCs.

Umbilical vein catheters (UVCs) are cared for in a similar manner as described earlier for UACs. Fluids are maintained at a minimum of 1.0 mL/hour to ensure line patency. Lines are flushed in a similar manner, and the length and position of the catheter are documented with radiographs after the initial placement (ideal placement is at the junction of the inferior vena cava [IVC] and the right atrium), as is their length every shift by the bedside nurse. Connections are checked hourly, and padded hemostats are available at the bedside for accidental disconnections. All fluids and tubing are changed in a similar manner to UACs. Discontinuation of either the UAC or UVC is performed by the physician, nurse practitioner, or qualified bedside nurses. Only 3–5 minutes of firm pressure is needed to maintain hemostasis.

Percutaneous and tunneled catheters are maintained in a similar manner. Access to the CVC via the hub, cap, or manifold is preceded by a 30-second scrub and 30-second air-dry time with 2% chlorhexidine gluconate with isopropyl alcohol (ChloraPrep). Heparin volumes for unused ports vary depending on the size of the line. We utilize the Biopatch protective disk (Ethicon) to cover and surround all insertion sites for CVCs. This disk and dressing is changed at a maximum of every 7 days or if the site appears erythematous or the dressing is compromised. The Biopatch should be used with caution in neonates under 1000 g as there has been reported a 15% incidence of contact dermatitis versus a 1.5% incidence in neonates ≥1000 g.[9] The site is cleansed with a 30-second ChloraPrep or 60-second povidone scrub. A new Biopatch and transparent occlusive dressing (Tegaderm or Opsite) is then applied after the site has completely dried. All CVCs are checked hourly and documented by the bedside nurse. Each shift, the nurse documents the position of any sutures, skin integrity, redness or induration, the position of the cuff in tunneled lines, occlusiveness of the dressing, changes in the extremity, and any site of pain or discomfort. Cut-down sites are maintained in a similar manner. Although uncommon, intraosseous (IO) needle sets can be placed in an emergency situation but are removed within 24 hours of placement. Povidone iodine–soaked gauze is placed around the insertion site and is changed every 2–3 hours or when the gauze is dry. Particular attention is paid to the hemodynamic status of the limb for any signs of compartment syndrome.

Complications

Complications associated with central lines are numerous, but most can be avoided with careful placement techniques and nursing care. Pneuomothorax, chylothorax, lung injury, malposition of the line, and perforation of the vessel are but a few of the many issues that can arise during the initial placement.[10] Cardiac arrhythmias can occur due to stimulation of the endocardium in those patients whose line is placed deeper than the superior vena cava/right atrial junction. This can be avoided in most cases by using fluoroscopy when placing subclavian or jugular venous access lines. Tunneled line expulsion is very uncommon when using Dacron cuffed tunneled lines.

Neonates in particular are susceptible to thrombosis near the catheter tip of CVCs given their small vessel. Even with continuous heparin infusion, up to 30% of neonates with CVCs have some form of thrombosis detected.[11,12] Most episodes of thrombosis are asymptomatic and generally present as inability to flush or withdraw blood from the CVC. tPA can be utilized to remove clot buildup on the catheter tip. This is usually successful and can be repeated for stable clots. Continued buildup of clot demonstrated by ultrasonography may necessitate removal of the line. Several papers have documented an increased rate of thrombosis in infants with abdominal pathology, particularly gastroschisis, who have lower extremity PICC placement.[13,14] In these patients, consideration should be made of placing only upper extremity or jugular access. One should be weary of removing lines in neonates unless the child is symptomatic due to the relative difficulty in placing and maintaining these lines. Rarely do neonates require heparin therapy following removal.[15]

The most common complication of any central catheter is infection. Historically, rates of central line–associated blood stream infection (CLABSI) as high as 29% have been seen in neonates, with smaller infants at greatest risk.[12,16] Differences in infection rates can be attributed to differences in patient populations and practice guidelines.[12] CLABSI has received a lot of attention in the past 10 years, which has resulted in a significant decrease in the infection rate. Particularly, creation of care "bundles" to standardize care and enforce best practice policies has been shown to decrease CLABSI rates even in high-risk infants.[17] Coagulase-negative staphylococci continue to be the most common cause of central line infection and bacteremia. Numerous other bacteria including gram-negatives, anaerobes, and *Candida* species can cause line infection, especially in the postsurgical neonate. Although many authors advocate treatment with antibiotics for the clearance of central line infection, removal of the foreign body (CVC) associated with the infection may be needed in refractory cases. PICC lines can be inserted as a bridge to replacement of more permanent access during antibiotic treatment of the bacteremia. Insertion site infections can generally be treated with antibiotics alone and do not require removal of the catheter unless bacteremia is documented. With careful guidelines for the placement and maintenance of these catheters, very low infection rates can be achieved.

PERIPHERALLY INSERTED CENTRAL CATHETER

The majority of centrally placed lines in most neonatal units are PICC lines. These lines can be quickly placed by specially trained nursing personnel, radiologists, or pediatric surgeons at the bedside with little to no sedation. The catheters are made of silicone or polyurethane and come in sizes as small as 1.9 Fr. In contrast, the smallest surgically placed lines are usually 2.7 Fr catheters. This small size allows for placement in neonates as small as 500 g. Although the initial experience with PICC line placement used fluoroscopy for all cases.[18] This is now generally reserved for those infants who have failed multiple attempts at bedside placement.

Access technique

Sterile technique is maintained throughout the procedure. After the appropriate site is chosen (antecubital, saphenous, or scalp veins), the catheter is flushed with heparinized saline 2 units/mL. The proposed length of the catheter is then measured. The site is cleansed with a surgical prep and draped in a sterile fashion, and a tourniquet is applied. Ultrasound is utilized to identify the target vein, and the introducer needle set is then inserted into the vein with

return of blood flow confirming position. The catheter is then advanced through the peel-away introducer in 1 cm increments to the premeasured length. The catheter can be flushed with normal saline to facilitate insertion. Once the desired length is reached, blood is aspirated, and the line is flushed with heparinized saline. The breakaway needle is released, and a securement device is placed. Steri-Strips are applied and a Biopatch placed over the insertion site with a transparent dressing as a covering. A chest radiograph confirms the position of the catheter tip.

UMBILICAL VEIN CATHETER

The majority of UVCs are placed by neonatologists at outside facilities prior to transfer. These lines can be used for emergency medications, fluids during resuscitation, transfusions, and longer-term central access for IV fluids. The complications are similar to other CVCs but do have an increased risk of infectious complications of the liver and heart.[3] The generally accepted optimal position for UVC placement is the tip at the level of the IVC/right atrial junction. Cardiac arrhythmia can occur with placement of the UVC within the heart itself and is the most common complication during insertion. Cardiac perforation with pericardial tamponade and subsequent demise has been reported with deep insertion.[19] Portal hypertension can occur with placement into the portal system secondary to extrahepatic portal vein thrombosis. Portal vein thrombosis is a known complication, I would not include hepatic necrosis. We have seen cardiac perforation with line advancement when ascites decreased (urinary ascites from perforated renal pelvis).

Access technique

The placement of the UVC catheter is similar to the previously described placement of the UAC. A 3.5 or 5 Fr catheter is used to gain access to the single umbilical vein. Catheters are advanced gently, usually only 1–2 cm beyond the point of blood return (generally only about 5 cm in a term infant). Radiographs confirm the position of the catheter preferably at the level of the diaphragm (Figure 17.1). The catheter is maintained similarly to the UAC.

Access can also be gained in emergency situations in the operating theater in the newborn by a supraumbilical incision with gentle dissection and cannulation of the vein along the abdominal wall. This site is usually only viable for a few days prior to closure.

PERCUTANEOUS CANNULATION

Multiple sites can be utilized for the percutaneous introduction of CVCs, including the internal jugular veins, subclavian veins, and femoral veins. Although these can be placed at the bedside in extreme conditions, they are more safely placed in the operating room under general anesthesia with ultrasound or fluoroscopic guidance. The technique of ultrasound-guided placement of central venous lines is particularly effective for the internal jugular vein[20] and is a helpful technique at any age. The improved safety with this placement technique is quickly establishing this as best standard practice. We utilize fluoroscopy liberally while placing any centrally dwelling catheter in the operating room. This not only helps to confirm placement but also allows direct vision while dilating vessels and advancing catheters into the correct position with the Seldinger technique.

Access technique

Percutaneous access for central line placement is accomplished by the use of the guidewire (Seldinger) technique. The patient is placed supine on the operating table, and a small towel roll or bump is placed under his/her shoulders to extend the neck with the head midline. Both sides of the neck and chest are prepped and draped in the standard fashion. The patient is then placed in the Trendelenburg position. The two standard infant-sized Broviac tunneled catheters are the 2.7 Fr and 4.2 Fr single-lumen catheters (Bard, Salt Lake City, Utah, USA). Temporary nontunneled 4 Fr double-lumen catheters are also available (Cook, Arrow). We prefer for the child to be at least 10 lb. before placing a double-lumen catheter given its size. Standard introducer sets contain introducer needles, guidewires, and introducer sheaths with dilators. In the central approach for internal jugular venous access, the vein lies at the apex of the sternal and clavicular heads of the sternocleidomastoid (SCM) muscle. Ultrasound guidance is particularly useful in identifying the vein. Once the vein has been accessed and the guidewire placed, fluoroscopy is utilized to confirm position. A site on the chest is chosen, and the catheter is tunneled from this site to the insertion site. We prefer to use live fluoroscopy to pass the dilator sheath complex over the guidewire and to measure the appropriate length of the catheter. The dilator and guidewire are then removed, and the catheter is placed via the peel-away sheath and into position. The final position of the line is confirmed with fluoroscopy. Incisions are closed, and a Biopatch and transparent, occlusive dressing are applied. This same technique can be used for percutaneous femoral vein catheterization. Subclavian vein access can be facilitated by ultrasound guidance, but the technical considerations are more difficult given the location of the clavicle. Generally, the landmarks of the mid angle of the clavicle and the sternal notch are used for subclavian venipuncture with fluoroscopy used in a similar manner as described.

The femoral vein can also be accessed at the bedside by first using a 24 Fr angiocatheter to gain access. A small guidewire (Cook 0.015" fixed-core guidewire) passes easily through this sheath. A larger angiocatheter can then be placed over the wire to facilitate the larger guidewire in the temporary central line set. Abdominal radiographs can then confirm position.

PERIPHERAL VEIN CUT-DOWN

With the significant increase in PICC lines placed at our institution, we have seen a dramatic decrease in the number of peripheral vein cut-downs performed. These now seem to be reserved for those small infants where percutaneous methods are impossible. The common facial vein, external jugular vein, internal jugular vein, and saphenous vein are the most commonly used sites. With excellent nursing care and sterile technique, the infection rates are comparable to the percutaneous route of cannulation.

Access technique

The saphenous vein can be accessed at numerous points along its course. The most distal site is just superior to the medial malleolus. This site is not useful for long-term access and is not central in its location. The saphenous vein drains into the femoral vein at the level of the femoral triangle and is an easy access point for central cannulation. The infant is placed in a supine position, and a rolled towel is placed under the pelvis to allow easier access. The groin is prepped and draped in the standard fashion. The length of the catheter can be measured by the length from the proposed incision to just superior to the umbilicus (iliac vein/IVC junction) (Figure 17.3) Ultrasound can be used

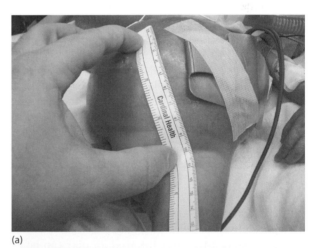

(a)

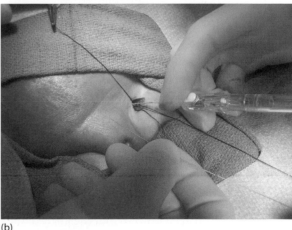

(b)

Figure 17.3 **(a)** Measurement for length of saphenous vein cut-down central line. **(b)** Access of the saphenous vein with 24 Fr angiocatheter.

to identify the vessels and aid in planning the location of the incision. A transverse incision is made inferior to the groin crease inferior to the inguinal ligament. Gentle dissection in carried out parallel to the expected path of the vessel with a hemostat until the saphenous vein is found. The vein is then elevated, and proximal and distal control is gained with 5-0 silk ties. At least 1 cm of the vein should be exposed to allow for easy cannulation. The distal control ligature is then elevated to put tension on the vessel. A 24 Fr angiocatheter is then used to gain access to the vessel and is advanced as the needle is removed (Figure 17.3). Care must be undertaken to avoid going through the back wall of the vein. A small guidewire (Cook 0.015" fixed-core guidewire) can then be advanced into the angiocatheter, allowing a 22 Fr angiocatheter to be placed, which is large enough to accommodate the guidewire found in most 3 or 4 Fr central line kits. The catheter is then advanced, and the proximal suture is tied down to secure the line and the vessel. The distal ligature can be removed or tied down if there is significant back-bleeding. The incision is then closed in the usual fashion, and the line site is dressed as previously described.

CENTRAL VEIN CUT-DOWN

Neck cut-down for access to the common facial vein or the internal jugular vein is also useful in neonates. This procedure can be performed bedside in the NICU with x-ray available to confirm line position. Typically, the right neck is used to take advantage of the drainage of the jugular vein directly into the superior vena cava. With a roll under the infant's shoulders and the head turned to the left, a transverse incision is made along the anterior border of the SCM one-third of the distance below the angle of the mandible and the clavicle. The SCM is exposed and retracted laterally to expose the vessels. The internal jugular vein is identified and the common facial vein branch dissected free. If the common facial vein is not useable (too small, aberrant anatomy, etc.), then the internal jugular can be used. Proximal and distal control is obtained around the target vein with silk or long-term absorbable suture. The distal side is tied off and a small venotomy made on the anterior vein wall. A vein pick may be helpful to better expose the vessel lumen. The catheter, which should be measured against the patient's body and is tunneled per the usual technique, is then introduced through the venotomy and advanced. Cutting the tip of the catheter in a beveled manner may assist with this process. The proximal tie can be secured lightly around the vessel and catheter with care to not occlude the small lumen. An x-ray should be obtained to confirm the position of the tip, and the catheter should draw blood and flush easily. Cannulation of the external jugular vein has also been utilized, but the angle of the vessel joining the subclavian may make passage of the small catheter difficult. The incision is then closed and the catheter dressed in the usual sterile fashion as described previously in the chapter.

INTRAOSSEOUS DEVICES

During trauma or emergency resuscitation, the venous system may be collapsed due to hypovolemia and shock. Gaining intervenous access in these cases can be quite challenging and time consuming. A quick and easy alternative is the placement of an intraosseous device. These devices come in a multitude of sizes, with the smallest available in our facility being 1.8 mm × 15 mm in length. Contraindications to their placement include fracture, absence of landmarks, infection at the proposed insertion site, and previous instrumentation of the extremity. These devices have gone through many evolutions and have a very low (<1%) complication rate.[1] The EZ-IO system (Vidacare, San Antonio, Texas, USA) allows for quick and stable access even in the newborn.

Access technique

For infants between 3 and 39 kg, the small, 15G needle system can be effectively used (Figure 17.4). The two most common insertion sites are the proximal tibia just below the tibial tuberosity and, less commonly in infants, the humerus at the level of the humeral head. Local anesthesia can be injected at the proposed insertion site once it is prepped and draped. The needle is inserted into the driver system, and the needle cap is removed. The needle and driver should be positioned at a 90-degree angle to the bone. The needle is then pressed into the skin until the tip touches the bone (ensure that at least 5 mm of the catheter is still visible at this point). The bone cortex is penetrated by squeezing the driver's trigger and applying gentle, steady downward pressure. Once a sudden give or pop is encountered, the medullary space has been entered. The driver and stylet are removed, and the catheter is flushed with at least 5 mL of normal saline. If the catheter flushes well, fluids and medications can be administered.[21] A dressing is placed around the device and changed on as needed. IO devices should be removed within 24 hours to avoid complications such as osteomyelitis and compartment syndrome.

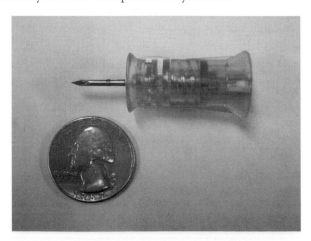

Figure 17.4 15G intraosseous needle (Vidacare, San Antonio, Texas, USA).

CONCLUSION

With smaller, critically ill neonates being managed in our intensive care units, reliable vascular access is a necessity. Improvements in techniques, miniaturization of catheters, and development of new materials allow for stable access and improved care in premature and newborn infants. As these catheters continue to evolve, newer and safer techniques will soon follow.

REFERENCES

1. Perlman, J et al. The International Liaison Committee on Resuscitation (ILCOR) consensus on science with treatment recommendations for pediatric and neonatal patients: Neonatal resuscitation. *Pediatrics* 2006; 117(5): e978–88.
2. Ramachandarappa A, Jain L. Iatrogenic disorders in modern neonatology: A focus on safety and quality of care. *Clin Perinatol* 2008; 35: 1–34.
3. Hermansen MC, Hermansen MG. Intravascular catheter complications in the neonatal intensive care unit. *Clin Perinatol* 2005; 32: 141–56.
4. Barrington KJ. Umbilical artery catheters in the newborn: Effects of position of the catheter tip. *Cochrane Database Syst Rev* 2000; (2): CD000505.
5. Inglis GD, Jardine LA, Davies MW. Prophylactic antibiotics to reduce morbidity and mortality in neonates with umbilical artery catheters. *Cochrane Database Syst Rev* 2007; (4): CD004697.
6. John Hopkins Hospital, Custer JW, Rau, RE. *The Harriet Lane Handbook: A Manual for Pediatric House Officers*, 18th edn. Philadelphia, PA: Elsevier Mosby, 2009.
7. Skukla H, Ferrara A. Rapid estimation of insertional length of umbilical catheters in newborns. *Am J Dis Child* 1986; 140: 786–8.
8. Wright IMR, Owers M. Wagner M. The umbilical arterial catheter: A formula for improved positioning in the very low birth weight infant. *Pediatr Crit Care Med* 2008; 9(5): 498–501.
9. Garland JS, Alex CP, Mueller CD et al. A randomized trial comparing povidone–iodine to a chlorhexidine gluconate–impregnated dressing for prevention of central venous catheter infections in neonates. *Pediatrics* 2001; 107(6): 1431–6.
10. Citak A, Karabocuoglu M, Ucsel R et al. Central venous catheters in pediatric patients—Subclavian approach as the first choice. *Pediatr Int* 202; 44(1): 83–6.
11. Shah PS, Kalyn A, Satodia P et al. A randomized, controlled trial of heparin versus placebo infusion to prolong the usability of peripherally placed percutaneous central venous catheters (PCVCs) in neonates: The HIP (Heparin Infusion for PCVC) study. *Pediatrics* 2007; 119(1): e284–91.
12. Ramasethu J. Complications of vascular catheters in the neonatal intensive care unit. *Clin Perinatol* 2008; 35: 199–222.
13. Ma M, Garingo A, Jensen AR et al. Complication risks associated with lower versus upper extremity peripherally inserted central venous catheters in neonates with gastroschisis. *J Pediatr Surg* 2015; 50(4): 556–8.
14. Kisa P, Ting J, Callejas A et al. Major thrombotic complications with lower limb PICCs in surgical neonates. *J Pediatr Surg* 2015; 50(5): 786–9.
15. Ramasethu J. Management of vascular thrombosis and spasm in the newborn. *NeoReviews* 2005; 6: e298–311.
16. Klein MD, Rood K, Graham P. Central venous catheter sepsis in surgical newborns. *Pediatr Surg Int* 2003; 19: 529–32.
17. Wang W, Zhao C, Ji Q et al. Prevention of peripherally inserted central line–associated blood stream infections in very low-birth-weight infants by using a central line bundle guideline with a standard checklist: A case control study. *BMC Pediatr* 2015; 18; 15: 69.
18. Crowley JJ, Pereira JK, Harris LS et al. Peripherally inserted central catheters: Experience in 523 children. *Radiology* 1997; 204: 617–21.
19. Nowlen TT, Rosenthal GL, Johnson GL et al. Pericardial effusion and tamponade in infants with central catheters. *Pediatrics* 2002; 110: 137–42.
20. Arul GS, Lewis N, Bromley P, Bennett J. Ultrasound-guided percutaneous insertion of Hickman line in children. Prospective study of 500 consecutive procedures. *J Pediatr Surg* 2009; 44: 1371–6.
21. Vidacare. EZ-IO intraosseous infusion system directions for use. 2006.

18

Radiology in the newborn

J. KELLEHER, IAN H. W. ROBINSON, AND ROISIN HAYES

INTRODUCTION

During the past decade, significant developments in surgical techniques, anesthesia, and intensive care have advanced and improved care of the sick newborn baby. All imaging modalities have reached a new higher level of sophistication, and the range of invasive and interventional radiology procedures has also greatly increased. These advances have placed greater demands on pediatric radiology departments, which must be well staffed, funded, and equipped to keep pace with these developments. Because of the plethora of available investigations, it is essential that both conventional radiographic and high-technology imaging facilities be used efficiently and rationally. A logical sequence of investigations should be applied, commencing with the simplest and least invasive, and where possible, minimizing exposure to ionizing radiation. At all times, the ALARA principle (as low as reasonably achievable) should be foremost in our mind. This approach may provide the diagnosis and obviate the need for more complex, invasive, and expensive studies, even if these additional modalities are readily available. Duplication of information obtained from these various imaging modalities, which does not improve or influence management of the patient, should be avoided.

CONVENTIONAL RADIOGRAPHY

Plain radiography is often the first and most useful study in the evaluation of the surgical neonate. Radiographic examinations should be directed to achieving the required information with the minimum of handling or disturbance while maintaining the infant's body temperature and employing measures to limit radiation exposure. Only relevant projections should be obtained in relation to the clinical problem and condition of the baby (Figure 18.1). There is no longer a place for routine lateral chest views.

Examination rooms should be kept warm—around 80°F (27°C)—and the baby should be removed from the warm protective environment of the incubator for the shortest possible time. The use of the newer generation of "giraffe"-type incubators has greatly facilitated the examination of fragile neonates.

High-frequency generators, added beam filtration, and digital image receptors all contribute significantly to reducing the radiation burden to the infant.[1] The beam should be collimated to cover only the relevant area, and gonad protection with lead shields should be used. Where repeated examination of the chest and mediastinum is anticipated, the use of thyroid shielding should be considered. Good radiographic technique is essential to produce radiographs of high quality, thus avoiding the unnecessary extra irradiation and disturbance of babies resulting from repeat exposure.[2] A sufficient number of well-trained and experienced radiographic technicians should be available to ensure that these high standards are maintained.

MOBILE EXAMINATIONS

In recent years, a great increase in demand for portable radiographic examinations has occurred. The position of vascular access catheters and endotracheal tubes may need to be repeatedly checked, and frequent examinations may be required in infants with severe respiratory problems on ventilation.[3] Mobile x-ray machines have become smaller and more maneuverable and give shorter exposure times. Incubators chosen for special or intensive care baby units should be user-friendly for radiography.

Lateral decubitus views of the chest or abdomen using a horizontal beam are easily performed on babies while in their incubators. They can be very useful in demonstrating pneumoperitoneum and in evaluating fluid levels in bowel (Figure 18.2). A dorsal decubitus view of the abdomen is perfectly adequate to either confirm or exclude pneumoperitoneum and is obtained without any re-positioning of the infant in the incubator (Figure 18.3a–c). Erect views should no longer be requested or performed.

Protocols should be in place to maximize the information obtained while minimizing the disturbance and distress to the infant. Our previous practice of performing

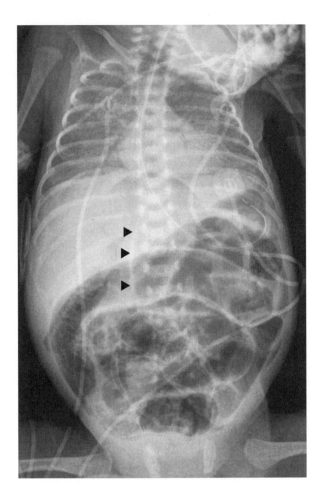

Figure 18.1 Supine chest and abdomen. Supine x-ray of the chest and abdomen in a premature neonate demonstrates abnormal increased lucency over the liver, with free intraperitoneal gas clearly outlining the falciform ligament (arrowheads). A decubitus x-ray is not required in this situation as the diagnosis of perforation is already made. Also evident is intramural gas in keeping with necrotizing enterocolitis and diffuse granular pulmonary parenchymal opacity with central air bronchograms, typical of surfactant deficiency syndrome.

inverted lateral radiographs for anorectal anomalies involved the baby being removed from the incubator and held upside down by its legs while the exposure was taken. Aside from the trauma to the infant, it is difficult to obtain a good true lateral view centered at the correct level. A prone lateral view with the buttocks elevated and using a horizontal x-ray beam is a far superior technique. The baby can be left comfortably in this position for a period of time to ensure that gas outlines the distal limit of the blind rectal pouch (Figure 18.4a,b).

FLUOROSCOPIC EXAMINATIONS

For investigations in neonates, the fluoroscopy room should be warm, with oxygen and suction outlets readily available. A fully equipped resuscitation trolley should be at hand. Procedures should be carried out quickly but carefully. Good

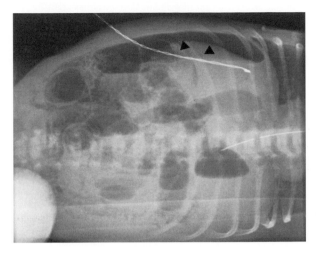

Figure 18.2 Left lateral decubitus. Decubitus x-ray in a neonate with perforated necrotizing enterocolitis. The free intraperitoneal gas rises, outlining the liver (arrowheads). Intramural gas in keeping with necrotising enterocolitis is also demonstrated. The decubitus x-ray is also useful in the detection of air–fluid levels.

venous access should be ensured before commencing any invasive or interventional procedure. The radiologist should concentrate on solving the clinical problem presented and tailor the study accordingly.

Developments in computerized digital fluoroscopy in recent years have resulted in the potential for a marked reduction in radiation exposure, more rapid performance of dynamic contrast studies, and greatly improved recorded images. Digital fluoroscopy units often have the facilities to provide a rapid series of exposures at up to 30 frames per second. While this can be very useful in studies of the swallowing mechanism or of the airway, the ability to store and review a *video loop* is much more valuable. The use of appropriate reduced-rate pulsed fluoroscopy greatly reduces radiation dose. A *last-image hold* facility allows relevant images to be saved, with no additional radiation. In most neonates, it should be possible to screen without a *grid*, thus further reducing radiation dose, and the use of magnification should be minimized. Modern installations provide image enhancement, processing, and digital subtraction facilities, which are very useful in angiography.[4]

Nonionic water-soluble contrast media are used for all intravascular studies in children. Such contrast agents can also be used for gastrointestinal examinations. They permit excellent anatomic delineation and may be safely used even where leakage into the mediastinum or peritoneal cavity, or gastrointestinal obstruction, is suspected. They are well tolerated even if pulmonary aspiration occurs, though some element of pulmonary edema may develop. If diluted, an iso-osmolar solution can be achieved for even greater tolerance in the airway. If a tracheoesophageal fistula is suspected, a feeding tube can be inserted into the proximal esophagus, through which nonionic contrast is injected under fluoroscopy, as demonstrated in Figure 18.5.

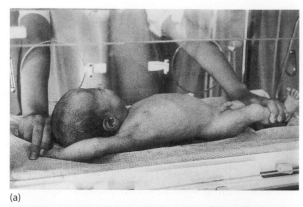

(a)

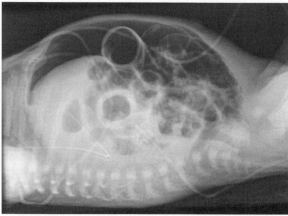

(b)

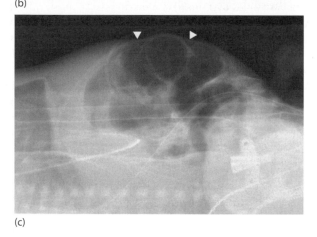

(c)

Figure 18.3 **(a)** Dorsal decubitus. Position of baby in incubator for horizontal beam exposure. **(b)** Dorsal decubitus—large amount of free gas. In the dorsal decubitus position, a large amount of free intraperitoneal gas clearly outlines the diaphragm, liver, and bowel loops. **(c)** Dorsal decubitus—small amount of free gas. Even small amounts of gas may be detected in the dorsal decubitus position, outlining the anterior abdominal wall and adjacent bowel, as in this case (arrowheads), or anterior to the liver.

Conventional ionic contrast agents, e.g., Urografin (Bayer) 30%, are less expensive and are appropriate for micturating cystourethrography (Figure 18.6). All infants should have appropriate antimicrobial cover during micturating cystourography (MCUG) to reduce the risk of infection. The contrast agent should be warmed to body temperature and may

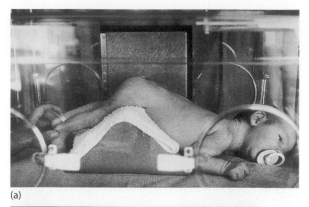

(a)

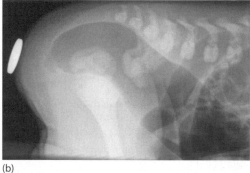

(b)

Figure 18.4 **(a)** Lateral rectum. Newborn with imperforate anus in prone position in incubator, with buttocks elevated for lateral view with horizontal beam. **(b)** Lateral rectum. Lateral x-ray of the rectum demonstrating the distal limit of the rectal pouch in this child with anorectal malformation. An assessment of the sacrum can also be made.

be diluted with sterile water. Either a 5F or a 6F feeding tube is used to catheterize the baby. In males, a steep oblique view of the urethra must be obtained during voiding to exclude the presence of posterior urethral valves. Screening time can be kept to a minimum by observing the flow of contrast from the bottle. When flow stops, the baby is usually ready to urinate.

ULTRASONOGRAPHY

This relatively inexpensive and widely available imaging modality has transformed neonatal diagnostic imaging. Lack of ionizing radiation, portability, and the freedom to do serial repeat studies make it especially suitable for this patient population. In premature or severely ill babies, ultrasonographic (US) scans can be performed satisfactorily without removing the infants from their incubators. The principles of minimal handling and maintenance of body temperature apply. Examinations should be carried out quickly and efficiently, aimed at achieving a diagnosis and not prolonged or repeated just to produce the "perfect picture."

Congenital structural abnormalities are being diagnosed with increasing frequency on antenatal scans. Many congenital brain malformations and spinal anomalies are easily recognized.[5] Prenatal recognition of anomalies such as cystic adenomatoid malformation, cystic renal disease, or

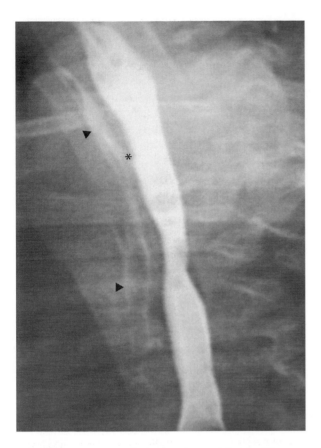

Figure 18.5 H-type tracheo-esophageal fistula. Water-soluble contrast fills the esophagus and passes through an H-type fistula (asterisk) into the trachea (arrowheads).

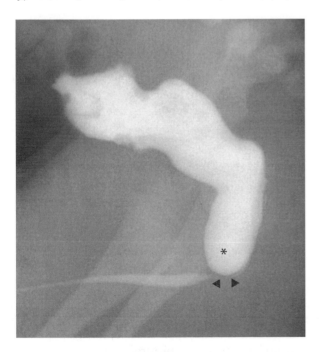

Figure 18.6 Micturating cystourethrography. Lateral image of the bladder and urethra in a male infant taken during micturition. The bladder is abnormal in contour, and the posterior urethra is markedly dilated (asterisk). The thin filling defect representing the membrane of the posterior urethra valve is visible (arrowheads).

intestinal tract obstructions alerts the neonatologist to the need for careful postnatal evaluation.

The identification of abdominal wall defects such as exomphalos and gastroschisis or of a diaphragmatic hernia on an antenatal scan allows the delivery to be arranged in or close to a major pediatric surgical center. Ex utero intrapartum treatment (EXIT surgery) can be planned if major airway problems are detected in utero. Antenatal interventional techniques can be performed under US guidance, e.g., the insertion of stents or drains in obstructed urinary tracts.

Cranial US is now an indispensible facility in any department dealing with newborn patients.[6] Using high-frequency transducers, images of excellent detail are obtained. Hydrocephalus secondary to intraventricular hemorrhage (IVH) or myelomeningocele can be accurately diagnosed and graded. Serial examinations are helpful in relation to the need for shunting. However, if the cause of the hydrocephalus is not evident, then further investigation using magnetic resonance imaging (MRI) may be necessary. One of the most important contributions of US is in the diagnosis and grading of IVH. Early diagnosis of minimal lesions can be achieved in infants at risk. The discovery of IVH can influence the decision to operate on a newborn with a congenital malformation if IVH is severe (Figure 18.7).

There is an increasing use of ultrasound in evaluating suspected anomalies of the spinal cord in infants. Ultrasound can demonstrate a broad spectrum of intraspinal anatomy, both normal and abnormal, and define pathological conditions with a high degree of accuracy in infants under 4 months of age.[7] It may obviate the need for MRI (Figure 18.8).

Sonography plays a significant role in the investigation of mass lesions in the neck and mediastinum. It permits localization, assessment of relationships to surrounding structures, and especially differentiation of cystic from solid

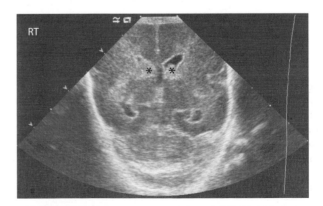

Figure 18.7 Cranial US. Coronal US image of the brain in a premature neonate. Hemorrhage is visible within both lateral ventricles (asterisk). The ventricle wall is echogenic. In addition, there is increased echogenicity within the periventricular parenchyma on the right, in keeping with infarction, indicating a Grade 4 intraventricular hemorrhage on this side. Note the relatively poor sulcation typical of a premature infant.

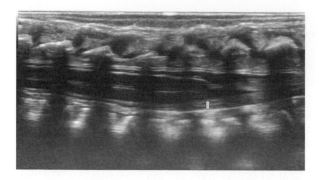

Figure 18.8 Ultrasound spine. This clearly depicts abnormal wedge-shaped truncation of the spinal cord (arrow) typical for caudal regression, in a newborn baby with anorectal malformation and lumbosacral dysgenesis.

lesions (Figure 18.9a,b). Real-time sonography is very useful in evaluating phrenic nerve paralysis.

Abdominal US is very frequently carried out in the newborn to diagnose or exclude renal disease. Lesions confined to the kidneys include multicystic dysplastic kidney, polycystic disease, and hydronephrosis. The latter may be due to obstruction at the pelviureteric or ureterovesical level or to severe reflux. In males, it may relate to the presence of posterior urethral valves. All of these conditions are readily diagnosed with US, and the severity of obstruction and renal damage can also be assessed. The kidneys are frequently involved in complex syndromes, e.g., VACTERL syndrome. The spectrum of renal anomalies varies from agenesis to crossed fused ectopic and duplex kidneys.

Ultrasound is well established as the optimal diagnostic tool in the routine evaluation of infantile pyloric stenosis. While pyloric stenosis is rare in the first 2 weeks of life, it has been reported, and the standard ultrasound measurement criteria may not be valid in this patient population.[8]

In the evaluation of mass lesions in the neonatal abdomen, US should be the first investigation. It can identify the organ of origin and help to characterize the lesion, differentiating cystic from solid. Figure 18.10 shows the typical cystic appearance of neonatal adrenal hemorrhage. In comparison, Figure 18.11 demonstrates a solid suprarenal mass, confirmed to be neuroblastoma, stage 4S. If a definitive diagnosis cannot be made on US, it should at least give a clear indication as to the next logical investigation.

In neonatal jaundice, US plays a key role in defining the anatomy of the biliary tract. Choledochal cyst may be diagnosed with confidence and biliary atresia excluded. It can demonstrate or exclude dilatation of the biliary duct system (Figure 18.12). Radionuclide imaging may have a complimentary role to play.

The development of Doppler, including color Doppler, has been a considerable advance with widespread application. The safe placement of vascular access lines is greatly aided by this technique. It can accurately map the vascular anatomy of abdominal masses or of arteriovenous

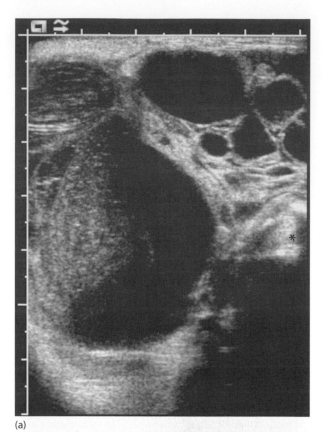

(a)

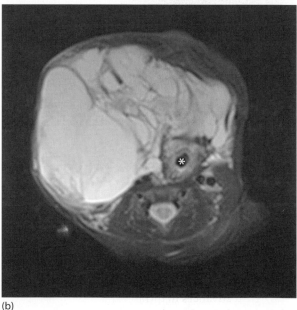

(b)

Figure 18.9 (a) Ultrasound of neck—cystic hygroma—plus accompanying (b) magnetic resonance imaging (MRI). US and MRI are complementary modalities. US has superior spatial resolution, for example, being able to detect thin septations. MRI, however, allows a more accurate assessment of the overall extent of a lesion and its relation to adjacent structures. In this example, the trachea is visible on both the US and MRI (asterisk).

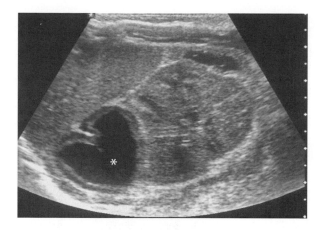

Figure 18.10 Ultrasound of adrenal hemorrhage. Cystic enlargement of the adrenal gland typical of an adrenal hemorrhage (asterisk).

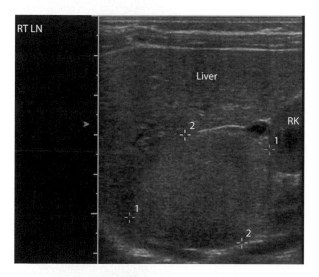

Figure 18.11 Ultrasound adrenal neuroblastoma. In contrast, this suprarenal mass is clearly solid and is typical for a neuroblastoma. (RK = right kidney.)

malformations in other sites. It allows noninvasive imaging of hepatic vascular structures.

NUCLEAR MEDICINE

With the great advances in ultrasound, computed tomography (CT), and MRI, the role of radionuclide examinations is very limited in the newborn period. Functional rather than morphological studies are usually required. Total and individual renal function can be assessed, but due to functional immaturity, imaging is less reliable than in the older infant or child. Technetium-99m-labeled mercaptoacetyl-triglycine (MAG 3) is used for assessment of obstruction, with technetium-labeled dimercaptosuccinic acid (DMSA) employed for static imaging and to demonstrate the functioning renal parenchyma. Either method will give an estimate of relative renal function. Excretory/intravenous urography or IVU has no place in modern neonatal imaging.

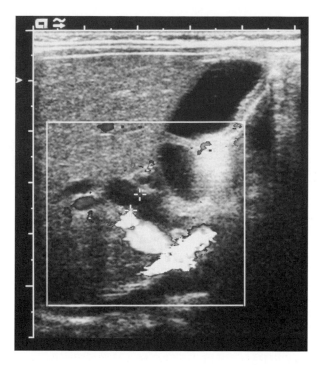

Figure 18.12 Ultrasound bile duct dilatation. US reveals dilatation of the common bile duct (calipers) in this neonate with gallstones. Color Doppler imaging is often used as in this instance to identify vascular structures separate from the bile duct.

Hepatobiliary scintigraphy is extremely useful in the investigation of neonatal jaundice where biliary atresia is a concern. The infant is given phenobarbital, 5 mg/kg per day divided into 2 equal doses, for 3 to 5 days prior to the scan, in order to induce liver enzyme activity. Mebrofenin labeled with technetium-99m (Choletec) is preferred in infants because of its greater hepatic extraction. The scan will usually differentiate between biliary atresia and neonatal hepatitis (Figure 18.13). If the biliary tract is patent, isotope should be detected in the intestine within 60 minutes.

Though uncommon, Meckel diverticulum may present with rectal bleeding in the newborn period. It can be elegantly demonstrated on technetium pertechnetate scintigraphy (Figure 18.14).

Isotope bone scanning is very unreliable in the diagnosis of osteomyelitis and/or septic arthritis in neonates and is rarely employed, US and MRI being much more sensitive.

Infants presenting with congenital hypothyroidism and absence of the thyroid gland from its normal location can be scanned using technetium-99m-pertechnetate looking for an ectopic or lingual thyroid (Figure 18.15).

COMPUTED TOMOGRAPHY

CT remains an established and vital imaging modality in pediatrics but has relatively limited application in the newborn, where ultrasound and MRI have many

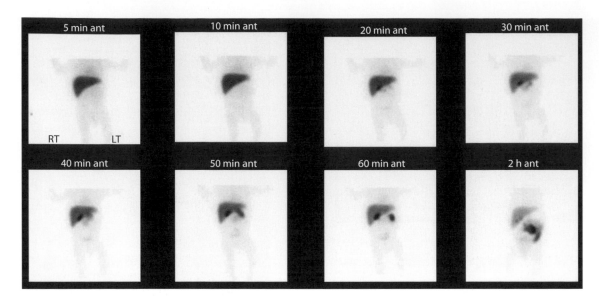

Figure 18.13 HIDA. Radioisotope rapidly appears within the liver. In this normal study, radioisotope is rapidly excreted into the gallbladder (20 minutes) and proximal small bowel (30 minutes). The delayed image at 2 hours shows radioisotope having largely passed through the liver and appearing within small bowel loops (RT = right, LT = left).

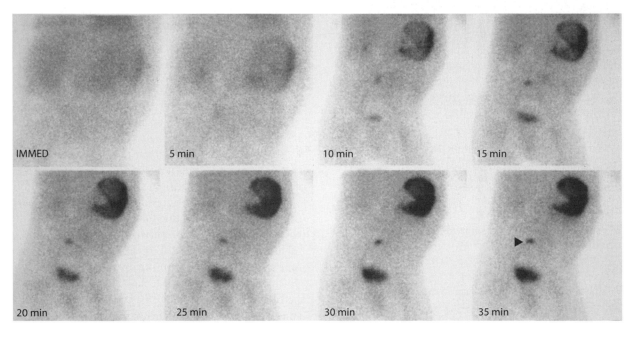

Figure 18.14 Meckel scan. Radioisotope is taken up by gastric mucosa within a Meckel diverticulum (arrowhead). Note the normal uptake by the gastric mucosa of the stomach. Also note the normal appearance of radioisotope within the bladder, having been excreted by the kidneys.

advantages. While CT can be useful in evaluating structural abnormalities in the thorax, such as congenital pulmonary adenomatoid malformations (CPAM) and congenital lobar emphysema (CLE), its usefulness in evaluating the neonatal abdomen is significantly limited by the lack of intra-abdominal fat. In general, abdominal MRI is more useful than CT when US fails to provide the diagnosis. While modern multislice scanning should be available on site in any specialized pediatric unit, radiation dose remains a major concern.[9] CT should be reserved in the newborn for specific indications where other modalities fail to provide sufficient information. These would include cranial CT scans in suspected head trauma; exclusion of intracranial calcification in congenital infection; and assessment of bony abnormality associated with severe choanal atresia (Figure 18.16). In all instances, protocols to reduce radiation dose must be in place as per the ALARA principle.[10]

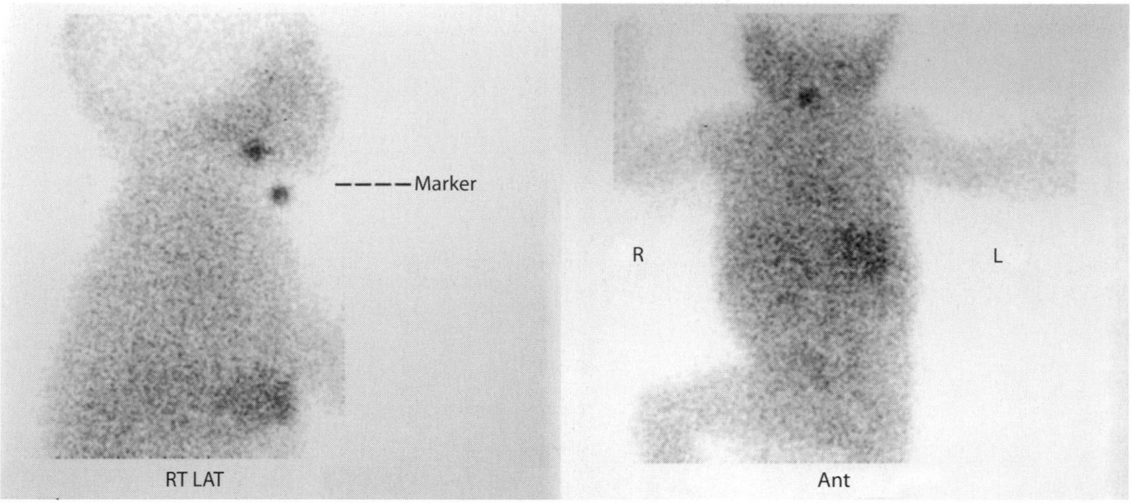

Figure 18.15 Lingual thyroid. Radioisotope accumulates within thyroid tissue, which is located at the base of the tongue. Its position can be determined relative to the chin and the marker at the sternal notch. On the anteroposterior view, the lingual thyroid has a rounded configuration, as opposed to the typical bilobed appearance expected of a normal thyroid gland.

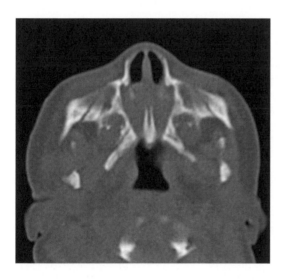

Figure 18.16 Computed tomography (CT) of choanal atresia. CT is the best modality for assessing the bony narrowing of the choanae. In this case there is severe bilateral narrowing of the posterior nasal cavity in a patient with bilateral choanal atresia.

MAGNETIC RESONANCE IMAGING

Increased access to MRI has transformed neonatal radiology. While US remains the mainstay of brain and spinal imaging in the neonate because of portability etc., MRI is used to clarify complex malformations and to provide vital functional and prognostic information. Hypoxic–ischemic brain injury (HIE) is a frequent and significant problem in the neonatal period. Regardless of the type of hypoxic injury, the imaging manifestations are related to the gestational maturity of the infant. Hypoxic injury to the premature brain affects primarily the germinal matrix and periventricular white matter, while in the term infant, damage to the cortical tissues and basal ganglia occurs (Figure 18.17). MRI with diffusion weighted imaging and spectroscopy is the diagnostic modality of choice in suspected neonatal HIE.[11]

Outside the central nervous system, the use of MRI is also increasing. In the evaluation of mass lesions of the neck and mediastinum, it offers exquisite anatomical detail. The ability to image in multiple planes facilitates surgical planning. In the abdomen, while US mostly reigns supreme, MRI is increasingly used to evaluate complex masses, to complement US in the biliary tract (magnetic resonance [MR] cholangiography), and to evaluate the renal tract (MR urography). However, its utilization continues to be limited by factors such as cost, availability, and motion artifacts, and in particular by its requirement of sedation or anesthesia.

Recent advances in MRI technology allow safe and accurate imaging of the fetus. Fetal MRI has become a useful adjunct to antenatal ultrasound.[12] It plays an important role in further evaluation of complex intracranial abnormalities. It is increasingly utilized in the antenatal assessment of complex thoracic and abdominal congenital abnormalities, such as congenital diaphragmatic hernia (CDH), where assessment of the severity of associated pulmonary hypoplasia, using volumetric lung measurements, can be useful in predicting fetal outcome. This information informs difficult decisions regarding management during pregnancy and following delivery. Figure 18.18 is a sagittal MRI scan showing a significant portion of the liver lying within the right hemithorax in a fetus with a right-sided CDH. Figure 18.19 shows MR imaging of a fetus with a large cystic hygroma of the neck. Assessment of the extent of the lesion, in particular its relationship to the airway, allowed planning for the EXIT procedure.[13]

INTERVENTIONAL TECHNIQUES

There has been a dramatic increase in recent years in the number, range, and complexity of interventional procedures

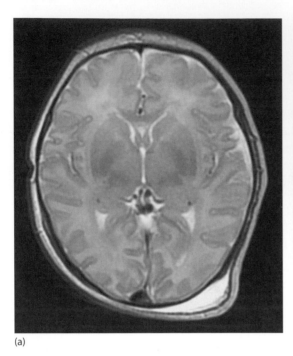
(a)

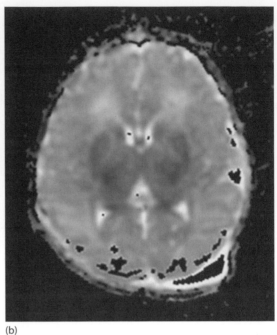
(b)

Figure 18.17 Magnetic resonance imaging of hypoxic–ischemic brain injury. **(a)** Axial T2 and **(b)** adjusted diffusion coefficient (ADC) map from the diffusion-weighted imaging (DWI). Signal abnormality in the newborn is often subtle on T1 and T2 imaging, and is influenced by gestation. DWI, when performed within an appropriate timeframe, is helpful in determining the extent of abnormality. In this term infant, extensive restricted diffusion is clearly evident within the basal ganglia (low signal on the ADC), in keeping with a profound hypoxic–ischemic event.

in pediatric as well as in adult radiology practice. Hospital stay may be shortened and patient outcome improved as these interventional procedures tend to be more cost-effective than the alternative conventional surgical approach. In the gastrointestinal tract, hydrostatic or pneumatic reduction of intussusception is a well-established technique. This, however, is a rare condition in the newborn. The nonoperative management of meconium ileus by gastrografin enema is almost universal (Figure 18.20). However, possible complications such as volvulus, peritonitis, and perforation must

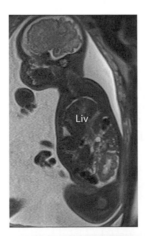

Figure 18.18 Fetal MRI of right CDH. Sagittal T2-weighted image shows a significant portion of liver (Liv) in right hemithorax.

be excluded before an enema is attempted. The fluoroscopy room should be warm, the infant well hydrated, and a functioning intravenous (IV) line in place. This author advocates the use of diluted gastrografin, one part contrast and two parts water, in order to reduce the risks of mucosal damage. Several attempts may be made over a period of days if the infant's condition permits.

Balloon catheter dilatation of postanastomosis esophageal strictures in neonates following repair of esophageal atresia is now established in major centers worldwide. The advantages of balloon dilatation over bougienage relate to the marked reduction in shear force with radial force mainly achieving the dilatation.

Balloon dilatation of colonic strictures complicating necrotizing enterocolitis is another useful, though infrequent, interventional procedure. Percutaneous gastrostomy and placement of a feeding tube in the jejunum are further useful techniques performed under fluoroscopy.

In urinary tract obstruction, percutaneous nephrostomy to relieve obstruction is widely practiced and should be performed under direct US guidance. Either a single-stab technique or a modified Seldinger approach may be used, and a pigtail catheter is left in place.

Percutaneous biopsy of organs or lesions under ultrasound, fluoroscopic, or CT guidance and the aspiration or drainage of abscesses or cysts are all part of the interventional radiologist's workload. The cumulative radiation burden to the infant must be borne in mind, and in general, ultrasound is the imaging modality of choice.[14]

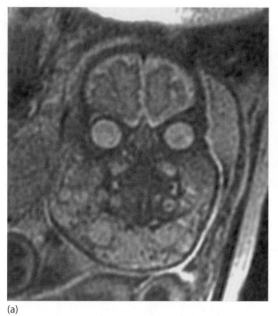

(a)

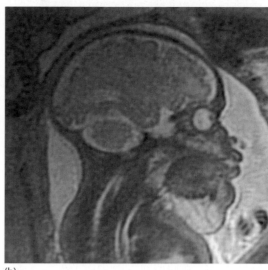

(b)

Figure 18.19 Magnetic resonance image (MRI) of fetus with a large cystic hygroma involving the floor of the mouth. Coronal and sagittal T2-weighted images showed the extent of this high-signal mass, and it's relationship to the airway, and facilitated planning for an elective EXIT procedure.

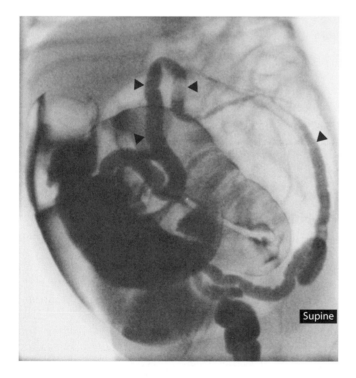

Figure 18.20 Meconium ileus. Contrast enema. Contrast fills a microcolon (arrowheads) before refluxing into markedly distended distal small bowel loops. Filling defects within these dilated loops are due to impacted meconium in this neonate with meconium ileus.

In the very-low-birth-weight (VLBW) infants, vascular access procedures are amongst the most common indications for radiological intervention and are not without complication.[15]

CONCLUSION

The role of the imaging department and of the pediatric radiologist in the management of the neonatal patient is continuously evolving and expanding. They should be involved as integral members of the *team*. Frequent consultation amongst all carers will avoid inappropriate requests for imaging. It will prevent duplication of examinations and the accumulation of redundant information, thus helping to reduce costs. The application of appropriate imaging techniques will also have the great virtue of reducing the infant's discomfort and morbidity.

REFERENCES

1. Willis CE. Optimizing digital radiography of children. *Eur J Radiol* 2009; 72: 266–73.
2. Gyll C, Blake NS. *Paediatric diagnostic imaging*. London: Heinemann, 1986: 44–62.
3. Narla LD, Hom M, Lofland GK, Moskowitz WB. Evaluation of umbilical catheter and tube placement in premature infants. *Radiographics* 1991; 11: 849–63.
4. Frush DP. Radiation safety. *Pediatr Radiol* 2009; 39(Suppl. 3): 385–90.

5. Pajkrt E, Chitty L. Prenatal sonographic diagnosis of congenital anomalies. In: De Bruyn R (ed). *Pediatric ultrasound: How, why and when.* London: Churchill Livingstone, 2005: 15–38.

6. Teele RL. Cranial ultrasonography. In: Hilton SVW, Edwards DK (eds). *Practical pediatric radiology.* Philadelphia: Saunders, 2006: 183–244.

7. Unsinn KM, Geley T, Freund MC, Gassner I. US of the spinal cord in newborns: Spectrum of normal findings, variants, congenital anomalies, and acquired diseases. *Radiographics* 2000; 20: 923–38.

8. Demian M, Nguyen S, Emil S. Early pyloric stenosis: A case control study. *Pediatr Surg Int* 2009; [epub ahead of print].

9. Rice HE, Frush DP, Farmer D et al. Review of radiation risks from computed tomography: Essentials for the pediatric surgeon. *J Pediatr Surg* 2007; 42: 603–7.

10. Goske MJ, Applegate KE, Boylan J et al. The Image Gently campaign: Working together to change practice. *AJR Am J Roentgenol* 2008; 190: 273–4.

11. Douglas-Escobar M, Weiss MD. Hypoxic-ischemic encephalopathy: A review for the clinician. *JAMA Pediatr* 2015; 169(4): 397–403.

12. Griffiths PD, Bradburn M, Campbell MJ et al. Use of MRI in the diagnosis of fetal brain abnormalities in utero (MERIDIAN): A multicentre, prospective, cohort study. *Lancet* 2017; 389(10068): 538–46.

13. Walz PC, Schroeder JW Jr. Prenatal diagnosis of obstructive head and neck masses and perinatal airway management: The ex utero intrapartum treatment procedure. *Otolaryngol Clin North Am* 2015; 48(1): 191–207.

14. Sidhu M, Coley BD, Goske MJ et al. Image Gently, Step Lightly: Increasing radiation dose awareness in pediatric interventional radiology. *Pediatr Radiol* 2009; 39: 1135–8.

15. Laffan EE, McNamara PJ, Amaral J et al. Review of interventional procedures in the very low birthweight infant (B1.5 kg): Complications, lessons learned and current practice. *Pediatr Radiol* 2009; 39: 781–90.

19

Immune system of the newborn

JUDITH MEEHAN, MURWAN OMER, FIONA O'HARE, DENIS J. REEN, AND ELEANOR J. MOLLOY

INTRODUCTION

The first line of defense against infection is the innate immune system, and activation occurs when a pathogen breaches the host's natural barriers (Figure 19.1).[1] The innate immune system developed before the separation of vertebrates from invertebrates and is the primary immune response for most multicellular organisms.[2] It responds instantaneously to microbes and is composed of both soluble (the alternative and mannan-binding lectin pathways of the complement system, acute phase proteins, and cytokines) and cellular elements (monocytes, macrophages, neutrophils, dendritic cells, and natural killer cells). Careful modulation of the innate immune system is vital to prevent either uncontrolled microbial growth or devastating inflammatory responses with tissue injury, vascular collapse, and multiorgan failure. Neonatal immunological research has concentrated on umbilical cord blood, and there is a paucity of detailed mechanistic research in neonatal postnatal samples due to the smaller blood volumes available. Recent developments in the analysis of microsamples including microarrays and multiplex assays have allowed rapid advances in the understanding of neonatal immunology during early development.

Detection of invading microorganisms is mediated by pattern recognition receptors expressed on the surface of innate immune cells, which recognize structures common to many microbial pathogens and are called pathogen associated molecular patterns (PAMPs). These include endotoxins (lipopolysaccharide: LPS), peptidoglycan, lipoteichoic acid, lipopeptides, flagellin, mannan, and viral RNA, which are essential for survival of the microorganisms and therefore do not undergo major mutations. Pattern recognition receptors have been evolutionarily conserved not to recognize any self-structure. Any receptor that bound to a self-ligand could lead to death of the organism that expressed such a receptor. Therefore, autoimmunity is prevented when the only available recognition system is the innate immune system.[3]

Several intracellular signaling pathways are activated when a PAMP binds to a pattern recognition receptor, resulting in activation of transcription factors (NF-kB, AP-1, Fos, Jun). These transcription factors control the expression of immune response genes and the release of numerous effector molecules, such as cytokines. Cytokines are chemical mediators with an essential role in orchestrating the innate and acquired immune responses to an invading pathogen.[4]

The acquired immune system has evolved relatively recently and is built upon the phylogenetically older innate immune system, by which it is controlled and assisted. The principal mediators of acquired immunity are the highly evolved lymphocytes, which express an enormous array of recombinant receptors, immunoglobulin and T-cell receptors (TCRs). They can recognize any potential pathogen with which the host may come in contact. This response takes from days to weeks to develop optimally. Newborns acquire passive immunity from their mothers by maternally derived IgG crossing the placenta. Transferable maternal immunologic memory is essential for the survival of the fetus, newborn, and infant. Moreover, the attenuation of infection by transferable maternal immunity permits microbial agents to immunize the child under optimal conditions. This provides protection for up to the first 6 months of life at which time neonatal acquired immunity has developed.[5]

The hygiene hypothesis states that exposure to allergens in the environment early in life reduces the risk of developing allergies by boosting immune system activity. Conversely, relatively clean environment in early life would sway the immune system toward allergy-promoting responses. The hygiene hypothesis may explain the rising incidence of allergic diseases and facts such as the lower incidence of allergy in those living on farms or in rural areas (due possibly to more exposure to bacteria); the lower incidence of allergy in younger children of large families

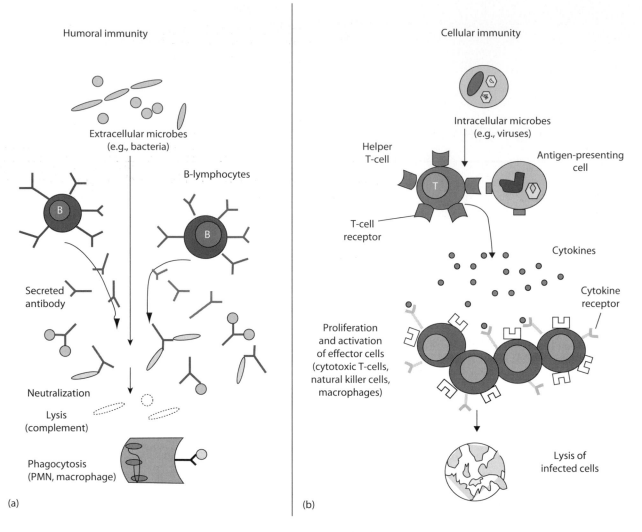

Figure 19.1 Immune function: humoral and cellular immunity. Humoral immunity is mediated by B-lymphocytes, which produce soluble antibody proteins. These antibodies can either **(a)** directly neutralize extracellular microbes or **(b)** activate complement, neutrophils, and macrophages to kill microorganisms. Cellular immunity is mediated by T-lymphocytes. Cytotoxic T-cells directly lyse pathogens. Helper T-cells produce cytokines, which stimulate other immune cells to remove microorganisms.

with three or more older siblings (due perhaps to repeated exposure to infection); and the lower incidence of asthma and wheezing in children attending day care (with more exposure to infections). The hygiene hypothesis, however, cannot explain the higher rates of allergic asthma among poor African Americans in inner city areas.[6,7]

CLINICAL OUTCOMES IN NEONATAL SEPSIS AND INFLAMMATION

Death and long-term complications are common sequelae of bacterial infections in newborns. Neonates undergoing intensive care have infection rates of 25%–50%,[8,9] and mortality has not changed from 15% to 20% over the last 20 years. Altered bactericidal mechanisms are responsible for the increased vulnerability to sepsis in this group and mirror the pattern seen in grossly neutropenic patients.[10] Neutropenia commonly develops in neonatal sepsis in

contrast to the leukocytosis in septic adults.[11] This may be mediated by a decreased neutrophil storage pool and a limited capacity for increased progenitor production in newborns especially preterms.[12]

There is increasing evidence that sepsis and inflammation are important in the pathogenesis of perinatal brain injury. In preterm infants, episodes of sepsis are associated with poorer neurodevelopmental outcomes.[13] In addition, an association between cerebral palsy and maternal peripartum infection in term infants has been well documented.[14] Elevated proinflammatory cytokines have also been demonstrated in retrospectively reviewed dried neonatal blood spots from children aged 3 years with cerebral palsy.[15] Activated leukocytes and infection have been implicated in the pathogenesis of neonatal brain damage.[16] Severe disruption of the blood brain barrier in severe asphyxia may exacerbate neuronal damage[17] allowing infiltration of activated immune cells and cytokines.

NEONATAL INNATE IMMUNITY

Newborns rely on their innate immune system initially following birth as there are deficiencies in the adaptive response due to lack of previous exposure to antigens *in utero*.[7] The intrauterine environment is usually sterile, and transition postnatally to the foreign antigen-rich external world starts with colonization of skin and gut with microorganisms. The fetus is considered to be immunologically naive and exists in a state of immune privilege *in utero* to prevent rejection by the maternal immune cells. The *in utero* defense system is largely unknown, although recent evidence hints at a powerful fetal system of innate immunity.[18] The antibacterial properties of vernix caseosa, the creamy white substance covering the skin of term babies, have also been recognized and in particular the presence of antimicrobial peptides including alpha defensins[19] and inflammatory mediators.[20] Antimicrobial peptides may be an adjunctive compensatory mechanism in the neonate as adaptive immunity evolves.[21] Neonates are immune competent but with a predominant Th2 profile being geared toward immune tolerance instead of toward defense from microbial infections (Th1-skewed).[22] Th1 responses are suppressed by placental products such as progesterone, prostaglandin E2, and cytokines such as IL-4 and IL-10.[23–25]

MONOCYTES

The crucial role of monocytes/macrophages in the immune response resides in their accessory cell and immunoregulatory functions of both humoral and cellular immunity. Human cord blood contains almost three times as many monocytes as adult blood, and major changes occur in the levels of monocytes during the first few weeks of life. Newborn macrophages show poor resistance against facultative intracellular organisms. Newborn monocytes exhibit marked heterogeneity with respect to density. This heterogeneity in density is reflected in functional responses in different populations of newborn monocytes.[26] The densest populations of newborn monocytes appear to have helper function for antibody production, while suppressor function resides in the less dense populations.[27] Neonatal blood monocytes are also characterized as having a much lower frequency of class II molecular expression than adult monocytes, which may be related to the selective incapacity of neonates to secrete significant levels of IFN-γ.[28] The precise role of the monocyte in the newborn's unique susceptibility to infections with various agents remains a challenging area for future study. Dendritic cells are the primary antigen-presenting cells for optimum sensitization of naive T-cells to antigen. Newborn dendritic cells have been shown to be deficient in IL-12 (p35) expression, a key regulator of Th1-type T-cell responses.[29]

The innate immune response relies on cell membrane (Toll-like receptors [TLR]) and intracellular (Nod-like receptors [NLR]) sensors to detect invading microbes. On sensing danger signals, some of the NLR can also trigger the activation of IL-1β by forming a large multiprotein complex called inflammasome.[144] The term inflammasome describes the caspase-activating complex that plays a major role in innate immune responses.[145] The NLRP3 inflammasome components are NLRP3 (NLR family, pyrin domain containing 3), ASC (apoptosis-related speck-like protein containing a caspase recruitment domain [CARD]), and procaspase-1.[146]

Sharma et al.[150] demonstrated crucial tight developmental mechanisms controlling IL-1β production by human monocytes in early gestation. While monocytes from preterm cord blood exhibit limited activation of caspase-1, preterm neonate's ability to secrete IL-1β is comparable to adult levels within 2 weeks postnatally, suggesting rapid maturation of these responses after birth.[150]

Neutrophils

The critical role of the neutrophil in host defenses against microbial infection has long suggested that defects in this particular cell type might be the cause of the increased susceptibility of the newborn to serious bacterial infections. Impaired neonatal neutrophil function at birth has also been implicated in neonatal inflammatory disorders.[11] Recent advances in our understanding of the molecular basis of cell adherence and phagocytosis have provided us with greater insight into the role of the neutrophil in the newborn's defense system. Numerous *in vitro* abnormalities include decreased chemotaxis, leukocyte adherence, bacterial killing, and depressed oxidative metabolism.[30,31] However, most of these neonatal neutrophil functions have been found in cord blood, which contains immature forms of the cells, and therefore care must be taken in interpreting some of the data. Oxidative metabolic function of cord blood monocytes, measured by chemoluminescence, has been shown to be depressed 12–36 hours after birth.[32] Cytoskeletal actin polymerization has also been shown to be altered in neonates.[33]

Decreased adherence of neonatal neutrophils may be caused, at least in part, by the decreased expression of adherence glycoproteins, or by decreased fibronectin content in the plasma membrane of neutrophils.[34] Humoral defects have also been found in neonates, which may help explain the decreased levels of chemotaxis reported in neonatal neutrophils. Such altered humoral factors include decreased levels of complement components and fibronectin.[35,36]

Neonatal neutrophils exhibit normal phagocytosis of opsonized particles as well as particles that required no opsonization. The major opsonic role of neutrophils for the uptake of antibody or complement-coated microorganisms is reflected in their expression of a number of receptors both for antibody (Fc-receptors) and complement (CR receptors). In newborn cord blood, the levels of these receptors are similar to those in adult neutrophils.[37–39] The level of expression of Fc receptors is significantly more upregulated in response to *in vitro* stimuli such as f-met-leu-phe (FMLP) on adult neutrophils compared to newborn neutrophils.[33]

Neonatal neutrophils have diminished function[40] and delayed apoptosis (programmed cell death) compared with adults.[41,42] In addition, neonatal neutrophil LPS responses are altered,[43,44] which may further increase susceptibility to sepsis in this population. The effects of granulocyte colony stimulating factor (GCSF) and granulocyte macrophage colony stimulating factor (GM-CSF) on neonatal neutrophils are altered compared with adults showing that GCSF may improve neutrophil survival, whereas GM-CSF augments function.[45]

Neutrophil extracellular traps (NETs) are lattices of extracellular DNA, chromatin, and antibacterial proteins that mediate extracellular killing of microorganisms and are thought to form via a unique death pathway signaled by nicotinamide adenine dinucleotide phosphate (NADPH) oxidase-generated reactive oxygen species (ROS). Neutrophils from term and preterm infants fail to form NETs when activated by inflammatory agonists—in contrast to leukocytes from healthy adults reflecting a deficit in extracellular bacterial killing.[46]

THE INFLAMMATORY RESPONSE SYNDROMES

One reason for the failure of anti-inflammatory strategies in patients with sepsis may be a change in the syndrome over time (Figure 19.2). Initially, sepsis may be characterized by increases in inflammatory mediators; but as sepsis persists, there is a shift toward an anti-inflammatory immunosuppressive state.[47,48] If the initial insult is sufficiently severe, the proinflammatory response can become intense and lead to a massive systemic inflammatory response syndrome (SIRS) and disrupts homeostasis.[49] If the delay is prolonged and the resolution of inflammation is blocked, the neutrophil[50] has a very high potential for causing extreme damage to healthy tissue due to the concentrated release of ROS and proteases.[51] This then forces the body to produce a massive compensatory anti-inflammatory response syndrome

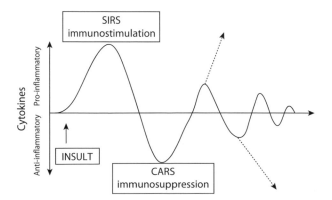

Figure 19.2 Pro-v anti-inflammatory responses. These responses eventually balance to produce homeostasis and recovery. If one or other response predominates, it may increase morbidity and mortality. SIRS: systemic inflammatory response syndrome; CARS: compensatory anti-inflammatory response syndrome.

(CARS) that may be inappropriate and result in tissue injury. If this occurs, the body develops "immune paralysis" and is more susceptible to infection. The final stage occurs when the overwhelming inflammation is not resolved causing multiple organ dysfunction syndrome and death of the patient.[52] Adjunctive immunomodulatory treatments for sepsis seek to balance these responses and restore homeostasis.[52] However, discovering which inflammatory phase is dominant in the patient at a certain time point remains difficult and hinders appropriate therapeutic immunomodulation. Anti-inflammatory treatment can increase mortality. Following a cecal ligation and puncture model of sepsis in a murine model, mortality was increased in mice pretreated with interleukin receptor antagonist (IL-1ra).[53]

Fetal and neonatal inflammatory responses (FIRS and NIRS) have been described. A systemic fetal inflammatory response as determined by increased interleukin-6 is an independent risk factor for severe neonatal morbidity.[54] Preterm neonates with systemic infection have elevated IL-6, IL-10, and TNF-α concentrations. Severe infection is signified by increased IL-10/TNF-α, and IL-6/IL-10 ratios. Transiently elevated IL-10 or IL-10/TNF-α levels are not invariably associated with a poor prognosis.[55]

Toll-like receptors

The TLR provide the critical link between microbial immune stimulants and initiation of host defense. TLR-4 is the transmembrane LPS receptor that initiates the innate immune response to common gram-negative bacteria.[56] Neonates have an equivalent if not enhanced capacity compared with adult white-blood cell TLR-mediated response to support Th17- and Th2-type immunity, which promotes defense against extracellular pathogens. However, neonates have reduced Th1-type responses, which promote defense against intracellular pathogens.[57] TLR-4, TLR-2, and CD14 are increased on neonatal immune cells, and cytokine release is decreased to a greater extent than adults with TLR-4 antagonists.[58] During infections, pathogens bind to TLR-4 and CD14 receptors and induce cytokine release, leading to inflammation. Neonatal IL-10 and TNF-α release depends on LPS binding not only to CD14/TLR-4 but also to CD14 associated with another TLR.[58] There is a differential expression of TLR-2 but not TLR-4 in the course of neonatal sepsis.[59] Although decreased levels of MyD88 have been described in neonatal monocytes in response to LPS,[60] there have been few studies on neonatal neutrophils. Wynn et al.[61] have recently demonstrated improved survival following polymicrobial sepsis induced by TLR-4 agonist pretreatment, which enhanced peritoneal neutrophil recruitment with increased oxidative burst production. Similarly, TLR-7/8 agonism also enhanced peritoneal neutrophil recruitment with increased phagocytic ability. However, these outcomes were independent of the adaptive immune system and type I interferon signaling.[61] Labor upregulates TLR-2 and TLR-4 on cord blood monocytes at the protein level, suggesting that labor may be immunologically beneficial to normal newborns.[62] Augmenting innate immune function using TLR signaling may be a potential future adjunctive therapy in neonatal sepsis.

MUCOSAL IMMUNITY, HUMAN MILK, AND NECROTIZING ENTEROCOLITIS

Although the intestinal tract of the fetus is considered to be sterile, recent studies suggest that many preterm infants are exposed to microbes found in the amniotic fluid, even without a history of rupture of membranes or culture-positive chorioamnionitis.[63] Infants are colonized during vaginal delivery and subsequent breastfeeding with maternal vaginal and fecal flora. The fecal microbial profile of infants delivered vaginally versus caesarean section showed no colonization with *Bacteroides* sp. before 2 months of age in infants in the latter group, and *Bacteroides* colonization that was half that of vaginally delivered infants by 6 months of age.[64] The common use of antibiotics, type of feeding (human milk versus formula), mode of delivery (vaginal versus caesarean section), decreased maternal–infant direct skin contact, and various manipulations in the neonatal intensive care unit (e.g., nursing in an incubator versus under radiant warmers) have the potential to alter the intestinal microbiota.[65] In response to pathogenic intestinal microbiota, proinflammatory cytokines can increase barrier permeability, facilitating bacterial translocation with elaboration of the SIRS and multiple organ failure.[66]

Necrotizing enterocolitis (NEC) is one of the most devastating diseases in newborns. It is associated with loss of gut integrity and immune dysfunction. NEC is also characterized by exaggerated TLR-4 signaling and decreased enterocyte proliferation through unknown mechanisms.[67] Delayed bacterial commensal gut colonization is common in preterm infants in intensive care and tends to render bacterial species virulent. This abnormally upregulates TLR-4 and is associated with activation of NF-kappa-B, promoting the transcription of genes for inflammation, and increased concentrations of inducible nitric oxide synthase, another potent proinflammatory regulator.[68] Increased intestinal expression of TLRs (especially TLR-2 and -4) and cytokines precedes histological injury in the experimental NEC.[69]

There is a dose-related association of human milk feeding with a reduction of risk of NEC or death after the first 2 weeks of life among extremely low birth weight infants.[70] Human milk influences neonatal microbial recognition by modulating TLR-mediated responses specifically and differentially.[71] Fresh human milk contains many immunoprotective factors, such as immunoglobulins (Igs), lactoferrin, neutrophils, lymphocytes, lysozyme, and PAF acetylhydrolase (which inhibits PAF). Human milk also is believed to promote intestinal colonization with *Lactobacillus*. The efficacy of banked human milk is less clear because freezing and pasteurization reduce the cellular components and immunoglobulins.[66]

NEONATAL ADAPTIVE IMMUNE RESPONSE

The adaptive immune system consists of B-cells, T-cells, and their products. T-cells or lymphocyte clones each bears a unique TCR that recognizes peptides, derived from foreign or self-proteins, bound in a molecular complex to the major histocompatibility complex (MHC) proteins on the surface of other cells. T-cells are divided into subsets based on their expression of different proteins, which are assigned cluster differentiation (CD) numbers. Killer T-cells express CD8 and are important to kill virally infected cells. Helper T-cells express CD4 and orchestrate the overall immune response by secreting cytokines and providing costimulatory signals to CD8+ cells and B-cells.

The basis of an adequate immune response resides in the capacity of individual cells of the immune system to recognize and react to the myriad of antigens in the environment. The hemopoietic system of pluripotent stem cells is the source of all the major cell types, which are involved in the immune response. These cells include various lymphocyte subsets, macrophages, natural killer cells, monocytes, and polymorphonuclear leukocytes. These cells are involved in a complex regulatory network of cell interactions, which constitute an immune response, and whose function is to eliminate both self-aberrant molecules and cells, as well as to protect the host from microbial attack (Figure 19.3).

Lymphocyte development occurs along two distinct pathways leading to the production of the two major lymphocyte populations, T-cells and B-cells, which have very different biological effector functions. The thymus is the site of development of T-cells, which are responsible for the range of effector functions collectively termed cell-mediated immunity. Cell-mediated immunity ranges from the release of soluble factors such as cytokines, which regulate the activity of all cells of the immune system, to direct cytopathic effect of cytotoxic lymphocytes on viruses or tumor cells. B-lymphocytes, on the other hand, have a more restricted effector function, confined to the synthesis and secretion of humoral antibodies in each of the immunoglobulin classes, IgG, A, M, D, and E. More recently, B-lymphocytes have been shown to be capable of presenting antigen to T-cells.[72] In man, the site of synthesis of B-lymphocytes is the bone marrow.

The different regulatory and effector functions mediated by cells of the immune system represent the capabilities of populations of cells that can be recognized by the presence of different patterns of expression of cell-surface antigens. The availability of monoclonal antibody reagents for the recognition of lineage, differentiation stage, activation phase, and effector function of different cell types has contributed enormously to our understanding of the extent of heterogeneity of different cell types within the immune system. This heterogeneity of cell types forms the basis for an international leukocyte typing classification system (CD), utilizing monoclonal antibodies that recognize specific cell-surface markers in order to define individual leukocyte subsets.[73]

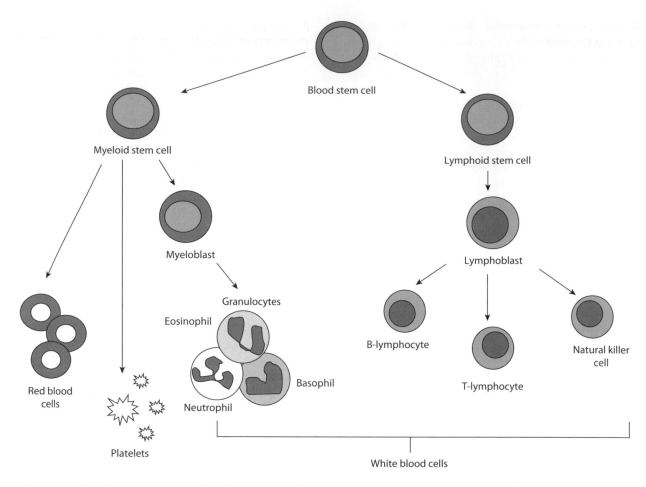

Figure 19.3 Blood cell development. Blood stem cells released from the bone marrow develop into mature blood cells over time. The blood stem cell may become a myeloid stem cell or a lymphoid stem cell. The myeloid stem can further differentiate into either red blood cells, white blood cells, or platelets. The lymphoid stem cell becomes a lymphoblast, which then differentiates into one of the following lymphocyte types: B-lymphocyte, T-lymphocyte, or natural killer cell.

The more widely used CD antigens, for classifying immune effector cell types, are described in Table 19.1.

It is now well established that T-lymphocytes do not recognize native antigen on any pathogen, but rather a processed form of the antigen, in association with self-major histocompatibility antigens (MHCs), or class I (HLA-A,B,C) or class II (HLA-DR/Ia) molecules.[74,75] This important processing of foreign antigen is carried out by one of a group of antigen-presenting cells which include macrophages, dendritic cells, Kupffer cells, and some B-cells. The proper functioning of these accessory cells is therefore as central to an adequate immune response as that of specific effector cells, such as the T-lymphocytes. When antigen becomes localized and processed by the antigen-presenting cell (APC), the complex interaction of APC, T-cells, and B-cells begins, which eventually leads to specific immunological memory, both of T-cells and B-cells, as well as to antibody production. Although B-cells can be directly activated by antigen, under experimental conditions, concomitant activation of T-cells is required for the clonal expansion of antigen-specific B-cells, leading to the generation of long-lived memory B-cells and immunoglobulin-secreting plasma cells.[76,77] In spite of their precipitous encounter with the environment, newborn infants cannot readily mount T helper type 1 (TH1) cell antibacterial and antiviral responses. Instead, they show skewing toward TH2 responses, which, together with immunoregulatory functions, are thought to limit the potential for inflammatory damage, while simultaneously permitting intestinal colonization by commensals. However, these collective capabilities account for relatively few T-cells.

T-cell responses

Several studies in the literature have questioned the stage of maturity of circulating lymphocytes in the newborn. Some parameters of T-cell function in cord blood, however, have been shown to be normal or similar to those of healthy older children. These include the quantity and proportion of T-lymphocytes,[78] lymphocyte response to mitogens,[79] and production of certain cytokines such as IL-2.[80] However, other newborn cellular immune functions have been reported to be depressed. These include PHA-induced cytotoxicity, lymphotoxin production, as well as reduced cAMP

Table 19.1 Cell surface antigens that identify leukocyte subtypes in the newborn

Antigen	Function
T-Cells	
CD2	LFA-3 receptor (adhesion)
CD3	Associated with cell receptor
CD4	Class II and HIV receptor
CD5	Costimulatory
CD7	Unknown
CD8	Class I receptor
B-Cells	
CD19	Signal transduction
CD20	Unknown
CD21	C3d and EBV receptor (CR2)
CD72	Ligand for CD5
NK Cells	
CD16	IgG receptor (FcRIII)
CD56	Isoform of N-CAM
CD94	Unknown
Myeloid/Monocytic Cells	
C14	Unknown
C15	Unknown
CD32	IgG receptor (FcRII)
CD35	C3b receptor (CRI)

levels.[81–83] The overall characteristic that distinguishes newborn T-cells from other T-cells at different stages of development is that they are recent thymic emigrants, not long after exiting the thymus.

Lymphocyte phenotype

There has been a reported incidence of up to 25% of cord blood lymphocytes coexpressing both CD4 helper T-cell and CD8 suppressor T-cell surface markers.[84] Cells of this double positive phenotype are common in the thymus, where they are considered to be the precursors of mature helper and suppressor T-cells. However, more recently, using more sensitive flow cytometry-based analytical techniques, workers investigating cord blood samples failed to detect the presence of doubly labelled CD4/CD8-labelled cells.[85] Other markers of an immature phenotype of newborn T-cells have been described. The CD38 antigen, which is a marker of immature thymus-derived T-cells, as well as activated lymphocytes, is present in the majority of newborn cord blood lymphocytes.[86] This thymocyte-like membrane phenotype can be modulated by the influence of thymic hormones *in vitro*.[87] In addition to the presence of CD38 thymocyte-associated antigen, human cord blood contains T-cells of the unusual phenotype, which include peanut agglutinin-positive/CD8-positive as well as some CD3-positive and CD1a-positive lymphocytes.[88] Like CD38, CD1a is a marker

present on early thymocytes.[88] CD1a-positive cells are especially present in preterm and antenatally stressed infants.[89] While the neonate has adequate numbers of CD4 helper T-cells, cord blood T-cells are deficient in their ability to provide help for antibody production, probably at the level of altered cytokine production.[90,91] The cellular basis for this functional defect is reflected in other phenotypic markers of functional activity. More than 90% of cord blood T-cells carry the CD45RA+ "virgin" cell phenotype marker, compared with 50% of adult T-cells, which express CD45RA+.[86] In contrast, less than 10% of cord blood lymphocytes express the CD45RA "memory" T-cell marker compared to a 50% level of expression in adult T-cells.[92] This major imbalance in the ratio of CD45RA+/CD45RA, CD4-positive T-cells in the newborn compared to adults may help explain some of the functional differences of newborn cells compared to adult lymphocytes.

A major T-cell effector function in human newborns is interleukin-8 (CXCL8) production, which may activate antimicrobial neutrophils and γδ T-cells. CXCL8 production was provoked by antigen receptor engagement of T-cells that are distinct from those few cells producing TH1, TH2, and TH17 cytokines, and was costimulated by TLR signaling. This was present in preterm infants especially those with neonatal infections and severe morbidities.[151] However, CXCL8-producing T-cells are infrequently found in adults, and no equivalent function was evident in neonatal mice. CXCL8 production counters the widely held view that T-lymphocytes in very early life are intrinsically anti-inflammatory, with implications for immune monitoring, immune interventions (including vaccination), and immunopathologies. This also highlights the qualitative differences among adult, cord, and neonatal immune function. Regulatory factors contributing to the differences in functional activity and the different phenotypic profiles of newborn T-cells compared to adults require further investigation in order to arrive at a fuller understanding of the mechanisms involved and using actual neonatal postnatal samples rather than cord blood.

B-cell responses

The newborn's capacity to produce antibody is significantly reduced, both quantitatively and qualitatively, compared to that of an adult. Newborn B-lymphocytes poorly differentiate into immunoglobulin-producing cells.[93,94] The mechanisms controlling this aspect of B-cell immunocompetence in the newborn are unknown. Many studies have focused on the ability of cord blood lymphocytes to terminally differentiate into IgG-, IgA-, and IgM-producing plasma cells in response to mitogens. However, a delay occurs in B-cell differentiation, resulting in decreased production of plasma cells, markedly diminishing the secretion of antibody, and restriction of secreted antibody to IgM isotype.[95] Cord blood B-lymphocytes, unlike adult B-cells, usually are unable to differentiate into immunoglobulin plaque-forming cells when cultured with pokeweed mitogen alone, or with killed *Staphylococcus aureus* Cowan 1 alone.[96] However, it appears that these two stimuli can act synergistically to induce a significant *in vitro* plaque-forming cell response in cord blood B-cells.

The relative inadequacy of IgG and IgA antibody synthesis cannot be attributed to the lack of precursor B-cells, since lymphocytes bearing these immunoglobulin classes on the surface are present in the fetus and on cord blood B-cells.[97,98] The impaired capacity to undergo IgG or IgA synthesis has been attributed to immaturity of cord blood B-cells, since their activation by polyclonal activators, like pokeweed mitogen, LPS, or Epstein–Barr virus, generally results in moderate or reduced levels of IgM synthesis with no IgA, IgG, or IgE production.[94] However, the question of T-cell immaturity as a significant factor in the restricted immunoglobulin isotype production of cord blood B-cells has to be taken into account.[99,100] Cord blood mononuclear cells produce normal levels of IgE *in vitro*, when cultured in the presence of IL-4, indicating that the B-cells are mature in their capacity to switch to IgE-producing cells.[99] The defect observed may be associated with the failure of cord blood T-cells to produce detectable levels of IL-4, which has been shown to be responsible for induction of IgE synthesis, both *in vitro* and *in vivo*.[100] An inadequacy of newborn T-cell help for plasma cell isotype switching to IgG and IgA immunoglobulin-producing cells is also suggested by the observation that IgG and IgA antibody responses are more dependent upon T-cell help than are IgM responses. In a series of experiments, coculturing adult T-cells and newborn T-cells with adult or newborn B-cells, the addition of adult T-cells greatly enhanced the pokeweed mitogen-driven responses of newborn mononuclear cells, which included IgG and IgA responses.[94,101] Cord blood T-cells, however, did not show augmentation of B-cell differentiation when cocultured with non-T-cells from adults. These data, looked at collectively, would indicate that deficient T-cell function as well as possible deficiencies of B-cell function exist in the newborn. The defect in immunoglobulin production may also be contributed, of course, by suppressor T-cell activity of newborn lymphocytes or even by enhanced suppressor activity of newborn monocytes. The newborn also possesses a major population of CD5-positive[94] B-cells, which are only commonly found in patients with autoimmune diseases. It appears that these cells, in the newborn, uniquely express the activation antigens 4F2 and CD25.[102] The significance of these activated CD5-positive B-lymphocytes is, however, unclear. A particular function of these cells is the production of natural polyspecific autoantibodies.[103] A possible role for these cells in the newborn may therefore be the influencing of emerging B-cell specificities. Preterm infants are susceptible to viral infection, and this is associated with impaired Toll-like receptor-3 and -7 expression on gamma delta cells compared with term babies, and they failed to optimize cytokine production in response to coincident TCR and TLR agonists.[104]

IMMUNOGLOBULINS

The presence of physiological hypogammaglobulinemia has been noted by several investigators in preterm and term infants. Neonates have low levels of IgA and IgM immunoglobulins because of the poor ability of these immunoglobulin classes to cross the placenta.[105] Furthermore, all IgG subclasses are not equally transferred across the placenta, especially the IgG2 and IgG_4 subclass levels, which are therefore also relatively low in the newborn.[54] The neonate is consequently very susceptible to pyogenic bacterial infections since most of the antibodies that opsonize capsular polysaccharide antigens of pyogenic bacteria are contained in the IgG2 subclass and IgM immunoglobulin subfraction. Neonates, even during overwhelming sepsis, do not produce type-specific antibodies.[57,106] This impairment in antibody production appears to be secondary to the defect in the differentiation of B-lymphocytes into immunoglobulin-secreting plasma cells and T-lymphocyte-mediated facilitation of antibody synthesis. There is a marked limitation in infant antibody responses to most bacterial capsular polysaccharides.[107] This limitation prevents successful infant immunization with Hib polysaccharide vaccines,[108] which fortunately can be circumvented by use of conjugate vaccines shown to be immunogenic in infants.[109]

CYTOKINES

Among the major molecular components of the immune system are the immunoglobulins, cytokines, and proteins of the acute phase response and complement system. The term "cytokine" is used to describe a group of peptides with potent immunoregulatory effects, which are produced and utilized by individual cells of the immune system, to communicate with each other and to control the environment in which they operate. A description of some of the major characterized cytokines is listed in Table 19.2.

Cytokines are of immense importance in controlling both local and systemic immune responses, inflammation, and the regulation of hematopoiesis.[110,111] Their most important function appears to be at the local level, modulating the behavior of adjacent cells in a paracrine fashion,[111] or the cells that secrete them, in an autocrine fashion.[112] In addition, especially in the case of TNF-α, IL-1, and IL-6, cytokines may effect endocrine-like activity on distant organs or tissues.[113] Cytokines have important biological activity, which can be of major clinical benefit, such as stimulation of antimicrobial function, promotion of wound healing, and myelostimulation.[114,115] With such diverse biological function, an exaggerated or prolonged secretion of these peptides may be detrimental for the host. Specifically, aberrant secretion of cytokines, such as TNF-α and IL-1, is thought to be responsible for the hemodynamic changes in the host during septic shock and in cachexia of chronic disease.[116,117] The availability of recombinant DNA techniques to produce cytokines in almost unlimited quantities and the production of specific antagonists such as soluble cytokine

Table 19.2 Cytokines

Name	Principal cellular source	Principal cellular target
IL-1α+β	Macrophages, fibroblasts, endothelial cells	Thymocytes, endothelial cells, neutrophils, T-cells, B-cells
IL-2	T-cells	T-cells, B-cells
IL-3	T-cells	Multipotential stem cells
IL-4	T helper cells	T-cells, B-cells, mast cells, macrophages
IL-5	T helper cells	B-cells, eosinophils
IL-6	Fibroblasts	B-cells, fibroblasts, hepatocytes
IL-7	Stromal cells	B-cells
IL-8	Macrophages	Neutrophils
IL-10	T-cells, activated monocytes	T-cell subsets, macrophages
IL-12	Macrophages	T-cells, NK cells
IL-13	T helper cells	B-cells
TNF	Macrophages, fibroblasts	Many cell types
TNF	T-cells	Many cell types
IFN	Macrophages, fibroblasts	Many cell types
IFN	Fibroblasts	Many cell types
IFN	T-cells, NK cells	Macrophages, T-cells, B-cells
TGF	T-cells, macrophages, platelets	Many cell types
GM-CSF	T-cells, endothelial cells	Multipotential stem cells

receptors and IL-1 receptor antagonists are leading to new and exciting therapeutic potential for these molecules.

Chronic lung disease may be associated with impairment in the transition from the innate immune response mediated by neutrophils to the adaptive immune response mediated by T-lymphocytes. The Neonatal Research Network of the National Institute of Child Health and Human Development recruited 1062 extremely low birth weight infants of whom 606 infants developed chronic lung disease or died. On the basis of results from all models combined, bronchopulmonary dysplasia/death was associated with higher concentrations of interleukin 1beta, 6, 8, and 10 and interferon gamma, and lower concentrations of interleukin 17, regulated on activation, normal T-cell expressed and secreted, and tumor necrosis factor beta.[118]

IMMUNOMODULATION

Neonates especially those preterms are particularly vulnerable to sepsis. Transplacental transfer of immunoglobulins from the mother to the fetus occurs after 32 weeks of gestation, and endogenous production commences at a few months of age. Administration of intravenous immunoglobulin provides IgG that can bind to cell surface receptors, provide opsonic activity, activate complement, promote antibody-dependent cytotoxicity, and improve neutrophilic chemoluminescence. Term neonates have low type-specific antibody and opsonin deficiencies.[39,119,120] Preterm neonates also have severe hypogammaglobulinemia[121] and deficient complement activity.[122,123]

Theoretically infectious morbidity and morbidity could be reduced by the administration of intravenous immunoglobulin (IVIG). Meta-analysis of small trials has suggested that IVIG may reduce the rate of neonatal death, but the Cochrane review could not recommend routine use of prophylaxis against nosocomial infections or for treatment in proven or suspected infection.[124,125] The International Neonatal Immunotherapy Study (INIS) was an international multicenter randomized controlled trial (RCT) studying the use of nonspecific IVIG in addition to antibiotics in babies with suspected or proven sepsis. This study was designed to confirm or refute the hypothesis that IVIG reduces the rate of mortality and major morbidity.[126] At 113 hospitals in nine countries, infants were enrolled if receiving antibiotics for suspected or proven serious infection (n = 3493) and randomly assigned to receive two infusions of either polyvalent IgG immune globulin or matching placebo 48 hours apart. There was no significant between-group difference in the rates of the primary outcome (death or major disability at 2 years of age), which occurred in 686 of 1759 infants (39%) who received IVIG and in 677 of 1734 infants (39%) who received placebo (relative risk: 1.00; 95% confidence interval [0.92–1.08]). Similarly, there were no significant differences in the rates of secondary outcomes, including the incidence of subsequent sepsis episodes. Therapy with IVIG had no effect on the outcomes of suspected or proven neonatal sepsis.[141]

The recently updated Cochrane review of IVIG for suspected or proven infection in neonates including nine studies of 3973 infants showed no reduction in mortality during hospital stay, or death or major disability at 2 years of age in infants with suspected or proven infection,[153] and therefore treatment with IVIG in this context was not recommended.

Infants with chylothorax postoperatively especially post-cardiothoracic surgery with prolonged, large-volume chyle loss have greater secondary immunodeficiency. Treatment with immunoglobulin is often used in this group of patients, although there is a paucity of detailed studies in this area, and Hoskote et al.[152] did not find any differences in infectious outcomes using IVIG.

COLONY STIMULATING FACTORS AND OTHER IMMUNOMODULATORY AGENTS

Neonates often become neutropenic when septic and therefore the use of GCSF and GM-CSF has been studied on this population. The Cochrane meta-analysis of trials has found no significant improvement in outcome when CSFs were used for prophylaxis or treatment of sepsis.[127]

The PROGRAMS Multicentre RCT of Prophylactic GM-CSF to Reduce Systemic Sepsis in Preterm Neonates included 280 infants <31 weeks. When GM-CSF 10 μg/kg/day was administered prophylactically for 5 days, neutrophil counts were higher on days 3–12 than controls. There were no significant differences in sepsis-free survival in infants who are neutropenic at recruitment, the number of infants experiencing one or more episodes of culture-positive sepsis, or survival to discharge. GM-CSF rapidly corrected neutropenia in preterm, growth-restricted neonates. Prophylactic GM-CSF and correction of neutropenia, even when severe, did not reduce sepsis or all-cause mortality.[128] Kuhn et al.[129] recently described a multicenter, randomized, double-blind, placebo-controlled trial of the prophylactic use of GCSF in neutropenic preterm infants <32 weeks (n = 200) and found no differences in survival free of confirmed infection for 4 weeks after treatment with either rG-CSF (10 mg/kg/day) or placebo for 3 days. However, activated leukocytes may mediate neonatal brain injury.[16] GM-CSF stimulates neonatal neutrophil activation unlike GCSF, and both prolong neutrophil survival.[45] The 2 year developmental outcomes of the PROGRAMS trial showed no improvement in neurodevelopmental or health outcomes at 2 or 5 years after prophylactic administration of GM-CSF.[142] This cohort of babies had lower developmental scores than expected for gestation. The suggestion of worse respiratory outcomes in the GM-CSF group at 2 years was replicated at 5 years.[155]

The 2003 Cochrane review of CSFs in neonatal sepsis included seven treatment studies of 257 infants and three prophylactic studies of 359 infants. The limited data suggesting that CSF treatment may reduce mortality when systemic infection is accompanied by severe neutropenia should be investigated further in adequately powered trials that recruit sufficient infants infected with organisms associated with a significant mortality risk. However, this has not yet been updated with recent trials.[127] APC (drotrecogin alfa [activated]) decreased death from any cause in patients with sepsis (absolute reduction in RR 6.1%), and there was 1 additional life saved for every 16 patients treated. There was a decrease in coagulopathy (D-dimers) and inflammation

(IL-6).[130] The RESOLVE (Researching Severe Sepsis and Organ Dysfunction in Children: A Global Perspective) trial evaluated sepsis for safety, pharmacokinetics, and pharmacodynamics of drotrecogin alfa (activated) in children with severe sepsis.[131] The patients ranged from term newborn to 18 years and similar pharmacokinetic profiles, effects on D-dimer levels, other coagulation parameters, and bleeding rates to PROWESS, although there was more gram-negative sepsis.

Pentoxifylline is a phosphodiesterase inhibitor and immunomodulatory agent. Pammi et al. recently updated the Cochrane review of pentoxyfylline for treatment of sepsis and NEC in neonates. They included six trials and 416 participants and found low-quality evidence suggesting that it could be used as an adjunct to antibiotics in neonatal sepsis and decreased mortality without any adverse effects.[156]

Lactoferrin, a normal component of human colostrum and milk, can enhance host defense and may be effective in the prevention of sepsis and NEC in preterm neonates. The recent Cochrane review of this subject included four RCTs, and evidence of moderate to low quality suggests that oral lactoferrin prophylaxis with or without probiotics decreases late-onset sepsis and NEC stage II or greater in preterm infants without adverse effects. Ongoing lactoferrin trials will provide evidence from more than 6000 preterm neonates and may clarify optimum dosing regimens, type of lactoferrin (human or bovine), and long-term outcomes.[156]

PREBIOTICS AND PROBIOTICS

Prebiotics are unique oligosaccharides that are not absorbed but facilitate colonization by probiotic organisms (bifidobacteria and lactic acid-producing bacteria). Use of probiotics has been shown to decrease the duration and severity of rotavirus-induced diarrhea, allergies to cow milk protein, atopic dermatitis, and some inflammatory intestinal diseases. A relative reduction in the risk of NEC, late-onset sepsis, and mortality has been demonstrated with probiotics (*Bifidobacterium infantis*, *Streptococcus thermophilus*, and *Bifidobacterium bifidum* in one study and *Lactobacillus acidophilus* and *B. infantis* in another).[131,132] A multicenter, double-blind, randomized, controlled trial of the probiotics *B. bifidum* and *L. acidophilus* showed a lower incidence of NEC in the study group than controls; but sepsis was more frequent in the study group,[133] although this difference was not significant on multivariate analyses and none of the affected patients developed sepsis with organisms used as probiotics. There are persistent concerns about the use of probiotics in immunosuppressed infants as there have been reports of preterm infants who had short gut syndrome developing *Lactobacillus* bacteremia while receiving this probiotic bacterium.[134] In adults, another multicenter, double-blind, randomized, controlled trial of probiotics to reduce infections in pancreatitis showed a more than twofold increase in mortality and no reduction in infections.[135] In addition to these immediate concerns about sepsis, the long-term effects of the use of probiotics, especially in preterm infants in terms of immune modulation in later life, development of immune disorders (such as insulin resistance, diabetes, obesity, and cancer), and neurodevelopmental outcomes are not known. In a recent multicenter, randomized controlled phase 3 study, The Probiotics in Preterm Infants Study Collaborative Group (the PIPS trial), infants born between 23 and 30 weeks gestational age were recruited within 48 hours of birth from 24 hospitals in southeast England. Infants were randomly assigned (1:1) to probiotic or placebo via a minimization algorithm randomization program. The probiotic intervention was *Bifidobacterium breve* BBG-001 suspended in dilute elemental infant formula given enterally in a daily dose of 8.2 to 9.2 $\log_{10}$ CFU; the placebo was dilute infant formula alone. Clinicians and families were masked to allocation. The primary outcomes were NEC (Bell stage 2 or 3), blood culture positive sepsis more than 72 hours after birth, and death before discharge from hospital.

Between July 1, 2010 and July 31, 2013, 1315 infants were recruited of whom 654 were allocated to probiotic and 661 to placebo. Five infants had consent withdrawn after randomization; thus, 650 were analyzed in the probiotic group and 660 in the placebo group. Rates of the primary outcomes did not differ significantly between the probiotic and placebo groups; 61 infants (9%) in the probiotic group had NEC compared with 66 (10%) in the placebo group (adjusted risk ratio 0.93 [95% CI 0.68–1.27]); 73 (11%) infants in the probiotics group had sepsis compared with 77 (12%) in the placebo group (0.97 [0.73–1.29]); and 54 (8%) deaths occurred before being discharged home in the probiotic group compared with 56 (9%) in the placebo group (0.93 [0.67–1.30]). No probiotic-associated adverse events were reported.[143]

The recent Cochrane review that predates the PIPS trial included 24 trials and concluded that enteral supplementation of probiotics prevented severe NEC and all-cause mortality in preterm infants. They strongly supported a change in practice.[157] However, there is a need for comparative studies to assess the most effective preparations, timing, and length of therapy to be utilized. This is especially valid in view of the negative results of the PIPS trial.

IMMUNE DEFICIENCY DISEASES IN THE NEWBORN

Although there are many forms of primary immunodeficiency in the newborn, there are several well-described clinical conditions, two of which we will mention in this chapter. Di George's syndrome (DGS) usually involves a hemizygous microdeletion in the chromosome 22q11.2 region characterized by the triad of conotruncal cardiac anomaly, thymic hypoplasia, and hypocalcemia. The syndrome encompasses a broad spectrum of congenital defects that have varying degrees of severity especially in the degree of immunodeficiency, and the incidence is 1 in 4000 births. Only <1% of patients have severe immunodeficiency, but early identification is essential to prevent and

treat life-threatening infections and to plan for immune reconstitution. Immunodeficient DGS patients present with profoundly decreased T-cell numbers (<50/mm³), depressed T-cell function (as measured by lymphocyte proliferation assays, such as with mitogens), and often concomitantly low Ig levels. These patients are at high risk for the development of disseminated and life-threatening infections with organisms that require an intact cell-mediated immune system for eradication, such as cytomegalovirus, adenovirus, or *Pneumocystis jiroveci* (formerly *Pneumocystis carinii*). Graft-versus-host disease also may be found due to transplacental transfer and engraftment of maternal T-cells, leading to the typical rash and diarrhea seen in other forms of graft-versus-host disease.[137]

Severe combined immunodeficiency (SCID) is a primary immune deficiency with a severe defect in both the T- and B-lymphocyte systems resulting in serious infections within the first few months of life. Newborn screening for SCID is advancing toward pilot trials as early diagnosis improves outcomes and facilitates bone marrow transplantation.[138] Persistent lymphopenia or leucopenia and recurrent infections in neonates warrant further investigation and immunology and infectious disease involvement.

NEONATAL AUTOINFLAMMATORY DISORDERS

Cryopyrin-associated periodic syndromes (CAPS) are a spectrum of autoinflammatory disorders; milder forms include familial cold autoinflammatory syndrome and Muckle–Wells syndrome, while the most severe form is represented by neonatal-onset multisystem inflammatory disease (NOMID), also known as chronic infantile neurologic, cutaneous, and arthritis.[159] CAPS results from gain-of-function mutations in the gene coding for NLRP3, a key component of NLRP3 inflammasome, which precipitates an overproduction of IL-1 beta.[149]

NOMID is essentially a clinical diagnosis, and a genetic diagnosis confirms the presence of NLRP3 germline missense mutations in approximately 60% of patients, while somatic mosaicism accounts for up to two thirds of the remainder (40%).[160–162] NOMID is characterized by persistent inflammation and tissue damage primarily affecting the nervous system, eyes, skin, and joints; patients present within the first few weeks of life with urticarial rash, followed by recurrent episodes of fever, arthropathy, and neurological manifestation such as chronic aseptic meningitis, raised intracranial pressure, cerebral atrophy, mental retardation, and seizures. Other clinical presentations include hepatosplenomegaly, eye inflammation, progressive hearing impairment, bony overgrowth, and short stature.[159–163]

The study of patients with NOMID demonstrated the role of IL1-β overproduction in precipitating inflammation-mediated organ damage and the subsequent resolution of symptoms and end-organ damage prevention with IL-1 blockade.[149,158]

CONCLUSION

In fetal and neonatal life, many aspects of the immune system are different to older children and adults. The molecular and cellular basis for these abnormalities, while partially explained by many of the observations described in this chapter, remains relatively unclear. The prospects for more specific and selective immunological intervention as part of the treatment of the immunocompromised neonate undergoing surgery will benefit enormously from ongoing research into the biological basis of immuno-incompetence of the newborn.

Designing new drugs to neutralize microbial products or block their interaction with a specific receptor on immune cells is an attractive concept.[139] Potential targets include LPS binding protein, CD14, TLR-4, and MD-2 for gram-negative sepsis, and CD14, TLR-2, and TLR-6 for gram-positive sepsis. Monoclonal antibodies against CD14 are being evaluated in phase II studies. Several intracellular signaling molecules such as MyD88 and the mitogen-activated protein kinase are other possible therapeutic targets. However, inactivating molecules that are pivotal to innate immunity can be harmful, as shown by the increased sensitivity to bacterial sepsis in mice with mutations of the Tlr4 gene.[140] Careful selection of patients with severe infections associated with a high probability of death will therefore be essential.

REFERENCES

1. Janeway Jr CA, Medzhitov R. Innate immune recognition. *Annu Rev Immunol* 2002; 20:197–216.
2. Kimbrell DA, Beutler B. The evolution and genetics of innate immunity. *Nat Rev Genet* 2001 Apr; 2(4):256–67.
3. Janeway CA. How the immune system works to protect the host from infection: A personal view. *Proc Natl Acad Sci USA* 2001; 98:7461–8.
4. Calandra T. Pathogenesis of septic shock: Implications for prevention and treatment. *J Chemother* 2001; 13:173–80.
5. Zinkernagel RM. Maternal Antibodies, Childhood Infections, and Autoimmune Diseases. *N Engl J Med* 2001; 345:1331–5.
6. Vassallo MF, Walker WA. Neonatal microbial flora and disease outcome. *Nestle Nutr Workshop Ser Pediatr Program* 2008; 61:211–24.
7. Levy O. Innate immunity of the newborn: Basic mechanisms and clinical correlates. *Nat Rev Immunol* 2007 May; 7(5):379–90.
8. Stoll BJ, Hansen N, Fanaroff AA, Wright LL, Carlo WA, Ehrenkranz RA, Lemons JA, Donovan EF, Stark AR, Tyson JE, Oh W, Bauer CR, Korones SB, Shankaran S, Laptook AR, Stevenson DK, Papile LA, Poole WK. Changes in pathogens causing early-onset sepsis in very-low-birth-weight infants. *NEJM* 2002; 347(4):240–7.
9. Fanaroff AA, Martin RJ. *Neonatal-Perinatal Medicine: Diseases of the fetus and infant*, 7th edn. St Louis: Mosby, 2002; 407.
10. Stoll BJ, Gordon T, Korones SB et al. Early-onset sepsis in very low birth weight neonates: A report from the National Institutes of Child Health and Human Development Neonatal Research Network. *J Pediatr* 1996; 129:72–80.
11. Cairo MS. Neonatal neutrophil host defense. Prospects for immunologic enhancement during neonatal sepsis. *Am J Dis Child* 1989 Jan; 143(1):40–6.
12. Carr R, Huizinga TW. Low soluble FcRIII receptor demonstrates reduced neutrophil reserves in preterm neonates. *Arch Dis Child Fetal Neonatal Ed* 2000 Sep; 83(2):F160.
13. Stoll BJ, Hansen NI, Adams-Chapman I, Fanaroff AA, Hintz SR, Vohr B, Higgins RD. National Institute of Child Health and Human Development Neonatal Research Network. Neurodevelopmental and growth impairment among extremely low-birth-weight infants with neonatal infection. *JAMA* 2004 Nov 17; 292(19):2357–65.
14. Nelson KB, Willoughby RE. Infection, inflammation and cerebral palsy. *Curr Opin Neurol* 2000; 13:133–9.
15. Nelson KB, Dambrosia JM, Grether JK, Phillips TM. Neonatal cytokines and coagulation factors in children with cerebral palsy. *Ann Neurol* 1998; 44(4):665–75.
16. Dammann O, Durum S, Leviton A. Do white cells matter in white matter damage? *Trends Neurosci* 2001 Jun; 24(6):320–4.
17. Kumar A, Mittal R, Khanna HD, Basu S. Free radical injury and blood brain barrier permeability in hypoxic-ischaemic encephalopathy. *Pediatrics* 2008 Sep; 122(3):e722–7.
18. Zasloff M. Vernix, the newborn and innate defense. *Pediatr Res* 2003; 53:203–4.
19. Yoshio H, Tollin M, Gudmundsson GH, Lagercrantz H, Jornvall H, Marchini G, Agerbeth B. Antimicrobial polypeptides of human vernix caseosa and amniotic fluid: Implications for the newborn innate defense. *Pediatr Res* 2003; 53:211–6.
20. Davis JR, Miller HS, Feng JD. Vernix caseosa peritonitis: Report of two cases with antenatal onset. *Am J Clin Pathol* 1998; 109:320–3.
21. Dorschner RA, Lin KH, Murakami M, Gallo RL. Neonatal skin in mice and humans expresses increased levels of antimicrobial peptides: Innate immunity during development of the adaptive response. *Pediatr Res* 2003 Apr; 53(4):566–72.
22. Morein B, Abusugra I, Blomqvist G. Immunity in neonates. *Vet Immunol Immunopathol* 2002; 87:207–13.
23. Wegmann TG, Lin H, Guilbert L, Mosmann TR. Bidirectional cytokine interactions in the maternal-fetal relationship is successful pregnancy a TH2 phenomenon? *Immunol Today* 1993; 14:353–6.

24. Sacks GP, Studena K, Sargent K, Redman CW. Normal pregnancy and preeclampsia both produce inflammatory changes in peripheral blood leukocytes akin to those of sepsis. *Am J Obstet Gynecol* 1998; 179(1):80–6.

25. Rukavina D, Pdack ER. Abundant perforin expression at the maternal-fetal interface: Guarding the semiallogeneic transplant? *Immunol Today* 2000; 21:160–3.

26. Mills EL. Mononuclear phagocyte in the newborn: Their relation to the state of relative immunodeficiency. *Am J Pediatr Haematol Oncol* 1983; 5:189–98.

27. Khansari N, Fuiderberg HH. Functional heterogeneity of human cord blood monocytes. *Scand J Immunol* 1984; 19:337–42.

28. Byson YJ, Winter HS, Gardm SE et al. Deficiency of immune interferon production by leukocytes of normal newborns. *Cell Immunol* 1980; 58:191–206.

29. Sztein MB, Steeg PS, Stiehm R et al. Modulation of human cord blood monocyte DR antigen expression in vitro by lymphokines and interferons. In: Oppenheim JJ, Cohen S (eds). *Interleukins, Lymphokines and Cytokines*. New York: Academic Press, 1983:299–305.

30. Beltas S, Goetza B, Spere CP. Decreased adherence, chemotaxis and phagocytic activities of neutrophils from pre-term neonates. *Acta Paediatr Scand* 1990; 79:1031–8.

31. Anderson DC, Huges BJ, Edwards MS et al. Impaired chemotaxigenesis by Type III group B streptococci in neonatal sera: Relationship to diminished concentration of specific anticapsular antibody and abnormalities. *Pediatr Res* 1983; 17:496–520.

32. Miels EI, Thompson T, Bjorksten B et al. The chemiluminescence response and bactericidal activity of polymorphonuclear neutrophils from newborns and their mothers. *Paediatrics* 1979; 63:429–34.

33. Hilmo A, Howard TH. F-actin content of neonate and adult neutrophils. *Blood* 1987; 69:429–949.

34. Anderson DC, Becker-Freeman KL, Herdt, B. Abnormal stimulated adherence of neonatal granulocytes: Impaired induction of surface Mac-1 by chemotactic factors and secretagogues. *Blood* 1987; 70:740–50.

35. Thonson U, Trudsson L, Gustavis B. Complement components in 100 newborns and their mothers determined by electro-immunoassays. *Acta Path Microbiol Scand Immunol C* 1983; 91:148–50.

36. Gerdes JS, Douglas SD, Kolski GB et al. Decreased fibronectin biosynthesis by human cord blood mononuclear phagocyte in vitro. *J Leuk Biol* 1984; 34:91–9.

37. Fleit HB. Fc and complement receptor (CR1 and CR3) expression on neonatal human polymorphonuclear leukocytes. *Biol Neonate* 1989; 55:156–63.

38. Smith JB, Cambell EE, Ludomirsky A et al. Expression of the complement receptors CR1 and CR3 and the type III Fcγ receptor on neutrophils from newborn infants and from newborn infants and from fetuses with Rh disease. *Pediatr Res* 1990; 28:120–6.

39. Carr R. Neutrophil production and function in newborn infants. *Br J Haematol* 2000; 110:18–28.

40. Koenig JM, Stegner JJ, Schmeck AC, Saxonhouse MA, Kenigsberg LE. Neonatal neutrophils with prolonged survival exhibit enhanced inflammatory and cytotoxic responsiveness. *Pediatr Res* 2005; 57:424–9.

41. Luo D, Schowengerdt KO Jr, Stegner JJ, May WS Jr, Koenig JM. Decreased functional caspase-3 expression in umbilical cord blood neutrophils is linked to delayed apoptosis. *Pediatr Res* 2003; 53:859–64.

42. Molloy EJ, O'Neill AJ, Grantham J, Sheridan-Pereira M, Fitzpatrick JM, Webb DW, Watson RWG. Labour prolongs neonatal neutrophil survival and increases lipopolysaccharide responsiveness. *Pediatr Res* 2004 Jul; 56(1):99–103.

43. Henneke P, Osmers I, Bauer K, Lamping N, Versmold HT, Schumann RR. Impaired CD14-dependent and independent response of polymorphonuclear leukocytes in preterm infants. *J Perinat Med* 2003; 31(2):176–83.

44. Bonner S, Yan SR, Byers DM, Bortolussi R. Activation of extracellular signal-related protein kinases 1 and 2 of the mitogen-activated protein kinase family by lipopolysaccharide requires plasma in neutrophils from adults and newborns. *Infect Immun* 2001 May; 69(5):3143–9.

45. Molloy EJ, O'Neill AJ, Grantham J, Sheridan-Pereira M, Fitzpatrick JM, Webb DW, Watson RWG. Granulocyte colony stimulating factor and granulocyte macrophage stimulating factor have differential effects on neonatal and adult neutrophil function and survival in vivo and in vitro. *Pediatr Res* 2005 Jun; 57(6):806–12.

46. Yost CC, Cody MJ, Harris ES, Thornton NL, McInturff AM, Martinez ML, Chandler NB, Rodesch CK, Albertine KH, Petti CA, Weyrich AS, Zimmerman GA. Impaired neutrophil extracellular trap (NET) formation: A novel innate immune deficiency of human neonates. *Blood* 2009 Jun 18; 113(25):6419–27.

47. Lederer JA, Rodrick ML, Mannick JA. The effects of injury on the adaptive immune response. *Shock* 1999; 11:153–9.

48. Oberholzer A, Oberholzer C, Moldawer LL. Sepsis syndromes: Understanding the role of innate and acquired immunity. *Shock* 2001; 16:83–96.

49. Pinsky MR. Sepsis: A pro- and anti-inflammatory disequilibrium syndrome. *Contrib Nephrol* 2001; 132:354–66.

50. Jiminez MF, Watson RW, Parodo J, Evans D, Foster D, Steinburg M, Rotstein OD, Marshall JC. Dysregulated expression of neutrophil apoptosis in the systemic inflammatory response syndrome. *Arch Surg* 1997; 132(12):1263–9.

51. Clark RA. The human neutrophil respiratory burst oxidase. *J Infect Dis* 1990; 161:1140–7.

52. Bone RC. Sir Isaac Newton, sepsis, SIRS, and CARS. *Crit Care Med* 1996 Jul; 24(7):1125–8.

53. Gomez R, Romero R, Ghezzi F, Yoon BH, Mazor M, Berry SM. The fetal inflammatory response. *Am J J Obstet Gynecol* 1998; 179:194–202.

54. Ashare A, Powers LS, Butler NS, Doershug KC, Monick MM, Hunnunhake GW. Anti-inflammatory response is associated with mortality and severity of infection in sepsis. *Am J Physiol Lung Cell Mol Physiol* 2005; 288:L633–40.

55. Ng PC, Li K, Wong RP, Chui K, Wong E, Li G, Fok TF. Proinflammatory and anti-inflammatory cytokine responses in preterm infants with systemic infections. *Arch Dis Child Fetal Neonatal Ed* 2003; 88:F209–13.

56. Medzhitov R, Janeway CA. Innate immunity: Impact on adaptive immune response. *Curr Opin Immunol* 1997; 9:4–9.

57. Kollmann TR, Crabtree J, Rein-Weston A, Blimkie D, Thommai F, Wang XY, Lavoie PM, Furlong J, Fortuno ES 3rd, Hajjar AM, Hawkins NR, Self SG, Wilson CB. Neonatal innate TLR-mediated responses are distinct from those of adults. *J Immunol* 2009 Dec 1; 183(11):7150–60.

58. Levy E, Xanthou G, Petrakou E, Zacharioudaki V, Tsatsanis C, Fotopoulos S, Xanthou M. Distinct roles of TLR4 and CD14 in LPS-induced inflammatory responses of neonates. *Pediatr Res* 2009 Aug; 66(2):179–84.

59. Viemann D, Dubbel G, Schleifenbaum S, Harms E, Sorg C, Roth J. Expression of toll-like receptors in neonatal sepsis. *Pediatr Res* 2005; 58:654–9.

60. Yan SR, Byers DM, Bortolussi R. Role of protein kinase p53/56lyn in diminished lipopolysaccharide priming of formylleucyl-phenylalanine-induced superoxide production in human newborn neutrophils. *Infect Immun* 2004; 72:6455–62.

61. Wynn JL, Scumpia PO, Winfield RD, Delano MJ, Kelly-Scumpia K, Barker T, Ungaro R, Levy O, Moldawer LL. Defective innate immunity predisposes murine neonates to poor sepsis outcome but is reversed by TLR agonists. *Blood* 2008 Sep 1; 112(5):1750–8.

62. DiGiulio DB, Romero R, Amogan HP et al. Microbial prevalence, diversity and abundance in amniotic fluid during preterm labor: A molecular and culture-based investigation. *PLoS One* 2008; 3:e3056.

63. Biasucci G, Benenati B, Morelli L, Bessi E, Boehm G. Cesarean delivery may affect the early biodiversity of intestinal bacteria. *J Nutr* 2008; 138:1796S–800S.

64. Shen CM, Lin SC, Niu DM, Kou YR. Labour increases the surface expression of two Toll-like receptors in the cord blood monocytes of healthy term newborns. *Acta Paediatr* 2009 Jun; 98(6):959–62.

65. Nathan J, Neu J. Necrotising enterocolitis: Relationship to innate immunity, clinical features, and strategies for prevention. *NeoReviews* 2006; 7;e143–50.

66. Sharma R, Young C, Mshvildadze M, Neu J. Intestinal microbiota: Does it play a role in diseases of the neonate? *NeoReviews* 2009; 10;e166–79.

67. Sodhi CP, Shi XH, Richardson WM, Grant ZS, Shapiro RA, Prindle T Jr, Branca M, Russo A, Gribar SC, Ma C, Hackam DJ. Toll-like receptor-4 inhibits enterocyte proliferation via impaired beta-catenin signaling in necrotizing enterocolitis. *Gastroenterology* 2009 Sep 26. [Epub ahead of print]

68. Leaphart CL, Cavallo J, Gribar SC et al. A critical role for TLR4 in the pathogenesis of necrotizing enterocolitis by modulating intestinal injury and repair. *J Immunol* 20071; 179:4808–20.

69. Liu Y, Zhu L, Fatheree NY, Liu X, Pacheco SE, Tatevian N, Rhoads JM. Changes in intestinal Toll-like receptors and cytokines precede histological injury in a rat model of necrotizing enterocolitis. *Am J Physiol Gastrointest Liver Physiol* 2009 Sep; 297(3):G442–50.

70. Meinzen-Derr J, Poindexter B, Wrage L, Morrow AL, Stoll B, Donovan EF. Role of human milk in extremely low birth weight infants' risk of necrotizing enterocolitis or death. *J Perinatol* 2009 Jan; 29(1):57–62.

71. LeBouder E, Rey-Nores JE, Rushmere NK, Grigorov M, Lawn SD, Affolter M, Griffin GE, Ferrara P, Schiffrin EJ, Morgan BP, Labeta MO. Soluble forms of Toll-like receptor (TLR)2 capable of modulating TLR2 signaling are present in human plasma and breast milk. *J Immunol* 2003; 171:6680–9.

72. Myers CD. Role of B-cell antigen processing and presentation in the humoral immune response. *FASEB J* 1991; 5:2547–53.

73. Schlossman ST, Boumsell L, Gilks W et al. *Leukocyte Typing V*. Oxford: Oxford University Press, 1995.

74. Meuer SC, Schlossman SG, Reinherz EL. Clonal analysis of human cytotoxic T lymphocytes: T4+ and T8+ effector T-cells recognise products of different major histo-compatibility complex regions. *Proc Natl Acad Sci USA* 1982; 79:4395–9.

75. Germain RN. The ins and outs of antigen presentation. *Nature* 1986; 322:687–9.

76. Melchers F, Anderson J, Curbel CM et al. Regulation of B lymphocyte replication and maturation. *J Cell Biochem* 1982; 19:315–21.

77. Singer A, Hodes RJ. Mechanisms of T-cell–B-cell interaction. *Ann Rev Immunol* 1983; 1:211–42.

78. Tosato G, Magrath IT, Koski IR, Dooley NJ, Blaese RM. B-cell differentiation and immunoregulatory T-cell function in human cord blood lymphocytes. *J Clin Invest* 1980; 66:383–8.

79. Puri P, Blacke P, Ren DJ. Lymphocyte transformation after surgery in the neonate. *J Paediatr Surg* 1980; 15:175–7.

80. Hayward AR, Kurnick J. Newborn T-cell suppression: Early appearance, maintenance in culture and lack of growth factor suppression. *J Immunol* 1981; 125:50–3.

81. Lubens RG, Gard SE, Soderberg-Warner M, Stiehm R. Lectin dependent T lymphocytes and natural killer cytotoxic deficiencies in human newborn. *Cell Immunol* 1982; 74:40–3.

82. Eife RF, Eife G, August CS et al. Lymphotoxin production and blast cell transformation by cord blood lymphocytes: Dissociated lymphocyte function in newborn infants. *Cell Immunol* 1974; 14:435–9.

83. Gupta S, Shwartz SA, Good RA. Subpopulation of human T-cell lymphocytes. VII cellular basis of con-canavalin A induced T-cell mediated suppression of immunoglobulin production by B-lymphocytes from normal humans. *Cell Immunol* 1978; 44:242–9.

84. Foa R, Giubellino M, Fierro M et al. Immature T-Lymphocytes in human cord blood identified by monoclonal antibodies: A model for the study of the differentiation pathway of T-cells in humans. *Cell Immunol* 1984; 89:194–201.

85. Reason DC, Ebiasawaaa M, Saito H et al. Human cord blood lymphocytes do not simultaneously express CD4 and CD8 cell surface markers. *Biol Neonate* 1990; 58:87–90.

86. Clement LT, Vink PE, Bradley GE. Novel immu-noregulatory functions of phenotypically distinct subpopulations of CD4+ cells in the human neonate. *J Immunol* 1990; 145:102–8.

87. Gerli R, Bertotto A, Spinozzi F et al. Thymic modu-lation of CD38 (T10) antigen on human cord blood lymphocytes. *Clin Immunol Immunopathol* 1987; 45:323.

88. Maccario R, Ferrari FA, Ciana S et al. Receptors for peanut agglutinin on a high percentage of human cord blood lymphocytes: Phenotype characterisa-tion of peanut positive cells. *Thymus* 1981; 2:239.

89. Meccario R, Nespoli IO, Mingrat G et al. Lymphocyte subpopulations in the neonate: Identification of an immature subset of OKT8-positive, OKT3-negative cells. *J Immunol* 1983; 130:1129–32.

90. Splawski JB, Lipsky PE. Cytokine regulation of immu-noglobulin secretion by neonatal lymphocytes. *J Clin Invest* 1991; 88:967–77.

91. Watson W, Oen K, Ramdahin R et al. Immunoglobulin and cytokine production by neona-tal lymphocytes. *Clin Exp Immunol* 1991; 83:169–74.

92. Erkeller-Yuuksel FM, Deneys V, Yuksel B et al. Age-related changes in human blood lymphocyte subpopulation. *J Pediatr* 1992; 120:216–22.

93. Wu LYF, Blanco A, Cooper MA et al. Ontogeny of B lymphocyte differentiation induced by poke-weed mitogen. *Clin Immunol Immunopathol* 1976; 5:208–17.

94. Hayward AR, Lawton AR. Induction of plasma cell differentiation of human fetal lymphocytes: Evidence for functional immaturity of T and B cell. *J Immunol* 1977; 115:1213.

95. Bird AG, Britton S. A new approach to the study of B lymphocyte function using an indirect B cell activa-tor. *Immunol Rev* 1984; 45:41.

96. Miller KM, Pittart WB, Sorenson RU. Cord blood B cell differentiation: Synergistic effect of pokeweed mitogen and *Staphylococcus aureus* on in vitro dif-ferentiation of B cells from human neonates. *Clin Exp Immunol* 1984; 56:415.

97. Andersson U, Bird AG, Britton S et al. Humoral and cellular immunity in humans studies at the cell level from birth to 2 years of age. *Immunol Rev* 1981; 57:5.

98. Durandy A, Fisher A, Griscelli C. Active suppression of B lymphocyte maturation by two different unborn T lymphocyte subsets. *J Immunol* 1979; 123:2646.

99. Pastorelli G, Rousset F, Pene J et al. Cord blood B-cells are mature in their capacity to switch to IgE producing cells in response to interleukin-4 in vitro. *Clin Exp Immunol* 1990; 82:114–9.

100. Finkelman SD, Katona IM, Urban JF et al. IL4 is required to generate and sustain in vivo IgE responses. *J Immunol* 1988; 141:2335–41.

101. Clough JD, Mims LH, Strober W. Deficient IgA antibody responses to arsanilic acid bovine serum albumin (BSA) in neonatally thymectomised rabbits. *J Immunol* 1971; 107:1624–9.

102. Durandy A, Thuillier S, Forbveille M et al. Phenotypic and functional characteristics of human newborns B-lymphocytes. *J Immunol* 1990; 144:60–5.

103. Raveche ES. Possible immunoregulatory role for CD5+B cells. *Clin Immunol Immunopathol* 1990; 56:135–50.

104. Gibbons DL, Haque SF, Silberzahn T, Hamilton K, Langford C, Ellis P, Carr R, Hayday AC. Neonates harbour highly active gammadelta T cells with selec-tive impairments in preterm infants. *Eur J Immunol* 2009 Jul; 39(7):1794–806.

105. Cates KL, Rowe JC, Ballow M. The premature infant as a comprised host. *Curr Probl Pediatr* 1983; 13:5–63.

106. Rijkers GT, Sanders EA, Breukels MA, Zegers BJ. Infant B cell responses to polysaccharide determi-nants. *Vaccine* 1998; 16:1396–4000.

107. Holmes SJ, Granoff DM. The biology of *Haemophilus influenzae* type b vaccination failure. *J Infect Dis* 1992; 165 Suppl A:S121–8.

108. Eskola J, Ward J, Dagan R, Goldblatt D, Zepp F, Fiegrist CA. Combined vaccination of *Haemophilus influenzae* type b conjugate and diphtheria-tetanus-pertussis containing acellular pertussis. *Lancet* 1999; 354:2063–8.

109. Goriely S, Vincart B, Stordeur P, Vekemans J, Willems F, Goldman M, De Wit D. Deficient IL-12 (p35) gene expression by dendritic cells derived from neonatal monocytes. *J Immunol* 2001; 166:2141–6.

110. Hamblin AS. *Lymphokines.* Oxford: IRL Press, 1988.

111. Whicker JT, Evans SW. Cytokines in disease. *Clin Chem* 1990; 36/7:1269–81.

112. Lucas C, Bald LN, Fandly BM et al. The autocrine production of transforming growth factor during lymphocyte activation: A study with a monoclonal antibody based ELISA. *J Immunol* 1990; 145:1415–22.

113. Nijsten MW, de Groot ER, ten Duis HJ et al. Serum levels of interleukin-6 and acute phase responses. *Lancet* 1987; 2:921.

114. Fong Y, Moldawer L, Shires GT et al. The biological characteristics of cytokines and their implication in surgery injury. *Surg Gynec Obstet* 1990; 170:363–78.

115. Leary AG, Ikeubuchi K, Hirai T. Synergism between interleukin-6 and interleukin-3 in supporting proliferation of human hematopoietic stem cells: Comparison with interleukin-1a. *Blood* 1988; 71:1759–63.

116. Beytler B, Mylsark IW, Cerami A. Passive immunisation against cachectin/tumor necrosis factor protects mice from the lethal effect of endotoxin. *Science* 1985; 229:869–71.

117. Schoham S, Davernne D, Cady AB et al. Recombinant tumor necrosis factor and interleukin-1 enhance slow-wave sleep. *Am J Phys* 1987; 253:142–9.

118. Ambalavanan N, Carlo WA, D'Angio CT, McDonald SA, Das A, Schendel D, Thorsen P, Higgins RD. Eunice Kennedy Shriver National Institute of Child Health and Human Development Neonatal Research Network. Cytokines associated with bronchopulmonary dysplasia or death in extremely low birth weight infants. *Pediatrics* 2009 Apr; 123(4):1132–41.

119. Geelen SPM, Fleer A, Bezemer AC, Gerards LJ, Rijkers GT, Verhoef J. Deficiencies in opsonic defense to pneumococci in the human newborn despite adequate levels of complement and specific IgG antibodies. *Pediatr Res* 1990; 27:514–8.

120. Drossou V, Kanakoudi F, Diamanti E, Tzimouli V, Konstantinidis T, Germenis A, Kremenopoulos G, Katsougiannopoulos V. Concentrations of main serum opsonins in early infancy. *Arch Dis Child* 1995; 72:F172–5.

121. Ballow M, Cates KL, Rowe JC, Goetz C, Desbonnet C. Development of the immune system in very low birth weight (less than 1500 g) premature infants: Concentrations of plasma immunoglobulins and patterns of infection. *Pediatr Res* 1986; 20:899–904.

122. Kovar I, Ajina NS, Hurley R. Serum complement and gestational age. *J Obstet Gynaecol* 1983; 3:182–6.

123. Notarangelo LD, Chirico G, Chiara A, Colombo A, Rondini G, Plebani A, Martini A, Ugazio AG. Activity of classical and alternative pathways of complement in preterm and small for gestational age infants. *Pediatr Res* 1984; 18:281–5.

124. Ohlsson A, Lacy JB. Intravenous immunoglobulin for suspected or subsequently proven infection in neonates. *Cochrane Database Syst Rev* 2004; (1):CD001239.

125. Ohlsson A, Lacy JB. Intravenous immunoglobulin for preventing infection in preterm and/or low-birth-weight infants. *Cochrane Database Syst Rev* 2004; (1):CD000361.

126. INIS Study Collaborative Group. The INIS Study. International Neonatal Immunotherapy Study: Non-specific intravenous immunoglobulin therapy for suspected or proven neonatal sepsis. An international, placebo controlled, multicentre randomised trial. *BMC Pregnancy Childbirth* 2008 Dec 8; 8(1):52.

127. Carr R, Modi N, Dore C. G-CSF and GM-CSF for treating or preventing neonatal infections. *Cochrane Database Syst Rev* 2003; (3):CD003066.

128. Carr R, Brocklehurst P, Doré CJ, Modi N. Granulocyte-macrophage colony stimulating factor administered as prophylaxis for reduction of sepsis in extremely preterm, small for gestational age neonates (the PROGRAMS trial): A single-blind, multicentre, randomised controlled trial. *Lancet* 2009; 373;226–33.

129. Kuhn P, Messer J, Paupe A, Espagne S, Kacet N, Mouchnino G, Klosowski S, Krim G, Lescure S, Le Bouedec S, Meyer P, Astruc D. A multicenter, randomized, placebo-controlled trial of prophylactic recombinant granulocyte-colony stimulating factor in preterm neonates with neutropenia. *J Pediatr* 2009; 155(3):324–30.e1.

130. Bernard GR, Ely EW, Wright TJ, Fraiz J, Stasek JE Jr, Russell JA, Mayers I, Rosenfeld BA, Morris PE, Yan SB, Helterbrand JD. Safety and dose relationship of recombinant human activated protein C for coagulopathy in severe sepsis. *Crit Care Med* 2001 Nov; 29(11):2051–9.

131. Nadel S, Goldstein B, Williams MD, Dalton H, Peters M, Macias WL, Abd-Allah SA, Levy H, Angle R, Wang D, Sundin DP, Giroir B. Researching Severe Sepsis and Organ Dysfunction in Children: A Global Perspective (RESOLVE) Study Group. Drotrecogin alfa (activated) in children with severe sepsis: A multicentre phase III randomised controlled trial. *Lancet* 2007 Mar 10; 369(9564):836–43.

132. Neu J. Perinatal and neonatal manipulation of the intestinal microbiome: A note of caution. *Nutr Rev* 2007; 65:282–285.

133. Parracho H, McCartney AL, Gibson GR. Probiotics and prebiotics in infant nutrition. *Proc Nutr Soc* 2007; 66:405–411.

134. Lin HC, Hsu CH, Chen HL et al. Oral probiotics prevent necrotizing enterocolitis in very low birth weight preterm infants: A multicenter, randomized, controlled trial. *Pediatrics* 2008; 122: 693–700.

135. Kunz AN, Noel JM, Fairchok MP. Two cases of *Lactobacillus* bacteremia during probiotic treatment of short gut syndrome. *J Pediatr Gastroenterol Nutr* 2004; 38:457–8.

136. Besselink MG, van Santvoort HC, Buskens E et al. Acute Pancreatitis Work Group Netherland. Probiotic prophylaxis in patients with predicted severe acute pancreatitis: A randomised, double-blind, placebo-controlled trial. *Lancet* 2008; 23:1651–9.

137. Bobey-Wright NAM, Tcheurekdjian H, Wara D, Lewis DB. Immunologic aspects of DiGeorge syndrome. *NeoReviews* Oct 2005; 6:e471–8.

138. Puck JM. Neonatal screening for severe combined immune deficiency. *Curr Opin Allergy Clin Immunol* 2007 Dec; 7(6):522–7.

139. Wynn JL, Neu J, Moldawer LL, Levy O. Potential of immunomodulatory agents for prevention and treatment of neonatal sepsis. *J Perinatol* 2009 Feb; 29(2):79–88.

140. Poltorak A, Smirnova I, He X, Liu MY, Van Huffel C, McNally O, Birdwell D, Alejos E, Silva M, Du X, Thompson P, Chan EK, Ledesma J, Roe B, Clifton S, Vogel SN, Beutler B. Genetic and physical mapping of the Lps locus: Identification of the toll-4 receptor as a candidate gene in the critical region. *Blood Cells Mol Dis* 1998 Sep; 24(3):340–55.

141. Brocklehurst P et al. Treatment of neonatal sepsis with intravenous immune globulin. The INIS Collaborative Group. *New Engl J Med* 2011 Sep 29; 365(13):1201–11.

142. Marlow N, Morris T, Brocklehurst P et al. A randomized trial of granulocyte-macrophage colony-stimulating factor for neonatal sepsis: Outcomes at 2 years. *Arch Dis Child Fetal Neonatal Ed* 2013; 98:F46–53.

143. Costeloe K et al. on behalf of The Probiotics in Preterm Infants Study Collaborative Group. *Bifidobacterium breve* BBG-001 in very preterm infants: A randomised controlled phase 3 trial. *Lancet* Vol(10019):649–60.

144. Martinon F, Mayor A, Tschopp J. The inflammasomes: Guardians of the body. *Annu Rev Immunol* 2009; 27:229–65.

145. Martinon F, Burns K, Tschopp J. The inflammasome: A molecular platform triggering activation of inflammatory caspases and processing of proIL-beta. *Mol Cell* 2002; 10:417–26.

146. Ozaki E, Campbell M, Doyle SL. Targeting the NLRP3 inflammasome in chronic inflammatory diseases: Current perspectives. *J Inflamm Res* 2015; 8:15–27.

147. Karmakar M, Katsnelson M, Malak HA et al. Neutrophil IL-1β processing induced by pneumolysin is mediated by the NLRP3/ASC inflammasome and caspase-1 activation and is dependent on K+ efflux. *J Immunol Baltim Md 1950* 2015; 194:1763–75.

148. Mankan AK, Dau T, Jenne D, Hornung V. The NLRP3/ASC/caspase-1 axis regulates IL-1β processing in neutrophils. *Eur J Immunol* 2012; 42:710–17.

149. Yu JR, Leslie KS. Cryopyrin-associated periodic syndrome: An update on diagnosis and treatment response. *Curr Allergy Asthma Rep* 2010; 11:12–2.

150. Sharma AA, Jen R, Kan B, Sharma A et al. Impaired NLRP3 inflammasome activity during fetal development regulates IL-1β production in human monocytes. *Eur J Immunol* 2015; 45:238–49.

151. Gibbons D, Fleming P, Virasami A, Michel ML, Sebire NJ, Costeloe K, Carr R, Klein N, Hayday A. Interleukin-8 (CXCL8) production is a signatory T cell effector function of human newborn infants. *Nat Med* 2014 Oct; 20(10):1206–10.

152. Hoskote AU1, Ramaiah RN, Cale CM, Hartley JC, Brown KL. Role of immunoglobulin supplementation for secondary immunodeficiency associated with chylothorax after pediatric cardiothoracic surgery. *Pediatr Crit Care Med* 2012 Sep; 13(5):535–41.

153. Ohlsson A1, Lacy JB. Intravenous immunoglobulin for suspected or proven infection in neonates. *Cochrane Database Syst Rev* 2015 Mar 27; 3:CD001239.

154. Pammi M, Haque KN. Pentoxifylline for treatment of sepsis and necrotizing enterocolitis in neonates. *Cochrane Database Syst Rev* 2015 Mar 9; 3:CD004205.

155. Marlow N, Morris T, Brocklehurst P, Carr R, Cowan F, Patel N, Petrou S, Redshaw M, Modi N, Doré CJ. A randomised trial of granulocyte-macrophage colony-stimulating factor for neonatal sepsis: Childhood outcomes at 5 years. *Arch Dis Child Fetal Neonatal Ed* 2015 Jul; 100(4):F320–6.

156. Pammi M, Abrams SA. Oral lactoferrin for the prevention of sepsis and necrotizing enterocolitis in preterm infants. *Cochrane Database Syst Rev.* 2015 Feb 20; 2:CD007137.

157. AlFaleh K, Anabrees J. Probiotics for prevention of necrotizing enterocolitis in preterm infants. *Cochrane Database Syst Rev* 2014 Apr 10; 4:CD005496.

158. Goldbach-Mansky R, Dailey NJ, Canna SW et al. Neonatal-onset multisystem inflammatory disease responsive to interleukin-1beta inhibition. *N Engl J Med* 2006; 355:581–92.

159. Goldbach-Mansky R. Current status of understanding the pathogenesis and management of patients with NOMID/CINCA. *Curr Rheumatol Rep* 2011; 13:123–31.

160. Almeida de Jesus A1, Goldbach-Mansky R. Monogenic autoinflammatory diseases: Concept and clinical manifestations. *Clin Immunol* 2013 Jun; 147(3):155–74.

161. Tanaka N, Izawa K, Saito MK, Sakuma M, Oshima K, Ohara O, Nishikomori R, Morimoto T, Kambe N, Goldbach-Mansky R, Aksentijevich I, de Saint Basile G, Neven B, van Gijn M, Frenkel J, Aróstegui JI, Yagüe J, Merino R, Ibañez M, Pontillo A, Takada H, Imagawa T, Kawai T, Yasumi T, Nakahata T, Heike T. High incidence of NLRP3 somatic mosaicism in patients with chronic infantile neurologic, cutaneous, articular syndrome: Results of an International Multicenter Collaborative Study. *Arthritis Rheum* 2011 Nov; 63(11):3625–32.

162. Izawa KI, Hijikata A, Tanaka N, Kawai T, Saito MK, Goldbach-Mansky R, Aksentijevich I, Yasumi T, Nakahata T, Heike T, Nishikomori R, Ohara O. Detection of base substitution-type somatic mosaicism of the NLRP3 gene with >99.9% statistical confidence by massively parallel sequencing. *DNA Res* 2012; 19(2):1–10.

163. Wilson SP, Cassel SL. Inflammasome mediated auto-inflammatory disorders. *Postgrad Med* 2010 Sep; 122(5):125–33.

20

Neonatal sepsis

JAMIE GOLDEN, JESSICA A. ZAGORY, CHRISTOPHER P. GAYER, TRACY C. GRIKSCHEIT, AND HENRI R. FORD

INTRODUCTION

Neonatal sepsis remains one of the most common and potentially preventable causes of mortality and long-term morbidity in the world. Although associated mortality is decreasing, over 400,000 neonates worldwide died from sepsis and other infectious conditions in 2015.[1] Compared with uninfected infants, those who develop infections in the neonatal period are significantly more likely to have adverse neurodevelopmental outcomes at follow-up. These include cerebral palsy, poor vision, delayed psychomotor development, low Bayley Scales of Infant Development II scores on the mental development index, as well as impaired head growth, a known predictor of poor neurodevelopmental outcome.[2] This chapter will examine the definition, epidemiology, pathophysiology, diagnosis, management, and outcome of neonatal sepsis.

DEFINITION AND CLASSIFICATIONS

Sepsis was classically described in the adult patient with a Gram-negative infection who subsequently developed fever, hypotension with poor tissue perfusion, and ultimately multiple organ failure. Subsequently, bench and clinical research demonstrated that a number of initial insults, including significant infection, toxin exposure, severe tissue necrosis, and open burn wounds, were capable of inducing these signs and symptoms. Therefore, the term systemic inflammatory response syndrome (SIRS) was introduced to describe a constellation of inflammatory symptoms that include fever, tachycardia, tachypnea, and abnormal white blood cell (WBC) count. A number of proinflammatory as well as regulatory (or anti-inflammatory) cytokines and hormones have been identified in association with the SIRS response. Investigators have grouped various patterns of cytokine response with specific clinical signs and symptoms. Thus, in addition to SIRS, the concept of a compensatory anti-inflammatory response

syndrome (CARS) or a mixed anti-inflammatory response syndrome (MARS)[3,4] has also evolved (Figure 20.1).[5]

Until recently, sepsis was defined as the presence of a SIRS response coupled with a causative infection. The surviving sepsis campaign defined severe sepsis as sepsis plus sepsis-induced organ dysfunction or tissue hypoperfusion, and defined septic shock as sepsis-induced hypoperfusion persisting despite adequate fluid resuscitation.[6] In pediatric patients, these definitions depend on age-specific vital signs and WBC cutoff values. More recently, a task force redefined sepsis in the Third International Consensus Definitions for Sepsis and Septic Shock. Sepsis is currently defined as "life-threatening organ dysfunction caused by a dysregulated host response to infection," thus making the term "severe sepsis" redundant.[7] However, these guidelines, published in 2016, do not specifically address the neonatal population (Figure 20.2).

Neonatal sepsis occurs within the first 28 days of life or up to 4 weeks beyond the expected delivery date in premature infants.[8] It is further subdivided into two categories: early onset sepsis (EOS) and late onset sepsis (LOS). EOS is characterized by the development of sepsis in the first 72 hours of life, while LOS occurs between 72 hours and 28 days of life. EOS and LOS have different etiologies, risk factors, and associated pathogens.

There are multiple criteria for defining or diagnosing sepsis. Clinicians can apply these criteria to determine if sepsis is likely, guide subsequent workup and antibiotic therapy, or document the presence of sepsis for outcome analysis. One of the important early criteria, for example, is the Rochester criteria.[9,10] These criteria predict serious bacterial infection and high risk of sepsis in a population of healthy term infants, less than 3 months of age. However, the Rochester criteria neither effectively define sepsis nor assist in the management of complicated perinatal or preterm infants.[11] Pediatric criteria,[12] developed from large-scale pediatric databases to parallel adult criteria, are useful in defining sepsis for outcome analysis but lack characteristics that

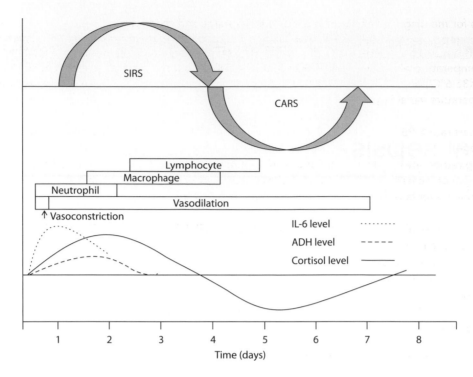

Figure 20.1 Following onset of sepsis, there are predictable phases of systemic inflammatory response syndrome (SIRS) and compensatory anti-inflammatory response syndrome (CARS). This figure is not meant to be comprehensive but representative of several of the most well understood components of each phase.

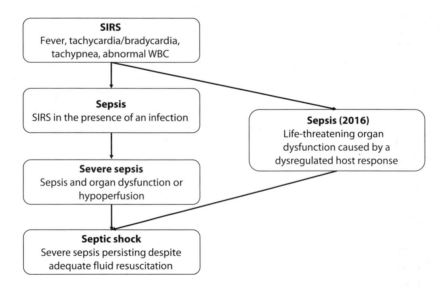

Figure 20.2 Classification of neonatal inflammatory responses including the most recent definition of sepsis. SIRS= systemic inflammatory response syndrome, WBC=white blood cell count.

make it applicable to the neonatal population. In addition, some criteria are strictly biochemical[13] rather than clinical, in contrast to the more classic "Bone" criteria.[14,15] Table 20.1 shows a useful list of criteria that help define the sepsis syndrome in the neonate.[16–19]

EPIDEMIOLOGY

The incidence of neonatal sepsis has increased in recent years, likely due to advances in neonatology, which allow the most susceptible premature and very low birth weight (VLBW) infants to survive the perinatal period. Rates of infection vary by geographic region, available health care resources, and maternal and infant risk factors.[20] Approximately 75% of neonatal deaths globally occur in the first week of life, and most occur in low- and middle-income countries due to lack of resources, limited access to care, and poor hygiene.[21,22] Recent figures for the overall incidence of neonatal sepsis range from 1 to 170 per 1000 live births, and 4 out of 10 neonates with sepsis die or experience

Table 20.1 Criteria for the diagnosis of sepsis in critically ill neonates and children

Physiologic criteria	Laboratory criteria	Biochemical criteria
1. Fever (rectal temperature >38°C), hypothermia (<35.6°C), or increased temperature variability in Isolette	1. WBC count >12,000 cell/cc or <4000 cell/cc	1. Elevated CRP (>3 mg/cc with physiologic symptoms, >10 mg/cc without symptoms)
2. Tachycardia (heart rate > 95th percentile for age)	2. Bandemia (>10% bands)	2. Elevated interleukin-6 (IL-6 >44.4 pg/mL)
3. Tachypnea (respiratory rate > 95th percentile for age) or increasing frequency of apneic events with bradycardia	3. Ratio of immature to total neutrophils (>0.2 for infection, >0.8 for bone marrow depletion)	3. Elevated procalcitonin (PCT >6.1 ng/mL)
4. Hypotension (mean arterial blood pressure <5th percentile for age)	4. Thrombocytopenia (<50,000 per cc)	4. Elevated lipopolysaccharide binding protein (LBP >25 mg/mL)
5. Poor peripheral perfusion (delayed capillary refill or central-peripheral temperature disparity)	5. Metabolic acidosis (pH <7.25 or base excess <−5)	
6. Oliguria (urine output <1 mL/kg/hour after day of life 1)	6. Elevated lactate (>4 mmol/cc)	
7. Poor feeding		

major disability, including significant neurodevelopmental impairment.[23,24]

Rates of neonatal sepsis vary based on gestational age and birth weight (Tables 20.2 and 20.3). The incidence of EOS and LOS increases with decreasing gestational age and is highest in preterm and extreme preterm infants.[25] Birth weight is defined relative to gestational age and is an independent risk factor for a number of outcomes, including neonatal sepsis. However, age-matched birth weight is a confounding variable. Thus, rate of sepsis for non-age-matched birth weight has been reported as well (Tables 20.3 and 20.4). Unfortunately, birth weight does not capture an additional important variable—the trajectory of intrauterine weight gain. A trajectory of normal weight gain for a small for gestational age fetus is significantly less concerning than a sudden change in the trajectory of weight gain for an appropriate weight fetus. Falling off an intrauterine growth curve can indicate either primary placental insufficiency or increased fetal demand due to maternal–fetal infection. Therefore, an abnormal growth curve is concerning for prenatal infection.

The epidemiology of neonatal sepsis differs between EOS and LOS. EOS is typically transmitted from the mother intrapartum through an ascending infection before or during labor. This includes transmission through hematogenous routes, chorioamnionitis, or during delivery through direct contact with or aspiration/ingestion of invasive organisms. The most commonly identified causative organisms are from the maternal vaginal flora. It is estimated that EOS occurs in 1–2/1000 live births and accounts for 9/1000 neonatal admissions,

Table 20.2 Rate of EOS and LOS by gestational age

	Extreme preterm (23–27 weeks)	Preterm (<37 weeks)	Late preterm (34–36 weeks)	Term (>37 weeks)
EOS	Not reported by gestational age	0.56%	0.44%	0.02%–0.35%
LOS	22%–48%	16%	6.3%	1.4%

Table 20.3 Rates of EOS and LOS sepsis by birth weight

	Extremely low birth weight (<1000 g)	Very low birth weight (1000–1500 g)	Low birth weight (1500–2500 g)	Appropriate birth weight (>2500 g)
EOS	Not reported	0.19%–0.59%	Not reported by weight	0.12%–0.66%
LOS	22%–33% mean, (38% 750–1000 g, 48% 500–750 g)	16%–22% mean, (7% 1250–1500 g, 18% 1000–1250 g)	5%–16%	1.4%–5.6%

Note: This table does not take into account large for gestational age (greatest 10th percentile).

Table 20.4 National surveillance and rates of nosocomial infection in neonatal intensive care units

Type of nosocomial infection	PPN	NNIS
BSI/1000 CVC-day	Not reported	8.6%
<1000 g	12.8%	9.1%
>1000 g	4.7%	4.1%
VAP/1000 vent-day	Not reported	2.5%
<1000 g	4.9%	1.5%
>1500 g	1.1%	1.4%
Overall PNA/1000 pt-day	12.9%	Not reported
UTI/1000 pt-day	8.6%	Not reported

Abbreviations: PPN = Pediatric Prevention Network, NNIS = National Nosocomial Infections Surveillance, BSI = blood stream infection, CVC = central venous catheter, VAP = ventilator-associated pneumonia, PNA = pneumonia, UTI = urinary tract infection.

carrying an associated mortality of 3% in term newborns and 16% in VLBW neonates.[26–29] In the United States, approximately 3300 cases of EOS and 400 deaths occur each year.[20]

In contrast, LOS is transmitted via postnatal acquisition from nosocomial or community pathogens.[30] It is much more common than EOS, with a reported incidence as high as 300/1000 neonates, contributing to up to 7% of neonatal intensive care unit (NICU) admissions.[29] Nursery-acquired sepsis has a national incidence of 1.4%, and NICU-acquired sepsis ranges from 5% to 30%, depending on the level of acuity of the unit.[31] It is a major contributor to morbidity and mortality in the NICU.[32] LOS is associated with indwelling devices commonly used in the NICU, including central venous catheters, endotracheal tubes, and urinary catheters (see Table 20.4).[33] Further, VLBW preterm neonates are at high risk of LOS (16%–30%, increasing to almost 50% in neonates <1000 g) and are the most likely to develop infection.[29]

RISK FACTORS

Risk factors for neonatal sepsis can be divided into maternal and neonatal factors (Table 20.5). Maternal contributors are more likely to be involved in EOS than LOS and have been divided into three categories: infection, colonization, and risk factors.[26] Maternal infection is defined as laboratory-confirmed bacterial infection with clinical signs such as peripartum fever. Colonization is characterized as positive reproductive tract or genital bacterial cultures with or without signs and symptoms of infection (such as group B *Streptococcus* or GBS) and can be associated with a 2% chance of developing invasive disease.[20] Risk factors include prematurity (<37 weeks), preterm labor, or prolonged rupture of membranes (>18 hours), and can lead to an increased risk of ascending infection. Low socioeconomic status or a history of an infant with GBS has also been shown to be strongly associated with EOS. Maternal factors are not thought to contribute strongly to LOS, except for prematurity and low birth weight.[34]

Neonatal factors are more commonly associated with LOS and include VLBW, newborn jaundice, intraventricular hemorrhage, prematurity, indwelling catheters and invasive procedures.[30] Alterations of the innate immune response, lack of passively acquired immunoglobulins from the mother, male sex, low Appearance, Pulse, Grimace, Activity, and Respiration (APGAR) scores, neonatal distress, anemia, hypothermia, and metabolic disorders are also considered neonatal risk factors for sepsis.[30]

Risk factors that predispose infants to nosocomial infection include admission to an intensive care unit, lack of enteral feeds, lack of maternal breast milk, indwelling devices, parenteral nutrition, and intestinal surgery or pathology. Additionally, widespread or prolonged use of broad spectrum antibiotics can lead to transmission of opportunistic or drug-resistant pathogens.[8] Hospitalized infants are also at risk of developing fungal infections such as candidiasis. Putative risk factors for such infections include low birth weight (<1500 g), parenteral nutrition, indwelling catheters, lack of enteral nutrition, mechanical ventilation, H-2 receptor antagonists, abdominal surgery, peritoneal dialysis, and exposure to broad spectrum or antenatal antibiotics.[8]

PATHOPHYSIOLOGY, PATHOGENS, AND BIOMARKERS

Sepsis was most recently defined as life-threatening organ dysfunction caused by a dysregulated host response to infection.[7] Therefore, sepsis involves both bacterial virulence and failure of the host defense system.

Bacterial virulence involves the pathogen's ability to adhere to epithelia, invade through the basement membrane into host tissues, and evade the host defense mechanisms. Microbial invasion depends on bacterial fimbriae or pili binding or adhering to host structural proteins or cellular integrins followed by internalization.[35] Bacteria then use different enzymes and toxins to neutralize intracellular, cell-mediated, and humoral host responses. These include enzymes such as hyaluronidase, collagenase, lecithinase, and proteinases, endotoxins such as lipopolysaccharide (LPS), and exotoxins.

Many pathogens that cause neonatal sepsis have been identified. *Escherichia coli* (*E. coli*) and group B *Streptococcus* (GBS) are the organisms most commonly involved in EOS. Other organisms that have been implicated in EOS include other *Streptococcus* species, *Staphylococcus aureus*, *Enterococcus* species, Gram-negative enteric bacilli,

Table 20.5 Risk factors for neonatal sepsis

	EOS	LOS
Maternal risk factors	• Bacterial infection • GBS colonization • Peripartum fever • Prematurity • Preterm labor • Prolonged rupture of membranes (>18 hours) • Low socioeconomic status	• Prematurity • Low birth weight
Neonatal risk factors	• Prematurity	• VLBW • Newborn jaundice • Intraventricular hemorrhage • Prematurity • NICU admission • Indwelling catheters • Invasive procedures
Nosocomial risk factors		• Admission to ICU • Lack of enteral feeds • Lack of maternal breast milk • Parenteral nutrition • Intestinal surgery or pathology • Prolonged broad spectrum antibiotics

Abbreviations: VLBW = very low birth weight, ICU = intensive care unit.

Haemophilus influenzae, and *Listeria monocytogenes*.[36] Viral infections can also cause EOS, including herpes simplex virus, enteroviruses, and parechovirus. Rarely, EOS can be caused by fungal pathogens with *Candida* species as the most common causative fungus.[36] In contrast, LOS is most often caused by Gram-positive organisms (70%) followed by Gram-negative organisms (25%) and fungi (5%). Pathogens responsible for LOS sepsis include coagulase negative *Streptococcus* (42%), *S. aureus* (10%), *Enterococci* (9%), GBS (5%), *E. coli* (8%), *Klebsiella* (5%), *Enterobacter* (5%), and *Pseudomonas* (3%).

The neonatal immune system is quite different from that of pediatric and adult patients. An infant's immune system is relatively immature and experiences a period of immunosuppression as it transitions from fetal to neonatal life. It consists of both innate and adaptive components and can generate both humoral and cellular responses (Figure 20.3). However, adaptive immune response requires 5–7 days from delivery for maturity,[30] while normal complement levels and opsonization do not occur until 6 months of life.[37] The adaptive humoral system is dependent on maternal production of antibodies supplied during the peripartum period through placental transfer and during the postpartum period through maternal colostrum and breast milk. Cellular innate and adaptive defense mechanisms are present as early as 13 weeks gestation, but significant production of leukocytes does not occur until nearly the 30th week.[38]

Barrier function of the skin and mucus membranes is also diminished in the neonatal population and is additionally compromised by invasive procedures such as intravenous access, intubation, and indwelling catheters.[36] The intestinal barrier in infants is particularly vulnerable and especially prone to colonization with pathogens leading to gut origin sepsis. The neonatal gut barrier has decreased motility, decreased acid secretion, and low levels of protective mucous, secretory IgA, and

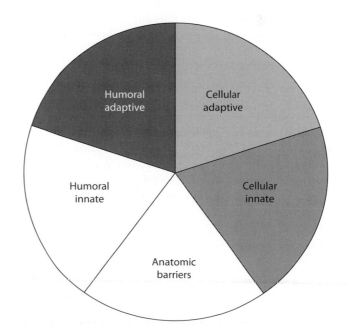

Figure 20.3 Five components of neonatal host defense against pathogens: anatomic barriers including skin and mucosa, innate and adaptive humoral response, and innate and adaptive cell-mediated response.

leaky tight junctions resulting in bacterial translocation from the gastrointestinal tract to normally sterile tissues.[22] Neonates who are delivered vaginally are colonized first with maternal fecal and vaginal flora, while neonates delivered by caesarean section are colonized first with skin flora or bacteria originating from the hospital. However, neonates in the ICU tend to acquire antibiotic-resistant and nosocomial pathogens suggesting that the environment has a strong effect on bacterial flora, patterns of colonization, and susceptibility to gut origin sepsis.[22] Additionally, other internal barriers, such as the meninges and the blood–brain barrier, are immature and allow for active translocation of bacteria to normally sterile areas during bacteremia.[39]

Bacterial invasion followed by stimulation of the host immune response leads to systemic inflammation and production of various inflammatory mediators including cytokines, chemokines, acute-phase proteins, adhesion molecules, components of the complement cascade, and cell surface markers.[40] Cytokines play a central role in neonatal sepsis and can be either proinflammatory or anti-inflammatory. Proinflammatory cytokines such as TNF-α, INF-γ, IL-1β, IL-6, and IL-8 induce a systemic inflammatory response favoring the migration and activation of immune cells. The proinflammatory response is counteracted by anti-inflammatory cytokines, such as IL-10, TGF-β, and IL-4.[40] Acute phase reactants, C reactive protein (CRP) and procalcitonin, are also involved in neonatal sepsis. IL-6 stimulates an increase in CRP concentrations, and levels rise within 6 to 8 hours after inflammation.[41] CRP can be used as a specific and late biomarker of neonatal infection but can also be elevated in noninfectious inflammatory conditions. Procalcitonin is produced by monocytes and hepatocytes 4 to 6 hours after infection.[42] Procalcitonin has a high diagnostic accuracy in the evaluation of neonatal sepsis and has a higher specificity and sensitivity for LOS compared with EOS.[42]

DIAGNOSIS AND WORKUP

Neonatal sepsis can have an extremely subtle initial presentation, and laboratory tests have limited diagnostic accuracy. The first signs of infection in a preterm infant are often apnea, bradycardia, and cyanosis followed by lethargy and increased respiratory effort. A term infant will likely present with respiratory distress.[36] Infants may also present with hyperthermia (>37.8°C) or hypothermia (<36°C), feeding intolerance, or abdominal distention.[8] Physical exam in these infants should evaluate for abnormalities in tone, posture, activity, color, skin changes, tachypnea, and capillary refill. Tachycardia is a nonspecific finding, and bradycardia is often a sign of more advanced sepsis. Meningitis may present with a high pitched cry, abnormal movements, arching of the back, and tense fontanels.[8]

If sepsis is suspected, a thorough history should be obtained to evaluate for exposure to pathogens and risk factors for neonatal sepsis. The Royal College of Obstetricians and Gynaecologists and the National Institute for Health and Care Excellence (NICE) published guidelines focused on the prevention of neonatal sepsis in the United Kingdom. The guidelines were updated in 2012 and include "red flag" indicators that are strongly suggestive of sepsis as well as "non-red flag" risk factors (Table 20.6). Red flags include parenteral antibiotics given to the mother, suspected or confirmed infection in another baby if there is a multiparous pregnancy, respiratory distress starting more than 4 hours after birth, seizures, mechanical ventilation in a term infant, and signs of shock.[43] The NICE guidelines are used to guide further workup and management of neonates with suspected sepsis.

While there are physiologic, laboratory, and biochemical criteria to aid in the diagnosis of sepsis (Table 20.1), the gold standard is a positive blood culture.[44] However, many infants have negative cultures but still have signs of sepsis. These infants may be considered to have "clinical sepsis."[24] Diagnostic workup in sepsis consists of a complete WBC count with differential, blood culture, urine culture, and lumbar puncture (LP) with the addition of tracheal aspirates, acute-phase reactants, and radiographs as indicated (Figure 20.4).

Cultures

One blood culture from a sterile site using at least 1 mL of blood in a single culture bottle is an adequate volume for bacterial detection. Up to 25% of infants with sepsis have low colony count bacteremia, and blood cultures with adequate volume are twice as likely to yield a positive result. Blood is most frequently drawn from a peripheral vein, but a sample from a recently placed umbilical artery catheter is also acceptable.[36,45] Most significant blood cultures are positive by 48 hours.[8]

EOS does not require a urine sample since positive cultures will likely be due to hematogenous seeding of the kidney.[36,45] Urine culture should be considered in older infants and should be from an uncontaminated urine specimen ideally from a suprapubic aspiration or fresh catheter specimen.

Body surface cultures and gastric aspirates are of limited value in the evaluation of sepsis. Tracheal aspirates may be of value in intubated neonates shortly after birth and immediately after endotracheal tube placement.[8,36,45]

Lumbar puncture

LP to obtain cerebrospinal fluid (CSF) is important in the evaluation of meningitis yet remains controversial. The incidence of meningitis in healthy-appearing infants is low, but the incidence is up to 23% in bacteremic patients. Further, up to 38% of infants with meningitis can have negative blood cultures.[45] A LP should be delayed or cancelled in infants with cardiorespiratory distress, tense or bulging anterior fontanel, severe thrombocytopenia, or infection at the LP site.[36]

Table 20.6 NICE risk factors and clinical indicators of possible infection

	Red flags	Non-red flags
Risk factors	• Parenteral antibiotics given to mother for confirmed or suspected bacterial infection during labor or within 24 hours before or after birth (excluding prophylactic antibiotics) • Suspected or confirmed infection in another baby in the case of a multiparous pregnancy	• Invasive GBS infection in a previous baby • Maternal GBS colonization, bacteriuria, or infection in the current pregnancy • Pre-labor rupture of membranes • Preterm birth following spontaneous labor (<37 weeks gestation) • Suspected or confirmed rupture of membranes for more than 18 hours in a preterm birth
Clinical indicators	• Respiratory distress starting >4 hours after birth • Seizures • Need for mechanical ventilation in a term baby • Signs of shock	• Altered muscle tone, behavior, or responsiveness • Feeding difficulties or intolerance • Abnormal heart rate • Signs of respiratory distress, apnea, or hypoxia • Jaundice within 24 hours of birth • Signs of neonatal encephalopathy • Need for CPR • Need for mechanical ventilation in a preterm baby • Persistent pulmonary hypertension • Temperature abnormality unexplained by environmental factors • Coagulopathy (excessive bleeding, thrombocytopenia, INR > 2) • Oliguria persisting beyond 24 hours after birth • Hypo/hyperglycemia • Metabolic acidosis • Local signs of infection

Source: Adapted from NICE Clinical Guidelines for Neonatal Infection, Excellence NIfHaC. Neonatal Infection: antibiotics for prevention and treatment 2012 [cited February 20, 2016]. Available from https://www.nice.org.uk/guidance/cg149.
Note: Red flags are considered strongly suggestive of sepsis.
Abbreviations: CPR = cardiopulmonary resuscitation, INR = international normalized ratio.

CSF parameters in neonates are also controversial. Levels are age-dependent and altered in premature infants. Additionally, if analysis is delayed greater than 2 hours, values may change significantly. Positive findings in CSF include age-adjusted elevated WBC, low glucose concentration, and elevated protein levels.[45]

Radiographs

Chest x-ray may be useful in the evaluation of pneumonia or to evaluate for anatomic causes of respiratory distress. Abdominal x-ray can be used to evaluate intra-abdominal causes of sepsis, such as pneumatosis intestinalis in infants suspected of having necrotizing enterocolitis.

Hematologic evaluation

A WBC count with differential along with neutrophil counts or ratios of immature to total neutrophils (I:T ratio) have relatively poor positive predictive accuracy in the evaluation of neonatal sepsis.[36] Neutropenia may be more specific for neonatal sepsis since only a few other conditions decrease neutrophils in neonates (maternal pregnancy-induced hypertension, asphyxia, and hemolytic disease). However, normal neutrophil counts vary with type of delivery, gestational age, site of sampling, and altitude.[45] I:T ratio has a poor positive predictive value for neonatal sepsis but a very high negative predictive value and can be elevated in up to 50% of uninfected infants.[36,45]

Thrombocytopenia is common in neonatal sepsis but is not sensitive or specific, is often a late indicator of sepsis, and is not useful in evaluating response to therapy.[36,45]

Acute phase reactants and biomarkers

Acute phase reactants and biomarkers can be measured in the evaluation of neonatal sepsis. The most commonly measured acute phase reactants are CRP and procalcitonin. CRP levels typically rise within 6–8 hours of infection and peak at 24 hours. An elevated CRP within 24–48 hours has the best positive predictive value, and two normal CRP values measured at 8–24 hours after birth and again 24 hours later have a negative predictive value of 99.7% for neonatal sepsis.[36,45,46] Procalcitonin is also commonly measured in neonatal sepsis and is more specific and sensitive for infection.[8] It is produced by monocytes and hepatocytes, and levels peak at 12 hours after an infectious episode.[36,45] Procalcitonin is more sensitive and specific for LOS as compared with EOS.[42]

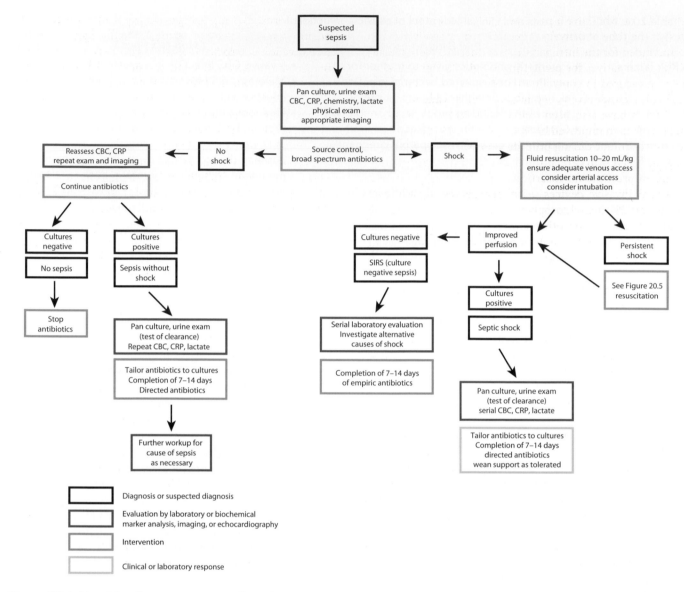

Figure 20.4 Algorithm for management of sepsis.

There is no single biomarker that can be used to reliably diagnose neonatal sepsis. One study evaluated 13 clinical and laboratory signs of sepsis and found that the maximum positive predictive value of any sign studied was 31.3%.[24] Combinations of biomarkers have been evaluated in neonatal sepsis to increase diagnostic accuracy. However, reports on the utility of biomarkers such as CRP, IL-6, serum amylase A, IL-8, procalcitonin, and TNF-α are inconsistent, and no standard biomarker guidelines have been accepted in the screening for neonatal sepsis.[42,47,48]

MANAGEMENT

Prevention strategies

Given the profound morbidity and mortality associated with neonatal sepsis, management should begin with prevention. Significant advances have been made in the prevention of sepsis in both the perinatal and peripartum period as well as in the early postpartum management of neonates. The most significant prevention strategy has been the implementation of prenatal screening and administration of intrapartum antibiotics for GBS infection. The Centers for Disease Control and Prevention published guidelines in 1996 on the prevention of perinatal GBS disease. The 2010 revised guidelines advocate for universal screening for maternal vaginal and rectal GBS at 35–37 weeks gestation and intrapartum antibiotics for women with GBS isolated from urine at any time during the pregnancy, who have a previous infant with invasive GBS disease, or who have tested positive for GBS colonization. Additionally, intrapartum antibiotics are recommended for women whose GBS screening is unavailable at the time of delivery, who deliver at less than 37 weeks gestation, who have a prolonged duration of membrane rupture (>18 hours), who have an intrapartum temperature

(>38°C), or who have a positive nucleic acid amplification test at the time of delivery.[49] Penicillin or ampicillin is recommended for the intrapartum treatment of mothers with GBS. Alternatives for penicillin allergic mothers have not been measured in controlled trials for efficacy but include cefazolin, clindamycin, erythromycin, and vancomycin.[49]

Efforts have also been made in the prevention of LOS sepsis through improved hand hygiene, umbilical cord care, sterile technique during procedures, early breast milk feeding, neonatal skin care, limited use of invasive devices, and uniform practices for insertion, care, and manipulation of essential invasive devices. Although aggressive skin care, including 3% hexachlorophene bathing, can significantly reduce S. aureus and other Gram-positive cocci colonization, the significant skin permeability of the neonate leads to absorption and associated neurotoxicity.[50] The World Health Organization recommends dry skin care in developed countries and antiseptic use in developing countries,[51] although many centers routinely apply small amounts of antimicrobials to the umbilicus and circumcision sites. Indeed, a recent randomized controlled trial investigating umbilical cord care demonstrated superiority and safety of chlorhexidine powder to dry care.[52] Additionally, prevention of colonization and infection in nurseries requires adequate space and personnel. Recommendations of space range from 36 to 100 square feet and nurse to patient ratio of 1:4 to1:1, depending on acuity. Although good outcome studies of individual interventions are not possible due to power restrictions, quality assurance and intervention bundle studies indicate that combined implementation of infection control techniques reduces the risk of nosocomial infections. This includes frequent hand hygiene, gowns and gloves, care of invasive devices, sterilization of equipment, and epidemic control techniques.[53,54] Despite the success of these environmental techniques, several well-designed Cochrane reviews failed to produce evidence in favor of prophylactic systemic antibiotics in ventilated newborn infants[55] or neonates with central venous[56] or umbilical catheters.[55] Additional strategies to prevent hospital associated infections include the administration of lactoferrin and probiotic supplementation.[20]

Treatment

Management of neonatal sepsis includes supportive care, source control, and administration of appropriate antibiotics. Significant improvement in the morbidity and mortality of adult and pediatric sepsis has been achieved through goal-directed resuscitation (see Figure 20.5).[57] Unfortunately, the "goal" of resuscitation is not as clear in the neonatal population as it is in adults.[58] At birth, newborns carry a "backpack" of extra salt and water to carry them through the transition to extrauterine life.[59] During this transition and early neonatal life, many hemodynamic parameters such as blood pressure do not have clear "normal" values.[60] In addition, immature cardiovascular and endocrine systems may blunt the appropriate stress response

in newborns, making vasopressor, inotrope, calcium, and hormone replacement necessary.[61] Finally, aggressive fluid resuscitation is associated with a significant risk of reopening the ductus arteriosus and potentially worsening perfusion.[62] Nevertheless, fluid resuscitation, vasopressor use, calcium replacement, and endocrine replacement are key components of the therapeutic armamentarium for achieving adequate tissue perfusion.[63,64]

There are no validated clinical signs of shock or poor tissue perfusion without end organ damage. The Surviving Sepsis Campaign guidelines now include pediatric considerations in the management of severe sepsis but do not distinguish between neonates and children. Carcillo et al.[65] provided newborn-specific clinical practice parameters for resuscitation and stabilization of neonates in septic shock (Table 20.7). Resuscitation should include (1) maintaining the airway and attaining adequate oxygenation and ventilation, (2) maintaining circulation defined as normal perfusion and blood pressure, and (3) maintaining threshold heart rates. Therapeutic endpoints include capillary refill of less than 2 seconds, normal pulses with no difference in central and peripheral pulses, warm extremities, urine output of greater than 1 mL/kg/h, normal mental status, normal blood pressure for age, preductal and postductal oxygen saturation difference of less than 5%, and oxygen saturation of >95%.[66] Though frequently assessed for management, studies have demonstrated no association between blood pressure and tissue perfusion,[67] and a weak association among color,[68] capillary refill,[69] and tissue perfusion. Significantly decreased tissue perfusion has several measurable laboratory and biochemical effects in the neonate. In particular, metabolic acidosis, base deficit, and serum lactate can be utilized as markers of poor perfusion.[70] Therefore, improvement in these laboratory markers along with urine output can be used as putative "goals" for resuscitation.

During resuscitation, need for intubation and vascular access should be assessed. Fluid boluses of 10 mL/kg should be given up to 60 mL/kg in the first hour to attain normal perfusion and blood pressure. Vasoactive support may be required, but pulmonary vascular resistance should be considered when selecting a vasopressor and support for persistent pulmonary hypertension of the newborn should be initiated if needed.[66] The most commonly studied and prescribed adrenergic medications include dopamine, dobutamine, and epinephrine. In addition, milrinone is a frequently used phosphodiesterase inhibitor. Due to the differing proportions of alpha- and beta-adrenergic receptors in the neonate, there has been significant skepticism regarding the utility of alpha-specific medications such as phenylephrine or norepinephrine, although they are used routinely in older patients. Nevertheless, a prospective trial evaluating norepinephrine demonstrated improved tissue perfusion and relative safety in the neonate with shock refractory to fluid and classic vasopressors.[71] Similarly, several reports of neonatal use of vasopressin agonists in refractory shock and post cardiopulmonary bypass stun

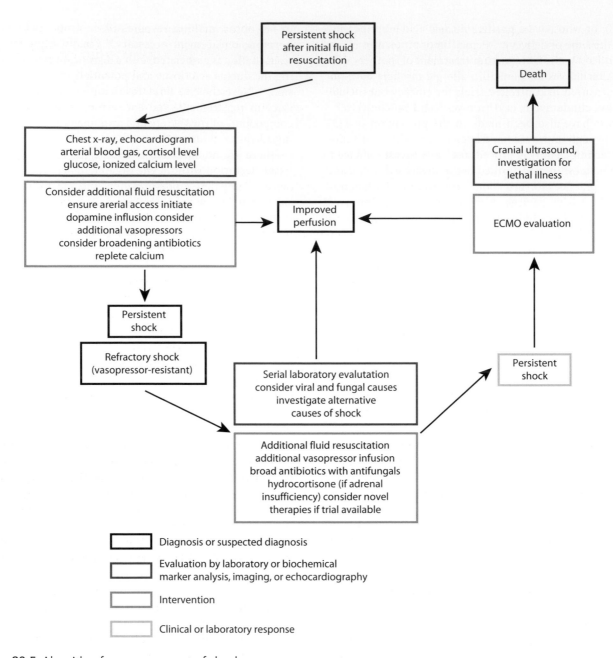

Figure 20.5 Algorithm for management of shock.

suggest that vasopressin[72] and terlipressin[73] appear to be effective and relatively safe. Nonetheless, current neonatal guidelines generally favor dopamine over dobutamine as an initial choice of vasopressor, and epinephrine as a rescue medication for dopamine-refractory shock, despite ongoing debate about the optimal pressor for different types of shock.[61] Because neonatal sarcomeres are immature, sarcoplasmic calcium stores are significantly less[74]; this results in a profound dependence on serum calcium for successful contractility of the myocardium and tone of the arteriolar vascular tree. Calcium chloride infusions, along with various other forms of calcium replacement, have been strongly advocated in the pediatric and anesthesia communities,[75] but safety and intravenous access issues have not been studied in the setting of calcium infusion for septic shock.

Nevertheless, most units prefer to add calcium to intravenous fluid and parenteral nutrition, as well as intravenous calcium boluses to maintain calcium in the normal range.

Evidence supports endocrine replacement therapy in the setting of neonatal shock refractory to vasopressor treatment.[76] Although there is inadequate evidence to support empiric corticosteroid use,[77,78] measurement of serum cortisol concentrations and absolute and relative adrenal insufficiency can identify neonates who will benefit from hydrocortisone replacement therapy.[79] Corticosteroids have two main classes of effects: genomic and nongenomic. Late effects, such as alterations in IL-2 production and secretion, are due to changes in leukocyte gene regulation. Early nongenomic effects, on the other hand, are responsible for the efficacy of endocrine

Table 20.7 Neonatal sepsis goals and therapeutic endpoints for resuscitation and stabilization

	Goals	Therapeutic endpoints
Initial resuscitation (first hour)	• Maintain airway • Maintain circulation • Maintain threshold heart rate	• Capillary refill ≤2 seconds • Normal pulses • No difference between peripheral and central pulses • Warm extremities • UOP >1 mL/kg/hour • Normal mental status • <5% difference in preductal and postductal oxygen saturation • Oxygen saturation of >95%
Stabilization	• Maintain threshold heart rate • Maintain perfusion and blood pressure • $ScvO_2$ >70% • CI >3.3 L/min/m^2 • SVC flow >40 mL/kg/min	• Maintain endpoints for initial resuscitation • Absence of right to left shunting, tricuspid regurgitation, or right ventricular failure • Normal glucose and calcium levels • Normal INR • Normal anion gap and lactate • Fluid overload <10%

Source: Adapted from Carcillo et al., J. Pediatr. (Rio J), 78(6), 449–66, 2002.
Abbreviations: UOP = urine output, $ScvO_2$ = central venous oxygen saturation, CI = cardiac index, SVC = superior vena cava, INR = international normalized ratio.

replacement in shock. In particular, corticosteroids lead, in a nongenomic, rapid fashion, to the prevention of endocytosis of adrenergic receptors and downregulation of secondary messenger systems that lead to tachyphylaxis to both autologous and extrinsically infused adrenergic vasopressors.[76] Successful response to hydrocortisone therapy generally is immediate (minutes to hours)[80] and requires replacement of stress dose cortisol levels only, or hydrocortisone 1 mg/kg every 6 hours. There are currently no evidence-based guidelines on weaning hydrocortisone in neonates.[81]

Therapeutic endpoints for neonatal stabilization beyond the first hour include maintaining the initial resuscitation targets and maintaining a central venous oxygen saturation (ScvO$_2$) of greater than 70%, normal glucose and ionized calcium levels, superior vena cava flow greater than 40 mL/kg/min, cardiac index greater than 3.3 L/min/m^2, normal INR, normal anion gap, normal lactate, fluid overload of less than 10%, and absence of right to left shunt, tricuspid regurgitation, or right ventricular failure. In the case of refractory shock, pericardial effusion, pneumothorax, blood loss, hypoadrenalism, hypothyroidism, inborn errors of metabolism, or heart disease should be evaluated and treated as discussed above. If these causes are excluded, practitioners should consider extracorporeal membrane oxygenation (ECMO).[65,66]

Source control is essential in the treatment of neonatal sepsis. EOS is most commonly caused by an ascending or transplacental transmission of infection, while LOS is most commonly related to indwelling catheters, ventilator-associated pneumonia, or urinary tract infections. For EOS,

source control consists of clamping and cutting the umbilical cord. For LOS, source control should include removal of catheters and extubation as early as clinically possible. Patients should also be evaluated for other causes of infection, and aggressive source control should be initiated for infected or necrotic tissue.

Selection of initial antibiotic therapy can be difficult. Blood cultures should be obtained, and empiric antibiotics should be administered within 1 hour of the identification of sepsis.[6] The epidemiology of EOS continues to change rapidly, and while a penicillin and aminoglycoside appear to be optimal peripartum therapy, integration of individual unit antibiograms and ongoing surveillance are necessary for treating LOS. Furthermore, decreasing Gram-negative and Gram-positive sepsis has led to a commensurate rise in anaerobic, fungal, and viral sepsis. There is inadequate evidence from randomized trials to support any particular antibiotic regimen in the initial treatment of suspected LOS in the newborn.[82] Although variations on penicillins (such as antipseudomonal penicillins or beta-lactamase inhibitors) and low cross resistance between aminoglycosides help individual units develop broad spectrum strategies, increasing rates of methicillin-resistant Staphylococcus aureus (MRSA) and multidrug resistant Gram-negative infections make optimal broad spectrum coverage a moving target. Increasingly, initial therapy includes vancomycin in units highly colonized with MRSA as well as an antifungal agent due to the increased incidence of Candida spp. sepsis as well.[83] Indeed, there are randomized controlled trials that support prophylactic,[84] initial, and completion antifungal therapy.[85,86]

Once culture-proven sepsis is documented, it is safe and appropriate to narrow the spectrum of initial antibiotic therapy toward the pathogen identified. The treatment duration varies from 10 to 14 days depending on the pathogen, while treatment for meningitis is usually longer. Duration should be adjusted based on response to therapy or complications including abscesses, osteomyelitis, or endocarditis.[36] For infants with neonatal sepsis and negative blood cultures, antibiotic duration should be determined by the clinical course and the risk of prolonged antibiotic therapy.[45] Monitoring response to antibiotic therapy should be performed with repeat blood cultures and laboratory values to document bacterial clearance. Trends in inflammatory biomarkers have been evaluated to determine response to antibiotic therapy and may allow for the early discontinuation of antibiotics in healthy appearing neonates.[42] However, further investigations are needed on targeted antibiotics and biomarkers to guide duration of therapy.

New therapies and preventive strategies

Several new therapies have been proposed for the management of neonatal sepsis. Intravenous immunoglobulin (IVIG) was evaluated due to its potential to supplement the immune system by augmenting antibody-dependent cytotoxicity and improving neutrophil function. An international study group of 113 hospitals and a Cochrane review of 10 controlled trials found no effect on morbidity or mortality with IVIG administration.[20] Recombinant granulocyte colony-stimulating factor was also evaluated in neonatal sepsis and was found to have no effect on severity of illness, morbidity, or mortality.[36,87] Pentoxifylline, an agent that improves microcirculation and decreases TNF-α, was studied in culture positive neonatal sepsis and may have potential for improved survival.[20,88] However, this response needs to be evaluated in a large multicenter trial.

MULTIDRUG RESISTANCE AND OPPORTUNISTIC INFECTIONS

Intrapartum antibiotic prophylaxis for maternal GBS has significantly decreased vertical transmission and the incidence of EOS due to GBS.[89] However, the use of prophylactic and broad spectrum antibiotics has caused a shift in the causative organisms and has increased the proportion of non-GBS organisms. E. coli has emerged as a leading non-GBS cause of EOS.[23] Gram-negative sepsis is linked to increased severity of disease and death in newborns, and raises significant concerns about the effect of widespread antibiotic use for prophylaxis and optimal prevention and treatment approaches.[34,89]

Previous studies have shown rapid development of and increased rates of resistance with the use of cefotaxime for the routine treatment of EOS.[45,90] Therefore, cefotaxime use should be restricted for infants with meningitis caused by Gram-negative bacteria.[91]

Candida species are the most common fungal infectious agents encountered in the NICU. *Candida* infections account for 1%–4% of all NICU admissions and approximately 10% of nosocomial sepsis in VLBW neonates.[92–94] However, colonization by *Candida* does not necessarily lead to invasive infection. A retrospective review by Manzoni et al.[95] found that colonization occurred in 32% of VLBW neonates at a single institution. The median age for the invasive fungal infections in this study was 21 days. The Neonatal Research Network prospectively collected data on neonates weighing <1000 g to study risk factors, causes, and outcomes of extremely low birth weight (ELBW) neonates with candidiasis in the NICU.[93] They found that invasive candidiasis was documented in 7% of ELBW neonates, with 68% survival. *C. albicans* and *C. parapsilosis* were the most commonly identified species with similar rates and mortality in blood infections and meningitis, with *C. albicans* having an increased mortality rate at 42% versus 20% overall. Furthermore, neonates with birth weight between 401 and 750 g and the use of a third-generation cephalosporin were found to increase the risk of developing candidiasis, while enteral feeding appeared protective.[93] Other factors associated with invasive fungal infections in colonized patients were: colonization of central venous catheter, colonization in multiple sites, low birth weight, prematurity, days on supplemental oxygen, positive gastric culture, positive endotracheal culture, intubation, and presence of bacterial sepsis.[95]

VIRAL SEPSIS

Neonatal viruses have been increasingly identified in infants evaluated for bacterial sepsis despite the lack of clinical indicators.[96,97] The VIRIoN-I study prospectively evaluated the incidence of respiratory viral infections and found that 6% of NICU sepsis evaluations had a viral infection detected.[96] Infants diagnosed with a respiratory virus had a longer hospital stay and were more commonly diagnosed with bronchopulmonary dysplasia (BPD).[97] Neonatal viral infections include coronavirus, enterovirus, human metapneumovirus, influenza, parainfluenza virus, respiratory syncytial virus, rhinovirus, herpes simplex virus, coxsackievirus, echovirus, cytomegalovirus, human immunodeficiency virus, varicella-zoster, rubella virus, influenza, and parechovirus.[28,36] Antivirals such as acyclovir, ganciclovir, and oseltamivir can be used in the treatment of infected neonates and have improved the morbidity and mortality associated with viral infection.[28,36]

OUTCOMES

Neonatal sepsis and its associated mortality is declining.[1] However, survival can be associated with adverse long-term outcomes. These include cerebral palsy, visual impairment, delayed psychomotor development, low Bayley Scales of Infant Development scores, overall poor neurodevelopment, and impaired growth.[2,20] Recurrent postnatal infection was found to be a risk factor for progressive white matter injury in premature infants, which may be related to the adverse neurodevelopmental sequelae observed after neonatal sepsis.[98] Preterm infants exposed to chorioamnionitis and subsequent EOS have an increased incidence of BPD resulting in chronic lung disease and poor developmental outcomes. Sepsis-induced endocarditis and thrombosis can cause rare complications such as pulmonary embolism, valvular damage, and infectious thromboembolism.[36]

CONCLUSIONS

Neonatal sepsis continues to be a major cause of long-term morbidity and mortality. As the prevention, identification, and therapy of sepsis advance, the epidemiology and bacteriology of the disease shift making optimal treatment of sepsis an evolving process.[6] Continued evaluation of current management guidelines and the development of preventive, diagnostic, and therapeutic measures for neonatal sepsis are essential.

REFERENCES

1. The World Health Organization Global Health Observatory Data Repository: World Health Organization; 2015 [cited 2015 February 24]. Available from: http://apps.who.int/gho/data/view .main.CM1002015WORLD-CH12?lang=en.
2. Stoll BJ, Hansen NI, Adams-Chapman I, Fanaroff AA, Hintz SR, Vohr B et al. Neurodevelopmental and growth impairment among extremely low-birth-weight infants with neonatal infection. *JAMA* 2004; 292(19):2357–65.
3. Rivers E, Nguyen B, Havstad S, Ressler J, Muzzin A, Knoblich B et al. Early goal-directed therapy in the treatment of severe sepsis and septic shock. *N Engl J Med* 2001; 345(19):1368–77.
4. Otero RM, Nguyen HB, Huang DT, Gaieski DF, Goyal M, Gunnerson KJ et al. Early goal-directed therapy in severe sepsis and septic shock revisited: Concepts, controversies, and contemporary findings. *Chest* 2006; 130(5):1579–95.
5. Rivers EP, Kruse JA, Jacobsen G, Shah K, Loomba M, Otero R et al. The influence of early hemodynamic optimization on biomarker patterns of severe sepsis and septic shock. *Crit Care Med* 2007; 35(9):2016–24.
6. Dellinger RP, Levy MM, Rhodes A, Annane D, Gerlach H, Opal SM et al. Surviving Sepsis Campaign: International guidelines for management of severe sepsis and septic shock, 2012. *Intensive Care Med* 2013; 39(2):165–228.
7. Singer M, Deutschman CS, Seymour CW, Shankar-Hari M, Annane D, Bauer M et al. The Third International Consensus Definitions for Sepsis and Septic Shock (Sepsis-3). *JAMA* 2016; 315(8):801–10.
8. Bedford Russell AR. Neonatal sepsis. *Paediatr Child Health* 2015; 21(6):265–9.
9. Dagan R, Powell KR, Hall CB, Menegus MA. Identification of infants unlikely to have serious bacterial infection although hospitalized for suspected sepsis. *J Pediatr* 1985; 107(6):855–60.
10. Jaskiewicz JA, McCarthy CA, Richardson AC, White KC, Fisher DJ, Dagan R et al. Febrile infants at low risk for serious bacterial infection—An appraisal of the Rochester criteria and implications for management. Febrile Infant Collaborative Study Group. *Pediatrics* 1994; 94(3):390–6.
11. Bachur RG, Harper MB. Predictive model for serious bacterial infections among infants younger than 3 months of age. *Pediatrics* 2001; 108(2):311–6.
12. Goldstein B, Giroir B, Randolph A, Sepsis ICCoP. International pediatric sepsis consensus conference: Definitions for sepsis and organ dysfunction in pediatrics. *Pediatr Crit Care Med* 2005; 6(1):2–8.
13. Groselj-Grenc M, Ihan A, Pavcnik-Arnol M, Kopitar AN, Gmeiner-Stopar T, Derganc M. Neutrophil and monocyte CD64 indexes, lipopolysaccharide-binding protein, procalcitonin and C-reactive protein in sepsis of critically ill neonates and children. *Intensive Care Med* 2009; 35(11):1950–8.
14. Bone RC. The sepsis syndrome. Definition and general approach to management. *Clin Chest Med* 1996; 17(2):175–81.
15. Bone RC, Balk RA, Cerra FB, Dellinger RP, Fein AM, Knaus WA et al. Definitions for sepsis and organ failure and guidelines for the use of innovative therapies in sepsis. The ACCP/SCCM Consensus Conference Committee. American College of Chest Physicians/Society of Critical Care Medicine. *Chest* 1992; 101(6):1644–55.
16. Levy MM, Fink MP, Marshall JC, Abraham E, Angus D, Cook D et al. 2001 SCCM/ESICM/ACCP/ATS/SIS International Sepsis Definitions Conference. *Intensive Care Med* 2003; 29(4):530–8.
17. Prinsen JH, Baranski E, Posch H, Tober K, Gerstmeyer A. Interleukin-6 as diagnostic marker for neonatal sepsis: Determination of Access IL-6 cutoff for newborns. *Clin Lab* 2008; 54(5–6):179–83.
18. Enguix A, Rey C, Concha A, Medina A, Coto D, Diéguez MA. Comparison of procalcitonin with C-reactive protein and serum amyloid for the early diagnosis of bacterial sepsis in critically ill neonates and children. *Intensive Care Med* 2001; 27(1):211–5.
19. Pavcnik-Arnol M, Hojker S, Derganc M. Lipopolysaccharide-binding protein, lipopolysaccharide, and soluble CD14 in sepsis of critically ill neonates and children. *Intensive Care Med* 2007; 33(6):1025–32.
20. Shane AL, Stoll BJ. Neonatal sepsis: Progress towards improved outcomes. *J Infect* 2014; 68 Suppl 1:S24–32.
21. Lawn JE, Cousens S, Zupan J, Team LNSS. 4 million neonatal deaths: When? Where? Why? *Lancet* 2005; 365(9462):891–900.

22. Basu S. Neonatal sepsis: The gut connection. *Eur J Clin Microbiol Infect Dis* 2015; 34(2):215–22.

23. Shah BA, Padbury JF. Neonatal sepsis: An old problem with new insights. *Virulence* 2014; 5(1):170–8.

24. Wynn JL. Defining neonatal sepsis. *Curr Opin Pediatr* 2016 Apr; 28(2):135–40.

25. Raju TN, Higgins RD, Stark AR, Leveno KJ. Optimizing care and outcome for late-preterm (near-term) infants: A summary of the workshop sponsored by the National Institute of Child Health and Human Development. *Pediatrics* 2006; 118(3):1207–14.

26. Chan GJ, Lee AC, Baqui AH, Tan J, Black RE. Risk of early-onset neonatal infection with maternal infection or colonization: A global systematic review and meta-analysis. *PLoS Med* 2013; 10(8):e1001502.

27. Jiang Z, Ye GY. 1:4 matched case-control study on influential factor of early onset neonatal sepsis. *Eur Rev Med Pharmacol Sci* 2013; 17(18):2460–6.

28. Santos RP, Tristram D. A practical guide to the diagnosis, treatment, and prevention of neonatal infections. *Pediatr Clin North Am* 2015; 62(2):491–508.

29. Bedford Russell AR, Kumar R. Early onset neonatal sepsis: Diagnostic dilemmas and practical management. *Arch Dis Child Fetal Neonatal Ed* 2015; 100(4):F350–4.

30. Cortese F, Scicchitano P, Gesualdo M, Filaninno A, De Giorgi E, Schettini F et al. Early and late infections in newborns: Where do we stand? A review. *Pediatr Neonatol* 2016 Aug; 57(4):265–73.

31. Yancey MK, Duff P, Kubilis P, Clark P, Frentzen BH. Risk factors for neonatal sepsis. *Obstet Gynecol* 1996; 87(2):188–94.

32. Srinivasan L, Kirpalani H, Cotten CM. Elucidating the role of genomics in neonatal sepsis. *Semin Perinatol* 2015; 39(8):611–6.

33. Banerjee SN, Grohskopf LA, Sinkowitz-Cochran RL, Jarvis WR, System NNIS, Network PP. Incidence of pediatric and neonatal intensive care unit-acquired infections. *Infect Control Hosp Epidemiol*. 2006; 27(6):561–70.

34. Stoll BJ, Hansen N, Fanaroff AA, Wright LL, Carlo WA, Ehrenkranz RA et al. Changes in pathogens causing early-onset sepsis in very-low-birth-weight infants. *N Engl J Med* 2002; 347(4):240–7.

35. Westerlund B, Korhonen TK. Bacterial proteins binding to the mammalian extracellular matrix. *Mol Microbiol* 1993; 9(4):687–94.

36. Simonsen KA, Anderson-Berry AL, Delair SF, Davies HD. Early-onset neonatal sepsis. *Clin Microbiol Rev* 2014; 27(1):21–47.

37. Kenzel S, Henneke P. The innate immune system and its relevance to neonatal sepsis. *Curr Opin Infect Dis* 2006; 19(3):264–70.

38. Fadel S, Sarzotti M. Cellular immune responses in neonates. *Int Rev Immunol* 2000; 19(2–3):173–93.

39. Stoll BJ, Hansen N, Fanaroff AA, Wright LL, Carlo WA, Ehrenkranz RA et al. To tap or not to tap: High likelihood of meningitis without sepsis among very low birth weight infants. *Pediatrics* 2004; 113(5):1181–6.

40. Machado JR, Soave DF, da Silva MV, de Menezes LB, Etchebehere RM, Monteiro ML et al. Neonatal sepsis and inflammatory mediators. *Mediators Inflamm* 2014; 2014:269681.

41. Fjalstad JW, Stensvold HJ, Bergseng H, Simonsen GS, Salvesen B, Rønnestad AE et al. Early-onset sepsis and antibiotic exposure in term infants: A nationwide population-based study in Norway. *Pediatr Infect Dis J* 2016; 35(1):1–6.

42. Deleon C, Shattuck K, Sunil JK. Biomarkers in neonatal sepsis. *NeoReviews* 2015; 16(5):e297–e308.

43. Excellence NIfHaC. Neonatal Infection: Antibiotics for prevention and treatment 2012 [cited 2016 February 20]. Available from: https://www.nice.org.uk/guidance/cg149.

44. Wynn JL, Wong HR, Shanley TP, Bizzarro MJ, Saiman L, Polin RA. Time for a neonatal-specific consensus definition for sepsis. *Pediatr Crit Care Med* 2014; 15(6):523–8.

45. Polin RA, Newborn CoFa. Management of neonates with suspected or proven early-onset bacterial sepsis. *Pediatrics* 2012; 129(5):1006–15.

46. Benitz WE, Wynn JL, Polin RA. Reappraisal of guidelines for management of neonates with suspected early-onset sepsis. *J Pediatr* 2015; 166(4):1070–4.

47. Hedegaard SS, Wisborg K, Hvas AM. Diagnostic utility of biomarkers for neonatal sepsis—A systematic review. *Infect Dis (Lond)* 2015; 47(3):117–24.

48. Albrich WC, Harbarth S. Pros and cons of using biomarkers versus clinical decisions in start and stop decisions for antibiotics in the critical care setting. *Intensive Care Med* 2015; 41(10):1739–51.

49. Prevention CfDCa. Prevention of Perinatal Group B Streptococcal Disease Revised Guidelines Morbidity and Mortality Weekly Report2010 [cited 2016 February 20]. Available from: http://www.cdc.gov/mmwr/pdf/rr/rr5910.pdf.

50. Shuman RM, Leech RW, Alvord EC. Neurotoxicity of hexachlorophene in humans. II. A clinicopathological study of 46 premature infants. *Arch Neurol* 1975; 32(5):320–5.

51. Zupan J, Garner P, Omari AA. Topical umbilical cord care at birth. *Cochrane Database Syst Rev* 2004; (3):CD001057.

52. Kapellen TM, Gebauer CM, Brosteanu O, Labitzke B, Vogtmann C, Kiess W. Higher rate of cord-related adverse events in neonates with dry umbilical cord care compared to chlorhexidine powder. Results of a randomized controlled study to compare efficacy and safety of chlorhexidine powder versus dry care in umbilical cord care of the newborn. *Neonatology* 2009; 96(1):13–8.

53. Lachman P, Yuen S. Using care bundles to prevent infection in neonatal and paediatric ICUs. *Curr Opin Infect Dis* 2009; 22(3):224–8.

54. Gardner SL. Sepsis in the neonate. *Crit Care Nurs Clin North Am* 2009; 21(1):121–41, vii.

55. Inglis GD, Jardine LA, Davies MW. Prophylactic antibiotics to reduce morbidity and mortality in ventilated newborn infants. *Cochrane Database Syst Rev* 2007; (3):CD004338.

56. Jardine LA, Inglis GD, Davies MW. Prophylactic systemic antibiotics to reduce morbidity and mortality in neonates with central venous catheters. *Cochrane Database Syst Rev* 2008; (1):CD006179.

57. Levy MM, Dellinger RP, Townsend SR, Linde-Zwirble WT, Marshall JC, Bion J et al. The Surviving Sepsis Campaign: Results of an international guideline-based performance improvement program targeting severe sepsis. *Crit Care Med* 2010; 38(2):367–74.

58. Seri I, Noori S. Diagnosis and treatment of neonatal hypotension outside the transitional period. *Early Hum Dev* 2005; 81(5):405–11.

59. Avery GB, MacDonald MG, Seshia MMK, Mullett MD. *Avery's Neonatology Pathophysiology and Management of the Newborn*, 5th edn. Philadelphia: Lippincott, Williams, and Wilkins, 2005.

60. Evans N. Assessment and support of the preterm circulation. *Early Hum Dev* 2006; 82(12):803–10.

61. Seri I. Inotrope, lusitrope, and pressor use in neonates. *J Perinatol* 2005; 25 Suppl 2:S28–30.

62. Weiss H, Cooper B, Brook M, Schlueter M, Clyman R. Factors determining reopening of the ductus arteriosus after successful clinical closure with indomethacin. *J Pediatr* 1995; 127(3):466–71.

63. Schmaltz C. Hypotension and shock in the preterm neonate. *Adv Neonatal Care* 2009; 9(4):156–62.

64. Seri I. Circulatory support of the sick preterm infant. *Semin Neonatol* 2001; 6(1):85–95.

65. Carcillo JA, Fields AI, Força-Tarefa Cd. [Clinical practice parameters for hemodynamic support of pediatric and neonatal patients in septic shock]. *J Pediatr (Rio J)* 2002; 78(6):449–66.

66. Carcillo JA. A synopsis of 2007 ACCM clinical practice parameters for hemodynamic support of term newborn and infant septic shock. *Early Hum Dev* 2014; 90 Suppl 1:S45–7.

67. Osborn DA, Evans N, Kluckow M. Clinical detection of low upper body blood flow in very premature infants using blood pressure, capillary refill time, and central-peripheral temperature difference. *Arch Dis Child Fetal Neonatal Ed* 2004; 89(2):F168–73.

68. De Felice C, Flori ML, Pellegrino M, Toti P, Stanghellini E, Molinu A et al. Predictive value of skin color for illness severity in the high-risk newborn. *Pediatr Res* 2002; 51(1):100–5.

69. Miletin J, Pichova K, Dempsey EM. Bedside detection of low systemic flow in the very low birth weight infant on day 1 of life. *Eur J Pediatr* 2009; 168(7):809–13.

70. Dempsey EM, Barrington KJ. Evaluation and treatment of hypotension in the preterm infant. *Clin Perinatol* 2009; 36(1):75–85.

71. Tourneux P, Rakza T, Abazine A, Krim G, Storme L. Noradrenaline for management of septic shock refractory to fluid loading and dopamine or dobutamine in full-term newborn infants. *Acta Paediatr* 2008; 97(2):177–80.

72. Meyer S, Gottschling S, Baghai A, Wurm D, Gortner L. Arginine-vasopressin in catecholamine-refractory septic versus non-septic shock in extremely low birth weight infants with acute renal injury. *Crit Care* 2006; 10(3):R71.

73. Filippi L, Poggi C, Serafini L, Fiorini P. Terlipressin as rescue treatment of refractory shock in a neonate. *Acta Paediatr* 2008; 97(4):500–2.

74. Fisher DJ, Towbin J. Maturation of the heart. *Clin Perinatol* 1988; 15(3):421–46.

75. Forsythe RM, Wessel CB, Billiar TR, Angus DC, Rosengart MR. Parenteral calcium for intensive care unit patients. *Cochrane Database Syst Rev* 2008; (4):CD006163.

76. Seri I. Hydrocortisone and vasopressor-resistant shock in preterm neonates. *Pediatrics* 2006; 117(2):516–8.

77. Efird MM, Heerens AT, Gordon PV, Bose CL, Young DA. A randomized-controlled trial of prophylactic hydrocortisone supplementation for the prevention of hypotension in extremely low birth weight infants. *J Perinatol* 2005; 25(2):119–24.

78. Subhedar NV, Duffy K, Ibrahim H. Corticosteroids for treating hypotension in preterm infants. *Cochrane Database Syst Rev* 2007; (1):CD003662.

79. Masumoto K, Kusuda S, Aoyagi H, Tamura Y, Obonai T, Yamasaki C et al. Comparison of serum cortisol concentrations in preterm infants with or without late-onset circulatory collapse due to adrenal insufficiency of prematurity. *Pediatr Res* 2008; 63(6):686–90.

80. Krediet T, van der Ent K. Rapid increase of blood pressure after low dose hydrocortisone in low birth weight neonates with hypotension refractory to high doses of cardiac inotropes. *Pediatr Res* 1998; 38:210.

81. Fernandez EF, Watterberg KL. Relative adrenal insufficiency in the preterm and term infant. *J Perinatol* 2009; 29 Suppl 2:S44–9.

82. Gordon A, Jeffery HE. Antibiotic regimens for suspected late onset sepsis in newborn infants. *Cochrane Database Syst Rev* 2005; (3):CD004501.

83. Fanos V, Cuzzolin L, Atzei A, Testa M. Antibiotics and antifungals in neonatal intensive care units: A review. *J Chemother* 2007; 19(1):5–20.

84. Manzoni P, Stolfi I, Pugni L, Decembrino L, Magnani C, Vetrano G et al. A multicenter, randomized trial of prophylactic fluconazole in preterm neonates. *N Engl J Med* 2007; 356(24):2483–95.

85. Driessen M, Ellis JB, Cooper PA, Wainer S, Muwazi F, Hahn D et al. Fluconazole vs. amphotericin B for the treatment of neonatal fungal septicemia: A prospective randomized trial. *Pediatr Infect Dis J* 1996; 15(12):1107–12.

86. Frattarelli DA, Reed MD, Giacoia GP, Aranda JV. Antifungals in systemic neonatal candidiasis. *Drugs* 2004; 64(9):949–68.

87. Marlow N, Morris T, Brocklehurst P, Carr R, Cowan F, Patel N et al. A randomised trial of granulocyte-macrophage colony-stimulating factor for neonatal sepsis: Childhood outcomes at 5 years. *Arch Dis Child Fetal Neonatal Ed* 2015; 100(4):F320–6.

88. Shabaan AE, Nasef N, Shouman B, Nour I, Mesbah A, Abdel-Hady H. Pentoxifylline therapy for late-onset sepsis in preterm infants: A randomized controlled trial. *Pediatr Infect Dis J* 2015; 34(6):e143–8.

89. Stoll BJ, Hansen NI, Sanchez PJ, Faix RG, Poindexter BB, Van Meurs KP et al. Early onset neonatal sepsis: The burden of group B Streptococcal and E. coli disease continues. *Pediatrics* 2011; 127(5):817–26.

90. Bryan CS, John JF, Jr., Pai MS, Austin TL. Gentamicin vs cefotaxime for therapy of neonatal sepsis. Relationship to drug resistance. *Am J Dis Child (1960)* 1985; 139(11):1086–9.

91. Begue P, Floret D, Mallet E, Raynaud EJ, Safran C, Sarlangues J et al. Pharmacokinetics and clinical evaluation of cefotaxime in children suffering with purulent meningitis. *J Antimicrob Chemother* 1984; 14 Suppl B:161–5.

92. Stoll BJ, Hansen N, Fanaroff AA, Wright LL, Carlo WA, Ehrenkranz RA et al. Late-onset sepsis in very low birth weight neonates: The experience of the NICHD Neonatal Research Network. *Pediatrics* 2002; 110(2 Pt 1):285–91.

93. Benjamin DK, Jr., Stoll BJ, Fanaroff AA, McDonald SA, Oh W, Higgins RD et al. Neonatal candidiasis among extremely low birth weight infants: Risk factors, mortality rates, and neurodevelopmental outcomes at 18 to 22 months. *Pediatrics* 2006; 117(1):84–92.

94. Botero-Calderon L, Benjamin DK Jr, Cohen-Wolkowiez M. Advances in the treatment of invasive neonatal candidiasis. *Expert Opin Pharmacother* 2015; 16(7):1035–48.

95. Manzoni P, Farina D, Leonessa M, d'Oulx EA, Galletto P, Mostert M et al. Risk factors for progression to invasive fungal infection in preterm neonates with fungal colonization. *Pediatrics* 2006;118(6):2359–64.

96. Ronchi A, Michelow IC, Chapin KC, Bliss JM, Pugni L, Mosca F et al. Viral respiratory tract infections in the neonatal intensive care unit: The VIRIoN-I study. *J Pediatr* 2014; 165(4):690–6.

97. Bennett NJ, Tabarani CM, Bartholoma NM, Wang D, Huang D, Riddell SW et al. Unrecognized viral respiratory tract infections in premature infants during their birth hospitalization: A prospective surveillance study in two neonatal intensive care units. *J Pediatr* 2012; 161(5):814–8.

98. Glass HC, Bonifacio SL, Chau V, Glidden D, Poskitt K, Barkovich AJ et al. Recurrent postnatal infections are associated with progressive white matter injury in premature infants. *Pediatrics* 2008; 122(2):299–305.

21

Hematological problems in the neonate

ANDREA M. MALONE AND OWEN P. SMITH

INTRODUCTION

Hematopoiesis in the fetus and neonate is in a constant state of flux and evolution as the newborn adapts to a new physiological milieu. Hematological problems may present during this period as a result of a genetic defect, immaturity, or stress, and present a major diagnostic and therapeutic challenge to the neonatologist and hematologist alike. Advances in molecular techniques have allowed the elucidation of the cellular mechanisms that give rise to some of these disorders of the hematopoietic system. It is hoped that this chapter will give the reader a broad understanding of the major hematological disorders seen in the neonatal period, especially those involving platelets, white cells, red cells, and clotting proteins.

PLATELETS

The normal range of the platelet count is similar in fetal life to that seen in adulthood, being in the range of 150×10^9/L to 400×10^9/L. Thrombocytopenia, defined as a blood platelet count of below 150×10^9/L, is the most common hematological abnormality encountered in the neonatal period, with a reported frequency approximating 0.1%–0.2% in unselected newborns and up to 35% in infants in intensive care units.[1-3] Platelet counts increase with advancing postnatal age, with thrombocytopenia present in about 30% of small for gestational age infants.[4] Severe thrombocytopenia (platelet count less than 50×10^9/L) is uncommon in the healthy newborn population, but has an incidence in neonates admitted to the neonatal intensive care unit of between 2.4 and 5%.[5] The differential diagnosis of thrombocytopenia in the neonatal period is similar to thrombocytopenia in older children with a number of additions that include inherited disorders, and those that arise due to pathophysiological events unique to the antenatal and perinatal periods. Although most automated counters in the laboratory are designed to detect platelet clumps, it is essential to confirm that the low platelet count is genuine by visual inspection of the blood smear before initiating further investigations. Pseudo thrombocytopenia due to platelet clumping is not associated with bleeding and does not require treatment. The approach to the investigation of thrombocytopenia should be tailored to the individual infant and mother. Assessment of the baby's general condition is very important as healthy neonates with thrombocytopenia usually have an immune or an inherited etiology, whereas the presence of hepatosplenomegaly, mass lesions, hemangiomas, and congenital anomalies will point toward a totally different spectrum of causes. A detailed maternal history should always be obtained, with specific focus on bleeding problems, hypertension, and drug ingestion, and also with respect to viral infections or connective tissue diseases. The causes of thrombocytopenia are divided into two broad categories: those due to increased platelet destruction and those due to decreased platelet production. Occasionally, both mechanisms contribute to the thrombocytopenia.

Increased destruction

Increased destruction of platelets is seen in a number of neonatal conditions. It encompasses immune-mediated platelet destruction or consumption.

AUTOIMMUNE THROMBOCYTOPENIA

This is seen in term babies that are generally clinically well and is mediated by the passive transfer of maternal autoantibodies in mothers with autoimmune disorders such as immune thrombocytopenic purpura (ITP), systemic lupus erythematosis, and hypothyroidism.[6] Thrombocytopenia is seen in about 10% of the infants born to mothers with ITP. The diagnosis is usually apparent from the mother's medical history. The risk of significant morbidity and mortality is minimal as the infant platelet count is rarely $<50 \times 10^9$/L. The nadir typically occurs between 2 and 5 days of age; therefore, affected infants need to be carefully monitored. The most feared complication of neonatal thrombocytopenia is intracranial hemorrhage; however, this very rarely happens in autoimmune thrombocytopenia[7] and is generally not related to the mode of delivery of the infant.[8] Symptomatic infants can be effectively treated with intravenous immunoglobulin (IVIG). Platelet transfusion should be restricted to treat hemorrhage or severe thrombocytopenia.

NEONATAL ALLOIMMUNE THROMBOCYTOPENIA

Neonatal alloimmune thrombocytopenia (NAIT) is characterized by marked thrombocytopenia in the fetus and neonate. It occurs following maternal sensitization to a paternally inherited fetal platelet antigen that is lacking in the mother. The mother forms an IgG antibody that crosses the placenta and destroys fetal platelets. In contrast to hemolytic disease of the newborn (the red blood cell analog of NAIT), NAIT may occur during the first pregnancy. It complicates between 1 in 100 and 1 in 2000 births.[9] NAIT typically presents as an isolated severe thrombocytopenia in an otherwise healthy child at birth. The most serious complication is intracranial hemorrhage, which occurs in 10%–20% of affected newborns.[10] The risk of severe thrombocytopenia and intracranial hemorrhage is greater in alloimmune than in autoimmune thrombocytopenia. For testing to confirm NAIT, it must reveal both a platelet antigen incompatibility between the parents and a maternal antibody derived against that antigen. The most commonly involved antigen is HPA-1a. The mainstay of treatment is transfusion of donor-matched, antigen negative platelets with neonatal specification, and IVIG. Initial evaluation should include a cranial ultrasound to detect hemorrhage. The thrombocytopenia typically resolves over 3–6 weeks. NAIT is very likely to recur in subsequent pregnancies, and the thrombocytopenia is often more severe in the next child.

Peripheral consumption

Increased destruction of platelets leading to thrombocytopenia may also occur from increased peripheral consumption of platelets.

HYPERSPLENISM

This is an uncommon cause of thrombocytopenia in the neonate due to splenic sequestration of platelets. It can be associated with an enlarged spleen. Underlying disorders include hemolytic anemia, congenital viral infection, congenital hepatitis, and portal vein thrombosis. Management is directed at the underlying cause, and platelet transfusions are used supportively.

KASABACH–MERRITT PHENOMENON

Kasabach–Merritt syndrome (KMS) is the association of a giant cavernous hemangioma and disseminated intravascular coagulation. Thrombocytopenia results from shortened platelet survival caused by the sequestration of platelets in the vascular formation. The vascular tumors associated with the KMS are usually kaposiform hemangioendotheliomas (KHE) and not the more usual infantile hemangiomas that are seen in early childhood. The KHE lesions have a predilection for the trunk, retroperitoneum, and proximal extremities, and

less frequently the cervicofacial region. Like other tumors, a KHE is dependent on the formation of new blood vessels from preexisting vasculature (angiogenesis), and this process is regulated by several proangiogenic and anti-angiogenic molecules. Because of their large size and infiltrative nature, complications such as hemorrhage, airway obstruction, and congestive cardiac failure are not uncommon in a small subset of these patients. The consumptive coagulopathy, which is seen in approximately 25% of cases, is usually low grade and compensated. Fortunately, spontaneous regression of the tumor occurs in the majority of cases.

Over the past three decades, medical treatment for these potentially life-threatening lesions has included the use of corticosteroids alone or in combination with vincristine and/or interferon-alpha, together with the judicious use of blood products and clotting factor concentrates. More recently, because of their role in tumor growth, there has been a move to target the platelet by using antiplatelet agents and withholding platelet infusions even in those patients who have significant thrombocytopenia and are coagulopathic. Excellent response rates have been achieved using antiplatelet therapy with vincristine.[11]

THROMBOSIS

Thrombocytopenia can be caused by hypercoagulability and associated consumption of platelets. A low platelet count may be the presenting sign of arterial or venous thrombosis in the neonate.

TYPE 2B VON WILLEBRAND DISEASE

In this type of von Willebrand disease (vWD), the structurally abnormal von Willebrand factor (vWF) has increased affinity for the glycoprotein 1b receptor on the platelet surface. This may lead to platelet aggregation and thrombocytopenia.[12]

Decreased production

Neonatal thrombocytopenia due to decreased platelet production encompasses the inherited disorders and diseases associated with bone marrow infiltration or suppression.

INHERITED BONE MARROW FAILURE SYNDROMES

The inherited bone marrow failure syndromes (IBMFSs) are a rare yet clinically important cause of neonatal hematological manifestations. It is of vital importance to identify them as many of these syndromes confer risks of multiple medical complications, including an increased risk of cancer. Some IBMFSs may present with cytopenias in the neonatal period, whereas others may present only with congenital physical anomalies and progress to pancytopenia later in life.

Thrombocytopenia with absent radii (TAR) is a rare, autosomal recessive disorder that is usually diagnosed at birth as the vast majority of these patients are thrombocytopenic and have the pathognomonic physical sign of bilateral absent radii. Other skeletal abnormalities involving the ulnae, fingers, and lower limbs are less commonly seen.

TAR differs from Fanconi anemia (FA) in several ways: the absent radii are accompanied by the presence of thumbs, the thrombocytopenia is the only cytopenia, and evolution to aplastic anemia and leukemia is rare.[13] The majority of children with TAR have severe thrombocytopenia and recurrent significant bleeding episodes in the first 6 months of life. The genetics of TAR were unknown until recently; however, next-generation sequencing has revealed that TAR patients inherit a deletion of chromosome band 1q21.1 from one parent and a single nucleotide variant in the RBM8A gene from the other parent, thus following an autosomal pattern of inheritance. The mainstay of treatment is judicious transfusion of single donor platelet concentrates as required for thrombocytopenia and orthopedic intervention for functional optimization of the upper limbs. The thrombocytopenia tends to improve over time.[14]

Congenital amegakaryocytic thrombocytopenia (CAMT) is an extremely rare autosomal recessively inherited disorder of infancy and early childhood. Of all the IBMFS, it is the one most likely to present in the neonatal period. Affected newborns show no physical abnormalities. The thrombocytopenia is non-immune and usually severe, and pancytopenia can ensue. The condition results from a mutation in the c-MPL gene that encodes the thrombopoietin (TPO) receptor. Management is largely symptomatic with platelet transfusions and antifibrinolytics for patients with bleeding. Currently, the only curative option for CAMT is hematopoietic stem cell transplantation (HSCT).[14]

FANCONI ANEMIA

FA is a chromosomal instability disorder caused by genetic defects in DNA repair. Bone marrow failure is rarely present in infancy. It is characterized by physical abnormalities (commonly short stature, skin hyper- or hypopigmentation, upper limb and thumb abnormalities), bone marrow failure, and an increased risk of malignancy. Progressive bone marrow failure with pancytopenia typically presents in the first decade. Thrombocytopenia is usually the first cytopenia to appear but rarely the neonatal period. The diagnosis of FA rests upon the detection of increased chromosomal breakage in lymphocytes after exposure to DNA cross-linking agents such as di-epoxybutane or mitomycin C. Recent advances in genomic technology, including next-generation sequencing and whole exome analysis, have accelerated gene discovery efforts. Whereas the first genetic mutation causing FA was discovered more than 20 years ago, there are currently 16 known genes that cause FA. Abnormalities of FA genes are inherited in an autosomal recessive manner except for pathogenic variants in *FANCB*, which are inherited in an X-linked manner.[15] A multidisciplinary team approach is required in the management of infants with FA. HSCT is the only curative treatment for the hematological manifestations of FA.

INHERITED PLATELET DISORDERS

The inherited thrombocytopenias comprise a group of disorders in which platelet numbers are reduced. In the vast majority of patients, the platelet count is only mild to moderately reduced, and therefore, significant spontaneous hemorrhage tends not to be problematic. Spontaneous bleeding is, however, a prominent clinical feature of Bernard–Soulier syndrome (BSS) and Wiskott–Aldrich syndrome (WAS). Immune-mediated thrombocytopenia is a major differential diagnosis in children with low platelet counts, and therefore, making the correct diagnosis of these conditions will prevent the useless and potentially dangerous prescribing of immunosuppressants such as corticosteroids.[12]

BERNARD–SOULIER SYNDROME

This is an autosomal recessive disorder of platelet function and number. It presents with moderate to severe thrombocytopenia, circulating "giant" platelets on the blood smear, and bleeding. On laboratory testing, platelets fail to aggregate with ristocetin. The underlying molecular defect results in an absent or nonfunctioning platelet membrane receptor for vWF. In the affected infant with BSS, platelets should be transfused if there is bleeding, or if the thrombocytopenia is severe in order to prevent spontaneous hemorrhage.[16]

PSEUDO-vWD

This is an autosomal dominant disorder characterized by mild intermittent thrombocytopenia, mild bleeding, absence of high molecular weight vWF multimers, and increased ristocetin-induced platelet aggregation. It can be differentiated from type 2B vWD, where the mutation resides in the vWF protein by spontaneous aggregation of the patients' platelets with normal plasma.[12]

TYPE 2B vWD

In this type of vWD, the structurally abnormal vWF has increased affinity for the glycoprotein 1b receptor on the platelet surface. This may lead to platelet aggregation and thrombocytopenia. It is clinically and biochemically very similar to pseudo-vWD. Type 2B is diagnosed by demonstrating enhanced platelet agglutination induced by low concentrations of ristocetin.[12]

Montreal platelet syndrome

This syndrome is characterized by thrombocytopenia, large platelets, spontaneous platelet aggregation, and a reduced response to thrombin-induced aggregation. It can be distinguished from BSS by its autosomal dominant inheritance and normal platelet response to ristocetin.[12]

Gray platelet syndrome

An extremely rare mild bleeding disorder for which both autosomal dominant and recessive inheritance have been described, gray platelet syndrome is characterized by the platelet's inability to store alpha granule proteins.[17] Thrombocytopenia is mild, platelets are large, and the absence of alpha granule content gives the platelets a gray appearance on blood smears.

Paris–Trousseau syndrome

This is an autosomal dominant syndrome composed of mild thrombocytopenia, a mild bleeding tendency, giant alpha-granules in a subpopulation of platelets, bone marrow micromegakaryocytes, and a deletion of the long arm of chromosome 11q that includes the FLI1 gene that is essential for megakaryocyte production.[18] There are several other congenital anomalies, including mental retardation, cardiac anomalies, and craniofacial abnormalities.

Wiskott–Aldrich syndrome

The WAS is inherited as an X-linked recessive trait and is characterized by moderate to severe thrombocytopenia, eczema, and a predisposition to infection. Platelets in WAS are typically small. It is often fatal in the early teens due to infection, lymphoreticular malignancy, or bleeding. Hemorrhagic events in this syndrome are common during the first 2 years of life.[12]

WAS VARIANTS (X-LINKED THROMBOCYTOPENIA)

This is a heterogeneous group of thrombocytopenic disorders with X-linked inheritance. The thrombocytopenia is usually less severe in WAS variants and requires no treatment.

Oculocutaneous Albinism—Hermansky–Pudlak and Chediak–Higashi syndromes

Oculocutaneous albinism denotes a group of inherited disorders characterized by reduced or absent pigmentation of the skin, hair, and eyes. While the majority of these patients have an isolated platelet storage pool defect, in some, accompanying low platelet counts can occur.

The Hermansky–Pudlak syndrome is an autosomal recessive disorder with oculocutaneous albinism and a platelet dense-granule defect. The bleeding tendency is usually mild and is related to a platelet function defect and not thrombocytopenia.

Like the Hermansky–Pudlak syndrome, the Chediak–Higashi syndrome is also an autosomal recessive condition with a platelet dense-granule defect and associated partial oculocutaneous albinism. Features of the syndrome may also include neutropenia and peripheral neuropathy. Thrombocytopenia usually occurs during the accelerated phase of the disease, which involves the development of pancytopenia, hepatosplenomegaly, lymphadenopathy, and extensive tissue infiltration with lymphoid cells.[12]

MYH9-related thrombocytopenia syndromes

May–Hegglin anomaly (MHA), Fechtner syndrome, Sebastian platelet syndrome, and Epstein syndrome constitute a group of related disorders with autosomal dominant inheritance and giant platelets.[19] Thrombocytopenia is mild; bleeding is infrequent and rarely life-threatening. Döhle-like inclusions within granulocytic cells are often seen on the blood smear. These disorders can also be associated with sensorineural deafness, glomerulonephritis, and cataracts. Platelet function has been reported to be normal in some and impaired in others.

CONGENITAL INFECTIONS

Thrombocytopenia may occur with congenitally acquired viral infections, including rubella, herpes virus, enterovirus, human immunodeficiency virus, and cytomegalovirus. They rarely produce severe thrombocytopenia, and therefore, therapeutic intervention in the form of platelet transfusion is only indicated when there is severe thrombocytopenia or active bleeding, or surgical intervention is being considered.[20]

NEONATAL INFECTIONS

Late onset thrombocytopenia is most often caused by neonatally acquired infections. Sepsis due to gram-negative bacteria results in particularly severe thrombocytopenia.

NECROTIZING ENTEROCOLITIS

Necrotizing enterocolitis (NEC) is a common and serious gastrointestinal disorder that predominantly affects premature infants. Ninety percent of neonates with NEC develop late onset thrombocytopenia. It is often severe and associated with bleeding.[21]

MISCELLANEOUS CONDITIONS

Other associations of neonatal thrombocytopenia include birth asphyxia; maternal pregnancy-induced hypertension; maternal drug use; disseminated intravascular coagulation; primary microangiopathic hemolytic anemia, including hemolytic uremic syndrome; transient abnormal myelopoiesis associated with Down's syndrome (discussed later); trisomies 21, 18, and 13; hemophagocytic lymphohistiocytosis (HLH; discussed in the section on coagulation); osteopetrosis; bone marrow infiltration with congenital leukemia or neuroblastoma; and inborn errors of metabolism.

DEVELOPMENTAL HEMOSTASIS

Neonates and infants have a rapidly developing hemostatic system, with developmental changes occurring over months, weeks, or even days.[22] Plasma levels of many of the hemostatic coagulation factors are lower in newborns than in older children and adults.[23] Both full-term and preterm neonates are born with low levels of most procoagulant factors, including all of the contact activation factors (XII, XI, prekallikrein, and high molecular weight kininogen) and vitamin K-dependent factors (II, VII, IX, X). In preterm infants, these levels are even lower. The natural anticoagulants, antithrombin, protein S, and protein C are also low at birth. The plasma levels of the procoagulant cofactors, factor V and factor VIII, and fibrinogen are the same in term infants as in adults. Like the coagulation system, the fibrinolytic system, of which plasminogen is the major protein, is also physiologically immature in the neonate.[24] Elevated levels of tissue plasminogen activator and plasminogen activator inhibitor also reflect the reduced fibrinolytic activity in neonates.

Despite the deficiencies of multiple hemostatic factors, healthy neonates have normal hemostasis. Although often characterized as "immature," the neonatal hemostatic system is functionally balanced with no tendency toward coagulopathy or thrombosis.

Inherited bleeding disorders

Deficiencies of factor VIII and IX are known as hemophilia A and B, respectively. The incidence is 1:5000 male births (FVIII) and 1 in 20,000 males (FIX). They are inherited in an X-linked manner; thus, females are carriers of the defect, and males with the abnormal gene express the disease. Persons with hemophilia are classified based on their plasma factor activity [severe (<1%), moderate (<5%), or mild (>5%)]. When there is a family history of hemophilia, newborns are usually diagnosed early with cord blood sampling as the condition is anticipated. Making the diagnosis of severe or moderate hemophilia A in the neonate is usually straightforward. However, making the diagnosis of mild hemophilia can be challenging due to increased FVIII activity resulting from the stress of delivery. Levels should be repeated at 6–12 months of age if mild FVIII deficiency is expected. However, 30% of all individuals with hemophilia A and B arise from *de novo* mutations, and it may be some time before a firm diagnosis is made as a significant number of these children may be seen in the general pediatric setting. Hemophilia A and B are clinically indistinguishable. In the severe form, the phenotype is characterized by bleeding into the joints and soft tissues. In the neonate, bleeding may present as a postprocedural bleed or an intracranial hemorrhage. Both the factor VIII and factor IX genes were sequenced and cloned over 20 years ago, and as a result, recombinant factor concentrates are now the treatment of choice in these conditions.[25]

Hemorrhagic complications in moderate and severe hemophilia A and B may become obvious after birth especially if the child is circumcised. The incidence of intracranial hemorrhage in neonates with severe hemophilia is estimated to be between 1% and 4%.[26,27] The severity and type of bleeding are related to the absolute level of circulating plasma VIII:C. A minimal effective level for hemostasis is about 25%–30% for hemophilia A and 20%–25% for hemophilia B. Those with severe deficiency (less than 1%) usually experience repeated and often spontaneous hemorrhages. While muscular bleeding is by far the commonest clinical event, other spontaneous hemorrhagic manifestations frequently occur and may be life-threatening. Successful treatment in acute or potentially acute (pre-surgery) bleeding is usually achieved with adequate and prompt factor replacement therapy. The level of factor concentrate required to achieve adequate hemostasis will depend on the type of bleeding.[28]

VON WILLEBRAND DISEASE

vWD is the most frequently inherited bleeding disorder, affecting approximately 1% of the population, and is transmitted in autosomal dominant or recessive patterns. Bleeding tends to be predominantly mucocutaneous. There are three main categories of vWD based on the quantitative level or function of vWF: type 1, 2, or 3. Type 2 is further divided into four separate subtypes: 2A, 2B, 2M, and 2N. There is significant phenotypic heterogeneity even among members of the same family. The majority of individuals have type 1 vWD with type 3 vWD being the rarest form of the disease and having the most severe bleeding phenotype due to complete or almost complete deficiency of vWF. Typically, only patients with type 3 or some type 2 vWD present with bleeding as neonates.[29] Bleeding can occur after surgery or trauma. Bleeding into joints is rare and typically only seen in individuals with severe type 3 disease. The diagnosis of vWD is based on three main laboratory assays: (i) quantitative measurement of vWF in plasma, (ii) activity of vWF and its ability to bind platelets, (iii) FVIII activity. High molecular weight multimer analysis can be performed to help differentiate type 2 varieties.[25]

The management of bleeding in a neonate with vWD is typically with plasma-derived FVIII products that contain vWF. Desmopressin can be used to stimulate endogenous vWF release; however, there is a significant risk of hyponatremia and consequent seizures, especially in very young children.[28] Its use in neonates is not recommended.

OTHER COAGULATION FACTOR DEFICIENCIES

Deficiencies of all coagulation factors have been described. However, it should be remembered that the number of patients with hemophilia A greatly outnumbers all of these put together. Common features of these rarer forms of coagulation factor deficiencies are variable bleeding tendencies and autosomal recessive inheritance.[25,28]

Acquired bleeding disorders

The acquired coagulation disorders are far more common than the inherited disorders and are usually associated with multiple coagulation factor deficiencies.

HEMOPHAGOCYTIC LYMPHOHISTIOCYTOSIS

HLH is a rare syndrome of infancy and childhood that manifests as a hyperinflammatory state resulting from pathologic immune activation. HLH can present as both a familial disorder and as an acquired one, in association with infection, malignancies, or rheumatologic disorders. The classical clinical features include fever, splenomegaly, cytopenias, hypertriglyceridemia, hypofibrinogenemia, hyperferritinemia, lymphadenopathy, skin rash, jaundice, and edema.Elevation of ferritin > 10,000 g/dL has been shown to be highly sensitive and specific for HLH.[30] Although it can occur in all age groups, neonatal-onset HLH is rare. Identified genetic defects are present in 45% of patients that present with HLH less than 1 month of age.[31] Therefore, mutational analyses for UNC13D and perforin gene (PRF1) should be performed in neonates suspected of having HLH. Early recognition and treatment is necessary to prevent disease progression. Remission can be achieved with the use of etoposide-based chemotherapy regimens in conjunction with immune modulating medications such as ciclosporin and corticosteroids. The only definitive cure, however, for patients with familial HLH is HSCT.[31]

VITAMIN K

Vitamin K is crucial for the production of procoagulant proteins II, VII, IX, and X and the natural anticoagulants protein C and protein S. It is essential for the γ-carboxylation of these clotting factors, which is required for their functionality. Vitamin K itself is recycled, and when this process is blocked as with warfarin administration, these vitamin K-dependent factors are not produced in adequate amounts.

VITAMIN K DEFICIENCY BLEEDING

Vitamin K deficiency bleeding (VKDB) is classified as early, classical, or late. Classical VKDB usually occurs on the second to seventh day of life as a result of decreased synthesis of vitamin K-dependent factors. The etiology of vitamin K deficiency in newborns is multifactorial and includes reduction of storage, functional immaturity of the liver, lack of bacterial synthesis of vitamin K in the gut, and low amounts of vitamin K in breast milk.[32] Early VKDB is due to the placental passage of compounds that interfere with vitamin K metabolism, such as maternal anticonvulsant medications, vitamin K antagonists (warfarin), and drugs used to treat tuberculosis. This usually presents within 24 hours of life and may cause a cephalohematoma, intracranial hemorrhage, or bleeding from the umbilical stump. Late VKDB is again due to inadequate vitamin K content in breast milk and occurs almost exclusively in breastfed infants. The diagnostic evaluation of VKDB is straightforward as the prothrombin time (PT) is always prolonged, and the activated partial thromboplastin time (aPTT) is nearly always prolonged. Typically, the PT is prolonged out of proportion to the aPTT. The most effective management of VKDB is prevention, and all newborns should receive vitamin K at birth. Exceptions to the rule are those children with known G6PD deficiency in the family, as a significant number of these patients will develop frank hemolysis. In those children who present with frank bleeding due to VKDB, parenteral vitamin K and plasma or prothrombin complex concentrates can be given to arrest the blood loss.[25]

LIVER DISEASE

The liver is responsible for the synthesis of most pro- and anticoagulant proteins, and TPO, which stimulates platelet production. A disruption in liver function may have a significant impact on the coagulation system in neonates, exacerbating the already delicately balanced system.

Laboratory abnormalities seen in liver failure are elevations in the PT, aPTT, and d-dimer, decreased fibrinogen, and a decreased platelet count. Furthermore, these patients have a functional defect in circulating platelets. The treatment of bleeding in liver failure is difficult due to the concomitant risk of fluid overload with large volumes of plasma and the risk of thrombosis. Correcting the coagulopathy involves replacement of vitamin K and infusion of fresh frozen plasma and platelets. In certain circumstances, off-label use of factor concentrates such as recombinant factor VIIa and prothrombin complex concentrate may be appropriate; however, it must be remembered that these concentrates carry a risk of thrombosis.

EXTRACORPOREAL LIFE SUPPORT

The coagulopathy associated with cardiopulmonary bypass and extracorporeal membrane oxygenation is multifactorial involving activation of the contact pathway, fibrinolytic pathway, tissue factor pathway, and an acquired platelet function defect.[28]

CONGENITAL HEART DISEASE

A significant number of children with congenital heart disease will have coagulation defects. It should be remembered, however, that in children with cyanotic heart disease with associated polycythemia, the elevation in PT/aPTT may be spurious and secondary to a sampling defect as there will be an alteration in the plasma anticoagulant ratio when the hematocrit is greater than 60%.[28]

Thrombotic states

The fetus and neonate are less efficient in generating thrombin, and thus, thrombotic disease in early childhood is rare and generally secondary to an acquired prothrombotic state or an inherited gene defect predisposing to clot formation. When it does occur in childhood, it can be fatal or associated with several sequelae such as amputation, organ dysfunction, and postphlebitic syndrome. The peak incidence for these thrombotic events is undoubtedly the neonatal period where the use of vascular access devices in tertiary care pediatrics is almost the norm. Preterm infants are at a greater risk than older children for thrombosis. When the delicate hemostatic balance is disrupted, in particular with vascular access devices and septicemia, the risk of developing thromboembolism increases significantly.

Acquired states

CENTRAL VENOUS CATHETER DEVICES

Central venous access devices have revolutionized the intensive care management of neonates. Unfortunately, thrombosis related to their placement continues to be a therapeutically challenging complication. It occurs in up to 10%

of neonates with central venous catheters; however, most of these are asymptomatic.[33] The presenting sign may be loss of patency of the catheter or swelling. Central venous lines or umbilical venous catheters associated with thrombus should be removed wherever possible. If the thrombosis is symptomatic, then a period of anticoagulation is necessary.[34] It should be remembered that although uncommon, death from venous thromboembolic disease in young children does occur. Therefore, early detection and adequate treatment are absolutely mandatory in this group of children.

RENAL ARTERY AND VEIN THROMBOSIS

Renal artery thrombosis in the neonatal period is associated with umbilical artery catheters (UAC). Risk factors for UAC-related thrombosis include hypoxia, hyperviscosity, sepsis, longer duration of UAC placement, the presence of calcium in the infused fluids, hypertonic saline, smaller umbilical artery caliber, and low UAC position. It may be difficult to diagnose, and hypertension and heart failure may be the presenting clinical features. There can be extension of the thrombus to other vascular beds such as the aorta. Recent clinical guidelines recommend high UAC placement to reduce thrombotic risk. Catheter removal, supportive care, anticoagulation, fibrinolytic therapy, and surgical approaches are all used in management of UAC thrombosis based on the severity of the clinical presentation.[35] Renal vein thrombosis (RVT) is more common than renal arterial thrombosis in the newborn period. It is associated with perinatal asphyxia, dehydration, sepsis, hypotension, cyanotic heart disease, polycythemia, babies born to diabetic mothers, and the presence of an indwelling umbilical venous catheter. The commonest presenting features are a palpable flank swelling, hematuria, and thrombocytopenia. Usually ultrasound will reveal renal enlargement with or without evidence of venous thrombosis. The use of anticoagulants and thrombolytic agents in this condition continues to be evaluated. There are no randomized controlled trials in the treatment of RVT. Either anticoagulant therapy or supportive care with close monitoring is an acceptable approach in unilateral RVT without renal impairment or clot extension into the inferior vena cava.[34] Acute complications of RVT include clot extension, adrenal hemorrhage, and acute renal failure. Survival rates in babies are as high as 80%, and renal status after recovery ranges from normal function to systemic hypertension and chronic renal insufficiency.

ACQUIRED PROTEIN C/S DEFICIENCY

Purpura fulminans in newborns is a rare life-threatening condition characterized by disseminated intravascular coagulation and hemorrhagic skin necrosis.[36] Affected infants present on the first day of life with ecchymosis, extensive venous and arterial thromboses, disseminated intravascular coagulation (DIC), and markedly low levels of protein C or protein S. It can result from inherited and acquired abnormalities of the protein C pathway. Acquired protein C deficiency can occur in conditions such as meningococcal septicemia. Early identification of the disorder and

treatment with protein C replacement is essential to prevent serious morbidity and death.

ACQUIRED ANTITHROMBIN DEFICIENCY

Antithrombin inhibits coagulation. Its activity is potentiated by heparin. Severe congenital antithrombin deficiency is a rare autosomal recessive condition with a tendency to thrombosis in the neonatal period or early infancy. Acquired deficiencies of antithrombin have been associated with a large number of diseases such as DIC and microangiopathic hemolytic anemias (i.e., hemolytic uremic syndrome). Antithrombin concentrates are available and are the treatment of choice during the acute phase of the disease.

MISCELLANEOUS CONDITIONS

Other associations of neonatal thrombosis include NEC, respiratory distress syndrome, heparin-induced thrombocytopenia/thrombosis syndrome (extremely rare in neonates), antiphospholipid antibodies, extra corporeal membrane oxygenation (ECMO), hemolytic uremic syndrome, and birth asphyxia.

Inherited thrombotic states

Genetic defects within the protein C pathway account for the majority of cases of inherited thrombophilia.[37]

PROTEIN C AND PROTEIN S DEFICIENCY

Hereditary protein C (PC) and protein S (PS) deficiency (homozygosity or compound heterozygosity) are associated with a high venous thromboembolic risk at birth or in the first few months of life. The first clinical manifestation is usually skin purpura mainly affecting extremities, and in some cases, massive large vessel thrombosis can also be a presenting feature. Optimum therapy involves factor replacement (protein C concentrate or fresh frozen plasma in protein S deficiency) and heparin in the acute phase and oral anticoagulation in the long term.[37]

ANTITHROMBIN DEFICIENCY

Homozygous antithrombin deficiency is extremely rare and appears to be incompatible with life. Presentations of antithrombin deficiency in neonates include myocardial infarction at birth, aortic thrombosis, sagittal sinus thrombosis, and cerebral thrombosis.

OTHER INHERITED THROMBOPHILIAS

Several other inherited gene defects have been associated with increased propensity to clot formation, the commonest being activated protein C resistance and factor V Leiden, factor II gene variant (prothrombin^{G20210A}), and hyperhomocysteinemia.

Management

The primary goal of treatment in this age group is to prevent clot extension, which can result in end-organ damage.

Because the triggers for thrombosis, such as in-dwelling catheters, are usually transient, the recurrence risk is low. The approach to an individual infant must balance the risks of anticoagulation against the benefits of such treatment. The indications for use of anticoagulants in infants and children have changed dramatically over the past 20 years with major advances in tertiary pediatric care such as ECMO, cardiopulmonary bypass, hemodialysis, and the use of intra-arterial and intravenous indwelling catheters. The choice of anticoagulant is dependent upon the duration of anticoagulation and comorbidities such as renal failure. In the acute phase, either unfractionated heparin (UFH) or low molecular weight heparin (LMWH) is used. The advantages of UFH are its rapid reversibility and low cost. However, due to its unpredictable pharmacokinetic response, it requires frequent monitoring and dedicated central venous access. LMWH, on the other hand, is administered subcutaneously and requires less laboratory monitoring and dose adjustments. However, an antifactor Xa assay to monitor its anticoagulant effect must be readily available. It should be remembered that because the hemostatic system in infancy and childhood is constantly maturing, the anticoagulant effects of heparin are not predictable and therefore are deemed age dependent.

Surgical thrombectomy is rarely performed in neonates as this procedure is generally limited by the small size of blood vessel and the clinical instability of newborns with thrombosis.

As regards the new oral anticoagulants, argatroban, bivalirudin (both direct thrombin inhibitors), and rivaroxaban (factor Xa inhibitor), there is insufficient evidence to support their routine use in the management of thrombosis in neonates at this time.[34]

ANEMIA

Immediately following birth, all infants experience a decrease in hemoglobin (Hb) that results in varying degrees of anemia. There follows a progressive decline in Hb concentration during the 8–10 weeks following birth. In healthy term infants, clinical signs and symptoms of anemia are absent. This is termed "physiological anemia," and it is a direct consequence of physiologic processes related to birth and the transition to extrauterine life. It arises due to the switch in oxygen dependency from placenta-based to lung-based, and the increase in arterial Hb oxygen saturation that occurs when infants take their first breath, together with redistribution of blood flow following birth, and changes in red cell production due to the downregulation of erythropoietin production.[38] When the level of Hb is below the "physiological anemia" range, then a pathological neonatal anemia is present. While the majority of cases of anemia occurring in the neonatal period are acquired, a number of inherited disorders that involve gene defects of Hb, red cell membrane, and enzymes also present during this period. Anemia, whether it be acquired or inherited, may present as an incidental finding on a blood count performed for

other reasons, with nonspecific signs of pallor, tachypnea, tachycardia, failure to thrive, jaundice, splenomegaly, or bleeding. If the anemia is due to a hemolytic process, then jaundice is almost always present. Like thrombocytopenia, the causes of neonatal anemia can be thought of in terms of decreased erythrocyte production and increased erythrocyte destruction.

Acquired anemia

ALLOIMMUNE HEMOLYTIC ANEMIA

Hemolytic disease of the fetus and newborn (HDFN) is the immune-mediated destruction of fetal red cells by a maternal antibody, formed when fetal red cells expressing a paternally derived red cell antigen enter the maternal circulation through a sensitizing event (e.g., via fetomaternal hemorrhage). The disease is mediated by the transplacental passage of a maternal IgG alloantibody. The spectrum of illness ranges from clinically insignificant to a severely affected anemic, hydropic fetus with jaundice, pleural and pericardial effusions, edema, and ascites. The D antigen from the Rhesus system (RhD) continues to be the most commonly identified antigenic stimulus for HDFN.[39] Other alloantibodies implicated in HDFN are anti-c and anti-Kell, which produce hemolysis in fetuses that carry the c and Kell antigens, respectively. The alloantibodies are acquired either as a result of prior blood transfusion or as a result of alloimmunization during the pregnancy itself. RhD negative mothers give birth to RhD positive fetuses in 0.9% of European ancestry pregnancies. In a first pregnancy, without prophylaxis, 15% of these mothers will become immunized against the RhD, and 0.7% will have infants affected with HDFN.[39] The diagnosis HDFN is confirmed by testing the blood group of the mother and baby together with the detection of maternal alloantibodies and a positive Coombs test. Thrombocytopenia may be present in those severely affected. Introduction of anti-D immunoglobulin prophylaxis has drastically decreased the prevalence of D antibodies and of anti-D mediated HDFN.

HDFN can also occur due to ABO blood group incompatibility. This tends to be more common and less severe than Rh incompatibility. It primarily affects group A or B newborns born to group O mothers. In this scenario, the Hb is often normal.

AUTOIMMUNE HEMOLYTIC ANEMIA

This is a very uncommon cause of neonatal anemia, and it arises when autoantibodies produced in the mother are directed against fetal red cell antigens causing hemolysis in a similar fashion to neonatal thrombocytopenia secondary to maternal ITP.

Infantile pyknocytosis

Hemolytic disease of the newborn has several generally well-known causes (Rh incompatibility, ABO incompatibility, red cell enzyme, and membrane defects), all of which are discussed in more detail in individual sections of this chapter. A rare cause is infantile pyknocytosis. It can cause early neonatal jaundice with transient hemolytic anemia. It earns its name from the diagnostic red blood cell appearances (pyknocytes) on the peripheral blood smear. The cause remains unknown, but there is probably a familial susceptibility, which may promote the occurrence under certain circumstances. Whether the trigger is environmentally acquired or intrinsic remains to be determined. Its management is largely supportive consisting of phototherapy and red cell transfusion before the condition resolves spontaneously around 4–6 months of age.[40]

Blood loss

Anemia due to blood loss is the commonest cause of neonatal anemia in preterm infants. In most cases, this is iatrogenic and due to frequent blood sampling. Blood loss may occur peri-delivery due to fetomaternal hemorrhage, in a twin-twin transfusion syndrome, as a result of bleeding from a ruptured cord or abnormal placenta, or as a result of a giant cephalohematoma, an intracranial, gastrointestinal, or retroperitoneal bleed.

ANEMIA OF PREMATURITY

Anemia of prematurity (AOP) is an exaggeration of the normal physiologic anemia. Almost all preterm infants have anemia, and several factors contribute to this. Erythropoietin (EPO) levels in premature infants are low partly due to the liver, which remains as the primary site of EPO production. The liver is less sensitive to tissue hypoxia as a stimulus to EPO production than the kidney. As the fetus transitions from the hypoxic intrauterine environment to the oxygen-rich postnatal environment, EPO production is downregulated. EPO clearance is higher in neonates, and the increased growth rate compared to that of term infants is also an endogenous factor causing AOP. Exogenous factors contributing to AOP include iatrogenic blood loss due to frequent phlebotomy, nutritional deficiencies, inflammation, infections, and chronic illness.[41] The goal of treatment is to maintain adequate oxygen delivery to tissue. Transfusion has a clear indication in the case of blood loss or shock for the restoration of blood volume. In the remaining situations, it is imperative to take into account the clinical signs and physiologic needs of the infant as well as laboratory parameters when making the decision to transfuse.[41] The amount of allogeneic red cell exposure can be significantly reduced by limiting phlebotomy in the baby, administering folate and iron to all preterm infants, using erythropoietin appropriately, and complying with peer-reviewed transfusion guidelines.

Approach to management

Only severe or moderate neonatal anemia should be treated with blood transfusion, and this decision is made on clinical grounds as well as the Hb in accordance with peer-reviewed guidelines.[42] Hemolytic disease of the newborn (HDN) always

resolves albeit it may take 1–2 months. In the first couple of weeks of life, the hemolytic process may be so brisk that the hyperbilirubinemia necessitates phototherapy to prevent kernicterus. Blood transfusion may also be required for infantile pyknocytosis and for neonatal anemia due to blood loss.

Inherited anemia

If the anemia is due to a hemolytic process, then jaundice is almost always present. When the hemolytic process is secondary to a red cell membrane defect, the abnormally shaped red blood cells are removed from the peripheral circulation, and the jaundice is usually accompanied by mild to moderate splenomegaly. Jaundice is also frequently seen in neonates with inherited red cell enzyme deficiencies, which can cause significant damage to the erythrocytes. Most of the hemoglobinopathies, apart from alpha-thalassemia major and hemoglobin-H (HbH) disease, do not cause neonatal jaundice.[43]

RED CELL MEMBRANE DEFECTS

These can be difficult to diagnose in the neonatal period especially in the case of the commonest type, hereditary spherocytosis (HS), where the classic blood film morphology of numerous spherocytes is indistinguishable from that seen in ABO incompatibility. Spherocytes are also seen in neonatal period with consumptive coagulopathy, birth asphyxia, and significant placental insufficiency. A positive family history of HS is very helpful in confirming the diagnosis, as osmotic fragility testing in this age group is not reliable and should be postponed until the child is between 6 and 12 months of age. It is predominantly a disease of autosomal dominant inheritance.

Hereditary elliptocytosis is also a disease of autosomal dominant inheritance caused by defects in various structural proteins, resulting in elliptical shaped red cells. The elliptocytes are unstable and nondeformable, and thus hemolyzed by the reticuloendothelial system. It is straightforward to diagnose by the presence of elliptocytes on the peripheral blood smear.[43]

Hemoglobinopathies

These are uncommon causes of anemia in neonates. As globin chain synthesis is in a state of flux between late fetal life and following birth, diagnosing hemoglobinopathy is fraught with difficulty in the neonatal period.

The hemoglobinopathies that cause significant neonatal anemia include homozygous α-thalassemia (Hb Barts hydrops fetalis) where there is deletion of all four α globin genes, and HbH disease where there is deletion of three of the regulatory α globin genes. In sickle cell syndromes, the Hb is normal in the neonate.[43]

Red cell enzyme deficiencies

These are usually straightforward to diagnose in the neonatal period. G6PD deficiency is an X-linked recessive disorder. It is active in the metabolic pathway of the erythrocyte that protects the cell from free radical damage. Defects in G6PD can result in accumulation of damaging agents, leading to hemolysis. A G6PD assay should be performed in any cases of prolonged or severe jaundice unless there is an obvious alternative cause.

Pyruvate kinase is an enzyme in the erythrocyte that is responsible for cellular energy production. A deficiency of PK can therefore result in premature cell death. It is an autosomal recessive disorder. It is diagnosed by assaying red cell enzyme levels; PK assays should be performed in cases of unexplained hydrops, those with hemolytic anemia of unknown cause, and where there is a family history.[43]

DIAMOND–BLACKFAN ANEMIA

Diamond–Blackfan anemia frequently presents in infancy with an isolated macrocytic anemia due to pure red cell aplasia. It classically causes reticulocytopenia. About half of these infants also have a variety of congenital anomalies. It is inherited in an autosomal dominant fashion, and the first causative gene, RPS19, was discovered more than 15 years ago. To date, 13 mutations in ribosomal genes have been identified. Red blood cell transfusions are the mainstay of treatment with careful monitoring of iron status to avoid visceral iron overload. HSCT may be considered.[14]

MISCELLANEOUS

Other inherited conditions that can present as anemia in the neonatal period include Pearson's syndrome, congenital dyserythropoietic anemia, Aase syndrome, and osteopetrosis. Congenital infection in newborns, such as parvovirus, and acquired nutritional deficiencies, such as iron, copper, folate, B12, B6, vitamin A, vitamin C, and vitamin E deficiencies, can result in reduced red blood cell production.[44]

Polycythemia in the neonatal period

Polycythemia occurs in 1%–5% of neonates. It is more common in infants who are small for gestational age, who are large for gestational age, who are born to diabetic mothers, who have delayed cord clamping, who are the recipient in a twin-twin transfusion syndrome, and with chromosomal disorders.

NEUTROPHILS

Neutropenia can be secondary to decreased production of neutrophils, increased destruction, or a combination of these two mechanisms. Congenital neutropenia is characterized by chronic neutropenia due to a constitutional defect. Neonatal neutropenia occurs most frequently in association with maternal hypertension, sepsis, twin-twin transfusion syndrome, alloimmunization, and hemolytic disease.

Alloimmune neutropenia

Like HDFN, alloimmune neutropenia occurs as a result of the transplacental passage of maternal antineutrophil antibodies that attack a paternally derived antigen on fetal neutrophils. In a well-appearing infant with persistent isolated neutropenia, an immune-mediated etiology should be considered. The condition is diagnosed by the demonstration of antineutrophil antibodies in the mother and the baby. It is confirmed by human neutrophil antigen genotyping of the mother and the father.[45] In general, the outcome is good with resolution of the neutropenia by 3 months after birth. Treatment is still a matter of debate, but granulocyte colony-stimulating factor (G-CSF), IVIG, corticosteroids, and antibiotics have all been used.

Autoimmune neutropenia

Neonatal autoimmune neutropenia results from the transmission of preexisting maternal antineutrophil autoantibodies into the fetus. This can occur in autoimmune conditions such as maternal systemic lupus erythematosus.

Autoimmune neutropenia of infancy

This is a transient autoimmune phenomenon where the infant's own immune system produces an antineutrophil antibody.

Miscellaneous

Various other conditions can lead to neutropenia in the neonate. In a critically ill infant, sepsis should be part of the differential diagnosis. NEC can lead to neutropenia. Copper deficiency is a consideration in infants with short bowel syndrome who are dependent on parenteral nutrition. Congenital bone marrow failure syndromes can rarely present early, and the presence of other phenotypic anomalies should raise this possibility. Neutropenia in association with cardiomyopathy and skeletal myopathy in a male infant is seen in Barth syndrome. Inborn errors of metabolism usually present late in the first week of life and beyond. Certain drugs may be implicated in neonatal neutropenia (thiazides, β-lactam antibiotics).[46]

Severe congenital neutropenia

Severe congenital neutropenia (SCN) is a heterogenous group of disorders characterized by severe neutropenia, maturation arrest of bone marrow myeloid precursors, and recurrent bacterial infections. Diagnosis is made on bone marrow biopsy and confirmed with genetic testing. Originally described by Kostmann with autosomal recessive inheritance, genetic discovery has broadened the spectrum of SCN inheritance. Autosomal dominant, X-linked, and sporadic causative mutations exist with 50%–60% of patients having a mutation in the neutrophil elastase gene ELA2 (ELANE). Other mutations reported to cause SCN include mutations in the HAX1, G6PC3, WAS, GFI1, and JAGN1.[14] Before the introduction of modern therapies, SCN was highly fatal. Treatment with G-CSF is standard, although development of myelodysplastic syndrome or leukemia is a concern with long-term use. For the minority who fail to respond adequately to G-CSF, HSCT should be considered.[14]

Shwachman–Diamond syndrome

Shwachman–Diamond syndrome (SDS) usually presents with isolated neutropenia that may progress to bone marrow failure. It is characterized by exocrine pancreatic insufficiency leading to malabsorption and steatorrhea in the first few months of life. Infants develop growth retardation, frequent bacterial infections, and failure to thrive. They have pathognomonic skeletal abnormalities including metaphyseal widening and dysostosis. The hematological features of SDS vary, but typically, severe intermittent neutropenia is the initial finding. It is inherited in an autosomal recessive fashion, with germline mutations in the SDS gene accounting for about 95% of patients. Management is multidisciplinary in approach based on the affected organ systems.[14]

HEMATOLOGICAL DISORDERS IN THE NEONATE WITH DOWN SYNDROME

Down syndrome (DS) is the most common chromosomal abnormality in the live newborn. It is caused by an extra whole or partial copy of chromosome 21. A number of hematological abnormalities are recognized in neonates with this condition. Up to 80%, 66%, and 34% of newborns with DS have neutrophilia, thrombocytopenia, and polycythemia, respectively.[47]

In general, these abnormalities are mild, the clinical course is benign, and they spontaneously resolve.

Transient myeloproliferative disorder (TMD) is a disease entity that is unique to DS or those with T21 mosaicism and is defined as the morphologic detection of blasts in the peripheral blood in newborns with DS less than 3 months of age. Typically, it is detected within the first week of life and spontaneously resolves within 6 months of birth. It is estimated to occur in up to 10% of all newborns with DS. TMD has a variable presentation in the fetus and newborn from mild disease to disseminated leukemic infiltration with pleural and pericardial effusions and fulminant hepatic fibrosis. However, it commonly presents with the isolated finding of circulating blasts without any clinical symptoms. It can cause neonatal death secondary to liver failure, heart failure, sepsis, hemorrhage, hyperviscosity, and DIC. All TMD blasts have a somatic mutation in the X-linked GATA-1 gene. TMD should be considered in the differential even if DS is not suspected because it can occur in neonates who are mosaic for trisomy 21. Most neonates with TMD do not need treatment. The outcome for those who have progressive life-threatening signs such as hepatic, renal, and/or cardiac failure may be improved by the administration of low-dose cytosine arabinoside.

Identifying TMD in the neonatal period is important since 20%–30% of cases later develop acute myeloid leukemia.[48]

REFERENCES

1. Castle V, Andrew M, Kelton J et al. Frequency and mechanism of neonatal thrombocytopenia. *J Pediatr* 1986; 108:749–55.
2. Mehta P, Vasa R, Neumann L et al. Thrombocytopenia in the high risk infant. *J Pediatr* 1980; 97:791–4.
3. Sainio S, Jarvenpaa AL, Renlund M et al. Thrombocytopenia in term infants: A population-based study. *Obstet Gynecol* 2000; 95:441–6.
4. Christensen RD, Baer VL, Henry E et al. Thrombocytopenia in small-for-gestational-age infants. *Pediatrics* 2015; 136(2):e361–70.
5. Baer VL, Lambert DK, Henry E, Christensen RD. Severe thrombocytopenia in the NICU. *Pediatrics* 2009; 124:e1095.
6. Cohen DL, Baglin TP. Assessment and management of immune thrombocytopaenia in pregnancy and in neonates. *Arch Dis Child* 1195; 72:71–5.
7. Burrows RF, Kelton JG. Pregnancy in patients with idiopathic thrombocytopenic purpura: Assessing the risks for the infant at delivery. *Obstet Gynecol Surv* 1993; 48(12):781–8.
8. Cines DB, Bussel JB. How I treat idiopathic thrombocytopenic purpura (ITP). *Blood* 2005; 106(7): 2244–51.
9. Kjeldsen-Kragh J, Killie MK, Tompter G et al. A screening and intervention programme aimed to reduce mortality and serious morbidity associated with severe neonatal alloimmune thrombocytopenia. *Blood* 2007; 110:833–9.
10. Bussel JB, Zabusky MR, Berkowitz RL et al. Fetal alloimmune thrombocytopenia. *N Engl J Med* 1997; 337:22.
11. O'Rafferty C, O'Regan GM, Irvine AD et al. Recent advances in the pathobiology and management of Kasabach–Merritt phenomenon. *Br J Haematol* 2015; 171(1):38–51.
12. Smith OP. Inherited and congenital thrombocytopenia. In: Arceci RJ, Hann IM, Smith OP (eds). *Pediatric Hematology*, 3rd edn. Massachusetts: Blackwell Publishing, 2006:507–26.
13. Geddis AE. Inherited thrombocytopenia: Congenital amegakaryocytic thrombocytopenia and thrombocytopenia with absent radii. *Semin Hematol* 2006; 43(3):196–203.
14. Khincha PP, Savage SA. Neonatal manifestations of inherited bone marrow failure syndromes. *Semin Fetal Neonatal Med* 2016; 21:57–65.
15. Alter BP, Kupfer G. In: Pagon RA, Adam MP, Ardinger HH et al. (eds). *Fanconi Anemia Gene Reviews*. Seattle: University of Washington, Feb 2013.
16. Bolton-Maggs PH, Chalmers EA, Collins PW et al. A review of inherited platelet disorders with guidelines for their management on behalf of the UKHCDO. *Br J Haematol* 2006; 135:603–33.

17. Nurden AT, Nurden P. The gray platelet syndrome: Clinical spectrum of the disease. *Blood Rev* 2007; 21:21–36.

18. Raslova H, Komura E, Le Couedic JP et al. FLI1 monoallelic expression combined with its hemizygous loss underlies Paris-Trousseau/Jacobsen thrombopenia. *J Clin Invest* 2004; 114:77–84.

19. Drachman JG. Inherited thrombocytopenia: When a low platelet count does not mean ITP. *Blood* 2004; 103;390–8.

20. Beutler E. Platelet transfusion, the 20,000/microL trigger. *Blood* 1993; 81:1411–2.

21. Kenton AB, O'Donovan D, Cass DL et al. Severe thrombocytopenia predicts outcome in neonates with necrotizing enterocolitis. *J Perinatol* 2005; 25:14–20.

22. Andrew M, Paes B, Milner R et al. Development of the human coagulation system in the full-term infant. *Blood* 1987; 70:165–72.

23. Attard C, Van Der Straaten T, Karlaftis V et al. Developmental hemostasis: Age-specific differences in the levels of hemostatic proteins. *J Thromb Haemost* 2013; 11:1850–4.

24. Parmar N, Albisetti M, Berry LR et al. The fibrinolytic system in newborns and children. *Clin Lab* 2006; 52(3–4):115–24.

25. Jaffray J, Young G, Ko Richard H et al. The bleeding newborn: A review of presentation, diagnosis, and management. *Semin Fetal Neonatal Med* 2016; 21:44–49.

26. Kulkarni R, Soucie JM, Lusher J et al. Sites of initial bleeding episodes, mode of delivery and age of diagnosis in babies with haemophilia diagnosed before the age of 2 years: Report from the disease control and prevention's (CDC) universal data collection project. *Haemophilia* 2009; 15:1281–90.

27. Richards M, Lavigne LG, Combescure C et al. Neonatal bleeding in haemophilia: A European cohort study. *Br J Haematol* 2012; 156(3):374–82.

28. Smith OP. Secondary haemostatic disorders. In: Smith OP, Hann IM (eds). *Essential Paediatric Haematology*, 1st edn. London: Martin Dunitz, 2002:96–115.

29. Donner M, Holmberg L, Nilsson IM. Type IIB von Willebrand's disease with probable autosomal recessive inheritance and presenting as thrombocytopenia in infancy. *Br J Haematol* 1987; 66:349–54.

30. Allen CE, Yu X, Kozinetz CA et al. Highly elevated ferritin levels and the diagnosis of hemophagocytic lymphohistiocytosis. *Pediatr Blood Cancer* 2008; 50:1227–35.

31. Jordan MB, Allen CE, Weitzman S et al. How I treat hemophagocytic lymphohistiocytosis. *Blood* 2011; 118:4041–52.

32. Sutor AH. Vitamin K deficiency bleeding in infants and children. *Semin Thromb Hemost* 1995; 21:317–29.

33. Haddad H, Lee KS, Higgins A et al. Routine surveillance ultrasound for the management of central venous catheters in neonates. *J Pediatr* 2014; 164:118.

34. Monagle P, Chan AK, Goldenberg NA et al. Antithrombotic therapy in neonates and children: Antithrombotic Therapy and Prevention of Thrombosis, 9th edn: American College of Chest Physicians Evidence-Based Clinical Practice Guidelines. *Chest* 2012; 141:e737S.

35. Saxonhouse MA, Burchfield DJ. The evaluation and management of postnatal thrombosis. *J Perinatol* 2009; 29:467–78.

36. Price VE, Ledingham DL, Krumpel A et al. Diagnosis and management of neonatal purpura fulminans. *Semin Fetal Neonatal Med* 2011; 16:318.

37. Aiach M, Borgel D, Gaussem P et al. Protein C and protein S deficiencies. *Semin Hematol* 1997; 34:205–16.

38. Bifano EM, Smith F, Borer J. Relationship between determinants of oxygen delivery and respiratory abnormalities in preterm infants and anemia. *J Pediatr* 1992; 120:292–7.

39. Ross ME, Waldron PE, Cashore WJ, de Alarcon PA. Erythrocyte disorders. In: de Alarcón PA, Werner EJ, Christensen RD (eds). *Neonatal Hematology*, 2nd edn. New York; Cambridge University Press, 2013:65–90.

40. El Nabouch M, Rakotoharinandrasana I, Ndayikeza A et al. Infantile pyknocytosis, a rare cause of hemolytic anemia in newborns: Report of two cases in twin girls and literature overview. *Clin Case Rep* 2015; 3(7):535–8.

41. Colombatti R, Sainati L, Trevisanuto D. Anemia and transfusion in the neonate. *Semin Fetal Neonatal Med* 2016; 21:2–9.

42. Venkatesh V, Khan R, Curley A et al. How we decide when a neonate needs a transfusion. *Br J Haematol* 2013; 160:421–33.

43. Aher S, Malwatkar K, Kadam S. Neonatal anemia. *Blood Rev* 2008; 13:239–47.

44. Gallagher PG, Ehrenkranz RA. Nutritional anemia in infancy. *Clin Perinatol* 1995; 22(3):671–92.

45. Maheshwari A. Neutropenia in the newborn. *Curr Opin Hematol* 2014; 21(1):43–9.

46. Nittala S, Subbarao GC, Masheshwari A. Evaluation of neutropenia and neutrophilia in preterm infants. *J Matern Fetal Neonatal Med* 2012; 25(0 5): 100–3.

47. Choi JK. Hematopoietic disorders in Down syndrome. *Int J Clin Exp Pathol* 2008; 1:387–95.

48. Roy A, Roberts I, Vyas P. Biology and management of transient abnormal myelopoiesis (TAM) in children with Down syndrome. *Semin Fetal Neonatal Med* 2012; 17:196–201.

22

Genetics in neonatal surgical practice

ANDREW GREEN

NATURE AND STRUCTURE OF A GENE

Genetics is traditionally defined as the science of biologic variation and has been a scientific discipline for over 100 years. Human genetics makes up a large part of the field of genetics, but the principal laws of genetics are universal, and apply equally to all species, including humans. Mendel's studies in the nineteenth century were originally felt to have no relevance to humans, and it is only in retrospect that their importance can be seen. Many of the principles of genetics were discovered through the study of smaller organisms, such as bacteria, yeast, and fruit flies. The basic genetic mechanisms of cell division, development, and differentiation happen in the same way in widely divergent species. Therefore, it is impossible to look at human genetics in isolation, and there are large amounts of information from lower species that have bearing on human disorders. The study of the genetics of small organisms has had a profound impact on our understanding of human development and of how human diseases develop. It is likely that such basic science will continue to contribute significantly to the understanding of human genetic disease. This chapter will attempt to outline the basic elements of genetics, describe the types of genetic tests now available to help in neonatal diagnosis, and give an approach to the diagnosis of congenital abnormalities.

The basic unit of inheritance for any species is the gene. The original concept of a gene arose long before the relationship between genes and nucleic acids was ever understood. A gene was considered to be a stable heritable element, which conferred a particular property or phenotype onto an individual organism. This element was passed on to subsequent generations of a particular species, and the nature of the phenotype varied according to the nature of the gene. The concept of dominant and recessive traits, which will be discussed later, was derived from studies of inheritance patterns, long before the molecular basis of the gene was understood.

A gene can also be considered in another way as a specific length of deoxyribonucleic acid (DNA), which encodes a particular function, in most cases the synthesis of a protein. This also is a stable heritable unit. Each cell in an organism, regardless of its function, has the entire set of genes for that particular organism, but only a proportion of those genes will be active. DNA is found in the nucleus of every cell of an organism as a double helix (Figure 22.1).

Each strand of the double helix has a backbone of alternating phosphate and deoxyribose sugar molecules, with the sugars attached to the 5′ and 3′ hydroxyl groups of the phosphate group. Attached to the sugar molecule, lying within the helix, is one of four nitrogen-containing nucleic acid bases. Two of these bases, adenine (A) and guanine (G), are purines, and two are the smaller pyrimidines, cytosine (C) and thymine (T). The A and T bases pair together by hydrogen bonding, and the G and C bases similarly pair by hydrogen bonds (Figure 22.2). The two strands of the double helix are held together by paired A–T or G–C bases of opposite strands of the double helix. The DNA strand can be read in only one direction from 5′ (left hand) to 3′ (right hand). The two strands of DNA are complementary to each other, and the sequence of one strand can be predicted from its opposite. If one strand reads 5′-CAGCGTA-3′, then the opposite strand must read 5′-TACGCTG-3′. The double-stranded sequence would then be written as follows:

5′-CAGCGTA-3′
3′-GTCGCAT-5′

The simplicity of the double helix structure allows for several important functions for DNA.

Firstly, huge amounts of information can be stored in the strand of DNA. If a molecule of DNA is 1 million bases long, then there are $4^{1,000,000}$ possible sequences for that stretch of DNA. A genome is the complete DNA sequence of an organism. In humans, the estimated genome size is 3×10^9 base pairs (bp). The human genome contains a huge

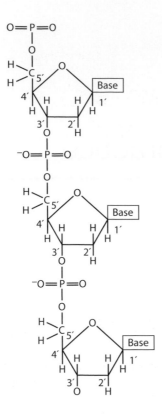

Figure 22.1 Structure of a DNA chain. The deoxyribose and phosphate residues are linked to form the sugar-phosphate backbone of DNA.

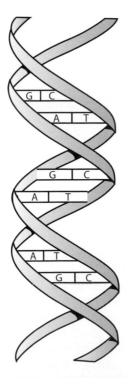

Figure 22.2 Double-helix structure of DNA. The double helix of deoxyribose and phosphate molecules is held together by paired purine and pyrimidine bonds.

amount of coded information, of which as yet only a small part is known.

Secondly, the double helix provides a framework for DNA replication. One strand of DNA acts as a template for the synthesis of a new strand of DNA. The double helix unwinds, allowing DNA replication enzymes access to the template strand of DNA. The replication system builds a new strand of DNA based on the template. The new double helix formed as a result will contain one original strand and a newly synthesized complementary second strand. This is the basic mechanism of DNA replication in all species.

Thirdly, the double helix provides a basis for repair of damaged DNA. A damaged base can be replaced, knowing its complementary base is present on the opposite strand. Damage to the sugar-phosphate backbone can also be repaired using the opposite strand as a template.

DECODING THE INFORMATION IN DNA

About 90% of the DNA in the human genome does not code for any specific property. Only about 10% of the genome actually contains coding information in the form of a gene. In simple terms, the genetic code in DNA is transcribed into a molecule called messenger RNA (mRNA). The mRNA is then translated into a protein, which carries out the function encoded by the specific DNA.

A gene has several distinct elements (Figure 22.3). The major part of the gene is divided into coding regions, called exons, and noncoding regions, called introns. Just before (5′) the first exon, there is a promoter that indicates where transcription of a gene should start. There can be several promoters for one gene, and different promoters can be used according to the tissue in which the gene is being expressed; in other words, the promoter is tissue specific. Further 5′ of the promoter, there can also be enhancers or suppressors, which can increase or decrease the level of transcription of the gene. Not all of the mRNA will code for protein, as some exons will code for mRNA that does not directly encode protein. These areas, known as untranslated regions, can be either at the start (5′) or the end (3′) of the mRNA.

To express the DNA code, mRNA is used. There are several different types of RNA, but mRNA is the most important in decoding DNA. There are three differences between RNA and DNA. Firstly, the sugar backbone of RNA contains ribose rather than deoxyribose. Secondly, mRNA exists as a single strand and remains more unstable. Thirdly, in RNA, the base uracil (U) is used instead of thymine (T), whereas the other three nucleic acids remain the same.

The DNA code in most genes is expressed as a protein, which is a peptide made of the building blocks of individual amino acids. Each amino acid is coded for by a sequence of three DNA bases, known as a codon. For some amino acids, there is more than one codon (see Table 22.1). A long series of DNA codons in a gene will thus code for an entire protein. The mRNA codons coding for amino acids are identical to DNA codons, with the substitution of uracil (U) for

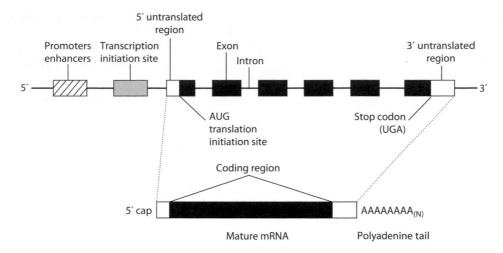

Figure 22.3 Idealized gene.

thymine (T). There is a tightly controlled mechanism for the generation of protein from a DNA template.

To decode a gene into protein, the DNA is first transcribed into mRNA. A strand (the "sense" strand) of the DNA double helix is used by the enzyme RNA polymerase to synthesize a complementary strand of mRNA. Transcription of mRNA starts from the 5′ end of the first exon of the gene until the end of the most 3′ exon. The intervening introns are initially included, and the first molecule is known as pre-mRNA. The intronic RNA sequences are spliced out, and a 3′ polyadenine tail is added, producing mature mRNA. The mature mRNA is then transferred from the nucleus to the ribosome to be used as a template for the production of protein. The mature mRNA has both 5′ and 3′ untranslated regions.

Protein synthesis does not begin at the 5′ end of the mRNA, but at the first 5′ AUG codon, which codes for the amino acid methionine. Protein translation stops at the first truncation codon (usually UGA) thereafter (Figure 22.3). In the ribosome, amino acid-specific RNA molecules, called transfer RNAs, bind a free molecule of their specific amino acid. The binding is carried out by an anti-codon in the tRNA, which is complementary to the mRNA that codes for that specific amino acid. Using its anti-codon, the tRNA binds the specific mRNA codon for its amino acid. By complex machinery, the amino acid is then added to a growing peptide chain, which will eventually form the mature protein (Figure 22.4). The 5′ end of the mRNA corresponds to the NH_2 (amino terminus) of the protein, and the 3′ end of the mRNA corresponds to the COOH (carboxyl terminus)

Table 22.1 Genetic code

First position	U amino acid		C amino acid		A amino acid		G amino acid		Third position
			Second position						
U	UUU	Phe	UCC	Ser	UAU	Tyr	UGU	Cys	U
	UUC	Phe	UCU	Ser	UAC	Tyr	UGC	Cys	C
	UUA	Leu	UCA	Ser	UAA	Stop	UGA	Stop	A
	UUG	Leu	UCG	Ser	UAG	Stop	UGG	Trp	G
C	CUU	Leu	CCU	Pro	CAU	His	CGU	Arg	U
	CUC	Leu	CCC	Pro	CAC	His	CGC	Arg	C
	CUA	Leu	CCA	Pro	CAA	Gln	CGA	Arg	A
	CUG	Leu	CCG	Pro	CAG	Gln	CGG	Arg	G
A	AUU	Ile	ACU	Thr	AAU	Asn	AGU	Ser	U
	AUC	Ile	ACC	Thr	AAC	Asn	AGC	Ser	C
	AUA	Ile	ACA	Thr	AAA	Lys	AGA	Arg	A
	AUG	Met	ACG	Thr	AAG	Lys	AGG	Arg	G
G	GUU	Val	GCU	Ala	GAU	Asp	GGU	Gly	U
	GUC	Val	GCC	Ala	GAC	Asp	GGC	Gly	C
	GUA	Val	GCA	Ala	GAA	Glu	GGA	Gly	A
	GUG	Val	GCG	Ala	GAG	Glu	GGG	Gly	G

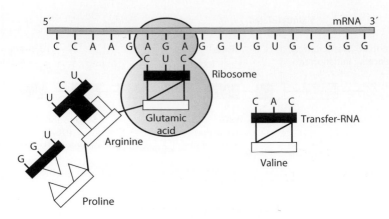

Figure 22.4 Diagram of protein synthesis from mRNA.

of the protein. Many proteins in higher species are modified after translation by the addition of phosphate or lipid groups.

CHROMOSOMES AND CELL DIVISION

To successfully package vast amounts of DNA into each cell nucleus, it must be compressed and compacted. The first coiling of DNA is in the form of the double helix. The negatively charged DNA double helix is then bound tightly to and wound 1.65 times around a core of eight positively charged *histone* proteins to form a *nucleosome*. The addition of another histone completes the second winding of DNA about the histone core to form a *chromatosome*. These units stack up and form loops of approximately 300 nm. These are stacked, compressed, and folded into fibers of 250 nm wide. These fibers are then tightly coiled to form a *chromatid*. Two sister chromatids make up a single chromosome, joined by a *centromere*. The centromere represents a division along the chromatids in a chromosome, creating a short arm "p" and a long arm "q."

Nonsex chromosomes are termed *autosomes*. Humans are *diploid*, carrying two copies of each autosome. The normal human chromosome complement in nonsex cells is 46, comprising 22 pairs of autosomes and two sex chromosomes. Females carry two copies of the X chromosome, while males have one copy each of chromosomes X and Y. Each member of a pair of autosomes contains the same genetic information. The two X chromosomes in a female contain the same genetic information. The X and Y chromosomes in a male only have a small amount of genes in common, with the Y chromosome bearing a number of genes encoding male-specific genetic information. A normal human metaphase karyotype is shown in Figure 22.5.

Cells involved in production of gametes are termed germ cells, while all other cells are termed somatic cells. The process of cell division and replication in somatic cells is termed mitosis. During this process, the parent cell should divide to produce two genetically and morphologically identical daughter cells. This process allows the formation of a complete human being from a single fertilized egg,

and is the process by which cells are constantly renewed. Genetic variation can arise as a result of spontaneous mutation during this process.

Mitosis is one short period during a carefully programmed cell cycle (Figure 22.6). Before commencing the process of cell division (M phase), the cell is said to be in interphase transitioning through different stages of DNA replication, chromosome elongation, and rest. After a mitotic event, nondividing cells enter a phase of rest (G0), while dividing cells commence a new cell cycle and enter the G1 phase. Upon entering G1, the cell grows and commences replication of DNA (S phase). Following the S phase, the cell enters G2, a resting phase, in preparation for cell division, thereafter entering the M phase.

The M phase itself comprises a number of stages—prophase, metaphase, anaphase, telophase, and cytokinesis—and involves interplay between the chromosomes and specialized tubulin-based microtubules. The mitotic spindle is composed of microtubules and microtubule-associated proteins. In metaphase, the condensed chromatids line up along the equatorial plane of a cell. In anaphase, spindle tubules extend from the centrioles located at each pole of

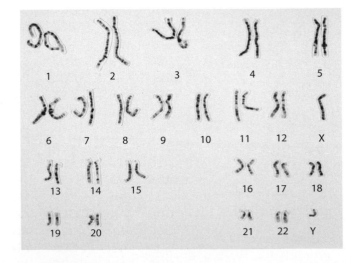

Figure 22.5 Normal male karyotype.

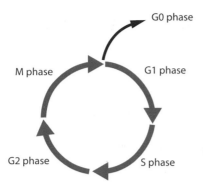

Figure 22.6 Cell cycle.

the cells to the chromosomal centromeres. As these tubules move back toward the centriole, they pull one chromatid with them to opposite poles of the cell. The splitting of the centromere and separation of sister chromatids toward two poles is termed anaphase. By the telophase, the chromatids have reached opposite poles of the dividing cell. The nuclear membrane starts to reform, completing mitosis, and the cytoplasm also divides. Cell division is completed by cytokinesis, during which the parent cell completely divides into two identical daughter cells.

Meiosis is a specific form of cell division, required to produce gametes (sperm or oocyte). Gametes are haploid, with only one copy of each chromosome, to give a total complement of 23 chromosomes. The process of fertilization results in the formation of a new diploid organism from two haploid gametes. In the parent, formation of a haploid gamete requires two successive divisions of a specialized diploid germ cell, namely the primary oocyte or primary spermatocyte, in stages termed *meiosis I* and *meiosis II*. In males, the products of these two divisions are four spermatozoa. In females, the products of meiosis I are one secondary oocyte and a small *polar body*. Meiosis I may last several years, arrested from the first stage in the fetus until the completion of meiosis I at puberty. The secondary oocyte then undergoes *meiosis II* to produce a large mature egg cell and second polar body.

Meiosis I produces two haploid daughter cells, with a total of 23 chromosomes each. One daughter cell contains the paternal homolog of each chromosome pair, and the maternal homolog is contained in the other daughter cell. This process is random for each chromosome pair, and each gamete has different contributions from paternal and maternal lineages depending on which chromatid of each of the 23 chromosome pairs ended up in that particular daughter cell. This independent assortment ensures variation between gametes, and therefore between fraternal siblings. Furthermore, *crossing over* of genetic material from one chromatid to another is possible. Approximately one or two crossovers occur per chromosome per meiosis. This process introduces further genetic diversity.

The first phase of meiosis I, *prophase I*, is similar to prophase in mitosis. Homologous chromosome pairs align. This process facilitates recombination between chromatids, and between maternal and paternal homologs, allowing *crossing*

over of material. In *metaphase I*, homologous chromosomes line up opposite each other along the metaphase plate. In *anaphase I*, these chromosome pairs are separated, moving to opposite cellular poles. Within each chromosome, sister chromatids remain united during this process. In *telophase I*, nuclear envelopes form to enclose the two separate groups of chromosomes. The cytoplasm around the two nuclei is then divided to form two distinct haploid daughter cells, each with only one set of chromosomes ($n = 23$), in a process called *cytokinesis*. Failure of the daughter cells to completely separate is termed *nondisjunction*, which can manifest as chromosomal aneuploidy in offspring. The frequency of nondisjunction events increases in direct relation to increasing maternal age, and is a common cause of chromosomal syndromes such as Down syndrome or Edward syndrome.

Meiosis II is analogous to mitotic division of each of the haploid daughter cells. Chromatids condense again in *prophase II* and line up along the axis of the dividing cell in *metaphase II*. The chromatids then separate, passing to opposite ends of the cell in *anaphase II*. The chromatids elongate into thin strands in *telophase II*. Meiosis II concludes with cytokinesis, resulting in four new cells that represent precursor gametes.

In males, all four cells are identical precursor spermatogonia. In females, although division of genetic material between the four daughter cells is equal, the division of cytoplasm in both cytokinesis I and cytokinesis II is unequal. In meiosis I, this results in one primary oocyte and smaller polar bodies, and in meiosis II, one secondary oocyte and three polar bodies. These polar bodies generally cannot be fertilized and often apoptose spontaneously. Spermatogenesis in males begins at puberty, producing four gametes per spermatocyte on a continuous basis throughout a male lifetime. In females, the process of oogenesis begins even before birth, arrested at meiosis I until puberty, at which stage some arrested oocytes proceed through the first stages of metaphase II. Only one ovum will be produced per oocyte.

CHROMOSOME ANOMALIES AND ANALYSIS

Chromosome abnormalities can broadly be classified into abnormalities of chromosome number or a rearrangement of a normal number of chromosomes. Problems can arise clinically if there is addition or loss of vital genetic material, or indeed if genetic material is moved in such a way that it loses proximity to regulatory regions.

Abnormalities of chromosome number are relatively common, but many are not recognized, as they may result in the early loss of a pregnancy. Triploidy (69 chromosomes) and tetraploidy (92 chromosomes) are relatively common causes of early pregnancy loss. Trisomy, the presence of a single extra chromosome (47 chromosomes), is also a common cause of miscarriage. Specific trisomies may be compatible with life, the commonest being trisomy 21 (Down syndrome), trisomy 13 (Patau's syndrome), and trisomy 18 (Edwards' syndrome). The most common cause of these trisomies is autosomal nondisjunction in meiotic division of the oocyte. In nondisjunction, the chromatids in question fail to separate, resulting in an extra chromosome in one oocyte and no chromosome in the opposite gamete (nullisomy). Nondisjunction tends to occur more frequently with increasing maternal age. Nondisjunction can occur in the male germline, but rarely produces viable offspring.

Fertilization of the oocyte with the extra chromosome will therefore result in an embryo that is trisomic for that particular chromosome. Conversely, fertilization of a nullisomic oocyte will result in an embryo that is monosomic for the chromosome in question; and generally, this is not compatible with life.

There are numerous types of chromosome rearrangements, the commonest of which are shown in Figure 22.7. Inversions refer to rotation of a section of a chromosome by 180°. Pericentric inversions (involving the centromere) and paracentric chromosome inversions (not crossing the centromere) are usually balanced, without any loss or gain of genetic material. These types of chromosomal anomalies may be inherited without any phenotypic effect. Paracentric inversions are usually associated with a low risk of producing a live-born with an unbalanced karyotype, but this risk is higher for inversions involving the centromere. Insertions, duplications, deletions, isochromosomes, and ring chromosomes are all usually aneuploid and associated with significant clinical abnormalities.

Reciprocal translocation refers to the exchange of genetic material from one arm of a chromosome in return for genetic material from a different chromosome. Reciprocal translocations are usually balanced, without clinical effect; but carriers of such translocations do carry the risk of producing offspring with an unbalanced number of chromosomes. Unbalanced reciprocal translation carriers can have a severe clinical phenotype.

Robertsonian translocation is a particular type of translocation involving chromosomes that bear very short p arms with little genetic information, termed *acrocentric* chromosomes (13, 14, 15, 21, and 22). In Robertsonian translocations, the two q arms of any of these acrocentric chromosomes fuse, with loss of the two respective p arms. Robertsonian translocations are one of the commonest human chromosome translocations, the most common of which is between chromosomes 13 and 14. Balanced Robertsonian translocations are of no clinical consequence to the carrier directly, but may have profound consequences for their offspring. A Robertsonian translocation involving chromosomes 14 and 21 is shown in Figure 22.8. Those who carry a Robertsonian translocation involving chromosome 21 may be at significantly higher risk of having a child with Down syndrome as an unbalanced product of the translocation. The same applies to a lesser extent for those carrying a Robertsonian translocation involving chromosome 13, and a subsequent risk of a child with Patau's syndrome.

Analysis of chromosomes involves close interrogation of chromosome number and structure, and can be carried out in two main ways: by karyotype or by array comparative genomic hybridization (array CGH, microarray).

As part of karyotype analysis, dividing cells in culture must be examined. These cells are usually lymphocytes (collected in lithium heparin), amniotic fluid cells, or fibroblasts. Cells are arrested in the metaphase stage of mitosis and stained in such a way that the chromosomes are easily

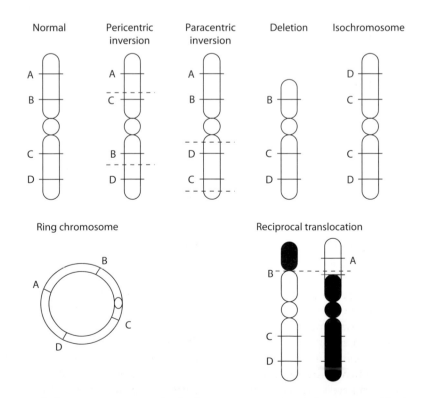

Figure 22.7 Different types of chromosome anomaly. A–D represent notional chromosomal loci.

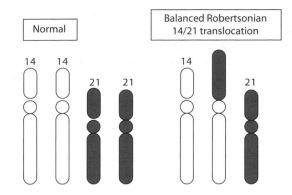

Figure 22.8 Robertsonian translocation.

visualized. The usual technique used is G-banding (using a Giemsa stain), which gives a characteristic positive and negative banding pattern to each chromosome. Each chromosome has a constriction, called a centromere, dividing the chromosome into a short arm (p) and a long arm (q). Each arm has a number of prominent bands, which can then be subdivided into smaller bands. The gene for the ABO blood group is localized to chromosome 9q34. The gene thus lies in the fourth subband from the centromere (q3<u>4</u>) of the third band from the centromere (q<u>3</u>4) on the long arm (<u>q</u>34) of chromosome 9 (<u>9</u>q34).

Karyotype analysis is useful for the analysis of chromosome structure as well as number, and can identify translocations or inversions, which may be missed by other types of chromosome studies.

The nomenclature for reporting a chromosome analysis is strict and needs to be read carefully. A karyotype is reported initially as the number of chromosomes, regardless of whether those chromosomes are normal or not, followed immediately by the sex chromosome, completing a normal report. Any abnormalities are added after the sex chromosomes. A normal male karyotype is reported as **46,XY**. A male with nondisjunctional Down syndrome will have the karyotype **47,XY, +21**, an extra unattached chromosome 21. In the case of a Robertsonian translocation between chromosomes 14 and 21, the parent will have a balanced complement, with inconsequential loss of 14p and 21p and fusion of 14q and 21q, leaving a total complement of 45 chromosomes. Her karyotype will be reported as **45, XX, t(14;21)**. She is at risk of having a child with an unbalanced translocation and Down syndrome. In this case, her child will have 46 chromosomes, but this includes three copies of 21q, leading to Down syndrome. A son with this rearrangement will have a karyotype 46,XY, der (14;21), +21.

However, recombinant DNA technology has allowed new techniques for chromosome analysis based on the hybridization of fluorescently labelled fragments of DNA to the DNA of chromosomes, prepared in a standard fashion, immobilized on a glass slide. The slides can then be visualized by eye using a fluorescent microscope, or indirectly by generating an image of the hybridization on a computer. This technique is known as fluorescent in situ hybridization

(FISH). The information that can be gained from this technique depends on the origin of the fragments of DNA hybridized to the chromosome preparation. Labelled whole chromosome "paints," consisting of DNA exclusively from one chromosome, are now commercially available. For example, whole chromosome paints can be used to identify the origin of extra chromosomal material that cannot be identified using G-banding techniques. Whole chromosome paints are also helpful in determining the origin of subtle complex translocations. It is also now technically possible to use a chromosome 21 paint on uncultured cells in interphase to look for trisomy 21. A cell would show three fluorescent nuclear dots, representing three chromosomes 21, as opposed to two in the normal situation.

Fluorescently labeled small DNA fragments, corresponding to 40–50 kb of DNA from a specific chromosomal region, can also be hybridized to metaphase chromosomes. Chromosomal deletions that cannot be detected within the resolution of conventional cytogenetic analysis can be detected by the FISH method. A normal karyotype will give two hybridization signals: one from the same part of each chromosome. A karyotype containing a submicroscopic chromosomal deletion involving the segment of the chromosome corresponding to the 50 kb DNA fragment will only give one hybridization signal. An example would be the submicroscopic deletion of chromosome 22q11, which occurs in most cases of the Di George spectrum, which can only be seen by FISH analysis of chromosomes.

GENOMIC ARRAY ANALYSIS

Array comparative genomic hybridization (array CGH or microarray) has become increasingly important in diagnosis of chromosomal anomalies. As part of this analysis, probes corresponding to tens of thousands of recognizable pieces of DNA are applied to slides of silicone or glass (microarrays). The patient DNA and a reference DNA sample are differentially labelled and are then applied to this microarray. Differences in the ratio of hybridization between the probes and patient DNA compared to that of the probes and reference genome are interrogated to identify loss or gain of genetic material. This genomic array technology can permit analysis of thousands of individual loci simultaneously and gives chromosome analysis at a resolution at least 100 times greater than conventional G-banded chromosome analysis. Array CGH is sometimes referred to as a "molecular karyotype." Genomic array technology will identify pathogenic chromosomal anomalies in 20%–25% of infants in whom no underlying diagnosis had been identified previously. There is a drawback in that genomic array technology will often find genetic variants of unknown significance (VUS), and the current understanding of the role of such variants in disease pathogenesis is limited. Genomic array technology is now becoming available in an increasing number of diagnostic cytogenetic laboratories. It is likely to replace standard G-banded chromosome analysis for a wide variety of indications over the next few years.

Single nucleotide polymorphisms (SNPs) refer to changes in a single base pair of DNA and are the most frequently occurring form of human variation, occurring once every 300 bases. The human genome contains millions of SNPs, and this knowledge can be applied to development of SNP microarrays. In this case, hybridization of the patient DNA to probes for the different alleles at known SNPs is analyzed. Utilities of SNP microarrays above conventional microarrays include detection of uniparental disomy, an unusual situation in which the two copies of a chromosome in an offspring are derived from only one parent.

PATTERNS OF INHERITANCE

Single-gene disorders have one of three principal modes of inheritance: autosomal dominant, autosomal recessive, and X-linked recessive. Other rare forms of inheritance include X-linked dominant and mitochondrial disorders, as well as disorders due to abnormalities of genetic imprinting. Disorders caused by inheritance of unstable elements of DNA are now increasingly being recognized (see later).

Autosomal dominant inheritance

Autosomal dominant disorders are characterized by vertical transmission from parent to child, and the hallmark of these conditions is that male-to-male transmission of the disease is possible (Figure 22.9).

Those affected with an autosomal dominant disorder have an alteration in one or other copy of their two genes responsible for that condition. Each child of a person with an autosomal dominant disorder has a 50:50 chance of inheriting the gene responsible for the condition from its parent.

There are many examples of autosomal dominant disorders, including neurofibromatosis 1 and 2, familial adenomatous polyposis coli, myotonic dystrophy, and Huntington's disease. There can often be variability in both *expression* and *penetrance* of autosomal dominant disorders. *Penetrance* refers to the development of a phenotype in an individual as a consequence of a particular genotype, while *expressivity* or *expression* refers to the severity of this

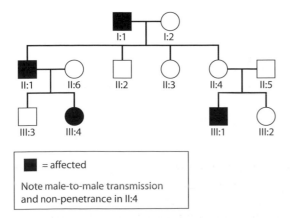

Figure 22.9 Autosomal dominant inheritance.

Table 22.2 Autosomal dominant disorders in neonatal surgical practice

System affected	Condition
Gastrointestinal	Hirschsprung's disease (some cases)
	Beckwith–Wiedemann syndrome with exomphalos (some cases)
	Pyloric stenosis (some cases)
Genitourinary	Vesicoureteric reflux
Skeletal	Stickler's syndrome
	Most craniosynostosis syndromes
	Achondroplasia
	Osteogenesis imperfecta
	Limb reduction defects (some cases)
Cardiac	Holt–Oram syndrome
	Noonan's syndrome
	22q11 microdeletion syndrome
Other	Retinoblastoma

phenotype. For example, neurofibromatosis 1, an autosomal dominant condition, will almost always manifest in someone who has an altered neurofibromatosis 1 gene. This means that the condition has almost complete penetrance. However, different people can manifest the condition in different ways, with some people showing mild skin lesions and others with severe intracerebral complications. This means that the expression or expressivity of the condition is very variable. In contrast, only 80% of those who have a single altered gene for the rare hereditary form of retinoblastoma will actually develop an eye tumor. The penetrance in this situation is 80%, but the expression of the altered gene is consistent, as manifested by a retinoblastoma.

Autosomal dominant disorders are not commonly seen in neonatal surgical practice. A list of the more frequent conditions is outlined in Table 22.2.

Autosomal recessive inheritance

When a child is diagnosed with an autosomal recessive disorder, both copies (alleles) of a particular gene responsible for the condition are altered. Generally, in this case, the child has inherited one mutated allele from each parent, meaning that the parents are unaffected *carriers* for the condition, with one normal and one altered gene. Carriers of autosomal recessive traits generally do not manifest features of the condition, as their normal copy of the gene can compensate for loss of function of the mutated allele. Two of an affected child's four grandparents are also carriers, and it is likely that many of the child's relatives are also unknowingly carriers (Figure 22.10). In most cases, being a carrier for an autosomal recessive condition has no effect on that person.

When both parents are carriers for an alteration in the same gene, then there is a 25% or 1 in 4 chance for each of their children to be affected by the condition. The risk of a healthy carrier sibling of having a child with the same

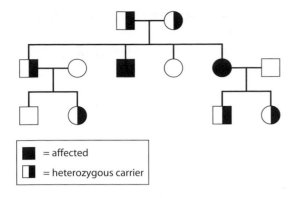

Figure 22.10 Autosomal recessive inheritance.

Table 22.3 Autosomal recessive disorders in neonatal surgical practice

System affected	Condition
Metabolic	Cystic fibrosis
	α-1-antitrypsin deficiency
Skeletal	Short-rib polydactyly syndrome
	Jeune's syndrome
	Robert's syndrome
Genitourinary	Infantile polycystic kidneys
	Meckel–Gruber syndrome
Endocrine	Congenital adrenal hyperplasia

condition depends on the chances of that sibling's partner also being a carrier. All children of a person with an autosomal recessive disorder will automatically be carriers. The chances of any of these children being affected will depend upon whether the other parent is a carrier for an alteration in the same gene.

Autosomal recessive disorders are commonly encountered in neonatal practice, and the nature of the disorder depends on the population being seen. Each regional population has its own recessive disorder, where the frequency of carriers for that disorder is the highest. For instance, cystic fibrosis is a very common autosomal recessive disorder in Western Europe, whereas sickle cell anemia is the commonest autosomal recessive disorder in West Africa. Common examples of autosomal recessive conditions include cystic fibrosis, sickle cell anemia, several of the mucopolysaccharidoses, beta-thalassemia, spinal muscular atrophy, and congenital adrenal hyperplasia (Table 22.3). Prenatal diagnosis is available for many of these conditions.

X-linked recessive inheritance

In X-linked recessive inheritance, the condition affects almost exclusively males, and females can be carriers (Figure 22.11). The classic examples of such conditions are hemophilia A and B, Duchenne and Becker muscular dystrophy, and Hunter syndrome.

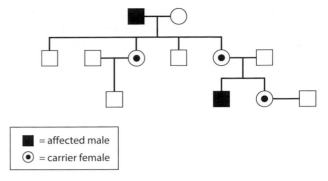

Figure 22.11 X-linked recessive inheritance.

Table 22.4 X-linked recessive disorders in neonatal surgical practice

System affected	Condition
Neurological	Hydrocephalus with aqueduct stenosis (some cases)
Hematological	Hemophilia
Skeletal	Amelogenesis imperfecta
Endocrine	Androgen insensitivity syndrome
Metabolic	Adrenoleukodystrophy

The daughters of a man with an X-linked recessive condition are all obligate carriers. The sons of a man with an X-linked condition are all normal, as they inherit his Y chromosome and not his X chromosome. When a woman is a carrier of an X-linked condition, each of her sons has a 50:50 chance of being affected, and each of her daughters has a 50:50 chance of being a carrier. There can be a relatively high mutation rate for some X-linked recessive conditions, and affected boys may not have any family history of the condition. About one-third of cases of boys with Duchenne muscular dystrophy occur as a result of new mutations. Prenatal diagnosis is available for a wide range of X-linked recessive diseases. The more common X-linked disorders in neonatal practice are shown in Table 22.4.

Polygenic inheritance

Many congenital conditions do not have a clear mode of inheritance and can be classed as polygenic or oligogenic, where a disease may arise as a result of the effects of several genes. A good example is cleft lip and palate, which usually occurs in the absence of a family history. However, monozygotic twins have a high concordance for cleft palate, suggesting a genetic influence. A similar model applies to the genetics of neural tube defects, which arise as a result of the combination of several environmental and genetic factors.

Other forms of inheritance

There are also much rarer forms of inheritance, including X-linked dominant. In X-linked dominant conditions, females may also be affected, despite having a second normal X chromosome. These conditions can be hard to distinguish from autosomal dominant, except that females will be more mildly affected, and there is no male-to-male transmission. An example of an X-linked dominant condition is hypophosphatemic rickets.

Mitochondrially inherited diseases show a very unusual pattern of inheritance. Most of the proteins in the mitochondria are encoded for by nuclear genes, but the mitochondria also contain their own small genome of 18 kb, with many copies per cell. The mitochondrial genome replicates independently and far more frequently than the nuclear genome. Several important mitochondrial proteins are encoded by the mitochondrial genome. Mitochondria are only inherited via oocytes and not sperm. Therefore, where a gene alteration is in the mitochondrial genome, it will pass exclusively down the female line, but both males and females can be affected. The children of an affected male will not inherit his mitochondrial gene alteration. Children with mitochondrial disorders can present with many varied symptoms, including myoclonic seizures, acute acidoses, muscle weakness, deafness, or diabetes. A number of point mutations and deletions in the mitochondrial genome have been described in patients with a wide variety of conditions, including MELAS (myoclonic epilepsy with lactic acidosis and stroke-like episodes) or MERRF (myoclonic epilepsy with ragged red fibers on muscle biopsy). To complicate matters further, Leber's hereditary ophthalmopathy is a mitochondrially inherited condition, with a characteristic mitochondrial mutation, but the expression appears to have an X-linked recessive influence.

Some conditions show a phenomenon known as genetic imprinting. An imprinted gene has been marked during meiosis to indicate the parent from which it comes. For some genes, it appears to be important not only to inherit two copies of that gene but also to inherit one from each parent. Some genes may be silenced, depending upon which parent has passed on that gene. A good example is the presence of a small deletion of chromosome 15q, which has a different effect, depending upon which chromosome 15 is deleted. If the deletion occurs on the chromosome inherited from a child's normal father, the child will develop Prader–Willi syndrome. If the deletion occurs on the chromosome inherited from a child's normal mother, the child will develop a completely different clinical condition, Angelman's syndrome. The genes in this area of chromosome 15 are therefore imprinted. In addition, if a child has two maternal copies of chromosome 15 (maternal disomy), but no paternal copy, he or she will also develop Prader–Willi syndrome. Other conditions that show imprinting effects include Russell–Silver syndrome, Beckwith–Wiedemann syndrome, and the rare condition of transient neonatal diabetes mellitus.

An unusual molecular mechanism for genetic disease is that of inherited unstable triplet repeat expansions. In one of these genes, an unaffected person has a stable number of a repetitive element of three bases of DNA (for example, 20 copies of a CAG repeat) in a particular gene. In that case, the gene functions normally and the children of that person have the same number of repeats in their gene. An affected person has an increased number of repeats (say, 100 copies) in that gene, and the affected children of that person have more serious disease, with perhaps 200 repeats in the gene. Increasing numbers of repeats can result in a nonfunctional protein product or can lead to toxic accumulation of mRNA in the cells depending on the location of the triplet repeat and on the gene in question. The molecular genetic findings appear to be the genetic correlate of the phenomenon of anticipation, where a condition appears to worsen from generation to generation. The most extreme example is that of congenital myotonic dystrophy, where a minimally affected mother can have a profoundly affected infant. In this case, there is a small repeat expansion of, say, 150 repeats in the mother, increasing to many hundreds of repeats in her affected infant.

This molecular mechanism is responsible for Fragile X syndrome, Huntington's disease, Friedreich's ataxia, several forms of spinocerebellar ataxia, and probably several other conditions.

MOLECULAR GENETIC ANALYSIS FOR SINGLE-GENE DISORDERS

Genetic technology is moving at a remarkably rapid rate and becoming increasingly affordable in line with Moore's law. In the case of a well-known and easily recognizable monogenic disorder, targeted gene analysis using Sanger sequencing and multiplex ligation-dependent probe amplication (MLPA) will detect the majority of responsible pathogenic genetic variants, for example, analysis of the RB1 gene in a child with a unilateral retinoblastoma. However, other disorders require more specialist testing because of the nature of the genetic variants responsible for the condition. For example, neurofibromatosis type I is generally diagnosed on a clinical basis; but if molecular diagnosis is required, DNA analysis by Sanger sequencing and MLPA will only detect 70% of mutations. These types of analyses examine the coding regions of the NF1 gene, while a number of NF1 mutations lie in the introns between the coding exons. Analysis of these regions by RNA sequencing can increase the detection rate.

Other disorders may have a recognizable clinical phenotype but may be genetically heterogeneous. For example, Noonan syndrome is most commonly caused by mutations in PTPN11, but may also be caused by mutations in SOS1, RAF1, and RIT1, among others. In such situations, it may be necessary to undertake sequencing of a number of genes. This can now be achieved by using next-generation sequencing, whereby a "panel" of multiple genes is analyzed simultaneously. This strategy has a number of advantages including faster turnaround time and technical ease. However, such an approach runs the risk of detection of VUS in more than one gene. In such a case, a genetic alteration may be detected that is not directly associated with the clinical phenotype. This can make interpretation extremely challenging. Hundreds of genes may be interrogated simultaneously using this technology, but the most prudent approach is to undertake only targeted analysis of those genes known to be associated with the clinical picture. A targeted approach limits the number of "incidental" findings of variants that may not be of clinical consequence, but that trigger significant workload in trying to delineate significance.

Genomic technology has developed to the stage whereby all coding regions of all known genes may be scrutinized contemporaneously, in the form of whole exome sequencing. Furthermore, all noncoding as well as coding regions may be sequenced as part of whole genome sequencing. Whole exome sequencing on average will detect 40,000–60,000 variants. Significant bioinformatics knowledge is then required to "filter" these variants to include only genes of interest. The interpretation of this type of data is highly dependent on the criteria used in filtering the available information, and therefore, close scrutiny of the phenotype and the pattern of inheritance in the family is required to produce meaningful and valid results.

Other laboratory tests for single-gene disorders have been available for a considerable amount of time. Hemoglobin electrophoresis for sickle cell anemia and thalassemia, and enzyme assays for Tay–Sachs' disease are very effective in resolving clinical issues in individual families. However, an increasing number of specific DNA-based tests can now be used in diagnosis and prediction of single-gene disorders.

The two major techniques used in molecular genetic analysis are the polymerase chain reaction (PCR) and Southern blotting techniques. PCR is a technique that allows amplification of a specific genetic region in large quantities from a small amount of DNA template (Figure 22.12). The DNA sequence of the region to be amplified must be known, so that synthetic pieces of single-stranded DNA (oligonucleotide primers) corresponding to the region can be designed and manufactured. The oligonucleotide primers are added in great excess to the DNA template, along with a thermostable DNA polymerase, and free nucleotides (A,C,T,G). The mixture is heated up to cause the two strands of template

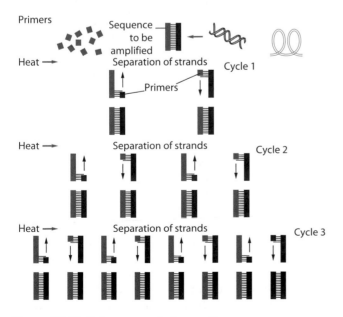

Figure 22.12 Polymerase chain reaction.

DNA to separate, and then cooled. As the DNA cools, the oligonucleotides bind to the template sequence and are extended by the polymerase. A new copy of the template DNA is thus produced. The cycle is repeated 30–40 times, with an exponential increase in the amount of the target sequence.

DNA generated by PCR can be used in many different ways to detect an abnormality in the sequence. If the test is aimed at detecting a known sequence abnormally, such as the common 3 base pair deletion on the cystic fibrosis gene Phe508del, the PCR product can be analyzed using mutation-specific oligonucleotide primers, or a DNA restriction enzyme test. If the search is for an unknown DNA mutation, such as those seen in hereditary breast and ovarian cancer, then many pieces of DNA generated by PCR from the patient can have their sequence analyzed using a semiautomated DNA analyzer.

Southern blotting is a more protracted procedure involving the digestion of a relatively large amount of DNA by a restriction enzyme. The digested DNA is then electrophoresed through an agarose gel, giving a smear of DNA of different sizes. The DNA is then transferred (blotted) and fixed to a membrane. The fixed DNA is then hybridized to a labelled DNA probe specific for the gene to be analyzed, and the specific sizes of DNA to which the probe binds allow determination of the "genotype" (Figure 22.13). This test is often superseded by PCR technology.

There are different degrees to which molecular genetic tests can contribute to clinical diagnosis. Some specific molecular genetic tests can be used to detect a known pathogenic DNA mutation and give a diagnosis, even without any knowledge of the patient's clinical status. For instance, the PCR detection of the Phe508del deletion in both copies of a person's cystic fibrosis (CFTR) gene immediately gives a diagnosis of cystic fibrosis. Such direct mutation tests are possible where the gene responsible for a condition has been isolated, and specific pathogenic mutations have been identified. Similarly, a PCR test detects a deletion of exons 7 and 8 in both alleles of a gene called SMN on chromosome 5q in almost all children with spinal muscular atrophy. Southern blot analysis of DNA from infants with congenital myotonic dystrophy shows a very large expansion in a triplet repeat DNA sequence in the myotonin kinase gene on chromosome 19, as described earlier under "Other Forms of Inheritance."

In other cases, molecular genetic diagnosis can point toward a diagnosis without confirming it. For instance, the presence of a single Phe508del CFTR gene mutation in a child with a history suggestive of cystic fibrosis increases the likelihood of the child being affected.

In some cases, where either a gene is not known or very few gene mutations have been identified in a known gene, gene tracking studies can be performed in a family to predict whether a person in that family is affected. This is known as linkage analysis. Such a study requires careful clinical examination of several family members to establish whether they are affected or unaffected. Where their clinical status is clear, DNA samples are then obtained.

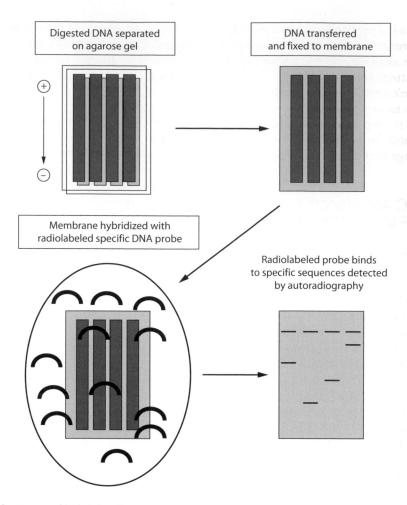

Figure 22.13 Southern blotting and hybridization.

Gene tracking analysis in the family uses the property of normal variation in a gene between different people. Some genetic areas show wide variation between individuals, and a DNA marker from such an area, which can detect many variations, is described as being polymorphic. Each variant of a polymorphic marker is known as an allele. There are now thousands of polymorphic markers covering most of the human genome, and such markers can be found very close to most known genes. There are several types of polymorphic DNA markers, including markers characterized by different numbers of specific DNA-cutting enzymes recognition sites or restriction fragment length polymorphisms (RFLPs). Other markers detect the variation in the number of anonymous elements of repetitive DNA and are called microsatellites or minisatellites.

If the two alleles of a polymorphic marker can be distinguished to discriminate between the two copies of that particular chromosome from where the marker comes, then the marker is informative in that individual. Where a gene location is known but the actual gene has yet to be found, the alleles of informative markers that lie on either side of the gene will be inherited along with each copy of the gene in question. This can be used to predict a child's clinical status.

If one set of alleles is found in the affected members of the family, but not in those unaffected, then the presence or absence of these alleles in the at-risk individual can be used to predict their chances of being affected. An example of linkage analysis for an autosomal recessive disorder is shown in Figure 22.14. This form of linkage analysis is often used in families with X-linked recessive conditions such as Duchenne muscular dystrophy to

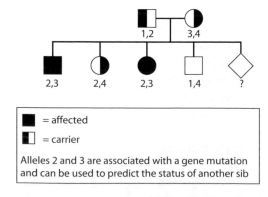

Figure 22.14 Linkage analysis in an autosomal recessive disorder using an intragenic polymorphic marker.

predict whether a woman is a carrier. Such linkage analysis can also be used in prenatal diagnosis.

Of its nature, linkage analysis is more prone to error than direct mutation testing. This can be due to difficulties in assessing a person's clinical status, and because of the possibility of recombination between the polymorphic markers. However, with the rapid advances in molecular genetics, many more mutations are being found in many different genes, and linkage analysis is often superseded by direct mutation testing.

CLINICAL GENETIC APPROACH TO DIAGNOSIS OF MALFORMATION SYNDROMES

Definitions

One child in 40 (2.5%) is born with a significant congenital anomaly, and 20%–25% of perinatal and childhood mortality is accounted for by congenital anomalies. Only a small number of these anomalies will occur as part of a specific genetic syndrome. A list of common congenital anomalies and approximate birth incidence is shown in Table 22.5.

Awareness of the possibility of a genetic or syndromal association for anomalies is very important for management of the patient and for advising the whole family. A distinction has also to be drawn between several different forms of abnormality, with appropriate definitions.

Table 22.5 Examples of major congenital anomalies

Type	Birth incidence (per 1000 births)
Cardiovascular	10
Ventricular septal defect	2.5
Atrial septal defect	1
Patent ductus arteriosus	1
Fallot's tetralogy	1
Central nervous system	10
Anencephaly	1
Hydrocephalus	1
Microcephaly	1
Lumbosacral spina bifida	2
Gastrointestinal	4
Cleft lip/palate	1.5
Diaphragmatic hernia	0.5
Esophageal atresia	0.3
Imperforate anus	0.2
Limb	2
Transverse amputation	0.2
Urogenital	4
Bilateral renal agenesis	2
Polycystic kidneys (infantile)	0.02
Bladder extrophy	0.03

A *disruption* can be defined as an anomaly that is caused by an interference in the structure of a normally developing organ. A good example would be the digital constrictions and amputations caused by amniotic bands.

A *deformation* can be defined as an anomaly that is caused by an external interference in the structure of a normally developing organ. An example would be talipes equinovarus caused by chronic oligohydramnios, perhaps from an amniotic leak.

A *malformation* can be defined as an anomaly that is caused by an intrinsic failure in the normal development of an organ. Common examples would be congenital heart disease, cleft lip and palate, and neural tube defects.

A *dysplasia* is an abnormal organization of cells in a tissue, often specific to a particular tissue. For example, achondroplasia is a skeletal dysplasia caused by a mutation in the FGFR3 gene. Most dysplasias are single-gene disorders.

A *sequence* can be defined as a group of anomalies that arise due to one single event. An example would be Potter's sequence. Potter's sequence (Figure 22.15) is the group of anomalies consisting of pulmonary hypoplasia, oligohydramnios, talipes, cleft palate, and hypertelorism. All of these anomalies arise as a result of the failure of urine production in the fetus. The cause of Potter's syndrome and failure of urine production could be posterior urethral valves, dysplastic or cystic kidneys, or renal agenesis, all of which can have genetic, nongenetic, or chromosomal origins. Pierre Robin sequence is the grouping of cleft palate, micrognathia, and glossoptosis, which can have at least 30 different causes. A sequence therefore does not have a specific cause or inheritance pattern.

An *association* can be defined as a clustering of anomalies, which is not a sequence, and which occurs more frequently than by chance, but has no prior assumption about causation. A good example is the association of VATER (vertebral anomalies, anal abnormalities, tracheoesophageal fistula, and radial or renal anomalies). There is no clear cause for VATER, although it can rarely occur in people with chromosome 22q11 microdeletions and can also rarely be mimicked by Fanconi's anemia.

A *syndrome* is a description of a group of symptoms and signs, and a pattern of anomalies, where there is often a known cause or an assumption about causation. The looser definition of "syndrome" to describe an anomaly should be avoided. The term can include chromosomal disorders such as Down syndrome or single-gene disorders such as van der Woude syndrome, which can cause cleft lip and palate with lower lip pits.

Approach to diagnosis

When a child is born with a congenital anomaly, several particular aspects of the history need to be explored. A good family history must be taken, with reference not only to a history of the same anomaly but other anomalies as well. A family history must include documentation of pregnancy losses, stillbirths and neonatal deaths. Any

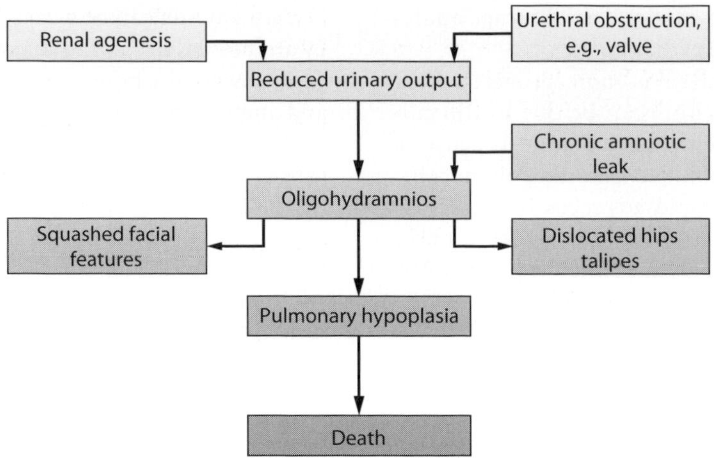

Figure 22.15 Potter's sequence.

history of potential teratogens in the pregnancy should be looked for, considering the likely embryological timing of the anomaly. Teratogens can include medications, recreational drugs, maternal diabetes, and prolonged maternal hyperthermia.

If a child has one congenital anomaly, a very careful examination should be carried out to check for any other more subtle abnormalities or for dysmorphic facial features, e.g., to check for hydrocephalus in an infant with a spinal meningomyelocele. If there is more than one malformation or significant dysmorphology, a chromosomal analysis should be requested, as chromosomal aneuploidy is a well-recognized cause of multiple malformations. A clinical genetic opinion should also be sought, as a clinical geneticist can often help greatly in achieving a diagnosis, as well as in counselling parents about the likelihood of recurrence of similar problems in other family members.

A diagnostic approach to congenital anomalies is outlined in Figure 22.16. Deformations and disruptions need to be excluded first. If the pattern of malformations fits into a well-described sequence, then a cause for that sequence should be sought. If the anomalies do not fit into a sequence, then a syndrome or association diagnosis should be attempted. If a syndrome diagnosis is achieved, it is important to remember that syndromes can be caused by chromosomal disorders, single-gene (monogenic) disorders, or environmental agents (teratogens).

The majority of congenital anomalies have a polygenic or multifactorial origin, and most are isolated (nonsyndromal). The causes of congenital abnormalities are outlined in Table 22.6, and it is important to note that about 50% do not have a clear cause. Nonetheless, parents and families want an explanation as to the origin of their child's anomaly, and it is therefore worthwhile to pursue a diagnosis wherever possible.

This chapter is an introduction to the concepts and principles of genetics in neonatal surgical practice. It is not intended to be a comprehensive review of syndromes. Further information can be obtained from the bibliography and many Internet sources.

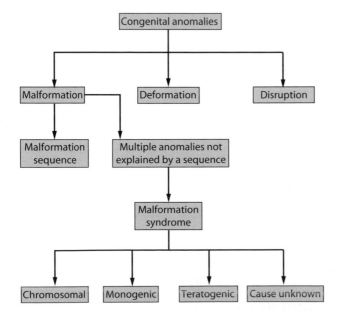

Figure 22.16 Diagnostic approach to congenital anomalies.

Table 22.6 Causes of congenital anomalies

Type	Relative frequency
Genetic	
Chromosomal	6%
Single gene	7.5%
Multifactorial/polygenic	20%–30%
Environmental	
Drugs, infections, maternal illness	5%–10%
Unknown	50%
Total	100%

FURTHER READING

Watson JD, Hopkins NH, Roberts JW, Steitz JA, Weiner AM. *Molecular Biology of the Gene*, 5th edn. Menlo Park, CA: Benjamin Cummings Publishing Company, 1993.

Strachan T, Read AP. *Human Molecular Genetics*. Oxford: BIOS Publishers, 1996.

Lewin B. *Genes V*. Oxford: Oxford University Press, 1994.

Connor M, Ferguson-Smith M. *Essential Medical Genetics*, 5th edn. Oxford: Blackwell Scientific, 1997.

Mueller RF, Young ID. *Emery's Elements of Medical Genetics*, 10th edn. Edinburgh: Churchill Livingstone, 2001.

Online Mendelian Inheritance in Man. A list of genetic disorders and the latest genetic developments for each condition. Website http://www3.ncbi.nlm.nih .gov/Omim.

GLOSSARY

3′ distal end of a gene, as indicated by the bond at the third hydroxyl group of the deoxyribose sugar.

5′ proximal end of a gene, as indicated by the bond at the third hydroxyl group of the deoxyribose sugar.

acrocentric a chromosome with effectively only a long arm—chromosomes 13, 14, 15, 21, and 22.

allele a genetic variation of a gene or DNA marker.

aneuploidy an excess or deficiency of chromosomal material.

anticodon an element of transfer RNA that binds a specific amino acid.

autosomal dominant inheritance pattern characterized by transmission through several generations, male-to-male transmission, and a 50:50 risk to the children of any affected person.

autosomal recessive inheritance pattern characterized by several affected members of the same generation, with carrier parents and a 1:4 recurrence risk where both parents are carriers.

base pair unit of double-stranded DNA.

centromere element of chromosome involved in chromosome replication, found as a constriction in the chromosome.

chromatid condensed chromosome found just before mitosis.

codon three base pair element of DNA encoding an amino acid.

diploid a complement of two copies of each chromosome per cell.

DNA marker a piece of DNA corresponding to a specific gene or chromosomal segment.

enhancers elements of DNA that are involved in increasing gene transcription.

exon a part of a gene that is transcribed into mRNA.

expression the way in which a gene fault manifests clinically.

FISH fluorescent in situ hybridization—a new and powerful technique for studying specific chromosomes or regions of chromosomes.

gamete a germ cell—sperm or oocyte.

genetic imprinting the marking of a gene according to which parent has passed the gene to its child.

haploid a complement of one copy of each chromosome per cell (as in sperm or oocyte).

haplotype a pattern of alleles of DNA markers representing one of the two copies of a chromosomal region.

histone a DNA-binding protein important in chromosomal folding.

interphase phase of mitosis in which the chromosomes are very elongated.

intron the part of a gene between the exons that is not transcribed into mRNA.

isochromosome an abnormal chromosome made up of two long or two short arms of a normal chromosome.

karyotype an analysis of the chromosome complement of a cell type.

linkage analysis the use of polymorphic DNA markers to perform gene tracking studies within a family.

meiosis the process of cell division to give haploid germ cells.

metaphase phase of mitosis in which the chromosomes are very condensed and easier to analyze.

microsatellite marker a DNA marker that detects variation in number of an anonymous small repetitive element of DNA.

minisatellite marker a DNA marker that detects variation in number of an anonymous medium repetitive element of DNA.

mitosis the normal process of cell division to give two diploid copies of a cell.

nondisjunction a failure of meiosis, giving two copies of a chromosome in one gamete, and no copy of a chromosome in the other gamete.

nucleosome the combination of a histone and its bound DNA.

oligonucleotide primers small lengths of synthetic single-stranded DNA of a specific sequence.

paracentric inversion a rearrangement of chromosomal material within one arm of a chromosome.

PCR polymerase chain reaction—a method of generating large amounts of specific DNA from a small amount of target sequence.

penetrance the number of people known to carry a gene mutation who manifest the condition.

pericentric inversion a rearrangement of chromosomal material around the centromere of a chromosome.

promoter element of a gene that is necessary to activate gene transcription.

prophase phase of the cell cycle where condensation of the chromosomes occurs, just before metaphase.

reciprocal translocation exchange of chromosomal segments between different chromosomes.

restriction enzyme an enzyme that cuts double-stranded DNA at a specific unique short DNA sequence.

restriction fragment length polymorphism a genetic variation between two copies of the same gene, where one gene may have one copy of a restriction enzyme recognition site, and the other has two copies. This variation can be detected using PCR or Southern blotting.

ribosome area of the cell where mRNA is converted into protein.

ring chromosome an abnormal chromosome in which the tips of the long and short arms have fused.

robertsonian translocation a fusion of two acrocentric chromosomes.

southern blotting a process of immobilizing DNA to nylon membrane for genetic analysis.

suppressor a DNA element that reduces the expression of a gene.

telophase the last phase of mitosis.

telomere the end of a chromosome.

transcription the process of converting DNA into mRNA.

translation the production of protein from a DNA sequence.

triploidy three of each chromosome, i.e., 69 chromosomes in man.

trisomy one extra chromosome, i.e., 47 chromosomes in man.

X-linked recessive inheritance characterized by affected males in several generations, and by female carriers.

23

Ethical considerations in newborn surgery

DONNA A. CANIANO AND JACQUELINE J. GLOVER

INTRODUCTION

In the course of routine practice, a pediatric surgeon often encounters clinical situations involving ethical choices, such as the following:

1. Counseling the parents of an extremely premature infant who is unstable following peritoneal drainage for perforated necrotizing enterocolitis
2. Providing prenatal consultation to a pregnant woman and her partner whose fetus has a high-risk congenital diaphragmatic hernia (CDH)
3. Deciding whether to participate in a prospective clinical trial for management of gastroschisis

Through case examples, this chapter provides the pediatric surgeon with an ethical framework to utilize in clinical practice when decision making may contain conflict with parental wishes as in the first case, risks and uncertainty (maternal and fetal) represented in the second instance, and the exercise of professional duties in the third instance.

The authors propose a set of guidelines and an organized process of establishing all relevant information, including what is known about the infant's medical and surgical condition and the relevant cultural and religious values of the parents. The totality of this information will come to bear on application of the *best-interests* ethical standard together with respectful acknowledgement of the role of culture in achieving a decision acceptable to the parents and the pediatric surgeon.

CASE STUDY 23.1

MS is a 21-day-old infant born at 25 weeks' gestation, weighing 575 g. He was stable on 50% oxygen and minimal ventilatory settings. He was on continuous feedings using a premature formula. At 21 days of age, the infant developed acute abdominal distention, intolerance to feedings, and bloody stools. Urgent consultation with the pediatric surgeon was requested. A radiograph showed diffuse pneumatosis. He was mottled, acidotic, and hypotensive. His laboratory values showed a white blood cell count of 2000, hemoglobin of 7 mg%, and a platelet count of 6000. He received packed red cells and platelets. Blood cultures were drawn, and he was started on triple antibiotics. The parents agreed to bedside peritoneal drainage. After 12 hours, MS remained clinically unstable, with worsening respiratory status. Laparotomy was advised by the pediatric surgeon, and the parents refused the operation.

MS's parents are from Nigeria and are in the United States on student visas. They have two other healthy children, aged 3 and 5, and plan to return to their native country in 3 months. The parents visit daily and are concerned about their son. Both the father and mother speak English. They ask appropriate questions and seem to understand their son's medical condition, prognosis, and alternatives for treatment. They desire that their son live but are strongly opposed to

TPN, especially since this technology is not available in their small city in Nigeria.

They acknowledge that MS is gravely ill and are accepting of his probable death. They say that they agreed to the use of all the previous medical technology because they thought it would save their son's life. But a life dependent on medical technology is too burdensome. They were expecting that their son would be able to live normally once he got out of the hospital. The parents explain that they have a strong faith in God; God will decide if their son lives or dies, and they will accept whatever happens. They believe that it is not in their power to alter God's will by the continued use of technology to support a life "that was not meant to be" and that if the boy is not able to eat like a normal infant, then it is better that he go to God. They have clearly stated their intention to return to Nigeria, where life-sustaining technology, such as total parenteral nutrition (TPN) and specialized nutritional formulas, are unavailable. In addition, they will not have access to pediatric specialists when they return to their native country, and worry about how they will secure medical and surgical care for an infant with a poorly functioning intestine and other chronic disabilities. What should the pediatric surgeon do? What is the best course of treatment for MS? What is the role of culture in this case, and how should it influence decision making?

GUIDELINES FOR ETHICAL DECISION MAKING

Ethical dilemmas most often arise when there is disagreement about a proposed course of treatment, what constitutes an acceptable quality of life, or what is in the best interest of the infant as perceived by the parents and by the pediatric surgeon. The authors have found the following questions to be useful in initiating an open and frank conversation with parents. The questions are intended as subject guides only; each pediatric surgeon should adapt the questions into his or her own style:

1. What is your understanding of your baby's current condition?
2. How has your baby's illness affected your family?
3. What is most important in the care of your baby?
4. What do you fear the most? What would you like to avoid?
5. What are your family's sources of strength and support?

Pediatric surgeons can help insure that their ethical judgments are reliable through the application of an organized process.[1] There are multiple versions available in the ethics literature, but they generally all contain the following components:

1. Identify the decision makers. Are the parents involved? Are there nonparental legal guardians? Do the parents have the capacity to make a decision? Who are the involved clinicians?
2. Gather the relevant medical facts. What is the diagnosis? What is the prognosis? Are additional tests necessary for further clarification? Is there necessary information to be gathered from other clinicians?
3. Solicit value data from all involved parties. Do conflicts exist among the values of the parents, other family members, and the physicians? Has the basis for the conflict been identified?
4. Define the available treatment options. With each option, what is the likelihood of cure or amelioration? What are the risks of an adverse effect? What is the minimum level of professionally acceptable treatment?
5. Evaluate possible treatment options and make a recommendation. Justify your choice according to the values of various parties.
6. Achieve a consensus resolution. Have all parties articulated their viewpoint? Would more factual information help to resolve any disputes? Would a mediator (ethics consultant, ethics committee, or other trusted third party) be helpful?

THE BEST-INTERESTS STANDARD APPLIED TO NEONATAL SURGERY

Since neonates and infants cannot make decisions about the appropriate use of technology based on their own personal values, the central ethical question is framed in pediatrics as, "What is in the best interests of this infant?" An answer requires a unique and complex ethical framework that combines a concern for who makes the decision and what decision is appropriate. In the United States, parents are presumed to be the appropriate decision makers for their infants.[1] Parents and pediatric surgeons must work together to make decisions that are in the best interests of infants.[2,3] The term *best interests* is meant to capture a balancing of the benefits and burdens to this infant of a particular intervention.[4]

In the mainstream medical culture in the United States, the term *best interests* was developed to focus attention on the need to assess the benefits and burdens of treatment for a particular infant from the infant's perspective. In an effort to be as objective as possible, only the direct pain and suffering associated with an infant's condition and/or proposed treatment was to be considered in conjunction with the benefit of continued life. The standard was proposed as a very strict one, regarding treatment as beneficial and in the infant's best interest unless the infant was dying, the treatment was medically contraindicated, or continued life would be worse for the infant than an early death. A central feature of this narrow understanding of best interests includes its child-centeredness, understood to mean the exclusion from consideration of the negative effects of an impaired infant's life on other persons, including parents, siblings, and society.

A second key feature is its emphasis on the infant's concrete experience of burden in the form of pain and suffering. In addition to the difficulties associated with assessing the burdens experienced by an infant, a narrow best-interests standard cannot be applied to neonates and infants with neurological deficits so severe as to exclude the possibility of experience of any sort. Infants who are not responsive to outside stimuli, for example, cannot experience pain and therefore cannot be burdened in the same way as conscious infants.

Some ethicists have appropriately pointed out that absence of pain is not the only morally relevant feature.[5] A *relational-potential* standard is necessary to augment a best-interests standard. It is not morally obligatory to sustain life without any capacity for human relationship, even though life is not burdensome per se. Just as the presence of pain unable to be relieved can preclude the attainment of those basic human goods that make life worth living, so the absence of fundamental human capacity can render a life devoid of the same basic human goods.[6]

An expanded understanding of best interests must take into consideration several competing ethical values. One value is respect for family autonomy or self-determination. Families ought to have the freedom to make important choices about family welfare independent of others. It is not so much that families have a right to make important decisions for their infants as it is that families have the responsibility to make decisions and provide the necessary financial and other types of support. Families are an essential unit of care that is both valuable in itself and instrumentally valuable to meet the social goal of caring for children. Since families are presumed to love their children and desire to do what is best for them, they have a unique claim to the decision-making role. Also, families have to live with the consequences of the health care decisions that are made.[7]

In a very real sense, the families' interests are linked with the interests of the neonate or infant.[8] An attempt to starkly separate infant and family interests is artificial and diminishes rather than enhances an understanding of the infant's well-being. One can understand how the best-interests standard developed in the context of imperiled newborns, where there is great uncertainty and no one has a longstanding relationship with the infant. The objectivity sought is comprehensible only because the infant is a stranger to all. Yet even in the case of newborns, most authors agree that parents should be the primary decision makers.[9] If family interests were irrelevant, it would be difficult to make sense of such a presumption. Given this presumption in favor of parental decision making, and the fact that most infants are not strangers to their parents, a best-interests standard would be better understood to include a more comprehensive understanding of a child-centered decision, one made by a family whose daily lives involve the love and care of their infant.

Additionally, the search for the best interests of the infant apart from the family has several negative consequences. First of all, it can antagonize parents and turn all parties into adversaries. It can also cut off discussion and planning rather than improve it. Families may not feel free to discuss difficulties, and important needs may go unmet. Rather than search for some artificial "best" interest, all parties should acknowledge the complex goal of promoting the infant's well-being and the necessary interdependence of families in that endeavor. To exclude the family in a concept of child-centeredness is to reduce the infant to only a physiological organism and well-being to pathophysiological function.

Another value that is in tension with respect for family decision making is respect for professional integrity. Since *best interests* also contains an important focus on the uniquely medical interests of the infant, professional judgment plays an important role in describing and evaluating the benefits and burdens of health care interventions.[10] Pediatric surgeons have independent obligations to the infants who are their patients, to promote their well-being and protect them from harm. They have a professional obligation to promote life and quality of life, and to avoid such harms as killing, premature death, pain, and suffering. Yet even based on so-called medical facts, decisions are a complex amalgam of what the infant's alternative futures will be like, how likely it is that these futures can be gained, and what the infant has to endure to get there. An infant's present interests in being free from undue burdens must be weighed against all future interests.[11]

A third important value is that of justice as nondiscrimination.[12] How do we understand the interests of a child in himself or herself, independent of how others may value him or her? What does society owe its children as a matter of justice? Infants do not only belong to their families, but they also are members of their community. Communities have an obligation to protect the most vulnerable among them, especially if they are vulnerable to the neglect and abuse of their families. All infants deserve a certain level of health care, independent of what their families might choose for them.

The principle of justice also has another important component that is in direct conflict with the highly individualistic interpretation of best interests. In fact, a best-interests standard is an attempt to narrowly focus decisions on the patient himself or herself and to avoid greater issues of the just distribution of health care resources, but this is impossible. Families and communities struggle to consider what they owe each child, but also to consider what is fair for this child and all children together. Resources of time, effort, services, and money are limited within families and communities. Each must consider the impact of choices on the availability of resources for others. There is no doubt that questions of distributive justice are among the most difficult ethical issues that families, professionals, and communities must face. But they will never be resolved if they are simply ignored in the decision-making process. The authors agree that allocation decisions are best made at levels other than at the bedside, as in the formulation of insurance plans and governmental policies. But these corporate allocation decisions will always have implications for bedside care and must not be ignored.

An expanded best-interests standard is an attempt to balance the benefits and burdens of a health care intervention according to the values of the parents, pediatric surgeons, and the larger society. It should be clear that the model described represents its application in the dominant medical culture in the United States. Firstly, other cultures and countries may have a different understanding of what constitutes family and necessarily include others besides parents. Perhaps others, such as family elders, are the persons designated as decision makers. Secondly, this particular model is based on western notions of the importance of informed consent and respect for the autonomy (self-determination) of the patient, and the family in the case of pediatrics. In other cultures and countries, families may not see their role as decision makers at all, only in terms of doing what the doctor orders. Also, other cultures and countries may emphasize other core values such as responsibility to the larger family and community rather than autonomy (self-determination). Finally, the model described presumes a certain access to technology that is primarily available in developed nations. A concern for quality of life is different in developed nations, where the issue may be the result of technology that is able to save life of diminished quality, as opposed to developing nations, where diminished quality of life may be primarily a consequence of inadequate access to basic health care services or the lack of advanced technology to support infants with chronic illness.

ROLE OF CULTURE IN DECISION MAKING

The ethical concept of best interests that has been articulated is largely dependent upon the authors' own experiences in the medical culture in the United States. In the case study of MS, we are compelled to value and respect cultural differences. Both his parents and the pediatric surgeon are struggling to fulfill their role-specific obligations to be good parents and a good physician. But they literally see their roles quite differently. It is culture that provides the lens for each of us to view the world. One definition of culture states,

> Culture is a set of guidelines (both explicit and implicit) which individuals inherit as members of a particular society, and which tells them how to view the world, how to experience it emotionally, and how to behave in it in relation to other people, to supernatural forces or gods, and to the natural environment. It also provides them with a way of transmitting symbols, language, art and ritual. To some extent, culture can be seen as an inherited "lens," through which individuals perceive and understand the world that they inhabit, and learn how to live within it.

> Growing up within any society is a form of enculturation, whereby the individual slowly acquires the cultural "lens" of that society. Without such a shared perception of the world, both the cohesion and the continuity of any human group would be impossible.[13]

It seems obvious from this definition that there is no way to talk about best interests from outside a cultural perspective. All of our discussion, then, is in some sense cross-cultural. The narrow explication of best interests represents the perspective of the United States, and perhaps predominantly the powerful status of its medical and legal culture.

A Nigerian anthropologist commenting on this case might point out that the United States has several unique cultural features. People in the United States tend to think that there is nothing worse than death—at least for a child or young person. Children are to be viewed as little adults—as individuals first and then only secondarily as members of a family or community, essentially independent of their families rather than dependent. Their right to grow up and to ultimately make their own choices is primary. US culture is very action oriented: when in doubt—act. The United Stated is also obsessed by the development and perceived power of technology. Technology and knowledge are primary goods.

But the central question is not really whether or not we have a cultural perspective, but whether we can judge some perspectives as better than others. This raises the difficult ethical question of cultural relativity. Cultural relativity refers to the following claims: (1) all moral judgments are relative to the culture in which they arise; (2) moral judgments across cultures are significantly different; and (3) there is no way to rank moral judgments across cultures.[14]

The well-respected physician–ethicist Edmund Pellegrino accepts that culture is essential in the context of medical and ethical decisions but that there are also features of human beings as human beings according to which we can judge among cultures.[15] It can be argued that there are some universal features that all cultures either should or would accept. An example would be that moral communities must allow democratic processes and cannot be oppressive.[16] The philosopher Sara Ruddick identifies three universal maternal interests that are applicable regardless of the particular form they take in a culture. These maternal interests include the following: (1) preservation, (2) growth, and (3) acceptability.[17] Other ethicists identify universal moral principles that underlie our commitments to be tolerant of cultural diversity.[18,19] Without some principle of respect for persons, for example, there would be no reason to prefer tolerance of cultural differences.

A cultural perspective is particularly important to ethical theorists, who support the inclusion of context and relationship in an ethical analysis, and to those of us working in clinical settings. As Carl Elliot writes,

Ethical concepts are tied to a society's customs, manners, tradition, institutions—all of the concepts that structure and inform the ways in which a member of that society deals with the world. When we forget this, we are in danger of leaving this world of genuine moral experience for the world of moral fiction—a simplified, hypothetical creation less suited for practical difficulties than for intellectual convenience.[20]

The authors wish to support an ethical analysis that includes culture as an important feature but also acknowledges the role of the application of universal ethical principles. Like Pellegrino, the authors accept that there are some ethical principles that apply to all humans based on their humanity. Culture is necessary to understand what these principles mean and how they are applied with respect to each of the parties in the conflict. It is possible to be respectful of cultural differences and at the same time acknowledge that there are limits. What remains critical is the perceived degree of harm; some cultural practices may constitute violations of fundamental human rights. It is useful to return to case #1 and apply the process for ethical decision making with special attention to its cross-cultural features.

The family in this case clearly values their son's life and his quality of life. They also value the impact of this infant's life on their other children, the life of the family as a whole, and their plans to return to their native country. They accepted the initial use of technology in the care of their premature son, in the hope that it would deliver a "normal" infant, free of future dependence on medical technology. They are clear that for them, in a cultural and religious sense, a life dependent on TPN, specialized nutritional feedings, and the prospect of bowel transplantation is unacceptable.

For the pediatric surgeon and the other members of the health care team, the preservation of this infant's life is a goal, but the quality of his life is also a consideration. The laparotomy will allow the pediatric surgeon to assess the severity of the necrotizing enterocolitis (NEC), the amount of diseased bowel, and the prognosis for MS to have functional intestine without the need for prolonged TPN.

There are basically three options available in this situation. First, the pediatric surgeon can go forward with all the care that it takes to save this infant's life. This would include surgery, the use of TPN for as long as necessary, and all efforts to preserve the life of MS, including the possibility for bowel transplantation. This would more than likely include going to court to force the parents to consent to the operation and having a guardian appointed to make medical decisions for MS. This option could result in the permanent loss of parental rights and placement of the infant in the care of the state. In the second option, the pediatric surgeon performs the operation in the hope that there is sufficient residual bowel without the need for long-term TPN and bowel transplantation. If there is clearly not enough viable bowel, MS would be provided with comfort care

and allowed to die. If there is sufficient residual bowel, care would proceed as appropriate. A difficulty arises if there is a questionable amount of bowel, and a trial of TPN would seem to be appropriate. The pediatric surgeon could resect the diseased bowel and proceed with a trial of TPN, discontinuing the use of TPN when it is clear that the bowel is not going to function normally. The third option is not to perform the operation. The infant could be maintained on current levels of support to see whether his bowel will heal on its own, or a comfort care plan could be initiated that would allow the infant to die sooner rather than prolonging the dying process.

The authors think that the first option is outside the range of moral justification and should not be recommended. The infant is critically ill with a disease that carries high rates of mortality and morbidity. Nontreatment for MS does not rise to the standard of medical neglect. The strongest argument for insisting on treatment rests on the claim that this infant is a member of the community, not only a member of his family. If families will not or cannot take proper care of their children, then we will step in to do so. But who is this "we"? If there is no such community support, or insofar as the broader community fails in this responsibility, then the community's claim on the family's choice is diminished.

In this case, the Nigerian community (here or in Nigeria) does not make demands on the parents' choice. They do not see themselves as able, or obligated, to provide these services to MS. But in what sense is MS and his family a member of the US community? An argument can be made that they are community members by virtue of their residence. Yet they are planning to return to Nigeria. The argument that treatment must be forced because of community obligations seems diminished by their departure. We will not be around to provide the support we claim is necessary.

But will we provide the necessary support even if they stay? Is it possible for them to stay? Our community claims also seem diminished insofar as the family's student visa is not renewed, or access to health and social services is limited based on their foreign status. To claim that we are discharging our community obligations only by saving the child's life seems to greatly distort the notion of community.

But a final consideration needs to be mentioned. Couldn't we discharge our community responsibility by keeping the child here and placing him up for adoption? Then he certainly would become a full member of our community, and the concerns raised earlier would no longer apply. Such an action could clearly state that we believe the only appropriate parental choice is to try and save the infant's life. To choose anything else is to act as bad parents who should be replaced. Yet are they really bad parents? Such a judgment clearly raises serious concerns about cultural norms of parenting and fails to take culture into consideration. From the parents' cultural perspective, good parents would not choose surgery, and neither would good physicians. This is not the standard of care in Nigeria.

But how should culture figure into the deliberations of the pediatric surgeon? It obviously cannot simply be ignored in a grand act of medical and parental imperialism. Also, we should not pay lip service to cultural perspectives, accepting the unusual and exotic only when it also fits into our own value framework. For example, this family could make the choice based on their cultural values only if there were a much higher mortality rate associated with the infant's condition. Finally, respect for different cultures cannot simply be some kind of ultimate trump. Automatically deferring to any choices based on cultural differences is to ignore the central values of our own culture. Ironically, it would be a violation of respect for cultural diversity in that our own cultural values are ignored. An attempt at negotiation and compromise is to be preferred.

The authors think that the pediatric surgeon should recommend surgery under the second scenario, saving the infant if possible, letting the infant die if appropriate, and negotiating a trial of TPN if necessary. But if this is not acceptable to the parents, the pediatric surgeon should respect the parents' decision not to have surgery and proceed with a plan of care aimed at keeping the infant comfortable until he either improves or dies. A decision by a pediatric surgeon to conscientiously withdraw from this patient's care out of concern for his or her own central values should be respected.

The second option is supported by the health care professionals' and the family's values. Surgery could save the infant's life, which all parties value, but it would do so under conditions of a quality of life that are acceptable to the family. Some health care professionals may have problems with this option if a trial of TPN is necessary. It is difficult to establish how long a trial of TPN should last. This difficult negotiation must consider what is medically feasible and also acceptable to the family. Also, many believe that there is a distinction between decisions not to start treatments (withholding) and decisions to stop treatments (withdrawing). Although this distinction is psychologically powerful, it is not ethically or legally valid in the United States.[21] If health care professionals and parents have sufficient justification based on the balance of benefits and burdens not to start a treatment, then they have the same justification to stop a treatment once begun. There is a hidden danger in maintaining this distinction between not starting and stopping medical and surgical treatments. Sometimes trials of therapy are not initiated when they are appropriate out of fear that the therapy cannot be stopped once it has begun.

Others argue that the provision of nutrition and hydration is different from other medical interventions, such as ventilators and dialysis, which are "extraordinary" and ethically can be withheld or withdrawn. According to this view, the provision of nutrition and hydration is ordinary and is always morally required. The attempt to classify categories of interventions independent of their application to the care of an individual patient is misguided. So-called ordinary treatments like antibiotics and the medical provision of hydration and nutrition can be disproportionally burdensome to certain infants and may be ethically forgone (withheld or withdrawn).[22,23] Many physicians and parents have particular values around the importance of feeding, regarding feeding tubes and TPN as morally equivalent to bottle or breast feeding an infant or to sharing a meal. Yet the provision of TPN is not readily comparable to feeding an infant or to a shared family meal. There are important differences. When hydration and nutrition are provided through medical means, they must be assessed according to the same principles used to evaluate any medical intervention. Decisions must be based on a careful evaluation of the proportionality of the possible benefits and burdens. For this family, TPN is burdensome not only because of the risk of frequent infections and the likelihood of progressive liver disease, but also because of what feeding through technology means in their culture, and the financial and social burdens to the entire family. The health care team in the United States cannot allocate this family's scarce resources for them, or for their country of origin.

CASE STUDY 23.2

A 35-year-old pregnant woman whose fetus was diagnosed at 18 weeks of gestation with a CDH is seen for prenatal consultation. She attends the visit with her husband, a self-employed electrician. They are the parents of a healthy 2-year-old girl. She works part-time as a nurse's aide at an assisted living facility and is active in their Christian church. They relate that they hope to have four children. Their male fetus has an isolated high-risk CDH with the liver up and an observed-over-expected lung-to-head circumference ratio <25%. The distraught couple relates that, although they have limited financial resources and no immediate family living close to them, they wish to do anything necessary to save their baby. What ethical obligations should guide the pediatric surgeon during the prenatal consultation? Should the pediatric surgeon inform the couple about a clinical trial of fetoscopic endoluminal tracheal occlusion (FETO) at a fetal treatment center nearly 1000 miles from their home?

The diagnosis of structural fetal anomalies by high-resolution ultrasonography at or around the 18th week of pregnancy is part of routine prenatal care in most developed countries. Identification of a fetal malformation typically prompts referral of the prospective parents to a pediatric surgeon for consultation about treatment and prognosis. However, the prenatal surgical consultation differs from the typical encounter between the pediatric surgeon and the parents of a neonate with a congenital anomaly, in which decisions center around operative intervention(s) for their already born infant. In the prenatal surgical consultation, there is an *expectation* of a future patient if the fetus is brought to term.[24] The unique role of the pediatric surgeon may be characterized as both an expert adviser and an expert counselor to the prospective parents. Furthermore, the advent of fetal intervention for both life-threatening conditions (CHD) and serious, non-life-threatening conditions (myelomeningocele) has increased the complexity of the prenatal surgical consultation. No longer is the encounter between the pediatric surgeon and the prospective parents confined to an explanation of the malformation, postnatal treatment, prognosis, and expected quality of life. A discussion of all available prenatal interventions, including fetal surgery, should also be within the scope of the consultation.

Ethical guidelines for prenatal surgical consultation are rooted in the dominant field of genetic counseling, a field that developed in the late 1960s after the human chromosomes could be karyotyped and carrier status of inherited diseases, such as cystic fibrosis and sickle cell anemia, could be identified. Value neutrality emerged as the prevailing ethic for genetic counseling with objectivity for the counselor and promotion of autonomy for the patient/client.[25] Historically, genetic counselors strove to be nondirective and supportive in their approach, allowing the patient/client full latitude in decision making. However, the authors believe that value neutrality fails to encompass the entirety of the pediatric surgeon's professional moral obligation during the prenatal consultation. Prospective parents have an expectation that the pediatric surgeon will offer them expert advice about the next steps in management of the fetus. Failure to do so could be viewed as abdication of professional duty.

Another unique feature of the prenatal surgical consultation is the obligation of the pediatric surgeon to recognize the pregnant woman's right to make autonomous decisions about her pregnancy, including its continuation or termination. In our case study, the pregnant woman intends to continue the pregnancy, expressing the desire to do everything possible for a successful outcome. As noted by Chervenak and McCullough,[26] she thus confers on her fetus (although still previable) the moral status of a patient. Therefore, the pediatric surgeon assumes beneficence-based obligations for the fetal patient, but within the context of both beneficence and autonomy-based obligations to the pregnant woman. This tightly linked maternal–fetal ethical bond must be considered when the pregnant woman weighs the risks to her own health and well-being in undergoing a prenatal surgical intervention.

It must also be remembered that the prospective parents of a fetus with a significant congenital anomaly come to the prenatal surgical consultation with sorrow and grief, mourning the loss of an expected "perfect baby." As the esteemed physician Eric Cassel observed, "The relief of suffering is the fundamental goal of medicine."[27] While most individuals in western societies place high trust in advanced medical and surgical technology, the prospective parents also seek from the pediatric surgeon a palpable grasp of their suffering. During the prenatal surgical consultation, they want more than technical expertise; they hope for a sharing of empathy, and an understanding of their anxiety about the loss of the imagined future replaced by a new reality for their baby.

The ethical principle of justice should not be forgotten in the discussion of prenatal intervention. Justice requires all physicians to act in a fair and equitable manner in distributing medical care, and for the pediatric surgeon, in providing surgical care. In many countries including the United States, pregnant women who come from socially and financially disadvantaged backgrounds are at a higher likelihood of having limited access to and use of optimal prenatal services. There are limited data that describe the socioeconomic, racial, and cultural backgrounds of pregnant women who are referred for prenatal surgical consultation and for fetal treatment. We can assume that since fetal treatment centers in the United States and other developed countries are located in a few major metropolitan areas, pregnant women with limited financial resources and family/social support systems rarely have realistic options for prenatal intervention. As a society and as a community of pediatric surgeons, we should have both an interest and a concern that poverty, limited education, and other social barriers impact the future welfare of a fetus with a congenital malformation.

In addition to the usual surgical care for infants with CDH, the pediatric surgeon should inform the prospective parents about prenatal intervention with FETO, since their fetus may be a candidate for this procedure. The provision of this information to prospective parents raises additional ethical issues, since there are currently no agreed-upon guidelines among the pediatric surgical community for what constitutes requisite information during prenatal consultation for fetal CDH. Brown et al.[28] highlighted their concerns about the current lack of standardization in information for prenatal counseling for myelomeningocele, another fetal malformation for which prenatal repair may be an option. They cautioned that, in the absence of standardized counseling information, unintentional consultant bias may unduly influence the pregnant woman's ability to make fully informed decisions about fetal treatment. Bias may extend to the larger community in which the pediatric surgeon practices, including neonatal and perinatal specialists, local professional views toward referral away from the local children's hospital, and attitudes about the financial and psychological hardships associated with treatment at a remote fetal center. Furthermore, most prospective parents are unaware of the variation in the postnatal treatment of infants with prenatally diagnosed high-risk CDH (for example, ex utero intrapartum treatment (EXIT) to extracorporeal membrane oxygenation [ECMO], timing of operative repair, duration of ECMO therapy, etc.) among major pediatric centers in the United States.

The authors support an ethical framework that includes a standardized guideline for pediatric surgeons to use for counseling prospective parents with high-risk fetal CDH in which fetal intervention is an option. Information would include the full range of treatment options (prenatal and postnatal), expected outcomes, the local hospital's survival and morbidity statistics, long-term sequelae, and availability of clinical trials and treatment at a fetal center.

This information resource supports the pediatric surgeon's upholding both beneficence and autonomy-based ethical obligations. It also supports the ethical duty of justice and permits every pregnant woman/prospective parents, without regard to her/their socioeconomic, cultural, and ethnic background, to be in a better position to make informed decisions. In the present case, the authors support complete disclosure of all possible treatments, including referral to a fetal treatment center for possible prenatal intervention.

CASE STUDY 23.3

You have been invited to participate in a new prospective multicenter randomized clinical trial investigating the treatment of gastroschisis. Pediatric surgeons randomized to the experimental arm would be required to adhere to a standardized treatment protocol, including placement of a bedside silo, a certain type of abdominal wall closure, and a strict feeding schedule. Pediatric surgeons randomized to the control group would use their usual operative and feeding management. The primary outcomes of the study include hospital length of stay and age in days to achieve full enteral or breast feeding. The secondary outcomes are days on the ventilator, days of intravenous nutrition, number of days on antibiotics, bacteremia, and total hospital costs. Does the pediatric surgeon have an ethical obligation to participate in this research trial?

Nearly all significant advances in pediatric surgery have been achieved by the development of new operations and treatments or incremental modifications of existing procedures without professional oversight. In a field where congenital anomalies are relatively uncommon, each pediatric surgeon has been free to make individual choices about a preferred operative technique or management plan. Surgical innovation has historically occurred without significant prior investigation. A successful single patient outcome from a "new operative technique" often results in a limited patient series whose results are presented at a professional meeting. Whether or not the new technique achieves general utilization depends on several variables including the perceived need for a better technique by peers, reputation of the innovator, its ease of reproducibility, and results when performed by other surgeons. If the early results of the new technique or novel treatment are promising, it is typically followed by a plethora of presentations at professional meetings and peer-reviewed publications before it enters the realm of accepted practice. While surgical innovation is both necessary and noble, it may thwart the development of optimal treatments and operations and have the unintentional consequences of patient harm unless subjected to careful investigation.

Are there sufficient questions about the best management of an infant with gastroschisis that the pediatric surgeon should consider his or her ethical obligation to enter a clinical trial? Lusk et al.[29] have reported that there is considerable variability in the surgical and medical management of infants with gastroschisis among different pediatric centers and also among pediatric surgeons within the same institution. They also observed that there is no consensus among pediatric surgeons about the optimal management of infants with gastroschisis. In the current era of greater awareness for patient safety and health care costs, the authors propose that treatment variability without clear outcome benefits for infants with gastroschisis supports prospective clinical investigation.

The notion of equipoise describes the uncertainty about which treatment of surgical procedure results in the best outcome, given two or more alternatives.[30] At the personal level of a single pediatric surgeon, equipoise can be misunderstood because of thinking that a preferred surgical and/or treatment approach is superior to other methods, despite the lack of previous investigative support. Community and/or clinical equipoise provides a more inclusive view in which a state of uncertainty about optimal management of gastroschisis exists within the professional specialty of pediatric surgery regarding the merits of competing treatments and/or operations. The benefit of invoking community equipoise is that it permits an individual pediatric surgeon to retain strong preferences for his or her preferred management, and still agree that there is reasonable uncertainty within the profession about optimal treatment and/or operations.

Do the professional organizations in pediatric surgery expect their members to participate in clinical research trials? The principles of medical ethics in the bylaws of the American Pediatric Surgical Association list the following obligations of its members:

> Members shall strive to...acquire new medical and surgical knowledge through continuing practice in order to benefit patients.... Members shall recognize a responsibility to participate in activities benefiting the community.[31]

Nwomeh and Caniano[32] have pointed out that pediatric surgeons are uniquely advantaged to participate in prospective clinical trials because (1) the anatomic derangement and pathophysiology of uncomplicated gastroschisis is relatively uniform; (2) major children's hospitals with several pediatric surgeons on staff provide institutional support for clinical investigation; (3) community equipoise around optimal treatment for gastroschisis is achieved; (4) there is a history of major patient benefit derived from pediatric surgical participation in prospective clinical trials, such as the treatment of Wilms tumor and other solid malignancies; and (5) there is a very real possibility that prospective clinical trials with a substantial cohort of patients will uncover negative/suboptimal treatment consequences and unintended morbidities.

Ultimately, any research trial should satisfy certain ethical requirements as proposed by Emanuel and colleagues.[33]

1. Social or scientific value
2. Scientific validity
3. Fair subject selection
4. Favorable risk–benefit ratio
5. Independent review
6. Informed consent
7. Respect for potential and enrolled subjects

Since infants represent a special vulnerable group, additional procedures have been recommended to improve protection of pediatric research participants.[34] These include data and safety monitoring committees, a robust parental consent process, and decision monitoring that could verify the *informed* nature of the parental consent (that there was no coercion or undue incentive for participation).

Although not relevant to our study case, a final issue concerns the need for special protections for research in developing countries, as an increasing amount of research is, in fact, multinational. Emanuel and colleagues[35] have proposed an eighth principle—collaborative partnership—to be added to the seven requirements listed here. This principle emphasizes the need to develop partnerships among researchers, makers of health policies and communities. It recognizes the importance of respecting the community's values, culture, traditions, and social practices. And perhaps most importantly, this principle seeks to ensure that the recruited participants and communities receive benefits from the conduct and results of the research.

SUMMARY

In this chapter we have endeavored to address three realistic situations that involve ethical choices for the pediatric surgeon. In the first, case we highlighted the importance of using the best-interests standard for neonatal decision making, while respecting the place of the infant within his or her parental and familial cultural milieu. For the second case, we discussed the ethical obligations of beneficence, autonomy, and justice that the pediatric surgeon should maintain during prenatal consultation. Finally, we offered an ethical rationale for pediatric surgeons to participate in clinical research as a way to benefit their future infant patients.

REFERENCES

1. Glover JJ, Caniano DA. Ethical issues in treating infants with very low birth weight. *Sem Pediatr Surg* 2000; 9: 56–62.
2. President's Commission for the Study of Ethical Problems in Medicine and Biomedical and Behavioral Research. Deciding to Forego Life-Sustaining Treatment, 1983, 197–229.
3. American Academy of Pediatrics Committee on Bioethics. Ethics and the care of critically ill infants and children. *Pediatr* 1996; 98: 149–52.
4. The Hastings Center Research Project on the care of imperiled newborns. *Hastings Center Report* 1987; 17: 5–32.
5. McCormick R. To save or let die: The dilemma of modern medicine. *JAMA* 1974; 29: 172–6.
6. Arras JD. Toward an ethic of ambiguity. *Hastings Center Report* 1984; 14: 25–33.
7. American Academy of Pediatrics Committee on Hospital Care, Institute for Family-Centered Care. Family-centered care and the pediatrician's role. *Pediatr* 2003; 12: 691–6.
8. Nelson JL. Taking families seriously. *Hastings Center Report* 1992; 22: 6–12.
9. Ruddick W. Questions parents should resist. In: Kopelman LM, Moskop JC (eds). *Children and Health Care: Moral and Social Issues*. Dordrecht: Kluwer Academic Publishers, 1989: 221–9.
10. Baylis F, Caniano DA. Medical ethics and the pediatric surgeon. In: Oldham KT, Colombani PM, Foglia RP (eds). *Surgery of Infants and Children*. Philadelphia: Lipincott-Raven, 1997: 281–388.
11. Buchanan A, Brock D. *Deciding for Others: The Ethics of Surrogate Decision Making*. Cambridge: Cambridge University Press, 1989: 83–135.
12. Wilkinson D, Savulescu J. Disability, discrimination and death: Is it justified to ration life saving treatment for disabled newborn infants? *Monash Bioethics Rev* 2014; 32: 43–62.
13. Helman CG. *Culture, Health and Illness*. London: Wright Publishing, 1990: 2–3.
14. Garcia J. African-American perspectives, cultural relativism, and normative issues: Some conceptual questions. In: Flack HE, Pellegrino ED (eds). *African-American Perspectives in Biomedical Ethics*. Washington, DC: Georgetown University Press, 1992: 11–66.
15. Pellegrino ED. Intersections of western bio-medical ethics. In: Pellegrino ED, Corsi PMP (eds). *Transcultural Dimensions in Medical Ethics*. Frederick, Maryland: University Publishing Group, 1992: 13–19.
16. Sherwin SL. *No Longer Patient: Feminist Ethics and Health Care*. Philadelphia: Temple University Press, 1992: 248–9.
17. Ruddick S. Maternal thinking. In: Trebilcot J (ed). *Mothering: Essays in Feminist Theory*. Totowa, New Jersey: Rowan & Allanheld, 1983: 213–30.
18. Beauchamp T. Response to Garcia. In: Flack HE, Pellegrino ED (eds). *African-American Perspectives in Biomedical Ethics*. Washington, DC: Georgetown University Press, 1992: 67–8.
19. Macklin R. Ethical relativism in a multicultural society. *Kennedy Instit of Ethics J* 1998; 8: 1–22.

20. Elliot C. Where ethics comes from and what to do about it. *Hastings Center Report* 1989; 22: 28–35.

21. American Academy of Pediatrics Committee on Bioethics. Guidelines on foregoing life-sustaining medical treatment. *Pediatr* 1994; 93: 532–6.

22. Nelson LJ, Rushton CH, Cranford RE, Nelson RM, Glover JJ, Truog RD. Forgoing medically provided nutrition and hydration in pediatric patients. *J Law Med Ethics* 1995; 23: 33–46.

23. American Academy of Pediatrics Clinical Report. Diekema DJ, Botkin J, Committee on Bioethics. Forgoing medically provided nutrition and hydration. *Pediatr* 2009: 124: 813–22.

24. Caniano DA, Baylis F. Ethical considerations in prenatal surgical consultation. *Pediatr Surg Int* 1999; 15: 303–9.

25. Sorenson JR. Genetic counseling: Values that have mattered. In: Bartels DM. Leroy BS, Caplan Al (eds). *Prescribing Our Future: Ethical Challenges in Genetic Counseling*. New York: De Gruyter, 1993: 3–14.

26. Chervenak FA, McCullough LB. Ethics of fetal surgery. *Clin Perinatol* 2009; 237–246.

27. Cassell E. *The Nature of Suffering and the Goals of Medicine*. New York: Oxford University Press, 1991: 249.

28. Brown SD, Feudtner C, Truog RD. Prenatal decision-making for myelomeningocele: Can we minimize bias and variability? *Pediatr* 2015; 136: 409–11.

29. Lusk LA, Brown EG, Overcash RT, Grogan TR, Keller RL, Kim JH, Poulian FR, Shew SB, Uy C, DeUgarte DA. Multi-institutional practice patterns and outcomes in uncomplicated gastroschisis: A report from the University of California Fetal consortium (UfC). *J Pediatr Surg* 2014; 49: 1782–6.

30. Freedman B. Equipoise and the ethics of clinical research. *N Engl J Med* 1987; 317: 141–5.

31. Bylaws of the American Pediatric Surgical Association. Principles of medical ethics. http://www.eapsa.org. Accessed February 2, 2016.

32. Nwomeh B, Caniano DA. Emerging ethical issues in pediatric surgery. *Pediatr Surg Int* 2011; 27: 555–62.

33. Emanuel EJ, Wendler D, Grady C. What makes clinical research ethical? *JAMA* 2000; 283: 2701–11.

34. Flotte TR, Frentzen B, Humphries MR, Rosenbloom AL. Recent developments in the protection of pediatric research subjects. *J Pediatr* 2006; 149: 285–6.

35. Emanuel EJ, Wendler D, Killen J, Grady C. What makes clinical research in developing countries ethical? The benchmarks of ethical research. *J Infect Dis* 2004; 189: 930–7.

24

Patient safety

IAIN YARDLEY

INTRODUCTION

During the 1990s, a growing realization emerged amongst the medical community that patients were being harmed during the course of their care. This came about through several highly influential studies[1,2] and reports.[3,4] The statistics presented were truly shocking: 1 in 10 patients experiences an adverse incident during a hospital stay[3]; deaths due to complications attributable to the provision of care are equivalent to an airliner crashing every week.[4] The potentially preventable ways in which patients come to harm are many and varied, from the most obvious and shocking, such as operating on the wrong body part or even the wrong patient[5] or accidentally giving an massive drug overdose[6] to less obvious and potentially overlooked events such as catheter-related infections and postoperative wound infections.[3,4]

What constitutes safe care is rather hard to define and can only really be categorized by the absence of dangerous care, as in the World Health Organization (WHO) definition: "the prevention of errors and adverse effects to patients associated with health care."[7] It is not possible to completely eliminate all occurrences that are included in the definition of an *adverse event*, for example, surgical site infections, but it is likely that their incidence can be reduced. Patient safety has therefore concentrated on minimizing and subsequently eliminating potentially avoidable harm.

Once it was acknowledged that healthcare was a hazardous undertaking, with significant risk of causing harm to those it was trying to help, the concept of *patient safety* grew, and the mainstream media, policy makers, and clinicians all took up the issue with a real sense of outrage and urgency. Efforts to reduce the risks encountered during patients' care were given the highest possible priority.[8] With little experience in healthcare of improving safety across a system, early workers in patient safety looked to other high-risk industries, most notably the aviation industry, with its enviable safety record for inspiration and advice

on how healthcare could follow their lead in making care safer. Several concepts and ideas have been introduced to the healthcare setting following their successful implementation in other arenas, such as the use of checklists[9] and reporting and learning systems.[10] Since the 1990s, patient safety has developed into a specialty of its own with huge resources invested into it, its own terminology (Table 24.1), and scientific journals dedicated to its study.

A very early realization for those working to improve patient safety was that the traditional model in healthcare—the person approach, where individuals carried responsibility for their actions and behavior, so if something went wrong, someone was to blame—was flawed. It was recognized that uncaring or careless individuals were not (in the vast majority of cases) the cause of safety incidents. These incidents occurred due to flaws in the systems in which healthcare workers operated and patients were cared for.[11] Rather than attempting to change individuals' behavior, changing and strengthening the systems that staff work in is much more likely to lead to improvements in safety.

SYSTEM THINKING

This *systems approach* has been the philosophy underlying the vast majority of patient safety work. Highly influential in this approach is Reason's[12] "Swiss cheese model." In this model, the multiple layers of defense that an organization has are represented by slices of Swiss cheese. For example, when prescribing a drug in the neonatal unit, the layers of defense that are intended to ensure the baby receives the correct dose of the correct medication are as follows: the initial writing of the prescription by the doctor; the pharmacist in the unit checking the prescription; the nurse responsible for administering the drug checking the prescription and drawing up the medication; and the nurse and his or her colleague administering the drug to the patient. However, these layers of defense are not perfect. Like Swiss cheese, they contain holes, or *latent errors* that can allow *active errors* to pass through the system and reach the patient,

Table 24.1 Glossary of terms used in patient safety

Patient safety term	Definition
Patient safety incident	Any situation that causes, or has the potential to cause, a patient to experience an adverse outcome.
Adverse outcome	Any situation where the final result of an episode of healthcare is suboptimal.
Adverse event	Any event that leads to an undesirable outcome associated with healthcare. An adverse event does not necessarily have to be associated with an error. For example, surgical site infections can occur despite all appropriate measures to prevent them being in place.
Error	An action that leads to an undesirable outcome. Theses can be acts of commission, e.g., prescribing the wrong dose of an antibiotic leading to renal damage, or of omission, e.g., not prescribing antibiotic prophylaxis appropriately and increasing the risk of surgical site infection.
Latent error	An attribute of a system that makes an adverse event more likely, for example inadequate staffing levels leading to staff members being overworked and fatigued and more likely to make mistakes. These could be described as "accidents waiting to happen."
Active error	An incorrect action that occurs at the interface between the healthcare system and the patient whose effect is usually rapidly evident. Active errors are almost always associated with one or more latent errors.
Critical incident	An incident (usually undesirable) that is particularly significant. Studying critical incidents can help prevent future adverse events. This is the principle behind reporting and learning systems.
Reporting and learning system	A system enabling the study of incidents to learn lessons from them and implement measures to reduce the likelihood of their recurrence.
Root cause analysis	An incident investigation technique that aims to discover the factors that underlie the occurrence of an incident rather than focus on the actions of individuals.
Near miss	A patient safety incident that had the potential to lead to harm but did not, either through good fortune or due to the fact that it was identified before affecting the patient. Studying near misses can be as informative as studying incidents that lead to harm.
Never events	A list of patient safety incidents that are serious and preventable if adequate safety systems are in place. Never events related to surgical care are operating on the wrong patient or body part, inserting the wrong surgical implant, and leaving an item in a body cavity following surgery.
Sentinel event	A patient safety incident that is particularly egregious or serious and implies that the organization in which the event occurred has significant systemic failures. Never events are generally considered to be sentinel events.
Swiss cheese model	A conceptual model for safety. The basis of the model is that any organization will have layers of defense against harm, and any one of these layers can prevent harm from reaching the patient. However, all of these layers are imperfect and contain holes, like a Swiss cheese. Only when these holes align can harm penetrate the system's defenses and reach the patient.
Human approach	A way of approaching patient safety incidents that concentrates on the actions of individuals and tries to eliminate future incidents by changing behavior through training, reminders, or reprimands.
Systems approach	A way of approaching patient safety incidents that acknowledges that individual workers are fallible and will make mistakes. Prevention of harm is more likely to come about by improving the systems people work in to prevent or detect these mistakes before they cause harm than by trying to create perfect workers who never make mistakes.
Human factors	The area of study that applies to how individual workers interact with their environment. This approach has been hugely influential in the study of patient safety.
Safety culture	An organizational attribute where the hazardous nature of the organization's activities is acknowledged and safety takes a high priority at all levels of the organization.

causing harm. In the example of the drug prescription, the doctor might be distracted by an emergency in the labor ward while writing the prescription (a latent error) and write up 10 times the intended dose of the drug (the active error). That day, the ward pharmacist is off sick, and no cover is available, so the prescription is not checked before it is time to administer the drug (another latent error). The nurse drawing up the medication usually has a calculator to assist in checking drug doses, but the battery has run out, so it cannot be used (the third latent error). As he knows and trusts the doctor who wrote the prescription, he or she draws up the drug as prescribed without repeating the calculations used to derive the dose (an active error). The second nurse that she gets to check the drug is her junior colleague and does not like to challenge her work (the final latent error) and so countersigns the prescription without checking the quantities herself (an active error), and a fatal overdose is delivered to the neonate. Any one of the layers of defense could have recognized the error and prevented it from reaching the patient. It was only when several latent and active errors coincided that the holes in the cheese lined up, allowing the patient to be harmed (Figure 24.1).

The application of system thinking to patient safety relies on the acknowledgement that active errors will inevitably occur, through either omission or commission. Attempts to eliminate these errors by changing the behavior of individuals, for example, through education or reminders, are likely to fail. Instead, a systems approach looks to increase the number of ways in which an error can be detected (increasing the number of layers of cheese) and make these defenses as robust as possible (making the holes in the cheese smaller). In the example given, if a person approach to error were taken, the response to the event occurring would be to reprimand or discipline the doctor who wrote

the prescription. However, the doctor did not write up a massive overdose because he did not know or had forgotten that this was incorrect. It was a mistake, so telling him not to do it again is unlikely to prevent a recurrence. A systems approach to prevent a similar error recognizes this and so would include many changes, including the following: employing extra doctors so that emergencies in the labor ward do not distract doctors working in the neonatal unit; developing cross-covering arrangements within the pharmacy department so that sick leave does not leave a clinical area uncovered; providing solar-powered calculators in all drug preparation areas; and developing team training for the nursing staff to flatten hierarchies and allow appropriate challenge even to senior colleagues when checking drugs.

There are many barriers to the implementation of system thinking based approaches to patient safety. Perhaps the most significant is the cultural change that is required for healthcare to move from its traditional stance of individual blame to a systems approach. Other impediments are that system-based approaches are more expensive in terms of time and resources both in the investigation required to determine the underlying causes of an incident and in the actions needed to reduce the risk of recurrence. In the example given, it would be far quicker, simpler, and cheaper to simply reprimand the doctor than implement the actions described.

SAFETY CONCERNS SPECIFIC TO SURGERY

Adverse events in surgery often appear starker, and consequently receive more attention, than other types of safety incident. This is due to a surgical procedure being a well-defined and discrete event, whereas other stages in a patient's care, such as establishing a correct diagnosis, occur at less

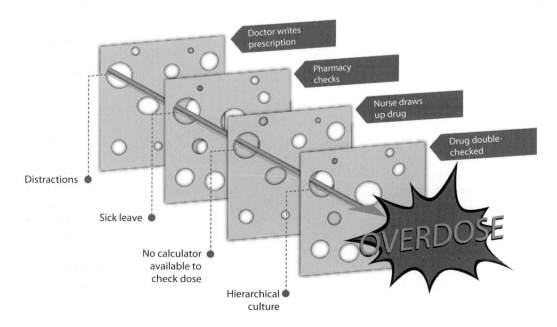

Figure 24.1 The "Swiss cheese model" of organizational defenses. (Adapted from Reason J., *Human Error*, Cambridge University Press, Cambridge, UK, 1990.)

distinct points in time. There are three surgery-specific incident types that have been termed *never events*. Never events are a group of safety events that are preventable using established safety procedures and so are considered inexcusable and should never happen. If they do happen, then it suggests there may be serious failings in the approach taken by the organization concerning patient safety.[13] The never events that relate specifically to surgical care are as follows: operating on the wrong patient or on the wrong body part, inserting the wrong implant, and leaving items inside the patient unintentionally following surgery.[14] Despite the term *never event*, these incidents still occur across healthcare settings and have shown little sign of decreasing in frequency.[15] Although it may seem hard to comprehend how such errors could occur with competent and conscientious medical staff on duty,[16] the systems in operation during surgical care are incredibly complex, and there are many opportunities for errors to occur, no matter how conscientious individual staff members are. For example, when performing a left inguinal herniotomy, the surgeon needs to make no fewer than eight mental steps after encountering the supine patient to fully transfer his or her understanding and concept of *left* to that of the patient's left groin and operate on the correct side.[17] An error in any one of these steps will potentially lead to operating on the incorrect side.

In addition to these clearly defined errors, there are many more subtle ways in which surgical patients can suffer harm during their care. These sources of harm can be preoperative, such as delays in diagnosis; intraoperative, such as allowing the patient's body temperature to drop below an acceptable limit; and during the postoperative period, such as developing surgical site infection. It is often impossible to identify one single cause of the adverse outcomes due to the complexity of the care provided and the multiplicity of factors affecting outcomes. No single distinct event, error, or omission will be responsible for an unexpected outcome, such as a surgical site infection. Rather, it is a combination of factors, including timely surgery, appropriate antibiotic prophylaxis, good temperature control intraoperatively, and so on, that is required to reduce the risk of infections.[18] Indeed, many adverse outcomes are not related to errors, of either omission or commission, and are unavoidable consequences of the patient's condition. Patient safety does not aim to eliminate adverse outcomes; rather, it aims to minimize them by eliminating those that are potentially preventable. For example, blood loss may be inevitable during surgery, so hemorrhage is not in itself necessarily due to an error. However, a failure to prepare for blood loss and not having adequate venous access for resuscitation or blood products for transfusion is a potentially preventable error.

Safety concerns specific to newborn surgery

The newborn surgical patient is susceptible to all of the same hazards as any other surgical patient, but in addition, these patients have unique attributes that increase their vulnerability to harm during their care.

SIZE

Newborn surgical patients are simply physically smaller than other surgical patients, sometimes extremely small.[19] This leads to increased risk from several sources. Firstly, decreasing the size of a body rapidly increases its surface area–to–volume ratio. In newborns, this means that they will lose heat far more rapidly than older patients and so are at risk of hypothermia and its attendant complications. Being small means newborns are more physically fragile than older patients and at risk of iatrogenic injury including fractures, particularly during transfer within or between healthcare facilities.[20] Physical fragility is also a source of risk when inserting tubes, as is common in the newborn surgical patient, for example, the danger of esophageal perforation with a nasogastric tube or bladder perforation with a urinary catheter.[21,22] Vascular access to deliver vital medications and fluids and to monitor the patient's condition is also more challenging in the newborn. Tiny, fragile veins make extravasation injuries a significant risk,[23] and the fine-bore catheters necessary for vascular access in the newborn make them more vulnerable to blockage and the need for replacement. A small circulating blood volume means that only minimal blood loss can lead to significant compromise of the neonatal circulation. Finally, when it comes to operating on newborns, their small size makes surgery more technically challenging and demanding, increasing the risk of complications such as wound breakdown and anastomotic leaks.[24]

ANATOMY

The anatomy of the newborn is not simply a smaller replica of the older child, as discussed elsewhere in this book. Several aspects of these anatomical differences create an increased risk when operating on the newborn. The liver and bladder are both relatively much larger than in older children, putting them in greater danger of iatrogenic injury during laparotomy or laparoscopy. The newborn liver also has a very tenuous capsule and friable parenchyma, which, coupled with an increased right heart pressure, makes liver injury and subsequent bleeding both more likely and harder to control than in the older child. As a baby completes the adjustment from the fetal to neonatal circulation, his or her cardiovascular system also presents specific risks to his or her surgical care. The foramen ovale and ductus arteriosus are commonly still patent, allowing shunting of blood from right to left, and hence, paradoxical emboli from the venous system can enter the arterial system and cause cerebral or other arterial infarcts. When combined with the patent umbilical vein, this can lead to major harm due to gas embolus during laparoscopy.[25]

IMMATURE ORGAN SYSTEMS

Many of a newborn's organ systems are still immature, especially for infants born prematurely; this makes their care more challenging and hazardous in several ways.[19] Perhaps most obviously, a premature baby's lung is not fully developed, necessitating ventilatory support. This will need careful management alongside the management of coexisting surgical conditions. In some specific newborn surgical conditions, notably diaphragmatic hernia, specific measures need to be undertaken to prevent iatrogenic damage to the immature or underdeveloped lung.[26] A newborn baby's skin is more permeable than the older child's, making bacterial translocation and subsequent sepsis more likely; transepidermal water loss is also increased, allowing both water and heat to escape.[27] Newborn surgical patients will therefore need careful attention paid to skin care perioperatively to reduce the risk of harm. The newborn kidney is also immature and less able to concentrate urine, making fluid balance potentially more challenging. During the newborn period, there is an exchange of hemoglobin from fetal to adult type; this creates bilirubin as a by-product that can overwhelm the neonatal liver, causing jaundice. The management of jaundice is a routine part of neonatal practice, but it is vital that it is not overlooked due to distractions from any concurrent surgical issues.[28] Glucose handling is commonly impaired in the neonate and requires careful monitoring and treatment to prevent serious complications.[29] In the newborn surgical patient, the stress of a surgical procedure and the prolonged fasting that is common during his or her perioperative course make careful glucose monitoring even more critical to prevent harm. The newborn brain is also relatively immature, especially following premature birth. This can create risks to the patient both directly and indirectly. Direct risk comes from the fragility of the blood vessels in the brain and bleeding leading to intraventricular or periventricular hemorrhage and the potential for the subsequent development of cerebral palsy.[30] Careful management of blood pressure and circulation is therefore vital in the newborn surgical patient, particularly intraoperatively. Indirect risk arises from a baby's inability to communicate with caregivers. Babies cannot tell the surgeon what symptoms they have, making accurate diagnosis and timely treatment more challenging. They are also unable to confirm what procedure they are due to undergo, potentially increasing the risk of wrong-site surgery.

ACUITY OF PROBLEMS

Many newborn surgical conditions require urgent or emergent operative intervention, for example, gastroschisis and perforated necrotizing enterocolitis (NEC). Even with antenatal diagnosis of a surgical condition, the timing of delivery is often unpredictable, and babies can be born at any time of the day or night. Similarly, babies with NEC can deteriorate at any time of the day or night, precipitating the need for surgical intervention. This acuity of newborn surgical conditions can lead to the need to operate outside normal working hours. This creates fatigue in healthcare workers, which is known to degrade both technical performance and decision making.[31] Staff can also become isolated when working out of hours when assistance may be harder to obtain during challenging or unexpected procedures.

COMORBIDITY

Although some newborn surgical patients will have an isolated condition that requires surgical correction, many will have other associated issues, especially those born prematurely. Some of these were mentioned previously, such as lung disease of prematurity, but there are others such as concomitant congential cardiac lesions found with the VACTERL (vertebral, anorectal, cardiac, tracheo-esophageal, renal and limb) association or other midline anomalies such as exomphalos. All need careful and coordinated multidisciplinary management and are not uncommonly the major determinants of outcome for newborn surgical patients.[32]

HEALTHCARE SYSTEM LIMITATIONS

The design of healthcare systems is often not optimized for the care of newborn infants with surgical issues. This is largely due to the relative rarity of these conditions, with systems appropriately focused on more common conditions. Newborn surgical expertise is concentrated in specialist centers, necessitating transfer from the place of birth in undiagnosed conditions. This need for transfer can create risks due to delays in care as well as the physical risks involved in interfacility transport.[20] Patient identification systems used in hospital usually include the patient's name. The requirement in hospital systems for a given name to be recorded means that it is not uncommon for newborn patients to be referred to as "Baby" until they are named by their parents. This creates the risk of misidentification and potentially wrong patient surgery.[33] The low volume of surgery carried out in newborns means the market for equipment designed for this type of surgery is limited, so manufacturers (with a few notable exceptions) have not produced tools specifically designed for small patients. This has led to the use of surgical equipment designed for adults in newborns, which can create the risk of harm.[34]

MEASURES TO IMPROVE SAFETY

As mentioned earlier, patient safety is now a specialty in its own right with an ever-growing evidence base. Unfortunately, very little work on patient safety has been done in pediatric surgery and even less in newborn surgery specifically. This leaves pediatric surgeons reliant on lessons learned in other surgical disciplines. There have been many studies published that investigate the nature of safety incidents in surgery but rather fewer that describe successful means to reduce their occurrence. Key safety interventions that have been developed for surgery include checklists, incident reporting, and training in nontechnical skills.

Checklists

Checklists have been used for many years by pilots to ensure that important steps are taken in preparation for key points during a flight, for example, immediately before and after takeoff or landing. The hope was that they would prove equally useful in ensuring that safety-critical steps were performed in healthcare.[35] The clearly defined event of performing surgery is an obvious moment at which a checklist could be deployed. Surgical checklists have taken several forms, the Joint Commission's Universal Protocol, introduced in 2003,[36] being one of the first to bring together standard safety steps into one document. In 2008, WHO's safe surgery checklist was launched as the centerpiece of the Safe Surgery Saves Lives project (Figure 24.2).[37] This project brought together international experts from the fields of surgery, anesthesia, and system safety to develop a means to improve the safety of surgical patients worldwide. Their work built on and expanded previous experience such as the Universal Protocol. The WHO surgical checklist is a 17-item checklist in three sections; before the induction of anesthesia, before commencing surgery, and before the patient leaves the operating room (Figure 24.2). A multicenter before-and-after trial of the use of the checklist in a variety of healthcare settings showed a dramatic reduction in surgical mortality and morbidity.[38] This reduction has been replicated in several studies of the checklist since the initial trial, including a randomized controlled trial.[39] A further expansion of the concept of checklists to cover the whole of a surgical patient's admission to the hospital has also been demonstrated to reduce surgical mortality and morbidity.[40] Away from surgery, another study demonstrated that by using a checklist when inserting central lines in a critical care unit catheter-related bloodstream infections could be almost eliminated.[41]

ADAPTING THE CHECKLIST FOR NEWBORN SURGERY

The WHO Guidelines for Safe Surgery that accompany the checklist encourage local adaption of the checklist to suit the circumstances (although not removing items, as they were all felt to be essential steps in performing safe surgery).[37] Useful adaptations when carrying out newborn surgery might include the following: ensuring adequate warming measures are in place as neonates are highly vulnerable to heat loss during surgery; creating the opportunity to review any relevant comorbidities, such as congenital cardiac lesions, that might affect surgery; checking that appropriate blood and blood products are available should they be needed rapidly during surgery; and ensuring that all intravenous lines are purged and flushed before leaving theatre to prevent later accidental administration of anesthetic agents.

The success of surgical checklists in early studies initially raised the hope that this would be a simple, quick, and cheap solution to many patient safety problems. However, replication of the results of these studies outside of clinical trials has been patchy, with limited uptake of the checklist[42] and improvements in outcome not necessarily related to the use of the checklist.[43] It appears from further study of both the WHO checklist and the central line checklist that complex social and cultural factors at play around the

implementation of the checklists were at least as important as the checklist itself in improving safety.[44,45] It is common for staff members, particularly surgeons,[42,46] to resist the use of the checklist in their daily practice. Successfully embedding checklist use in a department's routine requires a significant cultural change and takes time, even years to achieve.[47] Central mandates on checklist use from politicians or policy makers are unlikely to lead to effective use of the checklist.[48,49] Longer-term approaches are needed that take a more holistic view of the checklist and the environment that it is used in. Checklist implementation programs that involve the whole operating team in training have been shown to be more successful at achieving checklist use and reducing mortality.[50]

Reporting and learning

Another concept imported from the aviation industry to the healthcare arena is the idea that if patient safety incidents that do occur are identified and examined, then valuable lessons can be learned that may help reduce the risk of similar incidents happening again.[3,51] The intention of such *reporting and learning* systems is neatly described in Donaldson's "orange wire" analogy.[52] Here, the example was used that if a particular airplane were found to have a fault caused by a particular wire, then all planes of this type could be prevented from flying until the wire in question was replaced. The idea that this could be replicated in healthcare such that no incident became recurrent is highly attractive.

The potential benefits of a mechanism that could identify and prevent safety incidents from becoming recurrent led to the setting up of many systems for reporting of safety incidents around the world. One of the most notable is the National Reporting and Learning System in the British National Health Service (NHS), launched in 2004.[53] Over time this system has collected millions of reports of safety incidents and issued many reports, advisory notices, and alerts.[54] Unfortunately there is little sign that these have had any impact on patient safety, with reports of very similar incidents being received repeatedly.[55] The reasons for this lack of impact are multiple but include the volume of reports exceeding the resources available for investigation and analysis, the complex nature of the incidents and the number of factors that influence each one, and an absence in healthcare of the whole-system cultural change that went along with reporting and learning in the aviation arena.[56] Most safety incidents in healthcare are not amenable to a simple technical solution such as changing a wire. Rather, they require complex system-level interventions to reduce their likelihood of recurrence that are difficult to generalize from individual reports.

Despite these limitations, reporting and learning systems do play an important part in efforts to improve patient safety. Their availability to staff raises awareness of patient safety as an issue, and levels of reporting have been found to correlate with a positive safety culture within an organization.[57]

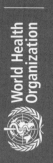

Surgical Safety Checklist

World Health Organization | **Patient Safety**
A World Alliance for Safer Health Care

Before induction of anaesthesia

(with at least nurse and anaesthetist)

Has the patient confirmed his/her identity, site, procedure, and consent?
☐ Yes

Is the site marked?
☐ Yes
☐ Not applicable

Is the anaesthesia machine and medication check complete?
☐ Yes

Is the pulse oximeter on the patient and functioning?
☐ Yes

Does the patient have a:

Known allergy?
☐ No
☐ Yes

Difficult airway or aspiration risk?
☐ No
☐ Yes, and equipment/assistance available

Risk of >500 ml blood loss (7 ml/kg in children)?
☐ No
☐ Yes, and two IVs/central access and fluids planned

Before skin incision

(with nurse, anaesthetist and surgeon)

Confirm all team members have introduced themselves by name and role.

Confirm the patient's name, procedure, and where the incision will be made.

Has antibiotic prophylaxis been given within the last 60 minutes?
☐ Yes
☐ Not applicable

Anticipated Critical Events

To Surgeon:
☐ What are the critical or non-routine steps?
☐ How long will the case take?
☐ What is the anticipated blood loss?

To Anaesthetist:
☐ Are there any patient-specific concerns?

To Nursing Team:
☐ Has sterility (including indicator results) been confirmed?
☐ Are there equipment issues or any concerns?

Is essential imaging displayed?
☐ Yes
☐ Not applicable

Before patient leaves operating room

(with nurse, anaesthetist and surgeon)

Nurse Verbally Confirms:
☐ The name of the procedure
☐ Completion of instrument, sponge and needle counts
☐ Specimen labelling (read specimen labels aloud, including patient name)
☐ Whether there are any equipment problems to be addressed

To Surgeon, Anaesthetist and Nurse:
☐ What are the key concerns for recovery and management of this patient?

This checklist is not intended to be comprehensive. Additions and modifications to fit local practice are encouraged.   Revised 1 / 2009

© WHO, 2009

Figure 24.2 The WHO safe surgery checklist. (Reprinted with permission from World Health Organization Patient Safety, *WHO Guidelines for Safe Surgery 2009: Safe Surgery Saves Lives*, Geneva: WHO Press, 2009, 98, available at http://apps.who.int/iris/bitstream/10665/44185/1/9789241598552_eng.pdf, accessed 8th March 2016.)

Improvements in the way in which reports are collected, investigated, and acted upon may lead to reporting and learning becoming a powerful tool in improving safety in healthcare.[56]

Nontechnical skills

Traditional surgical training has focused on the technical aspects of surgical practice. Surgical trainees are required to demonstrate that they have had exposure to sufficient numbers of cases relevant to their practice, especially important in a discipline such as newborn surgery that deals largely with a collection of rare conditions. They are expected to demonstrate their competency in specific procedural skills such as tissue dissection and bowel anastomosis. The mandatory examinations that they undertake test their knowledge of pathology, anatomy, and physiology and the application of this knowledge to clinical scenarios.

While all these are undeniably vital attributes for successful surgical practice, there is a growing recognition that safe surgical practice also requires the surgeon to have crucial cognitive and interpersonal skills.[58] These are known as *nontechnical* skills and can be grouped into four categories: situational awareness, decision making, communication and teamwork, and leadership.[59,60]

SITUATIONAL AWARENESS

Situational awareness relates to an individual's ability to gather and understand the information that is available to him or her and to use this awareness to predict a future state. In surgical practice, there are a huge number of sources of information, starting with clinical history taking and examination and progressing through investigation to a diagnosis and potentially surgical intervention. Intraoperatively, there are still many items of information being relayed to the surgeon that require processing. These include operative findings such as the condition of the intestine or the degree of blood loss and information from the anesthetic team on the patient's cardiorespiratory status. It is a vital skill for a surgeon to be able to remain focused on the task in hand while receiving and processing new information that may require a change to the initial plan.

DECISION MAKING

Good situational awareness allows, in turn, for sound decision making. Decision making requires the surgeon to use his or her situational awareness to consider the options available, select the most appropriate one, and then implement the chosen plan. Decision making in surgery is necessarily an ongoing process as new and changing information is made available. A combination of situational awareness and decision-making skills allows a surgeon to implement the correct management as a case develops. For example, when operating on a neonate, a choice may need to be made between attempting an intestinal anastomosis and forming a stoma, or between attempting primary closure of a gastroschisis and fashioning a silo. A safe surgeon will have the situational awareness skills to consider the operative findings, the current condition of the patient, and his or her own abilities in order to deploy his or her decision-making skills and take the correct path.

COMMUNICATION AND TEAMWORK

At all stages in the care of a newborn surgical patient, a key nontechnical skill is excellent communication. The surgeon must communicate with many different parties including the following; the patient's family, medical colleagues also caring for the patient, anesthetic colleagues, theatre staff, and surgical colleagues. Breakdown in communication is a common factor in many safety incidents, particularly those occurring intra-operatively,[61,62] and good communication is a skill that can be learned. There are several communication models that can be deployed to improve information exchange and ensure a shared understanding within the team.[63,64] Also vital to effective communication is ensuring that all team members can speak up when they have concerns.[65] This requires the surgeon to flatten traditional hierarchies and make himself or herself available to receive critical information, regardless of the source. The requirement of the WHO safe surgery checklist for all team members to introduce themselves by name and role is a simple way to promote open communication within the operating theatre.

LEADERSHIP

The final category of nontechnical skill, leadership, overarches situational awareness, decision making, and communication. An effective surgeon is, by necessity, the leader of a team caring for a patient, retaining the moral responsibility for the overall care of the patient. This calls for skill in setting and maintaining standards, supporting others in meeting these standards, and coping in an exemplary way as an individual, even under pressure.

SUMMARY AND CONCLUSIONS

Unfortunately, despite the vast amount of work done in the field of patient safety and our greater understanding of the nature of safety incidents, it is difficult to demonstrate a reduction in safety-related harm across healthcare provision as a whole.[66] There are just a few interventions that have robust evidence for improving safety in surgical practice.[67] These include the use of checklists and care pathways, as already described, particularly where this is linked to team training processes. Reporting surgical outcome data to a central audit is also associated with a reduction in adverse events, as is subspecializing within a surgical discipline, which is associated with fewer technical complications.

Every surgeon practicing newborn surgery has the responsibility to protect the safety of his or her patients. In order to do so, he or she should do the following:

- Ensure that surgery only takes place in an environment with the infrastructure required for this highly specialized work, including essential equipment, personnel, and other support services
- Engage proactively with measures to improve patient safety, including reporting and learning systems and safety checklists
- Take part in centralized data collection processes
- Undertake training in nontechnical skills that will complement their technical abilities
- Encourage and maintain open communication throughout the teams they work in
- Be honest and open about their own abilities and only practice within their limitations

REFERENCES

1. Brennan AT, Leape LL, Laird NM, Hebert L, Localio AR, Lawthers AG, Newhouse JP, Weiler PC, Hiatt HH. Incidence of adverse events and negligence in hospitalized patients—Results of the Harvard Medical Practice Study I. *N Engl J Med* 1991; 324: 370–6.
2. Leape LL, Brennan AT, Laird N, Lawthers AG, Localio AR, Barnes BA, Hebert L, Newhouse JP, Weiler PC, Hiatt H. The nature of adverse events in hospitalized patients—Results of the Harvard Medical Practice Study II. *N Engl J Med* 1991; 324: 377–84.
3. Department of Health. *An Organisation with a Memory: Report of an Expert Group on Learning from Adverse Events in the NHS Chaired by the Chief Medical Officer.* The Stationary Office, UK, 2000.
4. Institute of Medicine. *To Err Is Human: Building a Safer Health System.* USA: National Academy of Sciences, 1999.
5. Kwaan MR, Studdert DM, Zinner MJ, Gawande AA. Incidence, patterns and prevention of wrong site surgery. *Arch Surg* 2006; 141: 353–8.
6. Kaushal R, Bates DW, Landrigan C, McKenna KJ, Clapp MD, Federico F, Goldmann DA. Medication errors and adverse drug events in pediatric inpatients. *JAMA.* 2001; 285: 2114–20.
7. World Health Organization. *Patient Safety.* Available at http://www.euro.who.int/en/health-topics/Health-systems/patient-safety. Accessed March 8, 2016.
8. Fifty Fifth World Health Assembly. *WHA55.18 Quality of care: Patient Safety.* WHO, 2002. Available at http://apps.who.int/gb/archive/pdf_files/WHA55/ewha5518.pdf. Accessed March 8, 2016.
9. Borchard A, Schwappach DLB, Barbir A, Bezzola P. A systematic review of the effectiveness, compliance, and critical factors for implementation of safety checklists in surgery. *Ann Surg* 2012; 256: 925–33.
10. Shaw R, Drever F, Hughes H, Osborn S, Williams S. Adverse events and near miss reporting in the NHS. *Qual Saf Health Care* 2005; 14: 279–83.
11. Reason J. Human error: Models and management. *BMJ* 2000; 320: 768–70.
12. Reason J. *Human Error.* Cambridge University Press, Cambridge, UK, 1990.
13. Lembitz A, Clarke TJ. Clarifying "never events" and introducing "always events". *Patient Saf Surg* 2009; 3: 26.
14. Care Quality Commission. *Never Events.* Available at http://www.cqc.org.uk/content/never-events. Accessed March 8, 2016.
15. Mehtsun WT, Ibrahim AM, Diener-West M, Pronovost PJ, Makary MA. Surgical never events in the United States. *Surgery* 2013; 152: 465–72.
16. Dyer C. Doctors go on trial for manslaughter after removing wrong kidney. *BMJ* 2002; 324: 1476.
17. Seiden SC, Barach P. Wrong-side/wrong-site, wrong-procedure, and wrong-patient adverse events: Are they preventable? *Arch Surg* 2006; 141:931–9.
18. Wick EC, Hobson DB, Bennett JL, Demski R, Maragakis L, Gearhart SL, Efron J, Berenholtz SM, Makary MA. Implementation of a surgical comprehensive unit-based safety program to reduce surgical site infections. *J Am Coll Surg* 2012; 215: 193–200.
19. Committee on Understanding Premature Birth and Assuring Healthy Outcomes; Behrman RE, Butler AS (eds). *Preterm Birth: Causes, Consequences, and Prevention.* USA: National Academies Press, 2007. Available at http://www.ncbi.nlm.nih.gov/books/NBK11385/. Accessed March 8, 2016.
20. Madar RJ, Milligan DWA. Neonatal transport: Safety and security. *Arch Dis Child Fetal Neonatal Ed* 1994; 71: F147–8.
21. Gander JW, Berdon WE, Cowles RA. Iatrogenic esophageal perforation in children. *Pediatr Surg Int* 2009; 25: 395–401.
22. Basha M, Mersal MSA, Saedi SA, Williamson Balfe J. Urinary bladder perforation in a premature infant with Down syndrome. *Pediatr Nephrol* 2003; 18: 1189–90.
23. Wilkins CE, Emmerson AJB. Extravasation injuries on regional neonatal units. *Arch Dis Child Fetal Neonatal Ed* 2004; 89: F2745.
24. Chittmittrapap S, Spitz L, Kiely EM, Brereton RJ. Anastomotic leakage following surgery for esophageal atresia. *J Pediatr Surg* 1992; 27: 29–32.
25. Kudsi OY, Jones SA, Brenn BR. Carbon dioxide embolism in a 3-week-old neonate during laparoscopic pyloromyotomy: A case report. *J Pediatr Surg* 2009; 44: 842–5.
26. Logan JW, Cotten CM, Goldberg RN, Clark RH. Mechanical ventilation strategies in the management of congenital diaphragmatic hernia. *Semin Pediatr Surg* 2007; 16: 115–25.
27. Shwayder T, Akland T. Neonatal skin barrier: Structure, function, and disorders. *Dermatol Ther* 2005; 18: 87–103.

28. Bates D, Larizgoitia I, Prasopa-Plaizier N, Jha AK. Global priorities for patient safety research. *BMJ* 2009; 338: b1775.

29. Sweet CB, Grayson S, Polak M. Management strategies for neonatal hypoglycemia. *J Pediatr Pharmacol Ther* 2013; 18: 199–208.

30. Linder N, Haskin O, Levit O, Klinger G, Prince T, Naor N, Turner P, Karmazyn B, Sirota L. Risk factors for intraventricular hemorrhage in very low birth weight premature infants: A retrospective case-control study. *Pediatrics* 2003; 111: e590–5.

31. Hull L, Arora S, Aggarwal R, Darzi A, Vincent C, Sevdalis N. The impact of nontechnical skills on technical performance in surgery: A systematic review. *J Am Coll Surg* 2012; 214: 214–30.

32. Samangaya RA, Murphy F, McGlory S, Zaidi T, Gillham J, Morabito A. Outcomes of antenatally diagnosed exomphalos. *Arch Dis Child Fetal Neonatal Ed* 2011; 96: Fa73.

33. Racine A, Southern W, Rai A, Berger M, Reissman S, Parakkattu V, Chacko B, Adelman J, Aschner J, Schechter C, Angert R, Weiss J. Use of temporary names for newborns and associated risks. *Pediatrics* 2015; 136: 327–33.

34. Taylor SP, Sato TT, Balcom AH, Groth T, Hoffman GM. Gas analysis using Raman spectroscopy demonstrates the presence of intraperitoneal air (nitrogen and oxygen) in a cohort of children undergoing pediatric laparoscopic surgery. *Anesth Analg* 2015; 120: 349–54.

35. Kao LS, Thomas EJ. Navigating towards improved surgical safety using aviation-based strategies. *J Surg Res* 2008; 145: 327–35.

36. JCAHO's universal protocol released to widespread endorsement. *Jt Comm Perspect* 2004; 24: 1–4.

37. World Health Organisation Patient Safety. *WHO Guidelines for Safe Surgery 2009: Safe Surgery Saves Lives.* Geneva: WHO Press, 2009: 98. Available at http://apps.who.int/iris/bitstr eam/10665/44185/1/9789241598552_eng.pdf. Accessed March 8, 2016.

38. Haynes AB, Weiser TG, Berry WR, Lipsitz SR, Breizat A-HS, Dellinger EP, Herbosa T, Joseph S, Kibatala PL, Lapitan MCM, Merry AF,Moorthy K, Reznick RK, Taylor B, Gawande AA. A surgical safety checklist to reduce morbidity and mortality in a global population. *N Engl J Med* 2009; 360: 491–9.

39. Haugen AS, Søfteland E, Almeland SK, Sevdalis N, Vonen B, Eide G, Nortvedt MW Harthug S. Effect of the World Health Organization checklist on patient outcomes: A stepped wedge cluster randomized controlled trial. *Ann Surg* 2014; 261: 821–8.

40. de Vries EN, Prins HA, Crolla RMPH, den Outer AJ, van Andel G, Helden SH, Schlack WS, van Putten MA, Gouma DJ, Dijkgraaf MGW, Smorenburg SM, Boermeeste MA. Effect of a comprehensive surgical safety system on patient outcomes. *N Engl J Med* 2010; 363: 1928–37.

41. Pronovost P, Needham D, Berenholtz S, David Sinopoli D, Cosgrove S, Sexton B, Hyzy R, Welsh R, Roth G, Bander J, Kepros J, Goeschel C. An intervention to decrease catheter-related bloodstream infections in the ICU. *N Eng J Med* 2006; 355: 2725–32.

42. Pickering SP, Robertson ER, Griffin D, Hadi M, Morgan LJ, Catchpole KC, New S, Collins G, McCulloch P. Compliance and use of the World Health Organization checklist in UK operating theatres. *Br J Surg* 2013; 100: 1664–70.

43. Yuan CT, Walsh D, Tomarken JL, Alpern R, Shakpeh J, Bradley EH. Incorporating the World Health Organization Surgical Safety checklist into practice at two hospitals in Liberia. *Jt Comm J Qual Pt Saf* 2012; 38: 254–60.

44. Bosk CL, Dixon-Woods M, Goeschel CA, Pronovost PJ. Reality check for checklists. *Lancet* 2009; 374: 444–5.

45. Russ SJ, Sevdalis N, Moorthy K, Mayer EK, Rout S, Caris J, Mansell J, Davies R, Vincent C, Darzi A. A qualitative evaluation of the barriers and facilitators toward implementation of the WHO surgical safety checklist across hospitals in England: Lessons from the "Surgical Checklist Implementation Project". *Ann Surg* 2015; 261: 81–91.

46. Conley DM, Singer SJ, Edmondson L, Berry WR, Gawande AA. Effective surgery checklist implementation. *J Am Coll Surg* 2011; 212: 873–9.

47. Leitch J. The Healthcare Quality Strategy for the NHS in Scotland. Paper presented at the International Society for Quality in Healthcare 30th International Conference, Edinburgh, October 2013.

48. Urbach DR, Govindarajan A, Saskin R, Wilton AS, Baxter NN. Introduction of surgical safety checklists in Ontario, Canada. *N Engl J Med* 2014; 370: 1029–38.

49. van Klei WA, Hoff RG, van Aarnhem EE, Simmermacher RK, Regli LP, Kappen TH, van Wolfswinkel L, Kalkman CJ, Buhre WF, Peelen LM. Effects of the introduction of the WHO Surgical Safety Checklist on in-hospital mortality: A cohort study. *Ann Surg* 2012; 255: 44–9.

50. Neily J, Mills PD, Young-Xu Y, Carney BT, West P, Berger DH, Mazzia LM, Paull DE, Bagian JP. Association between implementation of a medical team training program and surgical mortality. *JAMA* 2010; 304: 1693–700.

51. Barach P, Small SD. Reporting and preventing medical mishaps: Lessons from non-medical near miss reporting systems. *BMJ* 2000; 320: 759–63.

52. Donaldson L. When will health care pass the orange-wire test? *Lancet* 2004; 364: 1567–8.

53. Katikireddi V. National reporting system for medical errors is launched. *BMJ* 2004; 328: 481.

54. Panesar SS, Cleary K, Sheikh A. Reflections on the National Patient Safety Agency's database of medical errors. *J R Soc Med* 2009; 102: 256–8.

55. Yardley IE, Donaldson LJ. Patient safety matters: Reducing the risks of nasogastric tubes. *Clin Med* 2010; 10: 228–30.

56. Macrae C. The problem with reporting and learning. *BMJ Qual Saf* 2016; 25: 71–5.

57. Snijders C, Kollen BJ, van Lingen RA, Fetter WPF, Molendijk H. Which aspects of safety culture predict incident reporting behavior in neonatal intensive care units? A multilevel analysis. *Crit Care Med* 2009; 37: 61–7.

58. Yule S, Flin R, Paterson-Brown S, Maran N. Nontechnical skills for surgeons: A review of the literature. *Surgery* 2006; 139: 140–9.

59. Yule S, Flin R, Maran N, Rowley D, Youngson G, Duncan J, Paterson-Brown S. Development and evaluation of the NOTSS behaviour rating system for intraoperative surgery (2003–2008). In: Flin R, Mitchell L (eds). *Safer Surgery*. CRC Press, Abdingdon, UK, 2009: 7–26.

60. Youngson G. Nontechnical skills in pediatric surgery: Factors influencing operative performance. *J Ped Surg* 2016; 51: 226–30.

61. Greenberg CL, Regenbogen SE, Studdart DM, Lipsitz SR, Rogers SO, Zinner MJ, Gawande AA. Patterns of communication breakdowns resulting in injury to surgical patients. *J Am Coll Surg* 2007; 204: 533–40.

62. Lingard L, Espin S, Whyte S, Regehr G, Baker GR, Reznick R, Bohnen J, Orser B, Doran D, Grober E. Communication failures in the operating room: An observational classification of recurrent types and effects. *Qual Saf Health Care* 2004; 13: 330–4.

63. Haig KM, Sutton S, Whittington J. SBAR: A shared mental model for improving communication between clinicians. *Jt Comm J Qual Pat Saf* 2006; 32: 167–75.

64. Amato-Vealey EJ, Barba MP, Vealey RJ. Hand-off communication: A requisite for perioperative patient safety. *AORN J* 2008; 88: 763–74.

65. Edmondson A. Speaking up in the operating room: How team leaders promote learning in interdisciplinary action teams. *J Manag Stud* 2003; 40: 1419–52.

66. Wachter RM. Patient safety at ten: Unmistakable progress, troubling gaps. *Health Affairs* 2010; 29: 165–73.

67. Howell A-M, Panesar SS, Burns EM, Donaldson LJ, Darzi A. Reducing the burden of surgical harm: A systematic review of the interventions used to reduce adverse events in surgery. *Ann Surg* 2014; 259: 630–41.

25

Minimally invasive neonatal surgery

RICHARD KEIJZER, OLIVER J. MUENSTERER, AND KEITH E. GEORGESON

INTRODUCTION

Gynecologists published the first reports on minimally invasive surgery in adults around 50 years ago. By then, it was mainly used for diagnostic procedures, because of the limitations in visualization and instrumentation. The introduction of chip cameras in the late 1980s enabled the surgeon and assistant to watch a screen and perform surgery at the same time, instead of holding a telescope and looking through a lens close to the patient. The development of better endosurgical instruments enabled surgeons to perform a variety of laparoscopic procedures including appendectomies, cholecystectomies, fundoplications, and more advanced operations. However, due to the lack of instruments, endoscopes, and trocars of appropriate size, the acceptance of minimally invasive surgery in the pediatric population in general, let alone in neonates, took longer than in adults. Recently, the development of smaller, shorter, and more durable instruments along with improved optical equipment has allowed pediatric surgeons to perform more complex endosurgical procedures in young children and newborns.[1]

This chapter reviews the current practice of minimally invasive neonatal surgery and reflects on potential future developments in this field.

THORACOSCOPY

The first experience with thoracoscopic procedures in children was published 30 years ago.[2] Biopsies of pulmonary lesions, both primary and metastatic in origin, are the most frequently performed thoracoscopic surgical procedure in children (reviewed in Karpelowsky[3]). With the advancement of experience and again, better equipment, more sophisticated procedures such as pulmonary resections and the repair of esophageal atresia (EA) with or without tracheoesophageal fistula (TEF) have been embraced by the pediatric surgical community. Compared to open thoracotomy, the potential advantages of a thoracoscopic approach are the muscle-sparing nature of the procedure, decreased the risk of nerve injury, and less secondary scoliosis in the long-term.[3]

Physiology and anesthetic considerations

The introduction of automatic carbon dioxide (CO_2) insufflation in the early 1960s created the necessary working domain to facilitate endoscopic surgical procedures. In most thoracoscopic cases, gentle insufflation of CO_2 to a maximum pressure of 4–5 mm Hg using a low flow of 1 L/min compresses the lung enough to allow access to most structures in the chest. Single-lung ventilation, which is more easily established and used in adult thoracoscopy, is rarely necessary in young children and neonates. In neonates, methods for single-lung ventilation are very limited. In those cases where single-lung ventilation is desired, a small Fogarty catheter has been placed into the ipsilateral main stem bronchus and gently inflated, blocking gas exchange to that lung.[4] Excellent communication between the surgeon and anesthesiologist is mandatory, as the establishment of an artificial capnothorax may change physiologic parameters. If anticipated, a higher end-tidal CO_2 can be overcome by increasing the ventilatory rate, and decreased venous return can be counteracted by appropriate volume replacement.[5] Although described in adults, the development of CO_2 embolism is exceedingly rare in the pediatric population.

Diagnostic thoracoscopy and biopsy or resection of pulmonary lesions

Improvement in the resolution of diagnostic imaging techniques, such as computerized tomography (CT) scanning and magnetic resonance imaging (MRI), along with the capability to produce multiplanar reconstructions in any three-dimensional plane, has made thoracoscopy almost obsolete for the mere assessment of intrathoracic anatomy. However, the good visualization and excellent access to nearly all intrathoracic lesions have resulted in the replacement of most open lung biopsies by the thoracoscopic technique. In fact, thoracoscopic lung biopsy and the resection of pulmonary lesions are the most commonly performed thoracoscopic operations in neonates. In many cases, small pulmonary lesions are readily identified and isolated from the rest of the lung using a Roeder loop (Endoloop, Ethicon San Angelo, Texas, USA). After placing the suture tightly around the base of the lesion, the tissue is excised sharply peripheral to the loop and retrieved through one of the trocar sites. In larger children, a stapler can be used to transect the lung central to the lesion. Larger pulmonary lesions, such as congenital cystadenomatoid malformations and congenital lobar emphysema, should be resected by respecting the lobar or segmental anatomy. Most of the time, this entails identifying the proprietary vessels and bronchus to the affected part of the lung, and using a vessel-sealing device such as the endoscopic Ligasure (Covidien, Dublin, Ireland) or Enseal (Ethicon, Cincinnati, Ohio, USA) to divide the vessels.[6] The bronchus can be stapled, sutured, or clipped. We prefer to leave a chest tube in place through one of the trocar sites for 24 hours after the procedure, but this is dependent on the surgeon's preference.

Mediastinum

The thoracoscopic approach to mediastinal masses such as esophageal duplication cysts, bronchogenic cysts, and extralobar sequestrations is very useful for several reasons. Visualization of adjacent anatomical structures is usually excellent due to the magnification of the video image (Figure 25.1). Furthermore, the anatomy of the mediastinum is usually well defined, and some lesions tend to be well vascularized.

During esophageal duplication cyst resection, opening of the esophagus is common, since the cyst and the esophagus often share a common wall. Therefore, the esophageal defect should be closed or reinforced using interrupted absorbable sutures. A dilator or endoscope can be placed inside the esophagus to decrease the risk of esophageal injury.

Closure of patent ductus arteriosus and aortopexy

The first reports on the thoracoscopic closure of patent ductus arteriosus (PDA) originate from the early 1990s.[7] Improvements in technique and instruments have made it possible to safely perform closure of a PDA thoracoscopically in neonates with a birth weight as low as 1500 grams. However, potential complications with the thoracoscopic approach and the safety and excellent outcome of open PDA ligation have prevented both the thoracoscopic and interventional approaches from being universally accepted.

Tracheomalacia, an intrinsic weakness of the tracheal wall causing the airways to collapse during expiration, is usually a benign, self-limiting condition that improves as the infant matures. In some cases, especially when associated with other intrathoracic lesions such as EA, the gas exchange is compromised, and the tracheomalacia should be treated with an aortopexy. It is important to rule out a vascular cause for the patient's stridor (such as a vascular ring or sling) by esophagram or angiography. Once all other causes are excluded, a thoracoscopic aortopexy can be performed using a triangular position of the camera and instruments in the anterior midline and anterior axillary line; the surgeon generally uses three interrupted sutures to pexy the aorta to the sternum.[8]

Esophageal atresia

Thoracoscopic repair of TEF and EA is considered one of the most technically challenging minimally invasive procedures in pediatric surgery due to the limited domain inside the neonatal thorax and the technical difficulty of making a good and trustworthy anastomosis between the proximal pouch and the distal fistula. Consequently, complications observed following thoracoscopic repair are often related to the anastomosis, such as anastomotic leakage and stricture.[9] Advocates of the thoracoscopic approach acclaim the excellent visualization of the anatomy and warn against the long-term disadvantages of repair using a thoracotomy, such as asymmetry of the chest wall, scoliosis, or a winged scapula as the consequence of nerve injury.[10] A recent randomized controlled clinical study comparing open versus thoracoscopic repair of TEF/EA expressed concerns about the effects of thoracoscopy on blood gases during the repair and recommended further evaluation.[11]

For EA and fistula repair, echocardiography is used to determine whether there is a right- or left-sided aorta. The esophagus is approached from the contralateral side. The patient is positioned in a lateral decubitus position, slightly prone, to allow gravitational retraction of the lungs away from the posterior mediastinum. Three triangulated trocars are used, with an additional access site if needed for retraction. In most cases, the azygos vein is divided, and the pleura is opened over the fistula. The fistula is suture-ligated or clipped, both ends of the esophagus are mobilized just enough to facilitate the anastomosis, and the anastomosis is performed (Figure 25.1a–d).

Congenital diaphragmatic hernia

In contrast to TEF repair, minimally invasive repair of congenital diaphragmatic hernia (most frequently Bochdalek hernias) has gained more popularity among pediatric surgeons during the past few years. Whereas the first reports of both laparoscopic and thoracoscopic repairs were mainly anecdotal and described the procedure in older infants and children, the indication for thoracoscopic repair has shifted to symptomatic congenital diaphragmatic hernias in newborns.[12] Even repair of the diaphragmatic defect using a patch has been well described with good results.[13] Most

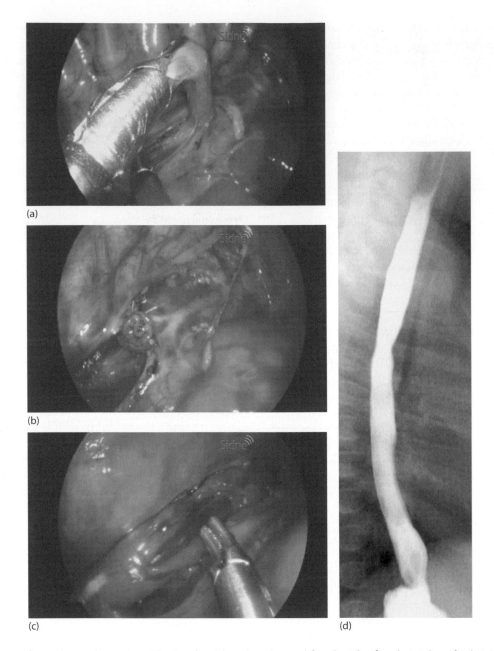

Figure 25.1 Repair of esophageal atresia with distal tracheoesophageal fistula. The fistula is identified, **(a)** dissected, ligated, **(b)** and divided. **(c)** Subsequently, the anastomosis is performed over an orogastric tube. **(d)** Postoperative results are generally excellent and comparable to those of the open technique.

likely, the positive outcomes in the latest studies reflect the completion of learning curves by those pediatric surgeons who perform the procedure frequently. The same randomized controlled trial expressing concerns about the thoracoscopic repair of TEF/EA recommended against the use of thoracoscopy with CO_2 insufflation for the repair of CDH as a result of the associated prolonged and severe hypercapnia and acidosis.[11] Due to the associated persistent pulmonary hypertension and pulmonary hypoplasia, many logical outcome measures to test the superiority of the open versus minimally invasive technique, such as ventilation days or length of stay, will be mainly influenced by the degree of any associated conditions.

The thoracoscopic approach is generally preferred over a purely laparoscopic repair of a congenital diaphragmatic hernia. In some cases, we have used simultaneous thoracoscopic and laparoscopic cameras to aid with the anatomic reduction of the viscera, and to rule out injury to the intraabdominal organs during suturing. The patient is positioned in a contralateral decubitus position, and an axillary triangulated trocar configuration is used. The most lateral suture often has the most tension, and a transcostal suture placed through a small stab incision through the lower chest is helpful in facilitating a complete and secure closure of the diaphragmatic defect. Figure 25.2 illustrates a standard diaphragmatic hernia repair.

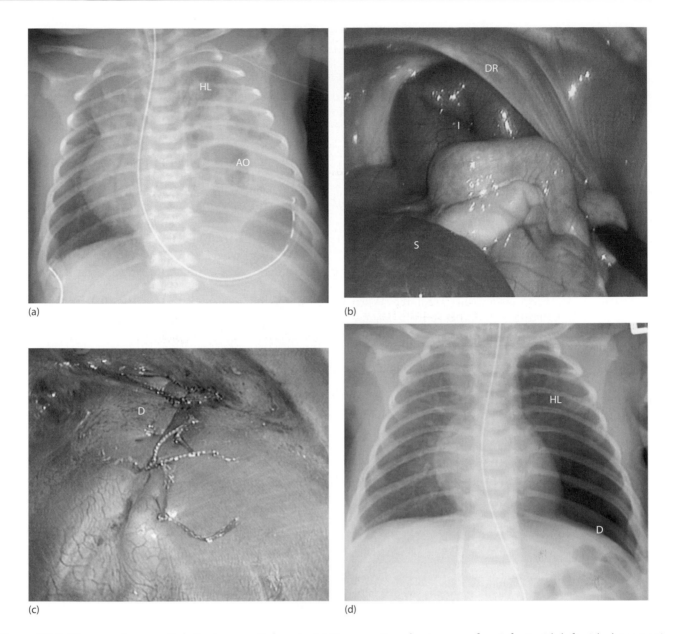

Figure 25.2 Closure of congenital diaphragmatic hernia: **(a)** Preoperative chest x-ray of an infant with left-sided congenital diaphragmatic hernia. **(b)** Thoracoscopic intraoperative view looking down on the abdominal organs (intestines and spleen) that herniated through the diaphragmatic defect into the thorax. **(c)** Diaphragmatic defect has been closed using interrupted sutures. **(d)** Postoperative chest x-ray. Note the hypoplastic lung in the top of the thorax and the reconstructed dome of the diaphragm. Abbreviations: AO, abdominal organs; D, diaphragm; DR, diaphragmatic rim; HL, hypoplastic lung; I, intestines; S, spleen.

LAPAROSCOPY

Physiology of pneumoperitoneum

While CO_2 insufflation into the thorax may be associated with considerable changes in the physiology, CO_2 insufflation to establish a capnoperitoneum is often very well tolerated by most neonatal patients. Still, the pressures and flows should be kept at the minimum necessary to guarantee adequate working space and visualization. In neonates, we use pressures of 6–8 mm Hg and flows between 1 and 2 L/min. Insufflated CO_2 is absorbed more readily into the bloodstream of infants, mainly due to smaller diffusion barriers and an increased peritoneal absorptive surface area in comparison to body weight. Hypercapnia and respiratory acidosis may result but can usually be overcome by increasing minute ventilation during the laparoscopic procedure.[5]

Potential adverse effects of increased intra-abdominal pressure include compression of the inferior caval vein resulting in a decrease in the venous return, as well as the upward displacement of the paralyzed diaphragm. This can result in pulmonary atelectasis that may only become clinically relevant after the resumption of spontaneous breathing. Some of these patients may require prolonged positive-pressure ventilation to recruit the collapsed pulmonary alveoli.

Abdominal access

There is no evidence that either the Veress needle technique or the Hasson techniques are safest for initial access to the abdomen in children. As long as one adheres to the fundamental principles of safe insertion, damage to intra-abdominal contents, including the large vessels, is rare. As in adults, abdominal access for laparoscopic procedures in newborns is usually obtained through the umbilicus. The umbilicus might be a potential source of infection after the umbilical cord has recently separated. Therefore, some surgeons prefer an incision above or below the umbilicus instead. Following the installation of local anesthetic, and after vertically incising the skin in the umbilical scar, we prefer to enter the abdomen using the naturally occurring small umbilical hernia defect to place a 5 mm radially expanding trocar. Reusable trocars can subsequently be inserted safely under direct vision where required. When placing the trocars, the surgeon should keep the triangulation principle in mind: left-hand instrument, camera, and right-hand instrument should form a triangle with the target organ in one axis with the surgeon and the camera.

Dislodgement of the trocars can be a major problem and nuisance during laparoscopic surgery in neonates and small children.[14] To prevent this, we place radially expanding 5 mm trocars through small incisions that hold them in place. Nonexpanding trocars are secured to the skin with a silk stitch in place using a red rubber cuff around the shaft of the trocar. The trocar can be moved in and out relative to the cuff using a mosquito clamp when required during the operation.

Pyloromyotomy

Laparoscopic pyloromyotomy is one of the few laparoscopic procedures that have recently been demonstrated in a large multicenter randomized clinical trial to be superior to the open classical approach. The conclusion of this hallmark study by Hall et al. was that both open and laparoscopic pyloromyotomy are safe, but that time to achieve full enteral feeding was better in the laparoscopic group. Therefore, the authors recommend laparoscopic pyloromyotomy in centers with sufficient laparoscopic experience. Interestingly, this trial was stopped by the data monitoring and ethics committee because of significant treatment benefit in the laparoscopy group at the interim analysis. Another prospective randomized trial concluded that the laparoscopic approach does not affect the length of recovery or complication rate.[15] However, the laparoscopic operation was associated with less pain and fewer episodes of emesis. Also, the authors mentioned the cosmetic benefit of the laparoscopic approach, when compared with a right upper quadrant incision.

Although the laparoscopic approach is associated with a considerable learning curve[16] that may have resulted in more incomplete pyloromyotomies in the first published patient series, recent randomized controlled clinical trials have failed to show a difference in this regard. In summary, the advantages of laparoscopic versus open pyloromyotomy appear to be less postoperative discomfort, a faster recovery, shorter length of stay, and better cosmesis.[17] Recently, a single-incision laparoscopic approach has been described.[18]

Gastrostomy

Gastrostomy placement to provide total or supplemental nutrition is a common procedure in infants and children. In many centers, gastroenterologists (sometimes in close collaboration with the pediatric surgeons) perform most of these feeding tube placements using the percutaneous endoscopic gastrostomy tube. The procedure combines flexible esophageal gastroduodenoscopy with percutaneous puncture of the stomach to place a gastrostomy tube that can later be replaced by a gastrostomy button device. However, the percutaneous endoscopic technique has significant drawbacks and a relatively high complication rate, including bowel perforation.[19] Therefore, we prefer the laparoscopic, single-incision technique for gastrostomy tube placement that has been developed in our center.[20] This procedure allows visualization of the stomach and abdominal wall during the entire process, avoiding injury of adjacent viscera. It also permits primary placement of a gastrostomy button device, which is preferred by the caregivers.

Fundoplication

The laparoscopic Nissen fundoplication quickly gained popularity for treatment of symptomatic gastroesophageal reflux disease (GERD). Good intraoperative visibility of the hiatus, excellent postoperative cosmesis, less pain, and reduced length of stay, as well as good efficacy combined with a low morbidity and mortality, have made this operation the standard of care. A recent randomized controlled trial demonstrated that laparoscopic fundoplication was associated with a higher recurrence rate of GERD.[21] In our practice, indications for a laparoscopic Nissen fundoplication are a failure of medical therapy for GERD and inability to tolerate gastric bolus feeds, either via the orogastric route or through an existing gastrostomy. The laparoscopic technique for gastrostomy placement described previously assures that it is in a good location on the anterior aspect of the stomach, close to the greater curvature, and about two-thirds down from the fundus to the antrum. In such cases, a later laparoscopic fundoplication is easily achieved if necessary. We perform a 360-degree wrap around the lower esophagus and the gastroesophageal junction with minimal dissection of the hiatus, as this has been shown to decrease failure rate.

Inguinal hernia

Inguinal hernia repair is one of the most common operations performed in newborns. The laparoscopic repair of an inguinal hernia involves the percutaneous or transabdominal suturing of the peritoneum of the internal inguinal ring. Randomized controlled trials have demonstrated that laparoscopic bilateral hernia repair is faster than open, whereas unilateral repair showed no difference.[22] Recurrence rates between open and laparoscopic repair do not differ. At this point, no strong recommendation based on the available literature can be made, and the results of prospective comparative studies are awaited.

Endorectal pull-through

Following a biopsy-proven diagnosis of Hirschsprung disease, a primary one-stage laparoscopic endorectal pull-through in the neonatal period is currently considered the standard of care by most pediatric surgeons.[23] A systematic review and meta-analysis did not show a difference between a laparoscopic and transanal endorectal pull-through for rates of enterocolitis, incontinence, or constipation.[24] Naturally, significant comorbidities or severe enterocolitis should be absent in this circumstance. The procedure is performed using three to four small abdominal ports, either in a triangular configuration or through the same skin incision in the umbilicus for a single-incision approach.[25] The transition zone is estimated by its morphology, and laparoscopic seromuscular biopsies are obtained. In patients with a rectosigmoid colon transition zone, the intraabdominal portion of the aganglionic bowel is devascularized using hook electrocautery. In patients with longer segments of an aganglionic colon, a pedicle preserving the marginal artery is fashioned as far proximal as necessary to bring the colon pedicle down without tension to form the neorectum. The rectal mobilization is performed transanally using an endorectal sleeve technique. The anastomosis is performed transanally 0.5 cm above the dentate line. Successful methods for performing laparoscopy-assisted Duhamel and Swenson pull-through procedures have also been reported in neonates. The laparoscopic-assisted endorectal pull-through has several advantages over a purely perineal approach. For one, the transition zone is histologically proven before the diseased bowel is resected. Furthermore, mobilization of the colon helps preserve a normal anorectal angle, which is essential for later continence.

Using similar principles, a minimally invasive technique for the correction of intermediate and high anorectal malformations (ARMs) has been developed in our institution: the laparoscopically assisted anorectoplasty (LAARP). Taking maximal advantage of the excellent visualization of the pelvic musculature from the inside using the laparoscope, the distal colon and fistula are dissected and divided. An expanding trocar is then placed through the muscle complex after identification using the electric nerve stimulator. Placement of the trocar is further aided by transillumination of the endoscope's light.[26] In comparative studies, functionality and continence for both the perineal and laparoscopic operation are comparable.[27]

Malrotation

Incomplete rotation or malrotation of the intestines results in a malposition and nonfixation of the duodenum and terminal ileum, and this situation predisposes the patient to midgut volvulus. Principles of the laparoscopic approach are similar to the open approach and include counterclockwise derotation of the intestines in case of a volvulus and release of the Ladd bands starting distal to the pylorus and continuing distally until the mesenteric stalk is widened; and the whole duodenum, as well as the jejunum, is located on the right side, and the cecum is allowed to fall over to the left side of the abdomen. This operation is usually performed with an incidental appendectomy as described by Ladd. One of the larger series comparing outcomes between treatment with laparotomy versus laparoscopy concluded that laparotomy was associated with a high rate of small bowel obstruction, more complications, and longer length of hospital stay, without an increased risk of recurrent volvulus.[28]

Duodenal atresia

Smaller laparoscopic surgical instruments have enabled pediatric surgeons to perform more sophisticated laparoscopic procedures such as duodenal atresia repair. The first reports of successful laparoscopic duodenal atresia repair were published at the beginning of this century. Using intracorporeal suturing, a diamond-shaped anastomosis is performed similarly to the open approach to open duodenal atresia repair. We prefer to use a running suture for the back wall and interrupted sutures in the front. Only a few small case series have been published so far, and a number of complications have been described. Therefore, this procedure should be reserved for very experienced pediatric endosurgeons, and a low threshold for conversion, in our view, is warranted.

Biliary pathology

Large series of laparoscopic choledochal cyst excision have been published in the literature with excellent results comparable to the open approach. The surgical principles are equivalent to those of the open procedure. Retraction of the gallbladder using a transabdominal suture in the upper right quadrant aids with the dissection. After resection of the cyst, a Roux-en-Y loop of bowel is created either intracorporeally or by exteriorizing the proximal small intestine through the umbilical incision. The anastomosis between the Roux loop and the proximal common bile duct is performed using an intracorporeal suturing technique (Figure 25.3a–d).

Although laparoscopic and robot-assisted Kasai procedures have been performed and reported, a higher failure rate has been reported compared to the open operation.[25] The reason for these findings is still unclear. In a sentinel vote at the 2007 IPEG (International Pediatric Endosurgery Group) meeting in Buenos Aires, the attending endoscopic

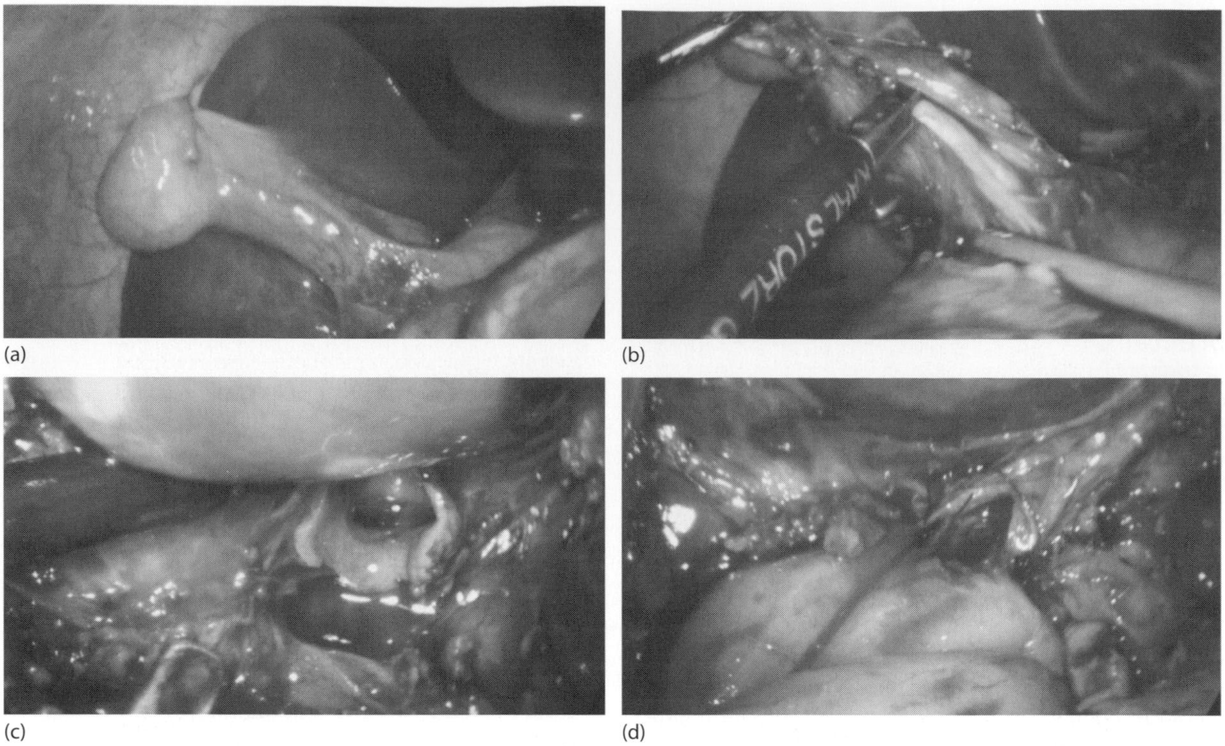

Figure 25.3 Resection of Type 1 choledochal cyst: **(a)** The gallbladder is restricted by a transabdominal suture, exposing the common bile duct below. **(b)** The common bile duct is transected proximally, and then **(c)** the cyst itself is resected. **(d)** After creation of a Roux-en-Y limb, an enterobiliary anastomosis is performed.

pediatric surgeons agreed to perform minimally invasive Kasai operations only in well-controlled study protocols until more information is available. A recent meta-analysis confirmed this recommendation.[29]

Pelvic pathology

With the improvement of prenatal ultrasound screening, pediatric surgeons see more neonates with enlarged ovarian cysts these days. Cysts with a complicated or complex ultrasound pattern and those over 4 cm in diameter that do not resolve spontaneously after several weeks of life warrant surgical exploration.[30] This is preferably done using laparoscopy. Serum alpha-fetoprotein (AFP) and beta-human chorionic gonadotropin (beta-HCG) levels should be checked preoperatively, and sound oncologic principles should be applied during surgery. Benign simple cysts may be drained by needle aspiration to facilitate removal through a trocar site. All other lesions can be removed using an endoscopic retrieval bag through the umbilicus or a separate, Pfannenstiel-type suprapubic incision.

Another pelvic pathology that can benefit from a laparoscopically assisted intrapelvic or intra-abdominal dissection is the resection of a sacrococcygeal teratoma.[31,32] More than 50% of the tumors have such an intracorporeal portion of the tumor, and dissection can be facilitated by the magnified view of the laparoscope. Control of the presacral veins can be achieved by laparoscopy, and the intra-abdominal portion of the tumor can be mobilized off surrounding structures.[33] Again, strict observance of oncologic principles is mandatory.

Future directions

In a period of only less than 25 years, minimally invasive surgery has become a major part of the practice of many pediatric surgeons. Many open procedures have been replaced or supplemented by comparable or even better minimally invasive procedures. It is hard to imagine that new developments in the field with even more minimally invasive procedures such as natural orifice transluminal endoscopic surgery (NOTES) or single-incision pediatric endosurgery (SIPES) are going to bring the same revolutionary advancement to general pediatric surgery that laparoscopic and thoracoscopic surgery have. Although the first large series of NOTES procedures (cholecystectomies through the vagina) in adults have been published recently, NOTES is still suffering from the technological difficulty of the perfect closure of the access organ that is used as the natural orifice.

In contrast, SIPES is slowly gaining more popularity, and series on several operations such as appendectomies, cholecystectomies, splenectomies, and pyloromyotomies have been published (reviewed in Bax and van der Zee,[33] Kozlov et al.[34] and Zhang et al.[35]). Introducing the camera and work instruments through the umbilicus, occasionally supplemented by a 2 mm percutaneous grasper in another location, we have been able to safely perform over 300 such procedures, including appendectomies, Nissen fundoplications, cholecystectomies, splenectomies, pyloromyotomies, and endorectal pull-throughs for Hirschsprung disease (Figure 25.4).[36] However, our experience demonstrates that the procedures are more technically demanding because of the loss of triangulation, instrument clashing, and limited visualization. Randomized clinical trials testing SIPES versus laparoscopic surgery regarding complications, postoperative recovery, length of stay, and postoperative pain should be awaited before this technically more demanding technique can be recommended universally.

CONCLUSION

Minimally invasive neonatal surgery has become an established tool in the palette of the modern pediatric surgeon. Although the number of controlled clinical trials testing

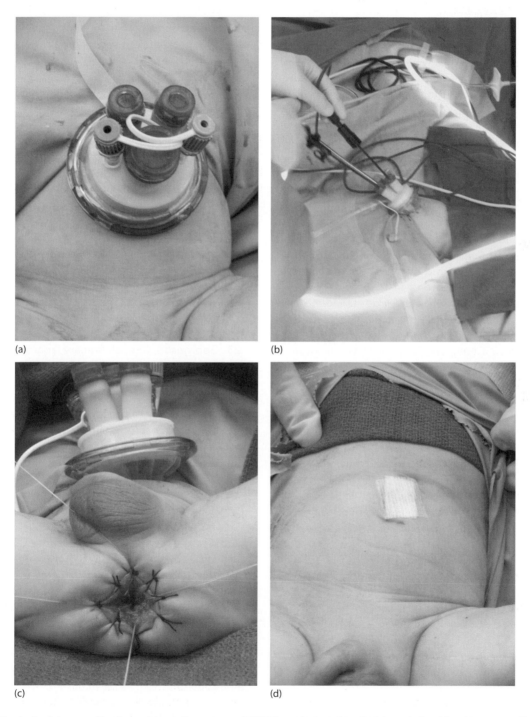

Figure 25.4 Single-incision pediatric endoscopic surgery (SIPES) endorectal pull-through for Hirschsprung disease. **(a)** Single incision port introduced through the umbilicus. **(b)** Intra-abdominal phase of operation via the umbilical port. **(c)** Perianal phase of operation while umbilical port is still in situ. **(d)** Umbilical incision leaves hardly any scar after surgery.

this relatively new approach is small, more and more publications are showing a benefit of the minimally invasive approach with regard to postoperative recovery, pain, and cosmesis. Whereas costs of minimally invasive surgery have always been a concern, the equipment has become cheaper over the past few years. In fact, when costs are considered on a macroeconomical scale, shorter length of stay after a minimally invasive procedure may level or offset the balance in favor of minimally invasive surgery. Eventually, it is likely that most surgical conditions in neonates will be corrected using these techniques.

REFERENCES

1. Blinman T, Ponsky T. Pediatric minimally invasive surgery: Laparoscopy and thoracoscopy in infants and children. *Pediatrics* 2012; 130: 539–49.
2. Rodgers BM, Moazam F, Talbert JL. Thoracoscopy in children. *Ann Surg* 1979; 189: 176–80.
3. Karpelowsky J. Paediatric thoracoscopic surgery. *Paediatr Respir Rev* 2012; 13: 244–51.
4. Rothenberg SS. Thoracoscopic repair of tracheo-esophageal fistula in newborns. *J Pediatr Surg* 2002; 37: 869–72.
5. Means LJ, Green MC, Bilal R. Anesthesia for minimally invasive surgery. *Semin Pediatr Surg* 2004; 13: 181–7.
6. Rothenberg SS et al. Two decades of experience with thoracoscopic lobectomy in infants and children: Standardizing techniques for advanced thoracoscopic surgery. *J Laparoendosc Adv Surg Tech A* 2015; 25: 423–8.
7. Rothenberg SS, Chang JH, Toews WH, Washington RL. Thoracoscopic closure of patent ductus arteriosus: A less traumatic and more cost-effective technique. *J Pediatr Surg* 1995; 30: 1057–60.
8. van der Zee DC, Straver M. Thoracoscopic aortopexy for tracheomalacia. *World J Surg* 2015; 39: 158–64.
9. Holcomb GW 3rd et al. Thoracsocopic repair of esophageal atresia and tracheoesophageal fistula: A multi-institutional analysis. *Ann Surg* 2005; 242: 422–8.
10. Dingemann C, Ure BM. Minimally invasive repair of esophageal atresia: An update. *Eur J Pediatr Surg* 2013; 23: 198–203.
11. Bishay M et al. Hypercapnia and acidosis during open and thoracoscopic repair of congenital diaphragmatic hernia and esophageal atresia: Results of a pilot randomized controlled trial. *Ann Surg* 2013; 258: 895–900.
12. Lansdale N, Alam S, Losty PD, Jesudason EC. Neonatal endosurgical congenital diaphragmatic hernia repair: A systematic review and meta-analysis. *Ann Surg* 2010; 252: 20–6.
13. Keijzer R et al. Thoracoscopic repair in congenital diaphragmatic hernia: Patching is safe and reduces the recurrence rate. *J Pediatr Surg* 2010; 45: 953–7.
14. Bax NM, van der Zee DC. Trocar fixation during endoscopic surgery in infants and children. *Surg Endosc* 1998; 12: 181–2.
15. St Peter SD et al. Open versus laparoscopic pyloromyotomy for pyloric stenosis: A prospective, randomized trial. *Ann Surg* 2006; 244: 363–70.
16. Handu AT et al. Laparoscopic pyloromyotomy: Lessons learnt in our first 101 cases. *J Indian Assoc Pediatr Surg* 2014; 19: 213–7.
17. Oomen MWN, Hoekstra LT, Bakx R, Ubbink DT, Heij HA. Open versus laparoscopic pyloromyotomy for hypertrophic pyloric stenosis: A systematic review and meta-analysis focusing on major complications. *Surg Endosc* 2012; 26: 2104–10.
18. Muensterer OJ et al. Single-incision laparoscopic pyloromyotomy: Initial experience. *Surg Endosc* 2010; 24: 1589–93.
19. Baker L, Beres AL, Baird R. A systematic review and meta-analysis of gastrostomy insertion techniques in children. *J Pediatr Surg* 2015; 50: 718–25.
20. Collins JB, Georgeson KE, Vicente Y, Hardin WD. Comparison of open and laparoscopic gastrostomy and fundoplication in 120 patients. *J Pediatr Surg* 1995; 30: 1065–70.
21. Fyhn TJ et al. Randomized controlled trial of laparoscopic and open nissen fundoplication in children. *Ann Surg* 2015; 261: 1061–7.
22. Esposito C et al. Laparoscopic versus open inguinal hernia repair in pediatric patients: A systematic review. *J Laparoendosc Adv Surg Tech A* 2014; 24: 811–8.
23. Georgeson KE et al. Primary laparoscopic-assisted endorectal colon pull-through for Hirschsprung's disease: A new gold standard. *Ann Surg* 1999; 229: 678–82.
24. Thomson D et al. Laparoscopic assistance for primary transanal pull-through in Hirschsprung's disease: A systematic review and meta-analysis. *BMJ Open* 2015; 5: e006063.
25. Muensterer OJ, Chong A, Hansen EN, Georgeson KE. Single-incision laparoscopic endorectal pull-through (SILEP) for hirschsprung disease. *J Gastrointest Surg* 2010; 14: 1950–4.
26. Georgeson KE, Inge TH, Albanese CT. Laparoscopic assisted anorectal pull-through for high imperforate anus—A new technique. *J Pediatr Surg* 2000; 35: 927–30.
27. Yang J et al. Comparison of clinical outcomes and anorectal manometry in patients with congenital anorectal malformations treated with posterior sagittal anorectoplasty and laparoscopically assisted anorectal pull through. *J Pediatr Surg* 2009; 44: 2380–3.
28. Ooms N, Matthyssens LEM, Draaisma JMt, de Blaauw I, Wijnen MHWA. Laparoscopic treatment of intestinal malrotation in children. *Eur J Pediatr Surg* 2016; 26: 376–81, doi:10.1055/s-0035-1554914.

29. Lishuang M et al. Laparoscopic portoenterostomy versus open portoenterostomy for the treatment of biliary atresia: A systematic review and meta-analysis of comparative studies. *Pediatr Surg Int* 2015; 31: 261–9.

30. Hermans AJ et al. Diagnosis and treatment of adnexal masses in children and adolescents. *Obstet Gynecol* 2015; 125: 611–5.

31. NMABax, van der Zee DC. The laparoscopic approach to sacrococcygeal teratomas. *Surg Endosc* 2004; 18: 128–30.

32. Lee KH et al. Laparoscopic-assisted excision of sacrococcygeal teratoma in children. *J Laparoendosc Adv Surg Tech A* 2008; 18: 296–301.

33. Bax KN, van der Zee DC. Laparoscopic ligation of the median sacral artery before excision of type I sacrococcygeal teratomas. *J Pediatr Surg* 2005; 40: 885.

34. Kozlov Y et al. Single-incision pediatric endosurgery in newborns and infants. *World J Clin Pediatr* 2015; 4: 55–65.

35. Zhang Z et al. Systematic review and meta-analysis of single-incision versus conventional laparoscopic appendectomy in children. *J Pediatr Surg* 2015; 50: 1600–9.

36. Hansen EN, Muensterer OJ, Georgeson KE, Harmon CM. Single-incision pediatric endosurgery: Lessons learned from our first 224 laparoendoscopic single-site procedures in children. *Pediatr Surg Int* 2011; 27: 643–8.

26

Fetal surgery

HANMIN LEE AND BENJAMIN PADILLA

INTRODUCTION

Birth defects have long captivated the human imagination. As Samuel Taylor Coleridge wrote, "The history of man for the nine months preceding his birth would be far more interesting and have events of far greater moment than all three-score and ten years that follow." Over the last 40 years, fetal diagnosis through imaging and fetal sampling has improved tremendously, allowing for earlier and more accurate diagnosis of birth defects. Surgeons are increasingly called upon for management of these anomalies before birth. In this chapter, we present general principles of fetal surgery, methods of fetal access, diseases that are amenable to fetal intervention, and a brief discussion of the future of fetal surgery.

GENERAL PRINCIPLES

Fetal intervention places both the fetus and the mother at risk. The mother gains nothing in terms of health benefits and is placed at risk of potential morbidity and mortality. The mother is an innocent bystander in the calculation of risk, with the possible benefit garnered by her unborn child. Our greatest responsibility is protecting the mother. In this light, fetal surgery is only considered for life-threatening or severely debilitating anomalies where fetal surgery shows promise of improving outcomes after thorough investigation in animal models.

A multidisciplinary approach is crucial to the success of any fetal treatment program. The team consists of perinatologists, anesthesiologists, radiologists, cardiologists, neonatologists, neurologists, geneticists, and pediatric surgeons working in concert. At the University of California, San Francisco (UCSF), all fetal referrals are discussed at a weekly meeting where imaging studies are reviewed and a consensus is reached regarding further diagnostic workup and treatment. Furthermore, the social and ethical aspects of each case are carefully weighed. A special institutional fetal treatment oversight committee reviews all fetal interventions, serving as both a quality control mechanism and ethical review body.

Since the first open fetal surgery at UCSF in 1982,[1] there have been no maternal mortalities following a fetal operation at UCSF.[2] Despite many technical advances, disruption of the membranes and preterm labor continue to be the Achilles heel of fetal surgery, resulting in premature delivery between 25 and 35 weeks gestation.[3] Multiport fetoscopic surgery has not significantly mitigated the risk of preterm labor, as membrane separation at the port sites is common.[2] Pulmonary edema associated with administration of tocolytics is the most common immediate maternal complication. Bleeding originating from the fetus, placenta, uterine wall, or maternal abdominal wall that requires transfusion is a serious although infrequent problem. Other complications include chorioamnionitis, pulmonary embolism, and deep venous thrombosis.[4] Importantly, fetal surgery does not adversely affect fertility or the ability to carry future pregnancies.[5] However, delivery of pregnancies after open fetal surgery requires cesarean section due to the risk of uterine rupture during labor.

FETAL DIAGNOSIS

Fetal ultrasound is the cornerstone of prenatal diagnosis and is a fundamental component of any fetal intervention. Routine anatomic surveys are generally conducted in the middle of the second trimester between 18 and 20 weeks gestation. Real-time fetal ultrasound identifies anatomic anomalies and provides physiologic information such as fetal heart rate, placental blood flow, and presence or absence of hydrops fetalis. Magnetic resonance imaging is increasingly used when high-resolution fetal imaging of the brain, spine, and body is needed. As many syndromes are associated with congenital heart defects, fetal echocardiography is an important diagnostic modality as well. The presence of a congenital heart defect precludes most fetal interventions (Figure 26.1).

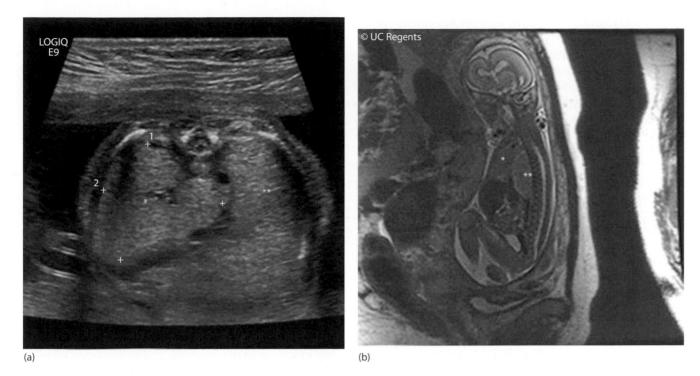

(a) (b)

Figure 26.1 Prenatally diagnosed congenital pulmonary airway malformation (CPAM). **(a)** Fetal ultrasound. **(b)** Fetal MRI. *CPAM; **normal lung.

Amniocentesis is the most widely used and accepted modality for karyotyping and DNA-based diagnosis of many genetic defects and inherited diseases. Although amniocentesis is safe, it cannot be used until the second trimester. Chorionic villus sampling can be performed between 10 and 13 weeks gestation, yet has a greater risk of pregnancy loss.[6] A number of noninvasive prenatal screening tests were developed to avoid the risk of pregnancy loss. A major breakthrough in noninvasive prenatal diagnosis came when cell-free DNA could be isolated from maternal blood and analyzed using polymerase chain reaction (PCR) technology for specific chromosomal sequences.[7] This technique allows for detection of paternally inherited and de novo genetic disorders as well as trisomy 21, 18, and 13, and fetal gender. Increasingly, microarrays are being used to gain further genetic information about fetuses.

FETAL ACCESS

There are three general methods of accessing the fetus: (1) percutaneous access, (2) minimally invasive fetoscopy, and (3) open hysterotomy. All three approaches require preoperative and intraoperative ultrasonography to define the anatomy, determine the position of the fetus, delineate the location of the placenta, and monitor the fetal heart rate and umbilical artery blood flow during the operation. In percutaneous and fetoscopic operations, ultrasound is of particular importance due to the lack of direct exposure of the fetus and uterus.

Maternal positioning is usually supine, with the left side down to minimize compression of the inferior vena cava.

Depending on the nature of the intervention, maternal anesthesia can be local, spinal, epidural, or general. Fetal anesthesia in the form of an intramuscular injection of an opiate and nondepolarizing muscle relaxant is given when operating directly on the fetus.[8,9]

Ultrasound-guided, percutaneous procedures are performed via small skin incision in the maternal skin. These require real-time ultrasound, as the only visualization of the fetal and maternal anatomy is via ultrasound images. Through this type of access, cystic structures, ascites, the bladder, or pleural fluid can be aspirated or drained into the amniotic space with the placement of a shunt. In addition, a radiofrequency ablation (RFA) probe can be deployed into the amniotic space for the treatment of various complications of twin gestation. The needles used to access the fetus are approximately 1.5–2 mm in diameter, resulting in minimal maternal morbidity.[10,11] Fetal cardiac valvuloplastes are also performed with ultrasound and echo guidance.[12]

Fetoscopic procedures are generally performed via a 3–4 mm port that accommodates a 3 mm fetoscope with a 1 mm working channel. Ultrasonography is essential for identifying a uterine "window" that is devoid of placenta in order to reduce the risk of maternal bleeding, placental abruption, and fetal morbidity. When using only the fetoscope, we usually make a 3 mm skin incision on the mother's abdomen to access the uterus rather than making a maternal laparotomy. Occasionally, the amniotic fluid is not clear enough to allow for a good image via a small endoscope. In these cases, the view is improved by performing amnioexchange with warmed crystalloid solution.[13]

Open fetal surgery requires general anesthesia and preoperative indomethacin and high-dose inhalational agents to maintain uterine relaxation.[8,9] The uterus is exposed through a low transverse abdominal incision. Ultrasonography is used to map out the placenta. A posteriorly positioned placenta allows for an anterior hysterotomy. An anteriorly positioned placenta requires elevation of the uterus out of the abdomen for a posterior hysterotomy. The hysterotomy should be a minimum of 5 cm from the edge of the placenta to prevent placental abruption and to facilitate closure of the hysterotomy. The hysterotomy is made with specially designed absorbable uterine staples that provide hemostasis and seal the membranes. Metallic stapling devices are not used as the metallic staples in the uterine wall act as in an intrauterine device and adversely affect future fertility after open fetal operations.[14] The fetus is monitored with continuous pulse oximetry and echocardiography. Warm saline solution is continuously infused around the fetus to prevent hypothermia and compression of the cord vessels. Fetal exposure is limited to the body part of interest. After completion of the fetal operation, the fetus is returned to the uterus, the amniotic fluid is replaced, and the hysterotomy is closed with running and interrupted absorbable suture. Postoperatively, tocolytics are administered, and the mother is monitored for contractions. The fetal heart rate is monitored, and daily echocardiogram is used to monitor for ductus arteriosus constriction and right-sided heart failure.

The ex utero intrapartum treatment (EXIT) procedure was developed as a bridge between fetal and postnatal therapy. Anesthesia is delivered to both mother and fetus, and a hemostatic hysterotomy is made. The uterus is completely relaxed to prevent placental separation, and the umbilical cord is not clamped. Fetal circulation is preserved, and the

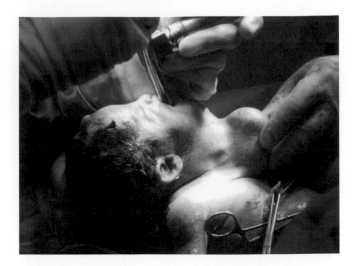

Figure 26.2 Fetal laryngoscopy after maternal hysterotomy during an EXIT procedure in a fetus with a large cervical neck mass.

fetus is maintained on full placental support until the airway can be secured (Figure 26.2). The EXIT procedure has been used to reverse tracheal occlusion and endotracheal intubation, repair the trachea, place a tracheostomy tube, resect large cervical tumors, and place cannulas for immediate extracorporeal membrane oxygenation (ECMO).[15]

ANOMALIES AMENABLE TO FETAL SURGERY

The current applications of fetal surgery are outlined in Table 26.1. Almost all fetal therapies are directed at lethal conditions, the notable exception being myelomeningocele (MMC).

Table 26.1 Fetal anomalies currently amenable to fetal intervention

Defect	Natural history	Fetal intervention
Urinary obstruction (urethral valves)	Renal failure, pulmonary hypoplasia	Percutaneous vesicoamniotic shunt
Congenital pulmonary airway malformation	Hydrops, death	Steroids, thoracoamniotic shunt, open pulmonary lobectomy
Congenital diaphragmatic hernia	Pulmonary hypoplasia, pulmonary hypertension	Temporary fetoscopic balloon tracheal occlusion
Sacrococcygeal teratoma	Hydrops, death	Open resection, vascular occlusion (RFA, alcohol)
Twin–twin transfusion syndrome[a]	Hydrops, death, neurologic damage to survivor	Fetoscopic laser ablation of placental vessels
Acardiac/anomalous twin (TRAP)	Death, neurologic damage to survivor	Cord occlusion/division, RFA
Cardiac valvular obstruction	Hypoplastic heart	Balloon valvuloplasty
Congenital high airway obstruction syndrome (CHAOS)	Hydrops, death	Fetoscopic tracheoplasty, EXIT
Cervical teratoma	Hydrops, death	Open resection, EXIT
Myelomeningocele[a]	Hydrocephalus, paralysis, neurogenic bowel/bladder	Open repair

[a] Intervention studied in large prospective randomized clinical trial.

Congenital diaphragmatic hernia

Despite advances in neonatal respiratory support, survival for children born with congenital diaphragmatic hernia (CDH) remains only 60%–70% throughout the United States. Herniation of the abdominal viscera into the chest interferes with normal lung development, resulting in pulmonary hypoplasia and pulmonary hypertension.[16,17] It was hypothesized that in utero intervention would allow for increased antenatal lung growth and improved survival postnatally.[18] In a fetal lamb model, compression of the lungs during the last trimester, either with an intrathoracic balloon or by creation of a diaphragmatic hernia, resulted in fatal pulmonary hypoplasia. In addition, removal of the compressing lesion allowed the lung to grow and develop sufficiently to permit survival at birth.[19]

It was important to identify the patients who might benefit the most from in utero CDH repair. Fetal ultrasound was used to stratify the severity of CDH. Liver herniation into the chest is the most important prognostic factor for CDH. In our experience, survival was 100% in fetuses with CDH without liver herniation and 56% in fetuses with CDH with liver herniation into the chest.[20,21] To further stratify risk in fetuses with liver herniation into the chest, the *lung-to-head ratio* (LHR) was developed. The LHR is calculated as the area of the contralateral lung at the level of the cardiac atria divided by the head circumference. This LHR value statistically correlated with survival in fetuses with liver herniation: 100% survival with an LHR greater than 1.35, 61% survival with an LHR between 0.6 and 1.35, and 0% survival with an LHR less than 0.6.[21]

Initial attempts at fetal surgery to treat CDH involved in utero diaphragmatic hernia repair. Although CDH repair via open hysterotomy proved feasible, there was no survival benefit. The benefit of in utero CDH repair was likely offset by the deleterious effect of premature delivery.[22] Efforts were redirected at finding a strategy for promoting in utero lung growth. The observation that fetuses affected by congenital high airway obstruction develop hyperplastic lungs[23] led to a series of animal studies that proved that tracheal occlusion leading to the accumulation of pressurized fluid in the airway results in lung growth.[24] The preliminary studies examined the effect of extrinsic tracheal occlusion by the in utero placement of an obstructing clip using both open and fetoscopic techniques. The tracheal occlusion group required an EXIT procedure to remove the clip at birth. In this small study, we found that fetoscopic tracheal occlusion in severe CDH conferred a survival advantage compared to open tracheal occlusion or standard postnatal therapy.[25] In 2003, the National Institutes of Health (NIH) sponsored a trial comparing fetoscopic tracheal occlusion with a clip to standard postnatal care in fetuses with severe CDH. Results of the trial showed survival of 75% with no difference between the tracheal occlusion group and the standard postnatal care group.[26] The survival in the postnatal care group was considerably greater than historical controls. Although this study did not demonstrate a difference in survival between the prenatal intervention group and the postnatal one, the results of this trial demonstrate the tremendous importance of proper randomized controlled trials for novel fetal surgical procedures.

Refinement of tracheal occlusion techniques has progressed from tracheal clipping to percutaneous, fetoscopic placement and retrieval of a detachable, intratracheal balloon. In utero retrieval of the balloon obviates the need for an EXIT procedure. Further data regarding tracheal occlusion suggest that short-term reversible tracheal occlusion may be preferable to longer-duration occlusion. Animal models of tracheal occlusion have demonstrated the benefits of short-term, reversible tracheal occlusion on fetal lung growth. Furthermore, long-term tracheal occlusion has been shown to be deleterious to type II pneumocytes: the cells that secrete surfactant.[27] In Europe, temporary fetal tracheal occlusion for CDH has been associated with survival of 50%. However, the unusually low survival of 15% in the standard therapy group has called the quality of postnatal care into question.[28] A prospective randomized trial of temporary tracheal occlusion versus standard therapy is underway in Europe, while safety and feasibility testing of the device is ongoing in the United States. Our group currently offers reversible, fetal tracheal occlusion for fetuses with liver herniation in the chest and an LHR of less than 1.0, as these patients continue to have greater than 60% mortality. We perform the initial procedure between 24 and 26 weeks gestation and remove the balloon between 32 and 34 weeks.

Tumors

Fetal tumors are rare and generally benign. When they do occur, most are best treated postnatally. However, very large tumors can impede venous return to the heart or create high-output heart failure via arteriovenous shunts that can lead to nonimmune hydrops in the fetus. Hydropic changes include polyhydramnios, placentomegaly, fetal skin and scalp edema, and pleural, pericardial, and peritoneal fluid accumulation. Left untreated, fetal hydrops is nearly always fatal; thus, the tumor must be addressed in utero.[29]

Congenital pulmonary airway malformation

Congenital pulmonary airway malformation (CPAM), previously referred to as congenital cystic adenomatoid malformation (CCAM), is characterized by an overgrowth of respiratory bronchioles with associated cyst formation.[30] Although most CPAMs can be managed postnatally, very large CPAMs can result in fetal hydrops and fetal demise. It is known that the size of the CPAM is the most important risk factor for developing fetal hydrops.[31] The most accepted method of predicting fetal hydrops is measurement of the CPAM volume ratio (CVR), defined as the product of the three longest measurements of the lesion on ultrasound, multiplied by the constant 0.52, divided by the head circumference. Crombleholme et al.[32] demonstrated that a CVR of 1.6 or greater is associated with an increased likelihood of hydrops.

CPAMs that are predominantly microcystic have a more predictable course than the macrocystic CPAMs. Microcystic CPAMs undergo steady growth and then plateau at 26–28 weeks gestation. In contrast, macrocystic CPAMs can abruptly enlarge due to rapid fluid accumulation within the cyst. For these reasons, patients with microcystic CCAMs are followed closely until 26–28 weeks gestation, and then the interval between ultrasound examinations can be lengthened, whereas macrocystic CPAMs require close follow-up throughout the duration of the pregnancy.[31,33]

Management of prenatally diagnosed CPAMs continues to evolve. A fetus of viable gestational age affected with a CPAM and associated hydrops should be delivered and undergo resection in the newborn period. In instances where a dominant macrocystic lesion is present in a previable fetus, thoracoamniotic shunt may reverse the hydrops fetalis.[34] Needle drainage is ineffective, as rapid reaccumulation of fluid is the norm. Fetal pulmonary lobectomy for microcystic CPAM with associated hydrops has been shown to reverse fetal hydrops but is associated with preterm labor and prematurity.[35] Interestingly, hydropic fetuses with large microcystic CPAMs can be successfully treated with administration of maternal steroids. This finding was discovered serendipitously at UCSF after several hydropic fetuses were treated with maternal steroids to enhance fetal lung maturity in preparation for fetal lung lobectomy. Subsequent fetal ultrasounds demonstrated resolution of the hydrops.[36] Several prospective studies have confirmed the effectiveness of maternal steroids for the fetal treatment of large microcystic CPAMs.[37] Macrocystic CPAMs do not respond to steroids and are still best managed with thoracoamniotic shunt placement or fetal surgery when fetuses develop hydrops (Figure 26.3).

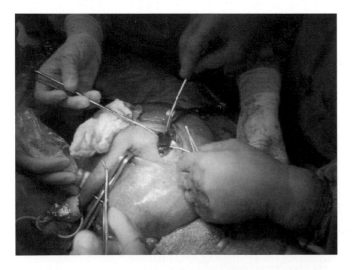

Figure 26.3 Fetal thoracotomy for CPAM. Note that only the right chest and arm are exposed for thoracotomy and pulse oximetry, while the remainder of the fetus is within the uterus.

Sacrococcygeal teratoma

Sacrococcygeal teratoma (SCT) is a rare tumor that is increasingly diagnosed in utero, allowing for greater understanding of the prenatal natural history of the disease. As with CPAM, fetuses with SCT can develop hydrops and in utero demise. SCT tumors can grow rapidly to a tremendous size in relation to the fetus, resulting in a vascular shunt and, in the extreme form, high-output cardiac failure and nonimmune hydrops. Rarely, tumors bleed either into the tumor or externally and can cause fetal anemia and hypovolemia. Other potential problems with a fetus with a large SCT are dystocia and preterm labor. Delivery can be particularly difficult when the diagnosis has not been made prenatally. Traumatic delivery may result in hemorrhage or tumor rupture. Most clinicians would favor cesarean delivery for fetuses with large SCTs. Thus, prenatal diagnosis and careful obstetrical planning are critical in the appropriate management of the fetus with an SCT.

Tumor morphology and tumor vascularity,[38] tumor growth rate,[39] and tumor metrics such as tumor volume-to–fetal weight ratio (TFR)[40] have all been defined as predictors of poor outcomes. The best predictors of risk for fetal hydrops and poor outcomes are solid tumor morphology and TFR >0.12.[40] Fetal resection of SCT in the face of hydrops reverses the pathophysiology if it is performed before mirror syndrome (maternal eclampsia) develops in the mother.

Among 15 fetuses with SCT and hydrops treated at UCSF, five survived (33%), five died in the neonatal period, and five died in utero. The most common method of fetal intervention is hysterotomy with resection or debulking of the tumor.[40] A predominantly cystic lesion may be amenable to percutaneous drainage or placement of a shunt. Attempts at ablating the tumor, either through alcohol injection or RFA, have been met with mixed success.[41]

ABNORMALITIES OF TWIN GESTATIONS

Identical twins may have separate placentas (dichorionic) or share a single placenta (monochorionic). Monochorionic twins may have unequal shares of placenta or blood flow and are at risk of discordant growth. More severe anomalies such as twin–twin transfusion syndrome (TTTS) or twin reversed arterial perfusion sequence (TRAP) can arise from monochorionic pregnancies. Complications arising from monochorionic twin gestations are the most common cause for referral to fetal diagnosis and treatment centers.[42]

Twin–twin transfusion syndrome

In monochorionic twins, there are connections on the placental surface between the umbilical arteries and veins arising from each twin. Normally, the blood flow between the twins is relatively balanced. TTTS occurs when there is net flow from one twin to the other. TTTS complicates about 10% of monochorionic pregnancies.[42] As a result of the transfusion of blood from the "donor" twin to the "recipient" twin, hemodynamic compromise can occur in either or both twins. The donor twin suffers from a low flow state and can sustain injuries to the brain and kidneys. Conversely, the recipient twin has fluid overload and can develop high-output heart failure and hydrops. The hallmark of TTTS is oligohydramnios in the donor twin and polyhydramnios in the recipient. In addition, often there is size discordance between the twins, with the donor being smaller than the recipient. Advanced disease is evidenced by progressive discordance in fluid volumes, with the donor becoming "stuck" in its amniotic sac due to a complete lack of fluid. In addition, worsening cardiac changes in the recipient portend a grave prognosis. If left untreated, TTTS carries 80%–90% mortality for both twins. In addition, if one twin dies, the other twin is at risk for neurologic injury due to a sump phenomenon in the placenta and demised fetus and from embolism.[43]

Previously, standard therapy for TTTS was serial high-volume amnioreduction of the polydraminiotic sac with the aim of decreasing the risk of preterm labor. The International Amnioreduction Registry showed that amnioreduction resulted in survival of 58%. However, survivors of TTTS treated with amnioreduction had an 18%–26% incidence of significant neurologic and cardiac morbidity. Additionally, serial amnioreduction does not confer a survival benefit in severe cases of TTTS.[44]

Fetoscopic laser photocoagulation of intertwin vascular connections has emerged as the gold standard for TTTS. This can be done nonselectively by ablating all inter-twin connections, or selectively, by ablating only Arterial-Venous (AV) connections with flow in the causative direction. Fetoscopic laser ablation is generally performed percutaneously using a 3–4 mm fetoscope with a side channel for irrigation and introduction of the laser. A large European prospective trial compared amnioreduction to selective laser ablation of intertwin vessels for the treatment of severe TTTS. The main outcome variable was survival of at least one twin. The trial was stopped early after interim analysis showed a clear survival advantage to laser therapy: 76% versus 51% for single survivor and 36% versus 26% for dual survivor.[45]

Twin reversed arterial perfusion

TRAP is a rare disease of monochorionic twins that occurs when one normal twin acts as a "pump" for an acardiac, acephalic one. As the acardiac, acephalic twin grows, the normal pump twin goes into high-output cardiac failure and hydrops. The blood flow in the acardiac twin is characteristically reversed, and thus, the acronym *TRAP* was coined to describe this anomaly. The natural history of TRAP is greater than 50% mortality in the pump twin due to hydrops.[46] The risk of hydrops increases as the mass of the acardiac twin increases relative to the normal twin. Generally, we choose

to intervene when there is evidence of hydrops in the pump twin, or when the estimated fetal weight of the acardiac twin is 50% or more relative to the pump one.

Multiple techniques have been used to separate the vascular supplies in TRAP pregnancies: open hysterotomy and delivery, fetoscopic ligation, bipolar cautery, harmonic scalpel division, thermal coagulation, and laser coagulation.[47] At UCSF, an RFA device is introduced percutaneously under ultrasound guidance to coagulate the umbilical cord insertion site on the acardiac twin's abdomen. RFA of TRAP pregnancies between 18 and 24 weeks gestation resulted in 92% survival with delivery at a mean gestational age of 36 weeks.[48]

Myelomeningocele

MMC, or spina bifida, is characterized by an open neural tube and exposed spinal canal elements. MMC can occur anywhere along the spine but most commonly occurs in the lumbar or cervical vertebral levels. Complications include neurologic deficits with motor and somatosensory abnormalities. In addition, bowel and bladder function is often deranged due to injury to the autonomic nervous system. Finally, nearly all patients with MMC develop the Arnold–Chiari II malformation of the hindbrain that results in noncommunicating hydrocephalus, and most will require ventriculoperitoneal (VP) shunting. Unlike previous patients considered for fetal intervention, fetuses with MMC have low perinatal mortality. Despite postnatal repair of the defect, the attendant morbidity from neurologic abnormalities is severe, and up to 30% of patients die before reaching adulthood.[49]

The rationale for fetal intervention in MMC is the "two-hit" hypothesis, where the first hit is the original neural tube defect that results in the open spinal canal. The second hit is postulated to be due to direct trauma to the exposed neural elements while the fetus is in utero.[50,51] It is this second hit that could potentially be ameliorated by fetal surgery. Animal models for fetal MMC proved this hypothesis and showed that in utero repair of the MMC improved distal neurologic function and reversed the Arnold–Chiari II malformation.[52]

These animal data led to pilot studies in human fetuses. MMC is the first nonlethal anomaly for which fetal surgery was undertaken (Figure 26.4).[53] Early attempts at fetal MMC repair showed promise in reversing the Arnold–Chiari II malformation and possibly decreasing the need for VP shunting.[54] The NIH sponsored a multicenter randomized trial (Management of Myelomeningocele Study [MOMS]) comparing fetal MMC repair at 19–26 weeks gestation versus postnatal repair. The success of the trial depended on the cooperation of all fetal centers in the country to place a moratorium on fetal MMC repair outside the context of the trial. The objectives of the trial were (1) to determine if fetal MMC repair improved survival or need for VP shunt by 1 year of life compared to standard postnatal repair and (2) to determine if fetal MMC repair improves motor and

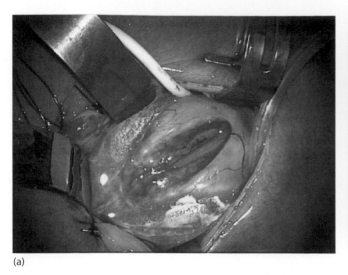
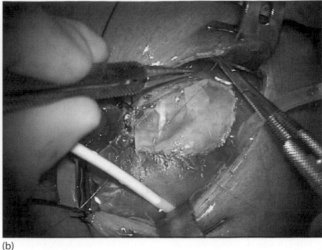

(a)   (b)

Figure 26.4 Fetal myelomeningocele repair. **(a)** MMC defect prior to repair. **(b)** MMC during placement of a patch to cover the skin defect.

cognitive function at 30 months of age compared to postnatal repair. The study closed early because of the superiority of fetal surgery. Fetal MMC repair reduced the need for ventricular shunting for hydrocephalus at 1 year (fetal group: 40% vs. postnatal group: 82%, $p < .001$) and improved motor function, including the ability to walk at 30 months of age (fetal group: 42% vs. postnatal group: 21%, $p < .01$). Fetuses treated prenatally were born at an average gestational age of 34.1 weeks, and 13% were born before 30 weeks gestation.[55]

THE FUTURE

The requirements for intervention to correct a fetal defect remain the same:

1. Experimental work to prove the pathophysiology of the defect
2. Careful study of the natural history of the untreated disease
3. Ability to select the fetus that will benefit from prenatal treatment

Stem cells and gene therapy

Gene therapy for prenatally identifiable diseases is currently experimental and is being actively pursued for specific disorders. In utero treatment with stem cells and/or virally directed genes may halt the progression of disease during gestation. The fetal immune system develops gradually, and prior to 15 weeks gestation, the fetus is in a preimmune state. Thus. in utero transplantation may avoid problems with rejection and graft-versus-host disease that are seen with postnatal transplantation.

Specific issues for in utero treatment of genetic diseases include timing of diagnosis, timing of therapy, delivery of stem cells or genes, sources for stem cells, and durability of treatment. With the advent of chorionic villus sampling, genetic diseases can be identified in the first trimester. Timing of potential treatments is crucial in order to take advantage of the possible preimmune status of the fetus, making fetuses potentially more receptive to exogenous genes or cells.[56] Several investigators have utilized hematopoietic stem cells (HSCs) as a vector to attempt to induce chimerism in order to treat the disease. Others have investigated the use of retroviral vectors in order to insert genetic material into fetal animals. This approach reduces the problem of obtaining the large numbers of stem cells needed to create even a modest amount of chimerism. Other approaches include use of maternal stem cells or genetic material as studies have demonstrated early cross-trafficking of maternal cells in the fetus. Candidate diseases include hematologic, immunologic, metabolic, and neurologic abnormalities.[57] To date, the only durable in utero HSC has been for severe combined immunodeficiency syndrome. Currently, in utero gene therapy and stem cell therapy are in their infancy but remain active topics of research and investigation.[58]

SUMMARY

Fetal surgery has progressed from an investigational therapy to an accepted mode of therapy for selected fetal diseases. The progress seen in the field of fetal surgery is a testament to the power of a rigorous investigational process, i.e., identifying clinical needs, understanding of the pathophysiology in the laboratory, the documentation of the natural history in the human fetus, and the push for less and less invasive procedures. Through these efforts, diseases with historically high perinatal mortality rates have shown improved survival with fetal surgery. Furthermore, NIH-funded, prospective trials have confirmed the value of fetal surgery for diseases such as TTTS and MMC and shown where fetal surgery remains investigational, as is the case for CDH. New areas of research include tissue engineering, stem cell therapy, and gene therapy. As always, maternal safety must remain paramount, and risk to the mother should be minimized at all times.

Many people have contributed to the development and success of fetal treatment and diagnosis. Collaborative, multidisciplinary teams are critical for the success of any fetal treatment program. It is also important to acknowledge the significant contributions of patients and their families to this enterprise. The brave families who chose to undergo early fetal therapies are the true pioneers on whose shoulders the success of fetal treatment rests.

REFERENCES

1. Harrison MR et al. Fetal surgery for congenital hydronephrosis. *N Engl J Med* 1982; 306(10): 591–3.
2. Golombek K et al. Maternal morbidity after maternal–fetal surgery. *Am J Obstet Gynecol* 2006; 194(3): 834–9.
3. Cortes RA, Farmer DL. Recent advances in fetal surgery. *Semin Perinatol* 2004; 28: 199–211.
4. Wu D, Ball RH. The maternal side of maternal–fetal surgery. *Clin Perinatol* 2009; 36: 247–53.
5. Farrell JA et al. Maternal fertility is not affected by fetal surgery. *Fetal Diagn Ther* 1999; 14(3): 190–2.
6. Akolekar R et al. Procedure-related risk of miscarriage following amniocentesis and chorionic villus sampling: A systematic review and meta-analysis. *Ultrasound Obstet Gynecol* 2015; 45(1): 16–26.
7. Wataganara T, Bianchi DW. Fetal cell-free nucleic acids in the maternal circulation: New clinical applications. *Ann NY Acad Sci* 2004; 1022: 90–9.
8. Rosen MA. Anesthesia for fetal procedures and surgery. *Yonsei Med J* 2001; 42(6): 669–80.
9. De Buck F, Deprest J, Van de Velde M. Anesthesia for fetal surgery. *Curr Opin Anaesthesiol* 2008; 21(3): 293–7.
10. Sydorak RM et al. Fetoscopic treatment for discordant twins. *J Pediatr Surg* 2002; 37(12): 1736–9.
11. Lee H et al. Efficacy of radiofrequency ablation for twin-reversed arterial perfusion sequence. *Am J Obstet Gynecol* 2007; 196(5): 459 e1–4.
12. Danzer E et al. Minimal access fetal surgery. *Eur J Obstet Genecol Reprod Biol* 2003; May 1; 108(1): 3–13.
13. Freud LR et al. Fetal aortic valvuloplasty for evolving hypoplastic left heart syndrome: Postnatal outcomes of the first 100 patients. *Circulation* 2014; 19(8): 638–45.
14. Adzick NS et al. Fetal surgery in the primate. III. Maternal outcome after fetal surgery. *J Pediatr Surg* 1986; 21(6): 477–80.
15. Hirose S et al. The ex utero intrapartum treatment procedure: Looking back at the EXIT. *J Pediatr Surg* 2004; 39: 375–80.
16. Logan JW et al. Congenital diaphragmatic hernia: A systematic review and summary of best-evidence practice strategies. *J Perinatol* 2007; 27(9): 535–49.
17. Moya FR, Lally KP. Evidence-based management of infants with congenital diaphragmatic hernia. *Semin Perinatol* 2005; 29(2): 112–7.
18. Adzick NS et al. Experimental studies on prenatal treatment of congenital anomalies. *Br J Hosp Med* 1985; 34(3): 154–9.
19. Adzick NS et al. Correction of congenital diaphragmatic hernia in utero. IV. An early gestational fetal lamb model for pulmonary vascular morphometric analysis. *J Pediatr Surg* 1985; 20(6): 673–80.
20. Albanese CT et al. Fetal liver position and perinatal outcome for congenital diaphragmatic hernia. *Prenat Diagn* 1998; 18: 1138–42.
21. Metkus AP et al. Sonographic predictors of survival in fetal diaphragmatic hernia. *J Pediatr Surg* 1996; 31(1): 148–51; discussion 151–2.
22. Harrison MR et al. Correction of congenital diaphragmatic hernia in utero. VII A prospective trial. *J Pediatr Surg* 1997; 32: 1637–42.
23. Hedrick MH et al. Congenital high airway obstruction syndrome (CHAOS): A potential for perinatal intervention. *J Pediatr Surg* 1994; 29(2): 271–4.
24. DiFiore JW et al. Experimental fetal tracheal ligation reverses the structural and physiological effects of pulmonary hypoplasia in congenital diaphragmatic hernia. *J Pediatr Surg* 1994; 29(2): 248–56; discussion 256–7.
25. Hedrick MH et al. Plug the lung until it grows (PLUG): A new method to treat congenital diaphragmatic hernia in utero. *J Pediatr Surg* 1994; 29(5): 612–7.
26. Harrison MR et al. A randomized trial of fetal endoscopic tracheal occlusion for severe fetal congenital diaphragmatic hernia. *N Engl J Med* 2003; 349(20): 1916–24.
27. Cannie MM et al. Evidence and patterns in lung response after fetal tracheal occlusion: Clinical controlled study. *Radiology* 2009; Aug; 252(2): 526–33.
28. Jani JC et al. Severe diaphragmatic hernia treated by fetal endoscopic tracheal occlusion. *Ultrasound Obstet Gynecol* 2009; 34(3): 304–10.
29. Grethel EJ et al. Fetal intervention for mass lesions and hydrops improves outcome: A 15-year experience. *J Pediatr Surg* 2007; 42: 117.
30. Adzick NS et al. Fetal cystic adenomatoid malformation: Prenatal diagnosis and natural history. *J Pediatr Surg* 1985; 20(5): 483–8.
31. Kunisaki SM et al. Large fetal congenital cystic adenomatoid malformations: Growth trends and patient survival. *J Pediatr Surg* 2007; 42(2): 404–10.
32. Crombleholme TM et al. Cystic adenomatoid malformation volume ratio predicts outcome in prenatally diagnosed cystic adenomatoid malformation of the lung. *J Pediatr Surg* 2002; 37(3): 331–8.

33. Miller JA, Corteville JE, Langer JC. Congenital cystic adenomatoid malformation in the fetus: Natural history and predictors of outcome. *J Pediatr Surg* 1996; 31(6): 805–8.

34. Wilson RD et al. Thoracoamniotic shunts: Fetal treatment of pleural effusions and congenital cystic adenomatoid malformations. *Fetal Diagn Ther* 2004; 19(5): 413–20.

35. Adzick NS et al. Fetal surgery for cystic adenomatoid malformation of the lung. *J Pediatr Surg* 1993; 28(6): 806–12.

36. Tsao K et al. Resolution of hydrops fetalis in congenital cystic adenomatoid malformation after prenatal steroid therapy. *J Pediatr Surg* 2003; 38(3): 508–10.

37. Curran PF et al. Prenatal steroids for microcystic congenital cystic adenomatoid malformations. *J Pediatr Surg* 2010; 45: 145–50.

38. Westerburg B et al. Sonographic prognostic factors in fetuses with sacrococcygeal teratoma. *J Pediatr Surg* 2000; 35(2): 322–5; discussion 325–6.

39. Hedrick HL et al. Sacrococcygeal teratoma: Prenatal assessment, fetal intervention, and outcome. *J Pediatr Surg* 2004; 39(3): 430–8; discussion 430–8.

40. Shue E et al. Tumor metrics and morphology predict poor prognosis in prenatally diagnosed sacrococcygeal teratoma: A 25-year experience at a single institution. *J Pediatr Surg* 2013; 48(6): 1225–31.

41. Van Mieghem T et al. Minimally invasive therapy for fetal sacrococcygeal teratoma: Case series and systematic review of the literature. *Ultrasound Obstet Gynecol* 2014; 43(6): 611–9.

42. Sebire NJ et al. The hidden mortality of monochorionic twin pregnancies. *Br J Obstet Gynaecol* 1997; 104(10): 1203–7.

43. Berghella V, Kaufmann M. Natural history of twin–twin transfusion syndrome. *J Reprod Med* 2001; 46(5): 480–4.

44. Roberts D et al. Interventions for the treatment of twin–twin transfusion syndrome. *Cochrane Database Syst Rev* 2008; (1): CD002073

45. Senat MV et al. Endoscopic laser surgery versus serial amnioreduction for severe twin-to-twin transfusion syndrome. *N Engl J Med* 2004; 351(2): 136–44.

46. Van Allen MI, Smith DW, Shepard TH. Twin reversed arterial perfusion (TRAP) sequence: A study of 14 twin pregnancies with acardius. *Semin Perinatol* 1983; 7(4): 285–93.

47. Tsao K et al. Selective reduction of acardiac twin by radiofrequency ablation. *Am J Obstet Gynecol* 2002; 187: 635–40.

48. Lee H et al. Efficacy of radiofrequency ablation for twin reversed arterial perfusion sequence. *Am J Obstet Gynecol* 2007; 196: 459.e1–e4.

49. Hirose S et al. Fetal surgery for myelomeningocele. *Clin Perinatol* 2009; 36(2): 431–8, xi.

50. Heffez DS et al. The paralysis associated with myelomeningocele: Clinical and experimental data implicating a preventable spinal cord injury. *Neurosurgery* 1990; 26(6): 987–92.

51. Meuli M et al. Creation of myelomeningocele in utero: A model of functional damage from spinal cord exposure in fetal sheep. *J Pediatr Surg* 1995; 30(7): 1028–32; discussion 1032–3.

52. Meuli M et al. In utero repair of experimental myelomeningocele saves neurological function at birth. *J Pediatr Surg* 1996; 31(3): 397–402.

53. Adzick NS et al. Successful fetal surgery for spina bifida. *Lancet* 1998; 352: 1675–6.

54. Farmer DL et al. In utero repair of myelomeningocele: Experimental pathophysiology, initial clinical experience, and outcomes. *Arch Surg* 2003; 138(8): 872–8.

55. Adzick NS et al. A randomized trial of prenatal vs postnatal repair of myelomeningocele. *N Engl J Med* 2011; 364: 993–1004.

56. MacKenzie TC. Fetal surgical conditions and the unraveling of maternal–fetal tolerance. *J Pediatr Surg* 2016; 51(2): 197–9.

57. Wagner AM, Schoeberlein A, Surbek D. Fetal gene therapy: Opportunities and risks. *Adv Drug Deliv Rev* 2009; 61(10): 813–21.

58. Nijagal A et al. In utero hematopoietic cell transplantation for the treatment of congenital anomalies. *Clin Perinatol* 2012; 39(2): 301–10.

27

Tissue engineering and stem cell research

PAOLO DE COPPI

INTRODUCTION

Congenital and acquired surgical conditions represent a major cause of morbidity and mortality during the first years of life and childhood. In those complex conditions, prosthetic materials are used because of the lack of biocompatible tissues able to replace or regenerate damaged organs. Besides the risk of infection, the major drawback of using a prosthetic patch closure is the risk of dislodgment and subsequent recurrence of the initial problem. Moreover, foreign body reactions and implant rejection occur when synthetic polymers are used. Regeneration of natural tissue from living cells to restore damaged tissues and organs is the main purpose of regenerative medicine. This relatively new field has emerged by the combination of tissue engineering and cell transplantation as a possible strategy for the replacement of damaged organs or tissues. So far, most of the attention has been focused on degenerative diseases such as Parkinson's or Alzheimer's, while very little has been done for the treatment of congenital conditions. However, the knowledge acquired in the last years from stem cell (SC) biology and regenerative medicine strategies could lead to new ways of repairing or replacing injured organs and systems, even during fetal development, and therefore, pediatric patients could largely benefit from the evolution of this new exciting field. In order to give rise to a new functional organ-like structure, several variables, such as local environment, nutrients, and metabolites, are pivotal. These variables, in the context of tissue engineering, are mainly dependent on the provision of a three-dimensional growth structure termed "scaffold."[1] Scaffolds can be either natural of synthetic. Natural scaffolds are essentially bioactive but lack mechanical strength. Synthetic scaffolds lack bioactivity, are mechanically strong and can be engineered with bespoke macrostructure and microstructure, which has the potential to enhance cellular growth and organogenesis.[2] Scaffolds could ultimately represent the exclusive tool required for tissue engineering, and several attempts to generate whole organs such as liver have been conducted using structures with vascular channels to ensure an adequate network of vascular supply.[3] Major developments in regenerative medicine have been achieved following the discovery of cells which can be isolated and expanded in number outside the body. SCs are unspecialized cells with the capacity to both self-renew, and give rise to multiple mature specialized cell types through asymmetric cell division.[4] There are three main sources of SCs in humans and animals: embryonic, fetal, and adult tissue. Adult SCs have a limited cellular regeneration, or turnover, this could represent a limitation for tissue engineering applications, where a large number of cells are necessary.[5] SCs they can be identified in many adult mammalian tissues, such as bone marrow (BM), skeletal muscle, skin, and adipose tissue, where they contribute to the replenishment of cells lost through normal cellular senescence or injury.[6–10] In contrast, SCs derived from embryonic sources have the ability to give rise to cells that not only proliferate and replace themselves indefinitely, but also have the potential to form any cell type.[11,12] Embryonic stem (ES) cells are derived from the inner cell mass of pre-implantation embryo, they are pluripotent, and demonstrate germ-line transmission in experimentally produced chimeras.[13,14] More recently, cells with intermediate potency have derived from the amniotic fluid (fetal SCs)[15] and from adult SCs which have been reprogrammed using various factors implicated in the maintenance of pluripotency in ES cells.[16] This chapter would like to offer an insight on the latest evolution of SCs, with a glance at their possible application for regenerative medicine, and recent clinical translations, particularly in the pediatric surgery field.

STEM CELLS

ES cells

ES cells derive from the inner cell mass of a blastocyst stage embryo.[17] They are pluripotent and give rise during development to all derivatives of the three primary germ layers: ectoderm, endoderm, and mesoderm; hence, they possess the potential to develop into most cell types within the body.[13,18,19] The field of ES cell research began with the study of teratocarcinoma cells in the 1950s, and continued in 1981 with first mouse ES cell lines derived from the inner cell mass of blastocysts using culture conditions (fibroblast feeder layers and serum). The field progressed further in 1998 when Thomson et al.[13,20,21] first isolated human ES (hES) cells. Optimal culture conditions have been developed for both mouse ES (mES) and hES cells to evaluate and maintain both their proliferative and differentiative capacities. mES cells are grown on a layer of gelatin and require the presence of leukemia inhibitory factor, while hES cells are grown on a feeder layer of mouse embryonic fibroblasts and require the presence of basic fibroblast growth factor.[18] The maintenance of pluripotency in the hES is assured by the presence of different transcription factors like Oct-4, Nanog, and SOX2, which are essential to ensure the suppression of genes that lead to differentiation.[22] The cell surface antigens most commonly used to identify hES cells are the glycolipids stem cells embryonic antigen-3 and -4 (SSEA3 and SSEA4) and the keratan sulfate antigens Tra-1-60 and Tra-1-81.[9] ES cells can be used to generate tissues but could also be employed as "cellular models" to study a range of human diseases, and to test new drug candidates for efficacy and toxicity (Figure 27.1).[23] ES cells, being pluripotent, require specific signals for correct differentiation, and if injected in vivo prior to commitment, they will give rise to many different types of cells, resulting in the formation of teratomas. So far, their potency, together with the difficulties related to their allogenic origin, have limited their possible clinical application.[24] In particular, the political debate surrounding SC research began suddenly after hES were created from a human embryo which was subsequently destroyed. Recently, researchers opened the possibility of generating ES cell lines without destroying embryos, by deriving cells from earlier stages of embryo development, and without impairing future development of the embryo.[25–27] Moreover, in the last few years, ES cells have been used as a model for tissue differentiation, and rudimental organs derived from ES cells have been engineered. Understanding the signaling necessary for

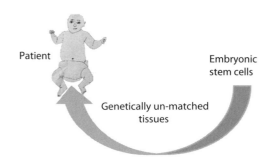

Figure 27.1 ES cells can be derived from culturing of fertilized eggs and differentiated into mature specialized tissues, which are, however, not matched to the recipient, and therefore ES cell transplantation must be associated to immunosuppression.

terminal differentiation has been important in defining the lineage-specific transcription factors, which can potentially be used to genetically engineer and terminally differentiate pluripotent SCs, increasing the chance of producing functionally differentiated tissues.

Somatic cell nuclear transfer

Somatic cell nuclear transfer (SCNT) has also been adopted to create patient-specific SCs, and avoid problems relating to the creation of allogenic tissue. This procedure specifically entails the removal of an oocyte nucleus in culture, followed by its replacement with a nucleus derived from a somatic cell obtained from a patient. SCNT technique was first reported by Briggs and King[28] and some years after was used to obtain the first vertebrate (a frog).[29] Cells yielded by this process are genetically identical to the donor and would not be rejected by the patient. SCNT can potentially be used for three purposes: (1) reproduction, leading to generation of an embryo for continuation of life (a notable example in 1996 was the generation of the first mammal, a sheep named Dolly, derived from an adult somatic cell using this technique[30]); (2) therapy, generating blastocysts for SC derivation; and (3) research and regenerative medicine. The first is scientifically and ethically condemned. The second has important implications for the future of ES therapies, allowing the production of nonimmunogenic ES lines. Besides, this cells could be stored and used subsequently for the treatment of future medical conditions. As a consequence, this could be relevant to the creation of autologous tissues for use in children who are born with complex malformations, in which tissue viability represents a problem and where patient-specific cells could be created *in vitro*. ES cells derived using SCNT would have the same genetic background as the patient who donated the initial genetic material, and the tissue created would not be rejected after transplantation. ES cells have, in fact, the advantage of being extremely plastic, facilitating the *in vitro* engineering of complex organs such as heart, liver, and kidney.[31–33] Nevertheless, in spite of the ethical considerations, the limitation of this technique is related both to the low efficiency, leading to a high loss in cell yield, and the inadequate supply of human oocytes.[34]

Induced pluripotent SCs

Since the major objection to hES research is their immunogenicity, it would be advantageous to develop a method of creating SCs from autologous tissue. Generation of induced pluripotent stem (iPS) cells, described by Yamanaka et al. in 2006, avoids both the immunological and ethical problems (Figure 27.2). iPS cells can be developed from nonpluripotent cells, usually adult somatic cells, by causing a forced expression of several genetic sequences such as Oct4 (POU5F1), the transcription factor Sox2, c-Myc proto-oncogene protein, and Klf4 (Krueppel-like factor 4). In 2007, successful iPS cells were obtained from human

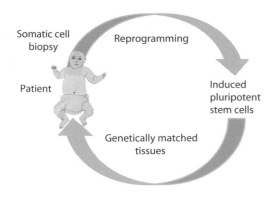

Figure 27.2 iPS cells can now be obtained from adult cells by reprogramming. It creates genetically matched tissues, but genetic manipulation of the cells during reprogramming can be teratogenic.

fibroblasts both using Oct3/4, Sox2, Klf4, and c-Myc with a retroviral transfection, and using OCT4, SOX2, NANOG, and a different gene LIN28 using a lentiviral system, improving transduction output.[36,37] The viral transfection systems used to insert the genes at random locations in the host's genome created concern for potential therapeutic applications of these iPS cells, because it might increase the risk of tumor formation.[38] To overcome these dangers, some studies have used adenovirus to transport the four sequences into the DNA of mouse somatic cells. Since the adenovirus does not combine any of its own genes with the targeted host, the danger of creating tumors is eliminated.[39] Yamanaka et al. have since demonstrated that reprogramming can be accomplished via plasmids without any virus transfection system at all, although at very low efficiencies.[38] iPS cells show morphological resemblance to hES cells, express typical human ES cell-specific cell surface antigens and genes, give rise to multiple lineages in vitro, and form teratomas when injected into immunocompromised mice. The efficiency of reprogramming adult fibroblasts has been low (<0.1%). However, since reprogrammed clones could consistently be recovered and expanded with existing gene combinations, for practical applications, the low reprogramming efficiency itself was not really considered an issue, unless reprogramming selects abnormal genetic or epigenetic events that were stably propagated in the resulting iPS cell lines.[40] Recently, Jaenisch's group found an elegant way to derive iPS from somatic cells of patients, free from reprogramming factors using Cre-recombinase excisable lentiviruses. The efficiency of reprogrammed iPS is very high with a low number of proviral vector integrations, and the cells maintain a gene expression profile more similar to hES than to hiPS these cells have been subsequently differentiated into dopaminergic neurons, demonstrating that Parkinson's disease patient-derived iPS cells can be free of viral reprogramming factors.[41] Interestingly, in the surgical community, the possibility to derive and isolate enteric nervous system (ENS) progenitors from human pluripotent SCs, and their further differentiation into functional enteric neurons, has been recently demonstrated.[42]

ENS precursors derived in vitro are capable of targeted migration in the developing chick embryo and extensive colonization of the adult mouse colon.[43] Moreover, iPS cells can be generated from fetal cells without any genetic manipulation. We have recently described that iPS cells can be easily derived from first trimester amniotic SCs when grown on Matrigel in hES cell medium, supplemented with the histone deacetylase inhibitor valproic acid.[44] It is possible that, because of their fetal origin, amniotic fluid stem cells (AFSC) (discussed in detail later) could be ideal for cell banking of patient-specific pluripotent cells and possible applications in pharmaceutical screening.

Fetal SCs

Fetal cells may represent the ideal source for therapy (Figure 27.2). Like ES cells, they are still plastic and easy to expand, and, in common with their adult counterparts, they are less controversial, not tumorigenic, and can be developed in an autologous setting. The latter is particularly important in the context of congenital malformation, as surgical treatment is often complicated by insufficient available tissue at time of repair. Regularly, artificial materials have been the only option for reconstruction in such cases, with high rates of morbidity. Recently, fetal tissue engineering has emerged as a promising concept in surgical reconstruction of birth defects. Redundant or purposely obtained fetal cells could be harvested, cultured, and manipulated in vitro during the remainder of pregnancy, and used later for tissue engineering of graft material that will be applied in postnatal reconstruction. Indeed, in the case of prenatal diagnosis of structural defects, there is the possibility of obtaining homologous cells at the time of invasive sampling such as chorionic villi biopsy, cordocentesis, or amniocentesis. Sampling of amniotic fluid is ideal for prenatal/neonatal applications with the following advantages: (i) relatively easy to perform, (ii) low risk for both the mother and the fetus, and (iii) a widely accepted method of prenatal diagnosis. AFSC's represent about 1% of all whole cells in cultures of human amniocentesis specimens, obtained for prenatal genetic diagnosis, these cells can be purified by immunoselection using c-Kit (CD117).[41] AFSC's are described as broadly multipotent SCs that can differentiate into adipogenic, osteogenic, myogenic, endothelial, neurogenic, and hepatogenic lineages, inclusive of all embryonic germ layers (Figures 27.3 and 27.4).[15,45–50] In contrast with mesenchymal cells, AFSC's show hematopoietic engraftment[51] and a functional and stable integration into the skeletal muscle SC niche, highlighting their value as the cell source for the treatment of muscular pathologies and skeletal muscle defects.[52] This group of cells can be steadily expanded in cultures without a feeder layer and has a typical doubling time of 36 hours. Subconfluent cells show no evidence of spontaneous differentiation; nevertheless, under specific inducing conditions, these cells are able to differentiate and, if injected in vivo, show no evidence of tumor growth in severe combined immunodeficient

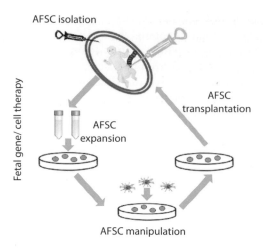

Figure 27.3 AFSC's can be used for *in utero* cell or cell/gene therapy in the same individual and therefore overcome the immunological problems, and they have higher potential than adult SCs.

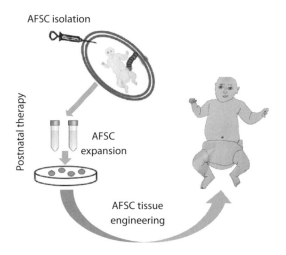

Figure 27.4 AFSC's can be used for engineering autologous tissue for postnatal transplantation and therefore overcome the immunological problems, and they have higher potential than adult SCs.

mice. AFSC's are positive for a number of surface markers commonly expressed by mesenchymal SCs (MSCs), but not by ES cells, such as CD29, CD44 (hyaluronan receptor), CD73, CD90, and CD105 (endoglin).[53] Human AFSC's are also positive for stage-specific embryonic antigen (SSEA)-4 which is expressed by previously used ES cells, and >90% of the cells express the transcription factor Oct4, which has been associated with the maintenance of the undifferentiated state and the pluripotency of ES and embryonic germ (EG) cells.[15,54] First trimester AFSC's can also be fully reprogrammed without using any genetic manipulation.[44] AFSC's can be used as a carrier for congenital monogenic disease, which theoretically could be corrected by a combined-approach gene-cell therapy (Figure 27.3). Following this approach, AFSC's could be isolated, the defect identified and corrected, and the cells injected back to the donor avoiding both fetal and maternal

immunorejection. Alternatively, in cases of structural anomalies, AFSC's could be expanded and used to engineer the missing tissue/organ (Figure 27.4). MSCs derived from amniotic fluid have already been used in large animal models for the repair of surgically created diaphragmatic defects,[55] and engineered diaphragmatic tendon graft using mesenchymal amniocytes has obtained preclinical validation and may soon become a clinical reality.[56]

Adult SCs

At the farthest end of the spectrum, we have SCs that are present in the postnatal life, are more differentiated/mature, and are classified as either multipotent or unipotent (Figure 27.5). Classically, hematopoietic SCs (HSCs) have successfully been used for more than 25 years, and transplantation of BM and cord blood (CB) HSCs is routinely performed for hematological/oncological disorders. Following preliminary studies by Friedenstein et al.,[57] other cells, defined as MSCs, distinguishable from HSCs because of the capacity to grow in adherent culture, were described. MSCs are multipotent SCs with fibroblast-like morphology, which can differentiate into osteogenic (bone), chondrogenic (cartilage), and adipogenic (BM stroma) lineages *in vitro*.[6,58] Their existence was first hypothesized when tissues biopsied (skeletal muscle, skin, heart, and even brain) from patients, who previously received a BM transplant, showed donor cell engraftment. To date, MSCs have been isolated both in the fetus and postnatally from blood, liver, and BM, amniotic fluid, lung, pancreas, dental pulp, and periosteum.[59–64] They have also been isolated from umbilical CB, Wharton's jelly, and placenta. These parts, previously considered a "biological waste," today are among the most interesting for MSC isolation.[65–67] Three major criteria to define MSCs have been introduced by the International Society for Cell Therapy[68]: (i) the cells must be plastic-adherent when maintained under standard culture conditions; (ii) >95% of the MSC population must express CD73 (ecto 5'-nucleotidase), CD90 (Thy-1), and CD105 (SH2 or MCAM or endoglin), LNGFR (low-affinity nerve growth factor receptor), CD166, ALCAM adhesion protein, CD146 (P1H12), CD29, and CD106 (vascular

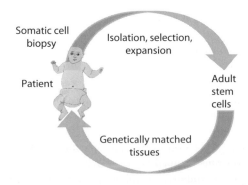

Figure 27.5 Adult SCs are relatively safer to use clinically, but they are limited in expansion and differentiation.

adhesion molecule-1 [VCAM-1]), and >98% MSC should be negative for hematopoietic cell surface antigens: CD45, a pan-leukocyte marker; CD34, a marker of primitive hematopoietic progenitors and endothelial cells; either CD11b or CD14, markers for monocytes; either CD19 or CD79a, B-cell markers; and human leukocyte antigen (HLA class 2); and (iii) MSC should be capable of differentiating into osteoblasts, chondroblasts, and adipocytes when placed into an appropriate induction/differentiation medium. Adult SCs or progenitors have already been used clinically to engineer urological constructs such as bladders and urethras, blood vessels, cornea, esophageal epithelium, bronchi, and tracheas. Moreover, MSCs have been tested for cellular therapy in pediatric patients for several clinical indications, such as inborn errors of metabolism (metachromatic leukodystrophy, Hurler syndrome, infantile hypophosphatasemia), osteogenesis imperfecta, and GVHD.[69–73] However, in contrast with the aforementioned cells, MSCs also have a limited lifespan and become senescent when cultured *in vitro*. This is a major problem for therapy since, regardless of the isolation procedure, the MSC quantity obtained from primary tissues is not sufficient for any downstream MSC application in clinical settings. *In vitro* expansion can affect biological properties of the cells, and MSCs go through very significant changes in phenotype and gene expression as a result of cell culture adaptation. Although considered a safer source compared with ES cells, the prospective clinical applications of MSCs require meticulous examination (Figure 27.5).

SCAFFOLDS

In order to develop a tissue-engineered construct to replace missing or damaged tissue, the combination of appropriate cellular engineering and material science is needed. Material science is concerned with the production of acellular scaffolds that can be seeded with cells, allowing and promoting their growth. General attributes that a scaffold must fulfill include

(i) Biocompatibility that does not lead to an immunogenic response from the host
(ii) Biodegradation in a suitable time period that permits sufficient cellular growth while not producing harmful degradation products
(iii) Mechanical properties that are in line with tissue growth; a significant amount of three-dimensional support in the early stages without obstructing cellular extracellular matrix production in the later stages

More specific scaffold attributes are related to the aim of recreating the nonmechanical attributes of the ECM. These properties include the mediation of cell adhesion via integrin receptors,[74] as well as positive influence on cell survival and proliferation by means of growth factors and cytokines.[75] What is more, the ECM has been argued to be

involved in mechanochemical transduction, as shown by the differentiation of MSCs to neurons, muscle cells, and osteoblasts when seeded on a substrate mimicking the elasticity of each of those host tissues respectively.[76]

Materials used, thus far, for tissue engineering have been traditionally divided into three categories: (i) naturally derived materials (e.g., collagen and elastin), (ii) synthetic materials (e.g., poly(L)-lactic acid [PLA], polyglycolic acid [PGA], and polylactic-co-glycolic acid [PLGA]), and (iii) natural acellular scaffolds.

Naturally derived materials

Materials composed of naturally occurring macromolecules, in particular those that formulate the ECM, have been tested for tissue engineering purposes. They have the advantage of having a specific structure with which cellular integrins bind well, promoting cellular adhesion. A classic example is collagen, the most abundant protein found in the ECM, making up a quarter of the total protein content in many animals.[77] So far, there have been 29 different types of collagen identified, though 90% of the collagen in the body are types I, II, III, and IV. In vertebrates, approximately 22% of the total protein content is of collagen type I, and in vascular tissue, such as the aorta, 80%–90% of the collagen content is of type I or III[2]. Collagen extracted from animal and human tissues has been used due to its influence in cell adhesion and proliferation[78] as well as low inflammatory and immunogenic responses.[79] Mechanical properties of the collagen-based scaffolds, including resorption rate, may be altered according to porosity, fiber orientation, and cross-linking conditions. Commercially available collagen has, for example, been cross-linked with 1-ethyl-3-[3-dimethylaminopropyl]carbodiimide hydrochloride (EDC) and N-hydroxysulfosuccinimide (NHS) and gellated on a nanopatterned polydimethylsiloxane (PDMS) surface.[80,81] Elastin is another ECM protein and is mainly found in blood vessels, making up a large part of the ECM content of arteries. It provides the arteries with their elastic properties and also has antithrombogenic properties.[82] Elastin scaffolds have developed using recombinant human elastin grown in *Escherichia coli* and then purified.[83,84] In order to optimize the environment, multiple ECM elements can be combined. For example, in vascular tissue engineering, production of a tubular scaffold containing both collagen and elastin allowed smooth muscle cells (SMCs) to orientate themselves in line with the fibers.[85–87]

Synthetic materials

Synthetic materials were considered as a possibility for tissue engineering following their use as biomaterials in other areas of medicine. They are advantageous because (i) they are easily cheaply manufactured, (ii) they can be formed into various shapes with the required dimensions (the microstructure and nanostructure can be well controlled), and (iii) they can be produced with a range of different mechanical properties and (iv) manufactured reproducibly. For all these reasons, synthetic polymers should be the best choice for clinical translation; however, it has been clearly very difficult to replicate in a laboratory the millions of years that evolution has taken to design the structure and composition of our tissues and organs. Some of those synthetic polymers, such as the polyester polymers, have been firstly used and already employed as sutures and orthopedic fixatives such as pins, rods, and screws.[88] The advantage of those scaffolds is related to scaffold degradation that occurs through hydrolytic attack of the ester bond, and its rate is affected by adjusting various properties of the scaffold including crystallinity, molecular weight, and porosity. The existing wide clinical application of polyesters supports their biocompatibility, although some studies have suggested that there can be problems due to their propensity to disintegrate into small particles[89] or toxicity associated with acidic degradation.[90] A commonly used biodegradable synthetic polymer is polyglycolic acid (PGA). Its degradation product, glycolic acid, is a natural metabolite and can therefore be readily metabolized without toxic effect, and is already in use as a material for resorbable sutures. PGA is a polyester with high crystallinity and as such is a stiff and brittle material.[91] It also has a fast degradation rate of 6 to 8 weeks[92] when fabricated as a mesh. Cao et al.[93] reported a 40% loss of mass over 8 weeks for a PGA mesh in pH 7.4 phosphate buffered saline (PBS) at 37°C and 5% CO_2, when pretreated with NaOH. The same group has cultured SMCs on a PGA mesh in a bioreactor and has seen almost complete loss of PGA after 8 weeks and production of ECM products like collagen.[94] PLA is a semicrystalline polymer with a similar rate of degradation to that of PGA and along with PGA is one of the few biodegradable polymers approved by the Food and Drug Administration for clinical use. It is often used in its L chiral form, PLLA, as this is preferentially metabolized. Lu et al.[95] isolated outgrowth endothelial cells from rabbit peripheral blood and grew them on an electrospun PLLA scaffold, where cells grew preferentially on aligned fibers. Polycaprolactone (PCL) is another semicrystalline polyester but with a much longer degradation time than PLA. As a homopolymer, it has shown degradation times of up to 2 to 3 years.[88] Taking inspiration from the mussel byssus, with its impressive adhesive qualities, that possesses a large number of catechol moieties, the pair posited that introducing catechol moieties via a poly(dopamine) coating would increase cellular attachment.[96] When compared with uncoated and gelatin-coated, the poly(dopamine)-coated PCL showed an increased number of live human umbilical cord endothelial cells (HUVECs) on the surface. Other groups have coated electrospun PCL with collagen,[97] fibroin and chitosan,[98] or PCL films with fibrin-based coating.[99] While electrospinning is still a very popular technique for fabricating PCL[100] and other scaffolds, related methods for creating nanofibers of a similar geometry to ECM fibers are being developed, such as jet-spraying.[101] When large amounts of tissue are to be engineered, vascular supply is an issue with synthetic materials since no means of attachment to the vascular tree

can be inherently designed to the scaffold. It is in these cases that mechanical properties such as porosity become important, affecting both cell motility and vascularization.[102]

Natural acellular matrix

Natural acellular matrices are organs from humans or animals that have been treated to remove cells and immunogenic material, producing natural scaffolds that maintain their architecture of origin. Following decellularization, these scaffolds may be implanted with or without prior cell seeding, aimed at regenerating a complete organ or improving tissue repair, respectively. The benefits of this technique include the preservation of the ECM, which favorably influences cell fate, as well as of the macro- and micro-architecture. The macro-architecture is important in recreating the three-dimensional structure of the organ to be tissue-engineered as well as maintaining a vascular tree that will allow for cell and nutrient delivery and waste removal. The micro-architecture is of value toward maintaining the mechanical properties and porosity of the tissue that will be optimal for cell seeding and growth. Since ECM components are preserved across species,[103] immunogenic responses are removed.[104,105] The decellularization process can be performed in a variety of manners including mechanical, chemical, and enzymatic methods. The aim is to remove cellular material while preserving the integrity and constituents of the ECM. Mechanical methods such as snap freezing, direct pressure, and sonication have been reported to disrupt ECM.[106] The major chemical methods used for decellularization include ionic detergents such as sodium dodecyl sulfate (SDS) and sodium deoxycholate, nonionic detergents such as Triton X-100, and zwitterionic detergents such as 3-[(3-cholamidopropyl)dimethylammonio]-1-propanesulfonate hydrate (CHAPS). Our experience with intestinal and bladder decellularization has suggested that a combination of milliQ water, sodium deoxycholate, and DNase is superior to the use of Triton X-100 in preserving ECM structure and collagen/glycosaminoglycan (GAG) content while removing cellular material.[105] Comparing the benefits of each method is beyond the scope of this review, and when they are looked at, they should be examined in a tissue-specific manner. They have the added hypothetical advantages over synthetic scaffolds of not producing potentially toxic degradation products or inducing inflammation, characteristics that may be important in the prevention of stenosis.[106] A successful example of natural acellular tissue currently used in the clinic is small intestinal submucosa (SIS) harvested from mammalian small intestine and treated with peracetic acid, followed by antibiotic or radioactive sterilization. Beyond preservation of the ECM structure, GAG, and collagen content, SIS has been demonstrated to contain growth factors such as vascular endothelial growth factor (VEGF),[107] fibroblast growth factor-2 (FGF-2), and tumor growth factor-β (TGF-β).[108] VEGF stimulates angiogenesis of the tissue, whereas TGF-β has immunomodulatory properties, suppressing T-helper response and reducing inflammatory or immune reactions.[109] Collectively, these properties provide an environment for tissue growth and vascularization while maintaining sufficient mechanical strength until endogenous ECM production occurs. Clinical uses of SIS include various types of hernia repair,[110–112] anal fistula closure,[113] and dural repair.[114] Similar materials that are being examined for clinical use in tissue repair include amniotic membrane tissue, cadaveric fascia, and acellular dermis (which has been used for full-thickness burns since 1995[115]). Decellularized esophageal scaffolds have been used with reportedly good results in both preclinical and clinical studies.[116,117] Significant heterogeneity exists among studies with respect to the type of scaffold, extent of surgery, and species used, which partly explains the range of results reported. Thus, regeneration of the muscularis propria layer is seen to take place in some studies.[118] Badylak et al.[117] laid sheets of SIS onto the raw internal surface of esophagus following endoscopic submucosal resection in five patients with superficial cancers. With a follow-up of 4–24 months, the scaffold promoted physiological remodeling as evidenced by endoscopy and histological characterization following biopsy. Strictures still formed, but only at areas outside those lined by SIS, suggesting possible technical improvements in scaffold delivery. In fact, when SIS was used to completely cover a 3 × 5 cm mucosal defect in the cervical esophagus, there was no stenosis or other complications and endoscopy at 4 weeks demonstrated good integration of the scaffold.[119] Hypothetically, decellularized esophageal tissue should retain the signals, both chemical and structural, that will direct the appropriate migration and differentiation of host cells, in a way that is unlikely to occur with scaffolds originating outside the esophagus, such as SIS. Ozeki et al.[120] compared two methods of decellularization of adult rat esophagus based on deoxycholate and Triton X-100, respectively, and assessed the resultant tissue using routine histology and biocompatibility. Those treated with deoxycholate showed superior mechanical properties, maintenance of the ECM, and a lower DNA content than those treated with Triton X-100. Bhrany et al.[121] found a combination of 0.5% SDS and Triton X-100 to be effective in decellularization, albeit with a loss of tensile strength as measured by burst pressure studies.[121]

Cell-derived ECM scaffolds

Instead of decellularizing blood vessels to obtain vascular ECM for cell seeding, some groups have taken the approach of culturing vascular cells to produce vascular ECM and then decellularizing. The cells can be allo- or xenogenic, and a much greater degree of control can be had over the manufacture, increasing reproducibility. This is an important factor in good manufacture practices (GMP), necessary if one wishes to take a tissue-engineered device from a lab to a clinic. The fibroblasts can produce a large amount of ECM, which autologous seeded SMCs seeded may not be able to do, depending on patient age, history, and site of extraction. The Niklason group at Yale has seeded SMCs from pigs,[122]

canines, or humans,[123] onto PGA scaffolds and cultured them in a biomimetic bioreactor for 10 weeks, before decellularizing the scaffold with a detergent treatment. The scaffolds can then be seeded with cells or implanted directly.

TISSUE ENGINEERING

In order to give rise to a new functional organ-like structure, several variables such as local environment, nutrients, and metabolites are pivotal. Major developments in the clinic have been achieved in the last few years using relatively simple scaffolds. Atala et al.[124] presented in 2006 a series of seven children with myelomeningocele, aged 4–19 years, with high-pressure or poorly compliant bladders, who successfully received an engineered bladder tissues. Briefly, after undergoing a bladder biopsy, urothelial and muscle cells were grown and then seeded onto a biodegradable bladder-shaped scaffold made of collagen, or a composite of collagen and PGA. About 7 weeks after the biopsy, the autologous engineered bladder constructs were implanted and wrapped in omentum with good long-term (mean 46 months) results.[124] The same group described in 2011 their experience with five boys who, following trauma, between 2004 and 2007 underwent urethral reconstruction using tubularized urethras seeded with autologous cells that remained functional for up to 6 years.[125] Macchiarini et al.[126] in 2008, using a decellularized human trachea seeded with autologous epithelial and MSC-derived chondrocytes, successfully transplanted a 30-year-old woman with end-stage bronchomalacia. The engineered left bronchus, at 4 months, functioned normally and was free from the risks of rejection. Using a similar approach, we have recently reported the first child who received a stem-cell-based tracheal replacement with a good functional outcome after 2 years of follow-up (Figure 27.6).[127] Interestingly, for this case, the scaffold was transplanted right after seeding without bioreactor conditioning, and SC engraftment was encouraged both by systemic granulocyte colony stimulating factor and human recombinant erythropoietin, associated with topical human recombinant erythropoietin and transforming growth factor β. Differently, endothelial and smooth muscle cells differentiated from the BM of the recipient were seeded on a decellularized donor iliac vein graft prior to transplantation in a 10-year-old girl with extrahepatic portal vein obstruction.[128] The graft was initially successful, but it was substituted after a year by a second tissue-engineered construct, which restored portal circulation. Decellularized tissue may, however, be not always the best. In 2001, a 4-year-old girl with a single right ventricle and pulmonary atresia, who underwent the Fontan procedure at the age of 3 years, was transplanted with a PCL–PLA copolymer (weight ratio, 1:1) reinforced with woven PGA seeded with autologous cells to bypass the total occlusion of the right intermediate pulmonary artery. Ten days after seeding, the graft was transplanted with no postoperative complications, and at 7 months the patient was doing well, with no evidence of graft occlusion or aneurysmal changes on chest radiography.[129]

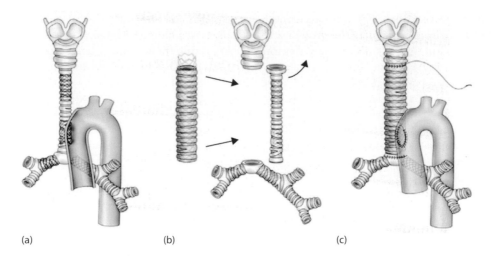

(a)   (b)   (c)

Figure 27.6 Schematic representation of the tissue-engineered trachea transplanted at Great Ormond Street Hospital in 2010. During surgery, the airway was found to be severely stenotic with multiple stents including one entering the ascending aorta **(a)**. The old homograft trachea was removed and replaced by the engineered graft. **(b)** The aortic defect was closed with a bovine pericardial patch and air leaks sealed **(c)**. (From Elliott, M. J. et al., *Lancet*, 380, 994–1000, 2012.)

More recently, a 36-year-old man, with recurrent primary cancer of the distal trachea and main bronchi, underwent excisional surgery followed by a reconstruction of his airway with a tailored bioartificial nanocomposite previously seeded with autologous BM mononuclear cells via a bioreactor for 36 hours.[130] More complex organs, such as the liver or the kidney, may require more time before being applied for therapy. Atala's group has described a perfusion decellularization technique for the liver and kidney generating decellularized organ scaffolds for organ bioengineering.[131] In an analogous fashion, Uygun et al.[132,133] have reported a successful approach of decellularizing rat livers and recellularizing them with rat primary hepatocytes, showing promising hepatic function and the ability to transplant heterotopically these bioengineered livers into animals for up to 8 hours. The decellularization approach was pioneered in the heart by Ott et al.[134] who showed that not only it was possible to generate whole organ scaffolds using a perfusion decellularization system but also that neonatal rat cardiomyocytes (delivered through transmural injection) and endothelial cells (injected through the aorta) could generate a contractile construct. Using a similar approach, lungs have also been regenerated through the seeding of pulmonary epithelium and vascular endothelium on rat lung ECM.[135] Among unmet clinical needs, intestinal engineering is particularly relevant, especially because of the relatively poor outcome of intestinal transplantation. However, although pioneering investigations in the field of intestinal bioengineering date back to the 1980s,[136] initial excitement has been blunted by the considerable limitations and roadblocks encountered in the course of experimental investigations. The main culprit of such stagnation is the complexity of intestinal anatomy and the various functions of the intestine. Vacanti's group showed that rodent organoid units seeded on a nonwoven PGA fiber and implanted in rats

having undergone the resection of 85% of their native intestine were able to partially replace gut function.[137–139] Bioengineered intestinal constructs were also successfully transplanted in pigs (Figure 27.7),[140] but this technology is inefficient because several centimeters of bowel are needed to obtain a sufficient number of organoid units that are able to repopulate just a few centimeters of engineered intestine.[141] Intestinal SCs, which reside in the base of Lieberkuhn crypts and express Lgr5,[20,142] have been shown to be capable of building crypt–villus structures in vitro without any mesenchymal niche.[143] As these cells could be reliably expanded in culture, they could represent the ideal source of progenitor cells for intestinal bioengineering. Although representing only an initial step toward the ultimate goal of generating fully functional organs, decellularized matrices may help in understanding the functional structure of complex organs and may represent in the midterm the bridge for transplantation since some of these structures may be difficult to mimic artificially.[104] Those barriers could be overcome by producing three-dimensional vascularized cellular constructs of clinically relevant size, shape, and structural integrity. Very recently, we have witnessed the first report of an integrated tissue-organ printer that could fabricate stable, human-scale tissue constructs of any shape. Biodegradable polymers and hydrogels could be printed to the correct shape by representing clinical imaging data as a computer model of the anatomical defect and translating the model into a program that controls the motions of the printer nozzles, which dispense cells to discrete locations.[144] Using this integrated tissue-organ printer (ITOP) technology, the authors could demonstrate capabilities of the ITOP by fabricating mandible and calvarial bone, cartilage, and skeletal muscle. Future development of the ITOP may lead to the production of tissues for human applications and to the building of more complex tissues and solid organs.

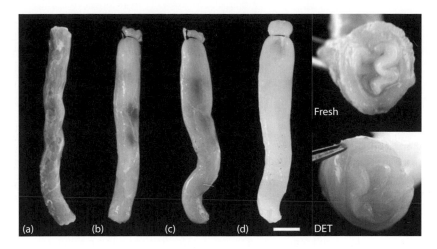

Figure 27.7 Decellularization of pig esophagus with detergent enzymatic treatment (DET) **(a–d)**. Macroscopic appearance of the esophagus during the decellularization process at cycle 0 **(a)**, 1 **(b)**, 2 **(c)**, and 3 **(d)**. The esophagus was perfused through the lumen with continuous fluid delivery, as described in the methods. The esophageal wall of the treated samples appeared gradually more translucent than the fresh tissue. Scale bar, 14 mm. (From Totonelli, G. et al., *Pediatric Surgery International* 29, 87–95, 2013.)

CONCLUSION

We are leading a very exciting time in medicine. Tissue and organ regeneration will revolutionize the treatment of diseases. It will be particularly interesting to observe the evolution of surgical approaches to malformations and organ transplantation, and the totally new possibility of correcting them using autologous tailor-made functional tissue.

REFERENCES

1. Placzek MR et al. Stem cell bioprocessing: Fundamentals and principles. *J R Soc Interface/ The Royal Society* 2009; 6:209–32, doi:10.1098 /rsif.2008.0442.
2. Safinia L, Datan N, Hohse M, Mantalaris A, Bismarck A. Towards a methodology for the effective surface modification of porous polymer scaffolds. *Biomaterials* 2005; 26:7537–47, doi:10.1016/j .biomaterials.2005.05.078.
3. Carraro A et al. In vitro analysis of a hepatic device with intrinsic microvascular-based channels. *Biomed Microdevices* 2008; 10:795–805, doi:10.1007 /s10544-008-9194-3.
4. Nagy RD et al. Stem cell transplantation as a therapeutic approach to organ failure. *J Surg Res* 2005; 129:152–60, doi:10.1016/j.jss.2005.04.016.
5. Jiang Y et al. Pluripotency of mesenchymal stem cells derived from adult marrow. *Nature* 2002; 418:41–9, doi:10.1038/nature00870.
6. Pittenger MF et al. Multilineage potential of adult human mesenchymal stem cells. *Science* 1999; 284:143–147.
7. McKinney-Freeman SL et al. Muscle-derived hematopoietic stem cells are hematopoietic in origin. *Proc Natl Acad Sci USA* 2002; 99:1341–6, doi:10.1073 /pnas.032438799.
8. Schwartz RE et al. Multipotent adult progenitor cells from bone marrow differentiate into functional hepatocyte-like cells. *J Clin Investig* 2002; 109:1291–302, doi:10.1172/JCI15182 .
9. LaBarge MA, Blau HM. Biological progression from adult bone marrow to mononucleate muscle stem cell to multinucleate muscle fiber in response to injury. *Cell* 2002; 111:589–601.
10. Ferrari G et al. Muscle regeneration by bone marrow-derived myogenic progenitors. *Science* 1998; 279:1528–30.
11. Shamblott MJ et al. Human embryonic germ cell derivatives express a broad range of developmentally distinct markers and proliferate extensively in vitro. *Proc Natl Acad Sci USA* 2001; 98:113–8, doi:10.1073/pnas.021537998.
12. Kofidis T et al. Myocardial restoration with embryonic stem cell bioartificial tissue transplantation. *J Heart Lung Transplant* 2005; 24:737–44, doi:10.1016/j.healun.2004.03.023.
13. Thomson JA et al. Embryonic stem cell lines derived from human blastocysts. *Science* 1998; 282:1145–7.
14. Markel TA et al. Stem cells as a potential future treatment of pediatric intestinal disorders. *J Pediatr Surg* 2008; 43:1953–63, doi:10.1016/j .jpedsurg.2008.06.019.
15. De Coppi P et al. Isolation of amniotic stem cell lines with potential for therapy. *Nat Biotechnol* 2007; 25:100–6, doi:10.1038/nbt1274.

16. Takahashi K, Yamanaka S. Induction of pluripotent stem cells from mouse embryonic and adult fibroblast cultures by defined factors. *Cell* 2006; 126:663–76, doi:10.1016/j.cell.2006.07.024.

17. Odorico JS, Kaufman DS, Thomson JA. Multilineage differentiation from human embryonic stem cell lines. *Stem Cells* 2001; 19:193–204, doi:10.1634/stemcells.19-3-193).

18. Amit M, Shariki C, Margulets V, Itskovitz-Eldor J. Feeder layer- and serum-free culture of human embryonic stem cells. *Biol Reprod* 2004; 70:837–45, doi:10.1095/biolreprod.103.021147.

19. Richards M, Fong CY, Chan WK, Wong PC, Bongso A. Human feeders support prolonged undifferentiated growth of human inner cell masses and embryonic stem cells. *Nat Biotechnol* 2002; 20:933–6, doi:10.1038/ nbt726.

20. Evans GS, Flint N, Somers AS, Eyden B, Potten CS. The development of a method for the preparation of rat intestinal epithelial cell primary cultures. *J Cell Sci* 1992; 101(Pt 1):219–31.

21. Martin GR. Isolation of a pluripotent cell line from early mouse embryos cultured in medium conditioned by teratocarcinoma stem cells. *Proc Natl Acad Sci USA* 1981; 78:7634–8.

22. Fong H, Hohenstein KA, Donovan PJ. Regulation of self-renewal and pluripotency by Sox2 in human embryonic stem cells. *Stem Cells* 2008; 26:1931–8, doi:10.1634/stemcells.2007-1002.

23. Lott JP, Savulescu J. Towards a global human embryonic stem cell bank. *Am J Bioeth* 2007; 7:37–44, doi:10.1080/15265160701462426.

24. Hipp J, Atala A. Sources of stem cells for regenerative medicine. *Stem Cell Rev* 2008; 4:3–11, doi:10.1007/s12015-008-9010-8.

25. Klimanskaya I, Chung Y, Becker S, Lu SJ, Lanza R. Human embryonic stem cell lines derived from single blastomeres. *Nature* 2006; 444:481–5, doi:10.1038/nature05142.

26. Chung Y et al. Embryonic and extraembryonic stem cell lines derived from single mouse blastomeres. *Nature* 2006; 439:216–9, doi:10.1038/nature04277.

27. Deb KD, Sarda K. Human embryonic stem cells: Preclinical perspectives. *J Transl Med* 2008; 6:7, doi:10.1186/1479-5876-6-7.

28. Briggs R, King TJ. Transplantation of living nuclei from blastula cells into enucleated frogs' eggs. *Proc Natl Acad Sci USA* 1952; 38:455–463.

29. Gurdon JB, Laskey RA. The transplantation of nuclei from single cultured cells into enucleate frogs' eggs. *J Embryol Exp Morphol* 1970; 24:227–48.

30. Campbell KH, McWhir J, Ritchie WA, Wilmut I. Sheep cloned by nuclear transfer from a cultured cell line. *Nature* 1996; 380:64–6, doi:10.1038/380064a0.

31. Franco D, Moreno N, Ruiz-Lozano P. Non-resident stem cell populations in regenerative cardiac medicine. *Cell Mol Life Sci* 2007; 64:683–91, doi:10.1007/s00018-007-6521-4.

32. Dalgetty DM, Medine CN, Iredale JP, Hay DC. Progress and future challenges in stem cell-derived liver technologies. *Ame J Physiol Gastrointest Liver Physiol* 2009; 297:G241–8, doi:10.1152/ajpgi.00138.2009.

33. Anglani F et al. In search of adult renal stem cells. *J Cell Mol Med* 2004; 8:474–87.

34. Lerou PH et al. Human embryonic stem cell derivation from poor-quality embryos. *Nat Biotechnol* 2008; 26:212–4, doi:10.1038/nbt1378.

35. Yu J et al. Induced pluripotent stem cell lines derived from human somatic cells. *Science* 2007; 318:1917–20, doi:10.1126/science.1151526.

36. Takahashi K et al. Induction of pluripotent stem cells from adult human fibroblasts by defined factors. *Cell* 2007; 131:861–72, doi:10.1016/j.cell.2007.11.019.

37. Okita K, Nakagawa M, Hyenjong H, Ichisaka T, Yamanaka S. Generation of mouse induced pluripotent stem cells without viral vectors. *Science* 2008; 322:949–53, doi:10.1126/science.1164270.

38. Meissner A, Wernig M, Jaenisch R. Direct reprogramming of genetically unmodified fibroblasts into pluripotent stem cells. *Nat Biotechnol* 2007; 25:1177–81, doi:10.1038/nbt1335.

39. Yu J, Thomson JA. Pluripotent stem cell lines. *Genes Dev* 2008; 22:1987–97, doi:10.1101/gad.1689808.

40. Zsebo KM et al. Stem cell factor is encoded at the Sl locus of the mouse and is the ligand for the c-kit tyrosine kinase receptor. *Cell* 1990; 63:213–24.

41. Burns AJ, Goldstein AM, Newgreen DF et al. White paper on guidelines concerning enteric nervous system stem cell therapy for enteric neuropathies. *Dev Biol* 2016; 417:229–251.

42. Fattahi F et al. Deriving human ENS lineages for cell therapy and drug discovery in Hirschsprung disease. *Nature* 2016; 531:105–9, doi:10.1038/nature16951.

43. Moschidou D et al. Valproic acid confers functional pluripotency to human amniotic fluid stem cells in a transgene-free approach. *Mol Ther* 2012; 20(10):1953–67, doi:10.1038/mt.2012.117.

44. Bollini S et al. In vitro and in vivo cardiomyogenic differentiation of amniotic fluid stem cells. *Stem Cell Rev* 2011; 7:364–80, doi:10.1007/ s12015-010-9200-z.

45. Decembrini S et al. Comparative analysis of the retinal potential of embryonic stem cells and amniotic fluid-derived stem cells. *Stem Cells Dev* 2011; 20:851–63, doi:10.1089/scd.2010.0291.

46. Bollini S et al. Amniotic fluid stem cells are cardioprotective following acute myocardial infarction. *Stem Cells Dev* 2011; 20:1985–94, doi:10.1089/scd.2010.0424.

47. Chiavegato A et al. Human amniotic fluid-derived stem cells are rejected after transplantation in the myocardium of normal, ischemic, immuno-suppressed or immuno-deficient rat. *J Mol Cell Cardiol* 2007; 42:746–59, doi:10.1016/j.yjmcc.2006.12.008.

48. Rota C et al. Human amniotic fluid stem cell preconditioning improves their regenerative potential. *Stem Cells Dev* 2012; 21:1911–23, doi:10.1089/scd.2011.0333.

49. De Coppi P et al. Amniotic fluid and bone marrow derived mesenchymal stem cells can be converted to smooth muscle cells in the cryo-injured rat bladder and prevent compensatory hypertrophy of surviving smooth muscle cells. *J Urol* 2007; 177:369–76, doi:10.1016/j.juro.2006.09.103.

50. Ditadi A et al. Human and murine amniotic fluid c-Kit+Lin- cells display hematopoietic activity. *Blood* 2009; 113:3953–60, doi:10.1182/blood-2008-10-182105.

51. Piccoli M et al. Amniotic fluid stem cells restore the muscle cell niche in a HSA-Cre, Smn(F7/F7) mouse model. *Stem Cells* 2012; 30:1675–84, doi:10.1002/stem.1134.

52. Cananzi M, Atala A, De Coppi P. Stem cells derived from amniotic fluid: New potentials in regenerative medicine. *Reprod Biomed Online* 2009; 18 Suppl 1:17–27.

53. Pan GJ, Chang ZY, Scholer HR, Pei D. Stem cell pluripotency and transcription factor Oct4. *Cell Res* 2002; 12:321–9, doi:10.1038/sj.cr.7290134.

54. Fuchs JR et al. Diaphragmatic reconstruction with autologous tendon engineered from mesenchymal amniocytes. *J Pediatr Surg* 2004; 39:834–8; discussion 834–838.

55. Turner CG et al. Preclinical regulatory validation of an engineered diaphragmatic tendon made with amniotic mesenchymal stem cells. *J Pediatr Surg* 2011; 46:57–61, doi:10.1016/j.jpedsurg.2010.09.063.

56. Friedenstein AJ, Petrakova KV, Kurolesova AI, Frolova GP. Heterotopic of bone marrow. Analysis of precursor cells for osteogenic and hematopoietic tissues. *Transplantation* 1968; 6:230–47.

57. Friedenstein AJ et al. Precursors for fibroblasts in different populations of hematopoietic cells as detected by the in vitro colony assay method. *Exp Hematol* 1974; 2:83–92.

58. Campagnoli C et al. Identification of mesenchymal stem/progenitor cells in human first-trimester fetal blood, liver, and bone marrow. *Blood* 2001; 98:2396–402.

59. In't Anker PS et al. Amniotic fluid as a novel source of mesenchymal stem cells for therapeutic transplantation. *Blood* 2003; 102:1548–9, doi:10.1182/blood-2003-04-1291.

60. Tsai MS, Lee JL, Chang YJ, Hwang SM. Isolation of human multipotent mesenchymal stem cells from second-trimester amniotic fluid using a novel two-stage culture protocol. *Hum Reprod* 2004; 19:1450–6, doi:10.1093/humrep/deh279.

61. Fan CG et al. Characterization and neural differentiation of fetal lung mesenchymal stem cells. *Cell Transplant* 2005; 14:311–21.

62. Waddington RJ, Youde SJ, Lee CP, Sloan AJ. Isolation of distinct progenitor stem cell populations from dental pulp. *Cells Tissues Organs* 2009; 189:268–74, doi:10.1159/000151447.

63. Eyckmans J, Luyten FP. Species specificity of ectopic bone formation using periosteum-derived mesenchymal progenitor cells. *Tissue Eng* 2006; 12:2203–13, doi:10.1089/ten.2006.12.2203.

64. Erices A, Conget P, Minguell JJ. Mesenchymal progenitor cells in human umbilical cord blood. *Br J Haematol* 2000; 109:235–42.

65. Romanov YA, Svintsitskaya VA, Smirnov VN. Searching for alternative sources of postnatal human mesenchymal stem cells: Candidate MSC-like cells from umbilical cord. *Stem Cells* 2003; 21:105–10, doi:10.1634/stemcells.21-1-105.

66. Igura K et al. Isolation and characterization of mesenchymal progenitor cells from chorionic villi of human placenta. *Cytotherapy* 2004; 6: 543–53.

67. Horwitz EM et al. Clarification of the nomenclature for MSC: The International Society for Cellular Therapy position statement. *Cytotherapy* 2005; 7:393–5, doi:10.1080/14653240500319234.

68. Horwitz EM et al. Isolated allogeneic bone marrow-derived mesenchymal cells engraft and stimulate growth in children with osteogenesis imperfecta: Implications for cell therapy of bone. *Proc Natl Acad Sci USA* 2002; 99:8932–7, doi:10.1073/pnas.132252399.

69. Horwitz EM et al. Transplantability and therapeutic effects of bone marrow-derived mesenchymal cells in children with osteogenesis imperfecta. *Nat Med* 1999; 5:309–13, doi:10.1038/6529.

70. Koc ON et al. Allogeneic mesenchymal stem cell infusion for treatment of metachromatic leukodystrophy (MLD) and Hurler syndrome (MPS-IH). *Bone Marrow Transplant* 2002; 30:215–22, doi:10.1038/sj.bmt.1703650.

71. Whyte MP et al. Marrow cell transplantation for infantile hypophosphatasia. *J Bone Miner Res* 2003; 18:624–36, doi:10.1359/jbmr.2003.18.4.624.

72. Le Blanc K et al. Fetal mesenchymal stem-cell engraftment in bone after in utero transplantation in a patient with severe osteogenesis imperfecta. *Transplantation* 2005; 79:1607–14.

73. Giancotti FG, Ruoslahti E. Integrin signaling. *Science* 1999; 285:1028–32.

74. Hynes RO. The extracellular matrix: Not just pretty fibrils. *Science* 2009; 326:1216–9, doi:10.1126/science.1176009.

75. Engler AJ, Sen S, Sweeney HL, Discher DE. Matrix elasticity directs stem cell lineage specification. *Cell* 2006; 126:677–89, doi:10.1016/j.cell.2006.06.044.

76. Bailey AJ. The nature of collagen. In: Florkin M, Stotz EH (eds). *Comprehensive Biochemistry*. New York: Elsevier, 1968:297–424.

77. Staatz WD et al. Identification of a tetrapeptide recognition sequence for the alpha 2 beta 1 integrin in collagen. *J Biol Chem* 1991; 266:7363–7.

78. DeLustro F, Condell RA, Nguyen MA, McPherson JM. A comparative study of the biologic and immunologic response to medical devices derived from dermal collagen. *J Biomed Mater Res* 1986; 20:109–20, doi:10.1002/jbm.820200110.

79. Zorlutuna P, Elsheikh A, Hasirci V. Nanopatterning of collagen scaffolds improve the mechanical properties of tissue engineered vascular grafts. *Biomacromolecules* 2009; 10:814–21, doi:10.1021/bm801307y.

80. Zorlutuna P, Vadgama P, Hasirci V. Both sides nanopatterned tubular collagen scaffolds as tissue-engineered vascular grafts. *J Tissue Eng Regen Med* 2010; 4:628–37, doi:10.1002/term.278.

81. Waterhouse A, Wise SG, Ng MK, Weiss AS. Elastin as a nonthrombogenic biomaterial. *Tissue Eng Part B, Rev* 2011; 17:93–9, doi:10.1089/ten.TEB.2010.0432.

82. Bozzini S et al. Enzymatic cross-linking of human recombiat elastin (HELP) as biomimetic approach in vascular tissue engineering. *J Mater Sci Mater Med* 2011; 22:2641–50, doi:10.1007/s10856-011-4451-z.

83. McKenna KA et al. Mechanical property characterization of electrospun recombinant human tropo-elastin for vascular graft biomaterials. *Acta Biomater* 2012; 8:225–33, doi:10.1016/j.actbio.2011.08.001.

84. Koens MJ et al. Controlled fabrication of triple layered and molecularly defined collagen/elastin vascular grafts resembling the native blood vessel. *Acta Biomater* 2010; 6:4666–74, doi:10.1016/j.actbio.2010.06.038.

85. Caves JM et al. The use of microfiber composites of elastin-like protein matrix reinforced with synthetic collagen in the design of vascular grafts. *Biomaterials* 2010; 31:7175–82, doi:10.1016/j.biomaterials.2010.05.014.

86. Kumar VA et al. Collagen-based substrates with tunable strength for soft tissue engineering. *Biomater Sci* 2013; 1, doi:10.1039/C3BM60129C.

87. Gunatillake PA, Adhikari R. Biodegradable synthetic polymers for tissue engineering. *Eur Cell Mater* 2003; 5:1–16; discussion 16.

88. Verheyen CC, de Wijn JR, van Blitterswijk CA, Rozing PM, de Groot K. Examination of efferent lymph nodes after 2 years of transcortical implantation of poly(L-lactide) containing plugs: A case report. *J Biomed Mater Res* 1993; 27:1115–8, doi:10.1002/jbm.820270817.

89. Taylor MS, Daniels AU, Andriano KP, Heller J. Six bioabsorbable polymers: In vitro acute toxicity of accumulated degradation products. *J Appl Biomater* 1994; 5:151–7, doi:10.1002/jab.770050208.

90. Hajiali H, Shahgasempour S, Naimi-Jamal MR, Peirovi H. Electrospun PGA/gelatin nanofibrous scaffolds and their potential application in vascular tissue engineering. *Int J Nanomedicine* 2011; 6:2133–41, doi:10.2147/IJN.S24312.

91. Kakisis JD, Liapis CD, Breuer C, Sumpio BE. Artificial blood vessel: The Holy Grail of peripheral vascular surgery. *J Vasc Surg* 2005; 41:349–54, doi:10.1016/j.jvs.2004.12.026.

92. Cao Y et al. Forty-year journey of angiogenesis translational research. *Sci Transl Med* 2011; 3:114rv113, doi:10.1126/scitranslmed.3003149.

93. Huang AH, Niklason LE. Engineering biological-based vascular grafts using a pulsatile bioreactor. *J Vis Exp* 2011; (52), doi:10.3791/2646.

94. Lu H, Feng Z, Gu Z, Liu C. Growth of outgrowth endothelial cells on aligned PLLA nanofibrous scaffolds. *J Mater Sci Mater Med* 2009; 20:1937–44, doi:10.1007/s10856-009-3744-y.

95. Ku SH, Park CB. Human endothelial cell growth on mussel-inspired nanofiber scaffold for vascular tissue engineering. *Biomaterials* 2010; 31:9431–7, doi:10.1016/j.biomaterials.2010.08.071.

96. Tillman BW et al. The in vivo stability of electrospun polycaprolactone-collagen scaffolds in vascular reconstruction. *Biomaterials* 2009; 30:583–8, doi:10.1016/j.biomaterials.2008.10.006.

97. Zhao J et al. Development of nanofibrous scaffolds for vascular tissue engineering. *Int J Biol Macromol* 2013; 56:106–13, doi:10.1016/j.ijbiomac.2013.01.027.

98. Mathews A, Colombus S, Krishnan VK, Krishnan LK. Vascular tissue construction on poly(epsilon-caprolactone) scaffolds by dynamic endothelial cell seeding: Effect of pore size. *J Tissue Eng Regen Med* 2012; 6:451–61, doi:10.1002/term.449.

99. Fioretta ES, Simonet M, Smits AI, Baaijens FP, Bouten CV. Differential response of endothelial and endothelial colony forming cells on electrospun scaffolds with distinct microfiber diameters. *Biomacromolecules* 2014; 15:821–9, doi:10.1021/bm4016418.

100. Sohier J, Corre P, Perret C, Pilet P, Weiss P. Novel and simple alternative to create nanofibrillar matrices of interest for tissue engineering. *Tissue Eng. Part C, Methods* 2014; 20:285–96, doi:10.1089/ten.TEC.2013.0147.

101. Brauker JH et al. Neovascularization of synthetic membranes directed by membrane microarchitecture. *J Biomed Mater Res* 1995; 29:1517–24, doi:10.1002/jbm.820291208.

102. Bernard MP et al. Structure of a cDNA for the pro alpha 2 chain of human type I procollagen. Comparison with chick cDNA for pro alpha 2(I) identifies structurally conserved features of the protein and the gene. *Biochemistry* 1983; 22:1139–45.

103. Totonelli G et al. A rat decellularized small bowel scaffold that preserves villus-crypt architecture for intestinal regeneration. *Biomaterials* 2012; 33:3401–10, doi:10.1016/j.biomaterials.2012.01.012.

104. Totonelli G et al. Detergent enzymatic treatment for the development of a natural acellular matrix for oesophageal regeneration. *Pediatr Surg Int* 2013; 29:87–95, doi:10.1007/s00383-012-3194-3.

105. Gilbert TW, Sellaro TL, Badylak SF. Decellularization of tissues and organs. *Biomaterials* 2006; 27:3675–83, doi:10.1016/j.biomaterials.2006.02.014.

106. Hodde JP, Record RD, Liang HA, Badylak SF. Vascular endothelial growth factor in porcine-derived extracellular matrix. *Endothelium* 2001; 8:11–24.

107. Voytik-Harbin SL, Brightman AO, Kraine MR, Waisner B, Badylak SF. Identification of extractable growth factors from small intestinal submucosa. *J Cell Biochem* 1997; 67:478–91.

108. Palmer EM et al. Human helper T cell activation and differentiation is suppressed by porcine small intestinal submucosa. *Tissue Eng* 2002; 8:893–900, doi:10.1089/10763270260424259.

109. Oelschlager BK et al. Biologic prosthesis reduces recurrence after laparoscopic paraesophageal hernia repair: A multicenter, prospective, randomized trial. *Ann Surg* 2006; 244:481–90, doi:10.1097/01.sla.0000237759.42831.03.

110. Helton WS et al. Short-term outcomes with small intestinal submucosa for ventral abdominal hernia. *Arch Surg* 2005; 140:549–60; discussion 560–42, doi:10.1001/archsurg.140.6.549.

111. Franklin ME Jr et al. The use of porcine small intestinal submucosa as a prosthetic material for laparoscopic hernia repair in infected and potentially contaminated fields: Long-term follow-up. *Surg Endosc* 2008; 22:1941–6, doi:10.1007/s00464-008-0005-y.

112. Champagne BJ et al. Efficacy of anal fistula plug in closure of cryptoglandular fistulas: Long-term follow-up. *Dis Colon Rectum* 2006; 49:1817–21, doi:10.1007/s10350-006-0755-3.

113. Bejjani GK, Zabramski J, Durasis Study Group. Safety and efficacy of the porcine small intestinal submucosa dural substitute: Results of a prospective multicenter study and literature review. *J Neurosurg* 2007; 106:1028–33, doi:10.3171/jns.2007.106.6.1028.

114. Wainwright DJ. Use of an acellular allograft dermal matrix (AlloDerm) in the management of full-thickness burns. *Burns* 1995; 21:243–8.

115. Badylak S, Meurling S, Chen M, Spievack A, Simmons-Byrd A. Resorbable bioscaffold for esophageal repair in a dog model. *J Pediatr Surg* 2000; 35:1097–103, doi:10.1053/jpsu.2000.7834.

116. Badylak SF et al. Esophageal preservation in five male patients after endoscopic inner-layer circumferential resection in the setting of superficial cancer: A regenerative medicine approach with a biologic scaffold. *Tissue Eng Part A* 2011; 17:1643–50, doi:10.1089/ten.TEA.2010.0739.

117. Nieponice A, Gilbert TW, Badylak SF. Reinforcement of esophageal anastomoses with an extracellular matrix scaffold in a canine model. *Ann Thorac Surg* 2006; 82:2050–8, doi:10.1016/j.athoracsur.2006.06.036.

118. Clough A, Ball J, Smith GS, Leibman S. Porcine small intestine submucosa matrix (Surgisis) for esophageal perforation. *Ann Thorac Surg* 2011; 91:e15–6, doi:10.1016/j.athoracsur.2010.10.011.

119. Ozeki M et al. Evaluation of decellularized esophagus as a scaffold for cultured esophageal epithelial cells. *J Biomed Mater Res Part A* 2006; 79:771–8, doi:10.1002/jbm.a.30885.

120. Bhrany AD et al. Development of an esophagus acellular matrix tissue scaffold. *Tissue Eng* 2006; 12:319–30, doi:10.1089/ten.2006.12.319.

121. Gui L et al. Development of novel biodegradable polymer scaffolds for vascular tissue engineering. *Tissue Eng Part A* 2011; 17:1191–200, doi:10.1089/ten.TEA.2010.0508.

122. Dahl SL et al. Readily available tissue-engineered vascular grafts. *Sci Transl Med* 3, 68ra69, doi:10.1126/scitranslmed.3001426.

123. Atala A, Bauer SB, Soker S, Yoo JJ, Retik AB. Tissue-engineered autologous bladders for patients needing cystoplasty. *Lancet* 2006; 367:1241–6, doi:10.1016/S0140-6736(06)68438-9.

124. Raya-Rivera A et al. Tissue-engineered autologous urethras for patients who need reconstruction: An observational study. *Lancet* 2011; 377:1175–82, doi:10.1016/S0140-6736(10)62354-9.

125. Macchiarini P et al. Clinical transplantation of a tissue-engineered airway. *Lancet* 2008; 372:2023–30, doi:10.1016/S0140-6736(08)61598-6.

126. Elliott MJ et al. Stem-cell-based, tissue engineered tracheal replacement in a child: A 2-year follow-up study. *Lancet* 2012; 380(9846):994–1000, doi:10.1016/S0140-6736(12)60737-5.

127. Olausson M et al. Transplantation of an allogeneic vein bioengineered with autologous stem cells: A proof-of-concept study. *Lancet* 2012; 380:230–7, doi:10.1016/S0140-6736(12)60633-3.

128. Shin'oka T, Imai Y, Ikada Y. Transplantation of a tissue-engineered pulmonary artery. *New Engl J Med* 2001; 344:532–3, doi:10.1056/NEJM200102153440717.

129. Jungebluth P et al. Tracheobronchial transplantation with a stem-cell-seeded bioartificial nanocomposite: A proof-of-concept study. *Lancet* 2011; 378:1997–2004, doi:10.1016/S0140-6736(11)61715-7.

130. Baptista PM et al. The use of whole organ decellularization for the generation of a vascularized liver organoid. *Hepatology* 2011; 53:604–17, doi:10.1002/hep.24067.

131. Uygun BE et al. Organ reengineering through development of a transplantable recellularized liver graft using decellularized liver matrix. *Nat Med* 2010; 16:814–20, doi:10.1038/nm.2170.

132. Uygun BE et al. Decellularization and recellularization of whole livers. *J Vis Exp* 2011; (48), doi:10.3791/2394.

133. Ott HC et al. Perfusion-decellularized matrix: Using nature's platform to engineer a bioartificial heart. *Nat Med* 2008; 14:213–21, doi:10.1038/nm1684.

134. Ott HC et al. Regeneration and orthotopic transplantation of a bioartificial lung. *Nat Med.* 2010; 16:927–33, doi:10.1038/nm.2193.

135. Vacanti JP et al. Selective cell transplantation using bioabsorbable artificial polymers as matrices. *J Pediatr Surg* 1988; 23:3–9.

136. Choi RS, Vacanti JP. Preliminary studies of tissue-engineered intestine using isolated epithelial organoid units on tubular synthetic biodegradable scaffolds. *Transplant Proc* 1997; 29:848–51.

137. Kim SS et al. Regenerative signals for tissue-engineered small intestine. *Transplant Proc* 1999; 31:657–60.

138. Grikscheit TC et al. Tissue-engineered small intestine improves recovery after massive small bowel resection. *Ann Surgery* 2004; 240:748–54.

139. Sala FG, Kunisaki SM, Ochoa ER, Vacanti J, Grikscheit TC. Tissue-engineered small intestine and stomach form from autologous tissue in a preclinical large animal model. *J Surg Res* 2009; 156:205–12, doi:10.1016/j.jss.2009.03.062.

140. Dunn JC. Is the tissue-engineered intestine clinically viable? *Nat Clin Pract Gastroenterol Hepatol* 2008; 5:366–7, doi:10.1038/ncpgasthep1151.

141. Li L, Clevers H. Coexistence of quiescent and active adult stem cells in mammals. *Science* 2010; 327:542–5, doi:10.1126/science.1180794.

142. Barker N et al. Identification of stem cells in small intestine and colon by marker gene Lgr5. *Nature* 2007; 449:1003–7, doi:10.1038/nature06196.

143. Kang HW et al. A 3D bioprinting system to produce human-scale tissue constructs with structural integrity. *Nat Biotechnol* 2016; 34:312–9, doi:10.1038/nbt.3413.

28

Surgical aspects of HIV infection

ALASTAIR J. W. MILLAR, BRIAN ELEY, AND SHARON COX

INTRODUCTION

Pediatric HIV (human immunodeficiency virus) infection occurs predominantly in sub-Saharan Africa (SSA). Approximately 2.3 million HIV-infected children under 15 years reside in SSA, representing 88% of the 2.6 million children living with HIV in the world.[1,2] More than 90% of all HIV-infected children less than 15 years of age have acquired HIV through mother-to-child transmission during the antenatal period, at the time of delivery, or through breastfeeding. The risk of transmission can be substantially reduced by prevention of mother-to-child transmission (PMTCT) intervention programs that include the administration of antiretroviral therapy (ART) to all HIV-infected women during pregnancy and throughout breastfeeding, and antiretroviral prophylaxis to their newborn infants during the first 6–12 weeks of life[3,4] In 2015, the World Health Organization recommended that all HIV-infected pregnant and breastfeeding women should commence lifelong ART.[5,6] Substantial progress has been made in extending the coverage of PMTCT intervention programs. At the end of 2014, 73% of all pregnant and breastfeeding women with HIV infection throughout the world were receiving antiretrovirals to prevent mother-to-child transmission.[1] Despite the advances in preventing pediatric HIV infection, many HIV-infected and HIV-exposed but uninfected (HEU) children can be expected to require surgical procedures for the following reasons:

1. Emergency procedures to deal with a non-HIV-related life-threatening condition
2. Emergency procedures to deal with an HIV-related complication or disease
3. Nonemergency procedures where surgery is required to assist in the diagnosis of an HIV-related condition
4. Elective surgery for routine childhood procedures

Most studies on the outcome of HIV-infected patients undergoing surgery have been in adults.[7–10] These studies have reported conflicting results, but several suggested increased morbidity associated with HIV infection with little or no impact on mortality. In contrast, there is limited information on surgical presentations and outcomes in HIV-infected children.

For HIV-infected children presenting with life-threatening diseases for which surgery is urgently indicated, the emergent nature of these events does not allow preoperative correction of comorbidities such as malnutrition or the management of the immune deficiency with ART in children who are antiretroviral-naive. However, antimicrobial therapy may be started for those with coinfections and appropriate perioperative antibiotic prophylaxis prescribed.

Surgical procedures are frequently undertaken to assist in the diagnosis of an HIV-related pathology or complication. Most of these procedures allow time for preoperative treatment of premorbid conditions and coinfections, and initiation of cotrimoxazole prophylaxis and ART.[8,9,11]

Lastly there are increasing numbers of HIV-infected children who require routine, elective surgical procedures. The health status and life expectancy of these children should be taken into account when considering the timing and need for surgery. If surgery can be delayed, then comorbidities such as malnutrition and coinfections may be treated, cotrimoxazole prophylaxis commenced, and ART initiated. Treatment with ART for a period of 2–3 months or longer prior to the surgical procedure will suppress viral replication, will permit partial reversal of the HIV-related immunodeficiency, and may aid healing and lower the risk of postoperative infection, thus improving the overall surgical outcome.

Surgical problems associated with HIV infection may be classified into four major categories (Table 28.1):

1. Soft tissue or organ-specific infections requiring drainage or debridement
2. GI tract disease and complications
3. Infections in the perineal area
4. Malignancies

Table 28.1 Presentation, etiology/differential diagnosis, and indications for surgery in HIV-infected children

	Clinical presentation	Etiology/differential diagnosis	Surgical indications

Surgical infection	Abscess
	Necrotizing fasciitis
	Bloodstream infection
		Staphylococcus aureus
		Streptococcus species
		Candida species
		Herpes simplex virus (HSV)
		Cytomegalovirus (CMV)
		Tuberculosis (TB)
		Molluscum contagiosum
		Gram-negative bacteria, e.g.,
		  Pseudomonas species
			Drain pus
			Debride necrotic tissue
			Obtain culture to direct
			  antibiotic therapy

Gastrointestinal disease and complications			

Esophageal diseases	Esophagitis
	Esophageal stricture
		Candida species
		CMV
		HSV
		Idiopathic ulcers (HIV related)
		Malignancy, e.g., Kaposi sarcoma
		Non-HIV-related pathogens
		Gastroesophageal reflux
			Contrast swallow to identify
			  strictures
			Endoscopy with biopsy for
			  histology and culture

Intra-abdominal problems	Gastrointestinal bleeding
	Gastrointestinal perforation
	Gastrointestinal obstruction
		CMV
		TB
		Mycobacterium avium-intracellulare
		Candida species
		Malignancy, e.g., non-Hodgkin
		  lymphoma
			Endoscopy to diagnose GI
			  bleeding
			Surgery for perforation and
			  obstruction

Perineal disease	Anocutaneous fistula
	Condyloma
	Rectovaginal fistula
	Rectourethral fistula
		CMV
		Human papillomavirus
			Colostomy for sepsis with
			  rectovaginal, rectourethral
			  fistulae
			Cryotherapy or laser for
			  condylomata

Malignancy	Depends on site and extent of disease	Non-Hodgkin lymphoma Karposi sarcoma Leiomyosarcoma	Biopsy of mass Surgical excision

INFECTIONS

Approximately 90% of HIV-infected children will develop mucocutaneous disease, which may be infectious or noninfectious.[11] Children with symptomatic HIV infection have an increased incidence of soft tissue infections (Figure 28.1). The cutaneous manifestations of HIV are indicators of underlying immune status. Bacterial skin infections are often recurrent, in atypical sites or due to atypical organisms (Figure 28.2).[12] The most common organisms causing skin infections are *Staphylococcus aureus* and *Streptococcus* species. These usually present as cellulitis, ecthyma, erysipelas, furunculosis (occasionally of disseminated nature), persistent and recurrent folliculitis, and impetigo. Pyomyositis is also increasingly reported, possibly associated with an increased risk of *Staphylococcus aureus* colonization. Gram-negative organisms may also cause severe, deep-seated skin infection in HIV-infected children. In particular, *Pseudomonas* species may produce cutaneous manifestations, including ecthyma gangrenosum and a papular rash, often in the perineal area.[13] Lethal mucormycosis infection can produce similar features (Figure 28.3a,b,c).[14]

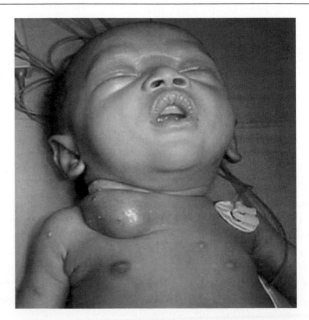

Figure 28.1 Extensive suppurative cervical lymphadenitis with multiple anterior chest wall and upper limb soft tissue abscesses.

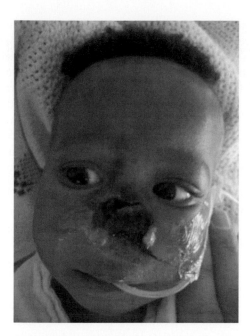

Figure 28.2 Noma (cancrum oris) polymicrobial necrotizing soft tissue infection of the face.

The principles of management of bacterial skin infection are as for HIV-unexposed children, including appropriate antibiotics and surgical drainage or debridement when needed. A high index of suspicion for rapidly spreading infection or necrotizing fasciitis must be maintained,[15] as the immune-compromised patient may not be able to mount an effective systemic response which is required to contain the infection.

Infection with molluscum contagiosum (Figure 28.4), a common viral infection due the DNA poxvirus, is frequent and is identical in appearance to that in HIV-unexposed patients but tends to be more extensive and recurrent, usually occurring on the face and neck.[16]

Immunization with live-attenuated bacillus Calmette–Guérin (BCG) vaccine soon after birth is widely practiced in low- and middle-income countries. This vaccine is typically administered intradermally on the right upper arm at the insertion of the deltoid muscle. Complications after immunization are common.[17] In healthy immunocompetent infants, a local reaction at the site of inoculation and nonprogressive ipsilateral axillary lymphadenopathy may occur. In HIV-infected children, site ulceration or abscess formation, suppurative ipsilateral axillary lymphadenopathy with or without fistulation (Figure 28.5a and b), and disseminated BCG infection may develop, especially after ART is commenced due to immune reconstitution inflammatory syndrome.[18] South African studies have shown that 6% of HIV-infected children develop BCG complications a median of 34 days after commencing ART, and 1% will develop disseminated BCG infection.[19,20] Vaccine site and regional lymphadenopathy complications follow a prolonged course but usually resolve spontaneously without specific intervention. Abscess drainage or surgical excision may be required. Disseminated BCG infection is treated with combination antimycobacterial therapy.[19,21]

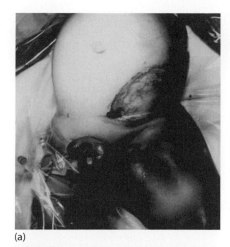

(a)

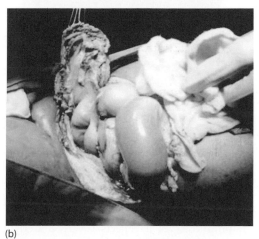

(b)

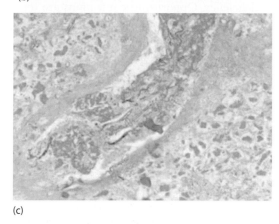

(c)

Figure 28.3 Mucormycosis. (a) Acute rapidly spreading soft tissue infection of the anterior abdominal wall with arterial thrombosis of the femoral and inferior epigastric vessels. (b) Surgical resection revealed abdominal wall and bowel necrosis. (c) Extensive invasion of branched hyphae of mucormycosis in the blood vessels seen on histology of resected tissue.

GI TRACT DISEASE

Esophagitis is a common problem in HIV-infected children that can cause prolonged discomfort and malnutrition, compromise adherence to ART, and lead to increased morbidity

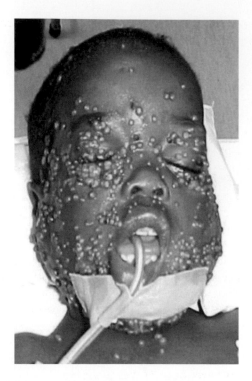

Figure 28.4 Extensive molluscum contagiosum on the face of an HIV-positive child.

and mortality.[22] Esophageal symptoms rank second only to diarrhea in frequency of GI complaints in HIV-infected children.[22] Esophageal disease may be a predictor of poor long-term prognosis, as it reflects severe underlying HIV immunodeficiency. Opportunistic infections are the leading cause of esophageal complaints. Treatment for most etiologies of esophagitis generally has a high degree of success, with a resultant improvement in quality of life especially with ART.[23]

The differential diagnosis for esophageal disease includes the following:

1. *Esophagitis or ulceration.* The causes are usually infective in origin, *Candida* species being the most frequent infection, followed by cytomegalovirus (CMV), herpes simplex virus, and idiopathic infective ulceration. Due to overlap of symptoms, endoscopy and biopsy are essential in identifying the pathology.[23] The growing number of effective antiviral and antifungal agents has mandated a more goal directed approach to therapy.

2. *Esophageal strictures.* The end result of untreated or extensive ulceration is likely to be stricture formation, occurring in approximately 10% of patients.[23] Strictures can be difficult to treat as they respond poorly to dilation and may require esophageal replacement surgery.[24]

Intra-abdominal pathology

The diagnosis and management of children with intra-abdominal surgical pathology can be challenging. Localizing signs and symptoms are frequently misleading due to underlying immunosuppression, debilitation, and antibiotic use. GI bleeding, distension, obstruction, perforation with abdominal pain, and tenderness are the most common clinical presentations associated with intra-abdominal diseases in HIV-infected children.[25]

GI bleeding represents an important source of morbidity and can result from opportunistic infections (CMV or *Candida* infection), HIV-associated malignancies (Kaposi sarcoma, leiomyosarcoma, or lymphoma) or may be unrelated to HIV infection.[26] Lower GI bleeding may be caused by CMV colitis, tuberculosis (TB), malignancy, or idiopathic colonic ulceration. Aggressive investigation with endoscopy to find the source of bleeding is required due to the wide differential diagnosis.[27]

Abdominal distension may occur secondary to chronic diarrhea, ileus, or obstruction. There are many causes for obstruction including inflammatory and infective causes, with TB predominating. Less commonly, neoplastic obstruction occurs secondary to lymphoma or Kaposi sarcoma. The obstruction may present due to invasive bowel infiltration by the tumor or from more localized disease and intussusception.[28] In neonates, the use of ART may mimic functional bowel obstruction.

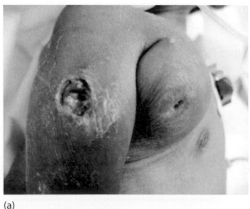
(a)

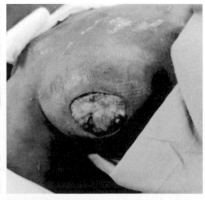
(b)

Figure 28.5 BCGosis. **(a)** Ulceration at the site of the BCG with surgically incised nodal abscess and **(b)** ulcerating nodal inflammation requiring surgical curettage.

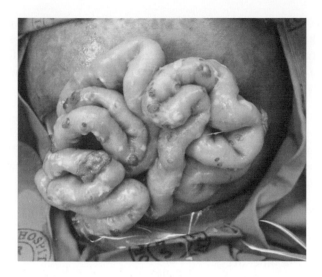

Figure 28.6 Multiple antemesenteric small bowel perforations due to CMV in a child with HIV.

GI perforations may be secondary to CMV (Figure 28.6), TB, or lymphoma. Infants with chronic diarrhea may develop peritonitis due to intestinal perforation.[29] HIV-infected and HEU neonates with necrotizing enterocolitis may have a higher mortality and develop more extensive disease than unexposed infants.[30] Likewise, infants outside the neonatal period may develop necrotizing enterocolitis–type pathology after acute gastroenteritis with shock, which may result in extensive small and large bowel necrosis.

Abdominal pain as a presenting symptom may be due to medical or surgical causes. Infective and neoplastic conditions may present with abdominal pain. Several unique problems arise, however. Nucleoside reverse transcriptase inhibitors, used in ART regimens, may cause abdominal pain due to pancreatitis or lactic acidosis. Pain in the HIV-infected child must be fully investigated for medical and other drug-induced or surgical causes.

PERINEAL DISEASE

HIV-infected children have an increased rate of perirectal abscess and anocutaneous fistula. There are several reports of rectovaginal fistula and rectourethral fistulae or multiple fistulae with an increased rate of sepsis.[29,31,32] Management includes debridement and antibiotics, and on occasion, stool diversion with proximal divided colostomy. Definitive repair has been reported to have poor results but may be successful if preceded by initiation of ART.

Anal condylomata are rare in children, but an increased incidence occurs in HIV-infected children, who may present with extensive and/or recurrent lesions. Anal condylomata may or may not be associated with sexual abuse in HIV-infected children. Most cases of anal condylomata can be managed with cryotherapy, electrocoagulation, or ideally, CO_2 laser ablation under general anesthesia, taking care not to include the whole anal circumference to avoid

anal stricture. A staged approach may be indicated if the lesions are very extensive.[33]

MALIGNANCY

HIV-infected children are at higher risk for malignancy than HIV-unexposed children, with tumors representing 2% of AIDS-defining events.[34] Kaposi sarcoma (Figure 28.7), non-Hodgkin lymphoma (NHL), and cervical cancer are AIDS-defining events.[35] Although rates of leiomyosarcoma and leiomyoma are higher in HIV-infected patients, they are regarded as non-AIDS-defining tumors. Kaposi sarcoma is the most common malignancy in HIV-infected individuals in Africa because human herpes virus-8 infection is highly prevalent in Africa and precedes the development of Kaposi sarcoma. NHL is the second most common HIV-associated malignancy in Africa but the most frequent HIV-associated malignancy in other parts of the world. Epstein–Barr virus infection often precedes the development of NHL. A recent South African study confirmed that Karposi sarcoma and NHL are the most frequently occurring malignancies in HIV-infected children. Furthermore, the risk of developing cancer was lower on ART, but increased with age and the degree of immunodeficiency.[36] These malignancies are treated with a combination of ART, chemotherapy, and radiotherapy. Surgery is usually limited to tissue biopsy or to the treatment of complications.

Incidental solid tumors must be treated as for HIV-unexposed children, although coexisting disease, specifically TB, should be considered during the investigation of solid tumors for metastatic spread.[34] This group of coinfected patients has been reported to have a high mortality independent of the primary tumor type. An HIV-infected child with malignancy should be started on ART as soon as possible. The widespread introduction of ART has lengthened life expectancy, which may result in an increased lifetime incidence of solid organ malignancy in HIV-infected children.[37,38]

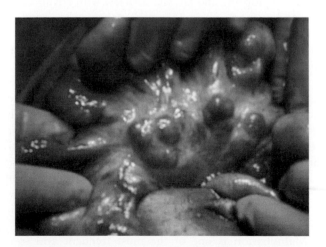

Figure 28.7 Mesenteric nodal involvement with Kaposi sarcoma in a child presenting with intussusception due to small bowel Kaposi sarcoma lesions.

MEDICAL ASPECTS OF PEDIATRIC HIV INFECTION AND THEIR EFFECT ON SURGERY

HIV-infected children have a greater risk of community- and hospital-acquired bacterial infections. These infections may be more severe, follow a protracted course, or result in a worse outcome compared to their HIV-unexposed counterparts. Bacterial infection can involve any organ system or present as bloodstream infection without a clinical focus. Infections may be polymicrobial or caused by drug-resistant pathogens, which has implications for the selection of perioperative prophylactic antibiotics.[39,40]

Reduced pulmonary reserve and an increase in pulmonary complications are of concern after major surgery.[39] HIV-infected children have a high incidence of pulmonary complications, which may be infective or noninfective. Respiratory involvement in HIV-infected children can involve either the upper or lower airway, with implications for airway management during anesthesia.[41] Adenotonsillar enlargement can cause upper airway obstruction and difficult endotracheal intubation. There is an increased incidence of chronic lung disease in HIV-infected children; this may impact on the anesthetic and perioperative management.[42] Lastly, the increased risk of infection may lead to nosocomial pneumonia complicating the postoperative course.

TB coinfection is common in HIV-infected children in low- and middle-income countries. Drug–drug interactions between rifampicin-containing TB drug regimens and other therapies including antiretroviral drugs create pharmaceutical challenges that may impact on the selection of drugs including anesthetic agents and analgesics for children requiring surgery.[5]

Hematological manifestations of HIV include anemia, neutropenia, lymphopenia and thrombocytopenia.[3,43] Anemia has been repeatedly identified as a strong, independent risk factor for HIV disease progression and death. Severe thrombocytopenia and anemia correlate with advanced disease and poor prognosis. Thrombocytopenia can complicate surgical procedures by increasing bleeding and the need for blood products, leading to increased complications in the perioperative period.

GI dysfunction including diarrhea, nausea and vomiting, dysphagia, or odynophagia causes significant morbidity among HIV-infected children. Abdominal surgery may result in a postoperative ileus. This together with pre-existing intestinal dysfunction can make postoperative fluid management and feeding challenging. Furthermore, odynophagia and dysphagia may be secondary to lesions, which are friable and thus easily traumatized during airway instrumentation or insertion of a nasoenteric tube, causing bleeding or perforation.

Malnutrition is one of the most frequent and severe complications of pediatric HIV infection, increasing morbidity and mortality. Analysis of approximately 18,000 HIV-infected children in five southern African countries showed that at the start of ART, 50% were underweight, 66% stunted, and 16% wasted.[44] Malnutrition has been reported to be an independent risk factor for an adverse surgical outcome.

HIV-infected children are at risk for the development of metabolic complications, some of which may be secondary to HIV infection or ART. The surgical and anesthetic implications of such complications must be considered in the overall management of HIV-infected children, including during the perioperative period.[41,42]

Postoperative pain control in HIV-infected children can be challenging. For adequate pain control, a combination of medications may be needed, increasing the potential for drug–drug interactions in children who are often receiving ART or other drugs.[45]

OUTCOMES OF HIV-INFECTED CHILDREN UNDERGOING SURGERY

Few prospective data exist on the outcomes in HIV-infected children undergoing surgery.[46,47] The first reports of surgical outcomes in children with HIV infection were brief, focusing on the procedures performed and risk of transmission of HIV to health care workers. Subsequently, a few case series reported HIV-specific surgical conditions in children without describing the outcome or complications of surgical intervention, although a neonatal subgroup was reported to have a high postoperative mortality of 30%. Most of these children reported on did not receive ART.

Several case reports or case series of procedures have been published, raising concerns of poor wound healing and complications.[46,48,49] A recent series of 48 HIV-infected children undergoing minimally invasive surgery (MIS) for diagnostic and therapeutic procedures concluded that MIS could be safely performed on HIV-infected children but that certain routine procedures such as fundoplication were more difficult and prone to complication.[50] The largest series of HIV-infected and HIV-exposed children undergoing surgery was published in 2009, but this report focused on the disease presentations and only alluded to a higher morbidity; furthermore, no control group existed in that study.[51] There is only one prospective cohort study undertaken comparing the outcomes of HIV-infected and HIV-unexposed children, which noted that HIV infection was the most important risk factor for development of a complication postsurgery, associated with an almost 12-fold higher risk. There was also a significantly higher mortality and longer length of stay.[2]

FACTORS INFLUENCING POSTSURGICAL COMPLICATIONS

Several factors may impact on the rate of postoperative complications in HIV-infected children.[2,52] ART has reduced mortality and morbidity, improved the quality of life, and slowed disease progression of HIV-infected children.[53,54] It suppresses viral replication, leading to a reduced plasma HIV viral load, reversal of CD4 cell attrition, improved overall immune function, and lower risks for infection and HIV-associated malignancy. Two adult studies have investigated the use of ART as an independent predictor of surgical complications. In both studies, three-drug ART regimens were administered for at least 2–3 months prior to surgery. Neither study found that ART reduced postoperative complications. Similarly, in pediatric studies, short-term perioperative ART was not found to be associated with a statistically significant decreased risk of postoperative complications. Thus, delaying elective surgery for the institution of short-term ART may not seem sensible.[55] However, whether or not a longer period of preoperative ART resulting in a greater degree of immune recovery will improve surgical outcomes has not been subjected to rigorous scientific evaluation.

A study that assessed the outcome of anorectal surgery in HIV-infected adults showed that only 40% of patients had healed their wounds by 3 months postsurgery. Wound healing was significantly delayed when the absolute CD4 count was <50 cells/μL. However, clinical stage of HIV infection, age of the patient, and serum albumin concentration were not significant predictors of wound healing.[56] In another study that evaluated the outcome of HIV-infected adults requiring invasive or surgical procedures, preoperative total white blood count, postoperative absolute CD4 count, and postoperative plasma viral load were associated with mortality, postoperative CD4 count was an independent predictor of both postoperative infection and other complications, and a decrease in CD4 percentage was an independent predictor of postoperative complications other than infection.[57]

Only one pediatric study has assessed predictors of postoperative complications in HIV-infected children undergoing surgery. Although this study was limited by sample size and a high proportion of children with advanced HIV disease, it found that only age less than 1 year and major surgery were predictors of postoperative complications. Malnutrition, clinical stage of HIV infection, ART, and type of surgery were not associated with postoperative complications.[55]

HIV-EXPOSED BUT UNINFECTED CHILDREN

A consequence of the success of PMTCT intervention programs is that there are now countless numbers of HEU infants and children in the world, primarily located in low- and middle-income countries. Compared to HIV-unexposed children, HEU infants and young children are at an increased risk of morbidity and mortality, primarily from infectious causes.[30,58] A recent study showed that HEU children are twice as likely to require hospitalization for invasive pneumococcal disease and those less than 6 months of age are less likely to survive an episode of invasive pneumococcal disease than HIV-unexposed children.[59] Reasons for the increased risk of infection in HEU infants are multifactorial, including adverse social factors associated with being born into an HIV-affected household, often shortened duration of breastfeeding, and higher risk of malnutrition. In addition, a range of immunological changes have been reported in HEU infants predisposing them to a spectrum of infections.[60] Susceptibility to infections may increase the risk for developing complications in the postoperative period. Poor growth and malnutrition may also impact on outcomes postsurgery, increasing the risk for infections and delayed wound healing. In a prospective study, it was noted that HEU children had a higher risk of developing postoperative complications and mortality than HIV-unexposed children, but this risk was lower than in HIV-infected children.[30]

CONCLUSION

HIV-infected children may present with conditions unique to HIV infection and common surgical conditions. HIV exposure confers an increased risk of complications and mortality for all children following surgery, whether or not they are HIV-infected. However, the risk of complications is much higher in HIV-infected patients. These findings seem to be independent of whether patients undergo an elective or emergency procedure, but the risk of an adverse outcome is higher after a major surgical procedure. Early treatment with ART is associated with reduced mortality in HIV-infected infants and children. However, further studies are required to optimize the duration of ART prior to surgery.

REFERENCES

1. UNAIDS. How AIDS changed everything. MDG6: 15 years, 15 kessons of hope from the AIDS response, 2015. Available from http://www.unaids.org/sites/default/files/media_asset/MDG6Report_en.pdf

2. Karpelowsky JS et al. Comparison of in-hospital morbidity and mortality in HIV-infected and uninfected children after surgery. Pediatr Surg Int 2012; 28(10): 1007–14.

3. Eley BS et al. A prospective, cross-sectional study of anaemia and peripheral iron status in antiretroviral naive, HIV-1 infected children in Cape Town, South Africa. BMC Infect Dis 2002; 2: 3.

4. World Health Organization. Consolidated guidelines on the use of antiretroviral drugs for treating and preventing HIV infection: Recommendations for a public health approach, June 2013. Available from http://apps.who.int/iris/bitstream/10665/85321/1/9789241505727_eng.pdf?ua=1

5. World Health Organization. Antiretroviral therapy of HIV infection in infants and children: Towards universal access. Recommendations for a public

health approach, 2010 revision. January 12, 2011. Available from http://whqlibdoc.who.int/publications /2010/9789241599801_eng.pdf

6. *World Health Organization Guideline on when to start antiretroviral therapy and on pre-exposure prophylaxis for HIV, September 2015.* Available from http://apps.who.int/iris/bitstream /10665/186275/1/9789241509565_eng.pdf?ua=1

7. Yii MK, Saunder A, Scott DF. Abdominal surgery in HIV/AIDS patients: Indications, operative management, pathology and outcome. *Aust N Z J Surg* 1995; 65(5): 320–6.

8. Shelburne SA et al. Incidence and risk factors for immune reconstitution inflammatory syndrome during highly active antiretroviral therapy. *AIDS* 2005; 19(4): 399–406.

9. Madiba TE, Muckart DJ, Thomson SR. Human immunodeficiency disease: How should it affect surgical decision making? *World J Surg* 2009; 33(5): 899–909.

10. Horberg MA et al. Surgical outcomes in human immunodeficiency virus-infected patients in the era of highly active antiretroviral therapy. *Arch Surg* 2006; 141(12): 1238–45.

11. Stefanaki C, Stratigos AJ, Stratigos JD. Skin manifestations of HIV-1 infection in children. *Clin Dermatol* 2002; 20(1): 74–86.

12. Prose NS. Cutaneous manifestations of HIV infection in children. *Dermatol Clin* 1991; 9(3): 543–50.

13. Flores G, Stavola JJ, Noel GJ. Bacteremia due to Pseudomonas aeruginosa in children with AIDS. *Clin Infect Dis* 1993; 16(5): 706–8.

14. Machoki S, Mugambia AT, Coxa S, Pillayb K, Numanoglua AJWMaA. Disseminated mucormycosis and necrotizing fasciitisin immune-compromised patients: Two case reports. *Ann Ped Surg* 2015; 11: 35–7.

15. Pijnenburg MW, Cotton MF. Necrotising fasciitis in an HIV-1-infected infant. *S Afr Med J* 2001; 91(6): 500–1.

16. Prose NS. Cutaneous manifestations of pediatric HIV infection. *Pediatr Dermatol* 1992; 9(4): 326–8.

17. Alexander A, Rode H. Adverse reactions to the bacillus Calmette–Guerin vaccine in HIV-positive infants. *J Pediatr Surg* 2007; 42(3): 549–52.

18. Puthanakit T et al. Immune reconstitution syndrome from nontuberculous mycobacterial infection after initiation of antiretroviral therapy in children with HIV infection. *Pediatr Infect Dis J* 2006; 25(7): 645–8.

19. Nuttall JJ et al. Bacillus Calmette–Guerin (BCG) vaccine-induced complications in children treated with highly active antiretroviral therapy. *Int J Infect Dis* 2008; 12(6): e99–105.

20. Hesseling AC et al. Disseminated bacille Calmette–Guerin disease in HIV-infected South African infants. *Bull World Health Organ* 2009; 87(7): 505–11.

21. Hesseling AC et al. Bacille Calmette–Guerin vaccine-induced disease in HIV-infected and HIV-uninfected children. *Clin Infect Dis* 2006; 42(4): 548–58.

22. Fantry L. Gastrointestinal infections in the immuno-compromised host. *Curr Opin Gastroenterol* 2003; 19(1): 37–41.

23. Cooke ML, Goddard EA, Brown RA. Endoscopy findings in HIV-infected children from sub-Saharan Africa. *J Trop Pediatr* 2009; 55(4): 238–43.

24. Issa RA et al. Esophagectomy in a patient with AIDS. *Dis Esophagus* 2004; 17(3): 270–2.

25. Bowley DM et al. Surgeons are failing to recognize children with HIV infection. *J Pediatr Surg* 2007; 42(2): 431–4.

26. Balderas V, Spechler SJ. Upper gastrointestinal bleeding in a patient with AIDS. *Nat Clin Pract Gastroenterol Hepatol* 2006; 3(6): 349–53, quiz following 353.

27. Zanolla G et al. Massive lower gastrointestinal hemorrhage caused by CMV disease as a presentation of HIV in an infant. *Pediatr Surg Int* 2001; 17(1): 65–7.

28. Cairncross LL et al. Kaposi sarcoma in children with HIV: A clinical series from Red Cross Children's Hospital. *J Pediatr Surg* 2009; 44(2): 373–6.

29. Kahn E. Gastrointestinal manifestations in pediatric AIDS. *Pediatr Pathol Lab Med* 1997; 17(2): 171–208.

30. Karpelowsky JS et al. Outcome of HIV-exposed uninfected children undergoing surgery. *BMC Pediatr* 2011; 11: 69.

31. Wiersma R. HIV-positive African children with rectal fistulae. *J Pediatr Surg* 2003; 38(1): 62–4; discussion 62–4.

32. Banieghbal B, Fonseca J. Acquired rectovaginal fistulae in South Africa. *Arch Dis Child* 1997; 77(1): 94.

33. Johnson PJ, Mirzai TH, Bentz ML. Carbon dioxide laser ablation of anogenital condyloma acuminata in pediatric patients. *Ann Plast Surg* 1997; 39(6): 578–82.

34. Hadley GP, Naude F. Malignant solid tumour, HIV infection and tuberculosis in children: An unholy triad. *Pediatr Surg Int* 2009; 25(8): 697–701.

35. Stefan DC et al. Infection with human immunodeficiency virus-1 (HIV) among children with cancer in South Africa. *Pediatr Blood Cancer* 2011; 56(1): 77–9.

36. Bohlius J et al. Incidence of AIDS-defining and other cancers in HIV-infected children on South Africa: Record linkage study. *Pediatr Infect Dis J*, 2016; 35(6): e164–70.

37. Caselli D et al. Human immunodeficiency virus–related cancer in children: Incidence and treatment outcome—Report of the Italian Register. *J Clin Oncol* 2000; 18(22): 3854–61.

38. Biggar RJ, Frisch M, Goedert JJ. Risk of cancer in children with AIDS. AIDS–Cancer Match Registry Study Group. *JAMA* 2000; 284(2): 205–9.

39. Zar HJ. Pneumonia in HIV-infected and HIV-uninfected children in developing countries: Epidemiology, clinical features, and management. *Curr Opin Pulm Med* 2004; 10(3): 176–82.

40. George R et al. Pulmonary infections in HIV-positive children. *Pediatr Radiol* 2009; 39(6): 545–54.

41. Bosenberg AT. Pediatric anesthesia in developing countries. *Curr Opin Anaesthesiol* 2007; 20(3): 204–10.

42. Leelanukrom R, Pancharoen C. Anesthesia in HIV-infected children. *Paediatr Anaesth* 2007; 17(6): 509–19.

43. Calis JC et al. HIV-associated anemia in children: A systematic review from a global perspective. *AIDS* 2008; 22(10): 1099–112.

44. Gsponer T et al. Variability of growth in children starting antiretroviral treatment in southern Africa. *Pediatrics* 2012; 130(4): e966–77.

45. Abuzaitoun OR, Hanson IC. Organ-specific manifestations of HIV disease in children. *Pediatr Clin North Am* 2000; 47(1): 109–25.

46. Nelson L, Fried M, Stewart K. HIV-infected patients: The risks of surgery. *J Perioper Pract* 2009; 19(1): 24–30.

47. Mattioli G et al. Risk management in pediatric surgery. *Pediatr Surg Int* 2009; 25(8): 683–90.

48. Kleinhaus S et al. The management of surgery in infants and children with the acquired immune deficiency syndrome. *J Pediatr Surg* 1985; 20(5): 497–8.

49. Beaver BL et al. Surgical intervention in children with human immunodeficiency virus infection. *J Pediatr Surg* 1990; 25(1): 79–82; discussion 82–4.

50. Banieghbal B. Minimally invasive surgery for children with HIV/AIDS. *J Laparoendosc Adv Surg Tech A* 2009; 19(1): 97–101.

51. Karpelowsky JS et al. Outcomes of human immunodeficiency virus-infected and -exposed children undergoing surgery—A prospective study. *J Pediatr Surg* 2009; 44(4): 681–7.

52. Desfrere L et al. Increased incidence of necrotizing enterocolitis in premature infants born to HIV-positive mothers. *AIDS* 2005; 19(14): 1487–93.

53. Violari A et al. Early antiretroviral therapy and mortality among HIV-infected infants. *N Engl J Med* 2008; 359(21): 2233–44.

54. Davies MA et al. Outcomes of the South African National Antiretroviral Treatment Programme for children: The IeDEA Southern Africa collaboration. *S Afr Med J* 2009; 99(10): 730–7.

55. Karpelowsky JS et al. Predictors of postoperative complications in HIV-infected children undergoing surgery. *J Pediatr Surg* 2011; 46(4): 674–8.

56. Lord RV. Anorectal surgery in patients infected with human immunodeficiency virus: Factors associated with delayed wound healing. *Ann Surg* 1997; 226(1): 92–9.

57. Tran HS et al. Predictors of operative outcome in patients with human immunodeficiency virus infection and acquired immunodeficiency syndrome. *Am J Surg* 2000; 180(3): 228–33.

58. Slogrove AL, Cotton MF, Esser MM. Severe infections in HIV-exposed uninfected infants: Clinical evidence of immunodeficiency. *J Trop Pediatr* 2010; 56(2): 75–81.

59. von Mollendorf C et al. Increased risk for and mortality from invasive pneumococcal disease in HIV-exposed but uninfected infants aged <1 year in South Africa, 2009–2013. *Clin Infect Dis* 2015; 60(9): 1346–56.

60. Mofenson LM. Editorial commentary: New challenges in the elimination of pediatric HIV infection: The expanding population of HIV-exposed but uninfected children. *Clin Infect Dis* 2015; 60(9): 1357–60.

29

Liver transplantation

ALASTAIR J. W. MILLAR AND CWN SPEARMAN

INTRODUCTION

History

One of the prime stimuli for the development of liver transplantation was the inevitable mortality from infant liver disease, and many of the advances in liver transplantation techniques were prompted by the need to tailor the procedure for the pediatric patient. The first ever human transplant was attempted in 1963 by Starzl[1] on a 3-year-old child with biliary atresia. The infant did not survive the operation, and it was not until 4 years later that he obtained "success" in achieving survival for 400 days in an 18-month-old girl with a malignant liver tumor. She died from disseminated metastases. Over the next decade, 1-year mortality remained high at around 50%, and it was not until cyclosporine was introduced in 1980 that survivals dramatically increased. In June 1983 at the National Institutes of Health Consensus Development Conference, liver transplantation was declared a valid treatment for end-stage liver disease. The introduction a decade later of tacrolimus, a more potent calcineurin inhibitor, pushed the boundaries of success even further. Technical advances included reduced-size liver transplantation,[2] split-liver, transplants,[3] and living related transplants.[4]

Advances in patient selection, organ preservation, surgical technique, anesthetic management, preoperative and postoperative care, and refinements in immunosuppression and management of the immunosuppressed patient over the last four decades have resulted in a much improved outcome with an ever-increasing list of indications being identified (Table 29.1).[5]

In infancy, the most frequent reasons for liver transplantation are infantile liver failure due to neonatal hemochromatosis and biliary atresia.

The current United Network for Organ Sharing pediatric Kaplan–Meier predicted overall patient and graft survival at 1 year is 86%–93% and 78%–87%; at 5 years, 77%–86% and 63%–75%; and at 10 years, 75% and 61%, respectively.

The survival figures vary according to recipient age at time of transplant: Overall 1-year patient and graft survival were 89% and 81%, respectively, in recipients aged <1 year; 86% and 78%, respectively, in recipients aged 1–5 years; 91% and 84%, respectively, in recipients aged 6–10 years; and 93% and 87%, respectively, in recipients aged 11–17 years. Overall 5-year patient and graft survival was 78% and 63%, respectively, in recipients aged <1 year; 77% and 67%, respectively, in recipients aged 1–5 years; 86% and 75%, respectively, in recipients aged 6–10 years; and 81% and 67%, respectively, in recipients aged 11–17 years.[5,6]

Excellent quality of life is the rule rather than the exception but does, to some extent, depend on pretransplant morbidity, particularly from the nutritional deprivation, which occurs with chronic liver function impairment and cholestasis, leading to neurodevelopmental delay. The longest survivor is in good health 46 years after transplantation. Current anxieties over organ donor scarcity militating against timely transplant, the long-term side effects of the immunosuppressive therapy, financial implications, and some ethical issues remain. The focus of attention has now shifted from an initial target of early posttransplant survival to quality of life in the long term. Shortage of donor organs has been tackled in an imaginative way with increasing use being made of size reduction of the donor liver even into a single segment, splitting the liver into two functioning units for two recipients, as well as the use of living related donors and non-heart-beating donors.

INDICATIONS

Liver disease has been generally underestimated as a cause of death in infants and children. This is probably because many liver conditions in children have led to rapid deterioration and death in the past. Pediatric liver transplantation is now established as routine treatment for children dying of end-stage chronic liver disease and acute/subacute liver failure in both developed and developing countries (Table 29.1). Almost all forms of liver disease in children

Table 29.1 Indications for which liver transplantation has been performed in children

I. Metabolic (inborn errors of metabolism)
(a) Alpha-1 antitrypsin
(b) Tyrosinemia
(c) Glycogen storage disease types III and IV
(d) Wilson disease
(e) Perinatal hemochromatosis
(f) Hypercholesterolemia
(g) Cystic fibrosis
(h) Hyperoxaluria (preemptive or with renal transplant)
(i) Hemophilia A + B
(j) Protein C deficiency
(k) Crigler–Najjar syndrome
(l) Urea cycle defect

II. Acute and chronic hepatitis
(a) Fulminant hepatic failure (viral, toxin, or drug induced)
(b) Chronic hepatitis (B, C, etc.; toxin, autoimmune, idiopathic)

III. Intrahepatic cholestasis
(a) Neonatal hepatitis
(b) Alagille syndrome
(c) Biliary hypoplasia
(d) Familial cholestasis
(e) Primary sclerosing cholangitis

IV. Obstructive biliary tract disease
(a) Biliary atresia
(b) Choledochal cyst with cirrhosis

V. Neoplasia
(a) Hepatoblastoma
(b) Hepatocellular carcinoma
(c) Sarcoma
(d) Hemangioendothelioma

VI. Miscellaneous
(a) Cryptogenic cirrhosis
(b) Congenital hepatic fibrosis
(c) Caroli disease
(d) Budd–Chiari syndrome
(e) Cirrhosis from prolonged parenteral nutrition

can be complicated by hepatocellular failure. These include acute and subacute liver failure from metabolic, toxic, or viral insults, and chronic parenchymal disease of varying causes, of which biliary atresia, biliary hypoplasia, autoimmune hepatitis, viral hepatitis, and some metabolic diseases are the most common.[5] The widespread introduction of vaccines for both hepatitis A and B has significantly reduced the incidence of acute liver failure. In some metabolic diseases, the manifestations are hepatocellular, and in others, there may be more widespread systemic effects such as with tyrosinemia, Wilson's disease, hyperglycoproteinemia, some glycogen storage diseases, and primary hyperoxaluria.

New treatments for acute liver failure due to neonatal hemochromatosis using antenatal intravenous immunoglobulin (IVIG) for the mother and exchange transfusion and IVIG for the newly diagnosed neonate may reduce the need for liver transplantation in this group of patients.[7,8]

In infants with type 1 primary hyperoxaluria, an innovative strategy may be that of early preemptive liver transplantation, perhaps preventing the need for later renal transplantation.[9]

Hemangioendothelioma in infancy is an occasional indication, if medical treatment with steroids, propranolol, and surgical treatment with resection, hepatic artery ligation, or embolization fails, but outcome is guarded.[10]

Children with cystic fibrosis with good respiratory reserve may require an isolated liver transplant for early-onset progressive liver disease.

Intestinal failure–associated liver disease (IFALD) develops in 40%–60% of infants who require long-term total parenteral nutrition. Isolated liver transplantation may be a lifesaving option for infants with short bowel syndrome and IFALD, when adaptation can be expected. Revised criteria for isolated liver transplantation include the following: progressive IFALD; 50 cm functional bowel in absence of the ileocecal valve (ICV) or 30 cm with ICV; and 50% daily energy intake tolerated enterally for 4 weeks with satisfactory growth. Children with a dysmotile bowel should be assessed for a combined liver–bowel transplant unless the dysmotility is resolved and associated with minimal line infections. Nontransplant surgery may be required to facilitate full adaptation, but a >50% long-term survival can be expected.[11]

ASSESSMENT

In general, liver transplantation should be considered as a therapeutic option in all cases of chronic liver disease before the complications of end-stage liver disease arise and in acute liver failure with defined parameters indicating a poor prognosis.

There are indeed few contraindications to liver transplantation (Table 29.2). These include uncontrolled systemic bacterial, viral, or fungal infections; malignancy outside the liver; cyanotic pulmonary arteriovenous shunting with pulmonary hypertension; active chronic hepatitis B; HIV/AIDS not controlled with antiviral treatment; as well as other major cardio-respiratory and/or neurological disease, which would be incompatible with quality long-term survival. To a certain extent, these are all relative contraindications. Psychosocial factors may be a reason for refusal. Parental substance abuse, severe psychiatric problems, and poor preoperative adherence with therapy are factors that need to be carefully examined. In developing countries, the socioeconomic factors such as poor sanitation and lack of access to adequate medical follow-up are often contraindications to transplantation.

Adherence is more difficult to predict in families of children with acute liver failure, as time from presentation to

Table 29.2 Contraindications to liver transplantation

- Poor socioeconomic circumstances—no access to electricity, running water—social worker evaluation required
- History of poor compliance with medications and medical follow-up—social work evaluation required
- No access to ongoing medical care and monitoring of graft function and immunosuppressive drug levels
- Severe cardiopulmonary disease
- Concomitant end-stage organ failure that cannot be corrected by a combined transplant
- Severe multisystem mitochondrial disease
- Irreversible serious neurological damage
- Uncontrolled sepsis
- HIV/AIDS—requires special evaluation and control of infection with HAART
- HBV infection unless prophylaxis with HBIG and antivirals available
- Extrahepatic malignancy (exception: Hepatoblastoma with isolated pulmonary metastases responsive to chemotherapy)
- HCC outside Milan criteria
- Cholangiocarcinoma

Relative contraindications

- Portal vein thrombosis (extensive splanchnic venous thrombosis)
- Previous extensive upper abdominal surgery
- Hemophagocytic lymphohistiocytosis
- Parents with life-threatening illnesses, unless there is an appropriate long-term substitute caregiver for pediatric transplant patients

Table 29.3 Investigation of the liver transplant candidate

A. Full symptom history and physical examination	
B. Hematology:	Complete blood count, clotting profile
	Blood group and tissue typing
	Serum biochemistry and liver function tests
C. Radiology:	Chest and abdominal x-ray
	X-ray wrists and long bones
D. Imaging:	Ultrasound with Doppler for size and flow in the portal vein and unusual anatomy. CT with contrast or magnetic resonance angiogram if a vascular anomaly is suspected
E. Renal function:	Urine analysis, biochemistry, and creatinine clearance
F. Cardiopulmonary:	Full evaluation, particularly if hepato-pulmonary syndrome is clinically evident
G. Serology:	Hepatitis A, B, C, CMV, EBV, HSV, HIV, measles, and varicella
H. Infection screen:	Cultures of urine, sputum, blood, stool, ascites fluid, and swabs from nose and throat. Dental check
I. Nutritional evaluation:	Micronutrients: iron, zinc, selenium, manganese, and vitamin levels A and E
J. Developmental assessment	
H. Psycho-social assessment	

decision to transplant is much shorter. Good adherence is one of the factors thought to contribute to the slightly better outcome after living-donor transplantation as the bond and responsibilities between donor and recipient are that much greater.

As the outcome of the operation is so much better in recent years, indications for early transplant in patients with chronic liver disease would be evidence of impaired synthetic function, including prolonged prothrombin time, reduced serum cholesterol levels, and low serum albumin. Clinical indicators include presence of ascites, bleeding from esophageal varices not controlled by sclerotherapy/banding, and poor response to nutritional resuscitation. Those with acute liver failure who develop encephalopathy, hypoglycemia, a prothrombin time of greater than 50 seconds, and a factor V level of less than 20% should be considered for transplant, as almost all of these children die without transplantation.

All patients require initial confirmation of the diagnosis, intensive medical investigation, nutritional resuscitation, and active treatment of the complications of the liver disease, portal hypertension, and nutritional deprivation (Tables 29.3 and 29.4). Immunization status must

be reviewed and supplemented as required with hepatitis A and B, hemophilus influenza, pneumococcal, varicella, meningococcal, and human papilloma virus immunizations. It is important that live attenuated vaccines are given pretransplant, as these are contraindicated posttransplantation. Blood group–identical or –compatible donors are much preferred as the long-term survival with blood group–incompatible donors has been significantly less, but there have been recent reports of excellent outcomes with blood group incompatibility particularly in infants under 1 year of age.[12] If urgent transplantation is required, an incompatible ABO blood group donor organ can be considered. There are also specific strategies to reduce the potential adverse immune consequences of a blood group–incompatible organ including the use of a CD20 monoclonal antibody, IVIG, and plasma exchange.[13]

Table 29.4 Evaluation of the patient pre-transplant

- Confirm the indication for transplant
- Determine severity of the liver disease and nutritional status
- Consider alternative treatments to transplant
- Identify and treat active infections
- Identify cardiac malformations that need correction pre-transplant
- Ensure that immunizations are up to date, especially live vaccines (measles and varicella) that are contraindicated post-transplantation
- Dental care
- Evaluate psycho-socioeconomic factors and logistics

Educate and counsel parents and medical caregivers about

- Pre-transplant waiting period and potential death on the waiting list
- Transplant procedure regarding the risk of surgery, especially technical complications such as vascular thrombosis and biliary complications
- Post-transplant complications of rejection, risks of immunosuppression, malignancy, and recurrent disease

Children with chronic liver disease are prioritized for liver transplantation according to the PELD (Pediatric End-Stage Liver Disease) (under 12 years) or MELD (Model for End-Stage Liver Disease) (12 years and older) score. Children presenting with acute liver failure are listed as UNOS Status 1a (this includes children <18 years old presenting with fulminant liver failure, primary graft nonfunction, hepatic artery thrombosis, acute decompensated Wilson's disease, and nonmetastatic hepatoblastoma). Children with chronic liver disease (PELD > 25) who are in the ICU and who have at least one of the following: on ventilator; gastrointestinal bleeding requiring at least 30 mL/kg packed red cell transfusion in previous 24 h; renal failure requiring dialysis; Glasgow coma scale < 10 are classified as UNOS Status 1b.

Young age (<6 months), creatinine clearance (<90 mL/1.73 m²), pretransplant hospitalization, pretransplant ventilation, retransplantation, and transplant for reasons other than cholestatic disease have been associated with a reduced survival.[14] Predictors of graft loss include the type of graft (split graft and reduced-size graft), donor age <5 months, prolonged warm ischemia time, and fulminant liver failure as indication for liver transplantation.[15]

SURGICAL TECHNIQUE

Donor organ suitability and function are difficult to predict. Increasingly, marginal donors are being used with a surprisingly low incidence of primary poor function or nonfunction. Age limits are being extended. However, stable donors aged under 45 years with a short intensive care unit stay (less than 3 days), little requirement for inotropic support and normal, or near-normal liver function are preferred, with an expected <5% incidence of impaired function after transplant. Liver biopsy is useful if steatosis is suspected. Greater than 50% fatty infiltration would preclude the use of the liver in most centers. Viral screening of the donors is essential and includes the following: hepatitis B (HBsAg, anti-HBV IgG core, and nucleic acid test [NAT]); hepatitis C (hepatitis C antibody and NAT); cytomegalovirus [CMV] IgG Ab; Epstein–Barr virus [EBV] IgG Ab; and HIV (HIV combined Ag/Ab test and NAT) screening. Use of hepatitis C virus (HCV)-positive donor livers should only be considered for HCV-positive recipients, as HCV transmission is universal.

Surgical techniques used for donor retrieval and recipient liver removal and engraftment have evolved over the last 40 years.[5,16,17] The majority of donor livers are removed as part of a multiorgan procurement procedure, which would include various combinations of kidneys, liver, heart or heart and lungs, small bowel, and pancreas. University of Wisconsin solution and histidine–tryptophan–ketoglutarate solution (HTK) are both widely used as the preservation solutions of choice.[18]

The principle two techniques is a careful dissection and excision technique or the so-called rapid technique described by Starzl.[17,19]

Donation after cardiac death has been an established practice for many years for renal transplantation, but recently, in an effort to expand the donor pool, this has been extended to other organs. The concept of cardiac death may be more acceptable to some and could increase the number of potential donors. Although there are considerable logistic problems to overcome, some success has been achieved with acceptable graft function even in segmental liver transplantation using a "super-rapid" technique and keeping both cold and warm ischemic times to a minimum.[20]

The graft should be of an appropriate size to provide adequate function but not too large to compromise the abdominal compartment domain. A minimum graft size should be >0.8% of body mass (normal ~2%), i.e., 40% of estimated standard liver volume. Grafts of smaller size have a poorer outcome from graft failure due to small-for-size (SFS) syndrome.

The *recipient operation* is commenced so that the estimated hepatic graft cold ischemic time is less than 12 hours. Much longer preservation times have been recorded, but this leads to an increased incidence of cholestasis and graft dysfunction.

Careful dissection of the graft is required when split-liver transplantation is being used, that is, when the liver is divided into two functional units for two recipients, and decisions must be made as to which porta hepatis structures will go with which graft. It is advisable to perform a portable cholangiogram to confirm bile duct anatomy, as there are many variations in biliary anatomy. Depending on local preference, many centers opt to export the right-sided graft with the full complement of structures of bile duct, portal vein, and hepatic artery, keeping the left lateral segment as the graft for a pediatric recipient in much the same way as a living-donor transplant. Where a reduced-size liver is used, the caudate lobe is always excised. The division of liver tissue may be performed using the standard forceps clamp or bipolar diathermy technique with titanium clip and/or suture and ligation of vascular and biliary structures. The ultrasonic dissector (Cavitron Ultrasonic Surgical Aspirator), Ligasure or Harmonic Scalpel may also be used. The cut edge of the liver is then sprayed with two layers of tissue glue. If the recipient inferior vena cava is to be preserved, this is simply done by carefully excising the diseased liver clear of the cava and, when the liver has been removed, individually suturing closed all small areas of leakage from divided direct caudate lobe hepatic veins. The IVC is prepared for the donor liver by dividing the bridges between the separate hepatic veins. This creates a wide orifice for the hepatic vein-to-cava anastomosis. The inferior vena cava should also be incised distally for approximately 1–2 cm to make a triangular orifice for the piggy-back graft.[21]

Engraftment should begin with the upper caval anastomosis taking into account the need to rotate the liver anticlockwise about 60 degrees with reduced-size liver grafts. Split grafts and living-donor segmental grafts may need to lie in an orthotopic anatomical position, and a number of techniques of stabilizing the graft have been used so as to avoid torsion at the hepatic vein-to-caval anastomosis and to facilitate vascular anastomoses without using interposition grafts. Prior to completion of the anastomosis, the liver is flushed of preservation solution via the portal vein with recipient blood, normal saline, or a colloid solution. It is important for the portal vein to be of adequate size and length, and it should lie without tension. If the recipient vein is too narrow and sclerotic, interposition of a donor iliac vein is indicated.[17] Likewise with the arterial anastomosis, if the recipient vessel is too small or the donor artery too short, an interposition graft is placed onto the supraceliac or infrarenal aorta. The bile duct is trimmed back and spatulated in pediatric donors such that there is good bleeding from the cut edge and a wide anastomosis is obtained. With reduced- and variant-size grafts, a Roux-en-Y choledochojejunostomy is always performed using fine absorbable sutures.[5]

Occasionally in pediatric cases, a duct-to-duct anastomosis may be performed with a whole liver graft in a recipient with a normal extrahepatic biliary system or for infants with short bowel syndrome undergoing isolated liver transplant. Stents or T tubes are optional but less used as there is some evidence of an increased incidence of biliary complications associated with their use.

SPLIT-LIVER TRANSPLANTATION AND LIVING DONATION

In split-liver transplantation, a whole cadaver donor organ is divided into two functional units. Segments 2 and 3 are used for an infant and the right liver for an adult recipient. The graft can be further reduced in size by removing segment 2, or alternatively, segment 2 is used as the graft, and segment 3 is resected and discarded. The disadvantage

of using a segment 3 graft is the greater anterior posterior dimension, which may be difficult to accommodate in an infant abdomen (Figure 29.1).[22] Living related donation of the left lateral segment, first successfully performed by Strong, has become widely accepted as a method of acquiring a liver graft in the face of severe donor shortages, particularly in countries with cultural or religious reticence to accept brain death in a ventilated heart-beating donor. There are clear advantages in the planned nature of the procedure preferably before end-stage liver disease in the recipient, the excellent quality of the graft, and short ischemic time. The use of a living donor also increases the availability of donor organs in general for other patients on the waiting list. The only advantage to the donor is a psychological one, and there is a current morbidity of around 10% (wound sepsis, hernia, bile leak, and adhesive bowel obstruction). There is also a reported mortality of around 0.2%, although in one center in Japan, more than 1000 of these operations were done without donor mortality.[23] There are ethical concerns, which appear justified, as with more widespread transplant activity, increasing mortality and morbidity have been recorded in adult-to-adult donation, but adult-to-child donation has a very low morbidity and mortality. The donor should first undergo a thorough screening both clinical and psychological without coercion and be given an option to withdraw from the procedure at any time before the transplant.[24,25] This process may have to be accelerated where donation is for fulminant hepatic failure. Cholangiography is essential as there is considerable variety in the intrahepatic biliary anatomy. Angiography is desirable but not essential.

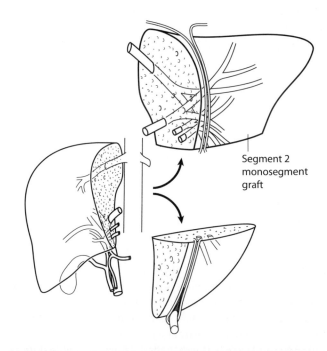

Segment 2 monosegment graft

Figure 29.1 Left lateral segment transplant from a living donor or split liver, further reduced in size to a monosegment graft by resection of segment 3. (From Oliveira P, Biliary complications after paediatric liver transplantation, *Pediatr Transplant* 2010 May;14(3): 437–8.)

Magnetic resonance (MR) imaging has made interventional radiographic techniques obsolete.

MEDICAL MANAGEMENT

Immunosuppression

There is no standard-of-care immunosuppression regimen, and chosen regimens are often determined by cost, particularly in resource-constrained countries, where the cost of induction agents, tacrolimus, and mycophenolate mofetil is often prohibitive.

Immunosuppressive regimens should, in addition to preventing acute and chronic rejection, promote good quality of life and be free of significant long-term side effects. Calcineurin inhibitors remain the cornerstone of immunosuppression, with tacrolimus being the preferred agent.[26] Tacrolimus is associated with lower incidences of both acute and chronic rejection,[27,28] hypertension, and hyperlipidemia, and does not cause hirsutism and gingival hyperplasia.[27,29]

Induction immunosuppressive regimens are usually a combination of calcineurin inhibitors (cyclosporin or tacrolimus) and steroids with variable use of an antimetabolite (azathioprine or mycophenolate mofetil). Maintenance monotherapy with tacrolimus or cyclosporine is the target, and attempts should be made to wean steroids by 3–6 months, but there is a risk of developing de novo autoimmune hepatitis following the cessation of steroids.[30,31] If steroids are required, aim for low-dose alternate-day steroids to encourage growth, as short stature is a significant side effect in young children.[32]

According to the Organ Procurement and Transplant Network (OPTN)/Scientific Registry of Transplant Recipients (SRTR) 2014 annual report, the most commonly used initial immunosuppression agents in North America were tacrolimus (94.8%), steroids (82.1%), and mycophenolate mofetil (39.7%). Only 31.8% received induction therapy (18.3% IL-2 [interleukin 2] receptor antagonists and 13.5% a T-cell-depleting agent). Among recipients, 1.4% were reported to have received a mammalian target of rapamycin (mTOR) inhibitor at the time of transplantation, but this increased to 8.2% at 1 year posttransplantation. Despite the long-term side effects, 55% of recipients were still on maintenance steroid therapy at 1 year.[6]

Both cyclosporin and tacrolimus cause a 30% reduction in renal function, and up to 5% of pediatric transplants develop severe chronic renal failure.[33] Renal-sparing regimens with IL-2 receptor blockers as induction therapy often in combination with mycophenolate mofetil enable delayed introduction of calcineurin inhibitors in the setting of pretransplant renal dysfunction, use of low-dose tacrolimus, as well as enabling the more rapid weaning or even avoidance of steroids.[34–38]

Sirolimus, an mTOR inhibitor has also been used as a renal-sparing and an immunological rescue agent[39] but is potentially hepatotoxic, can cause proteinuria, and increases serum triglyceride levels. Other side effects include a delay in wound healing and hepatic artery thrombosis, and it is thus not recommended in the early postoperative period. Children with posttransplant lymphoproliferative disease or hepatoblastoma may benefit from immune suppression with sirolimus.[40] Everolimus has not been registered for use in pediatric liver transplantation.

Postoperative care

Patients are monitored intensively postoperatively and usually require ventilation for a period of 24–48 hours. Liver ultrasound with color flow Doppler is performed frequently to confirm vascular patency and the absence of biliary dilatation.

Acute postoperative hypertension is almost universal in pediatric transplantation and persists in 25% of recipients. It is usually initially managed with oral amlodipine in titrated doses. Subsequently, ACE (angiotensin-converting enzyme) inhibitors and beta-blockers may be given in appropriate dosage. Aspirin 3 mg/kg given on alternate days is used as prophylaxis against arterial thrombosis, and a proton pump inhibitor is given for gastric mucosal protection.

Early enteral feeding and vitamin supplementation is advised, and if delayed beyond 48 hours of surgery, parenteral nutrition should be commenced. Phosphate and magnesium deficiency is common and requires replacement therapy in nearly all patients.

Liver biopsies are performed if indicated by increasing serum liver enzyme activity or by bilirubin levels, using the Menghini technique (Hepafix needle [Braun], diameter 1.4 mm), unless biliary dilatation is observed on ultrasonography. Biopsies are routinely assayed for viral and bacterial activity.

Diagnosis of rejection can be made on the basis of clinical, biochemical, and histologic changes and usually presents in the first few weeks after transplant with fever, malaise, a tender graft, and loose stools. The grade of rejection is assessed according to established histological criteria (lymphocyte- predominant portal infiltrates, cholangiolar damage, and endotheliitis) according to the Banff schema.[41]

Management of acute cellular rejection in the early postoperative period depends on the induction immunosuppressive regimen but is less problematic in children who are on Tacrolimus-based regimens and have received induction therapy with IL-2 receptor blockers. It is important to ensure adequate trough tacrolimus levels (10–15 ng/mL), substituting mycophenolate mofetil for azathioprine. If there is ongoing rejection, pulsing with intravenous methylprednisone can be used, but this is seldom necessary with present-day immunosuppressive regimens. The patient should be given four doses of methyl prednisolone at 10 mg/kg, the first three doses on successive days and the fourth dose on the fifth day after commencing treatment. IL-2 receptor blockers and T-cell-depleting agents are very rarely used for steroid resistant rejection. Once rejection is under control and liver function tests have returned to normal, steroids are weaned, and the tacrolimus dosage can be reduced, aiming for a trough level of 5–10 ng/mL at

6–12 months posttransplant, 3–8 ng/mL at 13–24 months posttransplant, and 2–4 ng/mL after 2 years.

Anti-infection agents

Immunosuppression naturally leads to increased susceptibility to bacterial, fungal, protozoal, and viral infections. Antibiotics are given as prophylaxis and according to culture and sensitivity of blood, sputum, and body fluid. In infants, there is a low threshold for antifungal therapy with either amphotericin or fluconazole. Caspofungin can be considered in children with impaired renal function. Ganciclovir is given as prophylaxis against CMV and EBV infections for 100 days, initially intravenously, but once stable, valganciclovir can be given orally.

Trimethoprim/sulfamethoxazole is routinely given for 6 months for pneumocystis jirovecci prophylaxis and can be restarted at times of increased immunosuppression.

Antituberculosis prophylaxis is given only if the reason for transplant is a reaction to antituberculosis drugs with fulminant hepatic failure, where evidence of tuberculosis is found before surgery and if a close family contact has tuberculosis.

First-line antituberculous therapy (isoniazid, rifampicin, ethambutol, and pyrazinamide) can be used in children with normal graft function, but regular monitoring of liver function tests is required as these drugs are potentially hepatotoxic. It is important to monitor tacrolimus/cyclosporin levels as rifampicin induces the cytochrome P450 system, resulting in increased drug metabolism. Tacrolimus or cyclosporin dosage should empirically be increased by 30% at the start of antituberculous therapy.

Surgical complications

Surgical complications may be reduced to an absolute minimum with meticulous technique (Table 29.5).[5,20] These may present early and late. Biliary complications continue to be a significant problem with an overall incidence of 10%–20%, particularly in living related left lateral segment grafts.[42] A proactive management approach is taken with close monitoring of vascular patency using Doppler ultrasound scanning and computed tomography (CT) or MR angiogram if there is any doubt. Radiological intervention techniques have been used successfully for later complications of biliary strictures and portal vein stenosis. SFS syndrome is a recognizable clinical scenario where the liver graft size is unable to meet the functional demands of the recipient in the absence of other causes for graft dysfunction. Grafts of less than 35% graft volume relative to standard liver volume or 0.8% of graft:recipient weight ratio (GRWR) are considered small for size. The liver failure presents toward the end of the first posttransplant week with coagulopathy, ascites, cholestasis, and encephalopathy and is often associated with pulmonary and renal dysfunction. The underlying pathophysiology is complex but is universally associated with a high portal vein blood flow (usually >250 mL/minute per

Table 29.5 Summary of common postoperative problems

1. **Biliary tract**
   (a) Stenosis or stricture
   (b) Anastomotic leak—often associated with hepatic artery thrombosis
   (c) Cholangitis
2. **Rejection**
   (a) Acute
   (b) Chronic (vanishing bile duct syndrome)
3. **Infection**—bacterial, viral (CMV, EBV, herpes zoster, hepatitis B), fungal (candida, aspergillus), parasitic (pneumocystis)
   (a) Abdominal (perihepatic or intrahepatic abscess)
   (b) Biliary tree
   (c) Pulmonary
   (d) Reactivated virus
   (e) Gastrointestinal tract
   (f) Catheter associated (intravenous, urinary tract)
4. **Vascular (thrombosis, stenosis)**
   (a) Hepatic artery
   (b) Portal vein
   (c) Inferior vena cava (suprahepatic and infrahepatic)
   (d) Hepatic vein (left lateral segment grafts), Budd–Chiari recurrence
5. **Renal dysfunction**
   (a) Calcineurin inhibitor–induced or other drug-induced injury
   (b) Tubular necrosis due to hypoperfusion
   (c) Preexisting disease (hepatorenal syndrome)
   (d) Hypertension
6. **Miscellaneous**
   (a) Encephalopathy (cyclosporin, tacrolimus, hypertensive, metabolic)
   (b) Bowel perforation (steroid, diathermy, hypoxia)
   (c) Diaphragm paresis/paralysis
   (d) Gastrointestinal hemorrhage (peptic ulceration, variceal)
   (e) Obesity (steroids)
   (f) Other drug side effects

100 g graft weight) and is aggravated by any hepatic vein outflow obstruction. The histological appearance shows marked congestion, dilatation of sinusoids and portal veins, scattered areas of necrosis, and severe cell denudation with neutrophilic inflammatory cell infiltrate. Strategies for avoiding SFS syndrome include avoiding small grafts, ensuring short ischemic times, and modulating portal vein flow. Splenic artery ligation at the time of transplant or embolization in the early postoperative period has been efficacious in reducing portal hypertension and improving outcomes.[43–45] Various types of partial portal vein decompression maneuvers have been tried both experimentally and in small clinical series. Medical management to reduce splanchnic flow includes somatostatin infusion and propranolol. Intraportal

infusion of prostaglandin E1 and thromboxane A2 have also been used.[46]

Medical follow-up and late complications

Most patients can be discharged from the intensive care unit within the first week after transplantation.[5,20] The majority of infections can be prevented. However, should the patient require excessive immunosuppression for persistent rejection, almost inevitably, he/she will develop some opportunistic infections.

In this situation, not only must specific therapy be directed at the pathogen, but also, immunosuppression must be reduced. CMV and EBV are best monitored with quantitative polymerase chain reaction (PCR) measurement of the virus.

Posttransplantation lymphoproliferative disorder (PTLD) presents from the first few weeks after transplant to several years later with a mean time of onset around 9 months. Risk of PTLD relates to the intensity of immunosuppression (5%–7% in liver transplant recipients) and pretransplant EBV status. Regular EBV PCR monitoring and appropriate reduction in immunosuppression reduces the risk.[47] A typical presentation is initially with acute membranous tonsillitis and associated cervical lymphadenopathy, which is resistant to antibiotic therapy. However, the disease may be widespread, and gastrointestinal and central nervous system involvement is common. Management strategies include reduction of immunosuppression, which may require complete withdrawal along with chemotherapy, anti-CD20 monoclonal antibodies, and adoptive immunotherapy, particularly with the monoclonal PTLD.[48] Mortality varies from 20% to 70% or more. Prophylactic ganciclovir initially intravenously followed by oral valganciclovir given for 3 months may be effective in preventing EBV activation, which is the promoter of PTLD in most cases.

The rates of de novo hepatitis B associated with the use of hepatitis B IgG core antibody–positive donors in the absence of HBV prophylaxis are 58% in HBV non-immune, 18% in previously vaccinated, 14% in isolated anti-HBV IgG core positive, and 4% in naturally immune (HBsAb and anti-HBV IgG core positive) individuals.[49] Lifelong Lamivudine is recommended as the most cost-effective option to prevent de novo hepatitis B from the use of hepatitis B IgG core antibody–positive donors.[50]

If children are transplanted for hepatitis B, then prophylaxis with hepatitis B hyperimmunoglobulin (HBIG) and an antiviral with high genetic barrier to resistance such as tenofovir or entecavir is recommended. Entecavir is recommended for children aged 2–11 years and tenofovir in children ≥12 years and weighing at least 35 kg. Lamivudine has to be used in children under the age of 2 years. There is no consensus regarding the duration, dosage, and mode of administration of intravenous injection [IVI] or intramuscular injection [IMI] HBIG, but antivirals should be given lifelong to prevent recurrence of chronic hepatitis, which is inevitable without prophylaxis.[51]

Children are frequently hypertensive and require antihypertensive therapy for a period of time posttransplant. A degree of renal impairment is almost inevitable in those patients suffering from chronic liver disease with cholestasis. With the additional burden of the use of nephrotoxic immunosuppressive drugs such as cyclosporin and tacrolimus, many have significant impairment of renal function in the long term. The importance of renal-sparing strategies in immunosuppression is becoming increasingly evident as 4%–5% long-term survivors present with drug-induced renal failure requiring renal replacement therapy.

Chronic rejection is an irreversible phenomenon, which is chiefly intrahepatic and ductular rather than a vascular phenomenon, in contrast to other organ transplants. This is usually manifested by disruption of bile duct radicals with development of the vanishing bile duct syndrome. The incidence seems less frequent with tacrolimus-based immunosuppressive regimens as opposed to cyclosporine, where an incidence of up to 10% has been recorded. Late chronic rejection may also be associated with a vasculopathy affecting larger arteries.

RETRANSPLANTATION

Retransplantation rates have improved, with OPTN/SRTR reporting rates as low as 8.8% for the period 2012–2014.[6] Early indications include primary graft nonfunction; early hepatic arterial thrombosis, and refractory acute cellular rejection; and later-established chronic ductopenic rejection. Early retransplantation is technically a much less traumatic procedure than the original transplant, although the patient may be in a poorer condition. Outcome largely depends on the indication for retransplantation and is quite good for technical causes but less satisfactory for rejection and infection. An increasingly poorer outcome can be expected after the third and fourth retransplants, and the efficacy and ethics of these interventions are in question.

LONG-TERM SURVIVAL AND QUALITY OF LIFE

One-year patient survival of >95% is being achieved in the best centers, with predicted 10-year patient survivals of around 70%–75%.[5,6] Patients grafted for acute liver failure have done less well, with a higher early death rate usually associated with cerebral complications and multiorgan failure. Overall, excellent quality of life can be achieved, and most children are fully rehabilitated.[52,53]

It is, however, increasingly evident that prolonged cholestatic jaundice and malnutrition in infancy may have late effects, and despite good physical rehabilitation, evidence of significant cognitive deficits, which present during early schooling as learning difficulties and attention deficit disorders, is common.[54]

Catch-up growth post liver transplant improves if steroids are reduced, used on alternate days, or withdrawn.[32] But with steroid withdrawal comes the risk of development of chronic rejection or de novo hepatitis.[30,31,55] As with any immunosuppressed patient, the incidence of neoplasia in a lifetime is greatly increased (12% skin and other malignancies).[56] Renal function impairment aggravated by hypertension and calcineurin inhibitor and antibiotic toxicity is frequent, with up to 25% developing chronic renal failure at 10 years posttransplant.[57]

Fibrosis on histology is an increasingly recognized phenomenon, which seems to be more related to factors at the time of the transplant (cold ischemic time, young age, donor:recipient weight ratio, use of partial grafts) rather than immunological or infective factors.[58]

At a workshop on long-term outcomes, the following factors were identified as requiring further research: risk factors associated with long-term immunosuppression complications; development of tolerance-inducing regimens; definition of biomarkers that reflect the level of clinical immunosuppression; development of instruments for the measurement of health wellness; identification of risk factors that impede growth and intellectual development before and after liver transplantation; and identification of barriers and facilitators that impact nonadherence and transition of care for adolescents.[59]

ADOLESCENCE

Nonadherence in adolescent transplant recipients (~20%) is a particular concern[60] In addition to coping with the usual issues of autonomy, peer pressure with regard to alcohol, recreational drugs, and sex, the transplant teenager has to cope with the cosmetic side effects of immunosuppression, regular medical monitoring, and strict adherence to drug regimens.[61] These issues often occur at the time of transfer to an adult unit. It is important to actively involve teenagers in the decision making, and discuss issues of sexuality, risks of pregnancy, and appropriate contraception. A planned transfer to an adult program is essential as the risk of nonadherence and graft loss is great during this period. Adolescents who have undergone transfer to the adult transplant services at a median age of 18.6 years have had good long-term outcomes.[62]

Transplantation in infancy appears to result in a reduced incidence of nonadherence in adolescence compared with later transplantation. Use of mobile phone text messaging has been shown in one study to reduce nonadherence amongst teenagers.[63]

CONCLUSION

Careful planning, extensive preparation of personnel, and a broad base of skills along with good teamwork between health professionals are required for the development of a successful pediatric transplant program. Surgical technique, anesthetic skills, and medical care of the highest order are essential. Size of the recipient is only important insofar as making the graft fit the recipient abdomen but long-term outcomes are excellent.

A patient with a liver transplant is a patient for life and requires complete commitment from the transplant medical and surgical team, which cannot be abrogated after discharge from hospital. However, it is essential to set up an effective shared care program with the referring medical caregiver, as many recipients will reside far from the transplant center.

The need for pediatric liver transplants has been assessed at approximately 1 to 2 children per million per year. Thus, transplant activity should be concentrated in specific centers with pediatric surgical and medical expertise. The shortage of donor organs will continue, and future efforts must be focused on maximum use of cadaver donors and increasing living related donation. No child with end-stage liver disease should be denied the opportunity of receiving appropriate treatment.

These challenges must be met to offer any infant or child requiring liver replacement a chance at a life. The ultimate aim is to restore the child to normal health such that he/she can grow up into a productive healthy adult who can make his/her contribution to society and develop all of his/her human potential.

REFERENCES

1. Starzl TE. *The Puzzle People: Memoirs of a Transplant Surgeon*. Pittsburgh: University of Pittsburgh Press, 1992. ISBN 0-8229-3714-X.
2. Bismuth H, Houssain D. Reduced-sized orthotopic liver graft in hepatic transplantation in children. *Surgery* 1984; 95(3): 367–70.
3. Pichlmayr R, Ringe B, Gubernatis G et al. [Transplantation of a donor liver to 2 recipients (splitting transplantation)—A new method in the further development of segmental liver transplantation]. *Langenbeck's Arch Chir* 1988; 373(2): 127–30.
4. Strong RW, Lynch SV, Ong TH et al. Successful liver transplantation from a living donor to her son. *N Engl J Med* 1990; 322(21): 1505–7.
5. Spada M, Riva S, Maggiore G et al. Pediatric liver transplantation. *World J Gastroenterol* 2009; 15(6): 648–74.
6. Kim WR, Lake JR, Smith JM et al. Liver. *Am J Transplant* 2016 Jan; 16 Suppl 2: 69–98.
7. Rand EB, Karpen SJ, Kelly S et al. Treatment of neonatal hemochromatosis with exchange transfusion and intravenous immunoglobulin. *J Pediatr* 2009; 155(4): 566–71.
8. Whitington PF, Kelly S. Outcome of pregnancies at risk for neonatal hemochromatosis is improved by treatment with high-dose intravenous immunoglobulin. *Pediatrics* 2008; 121(6): e1615–21.
9. Malla I, Lysy PA, Godefroid N et al. Two-step transplantation for primary hyperoxaluria: Cadaveric liver followed by living donor related kidney transplantation. *Pediatr Transplant* 2009; 13(6): 782–4.
10. Grabhorn E, Richter A, Fischer L et al. Neonates with severe infantile hepatic hemangioendothelioma: Limitations of liver transplantation. *Pediatr Transplant* 2009; 13(5): 560–4.

11. Dell-Olio D, Beath S, de Ville de Goyez J et al. Isolated liver transplant in infants with short bowel syndrome: Insights into outcomes and prognostic factors. *J Pediatr Gastroenterol Nutr* 2009; 48(3): 334–40.

12. Gelas T, McKiernan PJ, Kelly DA et al. ABO-incompatible pediatric liver transplantation in very small recipients: Birmingham's experience. *Pediatr Transplant* 2011 Nov; 15(7): 706–11.

13. Ikegami T, Taketomi A, Soejima Y et al. Rituximab, IVIG, and plasma exchange without graft local infusion treatment: A new protocol in ABO incompatible living donor liver transplantation. *Transplantation* 2009; 88(3): 303–7.

14. McDiarmid SV, Anand R, Lindblad AS, The SPLIT Research Group. *Studies of Pediatric Liver Transplantation (SPLIT) Annual Report*. Rockville, MD: SPLIT, 2004: 1–27.

15. Diamond IR, Fecteau A, Millis JM et al. Impact of graft type on outcome in pediatric liver transplantation: A report from Studies of Pediatric Liver Transplantation (SPLIT). *Ann Surg* 2007; 246(2): 301–10.

16. Christophi C. A comparison of standard and rapid infusion methods of liver preservation during multi-organ procurement. *Aust N Z J Surg* 1991; 61(9): 692–4.

17. de Ville de Goyet J, Reding J, Hausleithner V et al. Standardized quick en bloc technique for procurement of cadaveric liver grafts for pediatric liver transplantation. *Transpl Int* 1995; 8(4): 280–5.

18. Feng L, Zhao N, Yao X et al. Histidine–tryptophan–ketoglutarate solution vs. University of Wisconsin solution for liver transplantation: A systematic review. *Liver Transpl* 2007; 13(8): 1125–36.

19. Miller CM. Rapid flush technique for donor hepatectomy: Safety and efficacy of an improved method of liver recovery for transplantation. *Transplant Proc* 1988; 20(1): 948–50.

20. Hackl C, Schlitt HJ, Melter M et al. Current developments in pediatric liver transplantation. *World J Hepatol* 2015; 7(11): 1509–20.

21. Emond JC, Heffron TG, Whitington PF, Broelsch CE. Reconstruction of the hepatic vein in reduced size hepatic transplantation. *Surg Gynecol Obstet*, 1993; 176(1): 11–7.

22. de Santibanes E, McCormack L, Mattera J et al. Partial left lateral segment transplant from a living donor. *Liver Transpl* 2000; 6(1): 108–12.

23. Tanaka K, Kiuchi T. Living-donor liver transplantation in the new decade: Perspective from the twentieth to the twenty-first century. *J Hepatobiliary Pancreat Surg* 2002; 9(2): 218–22.

24. Krenn CG, Faybik P, Hetz H. Living-related liver transplantation: Implication for the anaesthetist. *Curr Opin Anaesthesiol* 2004; 17(3): 285–90.

25. Baker A, Dhawan A, Devlin J et al. Assessment of potential donors for living related liver transplantation. *Br J Surg* 1999; 86(2): 200–5.

26. McDiarmid SV, Anand R, Martz K et al. A multivariate analysis of pre-, peri-, and post-transplant factors affecting outcome after pediatric liver transplantation. *Ann Surg* 2011; 254(1): 145–54.

27. Kelly D, Jara P, Rodeck B et al. Tacrolimus and steroids versus ciclosporin microemulsion, steroids, and azathioprine in children undergoing liver transplantation: Randomised European multicentre trial. *Lancet* 2004; 364(9439): 1054–61.

28. Kelly D. Safety and efficacy of tacrolimus in pediatric liver recipients. *Pediatr Transplant* 2011; 15(1): 19–24.

29. Post DJ, Douglas DD, Mulligan DC. Immunosuppression in liver transplantation. *Liver Transpl* 2005; 11(11): 1307–14.

30. Kerkar N, Hadzic N, Davies ET et al. De-novo autoimmune hepatitis after liver transplantation. *Lancet* 1988; 351: 409–13.

31. Andries S, Casamayou L, Sempoux C et al. Posttransplant immune hepatitis in pediatric liver transplant recipients: Incidence and maintenance therapy with azathioprine. *Transplantation* 2001; 72: 267–72.

32. Kelly DA. Posttransplant growth failure in children. *Liver Transplant Surg* 1997; 3: S32–9 (Suppl 1).

33. Kelly DA. Current issues in pediatric transplantation. *Pediatr Transplant* 2006; 10: 712–20.

34. Arora N, McKiernan PJ, Beath SV et al. Concomitant basiliximab with low-dose calcineurin inhibitors in children post-liver transplantation. *Pediatr Transplant* 2002; 6(3): 214–8.

35. Reding R, Gras J, Sokal E et al. Steroid-free liver transplantation in children. *Lancet* 2003; 362(9401): 2068–70.

36. Reding R, Bourdeaux C, Gras J et al. The paediatric liver transplantation program at the Universite catholique de Louvain. *Acta Gastroenterol Belg* 2004; 67(2): 176–8.

37. Spada M, Petz W, Bertani A et al. Randomized trial of basiliximab induction versus steroid therapy in pediatric liver allograft recipients under tacrolimus immunosuppression. *Am J Transplant* 2006; 6(8): 1913–21.

38. Evans HM, McKiernan PJ, Kelly DA. Mycophenolate mofetil for renal dysfunction after pediatric liver transplantation. *Transplantation* 2005; 79(11): 1575–80.

39. Basso MS, Subramaniam P, Tredger M et al. Sirolimus as renal and immunological rescue agent in pediatric liver transplant recipients. *Pediatr Transplant* 2011; 15(7): 722–7.

40. Jiménez-Rivera C, Avitzur Y, Fecteau AH et al. Sirolimus for pediatric liver transplant recipients with post-transplant lymphoproliferative disease and hepatoblastoma. *Pediatr Transplant* 2004; 8(3): 243–8.

41. Hubscher S. Diagnosis and grading of liver allograft rejection: A European perspective. *Transplant Proc* 1996; 28(1): 504–7.

42. Oliveira P. Biliary complications after paediatric liver transplantation. *Pediatr Transplant* 2010 May; 14(3): 437–8.

43. Gruttadauria S, Mandala L, Miraglia R et al. Successful treatment of small for size syndrome in adult to adult living related liver transplantation: Single centre series. *Clin Transplant* 2007; 21(6): 761–6.

44. Umeda Y, Yagi T, Sadamori H et al. Preoperative proximal splenic artery embolization: A safe and efficacious portal decompression technique that improves the outcome of live donor liver transplantation. *Transplant Int* 2007; 20(11): 947–55.

45. Noujaim HM, Mayer D, Buckles JA et al. Techniques for and outcome of liver transplantation in neonates and infants weighing up to 5 kilograms. *J Pediatr Surg* 2002; 37(2): 159–64.

46. Suehiro T, Shimada M, Kishikawa K et al. Effect of intraportal infusion to improve small for size graft injury in living donor adult liver transplantation. *Transpl Int* 2005; 18(8): 923–8.

47. Lee TC, Savoldo B, Barshes NR et al. Use of cytokine polymorphisms and Epstein–Barr virus viral load to predict development of post-transplant lymphoproliferative disorder in paediatric liver transplant recipients. *Clin Transplant* 2006; 20(3): 389–93.

48. Choquet S, Leblond V, Herbrecht R et al. Efficacy and safety of rituximab in B-cell post-transplantation lymphoproliferative disorders: Results of a prospective multicenter phase 2 study. *Blood* 2006; 107(8): 3053–7.

49. Skagen CL, Jou JH, Said A. Risk of de novo hepatitis in liver recipients from hepatitis-B core antibody-positive grafts—A systematic analysis. *Clin Transplant* 2011; 25(3): E243–9.

50. Huprikar S, Danziger-Isakov L, Ahn J et al. Solid organ transplantation from hepatitis B virus-positive donors: Consensus guidelines for recipient management. *Am J Transplant* 2015 May; 15(5): 1162–72.

51. Wong TCL, Fung JYY, Mau Lo C. Prevention of recurrent hepatitis B infection after liver transplantation. *Hepatobil Pancreat Dis Int* 2013; 12: 465–72.

52. Duffy JP, Kao K, Ko CY et al. Long-term patient outcome and quality of life after liver transplantation: Analysis of 20-year survivors. *Ann Surg* 2010; 252(4): 652–61.

53. Avitzur Y, De Luca E, Cantos M et al. Health status ten years after pediatric liver transplantation—Looking beyond the graft. *Transplantation* 2004; 78(4): 566–73.

54. Gilmour S, Adkins R, Liddell GA et al. Assessment of psychoeducational outcomes after pediatric liver transplant. *Am J Transplant* 2009; 9(2): 294–300.

55. Evans HM, Kelly DA, McKiernan PJ et al. Progressive histological damage in liver allografts following pediatric liver transplantation. *Hepatology* 2006; 43(5): 1109–17.

56. Haagsma EB, Hagens VE, Schaapveld M et al. Increased cancer risk after liver transplantation: A population-based study. *J Hepatol* 2001; 34(1): 84–91.

57. Harambat J, Ranchin B, Dubourg L et al. Renal function in pediatric liver transplantation: A long-term follow-up study. *Transplantation* 2008; 86(8): 1028–34.

58. Scheenstra R, Peeters PM, Verkade HJ et al. Graft fibrosis after pediatric liver transplantation: Ten years of follow-up. *Hepatology* 2009; 49(3): 880–6.

59. Bucuvalas JC, Alonso E, Magee JC et al. Improving long-term outcomes after liver transplantation in children. *Am J Transplant* 2008; 8(12): 2506–13.

60. Falkenstein K, Flyn L, Kirkpatrick B et al. Non-compliance in children post-liver transplant. Who are the culprits? *Pediatr Transplant* 2004; 8(3): 233–6.

61. Wright J, Elwell L, McDonagh JE et al. 'It's hard but you've just gotta get on with it'—The experiences of growing-up with a liver transplant. *Psychol Health* 2015; 30(10): 1129–45.

62. Sagar N, Leithead JA, Lloyd C et al. Pediatric liver transplant recipients who undergo transfer to the adult healthcare service have good long-term outcomes. *Am J Transplant* 2015; 15(7): 1864–73.

63. Miloh T, Annunviato R, Arnon R et al. Improved adherence and outcomes for pediatric liver transplant recipients by using text messaging. *Pediatrics* 2009; 124(5): e844–50.

Head and neck

30

Choanal atresia

MIRA SADADCHARAM AND JOHN D. RUSSELL

INTRODUCTION

Choanal atresia is a well-recognized congenital defect characterized by obstruction in the posterior nasal apertures, usually by bone or soft tissue, secondary to failed recanalization of the nasal fossae during fetal development (Figure 30.1). This defect was first reported by Johann George Roederer in 1755 and was later characterized as an anatomic deformity of palatine bone by Adolf Otto in 1854.[1] The condition may be either unilateral or bilateral. Bilateral choanal atresia presents acutely in the neonatal period as an airway emergency, in view of the fact that neonates are obligate nasal breathers. The classic clinical scenario is one of increasing respiratory distress that improves when the child starts to cry, since he/she takes in air through the mouth, thus bypassing the obstructed choanal airway. A unilateral defect may go undetected for months or even years prior to diagnosis. Treatment may be divided into emergent and elective definitive categories and involves surgical repair of the defect. Following the first successful transnasal corrective surgery by Carl Emmert in 1854, surgical techniques have evolved from transmaxillary, transseptal, transpalatine, and sublabial intranasal approaches to modern endoscopic techniques. Despite the acceptance of the endoscopic approach as the current gold standard, controversies still exist on how to best manage patients with this condition, particularly regarding the use of adjuvant topical medications following surgical repair and the use and duration of postoperative stenting.[2]

EPIDEMIOLOGY

Choanal atresia occurs in approximately 1 in 5000–8000 live births. The ratio of unilateral to bilateral choanal atresia is 2:1, with the right side being more commonly affected in unilateral cases. Although choanal atresia does not appear to have a particular racial demographic, studies report that the female-to-male ratio for infants with choanal atresia is 2.2:1.[3] In addition, while no correlation appears to exist between maternal age and parity, there does appear to be a slightly increased incidence in twin births. Approximately 50% of all patients have other associated congenital abnormalities, which rises to approximately 75% in patients with bilateral disease.[4] The atretic plate may be either mixed, bony, or membranous in nature. A 90% rate of bony stenosis and 10% rate of membranous stenosis were classically reported, but modern imaging suggests a mixed bony/membranous obstruction in 70% and a pure bony obstruction in 30%.[5] Associated syndromes include CHARGE (coloboma, heart defect, atresia choanae, growth and mental retardation, genital hypoplasia, ear anomalies); Crouzon; DiGeorge; amniotic band syndrome; fetal alcohol syndrome; and Treacher Collins.

EMBRYOLOGY AND THEORIES OF CAUSATION

In humans, development of the face and cranial structures occurs in the first 12 weeks of gestation. Specifically, the choanae develop between the 4th and 11th weeks.[6] At 4 weeks' gestation, nasal development begins with the formation of nasal pits. At approximately 5 weeks' gestation, these nasal pits deepen and invaginate into the surrounding mesenchyme to form the nasal sacs, separated from the primitive oral cavity by oronasal membranes. At about 8 weeks' gestation, these membranes rupture to create a nasal cavity and primitive choanae located at the junction between the nasal cavities and the nasopharynx. By the end of the 10th week of gestation, the nasal septum and the developing palate fuse and the primitive choanae undergo alteration and are pushed posterior. At this stage, the choanae are termed secondary choanae. In a normal fetus, secondary choanae are patent, allowing for a functionally patent airway between the anterior part of the nose and the inner nasopharynx.[6]

In choanal atresia, the abnormality is complex, representing more than just an obstruction membrane across the posterior choanae. The lateral nasal wall and medial pterygoid plates form part of the obstruction and need to be addressed during the surgical repair.[7] The boundaries of the atretic plate are composed of the undersurface of the

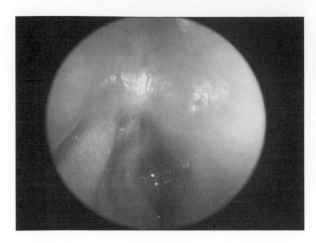

Figure 30.1 Endoscopic view of a right-sided choanal atresia as viewed from the nose.

sphenoid body superiorly, the medial pterygoid laterally, the vomer medially, and the horizontal portion of the palatine bone inferiorly.

Over the past two decades, four theories have gained prominence when investigating the etiology of choanal atresia. These are as follows: (1) persistence of the buccopharyngeal membrane from the foregut; (2) abnormal persistence or location of mesoderm-forming adhesions in the nasochoanal region; (3) abnormal persistence of the nasobuccal membrane of Hochstetter; and (4) misdirection of neural crest cell migration and subsequent mesodermal flow.

Currently, the theory of misdirection of neural crest migration and subsequent mesodermal flow is thought to offer the strongest evidence. During embryogenesis, the ectoderm at the neural plate margin produces neural crest cells. These cells subsequently migrate to form the skeletal and connective tissue framework of the face and portions of the cranium. Neural crest cell deficiencies have been associated with defects in the frontonasal parts of the face. Furthermore, disordered migration patterns have been found to be associated with caudal maxillary process and visceral arch derivatives as seen in choanal atresia.[8] Craniofacial anomalies with mesenchymal damage and cell disruption were found in offspring of mothers who took high doses of vitamin A, and these changes were associated with embryonic pathways involving the migration of neural crest cells in early fetal life.

Environmental risk factors for choanal atresia have not been well studied. Maternal behaviors, including lifestyle and nutritional intake during pregnancy, play an important role in optimal fetal development and outcomes. Women of reproductive age may be exposed to cigarette smoke, alcohol, caffeine, suboptimal nutrition, and medications, each of which has been associated with birth defects.

Barbero et al.[9] suggested that prenatal use of antithyroid medications, e.g., methimazole and carbimazole, were linked to choanal atresia. In addition, Lee et al.[10] evaluated the association between continuous and categorical infant T_4 levels and nonsyndromic choanal atresia and suggested a role of low thyroid hormone levels in the development of choanal atresia. They further suggested that low newborn T_4 levels could potentially be used as a proxy measure of risk.

The CHARGE association is associated with choanal atresia in approximately 30% of cases.[11] All patients diagnosed with choanal atresia should have a systematic examination for other features of the CHARGE association.

CLINICAL PRESENTATION

The clinical presentation of choanal atresia is dependent on whether the deformity is unilateral or bilateral and the presence of other coexisting comorbidities. Bilateral choanal atresia presents as an airway emergency at birth, since neonates are obligate nasal breathers for the first 6 weeks of life. Physical examination often demonstrates a bony and/or membranous obstruction in the nasal cavity, stridor, marked retraction of the chest, and paradoxical cyanosis (blueness of skin relieved by crying). Acute airway stabilization including insertion of an oral (Guedel) airway, use of a McGovern nipple (a nipple from a feeding bottle with the end opened to allow respiration), or even intubation is required in the first instance. Once the airway has been secured, it is important to consider differential diagnoses including pyriform aperture stenosis and severe neonatal rhinitis. Subsequent investigations should be targeted at both confirming the diagnosis and assessing for the presence or absence of associated comorbidity.

Unilateral atresia may be picked up in the newborn period during routine nasal catheter screening. However, if the catheter rolls up in the nasal cavity, choanal atresia may not be diagnosed until later, when the child presents with unilateral nasal obstruction (no misting of mirror) and an associated thick unilateral foul-smelling nasal discharge.

RADIOLOGIC INVESTIGATIONS

Traditional plain radiography in the supine position with the nasal cavity filled with radiopaque contrast has been replaced by computed tomography (CT). CT of the paranasal sinuses and skull base is recognized as the investigation of choice. Ideally, the nasal cavity should be suctioned prior to the scan as thick mucus can be hard to differentiate from a membranous atretic plate. Thin-section (1–2 mm) axial images provide the best view of the obstruction, but coronal reconstructions should also be provided to identify intraoperative landmarks. CT helps to accurately delineate the location of obstruction within the nasal passages, the position (anterior, posterior), laterality (unilateral, bilateral), and histological characteristics (bony, membranous, or mixed) of each affected choana. Prior to the availability of CT, the histological distribution of choanal atresia cases was estimated as 90% bony and 10% membranous.[12] More recent findings using CT and tissue specimens suggest that about 30% of choanal atresia is pure bone and 70% is mixed (membranous and bone), with no pure membranous occurrence.[13,14]

MANAGEMENT

Treatment of choanal atresia aims at establishing the patency of the airway, preventing further damage to the surrounding structures, and a short intervention with limited hospitalization. Infants with bilateral choanal atresia will require airway stabilization with at least an oropharyngeal airway as outlined previously. Such devices need to be carefully taped in place and an orogastric tube passed to facilitate feeding until definitive surgical repair can be attempted. Surgical repair should be performed early (even in the first week of life) in patients with bilateral atresia. The only contraindication to early correction is the presence of associated comorbidities, e.g., cardiac anomalies in those patients with the CHARGE association. Children with unilateral atresia can generally wait until 1 year of age, when the risk of general anesthetic has diminished. Occasionally, patients with unilateral atresia have significant airway difficulties and will require earlier intervention.

Since the first reported repair of choanal atresia by Carl Emmert in 1854, a number of surgical techniques have been described. Transnasal puncture of the atretic plate using urethral dilators was initially performed blindly. However, this technique has now largely been superseded by endoscopic resection using powered instruments.[1]

Endoscopic resection

This approach is preferred by the authors as it allows excellent visualization of the operative field. A tonsil (Boyle–Davis) mouth gag is inserted and a Vicryl suture placed through the uvula and clipped to facilitate retraction of the soft palate. A 120° 4 mm endoscope is passed through the mouth into the nasopharynx and a view of the posterior surface of the obstructed choanae obtained (Figure 30.2). The nasal cavity is decongested with 1:10,000 adrenaline patties, and the atretic plate injected with 1% lignocaine with 1:200,000 adrenaline. If present, the membranous component of the atretic plate is then perforated with a small suction catheter or urethral dilator. The 120° telescope is passed through the mouth to view the atretic plate at the time of perforation (Figure 30.3). The senior author then uses the Acclarent sinuplasty balloon for further atraumatic dilatation. The drill is then inserted through the nose until it reaches the nasopharynx. The senior author uses a specialized drill (Medtronic), which has a protective sheath over the shaft, preventing trauma to the nasal cavity. The drilling is performed medially over the vomer and laterally over the medal pterygoid plates. The posterior aspect of the vomer is then removed using a back-biting forceps into the nasopharynx and removing the posterior half of the vomer. This creates a common cavity posteriorly, which minimizes the chance of restenosis. Beclomethasone drops are applied in the immediate postoperative period to minimize edema. The child is electively taken back to the theatre 6 weeks postoperatively, at which point any granulations present are removed with a microdebrider and any restenosis dilated.

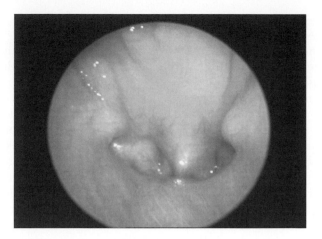

Figure 30.2 Endoscopic view of choanal atresia from the nasopharynx as viewed through a 120° telescope.

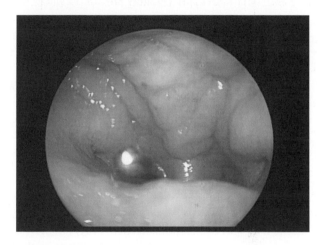

Figure 30.3 Endoscopic view of urethral dilator being passed through an atretic plate as viewed from the nasopharynx using a 120° telescope.

Multiple procedures for further microdebridement and dilatations are often required, with one large series reporting an average of 4.9 procedures.[12] A number of variations of the endoscopic technique are reported.[1] The most common variation from our technique is a complete transnasal approach using the 0° 4 mm (or 2.7 mm in neonates) telescope. We find the sole use of the transnasal approach to be associated with difficulty using two instruments in the same nasal cavity, particularly within the context of limited space available in the neonate. Similarly, mucosal-sparing flaps are advocated by some surgeons in an attempt to improve re-epithelialization.[13,14] However, the authors' experience is that these flaps are difficult to perform in the limited space of a neonatal nose, and they are generally not viable at the end of the procedure. CT-based image guidance systems are now widely used in pediatric endoscopic nasal surgery.[15] While not mandatory, we advocate their use in this procedure if available.

Transpalatal resection

The transpalatal approach was the first approach to the choanal abnormality that provided good exposure of the operative field. Together with simple blind dilatation, it remained the mainstay of surgical repair until the advent of endoscopic technology and techniques. In this procedure, a U-shaped incision is made over the hard palate 5 mm from the dental arch. A posteriorly based subperiosteal flap is elevated to gain access to the nasopharynx. The inferior vomer is encountered and removed prior to drilling of the lateral atretic plate. This technique remains useful in patients with a small nasopharynx and low skull base, such as infants with Treacher Collins syndrome, or where an endoscopic approach has failed. The transpalatal approach is associated with a higher complication rate compared to endoscopic techniques. Potential complications include postoperative pain, palatal fistula, and reduced midface face growth leading to a high arched palate and associated dental malocclusion, which occurs in approximately 50% of patients.[5]

Adjuncts to surgery

STENTS

The use of postoperative nasal stents continues to be controversial. Significant debate exists in the literature as to whether placing stents in the operative site after the procedure provides improved outcomes. Portex and manipulated endotracheal tubes are often used. When stents are used, the optimum duration of use is unclear with the literature reporting a range of 24 hours to 12 weeks.[1]

As a proponent of stenting, Friedman et al. reviewed 46 cases of choanal atresia and reported a favorable prognosis (defined as fewer operations needed) with children who had stents in for greater than 12 weeks.[16] Following this in 2004, Gujrathi et al.[17] performed a study on 52 patients who had stents in place for a median of 12 weeks. They found that only 2 of 52 (3.8%) patients required a revision operation. Despite this, stents are not without potential side effects, with necrosis of the external nose, septum, and palate reported.[17] Furthermore, stents have a tendency to become blocked with secretions, requiring lavage and suctioning on a routine basis by both the parents and the nursing staff. Several opponents to stenting make claims against its efficacy, often citing how there is a significant foreign body tissue reaction with the stent in place, leading to more granulation tissue and scarring down of the tissues. Schoem[18] demonstrated this in a study of 13 patients who did not have stents placed, with 4 of the subjects requiring no further operations and 9 of them requiring only one additional operation. More recently in 2013, Llorente et al.[19] demonstrated similar outcomes without stents, having 100% patency in their test subjects at 27 months' follow-up.

MITOMYCIN C

In addition to stents, the antineoplastic agent mitomycin C has been used as a treatment adjunct to try to decrease stenosis. Mitomycin C is an aminoglycoside that is produced by the bacteria streptomyces. It works by inhibiting fibroblast growth and proliferation, which may help minimize the granulation tissue. This drug is already commonly used in other areas of head and neck surgery. It is typically applied as a topical agent on a cotton pledget for a few minutes in the nose to achieve the desired effect. A study by Holland and McGuirt[20] demonstrated promising outcomes with the use of the drug. The study involved 8 test subjects and 15 controls. The primary outcome measure was the number of dilations required after initial surgery. They found that patients treated with adjunctive mitomycin C therapy required significantly fewer dilations than the control group.

CONCLUSIONS

When faced with a neonate or older child with signs of nasal/upper airway obstruction or respiratory distress, it is important to consider the possibility of a unilateral or bilateral choanal atresia. If choanal atresia is identified, it is necessary for the physician to investigate for the coexistence of associated conditions. If bilateral atresia is identified, this should be managed as an airway emergency and appropriate measures taken to secure the airway prior to considering surgical intervention.

When undergoing surgical treatment, one must consider the most effective approach and possible treatment adjuncts to give the patient the best outcome possible. A considerable array of surgical techniques (including adjuvant therapies) exist for the management of choanal atresia in the newborn.

The primary outcome measure is restenosis as evidenced by a need for reoperation. Reported revision rates for endoscopic resection vary from 0% to 36%.[1,11] Restenosis appears more likely to be required in patients who undergo surgery in the neonatal period for bilateral disease and suffer from gastroesophageal reflux. Favorable outcomes may be predicted by the absence of associated facial anomalies, higher weight at the time of surgery (>2.3 kg), and larger stent size.[21,22] One long-term study has demonstrated moderate hyposmia in adults who underwent bilateral choanal atresia repair as a child.[23]

To date, no randomized control trials exist to determine optimum treatment protocols, even for the more controversial questions such as the role of postoperative stenting. Unfortunately, due to overall rarity of the condition, this absence of evidence is likely to remain unchanged, and management guidelines will continue to be based on personal reports and case series.

REFERENCES

1. Ramsden JD, Campisi P, Forte V. Choanal atresia and choanal stenosis. *Otolaryngol Clin North Am* 2009; 42(2): 339–52, x.
2. Corrales CE, Koltai PJ. Choanal atresia: Current concepts and controversies. *Curr Opin Otolaryngol Head Neck Surg* 2009; 17(6): 466–70.
3. Michalski AM, Richardson SD, Browne ML et al. Sex ratios among infants with birth defects, National Birth Defects Prevention Study, 1997–2009. *Am J Med Genet A* 2015 May; 167A (5): 1071–81.
4. Keller JL, Kacker A. Choanal atresia, CHARGE association, and congenital nasal stenosis. *Otolaryngol Clin North Am* 2000; 33(6): 1343–51, viii.
5. Brown OE, Pownell P, Manning SC. Choanal atresia: A new anatomic classification and clinical management applications. *Laryngoscope* 1996; 106(1 Pt 1): 97–101.
6. Dunham ME, Miller RP. Bilateral choanal atresia associated with malformation of the anterior skull base: Embryogenesis and clinical implications. *Ann Otol Rhinol Laryngol* 1992 Nov; 101(11): 916–9.
7. Hasegawa M, Oku T, Tanaka H et al. Evaluation of CT in the diagnosis of congenital choanal atresia. *J Laryngol Otol* 1983; 97(11): 1013–5.
8. Johnston MC. The neural crest in abnormalities of the face and brain. *Birth Defects Orig Artic Ser* 1975; 11(7): 1–18.
9. Barbero P, Valdez R, Rodríguez H et al. Choanal atresia associated with maternal hyperthyroidism treated with methimazole: A case–control study. *Am J Med Genet A* 2008 Sep 15; 146A(18): 2390–5.
10. Lee LJ, Canfield MA, Hashmi SS et al. Association between thyroxine levels at birth and choanal atresia or stenosis among infants in Texas, 2004–2007. *Birth Defects Res A Clin Mol Teratol* 2012 Nov; 94(11): 951–4.
11. Hengerer AS, Brickman TM, Jeyakumar A. Choanal atresia: Embryologic analysis and evolution of treatment, a 30-year experience. *Laryngoscope* 2008; 118(5): 862–6.
12. Samadi DS, Shah UK, Handler SD. Choanal atresia: A twenty-year review of medical comorbidities and surgical outcomes. *Laryngoscope* 2003; 113(2): 254–8.
13. Dedo HH. Transnasal mucosal flap rotation technique for repair of posterior choanal atresia. *Otolaryngol Head Neck Surg* 2001; 124(6): 674–82.
14. Nour YA, Foad H. Swinging door flap technique for endoscopic transseptal repair of bilateral choanal atresia. *Eur Arch Otorhinolaryngol* 2008; 265(11): 1341–7.
15. Benoit MM, Silvera VM, Nichollas R et al. Image guidance systems for minimally invasive sinus and skull base surgery in children. *Int J Pediatr Otorhinolaryngol* 2009; 73(10): 1452–7.
16. Friedman, NR, Mitchell RB, Bailey CM et al. Management and outcome of choanal atresia correction. *Int J Pediatr Otorhinolaryngol* 2000; 52: 45–51.
17. Gujrathi, CS, Daniel SJ, James AL, Forte V. Management of bilateral choanal atresia in the neonate: An institutional review. *Int J Pediatr Otorhinolaryngol* 2004; 68: 399–407.
18. Schoem SR. Transnasal endoscopic repair of choanal atresia: Why stent. *Otolaryngol Head Neck Surg* 2004; 131: 362–6.
19. Llorente JL, Lopez F, Morato M, Suarez V. Endoscopic treatment of choanal atresia. *Acta Otorrinolaringol Esp* 2013; 64: 389–95.
20. Holland BW, McGuirt WF. Surgical management of choanal atresia: Improved outcome using mitomycin. *Arch Otolaryngol Head Neck Surg* 2001; 127: 1375–80.
21. Kubba H, Bennett A, Bailey CM. An update on choanal atresia surgery at Great Ormond Street Hospital for Children: Preliminary results with Mitomycin C and the KTP laser. *Int J Pediatr Otorhinolaryngol* 2004; 68(7): 939–45.
22. Teissier N, Kaguelidou F, Couloigner V et al. Predictive factors for success after transnasal endoscopic treatment of choanal atresia. *Arch Otolaryngol Head Neck Surg* 2008; 134(1): 57–61.
23. Leclerc JE, Leclerc JT, Bernier K. Choanal atresia: Long-term follow-up with objective evaluation of nasal airway and olfaction. *Otolaryngol Head Neck Surg* 2008; 138(1): 43–9.

31

Pierre Robin sequence

UDO ROLLE, ARANKA IFERT, AND ROBERT SADER

INTRODUCTION

The condition is originally named after the French dental surgeon Pierre Robin (1867–1950). He described micrognathia (firstly named "mandibular hypotrophy"), glossoptosis, and respiratory distress in his first paper.[1] In a later publication, Pierre Robin added cleft palate to the list of clinical signs.[2] There had been previous reports of the triad micrognathia, cleft palate, and glossoptosis resulting in dyspnea and cyanosis.[3–5] Pierre Robin added the term "glossoptosis" to better characterize the tendency for the tongue to fall back and cause pharyngeal obstruction.

The traditional name for the condition used to be "Pierre Robin syndrome," but after 1975, a series of nosologic changes took place, including Robin anomalad,[6] Robin malformation complex,[7] and then Robin sequence (PRS).[8]

The term "sequence" is used to reflect the hypothesis that the three cardinal symptoms develop sequentially, though it is still not proven what the correct sequence is. The traditional hypothesis states that a mandibular anomaly leads to an anomalous palate (cleft palate) and subsequent airway obstruction.[9] Even if this concept seems to be supported by animal experiments,[10] actual functional therapy results also support the opposite hypothesis that a malpositioned tongue leads to altered mandibular growing patterns.[11–13]

ETIOLOGY, PATHOPHYSIOLOGY

The most accepted etiological hypothesis is the hypoplasia or abnormal development of the mandible around 7–11 weeks gestational age displaces the tongue high within the nasopharynx.[14] Others comprise oropharyngeal and muscular deficiency or mandible compression in utero.[15] In mandible hypoplasia, the tongue, unable to descend because of either the lack of mandibular growth or severe retropositioning of the mandible, obstructs the palatal shelves from fusing. The cause of the growth insult to the mandible is uncertain and, presumably, is of heterogeneous etiology. Reported possible causes included (1) positional or mechanical deformation, as in oligohydramnios, which can be caused by a number of factors; (2) intrinsic mandibular hypoplasia, as in numerous congenital malformation syndromes; (3) neurological or neuromuscular abnormalities, such as myotonic dystrophy or arthrogryposis; and (4) connective tissue disorders, such as Larsen syndrome.

In all these cases, sequential events would lead to the changes seen in PRS. A logical assumption is that a variety of factors may lead to persistent mandibular hypoplasia with the resulting postnatal manifestations.[16] Since mandibular abnormalities might have numerous causes, PRS cannot be regarded as a specific disease entity. A differentiation should be made between isolated PRS and patients in which PRS is part of a recognized syndrome, part of a complex of multiple anomalies, or part of an unrecognized syndrome.

GENETICS, INCIDENCE

There is a high incidence of twins with PRS. Furthermore, family members of PRS patients have a higher incidence of cleft lip and palate.[17] Cleft palate is associated with deletions of 2q and 4p, and duplications of 3p, 3q, 7q, 78q, 10p, 14q, 16p, and 22q. Micrognathia is associated with deletions of 4p, 4q, 6q, and 11q, and duplications of 10q and 18q.

The proportion of the number of cases with isolated PRS varies in different studies from 40% to 74%.[18] There are more cases in females, with a male-to-female ratio of 3:2,[16] which is equal to the ratio comparing male and female children with cleft palate.[19]

The most common PRS syndromes are Stickler syndrome (20%–25% of all cases) and velocardiofacial syndrome (15% of all cases). Nager syndrome, spondylo-epiphyseal dysplasia congenital, and other recognized syndromes comprise the rest of the syndromic PRS cases.

The severity and persistence of the clinical pathology are probably related to the nature of the insult, as illustrated by the difference in outcome between "syndromic" and "non-syndromic" micrognathia.[20]

The previously reported incidence of PRS varies from 1 in 2000 to 1 in 30,000 live births.[21] The highest incidence has been reported for the United States with 1/3120 cases per live birth, followed by Germany with 1/8060, United Kingdom with 1/8500, and Denmark with 1/14,000.[15] The reported differences in the prevalence of PRS at birth are due to the variations of the case definitions and the different time periods of data collection, as well as the different data collection methods.[15]

Prenatal diagnosis or even prediction of severity of PRS has not been established yet.[22]

CLINICAL FEATURES (NEW CLASSIFICATION 2015)

PRS consists of three essential components.

1. Micrognathia or retrognathia
2. Glossoptosis, possibly accompanied by airway obstruction
3. Cleft palate (usually U-shaped, but V-shape also possible)

It should be mentioned that cleft palate does not have a complete penetrance and can only be seen in about 80% of the Pierre Robin patients.[9]

The airway obstruction in PRS requires early and proper management, since it may lead to hypoxia, cor pulmonale, failure to thrive, and cerebral impairment. Generally, syndromic cases are more severe and have worse prognosis than nonsyndromic PRS.

Usually, it is expected that patients with nonsyndromic PRS will show catch-up growth of the mandible.

AIRWAY MANAGEMENT

Airway obstruction due to glossoptosis can occur at or immediately after birth, but may take much longer (up to 3 weeks) to become apparent.[23] Most neonates present with an isolated PRS and not one of the syndromes, which typically present more significant clinical problems, i.e., airway and feeding difficulties. The airway obstruction in PRS is due to the narrowing or complete obstruction of the pharyngeal space by the posteriorly displaced tongue. This airway obstruction could be intermittent. Most of the complications and unfavorable outcomes of PRS are directly related to delayed or inappropriate airway management.[24] Therefore, special vigilance is required, even in patients with only minor defects. Typical clinical signs of upper airway obstruction are increased respiratory effort, stridor, subcostal retractions, and cyanotic or apneic spells. In an otherwise asymptomatic child, choking attacks, cyanosis during feeding, or repeated aspiration events may be due to intermittent airway problems.

Since PRS infants may also have short or collapsing epiglottis, laryngomalacia, and/or segmental tracheal stenosis, nasoendoscopy and bronchoscopy might be necessary to assess the child.

Every child with symptoms of airway obstruction should be nursed prone with the head to one side. The head should be maintained in level position to prevent either glossoptosis or gastroesophageal reflux. Usually, affected children can be successfully fed by mouth in this position.

Persistence of airway difficulties requires further intervention.

Nasopharyngeal tube

The nasopharyngeal airway bypasses the oral pharynx and the obstruction due to the glossoptosis. A regular endotracheal tube, cut to the appropriate length, is inserted by nasal route and securely strapped in place. The nasopharyngeal airway is a very effective, temporary form of airway management within the intensive care unit. Usually, patients with nasopharyngeal tubes in place would not be sent home, as dislodgement of the tube can result in an acute airway obstruction.

Endotracheal tube

Endotracheal intubation serves as a short-term support if the nasopharyngeal airway is not successful or during resuscitation or anesthesia.

Tongue–lip adhesion/glossopexy

Essentially, in this technique, the tongue is sutured to the lower lip. After the child has demonstrated catch-up growth, the tongue–lip adhesion can be released. The efficacy of the tongue–lip adhesion technique remains a controversial issue.

Glossopexy consists of suturing the tongue base to the mandible. Due to the relatively soft consistency of the mandible, a permanent glossopexy is difficult to achieve; therefore, this technique is also controversial.

Tracheostomy

Tracheostomy should be avoided if possible, and it should only be employed if all other techniques fail. It should be performed by an appropriately skilled surgeon who is familiar with infantile airways. Tracheostomy requires closed monitoring but enables oral feeding. It could be removed after the child's airway obstruction has resolved, which usually happens within the first year of life.

Distraction osteogenesis of the mandible

Distraction osteogenesis comprises a relatively new technique. The mandible needs to be cut near the angle of the mandible on both sides. A specialized mechanical device distracts these two portions every day by approximately 1.5–2 mm. Using this technique, the mandible gradually elongates over a period of 2–3 weeks. Timing of performing a mandibular distraction can be in newborns to prevent tracheostomy or at a later stage to remove a tracheostomy tube.

Distraction osteogenesis has been carried out only during the last 5–10 years. Therefore, long-term follow-up results of this promising technique are not available. Nevertheless, the distraction osteogenesis technique should be reserved for severe cases of nonsyndromic Pierre Robin and syndromic PRS, since in most cases of nonsyndromic PRS, physiologic catch-up growth of the mandible occurs.

Tongue positioning and stimulation plate

During the last decade, a new, nonsurgical technique was developed by orthodontists that guarantees, in most cases, a free airway space and treats the hypoplastic mandible causally. Immediately, a palatal plate is produced, similar to the feeding plate for cleft palate newborns, but with a dorsal spur that goes shortly to the epiglottis (Figure 31.1a–c). Sometimes endoscopic control is necessary during positioning to avoid irritation of the epiglottis. To accomplish this, the tongue is positioned anteriorly and the airway is kept patent. Moreover, via functional stimulation of the tongue, the mandible starts to grow during the following months and will be quite normal when the palatal closure is performed at the age of about 6 months (Figure 31.2a–e). Feeding is also supported, but problems remain in some cases.[25]

Noninvasive ventilation

There is growing evidence that noninvasive respiratory support could improve breathing patterns and respiratory outcomes for infants with severe upper airway obstruction due to PRS. Subsequently, the rate of necessary tracheostomies was reduced. Some authors consider this the first line treatment.[26]

NUTRITIONAL MANAGEMENT

Children with PRS have feeding difficulties in 38%–62%.[27] Initial treatment consists of bottle-feeding in a prone position with the head slightly elevated. This method of feeding is appropriate in children with catch-up growth of the mandible.

If this is not satisfactory, gavage or feeding tubes can be used temporarily to improve nutrition. If the feeding is still not successful, the child might need a gastrostomy, which could be removed after gaining the ability to be fed orally.

It has been shown clearly that infants with PRS require adequate caloric intake. It is important to achieve the maximum growth rate of the mandible since the resolution of the airway problems is directly related to mandibular growth. Only recently has increased work of breathing

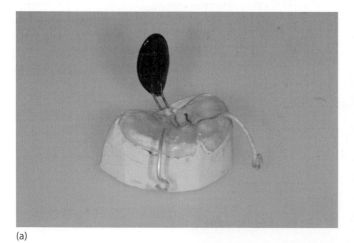

(a)

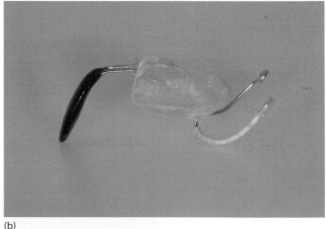

(b)

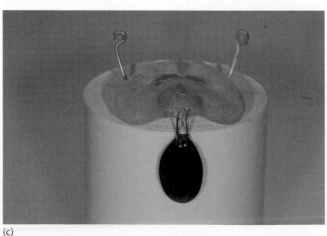

(c)

Figure 31.1 **(a–c)** Stimulation plate.

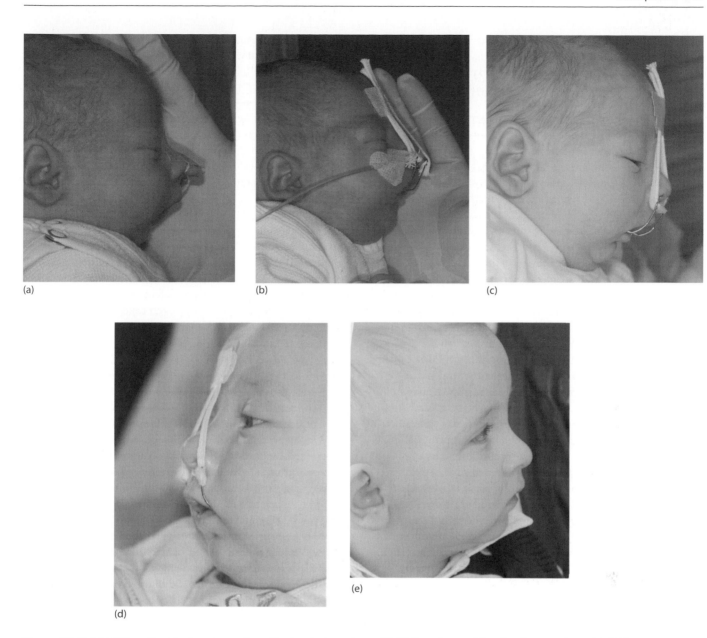

Figure 31.2 **(a)** PRS patient before insertion of stimulation plate. **(b)** PRS patient with stimulation plate. **(c)** PRS patient after 2 months of treatment with stimulation plate. **(d)** PRS patient after 4 months of treatment with stimulation plate. **(e)** PRS patient after closure of cleft palate at the age of 8 months.

been appreciated as an important component of calorie consumption. It may be necessary to provide these children with several times the normal caloric requirement of an infant to compensate for up to a 10-fold increase in respiratory work. Indeed, failure to gain weight despite maximum nutritional intake should suggest the need for more aggressive airway management. The availability of total parenteral nutrition should prevent any instances of failure to thrive, but it is rarely needed if other aspects of the condition are managed correctly.

It has been additionally proven that that PSR infants have a higher incidence of gastroesphageal reflux (GER), and even empiric reflux treatment may be indicated to improve breathing and feeding.

CLEFT PALATE

Cleft palate is present in at least 80% of patients with PRS. Cleft palates are typically repaired while patients are infants. A palatal plate can be used in patients with a cleft of the hard palate to improve feeding. The plate also corrects the tongue position by moving it anteriorly. In patients with a cleft of the soft palate alone, a palatal plate has no positive effect on feeding, but it can improve the tongue position and stimulate mandibular growth. To enhance this effect, the plate can be modified by an anterior stimulus according to Castillo-Morales.[28]

Surgical protocols differ from center to center, and cleft closure is performed not only by different techniques (i.e.,

Langenbeck, Furlow, Wardill) but also at different ages, ranging from 4 to 36 months.

It is currently assumed that early surgery will provide a better chance of normal palatal function and speech development.

MICROGNATHIA/RETROGNATHIA

The first described functional therapy for micrognathia was the use of the orthodontic palatal plate to achieve growth stimulation of the mandible. It was not clear until today whether the growth potential of the mandible after this stimulation is sufficient to achieve the normal dimensions. However, it has been shown, based on physical examinations until age 5, that the mandible can barely regain its growth in relation to a normal population.[29] A retrospective longitudinal study by cephalograms and lateral photographs of American patients with PRS and cleft of the soft palate showed that the mandible achieved only partial catch-up growth and, in adults, a smaller maxilla, mandible, and a narrow respiratory airway space persisted.[30] Studies in the Finnish population showed the same result.[31] An increased mandibular growth was seen during the first 2 years of life, but normal craniofacial dimensions were never achieved. At the young adult stage, even if the patient's profile appeared less retrognathic due to masking by the overlying soft tissues or the patient's teeth showed neutral occlusion, cephalograms revealed retrognathia and caudal–dorsal rotation of the mandible. Thus, it seems in accordance with today's knowledge that the microgenia in PRS can be balanced only partially by growth processes. Frequently, orthodontic therapy is necessary in childhood. In severe cases, surgical advancement of the mandible combined with a genioplasty can be beneficial, as well.

SKELETAL ANOMALIES

Around 11%–21% of children with PRS have limb defects.[18] Common anomalies are talipes equinovarus, syndactyly, short or absent digits, and hypoplastic long bones. Occipitoatlanto-axial instability has also been described, emphasizing the need for very experienced clinicians to undertake the intubation of such patients. Orthopedic and radiological consultation should be sought in children with suspected skeletal problems. Rare neuromuscular defects can also occur, resulting in a tendency for glossoptosis to persist despite mandibular growth.[11]

EAR PROBLEMS

Malformations of the ear have a frequency of 10.5% and consist of defects in the auditory capacity and anomalies of the shape of the ear. One main concern is the frequently recurring infections of the middle ear, which also occur in patients with a cleft palate and are based on disturbed function of the Eustachian tube. Therefore, a hearing screening has to be performed at birth. At a later date, control of the middle ear tube function has to be achieved and grommets placed, if necessary.[32]

CARDIOVASCULAR ANOMALIES

Intrinsic cardiac defects are found in up to 20% of infants with PRS.[33] Septal defects are common, but more complex lesions can also occur. A thorough cardiovascular examination should be performed in PRS babies, particularly since airway difficulties may aggravate the cardiac status.[34]

OCULAR ANOMALIES

Retinal detachment and micrognathia occur as part of Stickler syndrome,[35] but 10% of infants with nonsyndromic PRS also have eye defects, such as strabismus, ptosis, and microphthalmia. More severe defects such as cataract and congenital glaucoma have also been reported, and ophthalmologic consultation is recommended in all cases.[36]

NASAL OBSTRUCTION

Choanal atresia is a rare accompaniment of PRS,[37] but it may complicate the respiratory difficulties in small infants who do not mouth-breathe. It is important to ensure nasal patency, especially if one nostril is to be utilized for a nasogastric feeding tube. Choanal obstruction by itself can lead to glossoptosis, with consequences identical to those of PRS.[38]

CONCLUSION AND FUTURE DIRECTIONS

In isolated PRS, the long-term outcome is directly related to the quality of the management at the onset of symptoms. With adequate nutrition, mandibular growth will achieve normal or near-normal proportions, and the glossoptosis will resolve. To date, nonsurgical treatment is preferred for infants with PRS.[39]

The previously documented high incidence of mental retardation in PRS patients was almost certainly due to unrecognized episodes of hypoxia, and with good airway management, this complication is uncommon.

Undiagnosed hypoxia may also lead to pulmonary vasoconstriction, with resultant pulmonary hypertension and cor pulmonale. Some instances of sudden death in PRS were likely due to this problem. The presence of cardiomegaly on a chest x-ray should alert the physician to the possibility that hypoxic episodes have been overlooked, and appropriate steps should be taken immediately.

Although airway patency improves with growth, there remains a potential for obstruction, particularly after invasive procedures such as intubation or cleft palate repair.[40] In some children, obstruction may occur during sleep, causing occasional apnea with potentially hazardous consequences.[41] A degree of mandibular hypoplasia may persist for several years, resulting in malocclusion and the need for dental treatment.[42]

The overall mortality rate in infants with PRS is approximately 25%. The majority of deaths occur in children with associated anomalies, particularly those with cardiac defects or an underlying syndrome with two or more organ anomalies.[43] These facts must be considered when counselling parents of affected children. With good medical and nursing care, the prognosis for children with isolated PRS should be excellent.[44]

REFERENCES

1. Robin P. La chute de la base de la langue consideree comme une nouvelle cause de gene dans larespiration naso-pharyngienne. *Bull Acad Med Paris* 1923; 89: 37–41.
2. Robin P. Glossoptosis due to atresia and hypotrophy of the mandible. *Am J Dis Child* 1934; 48: 541–7.
3. St. Hilaire H. Sphenocephalus. *Philos Anat* 1822; 2: 97–8.
4. Fairbairn P. Suffocation in an infant from retraction of the base of the tongue, connected with defect of the frenum. *Month J Med Sci* 1846; 6: 280–1.
5. Shukowsky WP. Zur aetiologie des stridor inspiratorius congenitus. *Jahrb Kinderheilk* 1911; 73: 459–74.
6. Hanson JW, Smith DW. U-shaped palatal defect in the Robin anomalad: Developmental and clinical relevance. *J Pediatr* 1975; 87: 30–3.
7. Cohen MM. Syndromes with cleft lip and cleft palate. *Cleft Palate J* 1978; 15: 306–28.
8. Smith DW. *Recognizable Patterns of Human Malformation*, 3rd edn. Philadelphia: WB Saunders, 1982.
9. Sadewitz VL. Robin sequence: Changes in thinking leading to changes in patient care. *Cleft Palate Craniofac J* 1992; 29(3): 236–53.
10. Schubert J, Jahn H, Berginski M. Experimental aspects of the pathogenesis of Robin sequence. *Cleft Palate Craniofac J* 2005; 42: 372–6.
11. Carey JC, Fineman RM, Ziter FA. The Robin sequence as a consequence of malformation, dysplasia, and neuromuscular syndromes. *J Pediatr* 1982; 101: 858–64.
12. Bacher M, Bacher U, Göz G, Pham T, Cornelius CP, Speer CP, Goelz R, Arand J, Wendling F, Buchner, P, Bacher A: Three-dimensional computer morphometry of the maxilla and face in infants with Pierre Robin sequence—A comparative study. *Cleft Palate-Craniofac J* 2000; 37: 292–302.
13. Ludwig B, Glasl B, Sader R, Schopf P. Conservative orthodontic primary care of four newborns with the Pierre–Robin sequence triad. *J Orofac Orthoped* 2007; 68: 56–61.
14. Tan TY, Kilpatrick N, Farlie PG. Developmental and genetic perspectives on Pierre Robin sequence. *Am J Med Genet C* 2013; 163C: 295–305.
15. Cote A, Fanous A, Almajed A, Lacroix Y. Pierre Robin sequence: Review of diagnostic and treatment challenges. *Int J Pediatr Otorhinolaryng* 2015; 79: 451–64.
16. Pashayan HM, Lewis MB. Clinical experience with the Robin sequence. *Cleft Palate J* 1984; 21: 270–6.
17. Gangopadhyay N, Mendoonca DA, Woo AS. Pierre Robin sequence. *Sem Plast Surg* 2012; 26: 76–82.
18. Williams AJ, Williams MA, Walker CA, Bush PG. The Robin anomalad (Pierre Robin syndrome)—A follow up study. *Arch Dis Child* 1981; 45: 663–8.
19. Elliot M, Studen-Pavlovich D, Ranalli DN. Prevalence of selected pediatric conditions in children with Pierre Robin syndrome. *Pediatr Dent* 1995; 17: 106–11.
20. Cohen MM Jr. Robin sequences and complexes: Causal heterogeneity and pathogenetic/phenotypic variability. *Am J Med Genet* 1999; 84: 311–15.
21. Bush PG, Williams AJ. Incidence of the Robin anomalad (Pierre Robin syndrome). *Br J Plast Surg* 1983; 36: 434–7.
22. Lind K, Aubry MC, Belarbi N, Chalouhi C, Couly G, Benachi A, Lyonnet S, Abadie V. Prenatal diagnosis of Pierre Robin sequence: Accuracy and ability to predict phenotype and functional severity. *Prenat Diagn* 2015; 35: 853–8.
23. Ogborn MR, Pemberton PJ. Late development of airway obstruction in the Robin anomalad (Pierre Robin syndrome) in the newborn. *Aust Paediatr J* 1985; 21: 199–200.
24. Myer CM, Reed JM, Cotton RT, Willging JP, Shott SR. Airway management in Pierre Robin sequence. *Otolaryngol Head Neck Surg* 1998; 118: 630–5.
25. Brosch S, Flaig S, Bacher M, Michels L, de Maddalena H, Reinert S and Mauz P. The influence of the Tübingen soft palate plate and early cleft closure on swallowing and Eustachian tube function in children with Pierre Robin sequence. *HNO* 2006; 54: 756–60.
26. Leboulanger N, Picard A, Soupre V, Aubertin G, Denoyelle F, Galliani E, Roger G, Garabedian EN, Fauroux B. Physiologic and clinical benefits of noninvasive ventilation in infants with Pierre Robin sequence. *Pediatrics* 2010; 126: e1056–63.
27. Evans KN, Sie KC, Hopper RA, Glass RP, Hing AV, Cunningham ML. Robin Sequence. From diagnosis to development of an effective management plan. *Pediatrics* 2011; 127: 936–48.
28. Hohoff A, Ehmer U. Short-term and Long-term results after early treatment with the Castillo Morales stimulating plate—A longitudinal study. *J Orofac Orthop* 1999; 60: 2–12.

29. Daskalogiannakis J, Ross RB, Tompson BD. The mandibular catch-up growth controversy in Pierre Robin sequence. *Am J Orthod Dentofacial Orthop* 2001; 120: 280–5.

30. Figueroa AA, Glupker TJ, Fitz MG, BeGole EA. Mandible, tongue, and airway in Pierre Robin sequence: A longitudinal cephalometric study. *Cleft Palate-Craniofac J* 1991; 28: 425–34.

31. Laitinen SH, Heliövaara A, Ranta, RE. Craniofacial morphology in young adults with the Pierre Robin sequence and isolated cleft palate. *Acta Odontol Scand* 1997; 55: 223–8.

32. Handžić J, Ćuk V, Rišavi R, Katić V, Katušić D, Bagatin M, Štajner-Katušić S, Gortan D. Pierre Robin syndrome: Characteristics of hearing loss, effect of age on hearing level and possibilities in therapy planning. *J Laryngol Otol* 1996; 110: 830–5.

33. Pearl W. Congenital heart disease in the Pierre Robin syndrome. *Pediatr Cardiol* 1982; 2: 307–9.

34. Dykes EH, Raine PAM, Arthur DS, Drainer IK, Young DG. Pierre Robin syndrome and pulmonary hypertension. *J Pediatr Surg* 1985; 20: 49–52.

35. Opitz JM, France T, Herrman J, Spranger JW. The Stickler syndrome. *N Eng J Med* 1972; 286: 546–7.

36. Smith JL, Stowe FR. The Pierre Robin syndrome (glossoptosis, micrognathia, cleft palate). *Pediatrics* 1961; 27: 128–33.

37. Borovik HR, Kveton JF. Pierre Robin syndrome combined with unilateral choanal atresia. *Otolaryngol Head Neck Surg* 1987; 96: 67–70.

38. Cozzi F, Pierro A. Glossoptosis-apnoea syndrome in infancy. *Pediatrics* 1985; 75: 836–43.

39. Maas C, Poets CF. Initial treatment and early weight gain of children with Robin sequence in Germany: A prospective, epidemiological study. *Arch Dis Child Fetal Neonatal Ed* 2014; 99: F491–4.

40. Hatch DJ. Anaesthesia for paediatric surgery. In: Summer E, Hatch DJ (eds). *Textbook of Paediatric Anaesthesia Practice*. London: Baillière Tindall, 1989: 275–304.

41. Frohberg U, Lange RT. Surgical treatment of Robin sequence and sleep apnea syndrome: Case report and review of the literature. *J Oral Maxillofac Surg* 1993; 51: 1274–7.

42. Sheffield LJ, Reiss JA, Strohm K, Gilding M. A genetic follow-up study of 64 patients with the Pierre Robin complex. *Am J Med Genet* 1987; 28: 25–36.

43. Costa MA, Tu MM, Murage KP, Tholpady SS, Engle WA, Flores RL. Robin Sequence: Mortality, cause of death and clinical outcomes. *PRS J* 2014; 134 (4): 738–45.

44. Bull MJ, Givan DC, Sadove AM, Bixler D, Hearn D. Improved outcome in Pierre Robin sequence: Effect of multidisciplinary management. *Pediatrics* 1990; 86: 294–301.

32

Macroglossia

THAMBIPILLAI SRI PARAN AND GEORGE G. YOUNGSON

INTRODUCTION

Macroglossia (primary form) is defined as a resting tongue that protrudes beyond the teeth, or in the case of the neonate, the alveolar ridge.[1] Pseudomacroglossia arises when the tongue itself is normal but relative protrusion occurs because of a small mandible.[2]

ETIOLOGY

Primary macroglossia can be due to an intralingual lesion such as lymphangioma, hemangioma, dermoid cyst, or hyperplasia associated with systemic disorders such as chromosomal abnormalities, hypothyroidism, amyloidosis, or simply may be idiopathic. Secondary macroglossia is due to a lesion within the oral cavity adjacent to the tongue such as tumor (rhabdomyosarcoma), neurofibromatosis, lingual thyroglossal cyst, lingual thyroid, ranula, or myositis. Macroglossia is one of the most constant features of Beckwith–Wiedemann syndrome, which is characterized by an omphalocele or umbilical hernia, with associated visceromegaly, somatic gigantism or hemihypertrophy, and hypoglycemia.[3] Intraoral and intralingual enteric duplication cysts have been detected in utero.[4–6]

PATHOLOGY

The histological features depend upon the underlying disorder. In addition to the aforementioned conditions, macroglossia can also be found in the triad of intrauterine growth retardation, transient diabetes mellitus, and macroglossia.[7] It is also seen in a number of syndromes including Behmel, Hurler, Laband, and Tollner syndrome.

PRESENTATION

Lymphangioma is the most common cause of macroglossia to present in the neonatal period (Figure 32.1a and b), and prenatal diagnosis by ultrasound is possible when associated with Beckwith–Wiedemann syndrome[8] and some of the intraoral cystic lesions discussed earlier. The physical presentation will be obvious and may also be accompanied by noisy breathing, difficulty feeding, and drooling. When feeding difficulties are profound, then failure to thrive and poor weight gain will be evident. Macroglossia secondary to lymphangioma may lead to verrucous lesions on the surface of the tongue, and these can ulcerate and exude a serous discharge.

If unrecognized or untreated in the neonatal period, the lesion may become more problematic in infancy or later in childhood, when it may present with minor trauma, e.g., to a lingual lymphangioma. This can then result in intralesional hemorrhage and/or sepsis (usually cellulitis from group B hemolytic *Streptococcus*). In this event, abrupt enlargement may compromise the airway and produce a life-threatening emergency, necessitating tracheostomy and gastrostomy until definitive tongue reduction can be carried out (Figure 32.2).

If treatment is inappropriately delayed, protracted dental defects develop, including prognathism, anterior open bite, and an increased angle between the ramus and body of the mandible.[9] Speech defects occur, and articulation is subsequently defective, especially expression of consonants, which are precluded by inadequate tongue movement as a consequence of the increased bulk in a limited cavity. Regression of macroglossia is not a regular feature when due to lymphangioma, and a conservative approach to the lesion has little merit.

DIAGNOSIS

Investigation, following thorough physical examination for secondary causes of macroglossia, comprises thyroid function testing, echocardiography, and karyotype analysis. Magnetic resonance imaging to detail the extent of tongue involvement is indicated particularly when the volume of lingual tissue affected is not clinically apparent.

MANAGEMENT

Mild macroglossia as seen in most children with Beckwith–Wiedemann syndrome and smaller oral lesions does not need any special care. When associated with systemic disorders such as hypothyroidism, management of the primary

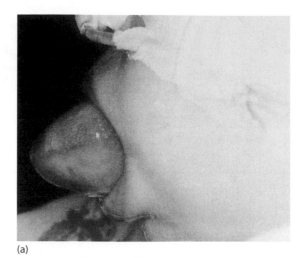

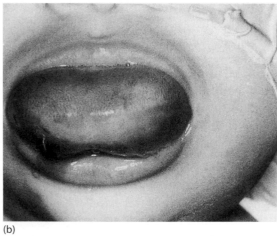

Figure 32.1 **(a, b)** Lymphangioma of the tongue occluding the oral cavity in a 4-week-old neonate.

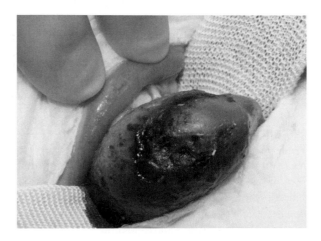

Figure 32.2 Intralesional hemorrhage into a lingual lymphangioma producing respiratory obstruction.

condition alone is what is needed. Moderate enlargements can be managed by nursing the infant in the lateral or prone position to assist the airway and drooling. A multidisciplinary approach including a dietician, speech therapist, and pediatric dentist will be useful.

However, when severe macroglossia with airway compromise is present, early involvement of an anesthetist or intensivist and otolaryngologist is necessary. The airway may have to be secured by a tracheostomy and feeding commenced via a formal gastrostomy. Biopsy is rarely indicated, with histology becoming available on the resected specimen. Needle aspiration of intralingual cystic lesions, however, may be a useful temporizing procedure[5] but requires confident exclusion of vascular anomalies by prenatal or postnatal imaging.

Intravascular photocoagulation[10] and embolism of vascular tongue anomalies[11] are useful in the management of some children. Steroid treatment may confer temporary benefit during an acute airway obstruction early in life. Glossitis and/or sepsis from tongue lesions is seen later in life and will need penicillin-based antibiotic treatment. Surgery with glossectomy, preferably before 7 months of age, confers optimal opportunity for rehabilitation of tongue movement and will avoid complications such as glossitis, hemorrhage, and secondary speech and maxillofacial abnormalities.[12] However, surgery is best avoided during the newborn period in order to minimize unnecessary morbidity.

SURGERY

Reduction glossectomy is the mainstay of treatment, and options include central wedge resection, circumferential wedge resection, or a combined transoral and transcervical approach for a massive infiltrative lymphangioma.[13]

The aims of reduction are to allow intraoral position of the tongue in the floor of the mouth, to restore normal tongue movement, and to permit speech and deglutition. Implicit in these objectives is the fact that surgery should be conservative and a repeat tapering procedure is preferable to removal of excess tissue. The principles involve careful hemostasis by use of a tourniquet or, alternatively, by use of an yttrium aluminium garnet (YAG) laser, CO_2 laser,[14] or harmonic scalpel. We recommend a V-shaped resection of the anterior tongue as has been previously described.[15,16]

Nasal intubation or tracheostomy secures airway protection. The head is placed in a silicone ring and the neck extended. A suture placed on the apex of the tongue and two hemostatic/traction sutures tied over silicone rubber dams at the base of the tongue provide the requisite traction (Figure 32.3). Traction on these three sutures delivers the necessary exposure and hemostasis sufficient for central wedge resection. The resection should not usually extend into the posterior one-third, where the extrinsic muscles of the tongue are inserted. The lateral margins of the incision extend from the level of the anterior gum, with the tongue in a resting position, to the apex, and this incision is beveled such that more ventral than dorsal tissue is removed. This re-creates the natural concavity of the central tongue (Figure 32.4). A straight needle is a useful adjunct to creating this bevel.

The divided lingual arteries are ligated. Restoration of the tongue flaps at the midline is performed incorporating mucosa and a few millimeter of muscle (Figure 32.5).

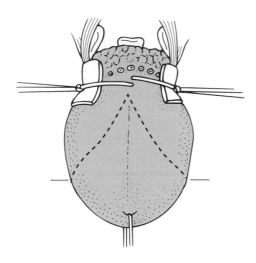

Figure 32.3 Traction sutures allow good exposure and good hemostasis during reduction glossectomy.

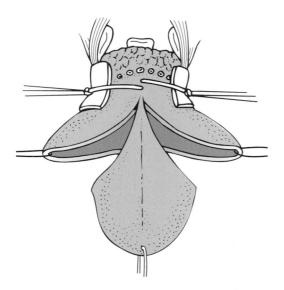

Figure 32.4 Wedge of tissue incorporating more of the dorsal than the ventral aspect of the tongue is removed.

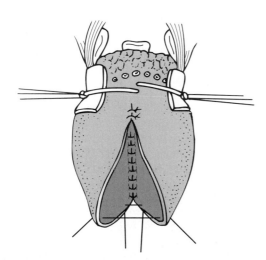

Figure 32.5 The remaining lateral segments of the tongue approximated in the midline.

The opportunity to place a percutaneous gastrostomy should be taken if protracted delay in feeding is anticipated. Antibiotics should be continued into the postoperative period to provide prophylaxis against sepsis in the floor of the mouth. Oral hygiene is maintained with chlorhexidine or saline oral toilet. The appropriate tracheostomy care, if required, is given and secondary orthodontic and speech therapy follow-up arranged.

REFERENCES

1. Gupta OP. Congenital macroglossia. *Arch Otolaryngol* 1971; 98: 378–83.
2. Murthy P, Laing M. Macroglossia. *Br Med J* 1994; 309: 1387.
3. Vogel JE, Mulliken JB, Kaban LB. Macroglossia: A review of the condition and a new classification. *Plast Reconstruct Surg* 1986; 78: 715–23.
4. Chen MK, Gross E, Lobe TE. Perinatal management of enteric duplication cyst of the tongue. *Am J Perinatol* 1997; 14: 161–3.
5. Eaton D, Billings K, Timmons C, Botth T, Biavati MJ. Congenital foregut duplication cyst of the anterior tongue. *Arch Otolaryngol Head Neck Surg* 2001; 127: 1484–7.
6. Surana R, Losty P, Fitzgerald R. Heterotopic gastric cyst of the tongue in a newborn. *Eur J Pediatr Surg* 1993; 3: 110–1.
7. Dacou-Voutetakis C, Anagnostakis D, Xanthou M. Macroglossia, Transient neonatal diabetes mellitus and intrauterine growth failure. A new distinct entity. *Pediatrics* 1975; 55: 127–31.
8. Harker CP, Winter T, Mack L. Prenatal diagnosis of Beckwith–Wiedemann syndrome. *Am J Radiol* 1997; 168: 520–2.
9. Rizer FM, Scheckter GL, Richardson MA. Macroglossia: Aetiological considerations and management techniques. *Int J Pediatr Otorhinolarygol* 1985; 81: 225–36.
10. Chang CJ, Fisher DM, Chen YR. Intralesional photocoagulation of vascular anomalies of the tongue. *Br J Plast Surg* 1999; 52: 178–81.
11. Slaba S, Herbreteau D, Jhaveri HS et al. Therapeutic approach to arterio-venous malformations of the tongue. *Eur Radiol* 1998; 8: 280–5.
12. Shafer AD. Primary macroglossia. *Clin Pediatr* 1968; 7: 357–65.
13. Dinerman WS, Myers EN. Lymphangiomatous macroglossia. *Laryngoscope* 1976; 86: 291–6.
14. Yilmaz N, Mercan H, Karaman E, Kaytaz A. Tongue reduction in Beckwith–Wiedemann syndrome with CO_2 laser. *J Craniofac Surg* 2009; 20: 1202–3.
15. Upadhyaya P, Upadhyaya P. Partial glossectomy for macroglossia. *J Pediatr Surg* 1986; 21: 457.
16. Davalbhakta A, Lamberty BGH. Technique for uniform reduction of macroglossia. *Br J Plast Surg* 2000; 53: 294–7.

33

Tracheostomy in infants

JEYANTHI KULASEGARAH, THOM LOBE, AND JOHN D. RUSSELL

INTRODUCTION

The indications for tracheostomy have changed over time owing to advancements in treatment and technology. In the early 1980s, many tracheostomies were performed as a result of upper airway infection.[1] With the introduction of vaccines against *Haemophilus influenza* and *Corynebacterium diphteriae* and improvements in intensive care units (ICUs) in the 1980s and 1990s, the number of tracheostomies required for infectious diseases has decreased.[2] Several series have documented the changing indications for tracheostomy in children over the past decade. Also, there are regional differences in tracheostomy indications. In the United Kingdom, three large series[3–5] have reported long-term ventilation as the most common indication for tracheostomies. Research from France,[6] Singapore,[7] and Spain[8] also reports a greater number of tracheostomies being done for ventilator dependency. However, some centers have reported a reversal back to upper airway obstruction as the most common indication, although it is most often owing to acquired or congenital causes rather than infection. Mahadevan and colleagues[9] from New Zealand published their experience from 1987 to 2003 and found that upper airway obstruction was the most common indication for tracheostomy. More recent studies from United States,[10] Canada,[11] and Switzerland[12] have also found upper airway obstruction as the most common indication.

This chapter will discuss the indications, techniques for insertion, and maintenance of a tracheostomy in infants.

INDICATIONS FOR TRACHEOSTOMY

The indications for tracheostomy in neonates and infants can be broadly divided into three categories: (1) prolonged ventilation, (2) upper airway obstruction (congenital or acquired), and (3) pulmonary toilet for mainly neurological patients with aspiration (Table 33.1).[2,6,9,12,13]

Tracheostomy is recommended for patients requiring extended periods of ventilation to manage lung disease, such as bronchopulmonary dysplasia in premature infants, as well as to manage respiratory failure directly or indirectly, as a result of congenital neurologic, pulmonary and cardiovascular abnormalities. There has also been a trend toward patients with significantly complex medical problems surviving long term, and these patients often require long-term ventilation via a tracheostomy.[3,4]

Airway obstruction, caused by congenital or acquired lesions, can lead to insertion of tracheostomy. The immature airway manifests itself as laryngomalacia, tracheomalacia, or a combination of the two conditions. Patients with a congenitally stenotic airway or tracheal agenesis are special cases. In the case of agenesis, an emergency tracheostomy may be necessary where the trachea reestablishes distally. Usually, however, these patients can be ventilated best using a mask because the bronchi come off the esophagus and an esophageal tube can cause obstruction. Technology today allows bedside bronchoscopy in such infants with tenuous airway status so that proper decisions can be made before one risks transporting the infant to the operating theatre.

Occasionally the management of a tumor such as a cervical teratoma or sarcoma in infancy will mandate a tracheostomy. More likely, a hemangioma or lymphangioma will compromise the airway to the extent that a more stable airway is needed. Infants with congenital high airway obstruction (CHAOS), often are diagnosed in utero today, and an ex utero intrapartum therapy (EXIT) procedure, where a tracheostomy is performed with maternal–fetal circulation intact, may be required.[14]

There are several acquired airway conditions that require tracheostomy, including infection, papillomatosis, neuromuscular failure, chronic aspiration, and subglottic stenosis.

Other related conditions are congenital or acquired vocal cord paralysis, which is usually due to a central nervous system deficit; phrenic nerve injury, which may be associated with a difficult delivery; and recurrent laryngeal nerve injury, which may occur after ligation of a patent ductus arteriosus.

Table 33.1 Indications for tracheostomy

Category		Indications
Prolonged ventilation	Respiratory	Bronchopulmonary dysplasia
		Pneumonia
		Restrictive lung disease
	Cardiac	Congenital heart disease
	Neuromuscular disease	Spinal muscular atrophy
		Myasthenia gravis
	Central	Encephalopathy
		Intracranial hemorrhage
		Status epilepticus
		Brainstem tumors
		Guillain–Barré syndrome
		Ondine syndrome
		Silvermann syndrome
	Others	Sepsis
		Trauma
Upper airway obstruction	Craniofacial anomalies	Mandibular hypoplasia
		Pierre Robin
		Crouzon syndrome
		CHARGE syndrome
		Treacher Collins
		Apert syndrome
		Freeman–Sheldon syndrome
	Nose/postnasal space	Choanal atresia/stenosis
	Larynx	Laryngeal atresia
		Laryngeal cleft
		Laryngeal stenosis
		Subglottic stenosis
	Trachea/bronchus	Tracheomalacia/bronchomalacia
		Tracheal stenosis
		Tracheal atresia
	Bilateral vocal cord paralysis	Congenital
		Arnold–Chiari malformation
		Brain tumor
		Prolonged intubation
	Tumor (airway/neck)	Giant cervical teratoma
		Laryngotracheal hemangioma
		Cervicofacial hemangioma
		Lymphangioma
	Trauma	Cranial/neck/vertebrae
Pulmonary toilet	Neurological patients with aspiration	
	Chronic aspiration syndrome	

Sources: Ozmen, S. et al., Pediatric tracheotomies: A 37-year experience in 282 children, *Int J Pediatr Otorhinolaryngol* 2009, 73, 959–961. Butnaru, C.S. et al., Tracheotomy in children: Evolution in indications, *Int J Pediatr Otorhinolaryngol* 2006, 70, 115–119. Mahadevan, M. et al., Pediatric tracheotomy: 17 year review, *Int J Pediatr Otorhinolaryngol* 2007, 71, 1829–1835. de Trey, L. et al., Pediatric tracheotomy: A 30-year experience, *J Pediatr Surg* 2013, 48, 1470–1475. Davis, G.M., Tracheostomy in children, *Paediatr Respir Rev* 2006, 7 Suppl 1, S206–209.
Note: CHARGE-Coloboma of the eye, heart defects, atresia of the nasal choanae, retardation of growth and/or development, genital and urinary abnormalities, ear abnormalities and deafness.

Some patients with craniofacial anomalies, such as choanal atresia and Pierre Robin syndrome, may require a tracheostomy.

Rarely, trauma will prompt the surgeon to perform a tracheostomy. This can be related to birth trauma, child abuse, burns, or accidents.

Majority of patients requiring a tracheostomy are under the age of 1, as shown in many series.[3,8,9,11,12]

PREOPERATIVE EVALUATION

Although originally, tracheostomy was developed as an emergency procedure for acute airway difficulties, in many settings, most infants who need a tracheostomy already have an endotracheal tube in place. Infants will require direct laryngoscopy and bronchoscopy to assess the airway.

Following an airway assessment of neonates and infants, especially patients in the neonatal intensive care unit (NICU) with complex malformations, extreme prematurity, complex syndromes, cardiac anomalies, or neurological deficit, a multidisciplinary team (MDT) consisting of a pediatric otolaryngologist, a pulmonologist, a neonatologist, an intensivist, pediatric surgeons, cardiothoracic surgeons, a neurologist, a tracheostomy nurse specialist, a speech and language therapist, and a dietician should meet and discuss the clinical situation and make appropriate recommendations to parents or caretakers prior to proceeding with tracheostomy. The MDT also gives an opportunity for family and caretakers to discuss the risks and benefits of the procedure, how the procedure is performed, and short- and long-term goals for the patient. A growing body of literature has demonstrated that an MDT approach gives the best results in terms of clinical outcome for the patients and cost effectiveness for the National Health Care System.[15,16]

When an infant is not intubated, but is under consideration for tracheostomy, the extent to which the child maintains oxygenation and demonstrates adequate ventilation as judged by the PCO_2 measured by transcutaneous monitoring will determine the need for a more direct assessment before a decision for tracheostomy is made.

The surgeon should make certain of the coagulation status, hemoglobin level, and electrolytes as indicated by the patient's condition. The nutritional status of the patient should also be taken into consideration. Poor nutrition will complicate nearly any condition in infancy and may weigh in favor of an earlier tracheostomy than would be indicated otherwise. Finally, patients with persistent aspiration, despite correction of any gastroesophageal reflux, may necessitate a tracheostomy to prevent severe pulmonary consequences.

Choosing the appropriate tube size is the key element when planning for tracheostomy. An extensive selection of neonatal and pediatric tracheostomy tubes are currently available, produced in response to a variety of specific clinical requirements.[17] The optimal size of the tracheostomy depends on the clinical indication for the procedure, the size of the airway, and the age of the patient. The size

designations of pediatric tracheostomy tubes are based on the inner diameter (ID). Neonatal tubes are similar to pediatric tubes in their ID and outer diameter (OD) but shorter in length.

There are several ways to determine the appropriate tracheostomy tube to be used. Tweedie and colleagues[17] at Great Ormond Street Hospital for Children in London have produced a sizing chart as a guide to determine appropriate tube selection prior to tracheostomy. Behl and Watt,[18] on the other hand, developed a simplified formula to calculate tracheostomy tube size from the age of the child, as follows:

$$ID\,(mm) = (Age/3) + 3.5$$

$$OD\,(mm) = (Age/3) + 5.5$$

The ID and OD of the tracheostomy tube also correlates well with patient weight, as follows[18]:

$$ID\,(mm) = [Weight\,(kg) \times 0.08] + 3.1$$

$$OD\,(mm) = [Weight\,(kg) \times 0.1] + 4.7$$

TECHNIQUE

The infant is placed supine on the operating table, sufficiently toward the head of the table so that the surgeon can access the infant's neck easily and also the anesthesiologist can gain access to the patient to manipulate the endotracheal tube when required during the procedure.

These cases should be done under a general anesthetic unless the infant is so ill as to be unable to tolerate the drugs. Even so, an anesthesiologist should maintain control of the airway while the surgeon is exposing and manipulating the trachea.

The patient's cardiorespiratory status should be monitored during the case. This should consist of a cardiac monitor for heart rate, a blood pressure monitor, and ideally, a pulse oximeter to assess the infant's oxygenation. A rigid bronchoscope should be available throughout the procedure, in case there is any need to manipulate and control the airway.

If the infant has not had prior laryngoscopy and bronchoscopy, a diagnostic examination is performed prior to tracheostomy to confirm the diagnosis and to assure that the tracheal lumen will accept a tracheostomy without difficulty. Special issues, such as a tracheostomy to stent an airway for severe tracheomalacia, can be assessed by bronchoscopy to determine the proper length of the proposed cannula, which may have to be specially ordered. In some cases, it may be necessary to use an ordinary endotracheal tube placed through the cervical incision and secured to the skin of the neck until this temporary tracheostomy cannula can be replaced with the specially ordered device.

When positioning the infant on the operating table, the neck should be extended sufficiently to allow complete access to the neck. Sometimes, in chubby infants, it is still difficult to see the entire neck, despite best attempts. A roll should be placed under the infant's shoulders to facilitate proper positioning (Figure 33.1).

The endotracheal tube should be secured so that the anesthesiologist can easily remove the tube at the appropriate time. This means that any tape should be loosened beforehand. If there is a feeding tube in place, it should be removed so that it does not interfere with endotracheal tube manipulation.

When the infant is properly positioned and monitored, the entire neck from the lower lip to below the nipples should be prepped with a suitable surgical prep and draped. The superior most surgical drape should allow easy access to the patient by the anesthesiologist.

Once prepped and draped, the surgeon should carefully palpate the infant's neck to locate the trachea that hopefully is in the midline. The surgeon must remember that the infant's trachea is quite mobile and compressible, and may be difficult to palpate. The anesthesiologist can jiggle the endotracheal tube from above to assist with its location.

A transverse skin incision is best. We make our incision in the lower neck crease, about the width of one finger above the jugular notch. If the incision is too low, you will end up in the mediastinum, and the cannula will be placed too low in the trachea. We first score the skin with a scalpel and then use a bipolar diathermy (electrocautery) device to deepen the incision, taking care not to burn the skin. This incision is extended through the subcutaneous fascia and platysma muscle, which is quite thin in the small infant. A pad of subcutaneous fat is excised. This shortens the tracheostomy tract and allows immediate exposure of the strap muscles. It is helpful to insert two right-angled retractors in the corners of this incision to better expose the operative site.

Next, we use two atraumatic forceps to grasp the anterior cervical fascia on either side of the midline and open it vertically in the midline. We extend this incision inferiorly to the jugular notch and superiorly to the thyroid gland.

The strap muscles, immediately beneath the anterior cervical fascia, similarly are separated in the midline. Usually, there are few to no blood vessels in the dissection thus far. Occasionally, the surgeon will encounter a few small vessels that cross the midline. These should be cauterized and divided as they are encountered.

Once these muscles are separated, we place the two retractors deep into the muscle edges and gently retract laterally to better expose the trachea below. Sometimes it is necessary to free the muscle edges sufficiently to allow room for the blade of the retractor to gain a secure purchase. The trachea should be visualized easily. If not, then palpation in the wound with manipulation of the endotracheal tube by the anesthesiologist will help locate the trachea.

The proposed tracheostomy cannula should be selected and opened and its OD visually checked against the exposed trachea to judge the correctness of its size. If it seems that the initial selection was incorrect, then a tracheostomy cannula of a more appropriate size should be selected.

The pretracheal fascia should be lightly scored with the cautery to coagulate any tiny vessels on the surface of the trachea in the midline. Again, the blades of the retractors should be deep in the wound on either side of the trachea for optimal exposure.

A suture of 4-0 Prolene or its equivalent should be placed on either side of the midline scored anterior trachea (Figure 33.2). Each suture incorporates one or two tracheal rings. These sutures are not tied onto the tracheal wall, but can be tied at their ends and should be left 6–8 cm in length. At the end of the case, these sutures should be taped securely to the anterior chest wall and used to locate the tracheal incision in the event of a postoperative emergency in which the newly placed tracheostomy cannula dislodges. These sutures also can be used to hold open the edges of the

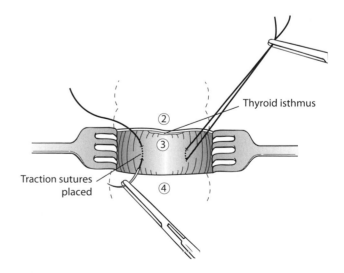

Figure 33.2 Traction sutures of fine silk are placed around the third tracheal ring to stabilize the trachea before incision. The sutures are tied in loose loops and later taped to the anterior chest wall. The sutures are left in place for 4 days as a precaution against accidental decannulation postoperatively.

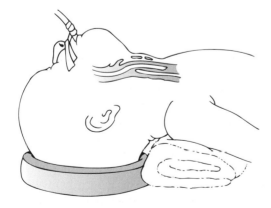

Figure 33.1 Position of infant for tracheostomy. The shoulders are elevated on a roll; the head is hyperextended on the neck and supported by a doughnut-form support.

tracheal incision for ease of placement of the tracheostomy cannula at operation.

In most tertiary centers, maturation sutures are used, and this involves the placement of sutures between the anterior tracheal wall and skin, which hastens the formation of a mature stoma and has the potential of decreasing the risk of accidental decannulation and the formation of granulation tissue.[19,20]

The surgeon should request that the endotracheal tube be loosened and prepared for removal. Using a No. 11 blade, a vertical incision is made through the tracheal wall along the score mark (Figure 33.3). Two or three tracheal rings should be divided, usually rings 2, 3, and 4. Rarely, it is necessary to divide the isthmus of the thyroid gland for proper tracheostomy positioning. In some centers, a transverse tracheal incision is used instead of a vertical incision.[21] Removal of a tracheal ring is likely to result in a tracheal deformity and thus should be avoided. Similarly, unless one is dealing specifically with a localized stenosis or deformity, tracheal wall resection is to be avoided.

Suction should be available in case blood or secretions interfere with the surgeon's view of the tracheal lumen. The tip of the cannula to be inserted should be lubricated with a water-soluble surgical lubricant and positioned over the incision, poised for insertion when the endotracheal tube is withdrawn.

The surgeon should then ask the anesthesiologist to withdraw the endotracheal tube sufficiently to clear the lumen so that the tracheostomy cannula can be inserted and directed caudally toward the carina.

One way to avoid misplacement is to insert a suction catheter through the lumen, beyond the tip of the cannula (Figure 33.4). The suction catheter then can be inserted into

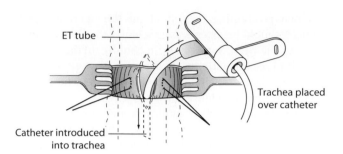

Figure 33.4 Tube insertion into the trachea is accomplished by shifting the endotracheal tube up to the cephalic margin of the new stoma, inserting a tracheal suction catheter into the trachea through the newly established opening, and then advancing the tracheostomy tube over the catheter in the trachea. This is safer than using the tube obturator, the short tip of which sometimes slips out of the stoma and allows the tracheostomy tube to pass anterior to the trachea and into the mediastinum. ET, endotracheal tube.

the tracheal lumen first and serve as a guide over which the cannula can be passed. This technique also is useful should the cannula become dislodged after the procedure.

If, for any reason, the tracheostomy cannula does not fit easily into the trachea, it should be removed and the endotracheal tube advanced beyond the tracheal incision so that ventilation will not be compromised. This might occur if the diameter of the tracheal lumen has been overestimated and the previously selected tracheostomy is too large to fit into the trachea. In the latter case, a smaller cannula should be selected.

As soon as the cannula is in place, the obturator or suction catheter should be removed, and the anesthesiologist should disconnect the ventilator hose from the endotracheal tube and connect it to the tracheostomy cannula. Once that is done, the anesthesiologist should administer several deep breaths to the patient to confirm that the cannula is in the proper place by auscultation of the lungs and that the infant can be ventilated satisfactorily. A flexible bronchoscope is used to confirm the position of the tracheostomy tube. If it appears that although the cannula width is appropriate, it is too long and its tip rests on the carina, then a shorter neonatal tube should be used instead of a pediatric tube. Once adequate ventilation is confirmed, then the endotracheal tube can be removed completely.

Once the cannula is connected to the ventilator, the cervical wings of the body of the cannula need to be secured to the patient. We don't rely on a tie placed around the neck, but accomplish this with the aid of sutures.

For each wing, a suture of 3-0 silk or its equivalent is passed through the skin of the neck, then through the upper edge of the wing of the cannula (midway between the midline and the end of the wing), through the lower edge of the wing, and then again through the skin. When this suture is tied, the skin will be drawn over the wing and usually will cover it. After these sutures are placed, both wings will be securely fixed to the skin of the neck.

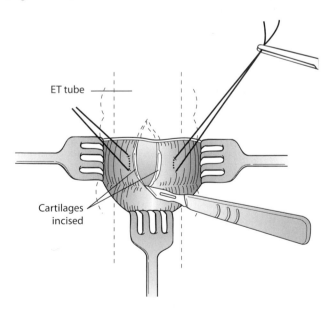

Figure 33.3 The trachea should be opened through a midline vertical incision across 2–3 tracheal rings. The incision must be long enough to avoid excess tube pressure against the cartilages. A tight tube can result in pressure deformity and reabsorption of cartilage. ET, endotracheal tube.

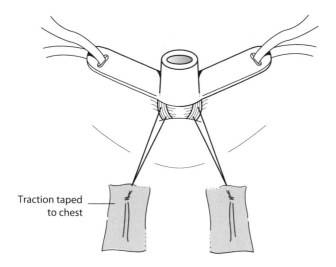

Figure 33.5 Prevention of accidental decannulation is the surgeon's responsibility. The tube should be taped to the anterior chest for 4 days in case an unexpected tube change should become necessary.

The two ties that were placed in the anterior tracheal wall should now be taped securely to the anterior chest wall in such a fashion that ensures that their ends are easily accessible in case they are needed in an emergency to reinsert the cannula (Figure 33.5).

Finally, the cotton tape or tie that usually comes with the cannula is passed through the holes in the end of the wings and tied around the neck to further secure the cannula. This should be tied in the back of the neck. Simple gauze dressing with antibiotic ointment applied is placed underneath the wings of the cannula over the cervical incision to complete the procedure.

We send our infants to the ICU after a fresh tracheostomy in case of emergency.

PERIOPERATIVE MANAGEMENT

If the skin of the patient's neck is infected with a bacterial or fungal infection, this should be cleared before any operation is undertaken unless emergency tracheostomy is required to save an infant's life.

In patients with short, fat necks, it may be necessary to place the infant in a position of neck extension to facilitate clearing any skin infection or breakdown that is due to chronic moisture. Simply exposing the infant's neck to air for drying often is sufficient to clear any problem.

Immediately after the tracheostomy is secured, the roll under the patient's neck should be removed, and a radiograph of the chest should be reviewed before the patient is transferred to the ICU. This is important to make certain that the tip of the cannula is sufficiently clear of the carina and will not become obstructed as the patient's neck is manipulated.

A bed-head notice completed by the ear, nose, and throat (ENT) surgeon or the tracheostomy nurse specialist must be placed on the patients' cot or bed, with details of the type and size of tracheostomy tube used, size and depth of suction catheter appropriate for the tube, any airway problems noted at laryngoscopy, and date of estimated first tube change.

The fresh tracheostomy should be left in place until the first tube change, which varies in different centers anywhere from 3 to 7 days.[22,23] At least once a day, the site should be cleaned using aseptic technique with gauze dampened in a solution of 0.9% normal saline.

Adequate humidification is mandatory to prevent crusting within the tracheostomy tube, as is gentle suctioning using the appropriate-sized suction catheter and adhering to precise depth measurement to prevent trauma to the tracheal mucosa. Suction catheters have numbered graduations for accurate insertion lengths.

The sutures securing the tracheostomy should be left untouched until the first tube change. The surgeon does the first tracheostomy tube change with the tracheostomy nurse specialist. The sutures to the edges of the tracheal incision should also be left until the first tube change.

If the patient is unusually agitated or the ventilator tubing is so heavy that dislodging the cannula is highly likely, then sedation or paralysis may be helpful until the wound has matured and reinsertion can be done more safely.

After the cannula is free and the cotton neck tape is untied, the cannula can be removed and replaced. If a temporary endotracheal tube is being replaced with a specially ordered tracheostomy cannula, the new cannula should be inserted as described earlier.

HOME INSTRUCTION AND CARE

Patients should be discharged home with an emergency case containing essential equipment (spare tracheostomy tubes, Ambu bag) and supplies required in case of accidental decannulation or for emergency tube change, and this case accompanies the child at all times. Parents and caretakers are taught basic life support (BLS) or cardiopulmonary resuscitation (CPR) prior to discharge. They should be familiar with emergency algorithms, mainly for blocked tube and when the tracheostomy tube cannot be replaced.

The tracheostomy tube is held in place with cotton tapes around the neck, and it is changed on a daily basis or twice daily when required. Two people are required to change the cotton tapes to prevent accidental decannulation. Parents and caretakers are trained prior to discharge not only on how to change the tube holder but also on how to clean the stoma and neck. It is important to ensure the skin around the tracheostomy tube and neck is not traumatized.

Precise suctioning is crucial in pediatric tracheostomy care and is only recommended when there are clear indications that the patency or ventilation of the patient is compromised. Parents or caretakers are sent home with a suction machine and are taught suction technique. They should also know how to use an Ambu bag for ventilation in conjunction with suctioning.

An air filter and humidification device, either heat moisture exchange (HME) or Swedish nose of appropriate size, should be attached to the tracheostomy cannula if a ventilating device or some other humidification device is not connected. Of course, the family or caretakers must know how to use and troubleshoot in case of problems with using any of the devices chosen, especially the cannula and its attachments.

Tracheostomy tube change is only performed by trained and competent staff[24] and is planned on a weekly or monthly basis depending on the type of tube used.

It is often helpful to arrange for home nursing visits until the family becomes familiar and comfortable with the new devices; this is especially true when it comes time for the first scheduled tracheostomy change if it is to be done at home.

COMPLICATIONS

The potential complications of tracheostomy are listed in Table 33.2. Pediatric patients have a higher reported morbidity and mortality rate, particularly preterm infants, compared to the adult population.[25,26] Published rates of complications range from 19% to 57% in several case series, with overall mortality rate attributed to underlying medical condition ranging from 10% to 21%, and tracheostomy related mortality was 0.9%–3.2%.[2,3,6,8,9,11,12,26]

Pneumothorax is a potential intraoperative complication because in infants, the apex of the lung extends into the root of the neck, and this can be violated if the surgeon fails to stay in the midline of the neck during the procedure.

Hemorrhage is an unusual complication that can occur at the time of operation or as a delayed event. When hemorrhage occurs at operation, it can be controlled easily with electrocautery or vessel ligation. Rarely, especially in the smaller newborn, the thyroid gland is near the incision site on the anterior trachea and is inadvertently divided or lacerated. The resultant hemorrhage usually can be controlled with sutures or electrocautery.

Late hemorrhage often is more problematic and can be more serious. First, it must be ascertained whether the hemorrhage is from the tracheal lumen or from the incision. Suctioning the cannula, inspecting the wound, and using a flexible bronchoscope through the tracheostomy tube can accomplish this.

More problematic is the possibility of hemorrhage from one of the great vessels, such as the innominate vein or artery. This can occur from erosion of the vessels when the cannula fits too snugly in the thoracic inlet and partially compresses the vessels against the manubrium or clavicle. This type of hemorrhage often presents with a so-called herald bleed, which starts briskly but stops, and usually requires a trip to the operating room to repair the damaged vessel.

Aside from hemorrhage, the cannula can become dislodged. We are compulsive about securing the cannula in

Table 33.2 Tracheostomy complications

Complications	
Intraoperative risk	Hemorrhage
	Recurrent laryngeal nerve injury
	Posterior tracheal wall tear
	Pneumothorax
	Esophageal injury
	Inability to ventilate
	Creation of false passage
	Cardiac arrest, death
Early postoperative risk	Accidental decannulation
	Respiratory arrest
	Inability to replace tracheostomy tube
	Stomal breakdown
	Skin erosion
	Ventilation problem
	Stomal bleeding
	Pneumothorax, pneumomediastinum
Long-term risk	Stomal granulation
	Tracheocutaneous fistulae
	Stomal infection/cellulitis
	Subglottic stenosis
	Suprastomal collapse
	Stomal bleeding
	Tracheitis
	Tracheomalacia
	Decannulation
	Tube occlusion

Sources: Ozmen, S. et al., Pediatric tracheotomies: A 37-year experience in 282 children, *Int J Pediatr Otorhinolaryngol* 2009, 73, 959–961. Douglas, C.M. et al., Paediatric tracheostomy—An 11 year experience at a Scottish paediatric tertiary referral centre, *Int J Pediatr Otorhinolaryngol* 2015, 79, 1673–1676. Mahadevan, M. et al., Pediatric tracheotomy: 17 year review, *Int J Pediatr Otorhinolaryngol* 2007, 71, 1829–1835. Davis, G.M., Tracheostomy in children, *Paediatr Respir Rev* 2006, 7 Suppl 1, S206–209. Carr, M.M. et al., Complications in pediatric tracheostomies, *Laryngoscope* 2001, 111, 1925–1928.

place using the techniques described earlier in order to avoid this complication. Even so, despite our best efforts, a suture will pull loose, or one of the plastic wings will tear, allowing the cannula to dislodge. We prefer to keep our infants in the ICU during the immediate postoperative period. We anticipate that if the cannula becomes dislodged, it will be noticed immediately. Replacing the cannula in the immediate postoperative period can be a treacherous ordeal that, under ideal circumstances, should be done by someone familiar with cannula insertion. If a surgeon or intensivist is readily available, then one of them should replace the cannula and resecure the device.

Injury to the vagus nerves or, more likely, the recurrent laryngeal nerves can occur. In experienced hands with a surgeon well versed in the anatomy of the infant's neck, this injury should be rare.

While unlikely, it is possible to place the cannula into the esophagus. This can occur if the trachea is retracted laterally, out of the field, and the esophagus is entered in error. If this occurs, the esophagus should be repaired primarily, and a drain should be left in place. The tracheostomy cannula can then be inserted properly.

Infection is an unusual complication and should be treated with the appropriate antimicrobials according to culture results.

Endotracheal granulation tissue can result from the chronic irritation of the tip of the tracheostomy cannula against the tracheal wall or from the repeated suctioning of the trachea. It is common for granulation tissue to develop at the stoma. This can be exophytic at the level of the skin or can be intraluminal. The exophytic granulation tissue at the skin should be cauterized with silver nitrate during an outpatient visit. This may need to be carried out every month or so if bothersome hemorrhage or chronic irritation with infection is present.

If the granulation tissue develops immediately within the trachea at the stoma, it usually can be left alone until it is time for decannulation. Only if the granulation tissue is so bulky that it interferes with routine tracheostomy changes or causes significant hemorrhage should it be removed before decannulation is contemplated.

The development of granulation tissue at the tip of the cannula can present with obstruction, sometimes resulting in a "ball-valve" effect, with trapped air and difficulty with ventilation. This can be diagnosed by slipping a flexible bronchoscope through the cannula to visualize the tracheal lumen beyond the tip of the cannula. If the results of this diagnostic maneuver are unclear, rigid bronchoscopy may be necessary.

Tracheostomy tube obstruction can be prevented with appropriate tube care. This is a more common problem among premature and newborn babies, with a rate of up to 72%, and less frequently in children 1 year and older, with a rate of up to 14%.[13] Suprastomal collapse, tracheal stenosis, and tracheomalacia are other potential long-term complications of tracheostomy. Prior to decannulation, patients should have an airway assessment to rule out these potential complications. If a tracheostomy tube has been in place for a prolonged period of time, following decannulation, there is a risk the stoma does not close completely, leaving a tracheocutaneous fistula. This can be surgically closed after waiting a suitable amount of time.

SPECIAL SITUATIONS

Occasionally, there exist special circumstances that require careful thought and planning. Such is the case with tracheal stenosis. Simple acquired subglottic stenosis can be easily managed with a tracheostomy inserted as described except for the size of the endotracheal tube. A small endotracheal tube may be difficult to palpate, however; thus, locating the trachea may be difficult.

With a particularly stenotic airway, mask ventilation may be the only way to maintain ventilation. The most difficult part of the case is locating the trachea without an endotracheal tube.

For patients with distal tracheal stenosis, tracheostomy insertion may be inappropriate. While beyond the scope of this discussion, the infant should be carefully studied if this diagnosis is suspected. Usually, plain radiographs of the chest may lead one to suspect the diagnosis. Computerized tomography or bronchoscopy may be required for confirmation. When the distal trachea is stenotic in an infant who is difficult to ventilate, a conventional tracheostomy cannula is inappropriate and may interfere with tracheal reconstruction.

Patients who are candidates for congenital heart surgery and in whom the ultimate need for a tracheostomy is anticipated may be best managed by completing the cardiac surgery before tracheostomy is performed. Otherwise, the sternal incision is so close to the tracheostomy site that the risk of cardiac infection is greatly increased.

DECANNULATION

Decannulation usually is anticipated well in advance. Its timing depends largely on the indication for the tracheostomy. Decannulation is considered for the following:

1. Resolution of underlying airway abnormality
2. Natural expansion of the airway with growth
3. Surgical procedures designed to open narrowed airways

There are slight variations in decannulation protocol in different pediatric units around the world, and we use the protocol in Figure 33.6.

Patients with severe subglottic stenoses may have their tracheostomy removed at the time of their laryngotracheal reconstruction or cricotracheal resection. The timing of this procedure, then, depends on the surgeon and may occur any time between 4–6 months and 2 years, or later.

In patients whose tracheostomy was placed because of tracheomalacia, it would be unusual to attempt decannulation before the infant is 1 year of age. The infant should undergo periodic bronchoscopic examination to assess the

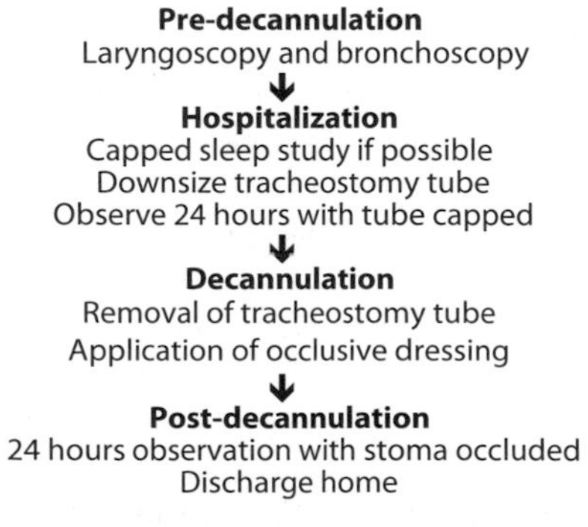

Pre-decannulation
Laryngoscopy and bronchoscopy
↓
Hospitalization
Capped sleep study if possible
Downsize tracheostomy tube
Observe 24 hours with tube capped
↓
Decannulation
Removal of tracheostomy tube
Application of occlusive dressing
↓
Post-decannulation
24 hours observation with stoma occluded
Discharge home

Figure 33.6 Decannulation protocol.

status of the malacia. Once it is certain that the airway is sufficiently mature as to be able to maintain its patency, decannulation can be attempted.

The first step is to make certain that the airway is mature and free of any potential obstructing lesions such as granulation tissue. This is best accomplished with rigid bronchoscopy. Any residual malacia or granulation tissue can be documented and dealt with as needed.

At the time of attempted decannulation, we bring the patient to the operating room, positioned as described earlier for insertion of the cannula with the neck extended, and perform the bronchoscopy. In order to assess whether malacia is present, the patient should not be paralyzed, and the anesthesia should be light. This is to determine whether the airway remains patent, with the patient breathing spontaneously.

Once committed to decannulation, the bronchoscope and neck roll should be removed, and the patient is observed for any difficulty such as severe chest retraction or deoxygenation that would suggest the continued need for the tracheostomy. If, on the other hand, the patient ventilates with ease, then the patient should be fully awakened and allowed to recover in a unit that permits careful observation.

We usually keep these patients in the hospital overnight, or longer if there is any concern, to assure that the tracheostomy is no longer required.

Once the cannula is removed, a snug dressing of plain or petroleum jelly–saturated gauze is secured over the tracheostomy stoma to occlude it. The caretakers or parents should be instructed on how to change this dressing until the stoma closes completely.

Occasionally, we encounter a stoma that does not close spontaneously. If the stoma remains open after several months, then operative closure of the stoma can be performed as an outpatient procedure. Usually, this is simply a matter of excising the stoma and placing a simple stitch or two in the anterior trachea. A larger persistent opening may require an anterior wedge excision for proper repair. This may necessitate admission to the hospital.

If, after the patient leaves the operating room decannulated, he/she becomes fatigued or demonstrates other signs of respiratory distress, the dressing can be removed, and another cannula should be reinserted. A smaller cannula size can be inserted if desired.

This technique often is used to serially wean a patient to progressively smaller-sized cannulas until decannulation is certain to be successful.

If, after decannulation, it is necessary to reinsert a tracheostomy, the procedure should be done in the operating room. While this is usually done with an endotracheal tube in place, there are some patients for whom it may be undesirable to insert an endotracheal tube. This avoids airway irritation and prevents restenosis. That being the case, the surgeon can inject a local anesthetic around the stoma, dilate the stoma with Hegar dilators (or possibly make a small incision with a No. 11 scalpel blade), and reinsert a cannula of an appropriate size. This maneuver should only

be attempted if the anesthesiologist can maintain an adequate airway during the procedure.

Reported decannulation failure rates in children range from 5% to 21.4% according to several series.[9,12,28,29]

REFERENCES

1. Prescott CA, Vanlierde MJ. Tracheostomy in children—The Red Cross War Memorial Children's Hospital experience 1980–1985. *Int J Pediatr Otorhinolaryngol* 1989; 17: 97–107.
2. Ozmen S, Ozmen OA, Unal OF. Pediatric tracheotomies: A 37-year experience in 282 children. *Int J Pediatr Otorhinolaryngol* 2009; 73: 959–61.
3. Douglas CM, Poole-Cowley J, Morrissey S, Kubba H, Clement WA Wynne D. Paediatric tracheostomy—An 11 year experience at a Scottish paediatric tertiary referral centre. *Int J Pediatr Otorhinolaryngol* 2015; 79: 1673–6.
4. Corbett HJ, Mann KS, Mitra I, Jesudason EC, Losty PD, Clarke RW. Tracheostomy—A 10-year experience from a UK pediatric surgical center. *J Pediatr Surg* 2007; 42: 1251–4.
5. Hadfield PJ, Lloyd-Faulconbridge RV, Almeyda J, Albert DM, Bailey CM. The changing indications for paediatric tracheostomy. *Int J Pediatr Otorhinolaryngol* 2003; 67: 7–10.
6. Butnaru CS, Colreavy MP, Ayari S, Froehlich P. Tracheotomy in children: Evolution in indications. *Int J Pediatr Otorhinolaryngol* 2006; 70: 115–9.
7. Ang AH, Chua DY, Pang KP, Tan HK. Pediatric tracheotomies in an Asian population: The Singapore experience. *Otolaryngol Head Neck Surg* 2005; 133: 246–50.
8. Perez-Ruiz E, Caro P, Perez-Frias J, Cols M, Barrio I, Torrent A, Garcia MA, Asensio O, Pastor MD, Luna C et al. Paediatric patients with a tracheostomy: A multicentre epidemiological study. *Eur Respir J* 2012; 40: 1502–7.
9. Mahadevan, M, Barber C, Salkeld L, Douglas G, Mills N. Pediatric tracheotomy: 17 year review. *Int J Pediatr Otorhinolaryngol* 2007; 71: 1829–35.
10. Lawrason A, Kavanagh K. Pediatric tracheotomy: Are the indications changing? *Int J Pediatr Otorhinolaryngol* 2013; 77: 922–5.
11. Ogilvie LN, Kozak JK, Chiu S, Adderley RJ, Kozak FK. Changes in pediatric tracheostomy 1982–2011: A Canadian tertiary children's hospital review. *J Pediatr Surg* 2014; 49: 1549–53.
12. de Trey L, Niedermann E, Ghelfi D, Gerber A, Gysin C. Pediatric tracheotomy: A 30-year experience. *J Pediatr Surg* 2013; 48: 1470–5.
13. Davis GM. Tracheostomy in children. *Paediatr Respir Rev* 2006, 7 Suppl 1: S206–9.
14. Abraham RJ, Sau A, Maxwell D. A review of the EXIT (Ex utero Intrapartum Treatment) procedure. *J Obstetr Gynaecol* 2010; 30: 1–5.

15. Kocyildirim E, Kanani M, Roebuck D, Wallis C, McLaren C, Noctor C, Pigott N, Mok Q, Hartley B, Dunne C et al. Long-segment tracheal stenosis: Slide tracheoplasty and a multidisciplinary approach improve outcomes and reduce costs. *J Thorac Cardiovasc Surg* 2004; 128: 876–82.

16. Torre M, Carlucci M, Avanzini S, Jasonni V, Monnier P, Tarantino V, D'Agostino R, Vallarino R, Della Rocca M, Moscatelli A et al. Gaslini's tracheal team: Preliminary experience after one year of paediatric airway reconstructive surgery. *Ital J Pediatr* 2011; 37: 51.

17. Tweedie DJ, Skilbeck CJ, Cochrane LA, Cooke J, Wyatt ME. Choosing a paediatric tracheostomy tube: An update on current practice. *J Laryngol Otol* 2008; 122: 161–9.

18. Behl S, Watt JW. Prediction of tracheostomy tube size for paediatric long-term ventilation: An audit of children with spinal cord injury. *Br J Anaesth* 2005; 94: 88–91.

19. Park JY, Suskind DL, Prater D, Muntz HR, Lusk RP. Maturation of the pediatric tracheostomy stoma: Effect on complications. *Ann Otol Rhinol Laryngol* 1999; 108: 1115–9.

20. Craig MF, Bajaj Y, Hartley BE. Maturation sutures for the paediatric tracheostomy—An extra safety measure. *J Laryngol Otol* 2005; 119: 985–7.

21. Song JJ, Choi IJ, Chang H, Kim DW, Chang HW, Park GH, Kim MS, Sung MW, Hah JH. Pediatric tracheostomy revisited: A nine-year experience using horizontal intercartilaginous incision. *Laryngoscope* 2015; 125: 485–92.

22. Van Buren NC, Narasimhan ER, Curtis JL, Muntz HR, Meier JD. Pediatric tracheostomy: Timing of the first tube change. *Ann Otol Rhinol Laryngol* 2015; 124: 374–7.

23. Mitchell RB, Hussey HM, Setzen G, Jacobs IN, Nussenbaum B, Dawson C, Brown CA, 3rd Brandt C, Deakins K, Hartnick C et al. Clinical consensus statement: Tracheostomy care. *Otolaryngol Head Neck Surg* 2013; 148: 6–20.

24. Roberts FE Consensus among physiotherapists in the united kingdom on the use of normal saline instillation prior to endotracheal suction: A Delphi study. *Physiother Can* 2009; 61: 107–15.

25. Kenna MA, Reilly JS, Stool SE. Tracheotomy in the preterm infant. *Ann Otol Rhinol Laryngol* 1987; 96: 68–71.

26. Wetmore RF, Handler SD, Potsic WP. Pediatric tracheostomy. Experience during the past decade. *Ann Otol Rhinol Laryngol* 1982; 91: 628–32.

27. Carr MM, Poje CP, Kingston L, Kielma D, Heard C. Complications in pediatric tracheostomies. *Laryngoscope* 2001; 111: 1925–8.

28. Prickett KK, Sobol SE. Inpatient observation for elective decannulation of pediatric patients with tracheostomy. *JAMA Otolaryngol Head Neck Surg* 2015; 141: 120–5.

29. Leung R, Berkowitz RG. Decannulation and outcome following pediatric tracheostomy. *Ann Otol Rhinol Laryngol* 2005; 114: 743–8.

34

Congenital cysts and sinuses of the neck

YOUSEF EL-GOHARY, JOSEPH FUSCO, AND GEORGE K. GITTES

INTRODUCTION

Pediatric surgeons frequently encounter cervical masses with intriguing clinical presentations in infants and children. Some can be easily diagnosed with a good history and physical examination, such as the thyroglossal cyst. Others require more extensive investigation and imaging to accurately diagnose and treat. The vast majority are benign in origin; however, rarely, they can be malignant.[1] They frequently form from residual embryologic structures that have failed to resorb completely, or failed to mature. Knowledge of the embryological origins of these cysts and sinuses, along with a detailed knowledge of neck anatomy, is essential for proper management and for successful dissection and excision. Thyroglossal duct cysts are the most congenital neck masses to be encountered in practice, followed by branchial cleft anomalies and dermoid cysts.[2] We will discuss in this chapter the embryology of the neck, followed by a brief review of the common neck cysts and sinuses, along with their management.

EMBRYOLOGY

During early embryonic stages, the primitive gut tube, which is derived from the endodermal germ layer during gastrulation, is divided into the foregut, midgut, and hindgut domains, each of which will give rise to specialized regions due to the regional specification of the gut tube.[3] The foregut, which includes the pharyngeal (branchial) apparatus, extends between the buccopharyngeal membrane and ends at the origin of the liver bud.

The pharyngeal apparatus, which consists of arches, pouches, and clefts, will eventually give rise to the various muscles, nerves, bones, and cartilage in the head and neck region, as illustrated in Figure 34.1 and Table 34.1. There are six pharyngeal (branchial) arches, each consisting of a core of mesoderm, with its own nerve and arterial supply, surrounded by an outer ectodermal and inner endodermal lining. The mesoderm of the second pharyngeal arch proliferates and causes the arch to grow caudally, overlapping the third and fourth arches, and in the process burying the second, third, and fourth pharyngeal clefts and creating a temporary cervical sinus, which normally disappears (illustrated in Figure 34.2). The first pharyngeal cleft will give rise to the external auditory meatus, and the fifth arch disappears. It is the incomplete closure or obliteration of these ectodermal portions of the second, third, and fourth pharyngeal clefts that leads to the various neck anomalies, including cartilaginous remnants, that pediatric surgeons encounter today.[4] The remnants of these clefts form the cervical sinus, which remains connected to the surface via a narrow canal called the "external" branchial fistula, which may drain a branchial cyst. Rarely does the branchial fistula connect to the pharynx, near the tonsil area, via the "internal" branchial fistula.[5]

INCIDENCE

Branchial clefts and fistulae represent about 23% of cervical masses in children.[6] The "rule of 80" is often applied in adults, which states that 80% of nonthyroid neck masses in adults are neoplastic and that 80% of these masses are malignant. A neck mass in a child, on the other hand, has a 90% probability of being benign.

BRANCHIAL ANOMALIES

First-branchial-cleft anomalies account for less than 10% of all of the branchial cleft defects.[7] They have a wide range of presentations, manifesting in a sinus, fistula, or cyst anywhere between the floor of the external auditory meatus and the submandibular region (Figure 34.3).[8] Clinically, they can present with either a persistent purulent discharge from the ear, preauricular swelling in the parotid area, or fistula in the neck above the hyoid bone. However, they are most commonly associated with an infection, often being initially treated with a course of antibiotics or unnecessary repeated incision and drainage of an abscess.[7,9] The relationship of

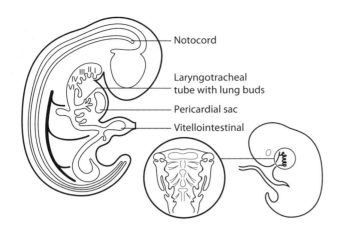

Figure 34.1 Schematic illustration of the embryo with the pharyngeal arches (I–VI).

Table 34.1 Summary of the derivatives of the pharyngeal arches

Arch	Muscles	Nerve	Cartilage, bone, and ligament
I	Muscles of mastication	Mandibular division of trigeminal nerve	Malleus, incus Sphenomandibular ligament
II	Muscles of face and scalp	Facial nerve	Stapes Styloid process Styloid ligament Lesser horn and upper part of body of hyoid bone
III	Stylopharyngeus	Glossopharyngeal nerve	Greater horn and lower part of body of hyoid bone
IV	Cricothyriod	Superior laryngeal branch of vagus nerve	Thyroid cartilage
VI	Intrinsic muscles of larynx	Recurrent laryngeal branch of vagus nerve	All laryngeal cartilages *except* thyroid cartilage

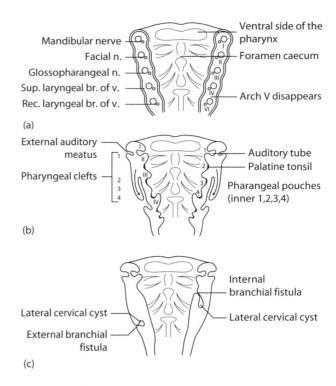

Figure 34.2 Illustration of the pharyngeal arches (I–VI) with their own nerve supply. **(a,b)** The mesoderm of the second pharyngeal arch grows downward, burying in the process the second, third, and fourth pharyngeal clefts. **(c)** Incomplete closure of these pharyngeal clefts leads to the formation of branchial anomalies such as a cyst or fistula.

the facial nerve to the anomaly is variable, with careful and meticulous surgical dissection needed to avoid nerve paralysis.[10] In a series of 39 patients with first-branchial-cleft anomalies reported, 6 patients developed temporary facial nerve paralysis, and only 1 (2.5%) patient developed permanent damage.[11] Diagnosing first-cleft anomalies can be challenging, with the anomaly often closely related to the parotid gland. Examining the external auditory meatus may reveal a fistula, thus linking the parotid swelling or lateral neck mass to a first-cleft anomaly. Preoperative imaging with magnetic resonance imaging (MRI) allows assessment of the extent of the anomaly, especially in the parotid area, and high-resolution computed tomography (CT)

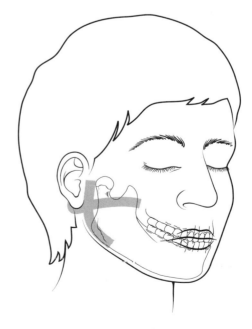

Figure 34.3 Shaded area on the face represents locations where the first-branchial-cleft anomalies would be generally located.

imaging shows its exact relationship to the external auditory canal and the middle ear.[11] Complete surgical excision is the treatment of choice, which often necessitates a superficial parotidectomy, with careful preservation of the facial nerve. Methylene blue injection into a draining tract prior to excision may facilitate removal. Recurrent infections or previous surgical interventions will increase the morbidity of the operation.[12] That is why it is essential to have an adequate preoperative workup prior to any surgical intervention.

Second-branchial-cleft anomalies are the most common (95%),[13] often presenting along the anterior border of the sternocleidomastoid muscle as a sinus, fistula or cyst, typically at the junction of the upper two-thirds and lower third of the muscle. The fistula typically travels deep to the platysma muscle along the carotid sheath between the external and internal carotid artery, above the hypoglossal and glossopharyngeal nerves, and ends near the tonsillar fossa (Figure 34.4).[8] Deep fistulas or sinuses would generally necessitate two or three "stepladder" or McFee incisions in order to completely remove the entire tract. However, the majority of the anomalies manifest as cysts[14] and rarely present as a full fistula tract.[13]

Bailey[15] described four types of cysts. Type 1 is superficial and lies beneath the platysma and cervical fascia, but anterior to sternocleidomastoid process. Type 2 cysts, which are the most common, characteristically lie on the great vessels and may be adherent to the internal jugular vein. Type 3 cysts course between internal and external carotid artery and extend to the lateral wall of the pharynx. Type 4 cysts lie against the pharyngeal wall.

Studies of less invasive procedures are promising, including sclerotherapy[16,17] and endoscopic excision.[18] However,

complete surgical excision is the treatment of choice, with recurrence being the most common postoperative surgical complication. A large series of 208 cases showed recurrence in 21% of those with a history of prior surgical intervention, 14% with a history of infection, and 3% with a history of neither.[19]

Third- and fourth-branchial-cleft anomalies are rare, accounting for 2%–8% and 1%–2% of all branchial anomalies, respectively.[7,20] Clinically and radiologically, it can be difficult to distinguish between the two, as both types begin at the pyriform sinus and end blindly in the paratracheal or thyroid region. Ninety-seven percent of the lesions occur on the left side.[19] Although rare anomalies, they can have devastating respiratory consequences, presenting with acute stridor,[21,22] or acute thyroiditis.[23,24] Diagnosis can be quite challenging, as these cysts are generally subjected to repeated incision and drainage, being mistaken for a simple abscess. A plain film showing air or fluid levels within the cyst can help differentiate a branchial anomaly from other causes of pediatric neck masses. The pharyngeal opening may be visualized by flexible fiber-optic nasopharyngoscopy or demonstrated using a barium meal.[25] In a series of 43 patients with acute suppurative thyroiditis, nearly 88% of the patients were documented to have a pyriform sinus fistula.[24] Therefore, it should be a consideration for any patient presenting with acute thyroiditis to have a potential third- or fourth-branchial anomaly as an underlying cause, and to promote a search for it. The only definitive way of distinguishing an anomaly as being a third or fourth arch is through surgical dissection, which is the treatment of choice, ensuring that the tract is completely excised to avoid risk of recurrence. This is done by demonstrating the relationship of the tract to the recurrent and superior laryngeal nerves. A tract that goes inferior to the superior laryngeal nerve (fourth arch) and superior to the recurrent nerve (sixth arch) is derived from the fourth pouch. However, if the tract passes superior to the superior laryngeal nerve (fourth arch), then a third-pouch origin is likely. Vocal cord paralysis is a potential complication as a result of the dissection.

CT scan and MRI are the imaging modalities of choice to assess the extent and depth of any branchial cleft cysts.[26]

Endoscopic-assisted branchial cleft excision has been recently advocated by several recent case reports and case series to improve cosmetic results,[27] with almost identical recurrence rates particularly for third and fourth branchial anomalies.[28,29] Surgical approaches include the axilloareolar, retroauricular, posterior occipital, and transcervical approach. Teng et al.[27] reported a series of 24 patients undergoing branchial cleft excision, 8 of whom underwent a transcervical endoscopic approach using gasless 4 mm endoscopic technique through an average 2.1 ± 0.2 cm skin incision versus the standard open approach via 4.1 ± 1.5 cm incision. Two out of the eight patients encountered transient weakness of the greater auricular nerve and marginal mandibular nerve.[27]

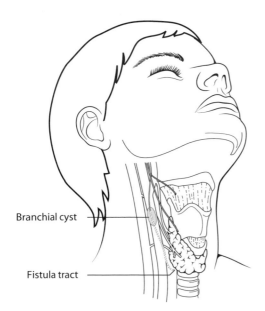

Branchial cyst

Fistula tract

Figure 34.4 Second branchial cleft cyst and fistula tract coursing between the internal and external carotid arteries, above nerves IX and XII, ending near the tonsillar fossa.

THYROGLOSSAL DUCT CYSTS AND SINUSES

Thyroglossal duct anomalies are the most common congenital anomalies of the neck, constituting nearly 70% of all cervical neck masses in children.[30] They represent remnants from the embryological migration of thyroid tissue from the foramen cecum to the thyroid fossa. Clinically, they usually present as a palpable, nontender midline neck mass that elevates with swallowing or protrusion of the tongue (Figure 34.5). It is important to note that 10%–24% of these cysts are located laterally, often to the left.[31]

Ultrasonography is the imaging technique of choice for these lesions, especially to document the presence of a normal thyroid and to rule out thyroid ectopia.[32] The reported incidence of an ectopic thyroid being misdiagnosed as a thyroglossal cyst is 1%–2%.[33]

The Sistrunk procedure, with dissection of the tract up to the hyoid bone, including its midportion, is accepted as the main operation of choice with the lowest recurrence rate of around 3%.[32,34] Malignancy of the thyroglossal duct cysts is rare (1%),[33,35] with the majority (80%) of histological examination revealing a papillary adenocarcinoma.[36,37]

CONGENITAL MIDLINE CERVICAL CLEFTS

Congenital midline cervical clefts (CMCCs) are rare developmental anomalies, with variable severity from patient to patient and with variable length and width.[38] The embryological origins have not been fully elucidated, but they are thought to be a result of failed mesodermal fusion of the first or second branchial arches in the midline.[39] There has been no observed familial inheritance pattern. Affected

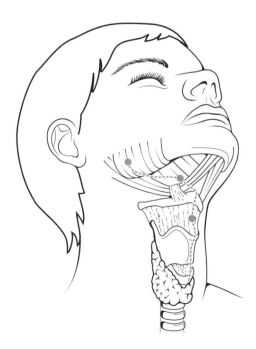

Figure 34.5 Illustration for the thyroglossal duct tract.

patients present soon after birth, with common characteristic features including midline fissure or atrophic skin, a caudal-directed sinus that may have mucoid discharge, subcutaneous fibrous cord, and a thickened nipple-like projection at the superior aspect of the lesion.[40] There is often a subcutaneous fibrous cord of variable length spanning anywhere along the midline of the neck from the symphysis of the mandible to the suprasternal notch. It is occasionally seen in conjunction with thyroglossal and bronchogenic cysts. CMCC presenting with a midline cervical sinus can be differentiated from a sinus associated with a thyroglossal cyst based on the orientation of the sinus. The sinus in CMCC is generally caudally directed, whereas with thyroglossal duct cysts, the associated sinus will tend to be directed cranially. The distinction between these two clinical entities is important since the surgical approach is vastly different. Thyroglossal duct cyst excision involves removal of the central portion of the hyoid bone (Sistrunk operation), whereas CMCC does not involve the hyoid bone.[40]

Diagnosis of CMCC is mainly clinical, but imaging studies such as ultrasound may be obtained to evaluate the thyroid gland and hyoid bone to rule out any associated anomalies. CT or MRI can be done for a more thorough assessment of involvement of any deeper neck structures.

Midline cervical clefts need to be completely excised because if left untreated, the cleft will cause cicatrical skin contracture, limiting neck extension and causing webbing of the neck. It is recommended to excise the cleft between 10 and 12 weeks of age, before tethering of the anterior skin occurs.[41] Simple linear closure has been reported to result in hypertrophic scarring and recurrent neck contracture.[42] As a result, a step Z-plasty lengthening procedure is the preferred surgical management of this congenital anomaly, as it provides a superior cosmetic result compared to linear closure and adds the lengthening effect on the anterior neck skin that aids in preventing recurrent contracture.[40] Depending upon the angle of the Z-plasty chosen, a 30°, 45°, or 60° angle will result in 25%, 50%, and 75% gain of length, respectively. Any smaller angle results in risk of necrosis of the tip of the flap, and any broader angle will make flap rotation difficult (Figure 34.6).[40]

DERMOID CYSTS

Cervical dermoid cysts are benign tumors that are frequently mistaken for a thyroglossal duct cyst due to similar presentation and location. They are of ectodermal and mesodermal origin, and a definitive diagnosis is usually made during histologic examination revealing hair follicles, smooth muscle, sebaceous glands and connective tissue elements.[43] They are thought to arise due to trapping of epithelial rests during midline fusion of the first and second branchial arches.[44] Surgical excision is the treatment of choice.

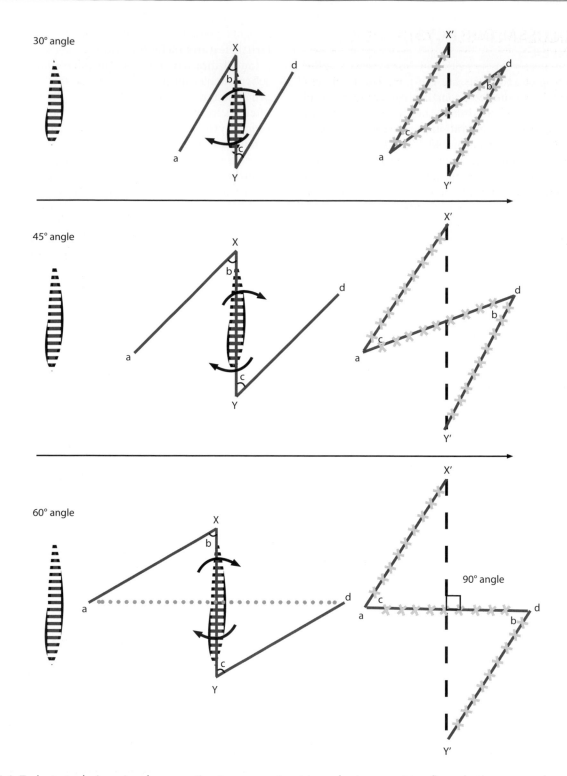

Figure 34.6 Z-plasty technique involves creating two opposing triangular transposition flaps that are rotated synchronously to close central defect. Lateral limbs are equal in length to central limb tissue defect. Angles vary from 30° to 60° depending on desired length gain. Z-plasties may be single, especially for lesions that are equal to 2 cm or less, or arranged in series with multiple flaps to allow shortening of the lateral limbs so as to avoid anesthetic boundaries. Central defect (X–Y) with flap reference points (a–d) resulting in lengthening of wound (X′–Y′).

PREAURICULAR SINUSES AND CYSTS

Preauricular sinuses are congenital malformations, usually noted during physical examination as small pits adjacent to the external ear, usually at the anterior margin of the ascending limb of the helix.[45] The incidence varies between different races, with the reported incidence ranging between 0.02% and 5%, with higher incidence amongst African American and Asian populations.[46-49] They are mostly unilateral with usually an asymptomatic presentation; however, they can present with purulent discharge from the sinus opening, resulting in facial cellulitis or abscess formation, which is the most common indication for a fistulectomy. Surgery should be performed once the infection has resolved, whenever possible, with the recurrence rate after surgery being reported between 3.7% and 36%, with the rate much higher if infection preceded surgery.[49-51] In the process of excising the sinus tract, various techniques can be used to identify its extension, but it is recommended to combine the use of dye injection with probing using a fine lacrimal duct probe at the time of surgery.[47,49] Use of microscope guidance for sinus excision has been reported to have a lower recurrence (0.9%) compared to the standard methylene blue dye and probe guidance (4.3%).[52]

RANULA

Ranulas are divided into simple and plunging ranulas. Simple ranulas are either mucus retention cysts that are restricted to the oral cavity floor or else mucus extravasation pseudocysts. Plunging ranulas are mucus extravasation pseudocysts that originate from the sublingual glands and herniate through the mylohyoid muscle to present as a cervical neck swelling, which may be confused with a submandibular mass when there is no intraoral component.[53] The ideal management for both of these lesions remains controversial, ranging from injecting sclerosing agents to different surgical techniques. Although most would agree to surgically excise them, a consensus on the ideal technique and approach is lacking.

Injecting simple and plunging ranulas with OK-432 (a mixture of a low-virulence strain of *Streptococcus pyogenes* incubated with benzylpenicillin) has a reported success rate of 74% and 100%, respectively, but only after multiple injections.[54,55] Most advocate marsupialization of the oral ranula, as illustrated in Figure 34.7, which is associated with a recurrence rate of around 20%.[56] Others advocate surgical excision of the cyst alone, which has a recurrence rate of 12%.[56] Some authors prefer to remove the sublingual gland, seen as the definitive treatment with the lowest recurrence rate, along with the cyst. This, however, is associated with a low incidence of lingual nerve and submandibular duct damage due to the more invasive intervention. Others simply excise the sublingual gland transorally along with evacuation of the ranula, which is seen as the modality yielding the lowest recurrence (1%–2%) and lowest complication rates for both oral and plunging ranulas.[56,57] A transoral

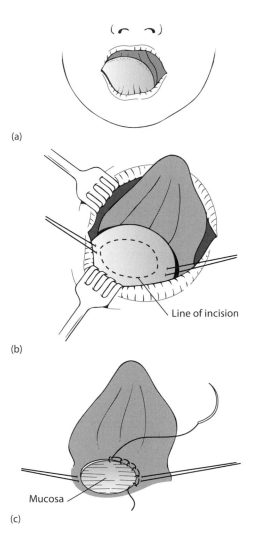

Figure 34.7 **(a)** Large ranula occupying the floor of the mouth. **(b)** Line of incision. **(c)** Continuous 4-0 Vicryl stitch to complete marsupialization.

approach for plunging ranulas is associated with a lower morbidity and complication rate compared to the cervical approach, as the latter places the marginal mandibular and hypoglossal nerves at risk of damage.[58,59] Removing the origin of the disease, usually the sublingual gland, is the key to successful treatment of simple and plunging ranulas.

CYSTIC HYGROMA (CYSTIC LYMPHANGIOMA)

Cystic hygromas or lymphangiomas are nonmalignant cystic (unilocular or multilocular) abnormalities of the lymphatic system, mostly occurring in the cervicofacial region with a predilection to the left side, and with a prevalence of 1 in every 6000 live births.[60] They can occur in the axilla, mediastinum, retroperitoneum, and rarely in the extremities with variable sizes, ranging from a few centimeters in diameter to large masses, potentially filling a large portion of the thorax.[61,62]

The term *hygroma* is derived from Greek, meaning moist or watery tumor. Hygromas have equal sex distribution. They rarely self-resorb after aspiration of the cystic fluid, which is usually clear or amber-colored, and occasionally hemorrhagic,[62] usually resulting in rapid reaccumulation. They can present as a congenital birth defect or be acquired at a later stage in life, with the majority (80%–90%) presenting by 2 years of age.[63,64]

They are thought to arise due to the failure of lymph vessels to communicate with the venous system, with abnormal budding and/or sequestrations of primitive embryonic lymphatic tissue.[65] Lymphangiomas are often classified into three types based on histology: capillary lymphangioma or lymphangioma simplex, composed of small thin-walled lymphatics; cavernous lymphangioma, consisting of larger lymphatic channels with adventitial coats; and cystic lymphangioma (hygroma), made up of larger macroscopic lymphatic spaces.[66,67] Immunocytochemical staining for CD31 (platelet endothelial cell adhesion molecule-1), a stain that is intended to reveal the endothelium of small vessels, confirms the diagnosis.

Diagnosis can be made with a good history and clinical examination, due to the characteristic clinical appearance, usually soft, compressible, and transilluminates with light. In a series of 168 patients with lymphangiomas, 41% were diagnosed based on clinical examination alone. Ultrasonography is a useful aid in diagnosis, revealing a cystic structure rather than solid. However, CT or MRI can show the full extent of the lesion and its relationship with the surrounding structures.[63,68] The radiologic characteristics of cystic hygroma are consistent with a fluid-filled, multiseptate mass with enhancing septal walls.[61]

Malignant transformation has not been reported; however, complete surgical excision is the surgical treatment of choice. It is generally recommended to remove the mass due to its potential for growth, which can compromise the airway if in the cervicofacial area, as well as disfigurement and recurrent bouts of inflammation, which unfortunately does not induce regression.[69] Aspirating the lesion may be useful for emergency decompression. Complete surgical resection can be difficult in the infiltrative form. Hygromas can be complicated with recurrences after surgical excision, reported to be 12% in patients who have undergone complete excision for neck lesions,[63] as well as with lymphangitis and cellulitis, which can lead to sepsis, prompting the need for intravenous antibiotics. It is advised that the initial approach for patients with recurrences after complete excision is to observe and wait, as spontaneous regression has been reported in up to 12% of patients after surgery. Other alternative treatments include intralesional injection with bleomycin or OK-432, with a reported response rate of 55%–60%,[70,71] and argon beam ablation and laser treatment. These modalities may be useful in patients with complex diffuse lesions when surgical therapy may be difficult to achieve a complete cure, or when vital structures are involved with the lesion.[72–74]

TORTICOLLIS

Torticollis or "sternocleidomastoid tumor" results from shortening of the sternocleidomastoid muscle, which may lead to limitation of neck movement and craniofacial deformity. The term *torticollis* is derived from two Latin roots, *tortus*, meaning twisted, and *collum*, which means neck.[75] It is considered one of the most common congenital musculoskeletal anomalies after developmental dysplasia of the hip and clubfoot, with an incidence of 0.3%–2%.[75–77] Although various theories have been proposed with regard to its etiology, such as birth trauma, intrauterine malposition, infectious myositis, and compartment syndrome, an exact cause has not been identified.[75] Diagnosis is usually established on clinical examination of a firm, spindle-shaped mass within the sternocleidomastoid muscle. Ultrasonography is the imaging modality of choice to confirm the diagnosis, usually hypoechoic compared to muscle.[78] This unilateral contraction of the muscle results in the head tilting toward the affected side and the face rotating to the opposite side, as is seen in Figure 34.8. This therefore can induce plagiocephaly and facial asymmetry at presentation. Treatment includes physical therapy, which is the primary treatment modality, with over 95% achieving passive cervical rotation after physiotherapy.[79] Physiotherapy involves stretching the affected muscle to an overcorrected position by gentle, even, and persistent motion with the infant lying in a supine position. The head is flexed forward and away form the affected side, and the chin is rotated toward the affected side. Some use botulinum toxin injection as an adjunct to physical therapy in those who have not responded to 3 months of conservative management.[80] Failure to respond to conservative treatment after the age of 1 year may necessitate the need for surgical intervention. Surgical options include

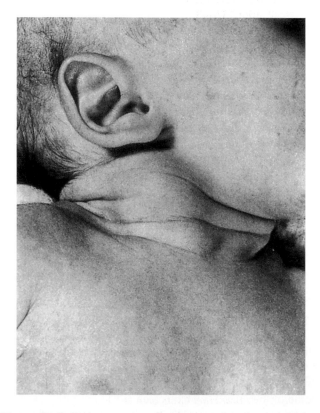

Figure 34.8 Right sternomastoid tumor in a 3-week-old infant.

unipolar or bipolar release, release with Z-plasty, transaxillary endoscopic release, and muscle resection. The transaxillary subcutaneous endoscopic approach has recently been developed to avoid the potential for poor cosmesis from neck scars.[81] The overall outcome from all these treatment modalities is excellent.

REFERENCES

1. Good GM, Isaacson G. Hodgkin's disease simulating a pediatric thyroglossal duct cyst. *Am J Otolaryngol* 2000; 21: 277–80.
2. LaRiviere CA, Waldhausen JH. Congenital cervical cysts, sinuses, and fistulae in pediatric surgery. *Surg Clin North Am* 2012; 92: 583–97, viii.
3. Grapin-Botton A. Antero-posterior patterning of the vertebrate digestive tract: 40 years after Nicole Le Douarin's PhD thesis. *Int J Dev Biol* 2005; 49: 335–47.
4. Bajaj Y, Tweedie D, Ifeacho S et al. Surgical technique for excision of first branchial cleft anomalies: How we do it. *Clin Otolaryngol* 2011; 36: 371–4.
5. Gaddikeri S, Vattoth S, Gaddikeri RS et al. Congenital cystic neck masses: Embryology and imaging appearances, with clinicopathological correlation. *Curr Probl Diagn Radiol* 2014; 43: 55–67.
6. Moussatos GH, Baffes TG. Cervical masses in infants and children. *Pediatrics* 1963; 32: 251–6.
7. Ford GR, Balakrishnan A, Evans JN, Bailey CM. Branchial cleft and pouch anomalies. *J Laryngol Otol* 1992; 106: 137–43.
8. Bajaj Y, Ifeacho S, Tweedie D et al. Branchial anomalies in children. *Int J Pediatr Otorhinolaryngol* 2011; 75: 1020–3.
9. Finn DG, Buchalter IH, Sarti E et al. First branchial cleft cysts: Clinical update. *Laryngoscope* 1987; 97: 136–40.
10. Chen Z, Wang Z, Dai C. An effective surgical technique for the excision of first branchial cleft fistula: Make-inside-exposed method by tract incision. *Eur Arch Otorhinolaryngol* 2010; 267: 267–71.
11. Triglia JM, Nicollas R, Ducroz V et al. First branchial cleft anomalies: A study of 39 cases and a review of the literature. *Arch Otolaryngol Head Neck Surg* 1998; 124: 291–5.
12. Chan KC, Chao WC, Wu CM. Surgical management of first branchial cleft anomaly presenting as infected retroauricular mass using a microscopic dissection technique. *Am J Otolaryngol* 2012; 33: 20–5.
13. Ang AH, Pang KP, Tan LK. Complete branchial fistula. Case report and review of the literature. *Ann Otol Rhinol Laryngol* 2001; 110: 1077–9.
14. Brown RL, Azizkhan RG. Pediatric head and neck lesions. *Pediatr Clin North Am* 1998; 45: 889–905.
15. Bailey H. *Branchial Cysts and Other Essays on Surgical Subjects in the Facio-cervical Region*. London: Lewis, 1929.
16. Kim MG, Lee NH, Ban JH et al. Sclerotherapy of branchial cleft cysts using OK-432. *Otolaryngol Head Neck Surg* 2009; 141: 329–34.
17. Roh JL, Sung MW, Hyun Kim K, Il Park C. Treatment of branchial cleft cyst with intracystic injection of OK-432. *Acta Otolaryngol* 2006; 126: 510–4.
18. Chen LS, Sun W, Wu PN et al. Endoscope-assisted versus conventional second branchial cleft cyst resection. *Surg Endosc* 2012; 26: 1397–402.
19. Houck J. Excision of branchial cysts. *Operat Tech Otolaryngol* 2005; 16: 213–22.
20. Choi SS, Zalzal GH. Branchial anomalies: A review of 52 cases. *Laryngoscope* 1995; 105: 909–13.
21. Rosenfeld RM, Biller HF. Fourth branchial pouch sinus: Diagnosis and treatment. *Otolaryngol Head Neck Surg* 1991; 105: 44–50.
22. Chin AC, Radhakrishnan J, Slatton D, Geissler G. Congenital cysts of the third and fourth pharyngeal pouches or pyriform sinus cysts. *J Pediatr Surg* 2000; 35: 1252–5.
23. Narcy P, Aumont-Grosskopf C, Bobin S, Manac'h Y. Fistulae of the fourth endobranchial pouch. *Int J Pediatr Otorhinolaryngol* 1988; 16: 157–65.
24. Miyauchi A, Matsuzuka F, Kuma K, Takai S. Piriform sinus fistula: An underlying abnormality common in patients with acute suppurative thyroiditis. *World J Surg* 1990; 14: 400–5.
25. Tyler D, Effmann E, Shorter N. Pyriform sinus cyst and fistula in the newborn: The value of endoscopic cannulation. *J Pediatr Surg* 1992; 27: 1500–1.
26. LaPlante JK, Pierson NS, Hedlund GL. Common pediatric head and neck congenital/developmental anomalies. *Radiol Clin North Am* 2015; 53: 181–96.
27. Teng SE, Paul BC, Brumm JD et al. Endoscope-assisted approach to excision of branchial cleft cysts. *Laryngoscope* 2016; 126(6): 1339–42.
28. Nicoucar K, Giger R, Jaecklin T et al. Management of congenital third branchial arch anomalies: A systematic review. *Otolaryngol Head Neck Surg* 2010; 142: 21–8 e22.
29. Nicoucar K, Giger R, Pope HG, Jr. et al. Management of congenital fourth branchial arch anomalies: A review and analysis of published cases. *J Pediatr Surg* 2009; 44: 1432–9.
30. Foley DS, Fallat ME. Thyroglossal duct and other congenital midline cervical anomalies. *Semin Pediatr Surg* 2006; 15: 70–5.
31. Pollock WF, Stevenson EO. Cysts and sinuses of the thyroglossal duct. *Am J Surg* 1966; 112: 225–32.
32. Kepertis C, Anastasiadis K, Lambropoulos V et al. Diagnostic and surgical approach of thyroglossal duct cyst in children: Ten years data review. *J Clin Diagn Res* 2015; 9: PC13–5.
33. Allard RH. The thyroglossal cyst. *Head Neck Surg* 1982; 5: 134–46.
34. Sistrunk WE. The surgical treatment of cysts of the thyroglossal tract. *Ann Surg* 1920; 71: 121–2.

35. Kennedy TL, Whitaker M, Wadih G. Thyroglossal duct carcinoma: A rational approach to management. *Laryngoscope* 1998; 108: 1154–8.

36. Boswell WC, Zoller M, Williams JS et al. Thyroglossal duct carcinoma. *Am Surg* 1994; 60: 650–5.

37. Van Vuuren PA, Balm AJ, Gregor RT et al. Carcinoma arising in thyroglossal remnants. *Clin Otolaryngol Allied Sci* 1994; 19: 509–15.

38. Ercocen AR, Yilmaz S, Aker H. Congenital midline cervical cleft: Case report and review. *J Oral Maxillofac Surg* 2002; 60: 580–5.

39. Minami RT, Pletcher J, Dakin RL. Midline cervical cleft. A case report. *J Maxillofac Surg* 1980; 8: 65–8.

40. McInnes CW, Benson AD, Verchere CG et al. Management of congenital midline cervical cleft. *J Craniofac Surg* 2012; 23: e36–8.

41. Cochran CS, DeFatta RJ, Brenski AC. Congenital midline cervical cleft: A practical approach to Z-plasty closure. *Int J Pediatr Otorhinolaryngol* 2006; 70: 553–9.

42. Maschka DA, Clemons JE, Janis JF. Congenital midline cervical cleft. Case report and review. *Ann Otol Rhinol Laryngol* 1995; 104: 808–11.

43. Cunningham MJ. The management of congenital neck masses. *Am J Otolaryngol* 1992; 13: 78–92.

44. Ro EY, Thomas RM, Isaacson GC. Giant dermoid cyst of the neck can mimic a cystic hygroma: Using MRI to differentiate cystic neck lesions. *Int J Pediatr Otorhinolaryngol* 2007; 71: 653–8.

45. Shim HS, Ko YI, Kim MC et al. A simple and reproducible surgical technique for the management of preauricular sinuses. *Otolaryngol Head Neck Surg* 2013; 149: 399–401.

46. Moll M. Congenital earpits or auricular sinuses. *Apmis* 1991; 99: 96–8.

47. Chami RG, Apesos J. Treatment of asymptomatic preauricular sinuses: Challenging conventional wisdom. *Ann Plast Surg* 1989; 23: 406–11.

48. Emery PJ, Salama NY. Congenital pre-auricular sinus. A study of 31 cases seen over a ten year period. *Int J Pediatr Otorhinolaryngol* 1981; 3: 205–12.

49. Gur E, Yeung A, Al-Azzawi M, Thomson H. The excised preauricular sinus in 14 years of experience: Is there a problem? *Plast Reconstr Surg* 1998; 102: 1405–8.

50. Yeo SW, Jun BC, Park SN et al. The preauricular sinus: Factors contributing to recurrence after surgery. *Am J Otolaryngol* 2006; 27: 396–400.

51. Gohary A, Rangecroft L, Cook RC. Congenital auricular and preauricular sinuses in childhood. *Z Kinderchir* 1983; 38: 81–2.

52. Gan EC, Anicete R, Tan HK, Balakrishnan A. Preauricular sinuses in the pediatric population: Techniques and recurrence rates. *Int J Pediatr Otorhinolaryngol* 2013; 77: 372–8.

53. Seo JH, Park JJ, Kim HY et al. Surgical management of intraoral ranulas in children: An analysis of 17 pediatric cases. *Int J Pediatr Otorhinolaryngol* 2009; 74: 202–5.

54. Roh JL. Primary treatment of ranula with intracystic injection of OK-432. *Laryngoscope* 2006; 116: 169–72.

55. Fukase S, Ohta N, Inamura K, Aoyagi M. Treatment of ranula with intracystic injection of the streptococcal preparation OK-432. *Ann Otol Rhinol Laryngol* 2003; 112: 214–20.

56. Patel MR, Deal AM, Shockley WW. Oral and plunging ranulas: What is the most effective treatment? *Laryngoscope* 2009; 119: 1501–9.

57. Huang SF, Liao CT, Chin SC, Chen IH. Transoral approach for plunging ranula—10-year experience. *Laryngoscope* 120: 53–7.

58. Hidaka H, Oshima T, Kakehata S et al. Two cases of plunging ranula managed by the intraoral approach. *Tohoku J Exp Med* 2003; 200: 59–65.

59. Zhao YF, Jia J, Jia Y. Complications associated with surgical management of ranulas. *J Oral Maxillofac Surg* 2005; 63: 51–4.

60. Gedikbasi A, Gul A, Sargin A, Ceylan Y. Cystic hygroma and lymphangioma: Associated findings, perinatal outcome and prognostic factors in live-born infants. *Arch Gynecol Obstet* 2007; 276: 491–8.

61. Carpenter CT, Pitcher JD, Jr., Davis BJ et al. Cystic hygroma of the arm: A case report and review of the literature. *Skeletal Radiol* 1996; 25: 201–4.

62. Kostopoulos GK, Fessatidis JT, Hevas AL et al. Mediastinal cystic hygroma: Report of a case with review of the literature. *Eur J Cardiothorac Surg* 1993; 7: 166–7.

63. Alqahtani A, Nguyen LT, Flageole H et al. 25 years' experience with lymphangiomas in children. *J Pediatr Surg* 1999; 34: 1164–8.

64. Hunt I, Eaton D, Dalal P et al. Minimally invasive excision of a mediastinal cystic lymphangioma. *Can J Surg* 2009; 52: E201–2.

65. Brown LR, Reiman HM, Rosenow EC 3rd et al. Intrathoracic lymphangioma. *Mayo Clin Proc* 1986; 61: 882–92.

66. Limmer S, Krokowski M, Kujath P. Pulmonary lymphangioma. *Ann Thorac Surg* 2008; 85: 336–9.

67. Weiss SW, Goldblum JR, Enzinger FM. *Enzinger and Weiss' Soft Tissue Tumors*. Philadelphia, PA: Mosby Elsevier, 2008.

68. Pui MH, Li ZP, Chen W, Chen JH. Lymphangioma: Imaging diagnosis. *Australas Radiol* 1997; 41: 324–8.

69. Hancock BJ, St-Vil D, Luks FI et al. Complications of lymphangiomas in children. *J Pediatr Surg* 1992; 27: 220–4; discussion 224–6.

70. Fujino A, Moriya Y, Morikawa Y et al. A role of cytokines in OK-432 injection therapy for cystic lymphangioma: An approach to the mechanism. *J Pediatr Surg* 2003; 38: 1806–9.

71. Okada A, Kubota A, Fukuzawa M et al. Injection of bleomycin as a primary therapy of cystic lymphangioma. *J Pediatr Surg* 1992; 27: 440–3.

72. Schmidt B, Schimpl G, Hollwarth ME. OK-432 therapy of lymphangiomas in children. *Eur J Pediatr* 1996; 155: 649–52.

73. Papsin BC, Evans JN. Isolated laryngeal lymphangioma: A rare cause of airway obstruction in infants. *J Laryngol Otol* 1996; 110: 969–72.

74. Rothenberg SS, Pokorny WJ. Use of argon beam ablation and sclerotherapy in the treatment of a case of life-threatening total abdominal lymphangiomatosis. *J Pediatr Surg* 1994; 29: 322–3.

75. Lee IJ, Lim SY, Song HS, Park MC. Complete tight fibrous band release and resection in congenital muscular torticollis. *J Plast Reconstr Aesthet Surg* 2009; 63(6): 947–53.

76. Do TT. Congenital muscular torticollis: Current concepts and review of treatment. *Curr Opin Pediatr* 2006; 18: 26–9.

77. Dudkiewicz I, Ganel A, Blankstein A. Congenital muscular torticollis in infants: Ultrasound-assisted diagnosis and evaluation. *J Pediatr Orthop* 2005; 25: 812–4.

78. Chan YL, Cheng JC, Metreweli C. Ultrasonography of congenital muscular torticollis. *Pediatr Radiol* 1992; 22: 356–60.

79. Cheng JC, Wong MW, Tang SP et al. Clinical determinants of the outcome of manual stretching in the treatment of congenital muscular torticollis in infants. A prospective study of eight hundred and twenty-one cases. *J Bone Joint Surg Am* 2001; 83-A: 679–87.

80. Collins A, Jankovic J. Botulinum toxin injection for congenital muscular torticollis presenting in children and adults. *Neurology* 2006; 67: 1083–5.

81. Dutta S, Albanese CT. Transaxillary subcutaneous endoscopic release of the sternocleidomastoid muscle for treatment of persistent torticollis. *J Pediatr Surg* 2008; 43: 447–50.

35

Stridor in infants

SAM J. DANIEL AND FAISAL ZAWAWI

INTRODUCTION

Stridor refers to the abnormal noisy breathing that occurs due to turbulent airflow passing through the narrow lumen of a partially obstructed airway. The degree of stridor is dictated by the amount of reduction in lumen size, whereas the type of stridor is determined by the location of the obstruction.

Stridor can be classified as inspiratory, expiratory, or biphasic. Inspiratory stridor is classically caused by a supraglottic obstruction (above the level of the vocal cords), and expiratory stridor is caused by tracheal and bronchial obstruction. At these levels, often, the issue is a dynamic obstruction. This is the reason behind single-phase stridor. At the level of the vocal folds and subglottis, there is usually a fixed obstruction. This explains why at these locations, a biphasic stridor occurs.

There are many causes for stridor in a newborn. These can be classified either by location (supraglottic, glottic, subglottic, and tracheal) or by the type of disorder causing the airway obstruction (congenital, infectious, neoplastic, etc.) (Table 35.1).

In this chapter, we will review the most common and important differential diagnoses.

SUPRAGLOTTIC DISORDERS

Laryngomalacia

This is the most common cause of stridor in neonates. It is usually caused by an immature neuromuscular tone and/or weak and immature cartilages of the larynx. This leads to a dynamic obstruction with inspiration. Classically, laryngomalacia does not become symptomatic until 6–8 weeks after birth.[1,2] This is because at birth, the inspiratory pressures are not enough to collapse the supraglottic immature structures. As the child grows, the lungs mature and become able to generate enough pressure that can overcome the supraglottic cartilage strength.[3]

There are numerous classifications for laryngomalacia based on either anatomy or severity. The features of laryngomalacia by anatomic designation are collapse of the cuneiform and corniculate cartilages, posterior inspiratory displacement of the epiglottis, short aryepiglottic folds (AE folds), and long tubular (omega-shaped) epiglottis.[3–10] In severe cases, the vocal cords cannot be visualized.

Laryngomalacia usually presents with stridor that worsens in the supine position, with crying, and with feeding. Findings that should prompt a more urgent evaluation by an airway specialist (red flags) include apnea, tachypnea, cyanosis, feeding difficulties despite adequate acid suppression and food texture modification, failure to thrive, weight loss, evidence of aspiration or pneumonia, and cor pulmonale. Gastroesophageal reflux disease (GERD) is associated with laryngomalacia.[11] In fact, symptoms of GERD should be carefully sought while taking history to assess the severity of the reflux and the need for treatment. These symptoms include back arching after feeds, spit-ups, and recurrent emesis.

A complete physical examination including a flexible laryngoscopy on an awake child is performed routinely to confirm the diagnosis. Findings on physical examination tend to vary according to the severity of the condition. Red flags listed previously as well as suprasternal tug or retraction are suggestive of a more severe obstruction. During the endoscopy, features of laryngomalacia should be documented alongside signs of reflux.[12]

Laryngomalacia usually resolves spontaneously by the age of 12–18 months. In mild to moderate cases, medical therapy with aggressive GERD treatment is usually all that is needed to control the patients' symptoms. However, severe laryngomalacia resulting in failure to thrive, apneas, cyanotic spells, and/or cor pulmonale is likely to require surgical treatment.

Supraglottoplasty is the surgery of choice. It addresses the various contributing factors of the supraglottic collapse or obstruction. Usually, all that is needed is an AE fold release, although occasionally, addressing the redundant cuneiform

Table 35.1 Etiologies of airway obstruction in the newborn

Congenital	Laryngomalacia, subglottic stenosis, laryngeal cysts, laryngeal stenosis/web, local fold immobility, subglottic cysts, tracheal stenosis, complete tracheal rings, tracheomalacia, vascular anomalies, thymic masses
Infections	Epiglottitis (rare), angioedema, laryngotracheobronchitis, bacterial tracheitis
Neoplasm	Vascular tumors, recurrent respiratory papillomas, thyroid and mediastinal tumors
Other	Acquired vocal fold immobility (scar), foreign body, post-intubation trauma

or corniculate cartilages, the arytenoid mucosa, and a long epiglottis are necessary.[13] In some cases, an epiglottopexy is required, to lift the epiglottis forward and attach it to the base of tongue or hyoid bone. Also in very rare occasions, a tracheostomy is needed.

It is important after a supraglottoplasty to monitor the child's breathing and feeding. Opening up the airway may increase the risk of airway penetration or aspiration.[6,13]

Laryngeal cysts

Congenital laryngeal cysts are rare findings in an infant. When they occur, the infant usually presents with upper airway obstructive symptoms. They can be extralaryngeal (vallecular cysts) or endolaryngeal (saccular cysts).[14]

Vallecular cysts are unilocular cysts that arise from the lingual surface of the epiglottis. The pathogenesis of their development is thought to be due to mucus gland obstruction or developmental malformation during the gestational period. Infants with vallecular cysts present with symptoms of supraglottic airway obstruction that are similar to laryngomalacia. Flexible laryngoscopy is usually able to diagnose these cysts. Therefore, a focused laryngoscopy examination is encouraged while assessing infants with laryngomalacia-like picture. In almost all cases, these infants are treated surgically using an endoscopic approach. Complete excision of the cyst is often feasible, especially in older children, but when not feasible, marsupialization of the cyst is performed.

Congenital saccular cysts are rare anomalies that are believed to form due to failure of maintaining a saccular orifice. They develop into an abnormal herniation of the saccule but without an opening at the ventricle. These cysts are filled with mucus.[14]

There are two types of saccular cysts, anterior and lateral saccular cysts. Anterior cysts enlarge medially and posteriorly between the true and false cords, protruding into the lumen of the larynx. Lateral cysts progress in a posterosuperior direction, causing distension of the false vocal cord and AE fold. The growth of such cysts is restricted by the thyroid cartilage, but lateral extension through the thyrohyoid membrane may occur, resulting in a neck mass. Saccular cysts can also be divided into endolaryngeal (type 1) and extralaryngeal (type 2). The second type is further classified into endodermal elements only (2a) and endodermal and mesodermal elements (2b).[15]

Saccular cysts present with inspiratory stridor and respiratory distress at birth. Weak or muffled cry and dysphagia can also occur. A flexible fiber-optic laryngoscopy allows the visualization of fullness at the level of the ventricle, and in larger cysts, a round swelling protruding into the laryngeal lumen. Imaging is recommended to determine the extent of the cyst and plan the intervention after securing the airway.[14-18]

Endolaryngeal cysts are usually excised endoscopically. Extralaryngeal cysts often require an open approach that involves either dissecting through the thyrohyoid membrane or creating a thyroid ala window to approach the ventricle. Preoperative careful assessment with cross-sectional studies can help reduce the risk of recurrence.[14-18]

GLOTTIC AND SUBGLOTTIC DISORDERS

Vocal fold immobility

There are several causes for vocal fold immobility. These include traumatic causes such as injury during thoracic and cardiac surgery, trauma during delivery that could result in nerve stretch injury, or trauma from endotracheal intubation. Other important causes are neurologic such as hydrocephalus and Arnold–Chiari malformation.[19-22]

There are two different presentations of vocal fold immobility. In unilateral vocal fold immobility, the children often present with episodes of choking with feeds, aspiration, and weak voice and cry. Stridor in these patients could be due to a coexistent disorder, e.g., laryngomalacia. On the other hand, infants with bilateral vocal fold immobility can present with stridor that could be either uniphasic (inspiratory only) or biphasic, and tend to have a strong cry.[19-22]

Physical examination is the key to diagnose these conditions, with awake flexible laryngoscopy being the gold standard. Despite that, findings can be challenging to interpret. This is due to the movement that is caused by the Bernoulli effect of air passing through the vocal folds. Other causes of difficult examination include laryngomalacia covering the view of the cords and supraglottic hyperfunction.

Once vocal fold immobility is diagnosed, cross-sectional imaging of the head down to the chest should be performed looking at the whole course of the recurrent laryngeal nerve. The child should be assessed for swallowing function. Also in bilateral immobility, it is imperative to assess the patient's ability to ventilate well. Overnight oximetry and polysomnography may be warranted depending on the severity of the case.

Laryngeal electromyogram (LEMG), although challenging to perform in neonates, can provide useful information to differentiate paralysis from ankyloses or cord fixation. This could guide the therapeutic intervention needed.[23]

Some causes of immobility are fully reversible. For an example, when a Chiari malformation is decompressed, vocal cold mobility tends to return to normal. If the cause cannot be determined, as in idiopathic cases, the patient should be carefully observed, as most cases recover in the first 2–3 years of life. There are reports for even further delays in recovery in some children with vocal fold paralysis which makes identifying a precise time of potential recovery challenging.[19–21,24–26]

If the patient is unable to ventilate appropriately, a tracheostomy is usually necessary.[24] Recently, new studies have looked at the use of botulinum toxin injection into the laryngeal muscles in order to gain a few millimeters that could prevent the need for a tracheostomy.[27]

There are also several procedures that can be performed to help open up the glottic airway in children with bilateral vocal fold immobility. Most of these procedures are irreversible; hence, they should not be performed early on in life until the immobility has been persistent for few years and the chances of spontaneous recovery are deemed negligible. Vocal fold lateralization, posterior cordotomy, arytenoidectomy, posterior cricoid graft, and anterior and posterior cricoid splits with balloon dilatation are a few of many procedures that can be performed to help a child with bilateral vocal fold immobility.[19,21,22,27–35]

Glottic stenosis

Glottic stenosis is defined as a narrowing of the lumen at the level of the vocal folds. The narrowing can be due to fibrosis, scarring, or webbing. The cause of the stenosis (whether anterior or posterior) is either congenital or acquired, with the latter being much more common. Acquired conditions can be posttraumatic, infectious, inflammatory, or iatrogenic in origin. The risk of developing a posterior glottis stenosis is about 15% in patients who have been intubated for more than 10 days. Factors that increase the risk even further are traumatic intubation, multiple extubations and reintubations, oversized endotracheal tube, GERD, and infections.[36]

Congenital laryngeal web is due to failure of complete recanalization of the larynx during embryogenesis. This accounts for 5% of all laryngeal anomalies, with 75% of those webs occurring at the level of the vocal folds.[37] Patients who are diagnosed to have anterior glottic web should be worked up genetically to rule out other syndromes, most importantly velocardiofacial syndrome.[38]

Glottic webs typically present with airway obstructive symptoms, biphasic stridor, weak voice, and occasionally aphonia. Most of the congenital glottic webs are located anteriorly.

Flexible laryngoscopy is able to identify most of the anterior glottic webs. These patients should undergo a rigid bronchoscopy for further assessment of the airway especially to identify the thickness of the web and to rule out other airway anomalies. Cohen's classification can be useful to classify glottic webs according to their severity. Grade 1 consists of a thin anterior web involving less than 35% of the glottis with no subglottic extension. In grade 2, there is up to 50% glottic stenosis with some subglottic extension. In grade 3, up to 75% of the glottis is involved with subglottic extension (potentially cartilaginous), and in grade 4, there is more than 75% glottic stenosis with thick subglottic cartilaginous involvement.

Infants with glottic stenosis are managed according to the severity of their airway blockage. Infants with grades 1 and 2 are usually observed until 3 years of age prior to surgical intervention.[36,37,39] Infants with grades 3 and 4 usually have breathing difficulties requiring a more urgent airway intervention.[37] This may include a temporary tracheostomy.

There are several surgical options to repair a web. The choice is based on the infant's clinical picture, the degree of stenosis, as well as the surgeon's preference. Open approaches involve performing a complete laryngofissure, cutting the web, and placing a keel. Endoscopic approaches can also be used, severing the web with various types of mucosal flaps to reduce the risk of restenosis. Dedo and Lichtenberger described a procedure in which the web is severed and a keel is placed endoscopically, using a specialized endo-extralaryngeal needle carrier.[37,39–42]

The most common complication is restenosis, and for that reason, these infants are followed closely to detect symptoms and signs of restenosis.[40]

Subglottic stenosis

The subglottis extends from the under surface of the vocal folds to the inferior edge of the cricoid cartilage. It is the narrowest area of an infant airway, measuring normally 4.5–7 mm in a full-term newborn. A preterm newborn's subglottis measures approximately 3–4 mm in diameter. Narrowing of the subglottis, i.e., subglottic stenosis, can be congenital or acquired, the latter being more common. This is due to the improved neonatal intensive care units with improved survival of premature infants, who would require prolonged ventilation and intubation due to premature lung disease. Most of the acquired form is secondary to prolonged intubation, laryngeal trauma, or iatrogenic subglottic damage from an airway procedure. Risk factors for developing subglottic stenosis include recurrent intubation, use of a large endotracheal tube, tracheitis, and infection while the patient is intubated.

Congenital subglottic stenosis is a diagnosis of exclusion. The hypothesis behind its development is failure of recanalization of the tracheal lumen.[43] It can be classified into two types: The first is a cartilaginous type where the abnormality is in the cricoid cartilage, i.e., an elliptical cricoid that causes the subglottic lumen to be narrower than it should be. The other type is membranous, in which there is a thin soft tissue narrowing the lumen.[44,45]

Children with subglottic stenosis present with biphasic stridor and respiratory distress. Another presentation is failure of extubation due to increased work of breathing and stridor in an otherwise fit patient to be extubated. Milder forms of subglottic stenosis can present with a barking cough and early onset of recurrent croup.[46]

While assessing these patients, a thorough history should be obtained with a focus on prematurity, comorbidities, and a prior history of intubation, in addition to choking spells, feeding issues, reflux, and failure to thrive.[46]

General examination of the infant will give the physician a hint as to the level of the obstruction. Biphasic stridor is a classic finding in patients with subglottic stenosis. Increased work of breathing or shallow breathing indicates that the patient is tiring out and about to decompensate.[46]

In patients with only subglottic stenosis, flexible laryngoscopy will show normal anatomy, though on some occasions and in more severe cases, a subglottic narrowing can be visualized. If subglottic stenosis is not diagnosed on a flexible laryngoscopy, it is not recommended to pass the scope through the vocal cord, as this may result in life-threatening airway obstruction due to laryngospasm.[46]

The gold standard diagnostic and evaluation tool is a rigid bronchoscopy performed in the operating room. This also allows the identification of secondary airway lesions and deformities if present. To complete the assessment, airway sizing should also be performed. This can be done using serial endotracheal tubes according to the Myer–Cotton staging system. In this method, a size-appropriate endotracheal tube is chosen according to age. After intubation and confirmation of the position, an air leak is tested. The endotracheal tube that will pass through the lumen, if one exists, and tolerate normal leak pressures (10–25 cm H_2O) can be compared to the expected age-appropriate endotracheal tube size. If the leak is found at less than 10 cm H_2O, then the tube is considered too small, and the procedure is repeated with the next size up. When the leak is found to be absent or present only at higher than 25 cm H_2O, the tube is deemed to be too big, and the test is repeated with a smaller tube. An appropriate tube to lumen should have an air leak between 10 and 25 cm H_2O. That size is then compared to the Myer–Cotton scale to determine the narrowing of the lumen. Based on that grading system, a grade 1 has less than 50% obstruction of the lumen, grade 2 is 51–70%, grade 3 is 71–99% obstruction, and grade 4 is when there is no lumen to be detected (complete obstruction).[47] Cross-sectional imaging, i.e., computed tomography (CT) and magnetic resonance imaging (MRI), are rarely necessary in these cases but may be of help to quantify the length of the narrowed segment, especially in cases with grade 3 or 4 subglottic stenosis.

The management of infants with subglottic stenosis is dictated by the presentation, symptoms, and severity of the stenosis. In milder forms, observation and GERD control can be sufficient.

In patients who failed extubation due to subglottic stenosis, management options include an anterior cricoid split.

Table 35.2 Candidacy criteria for anterior cricoid split in neonates

2 or more failed extubations due to a laryngeal cause
Weight > 1500 g
No ventilation requirement for >10 days
FiO_2 < 30%
No congestive heart failure for >1 month
No acute respiratory illness
No antihypertensive medications for >10 days

For infants to be candidates, they have to meet certain criteria to improve the outcome and the benefit of the procedure (Table 35.2). The procedure involves splitting the cricoid cartilage anteriorly and placing a larger endotracheal tube to stent the airway. On some occasions, a thyroid alar cartilage graft is used if the gap after the cricoid split is more than 3 mm. The patient is then extubated 5–7 days later.[48]

The surgical approach is determined based on the level and length of the segment, the involvement of the vocal folds, the mobility of the vocal folds, the swallowing assessment, and other comorbidities. Surgical options could be either endoscopic or open. Endoscopic approaches (e.g., balloon dilation and laser) are usually reserved for grades 1 and 2 stenosis, where as grades 3 and 4 would require an open approach.[49] Options include laryngotracheoplasty with rib grafts (anterior, posterior, or both) or cricotracheal resection and anastomosis.[44,46,50]

TRACHEAL DISORDERS

Tracheal anomalies, whether congenital or acquired, can be classified into three categories based on the patient's clinical presentation, endoscopic findings, and histological results. These categories are intrinsic tracheal anomalies, extrinsic tracheal anomalies, and acquired tracheal anomalies.[51]

Intrinsic tracheal anomalies are disorders involving the maturity of the tracheal cartilages, narrowed lumen due to complete tracheal rings, atresia, or webs. Extrinsic anomalies include vascular rings and aberrant innominate arteries. Acquired tracheal disorders occur with chronic tracheal infections, prolonged intubation, or inflammatory conditions like relapsing polychondritis.[52,53]

Tracheomalacia

Tracheomalacia is characterized by weakness of the tracheal cartilages, widening of the posterior wall, and reduced airway caliber. These result in tracheal collapse, which becomes more evident during increased airflow periods such as crying, feeding, or coughing.[51,53,54] Tracheomalacia can be associated with various airway defects (e.g., tracheoesophageal fistula and laryngeal clefts), cardiovascular defects, developmental delay, and GERD.[51,53,54]

Patients present with expiratory stridor (occasionally they could have biphasic stridor) that could resemble wheezing. During heavy breathing, the posterior wall advances

376 Stridor in infants

anteriorly, and on some occasions, it even touches the anterior wall, causing narrowing in the airway lumen. Initially, the symptoms start to get worse as the infant grows due to the increased respiratory movement.

Primary tracheomalacia is a rare disorder of the tracheal rings, whereas, more commonly, secondary tracheomalacia is when cartilage weakness results from a persistent external pressure. Frequent causes of secondary tracheomalacia include vascular compression, such as from a double aortic arche or innominate artery compression, and in association with a tracheoesophageal fistula. Even after vascular repair, the cartilages may not return to their normal appearance for many years, due to chronic changes of the cartilage from general sclerosis or scarring.

The gold standard in diagnosing tracheomalacia is using a flexible bronchoscopy. Other helpful tests include airway fluorography and also rigid bronchoscopy using either just a Hopkins telescope or a very small bronchoscope. The bronchoscopy has to be performed with the patient spontaneously ventilating; otherwise, the diagnosis might not be evident, due to the positive airway pressure stenting the airway, or if apneic techniques are adopted, the loss of the respiratory drive reduce, the severity of the tracheomalacia.

Tracheomalacia is generally self-limiting because adequate growth of the airway diameter eliminates the symptoms by the time the patient is 2–3 years old.[55,56] Therefore, treatment is aimed at preventing complications for tracheomalacia such as atelectasis. In severe cases, continuous positive airway pressure (CPAP) may be necessary until the infant outgrows the tracheomalacia. Furthermore, in some cases, a tracheostomy is performed to delivery CPAP to the distal trachea.[53]

When vascular compression is noted, aortopexy may be used to alleviate the pressure of the trachea and reduce the effect of tracheomalacia.[53,56,57] Internal airway stenting is another method but comes with a long list of downsides, including granulation tissue formation, risk of foreign body reaction, and extrusion, which could be fatal if the compression is from a major vessel. For that reason, caution is warrant while selecting patients for internal airway stenting.[58,59]

Vascular anomalies

In these disorders, the trachea is inherently normal. However, due to a large vessel extrinsically compressing it, the tracheal wall is deformed. Vascular anomalies are due to abnormal development of the branchial arches. They are rare anomalies and frequently coexist with other cardiac anomalies. Abnormalities that can occur in vessels include abnormal positioning of the aorta, anomalous branching, interrupted arches, or anomalous origin of the pulmonary artery.

The presenting symptoms depend on the degree of airway compression. Symptoms range from asymptomatic to severe life-threatening airway distress. Frequent presentations include recurrent pneumonias, stridor, dysphagia, and cough. Occasionally, these infants hyperextend their neck to stretch their trachea, which results in a widening of the diameter of the airway. Patients can also present as acute life-threatening events (ALTEs), reflex apnea, or cyanotic spells.[60,61]

When suspected on a bronchoscopy the diagnosis can be confirmed using an echocardiography, MRI, or CT scan. Additionally, angiography may help in the diagnosis.[62–64]

The most common vascular abnormality is an aberrant innominate artery compressing the anterior wall of the trachea.[65] The second most common is double aortic arch. This anomaly results in a double compression: on the trachea anteriorly and the esophagus posteriorly. Other anomalies include pulmonary artery sling in which the left pulmonary artery passes between the trachea and the esophagus, resulting in right bronchus and distal tracheal posterior compression. It is also associated with complete rings of the trachea. Aberrant right subclavian artery, which is also known as arteria lusoria, is a condition in which the right subclavian artery arises as a fourth branch (instead of being the first branch of the aortic arch). It passes posterior to the esophagus in 80% of cases to reach to the right side. It is associated with a right nonrecurrent laryngeal nerve.[66]

The treatment in these cases is dictated by the patient's airway and dysphagia symptoms. If not severe, the patient could be observed safely,[55] but occasionally, aortopexy, dividing the arches, or vascular rerouting can be performed to alleviate the compression if the patient's symptoms are severe.

Complete tracheal rings

Development of abnormal tracheal rings occurs after 8 weeks of gestation. The tracheal cartilages are fused posteriorly, and there is absence of the posterior membranous trachea and the typical C-shaped rings. It is a rare condition representing less than 1% of all laryngotracheal stenosis. This anomaly may involve a few rings up to the entire length of the trachea.[67]

Patients present with dyspnea, increased work of breathing, and biphasic or expiratory stridor (depending on the location and the length of the segment). In patients with <50% tracheal stenosis, symptoms may be mild, or the patient may be asymptomatic.[68]

Plain chest x-ray may provide clues as to the stenosis due to a narrow air column. Other radiological tests including CT and MRI are helpful especially when looking for associated disorders (e.g., pulmonary sling). The gold standard remains a rigid bronchoscopy to diagnose the anomalies and measure the length of the stenotic segment.[67,68]

Infants with mild symptoms can be treated medically by controlling their GERD and respiratory disorders. More severe cases generally require a surgical intervention. Surgical options vary depending on the symptoms, degree of stenosis, and location of the stenotic segment. Endoscopic approaches, using laser, dilation, and possibly stenting, are reserved for short segments.[69] Open procedures are used for failed endoscopic approach, severe stenosis, and thick or long segments.[67,70–72] Primary resection and anastomosis is a very good option for short segments with severe stenosis.

For longer segments, tracheoplasty with alloplastic or pericardial grafts was considered a classic technique, which is currently less utilized due to the higher risks of complications. Instead, slide tracheoplasty is currently the procedure of choice for most airway surgeons to treat long-segment complete tracheal rings. In these surgeries, extracorporeal myocardial oxygenation (ECMO) may be necessary while performing the procedure, especially in children with long- or distal-segment tracheal stenosis.[70-72]

Tracheal atresia and agenesis

This is a rare usually fatal anomaly of the airway. The tracheal is either completely absent (agenesis) or considerably underformed (atresia). This means that the communication between the lungs and larynx is missing. Therefore, newborns are only able to survive if there is an alternate way for the air to go to the lungs, e.g., bronchoesophageal fistula. Surgical repair can be attempted, but in general, the prognosis is poor.[73,74]

REFERENCES

1. Erickson B, Cooper T, El-Hakim H. Factors associated with the morphological type of laryngomalacia and prognostic value for surgical outcomes. *JAMA Otolaryngol Head Neck Surg* 2014; 140: 927–33.
2. Cooper T, Benoit M, Erickson B, El-Hakim H. Primary Presentations of Laryngomalacia. *JAMA Otolaryngol Head Neck Surg* 2014; 140: 521–6.
3. Kay DJ, Goldsmith AJ. Laryngomalacia: A classification system and surgical treatment strategy. *Ear Nose Throat J* 2006; 85: 328–31, 336.
4. Shah UK, Wetmore RF. Laryngomalacia: A proposed classification form. *Int J Pediatr Otorhinolaryngol* 1998; 46: 21–6.
5. Walner DL, Cotton RT, Willging JP, Bove KE, Toriumi DM. Model for evaluating the effect of growth factors on the larynx. *Otolaryngol Head Neck Surg* 1999; 120: 78–83.
6. Olney DR, Greinwald JH, Jr., Smith RJ, Bauman NM. Laryngomalacia and its treatment. *Laryngoscope* 1999; 109: 1770–5.
7. Holinger LD, Konior RJ. Surgical management of severe laryngomalacia. *Laryngoscope* 1989; 99: 136–42.
8. McSwiney PF, Cavanagh NP, Languth P. Outcome in congenital stridor (laryngomalacia). *Arch Dis Child* 1977; 52: 215–8.
9. Roger G, Denoyelle F, Triglia JM, Garabedian EN. Severe laryngomalacia: Surgical indications and results in 115 patients. *Laryngoscope* 1995; 105: 1111–7.
10. Lee KS, Chen BN, Yang CC, Chen YC. CO_2 laser supraglottoplasty for severe laryngomalacia: A study of symptomatic improvement. *Int J Pediatr Otorhinolaryngol* 2007; 71: 889–95.
11. Giannoni C, Sulek M, Friedman EM, Duncan NO, 3rd. Gastroesophageal reflux association with laryngomalacia: A prospective study. *Int J Pediatr Otorhinolaryngol* 1998; 43: 11–20.
12. van der Heijden M, Dikkers FG, Halmos GB. The groningen laryngomalacia classification system—Based on systematic review and dynamic airway changes. *Pediatr Pulmonol* 2015; 50: 1368–73.
13. Thompson DM. Laryngomalacia: Factors that influence disease severity and outcomes of management. *Curr Opin Otolaryngol Head Neck Surg* 2010; 18: 564–70.
14. DeSanto LW, Devine KD, Weiland LH. Cysts of the larynx—Classification. *Laryngoscope* 1970; 80: 145–76.
15. Forte V, Fuoco G, James A. A new classification system for congenital laryngeal cysts. *Laryngoscope* 2004; 114: 1123–7.
16. Abramson AL, Zielinski B. Congenital laryngeal saccular cyst of the newborn. *Laryngoscope* 1984; 94: 1580–2.
17. Booth JB, Birck HG. Operative treatment and postoperative management of saccular cyst and laryngocele. *Arch Otolaryngol* 1981; 107: 500–2.
18. Holinger LD, Barnes DR, Smid LJ, Holinger PH. Laryngocele and saccular cysts. *Ann Otol Rhinol Laryngol* 1978; 87: 675–85.
19. Cohen SR, Geller KA, Birns JW, Thompson JW. Laryngeal paralysis in children: A long-term retrospective study. *Ann Otol Rhinol Laryngol* 1982; 91: 417–24.
20. Emery PJ, Fearon B. Vocal cord palsy in pediatric practice: A review of 71 cases. *Int J Pediatr Otorhinolaryngol* 1984; 8: 147–54.
21. Gentile RD, Miller RH, Woodson GE. Vocal cord paralysis in children 1 year of age and younger. *Ann Otol Rhinol Laryngol* 1986; 95: 622–5.
22. Rosin DF, Handler SD, Potsic WP, Wetmore RF, Tom LW. Vocal cord paralysis in children. *Laryngoscope* 1990; 100: 1174–9.
23. Berkowitz RG. Laryngeal electromyography findings in idiopathic congenital bilateral vocal cord paralysis. *Ann Otol Rhinol Laryngol* 1996; 105: 207–12.
24. Murty GE, Shinkwin C, Gibbin KP. Bilateral vocal fold paralysis in infants: Tracheostomy or not? *J Laryngol Otol* 1994; 108: 329–31.
25. Zbar RI, Chen AH, Behrendt DM, Bell EF, Smith RJ. Incidence of vocal fold paralysis in infants undergoing ligation of patent ductus arteriosus. *Ann Thorac Surg* 1996; 61: 814–6.
26. Zbar RI, Smith RJ. Vocal fold paralysis in infants twelve months of age and younger. *Otolaryngol Head Neck Surg* 1996; 114: 18–21.
27. Daniel SJ, Cardona I. Cricothyroid onabotulinum toxin A injection to avert tracheostomy in bilateral vocal fold paralysis. *JAMA Otolaryngol Head Neck Surg* 2014; 140: 867–9.

28. Dennis DP, Kashima H. Carbon dioxide laser posterior cordectomy for treatment of bilateral vocal cord paralysis. *Ann Otol Rhinol Laryngol* 1989; 98: 930–4.

29. Laccourreye O, Paz Escovar MI, Gerhardt J, Hans S, Biacabe B, Brasnu D. CO_2 laser endoscopic posterior partial transverse cordotomy for bilateral paralysis of the vocal fold. *Laryngoscope* 1999; 109: 415–8.

30. Ossoff RH, Sisson GA, Duncavage JA, Moselle HI, Andrews PE, McMillan WG. Endoscopic laser arytenoidectomy for the treatment of bilateral vocal cord paralysis. *Laryngoscope* 1984; 94: 1293–7.

31. Eckel HE, Thumfart M, Wassermann K, Vossing M, Thumfart WF. Cordectomy versus arytenoidectomy in the management of bilateral vocal cord paralysis. *Ann Otol Rhinol Laryngol* 1994; 103: 852–7.

32. Eckel HE, Sittel C. [Morphometric studies at the level of the glottis as a principle in larynx enlarging microlaryngoscopic surgical procedures in bilateral recurrent nerve paralysis]. *Laryngo-rhino-otologie* 1994; 73: 417–22.

33. Su WF, Liu SC, Tang WS, Yang MC, Lin YY, Huang TT. Suture lateralization in patients with bilateral vocal fold paralysis. *J Voice* 2014; 28: 644–51.

34. Sztano B, Szakacs L, Madani S et al. Comparison of endoscopic techniques designed for posterior glottic stenosis—A cadaver morphometric study. *Laryngoscope* 2014; 124: 705–10.

35. Helmus C. Microsurgical thyrotomy and arytenoidectomy for bilateral recurrent laryngeal nerve paralysis. *Laryngoscope* 1972; 82: 491–503.

36. Sittel C. Pathologies of the larynx and trachea in childhood. *GMS Curr Topics Otorhinolaryngol Head Neck Surg* 2014; 13: Doc09.

37. Cohen SR. Congenital glottic webs in children. A retrospective review of 51 patients. *Ann Otol Rhinol Laryngol Suppl* 1985; 121: 2–16.

38. Miyamoto RC, Cotton RT, Rope AF et al. Association of anterior glottic webs with velocardiofacial syndrome (chromosome 22q11.2 deletion). *Otolaryngol Head Neck Surg* 2004; 130: 415–7.

39. Dedo HH, Sooy CD. Endoscopic laser repair of posterior glottic, subglottic and tracheal stenosis by division or micro-trapdoor flap. *Laryngoscope* 1984; 94: 445–50.

40. Lichtenberger G, Toohill RJ. New keel fixing technique for endoscopic repair of anterior commissure webs. *Laryngoscope* 1994; 104: 771–4.

41. Montgomery WW. Posterior and complete laryngeal (glottic) stenosis. *Arch Otolaryngol* 1973; 98: 170–5.

42. Zalzal GH. Posterior glottic fixation in children. *Ann Otol Rhinol Laryngol* 1993; 102: 680–6.

43. Walander A. The mechanism of origin of congenital malformations of the larynx. *Acta Oto-laryngol* 1955; 45: 426–32.

44. Fearon B, Cotton R. Surgical correction of subglottic stenosis of the larynx. Preliminary report of an experimental surgical technique. *Ann Otol Rhinol Laryngol* 1972; 81: 508–13.

45. Tucker GF, Ossoff RH, Newman AN, Holinger LD. Histopathology of congenital subglottic stenosis. *Laryngoscope* 1979; 89: 866–77.

46. Cotton RT. Management of subglottic stenosis. *Otolaryngol Clin North Am* 2000; 33: 111–30.

47. Myer CM, 3rd, O'Connor DM, Cotton RT. Proposed grading system for subglottic stenosis based on endotracheal tube sizes. *Ann Otol Rhinol Laryngol* 1994; 103: 319–23.

48. Silver FM, Myer CM, 3rd, Cotton RT. Anterior cricoid split. Update 1991. *Am J Otolaryngol* 1991; 12: 343–6.

49. Rutter MJ, Cohen AP, de Alarcon A. Endoscopic airway management in children. *Curr Opin Otolaryngol Head Neck Surg* 2008; 16: 525–9.

50. Rutter MJ, Hartley BE, Cotton RT. Cricotracheal resection in children. *Arch Otolaryngol Head Neck Surg* 2001; 127: 289–92.

51. Beasley SW, Qi BQ. Understanding tracheomalacia. *J Paediatr Child Health* 1998; 34: 209–10.

52. Berrocal T, Madrid C, Novo S, Gutierrez J, Arjonilla A, Gomez-Leon N. Congenital anomalies of the tracheobronchial tree, lung, and mediastinum: Embryology, radiology, and pathology. *Radiographics* 2004; 24: e17.

53. Carden KA, Boiselle PM, Waltz DA, Ernst A. Tracheomalacia and tracheobronchomalacia in children and adults: An in-depth review. *Chest* 2005; 127: 984–1005.

54. Gaissert HA, Burns J. The compromised airway: Tumors, strictures, and tracheomalacia. *Surg Clin North Am* 2010; 90: 1065–89.

55. McNamara VM, Crabbe DC. Tracheomalacia. *Paediatr Respir Rev* 2004; 5: 147–54.

56. Anton-Pacheco JL, Garcia-Hernandez G, Villafruela MA. The management of tracheobronchial obstruction in children. *Minerva Pediatr* 2009; 61: 39–52.

57. Kikuchi S, Kashino R, Hirama T, Kobayashi H, Abe T. Successful treatment of tracheomalacia associated with esophageal atresia without a tracheoesophageal fistula by aortopexy: Report of a case. *Surg Today* 1999; 29: 344–6.

58. Collard P, Freitag L, Reynaert MS, Rodenstein DO, Francis C. Respiratory failure due to tracheobronchomalacia. *Thorax* 1996; 51: 224–6.

59. Fayon M, Donato L, de Blic J et al. French experience of silicone tracheobronchial stenting in children. *Pediatr Pulmonol* 2005; 39: 21–7.

60. Boogaard R, Huijsmans SH, Pijnenburg MW, Tiddens HA, de Jongste JC, Merkus PJ. Tracheomalacia and bronchomalacia in children: Incidence and patient characteristics. *Chest* 2005; 128: 3391–7.

61. Sanchez MO, Greer MC, Masters IB, Chang AB. A comparison of fluoroscopic airway screening with flexible bronchoscopy for diagnosing tracheomalacia. *Pediatr Pulmonol* 2012; 47: 63–7.
62. Humphrey C, Duncan K, Fletcher S. Decade of experience with vascular rings at a single institution. *Pediatrics* 2006; 117: e903–8.
63. Baroni RH, Ashiku S, Boiselle PM. Dynamic CT evaluation of the central airways in patients undergoing tracheoplasty for tracheobronchomalacia. *AJR Am J Roentgenol* 2005; 184: 1444–9.
64. Baroni RH, Feller-Kopman D, Nishino M et al. Tracheobronchomalacia: Comparison between end-expiratory and dynamic expiratory CT for evaluation of central airway collapse. *Radiology* 2005; 235: 635–41.
65. Mahboubi S, Harty MP, Hubbard AM, Meyer JS. Innominate artery compression of the trachea in infants. *Int J Pediatr Otorhinolaryngol* 1996; 35: 197–205.
66. Atay Y, Engin C, Posacioglu H et al. Surgical approaches to the aberrant right subclavian artery. *Tex Heart Inst J* 2006; 33: 477–481.
67. Ho AS, Koltai PJ. Pediatric tracheal stenosis. *Otolaryngol Clin North Am* 2008; 41: 999–1021, x.
68. Rutter MJ, Willging JP, Cotton RT. Nonoperative management of complete tracheal rings. *Arch Otolaryngol Head Neck Surg* 2004; 130: 450–2.
69. Gotway MB, Golden JA, LaBerge JM et al. Benign tracheobronchial stenoses: Changes in short-term and long-term pulmonary function testing after expandable metallic stent placement. *J Comput Assist Tomogr* 2002; 26: 564–72.
70. Cunningham MJ, Eavey RD, Vlahakes GJ, Grillo HC. Slide tracheoplasty for long-segment tracheal stenosis. *Arch Otolaryngol Head Neck Surg* 1998; 124: 98–103.
71. Gallagher TQ, Hartnick CJ. Slide tracheoplasty. *Adv Oto-rhino-laryngol* 2012; 73: 58–62.
72. Rutter MJ, Cotton RT, Azizkhan RG, Manning PB. Slide tracheoplasty for the management of complete tracheal rings. *J Pediatr Surg* 2003; 38: 928–34.
73. Ergun S, Tewfik T, Daniel S. Tracheal agenesis: A rare but fatal congenital anomaly. *McGill J Med* 2011; 13: 10.
74. Lange P, Fishman JM, Elliott MJ, De Coppi P, Birchall MA. What can regenerative medicine offer for infants with laryngotracheal agenesis? *Otolaryngol Head Neck Surg* 2011; 145: 544–50.

PART 3

Chest

36

Congenital thoracic deformities

KONSTANTINOS PAPADAKIS AND ROBERT C. SHAMBERGER

INTRODUCTION

Congenital thoracic deformities present a wide spectrum of abnormalities. They include a myriad of complete and incomplete sternal defects: thoracic ectopia cordis, thoracoabdominal ectopia cordis (Cantrell pentalogy), and bifid sternum. The most frequent are the deformities of the ribs—including pectus excavatum, pectus carinatum, and Poland syndrome. Asphyxiating thoracic dystrophy (Jeune syndrome) and spondylothoracic dysplasia (Jarcho–Levin syndrome) pose the greatest surgical challenges.

ECTOPIA CORDIS

The first report as described of an exposed heart through a split sternum was described in 1671–1672, by N. Stensen.[1] Later reports, by Weese in 1818[2] and Todd in 1836,[3] proposed classifications of this disorder.

Infants with this anomaly are best classified by the precise location of the heart: cervical (3%), cervicothoracic, thoracic (60%), thoracoabdominal (7%), and abdominal types (30%).[2,3] In cervical ectopia cordis, the heart protrudes at the base of the neck and occurs in association with other severe deformities of the fetus. The cervical type is not compatible with life.

Thoracic ectopia cordis includes infants with an entirely bare heart that is outside the thorax, with cephalic orientation of the cardiac apex. It protrudes through a central sternal cleft and lacks a parietal pericardium and overlying skin. This condition may be associated with a separate epigastric omphalocele or upper abdominal wall defect. Thoracic ectopia cordis must be distinguished from cleft sternum, in which the heart is covered by normal skin in an orthotopic intrathoracic position and is anatomically normal.

In thoracoabdominal ectopia cordis, also known as pentalogy of Cantrell, the heart is covered by skin or an omphalocele-like membrane. It is associated with a constellation of anomalies. The classic pentalogy includes the following: (1) a midline, supraumbilical abdominal wall defect; (2) a defect of the lower sternum; (3) a deficiency of the anterior diaphragm (absence of septum transversum); (4) a defect in the diaphragmatic pericardium; and (5) congenital intracardiac defects. All five anomalies may not be present, and there can be an incomplete expression of the syndrome.[4] In contrast with thoracic ectopia cordis, the heart is covered and lacks severe anterior displacement and cephalic orientation. The world literature on ectopia cordis has been extensively reviewed previously.[5]

Ectopia cordis is diagnosed by prenatal ultrasound from early stages of gestation, which facilitates perinatal preparation.[6,7] Associated intrinsic cardiac anomalies and other anomalies can be defined by in utero studies in order to facilitate parental discussion regarding prognosis.

The cause is unknown. There has been a weak association with trisomy 18,[8-10] triploidy, and familial X-linked inheritance. The incidence is 5.5–7.9 per 1 million live births.

Thoracic ectopia cordis

The presentation of the heart, naked and beating upon the chest wall, has stimulated many case reports (Figure 36.1). Surgical repair has been described,[11,12] but long-term successes are limited by a combination of associated intrinsic cardiac malformations and abnormal rotation of the heart with the apex pointing cephalad.[13] The first successful repair of ectopia cordis was achieved by Koop in 1975, as reported by Saxena.[14] An infant with a normal heart had skin flap coverage at 5 hours of age, with inferior mobilization of the anterior attachments of the diaphragm. At 7 months of age, an acrylic resin of Dacron and Marlex mesh was inserted to widen the sternal cleft with primary skin closure. Necrosis of the skin flaps complicated the postoperative course; the infection of the prosthetic material required its subsequent removal. The child's long-term survival has been reported.[15] Lillehei (as reported by Hornberger et al.[16]) achieved successful repair of the only infant with an intrinsic cardiac

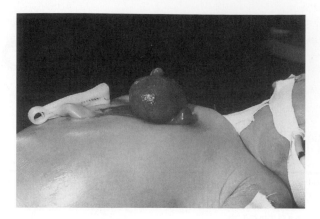

Figure 36.1 Infant with thoracic ectopia cordis. Heart lies anterior to the thoracic cavity, and apex is directed cephalad.

anomaly, tetralogy of Fallot with pulmonary atresia. A combination of thoracic ectopia cordis and separate omphalocele with an intervening bridge of normal skin can be particularly difficult to manage. In this group of patients, adequate skin and abdominal wall components, to cover both areas, are lacking, and no survivors exist. The unifying theme of successfully managed cases is construction of a partially anterior chest cavity surrounding the heart and avoidance of attempts to return the heart to an orthotopic location (Table 36.1).[16–18]

For a successful outcome in infants with thoracic ectopia cordis, early definition of the associated cardiac malformation is necessary. Prenatal workup with echocardiography and magnetic resonance imaging (MRI) is often more successful than postnatal attempted ultrasonography, which is complicated by direct motion artifact of the heart and interference by air. Cardiac catheterization with angiography may be required in infants not diagnosed by antenatal studies. If the cardiac malformation is correctable, the infant should be taken from the cath lab directly to the operating room for cardiac repair. Some form of cardiac enclosure must then be provided. Use of prosthetic materials is associated with a high incidence of sepsis and death, especially when prosthetic materials have been used inside the cardiac repair.

Thoracoabdominal ectopia cordis (Cantrell pentalogy)

In 1958, Cantrell and coworkers[19] reported a series of a previously described congenital syndrome characterized by the following: (1) a midline, supraumbilical abdominal defect; (2) a defect of the lower sternum; (3) a deficiency of the anterior diaphragm; (4) a defect in the diaphragmatic pericardium; and (5) congenital intracardiac defects (Figure 36.2). A complete summary of all reported cardiac anomalies has been presented.[5] All five anomalies may not be present, and there can be an incomplete expression of the syndrome.[4,20] This condition was precisely described by Wilson in 1798, with the first repair attempted by Arndt in 1896 and the first successful repair by Weiting in 1912.[21–23] The anomaly was reviewed by Major in 1953 and later by Cantrell et al. in 1958, for whom the anomaly has ironically been named.[19,24] The pathogenesis of the defects is unclear, but the occurrence of this syndrome is likely sporadic. X-chromosome recessive inheritance has been postulated. There have been associated cases with trisomy 13, 18, and 21, as well as posterior fossa anomalies, hemangioma, arterial lesions, cardiac abnormalities/coarctation of the aorta, and eye anomalies (PHACES) syndrome.[25] Multiple etiologies, including viral infection, maternal abuse of beta-aminopropionitrile, and chlorine inhalation, have also been implicated.[26,27] The occurrence rate is less than 1 out of 100,000 live births, and the condition more frequently affects males (2:1), while affected females have more severe symptoms. Due to the variable nature of expression, Toyama[4] suggested further subclassification of this syndrome: Class 1, definite diagnosis with all five defects present; Class 2, probable diagnosis with four defects noted (including intracardiac and ventral abdominal wall abnormalities); and Class 3, incomplete expression. Early prenatal diagnosis in the first trimester, with 2-D and 3-D sonography, is helpful for parental counseling.[28–30]

The successful management of thoracoabdominal ectopia cordis necessitates a multispecialty approach from the establishment of the antenatal diagnosis to the completed staged repairs. Immediate neonatal intervention is required in patients with a large upper omphalocele and lower sternal cleft (Figure 36.3).[31] In a staged repair, primary closure, split-thickness skin graft, cadaveric skin graft, or prosthetic material sutured to the skin edges must be achieved to prevent fluid

Table 36.1 Successful repairs of ectopia cordis

Author	Year	Cardiac lesion	Method of sternal closure
Koop	1975	None	Skin flap closure at 5 hours. Acrylic resin applied to sternal cleft at 7 months (Saxena[14]).
Dobell et al.[17]	1982	None	Perinatal skin closure in one stage. Second-stage repair with autologous rib grafts.
Amato et al.[18]	1988	None	Skin flaps mobilized; diaphragm moved inferiorly. Gortex membrane used to close defect with skin flaps over it. Child survived but died of aspiration at 11 months of age.
Lillehei	1996	Tetralogy of Fallot	Perinatal skin flap closure (Hornberger et al.[16]). Blalock–Taussig shunt at 4 days of life and complete repair at 2 years of age. No prosthetic tissue coverage.

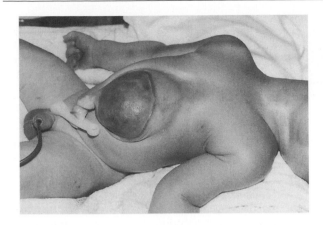

Figure 36.2 Newborn male with Cantrell pentalogy. Flaring of the lower thoracic cavity is present with a large epigastric omphalocele. The septum transversum and the inferior portion of the pericardium were absent. (From Welch K., Chest Wall Deformities, *Pediatr Surg* 1980, Eds. Holder TM and Ashcraft, KW:162–82. By permission of W.B. Saunders Co., Philadelphia.)

losses, cardiac dessication, or trauma to the heart. Subsequent intervention may be needed to gradually reduce the heart to a more anatomic position. Multiple procedures have been suggested to try to accommodate the heart; these include partial or total excision of the thymus, repair of the diaphragmatic defect, plication of a hemidiaphragm, or division of the costal cartilages. Some have even advocated that a left lower lobectomy be performed in order to better accommodate the heart in the left pleural space. In all procedures, care must be taken to prevent kinking of the great vessels and to avoid phrenic nerve damage. Other options include the use of alloplastic materials, such as creation of methyl methacrylate struts shaped as ribs and spaced to allow for future growth of ribs and thorax.

BIFID STERNUM

Sternal clefts are malformations caused by the failure of fusion of the sternal elements. The etiology of sternal cleft deformity is unknown. There are studies on ventral body

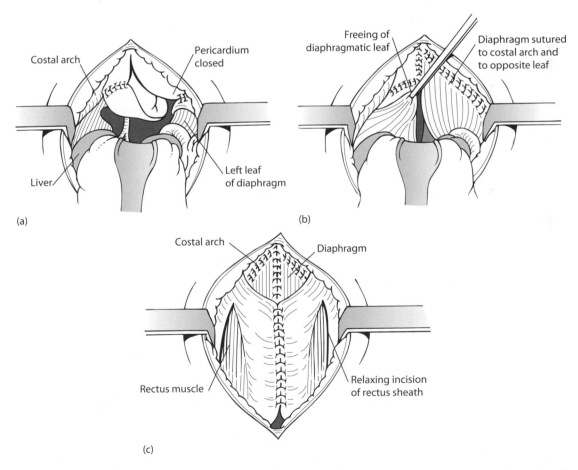

Figure 36.3 Repair of pentalogy of Cantrell is depicted. **(a)** The pericardium is closed after appropriate lateral and inferior dissection to the vena cava. The right and left dorsal leaves of the diaphragm, which are widely separated, are identified. The liver is retracted inferiorly after division of the falciform ligament. **(b)** Pedicles of the diaphragm are developed from each side and transposed medially. They are sutured together and to each costal arch. **(c)** After diaphragmatic closure, the falciform ligament is reconstructed. Closure continues by advancement of the anterior sheath of the rectus muscle to the midline. Lateral relaxing incisions are often required. Parietal repair can be accomplished at the time of cardiac correction. Prosthetic material may be required to obtain closure of the abdominal component of the repair. (From Welch K., Chest Wall Deformities, *Pediatr Surg* 1980, Eds. Holder TM and Ashcraft, KW:162–82. By permission of W.B. Saunders Co., Philadelphia.)

development in mice that indicate that impairment in Hoxb gene expression may be a possible factor.[32] Cleft sternum may be complete or incomplete and results from failure of the mesenchymal plate fusion process at the eighth week of gestation. No familial predisposition has been described. Alcohol intake and methylcobalamine deficiency have been implicated. There is a slight female predominance. Sternal clefts can be associated with cervicofacial hemangiomas (vascular dysplasia) and PHACES syndrome.[33,34]

In all cases, there is a sternal separation and skin coverage of the midline defect, intact pleural envelopes, and a normal diaphragm. Omphalocele does not occur in association with this anomaly, and the condition causes little difficulty other than a dramatic increase in the deformity with crying or Valsalva maneuver (Figure 36.4). The sternal defect involved an upper cleft in 46 patients, an upper cleft to the xiphoid in 33 patients, and a complete cleft in 23 patients.[5] The cleft involved the lower sternum in only five reported cases. A total of 69 repairs have been reported, 25 with primary closure. None of the infants and children had intrinsic congenital heart disease.

Most authors now recommend surgical treatment in the newborn period after all other anomalies are ruled out and addressed (Figure 36.5).[35,36] Recent studies have shown no difference in surgical outcome between primary closure and

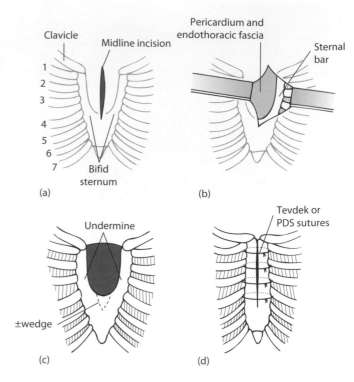

Figure 36.5 **(a)** Repair of bifid sternum is best performed through a longitudinal incision extending the length of the defect. **(b)** Directly beneath the subcutaneous tissues, the sternal bars are encountered with pectoral muscles present lateral to the bars. The endothoracic fascia and pericardium are just below these structures. **(c)** The endothoracic fascia is mobilized off the sternal bars posteriorly with blunt dissection to allow safe placement of the sutures. Approximation of the sternal bars may be facilitated by excising a wedge of cartilage inferiorly. Repair is best accomplished in the neonatal period because of the flexibility of the chest wall. **(d)** Closure of the defect is achieved with 2-0 Tevdek or PDS sutures. (With kind permission from Springer Science+Business Media: *Pediatr Surg Int*, Sternal Defects, 5, 1992, 156–64, Shamberger R. and Welch K.)

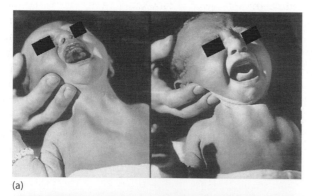

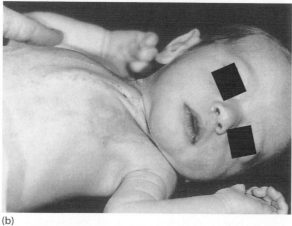

Figure 36.4 Newborn infant with a bifid sternum. **(a)** Vigorous crying produces retraction at the defect with inspiration (left) and protrusion with exhalation or Valsalva maneuver (right). **(b)** Following repair, normal configuration of the sternum is present.

treatment with prostheses.[37] No reports of recurrence or delayed healing have been encountered. In older children, reconstruction of the anterior chest wall using multiple oblique sliding chondrotomies leaving the perichondrium intact was reported by Sabiston[38] and subsequently by others.[39] This technique is useful in older infants and children with a less flexible chest wall and a wide defect. Closure employing composite cartilage grafts from the costal arch or reversed sternal plates[40] or prosthetic materials such as Marlex, Teflon, or Surgisis[41] mesh have also been reported, but these methods can be avoided with repair of the infants in a timely fashion.

Shamberger and Welch[5] reviewed their experience with sternal defects at Boston Children's Hospital, Massachusetts, USA. A total of 16 patients with sternal defects were identified, 5 with ectopia cordis, 8 with thoracoabdominal ectopia cordis, and 3 with cleft sternum. Thoracic ectopia cordis was uniformly fatal in their series; thoracoabdominal ectopia cordis was fatal in five of eight cases, and bifid sternum was successfully repaired in all three cases in infancy.

PECTUS EXCAVATUM

Pectus excavatum (funnel chest or *trichterbrust* [German]) is a depression of the sternum and lower costal cartilages. It is generally identified within the first year of life (in 86% of patients), and in many infants, it is noted at birth.[42] The extent of sternal and cartilaginous deformity is quite variable, but generally consists of posterior displacement of the sternum below the insertion of the second costal cartilage. The first and second costal cartilages are generally normal in contour, whereas the third to seventh are curved posteriorly to join the sternum. The ossified portion of the rib is normal in configuration in infancy. In infants, the extreme flexibility of the costal cartilages results in remarkable changes in the deformity with vigorous respiration or crying. Self-limited deformities are either gone or vastly improved by 3 years of age. Repairs should be avoided in all infants younger than 2 years of age. We generally delay open repair until children have achieved much of their chest wall growth to avoid the reported occurrence of acquired thoracic dystrophy in younger children following repair.

Pectus excavatum may occur as frequently as 1 in 300–400 live births.[43] The etiology of pectus excavatum is unknown. A family history of some type of anterior thoracic deformity is present in 37% of patients.[42] Scoliosis is identified in up to 15% of patients with pectus excavatum, usually in children with an asymmetric thoracic deformity, but it is generally not seen in infancy. Patients with Marfan syndrome have a high incidence of associated chest wall deformities, often in the most severe form and usually accompanied by scoliosis.

PECTUS CARINATUM

Pectus carinatum, the anterior protrusion deformity of the chest, is much less frequent than pectus excavatum, comprising 16% of our combined series.[44] A spectrum of protrusion deformities exist, and these are often divided into four types. The most frequent type consists of anterior displacement of the sternum with symmetric concavity of the costal cartilages laterally. Asymmetric deformities with anterior displacement of the costal cartilages on one side and a normally positioned or oblique sternum and normal cartilages on the contralateral side are less common. "Mixed" lesions have a carinate deformity on one side and a depression or excavatum deformity on the contralateral side, often with sternal obliquity. Most unusual are the upper "pouter pigeon" or chondromanubrial deformities, with protrusion of the manubrium and second and third costal cartilages and relative depression of the body of the sternum.

The etiology of pectus carinatum is unknown. There is overgrowth of the costal cartilages, with forward buckling and anterior displacement of the sternum. As with pectus excavatum, there is a clear-cut increased family incidence, suggesting a genetic basis. In a recent review, 26% of patients had a family history of chest wall deformity, and 12% had a family history of scoliosis.[44] Pectus carinatum is much more common in boys than girls, with a ratio of 4:1. Only the upper pouter pigeon deformity is associated with congenital heart disease, in 18% of cases.[45]

In contrast to pectus excavatum, patients with pectus carinatum have a much later appearance of the deformity. In a recent review, only one-sixth of the patients were noted to have a carinate deformity within the first year of life, and in almost half, it was noted after the onset of the pubertal growth spurt at 11 years of age.[44] The deformity, which may be mild at birth, often worsens rapidly during puberty. Because of mild deformity at birth and flexible costal cartilages, this deformity is rarely repaired during the first 2 years of life and is probably best repaired in the early teenage years. Bracing is effective in correcting the protrusion in the majority of patients, avoiding the need for surgical intervention.

POLAND SYNDROME

Poland, in 1841, described congenital absence of the pectoralis major and minor muscles, associated with syndactyly.[46] This is a diverse syndrome, often involving chest wall and breast deformity as well as serious ipsilateral hand and arm anomalies. A Poland–Möbius variant has been described, with dextrocardia and facial weakness.[47] The extent of thoracic involvement may range from hypoplasia of the sternal head of the pectoralis major and minor muscles with normal underlying ribs, to complete absence of the anterior portions of the second to fourth ribs and cartilages, often called the second to fourth rib syndrome. Breast involvement is significant in females, ranging from mild degrees of breast hypoplasia to complete absence of the breast (amastia) and nipple (athelia). Hand deformities are frequent and occurred in the patient described by Poland. They may include hypoplasia (brachydactyly), fused fingers (syndactyly), and mitten or claw deformity (ectromelia).

This condition is present at birth and has an estimated incidence of 1 in 30,000 to 1 in 32,000.[48] The etiology of this deformity is unknown, but it affects the developing somatic tissue for the entire limb bud and chest wall. Abnormalities in the breast can be recognized at birth by the absence of the underlying breast bud and hypoplastic, often superiorly displaced nipple. Males predominate by at least 3:1 and show a right-sided predilection. Females show less sidedness. Familial cases, in either gender, occur equally on the left and the right. In our series, chest wall reconstruction was required in 10 out of 41 cases, but never in infancy.[49]

THORACIC DEFORMITIES IN SKELETAL DISORDERS

Congenital asphyxiating thoracic dystrophy (Jeune disease)

Jeune, in 1954, first described a pair of siblings with a narrow rigid chest and multiple cartilage anomalies.[50] The syndrome is also known as asphyxiating thoracic dysplasia (ATD) and thoracic–pelvic–phalangeal dystrophy.[51] This is a rare autosomal recessive disorder.[52,53] Other manifestations include dwarfism with short ribs and short limbs—with radiographic changes in the ribs and pelvis. There is some association with abnormalities of the kidneys, liver, pancreas, and retina.[54] Variable skeletal and radiographic severity occurs in this syndrome. Its most prominent feature is a narrow "bell-shaped" thorax and protuberant abdomen. The thorax is narrow in both the transverse and sagittal axes and has little respiratory motion due to the horizontal direction of the ribs (Figure 36.6). The ribs are short and wide, and the splayed costochondral junctions barely reach the anterior axillary line. The costal cartilage is abundant and irregular like a rachitic rosary. Microscopic examination of the costochondral junction reveals disordered and poorly progressing endochondral ossification, resulting in decreased rib length.

The syndrome has variable expression and extent of pulmonary involvement, resulting in a wide range of survival.[55] Lung hypoplasia is due to a restricted thoracic cage and may be the cause of death in infancy. The most common presentation is hypoventilation, caused by impaired chest expansion. Frequency of the condition is approximately 1 per 100,000–130,000 live births.[56] Reports have described the ability to diagnose fetuses suspected to have Jeune syndrome with prenatal ultrasonography.[57,58] The pathological findings in autopsy cases are variable and show a range of pulmonary development; in most cases, the bronchial development is normal, and there is a variable decrease in alveolar divisions.[59]

There have been many surgical attempts to treat this disorder. The main goal of surgery is to expand thoracic volume and allow improved lung expansion. Early surgical interventions were reported by Barnes and colleagues, Karjoo and coworkers, and Mustard.[43,60,61] Early repairs reported attempts at thoracic enlargement by splitting the sternum, which was then held apart by a variety of graft materials. Authors used either autologous tissue, such as rib grafts or iliac crest bone, or synthetic materials including methyl methacrylate,[62] and stainless steel wires. There are multiple reports of initial improvement in lung ventilation, but subsequent growth failure of the chest resulted in recurrent respiratory distress.[62,63] Davis and coworkers,[64] in 1995, described a new lateral thoracic expansion (LTE) technique for ATD. New bone formation is documented 3 weeks after the procedure. LTE has been successfully performed on a preterm infant in the neonatal period.[65] Long-term follow-up for this procedure has not been reported, however.

Campbell and coworkers[66] have described a vertical expandable prosthetic titanium rib (VEPTR) procedure for use in a variety of pediatric conditions of "thoracic insufficiency syndrome." Vertically oriented titanium struts are attached to ribs and/or transverse processes of the spine and progressively lengthened with a series of surgical procedures to allow progressive expansion of the chest cavity. Computed tomography (CT) imaging studies have documented postoperative increase in chest volume; however, improvements in pulmonary function tests have not been demonstrated. Few patients with Jeune syndrome[67] have had VEPTR procedures. In one series, 9% of those treated

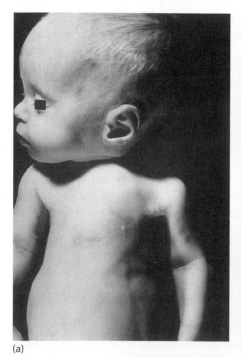
(a)

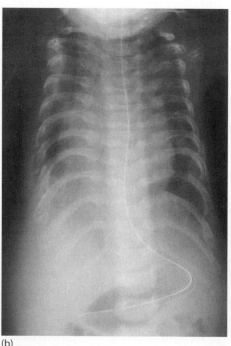
(b)

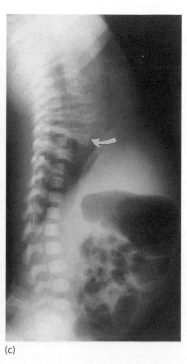
(c)

Figure 36.6 Infant with asphyxiating thoracic dystrophy (Jeune syndrome). **(a)** Clinical photograph demonstrates small size of thorax relative to infant. **(b)** Radiograph shows the short horizontal ribs and narrow thorax with limited lung volumes. **(c)** Lateral radiograph demonstrates the endings of the bony ribs at the midaxillary line and the abnormal costochondral junctions (arrow).

with VEPTR had Jeune syndrome, and all died within 2 years of the procedure—two from respiratory complications, one from renal failure, and one from liver failure.[68] The ultimate results of all surgical attempts will depend on the degree of underlying pulmonary parenchymal impairment of the infants. Respiratory failure is the most common cause of death for infants under 2 years of age and renal failure for deaths between the ages of 3 and 10 years of age.[69]

Spondylothoracic dysplasia (Jarcho–Levin syndrome)

Spondylothoracic dysplasia is an autosomal recessive deformity characterized by short-trunk dwarfism associated with multiple vertebral and rib malformations.[70] The ribs have a crab-like appearance (Figure 36.7). Death occurs early in infancy from respiratory failure and pneumonia. Patients have multiple alternating hemivertebrae, which affect most of the thoracic and lumbar spine. The ossification centers rarely cross the midline. Multiple posterior fusions of the ribs as well as remarkable shortening of the thoracic spine result in a crab-like radiographic appearance of the chest. One-third of the patients with this syndrome have associated malformations including congenital heart disease and renal anomalies. Its occurrence has been reported primarily in Puerto Rican families (15 out of 18 cases).[71] Bone formation is normal in these patients. Successful prenatal diagnosis can be established by sonographic examination.[72] Thoracic deformity is secondary to the spinal anomaly, which results in close posterior approximation of the origin of the ribs. The VEPTR procedure has been successfully performed in the neonatal period for this highly lethal syndrome.[73] Spondylothoracic dysplasia has a mortality rate approaching 50% from respiratory complications due to thoracic insufficiency syndrome. Most infants with this syndrome succumb before 15 months of age.[74] In spite of severe restrictive respiratory disease, adult survivors of spondylothoracic dysplasia appear to do well clinically for unknown reasons.[75]

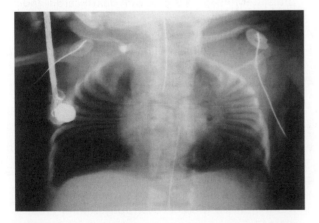

Figure 36.7 Radiograph of infant with spondylothoracic dysplasia (Jarcho–Levin syndrome). Severe abnormality of the spine is apparent with multiple hemivertebrae and the crab-like ribs with close approximation posteriorly and splaying out anteriorly.

REFERENCES

1. Stensen N. In: Bartholin T (ed). *Acta Medica et philosophica Hafniencia.* 1: 202–3, 1671–2. Reprinted in Stenonsis, Nicolai: *Opera Philosphica* 2: 49–53, edited by Vilhelm Maar, Copenhagen, 1910
2. Weese C. Des cordis ectopia. Inaugural dissertation. Starck, Berlin, 1818.
3. Todd R. Abnormal conditions of the heart. *Cyclopaed Anat Physiol* 1836; 2: 630–47.
4. Toyama W. Combined congenital defects of the anterior abdominal wall, sternum, diaphragm, pericardium and heart: A case report and review of the syndrome. *Pediatrics* 1972; 50: 778–86.
5. Shamberger R, Welch K. Sternal defects. *Pediatr Surg Int* 1992; 5: 156–64.
6. Tongson T, Wanapirak C, Sirivatanapa P et al. Prenatal sonographic diagnosis of ectopia cordis. *J Clin Ultrasound* 1999; 27: 440–5.
7. Harrison M, Filly R, Stanger P et al. Prenatal diagnosis and management of omphalocele and ectopia cordis. *J Pediatr* 1982; 17: 64–6.
8. Soper S, Roe L, Hoyme H et al. Trisomy 18 with ectopia cordis, omphalocele and ventricular septal defect: Case report. *Pediatr Pathol* 1986; 5: 481–3.
9. Bick D, Markowitz R, Horwich A. Trisomy 18 associated with ectopia cordis and occipital meningocele. *Am J Med Gent* 1988; 80: 805.
10. Fox J, Gloster E, Mirchandani R. Trisomy 18 with Cantrell pentalogy on a stillborn infant. *Am J Med Gent* 1988; 31: 391–4.
11. Ley E, Roth J, Kim K et al. Successful repair of ectopia cordis using alloplastic materials: 10 year follow-up. *Plast Reconstr Surg* 2004; 114: 1519–22.
12. Samir K, Ghez O, Metras D et al. Ectopia cordis, a successful single stage repair thoracoabdominal repair. *Interact Cardiovasc Thorac Surg* 2003; 2(4): 611–3.
13. Humpl T, Huggan P, Hornberger L et al. Presentation and outcomes of ectopia cordis. *Can J Cardiol* 1999; 15: 1353–7.
14. Saxena N. Ectopia cordis child surviving; prosthesis fails. *Pediatr News* 1976; 10: 3.
15. Van Praagh R, Weinberg P, Smith S et al. Malpositions of the heart. In: Adams FH Emmanouilides GC, Riememschneider TA (eds). *Moss's Heart Disease in Infants, Children, and Adolescents,* 4th edn. Baltimore: Williams and Wilkins, 1989: 530–80.
16. Hornberger L, Colan S, Lock J et al. Outcome of patients with ectopia cordis and significant intracardiac defects. *Circulation* 1996; 94: 1132–7.
17. Dobell A, Williams H, Long R. Staged repair of ectopia cordis. *J Pediatr Surg* 1982; 17: 353–8.

18. Amato J, Cotroneo J, Gladiere R. Repair of complete extopia corids (film). Presented at American College of Surgeons, Clinical Congress. Chicago, October 23–28, 1988.

19. Cantrell J, Haller J, Ravitch M. A syndrome of congenital defects involving the abdominal wall, sternum, diaphragm, pericardium, and heart. *Surg Gynecol Obstet* 1958; 107: 602–14.

20. Kaul B, Sheikh F, Zamora I et al. 5, 4, 3, 2, 1: Embryologic variants of pentalogy of Cantrell. *J Surg Res* 2015; 199: 141–8.

21. Wilson J. A description of a very unusual formation of the human heart. *Phil Trans Roy Soc Lond* 1798; Part II: 346–56.

22. Arndt C. Nabelschnurbruch mit Herzhernie: Operation durch Laparotomie mit Todlichem Ausgang. *Centralbl Gynakol* 1896 (20): 632–3.

23. Weiting K. Eine operative behandelte Hermissbildung. *Dtsch Z Chir* 1912; 114: 293–5.

24. Major J. Thoracoabdominal ectopia cordis. *J Thorac Surg* 1953; 26: 309–17.

25. Lopez-Gutierrez J. PHACES syndrome and ectopia cordis. *Interact Cardiovasc Thorac Surg* 2011; 12: 642–4.

26. Barrow M, Willis L. Ectopia cordis (ectocardia) and gastroschisis induced in rates by maternal administration of lathyrogen, betaaminopropionitrile (BAPN). *Am Heart J* 1972; 83: 518–26.

27. Sosa M. Pentologia de Cantrell con malformaciones multiples y asociada a inhalacion de cloro. *Ultrason Med* 1994; 10: 27–33.

28. Bognoni V, Quartuccio A, Quartuccio A. First-trimester sonographic diagnosis of Cantrell's pentalogy with exencephaly. *J Clin Ultrasound* 1999; 27: 276–8.

29. Ergenoglu M, Yeniel A, Peker N et al. Prenatal diagnosis of Cantrell pentology in first trimester screening: Case report and review of literature. *J Turk Ger Gynecologic Assoc* 2012; 13: 145–8.

30. Peer D, Moroder W, Delluca A. Prenatal diagnosis of pentalogy of Cantrell combined with exencephaly and amniotic band syndrome. *Ultraschall Med* 1993; 1494: 94–5.

31. Welch K. Chest wall deformities. In: Holder TM, Ashcraft, KW (eds). *Pediatric Surgery*. Philadelphia, WB Saunders, 1980: 162–82.

32. Forzano F, Daubeney P, White S. Midline raphe, sternal cleft and other midline abnormalities: A new dominant syndrome? *Am J Med Gent* 2005; 135A: 9–12.

33. Frieden I, Reese V, Cohen D. PHACE syndrome. The association of posterior fossa brain malformations, hemangiomas, arterial anomalies, coarctation of the aorta and cardiac defects and eye abnormalities. *Arch Dermatol* 1996; 132: 307–11.

34. James P, McGaughran J. Complete overlap of PHACE syndrome and sternal malformation–vascular dysplasia association. *Am J Med Gent* 2002; 110: 78–84.

35. Daum R, Zachariou Z. Total and superior sternal clefts in newborns: A simple technique for surgical correction. *J Pediatr* 1999; 34: 408–11.

36. Domini M, Cupaioli M, Rossi F et al. Bifid sternum: Neonatal surgical treatment. *Ann Thorac Surg* 2000; 69: 267–9.

37. Torre M, Rapuzzi G, Carlucci M. Phenotypic spectrum and management of sternal cleft: Literature review and presentation of a new series. *Eur J Cardiothorac Surg* 2012; 41: 4–9.

38. Sabiston D. The surgical management of congenital bifid sternum with partial ectopia cordis. *J Thorac Surg* 1958; 35: 118–22.

39. Muthialu N. Primary repair of sternal cleft in infancy using combined periosteal flap and sliding osteochondroplasty. *Interact Cardiovasc Thorac Surg* 2013; 16(6): 923–5.

40. Elsayed H, Soliman S. Reversed autogenous sternal plate flaps for treatment of sternal clefts: A novel technique. *J Pediatr Surg* 2015; 50: 1991–4.

41. Oliveira C, Zamakhshary M, Alfadda T et al. An innovative method of pediatric chest wall reconstruction using Surgisis and swinging rib technique. *J Ped Surg* 2012; 47: 867–73.

42. Shamberger R, Welch K. Surgical correction of pectus excavatum. *J Pediatr Surg* 1988; 23: 615–22.

43. Ravitch M (ed). Pectus excavatum. In Ravitch MM (ed). *Congenital Deformities of the Chest Wall and Their Operative Correction*. Philadelphia, WB Saunders, 1977: 78–205.

44. Shamberger R, Welch K, Sanders S. Mitral valve prolapse associated with pectus excavatum. *J Pediatr* 1987; 111(3): 404–7.

45. Lees R, Caldicott W. Sternal anomalies and congenital heart disease. *Am J Roentgenol* 1975; 124:423–7.

46. Poland A. Deficiency of the pectoral muscles. *Guy's Hosp Rep* 1841; 6 :191–3.

47. Flores A, Ross J, Tullius T, Jr. A unique variant of Poland–Mobius syndrome with dextrocardia and a 3q23 gain. *J Perinat* 2013; 33: 572–3.

48. McGillivray B, Lowry R. Poland syndrome in British Columbia: Incidence and reproductive experience of affected persons. *Am J Med Gent* 1977; 1: 65–74.

49. Shamberger R, Welch K, Upton J, III. Surgical treatment of thoracic deformity in Poland's syndrome. *J Pediatr Surg* 1989; 24: 760–6.

50. Jeune M, Beraud C, Carron R. Asphyxiating thoracic dystrophy with familial characteristics. *Arch Fr Pediatr* 1955; 12(8): 886–91.

51. Langer L. Thoracic–pelvis–phalangeal dystrophy: asphyxiating thoracic dystrohy of the newborn infantile thoracic dystrophy. *Radiol* 1968; 91:447–56.

52. Tahernia A, Stamps P. 'Jeune syndrome' (asphyxiating thoracic dystrophy): Report of a case, a review of the literature, and an editor's commentary. *Clin Pediatr* 1977; 16: 903–8.

53. Morgan N, Bacchelli C, Gissen P et al. A locus for asphyxiating thoracic dystrophy, ATD, maps to chromosome 15q13. *J Med Genet* 2003; 40(6): 431–5.
54. Oberklaid F, Danks D, Mayne V et al. Asphyxiating thoracic dysplasia: Clinical, radiological, and pathological information on 10 patients. *Arch Dis Child* 1977; 52: 758–65.
55. Kozlowski K, Masel J. As[hyxiating thoracic dystrophy without respiratory disease: Report of two cases of the latent form. *Pediatr Radiol* 1976; 5: 30–3.
56. Phillips J, van Aalst J. Jeune's syndrome (asphyxiating thoracic dystrophy): Congenital and acquired. *Semin Pediatr Surg* 2008; 17: 167–72.
57. Den Hollander N, Robben S, Hoogeboom A et al. Early prenatal sonographic diagnosis and follow-up of Jeune syndrome. *Ultrasound Obstet Gynecol* 2001; 18(4): 378–83.
58. Chen C, Lin S, Liu F et al. Prenatal diagnosis of asphyxiating thoracic dysplasia (Jeune syndrome). *Am J Perinatol* 1996; 13(8): 495–8.
59. Williams A, Vawter G, Reid L. Lung structure in asphyxiating thoracic dystrophy. *Arch Pathol Lab Med* 1984; 108: 658–61.
60. Barnes N, Hull D, Milner A et al. Chest reconstruction in thoracic dystrophy. *Arch Dis Child* 1971; 46: 833–7.
61. Karjoo M, Koop C, Cornfield D et al. Pancreatic exocrine deficiency associated with asphyxiating thoracic dystrophy. *Arch Dis Child* 1973; 48: 143–6.
62. Todd D, Tinguely S, Norberg W. A thoracic expansion technique for Jeune's asphyxiating thoracic dystrophy. *J Pediatr Surg* 1986; 21: 161–3.
63. Aronson D, VanNierop J, Taminiau A et al. Homologous bone graft for expansion thoracoplasty in Jeune's asphyxiating thoracic dystrophy. *J Pediatr Surg* 1999; 34: 500–3.
64. Davis J, Long F, Adler B et al. Lateral thoracic expansion for Jeune syndrome: Evidence of rib healing and new bone formation. *Ann Thorac Surg* 2004; 77(2): 445–8.
65. Andrade C, Cardoso P, Felicetti JC. Lateral thoracic expansion in a preterm baby with asphyxiating thoracic dystrophy. *Thorac Cardiovasc Surg* 2011; 59(1): 56–8.
66. Campbell R, Jr., Smith M, Mayes T et al. The effect of opening wedge thoracostomy on thoracic insufficiency syndrome associated with fused ribs and congenital scoliosis. *J Bone Joint Surg* 2004; 86A(8): 1659–74.
67. Waldhausen J, Redding G, Song K. Vertical expandable prosthetic titanium rib for thoracic insufficiency syndrome: A new method to treat an old problem. *J Pediatr Surg* 2007; 42(1): 76–80.
68. Betz R, Mulcahey M, Ramirez N et al. Mortality and life-threatening events after vertical expandable prosthetic titanium rib surgery in children with hypoplastic chest wall deformity. *J Ped Orthoped* 2008; 28(8): 850–3.
69. Keppler-Noreuil K, Adam M, Welch J et al. Clinical insights gained from eight new cases and review of reported cases with Jeune syndrome (asphyxiating thoracic dystrophy). *Am J Med Gent A* 2011; 155: 1021–32.
70. Jarcho S, Levin P. Hereditary malformation of the vertebral bodies. *Bull Johns Hopkins Hosp* 1938; 62: 216–26.
71. Heilbronner D, Renshaw T. Spondylothoracic dysplasia. *J Bone Joint Surg* 1984; 66A: 302–3.
72. Basaran A, Deren O, Onderoglu L. Prenatal diagnosis of Jarcho–Levin syndrome in combination with inguinoscrotal hernia. *Am J Perinatol* 2010; 27(3): 189–92.
73. Odehouri-Koudou T, Yaokreh R, Tembely S et al. Sporadic occurrence of Jarcho–Levin syndrome in an Ivorian newborn. *Case Rep Orthop* 2013; Article 129625.
74. Roberts A, Conner A, Tolmie J et al. Spondylothoracic and spondylocostal dysostosis: Hereditary forms of spinal deformity. *J Bone Joint Surg* 1988; 70B: 123–6.
75. Campbell R, Jr. Spine deformities in rare congenital syndromes: Clinical issues. *Spine* 2009; 34(17): 1815–27.

37

Mediastinal masses in the newborn

ISRAEL FERNANDEZ-PINEDA AND STEPHEN J. SHOCHAT

Mediastinal masses in the newborn represent a wide variety of congenital and neoplastic lesions, which can present interesting diagnostic and therapeutic challenges. However, despite the heterogeneous makeup of this group of lesions, an accurate preoperative diagnosis can usually be established on the basis of the location of the mass. Although many of these mediastinal masses may grow in utero and appear quite prominent on prenatal ultrasound, watchful waiting is recommended unless the fetus is severely compromised. Indications for prenatal intervention may include compression from the mass on the esophagus that may lead to polyhydramnios; compression on the mediastinal lymphatics, veins, and heart that may lead to hydrops and heart failure; and compression on the lungs that may lead to pulmonary hypoplasia and respiratory failure after birth.

DIFFERENTIAL DIAGNOSIS

The differential diagnosis of mediastinal masses in newborns and infants is simplified if the mediastinum is arbitrarily separated into three compartments (Figure 37.1). For the purpose of this discussion, the mediastinum will be partitioned as follows: the anterior mediastinum lies anterior to the heart and lung roots and contains the thymus, anterior mediastinal lymph nodes, and rarely, a substernal extension of the thyroid and parathyroid. The middle mediastinum contains the trachea, bronchi, mediastinal lymph nodes, heart, and great vessels. The posterior mediastinum lies behind the heart and lung roots and contains the esophagus and intercostal sympathetic nerves. Anterior mediastinal masses include prominent thymus, ectopic thymus, thymic cysts/hyperplasia/tumors, teratomas, lymphatic malformations (LMs), lipomas, and lymphomas. Masses within the middle mediastinum include congenital vascular lesions such as double aortic arch, bronchogenic cysts, esophageal duplication cysts, neuroenteric cysts, lymphomas, and granulomatous infections within the mediastinal lymph nodes. Posterior mediastinal lesions include the tumors of neurogenic origin, undifferentiated sarcomas, congenital foregut duplications, and extralobar sequestrations.

The age of the patient at the time of diagnosis is extremely important, since certain masses have a predilection for younger infants and others are predominantly seen in older children and adolescents. In newborns and children under 2 years of age, the most common mediastinal mass is the neuroblastoma within the posterior mediastinum. In addition, thymic hyperplasia and bronchogenic cysts are seen predominantly in children less than 2 years of age. The various lymphomas are the most common mediastinal masses seen in children older than 2 years.

The presenting signs and symptoms in newborns and infants with mediastinal masses are variable:

- Acute respiratory distress
- Fever
- Cough
- Shortness of breath
- Stridor
- Cervical adenopathy
- Superior vena cava syndrome
- Horner syndrome
- Asymptomatic

Infants under 2 years of age frequently present with signs of tracheal compression (Figure 37.2) and acute respiratory distress. This is due to the smaller, softer, more pliable tracheobronchial tree in infants as well as the fact that they do not have a fixed mediastinum, so that large mediastinal masses can cause a significant shift of the mediastinum with compromise of the contralateral hemithorax. Older children will present with symptoms of fever, cough, and shortness of breath. Superior vena cava obstruction is rare in children but is occasionally seen. Horner syndrome may be the presenting finding in infants with neurogenic tumors of the posterior mediastinum. Asymptomatic mediastinal masses are seen in children of all ages and are frequently noted on a chest x-ray performed for a mild upper respiratory infection or are discovered incidentally following imaging studies for symptoms unrelated to the mediastinal mass.

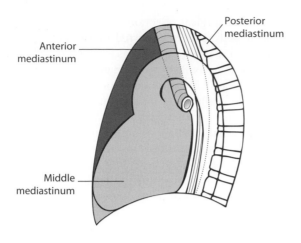

Figure 37.1 Compartments of mediastinum.

DIAGNOSIS

A systematic approach to the diagnosis of a mediastinal mass in the newborn is imperative and may include the following:

- Posteroanterior–lateral chest x-ray
- Barium swallow
- Ultrasonography (US)
- Computed tomography (CT)/angio-CT scan
- Magnetic resonance imaging (MRI)/magnetic resonance angiography (MRA)
- Bone marrow–lymph node biopsy
- Skin test—complement fixation
- Serum markers—alpha-fetoprotein (AFP), human chorionic gonadotropin (HCG)
- Urinary catecholamines
- Metaiodobenzylguanidine (MIBG)

The goals of diagnostic imaging evaluating a mediastinal mass include the following: (1) identifying the characteristics and origin of the mass within the mediastinum; (2) delineating the extension; and (3) providing a differential diagnosis. The most helpful diagnostic technique in this age group is still the chest x-ray in the posteroanterior and lateral projections, in order to localize the position of the mass. Vertebral anomalies associated with a mediastinal mass in a newborn or infant should raise suspicion of the so-called neuroenteric variety of enterogenous cyst, which communicates with the meninges. Calcification within a posterior mediastinal mass suggests the presence of a neuroblastoma, and anterior mediastinal teratomas frequently contain calcification and cystic areas. In cases of suspected enterogenous and bronchogenic cysts, the esophagogram may be of value. US of the chest can be particularly helpful in newborns and infants younger than 12 months. The unossified sternal and costal cartilages provide an acoustic window large enough to allow evaluation of anterior mediastinal masses such as thymic hyperplasia. Echocardiography should be performed to delineate the heart and great vessels if lesions of these structures are suspected. A CT scan should be reserved for difficult diagnostic dilemmas and for delineating anatomical boundaries in preparation for tumor resection. CT scan offers multiplanar reformations and 3-D reconstructions. MRI and MRA may be of help in differentiating masses of vascular origin from other mediastinal structures and may be helpful in infants with suspected thymic hyperplasia. In addition, MRI should be considered in cases of posterior mediastinal masses in order to detect intraspinous extension of dumbbell tumors. Cardiac MRI, with its excellent tissue characterization and wide field of view, may provide additional unique information.

A bone marrow aspiration/biopsy and cervical lymph node biopsy should be considered in children with middle mediastinal lesions and suspected lymphoma. Skin testing and complement fixation titers should be considered in infants with middle mediastinal masses to rule out granulomatous infections. AFP determination and HCG titers

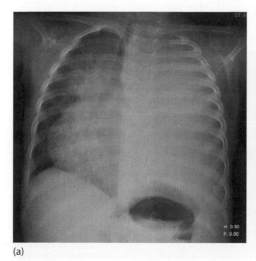

(a)

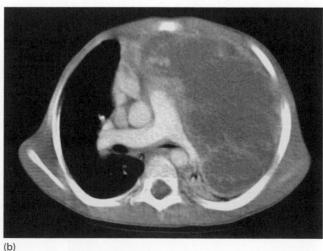

(b)

Figure 37.2 Mediastinal germ cell tumor with compression and displacement of the airway: **(a)** posteroanterior chest x-ray and **(b)** axial-view CT scan.

should be performed in children with anterior mediastinal masses if malignant germ cell tumors (GCTs) are suspected. Urinary catecholamine metabolites should be evaluated in infants with posterior mediastinal masses both for diagnosis and for postoperative follow-up in children with suspected neuroblastomas.

ANTERIOR MEDIASTINUM

The anterior mediastinum accounts for most of all mediastinal masses in newborns, with thymic hyperplasia as the most common anterior mediastinal mass (Figure 37.3). This diagnosis is usually not difficult as there is frequently a characteristic "sail" sign on routine chest x-ray. Recently, US has been very helpful in differentiating thymic hyperplasia from other mediastinal masses and should be considered in difficult cases. If definite confirmation of normal thymus cannot be made from radiographs and US imaging, a correct diagnosis can be confidently made with CT or MRI. Most GCTs in the newborn period and under 2 years of age are benign teratomas (Figure 37.4). CT or MRI typically shows well-encapsulated, complex masses with cystic and solid areas containing fat and irregular calcifications. These tumors tend to displace rather than invade adjacent

structures, and surgical resection through a posterolateral thoracotomy is usually the preferred approach. LMs (Figure 37.5) also are observed in newborns and infants but usually have a cervical or axillary component, which makes this diagnosis obvious. LMs at this location are at risk of airway obstruction in newborns. Ex utero intrapartum treatment (EXIT procedure) involves partial delivery of the fetus with the fetal–placental circulation maintained. This allows for management of the obstructed fetal airway via direct laryngoscopy, bronchoscopy, tracheostomy, or surgical intervention. The EXIT procedure should be available for newborns with prenatal diagnosis of cervicothoracic mass. Malignant GCTs of the anterior mediastinum are usually seen in older children and adolescents, and many have an endodermal sinus or yolk sac component with an elevated serum AFP. AFP and HCG levels should be obtained in children with anterior mediastinal masses as these markers are helpful not only in diagnosis but also in following response to therapy. When the tumor is nonresectable, a biopsy rather than partial resection is followed by chemotherapy and delayed primary excision.

MIDDLE MEDIASTINUM

Mediastinal foregut duplication cysts are uncommon congenital anomalies that result from developmental malformations of the embryonic foregut. They can be classified into three types: bronchogenic, esophageal duplication, and neuroenteric cysts. Bronchogenic cysts may be seen in all age groups but are the most frequent mass seen within the middle mediastinum in infants and children under 2 years of age (Figure 37.6). They are generally located in the subcarinal region and are frequently associated with a characteristic expiratory stridor due to accentuation of the obstruction of the lower trachea during expiration. Diagnosis may be difficult on routine chest x-ray, but there is usually a characteristic displacement of the esophagus on barium swallow (Figure 37.7). Bronchogenic cysts occasionally are intimately attached to the membranous

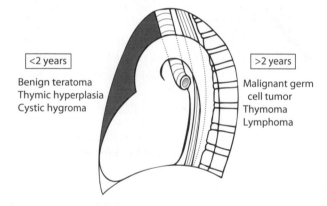

<2 years	>2 years
Benign teratoma	Malignant germ
Thymic hyperplasia	cell tumor
Cystic hygroma	Thymoma
	Lymphoma

Figure 37.3 Anterior mediastinum.

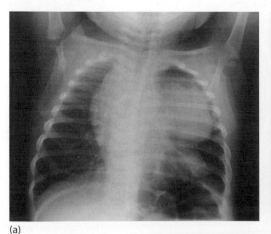
(a)

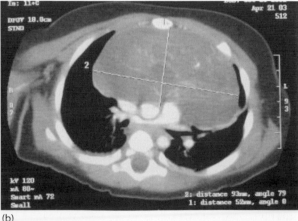
(b)

Figure 37.4 Anterior mediastinum teratoma: **(a)** posteroanterior chest x-ray and **(b)** axial-view CT scan.

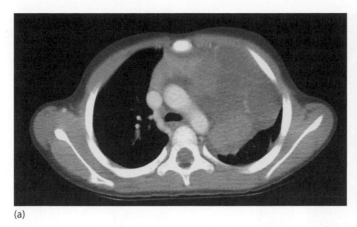
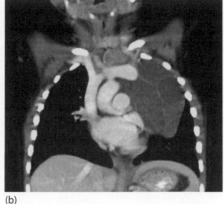

(a)

(b)

Figure 37.5 Anterior mediastinum lymphatic malformation: **(a)** axial-view CT scan and **(b)** coronal-view CT scan.

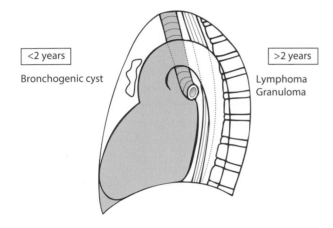

<2 years

Bronchogenic cyst

>2 years

Lymphoma
Granuloma

Figure 37.6 Middle mediastinum.

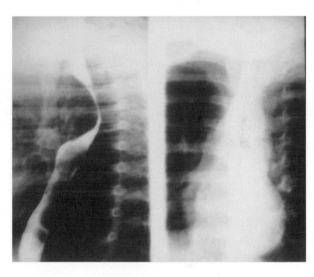

Figure 37.7 Bronchogenic cyst showing displacement of esophagus. Normal-appearing chest x-ray.

trachea, and if this is the case, a small portion of the cysts should be left attached to the trachea. Esophageal duplication cysts are typically located adjacent to the upper third of the esophageal wall, and dysphagia is the most common presenting symptom. Neuroenteric cysts, while rare, represent an interesting spectrum of lesions that may be seen in the middle and posterior mediastinum. They may be intimately associated with the esophagus and cause dysphagia, or they can contain gastric mucosa, which has been associated with peptic ulceration, perforation, and bleeding. Large cysts can have abdominal extensions and communicate with an intestinal duplication. Lymphadenopathy in the middle mediastinal compartment in children is most commonly due to either neoplastic or infectious processes. Lymphomas are the most frequent tumors involving the middle mediastinum over 2 years of age but are rarely seen in the newborn or infant. If the diagnosis of lymphoma is highly suspicious, one should be aware of the use of less invasive diagnostic tools, including examination of pleural fluid, bone marrow, or biopsy of peripheral lymphadenopathies. Granulomatous infections of the paratracheal, subcarinal, or hilar lymph nodes are occasionally seen and can usually be diagnosed by appropriate skin tests and complement fixation titers.

POSTERIOR MEDIASTINUM

The most common mass of the posterior mediastinum and in fact the most common mass in newborns is a posterior mediastinal neuroblastoma (Figure 37.8). Mediastinal neuroblastomas are interesting in that they seem to have a different biological behavior from intraabdominal tumors. The majority of mediastinal neuroblastomas are localized or low-stage disease and have a favorable outcome following resection. These tumors are more often occult and are diagnosed on x-ray examination for other complaints. Respiratory distress due to compression or deviation of trachea is a feature in some cases. Thoracic neuroblastomas with dumbbell extension may present with neurological symptoms due to spinal cord compression. While the treatment of mediastinal neuroblastomas in children is total excision if at all possible, this does not mean radical chest wall resection. In the rare case of a massive mediastinal neuroblastoma that cannot be resected without a radical operation, a biopsy to establish the diagnosis is followed by chemotherapy

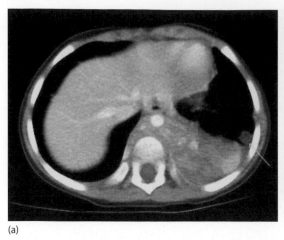
(a)

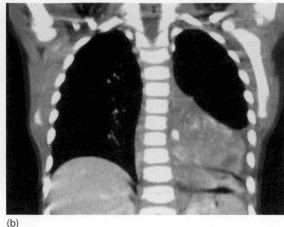
(b)

Figure 37.8 Left posterior mediastinum neuroblastoma: **(a)** axial view CT scan and **(b)** coronal-view CT scan.

and delayed primary excision. While this clinical situation is unusual, a tissue diagnosis can usually be obtained by a percutaneous core needle biopsy or a thoracoscopic approach avoiding formal thoracotomy. In children with disseminated neuroblastoma, the prognosis continues to be discouraging.

Children with posterior mediastinal neuroblastoma can also present with unusual symptoms. High thoracic and cervical tumors can be associated with Horner syndrome (unilateral ptosis, myosis, anhydrosis). Large thoracic tumors may cause vena cava syndrome. Paraspinal tumors may extend into the neural foramina of the vertebral bodies and cause neurological symptoms.

ANESTHETIC MANAGEMENT OF INFANTS WITH A MEDIASTINAL MASS

Respiratory compromise on induction of general anesthesia in children with large mediastinal masses is a well-recognized complication that must be considered in the preoperative evaluation of any child with a mediastinal mass. Newborns and small children have a small compressible airway, which is associated with significant increased airway resistance with even a modest degree of narrowing. In addition, the mediastinum is not fixed at this age, and large masses can easily displace the mediastinal structures with compression of the tracheobronchial tree, superior vena cava, or right ventricular outflow tract. Cardiac output may also be diminished due to pressure on the great vessels. Induction of anesthesia is associated with a decrease in the functional residual capacity, decrease in lung capacity, and increase in lung retractile force. These alterations are extenuated with the addition of paralysis. Narrowing of the trachea will also occur when the patient changes from spontaneous to positive-pressure ventilation. All of these factors lead to the sometimes critical condition that is associated with general anesthesia in these patients.

The most important factor in preventing anesthetic complications in children with mediastinal mass is a recognition of the aforementioned problems and the anticipation of a possible airway problem. A very thorough radiologic evaluation should be performed, and CT examination to determine the tracheal cross-sectional area maybe of help as well. Once the preoperative evaluation is completed, the anesthetic of choice can be determined depending upon the procedure that will be performed. Preoperative radiation therapy, corticosteroids, or chemotherapy may be required prior to primary excision or biopsy. Incisional biopsies can be performed under local anesthesia in older children, and needle biopsy with local anesthesia can be performed in younger children and infants. In children with benign lesions, one-lung anesthesia with placement of the endotracheal tube beyond the obstruction has been found to be helpful, and occasionally, ventilation through a rigid bronchoscope is necessary. While cardiopulmonary bypass or extracorporeal membrane oxygenation (ECMO) may be required, these techniques are usually not necessary in the majority of patients. A high index of suspicion, meticulous preoperative evaluation, and a multidisciplinary action plan decided upon by the surgeons, anesthesiologist, radiation therapist, hematology/oncologist, and pathologist can usually advert the potential catastrophe associated with general anesthesia in children with critical mediastinal masses.

OPERATIVE TECHNIQUE FOR REMOVAL OF MEDIASTINAL NEUROBLASTOMA

Resection of posterior mediastinal neuroblastoma has traditionally been approached via a posterolateral thoracotomy. However, in recent years, video-assisted thoracic surgery (VATS) (Figure 37.9) has become more popular among pediatric surgeons, resulting in shorter operative times, less postoperative pain, shorter hospital stay, and excellent cosmetic results. Outcomes for both procedures,

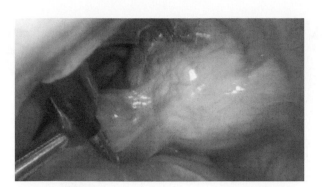

Figure 37.9 Thoracoscopic view of a posterior mediastinum neuroblastoma.

open thoracotomy and VATS, are similar. Surgical resection is facilitated by single-lung ventilation. During VATS, CO_2 insufflation may help to keep the lung out of the surgical field. The lung is retracted medially to reveal the tumor covered with pleura and arising from the sympathetic trunk; an assessment of the lymph node involvement in the tumor vicinity is performed. The pleura is incised around the tumor approximately 1 cm from it and the fascia and pleura mobilized toward the tumor. A plane of dissection can usually be developed superficial to the endothoracic fascia. The tumor is now mobilized from the ribs by sharp dissection, and intercostal vessels entering the tumor will need division. If the tumor extends far enough anteriorly, the azygos vein on the right side will need division. Care is taken to avoid damage to the first thoracic nerve passing laterally across the first rib to join the brachial plexus. The superior intercostal artery normally descends between the first nerve and the sympathetic trunk. Other intercostal nerves may be sacrificed if they are intimate with the tumor.

Depending on how far the tumor has extended anteriorly, it will need to be dissected off the main structures in the superior mediastinum. This is most likely to be the esophagus and the closely applied vagus nerve, but in a large tumor, the trachea may be involved. It may prove useful to have a large size nasogastric tube in the esophagus to aid dissection. On the left side, the thoracic duct and the arch of the aorta with subclavian and carotid branches, along with the vagus, will need protection.

It should now prove possible to dissect the tumor off the bodies of the vertebra, and any extension into the intravertebral foramen should be carefully dissected out. Titanium clips may prove useful to control hemorrhage in small vessels, and these will not interfere with subsequent CT scanning. They may also be used as markers if all tumor is not excised and radiation therapy is being considered. Any suspiciously involved lymph nodes locally should be taken for biopsy (staging).

FURTHER READING

Anghelescu DL, Burgoyne LL, Liu T, Li CS, Pui CH, Hudson MM, Furman WL, Sandlund JT. Clinical and diagnostic imaging findings predict anesthetic complications in children presenting with malignant mediastinal masses. *Paediatr Anaesth* 2007 November; 17(11): 1090–8.

Cass DL, Olutoye OO, Cassady CI, Zamora IJ, Ivey RT, Ayres NA, Olutoye OA, Lee TC. EXIT-to-resection for fetuses with large lung masses and persistent mediastinal compression near birth. *J Pediatr Surg* 2013; 48: 138–44.

Grosfeld JL, Skinner MA, Rescorla FJ, West KW, Scherer LR 3rd. Mediastinal tumors in children: Experience with 196 cases. *Ann Surg Oncol* 1994; 1: 121–7.

Hammer GB. Anaesthetic management for the child with a mediastinal mass. *Pediatr Anesthest* 2004; 14: 95–7.

Kang CH, Kim YT, Jeon SH, Sung SW, Kim JH. Surgical treatment of malignant mediastinal neurogenic tumors in children. *Eur J Cardiothorac Surg* 2007 April; 31(4): 725–30.

Lee EY. Evaluation of non-vascular mediastinal masses in infants and children: An evidence-based practical approach. *Pediatr Radiol* 2009; 39 Suppl 2: S184–90.

Malek MM, Mollen KP, Kane TD, Shah SR, Irwin C. Thoracic neuroblastoma: A retrospective review of our institutional experience with comparison of the thoracoscopic and open approaches to resection. *J Pediatr Surg* 2010; 45: 1622–6.

Patel R, Lim RP, Saric M, Nayar A, Babb J, Ettel M, Axel L, Srichai MB. Diagnostic performance of cardiac magnetic resonance imaging and echocardiography in evaluation of cardiac and paracardiac masses. *Am J Cardiol* 2016 Jan 1, 117(1): 135–40.

Perger L, Lee EY, Shamberger RC. Management of children and adolescents with a critical airway due to compression by an anterior mediastinal mass. *J Pediatr Surg* 2008 November; 43(911): 1990–7.

Saenz NC. Posterior mediastinal neurogenic tumors in infants and children. *Semin Pediatr Surg* 1999; 8: 78–84.

Williams HJ, Alton HM. Imaging of paediatric mediastinal abnormalities. *Paediatr Respir Rev* 2003; 4: 55–66.

Wright CD. Mediastinal tumors and cysts in the pediatric population. *Thorac Surg Clin* 2009 February; 19(1): 47–61, vi.

38

Congenital airway malformations

ALESSANDRO DE ALARCÓN AND RICHARD G. AZIZKHAN

INTRODUCTION

Congenital airway malformations encompass a broad array of disorders that occur at diverse anatomic levels. The presentation of these disorders varies widely and is influenced by the level at which obstruction occurs as well as the severity of the obstruction. In view of the distinct anatomy of the pediatric airway and the possibility of airway symptoms rapidly progressing to life-threatening airway compromise, early detection, diagnosis, and appropriate management are essential. The aim of this chapter is to present an overview of congenital anomalies extending from the larynx to the distal airway, briefly describing patient assessment, symptomatology, and contemporary management strategies.

ASSESSMENT

Medical history

The evaluation of an infant with respiratory compromise should begin with a thorough review of the infant's history of airway symptoms. Clinicians should explore circumstances that may elicit the onset of symptoms and question parents regarding the duration of symptoms and symptom progression. They should also explore possible swallowing or feeding problems, the nature of the child's cry, and the possibility of foreign-body aspiration. Additionally, any history of endotracheal intubation, trauma, or previous cardiac surgery should be carefully reviewed. All of this information may help to determine the underlying etiology and provide information that significantly impacts management decisions.

Signs and symptoms

Mild airway compromise may manifest with subtle symptoms such as irritability, restlessness, and feeding difficulties. Children with more severe obstruction frequently present with severe suprasternal and intercostal retractions, tachypnea, lethargy, and cyanosis. Stridor, defined as a sound of variable pitch that is produced by turbulent airflow through a partially obstructed laryngeal or tracheal airway, can manifest during either the expiratory or inspiratory phase of respiration or can be biphasic. Inspiratory stridor usually indicates an airway obstruction in the extrathoracic airway, whereas expiratory stridor usually indicates a problem in the intrathoracic airway. Biphasic stridor typically signifies a fixed glottic or subglottic lesion. The pitch of stridor, as well as its relationship to the respiratory cycle, is generally helpful in establishing a differential diagnosis and in establishing priorities for patient assessment. Clinicians should be mindful of the fact that that the degree of stridor does not necessarily reflect the severity of airway obstruction. More specifically, even minimal stridor can reflect the lack of airway movement across a critical airway.

Because stridor is produced by turbulent airflow through the airway, it is not normally seen in children who are intubated or tracheotomy dependent. If seen in a tracheotomized child, it is of particular concern, as it indicates obstruction distal to or within the tracheotomy tube (e.g., mucous plugging) or that the tracheotomy tube is not lying in the trachea.

Diagnostic studies

ENDOSCOPY

In view of the fact that 17% pediatric patients have a synchronous airway lesion, evaluation of the entire airway is imperative. The most critical component of the airway assessment is endoscopy. This may include three endoscopic procedures performed consecutively with the patient under a single anesthesia: (1) flexible bronchoscopy with bronchoalveolar lavage (BAL); (2) microlaryngoscopy and rigid bronchoscopy; and (3) esophagoduodenoscopy with biopsy. Each component of the endoscopic evaluation is aimed at identifying possible pathology and risk factors that can impact the success of airway reconstruction.

FLEXIBLE BRONCHOSCOPY

Flexible bronchoscopy offers several advantages over rigid bronchoscopy. It can identify particular areas that can cause airway obstruction and that may be missed with a rigid bronchoscope. More specifically, flexible bronchoscopy provides better assessment of disorders such as laryngomalacia, tracheomalacia, and bronchomalacia. Evaluation of the distal airway may provide additional information on vascular compression, bronchiectasis, and assessment of aspiration by BAL.

MICROLARYNGOSCOPY AND RIGID BRONCHOSCOPY

The primary aim of microlaryngoscopy and rigid bronchoscopy is to identify anatomic levels of airway obstruction from the larynx to the carina. The supraglottis is evaluated with attention given to the possibility of supraglottic obstruction such as laryngomalacia and supraglottic stenosis. The vocal fold level is then evaluated for posterior glottic stenosis, anterior glottic web, and laryngeal cleft. If vocal fold immobility is suspected or seen on the fiber-optic endoscopic evaluation of swallowing (FEES) or on voice evaluation, the cricoarytenoid joints should be palpated to determine if there is any fixation of the joint.

Rigid bronchoscopy is performed using a combination of Hopkins rod telescopes and rigid bronchoscopes. The subglottis is initially evaluated. If subglottic stenosis (SGS) is present, it is classified by the Myer–Cotton scale[1] and sized using appropriate endotracheal tubes. Additionally, the length of stenosis and the proximity to the vocal folds is assessed and documented. If a tracheotomy is in place, attention is paid to the evaluation of the suprastomal area, considering the possibility of suprastomal collapse, granuloma, intratracheal skin tract, and high tracheotomy. The trachea is evaluated to the level of the carina, looking for additional pathology, including tracheal stenosis, complete tracheal rings, tracheoesophageal fistula (TEF), TEF pouches, vascular compression, and tracheomalacia.

ESOPHAGODUODENOSCOPY

Evaluation of the upper gastrointestinal tract can provide information that is crucial in decision making as to future surgery. Inflammation in the laryngotracheal complex can be caused by conditions of the upper gastrointestinal tract, resulting in an "active" (i.e., inflamed) larynx. Poor wound healing and scarring are more likely to occur in this setting. The two gastrointestinal conditions associated with laryngeal inflammation are gastroesophageal reflux (GER) and eosinophilic esophagitis (EE). For patients in whom GER is suspected or in whom this condition would have negative consequences on subsequent management, objective evaluation of GER is strongly recommended. The diagnosis of EE is made on esophageal biopsy. Laryngeal inflammation may resolve with appropriate treatment of the underlying condition, permitting surgical reconstruction with a lower risk of complication.

Given that up to 45% of children with congenital airway obstruction also have significant nonairway anomalies, patients also require a thorough overall evaluation. Imaging studies are helpful in diagnosis as well as patient management. Computed tomography (CT) and magnetic resonance (MR) imaging studies provide a rapid and precise way of assessing and measuring the extent and length of airway narrowing or displacement. These investigations are also helpful in detecting associated mediastinal and pulmonary anomalies. Specifically, MR angiography is valuable in assessing the relationship of mediastinal great vessel anomalies (e.g., vascular rings, pulmonary artery slings) to the airway. Newer computer software allows for three-dimensional image reconstruction and is helpful in planning surgical procedures. Echocardiography is valuable in identifying intracardiac defects and most associated great vessel anomalies. Contrast swallow studies are valuable in assessing esophageal motility, aspiration, and some mediastinal lesions that affect the airway. FEES is performed to evaluate structural and functional disorders of swallowing and to identify functional problems of the larynx, pharynx, epiglottis, and proximal esophagus.

CONGENITAL LARYNGEAL ANOMALIES

Laryngomalacia

Laryngomalacia is the most common congenital laryngeal anomaly and is also the most common cause of stridor in neonates.[2] This symptom is usually evident soon after birth or within the first few days of life. It is generally mild but is typically exacerbated by feeding, crying, or lying in a supine position. In 50% of children, stridor worsens during the first 6 months of life. A small subset of children with severe laryngomalacia may present with a spectrum of symptoms, including apnea, cyanosis, severe retractions, and failure to thrive. Also, many patients suffer from clinically significant GER. In extremely severe cases, cor pulmonale is seen. The reported incidence of secondary airway lesions in infants with laryngomalacia varies, with some authors reporting rates as high as 50%[3] and 64%.[4]

Although 50% of children with laryngomalacia experience a worsening of symptoms during the first 6 months of life, laryngomalacia generally resolves by 1 year of age. When the disorder is severe, however, surgical intervention is required.

In most cases, the diagnosis is confirmed by transnasal flexible fiber-optic laryngoscopy. Pathognomonic findings include short aryepiglottic folds, with prolapse of the cuneiform cartilages. Because of the Bernoulli effect, collapse of the supraglottic structures is seen on inspiration, and inflammation indicative of reflux laryngitis is also frequently seen (Figure 38.1). In some patients, a tightly curled (omega-shaped) epiglottis is observed.

The decision as to whether to intervene surgically is based more so on symptom severity than on the endoscopic

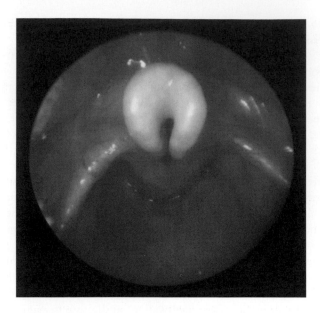

Figure 38.1 Endoscopic view of laryngomalacia in an infant showing partial collapse of the supraglottic structures during inspiration.

appearance of the larynx. For patients with severe symptoms, supraglottoplasty (also termed epiglottoplasty) is the preferred operative procedure, with a reported surgical success as high as 94%.[5-7] Both aryepiglottic folds are divided, and one or both cuneiform cartilages may be removed. If the aryepiglottic folds alone are divided, postoperative intubation is usually not required. Patients should be observed overnight in the intensive care unit. Reflux management with either an H2 antagonist or a proton pump inhibitor is advisable for helping to minimize laryngeal edema. This is especially important in patients with a synchronous airway lesion, as these patients are known to have a higher incidence of GER than those without a synchronous lesion.[3,5] Synchronous airway lesions as well as neurologic conditions and preexisting laryngeal edema can adversely affect operative outcomes.[8] Occasionally, an infant's obstructive symptoms continue despite an adequate postoperative appearance of the larynx. These infants may have an underlying neurologic problem that may become more evident over time. They are therefore far more likely to require tracheotomy placement.

Laryngeal webs

Laryngeal webs result from a failure of recanalization of the glottic airway in the early weeks of embryogenesis. In severe cases, as recanalization commences posteriorly and progresses anteriorly, complete laryngeal atresia may occur. In less severe cases, a thin anterior glottic web may be the only remnant of the recanalization process. The web is typically thickened anteriorly and thins out toward the posterior edge. Associated congenital anomalies are seen in up to 60% of children with webs, and there is a strong association between anterior glottic webs and velocardiofacial syndrome.[9]

Although webs have been described in the supraglottic, glottic, and subglottic regions and may occur anteriorly or posteriorly, anterior glottic webs are the most commonly seen. Some anterior glottic webs are gossamer-thin; however, most are thick and generally associated with a subglottic "sail" that compromises the subglottic lumen. Patients have varying degrees of glottic airway compromise, which usually manifests in an abnormal cry, aphonia, or respiratory distress. Thin webs may elude detection, as neonatal intubation for airway distress may lyse the web, which is curative.

Thick webs require open reconstruction with either reconstruction of the anterior commissure or placement of a laryngeal keel.[10] The presence of thick membranous webs requires placement of a tracheotomy in approximately 40% of patients.

Subglottic stenosis

SGS is an anomaly that involves a narrowing of the subglottic lumen. It can be either congenital or acquired; however, the latter is seen far more frequently and is generally a sequela of prolonged intubation of the neonate. Congenital SGS is thought to be caused by failure of the laryngeal lumen to recanalize during embryogenesis and is one of a continuum of embryologic failures that include laryngeal atresia, stenosis, and webs. It may occur as an isolated anomaly or may be associated with other congenital head and neck lesions and chromosomal anomalies such as a small larynx in a patient with Down syndrome. In the premature infant, SGS is considered present when this lumen measures 3.0 mm or less in diameter at the level of the cricoid, whereas in the full-term neonate, SGS is defined as a lumen of 4.0 mm or less in diameter at this level.

Levels of SGS severity range from mild to severe, and are graded based on the Myer–Cotton grading system (Table 38.1). Patients with mild SGS (no obstruction to 50% obstruction) may present with recurrent upper respiratory infections, often misdiagnosed as croup. In a young child, the greatest obstruction is usually 2 to 3 mm below the true vocal cords.[11] Patients with more severe narrowing (71%–99% obstruction) may present with acute airway compromise and require endotracheal intubation or tracheotomy placement at delivery (Figure 38.2). However, many of these infants, even those

Table 38.1 Myer–Cotton grading system for subglottic stenosis

Classification	Level of airway obstruction	
	From	To
Grade I	No obstruction	50% obstruction
Grade II	51% obstruction	70% obstruction
Grade III	71% obstruction	99% obstruction
Grade IV	No detectable lumen	

Source: Myer CM III et al., Proposed grading system for subglottic stenosis based on endotracheal tube sizes, *Ann Otol Rhinol Laryngol* 1994;103: 319–323.

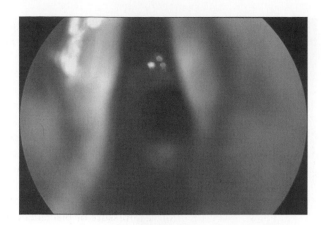

Figure 38.2 Very high-grade subglottic stenosis in a symptomatic neonate.

with grade III SGS (71%–99%), may not be symptomatic for weeks or months. When stridor is present, it initially occurs during the inspiratory phase of respiration. As SGS severity increases, stridor becomes biphasic.

Radiologic evaluation of the nonintubated airway may provide information regarding the site of the stenosis and its extent. Chest x-ray, inspiratory and expiratory lateral soft-tissue neck films, and fluoroscopy are helpful in revealing the dynamics of the trachea and larynx. High-kilovoltage airway films identify the classic steeplelike configuration seen in patients with SGS as well as possible tracheal stenosis, and are therefore of utmost importance. The latter condition is generally caused by complete tracheal rings, which may predispose the patient to a life-threatening situation during rigid endoscopy.

As discussed earlier in this chapter, endoscopic assessment is considered the gold standard. Flexible and rigid endoscopy are used in a complementary fashion for airway evaluation and are both essential. Precise evaluation of the endolarynx should be carried out, including grading of the SGS. Flexible endoscopy provides critical information regarding the structural dynamics of airflow in the hypopharyngeal and laryngeal airways, whereas rigid endoscopy provides an assessment of the entire laryngotracheobronchial airway. Stenosis caused by scarring, granulation tissue, submucosal thickening, or a congenitally abnormal cricoid can be differentiated from SGS with a normal cricoid, but endoscopic measurement with endotracheal tubes or bronchoscopies is required for accurate evaluation.

In children with mild to moderate disease (grade I or II), congenital SGS may improve with age. Children with a minor degree of SGS who experience mild symptoms may nevertheless benefit from endoscopic intervention. Endoscopic options include radial incisions (cold steel or laser) through the stenosis, laryngeal dilatation,[12] and the application of topical or injected steroids. Less than 50% of these patients require tracheotomy placement to maintain their airway. Children with more severe disease are best managed with open airway reconstruction. Laryngotracheal reconstruction using costal cartilage grafts placed through the split lamina of the cricoid cartilage is reliable and has withstood the test of time.[13,14] Costal cartilage grafts can be placed through either the anterior or posterior lamina of the cricoid cartilage or both. These procedures may be performed as a single-stage laryngotracheoplasty[15,16] or as a two-stage procedure, requiring stenting and placement of a temporary tracheostomy.[17] Higher decannulation rates have reportedly been achieved with cricotracheal resection than with laryngotracheal reconstruction in the management of children with severe SGS[18,19]; however, this is a demanding procedure that carries a significant risk of complications. Successful outcomes depend on the management of comorbidities such as GER, EE, and low-grade tracheal infection.

Subglottic hemangioma

Hemangiomas of infancy (also referred to as infantile hemangiomas) are the most common vascular tumors, affecting 1 in 10 white infants in North America[20] and occurring with a threefold female preponderance. These benign lesions usually follow a predetermined phase of growth (proliferation) and later tumor regression (involution). The involutive phase occurs at 12 to 18 months and is generally complete by the first decade of life.

Hemangiomas generally present cutaneously but can occur in any organ or anatomic site. Lesions within the tracheobronchial tree most commonly occur in the subglottis. Their natural history generally mirrors that of cutaneous lesions. More than 50% of children with a subglottic hemangioma also have cutaneous lesions. The latter may therefore provide an indication of the possible presence of a subglottic lesion. The highest-risk (65%) patients are those with a hemangioma occurring in a beard distribution[21] or those with PHACE association, which is characterized by *p*osterior fossa abnormalities, *h*emangiomas of the cervicofacial region that are usually plaque-like and segmental, *a*rterial defects, *c*ardiac and aortic arch defects, and *e*ye abnormalities.[22,23]

As a subglottic hemangioma undergoes proliferation, progressive worsening of the airway usually occurs. Symptoms typically include progressive biphasic stridor with retractions. The degree of obstruction varies and can be exacerbated by certain positions or crying, both of which increase venous pressure and lead to vascular engorgement. When airway narrowing is severe, apnea, cyanosis, and "dying spells" may result.

The diagnosis is based on medical history and findings on rigid bronchoscopy, and although radiologic evaluation (MR imaging with contrast enhancement) is indicated, it rarely reveals extension of the lesion beyond the subglottis. Lesions are typically asymmetric and may be covered by a normal smooth mucosa (Figure 38.3). Because of the risk of hemorrhage, biopsy is not advised. Most patients require treatment, and combining various treatment modalities is often essential.

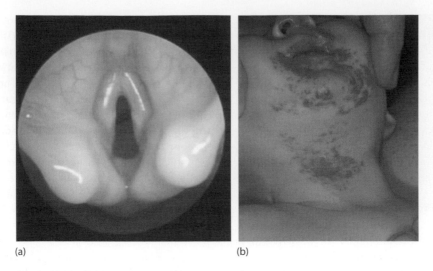

(a)   (b)

Figure 38.3 **(a)** Endoscopic view of a subglottic hemangioma in **(b)** a patient with infantile hemangioma in bearded distribution.

Depending on both the severity of the obstruction and the expertise of involved clinicians, early symptoms are managed with systemic steroids and, more recently, with propranolol—a nonselective beta-blocker. In a landmark article published in the *New England Journal of Medicine* (2008), Leaute-Labreze et al.[24] reported that a child with a large infantile hemangioma who was being treated with propranolol for an unrelated hypertrophic cardiomyopathy exhibited rapid regression of the hemangioma within days of initiating propranolol. These unexpected results spurred numerous investigations and case reports documenting excellent outcomes.[25–30] These outcomes have dramatically changed the paradigm of both pharmacologic and surgical treatment.[31–32]

Vocal cord paralysis

Vocal cord paralysis is the second most common cause of stridor in newborns and may be either congenital or acquired.[33] Congenital vocal cord paralysis generally manifests bilaterally. Although it is usually idiopathic, it is sometimes seen in children with central nervous system pathology (e.g., hydrocephalus and Chiari malformation of the brainstem). Although most children with bilateral paralysis present with significant airway compromise, they have an intelligible voice and do not aspirate.

Acquired disease is generally, though not always, a unilateral condition arising from iatrogenic injury to the recurrent laryngeal nerve. Because of the length and course of the left recurrent nerve, this is far more likely to be damaged than the right recurrent laryngeal nerve. As such, acquired disease usually affects the left vocal cord. Risk factors for acquired paralysis include patent ductus arteriosus repair, the Norwood cardiac repair, and esophageal surgery, particularly TEF repair. In older children, thyroid surgery is an additional risk factor. Unlike children with bilateral vocal cord paralysis, most children with unilateral disease have an acceptable airway but a breathy voice. These children are at a slightly higher risk of aspiration.

The diagnosis of vocal cord paralysis is established with awake flexible transnasal fiber-optic laryngoscopy and/or stroboscopy. Once paralysis has been confirmed, management depends on a number of factors. Children with acquired vocal cord paralysis (whether unilateral or bilateral) may experience spontaneous recovery several months after nerve injury; however, this occurs only if the nerve is stretched or crushed but is otherwise intact.

Children with unilateral paralysis can be initially managed with observation, temporary injection medialization, or speech and voice therapy. Determining the appropriate option is based on a discussion with the patient's family, taking into account the need for restoration of normal voice and improvement of aspiration. Regardless of which option is chosen, these children should be observed for at least 1 year prior to any permanent intervention. If paralysis persists after this period of time and there is a functional deficit, long-term interventions such as ansa cervicalis reinnervation, permanent medialization laryngoplasty, or long-term injection medialization (fat or Radiesse) are considered. These options are discussed with the family and are often influenced by the age of the child and the presence of comorbidities. Medialization laryngoplasty is best performed after puberty.

For patients with bilateral paralysis associated with an underlying disease process, successful treatment of that disease may reverse the paralysis; however, up to 90% of these infants ultimately require tracheotomy placement. Given that up to 50% of children with congenital idiopathic bilateral vocal cord paralysis have spontaneous resolution of their paralysis by 1 year of age,[34] surgical intervention to achieve decannulation is almost always delayed until patients are older than 1 year of age.

Several surgical options have been used for patients with bilateral paralysis, and no particular option offers a universally acceptable outcome. The aim of surgery is two-fold: (1) to achieve an adequate decannulated airway while maintaining voice and (2) to prevent aspiration. Surgical options include laser cordotomy, partial or complete arytenoidectomy (endoscopic or open), vocal process lateralization (open or endoscopically guided), and posterior cricoid cartilage grafting (open or endoscopic).[35–37] In a child with a tracheotomy, it is often prudent to maintain the tracheotomy to ensure an adequate airway prior to decannulation. In a nontracheotomized child, a single-stage surgical procedure can be carried out. Acquired bilateral vocal cord paralysis that does not resolve spontaneously is usually less responsive to treatment than idiopathic cord paralysis. In these cases, more than one operative intervention may be required to achieve decannulation. In patients who have undergone such interventions, postextubation stridor may respond to continuous positive airway pressure (CPAP) or high-flow nasal cannula. The postoperative risk of aspiration should be evaluated by a video swallow study before the child returns to a normal diet. During the initial postoperative weeks, some children have an increased risk of aspirating with certain textures, especially thin fluids.

Posterior laryngeal cleft

Posterior laryngeal cleft is a rare congenital anomaly that results from failure of the laryngotracheal groove to fuse during embryogenesis. This anomaly comprises four anatomic subtypes that differ with respect to involvement of the larynx and/or trachea (Figure 38.4).[38] Patients frequently have coexisting anomalies, many of which affect the airway. Associated airway anomalies include tracheomalacia (almost always present in varying levels of severity), TEF formation (20%), laryngomalacia, vocal cord paralysis, SGS, and innominate artery compression. Associated nonairway conditions include anogenital anomalies, cleft lip and palate, congenital heart defects, and GER, which affects most children. The most common associated syndrome is Opitz–Frias syndrome, which is characterized by hypertelorism, anogenital anomalies, and posterior laryngeal clefting.[39]

Diagnosis can be extremely difficult, as presenting symptoms vary greatly. In type I and type II clefts, symptoms are often subtle and may mimic those of other disorders such as GER. Nonetheless, aspiration is a hallmark clinical feature of this spectrum of disease. With more severe clefts, gross aspiration may occur with associated apnea, cyanosis, and even pneumonia. For milder clefts, the symptoms are those of microaspiration, with choking episodes, transient cyanosis, and recurrent chest infections.[11,39] Airway obstruction manifested by stridor may also be present and is caused by either redundant mucosa on the edge of the cleft or a small cricoid ring. In patients with severe tracheomalacia, especially those with an associated TEF, the airway may be significantly compromised. Contrast swallow studies may demonstrate aspiration; however, rigid laryngoscopy and bronchoscopy are essential for definitive diagnosis. The interarytenoid area is specifically probed to determine if a posterior laryngeal cleft is present.

In children who are symptomatic and do not have other more severe anomalies, repair of the posterior laryngeal cleft should be performed as soon as possible to prevent chronic microaspiration with long-term pulmonary sequelae. Depending on the extent of the airway anomaly, tracheotomy and gastrostomy tube placement may be required before definitive surgical repair of the airway. Because of the high incidence of GER, fundoplication is often required and is preferably performed prior to surgical repair. Most type I and some type II clefts are amenable to endoscopic surgical repair, whereas clefts that extend into the cervical or thoracic trachea often require open repair. A transtracheal approach is advised, as it provides optimal exposure of the cleft while protecting the recurrent laryngeal nerves. A two-layer closure is recommended, with the option of performing an interposition graft if warranted. Type IV long clefts, which extend to the carina or beyond and are often associated with multiple congenital anomalies, are exceedingly difficult to repair and are prone to anastomotic breakdown.[39] Reported success rates for cleft repair vary (50%–90%) depending on both the severity of the cleft and the presence of comorbidities; however, a recent study by de

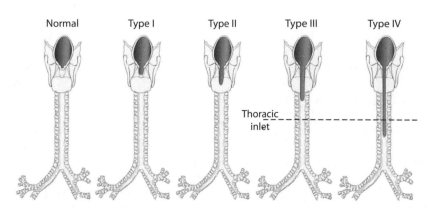

Figure 38.4 Posterior laryngeal cleft classification.

Alarcón et al.[40] reported a high success rate (>90%) despite the presence of additional airway anomalies.

Laryngeal atresia

CONGENITAL HIGH AIRWAY OBSTRUCTION SYNDROME

Congenital high airway obstruction syndrome (CHAOS) is a rare, life-threatening, prenatally diagnosed condition caused by complete or near-complete obstruction of the larynx and trachea. Fetal lung fluid becomes trapped, causing the lungs to become abnormally distended. This creates massive lung expansion that characteristically everts the hemidiaphragms.

This type of fetal airway obstruction may be caused by multiple etiologies, including laryngeal atresia, laryngeal web, tracheal atresia, and laryngeal cyst.[41] Airway atresia is sometimes an isolated anomaly but often is seen in association with genitourinary, vertebral, and cardiac anomalies as well as with hydrocephalus malformation of the aqueduct of Sylvius, bronchotracheal fistula, esophageal atresia, TEF, and syndactyly. Regardless of the etiology, the clinical features and presentation of CHAOS are the same. Prenatal findings on ultrasonography (US) include diffuse and enhanced echogenicity of the lungs, dilated airways, and flattened or everted diaphragms with associated fetal ascites and nonimmune hydrops (Figure 38.5). A fetus identified with these sonographic features is at significant risk of intrauterine death and faces a high likelihood of mortality should the pregnancy progress to delivery. Although US provides a good

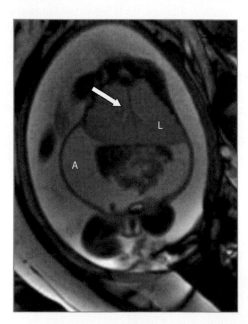

Figure 38.5 Fetal ultrasonography at 27 weeks gestation demonstrating findings consistent with the diagnosis of congenital high airway obstruction: enlarged echogenic lungs (L), dilated airway (white arrow), flattened or everted diaphragms, and fetal ascites (A) and hydrops. (Courtesy of Timothy Crombleholme, MD, Denver, Colorado.)

initial assessment of CHAOS, MR imaging is clearly superior in identifying severity and the level of airway obstruction, and optimizes planning for airway management at delivery.[42] These patients all require delivery by the ex utero intrapartum technique (EXIT) procedure. This procedure maintains placental circulation to the fetus while securing the airway at the time of delivery.[41] Securing the airway may include a full endoscopic diagnostic assessment and tracheostomy.

For the newborn diagnosed with CHAOS, securing and maintaining the airway is the highest priority. These patients are almost always extremely ill and require a prolonged period of critical care and ventilatory support. Once the infant's cardiorespiratory status is stable and other critical or potentially life-threatening anomalies are ruled out, careful endoscopic evaluation of the airway precedes elective laryngotracheal reconstruction; however, consensus has not been reached as to optimal timing of airway reconstruction. Although a functional airway can be constructed, patients do not always attain intelligible speech capabilities.

Diagnosis in the middle of the second trimester generally correlates with a poor perinatal outcome. A fetus presenting in the third trimester with CHAOS in the absence of associated anomalies or hydrops is likely to have incomplete obstruction, and is therefore more likely to survive.

ANOMALIES OF THE TRACHEA AND BRONCHI

Tracheal agenesis and atresia

Tracheal agenesis is a rare developmental anomaly that almost always results in death. Patients who are prenatally diagnosed and in whom the atresia involves only the proximal trachea occasionally survive with the use of an EXIT procedure and eventual tracheal reconstruction. In another form of tracheal agenesis, the entire trachea is absent, and the bronchi come directly off the esophagus. Neonates present at birth with severe respiratory distress, attempting ventilation through bronchoesophageal communications. Temporary ventilation may be possible with esophageal intubation of the esophagus, but this is typically unsustainable. If there is no communication between the airway and the esophagus, CHAOS will result.[41]

Tracheal stenosis and webs

Tracheal stenosis encompasses a broad spectrum of rare tracheal anomalies. Affected segments of the trachea differ in the degree and extent of stenosis, which can range from extremely thin webs to more severe long segments of stenosis affecting the entire airway.

TRACHEAL WEBS

Tracheal webs involve an intraluminal soft-tissue stenosis of the trachea. These webs may be membranous or consist of thick, relatively rigid tissue. Patients typically present with biphasic stridor or expiratory wheezing, and the severity of these symptoms depends on the degree of the stenosis. Thin webs can be easily managed by hydrostatic balloon dilatation. For thicker webs that are not associated with underlying cartilage deformity, laser ablation is often used.[43] The carbon dioxide (CO_2) or potassium titanyl phosphate (KTP) laser is beneficial for treating lesions in the proximal trachea. Lesions in the distal airway are best managed with the KTP laser, which can be used through small fiber-optic cables. For children with a web greater than 1 cm in length or those in whom the airway cartilage is thought to be structurally deficient or anomalous, operative treatment with segmental tracheal resection or slide tracheoplasty is usually carried out.

CARTILAGINOUS RING APLASIA

Cartilaginous ring aplasia is an extremely rare anomaly in which only a small region of the trachea lacks cartilage, creating a distinct anatomic area that is both malacic and stenotic. The remainder of the trachea is unaffected, and most children do not have coexisting congenital anomalies. Management entails segmental resection of the trachea or slide tracheoplasty,[44] which successfully restores the airway.

TRACHEAL CARTILAGINOUS SLEEVE

Tracheal cartilaginous sleeve is also extremely rare. In children with this anomaly, discrete cartilaginous rings are replaced by a fused cartilaginous cylinder, with or without a membranous portion. It is typically seen in children with craniosynostosis syndromes such as Pfeiffer, Apert, Crouzon, and Goldenhar.[45–47] Neonates usually exhibit respiratory illness. Patients presenting in early infancy often experience acute respiratory symptoms, which may include biphasic stridor with respiratory distress, cough, and frequent respiratory infections. Because of tracheal rigidity, the mechanism for clearing secretions is impaired.

On endoscopy, the anterior tracheal wall appears smooth, though the membranous posterior tracheal wall may be normal, stenotic, or absent. CT and MR imaging are sometimes useful in determining the extent of the lesion.

Tracheotomy placement may be used as a temporizing measure. In some cases, observation alone is appropriate. If surgical management is necessary, a slide tracheoplasty is the current gold standard.[48]

COMPLETE TRACHEAL RINGS

Although rare, complete tracheal rings are the most common congenital tracheal stenosis. With this spectrum of potentially life-threatening anomalies, either the trachea alone or both the trachea and bronchi are significantly narrowed. The tracheal cartilage in these patients is abnormally shaped and forms complete rings (Figure 38.6). More than 50% of infants have a segmental stenosis. The clinical manifestations of complete tracheal rings vary from life-threatening respiratory distress during the perinatal period to subtle symptoms of airway compromise in older children. Most symptomatic infants exhibit deterioration of respiratory function over the first few months of life. Symptoms include stridor, retractions, cough, and alterations of cry. Atypical and persistent wheezing and rhonchi and sudden death can also occur. More than 80% of children with complete tracheal rings have other and often multiple congenital anomalies[11]; 50% specifically have congenital heart disease with or without great vessel anomalies.

In some patients, placement of an endotracheal tube may further exacerbate respiratory distress by causing acute swelling and inflammation of the mucosa. Partially obstructing tracheal lesions also may become life threatening following the onset of a respiratory infection. In an infant or child with an abnormal trachea, the cross-sectional area of airway can be significantly decreased with as little as 1 mm of edema. This accounts for the rapid worsening of symptoms in some children with acute inflammatory conditions and coexisting tracheal narrowing.

Prompt diagnostic evaluation to define tracheobronchial anatomy is essential. An initial high-kilovolt airway film may indicate stenosis; however, bronchoscopy is required to reveal the precise location and extent of the stenosis. Bronchoscopy should be performed with extreme caution, using the smallest possible telescopes,

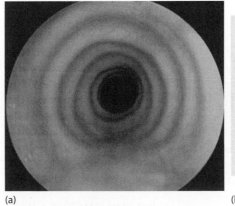
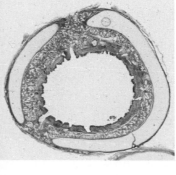

(a) (b)

Figure 38.6 Congenital tracheal stenosis. **(a)** Endoscopic view demonstrating complete tracheal rings. **(b)** Histology showing cartilaginous rings that are circumferential.

and any airway edema in the region of the stenosis may turn a narrow airway into a critical airway.[11] CT scans provide a rapid and precise method of measuring the extent and length of airway narrowing or displacement. Three-dimensional reconstruction of the airway and its relationship to the great vessels aids in operative planning. Furthermore, with new software enhancements, virtual bronchoscopic images can be obtained. These images are particularly useful in assessing the airway distal to the obstruction (Figure 38.7). MR imaging is also valuable in evaluating the relationship of the mediastinal great vessels to the airway. Echocardiography is used mainly to determine whether intracardiac defects are present, and can identify most coexisting pulmonary artery slings.

About 10% of patients with complete tracheal rings are minimally symptomatic and can be managed nonoperatively, though they require ongoing observation.[49] Most children must undergo tracheal reconstruction.[49] Repair of coexisting anomalies such as pulmonary artery sling or vascular ring should be carried out concurrent with the tracheal repair. Although patch tracheoplasty was historically the preferred procedure for long segments of narrowing, slide tracheoplasty is now the procedure of choice for both short- and long-segment stenosis (Figure 38.8).[50] This approach results in significantly less morbidity than other tracheal reconstruction techniques and is adaptable to all anatomic configurations of complete tracheal rings. Slide tracheoplasty uses only autologous tracheal tissue and is performed by transecting the trachea into two equal segments. The anterior wall of the lower half of the trachea and the posterior wall of the upper trachea are incised. These segments are then slid over each other and anastomosed with 5-0 monofilament and absorbable sutures. Postoperatively, the cross-sectional area of the airway has a fourfold increase, and the length of the involved airway decreases by half. Airflow is increased 16-fold.

Postoperatively, endotracheal intubation is generally required for 1 to 2 days, though some patients with parenchymal pulmonary disease require longer ventilatory support. During the perioperative period, unnecessary movements of the endotracheal tube or unplanned extubation must be avoided to minimize the risk of damage to the newly reconstructed airway. Nasotracheal intubation is preferred, as the endotracheal tube can be more securely stabilized. Patients require continuous monitoring, careful pulmonary toilet, and endoscopic removal of any obstructing granulation tissue. Immediately prior to extubation, the integrity and patency of the reconstructed airway are assessed by flexible fiber-optic endoscopy through the endotracheal tube, thus ensuring a safe extubation.

Although airway configuration following slide tracheoplasty may resemble a figure eight, this does not indicate airway obstruction. The trachea generally remodels to a normal oval shape within 1 year of reconstruction. In our experience, the long-term survival rate is 90%. Mortality is usually associated with severe comorbidities such as cardiac disease rather than airway complications.

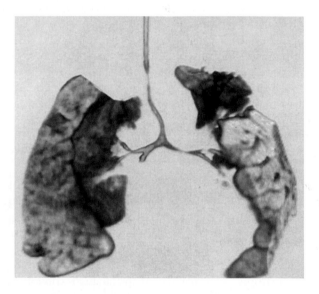

Figure 38.7 Computed tomographic (CT) scan with three-dimensional reconstruction to demonstrate anatomy of the trachea in a patient with congenital tracheal stenosis involving the majority of the tracheal length.

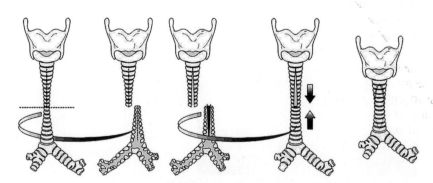

Figure 38.8 Slide tracheoplasty: The trachea is transversely divided at the midpoint of the tracheal stenosis. After proximal and distal tracheal mobilization, the posterior portion of the cephalic trachea segment and the anterior portion of the caudal tracheal segment are incised. The two tracheal segments are then overlapped and obliquely sutured together.

stenosis is more common than its congenital manifestation, and is a significant cause of morbidity and mortality in infants who have undergone prolonged intubation and respiratory support. Most such cases can be managed with endoscopic balloon dilatation or laser resection.

REFERENCES

1. Myer CM III, O'Connor DM, Cotton RT. Proposed grading system for subglottic stenosis based on endotracheal tube sizes. *Ann Otol Rhinol Laryngol* 1994; 103: 319–23.
2. Thompson DM. Abnormal sensorimotor integrative function of the larynx in congenital laryngomalacia: A new theory of etiology. *Laryngoscope* 2007; 117: 1–33.
3. Dickson JM, Richter GT, Meinzen-Derr J et al. Secondary airway lesions in infants with laryngomalacia. *Ann Otol Rhinol Laryngol* 2009; 118: 37–43.
4. Cohen SR, Eavey RD, Desmond MS et al. Endoscopy and tracheotomy in the neonatal period: A 10-year review, 1967–1976. *Ann Otol Rhinol Laryngol* 1977; 86: 577–83.
5. Richter GT, Thompson DM. The surgical management of laryngomalacia. *Otolaryngol Clin N Am* 2008; 41: 837–64.
6. Loke D, Ghosh S, Panarese A et al. Endoscopic division of the aryepiglottic folds in severe laryngomalacia. *Int J Pediatr Otorhinolaryngol* 2001; 60: 59–63.
7. Martin JE, Howarth KE, Khodaei I et al. Aryepiglottoplasty for laryngomalacia: The Alder Hey experience. *J Laryngol Otol* 2005; 119: 958–60.
8. Schroeder JW, Bhandarkar ND, Holinger LD. Synchronous airway lesions and outcomes in infants with severe laryngomalacia requiring supraglottoplasty. *Arch Otolaryngol Head Neck Surg* 2009; 135: 647–51.
9. Miyamoto RC, Cotton RT, Rope AF et al. Association of anterior glottic webs with velocardiofacial syndrome (chromosome 22q11.2 deletion). *Otolaryngol Head Neck Surg* 2004; 130: 415–7.
10. Wyatt ME, Hartlley BE. Laryngotracheal reconstruction in congenital laryngeal webs and atresias. *Otolaryngol Head Neck Surg* 2005; 132: 232–8.
11. Rutter MJ. Evaluation and management of upper airway disorders in children. *Semin Pediatr Surg* 2006; 15: 116–23.
12. Monnier P, George M, Monod ML et al. The role of the CO_2 laser in the management of laryngotracheal stenosis: A survey of 100 cases. *Eur Arch Otorhinolaryngol* 2005; 262: 602–8.
13. Cotton RT, Gray SC, Miller RP. Update of the Cincinnati experience in pediatric laryngotracheal reconstruction. *Laryngoscope* 1989; 99: 1111–6.
14. Santos D, Mitchell R. The history of pediatric airway reconstruction. *Laryngoscope* 2010; 120: 815–20.
15. White DR, Bravo M, Vijayasekaran S et al. Laryngotracheoplasty as an alternative to tracheotomy in infants younger than 6 months. *Arch Otolaryngol Head Neck Surg* 2009; 135: 445–7.
16. de Alarcon A, Rutter MJ. Revision pediatric laryngotracheal reconstruction. *Otolaryngol Clin N Am* 2008; 41: 959–80.
17. Monnier P. Airway stenting with the LT-Mold™: Experience in 30 pediatric cases. *Int J Pediatr Otorhinolaryngol* 2007; 71: 1351–9.
18. White DR, Cotton RT, Bean JA et al. Pediatric cricotracheal resection: Surgical outcomes and risk factor analysis. *Arch Otolaryngol Head Neck Surg* 2005; 131: 896–9.
19. Rutter MJ, Hartley BE, Cotton RT. Cricotracheal resection in children. *Arch Otolaryngol Head Neck Surg* 2011; 127: 289–92.
20. Mulliken JB, Fishman SJ, Burrows PE. Vascular anomalies. *Curr Probl Surg* 2000; 37: 517–84.
21. Orlow SJ, Isakoff MS, Blei F. Increased risk of symptomatic hemangiomas of the airway in association with cutaneous hemangiomas in a "beard" distribution. *J Pediatr* 1997; 131: 643–6.
22. Perkins JA, Duke W, Chen E et al. Emerging concepts in airway infantile hemangioma assessment and management. *Otolaryngol Head Neck Surg* 2009; 141: 207–12.
23. O-Lee TJ, Messner A. Subglottic hemangioma. *Otolaryngol Clin N Am* 2008; 41: 903–11.
24. Léaute-Labrèze C, Dumas de la Roque E, Hubiche T et al. Propranolol for severe hemangiomas of infancy. *N Engl J Med* 2008; 358: 2649–51.
25. Truong MT, Chang KW, Berk DR et al. Propranolol for the treatment of a life-threatening subglottic and mediastinal infantile hemangioma. *J Pediatr* 2010; 156: 335–8.
26. Jephson CG, Manunza F, Syed S et al. Successful treatment of isolated subglottic haemangioma with propranolol alone. *Int J Pediatr Otorhinolaryngol* 2009; 73: 1821–3.
27. Denoyelle F, Leboulanger N, Enjolras O et al. Role of propranolol in the therapeutic strategy of infantile laryngotracheal haemangioma. *Int J Pediatr Otorhinolaryngol* 2009; 73: 1168–72.
28. Fuchsmann C, Quintal MC, Giguere C et al. Propranolol as first-line treatment of head and neck hemangiomas. *Arch Otolaryngol Head Neck Surg* 2011; 137: 471–8.
29. Raol N, Metry D, Edmonds J et al. Propranolol for the treatment of subglottic hemangiomas. *Int J Pediatr Otorhinolaryngol* 2011; 75: 1510–4.
30. Leboulanger N, Fayoux P, Teissier N et al. Propranolol in the therapeutic strategy of infantile laryngotracheal hemangioma: A preliminary retrospective study of French experience. *Int J Pediatr Otorhinolaryngol* 2010; 74: 1254–7.

31. Bajaj Y, Kapoor K, Ifeacho S et al. Great Ormond Street Hospital treatment guidelines for use of propranolol in infantile isolated subglottic haemangioma. *J Laryngol Otol* 2013; 127: 295–8.

32. Elluru RG, Friess MR, Richter GT et al. Multicenter evaluation of the effectiveness of systemic propranolol in the treatment of airway hemangiomas. *Otolaryngol Head Neck Surg* 2015; 153: 452–60.

33. Hartnick CJ, Brigger MT, Willging JP et al. Surgery for pediatric vocal cord paralysis: A retrospective review. *Ann Otol Rhinol Laryngol* 2003; 112: 1–6.

34. Miyamoto RC, Parikh SR, Gellad W et al. Bilateral congenital vocal cord paralysis: A 16-year institutional review. *Otolaryngol Head Neck Surg* 2005; 133: 241–5.

35. Sipp JA, Kerschner JE, Braune N et al. Vocal fold medialization in children. *Arch Otolaryngol Head Neck Surg* 2007; 133: 767–71.

36. Chen EY, Inglis AF Jr. Bilateral vocal cord paralysis. *Otolaryngol Clin N Am* 2008; 41: 889–901.

37. Gerber ME, Modi VK, Ward RF et al. Endoscopic posterior cricoid split and costal cartilage graft placement in children. *Otolaryngol Head Neck Surg* 2013; 148: 494–502.

38. Benjamin B, Inglis A. Minor congenital laryngeal clefts: Diagnosis and classification. *Ann Otol Rhinol Laryngol* 1989; 98: 417–20.

39. Rutter MJ, Azizkhan RG. Posterior laryngeal cleft. In: Ziegler M, Azizkhan RG, Weber T, von Allmen D (eds). *Operative Pediatric Surgery*, 2nd edn, Chapter 21. New York: McGraw-Hill, 2014.

40. de Alarcón A, Osborn AJ, Tabangin ME et al. Laryngotracheal cleft repair in children with complex airway anomalies. *JAMA Otolaryngol Head Neck Surg* 2015; 141: 828–33.

41. Marwan A, Crombleholme TM. The EXIT procedure: Principles, pitfalls, and progress. *Semin Pediatr Surg* 2006; 15: 107–15.

42. Mong A, Johnson AM, Kramer SS et al. Congenital high airway obstruction syndrome: MR/US findings, effect on management, and outcome. *Pediatr Radiol* 2008; 38: 1171–9.

43. Azizkhan RG, Lacey SR, Wood RE. Acquired symptomatic bronchial stenosis in infants: Successful management using an argon laser. *J Pediatr Surg* 1990; 25: 19–24.

44. Manning PB, Rutter MJ, Lisec A et al. One slide fits all: The versatility of slide tracheoplasty with cardiopulmonary bypass support for airway reconstruction in children. *J Thorac Cardiovasc Surg* 2011; 141: 155–61.

45. Davis S, Bove KE, Wells TR et al. Tracheal cartilaginous sleeve. *Pediatr Pathol* 1992; 12: 349–64.

46. Hockstein NG, McDonald-McGinn D, Zackai E et al. Tracheal anomalies in Pfeiffer syndrome. *Arch Otolaryngol Head Neck Surg* 2004; 130: 1298–302.

47. Elloy MD, Cochrane LA, Wyatt M. Tracheal cartilaginous sleeve with cricoid cartilage involvement in Pfeiffer syndrome. *J Craniofac Surg* 2006; 17: 272–4.

48. Rutter MJ, de Alarcon A, Manning PB. Tracheal anomalies and reconstruction. In: da Cruz E, Ivy D, Jaggers J (eds). *Pediatric and Congenital Cardiology, Cardiac Surgery and Intensive Care*, Chapter 166. London: Springer-Verlag, 2014.

49. Rutter MJ, Willging JP, Cotton RT. Nonoperative management of complete tracheal rings. *Arch Otolaryngol Head Neck Surg* 2004; 130: 450–2.

50. Rutter MJ, Cotton RT, Azizkhan RG et al. Slide tracheoplasty for the management of complete tracheal rings. *J Pediatr Surg* 2003; 38: 928–34.

51. Cheng ATL, Gazali N. Acquired tracheal diverticulum following repair of tracheo-oesophageal fistula: Endoscopic management. *Int J Pediatr Otorhinolaryngol* 2008; 72: 1269–74.

52. Shah AR, Lazar EL, Atlas AB. Tracheal diverticula after tracheoesophageal fistula repair: Case series and review of the literature. *J Pediatr Surg* 2009; 44: 2107–11.

53. Johnson LB, Cotton RT, Rutter MJ. Management of symptomatic tracheal pouches. *Int J Pediatr Otorhinolaryngol* 2007; 71: 527–31.

54. McNamara VM, Crabbe DC. Tracheomalacia. *Paediatr Respir Rev* 2004; 5: 147–54.

55. Perger L, Kim HB, Jaksic T et al. Thoracoscopic aortopexy for treatment of tracheomalacia in infants and children. *J Laparoendosc Adv Surg Tech* 2009; 19 Suppl 1: S-249–254.

56. Tsugawa J, Tsugawa C, Satoh S et al. Communicating bronchopulmonary foregut malformation: Particular emphasis on concomitant congenital tracheobronchial stenosis. *Pediatr Surg Int* 2005; 21: 932–5.

57. Revillon MY, Salakos C, DeBlic J et al. Successful bronchotracheal reconstruction in esophageal bronchus: Two case reports. *J Pediatr Surg* 1997; 32: 739–42.

58. Chawla SC, Jha P, Breiman R et al. Congenital tracheobiliary fistula diagnosed with contrast-enhanced CT and 3-D reformation. *Pediatr Radiol* 2008; 38: 999–1002.

59. DiFiore JW, Alexander F. Congenital bronchobiliary fistula in association with right-sided congenital diaphragmatic hernia. *J Pediatr Surg* 2002; 37: 1208–9.

60. Tommasoni N, Gamba PG, Midrio P et al. Congenital tracheobiliary fistula. *Pediatr Pulmonol* 2000; 30: 149–52.

61. Egrari S, Krishnamoorthy M, Yee CA et al. Congenital bronchobiliary fistula: Diagnosis and postoperative surveillance with HIDA scan. *J Pediatr Surg* 1996; 31: 785–6.

62. Stocker JT. Cystic lung disease in infants and children. *Fetal Pediatr Pathol* 2009; 28: 155–84.

63. Koontz CS, Oliva V, Gow KW et al. Video-assisted thoracoscopic surgical excision of cystic lung disease in children. *J Pediatr Surg* 2005; 40: 835–7.

64. Hirose S, Clifton MS, Bratton B et al. Thoracoscopic resection of foregut duplication cysts. *J Laparoendosc Adv Surg Tech* 2006; 16: 526–9.

65. Morikawa N, Kuroda T, Honna T. Congenital bronchial atresia in infants and children. *J Pediatr Surg* 2005; 40: 1822–6.

66. Peranteau WH, Merchant AM, Hedrick HL et al. Prenatal course and postnatal management of peripheral bronchial atresia: Association with congenital cystic adenomatoid malformation of the lung. *Fetal Diagn Ther* 2008; 24: 190–6.

67. Antón-Pacheco JL, Galletti L, Cabezali D et al. Management of bilateral congenital bronchial stenosis in an infant. *J Pediatr Surg* 2007; 42: E1–3.

68. Grillo HC, Wright CD, Vlahakes G et al. Management of congenital tracheal stenosis by means of slide tracheoplasty or resection and reconstruction, with long term follow up of growth after slide tracheoplasty. *J Thorac Cardiovasc Surg* 2002; 123: 145–52.

39

Vascular rings

BENJAMIN O. BIERBACH, JOHN MARK REDMOND, AND CHRISTOPHER HART

INTRODUCTION

Vascular rings are unusual congenital anomalies that occur early in the development of the aortic arch and great vessels. The primary symptoms associated with vascular rings relate to the structures that are encircled by the ring, namely, the trachea and esophagus.

DEFINITION AND HISTORY

A vascular ring is a rare congenital condition in which an anomalous configuration of the aortic arch or associated vessels surrounds the trachea and esophagus, to form a complete compressing ring around them. Several other related vascular anomalies involving aortic arch vessels do not form complete rings but have been grouped descriptively with vascular rings because they can produce similar symptoms related to compression of the trachea and or esophagus. In common usage, however, the definition of a complete vascular ring is extended to include pulmonary artery slings, which do not completely surround the trachea and esophagus but may compress them. Both complete and incomplete rings and slings are discussed in this chapter.

The first vascular ring described was that of a double aortic arch by Hommel[1] in 1737. Subsequently, Bayford reported a retroesophageal right subclavian artery in 1794 after performing an autopsy on a woman who had experienced dysphagia for years and died of starvation. Maude Abbott described five cases of double aortic arch in 1932 and made the suggestion that surgical intervention should be undertaken in such cases.

The term *vascular ring* was first used by Dr. Robert Gross[2] in his report describing the first successful division of a double aortic arch.

Potts and Holinger coined the term *pulmonary artery sling* when they reported the first successful repair of this anomaly in a 5-month old with wheezing and intermittent episodes of dyspnea and cyanosis.[3] This anomaly was, however, first reported in a postmortem study in a 7-month-old infant with severe respiratory distress.[4]

Although innominate artery compression syndrome and pulmonary artery sling are not complete anatomic rings, they have been traditionally classified with classic vascular rings because of the similarities in patient presentation, diagnosis, and surgical therapy.

FREQUENCY

Vascular rings are uncommon anomalies and make up less than 1% of all congenital cardiac defects. They occur with about equal frequency in both sexes. No geographical or racial predominance exists. Some vascular rings are associated with other congenital heart defects, while others may be isolated malformations.

The two most common types of complete vascular rings are double aortic arch and right aortic arch with left ligamentum arteriosum. These make up 85%–95% of cases. Two other complete vascular rings that are extremely rare (<1%) include right aortic arch with mirror-image branching and left ligamentum arteriosum, and left aortic arch with retroesophageal right subclavian artery, right-sided descending aorta, and right ligamentum arteriosum.

Other anomalies that produce symptoms but do not form a complete anatomic vascular ring make up the remainder and include the anomalous innominate artery and the anomalous right subclavian artery with left-sided aortic arch and left ligamentum arteriosum.

The anomalous left pulmonary artery or pulmonary artery sling makes up about 10% of cases, and, although it is not associated with anomalies of the aortic arch or its branches, it arises from an abnormality of the sixth branchial arch and produces a complete ring. This anomaly is associated with intracardiac defects in 10%–15% of cases.

EMBRYOLOGY

In 1922, Congdon[5] reported his extensive experience with the study of the embryogenic development of the human aortic arch system. Edwards[6] developed a schematic model with a double aortic arch system and bilateral ductus arteriosus (Figure 39.1).

Vascular rings are a group of congenital anomalies caused by different regressions and involutions from the embryonic aortic arch system. Several recent papers report the close association of band 22q11 deletion with anomalies of the aortic arch as well as other congenital cardiac abnormalities. In the embryonic aortic arch system, the ventral and dorsal aortae are connected by six primitive aortic arches. The embryo then utilizes the mechanism of programmed cell death (apoptosis) to eliminate redundant and unnecessary components. The multiple branchial arches in the human embryo are an excellent example. They represent the blood supply of gill-breathing organisms, which lie in our phylogenetic past. They are transiently present during human development but either partially or completely disappear as the pulmonary circulation develops and connects with the heart. Only a few segments usually remain. In case unnecessary segments persist, anomalies such as vascular rings may result.

The paired right and left dorsal aortae, one of which will eventually become the descending thoracic aorta, are present in the embryo by approximately the 21st day of intrauterine life. Subsequently, the first to sixth branchial arteries form bilaterally, each with its own aortic arch communicating from the aortic sac to the dorsal aortas.

At this point in development, multiple vascular rings are present. The first and second arches largely resorb and contribute only to minor facial arteries, while the third arches form the carotid arteries. The left fourth arch forms the distal aortic arch and aortic isthmus from the origin of the left common carotid artery to the origin of the descending thoracic aorta, which itself represents a persistence of the left dorsal aorta. So, if the right fourth arch involutes, a normal left arch is formed, which results in the aorta passing from the anterior to the posterior mediastinum to the left of the trachea and esophagus. If the left fourth arch involutes, a right aortic arch is formed. In this case, the aorta courses to the right of the trachea and esophagus from the anterior to the posterior mediastinum.

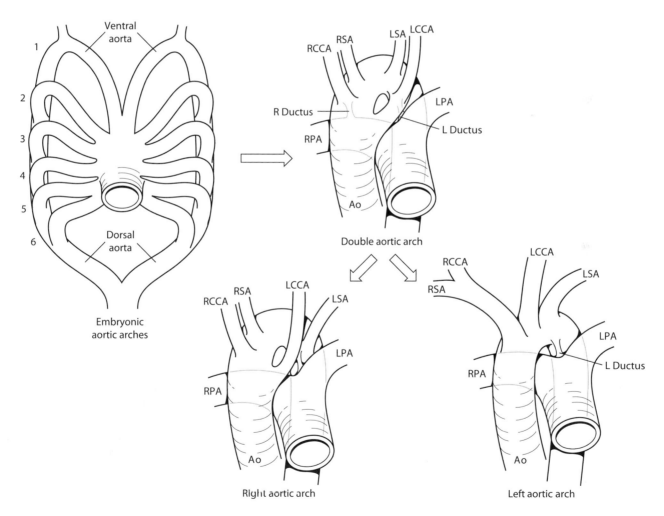

Figure 39.1 Diagram of the embryonic aortic arches. Six pairs of aortic arches originally develop between the dorsal and ventral aorta. The first, second, and fifth arches regress completely. Preservation or deletion of different segments of the rudimentary arches results in a double aortic arch, a right aortic arch, or the normal left aortic arch. Ao: aorta; LCCA, RCCA: left and right common carotid artery; LPA, RPA: left and right pulmonary artery; LSA, RSA: left and right subclavian artery.

Proximally, septation of the conotruncus produces the ascending aorta, which joins with the fourth left arch. The right dorsal aorta ultimately contributes to the right subclavian artery. The first, second, and fifth arches involute to form the Edwards classic double aortic arch.

Stewart et al.[7] summarized these pathologic, embryologic, and roentgenographic correlations of the lesions contributing to anomalies of the aortic arch.

FORMS

Different variations of vascular anomalies exist (listed by incidence):

1. Double aortic arch
2. Right aortic arch
3. Pulmonary artery sling
4. Vascular rings associated with left aortic arch
5. Cervical aorta

Double aortic arch

Double aortic arch is an anomaly in which both right and left arches are present and may be one of several variations (Figure 39.2a–c):

a. Both arches widely patent
b. Hypoplasia of one arch (usually the left)
c. Atresia of one arch (usually the left).

Double aortic arch represents a persistence of both right and left embryonic fourth branchial arches joining the aortic portion of the truncoaortic sac to their respective dorsal aorta. The ascending aorta bifurcates anterior to the trachea, and each arch courses either to the left or to the right of the trachea or esophagus. The larger of the two arches usually crosses posterior to the esophagus and joins with the other arch in the posterior mediastinum to form the unified descending aorta. Thus, a complete vascular ring is formed. Note that the right recurrent laryngeal nerve has to pass around the right aortic arch, rather than being in its usual position around the right subclavian artery. Double aortic arch is rarely associated with congenital heart disease, but when present, tetralogy of Fallot and transposition of the great vessels are most common.

Right aortic arch

In cases of individuals in whom the left fourth branchial arch involutes and the right remains, a right aortic arch is present (Figure 39.3a–c). Right aortic arch occurs less frequently than 1 in 100,000 times in the general population and may exist in the absence of any other anomalies. Its presence is suggestive of the existence of an associated anomaly. About 30% of patients with tetralogy of Fallot have an associated right aortic arch. Persistence of the right arch with involution of the left creates a situation in which the origins of the left subclavian artery and ductus arteriosus can vary. Several of these configurations can produce a vascular ring.

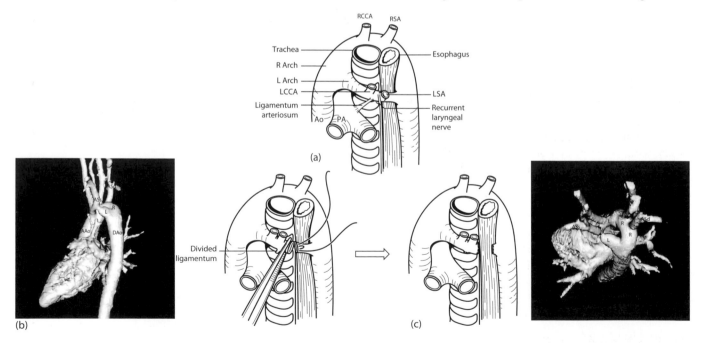

Figure 39.2 Division of a double aortic arch (a). Double aortic arch with a dominant right aortic arch. The lesser left aortic arch is divided between two applied vascular clamps. The stumps are oversewn, and this opens up the desired space for the trachea and esophagus. Ao: aorta; LCCA, RCCA: left and right common carotid artery; PA: pulmonary artery; LSA, RSA: left and right subclavian artery. 3-D rendered images from a contrast-enhanced MRI of a 4-year-old boy with tracheal compression by a double aortic arch. In (b), a left lateral view, and in (c), a cranial view is provided. Interrupted circle: ring formation from both arches; AAo: ascending aorta; DAo: descending aorta; R: right aortic arch; L: left aortic arch; ACs: left carotid artery; ACd: right carotid artery; ASs: left subclavian artery; ASd: right subclavian artery.

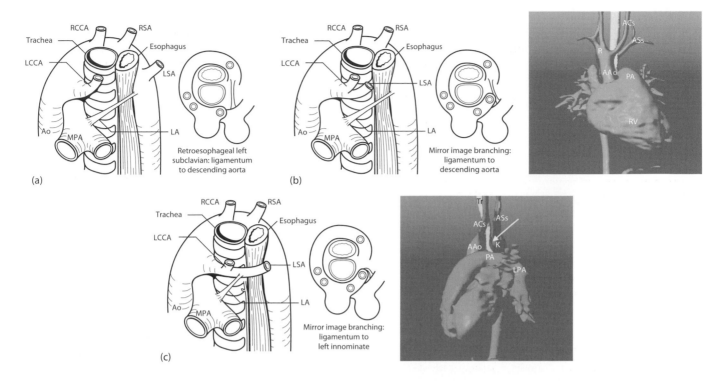

Figure 39.3 Right aortic arch types. **(a)** Retroesophageal left subclavian artery, ligamentum arteriosum to descending aorta. **(b)** Mirror-image branching, ligamentum arteriosum to descending aorta. **(c)** Mirror-image branching, ligamentum arteriosum to the left innominate artery. Ao: aorta; LCCA, RCCA: left and right common carotid artery; MPA: main pulmonary artery; LSA, RSA: left and right subclavian artery. 3-D rendered images from contrast-enhanced MRI of a 2½-year-old boy with tracheal compression by a right aortic arch and abnormal left subclavian artery originating from a large diverticulum of Kommerell. In **(b)**, an anterior view, and in **(c)**, a left lateral view is provided. Arrow: compression of trachea; Tr: trachea; AAo: ascending aorta; DAo: descending aorta; R: right aortic arch, ACs: left carotid artery; ASs: left subclavian artery; K: diverticulum of Kommerell; RV: right ventricle; PA: pulmonary artery; LPA: left pulmonary artery.

RIGHT AORTIC ARCH WITH ABERRANT LEFT SUBCLAVIAN ARTERY AND LEFT LIGAMENTUM ARTERIOSUM

In this anomaly, the right arch first gives off the left carotid artery, which travels anterior to the trachea. It then gives off the right carotid, followed by the right subclavian artery, and, lastly, the left subclavian artery, which courses in a retroesophageal position and gives rise to the ligamentum arteriosum from its base. The ligamentum arteriosum connects the left subclavian or descending aorta to the left pulmonary artery. The trachea and esophagus are surrounded by the ascending aorta anteriorly, the aortic arch on the right, the descending aorta posteriorly, and the ligamentum arteriosum and left pulmonary artery on the left (Figure 39.3b and c). Almost 10% of these defects are associated with an intracardiac defect.

RIGHT AORTIC ARCH WITH MIRROR-IMAGE BRANCHING AND RETROESOPHAGEAL LIGAMENTUM ARTERIOSUM

In these cases, only partial resorption of the distal left fourth arch occurs. The first brachiocephalic vessel originating from the right arch is the left innominate artery, which, in turn, branches into a left carotid and left subclavian artery.

These vessels course anterior to the trachea. Following these, a right carotid artery and then a right subclavian artery arise. The ligamentum arteriosum is the final structure arising from the arch in this sequence. It originates from an area called the Kommerell diverticulum, which represents the nonresorbed remnant of the left fourth arch and is situated at the point of merger between the right arch and the proximal descending thoracic aorta. The ligamentum passes leftward and behind the esophagus and then travels anteriorly to join with the left pulmonary artery and complete the ring.

More commonly, in cases of right aortic arch with mirror-image branching, the ligamentum arteriosum travels from the mirror-image innominate or left subclavian artery to the left pulmonary artery. A complete ring is not present in these cases. Most importantly, this type of vascular ring has a more than 90% association with intracardiac defects.

Pulmonary artery sling

Typically, the left pulmonary artery arises directly from the right pulmonary artery and passes leftward between the trachea and the esophagus (Figure 39.4).[8] The ligamentum arteriosum passes posteriorly from the origin of the right

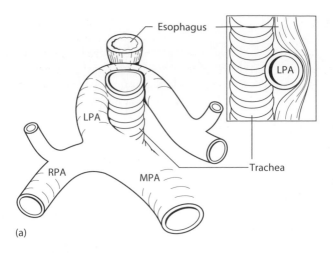

(a)

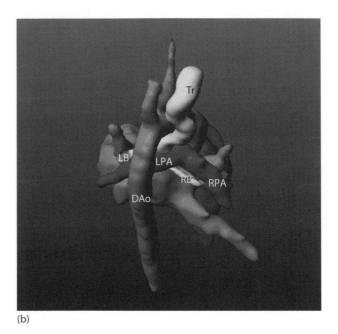

(b)

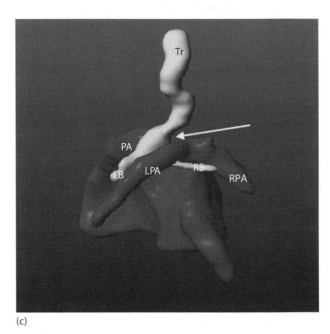

(c)

Figure 39.4 (a–c) Pulmonary artery sling. MPA, LPA, RPA: main pulmonary artery, left pulmonary artery, and right pulmonary artery; inset: lateral view of anterior compression of the esophagus. 3-D rendered images from contrast-enhanced MRI of a 2-week-old male newborn with severe tracheal/bronchial compression and air trapping by a pulmonary sling. In (b), a posterior view of all vascular structures, and in (c), a posterior view only on the pulmonary arteries is provided. Arrow: compression of trachea and right bronchus; Tr: trachea (airways); LB: left bronchus; RB: right bronchus; DAo: descending aorta; RV: right ventricle; PA: pulmonary artery; LPA: left pulmonary artery; RPA: right pulmonary artery.

pulmonary artery, where it arises from the main pulmonary artery to the undersurface of the aortic arch, thus creating a vascular ring surrounding the trachea but not the esophagus. The left pulmonary artery is often relatively hypoplastic. In contrast, the right pulmonary artery appears larger than normal and almost like a direct extension of the main pulmonary artery. The small calibre of the left pulmonary artery may explain the high incidence of anastomotic problems that have been observed in the past with attempts to reimplant the vessel at the main pulmonary artery.

This lesion is often associated with hypoplasia and other abnormalities of the tracheal and bronchial cartilages. Most patients are symptomatic by 1 month after birth. Respiratory symptoms predominate, as the most severe compression is on the trachea. More than 50% of infants also have severe tracheobronchial anomalies such as absence of the posterior membranous component, tracheomalacia, stenosis, webs, or complete tracheal rings. Although the presence of complete rings does not imply that high-graded stenosis will be observed, the trachea is often narrower than normal. The complete rings may be localized at the region where the sling passes around the trachea, although in some cases, the entire trachea consists of complete ringed cartilages. Severe stenosis can involve the carina and extend for a considerable distance into one or both mainstem bronchi. Intracardiac defects are also seen in 20% of these infants.

Vascular rings associated with left aortic arch

Two extremely rare complete rings occur in the presence of a left aortic arch, and both are associated with a right-sided descending thoracic aorta.

LEFT AORTIC ARCH WITH RIGHT DESCENDING AORTA AND RIGHT LIGAMENTUM ARTERIOSUM

The first arch vessel to exit the left aortic arch is the right common carotid, which passes anterior to the trachea. The left carotid is next, followed by the left subclavian artery. The right subclavian artery arises more distally as a branch of the proximal right-sided descending aorta. The ligamentum arteriosum arises from the base of the right subclavian artery or a nearby diverticulum and travels to the right pulmonary artery.

LEFT AORTIC ARCH, RIGHT DESCENDING AORTA, AND ATRETIC RIGHT AORTIC ARCH

The brachiocephalic vessels arise from the left-sided arch in a normal arrangement. The left arch passes behind the esophagus to join a right-sided descending aorta. An atretic right arch is present and completes the ring.

LEFT AORTIC ARCH AND LEFT LIGAMENTUM ARTERIOSUM WITH RETROESOPHAGEAL RIGHT SUBCLAVIAN ARTERY

This is the most common of the arch vessel anomalies, occurring in about 0.5% of the population (Figure 39.5). In these cases, the right subclavian artery does not arise from an innominate trunk with the right carotid artery but originates as the last brachiocephalic branch from the descending aorta and takes a retroesophageal route to its destination (Figure 39.5). In this case, the right subclavian artery is called *arteria lusoria*. A normally positioned

ligamentum arteriosum is present on the left. If a right ligamentum arteriosum were present instead of one on the left, its course would proceed from the base of this anomalous right subclavian artery to the right pulmonary artery, and a complete ring would exist. Instead, no true vascular ring is present in these cases. Most patients are symptomatic, but the occasional patient may present with dysphagia.

LEFT AORTIC ARCH WITH ANOMALOUS ORIGIN OF THE INNOMINATE ARTERY

The actual prevalence of this abnormality is widely debated (Figure 39.6). This is because in as many as 90% of cases in which symptomatic tracheal compression is produced by the innominate artery, the vessel is noted angiographically to have a normal origin from the aorta. When an anatomic abnormality is noted in these cases, the innominate artery appears to originate from a more distal and leftward position on the arch than normal. As it takes its course from left to right, it crosses the trachea anteriorly and in doing so may produce compression of the trachea.

Cervical aorta

This a rare anomaly in which the aorta ascends into the neck on the right or left side, forming a pulsatile mass in the supraclavicular region. Several morphological types have been described according to the side of the aortic arch (contralateral or ipsilateral) and the origin of the head and neck vessels.[9]

CLINICAL FINDINGS

Clinical manifestations are related to the nature of malformation and tightness of the ring. Most children with

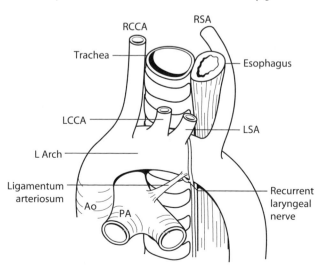

Figure 39.5 Left aortic arch with aberrant right subclavian artery compressing the esophagus. Ao: aorta; LCCA, RCCA: left and right common carotid artery; PA: pulmonary artery; LSA, RSA: left and right subclavian artery.

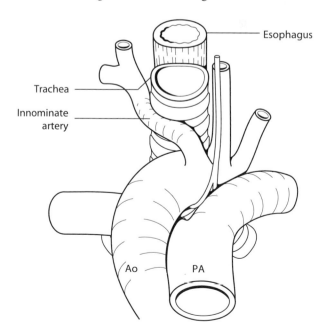

Figure 39.6 Innominate artery compression of the anterior trachea. Ao: aorta; PA: pulmonary artery.

vascular rings present with symptoms in the first few months of life and require surgery within the first year of life.[10] The classic sign of a child with a vascular ring is the "seal-bark" cough. In addition, noisy breathing may be heard during both inspiration and expiration (biphasic stridor), while in asthma, the noise is mainly at the end of expiration. A common finding in all forms of vascular rings is fact that recurrent respiratory infections occur.

In children with double aortic arches, if both arches are widely patent, the rings are tight, and patients present with biphasic stridor in the first weeks of life. In case one arch is hypoplastic or atretic, the rings are usually looser, with presentation at 3–6 months of age. Rarely does a double aortic arch present in adulthood. Children with double aortic arches are often small and poorly developed, and hold their head in hyperextension. Repeated severe respiratory infections may occur.

Children with a pulmonary artery sling and/or complete tracheal rings often have severe respiratory distress requiring emergent intubation and ventilation.

Children with the innominate artery compression syndrome often present with apnea as an initial symptom.

Feeding difficulties occur when solid feeding is attempted to be introduced to the infant. This results in dysphagia and only tends to occur in older children. Gastroesophageal reflux with concomitant pain or fear of food intake is observed. Cyanotic spells in these young patients may have caused episodes that are termed apparent life-threatening events (ALTE) or death spells, in which acute apneic or severe obstructive events are accompanied by cyanosis.

Physical exam may be within normal limits, but one may see coughing, dyspnea, drooling, or dysphagia. Infants will feed poorly due to respiratory distress and may have life-threatening episodes of apnea and cyanosis.

Cardiac exam will most often be normal. Lung exam may or may not show evidence of pneumonia.

ASSOCIATED SYNDROMES AND NONCARDIAC CONDITIONS

Double aortic arch is associated with a chromosome band 22q11 deletion in approximately 20% of patients. Band 22q11 deletion is responsible for *DiGeorge*, *velocardiofacial*, and conotruncal anomaly face syndromes, which are often referred to using the unified terms CATCH-22 syndrome and chromosome band 22q11 deletion syndrome. In patients with double aortic arch, the frequency of phenotypes satisfying the clinical criteria for these various syndromes is not known. Rather, the important point is that double aortic arch may be associated with band 22q11 deletion, which has various other possible manifestations. These include, but are not limited to, palatal abnormalities, laryngotracheal anomalies, speech and learning delay, characteristic facial features, *hypocalcemia*, abnormalities of T-cell-mediated immune function, and neurologic defects.

Occasionally, patients with double aortic arch may have anomalies consistent with either vertebral, anal, cardiac, tracheal, esophageal, renal, and limb (VACTERL) or posterior coloboma, heart defect, choanal atresia, retardation, genital, and ear (CHARGE) associations. Double aortic arch has also been reported in association with other chromosomal anomalies, such as trisomy 21 and other syndromes.

One of the more important noncardiac features that sometimes are found in association with double aortic arch is esophageal atresia, insofar as an undiagnosed arch anomaly may complicate repair of the esophageal atresia, which is usually recognized earlier than the double aortic arch.

Another noncardiac anomaly that may be associated with vascular rings is a congenital laryngeal web, which may present with the same symptoms and signs as a vascular ring. Accordingly, patients with persistent stridor or upper airway obstruction after repair of a vascular ring, particularly those with a chromosome 22q11 deletion, should be evaluated for the presence of a congenital laryngeal web.

DIAGNOSTIC TESTS

Laboratory studies

No laboratory screening or diagnostic study exists for this abnormality.

Chest radiography

Children usually present with symptoms of respiratory difficulty; therefore, chest radiography is always the first and most commonly performed test. Look for the position of the aortic arch, which is usually identifiable on the plain chest radiograph. The identification of a right aortic arch on chest radiograph in a child with airway difficulties, respiratory distress, or dysphagia should alert the clinician to a higher likelihood of a vascular ring. An ill-defined arch location is often observed in patients with double aortic arch. Such a finding should raise the suspicion of an arch anomaly in a symptomatic child. Other radiographic findings that may be noted with vascular rings include compression of the trachea and hyperinflation and or atelectasis of some of the lobes of either lung. A specific finding associated with anomalous left pulmonary artery is hyperinflation of the right lung. In general, chest radiography is not very sensitive in the diagnosis of vascular rings.

Barium esophagram

Most authorities consider barium esophagram to be the most important study in patients with a suspected vascular ring, and it is diagnostic in the vast majority of cases. However, in recent years, computer tomography and magnetic resonance imaging (MRI) have replaced this imaging modality as the primary source of information.

Double aortic arch (Figure 39.7) produces bilateral and posterior compressions of the esophagus, which remain constant regardless of peristalsis. The right indentation is

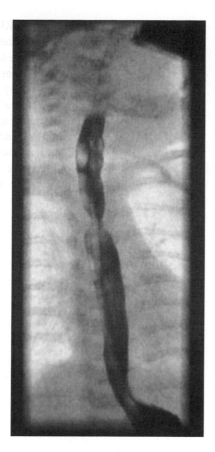

Figure 39.7 Barium esophagram in anteroposterior projection in a patient with double aortic arch.

usually slightly higher than the left, and the posterior compression is usually rather wide and courses in a downward direction as it goes from right to left. Patients having anomalies in which the right subclavian artery takes a retroesophageal course have a posterior defect slanting upward from left to right. The posterior defect in these cases is usually not as broad as that found in double aortic arch. In opposition, in patients with left aortic arch and aberrant subclavian artery, the oblique filling defect is mirror-imaged. An experienced radiologist can usually distinguish a double aortic arch from the retroesophageal subclavian artery based on the esophageal impression.[11]

An anterior indentation of the esophagus is, however, typical of an anomalous left pulmonary artery or so-called pulmonary artery sling. No posterior compression is present with this anomaly. Cases of abnormally located innominate artery causing tracheal compression have normal findings on esophagram.

Echocardiography and color-flow doppler

Echocardiographic studies have been increasingly used for the diagnosis of a vascular ring. This study has replaced pulmonary angiography at many centers to determine the presence of an anomalous left pulmonary artery. It is essential in the diagnostic workup of associated congenital cardiac defects. Some limitations in diagnosis using this study exist. Structures without a lumen, such as a ligamentum arteriosum or an atretic arch, have no blood flow and are difficult to identify with color-flow echocardiography. Also, identification of compressed midline structures and their relationship to encircling vascular anomalies may be difficult to detect, especially for the less experienced echocardiographer.

Computerized tomography scan, magnetic resonance imaging, and digital subtraction angiography

Computerized tomography (CT) scan, MRI, and digital subtraction angiography (DSA) can be useful diagnostic tools because they reveal the positions of vascular, tracheobronchial, and esophageal structures and their relationships to one another. These modalities provide excellent delineation of all of the associated structures. MRI has been proposed as an excellent substitute for angiography. All of these studies have drawbacks. CT scan and DSA expose the patient to radiation and require intravenous contrast. MRI requires patients to remain very still, so very young patients who are unable to understand verbal instructions require sedation. This may be particularly risky in young children with existing airway compromise. The expense encountered with these investigations must also be considered.

Aortic angiography and cardiac catheterization

In the past, diagnostic aortography was performed in selected cases to delineate the anomalous arch vasculature. It is generally agreed at present that echocardiography, CT scan, or MRI can usually provide the required information. However, reported cases exist of rare arch anomalies in which aortography was the only study from which the correct anatomic configuration was identified.[12] This study may be required in cases in which the diagnosis and arch configuration remain in question after other less invasive studies fail to provide a definitive answer. Cardiac catheterization is useful in cases in which associated cardiac abnormalities are known or suspected and echocardiography does not provide adequate diagnostic information.

Bronchoscopy

This diagnostic study has been used in the evaluation of children with symptoms of airway obstruction or compression. It is an essential part of the workup for congenital tracheal stenosis. It is rarely required in the diagnosis of the various types of complete vascular ring. In case a simple vascular ring was diagnosed by other tests, a bronchoscopy should not be performed, due to the added risks and costs.

In the presence of a vascular ring, pulsatile external tracheal compression is easily observed. Note that compression of the airway by a vascular structure in the pediatric patient does not represent an unyielding obstruction and should not pose a problem for passage of the bronchoscope. In cases of an abnormally placed innominate artery, obvious pulsation is observed in the anterior wall of the trachea corresponding to the area of compression. A Kommerell diverticulum produces a pulsating tracheal obstruction placed in the membranous part of the trachea.

INDICATION FOR INTERVENTION

Surgical division of the vascular ring is indicated in any patient who is symptomatic with airway or esophageal compression.

Medical therapy

No medical therapy exists for the definitive treatment of vascular rings. Preoperatively, the patient should be given adequate nutritional support as well as general respiratory care and appropriate treatment of any respiratory tract infection. Surgery should not be delayed in the presence of a respiratory tract infection, because the division of the ring allows more adequate and complete clearing of respiratory secretions.

Surgical therapy

Surgical division of vascular rings causing clinical signs is the only appropriate form of therapy (Table 39.1). Surgery should be performed promptly after the diagnosis is made, especially in patients with stridor, apnea, or other symptoms of respiratory distress. Delay in operative intervention can result in complications of a serious nature. Left thoracotomy is the surgical approach of choice for the division of a vascular ring in the majority of cases. Anomalous left pulmonary artery sling has been corrected using the left thoracotomy approach in the past. More recently, the use of median sternotomy and cardiopulmonary bypass has been shown to produce better long-term results. The extremely rare configurations associated with left aortic arch and right descending thoracic aorta are the lesions that should be approached via a right thoracotomy for division of the ring. General anesthesia with a single-lumen nasotracheal or orotracheal tube is used for infants and small children. Bilateral radial arterial lines and a femoral arterial line together with oxygen saturation probes on all extremities are ideal.

DIVISION OF A DOUBLE AORTIC ARCH

Traditional thoracotomy approach

The surgical approach to a double aortic arch is through a left thoracotomy in the fourth intercostal space with a muscle-sparing technique, and the components of the vascular ring are visualized. The pleura overlying the vascular ring should then be opened and careful dissection performed to clearly identify all the pertinent vascular structures (Figure

Table 39.1 Surgical management

Double Aortic Arch
Left thoracotomy in muscle-sparing technique—fourth interspace
Division of lesser of the two arches at insertion with descending aorta
Preserve blood flow to head and neck arteries
Ligate and divide ligamentum arteriosum
Leave pleura open
Right aortic arch with left ligamentum arteriosum
Left thoracotomy in muscle sparing technique—fourth interspace
Ligate and divide ligamentum arteriosum
If present, resect Kommerell diverticulum and transfer left subclavian to left carotid artery
Lyse adhesive bands
Leave pleura open

Pulmonary Artery Sling
Median sternotomy
Commence extracorporeal circulation
Resect left pulmonary artery (LPA) at its origin at the right pulmonary artery (RPA)
Oversew resulting defect in RPA
Reimplant LPA into main pulmonary artery anterior to trachea
Tracheal sling plasty for affected segment of trachealstenosis

Innominate Artery Compression Syndrome
Right anterolateral thoracotomy (left-sided thoracotomy also possible)—third or fourth interspace
Resect right lobe of thymus
Suspend innominate artery to posterior sternum
Postoperative bronchoscopy

39.8a). The right, or posterior, arch does not require mobilization unless it is the lesser of the two arches and is to be divided. In such cases, the proximal descending aorta should be reflected anteriorly to visualize the area where the right arch enters.

The goal of surgical therapy is to divide the smaller of the two arches at a site that does not compromise the blood flow to the head vessels. A likely site for division of the minor, or atretic, arch is at its point of juncture with the descending aorta. Identify and avoid the recurrent laryngeal and vagus nerves. Before dividing the arch, it should be temporarily occluded and the anesthesiologist asked to check right and left radial and carotid pulses. Arch division should always be done between vascular clamps with oversewing of the divided stumps with nonabsorbable sutures. Simple ligation and division has been associated with ligature slippage and subsequent catastrophic hemorrhage. The divided stumps typically separate by 1.5–2 cm and disappear into the posterior mediastinum, making precise hemostasis quite

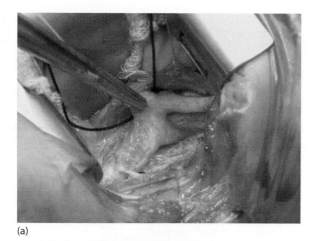

(a)

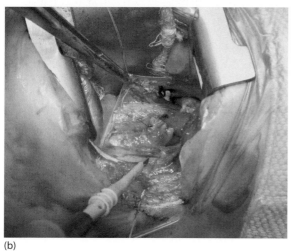

(b)

Figure 39.8 (a and b) Operative photograph taken during dissection after posterolateral thoracotomy in a patient with double aortic arch. The parietal pleura is opened, and the vascular structures are dissected. The left-sided ductus arteriosus is looped by a silk tie. The double aortic arch is divided by transaction and oversewing of the anterior arch at its junction with the descending aorta. The left-sided ductus arteriosus is tied, and only the aortic component is still visible. Note the resulting gap between the two stumps of the anterior aortic arch.

important. The operative repair is completed by freeing up all adhesive bands surrounding the esophagus in the area of the divided ring (Figure 39.8b).

Closure of the mediastinal pleura is not performed to avoid the development of adhesive scarring in the already affected area of the trachea and esophagus. The thoracotomy incision is closed without a chest tube by evacuating air from the pleural space with a small suction catheter. It may take up to 1 year for the child's noisy breathing to disappear as the tracheobronchomalacia caused by the ring resolves.

Video-assisted technique

A couple of groups advocate this technique as the method of choice for treatment of vascular rings, unless preoperative studies suggest that a patent segment of a double aortic arch is present.[13-15]

The patient is placed in right lateral decubitus position following single-lumen endotracheal intubation. Four small stab incisions are made in the posterolateral chest wall to admit from medial to lateral a grasping forceps, a lung retractor, a video scope, and an L-shaped cautery probe. Exposure is achieved by retracting the inflated left upper lobe inferiorly and medially. The mediastinal pleura is incised over the left subclavian artery, which leads to the other components of the vascular ring. The ring is dissected free from the esophagus and surrounding structures. The atretic segment of the vascular ring and ligamentum are identified. Clips are placed, and the ring and the ligamentum are divided between clips. Fibrous bands over the esophagus are also freed. A small chest tube is placed under direct vision, and the wounds are closed with Steri-Strips.[13,16]

RIGHT AORTIC ARCH

Surgical treatment of this condition also consists of dividing the ductus arteriosus or the ligamentum arteriosum. Division of the left subclavian artery is not generally necessary for relieving tracheal compression. Patients with an anomalous left subclavian artery and Kommerell[17] diverticulum are at risk of developing severe tracheal compression. Backer et al.[18-21] have recommended resection of the diverticulum and reimplantation of the left subclavian artery to the left carotid artery as a primary operation.[22] Surgery is performed through a muscle-sparing left lateral thoracotomy in the fourth intercostal space. As an alternative approach, the Kommerell diverticulum may be approached via median sternotomy. After dissection of the vascular structures and division of the ligamentum arteriosum, the patient is anticoagulated. Any adhesive bands are lysed, and the recurrent laryngeal and phrenic nerves are carefully identified and protected. The base of the Kommerell diverticulum is taken in a side-biting clamp, and the distal subclavian artery is occluded with a vascular clamp prior to its division. The diverticulum is resected and its base oversewn. The left subclavian artery is then anastomosed to the origin of the left carotid artery. This anastomosis may be performed more easily via the sternotomy approach.

PULMONARY ARTERY SLING

Although the traditional approach has been through a left-sided thoracotomy with reimplantation at the original site of the left pulmonary artery as performed in 1953 by Potts et al.[3] and then reimplantation of the left pulmonary artery on the left side of the main pulmonary artery as described by Hiller and MacLean,[23] currently, the preferred method is to undertake repair via median sternotomy. With this approach and utilizing cardiopulmonary bypass, reimplantation of the left pulmonary artery onto the left side of the main pulmonary artery without application of a side-biting clamp is carried out without aortic cross-clamping. If tracheal repair is necessary, it can be performed thereafter, or tracheal repair is performed on cardiopulmonary bypass and the left pulmonary artery is relocated in front of the trachea after extensive dissection of the left pulmonary artery into the left hilum. This technique was introduced by Kirklin and Barrat-Boyes.[24] Different techniques are utilized for tracheal repair depending on the length and site of the tracheal stenosis. Over recent years, many different types of repair have been undertaken, including simple end-to-end repair,[25,26] various forms of patch tracheoplasty,[27,28] tracheal homograft implantation,[29,30] and slide tracheoplasty.[31–36] In recent years, slide tracheoplasty has been favored by most groups.

A review of these methods is beyond the scope of this chapter, but more comprehensive reviews are available.[20,21,35–40]

LEFT AORTIC ARCH WITH ANOMALOUS ORIGIN OF THE INNOMINATE ARTERY

The surgical treatment of this anomaly is based on the suspension of the innominate artery from the posterior aspect of the sternum. This operation can be performed from either side.[41,42] The thymus lobe of the corresponding side is resected and the pericardium opened respecting the phrenic nerve. The ascending aorta or the innominate artery is approximated to the posterior aspect of the sternum by two or three interrupted pledget-supported heavy sutures. Bronchoscopy is then performed to confirm the tracheal relief. In order to relief the compression of the trachea it is essential not to dissect a plane between the great vessels and the trachea, so the tension applied by the suture on the vessels is transferred to the trachea's anterior wall.

Other authors have described using a median sternotomy with division of the innominate artery and reimplantation into the ascending aorta at a site more rightward and anterior to the native site.[43] This technique sacrifices the active suspending mechanism on the tracheal wall provided by the classical suspension maneuver. In addition, there seems to be some risk of cerebrovascular accident, although Grimmer et al.[44] report no cerebrovascular injury in a long-term follow-up study.

Results

TRADITIONAL THORACOTOMY APPROACH

One of the largest reports of vascular anomalies causing tracheoesophageal compression comes from Backer et al. from the Children's Memorial Hospital in Chicago, United States, published in 1989[10] and updated in 2005.[19] The authors described 204 infants and children with a mean age of 13 months who had undergone surgical procedures for tracheoesophageal obstruction. Of these, 113 patients had a vascular ring, 61 with a double aortic arch and 52 with a right aortic arch and left ligamentum. The operative mortality rate was 4.9% with a late mortality rate of 3.4%. However, there were no operative deaths within the last 28 years. At a mean follow-up of 8.5 years, 92% of the patients were essentially free of symptoms.

In 1994, Cordovilla Zurdo et al.[45] from Madrid, Spain, reported on a series of 43 patients with one hospital and one late death. Over a mean follow-up of 11 years, 90% of the patients were asymptomatic. Similarly, Anand et al.[46] from Atlanta, Georgia, United States, reported on 44 patients operated on for vascular ring or pulmonary artery sling in the period of 1977–1990. In this series, three deaths due to cardiac failure after repair of complex anomalies were reported.

Further studies report on good long-term results with low operative mortality. Mortality seems to be limited and only occurring in patients with complex cardiac anomalies.[47–50]

Video-assisted technique

At the moment, only a limited number of publications are available reporting on results after thoracoscopic division of vascular rings.[13–16] In these series, no mortality was observed. However, stay in the intensive care unit (ICU) and in the hospital was not different from the conventional technique. It should be taken into account that this technique offers only a limited amount of control, and in addition, the surgical times are much longer than the conventional procedures. In addition, the video-assisted technique is only applicable if the vascular structures to be divided are obliterated.

Pulmonary artery sling with tracheal repair

Kocyildirim from Great Ormond Street Hospital for Children, London, United Kingdom, reports in his study on 34 patients with long-segment tracheal stenosis (21 patients with pulmonary artery sling). Cardiopulmonary bypass was used in all operations. Before the establishment of the multidisciplinary tracheal team, pericardial patch tracheoplasty was performed in 15 of 19 patients. Twelve patients had a suspended pericardial patch tracheoplasty, 2 (17%) of whom died late after the operation. Of 3 patients who had had a simple unsuspended patch, 2 (67%) died early after the operation. Four patients were operated on with the tracheal autograft technique, 2 (50%) dying early in the postoperative period. After multidisciplinary tracheal team formation, in the era between 2001 and 2004, 15 patients were operated on with slide tracheoplasty, and there were 2 (13%) early postoperative deaths. A significant reduction in cost and duration of stay has been shown in both the ICU and the hospital.[51]

Backer from the Children's Memorial Hospital in Chicago, United States, reports on 28 infants after pericardial tracheoplasty for long-segment tracheal stenosis. Seven of these infants required reoperation or stenting for residual or recurrent tracheal or bronchial stenosis. Revisions were performed 2–6 months after the original procedure with cardiopulmonary bypass and bronchoscopic guidance. Two patients underwent repeat pericardial patch tracheoplasty, and four patients underwent insertion of a rib cartilage graft. Two of these patients required Palmaz wire expandable stents, and one other patient also underwent stent placement. There was one late death 1 year after cartilage graft insertion. The authors identified three risk factors for reoperation after tracheoplasty: younger age at initial surgery and associated pulmonary artery sling or tracheal right upper lobe bronchus. Good intermediate results are possible in this difficult group of children using a selective and inclusive strategy for tracheal enlargement that includes repeat pericardial tracheoplasty, autologous cartilage grafts, and expandable wire stents.[52,53]

CONCLUSION AND FUTURE DIRECTIONS

Nowadays, children presenting with tracheal or esophageal obstructions caused by congenital vascular malformations can be treated with low morbidity and a minute mortality. Conventional surgery involving thoracotomy or median sternotomy is still the standard of treatment. Minimally invasive approaches have been developed, but further technical advances are necessary to promote a wider dissemination of these techniques.

REFERENCES

1. Hommel TW. On irregularities of the pulmonary artery, arch of the aorta and primary branches of the arch with an attempt to illustrate their mode of origin by a reference to development. *Br Foreign Medico-Chirurg Rev* 1962; 30: 173.
2. Gross R. Surgical relief for tracheal obstruction from a vascular ring. *N Engl J Med* 1945; 233: 586–90.
3. Potts WJ, Holinger PH, Rosenblum AH. Anomalous left pulmonary artery causing obstruction to right main bronchus: Report of a case. *J Am Med Assoc* 1954; 155: 1409–11.
4. Glavecke H, Döhle W. Über eine seltene angeborene Anomalie der Pulmonalarterie. *München Med Wochenschr* 1897; 44: 950.
5. Congdon E. Transformation of the aortic arch system during the development of the human embryo. *Contrib Embryol* 1922; 14: 47.
6. Edwards J. Anomalies of the derivates of the aortic arch system. *Med Clin North Am* 1948; 32: 925.
7. Stewart J, Kincaid O, Edwards J. *An Atlas of Vascular Rings and Related Malformations of the Aortic Arch System.* Springfield, Illinois: Charles C. Thomas Publisher, 1964.
8. Wolman I. Congenital stenosis of the trachea. *Am J Dis Child* 1941; 61:1263.
9. Haughton VM, Fellows KE, Rosenbaum AE. The cervical aortic arches. *Radiology* 1975; 114: 675–81.
10. Backer CL, Ilbawi MN, Idriss FS, DeLeon SY. Vascular anomalies causing tracheoesophageal compression. Review of experience in children. *J Thorac Cardiovasc Surg* 1989; 97: 725–31.
11. Neuauser E. The roentgen diagnosis of double aortic arch and other anomalies of the great vessels. *Am J Roentgenol* 1946; 56: 1.
12. Singh GK, Greenberg SB, Balsara RK. Diagnostic dilemma: Left aortic arch with right descending aorta—A rare vascular ring. *Pediatr Cardiol* 1997; 18: 45–8.
13. Burke RP, Rosenfeld HM, Wernovsky G, Jonas RA. Video-assisted thoracoscopic vascular ring division in infants and children. *J Am Coll Cardiol* 1995; 25: 943–7.
14. Koontz CS, Bhatia A, Forbess J, Wulkan ML. Video-assisted thoracoscopic division of vascular rings in pediatric patients. *Am J Surg* 2005; 71: 289–91.
15. Kogon BE, Forbess JM, Wulkan ML, Kirshbom PM, Kanter KR. Video-assisted thoracoscopic surgery: Is it a superior technique for the division of vascular rings in children? *Congenit Heart Dis* 2007; 2: 130–3.
16. Burke RP, Wernovsky G, van der Velde M, Hansen D, Castaneda AR. Video-assisted thoracoscopic surgery for congenital heart disease. *J Thorac Cardiovasc Surg* 1995; 109: 499–507; discussion 508.
17. Kommerell B. Verlagerung durch eine abnorm verlaufende Arteria subclavia dextra (Arteria lusoria). *Fortschritte Gebiet Röntgenstr* 1936; 54: 590.
18. Backer CL, Hillman N, Mavroudis C, Holinger LD. Resection of Kommerell's diverticulum and left subclavian artery transfer for recurrent symptoms after vascular ring division. *Eur J Cardiothorac Surg* 2002; 22: 64–69.
19. Backer CL, Mavroudis C, Rigsby CK, Holinger LD. Trends in vascular ring surgery. *J Thorac Cardiovasc Surg* 2005; 129: 1339–47.
20. Backer CL, Hyde MR, Wurlitzer KC, Rastatter JC, Rigsby CK. Primary resection of Kommerell diverticulum and left subclavian artery transfer. *Ann Thorac Surg* 2012; 94: 1612–8.
21. Backer CL, Russell HM, Kaushal S, Rastatter JC, Rigsby CK, Holinger LD. Pulmonary artery sling: Current results with cardiopulmonary bypass. *J Thorac Cardiovasc Surg* 2012; 143: 144–51.
22. Shinkawa T, Greenberg SB, Jaquiss RDB, Imamura M. Primary translocation of aberrant left subclavian artery for children with symptomatic vascular ring. *Ann Thorac Surg* 2012; 93: 1262–5.
23. Hiller HG, Maclean AD. Pulmonary artery ring. *Acta Radiol* 1957; 48: 434–8.
24. Kirklin J, Barratt-Boyes B. *Cardiac Surgery.* Hoboken: John Wiley, 1986.
25. Jonas RA, Spevak PJ, McGill T, Castaneda AR. Pulmonary artery sling: Primary repair by tracheal resection in infancy. *J Thorac Cardiovasc Surg* 1989; 97: 548–50.
26. Cotter CS, Jones DT, Nuss RC, Jonas R. Management of distal tracheal stenosis. *Arch Otolaryngol Head Neck Surg* 1999; 125: 325–8.
27. Bando K, Turrentine MW, Sun K, Sharp TG, Matt B, Karmazyn B, Heifetz SA, Stevens J, Kesler KA, Brown JW. Anterior pericardial tracheoplasty

for congenital tracheal stenosis: Intermediate to long-term outcomes. *Ann Thorac Surg* 1996; 62: 981–9.

28. Idriss FS, DeLeon SY, Ilbawi MN, Gerson CR, Tucker GF, Holinger L. Tracheoplasty with pericardial patch for extensive tracheal stenosis in infants and children. *J Thorac Cardiovasc Surg* 1984; 88: 527–36.

29. Schlosshauer B. Zur Verhütung und Behandlung von Kehlkopf- und Luftröhrenstenosen im Kindesalter. *HNO* 1975; 23: 342–4.

30. Herberhold C, Stein M, von Falkenhausen M. Langzeitresultate von Homograftrekonstruktionen der Trachea im Kindesalter. *Laryngorhinootologie* 1999; 78: 692–6.

31. Grillo HC. Slide tracheoplasty for long-segment congenital tracheal stenosis. *Ann Thorac Surg* 1994; 58: 613–9; discussion 619–21.

32. Tsang V, Murday A, Gillbe C, Goldstraw P. Slide tracheoplasty for congenital funnel-shaped tracheal stenosis. *Ann Thorac Surg* 1989; 48: 632–5.

33. Dayan SH, Dunham ME, Backer CL, Mavroudis C, Holinger LD. Slide tracheoplasty in the management of congenital tracheal stenosis. *Ann Otol Rhinol Laryngol* 1997; 106: 914–9.

34. Elliott M, Hartley BE, Wallis C, Roebuck D. Slide tracheoplasty. *Curr Opin Otolaryngol Head Neck Surg* 2008; 16: 75–82.

35. Beierlein W, Elliott MJ. Variations in the technique of slide tracheoplasty to repair complex forms of long-segment congenital tracheal stenosis. *Ann Thorac Surg* 2006; 82: 1540–2.

36. Elliott M, Roebuck D, Noctor C, McLaren C, Hartley B, Mok Q, Dunne C, Pigott N, Patel C, Patel A, Wallis C. The management of congenital tracheal stenosis. *Int J Pediatr Otorhinolaryngol* 2003; 67 Supplement 1: S183–92.

37. Backer CL, Mavroudis C, Gerber ME, Holinger LD. Tracheal surgery in children: An 18-year review of four techniques. *Eur J Cardiothorac Surg* 2001; 19: 777–84.

38. Manning PB, Rutter MJ, Lisec A, Gupta R, Marino BS. One slide fits all: The versatility of slide tracheoplasty with cardiopulmonary bypass support for airway reconstruction in children. *J Thorac Cardiovasc Surg* 2011; 141:155–61.

39. Yong MS, d'Udekem Y, Brizard CP, Robertson T, Robertson CF, Weintraub R, Konstantinov IE. Surgical management of pulmonary artery sling in children. *J Thorac Cardiovasc Surg* 2013; 145: 1033–9.

40. Butler CR, Speggiorin S, Rijnberg FM, Roebuck DJ, Muthialu N, Hewitt RJ, Elliott MJ. Outcomes of slide tracheoplasty in 101 children: A 17-year single-center experience. *J Thorac Cardiovasc Surg* 2014; 147: 1783–9.

41. Gross RE, Neuhauser EB. Compression of the trachea by an anomalous innominate artery; An operation for its relief. *Am J Dis Child* 1948; 75: 570–574.

42. Moes CA, Izukawa T, Trusler GA. Innominate artery compression of the trachea. *Arch Otolaryngol* 1975; 101: 733–8.

43. Hawkins JA, Bailey WW, Clark SM. Innominate artery compression of the trachea. Treatment by reimplantation of the innominate artery. *J Thorac Cardiovasc Surg* 1992; 103: 678–82.

44. Grimmer JF, Herway S, Hawkins JA, Park AH, Kouretas PC. Long-term results of innominate artery reimplantation for tracheal compression. *Arch Otolaryngol Head Neck Surg* 2009; 135: 80–4.

45. Cordovilla Zurdo G, Cabo Salvador J, Sanz Galeote E, Moreno Granados F, Alvarez Diaz F. Anillos vasculares de origen aortico: Experiencia quirurgica en 43 casos. *Rev Esp Cardiol* 1994; 47: 468–75.

46. Anand R, Dooley KJ, Williams WH, Vincent RN. Follow-up of surgical correction of vascular anomalies causing tracheobronchial compression. *Pediatr Cardiol* 1994; 15: 58–61.

47. Ruzmetov M, Vijay P, Rodefeld MD, Turrentine MW, Brown JW. Follow-up of surgical correction of aortic arch anomalies causing tracheoesophageal compression: A 38-year single institution experience. *J Pediatr Surg* 2009; 44: 1328–32.

48. Sebening C, Jakob H, Tochtermann U, Lange R, Vahl CF, Bodegom P, Szabo G, Fleischer F, Schmidt K, Zilow E, Springer W, Ulmer HE, Hagl S. Vascular tracheobronchial compression syndromes— Experience in surgical treatment and literature review. *Thorac Cardiovasc Surg* 2000; 48: 164–74.

49. Yilmaz M, Ozkan M, Dogan R, Demircin M, Ersoy U, Boke E, Pasaoglu I. Vascular anomalies causing tracheoesophageal compression: A 20-year experience in diagnosis and management. *Heart Surg Forum* 2003; 6: 149–52.

50. van Son JA, Julsrud PR, Hagler DJ, Sim EK, Pairolero PC, Puga FJ, Schaff HV, Danielson GK. Surgical treatment of vascular rings: The Mayo Clinic experience. *Mayo Clin Proc* 1993; 68: 1056–63.

51. Kocyildirim E, Kanani M, Roebuck D, Wallis C, McLaren C, Noctor C, Pigott N, Mok Q, Hartley B, Dunne C, Uppal S, Elliott MJ. Long-segment tracheal stenosis: Slide tracheoplasty and a multidisciplinary approach improve outcomes and reduce costs. *J Thorac Cardiovasc Surg* 2004; 128: 876–82.

52. Backer CL, Mavroudis C, Dunham ME, Holinger LD. Reoperation after pericardial patch tracheoplasty. *J Pediatr Surg* 1997; 32: 1108–11; discussion 1111–2.

53. Backer CL, Mavroudis C, Dunham ME, Holinger L. Intermediate-term results of the free tracheal autograft for long segment congenital tracheal stenosis. *J Pediatr Surg* 2000; 35: 813–8; discussion 818–9.

40

Pulmonary air leaks

PREM PURI AND JENS DINGEMANN

INTRODUCTION

Pulmonary air leaks include urgent life-threatening neonatal emergencies like pulmonary interstitial emphysema (PIE), pneumomediastinum, pneumothorax (PT), or pneumopericardium.[1-4] The incidence of pulmonary air leaks in the neonates has increased in recent years, possibly because an increasing number of sick infants with respiratory distress on assisted ventilation are now surviving to develop this complication.[5] The sequence of events in the occurrence of pulmonary air leaks is similar regardless of whether it is caused by uneven alveolar ventilation, air trapping, and high transpulmonary pressure swings. The rupture of terminal air sacs causes air to escape into the pulmonary interstitium, resulting in pulmonary interstitial emphysema. The air tracks along the sheaths of pulmonary blood vessels to the lung hilum and air may then rupture into mediastinum, pleura, or pericardium.[6] It has also been suggested that air directly enters the pleural cavity following a rupture of a subpleural bleb.[7] Rarely systemic air embolism may be a terminal event of pulmonary air leaks.

PULMONARY INTERSTITIAL EMPHYSEMA

PIE is predominantly seen in preterm infants with respiratory distress syndrome (RDS) who are on assisted ventilation.[8] Occasionally, it follows vigorous resuscitative efforts. The lesion represents air that has dissected along perivascular sheath within pulmonary interstitium. The compression caused by interstitial "air conduits" interferes with ventilation and reduces pulmonary perfusion leading to CO_2 retention and hypoxemia.

The incidence of PIE increases with low birth weight (LBW) and prematurity. In one series, 20 out of 303 ventilated LBW babies developed PIE,[9] but significantly high incidences of 32% and 42% have been reported in other series.[10,11]

Presentation and diagnosis

PIE may be diffuse or localized. Transillumination of the chest with diffuse PIE will give the same appearance as a large pneumothorax.[12] However, chest x-ray is the method of choice to diagnose PIE. The radiological features consist of hyperinflation and multiple cyst-like lucencies that appear to radiate outward from the hilum of the lung (Figure 40.1). Suspect neonates should be monitored by daily chest x-ray for an earlier diagnosis of PIE. At a later stage, large bullae may appear. The localized form of PIE may be misdiagnosed as cystic adenomatoid malformation of the lung.

Treatment

PIE, diffuse or localized, makes ventilatory management difficult. It is mandatory to use appropriate ventilation strategies to prevent PIE or its deterioration, respectively. Ventilatory pressures should be kept at a safe minimum while aiming for acceptable blood gas values of $PaO_2 > 6-7$ kPa, pH > 7.25, and $PaCO_2 < 8$ kPa.[13]

No specific surgical treatment is indicated for diffuse PIE. Benefit has been demonstrated for both High Frequency Positive Pressure Mechanical Ventilation (HFPPV) and triggered ventilation with regard to a reduction in air leak and a shorter duration of ventilation.[13] Also the prophylactic application of surfactant has been shown to be beneficial for the outcome of preterm infants with PIE.[14] If the disease is unilateral or localized, selective partial or complete atelectasis of the desired segment can be achieved by selective bronchial intubation[15,16] or by placing the infant with his or her hyperinflated lung dependent in the lateral decubitus position at all times.[17]

An aggressive approach of decompressing the lungs and creation of artificial pneumothorax has been described for patients in whom conservative management fails. This approach has been shown to successfully remove interstitial gas, and after re-evacuation of the pneumothorax, ventilation could be discontinued shortly.[18]

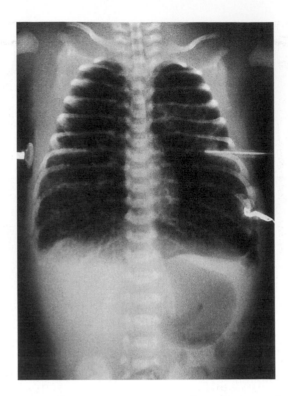

Figure 40.1 Diffuse PIE in a baby weighing 1200 g and requiring prolonged positive pressure ventilation for hyaline membrane disease. The lungs are grossly hyperinflated with a diffuse cystic pattern in this film at 7 days of life. Note narrow heart shadow due to tamponade effect of the distended lungs. A shallow pneumothorax is present in the left upper zone and a left chest drain has been inserted.

Surgery is reserved for patients in whom conservative or interventional therapy failed. However, localized PIE has been successfully treated by atypical wedge resection[19] and lobectomy.[20]

Prognosis

The mortality rate from diffuse PIE has been reported to be from 24% to as high as 60%.[9,21] There have been no significant differences in neonatal parameters between infants who died or survived. However, the survivors had a significantly lower maximal peak inspiratory pressure and FiO_2 on the first day of ventilation.[21]

PIE is invariably fatal in the group of neonates with RDS who weigh <1600 g at birth and who develop bilateral PIE within the first 48 hours of life, needing FiO_2 above 0.6 on the first day. High positive inspiratory pressure on day 1 was found to be the most significant parameter associated with fatal PIE. A cutoff level of 26 cmH$_2$O was found to be discriminant.[22] These criteria may be useful in selecting neonates who might benefit best from the new modes of ventilation. In preterm infants, additional application of surfactant significantly reduces the mortality of PIE.[14] In the survivors, diffuse PIE greatly increases the incidence of bronchopulmonary dysplasia, contributing to the long-term sequelae of RDS in preterm infants.[12]

PNEUMOMEDIASTINUM

Pneumomediastinum develops when interstitial air in PIE migrates to the mediastinum. Also spontaneous pneumomediastinum without any history of mechanical ventilation or concomitant lung disease has been reported.[23] If the collection of air is small, it remains asymptomatic. However, large collections of mediastinal air may produce respiratory distress.[23] Heart sounds are muffled and the sternum may appear bowed.

The diagnosis is made on chest x-ray. The anteroposterior views may show the characteristic "angel-wing" sign produced by air elevating the thymus gland (Figure 40.2a).

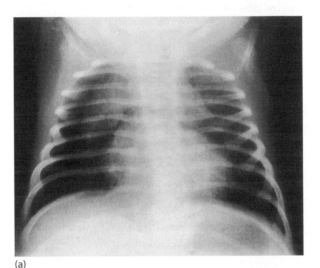

(a)

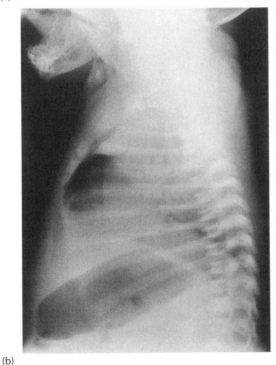

(b)

Figure 40.2 Pneumomediastinum. **(a)** Anteroposterior view demonstrates the characteristic "angel wing" sign produced by air elevating the thymus from the heart. **(b)** Lateral view confirms air in the anterior mediastinum.

It has also been described as having a crescentic configuration resembling a "spinnaker sail."[4] Lateral x-ray of the chest shows marked hyperlucency in the anterior mediastinum (Figure 40.2b). Ultrasound can be used to diagnose pneumomediastinum. It has been reported to be superior to x-ray under certain conditions and should be considered if a pneumomediastinum is clinically suspected and x-ray shows no typical findings.[24]

Retrocardiac pneumomediastinum has a strong association with other manifestations of extra-alveolar air leaks such as PIE, pneumothorax, dissection of air into the soft tissues of the neck, and pneumoperitoneum. Tension pneumomediastinum has also been described to cause isolated left ventricular inflow obstruction. Symptomatic pneumomediastinum is managed by ultrasound-guided needle aspiration of the anterior mediastinal compartment.[25] Successful chest tube insertion into the anterior mediastinum under ultrasound guidance has also been described in a preterm infant with tension pneumomediastinum in whom initial needle aspiration had not led to relief of symptoms. In asymptomatic cases, air is absorbed spontaneously and no treatment is indicated.

PNEUMOTHORAX

Pneumothorax is far more frequent in the newborn period than in any other period of life—symptomatic pneumothorax occurs in 0.08% of all live births[26] and in 5%–7% of infants with birth weight of ≤1500 g.[27,28] It is bilateral in about 20% of cases.[29] Pneumothorax in the newborn predominantly occurs in patients with hyaline membrane disease, meconium aspiration syndrome, pulmonary hypoplasia, and infants requiring vigorous resuscitation at birth.[29–31]

In ventilated preterm infants, it has been shown to be attributed to high peak inspiratory pressure low Fio_2, pulmonary hemorrhage, and high arterial CO_2, while a decreased risk was associated with high positive end-expiratory pressure.[32]

The overall incidence of pneumothorax in the newborn with respiratory difficulties has been reported to be as high as 34% of those who are ventilated.[33] Pneumothorax can also be caused as a complication of deep endotracheal tube suction[34] and by other iatrogenic perforation of the bronchus. A rare association of spontaneous pneumothorax with congenital cystic adenomatoid malformation[35] and early spontaneous pneumothorax with common pulmonary vein atresia[36] have been reported. The "surgical" cases of pneumothorax and/or pneumomediastinum at the Liverpool Neonatal Surgical Centre included infants with gross renal anomalies, large exomphalos, a rare type of vascular sling, and spontaneous perforation of esophagus. In half of the cases, the etiology was less obvious.[37]

PRESENTATION AND DIAGNOSIS

Pneumothorax should be suspected in infants with respiratory distress who suddenly deteriorate. Tachypnea is a uniform finding and is often accompanied by grunting, chest retractions, and cyanosis. Physical findings in unilateral pneumothorax include a shift of the cardiac impulse to the

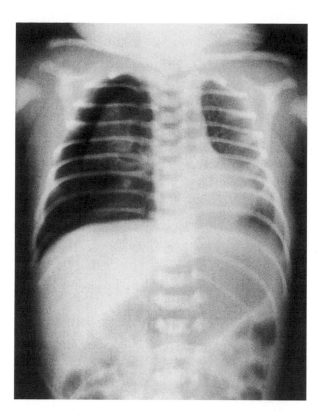

Figure 40.3 Right pneumothorax complicating interstitial emphysema in an infant with hyaline membrane disease. Note air lucency around right lung with absence of lung markings. The mediastinum is shifted to the left, indicating tension.

unaffected side, diminished or absent breath sounds, and a hyperresonant percussion note on the affected side. In tension pneumothorax, arterial hypotension, apnea, and bradycardia are usually the initial signs.

A large pneumothorax can be diagnosed by transillumination using a high-intensity light with fiber-optic probe.[38] The advantage of this method is the rapidity with which large life-threatening pneumothoraces can be diagnosed and treated. The gold standard for diagnosis is radiography of the chest. A large pneumothorax is easily recognizable in infants by identification of the visceral pleural line, which is most readily seen over the apex and along the costal surface of the lung (Figure 40.3). Other important observations in pneumothoraces are a mediastinal shift and absence of lung markings. Small volume pneumothoraces are more difficult to identify, and in these cases, lateral decubitus cross-table views are very helpful in showing the rise in pleural air to the lateral or medial side of the hemithorax (Figure 40.4). Rarely, lobar emphysema, congenital cystic adenomatoid malformation, or congenital diaphragmatic hernia may resemble pneumothorax in the chest x-ray.[12]

TREATMENT

Most small pneumothoraces with no symptoms need only close observation and monitoring in a neonatal intensive

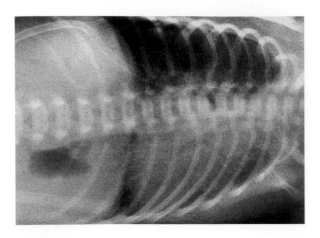

Figure 40.4 Small-volume pneumothorax demonstrated in the lateral decubitus view with the right side raised.

care unit.[39] The ventilatory management should aim to keep pressures at lower acceptable values including the use of patient-triggered ventilation and high-frequency positive pressure ventilation[13] such as adjuvant neuromuscular paralysis of the infant.[40] A pneumothorax should be drained in the following situations:

- Radiological signs of tension pneumothorax
- Cardiorespiratory symptoms
- Infants on intermittent positive pressure ventilation, even if asymptomatic

The infant should be temporarily disconnected from the ventilator during the introduction of a chest drain or aspiration of a pneumothorax to avoid the risk of lung damage.[41]

In a desperately ill neonate, a life-saving emergency needle aspiration of a tension pneumothorax can be done before formal insertion of a chest drain. A butterfly (18-gauge) or i.v. cannula with a three-way tap and a 20 ml syringe can be used for decompression. Aspiration is performed through the second intercostal space in the midclavicular line. The insertion of the needle is oblique through the muscle plane to avoid entry of air once the needle is removed. Occasionally a single aspiration may be enough, but all these babies must be closely observed and monitored clinically and radiologically as nearly all of them require a tube thoracostomy on follow-up.

Tube thoracostomy is required in the majority of cases. A chest drain (10–14 French gauge) is inserted through the second intercostal space in the midclavicular line or the sixth space in the mid-axillary line under local anesthesia. The tip of the chest tube should be placed anteriorly retrosternally for better drainage.[42] A purse-string stitch around the site of the catheter insertion is not necessary in neonates. The insertion site should be closed with a waterproof adhesive plastic film to avoid any air leak. After fixing the catheter firmly, it is connected to an underwater seal drain with or without a low-grade suction of 5–10 cmH$_2$O. Once the lung is expanded and stable, the tube can then be removed. A chest film after

removal of the tube to ensure that a pneumothorax has not recurred should only be done if this is clinically suspected.

Use of conventional chest drains is not free from complication as they can cause lung perforation[41] or phrenic nerve injury related to abnormal location of the medial end of the chest tube.[43]

There are pigtail pleural drainage catheters available, which have been designed to prevent iatrogenic damage of intrathoracic organs.[44] However, even these catheters made from softer material can be the cause of pulmonary injury in premature infants.[45] Another option is the insertion of ordinary 18G venous catheters, which have been proven to be a quick, effective, and safe alternative to drain neonatal pneumothorax. In the majority of cases, a properly sized ordinary chest drain with an underwater seal or with a vacuum-control unit should be adequate. The Heimlich flutter valve, though useful clinically, adds to the resistance of the system, especially if fluid accumulates in the valve.[46]

Prognosis

Cases with pneumothoraces without underlying lung disease have a good prognosis. The mortality, though not the incidence, varies with birth weight and is, in general, double that of babies who have RDS but no air leak.[12] In one series of infants presenting with pneumothoraces within the first 24 hours of life, the overall mortality rate was 52%.[47] The mortality rate is inversely proportional to the infant's birth weight: 53% in infants with birth weights <1 kg.[48] The incidence of grades 3 or 4 intraventricular hemorrhage in infants with pneumothoraces associated with arterial hypotension is 89% as compared with neonates with pneumothoraces associated with normal blood pressure, which is only 10%.[49] This can have a detrimental effect on the neurological outcome. Ventilatory parameters may be helpful in making a prognostic assessment. The survivor group responds well to a fraction of inspired oxygen of less than 70% and a PEEP of 6 cm or less. A CO_2 retention associated with pneumopericardium and PIE is an unfavorable sign.[47]

Pneumopericardium

Pneumopericardium is the least frequent pulmonary air leak. However, recently, it has been occurring with increasing frequency as a complication of ventilatory therapy. Pneumopericardium can develop while the patients are on high-frequency ventilation respiratory support.[50] Neonatal pneumopericardium has also been reported during nasal continuous positive airway pressure (CPAP) ventilation and in a full-term neonate following a forceps delivery and mild asphyxia. The exact etiology of pneumopericardium is not known; it is probably interstitial pulmonary air, secondary to alveolar rupture, which dissects into the mediastinum and then enters the pericardial space at the reflection of the pericardium onto the great vessels.

The pneumopericardium may be asymptomatic or symptomatic. Asymptomatic infants do well without any

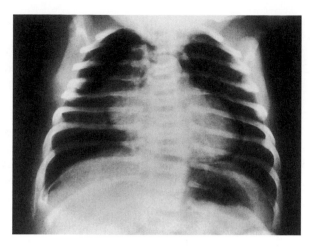

Figure 40.5 Pneumopericardium in a 2-day-old full-term infant with complicating meconium aspiration. Note right pneumothorax also.

treatment. The clinical signs in symptomatic patients are those of cardiac tamponade, i.e., a sudden onset of bradycardia, muffled heart sounds, cyanosis, and hypotension. Changes in ECG axis and/or voltage may be observed. The classic radiological finding is a continuous radiolucent band of air that conforms to the cardiac outline and does not extend beyond the level of the great vessels (Figure 40.5). Extra ventilatory air (PIE and pneumomediastinum) is present in over 90% of patients. Simple needle pericardiocentesis is the appropriate therapy for most cases with cardiac tamponade. However, a few babies with pneumopericardium uncontrolled by needle aspiration require placement of a pericardial catheter for continuous drainage of air.

Pneumopericardium can be masked by other pulmonary air leaks and should be considered if drainage of the primarily obvious site does not improve the cardiorespiratory status of the infant.[3] The mortality rate in infants with pneumopericardium is high, especially in preterm infants.[3,12]

REFERENCES

1. Jassal MS, Benson JE, Mogayzel PJ Jr. Spontaneous resolution of diffuse persistent pulmonary interstitial emphysema. *Pediatr Pulmonol* 2008 Jun; 43(6): 615–9. Review.
2. Katar S, Devecioğlu C, Kervancioğlu M, Ulkü R. Symptomatic spontaneous pneumothorax in term newborns. *Pediatr Surg Int* 2006 Sep; 22(9): 755–8. Epub 2006 Aug 3.
3. Cools B, Plaskie K, Van de Vijver K, Suys B. Unsuccessful resuscitation of a preterm infant due to a pneumothorax and a masked tension pneumopericardium. *Resuscitation* 2008 Aug; 78(2): 236–9. Epub 2008 May 15.
4. Lawal TA, Glüer S, Reismann M, Dördelmann M, Schirg E, Ure B. Spontaneous neonatal pneumomediastinum: The "spinnaker sail" sign. *Eur J Pediatr Surg* 2009 Feb; 19(1): 50–2. Epub 2008 Jun 17.
5. Hosono S, Ohno T, Kimoto H, Shimizu M, Harada K. Morbidity and mortality of infants born at the threshold of viability: Ten years' experience in a single neonatal intensive care unit, 1991–2000. *Pediatr Int* 2006 Feb; 48(1): 33–9.
6. Macklin CC. Transport of air along sheaths of pulmonic blood vessels from alveoli to mediastinum, clinical applications. *Arch Int Med* 1939; 64: 913–26.
7. Plenat F, Vert P, Didier F, Andre M. Pulmonary interstitial emphysema. *Clin Perinatol* 1978; 5: 351–75.
8. Miller JD, Carlo WA. Pulmonary complications of mechanical ventilation in neonates. *Clin Perinatol* 2008 Mar; 35(1): 273–81, x–xi.
9. Lerman-Sagie T, Davidson S, Wielunsky E. Pulmonary interstitial emphysema in low birth weight infants: Characteristics of survivors. *Acta Paediatr Hung* 1990; 30: 383–9.
10. Hart SM, McNair M, Gamsu HR, Price JF. Pulmonary interstitial emphysema in very low birth weight infants. *Arch Dis Child* 1983; 58: 612–15.
11. Yu VYK, Wong PY, Bajuk B, Symonowicz W. Pulmonary air leak in extremely low birth weight infants. *Arch Dis Child* 1986; 61: 239–41.
12. Greenough A, Milner AD. Acute respiratory disease. In: Rennie JM (ed). *Rennie and Robertson's Textbook of Neonatology*, 5th edn. London: Churchill Livingstone, 2012.
13. Greenough A, Dimitriou G, Prendergast M, Milner AD. Synchronized mechanical ventilation for respiratory support in newborn infants. *Cochrane Database Syst Rev* 2008 Jan 23; (1): CD000456.
14. Soll R, Ozek E. Prophylactic protein free synthetic surfactant for preventing morbidity and mortality in preterm infants. *Cochrane Database Syst Rev* 2010 Jan 20; (1): CD001079.
15. Chalak LF, Kaiser JR, Arrington RW. Resolution of pulmonary interstitial emphysema following selective left main stem intubation in a premature newborn: An old procedure revisited. *Paediatr Anaesth* 2007 Feb; 17(2): 183–6.
16. O'Donovan D, Wearden M, Adams J. Unilateral pulmonary interstitial emphysema following pneumonia in a preterm infant successfully treated with prolonged selective bronchial intubation. *Am J Perinatol* 1999; 16(7): 327–31.
17. Cohen RS, Smith DW, Stevenson DK, Moskowitz PS, Graham CB. Lateral decubitus position as therapy for persistent pulmonary interstitial emphysema in neonates: A preliminary report. *J Pediatr* 1984; 104: 441–3.
18. Dördelmann M, Schirg E, Poets CF, Ure B, Glüer S, Bohnhorst B. Therapeutic lung puncture for diffuse unilateral pulmonary interstitial emphysema in preterm infants. *Eur J Pediatr Surg* 2008 Aug; 18(4): 233–6. Epub 2008 Aug 14.

19. Messineo A, Fusaro F, Mognato G, Sabatti M, D'Amore ES, Guglielmi M. Lung volume reduction surgery in lieu of pneumonectomy in an infant with severe unilateral pulmonary interstitial emphysema. *Pediatr Pulmonol* 2001 May; 31(5): 389–93.

20. Matta R, Matta J, Hage P, Nassif Y, Mansour N, Diab N. Diffuse persistent interstitial pulmonary emphysema treated by lobectomy. *Ann Thorac Surg* 2011 Oct; 92(4): e73–5.

21. Greenough A, Dixon AD, Roberton NRC. Pulmonary interstitial emphysema. *Arch Dis Child* 1984; 59: 1046–51.

22. Morisot C, Kacet N, Bouchez MC, Rouland V, Dobos JP, Gremillet C, Lequien P. Risk factors for fatal pulmonary interstitial emphysema in neonates. *Eur J Pediatr* 1990; 149(7): 493–5.

23. Hauri-Hohl A, Baenziger O, Frey B. Pneumomediastinum in the neonatal and paediatric intensive care unit. *Eur J Pediatr* 2008 Apr; 167(4): 415–8. Epub 2007 May 30.

24. Megremis S, Stefanaki S, Tsekoura T, Tsilimigaki A. Spontaneous pneumomediastinum in a child: Sonographic detection in a case with minimal findings on chest radiography. *J Ultrasound Med* 2008 Feb; 27(2): 303–6.

25. Mohamed IS, Lee YH, Yamout SZ, Fakir S, Reynolds AM. Ultrasound guided percutaneous relief of tension pneumomediastinum in a 1-day-old newborn. *Arch Dis Child Fetal Neonatal Ed* 2007 Nov; 92(6): F458.

26. Trevisanuto D, Doglioni N, Ferrarese P, Vedovato S, Cosmi E, Zanardo V. Neonatal pneumothorax: Comparison between neonatal transfers and inborn infants. *J Perinat Med* 2005; 33(5): 449–54.

27. Fanaroff AA, Stoll BJ, Wright LL et al. Trends in neonatal morbidity and mortality for very low birth weight infants. *Am J Obstet Gynecol* 2007; 196(2): e1–e8.

28. Horbar JD, Carpenter JH, Buzas J et al. Collaborative quality improvement to promote evidence based surfactant for preterm infants: A cluster randomized trial. *BMJ* 2004; 329(7473):1004.

29. Sahn SA, Heffner JE. Spontaneous pneumothorax. *N Eng J Med* 2000; 342(12): 868–74.

30. Esme H, Doğru O, Eren S, Korkmaz M, Solak O. The factors affecting persistent pneumothorax and mortality in neonatal pneumothorax. *Turk J Pediatr.* 2008 May–Jun; 50(3): 242–6.

31. Basu S, Kumar A, Gupta AK. Complications associated with neonatal resuscitation. *Resuscitation* 2009 Jan; 80(1): 4–5.

32. Klinger G, Ish-Hurwitz S, Osovsky M, Sirota L, Linder N. Risk factors for pneumothorax in very low birth weight infants. *Pediatr Crit Care Med* 2008 Jul; 9(4): 398–402.

33. Madansky DL, Lawson EE, Chernick V, Taeusch HW Jr. Pneumothorax and other forms of pulmonary air leak in newborns. *Am Rev Respir Dis* 1979; 120(4): 729–37.

34. Thakur A, Buchmiller T, Atkinson J. Bronchial perforation after closed-tube endotracheal suction. *J Pediatr Surg* 2000 Sep; 35(9): 1353–5.

35. Laberge JM, Puligandla P, Flageole H. Asymptomatic congenital lung malformations. *Semin Pediatr Surg* 2005 Feb; 14(1): 16–33.

36. Sharda JK, Kurlandsky LE, Lacina SJ, Radecki LL. Spontaneous pneumothorax in common pulmonary vein atresia. *J Perinatol* 1990; 10(1): 70–4.

37. Irving IM. Neonatal Surgery. Malformations and acquired lesions of lungs, pleura and mediastinum. In: Lister J, Irving IM (eds). *Neonatal Surgery*, 3rd edn. London: Butterworths, 1990: 259–78.

38. Kulrus LR, Bednarek FJ, Wyman ML, Roloff DW, Borer RC. Diagnosis of pneumothorax or pneumomediastinum in the neonate by transillumination. *Pediatrics* 1975; 56: 355–60.

39. Litmanovitz I, Carlo WA. Expectant management of pneumothorax in ventilated neonates. *Pediatrics.* 2008 Nov; 122(5): e975–9. Epub 2008 Oct 13.

40. Cools F, Offringa M. Neuromuscular paralysis for newborn infants receiving mechanical ventilation. *Cochrane Database Syst Rev* 2005 Apr 18; (2): CD002773.

41. Moessinger AC, Driscoll JM Jr, Wigger HJ. High incidence of lung perforation by chest tube in neonatal pneumothorax. *J Pediatr* 1978; 92: 635–7.

42. Allen RW, Jung AL, Lester PD. Effectiveness of chest tube evacuation of pneumothorax in neonates. *J Pediatr* 1981; 99: 629–34.

43. Odita JC, Khan AS, Dincsoy M, Kayyali M, Masoud A, Ammari A. Neonatal phrenic nerve paralysis resulting from intercostal drainage of pneumothorax. *Pediatr Radiol* 1992; 22(5): 379–81.

44. Cates LA. Pigtail catheters used in the treatment of pneumothoraces in the neonate. *Adv Neonat Care* 2009 Feb; 9(1): 7–16. Review.

45. Brooker RW, Booth GR, DeMello DE, Keenan WJ. Unsuspected transection of lung by pigtail catheter in a premature infant. *J Perinatol* 2007 Mar; 27(3): 190–2.

46. Bakker JC, Liem M, Wijnands JB, Karsdon J, Berger HM. Neonatal pneumothorax drainage systems: In vitro evaluation. *Eur J Pediatr* 1989; 149(1): 58–61.

47. Mandal AK, Yamini S, Bean X. Arterial blood gas and expiratory pressure monitoring in infants with pneumothorax: Prognostic predictability. *J Natl Med Assoc* 1990; 82(1): 33–7.

48. Greenough A, Robertson NRC. Morbidity and survival in neonates ventilated for respiratory distress syndrome. *Br Med J* 1985; 290: 597–600.

49. Mehrabani D, Gowen CW Jr, Kopelman AE. Association of pneumothorax and hypotension with intraventricular haemorrhage. *Arch Dis Child* 1991; 66(1 Spec No): 48–51.

50. Neal RC, Beck DE, Smith VC, Null DM. Neonatal pneumopericardium with high frequency ventilation. *Ann Thorac Surg* 1989; 47(2): 274–7.

41

Chylothorax and other pleural effusions in neonates

MIHO WATANABE, BELINDA HSI DICKIE, AND RICHARD G. AZIZKHAN

INTRODUCTION

Pleural effusions in neonates and children can present as a spectrum from asymptomatic small accumulations of fluid to life-threatening collections that could result in compression of the lung parenchyma and/or mediastinal shift.

Pleural effusions in neonates are rare, at an estimated 5.5–220 per 10,000 deliveries. In fetuses and neonates, the most common cause of congenital effusions is a chylothorax. A well-established entity, chylothorax results from leakage of chyle from the thoracic duct into the pleural cavity. The most common etiology of acquired pleural effusion in newborns is iatrogenic (result of cardiac or thoracic surgery).[1–3] In the older child, parapneumonic effusions due to empyema are the leading cause of effusions, followed by congestive heart failure and malignancy.[4–6] It is very important to recognize the diagnosis early so as to provide appropriate treatment and limit morbidity.

This chapter presents a basic description of the pathophysiology of pleural effusion and chyle, the anatomy and embryology of the pleura and lymphatic system, and an overview of key clinical aspects of neonatal pleural effusions, especially chylothorax, as well as fetal pleural effusion, hemothorax, and empyema, to provide the foundation for understanding this disorder.

PATHOPHYSIOLOGY

Normally, with the thoracic cavity, there is a small amount of thin fluid (~0.3 mL/kg).[7] The function of the pleural fluid is to lubricate the pleura to allow for smooth lung movement and to provide surface tension of the lung to keep the appropriate distance from the thoracic wall. Fluid continuously moves from the parietal pleura though the pleural space to be absorbed by the visceral pleura.[8] The fluid then drains into the lymphatic system via the thoracic duct.[9] The volume of fluid in the pleural space is minimized by a balance of starling forces, oncotic pressure in the circulation, and negative pressure in the lymphatics of the thorax. Recently, another hypothesis states that the amount of fluid can be controlled and absorbed via a metabolically active transport system in the parietal pleural mesothelial cells.[10,11] Turnover of the pleural fluid is estimated to be about 0.15 mL kg/hour, and any interruption in the flow of the fluid may significantly increase the volume within the thoracic cavity. Therefore, accumulation can occur when the balance between the rate of filtration and lymphatic clearance is altered. This can be seen in increased systemic capillary or venous pressure, increased capillary vessel permeability due to infection or inflammation, decreased plasma colloid osmotic pressure, increased negative intrapleural pressure, obstructed lymphatic flow, or abnormality or injury of the lymphatic system.

Chyle is defined as a mixture of lymph and chylomicrons. Chylomicrons (emulsified fat globules) are absorbed from the small intestine, and are mixed with clear lymph from the pelvis and lower extremities, conducted centrally, and then drained into the venous system via the thoracic duct. At birth, chyle is clear and straw colored; soon after milk feeding begins, chylomicrons render it milky white. The fat content of the fluid varies between 0.4 and 4.0 g/100 mL, with a triglyceride content of >500 mg/100 mL. Variation is dependent on the amount of milk ingested. Lymphocyte counts in chyle are high (80%–100%) and are predominantly T cell.[12] The protein and electrolytes in chyle are similar to those in plasma. The volume of chyle loss per day can exceed 1.7 times the patient's blood volume, resulting in a serious state of depletion characterized by hyponatremia, hypoproteinemia, metabolic acidosis, and lymphocytopenia.[13]

ANATOMY

The lymphatic system is a one-directional circulatory system that transfers extracellular fluid, lymph, and chyle from peripheral tissues to the subclavian vein without a central pump. Lymph is collected in the cisterna chyli and reaches the venous system via the thoracic duct, which ascends in the posterior mediastinum between the azygos vein and the descending aorta. This duct crosses to the left at the level of the fifth thoracic vertebra, continues its ascent into the neck on the left of the esophagus, and opens into the venous system at the confluence of the internal jugular and subclavian veins. In the thorax, it receives lymph from the parietal pleura of both sides via several collecting trunks. Lymphatic branches from structures in the posterior mediastinum and from the left lung and its pleura join to form the left bronchomediastinal trunk; this trunk opens into the thoracic duct or directly into the great veins. There are also several potential lymphatic–venous communications that may function when the main duct is traumatized or blocked.

While the thoracic duct is usually a singular structure, its embryology underscores the potential for anatomic variations and congenital anomalies. It may develop in different anatomical patterns with several lymphaticovenous anastomoses. Variation in lymphatic pathways and the presence of accessory lymphatic channels can account for chylous effusions resulting from surgical procedures that do not expose the main thoracic duct. Trauma to the duct in the posterior mediastinum can produce a unilateral or bilateral chylothorax. Increased intraductal tension leads to drainage of chyle into the thorax. Rupture of the thoracic duct between the diaphragm and T5 usually produces a right-sided chylothorax, and above T5, a left-sided chylothorax. Rupture in the midline at T5 or as part of a more diffuse lymphatic condition causes bilateral chylothorax.

EMBRYOLOGY

The lymphatic system begins to develop at the end of week 5, approximately 2 weeks later than the cardiovascular system. One hypothesis states that lymphatics develop as diverticula of the endothelium of the adjacent veins, establishing venous endothelium as the primordial structure of the lining of the lymphatic system.[14] In weeks 6–9, the lymphatic channels are developed as outgrowths of the venous endothelium in six original lymph sacs and dilate locally—two jugular lymph sacs, two iliac lymph sacs, one retroperitoneal lymph sac, and one cisterna chyli dorsal to the retroperitoneal lymph sac. These sacs branch into the tissues to form the jugular sacs, iliac sacs, and retroperitoneal and cisternal sacs. The lymph sacs except the cisterna chyli are transformed into groups of lymph nodes around the third gestational month.

ETIOLOGY

Twenty-three to thirty-two percent of neonatal pleural effusions are congenital. The main cause of the effusions is chylothoraces, but other causes are associated with hydrops fetalis, congenital anomalies, and genetic abnormalities.[3,15]

Congenital chylothorax

Chylothorax can present in utero or in the neonatal period. Males are affected twice as frequently as females, and 60% of cases involve the right side of the chest.[16] The occurrence of congenital chylothorax in the absence of other disease suggests the existence of congenital malformation of the lymphatic system or the thoracic duct, resulting in the leakage of chyle into the pleural space.[17] The malformation can be congenital atresia of the thoracic duct or congenital fistula due to failure of peripheral lymphatic channels to communicate with the major lymphatic network. Congenital chylothorax can also be associated with other congenital malformations (76%), chromosomal anomalies (trisomy 21) (12%), and other syndromes (Noonan, Turner) (6%).[3] Congenital chylothorax is usually bilateral, with low Apgar score and occasional need for immediate thoracocentesis.

Congenital pleural effusion with associated diseases

Congenital pleural effusion is also associated with hydrops fetalis, other congenital anomalies, or genetic abnormalities.[3]

Hydrops fetalis is a serious fetal condition defined as abnormal fluid accumulation in two or more fetal compartments, including ascites, pleural effusion, pericardial effusion, and skin edema. The underlying cause is an imbalance of interstitial fluid production and subsequent lymphatic return. The causes of hydrops fetalis are (1) immune hydrops fetalis (Rhesus blood group isoimmunization of the fetus) and (2) nonimmune hydrops fetalis (major causes are cardiovascular disorder and lymphatic dysplasia, followed by thoracic disorder, hematologic disorder, twin pregnancy, infection, genetic syndromes, and chromosomal abnormalities). Nonimmune hydrops is more common than immune hydrops. The pathogenesis of pleural effusion in these diseases is incompletely understood, but multiple features for dysregulation of the net fluid movement would be involved. Pleural effusion in hydrops can be either chylous, transudate, or exudate. In contrast, pleural effusion with other congenital anomalies or genetic abnormalities is mostly transudate but can be chylous.

Acquired pleural effusions

IATROGENIC ACQUIRED PLEURAL EFFUSIONS

Acquired pleural effusion results primarily from iatrogenic insult, surgery, or trauma to the thorax (61%–74%).[3] Recent studies suggest an increase in the prevalence of postoperative chylothorax from the previously reported 1% or less to 2.5%–4.7%.[18–20] This has been attributed to the increased complexity of the surgery being performed and possibility of the earlier reintroduction of feeding after surgery. Iatrogenic injury can occur during surgery in the region of the aortic arch for conditions such as patent ductus arteriosus, coarctation of aorta, vascular ring, and other congenital cardiovascular anomalies[20,21] as well as during esophageal repair or repair of congenital diaphragmatic hernia.[22,23] Acquired iatrogenic pleural effusions are mainly chylothorax (65%). Acquired iatrogenic pleural effusions can also be a manifestation of a complication of subclavian and internal jugular venous cannulation and/or superior vena caval obstruction secondary to previous catheterization, chest tube insertion, and traumatic delivery. Acquired iatrogenic pleural effusion is often unilateral, on the left side.

NONIATROGENIC ACQUIRED PLEURAL EFFUSIONS

The etiology of noniatrogenic acquired pleural effusion includes empyema, superior vena cava syndrome, hypoproteinemia, heart failure, and renal failure. There have been rare reports of infantile chylothorax resulting from abdominal blunt trauma due to child abuse.[24,25] It is sometimes difficult to determine the cause of noniatrogenic acquired pleural effusion.

CLINICAL SYMPTOMS

Symptoms of pleural effusion are very broad depending on the volume, compression of the lung, and displacement of the mediastinum. Tachypnea, dyspnea, retraction of chest wall, and cyanosis are typical presenting signs and symptoms. On examination, dullness and diminution of breath sounds on the affected side and displacement of the heart and mediastinum to the opposite side can be found. Chest pain can be one of the symptoms in the older child due to irritation of the parietal pleura; however, it can also be referred pain to the thoracoabdominal wall (intercostal nerves) or to the shoulder (phrenic nerve).

In cases of congenital pleural effusion, symptoms of respiratory distress may be noted shortly after birth or at any time up to 2 weeks of life. In contrast, the interval between surgery and the occurrence of acquired pleural effusion can vary from 1 to 25 days. The time is shortest when there is a direct injury to the duct (5–7 days) and longest when there is high pressure or thrombosis of the vena cava (10–14 days). Chyle may accumulate in the mediastinum for several days before extravasating into the pleural space.

The loss of large quantities of chyle over a period of time produces nutritional failure, metabolic acidosis, sepsis, and renal failure. Significant loss of protein and lymphocytes can result in lymphocytopenia and hypogammaglobinemia, causing immune deficiencies and abnormal cell-mediated immune responses.

DIAGNOSIS

Radiology

Chest radiographs will typically show opacification of one or both hemithoraces, with or without compression of the lung and displacement of mediastinal structures in unilateral pleural effusion (Figure 41.1). Radiographic diagnosis in premature infants may, however, be difficult, because most of these infants already have significant pulmonary disease, and chest radiographs may appear to have areas of increasing consolidation rather than the more typical layering of pleural fluid seen in older children.

Ultrasonography is a reliable diagnostic method to detect pleural effusion in neonates and children. Its use in obstetric practice as the primary method of imaging the fetal chest has led to the increasing frequency with which in utero diagnosis can be made.

Other modalities such as computerized tomography (CT) scan, lymphangiography, and lymphoscintigraphy can be helpful. Lymphangiography involves injection of a contrast agent into the lymphatic system and following the lymphatic flow proximally. Simultaneous CT or magnetic resonance imaging (MRI) can better delineate the lymphatic anatomy and define the site of leak or obstruction. Lymphoscintigraphy uses injection of a radionuclide (commonly 99m-technetium) either intradermally or subcutaneously to outline the network of the lymphatics.

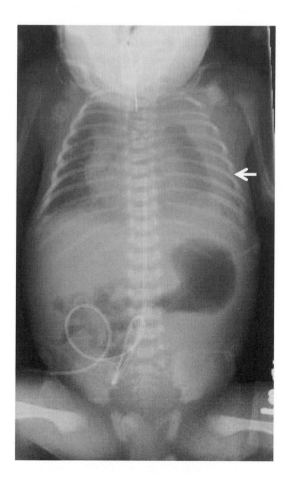

Figure 41.1 Radiographic images of fetal bilateral pleural effusions. X-ray (anteroposterior view) of neonate with unilateral pleural effusion (arrows), demonstrating a moderate left pleural effusion with mild rightward mediastinal shift.

Laboratory testing

Analysis of the pleural fluid is used to help diagnose the cause of pleural effusion and to differentiate types of pleural effusion (transudate, exudate, chylothorax, emphysema, hemothorax, total parenteral nutrition [TPN] leakage). Pleural effusion is drained by thoracentesis or chest tube placement. The fluid should be sent for diagnostic analysis including (1) microscopic examination for fluid characteristic and cell count, (2) pleural fluid biochemistry, (3) cytology, and (4) Gram stain and culture for bacterial or fungal infection. Normal pleural fluid is usually clear, with a composition of pH of 7.60–7.64, protein less than 1–2 g/dL, white blood cells (WBCs) fewer than 1000/mm^3, glucose similar to that of plasma, and lactate dehydrogenase (LDH) less than 50% of plasma.

Chylothorax is characterized by an absolute white cell count >1000 cells/μL with a lymphocyte fraction >80% and triglyceride level >110 mg/dL. It may also have elevated total protein and albumin levels (less than that of serum), a specific gravity of >1.012, and total fat levels if the infant is milk-fed.[26,27] In the unfed neonate, the fat content of the chylothorax may be quite low, and the fluid does not have the characteristic milky appearance.

Empyema is defined as an exudate purulent effusion with a total leukocyte count >5000/mm^3 and a predominance of polymorphonuclear cells. Hemothorax is characterized by a hematocrit value more than 50% serum hematocrit, but the presence of blood in the fluid is diagnostic in a traumatic hemothorax. Although rare, leakage of TPN though a central line into the pleural cavity has been documented. Analysis of the fluid will show a low leukocyte count and high concentrations of both glucose and potassium.

Transudates are effusions with a total protein level <3.0 g/dL or a pleural-to-serum protein ratio <0.5, and a total leukocyte count <1000/mm^3 with predominance of mononuclear cells. Exudate, on the other hand, has a protein level >3.0 g/dL with a pleural-to-serum protein ratio >0.5, pleural fluid LDH values >200 IU/L, or a pleural-to-serum LDH ratio >0.6.

MANAGEMENT

General management principles

Because neonatal pleural effusion is associated with a wide array of disorders and accompanying clinical circumstances, the management of patients with this condition varies considerably. Although there are some case series of neonatal pleural effusion,[3,15,28] clinical outcomes are still poorly understood, and there are no prospective or randomized trials regarding treatment. To date, there has been a lack of protocol regarding treatment approaches for neonatal pleural effusions, although two guidelines for management of pediatric chylothorax have been proposed.[27,29] The timing and type of operative intervention have been particularly controversial. There has been introduction of new medical therapies, but where in the treatment algorithm these medications are useful is yet to be determined.

Despite the differences between the pediatric population and neonatal population, it is generally agreed that the initial treatment should be nonoperative management. The duration of medical therapy can range from days to weeks, and the critical and unresolved issue is the early identification of babies for whom the morbidity of medical therapy will exceed that of early surgical therapy.[19]

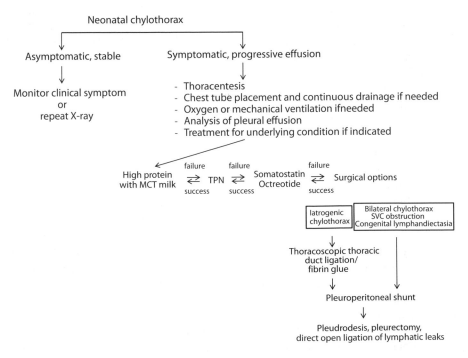

Figure 41.2 Algorithm of management principles for neonatal pleural effusions. MCT: medium-chain triglyceride; SVC: superior vena cava; TPN: total parenteral nutrition.

The main principles of nonoperative management of pleural effusions include the following (Figure 41.2)[29]:

1. Initial drainage and continuous drainage if needed
2. Dietary modification
3. The use of drugs to try and decrease the production of fluid (somatostatin [SST], octreotide [OCT])
4. Pleurodesis using agents such as OK-432 and doxycycline
5. Treatment of underlying cause
6. Supportive care as needed—ventilation, nutrition
7. Prevention and treatment of complications

Nonoperative management

Initial thoracentesis is diagnostic and provides immediate relief of respiratory failure. If the size of the pleural effusion compromises respiration, and/or there is a high likelihood of ongoing fluid production and reaccumulation, a chest tube should be inserted for continuous drainage to keep the lungs fully expanded. Adequate drainage is necessary for sealing chyle leakage. If there is a need for repeating thoracentesis after the initial drainage, a thoracostomy tube is usually placed because of increased risk of producing pneumothorax and introducing infection. Prophylactic antibiotics are given when chest tubes are in place, since many of these neonates have an acquired immune deficiency caused by the acquired lymphocytopenia.

An initial nonoperative management relies on adequate drainage of the effusion in conjunction with nutritional supplementation. Enteral feeding (high protein and fat-free) with medium-chain triglycerides (MCTs) should be given to reduce the flow of chyle through the thoracic duct while waiting for spontaneous healing. MCTs, which have a 6- to 12-carbon backbone, are the only fats to be absorbed directly via the portal system, bypassing the lymphatics. On the contrary, more than 60% of ingested fats travel to the bloodstream via the thoracic duct. Some investigators have observed no difference in MCT or TPN with regard to duration or amount of chylous drainage.[30] In recalcitrant or severe cases, patients may require TPN or a combination of both modalities. When superior vena caval thrombosis is present with chylothorax, the albumin, gamma-globulin, and fibrinogen that are contained in chyle, as well as fat-soluble vitamins, are adequately replaced. The majority of cases of congenital and iatrogenic chylothorax resolve spontaneously with nonoperative management with MCT-enriched diets and/or TPN.

SST and OCT are established but controversial medical treatment alternatives for congenital and iatrogenic chylothorax recalcitrant to nonsurgical therapies. Growing evidence from case studies suggests that SST and OCT exert a positive effect on persistent congenital and postoperative chylothorax.[31] SST is a polypeptide with mainly inhibitory actions on the release of various hormones (e.g., growth hormone and insulin) and lymph fluid excretion. OCT is a synthetic long-acting SST analogue with antisecretory properties similar to those of SST. It is thought that OCT may act directly on SST receptors in the splanchnic circulation

to reduce lymph fluid production. OCT also decreases the volume of gastric, pancreatic, and biliary secretions, thus reducing the volume and protein content of fluid within the thoracic duct, because thoracic duct lymphatic flow depends on splanchnic vascular tone as well as gastric motility. Current research suggests that OCT is well tolerated, even with several modes of administration. SST is usually administered as an intravenous infusion (a median dose of 204 μg/kg/day for a median duration of 9.5 days). OCT is administered either as an intravenous infusion (a median dose of 68 μg/kg/day for a median duration of 7 days) or subcutaneously (a median dose of 40 μg/kg/day for a median duration of 17 days).[31] Also, a different way of administration, such as initiation with 0.5 μg/kg/hour of OCT and gradually increasing the dose up to 10–12 μg/kg/hour, was reported.[31,32] Reduction of lymphatic flow rate is usually evident within 3–6 days after initiation of SST or OCT. Use of SST or OCT has been shown to shorten the duration of intensive care treatment, reduce the need for recurrent thoracentesis, and decrease the amount of fluid and plasma infusions, thereby reducing the risk of infection. To date, no randomized controlled trials have been identified; reported route of administration, dose, duration of therapy, and strategy for discontinuation of therapy vary; and the optimal way of administration is not known.[33] Unfortunately, specific pharmacokinetic data are not yet available regarding these agents in neonates and children. Both SST and OCT are considered safe with potential adverse effects, including cholelithiasis, liver impairment, renal impairment, transient glucose intolerance, hypothyroidism, and necrotizing enterocolitis. It is thus prudent for patients to undergo routine monitoring of liver function, blood glucose, and thyroid parameters during the course of treatment.

OK-432 (Picibanil) is a lyophilized incubation mixture of the group A *Streptococcus pyogenes* of human origin for use in pleurodesis. It is presently used to treat fetal chylothorax and congenital cases resistant to SST/OCT as well as adults with chylothorax. To date, information is sparse, and reports emanate primarily from centers in Japan, where OK-432 is manufactured and readily available.

Operative management

Surgical intervention is warranted when nonoperative management fails to significantly diminish lymphatic drainage, or if a patient's respiratory, nutritional, or metabolic status declines (Figure 41.2). There is no consensus on the timing of surgery, but the goal is to intervene prior to development of morbidity. Possible clinical conditions that have a high failure rate with nonoperative management include iatrogenic cases where there is injury to the thoracic duct and massive lymph leakage, vena caval obstruction or elevated central venous pressures, and congenital chylothorax associated with superior vena caval thrombosis in the premature neonate. Although there is no consensus on timing of surgery, many will consider early intervention in the high-risk cases.

The percentage of neonates requiring surgery with failure of nonoperative management and the timing of surgical intervention vary widely among reported series, dependent upon the patient population being studied, etiology, and the clinical status of the patients. There are several surgical approaches, and different options are often used in combination. They include thoracic duct ligation (open thoracotomy or thoracoscopy), pleurodesis (mechanical and chemical), pleurectomy, and pleuroperitoneal shunting.

THORACIC DUCT LIGATION

Direct surgical ligation of the thoracic duct is historically the most common surgical therapy and has been the most definitive and successful in resolving chylous leak if the site of rupture can be identified intraoperatively. It can be performed via an open thoracotomy or a thoracoscopic approach. Video-assisted thoracoscopic procedures are being used with increasing frequency. These procedures offer the advantage of access to the entire hemithorax, with excellent visualization of the mediastinal structures. This approach allows application of clips to the thoracic duct at the hiatus or to the thoracic duct at the level of the injury or pleural defects. It also facilitates mechanical or chemical pleurodesis and application of fibrin glue. Despite its advantages, its use is limited by an infant's size and pulmonary status. Also, it may be difficult to correctly visualize leaks in the presence of a massive chylous effusion. The thoracoscopic approach has been shown to have a lower rate of complications.[34,35]

Regardless of the surgical approach, visualization of the site of chyle leakage can be difficult. Giving cream or milk through the nasogastric tube several hours before the operation or injection of 1% Evans blue dye in the thigh helps to identify the sites of leakage by giving the lymphatic drainage a color. Major leaks from the thoracic ducts can be closed by direct suturing or by ligating the duct above and below the leak. If the thoracic duct or site of the leak is not identified, a mass ligation of the thoracic duct and its surrounding tissue can be done between the aorta, azygos vein, and esophagus, adjacent to the vertebral body.

PLEURODESIS AND PARIETAL PLEURECTOMY

Pleurodesis and parietal pleurectomy, which obliterate the pleural space, have been used when there is generalized weeping of chyle from parietal pleura. Mechanical pleurodesis is commonly performed with thoracoscopy with direct irritation of the parietal pleura. Chemical pleurodesis, with the administration of a sclerosing agent (tetracycline, talc, povidone–iodine, OK-432) is performed via a chest tube. Parietal pleurectomy has been reported as a successful option for the pediatric population in 1980s, but it is rarely performed now. It is an extensive surgical procedure that may increase the possibility of pulmonary lymphedema, fibrosis, and further pulmonary compromise.

Fibrin glue applied to the leakage site after patent ductus arteriosus ligation has been reported to successfully manage chylothorax in both a 3.5-month-old infant and a premature infant weighing 600 g.[36]

PLEUROPERITONEAL SHUNTS

Pleuroperitoneal shunts, first used by Azizkhan et al.[37] in 1983 to treat five ventilator-dependent infants with persistent chylothorax, are used as a surgical treatment option. The procedure avoids the risks associated with a more complicated open surgical procedure in high-risk infants and is considered safe, highly effective, and easy to perform. Pleuroperitoneal shunts provide a way of draining chyle from the pleural space to the peritoneal space but require manual compression of the shunt chamber.[37] During the immediate postoperative period, the pumping chamber is compressed 50–100 times per hour in order to completely clear the hemithorax of chyle. As the infant's clinical status improves, a gradual decrease in the frequency of shunt compression is begun. Resolution of pleural effusion often occurs within 2–3 weeks. The valve and pumping chamber sometimes become dysfunctional after several weeks due to an accumulation of fibrin and protein in the valve mechanism. Because it is less invasive, it is ideal for patients who require a relatively short or stabilizing procedure. Also, in case of both pleural effusion and intra-abdominal ascites, a combination of a pleuroperitoneal shunt and a peritoneovenous shunt may be required.

OUTCOME

In general, neonatal pleural effusion has a good prognosis, except in hydropic neonates. The mortality rate in hydrops is 53%. It has been reported that hydrops resulting from lymphatic dysplasia has a more favorable outcome. However, the causes of death were related to the underlying disease, such as respiratory failure due to pulmonary hypoplasia, multiorgan failure, or sepsis, and not to the pleural effusion. Neonates with acquired iatrogenic pleural effusion tend to have increasing needs for parenteral feeding, oxygen therapy, and diuretic regimen, as well as longer periods of mechanical ventilation and a longer stay in the neonatal intensive care unit (NICU), when compared to congenital primary pleural effusion. Recently, blood albumin level has been proposed to be predictive of prognosis for neonatal pleural effusion.[15]

FETAL PLEURAL EFFUSION

Fetal pleural effusion (or fetal hydrothorax) is a rare condition, with an incidence of 1/7300 to 1/15000.[2] Increased use of fetal sonography over the past decades has led to an increased frequency of diagnosis. Fetal pleural effusion is detected by prenatal ultrasound as a unilateral or bilateral anechoic space in the thorax surrounding the lungs (Figure 41.3). Pleural effusion can be an isolated finding or occur in association with other conditions.

The clinical course varies from complete spontaneous resolution to a progressive phenotype leading to the development of hydrops fetalis and perinatal death. If the pleural effusion is severe enough to increase intrathoracic pressure, it reduces cardiac output, leading to polyhydramnios and pulmonary hypoplasia. This results in potential cardiac failure, in utero

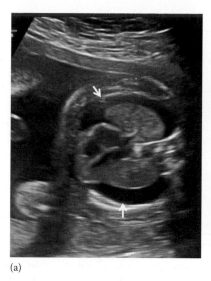 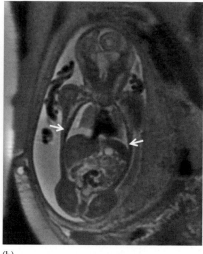

(a)   (b)

Figure 41.3 Radiographic images of fetal bilateral pleural effusions. **(a)** Ultrasound transverse view of fetal chest, demonstrating a fetus with bilateral pleural effusions (arrows) at 22 gestational weeks. **(b)** MRI coronal view of fetus, demonstrating a fetus with bilateral pleural effusions in thorax (arrows) in uterus at 25 gestational weeks. Lungs are partially compressed in the presence of large bilateral pleural effusions. The cardiothymic silhouette remains in normal position, no mediastinal shift. Also, there is no evidence of hydrops.

demise, premature delivery, and neonatal death. Fetal pleural effusion is usually detected around a gestation age of 21–24 weeks. Nine to twenty-two percent of fetuses will have spontaneous regression, often in the second trimester. In contrast to neonatal pleural effusions, fetal pleural effusions are associated with a high mortality rate. In those fetuses with progression, overall survival rate is 22%–53%. Lower survival rate is seen in pleural effusion associated with structural/chromosomal abnormalities or hydropic fetuses, younger gestational age at diagnosis, higher volume effusions, and bilateral disease.[2,38,39]

Diagnostic workup for a fetal pleural effusion should include fetal ultrasound, fetal MRI, fetal echocardiography, karyotyping, maternal blood count, type and screen with antibody status, and virology screening for Toxoplasmosis, Other Agents, Rubella, Cytomegalovirus, and Herpes Simplex (TORCH) and parvovirus B19.

The management of fetal pleural effusion has been controversial, and the optimal treatment approach remains unclear. Prenatal intervention for selected rapidly progressive cases with a high risk of perinatal morbidity and mortality is accepted (Figure 41.4). Current fetal interventions include (1) thoracocentesis using a 20G spinal needle to aspirate the pleural effusion, (2) thoracoamniotic shunting for reaccumulated fluid after aspiration, and (3) fetal intrapleural injection of OK-432. Therapeutic outcomes in the literature showed a 60%–65% overall survival rate irrespective of the different treatment options, with worse outcome if there is a presence of hydrops. However, as with any fetal therapy, there are the inherent risks of inducing preterm labor, preterm premature rupture of membrane, intrauterine infection, bleeding, and maternal or fetal organ trauma. In particular, with any shunt procedure, there are the risks of shunt displacement and blockage of the shunt.[40]

OTHER PLEURAL EFFUSIONS

Hemothorax

Although massive hemothorax is uncommon, accidental injury to the intercostal artery during thoracentesis or closed intercostal drainage can result it intrapleural bleeding. Hemothorax has been reported as a complication of a variety of congenital malformations (e.g., sequestration, patent ductus, and pulmonary arteriovenous malformation) and of subclavian vein catheters.[41] It is also an occasional manifestation of intrathoracic neoplasms, blood dyscrasias, and bleeding diatheses. Additionally, it can occur spontaneously in neonates, sometimes in association with a pneumothorax. Symptoms reveal respiratory embarrassment similar to that seen in tension pneumothorax. However, the percussion note is dull, and chest radiographs show opacification. More importantly, the infant may show signs of hypovolemic shock. Blood transfusion and urgent tube thoracostomy generally provide adequate control of bleeding. To avoid sudden circulatory collapse, transfusion should precede intercostal drainage. It is very rare in neonates; however, urgent thoracotomy and identification and securing of the bleeding site might be required, if massive blood loss continues.

Empyema

Owing primarily to improved antibiotic treatment of chest infections, empyema (purulent effusion) has become a rare condition in infants. The most common cause of empyema is a pneumonia caused by organisms such as *Staphylococcus aureus*, *Staphylococcus pneumoniae*, and *Staphylococcus*

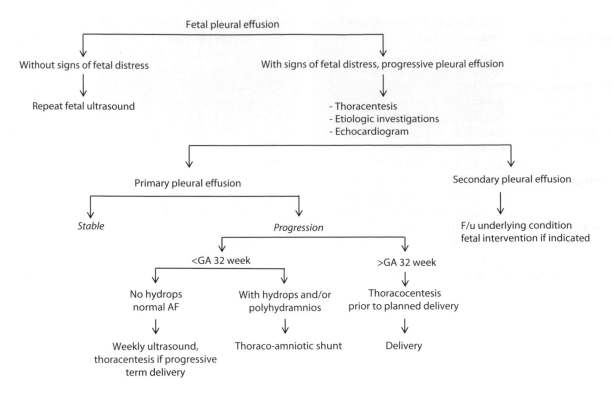

Figure 41.4 Algorithm of management principles for fetal pleural effusions. AF: amniotic fluid; f/u: follow-up; GA: gestation age.

pyogenes. It may, however, be incurred through the introduction of skin bacteria during thoracentesis or thoracotomy. Empyema may also be accompanied by anaerobic infection. Symptoms include indications of respiratory distress in addition to abdominal distension, lethargy, and at times, a septicemic state. Diagnosis is suspected by chest radiographs in which the effusion and pneumonic process are identified. Ultrasonography during diagnostic thoracentesis if helpful in specifically localizing loculated fluid collection. Prior to beginning a course of antibiotic therapy, a fluid specimen taken during thoracentesis is sent for a Gram stain and aerobic and anaerobic culture. Although most cases resolve with effective intercostal tube drainage, fibrinolysis, and a prolonged period of systemic administration of antibiotics, anaerobic infection tends to be multilocular and may thus require debridement and, in rare instances, decortication.

REFERENCES

1. Chernick V, Reed MH. Pneumothorax and chylothorax in the neonatal period. *J Pediatr* 1970; 76: 624–32.
2. Longaker MT, Laberge JM, Dansereau J, Langer JC, Crombleholme TM, Callen PW et al. Primary fetal hydrothorax: Natural history and management. *J Pediatr Surg* 1989; 24: 573–6.
3. Rocha G, Fernandes P, Rocha P, Quintas C, Martins T, Proenca E. Pleural effusions in the neonate. *Acta Paediatr* 2006; 95: 791–8.
4. Utine GE, Ozcelik U, Kiper N, Dogru D, Yalcn E, Cobanoglu N et al. Pediatric pleural effusions: Etiological evaluation in 492 patients over 29 years. *Turk J Pediatr* 2009; 51: 214–9.
5. Efrati O, Barak A. Pleural effusions in the pediatric population. *Pediatr Rev/Am Acad Pediatr* 2002; 23: 417–26.
6. Givan DC, Eigen H. Common pleural effusions in children. *Clin Chest Med* 1998; 19: 363–71.
7. Miserocchi G, Agostoni E. Contents of the pleural space. *J Appl Physiol* 1971; 30: 208–13.
8. Neergaard, KN. Zur Frage des Drukes in Pleuraspalt. *Beitr Klin Erforsch Tuberk Lungenkr* 1927; 65: 476–85.
9. Wiener-Kronish JP, Berthiaume Y, Albertine KH. Pleural effusions and pulmonary edema. *Clin Chest Med* 1985; 6: 509–19.
10. Miserocchi G. Physiology and pathophysiology of pleural fluid turnover. *Eur Respir J* 1997; 10: 219–25.
11. Zocchi L. Physiology and pathophysiology of pleural fluid turnover. *Eur Respir J* 2002; 20: 1545–58.
12. Strausser JL, Flye MW. Management of nontraumatic chylothorax. *Ann Thorac Surg* 1981; 31: 520–6.
13. Curci MR, Dibbins AW. Bilateral chylothorax in a newborn. *J Pediatr Surg* 1980; 15: 663–5.
14. Sabin FR. The method of growth of the lymphatic system. *Science* 1916; 44: 145–58.
15. Barbosa MR, G. Flor-de-Lima, F. Guimaraes, H. Neonatal pleural effusions in a level III neonatal intensive care unit. *J Pediatr Neonat Indiv Med* 2015; 4: e040123, 1–12.

16. Morphis LG, Arcinue EL, Krause JR. Generalized lymphangioma in infancy with chylothorax. *Pediatrics* 1970; 46: 566–75.

17. Arena Ansotegui J, Rey Otero A, Albisu Andrade J. [Spontaneous neonatal chylothorax. Apropos of 5 cases]. *Anal Esp Pediatr* 1984; 20: 49–54.

18. Verunelli F, Giorgini V, Luisi VS, Eufrate S, Cornali M, Reginato E. Chylothorax following cardiac surgery in children. *J Cardiovasc Surg* 1983; 24: 227–30.

19. Beghetti M, La Scala G, Belli D, Bugmann P, Kalangos A, Le Coultre C. Etiology and management of pediatric chylothorax. *J Pediatr* 2000; 136: 653–8.

20. Chan EH, Russell JL, Williams WG, Van Arsdell GS, Coles JG, McCrindle BW. Postoperative chylothorax after cardiothoracic surgery in children. *Ann Thorac Surg* 2005; 80: 1864–70.

21. Densupsoontorn NS, Jirapinyo P, Wongarn R, Thamonsiri N, Nana A, Laohaprasitiporn D et al. Management of chylothorax and chylopericardium in pediatric patients: Experiences at Siriraj Hospital, Bangkok. *Asia Pacific J Clin Nutr* 2005; 14: 182–7.

22. Kavvadia V, Greenough A, Davenport M, Karani J, Nicolaides KH. Chylothorax after repair of congenital diaphragmatic hernia—Risk factors and morbidity. *J Pediatr Surg* 1998; 33: 500–2.

23. Naik S, Greenough A, Zhang YX, Davenport M. Prediction of morbidity during infancy after repair of congenital diaphragmatic hernia. *J Pediatr Surg* 1996; 31: 1651–4.

24. Ichikawa Y, Sato A, Sato K, Nakamura K, Kitagawa N, Tanoue K et al. Chylothorax associated with child abuse. *Pediatr Int* 2015; 57: 1202–4.

25. Anderst JD. Chylothorax and child abuse. *Pediatric Crit Care Med* 2007; 8: 394–6.

26. Brodman RF. Congenital chylothorax. Recommendations for treatment. *NY State J Med* 1975; 75: 553–7.

27. Buttiker V, Fanconi S, Burger R. Chylothorax in children: Guidelines for diagnosis and management. *Chest* 1999; 116: 682–7.

28. Shih YS, PH. Chen, JY. Lee, IC. Hu, JM. Chang, HP. Common etiologies of neonatal pleural effusion. *Pediatr Neonatol* 2010; 52: 251–5.

29. Soto-Martinez M, Massie J. Chylothorax: Diagnosis and management in children. *Paediatr Respir Rev* 2009; 10: 199–207.

30. Allen EM, van Heeckeren DW, Spector ML, Blumer JL. Management of nutritional and infectious complications of postoperative chylothorax in children. *J Pediatr Surg* 1991; 26: 1169–74.

31. Roehr CC, Jung A, Proquitte H, Blankenstein O, Hammer H, Lakhoo K et al. Somatostatin or octreotide as treatment options for chylothorax in young children: A systematic review. *Intensive Care Med* 2006; 32: 650–7.

32. Kalomenidis I. Octreotide and chylothorax. *Curr Opin Pulmon Med* 2006; 12: 264–7.

33. Das A, Shah PS. Octreotide for the treatment of chylothorax in neonates. *Cochrane Database Syst Rev.* 2010: CD006388.

34. Graham DD, McGahren ED, Tribble CG, Daniel TM, Rodgers BM. Use of video-assisted thoracic surgery in the treatment of chylothorax. *Ann Thorac Surg* 1994; 57: 1507–11; discussion 1511–2.

35. Pego-Fernandes PM, Nascimbem MB, Ranzani OT, Shimoda MS, Monteiro R, Jatene FB. Video-assisted thoracoscopy as an option in the surgical treatment of chylothorax after cardiac surgery in children. *J Bras Pneumol* 2011; 37: 28–35.

36. Stenzl W, Rigler B, Tscheliessnigg KH, Beitzke A, Metzler H. Treatment of postsurgical chylothorax with fibrin glue. *Thorac Cardiovasc Surg* 1983; 31: 35–6.

37. Azizkhan RG, Canfield J, Alford BA, Rodgers BM. Pleuroperitoneal shunts in the management of neonatal chylothorax. *J Pediatr Surg* 1983; 18: 842–50.

38. Rustico MA, Lanna M, Coviello D, Smoleniec J, Nicolini U. Fetal pleural effusion. *Prenat Diag* 2007; 27: 793–9.

39. Ruano R, Ramalho AS, Cardoso AK, Moise K, Jr., Zugaib M. Prenatal diagnosis and natural history of fetuses presenting with pleural effusion. *Prenat Diagn* 2011; 31: 496–9.

40. Aubard Y, Derouineau I, Aubard V, Chalifour V, Preux PM. Primary fetal hydrothorax: A literature review and proposed antenatal clinical strategy. *Fetal Diagn Ther* 1998; 13: 325–33.

41. Feliciano DV, Mattox KL, Graham JM, Beall AC, Jr., Jordan GL, Jr. Major complications of percutaneous subclavian vein catheters. *Am J Surg* 1979; 138: 869–74.

42

Congenital malformations of the lung

SHANNON M. KOEHLER AND KEITH T. OLDHAM

INTRODUCTION

Congenital lung abnormalities are uncommon and diverse in their presentations. However, all those who care for infants and children must have an appreciation for the diagnosis and treatment of these anomalies because the potential consequences can be life threatening. In order to understand the pathophysiology of these malformations, one must have a basic understanding of the embryology of lung development as well as lung anatomy and respiratory physiology, which are presented below. Classical lesions including congenital lobar emphysema (CLE), congenital pulmonary airway malformation (CPAM), pulmonary sequestration, and bronchogenic cysts will be discussed along with several more uncommon lung anomalies.

Embryology

During the fourth week of gestation, the human embryo develops a diverticulum of the ventral foregut, which forms the primordium of the respiratory system.[1,2] This is mainly of endodermal origin; however, cartilaginous and muscular elements will be derived from the splanchnic mesoderm that surrounds the primitive foregut.[2] As the laryngotracheal diverticulum grows caudad, it becomes separated from the foregut by the lateral tracheoesophageal folds, which fuse to form the tracheoesophageal septum at the end of the fifth gestational week.[1,2] Thus, the dorsal esophagus and the more ventral trachea and lung buds are defined. The larynx, which is formed from the fourth and sixth branchial arches,[1] maintains communication between the pharynx and the trachea.

The lung buds penetrate the coelomic cavity by caudal growth, resulting in the formation of pericardioperitoneal canals on either side of the foregut.[1,2] The expanding lung buds eventually come to nearly fill these canals, with the small residual spaces becoming the primitive pleural cavities.[2] The right lung bud divides into three lobes, whereas the left forms two by the end of the embryo's fifth week.[2] The bronchi continue successive dichotomous division, and

by the end of the sixth month of gestation, 17 generations of subdivisions have formed.[2] This period is also the time at which terminal bronchioles and alveoli are forming. An additional six divisions of the terminal airways will occur during early postnatal life[2]; however, lung development probably does not cease until about 8 years of age.[2] Thus, development of conductive airways is essentially complete by the end of the second trimester, while terminal airways and alveoli, which are the site of gas exchange, continue to develop in late fetal life and early childhood. As one considers the various clinical lesions and their therapeutic options, this perspective is critical.

The pulmonary vascular system develops in parallel to the lung parenchyma. As the lung buds form, a pulmonary vascular plexus arises.[3] The lung buds branch to give rise to the pulmonary tree, while the mesenchymal tissue condenses to form the pulmonary vessels by vasculogenesis.[3] Over the course of fetal development, the pulmonary vasculature expands by vasculogenesis and angiogenesis.[3] It is not until 36 weeks gestational age that the pulmonary capillary networks remodel to position the capillary and alveoli in close proximity to allow optimal gas exchange.[3]

Anatomy

A brief discussion of clinically relevant anatomy is appropriate; several excellent references are available for a more detailed review.[4,5] As seen in early gestational development of the lungs, the mature right lung is composed of three lobes in contrast to the two lobes of the left.[4–7] The carina is positioned at the level of the fourth or fifth thoracic vertebral body in the term infant.[6] The mainstem bronchus of the right lung follows a straighter, more caudad course and is usually shorter and larger in diameter than that of the left.[4,6] This accounts for the preference of aspirated material to enter the right lower lobe or the posterior segment of the right upper lobe. Similarly, the configuration explains the propensity for right mainstem bronchus intubation during endotracheal tube placement.[6]

The vascular supply of the trachea, bronchi, and lung parenchyma is systemic in origin and separate from the pulmonary arterial circulation.[6] The trachea is supplied by branches of the paired inferior thyroid arteries, which anastomose with the bronchial blood supply derived from the aorta on the left and the third intercostal artery on the right.[6] Venous drainage is via the azygous and hemiazygous systems.[6] This systemic arterial supply and its accompanying venous drainage generally follow the segmental architecture of the lung and bronchi.[6]

The pulmonary arterial circulation is dedicated to gas exchange. Oxygen-depleted blood arrives at the lung through the pulmonary artery.[7] The blood travels through the lungs to the capillary network where it releases carbon dioxide and picks up oxygen during respiration.[7] The oxygenated blood then leaves the lungs through pulmonary veins, which return it to the left heart, completing the pulmonary cycle.[7]

Congenital lobar emphysema

CLE is characterized by air trapping and overdistention of one or more lobes, which are otherwise anatomically normal. This distention causes compression of adjacent normal lung parenchyma and can result in mediastinal shift and cardiorespiratory compromise (Figure 42.1).

A specific etiology of this disorder cannot be demonstrated in up to half of reported cases.[8–10] The underlying cause in the remaining 50% can be divided into extrinsic and intrinsic subtypes.[9] Extrinsic causes include compression from anomalous or enlarged blood vessels, congenital heart disease, mediastinal lymphadenopathy, bronchogenic and enteric cysts, and tumors.[6,8,9,11] Intrinsic causes encompass structural deficiency or absence of supportive cartilage in the affected lobar bronchus,[6,8,9,11] thereby causing expiratory collapse of the conducting airway with impedance to expiratory flow.[8] Partial obstruction from mucous plugging, extensive mucosal proliferation, inflammation, infection,

bronchial torsion, bronchial atresia, or aspirated materials are other possible intrinsic causes of CLE.[6,8,9,11]

CLE is a rare disorder with an incidence of 1 in 20,000 to 1 in 90,000 births.[12,13] Historically, it has been considered a disease of the Caucasian population with a male predominance (2:1 to 3:1)[6]; however, a more recent study suggested a higher incidence in non-whites,[14] and another study failed to show a male predominance.[15] It is most common in the left upper lobe (40%–50%), with other sites affected less frequently: right middle lobe (30%–40%), right upper lobe (20%), and lower lobes (1%).[8,11] In 14% of infants, CLE is associated with congenital heart disease.[13,16] The most common cardiac anomalies are large left-to-right shunts or pulmonary hypertension, but tetralogy of Fallot and patent ductus arteriosus have also been described.[16] Routine echocardiography is recommended in the screening evaluation of these patients. Rarely, other anomalies in the renal, gastrointestinal, musculoskeletal, or cutaneous systems may be seen.[10]

Presentation and diagnosis

CLE is rarely diagnosed on prenatal ultrasound.[10] The main finding on ultrasound is increased echogenicity of the lungs, but this is generally subtle and can also be seen in pulmonary sequestration, CPAM, or upper airway obstruction.[10] Also, similar to pulmonary sequestration and CPAM, there are reports of decreasing size of the lesion during pregnancy.[10] In more severe cases, mediastinal shift, polyhydramnios, or fetal hydrops can be appreciated on prenatal ultrasound.[10] Recently, reports of diagnosis of CLE with fetal magnetic resonance imaging (MRI) have been emerging and may prove useful in prenatally identifying the etiology in some cases.[17,18]

If symptomatic, patients with CLE typically present in the neonatal period with respiratory distress.[9,10,15,17] Only ~25% of patients are diagnosed at birth, ~50% by 1 month of age, and nearly all by 6 months of age.[8,11] Rarely, older children or adults may present with milder symptoms such as recurrent respiratory infections or cough, or may be asymptomatic altogether.[19,20] Depending upon the severity of adjacent lung compression, cyanosis and respiratory failure may occur, and this is noted in 12% of patients with CLE.[15]

On exam, the patient with CLE will demonstrate signs consistent with a hyperinflated lobe, including thoracic and respiratory asymmetry, decreased breath sounds, and percussive hyperresonance of the ipsilateral chest. Findings of mediastinal shift such as tracheal deviation and displacement of the cardiac apical impulse are relatively late clinical signs.

Chest roentgenography is the initial and often the sole diagnostic maneuver of choice (Figure 42.1).[9] There is increased radiolucency over the affected side, with accompanying atelectasis of adjacent compressed parenchyma and a flattened ipsilateral hemidiaphragm. Mediastinal displacement to the contralateral side may also be apparent. The chest radiograph should be inspected closely to

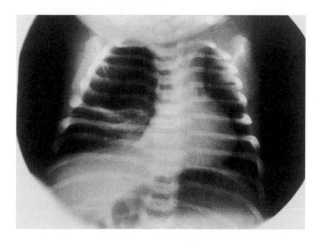

Figure 42.1 Congenital lobar emphysema. Chest x-ray in a 3-day-old infant who presented with respiratory distress, showing marked hyperinflation of right upper lobe.

differentiate between CLE and tension pneumothorax, which may have similar presentation and appearance but vastly different management. Contrary to CLE, tension pneumothorax has no peripheral lung markings. In the first hours after birth, the affected lobe may still be filled with fetal lung fluid and therefore have the appearance of a mass with fluid density.[11] Some authors advocate ventilation–perfusion radioisotope scanning as a useful adjunct to the chest radiograph.[11] Others advise the use of computed tomography (CT) or MRI.[11]

Treatment

Rapid and judicious bronchoscopy should also be employed to rule out intrinsic subtypes that may be treated without need for lobectomy. However, the surgeon must be available for emergent decompressive thoracotomy, particularly when positive-pressure ventilation is employed at procedures such as anesthesia induction or bronchoscopy.[11] If a source of endobronchial obstruction cannot be found and corrected, then the often-progressive nature of this lesion, as well as the risk of respiratory failure, dictate lobectomy of the affected lobe in infants. This is done via either muscle sparing thoracotomy or thoracoscopy. For the older child without symptoms, this approach can be reasonably tempered. Reconstructive procedures such as bronchoplasty or segmental bronchial resection are generally not appropriate, as the bronchial defects may not be focal or readily localized. In addition, lobectomy in the infant population is very well tolerated,[21-23] and bronchial reconstruction in the newborn is fraught with technical limitations.

Polyalveolar lobe

Polyalveolar morphology mimics CLE in its clinical presentation. This is a descriptive histologic term that refers to unusual and abnormal anatomic findings characterized by an increase in the number of alveoli in a particular lobe.[11] This is in contrast to CLE where alveolar histopathology is normal except for overdistention. Similar to CLE, polyalveolar lung results in expiratory air trapping and lobar overdistension with respiratory compromise.[11] The diagnosis and treatment of polyalveolar morphology are not different than for CLE. Likewise, because CLE and polyalveolar lung cannot be distinguished clinically or radiologically, these are often grouped together as congenital lobar overinflation.[11]

Congenital pulmonary airway malformations

CPAMs are a rare group of cystic lobar hamartomatous lesions, but represent up to 50%–70% of the bronchopulmonary foregut malformations in some reports.[24] The lesions are generally large, firm, multicystic masses that are composed of terminal respiratory structures, usually bronchiolar in origin and lacking normal alveoli.[9] They are typically unilobar and unilateral, and do not have a predilection for a certain side of the lung,[9] but are most common in the lower lobes.[11]

The precise pathogenesis of CPAM is unknown. Several theories exist regarding the origin of CPAM including anomalous or developmental arrest of terminal bronchiole maturation, while others believe it is due to focal pulmonary dysplasia.[25] Similar to the pathogenesis, the timing of development is debated with pathological and radiologic evidence at 5–22 weeks gestational age. Histology demonstrates ciliated cuboidal or columnar cells lining the cysts, with a lack of organized architecture; usually no cartilage is present (Figure 42.2). These malformations typically communicate with the normal bronchial tree and have a normal vascular supply, although aberrant systemic vasculature, sometimes derived from the aorta, has been described.[26]

The incidence of CPAM, in general, is reported at 1 to 10,000 to 1 in 35,000.[9] They do not have an increased incidence in a certain race or sex.[9] Associated anomalies are uncommon with CPAM.[11]

The classification of CPAMs has undergone constant modification in the past four decades. Adzick et al.[27] described macrocystic and microcystic or solid lesions based on prenatal ultrasound imaging. The contemporary classification scheme proposed by Stocker and colleagues grouped CPAMs into five distinct pathologic types (Table 42.1).[28,29] This classification system, which is based on the presumed site of development of the malformation, carries both descriptive and prognostic significance.[28,30] Type 0 CPAMs, previously termed acinar dysplasia, represent only 1%–3% of CPAMs.[29] The lesions appear solid on prenatal ultrasound and are composed of multiple small cysts less than 0.5 cm.[29] Unlike most other forms of CPAMs, these patients may have other congenital anomalies.[29] These patients have a poor prognosis, and some references even state that it is incompatible with life.[29]

Type 1 CPAMs are the most common subtype and account for about 65% of cases.[28,29] This form typically has one dominant cyst, in one lobe, measuring in size from 0.5 to 10 cm.[28,29] At birth, the cyst expands and compresses the adjacent healthy lung, flattens the diaphragm, and may cause mediastinal shift.[28] Thus, affected patients usually

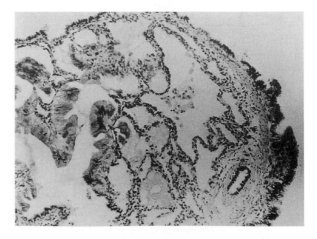

Figure 42.2 Type 1 CPAM. Histology specimen of lung showing mucinogenic cells, papillary epithelium, and disorganized, irregular alveoli.

Table 42.1 Pathologic features of CPAM

Stocker's type	0	1	2	3	4
Approximate frequency (%)	1–3	>65	20–25	8	2–4
Cyst size (max, cm)	0.5	10.0	2.5	1.5	7.0
Epithelial lining (cysts)	Ciliated; pseudostratified; tall columnar	Ciliated; pseudostratified; tall	Ciliated; cuboidal	Ciliated; cuboidal	Flattened; alveolar lining cells
Muscular wall thickness of cysts (in mm)	With goblet cells 100–500	Columnar 100–300	Or columnar 50–100	0–50	25–100
Mucous cells	Present in all cases	Present in 33%	Absent	Absent	Absent
Cartilage	Present in all cases	Present in 5%–10%	Absent	Absent	Absent
Skeletal muscle	Absent	Absent	Present in 5%	Absent	Absent

Source: Shimohira M et al. *J Thorac Imaging* 2007; 22: 149–53. With permission.

present with respiratory distress in the immediate postnatal period.[28] Type 1 CPAM patients usually have a good prognosis[29] with lobectomy.[28] If the lesion is small, patients may not present until later in life with recurrent infections.[28]

Type 2 CPAMs represent 10%–20% of CPAMs.[28,29] These lesions have multiple smaller cysts ranging in size from 0.5 to 2.0 cm. They can be seen in patients with pulmonary sequestration[30]; however, these lesions are also associated with other congenital anomalies (cardiovascular, genitourinary, and musculoskeletal) in up to 50% of patients.[28–30] The prognosis for these patients is often related to these associated anomalies, which may be severe, such as bilateral renal agenesis.[28] If patients do not have severe associated abnormalities, they may present with respiratory distress similar to Type 1 CPAMs, and treatment in this situation would be surgical resection.[28]

Type 3 lesions only represent ~5% of CPAMs and are more solid than cystic in nature.[29] Prenatally, these lesions often grow to a significant size, which leads to pulmonary hypoplasia and mediastinal shift. If this scenario progresses, it continues to polyhydramnios and hydrops, which can result in fetal demise.[30]

Type 4 CPAMs are also macrocystic and are made up of large cysts of size up to 10 cm.[28,29] This subtype represents 10–15% of all CPAMs, and also like Type 1 CPAMs, these patients have a generally good prognosis.[28] Unlike Type 1, which are bronchial, these lesions are peripherally oriented, and as a result, patients may present with respiratory distress in the neonatal period or with a pneumothorax in older children.[28,29] As with the other forms of CPAMs, the treatment of choice is surgical resection. It is important to examine these lesions closely intraoperatively as they can be confused with pleuropulmonary blastoma, which would have a solid component.[28]

Regardless of subtype, CPAM volume ratio (CVR) has been used as a prognostic indicator.[31,32] The volume of the lesion is calculated by measuring three dimensions of the CPAMs on prenatal ultrasound, and the ratio is determined by dividing by the head circumference to correct for gestational age.[32] Crombleholme et al.[32] demonstrated that a CVR ≤ 1.6 was low risk and >1.6 was at increased risk for developing hydrops.[32]

Presentation and diagnosis

Since the advent of routine ultrasound in obstetric practice, the majority of cystic lung lesions are now discovered prenatally in many institutions in the United States. The location of the stomach aids in differentiation between CPAM and congenital diaphragmatic hernia (CDH), although prenatal MRI may be needed for definitive diagnosis in difficult cases.[33] Serial ultrasonographic exams may demonstrate shrinkage or even spontaneous resolution in 15%–40% of fetal CPAMs.[22,34,35]

Physiologic consequences of CPAM can be seen antepartum and occur secondary to mediastinal shift and compression of normal lung tissue. Large masses, especially those involving type 2 or 3 lesions, can result in nonimmune hydrops fetalis and fetal demise. The polyhydramnios is thought to result from esophageal compression, preventing fetal swallowing of amniotic fluid; the hydrops results from mediastinal shift from the mass effect, diminishing cardiac output by vena caval obstruction.[22] Either finding during pregnancy is associated with poor outcome.

In the neonatal period, some infants will demonstrate tachypnea, dyspnea, cyanosis, or impending respiratory failure. Although this can be dramatic, numerous series in the literature have demonstrated that only 26%–45% of patients present in this manner.[36] Of the remaining patients, most will present within the first 2 years of life with recurrent or persistent respiratory infections, respiratory distress, pneumothorax, or chronic cough.[36]

As with all bronchopulmonary foregut malformations, the plain chest radiograph is the best initial diagnostic test in the neonate (Figure 42.3). Nasogastric tube position is often helpful to distinguish CPAM from CDH as an intrathoracic stomach

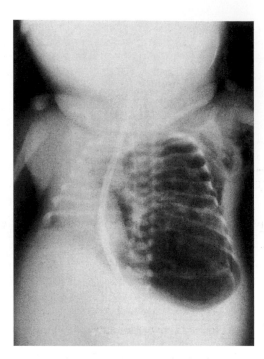

Figure 42.3 Congenital pulmonary airway malformation of the left lung with gross expansion of the lung, marked mediastinal shift to the right, and downward displacement of diaphragm. Note surgical emphysema of left axilla and chest wall, indicating rupture of a cyst.

is quite common with left CDH. The radiographic findings are variable; radiographs taken early in the neonatal period may demonstrate fluid within the lesion, whereas later films may show air-filled cysts.[37] Mediastinal shift, an ipsilateral flattened diaphragm, and compressed adjacent normal lung may also be present, depending on the severity of disease. It is advisable to obtain an axial imaging study, either a CT scan with intravenous contrast or MRI,[37] in all patients with cystic lesions of the chest in order to establish a diagnosis as well as delineate anatomic relationships prior to elective resection (Figure 42.4). Even those who have had spontaneous intrauterine resolution of an apparent CPAM demonstrated by serial prenatal ultrasound should be evaluated with axial imaging following birth, as residual parenchymal abnormalities may be present.[34,35,37]

Treatment

Maternal administration of betamethasone has been a subject of investigation in the fetal treatment of predominantly microcystic CPAM. While the exact mechanism is unknown, a recent study by Peranteau et al.[38] is one of the largest to demonstrate the benefit of prenatal betamethasone in congenital lung lesions. The majority of these fetuses had microcystic CPAM, but the study did include fetuses with large microcystic or solid non-CPAM congenital lung lesions (bronchopulmonary sequestration, CLE, and hybrid lesions). In this 11-year retrospective study, fetuses with a CVR > 1.6 or concern for hydrops were candidates for betamethasone administration.[38] The mothers of these fetuses

were given two doses of 12 mg intramuscular betamethasone 24 h apart. In some cases, this course was repeated one or two more times.[38] The majority of patients had reduction in the size of the lesion (82%) and resolution of hydrops (88%) in the single course cohort.[38] While the reduction was not as robust in the multiple course recipients (47% and 56%, respectively), it was still significant compared to nontreated historical controls. Furthermore, the survival rates were 93% and 86% in the single and multiple course patients, respectively, compared to historical controls where

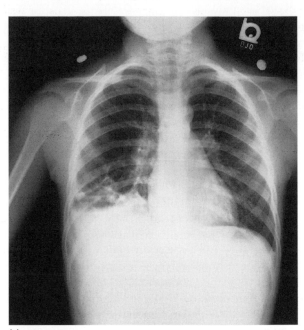

(a)

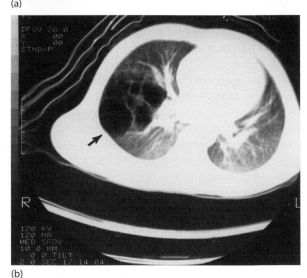

(b)

Figure 42.4 (a) Plain chest x-ray of a 9-year-old child who presented with fever, pleuritic chest pain, and cough. The lesion is an infected type 1 CPAM of the right lower lobe. (b) The lesion in (a) is shown on chest CT scan after treatment with antibiotics and before surgical resection of the right lower lobe. (From Coran AG, Oldham KT, The pediatric thorax. In: Greenfield LJ, Mulholland MW, Oldham KT et al. (eds). *Surgery: scientific principles and practice.* Philadelphia: JB Lippincott, 1993: 944. With permission.)

0% with hydrops survived and only 56% with a CVR > 1.6 survived.[38]

Prenatal treatment of macrocystic CPAM has also been advocated. Wilson et al.[39] have studied thoracoamniotic shunts for patients with macrocystic CPAM complicated by hydrops or at significant risk for pulmonary hypoplasia. In this population, they demonstrated increased survival after shunting compared to published reports.[39] Other groups recommend more liberal indications for shunting. Schrey et al.[40] offered thoracoamniotic shunting if fetuses had hydrops, ascites, polyhydramnios, large lesions, or lesions that were rapidly increasing in size. In this study, which included 11 fetuses, 1 hydropic fetus did not survive, but the rest were delivered alive at a mean gestational age of 38.2 weeks.[40] Thoracoamniotic shunting does appear to be a promising intrauterine treatment for macrocystic CPAM; however, further research will be required to determine the exact indications for this fetal intervention.

Ex utero intrapartum therapy (EXIT) procedures have also been utilized as treatment for high-risk CPAM. This involves resection of the CPAM via thoracotomy while maternal–placental–fetal circulation is maintained, followed by delivery of the infant.[41] Cass et al.[42] defined a population of patients with fetal hydrops or a CCAM-volume ratio > 1.6 and persistent mediastinal compression near birth who were selected for the EXIT procedure (*n* = 9) or standard delivery (*n* = 7). In this study, those patients who underwent EXIT procedures had favorable outcomes and survived to discharge, whereas all those in the standard delivery group developed respiratory distress requiring urgent resections and resulted in 28.6% mortality rate.[42] Larger studies are needed to confirm these results and clarify indications for procedure; however, like thoracoamniotic shunting, this procedure shows promise for improved outcomes in fetuses with high-risk CPAM.

Postnatally, the cornerstone of treatment in symptomatic patients with CPAM is complete resection of the abnormal tissue, which usually requires lobectomy. This is done via open, muscle sparing thoracotomy or thoracoscopy. Patients with multilobular disease may benefit from segmental resection if possible, and total pneumonectomy is occasionally required.[43] Prenatal diagnosis of CPAM should prompt referral to a tertiary care center, where critical care support and emergent pediatric surgical care are available. Like infants with CLE, the postnatal phenomenon of breathing or positive pressure ventilation may rapidly precipitate a crisis in CPAM patients if there is progressive distention of the affected lobe. Older children who present with pulmonary infection may be managed acutely with antibiotics, and then undergo subsequent elective lobectomy.

Treatment of asymptomatic patients with CPAMs is somewhat controversial. Some suggest that not all CPAMs require resection. They state that as prenatal imaging is improving, more CPAMs are being diagnosed leading to a new population of asymptomatic CPAM patients with smaller, previously unrecognized lesion. One report offers four arguments against surgery in asymptomatic infants:

(1) the natural history of CPAM is not well defined as until recently all were resected; (2) there is morbidity to surgery; (3) the malignant potential is overstated; and (4) there is the possibility of further regression with increasing age.[44] Similar arguments were proposed by Stanton[45] whose group had previously reported that only 5% of patients with congenital lung malformations (85% CPAM) went on to develop symptoms by age 5.[45,46]

Similar arguments were proposed by Ng whose group had previously reported that only 5% of patients with congenital lung malformations (86% CPAM) went on to develop symptoms by age 5.[46] In striking comparison to the Ng et al. study quoted above, Wong et al.[36] found that 86% of patients with asymptomatic CPAM at birth subsequently became symptomatic at a median age of 2 years. When surgical resection was performed electively at 1–3 months of age on patients with asymptomatic CPAM, there is minimal morbidity; however, there was a 47% complication rate when surgical resection was performed after the patients became symptomatic.[36] Likewise, two meta-analyses demonstrated significantly fewer operative complications when resection is performed prior to onset of symptoms.[47,48] Finally, operations performed in presymptomatic patients were associated with potentially parenchyma sparing resection such as segmentectomy with better long-term lung function.[49]

It was also thought that once discovered, these lesions should be removed regardless of symptomatology as malignant transformation with bronchioalveolar carcinoma was estimated to occur in 1% of CPAMs in general.[28,29,50] Furthermore, because bronchioalveolar carcinoma has been found in patients who have had their CPAM removed in infancy, a full lobectomy has been recommended to decrease the risk of bronchioalveolar carcinoma later in life.[28] Thus, for all of the above reasons, lobectomy has been advised in any patient with CPAM. Currently, there are no prospective studies comparing elective surgery with conservative management for asymptomatic patients,[45] and this will be necessary to completely resolve this debate.

Pulmonary sequestration

Pulmonary sequestrations make up 10%–30% of the cystic bronchopulmonary foregut malformations in most reports.[43,51] They are portions of the lung that are isolated from the surrounding parenchyma and have no communication with the normal tracheobronchial tree. In addition, the malformation receives its blood supply from aberrant systemic arterial vessels (Table 42.2).[52] They are classified by whether the sequestration resides within the visceral pleura of the normal lung (intralobar sequestration) or is invested by its own visceral pleura (extralobar sequestration).

Intralobar sequestrations make up the majority (75%) of pulmonary sequestrations, and most commonly involve the posterior basal segments of the left lower lobe.[53] As mentioned, these intralobar lesions are surrounded by normal lung parenchyma and pleura. The arterial supply is usually derived

Table 42.2 Characteristics of pulmonary sequestrations

Characteristic	Intralobar	Extralobar
Incidence	Uncommon	Rare
Incidence ratio	3	1
Sex	Equal	Male 80%
Side	60% left	90% left
Location	Usually in the posterior basal segment	Above the diaphragm, rarely below
Age at presentation and symptoms	Adolescent to young adults, 50% >20 years, recurrent pulmonary infections	Neonate 60%, B1 year, respiratory distress
Associated anomalies	Uncommon	Frequent (>50%), e.g., congenital diaphragmatic hernia (30%)
Diagnosis at neonatal autopsy	None	Frequent
Arterial supply	Systemic—from aorta, large vessels, often a single vessel	Systemic—from pulmonary or aorta, usually small vessels
Venous drainage	Pulmonary—inferior pulmonary vein	Systemic—azygos or hemiazygos vein; rarely portal vein
Anatomical relations	Not separate, within and part of normal lobe	Separate, has its own investment—visceral pleura
Connection with foregut	Very rare	More common
Bronchial communication	Present, small	None

Source: Shamji FM et al. Surg Clin North Am 1988; 68: 581–620. With permission.

from aberrant branches of the descending thoracic aorta.[53] Occasionally, intercostal, brachiocephalic, or abdominal aortic aberrant or multiple anomalous vessels are encountered.[53] Venous drainage is usually via the associated pulmonary vein.[53] Although sequestrations are, by definition, nonfunctional and sequestered from the respiratory tree, intralobar sequestrations may communicate with neighboring alveoli in the normal lung via abnormal air spaces, allowing some ventilation and air-trapping within the intralobar lesions.[53] Concomitant anomalies have been described in 11%–13.7% of patients with intralobar sequestration including musculoskeletal, renal, and cardiac anomalies or CDH.[53,54]

Extralobar sequestrations are completely separated from the normal lung and invested by an individual pleura. They are most commonly found on the left side (65%–90%) and in the lower chest (63%–77.4%), with the vast majority in the thoracic cavity (77%–91.7%) but may occur intra-abdominally (8.2%–15%).[52–54] These sequestrations also derive arterial blood supply from the thoracic or abdominal aorta,[54] with up to 20% having an aberrant vessel traversing the diaphragm. Venous drainage into systemic veins, such as the azygous, hemiazygous, or the inferior vena cava, is typical for extralobar sequestrations.[54] Aberrant air-space connections are not present; rather extralobar sequestrations are prone to hemorrhage or arterial-venous shunting, and the patients may present with high-output congestive heart failure.[54] Associated congenital anomalies are very common with extralobar sequestrations and are seen in ~60% of cases.[53,54] CDHs and CPAMs are the most commonly seen anomalies, but a variety of other congenital defects have also been described.[53,55] Unlike intralobar sequestrations, there is a 3 to 4:1 male predominance in most published series of extralobar sequestration.[54]

The embryologic origin of pulmonary sequestrations is unclear and controversial. Generally, extralobar sequestrations are thought to be congenital in origin and a result of either abnormal budding of the tracheobronchial tree or accessory budding of the foregut, or a combination of the two.[54] Some believe that intralobar sequestration has a similar etiology; however, others believe that it is an acquired disease caused by local infection.[54]

Presentation and diagnosis

Although diagnosis of intralobar sequestration is improving, patients with intralobar sequestration often present with pulmonary infections due to abnormal air-space connections with inadequate drainage, or from compressive atelectasis of adjacent parenchyma. This pathophysiology explains why diagnosis is uncommon in infancy, and presentation occurs later in childhood or adulthood with complaints of recurrent or refractory pneumonias, lung abscesses, or hemoptysis.

Extralobar sequestrations, on the other hand, are frequently diagnosed on prenatal ultrasound by identifying the pathognomonic aberrant arterial blood supply on Doppler. If the mass is large, shift of mediastinal structures, fetal hydrops, and fetal demise can occur. Ipsilateral pleural effusions are seen in 6%–10% of cases,[56] and the presence of a large pleural effusion puts the fetus at high risk for pulmonary hypoplasia.[57]

Infants with extralobar sequestration are often asymptomatic at birth. However, even if missed prenatally, due to the frequency of associated anomalies, they are often diagnosed early in infancy during evaluation for these other problems. Occasionally, these lesions will be identified during surgical repair of their associated CDH.[54] Those 25% that are symptomatic shortly after birth will present with respiratory distress or feeding difficulties.[54] The majority of symptomatic extralobar pulmonary sequestration patients will present with respiratory symptoms or congestive heart failure within the first 6 months of life.[54]

Plain radiographs of the chest will usually demonstrate an intralobar sequestration as a well-defined, triangular, non-aerated, atelectatic mass, or as a cyst with an air-fluid level (Figure 42.5a). Extralobar sequestrations are often difficult to visualize on chest x-ray but most often appear as a left posterior mediastinal mass or triangular retrocardiac density.[54]

In most infants and children with pulmonary sequestration, additional imaging beyond the initial radiographs is recommended. Ultrasound with Doppler (Figure 42.5b),

CT angiogram (Figure 42.5c), or MRI provide good anatomic detail and demonstrate relationships to neighboring structures. Importantly, all delineate the aberrant arterial vessels for purposes of diagnosis and preoperative planning. Preoperative upper gastrointestinal contrast study may assist in identifying the rare patients who have anomalous foregut communication with their sequestration, sometimes referred to as communicating bronchopulmonary foregut malformation.[54] Some experienced pediatric surgeons do not routinely do this, relying instead on intraoperative discovery.

Treatment

Fetal interventions are rarely required for pulmonary sequestration, but those complicated by massive pleural effusions may require early intervention. Thoracoamniotic

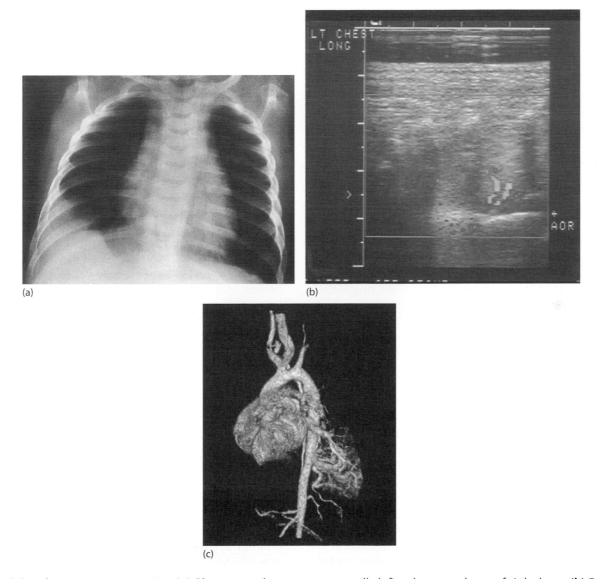

(a)

(b)

(c)

Figure 42.5 Pulmonary sequestration. **(a)** Chest x-ray demonstrates a well-defined mass at base of right lung. **(b)** Prenatal Doppler ultrasound demonstrating two aberrant arterial vessels to extralobar sequestration (arrow). **(c)** CT angiogram demonstrates an enlarged bronchial artery arising from the distal descending thoracic aorta, supplying an intrapulmonary sequestration.

shunts and laser ablation to interrupt the aberrant blood supply to the lesion have both been described.[58] Laser ablation has been shown to cause resolution of the associated pleural effusion and reduction or resolution of the sequestration itself.[57] A more recent retrospective study compared thoracoamniotic shunting to laser ablation and found laser ablation to be more effective, have fewer complications, and possibly reduce the need for postnatal surgery.[59] However, this study was retrospective and only had seven patients in the thoracoamniotic shunting arm and five in the laser ablation arm; thus, further studies are warranted to verify these results.

Postnatal treatment for pulmonary sequestrations consists of excision of the abnormal tissue. Although extralobar sequestrations may be asymptomatic, the cumulative risks of hemorrhage, infection, arteriovenous shunting, and late malignancy have generally been considered to be an indication for resection when diagnosed. This is a point of some controversy in recent years, as some have chosen to observe asymptomatic patients. In patients with extralobar sequestration, surgical resection is a relatively straightforward procedure performed via thoracotomy versus thoracoscopy, or laparotomy versus laparoscopy depending on the location of the lesion. Intralobar sequestration is treated with lobectomy via thoracotomy or thoracoscopy,[60] although in selected cases, segmentectomy may be appropriate. Segmentectomy may be more feasible in situations where prenatal discovery offers opportunity for resection prior to the onset of infectious complications.

A critical element in resection of a pulmonary sequestration is the identification and control of the anomalous systemic arterial blood supply. Reports of unrecognized or uncontrolled hemorrhage from accidental division of the aberrant arteries emphasize this point.[53] This is especially true of vessels with a subdiaphragmatic origin that course through the inferior pulmonary ligament and are prone to retraction into the abdomen when severed or avulsed. Current imaging techniques allow preoperative assessment of the arterial and venous anatomy associated with these lesions, and assist the surgeon in operative planning.

Other important technical points include particular care in identification of the phrenic nerve, which may travel adjacent and lateral to an extralobar sequestration. Abnormal foregut communications, whether diagnosed preoperatively or not, must be carefully sought and controlled appropriately intraoperatively.

More recently, reports have emerged in the literature regarding the use of endovascular embolization as treatment for pulmonary sequestration in infants and children. This is more frequently used in those patients who present with cardiac failure requiring closure of their shunt.[61] These patients will need to be followed long term to determine if they subsequently develop infections, recurrent shunts, or pulmonary hypertension. A randomized controlled trial would be ideal; however, given the selection bias inherent to the treatment of choice, this may prove difficult.

Bronchogenic cysts

Bronchogenic cysts are typically thick-walled, unilocular lesions, which are composed of smooth muscle, cartilage, and mucous glands lined by ciliated columnar epithelium.[60] They are usually simple and contain fluid or mucus.[9] However, air-fluid levels and infection may be seen if there is continuity with the tracheobronchial tree. In contrast to sequestrations, bronchogenic cysts have a normal bronchial blood supply. They arise from the trachea, bronchus, or other conducting airways but have usually lost their connection with the parent structure, although they often remain adjacent. Thus, the majority of bronchogenic cysts are found in the mediastinum (65%–86%).[9,37,62] Bronchogenic cysts can arise during any stage of airway development and can also migrate to subpleural, pericardial, paravertebral, cervical, or retroperitoneal locations if connections are lost with the parent structure; therefore, they can be found in many locations clinically.[9] Though benign, they generally progress to infectious, compressive, or hemorrhagic complications.[63] Rarely, bronchogenic cyst specimens have been shown to undergo malignant change[9,50] including rhabdomyosarcoma.[64]

Presentation and diagnosis

Prenatal diagnosis of bronchogenic cysts is occurring with increasing frequency. On ultrasound, these lesions appear as unilocular fluid-filled cysts in the middle or posterior mediastinum.[50]

Postnatally, if symptomatic, the presentation of bronchogenic cysts varies with age of initial symptoms.[60] Infants may present with respiratory symptoms such as dyspnea, cyanosis, or feeding difficulties.[60] These symptoms are related to compression of the adjacent conducting airway with partial obstruction or associated tracheomalacia. Older children generally present with pulmonary infections.[60] Hemoptysis may occur as a result of infection. Rarely, the cyst may enlarge to the point where the mass effect leads to mediastinal displacement, airway compression, compression of normal lung, and cardiorespiratory failure.

Plain chest radiographs typically demonstrate a smooth, spherical, paratracheal or hilar solid mass without calcifications (Figure 42.6). If airway communication or infection is present, an air-fluid level may be seen.[9] Displacement of adjacent airway structures is commonly observed. While these cysts are generally unilocular, a honeycomb appearance can be seen in some forms of this lesion. However, findings on radiographs are generally not specific enough to allow diagnosis. CT or MRI often is necessary to definitively diagnose a bronchogenic cyst and will assist in demonstrating anatomic relationships.[9,63] Contrast esophagram and bronchoscopy are additional modalities by which to identify foregut communication or extrinsic compression.

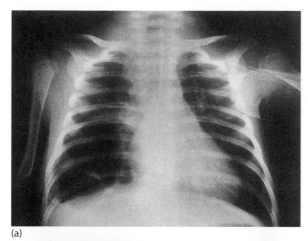

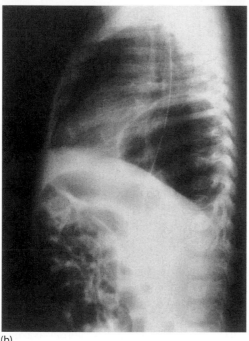

(a)

(b)

Figure 42.6 **(a)** Chest x-ray showing a large cyst occupying the lower half of the right thorax. **(b)** Lateral view localized the cyst to the lower lobe.

Treatment

If identified prenatally, postnatal excision is recommended. This can generally be done between 4 and 6 months of age.[63] However, acute respiratory decompensation from a large tense bronchogenic or lung cyst may necessitate needle or chest tube thoracostomy as a temporizing measure. Preexisting pneumonias should be treated with preoperative antibiotics. Thereafter, patients can be treated with surgical resection, enucleation, or lobectomy.[9] In patients with stable cysts, simple cystectomy should be performed with oversewing or stapling of any anomalous bronchial communications (Figure 42.7). If a bronchogenic cyst cannot be removed in its entirety, remaining portions of cyst wall may be destroyed with electrocautery. Generally, lateral thoracotomy or thoracoscopy is employed for management

of these lesions, although median sternotomy may be appropriate for certain central lesions.[62] The thoracoscopic approach has been used successfully in recent years and may be associated with shorter duration of thoracostomy drainage and hospital stay.[50,63]

Pulmonary hypoplasia, aplasia, and agenesis

Pulmonary hypoplasia refers to the abnormal development of an entire lung or both lungs, resulting in a diminutive and potentially dysfunctional gas exchange organ. The exact pathogenesis is not completely understood, but normal lung development requires a normal thoracic cavity, normal fetal breathing movements, as well as normal amniotic fluid volume and pressure.[65] Pulmonary tissue needs space to grow and expand in the thoracic cavity.[66] If expansion is prevented, developmental arrest during organogenesis sometime after the sixth gestational week will result in a reduction in the number and size of alveoli.[65] Varying degrees of pulmonary hypoplasia can occur, but it may be marked.[66] While primary pulmonary hypoplasia rarely occurs, it is most often a consequence of renal or urinary tract anomalies. Extrinsic compression during gestational development is also commonly seen.[65] A number of intrathoracic mass lesions may cause extrinsic compression of the lung; the most common are CDH, CPAM, and pleural effusions.[65] The physiologic consequences of pulmonary hypoplasia can be severe and include pulmonary hypertension, persistent fetal circulation, and respiratory failure. Extraordinary measures of clinical support are frequently required including high-frequency oscillation, the use of inhaled nitric oxide, and extracorporeal membrane oxygenation.[51,65–67]

Pulmonary agenesis is the complete absence of one or both lungs. This rare congenital anomaly has an estimated prevalence of 24–34 per 1,000,000 live births but is seen on 1 per 10,000–15,000 autopsies.[68,69] The specific cause of this accident of embryogenesis is unknown; however, there is apparent failure of organogenesis at about the time the trachea divides into the two lung buds, early in the fourth week of gestation.[69]

The diagnosis of pulmonary agenesis can often be suggested on prenatal ultrasound. With the addition of color Doppler to demonstrate the absence of the ipsilateral pulmonary artery, definitive diagnosis can be made.[69] Kuwashima and Kaji[70] have suggested that if prenatal ultrasound is indicative of unilateral pulmonary agenesis, fetal MRI should be performed. If (1) the lung is absent, (2) the ipsilateral main bronchus is absent, (3) the ipsilateral pulmonary artery is absent, (4) the unaffected lung has homogeneous, normal intensity, and (5) the abdominal contents are in the abdomen, the diagnosis of unilateral pulmonary agenesis can be made.[70]

Postnatally, bilateral pulmonary agenesis is exceedingly rare and is inevitably incompatible with life. Unilateral pulmonary agenesis may be asymptomatic; however, symptomatic patients may pose difficult neonatal management issues, not only from the standpoint of respiratory insufficiency but

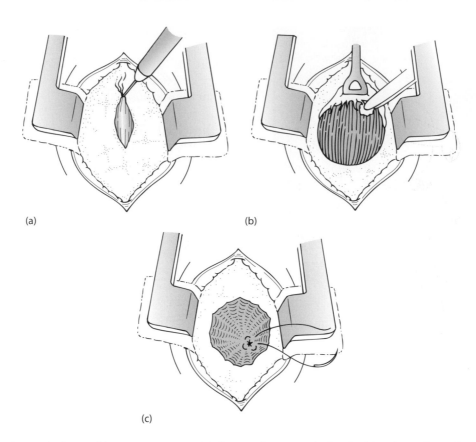

Figure 42.7 Operative technique of lung cystectomy. **(a)** Cyst wall exposed after incising lung tissue just above the cyst. **(b)** Dissection in the plane between the cyst and lung tissue. **(c)** Showing a small bronchus opening into the cyst—the opening is closed by oversewing it.

also because of a high incidence (50%–70%) of associated anomalies.[69] Older children may be asymptomatic or demonstrate nonspecific respiratory symptoms including a history of failure to thrive, exercise intolerance, recurrent respiratory infections, and chest asymmetry or scoliosis. A shift in the location of heart tones and absent ipsilateral breath sounds is demonstrable on physical examination. Chest roentgenograms will demonstrate hyperinflation of the contralateral lung and possibly a fluid-filled ipsilateral hemithorax in the setting of marked displacement of the mediastinum.[69] If the diagnosis had not yet been confirmed, again, the absence of the ipsilateral mainstem bronchus or the pulmonary artery is a definitive finding, and this can be established by endoscopy, echocardiography, axial imaging, or angiography. The prognosis reported in the literature is quite variable, but there is a worse prognosis for those patients with right-sided unilateral pulmonary agenesis. Kayemba-Kay et al.[69] suggest that a normal life can be expected for those patients with left-sided pulmonary agenesis, but this likely depends more on the concurrent congenital anomalies.

LUNG SURGERY IN NEWBORNS

Although a full discussion of thoracic surgery in children is beyond the scope of this chapter, a brief description of surgical technique in neonates is relevant. A number of comprehensive

texts are available.[71–73] Lung surgery in neonates is generally similar to that in adults except that the diminutive size, the associated lesions, and the unique pathologic entities require certain special considerations. Of course, the smaller the child is, the more care must be taken in order to avoid technical injury. As with all lung surgery, technical problems may result in serious and irreversible consequences. Collaboration with pediatric anesthesiologists familiar with the unique circumstances of pediatric chest surgery is essential.

Lobectomy

The patient is positioned in the lateral decubitus position, with the upper arm extended and placed over the head (Figure 42.8a). Rolled towels and other positioning devices may be placed in order to optimize stabilization and exposure of the operative field. As always in pediatric surgery, heat loss is a concern, and insulating coverings should be placed over exposed areas without interference to the surgical site. Convective and radiant warmers should also be employed.

Optimal exposure is gained by transverse or oblique incision over the fourth or fifth intercostal space, below and lateral to the nipple to avoid cosmetic and functional damage to the breast tissue. There should be some space between the tip of the scapula and the posterior extent of the incision. This becomes important during closure of the muscle layers, especially if the

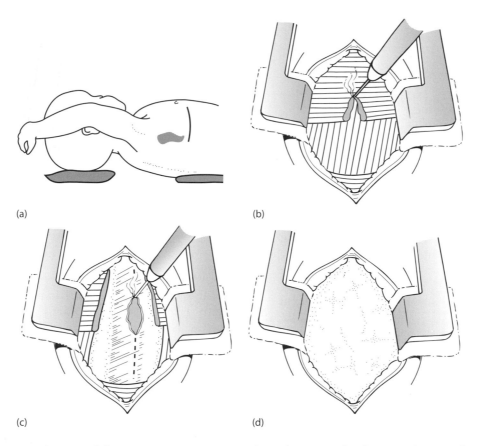

(a)

(b)

(c)

(d)

Figure 42.8 Operative technique of thoracotomy: **(a)** transverse lateral incision; **(b)** division of external intercostal muscles; **(c)** division of intercostal muscles along the upper border of the lower rib; and **(d)** retraction of ribs to expose the lung.

incision must be extended posterolaterally. Underlying muscle and subcutaneous tissue is divided along the line of incision (Figure 42.8b) by electrocautery. To limit postoperative morbidity from scoliosis, it is desirable and usually possible to employ a muscle sparing approach, which involves retraction of the serratus anterior and latissimus dorsi muscles, but leaves them intact. The scapula is elevated off the chest wall by retractor to gain exposure, and palpation is used to count the ribs to the correct interspace. In most situations in infants, the highest palpable rib is the second. Generally, the fourth interspace is used for a lobectomy, although the fifth can be used effectively as well. The incision is then continued with electrocautery just superior to the lower rib of the selected intercostal space to avoid damage to the neurovascular bundle that runs along the inferior border of each rib (Figure 42.8c). Care must be taken when entering the pleura to avoid injury to the lung parenchyma. A rib spreader is then placed to facilitate retraction (Figure 42.8d). The incision may then be extended anteriorly or posteriorly if further exposure is needed. It is clear that thoracoscopic techniques in practiced hands yield similar good results as do open techniques.

The following technique and illustrations are described for an left upper lobectomy; however, the principles are the same for any lobe resection. Gentle lateral and inferior traction on the lobe exposes the hilum. The visceral pleura is carefully incised circumferentially, exposing the hilar structures (Figure 42.9). Meticulous dissection reveals the left main pulmonary

artery as it courses under the aortic arch (Figure 42.10) and crosses the left upper lobe bronchus. Important structures to note are the left phrenic nerve anteriomedially along the mediastinum, and the recurrent laryngeal nerve branching from the vagus under the aortic arch. A review of segmental anatomy of the lung describes four main arterial branches supplying the left upper lobe; however, this can be variable. These are individually encircled, ligated, and divided. This is typically done with heavy silk and using double proximal

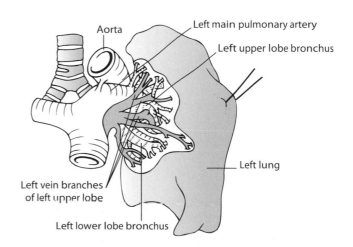

Figure 42.9 Normal anatomy of the left lung hilum containing the pulmonary artery, veins, and bronchus.

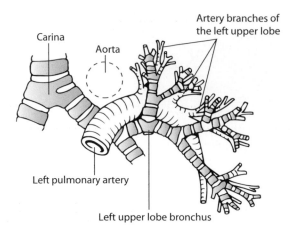

Figure 42.10 Main segmental pulmonary artery branches to the left upper lobe.

ligatures. Clips or stapling devices are suitable if appropriately sized. The bronchial blood supply traveling with the left upper lobe bronchus is likewise identified, controlled, and divided. Attention is then directed to the left upper lobe venous drainage. Again, individual branches are circumferentially dissected and ligated using the same approach as for the arterial circulation (Figure 42.11). The bronchus is then dissected, clamped, and divided. Closure of the bronchial stump with commercial surgical stapling devices is appropriate in older children; however, size and other technical limitations may make this undesirable or impractical in infants. If so, a simple sewn closure is best (Figure 42.12). Air leaks may be identified for suture repair by filling the chest with warm saline coincident with inflation of the residual lobe by the anesthesiologist. The inferior pulmonary ligament should be divided at this time to facilitate expansion of the left lower lobe, or it may be done early in the dissection to facilitate exposure. A tunneled chest tube is placed within the pleural space for drainage, and the wound or port site is closed in anatomical layers using absorbable suture. Postoperatively, the chest tube can be removed when there is no demonstrable air leak and output is minimal.

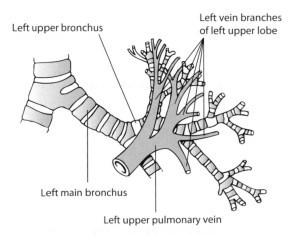

Figure 42.11 Segmental vein branches of the left upper lobe.

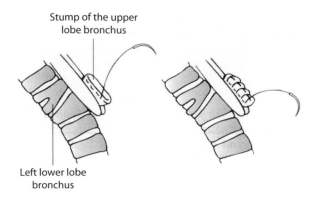

Figure 42.12 Vascular clamp placed across the left upper bronchus and the bronchus oversewn.

Wedge resections and lobectomies are remarkably well tolerated in the pediatric population, although age at resection is a factor. Older children demonstrate less compensatory growth than infants. Even so, most children will have little or no functional deficit after these procedures.[21,22,74]

The need for a pneumonectomy is limited in infants and children. Outcomes of pneumonectomy are generally good, yet children are more likely than adults to develop postpneumonectomy syndrome. This rare and potentially life-threatening complication occurs more frequently in children due to a more mobile mediastinum and greater tissue elasticity.[75] It is characterized by severe mediastinal shift, bronchial stretching, and respiratory failure.[75] Placement of an expandable intrathoracic prosthesis has been described as a strategy to manage this potential problem.[75,76]

REFERENCES

1. Carlson BM. Digestive and respiratory systems and body cavities. In: Carlson BM (ed). *Human Embryology and Developmental Biology*, 5th edn. Philadelphia: Elsevier Saunders, 2014:335.
2. Moore KL, Persaud TVN, Torchia ME. Respiratory system. In: *The Developing Human*, 10th edn. Philadelphia: Elsevier Saunders, 2016:195.
3. Woik N, Kroll J. Regulation of lung development and regeneration by the vascular system. *Cell Mol Life Sci* 2015; 72(14):2709–18.
4. Agur AMR, Dalley AF. Thorax. In: Agur AMR, Dalley AF (eds). *Grant's Atlas of Anatomy*, 13th edn. Philadelphia: Lippincott Williams & Walker, 2013:1.
5. Netter FH. Thorax. In: Brueckner JK, Carmichael SW, Gest TR, Granger NA, Hansen JT, Walji AH (eds). *Atlas of Human Anatomy*, 6th edn. Philadelphia: Elsevier, 2014:e49.
6. Pinkerton HJ, Oldham KT. Lung. In: Oldham KT, Colombani PM, Foglia RP, Skinner MA (eds). *Principles and Practice of Pediatric Surgery*, 2nd edn. Philadelphia: Lippincott Williams & Wilkins, 2005:951.

7. Weinberger SE, Cockrill BA, Mandel J. Pulmonary anatomy and physiology. In: Weinberger SE, Cockrill BA, Mandel J (eds). *Principles of Pulmonary Medicine*, 6th edn. Philadelphia: Elsevier Saunders, 2014:1.

8. Pearson EG, Flake AW. Congenital bronchopulmonary malformations. In: Holcomb GW, Murphy PJ, Ostlie DJ (eds). *Ashcraft's Pediatric Surgery*, 6th edn. Philadelphia: Elsevier Saunders, 2014:290.

9. Durell J, Lakhoo K. Congenital cystic lesions of the lung. *Early Hum Dev* 2014; 90(12):935–9.

10. Pariente G, Aviram M, Landau D, Hershkovitz R. Prenatal diagnosis of congenital lobar emphysema: Case report and review of the literature. *J Ultrasound Med* 2009; 28(8):1081–4.

11. Adzick NS, Farmer DL. Cysts of the lungs and mediastinum. In: Coran AG (ed). *Pediatric Surgery*, 7th edn. Philadelphia: Elsevier Saunders, 2012:825.

12. Ward CF. Diseases of infants. In: Katz J, Benumof JL, Kadis LB (eds). *Anesthesia and Uncommon Diseases*. Philadelphia: WB Saunders Co, 1990:199.

13. Kravitz RM. Congenital malformations of the lung. *Pediatr Clin North Am* 1994; 41(3):453–72.

14. Thakral CL, Maji DC, Sajwani MJ. Congenital lobar emphysema: experience with 21 cases. *Pediatr Surg Int* 2001; 17(2–3):88–91.

15. Cataneo DC, Rodrigues OR, Hasimoto EN, Schmidt Jr AF, Cataneo AJ. Congenital lobar emphysema: 30-year case series in two university hospitals. *J Bras Pneumol* 2013; 39(4):418–26.

16. Moideen I, Nair SG, Cherian A, Rao SG. Congenital lobar emphysema associated with congenital heart disease. *J Cardiothorac Vasc Anesth* 2006; 20(2):239–41.

17. Olutoye OO, Coleman BG, Hubbard AM, Adzick NS. Prenatal diagnosis and management of congenital lobar emphysema. *J Pediatr Surg* 2000; 35(5):792–5.

18. Liu YP, Shih SL. Congenital lobar emphysema: Appearance on fetal MRI. *Pediatr Radiol* 2008; 38(11):1264-008-0985-8. Epub 2008 Aug 26.

19. Pike D, Mohan S, Ma W, Lewis JF, Parraga G. Pulmonary imaging abnormalities in an adult case of congenital lobar emphysema. *J Radiol Case Rep* 2015; 9(2):9–15.

20. Toyoshima M, Suda T, Chida K. Asymptomatic congenital lobar emphysema in a young adult. *Intern Med* 2012; 51(19):2839–40.

21. McBride JT, Wohl ME, Strieder DJ et al. Lung growth and airway function after lobectomy in infancy for congenital lobar emphysema. *J Clin Invest* 1980; 66(5):962–70.

22. Frenckner B, Freyschuss U. Pulmonary function after lobectomy for congenital lobar emphysema and congenital cystic adenomatoid malformation. A follow-up study. *Scand J Thorac Cardiovasc Surg* 1982; 16(3):293–8.

23. Choudhury SR, Chadha R, Mishra A, Kumar V, Singh V, Dubey NK. Lung resections in children for congenital and acquired lesions. *Pediatr Surg Int* 2007; 23(9):851–9.

24. Adzick NS, Harrison MR, Crombleholme TM, Flake AW, Howell LJ. Fetal lung lesions: Management and outcome. *Am J Obstet Gynecol* 1998; 179(4):884–9.

25. Andrade CF, Ferreira HP, Fischer GB. Congenital lung malformations. *J Bras Pneumol* 2011; 37(2):259–71.

26. Rashad F, Grisoni E, Gaglione S. Aberrant arterial supply in congenital cystic adenomatoid malformation of the lung. *J Pediatr Surg* 1988; 23(11):1007–8.

27. Adzick NS, Harrison MR, Glick PL et al. Fetal cystic adenomatoid malformation: Prenatal diagnosis and natural history. *J Pediatr Surg* 1985; 20(5):483–8.

28. Stocker JT. Cystic lung disease in infants and children. *Fetal Pediatr Pathol* 2009; 28(4):155–84.

29. MacSweeney F, Papagiannopoulos K, Goldstraw P, Sheppard MN, Corrin B, Nicholson AG. An assessment of the expanded classification of congenital cystic adenomatoid malformations and their relationship to malignant transformation. *Am J Surg Pathol* 2003; 27(8):1139–46.

30. Shimohira M, Hara M, Kitase M et al. Congenital pulmonary airway malformation: CT-pathologic correlation. *J Thorac Imaging* 2007; 22(2):149–53.

31. Yong PJ, Von Dadelszen P, Carpara D et al. Prediction of pediatric outcome after prenatal diagnosis and expectant antenatal management of congenital cystic adenomatoid malformation. *Fetal Diagn Ther* 2012; 31(2):94–102.

32. Crombleholme TM, Coleman B, Hedrick H et al. Cystic adenomatoid malformation volume ratio predicts outcome in prenatally diagnosed cystic adenomatoid malformation of the lung. *J Pediatr Surg* 2002; 37(3):331–8.

33. Hubbard AM, Adzick NS, Crombleholme TM et al. Congenital chest lesions: Diagnosis and characterization with prenatal MR imaging. *Radiology* 1999; 212(1):43–8.

34. van Leeuwen K, Teitelbaum DH, Hirschl RB et al. Prenatal diagnosis of congenital cystic adenomatoid malformation and its postnatal presentation, surgical indications, and natural history. *J Pediatr Surg* 1999; 34(5):794–8; discussion 798–9.

35. Khalek N, Johnson MP. Management of prenatally diagnosed lung lesions. *Semin Pediatr Surg* 2013; 22(1):24–9.

36. Wong A, Vieten D, Singh S, Harvey JG, Holland AJA. Long-term outcome of asymptomatic patients with congenital cystic adenomatoid malformation. *Pediatr Surg Int* 2009; 25:479–85.

37. Winters WD, Effmann EL. Congenital masses of the lung: Prenatal and postnatal imaging evaluation. *J Thorac Imaging* 2001; 16(4):196–206.

38. Peranteau WH, Boelig MM, Khalek N et al. Effect of single and multiple courses of maternal betamethasone on prenatal congenital lung lesion growth and fetal survival. *J Pediatr Surg* 2016; 51(1):28–32.

39. Wilson RD, Baxter JK, Johnson MP et al. Thoracoamniotic shunts: Fetal treatment of pleural effusions and congenital cystic adenomatoid malformations. *Fetal Diagn Ther* 2004; 19(5):413–20.

40. Schrey S, Kelly EN, Langer JC et al. Fetal thoracoamniotic shunting for large macrocystic congenital cystic adenomatoid malformations of the lung. *Ultrasound Obstet Gynecol* 2012; 39(5):515–20.

41. Hedrick HL, Flake AW, Crombleholme TM et al. The ex utero intrapartum therapy procedure for high-risk fetal lung lesions. *J Pediatr Surg* 2005; 40(6):1038–43; discussion 1044.

42. Cass DL, Olutoye OO, Cassady CI et al. EXIT-to-resection for fetuses with large lung masses and persistent mediastinal compression near birth. *J Pediatr Surg* 2013; 48(1):138–44.

43. Ryckman FC, Rosenkrantz JG. Thoracic surgical problems in infancy and childhood. *Surg Clin North Am* 1985; 65(6):1423–54.

44. Fitzgerald DA. Congenital cyst adenomatoid malformations: Resect some and observe all? *Paediatr Respir Rev* 2007; 8(1):67–76.

45. Stanton M. The argument for a non-operative approach to asymptomatic lung lesions. *Semin Pediatr Surg* 2015; 24(4):183–6.

46. Ng C, Stanwell J, Burge DM, Stanton MP. Conservative management of antenatally diagnosed cystic lung malformations. *Arch Dis Child* 2014; 99(5):432–7.

47. Stanton M, Njere I, Ade-Ajayi N, Patel S, Davenport M. Systematic review and meta-analysis of the postnatal management of congenital cystic lung lesions. *J Pediatr Surg* 2009; 44(5):1027–33.

48. Kapralik J, Wayne C, Chan E, Nasr A. Surgical versus conservative management of congenital pulmonary airway malformation in children: A systematic review and meta-analysis. *J Pediatr Surg* 2016; 51(3):508–12.

49. Komori K, Kamagata S, Hirobe S et al. Radionuclide imaging study of long-term pulmonary function after lobectomy in children with congenital cystic lung disease. *J Pediatr Surg* 2009; 44(11):2096–100.

50. Wall J, Coates A. Prenatal imaging and postnatal presentation, diagnosis and management of congenital lung malformations. *Curr Opin Pediatr* 2014; 26(3):315–9.

51. Schwartz MZ, Ramachandran P. Congenital malformations of the lung and mediastinum—A quarter century of experience from a single institution. *J Pediatr Surg* 1997; 32(1):44–7.

52. Shamji FM, Sachs HJ, Perkins DG. Cystic disease of the lungs. *Surg Clin North Am* 1988; 68(3):581–620.

53. Savic B, Birtel FJ, Knoche R, Tholen W, Schild H. Pulmonary sequestration. *Ergeb Inn Med Kinderheilkd* 1979; 43:57–92.

54. Corbett HJ, Humphrey GM. Pulmonary sequestration. *Paediatr Respir Rev* 2004; 5(1):59–68.

55. Conran RM, Stocker JT. Extralobar sequestration with frequently associated congenital cystic adenomatoid malformation, type 2: Report of 50 cases. *Pediatr Dev Pathol* 1999; 2(5):454–63.

56. Stocker JT. Sequestrations of the lung. *Semin Diagn Pathol* 1986; 3(2):106–21.

57. Cavoretto P, Molina F, Poggi S, Davenport M, Nicolaides KH. Prenatal diagnosis and outcome of echogenic fetal lung lesions. *Ultrasound Obstet Gynecol* 2008; 32(6):769–83.

58. Wilson RD. In utero therapy for fetal thoracic abnormalities. *Prenat Diagn* 2008; 28(7):619–25.

59. Mallmann MR, Geipel A, Bludau M et al. Bronchopulmonary sequestration with massive pleural effusion: Pleuroamniotic shunting vs intrafetal vascular laser ablation. *Ultrasound Obstet Gynecol* 2014; 44(4):441–6.

60. Wesley JR, Heidelberger KP, DiPietro MA, Cho KJ, Coran AG. Diagnosis and management of congenital cystic disease of the lung in children. *J Pediatr Surg* 1986; 21(3):202–7.

61. Brown SC, De Laat M, Proesmans M et al. Treatment strategies for pulmonary sequestration in childhood: Resection, embolization, observation? *Acta Cardiol* 2012; 67(6):629–34.

62. Di Lorenzo M, Collin PP, Vaillancourt R, Duranceau A. Bronchogenic cysts. *J Pediatr Surg* 1989; 24(10):988–91.

63. Tolg C, Abelin K, Laudenbach V et al. Open vs thoracoscopic surgical management of bronchogenic cysts. *Surg Endosc* 2005; 19(1):77–80.

64. Murphy JJ, Blair GK, Fraser GC et al. Rhabdomyosarcoma arising within congenital pulmonary cysts: Report of three cases. *J Pediatr Surg* 1992; 27(10):1364–7.

65. Porter HJ. Pulmonary hypoplasia. *Arch Dis Child Fetal Neonatal Ed* 1999; 81(2):F81–3.

66. Parikh DH, Rasiah SV. Congenital lung lesions: Postnatal management and outcome. *Semin Pediatr Surg* 2015; 24(4):160–7.

67. Waszak P, Claris O, Lapillonne A et al. Cystic adenomatoid malformation of the lung: Neonatal management of 21 cases. *Pediatr Surg Int* 1999; 15(5–6):326–31.

68. Dinamarco PV, Ponce CC. Pulmonary agenesis and respiratory failure in childhood. *Autops Case Rep* 2015; 5(1):29–32.

69. Kayemba-Kay's S, Couvrat-Carcauzon V, Goua V et al. Unilateral pulmonary agenesis: A report of four cases, two diagnosed antenatally and literature review. *Pediatr Pulmonol* 2014; 49(3):E96–102.

70. Kuwashima S, Kaji Y. Fetal MR imaging diagnosis of pulmonary agenesis. *Magn Reson Med Sci* 2010; 9(3):149–52.

71. Kunisaki SM, Geiger JD. Thoracic surgery: General principles of access. In: Spitz L, Coran AG (eds). *Operative Pediatric Surgery*, 7th edn. Boca Raton, FL: Taylor & Francis Group, 2013:115.

72. Islam S, Geiger JD. Lung surgery. In: Spitz L, Coran AG (eds). *Operative Pediatric Surgery*, 7th edn. Boca Raton, FL: Taylor & Francis Group, 2013:207.

73. Sugarbaker DJ, DaSilva MC. Pulmonary resection. In: Fischer JE (ed). *Mastery of Surgery*, 6th edn. Philadelphia, PA: Lippincott, Williams & Wilkins, 2012:685.

74. Szots I, Toth T. Long-term results of the surgical treatment for pulmonary malformations and disorders. *Prog Pediatr Surg* 1977; 10:277–88.

75. Choi L, LaQuaglia MP, Cordeiro PG. Prevention of postpneumonectomy syndrome in children with prophylactic tissue expander insertion. *J Pediatr Surg* 2012; 47(7):1354–7.

76. Podevin G, Larroquet M, Camby C, Audry G, Plattner V, Heloury Y. Postpneumonectomy syndrome in children: Advantages and long-term follow-up of expandable prosthesis. *J Pediatr Surg* 2001; 36(9):1425–7.

43

Congenital diaphragmatic hernia

PREM PURI AND JULIA ZIMMER

INTRODUCTION

Congenital diaphragmatic hernia (CDH) is a common malformation characterized by a defect in the posterolateral diaphragm, the foramen of Bochdalek, through which the abdominal viscera migrate into the chest during fetal life. Population-based studies have reported the prevalence of CDH to be between 1 in 2500 and 1 in 3000 live births.[1,2] A recent study reported the prevalence of CDH in Europe to be 2.3 per 10,000 births for all cases and 1.6 per 10,000 births for isolated cases.[3] Approximately 80% of the CDH cases are left sided, 15% are right sided, and less than 5% are bilateral.[4,5] The size of the defect varies from small (2 or 3 cm) to vary large, involving most of the hemidiaphragm. The international committee of the Congenital Diaphragmatic Hernia Study Group (CDH Study Group), recently created a standardized four-grade (A to D) reporting system for CDH[6]: *A* defects are completely surrounded by muscle. *B* defects have a small and *C* defects a large portion of the chest wall devoid of diaphragm tissue. *D* defects present with a complete or near-complete absence of the diaphragm. The size of the diaphragmatic defect and also a potential severe cardiac anomaly were shown to worsen the outcome.[6] Despite advances in neonatal resuscitation and intensive care, newborn infants with CDH continue to have high mortality. Current survival rates in population-based studies are around 55%–80%.[4,5,7] Highly specialized centers report up to 90% survival but discount the hidden mortality, mainly in the antenatal period.[8] The high mortality and morbidity in CDH are mainly attributed to pulmonary hypoplasia and persistent pulmonary hypertension.[8–10]

EMBRYOGENESIS

The etiology of CDH is still not clearly understood. Although it is generally considered to be sporadic, there are reports of known chromosomal aberrations and autosomal recessive inheritance of unknown chromosomal origin.[11] The embryogenesis of CDH has been described as a failure of the pleuroperitoneal canals in the posterolateral aspect of the diaphragm to fuse during gestational week 8.[12] Consequently, the abdominal viscera including the liver and bowel migrate into the thorax, which is thought to cause pulmonary hypoplasia by compression of the growing lungs. The pulmonary hypoplasia associated with CDH extends to all aspects of the lung, resulting in fewer alveoli, thickened alveolar walls, increased interstitial tissue, and markedly diminished alveolar air space and gas-exchange area.[12] Parallel to airway changes, pulmonary vasculature is abnormal with a reduced number of vessels, adventitial thickening, medial hyperplasia, and peripheral extension of the muscle layer into the smaller intra-acinary arterioles.[13] The morphology of the CDH lung furthermore has an immature appearance.[12,13] The ipsilateral lung is the most severely affected, but the changes usually extend to the contralateral lung as well.

Experimental studies have suggested that the classical view of embryogenesis of CDH may have to be revised. A toxicological nitrofen model of CDH has shown that abnormalities in the contralateral lung as well as the ipsilateral side are present even before the diaphragm starts to develop.[14] Keijzer et al.[15] proposed the *dual-hit* hypothesis to explain the observations on pulmonary hypoplasia in this model. This hypothesis proposes that the early retardation in lung development that occurs before the development of the diaphragmatic defect is caused by nitrofen, whereas the late-gestational increase in lung hypoplasia is caused by mechanical compression from herniated viscera. Kluth et al.[16] have shown that pleuroperitoneal canals are not wide enough to allow herniation of gut loops in rats. Several groups have shown aberrant gene/protein expression of different growth factors and transcription factors in experimental models as well as in patients with CDH.[17–20] The retinoid signaling pathway and also its downstream target COUP transcription factor 2 (COUP-TFII) have been shown to be disrupted in the nitrofen model of CDH.[21–23] Beurskens et al.[24] reported significantly lower levels of cord retinol and retinol-binding protein in neonates with CDH. Vitamin

A–deficient rats display pulmonary hypoplasia with CDH.[25] Furthermore, the lungs in experimental models of CDH exhibit a response to retinoic acid different from normal lungs.[23,26] Furthermore, prenatal retinoic acid (RA) treatment has been shown to upregulate pulmonary expression levels of genes involved in lung morphogenesis in the nitrofen-induced hypoplastic lung.[27] Although prenatal use of RA has been controversial, these experimental data suggest that prenatal RA treatment may have a therapeutic potential to revert pulmonary hypoplasia associated with CDH.

Knockout models for Wt1,[28] Shh,[29] Slit3,[30] Gli2/Gl3,[31] Gata4/Gata6,[32,33] Fog2,[34] Pdgfrα,[35] COUP-TFII,[36] and retinoic acid receptors (RARs)[37] exhibit diaphragmatic hernia. So far, only mutations of Fog2 and WT1 have been identified in human patients with CDH.[35,38,39]

PATHOPHYSIOLOGY

The onset and severity of symptoms depends on the amount of abdominal viscera in the chest and the degree of pulmonary hypoplasia. Postnatally, the most severely affected babies present with respiratory distress (cyanosis, tachypnea, and sternal recession) at birth. Although the major cause of this is pulmonary hypoplasia, the resulting hypoxia and hypercarbia will result in pulmonary vasoconstriction and pulmonary hypertension. This in turn will cause reversal to right-to-left shunting through the ductus arteriosus and the foramen ovale, and the infant enters a vicious, self-perpetuating cycle.

Several factors have been known to contribute to the severe pulmonary hypertension in CDH. The pulmonary vascular bed is abnormal, with increased muscularization of arterioles in a manner similar to infants with idiopathic persistent pulmonary hypertension of the newborn (PPHN).[13] Increased thickness of the media as well as the adventitia of arteries of all sizes has also been demonstrated.[40] Furthermore, vasoactive substances such as endothelin-1 seem to be increased in infants with CDH. Kobayashi and Puri[41] found increased blood levels of endothelin, as well as increased expression of endothelin-1 in endothelial cells in the pulmonary vasculature. Endothelin-1 causes pulmonary vasoconstriction by binding to the endothelin A (ETA) receptor. The ETA receptor is ubiquitously present in the smooth muscle cells of the pulmonary vasculature,[42] and the increased endothelin-1 levels may thus adversely affect pulmonary vasoconstriction.

Hypoxia and hypercarbia may be further aggravated by a reported immaturity of the surfactant system in experimental animals and infants with CDH.[43] Others could, however, not confirm this deficiency,[44] and it has been postulated that the apparent surfactant deficiency may in fact be secondary to respiratory failure, rather than to a primary deficiency.[45]

Recently, Fleck et al.[46] reported that patients with CDH demonstrate proinflammatory and chemotactic signals in fetal blood at the time of birth. The authors suggested that these molecular signals lead to vascular changes resulting in pulmonary hypertension in these patients.[46]

DIAGNOSIS

CDH can be reliably diagnosed prenatally by ultrasonography at about 20 weeks of gestation. The diaphragm can be visualized, and its absence is indirectly suggested by the intrathoracic presence of abdominal viscera and compression of thoracic organs.[47] An important feature to look for is the presence of the liver in the thorax, if necessary using Doppler of the umbilical vein and hepatic vessels.[47]

Differential diagnosis with other intrathoracic pathologies, including congenital cystic adenomatoid malformation (CCAM), bronchopulmonary sequestration, diaphragmatic eventration, and bronchogenic cyst, needs to be made. It is also of vital importance to exclude the presence of other anomalies, including neural tube defects, cardiac malformations, and chromosomal aberrations A recent study demonstrated the prevalence of additional congenital disorders in 50% of the CDH patients.[48] Chromosomal aberrations are found in 5%–30%, with trisomy 21,18, and 13 as the most common anomalies.[1] Furthermore, the degree of pulmonary hypoplasia should be assessed. The presence of the liver in the chest in left-sided CDH indicates severe pulmonary hypoplasia.[49] The lung-to-head ratio (LHR—the area of the right lung at the level of the four-chamber view divided by the head circumference) has been shown to be a predictable estimation of the degree of pulmonary hypoplasia.[50] Additionally, the fetal lung volume and intrathoracic organs can be stratified by magnetic resonance imaging (MRI).[9]

Postnatally, CDH should be suspected in infants with severe respiratory distress at birth or within the first few hours of life. Physical examination reveals a scaphoid abdomen, an increased anteroposterior diameter of the thorax, and mediastinal shift. Breath sounds are absent on the affected side. Associated congenital anomalies may also be seen or revealed on further examination. The definitive diagnosis is made by plain radiography of the chest and abdomen by demonstration of air-filled loops of the bowel in the chest and a paucity of gas in the abdomen (Figure 43.1a,b). There is a mediastinal shift to the opposite side, and only a small portion of lung may be seen on the ipsilateral side.

TREATMENT

As recommended by the CDH Study Group,[51] nowadays, most centers perform endotracheal intubation and mechanical ventilation directly postnatally in order to perpetuate cardiopulmonary stability and delay the natural progression into severe hypoxemia and hypercapnia.[1] Mask ventilation should be avoided as it will distend the stomach and further compromise respiratory status. A baby with CDH should be sedated and have a nasogastric tube placed to prevent distension of the stomach and bowel. The usage of muscle relaxants should be avoided as part of the gentle ventilation strategy.[7,51]

CDH was previously considered a surgical emergency, where prompt surgery was performed with reduction of the

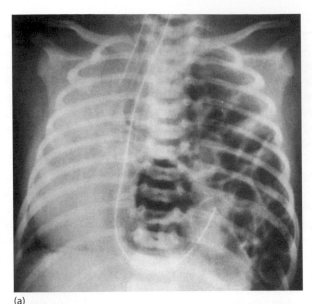

(a)

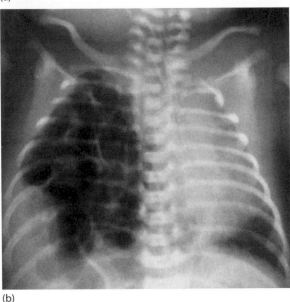

(b)

Figure 43.1 **(a)** Left CDH with viscera visible in the left chest, pulmonary hypoplasia, and significant mediastinal shift to the right. **(b)** Right CDH with viscera visible in the right chest and mediastinal shift to the left side.

abdominal viscera, thereby allowing the lungs to expand. The increased knowledge of the pathophysiology of CDH has led to a different approach, where prolonged preoperative stabilization has proven useful. Although it is now usual consensus to wait until the patient is cardiorespiratorily and hemodynamically stable, a Cochrane review provided no clear evidence preferring delayed (when stabilized) or immediate (within 24 hours of birth) surgical hernia repair.[52]

Preoperative treatment

An infant with respiratory distress requires endotracheal ventilatory support. Previously aggressive hyperventilation and hypocarbia were widely used, often causing barotrauma.[53,54] A new approach with gentle ventilation and permissive hypercarbia has been proven to decrease the mortality rate,[55–57] and several centers have shown improved survival as compared to historical controls, using a combination of gentle ventilation and delayed surgery.[53,56]

High-frequency oscillatory ventilation (HFOV) is a valuable tool in the treatment of infants with respiratory distress, since it provides effective ventilation while decreasing barotrauma. However, in CDH, HFOV has not been shown to improve the mortality or morbidity rates.[57–59] The impact of changes in HFOV settings must be monitored carefully, as high airway pressures may cause lung hyperinflation, with adverse effects on venous return, pulmonary vascular resistance, and ultimately cardiac output.[56]

European and American study groups recommend the following initial ventilation settings to achieve a target SaO_2 of >85% preductally and a pCO_2 of 45–60 mmHg.[51,57]

For pressure-controlled ventilation, the setting should comprise a peak inspiratory pressure (PIP) of 20–25 cm H_2O, a positive end-expiratory pressure (PEEP) of 2–5 cm H_2O, and a frequency (f) of 40–60/minute. Using HFOV, the mean airway pressure (MAP) should be 13–17 cm H_2O, with a frequency of 10 Hz and a pressure delta (Δp) of 30–50 cm H_2O, based on the extent of chest rise on the chest x-rays.[51,57]

Nitric oxide (NO) is a direct pulmonary vasodilator, and inhalation (5–20 parts per million) improves oxygenation,[1] but its relevance for CDH patients with CDH remains controversial.[1,60,61] NO can cause a short-term improvement in oxygenation in selected patients, which is beneficial for stabilizing the patient during transport or awaiting the extracorporeal membrane oxygenation (ECMO) cannulation; however, inhaled NO does not reduce the need for ECMO itself.[1,62,63]

ECMO is a life support system used in the treatment of CDH when conventional mechanical ventilation fails. ECMO employs partial heart–lung bypass, providing rest to the lungs for long periods of time, during which it is hoped that the lung and pulmonary vasculature will mature. Several centers advocate the use of ECMO only in patients with evidence of a "honeymoon period," i.e., patients with adequate gas exchange for a period preceding the deterioration in respiratory status. Others use preductal blood gases, where only patients with a period of normal preductal pO_2 and pCO_2 will be considered for ECMO.[56] Although widely used, a Cochrane review found that the ECMO benefit is unclear,[64] and also, other studies were unable to show a survival benefit of ECMO usage in CDH patients.[65,66]

Surfactant replacement has been tried as an adjunct to conventional mechanical ventilation or ECMO, but its administration is not without risk, and the benefits remain unclear.[56,67] Other ventilation strategies have been tried in CDH infants to provide efficient ventilation and protect the lung against barotrauma. Partial liquid ventilation has been shown to be beneficial in some cases, and some preliminary promising results have been obtained by the use of intratracheal pulmonary ventilation (ITPV).[68] However, none of these methods can improve the fundamental problem with the CDH lung, i.e., hypoplasia, and they therefore share the shortcomings of ECMO treatment.

Appropriate fluid management, as well as the use of inotropic agents, is crucial in the treatment of CDH. Adequate sedation and pain management should be used. Surgery should be performed when the infant is stable with minimal ventilator settings and is diuresing well, and the chest radiograph is improving. Routine administration of prenatal or postnatal glucocorticoids is not recommended.[57]

Several alternative therapies are in use for NO-resistant pulmonary hypertension. The phosphodiesterase inhibitor (PDE) 5 inhibitor sildenafil enhances NO-mediated vasodilatation,[1] and its use has been shown to improve oxygenation and outcome.[69,70] The efficacy of the PDE 3 inhibitor milrinone in neonates has been described in several case reports.[1] Other agents with proposed benefit are prostaglandins or Endothelin-1 (ET1) receptor antagonists, and also, novel agents like L-citrulline, Rho-kinase inhibitors, or proliferator-activated receptor-γ agonists are currently under investigation.[71]

Operative repair

An open approach (laparotomy or thoracotomy) or minimally invasive surgery (laparoscopic or thoracoscopic) is still a matter of discussion for the surgical repair of the diaphragmatic defect[72] (Figure 43.2). The most commonly preferred approach is abdominal, offering good exposure, easy reduction of the abdominal viscera, and recognition and correction of associated gastrointestinal anomalies.[68] The contents of hernia are gently reduced in the abdomen. On the right side, the small intestine and the colon are first reduced, and the liver is withdrawn last. After the hernia is reduced, an attempt is made to visualize the ipsilateral lung. Most diaphragmatic defects can be sutured by direct sutures of the edges of the defect. Although the anterior rim of the diaphragm is usually quite evident, the posterior rim may not be immediately apparent and may require dissection for delineation. There is usually a layer of peritoneum running from the retroperitoneum over the lower edge of the defect. Division of this tissue usually allows visualization of the posterior edge of the diaphragm. The defect is closed by interrupted nonabsorbable suture.

Sometimes, the posterior rim is absent altogether, in which case the anterior rim of the diaphragm is sutured to the lower ribs with either periosteal or pericostal sutures. In some cases, the defect is too large for primary closure, and prosthetic material is used (Figure 43.2f). Various patch types are commercially available (absorbable vs. nonabsorbable, natural vs. synthetic), but the ideal material has not been identified yet.[73]

An alternative is a muscle flap taken from the transversus abdominus, leaving the outer abdominal muscle layers intact. This technique should not be performed on patients on ECMO, or at risk of ECMO treatment, because of the risk of hemorrhagic complications. It also should be noted that the operations involving muscle flaps are too long and complex for critically ill patients and can lead to unsightly chest deformities. If the abdominal cavity is small, gentle stretching of the abdominal wall will enable safe closure in most patients. Whether a chest drain should be inserted prior to closure is controversial. The argument against the use of a chest drain is in avoidance of barotraumas as it increases the transpulmonary pressure gradient.

Minimally invasive surgery has been argued to reduce the trauma and physiological disturbance of surgery and cause a cosmetically better outcome. Although survival and patch usage are similar to open surgery, neonatal thoracoscopic CDH repair has been found to be associated with greater recurrence rates, longer operative times, and severe intraoperative hypercapnia and acidosis.[74–76]

Postoperative treatment

Postoperative care should be performed in the same manner as preoperatively, with a close watch on fluid management, ventilator, support and hemodynamic monitoring.[77] Some infants show improvement in oxygenation in the honeymoon period but usually deteriorate 6–24 hours later. This deterioration is due to pulmonary hypertension and persistent fetal circulation with an increase in pulmonary artery resistance, elevated pulmonary artery pressure, and right-to-left ductal and preductal shunting, leading to hypoxemia. Pulmonary hypertension is probably caused by multiple factors, such as increased abdominal pressure with impaired visceral and peripheral perfusion, limited diaphragmatic excursion, overdistension of the alveoli in the hypoplastic lungs with diminished alveolar-capillary blood flow, release of vasoactive cytokines, and deterioration in pulmonary compliance after surgical repair. Sudden deterioration in the patient's oxygenation status should raise the suspicion of pneumothorax. Infection complications including pneumonia and septicemia are not uncommon.

PRENATAL TREATMENT

A prenatal intervention that can reverse the lung hypoplasia might theoretically improve prognosis. Fetal surgery with primary repair of the defect seemed to be a promising approach, but clinical application of anatomical fetal CDH repair was abandoned once it became clear that it was not possible in fetuses with liver herniation and that those without did not benefit from the intervention.[78,79]

A fetoscopic tracheal occlusion (FETO) was then developed as it became clear from experimental studies that lung growth can also be triggered by tracheal occlusion. The effect on lung growth by tracheal occlusion and retention of pulmonary fluid seems to be exerted by pulmonary stretch itself, which in turn causes upregulation of different growth factors.[80–82] For FETO, currently, a one-port technique with endoscopic placement of a tracheal balloon is used.[50,83] A European group has achieved the best results

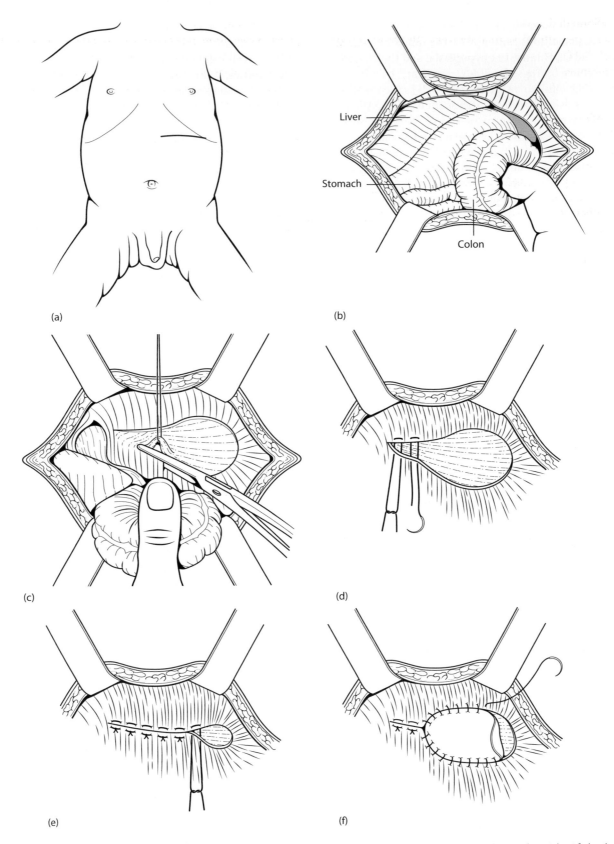

Figure 43.2 Operative repair of CDH. **(a)** A subcostal transverse muscle cutting incision is made on the side of the hernia. **(b)** The contents of hernia are gently reduced in the abdomen. **(c)** After inspecting the diaphragmatic defect, the posterior rim of the diaphragm is mobilized by incising the overlying peritoneum. **(d** and **e)** The defect is then closed by interrupted nonabsorbable sutures. **(f)** Large diaphragmatic defect is closed by using Surgisis soft tissue graft.

using balloon deflation by repeat tracheoscopy at 34 weeks' gestation,[50] permitting vaginal delivery. The most complication of FETO procedure is preterm premature rupture of the membranes (PPROM), which is probably iatrogenic in nature.[84] PPROM does have an impact on gestational age at delivery and complicates balloon removal.[84] In order to deliver infants with FETO, a special method of delivery had to be developed, the ex utero intrapartum treatment procedure (EXIT). Cesarean section is performed with maximal uterine relaxation, and while keeping the infant on placental support, the upper airway can be instrumented. However, a recent Cochrane analysis showed that there is currently only insufficient evidence to recommend in utero intervention for CDH fetuses as a routine clinical practice.[85] Neither an open nor a minimally invasive FETO approach delivered enough suitable data on perinatal mortality. Furthermore, antenatal corticosteroid treatment presented no clear benefit regarding perinatal mortality, days of mechanical ventilation, or days of hospital admission.[85]

Various other medical strategies for lung hypoplasia have been tested in the last decades in different CDH animal models.[9,86] These studies mainly focus on steroid administration with or without thyrotropin releasing hormone, vitamins, and stem cell therapy, but their future value for the human situation has yet to be addressed.[9,86]

PROGNOSIS

It is of vital importance to recognize variables that predict prenatal and perinatal mortality, since they will influence the information given to the family, as well as deciding eligibility for prenatal intervention. Firstly, other lethal malformations, as well as chromosomal aberrations, should be excluded. Intrathoracic herniation of both the liver and the stomach has been shown to be associated with a higher mortality.[9,87,88] The LHR can adequately predict outcome in CDH. LHR values <1 are associated with a worse prognosis with high risk of death, need for ECMO, and pulmonary hypertension at 1 month.[9,89] The observed-to-expected LHR (O/E LHR) is associated with death if the value is less than ~20%.[87] In MRI studies, the observed-to-expected total fetal lung volume (O/E TLV), percent predicted lung volumes (PPLV), and percent liver herniation have been found to correlate with survival, need for ECMO, and development of chronic lung disease.[9,90-92]

Several other factors have also been reported to be predictors for survival. In 2001, the CDH Study Group created a logistic equation using birth weight and 5-minute Apgar score to separate between high, intermediate, and low risk of death.[93] Later, they stratified the fetus risk using the factors very low birth weight, absent or low 5-minute Apgar score, presence of chromosomal or major cardiac anomaly, and suprasystemic pulmonary hypertension.[94]

Initial, $PaCO_2$ in nonsurvivors at 30 days has been found to be higher than the levels in survivors.[1,95] Furthermore, neonates with continuous hypercarbia had a worse prognosis than those who were stabilized to a normal $PaCO_2$.[95]

Further biomarkers to predict the patient's outcome are the best oxygenation index on day 1[96] and the simplified formula of postnatal blood gas (PaO_2–$PaCO_2$) to predict the need for ECMO or death.[97] Wynn et al.[8] found that low birth weight, patch repair, and need for ECMO correlate with more severe pulmonary hypertension at 1 month.

LONG-TERM OUTCOME

Improvement in the treatment of infants with CDH has increased the survival of more severely affected infants. Long-term follow up of those patients has led to the recognition of pulmonary and extrapulmonary morbidities that were not previously recognized. Pulmonary morbidity is the most common problem in CDH infants surviving beyond the neonatal period, which is even more distinct in patients treated with ECMO or requiring patch repair.[98] The prevalence of BPD was reported to be 41% in CDH neonates who survived until day 30.[99] Furthermore, the severity of chronic lung disease in CDH survivors may require prolonged ventilator support and tracheostomy.[98,100] CDH survivors also suffer from recurrent respiratory tract infections in infancy and early childhood.[101]

Some authors recommend palivizumab (Synagis) vaccination for CDH infants in the fall and winter.[102-104] However, there are currently no large clinical studies investigating the efficacy of palivizumab in depleting hospitalization rates for respiratory tract infections in these patients.[101]

Neurodevelopmental abnormalities have been abundantly described in CDH survivors presenting developmental delay; motor, cognitive, and behavioral disorders; as well as impaired language and neurocognitive skills.[101,105-107]

Sensorineural hearing loss (SNHL) has also been frequently reported in CDH survivors.[101] Potential predisposing factors, including the use of ototoxic medications and prolonged mechanical ventilations with high oxygen tensions, lead to SNH, which is found in CDH survivors treated with or without ECMO, suggesting that the use of ECMO is not the only predisposing factor for SNHL.[108] However, several retrospective studies found that the SNHL rate in both ECMO and non-ECMO CDH survivors is between 2.3% and 7.5%,[109-111] which is equivalent to the SNHL rate of all neonatal intensive care unit patients.[101,112]

A significant number of CDH survivors present gastrointestinal symptoms, including gastroesophageal reflux (GER), failure to thrive (defined as weight < 25th or 5th centile), and late bowel obstruction.[113,114] Gastrostomy tubes needed to be placed in one-third of patients in two survival cohorts due to nutritional morbidity.[101,115,116] Gastroesophageal reflux disease (GERD) treatment usually starts with H2-blockers, but if clinical problems like pulmonary infections or choking persist, fundoplication should be considered.[101] Nearly 40% of babies operated on for CDH will have symptomatic GER, half of which require antireflux surgery.[117] The most frequently reported predictor of antireflux surgery is the need of diaphragmatic patch repair.[98,116] Recurrence is more common in patients repaired with a prosthetic patch. Additionally, patients with patch repair have a higher risk for developing musculoskeletal deformities such as pectus excavatum or scoliosis.[118]

Although most survivors beyond the neonatal period are able to lead a normal life, children with CDH should be multidisciplinarily followed up and assessed for their pulmonary, neurodevelopmental, and nutritive outcome until adolescence.

CONGENITAL EVENTRATION OF THE DIAPHRAGM

Eventration of the diaphragm characterizes an atypically high or deviated position of all or parts of the hemidiaphragm, which can occur congenitally or be acquired as a result of phrenic nerve palsy. Congenital eventration is a developmental abnormality leading to muscular aplasia of the diaphragm, which primarily has fully developed musculature and becomes atrophic secondary to phrenic nerve damage and disuse. The incidence of congenital eventration of the diaphragm (CDE) is 1 per 1400 patients, with higher prevalence in males.[119] This paragraph deals with congenital eventration; however, clinical characteristics and management strategies are similar in congenital and acquired forms of eventration.

Clinical characteristics

Clinical characteristics of CDE vary widely from being asymptomatic to severe respiratory distress, bronchitis, pneumonia, or bronchiectasis. Gastrointestinal symptoms like vomiting or epigastric discomfort are also reported in later childhood. Patients with phrenic nerve palsy may have a history of difficult delivery, exhibiting tachypnea, respiratory distress, or cyanosis. During physical examination, breathing sounds may be reduced on the affected side, and a mediastinal shift during inspiration and a scaphoid abdomen are observed. Occasionally, CDE patients present with associated malformations such as hypoplastic lung, congenital heart disease, or cryptorchidism.[119]

Diagnosis

CDE is usually diagnosed via chest x-ray, revealing an elevated diaphragm with a smooth, unbroken outline on frontal and lateral chest x-rays (Figure 43.3a,b). Fluoroscopy is useful to distinguish a complete eventration from a hernia. Complete eventration can lead to paradoxical diaphragmatic movements. Ultrasound is the most useful tool in diagnosing CDE and to identify abnormal organs underneath the eventration. Other study modalities such as pneumoperitonography, contrast peritonography, radioisotope scanning, and computed tomography (CT) or MRI scans are rarely required.

Management

Asymptomatic patients without crucial pulmonary abnormalities may be treated observantly. Likewise, conservative

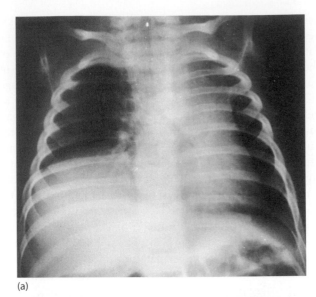

(a)

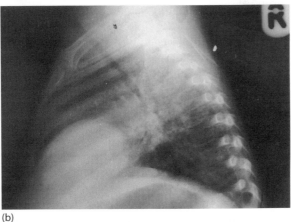

(b)

Figure 43.3 **(a)** Anterior-posterior (AP) x-ray image showing right CDE with liver visible in the right chest and mediastinal shift to the left. **(b)** Lateral x-ray image of right CDE with liver visible in the right chest.

treatment is recommended for patients with incomplete phrenic nerve palsy without paradoxical movement as normal function usually returns.

In contrast, symptomatic patients, especially those with respiratory distress, need prompt respiratory support and ventilation with humidified oxygen to minimize the diaphragmatic excursions. Intravenous fluids should be started, and a nasogastric tube helps to decompress the stomach. Surgery is undertaken once the patient's condition is stabilized.

Operative repair

Diaphragmatic plication is the method of choice, increasing both tidal volume and maximal breathing capacity (Figure 43.4). An abdominal approach trough a subcostal incision is useful for left-sided CDE. A thoracic approach with a posterolateral incision in the sixth space may be used for right-sided CDE. A transabdominal approach facilitates good visualization of the complete diaphragm and easier mobilization of

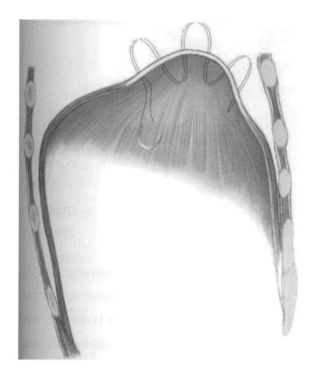

Figure 43.4 Plication repair of diaphragmatic eventration.

abdominal contents. Plications via laparoscopic and thoracoscopic approaches are also safe repair methods.

Outcome

Patients with CDE without underlying pulmonary hypoplasia commonly have an excellent prognosis. Mortality is related to pulmonary hypoplasia. A recent large single-center study showed that timely precise diagnosis and management of symptomatic CDE effectively prevents respiratory morbidity and diminishes complications,[119] including recurrence, renal insufficiency, as well as pneumonia and pleural effusions.[119]

REFERENCES

1. McHoney M. Congenital diaphragmatic hernia, management in the newborn. *Pediatr Surg Int* 2015; 31: 1005–13.
2. Morini F, Lally PA, Lally KP, Bagolan P. The Congenital Diaphragmatic Hernia Study Group Registry. *Eur J Pediatr Surg* 2015; 25: 488–96.
3. McGivern MR, Best KE, Rankin J, Wellesley D, Greenlees R, Addor M et al. Epidemiology of congenital diaphragmatic hernia in Europe: A register-based study. *Arch Dis Child Fetal Neonatal Ed* 2015; 100: F137–44.
4. Gallot D, Boda C, Ughetto S, Perthus I, Robert-Gnansia E, Francannet C et al. Prenatal detection and outcome of congenital diaphragmatic hernia: A French registry-based study. *Ultrasound Obstet Gynecol* 2007; 29: 276–83.
5. Colvin J, Bower C, Dickinson JE, Sokol J. Outcomes of congenital diaphragmatic hernia: A population-based study in Western Australia. *Pediatrics* 2005; 116: e356–63.
6. Lally KP, Lasky RE, Lally PA, Bagolan P, Davis CF, Frenckner BP et al. Standardized reporting for congenital diaphragmatic hernia—An international consensus. *J Pediatr Surg* 2013; 48: 2408–15.
7. Boloker J, Bateman DA, Wung J, Stolar CJH. Congenital diaphragmatic hernia in 120 infants treated consecutively with permissive hypercapnea/spontaneous respiration/elective repair. *J Pediatr Surg* 2002; 37: 357–66.
8. Wynn J, Krishnan U, Aspelund G, Zhang Y, Duong J, Stolar CJH et al. Outcomes of congenital diaphragmatic hernia in the modern era of management. *J Pediatr* 2013; 163: 114–9.e1.
9. Jeanty C, Kunisaki SM, MacKenzie TC. Novel nonsurgical prenatal approaches to treating congenital diaphragmatic hernia. *Semin Fetal Neonatal Med* 2014; 19: 349–56.
10. Coughlin MA, Werner NL, Gajarski R, Gadepalli S, Hirschl R, Barks J et al. Prenatally diagnosed severe CDH: Mortality and morbidity remain high. *J Pediatr Surg* 2015; 40(3): 160–73.
11. Wynn J, Yu L, Chung WK. Genetic causes of congenital diaphragmatic hernia. *Semin Fetal Neonatal Med* 2014; 19: 324–30.
12. Sadler TW. *Langman's Medical Embryology*, 11th edn. Baltimore: William & Wilkins, 2009.
13. Levin DL. Morphologic analysis of the pulmonary vascular bed in congenital left-sided diaphragmatic hernia. *J Pediatr* 1978; 92: 805–9.
14. Iritani I. Experimental study on embryogenesis of congenital diaphragmatic hernia. *Anat Embryol (Berl)* 1984; 169: 133–9.
15. Keijzer R, Liu J, Deimling J, Tibboel D, Post M. Dual-hit hypothesis explains pulmonary hypoplasia in the nitrofen model of congenital diaphragmatic hernia. *Am J Pathol* 2000; 156: 1299–306.
16. Kluth D, Keijzer R, Hertl M, Tibboel D. Embryology of congenital diaphragmatic hernia. *Semin Pediatr Surg* 1996; 5: 224–33.
17. Burgos CM, Uggla AR, Fagerstrom-Billai F, Eklof A, Frenckner B, Nord M. Gene expression analysis in hypoplastic lungs in the nitrofen model of congenital diaphragmatic hernia. *J Pediatr Surg* 2010; 45: 1445–54.
18. Goumy C, Gouas L, Marceau G, Coste K, Veronese L, Gallot D et al. Retinoid pathway and congenital diaphragmatic hernia: Hypothesis from the analysis of chromosomal abnormalities. *Fetal Diagn Ther* 2010; 28: 129–39.
19. Hofmann AD, Takahashi T, Duess J, Gosemann J, Puri P. Increased expression of activated pSTAT3 and PIM-1 in the pulmonary vasculature of experimental congenital diaphragmatic hernia. *J Pediatr Surg* 2015; 50: 908–11.

20. Takahashi T, Friedmacher F, Zimmer J, Puri P. Mesenchymal expression of the FRAS1/FREM2 gene unit is decreased in the developing fetal diaphragm of nitrofen-induced congenital diaphragmatic hernia. *Pediatr Surg Int* 2016; 32: 135–40.

21. Nakazawa N, Montedonico S, Takayasu H, Paradisi F, Puri P. Disturbance of retinol transportation causes nitrofen-induced hypoplastic lung. *J Pediatr Surg* 2007; 42: 345–9.

22. Noble BR, Babiuk RP, Clugston RD, Underhill TM, Sun H, Kawaguchi R et al. Mechanisms of action of the congenital diaphragmatic hernia-inducing teratogen nitrofen. *Am J Physiol Lung Cell Mol Physiol* 2007; 293: L1079–87.

23. Doi T, Sugimoto K, Puri P. Up-regulation of COUP-TFII gene expression in the nitrofen-induced hypoplastic lung. *J Pediatr Surg* 2009; 44: 321–4.

24. Beurskens, Leonardus W J E, Tibboel D, Lindemans J, Duvekot JJ, Cohen-Overbeek TE et al. Retinol status of newborn infants is associated with congenital diaphragmatic hernia. *Pediatrics* 2010; 126: 712–20.

25. Andersen DH. Incidence of congenital diaphragmatic hernia in the young of rats bred on a diet deficient in vitamin A. *Am J Dis Child* 1941; 62: 888–9

26. Sugimoto K, Takayasu H, Nakazawa N, Montedonico S, Puri P. Prenatal treatment with retinoic acid accelerates type 1 alveolar cell proliferation of the hypoplastic lung in the nitrofen model of congenital diaphragmatic hernia. *J Pediatr Surg* 2008; 43: 367–72.

27. Doi T, Sugimoto K, Ruttenstock E, Dingemann J, Puri P. Prenatal retinoic acid upregulates pulmonary gene expression of PI3K and AKT in nitrofen-induced pulmonary hypoplasia. *Pediatr Surg Int* 2010; 26: 1011–5.

28. Clugston RD, Klattig J, Englert C, Clagett-Dame M, Martinovic J, Benachi A et al. Teratogen-induced, dietary and genetic models of congenital diaphragmatic hernia share a common mechanism of pathogenesis. *Am J Pathol* 2006; 169: 1541–9.

29. Pepicelli CV, Lewis PM, McMahon AP. Sonic hedgehog regulates branching morphogenesis in the mammalian lung. *Curr Biol* 1998; 8: 1083–6.

30. Yuan W, Rao Y, Babiuk RP, Greer JJ, Wu JY, Ornitz DM. A genetic model for a central (septum transversum) congenital diaphragmatic hernia in mice lacking Slit3. *Proc Natl Acad Sci U S A* 2003; 100: 5217–22.

31. Motoyama J, Liu J, Mo R, Ding Q, Post M, Hui CC. Essential function of Gli2 and Gli3 in the formation of lung, trachea and oesophagus. *Nat Genet* 1998; 20: 54–7.

32. Jay PY, Bielinska M, Erlich JM, Mannisto S, Pu WT, Heikinheimo M et al. Impaired mesenchymal cell function in Gata4 mutant mice leads to diaphragmatic hernias and primary lung defects. *Dev Biol* 2007; 301: 602–14.

33. Molkentin JD. The zinc finger–containing transcription factors GATA-4, -5, and -6. Ubiquitously expressed regulators of tissue-specific gene expression. *J Biol Chem* 2000; 275: 38949–52.

34. Ackerman KG, Herron BJ, Vargas SO, Huang H, Tevosian SG, Kochilas L et al. Fog2 is required for normal diaphragm and lung development in mice and humans. *PLoS Genet* 2005; 1: 58–65.

35. Bleyl SB, Moshrefi A, Shaw GM, Saijoh Y, Schoenwolf GC, Pennacchio LA et al. Candidate genes for congenital diaphragmatic hernia from animal models: Sequencing of FOG2 and PDGFRalpha reveals rare variants in diaphragmatic hernia patients. *Eur J Hum Genet* 2007; 15: 950–8.

36. You L, Takamoto N, Yu C, Tanaka T, Kodama T, Demayo FJ et al. Mouse lacking COUP-TFII as an animal model of Bochdalek-type congenital diaphragmatic hernia. *Proc Natl Acad Sci U S A* 2005; 102: 16351–6.

37. Mendelsohn C, Lohnes D, Decimo D, Lufkin T, LeMeur M, Chambon P et al. Function of the retinoic acid receptors (RARs) during development (II). Multiple abnormalities at various stages of organogenesis in RAR double mutants. *Development* 1994; 120: 2749–71.

38. Devriendt K, Deloof E, Moerman P, Legius E, Vanhole C, Zegher F de et al. Diaphragmatic hernia in Denys–Drash syndrome. *Am J Med Genet* 1995; 57: 97–101.

39. Scott DA, Cooper ML, Stankiewicz P, Patel A, Potocki L, Cheung SW. Congenital diaphragmatic hernia in WAGR syndrome. *Am J Med Genet A* 2005; 134: 430–3.

40. Taira Y, Yamataka T, Miyazaki E, Puri P. Adventitial changes in pulmonary vasculature in congenital diaphragmatic hernia complicated by pulmonary hypertension. *J Pediatr Surg* 1998; 33: 382–7.

41. Kobayashi H, Puri P. Plasma endothelin levels in congenital diaphragmatic hernia. *J Pediatr Surg* 1994; 29: 1258–61.

42. Nobuhara KK, Wilson JM. Pathophysiology of congenital diaphragmatic hernia. *Semin Pediatr Surg* 1996; 5: 234–42.

43. Glick PL, Stannard VA, Leach CL, Rossman J, Hosada Y, Morin FC et al. Pathophysiology of congenital diaphragmatic hernia II: The fetal lamb CDH model is surfactant deficient. *J Pediatr Surg* 1992; 27: 382–7; discussion 387–8.

44. Sullivan KM, Hawgood S, Flake AW, Harrison MR, Adzick NS. Amniotic fluid phospholipid analysis in the fetus with congenital diaphragmatic hernia. *J Pediatr Surg* 1994; 29: 1020–3; discussion 1023–4.

45. IJsselstijn H, Zimmermann LJ, Bunt JE, Jongste JC de, Tibboel D. Prospective evaluation of surfactant composition in bronchoalveolar lavage fluid of infants with congenital diaphragmatic hernia and of age-matched controls. *Crit Care Med* 1998; 26: 573–80.

46. Fleck S, Bautista G, Keating SM, Lee T, Keller RL, Moon-Grady AJ et al. Fetal production of growth factors and inflammatory mediators predicts pulmonary hypertension in congenital diaphragmatic hernia. *Pediatr Res* 2013; 74: 290–8.

47. Deprest J, Jani J, Cannie M, Debeer A, Vandevelde M, Done E et al. Prenatal intervention for isolated congenital diaphragmatic hernia. *Curr Opin Obstet Gynecol* 2006; 18: 355–67.

48. Bojanic K, Pritisanac E, Luetic T, Vukovic J, Sprung J, Weingarten TN et al. Malformations associated with congenital diaphragmatic hernia: Impact on survival. *J Pediatr Surg* 2015; 50: 1817–22.

49. Metkus AP, Filly RA, Stringer MD, Harrison, Adzick NS. Sonographic predictors of survival in fetal diaphragmatic hernia. *J Pediatr Surg* 1996; 31: 148–51; discussion 151–2.

50. Deprest J, Jani J, van Schoubroeck D, Cannie M, Gallot D, Dymarkowski S et al. Current consequences of prenatal diagnosis of congenital diaphragmatic hernia. *J Pediatr Surg* 2006; 41: 423–30.

51. Reiss I, Schaible T, van den Hout L, Capolupo I, Allegaert K, van Heijst A et al. Standardized postnatal management of infants with congenital diaphragmatic hernia in Europe: The CDH EURO Consortium consensus. *Neonatology* 2010; 98: 354–64.

52. Moyer V, Moya F, Tibboel R, Losty P, Nagaya M, Lally KP. Late versus early surgical correction for congenital diaphragmatic hernia in newborn infants. *Cochrane Database Syst Rev* 2002: CD001695.

53. Masumoto K, Teshiba R, Esumi G, Nagata K, Takahata Y, Hikino S et al. Improvement in the outcome of patients with antenatally diagnosed congenital diaphragmatic hernia using gentle ventilation and circulatory stabilization. *Pediatr Surg Int* 2009; 25: 487–92.

54. Vitali SH, Arnold JH. Bench-to-bedside review: Ventilator strategies to reduce lung injury—Lessons from pediatric and neonatal intensive care. *Crit Care* 2005; 9: 177–83.

55. Conforti AF, Losty PD. Perinatal management of congenital diaphragmatic hernia. *Early Hum Dev* 2006; 82: 283–7.

56. Logan JW, Cotten CM, Goldberg RN, Clark RH. Mechanical ventilation strategies in the management of congenital diaphragmatic hernia. *Semin Pediatr Surg* 2007; 16: 115–25.

57. Puligandla PS, Grabowski J, Austin M, Hedrick H, Renaud E, Arnold M et al. Management of congenital diaphragmatic hernia: A systematic review from the APSA outcomes and evidence based practice committee. *J Pediatr Surg* 2015; 50: 1958–70.

58. Migliazza L, Bellan C, Alberti D, Auriemma A, Burgio G, Locatelli G et al. Retrospective study of 111 cases of congenital diaphragmatic hernia treated with early high-frequency oscillatory ventilation and presurgical stabilization. *J Pediatr Surg* 2007; 42: 1526–32.

59. Lago P, Meneghini L, Chiandetti L, Tormena F, Metrangolo S, Gamba P. Congenital diaphragmatic hernia: Intensive care unit or operating room? *Am J Perinatol* 2005; 22: 189–97.

60. Davis CF, Sabharwal AJ. Management of congenital diaphragmatic hernia. *Arch Dis Child Fetal Neonatal Ed* 1998; 79: F1–3.

61. Tiryaki S, Ozcan C, Erdener A. Initial oxygenation response to inhaled nitric oxide predicts improved outcome in congenital diaphragmatic hernia. *Drugs R D* 2014; 14: 215–19.

62. Oliveira CA, Troster EJ, Pereira CR. Inhaled nitric oxide in the management of persistent pulmonary hypertension of the newborn: A meta-analysis. *Rev Hosp Clin Fac Med Sao Paulo* 2000; 55: 145–54.

63. Inhaled nitric oxide and hypoxic respiratory failure in infants with congenital diaphragmatic hernia. The Neonatal Inhaled Nitric Oxide Study Group (NINOS). *Pediatrics* 1997; 99: 838–45.

64. Mugford M, Elbourne D, Field D. Extracorporeal membrane oxygenation for severe respiratory failure in newborn infants. *Cochrane Database Syst Rev* 2008: CD001340.

65. Davis PJ, Firmin RK, Manktelow B, Goldman AP, Davis CF, Smith JH et al. Long-term outcome following extracorporeal membrane oxygenation for congenital diaphragmatic hernia: The UK experience. *J Pediatr* 2004; 144: 309–15.

66. Morini F, Goldman A, Pierro A. Extracorporeal membrane oxygenation in infants with congenital diaphragmatic hernia: A systematic review of the evidence. *Eur J Pediatr Surg* 2006; 16: 385–91.

67. Lotze A, Knight GR, Anderson KD, Hull WM, Whitsett JA, O'Donnell RM et al. Surfactant (beractant) therapy for infants with congenital diaphragmatic hernia on ECMO: Evidence of persistent surfactant deficiency. *J Pediatr Surg* 1994; 29: 407–12.

68. Puri P. Congenital Diaphragmatic Hernia and Eventration. In: Puri P, Höllwarth ME (eds). *Pediatric Surgery*. Springer Surgery Atlas Series. Berlin: Springer, 2006: 115–24.

69. Rocha G, Baptista MJ, Correia-Pinto J, Guimaraes H. Congenital diaphragmatic hernia: Experience of 14 years. *Minerva Pediatr* 2013; 65: 271–8.

70. Bialkowski A, Moenkemeyer F, Patel N. Intravenous sildenafil in the management of pulmonary hypertension associated with congenital diaphragmatic hernia. *Eur J Pediatr Surg* 2015; 25: 171–6.

71. Lakshminrusimha S, Mathew B, Leach CL. Pharmacologic strategies in neonatal pulmonary hypertension other than nitric oxide. *Semin Perinatol* 2016.

72. Terui K, Nagata K, Ito M, Yamoto M, Shiraishi M, Taguchi T et al. Surgical approaches for neonatal congenital diaphragmatic hernia: A systematic review and meta-analysis. *Pediatr Surg Int* 2015; 31: 891–7.

73. Zani A, Zani-Ruttenstock E, Pierro A. Advances in the surgical approach to congenital diaphragmatic hernia. *Semin Fetal Neonatal Med* 2014; 19: 364–9.

74. Lansdale N, Alam S, Losty PD, Jesudason EC. Neonatal endosurgical congenital diaphragmatic hernia repair: A systematic review and meta-analysis. *Ann Surg* 2010; 252: 20–6.

75. Bishay M, Giacomello L, Retrosi G, Thyoka M, Garriboli M, Brierley J et al. Hypercapnia and acidosis during open and thoracoscopic repair of congenital diaphragmatic hernia and esophageal atresia: Results of a pilot randomized controlled trial. *Ann Surg* 2013; 258: 895–900.

76. Pierro A. Hypercapnia and acidosis during the thoracoscopic repair of oesophageal atresia and congenital diaphragmatic hernia. *J Pediatr Surg* 2015; 50: 247–9.

77. Puri P, Nakazawa N. Congenital diaphragmatic hernia. In: Puri P, Höllwarth ME (eds). *Pediatric Surgery: Diagnosis and Management*. Berlin: Springer, 2009: 307–13.

78. Harrison MR, Adzick NS, Flake AW, Jennings RW, Estes JM, MacGillivray TE et al. Correction of congenital diaphragmatic hernia in utero: VI. Hard-earned lessons. *J Pediatr Surg* 1993; 28: 1411–7; discussion 1417–8.

79. Harrison MR, Adzick NS, Bullard KM, Farrell JA, Howell LJ, Rosen MA et al. Correction of congenital diaphragmatic hernia in utero VII: A prospective trial. *J Pediatr Surg* 1997; 32: 1637–42.

80. Liao SL, Luks FI, Piasecki GJ, Wild YK, Papadakis K, Paepe ME de. Late-gestation tracheal occlusion in the fetal lamb causes rapid lung growth with type II cell preservation. *J Surg Res* 2000; 92: 64–70.

81. Nobuhara KK, DiFiore JW, Ibla JC, Siddiqui AM, Ferretti ML, Fauza DO et al. Insulin-like growth factor-I gene expression in three models of accelerated lung growth. *J Pediatr Surg* 1998; 33: 1057–60; discussion 1061.

82. Muratore CS, Nguyen HT, Ziegler MM, Wilson JM. Stretch-induced upregulation of VEGF gene expression in murine pulmonary culture: A role for angiogenesis in lung development. *J Pediatr Surg* 2000; 35: 906–12; discussion 912–3.

83. Harrison MR, Keller RL, Hawgood SB, Kitterman JA, Sandberg PL, Farmer DL et al. A randomized trial of fetal endoscopic tracheal occlusion for severe fetal congenital diaphragmatic hernia. *N Engl J Med* 2003; 349: 1916–24.

84. Deprest J, Nicolaides K, Done' E, Lewi P, Barki G, Largen E et al. Technical aspects of fetal endoscopic tracheal occlusion for congenital diaphragmatic hernia. *J Pediatr Surg* 2011; 46: 22–32.

85. Grivell RM, Andersen C, Dodd JM. Prenatal interventions for congenital diaphragmatic hernia for improving outcomes. *Cochrane Database Syst Rev* 2015; 11: CD008925.

86. Eastwood MP, Russo FM, Toelen J, Deprest J. Medical interventions to reverse pulmonary hypoplasia in the animal model of congenital diaphragmatic hernia: A systematic review. *Pediatr Pulmonol* 2015; 50: 820–38.

87. Ruano R, Takashi E, da Silva MM, Campos, J A D B, Tannuri U, Zugaib M. Prediction and probability of neonatal outcome in isolated congenital diaphragmatic hernia using multiple ultrasound parameters. *Ultrasound Obstet Gynecol* 2012; 39: 42–9.

88. Mann PC, Morriss FH, Klein JM. Prediction of survival in infants with congenital diaphragmatic hernia based on stomach position, surgical timing, and oxygenation index. *Am J Perinatol* 2012; 29: 383–90.

89. Garcia AV, Fingeret AL, Thirumoorthi AS, Hahn E, Leskowitz MJ, Aspelund G et al. Lung to head ratio in infants with congenital diaphragmatic hernia does not predict long term pulmonary hypertension. *J Pediatr Surg* 2013; 48: 154–7.

90. Walleyo A, Debus A, Kehl S, Weiss C, Schönberg SO, Schaible T et al. Periodic MRI lung volume assessment in fetuses with congenital diaphragmatic hernia: Prediction of survival, need for ECMO, and development of chronic lung disease. *AJR Am J Roentgenol* 2013; 201: 419–26.

91. Ruano R, Lazar DA, Cass DL, Zamora IJ, Lee TC, Cassady CI et al. Fetal lung volume and quantification of liver herniation by magnetic resonance imaging in isolated congenital diaphragmatic hernia. *Ultrasound Obstet Gynecol* 2014; 43: 662–9.

92. Barnewolt CE, Kunisaki SM, Fauza DO, Nemes LP, Estroff JA, Jennings RW. Percent predicted lung volumes as measured on fetal magnetic resonance imaging: A useful biometric parameter for risk stratification in congenital diaphragmatic hernia. *J Pediatr Surg* 2007; 42: 193–7.

93. Estimating disease severity of congenital diaphragmatic hernia in the first 5 minutes of life. *J Pediatr Surg* 2001; 36: 141–5.

94. Brindle ME, Cook EF, Tibboel D, Lally PA, Lally KP. A clinical prediction rule for the severity of congenital diaphragmatic hernias in newborns. *Pediatrics* 2014; 134: e413–9.

95. Abbas PI, Cass DL, Olutoye OO, Zamora IJ, Akinkuotu AC, Sheikh F et al. Persistent hypercarbia after resuscitation is associated with increased mortality in congenital diaphragmatic hernia patients. *J Pediatr Surg* 2015; 50: 739–43.

96. Ruttenstock E, Wright N, Barrena S, Krickhahn A, Castellani C, Desai AP et al. Best oxygenation index on day 1: A reliable marker for outcome and survival in infants with congenital diaphragmatic hernia. *Eur J Pediatr Surg* 2015; 25: 3–8.

97. Park HW, Lee BS, Lim G, Choi Y, Kim EA, Kim K. A simplified formula using early blood gas analysis can predict survival outcomes and the requirements for

extracorporeal membrane oxygenation in congenital diaphragmatic hernia. *J Korean Med Sci* 2013; 28: 924–8.

98. Jaillard SM, Pierrat V, Dubois A, Truffert P, Lequien P, Wurtz AJ et al. Outcome at 2 years of infants with congenital diaphragmatic hernia: A population-based study. *Ann Thorac Surg* 2003; 75: 250–6.

99. van den Hout L, Reiss I, Felix JF, Hop WCJ, Lally PA, Lally KP et al. Risk factors for chronic lung disease and mortality in newborns with congenital diaphragmatic hernia. *Neonatology* 2010; 98: 370–80.

100. Bagolan P, Casaccia G, Crescenzi F, Nahom A, Trucchi A, Giorlandino C. Impact of a current treatment protocol on outcome of high-risk congenital diaphragmatic hernia. *J Pediatr Surg* 2004; 39: 313–8; discussion 313–8.

101. Tracy S, Chen C. Multidisciplinary long-term follow-up of congenital diaphragmatic hernia: A growing trend. *Semin Fetal Neonatal Med* 2014; 19: 385–91.

102. Resch B. Respiratory syncytial virus infection in high-risk infants—An update on palivizumab prophylaxis. *Open Microbiol J* 2014; 8: 71–7.

103. Gaboli M, de la Cruz OA, de Aguero MI, Moreno-Galdo A, Perez GP, de Querol MS. Use of palivizumab in infants and young children with severe respiratory disease: A Delphi study. *Pediatr Pulmonol* 2014; 49: 490–502.

104. Masumoto K, Nagata K, Uesugi T, Yamada T, Kinjo T, Hikino S et al. Risk of respiratory syncytial virus in survivors with severe congenital diaphragmatic hernia. *Pediatr Int* 2008; 50: 459–63.

105. Friedman S, Chen C, Chapman JS, Jeruss S, Terrin N, Tighiouart H et al. Neurodevelopmental outcomes of congenital diaphragmatic hernia survivors followed in a multidisciplinary clinic at ages 1 and 3. *J Pediatr Surg* 2008; 43: 1035–43.

106. Danzer E, Hedrick HL. Neurodevelopmental and neurofunctional outcomes in children with congenital diaphragmatic hernia. *Early Hum Dev* 2011; 87: 625–32.

107. Danzer E, Gerdes M, Bernbaum J, D'Agostino J, Bebbington MW, Siegle J et al. Neurodevelopmental outcome of infants with congenital diaphragmatic hernia prospectively enrolled in an interdisciplinary follow-up program. *J Pediatr Surg* 2010; 45: 1759–66.

108. Robertson CMT, Tyebkhan JM, Hagler ME, Cheung P, Peliowski A, Etches PC. Late-onset, progressive sensorineural hearing loss after severe neonatal respiratory failure. *Otol Neurotol* 2002; 23: 353–6.

109. Partridge EA, Bridge C, Donaher JG, Herkert LM, Grill E, Danzer E et al. Incidence and factors associated with sensorineural and conductive hearing loss among survivors of congenital diaphragmatic hernia. *J Pediatr Surg* 2014; 49: 890–4; discussion 894.

110. Dennett KV, Fligor BJ, Tracy S, Wilson JM, Zurakowski D, Chen C. Sensorineural hearing loss in congenital diaphragmatic hernia survivors is associated with postnatal management and not defect size. *J Pediatr Surg* 2014; 49: 895–9.

111. Wilson MG, Riley P, Hurteau A, Baird R, Puligandla PS. Hearing loss in congenital diaphragmatic hernia (CDH) survivors: Is it as prevalent as we think? *J Pediatr Surg* 2013; 48: 942–5.

112. Hille ETM, van Straaten HI, Verkerk PH. Prevalence and independent risk factors for hearing loss in NICU infants. *Acta Paediatr* 2007; 96: 1155–8.

113. Sigalet DL, Nguyen LT, Adolph V, Laberge JM, Hong AR, Guttman FM. Gastroesophageal reflux associated with large diaphragmatic hernias. *J Pediatr Surg* 1994; 29: 1262–5.

114. Rais-Bahrami K, Robbins ST, Reed VL, Powell DM, Short BL. Congenital diaphragmatic hernia. Outcome of preoperative extracorporeal membrane oxygenation. *Clin Pediatr (Phila)* 1995; 34: 471–4.

115. Chiu PPL, Sauer C, Mihailovic A, Adatia I, Bohn D, Coates AL et al. The price of success in the management of congenital diaphragmatic hernia: Is improved survival accompanied by an increase in long-term morbidity? *J Pediatr Surg* 2006; 41: 888–92.

116. Muratore CS, Utter S, Jaksic T, Lund DP, Wilson JM. Nutritional morbidity in survivors of congenital diaphragmatic hernia. *J Pediatr Surg* 2001; 36: 1171–6.

117. Bagolan P, Morini F. Long-term follow up of infants with congenital diaphragmatic hernia. *Semin Pediatr Surg* 2007; 16: 134–44.

118. Jancelewicz T, Vu LT, Keller RL, Bratton B, Lee H, Farmer D et al. Long-term surgical outcomes in congenital diaphragmatic hernia: Observations from a single institution. *J Pediatr Surg* 2010; 45: 155–60; discussion 160.

119. Wu S, Zang N, Zhu J, Pan Z, Wu C. Congenital diaphragmatic eventration in children: 12 years' experience with 177 cases in a single institution. *J Pediatr Surg* 2015; 50: 1088–92.

44

Extracorporeal life support for neonatal cardiorespiratory failure

WILLIAM MIDDLESWORTH, JEFFREY W. GANDER, AND CHARLES J. H. STOLAR

INTRODUCTION

Extracorporeal membrane oxygenation (ECMO) is a life-saving technology that temporarily replaces the function of the heart and lungs. It is a supportive modality rather than a therapeutic tool that provides gas exchange and mechanical hemodynamic support for neonates with an acute, reversible respiratory or cardiac condition. This support spares the infant from the deleterious effects of high Fi02, high airway pressure, traumatic mechanical ventilation, and perfusion impairment. ECMO was first used in newborns in 1974. Since then, the Extracorporeal Life Support Organization (ELSO) has recorded approximately 36,000 newborns that have been supported with ECMO for a variety of cardio-respiratory disorders. The most common disorders in the newborn treated with ECMO are meconium aspiration syndrome (MAS), persistent pulmonary hypertension of the neonate (PPHN), congenital diaphragmatic hernia (CDH), sepsis, and cardiac support. Depending on the indication for ECMO, the outcome is varied, but overall, a cumulative survival rate of over 80% has been reported for newborns (reported to the ELSO registry since its inception) treated for respiratory failure.[1] This chapter will discuss the selection criteria for ECMO in neonates and the management of these babies while on ECMO. It will then discuss ECMO for use in difficult clinical scenarios, such as CDH, and finally review outcome and follow-up of neonates treated with ECMO.

SELECTION CRITERIA FOR NEONATAL ECMO

The selection criteria for newborns are based on historic experience from multiple institutions, patient safety, and mechanical limitations related to the biomedical devices.

Gestational age

The gestational age should be at least 34 weeks. In the early experience with ECMO, infants <34 weeks' gestation who were offered ECMO developed significant morbidity and mortality related to intracranial hemorrhage (ICH).[2] Despite refinement of ECMO techniques in the ensuing decades, premature infants continue to be at high risk for ICH. This may be due to inherent fragility of the germinal matrix vasculature of the premature infant's developing brain, making them susceptible to intracranial bleeding.[3] The incidence of ICH decreases with advancing gestational age. Hardart et al.[4] reported a 22% incidence of ICH at 32 weeks versus 12% at 36 weeks gestational age. The systemic anticoagulation necessary to maintain a thrombus-free ECMO circuit also increases the risk and severity of bleeding complications.

Birth weight

The birth weight should be nearly 2000 g, as children under this weight present unique anatomical challenges to cannulation. The smallest single-lumen ECMO cannula is 8 French (Fr.), and the vessels of very small infants may not accommodate commercially available cannulas. Furthermore, the radius of a tube greatly impacts flow. Poiseuille's law tells us that flow through a tube is related to the fourth power of the radius of the tube. If the vein is small, then the cannula will be small, resulting in flow that will be reduced by a fourth power. From historic experience, if the baby weighs less than 2 kg, then the difficulty of the placement of the cannulas in conjunction with the inadequate flow from small catheters makes ECMO in these small babies challenging.

Bleeding and coagulopathy

Active bleeding and major coagulopathy represent relative contraindications to ECMO support. Patients with uncorrectable coagulopathy, ongoing uncontrollable bleeding, or sepsis are at high risk of bleeding complications while on ECMO. The need for continuous systemic heparin therapy adds to this risk of bleeding.[4] Therefore, prior to initiating ECMO, bleeding should be controlled and coagulopathy should be corrected whenever possible.[5]

Preexisting intracranial hemorrhage

The infant should not have an ICH. Preexisting ICH may be exacerbated by the use of heparin and the altered cerebral blood flow while on ECMO. Infants with small interventricular hemorrhages (grade I–II) may be considered for ECMO on an individual case basis, but these patients should be closely monitored for worsening bleeding. Patients with previous intracranial bleeds, cerebral infarcts, and other risk factors (prematurity, coagulopathy, ischemic central nervous system injury, or sepsis) are particularly at high risk for severe neurologic consequences.[2,6] Discussion with parents in this circumstance, prior to cannulation, is especially important.

Reversible disease process

ECMO support is best suited to infants with reversible or transient cardiorespiratory failure. Ideally, ECMO candidates will have been supported by invasive mechanical ventilation for no longer than 10–14 days. Babies who have had prolonged exposure to high inspired oxygen concentration and positive-pressure ventilation develop bronchopulmonary dysplasia (BPD).[7] Recovery from this type of irreversible lung injury may take from weeks to months to occur, if it does at all. Support with ECMO can be beneficial for reversible lung disease over a relatively short period of time (2–3 weeks). However, even a lengthy ECMO course is unlikely to be sufficient to permit recovery of the irreversible fibrotic changes that occur to the lung following sustained barotrauma and/or oxygen toxicity. In addition, with a longer ECMO run, the chance of infection, bleeding complications, thromboembolic events, and mechanical failure increases.

In a retrospective case–control study, which reviewed the records of ECMO patients over 66 months, patients with oxygen dependency at 1 month of age and radiographic evidence of BPD were compared to patients without these findings.[8] Patients with BPD were placed on ECMO at an older mean age than non-BPD patients (135 versus 50 hours old). The BPD group had longer mean ECMO courses as well (203 versus 122 hours). The authors suggest that BPD from high levels of ventilatory support can occur with as few as 4 days of assisted ventilation.

ECMO is used with increasing frequency and success to support infants who develop myocardial dysfunction and hemodynamic instability in the period surrounding repair of congenital heart disease.[9] The transient myocardial dysfunction that is sometimes seen in the post cardiotomy period is an example of a reversible process well suited to ECMO support.

Coexisting anomalies

ECMO is not intended to prolong the process of an inevitable death, and therefore, candidates should have no lethal congenital or chromosomal anomalies such as trisomy 13 or 18. Other treatable conditions, such as total anomalous pulmonary venous return (TAPVR) and transposition of the great vessels (TOGV), may initially manifest with cardiorespiratory failure. When possible, an echocardiogram should be rapidly obtained to determine whether ECMO or surgical correction is most appropriate.

Bridge to diagnosis

Every effort should be made to establish a clear diagnosis before the initiation of ECMO. Circumstances arise, however, where clinical decompensation is rapid, and survival depends on immediate provision of mechanical hemodynamic support. In this situation, it is reasonable and appropriate to institute ECMO, with a plan to establish the diagnosis after achieving clinical stability during the course of ECMO. For example, pulmonary vein misalignment, a uniformly fatal anomaly of deficient alveolar capillaries and anomalous veins within the bronchoarterial bundles, presents with symptoms of persistent pulmonary hypertension unresponsive to pharmacologic treatment.[10] These infants are often placed onto ECMO. When pulmonary hypertension is intractable despite ECMO support, the diagnosis of alveolar capillary dysplasia should be entertained.[11] This diagnosis is made via lung biopsy. If alveolar capillary dysplasia is confirmed, then discussion with the family regarding withdrawal of ECMO support is appropriate. In addition, some important cardiac conditions such as TAPVR and TOGV with intact septum may present as respiratory failure, as mentioned previously. These patients are occasionally placed onto ECMO before an accurate diagnosis can be rendered. Once the diagnosis is established, appropriate treatment should be instituted.

Failure of medical management

Before institution of ECMO support, all medical means of managing cardiopulmonary failure should have been attempted. The precise definition of "failure of optimal medical management" is a subjective term, whose definition may vary among institutions. Different institutions have varying specialties, capabilities, and expertise. Current optimal medical management generally includes pharmacologic support with vasodilator or vasoconstrictive agents, inotropic agents, sedatives and analgesics, and correction of treatable conditions like pneumothorax. Ventilatory support usually begins with noninvasive and conventional invasive strategies, but may escalate to include exogenous surfactant administration, inhaled nitric oxide, or high-frequency oscillatory ventilation. The merits and drawbacks of these treatment strategies are beyond the scope of this chapter. While the concept may be difficult to quantify, a team of involved clinicians can usually reach consensus about when further medical treatment is unlikely to reverse clinical deterioration.

Innovations in medical management have obviated the need for ECMO in patients who, historically, would have required it. These innovations include high-frequency oscillatory ventilation, permissive hypercapnea with spontaneous ventilation, and nitric oxide. In 1985, Wung et al.[12] used a nontraditional approach to the management of patients with persistent pulmonary hypertension. Hyperventilation and hyperoxia were *not* emphasized, and muscle relaxants were *not* used. Permissive hypercapnea in conjunction with spontaneous ventilation was employed. In the reported series of 15 patients, a $PaCO_2$ of 50–80 mmHg and a PaO_2 of 40 mmHg were tolerated, and the minimal inspiratory pressure that provided adequate chest wall excursion was used. These patients, who otherwise met institutional criteria for ECMO, survived with this medical approach alone.

Other, more objective criteria have been established to quantify respiratory failure and aid in determining which infants should be placed on ECMO. High ventilator settings (PIP > 40 cm H_2O, PEEP > 7 cm H_2O, IMV > 100, and FiO_2 of 1.0) have correlated with mortality. In addition, other studies have identified arterial oxygen pressure (PaO_2 < 40 mmHg), alveolar–arterial oxygen gradient (A-aDO_2 > 625 mmHg for 4 hours), and oxygenation index (OI > 40) as predictors of mortality.[13–16] Some investigators have argued that the alveolar–arterial oxygenation gradient and oxygenation index should not be heavily weighted as indicators to implement ECMO support because they can be manipulated by altering ventilator settings.

CLINICAL MANAGEMENT OF NEONATES ON ECMO

Venovenous versus venoarterial ECMO

Venoarterial (VA) ECMO involves drainage of venous blood from the infant (typically from the right atrium, through a cannula placed in the right internal jugular vein) and return of oxygenated blood into the aorta (typically through a cannula placed in the right common carotid artery). This mode augments or replaces the function of both the heart and lungs. For infants with respiratory failure but preserved hemodynamics, venovenous (VV) ECMO support may be appropriate. VV ECMO is most often delivered through a dual lumen cannula directed into the right atrium through the right internal jugular vein. Venous blood is drained from the atrium to the circuit, and the oxygenated blood is returned to the atrium, with flow directed toward the tricuspid valve in an attempt to avoid mixing and recirculation through the circuit. Though cannula design is intended to minimize recirculation, cardiac output is the greatest determinant, and poor

cardiac function will cause the recirculation of oxygenated blood through the ECMO circuit, diminishing the delivery of oxygenated blood to the patient. Bicaval dual lumen cannulas are used extensively in adults and older children. These cannulas are positioned across the right atrium into the inferior vena cava, and blood is drained from the superior vena cava (SVC) and the inferior vena cava (IVC) and returned to the atrium, reducing recirculation. In infants, however, the rate of atrial perforation related to bicaval cannula use is considered by some practitioners to be unacceptably high,[17] and so dual lumen atrial, rather than bicaval, cannulas are preferred (Figure 44.1).

In distinction to VV ECMO, VA ECMO provides both respiratory and mechanical hemodynamic supports. It is the preferred mode of support when ECMO is instituted in the setting of cardiac arrest. VA ECMO is also useful in the event of progressive cardiac dysfunction and difficulty weaning from cardiopulmonary bypass after heart surgery, and when decompensation occurs following repair of congenital heart defects. In summary, VV ECMO provides respiratory support, is dependent on native cardiac output to avoid recirculation through the circuit, and does not involve carotid artery ligation. Oxygenated blood is directed toward the pulmonary circulation, which may be therapeutic in treating primary or secondary pulmonary artery hypertension. VA ECMO provides both cardiac and respiratory support, and delivers oxygenated blood more reliably to the systemic circulation. VA ECMO does, however, involve ligation of the right common carotid artery, decreases pulmonary blood flow, and increases left ventricular afterload. When instituting ECMO support, it is always critical to consider native cardiac anatomy and the potential effects of extracorporeal circulation, as certain congenital abnormalities may preclude certain kinds of support (VA

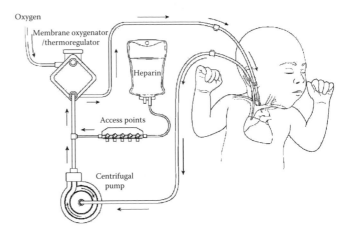

Figure 44.1 Schematic of completed VA ECMO circuit. Extrathoracic cannulation of the right atrium and ascending aorta allows venous drainage to a pump and arterial return directly to the heart and brain. A membrane oxygenator provides oxygenation and CO_2 removal. The blood is temperature-controlled before returning to the infant. All parenterally administered substances such as heparin, fluids, blood products, and drugs can be given directly into the circuit.

ECMO may be contraindicated, for example, in severe aortic coarctation).

Patient preparation and cannulation

The preferred site for cannula placement in an infant is in the vessels of the right neck, as the femoral vessels are too diminutive. The infant is positioned over a transverse shoulder roll with the head at the edge of the bed and turned to the left. After standard preparation of the skin and placement of sterile drapes, cannulation is achieved through open, percutaneous, or combined technique. For VV ECMO, the right internal jugular vein is accessed and the cannula is passed into the right atrium. Portable ultrasound, echocardiography, and x-ray are all useful tools in directing and confirming cannula placement. Percutaneous technique is thought to be associated with preserved vessel patency after decannulation, whereas open technique involves ligation of the vein cephalad to the venotomy. Surgical exposure of the carotid artery and jugular vein is performed to institute VA ECMO support. Adequate anesthetic support is essential. Heparin is administered after identification of the vessels and prior to cannulation. During the open procedure, muscle relaxants are given to prevent the inadvertent aspiration of air into the vein. After placement of the cannulas, they are de-bubbled, flushed, and connected to the circuit. ECMO flow is initiated, and the catheters are carefully secured with sutures to the blood vessel and skin (Figure 44.2a–c).

A chest radiograph is performed to demonstrate cannula position. The tip of the venous cannula should be within the right atrium, while the tip of the arterial cannula should be in the ascending aorta. Echocardiography is used to confirm that the flow of oxygenated blood is toward the tricuspid valve (for VV cannulations) and that the tip of the arterial cannula is cephalad to, and not impinging on, the aortic valve (for VA cannulations).

The ECMO circuit

ECMO circuits have several essential components. Among them are tubing, a pump, an oxygenator, and a heat exchanger that regulates the temperature of the blood as it passes through the circuit. In addition, there are several monitors on the circuit to confirm function and enhance safety. These include pressure and temperature monitors, flow probes to measure blood flow, an oxygen saturation monitor, and a bubble detector. Technological improvements in all circuit components are ongoing and beyond the scope of this chapter, but a general description of them is provided here.

PRIMING THE CIRCUIT

The tubing of the ECMO circuit is initially flushed with crystalloid and purged of all air bubbles. Twenty-five percent albumin solution is then added to coat the tubing, in an attempt to mitigate the inflammatory response that can be provoked by contact of the patient's blood with the tubing. Depending on the priming volume of an individual circuit, approximately 2 units of packed red blood cells are required for initial priming, which displaces the crystalloid and colloid in the circuit. Calcium is added to bring the calcium concentration of the circuit into the physiologic range. Perturbation of serum calcium can provoke arrhythmias during institution of ECMO support. Sodium bicarbonate and heparin are added to the circuit as well to bring pH, oxygen content, and carbon dioxide content of the circuit into the physiologic range. The heat exchanger warms the prime to normal body temperature. In sum, the primed circuit should be as

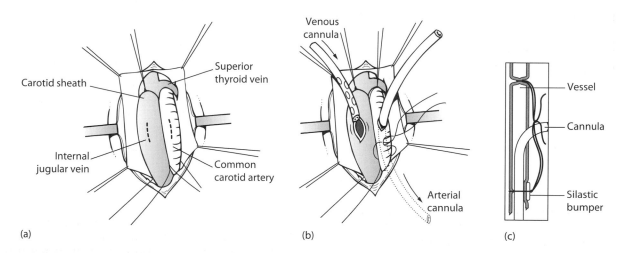

Figure 44.2 Details of the cannulation procedure for VA ECMO. **(a)** The carotid sheath is opened with the sternocleidomastoid muscle retracted. This exposes the common carotid artery and internal jugular vein. **(b)** The infant is anticoagulated after the vessels are dissected and controlled. The vessels are then ligated at the cephalad aspect. An arterial cannula is passed into the aorta through an arteriotomy in the carotid. A venous cannula is passed into the right atrium through the venotomy. **(c)** The cannulas are fixed in position by ligation over a Silastic bumper, de-bubbled and connected to the ECMO circuit. After the incision is closed, the cannulas are also sutured to the skin over the mastoid process.

physiologically normal as possible prior to initiating ECMO to maximize support and minimize metabolic derangement.

PUMP MANAGEMENT

The goal of ECMO is to provide, through augmented flow of oxygenated blood, the oxygen delivery needed to maintain organ function in the critically ill newborn. The pump regulates the flow of blood through the circuit. There are two basic pump configurations in use: roller pumps and centrifugal pumps. Blood flow through a roller pump is directly proportional to the speed, in rotations per minute (rpm) of the roller head as it propels the blood along the "raceway" (tubing within the roller pump housing). Centrifugal pumps, in distinction to roller pumps, contain an impeller that is magnetically coupled to a motor. As the impeller spins, a pressure differential is generated that draws blood through the pump. An important difference between the two types of pumps is that, while flow through a roller pump is proportional to the rpm of the roller head, the pressures at the inlet and outlet of the pump affect flow through a centrifugal pump. The flow driven by the pump should be adjusted to maintain adequate oxygen delivery. Confirmation of adequate oxygen delivery is achieved through standard means: monitoring pH, arterial lactate, urine output, hepatic and renal function, and mixed venous oxygen saturation. It is important to note that, when V V ECMO is used, the blood drawn from the venous limb of a dual lumen cannula may contain recirculated, oxygenated blood being delivered into the right atrium through the arterial limb. This will result in a measured mixed venous saturation that is artificially elevated and not truly reflective of the infant's mixed venous saturation. This is not a concern with VA support when cardiac anatomy is normal.

OXYGENATOR MANAGEMENT

The development of the original bubble oxygenator made open heart surgery possible, but caused too much damage to red blood cells and could therefore not provide support for an extended period of time. Prolonged extracorporeal support was made possible by the development of the membrane oxygenator, where blood was separated from gas by a semipermeable membrane, allowing diffusion of oxygen and carbon dioxide between the gas and the blood, mimicking the function of the human lung. Blood and gas (called "sweep gas") both flow across the oxygenator without coming into direct contact. The oxygen content and flow rate of the sweep gas are adjusted to meet the needs of the patient. Increasing gas flow enhances elimination of carbon dioxide from the blood (at a given blood flow rate), while increasing the oxygen content of the sweep gas enhances oxygenation. More recent and technologically advanced oxygenators (like the poly-methyl pentene hollow-fiber oxygenator currently in use) require lower prime volume, have less leakage of plasma across the membrane and reduced resistance to blood flow. Current oxygenators remain imperfect, however, and thrombus may form in the oxygenator over time. As a thrombus extends, the membrane surface area is decreased, resulting in decreased oxygen and carbon dioxide transfer.

Oxygenator function is monitored through the use of pre- and post-oxygenator pressure measurements. An increase in the pressure drop across the oxygenator, or ΔP, may herald oxygenator failure. To optimize performance, blood flow across the oxygenator should be maintained within the parameters suggested by the manufacturer. Pre- and post-oxygenator blood gas analysis is also tracked to monitor oxygenator function. The sweep gas is periodically purged to maintain clear flow across the gas phase of the oxygenator. Extended use during long ECMO runs may result in leakage of blood and plasma across into the gas phase. When evidence of oxygenator failure develops, the oxygenator can be replaced. Experienced ECMO teams are able to cut away and replace a failing oxygenator with a new, pre-primed oxygenator very rapidly. Ventilator and hemodynamic support is transiently escalated during the oxygenator change to support the patient through the brief interruption of ECMO.

Fluid management

Principles and goals of hemodynamic support do not differ substantially during ECMO. While on ECMO, maintenance fluid requirements for a term newborn under a radiant warmer are estimated to be 100 cc/kg/day. Daily insensible water loss through the oxygenator is related to the flow rate of the sweep gas and has been demonstrated by multiple authors in experimental models to be between 50 and 100 mL per liter per minute of sweep. Fluid losses from urine, stool, chest tubes, nasogastric tubes, ostomies, mechanical ventilation, radiant fluid loss, and blood sampling should be carefully recorded. Fluid management may be challenging early in the ECMO course, when capillary leak might occur. Fluid boluses are frequently needed in this period to maintain intravascular volume and circuit function. Meticulous recordings of the net fluid balance on ECMO should be maintained. Typically, there is positive fluid balance and weight gain in the first 1–3 days as the patient becomes increasingly edematous. On the third day of ECMO, spontaneous diuresis of the excess edema fluid frequently begins and can be facilitated with the use of furosemide. This diuretic phase is often a harbinger of recovery. In the event of renal failure on ECMO, hemofiltration or hemodialysis can be added to the ECMO circuit for removal of excess fluid and electrolyte correction. In a retrospective comparison of neonates on ECMO, use of hemofiltration was associated with shorter duration on ECMO and time on mechanical ventilation.[18]

Respiratory management on ECMO

Once the desired oxygen delivery is attained, the ventilator should be promptly weaned in order to avoid oxygen toxicity and barotrauma. Such "rest settings" have been studied and debated.[19] At the authors' institution, the FiO_2 is decreased to 0.21, PEEP to 5 cm H_2O, PIP to 20–25 cm H_2O, a rate of 12 breaths/minute, and inspiratory time of 0.5 seconds provided the infant's arterial and venous oxygenation are adequate.

If a baby remains hypoxic despite maximal pump flow, then higher ventilator settings may be temporarily required. Alternatively, neonates whose hypoxia is not correctible by VV ECMO may need to be converted to VA ECMO to achieve full and adequate cardiorespiratory support. On occasion, the chest x-ray will worsen in the first 24 hours, independent of ventilator settings, and will often improve after diuresis. As the patient improves on ECMO and the pump flow is weaned, ventilator settings are then modestly increased to support the baby off ECMO. In neonates, if the oxygen saturation is greater than 93%, the authors consider FiO_2 of 0.4, PIP < 28, PEEP of 5, and a respiratory rate of <30 breaths/minute as adequate settings for a trial off of ECMO.

During the course of ECMO, pulmonary toilet is essential to respiratory improvement and includes gentle chest percussion and postural drainage. Special attention should be made to the ECMO catheters and keeping the head and body aligned. Endotracheal suctioning is also recommended every 4 hours and as needed based on the amount of pulmonary secretions present.

Medical management

After the initiation of ECMO, vasoactive medications should be weaned and discontinued, provided the blood pressure remains stable. With VV support, improved oxygenation often results in improved cardiac function, and with VA support, the mechanical blood pressure support replaces pharmacologic agents. At the authors' institution, routine consultation from the neurology service and electroencephalography (EEG) monitoring are employed, as seizure activity in newborns is clinically evident only one third of the time.[19] When detected, seizures are treated with standard antiepileptic medication. Both cranial ultrasound and chest radiograph are obtained daily. Nasogastric decompression is maintained, and stress ulcer prophylaxis with an H_2-blocker is instituted. Fentanyl and midazolam are usually administered for analgesia and sedation; however, the use of paralytics is avoided. The baby's muscle activity is important not only for fluid mobilization of edema but also for monitoring of neurologic activity.

As is the case for all patients with central vascular catheters, infection is a constant concern; therefore, strict observance to aseptic technique when handling the ECMO circuit should be maintained. Routine blood, urine, and tracheal cultures are obtained to monitor for infection. At our center, infectious prophylaxis is provided by cefazolin, if antibiotics are not being given for specific treatment; many neonates who are placed on ECMO are already receiving broad-spectrum antibiotics at the time of cannulation.

The caloric intake on ECMO should be optimized using standard hyperalimentation. For a newborn, total parenteral nutrition (TPN) should be started at 100 kcal/kg/day. Normally, this should be supplied as 60% carbohydrates (14.6 g/kg/day) and 40% fat (4.3 g/kg/day). Intralipid infusions may be used as a fat source, although there is some

controversy with its use in the setting of severe lung disease. As a result, the percentage of fat in the hyperalimentation may be lowered. Amino acids are provided, with consideration given to impaired kidney function. With normal renal function, approximately 2.5 g protein/kg/day should be provided in the TPN mixture.

The benefits of enteral nutrition are increasingly recognized, and consensus guidelines support the use of enteral nutrition in newborns on ECMO support whose condition has stabilized.[20] Initial concern with feeding enterally on ECMO was that there was inadequate gut perfusion from the initial insult, which could lead to necrotizing enterocolitis when feeding was begun.[21] However, a retrospective study of 67 neonates supported with VA ECMO that were fed enterally did not show any significant adverse effects.[22] While septic complications of enteral feeding are infrequent, many of these patients will have a gastrointestinal ileus. Of the previously mentioned 67 neonates, 21% had enteral feeding temporarily discontinued due to high gastric residuals.

Electrolytes are closely monitored and repleted as necessary. Sodium and phosphorus are usually not repleted as they are often provided in blood products and volume expanders.

Coagulation management

Guidelines regarding the management of anticoagulation are institution-specific, and the intricacies of caring for complex ECMO patients have hindered widespread acceptance of any one specific protocol. At the authors' institution, a guideline for management of anticoagulation is developed for ECMO patients that have "bleeding" and "nonbleeding" arms to recognize the special circumstances involved when caring for an ECMO patient with active hemorrhage. Additionally, special care must be exercised in managing anticoagulation in the perioperative period, such as when a patient with CDH is repaired while on ECMO. Agents such as aminocaproic acid, which binds plasmin and inhibits fibrinolysis, are useful in this setting.

As noted previously, a heparin bolus of 50–100 units/kg is administered at the time of cannulation. When the activated clotting time (ACT) falls below 300 seconds, a continuous heparin infusion is begun at a dose of 28 units/kg/h and titrated to a goal heparin level (antifactor Xa assay) of 0.3–0.7 U/mL, which typically corresponds to an activated partial thromboplastin time (aPTT) of 60–80 seconds. Other useful parameters are the international normalized ratio (INR), prothrombin time, fibrinogen, and the antithrombin III (ATIII) level. Our practice is to maintain the INR at less than 1.5 with transfusion of fresh frozen plasma. Recombinant ATIII is administered to maintain the ATIII level above 50%, and cryoprecipitate is transfused (5 mL/kg) to keep the fibrinogen level greater than 150 mg/dL. While on ECMO, the baby's hemoglobin is maintained above 12 g/dL to maximize the oxygen-carrying capacity of the blood. Platelet consumption is commonly seen during

ECMO, and platelet transfusion is given to maintain a platelet count above 80,000/mm.[23] Point-of-care monitoring of anticoagulation is sometimes necessary when laboratory processing times do not meet clinical needs, and the ACT is useful in this setting. It must be stressed that management of anticoagulation is a highly individualized process that is affected by ECMO flow rate, existing thrombus in the circuit, individual risk of bleeding, and numerous other clinical concerns. Anticoagulation is stopped at the time of decannulation.

COMPLICATIONS ON ECMO

Mechanical complications

Interruption or impairment of blood flow through the ECMO circuit is perhaps the most frequent and one of the most urgent issues faced by the ECMO practitioner. Elevated negative venous pressures may alert the clinician to intravascular volume depletion, cannula malposition, or kinks in the cannula or circuit tubing. In addition, pneumothorax, cardiac tamponade, and abdominal compartment syndrome should be considered if there is no readily appreciated mechanical reason for poor venous return. Intravascular volume depletion may be treated with infusions of crystalloid or colloid, as clinically indicated. In some conditions such as sepsis, there may be capillary leakage, in which case administration of significant fluid and resulting anasarca may be unavoidable. Management of oxygenator failure has been discussed previously. Accidental cannula dislodgement and tubing rupture are catastrophic and sometimes fatal events.

Neurologic complications

ICH is the most devastating complication of ECMO. Cranial ultrasound should be performed daily and after any major event, such as equipment malfunction, sudden worsening in oxygenation status, change in heparin requirement, or unexplained drop in hematocrit. EEG, as noted previously, is also helpful in the neurologic evaluation of the neonate. Other serious, if less acute, complications observed in the ECMO patient include long-term neurologic impairment (e.g., learning disorders, motor dysfunction, cerebral palsy) and may be due to hypoxia and acidosis prior to ECMO. During the ECMO course, frequent neurological examinations are performed, and neuromuscular blocking agents are avoided. Physical exam consists of evaluation of alertness and interaction, fullness of the fontanels, reflexes, tone, spontaneous movements, pupillary response and eye movements, and presence of seizure activity.

Renal complications

Infants on ECMO may sustain acute kidney injury (AKI) marked by oliguria and increasing BUN and creatinine levels. A single-center study from the Netherlands published in 2013 reported that two-thirds of neonates who required ECMO sustained AKI.[24] The authors observed significantly lower survival in those babies whose RIFLE score was "F" (failure of kidney function) and concluded that, since AKI in childhood may predispose to chronic kidney disease in adulthood, all infants who develop AKI while on ECMO should receive long-term monitoring of kidney function. The mechanism of AKI is likely multifactorial and includes both inadequate organ perfusion associated with the need for ECMO and effects of the circuit. The authors of the Netherlands study observed that the severity of AKI was greatest in the first 2 days of ECMO support. Both hemofiltration and hemodialysis have been used in conjunction with ECMO support and may help manage fluid volume status and electrolyte abnormalities.

WEANING FROM ECMO

As a patient recovers native cardiopulmonary function, ECMO support is gradually withdrawn. With VA support, which essentially involves the oxygenation and shunting of blood from the right atrium to the aorta, pump flow is gradually decreased. This results in increased pulmonary blood flow and transfer of the "work" of gas exchange and blood flow back to the patient from the circuit. Arterial and mixed venous blood gas analysis, in addition to standard hemodynamic monitoring, is used to assess patient readiness for decannulation. From starting flows as high as 150 cc/kg/minute, the flow is decreased to 30–50 cc/kg/minute while maintaining adequate perfusion. The ACT should be maintained at a higher level during periods of slow flow to prevent thrombosis. For cardiac patients, inotropic support is frequently reinstituted as mechanical support is withdrawn. Ventilator support is also increased above the "rest" settings used during ECMO support. Prior to complete withdrawal of ECMO, the cannulas are clamped and flushed with heparin–saline, and the blood is recirculated for a period of several hours through a shunt built in the circuit. This is done to confirm patient readiness prior to cannula removal. An alternative strategy that is appropriate for neonates supported with VV ECMO is to wean by reducing the oxygen content and flow of the sweep gas, and the relative equivalent of a clamp trial is accomplished by shutting off the sweep gas while maintaining flow through the circuit.

If the recirculation is tolerated, then decannulation is performed. As with the insertion, decannulation should be performed as a sterile surgical procedure. The patient should be placed in the Trendelenburg position, and muscle relaxants should be administered to prevent air aspiration into the vein. Prior to decannulation, alternative vascular access must be secured through which vasoactive medication and hyperalimentation are administered. Once the cannula is removed, the vein is ligated and not repaired. This is also usually true for the artery in the case of VA ECMO. Percutaneously placed dual lumen VV cannulas can be withdrawn and pressure applied for adequate time to achieve hemostasis.

ECMO IN INFANTS WITH CDH

Overall survival of infants with CDH has improved significantly with the use of permissive hypercapnia, spontaneous respiration, delayed surgery, and avoidance of ventilator-induced lung injury, and now exceeds 80% in many centers.[25–32] Among the most severely affected babies, however, active investigation into the best treatment methods continues. Prenatal markers of severity have guided the selection of patients to undergo fetal interventions, such as temporary tracheal occlusion, which provokes distension and growth of the lung ipsilateral to the diaphragmatic defect. Attempts to identify optimal postnatal treatments to further improve survival are active and ongoing, as many questions remain: What is the optimal timing of surgery for the most severely affected CDH patients? When is ECMO appropriate, and when is it futile? Is repair best accomplished on ECMO, or should ECMO be discontinued prior to repair? Which is the preferred mode of ECMO support in CDH patients, VA or VV? Data needed to provide conclusive answers to these questions are lacking, though literature exists to support many treatment options.

While it is widely recognized that CDH patients who require ECMO have a far lower survival rate than those who do not (51% and 95%, respectively),[1,25] this reflects differential disease severity between these two groups and is likely not an *effect* of ECMO. A study by the Congenital Diaphragmatic Hernia study group concluded that ECMO support did convey a survival advantage among the group of patients with the greatest predicted mortality.[33] The literature on this subject is almost exclusively retrospective in nature, and it is therefore difficult to establish a causal relationship between any individual therapy or treatment plan and improved survival. What seems clear is that ECMO can effectively rescue CDH patients from the cycle of pulmonary vasospasm, pulmonary hypertension, right-to-left shunting of blood, and worsening hypoxemia, hypercarbia, and acidosis that can ensue in the initial days of life. VV support offers the benefits of delivering oxygenated blood to the pulmonary vascular bed (and hence reverse pulmonary hypertension) and preserving the carotid artery. It also seems likely that the volume–outcome relationships that are demonstrated in many areas of medical care hold true for ECMO and CDH: high-volume centers are likely to have better outcomes.[25]

OUTCOME AND FOLLOW-UP OF NEONATES TREATED WITH ECMO

Mortality

In 1987, 653 neonatal respiratory ECMO runs were reported to the ELSO registry, and survival was 85%. In 2015, 627 runs were reported, and survival was only 63%. These numbers reflect a steady decline in reported survival of respiratory ECMO since the registry's inception.[1] The average run length has nearly doubled over the same time period (from 121 to 203 hours), while the longest reported run each year has quadrupled (411 to 1662 hours). Annual case volume peaked in 1992 at 1516 cases, and the fewest number of cases reported in a single year was 627 in 2015. These trends—longer runs, fewer cases, and increasing mortality—may all be the result of improvements in the medical management of critically ill newborns, and thus a sicker population of ECMO patients. Chronic respiratory failure from pulmonary hypertension has been a major cause for hospital readmission and late deaths, but mortality has remained specific to the primary diagnosis prior to ECMO.[1] This is understandable, since ECMO is more of a supportive, temporary organ replacement therapy than it is a treatment for any specific disease. ECMO patients with the diagnosis of CDH have about a 50% mortality rate, while the diagnosis of MAS carries only a 5% mortality rate.[1,30] The overall survival rate for respiratory ECMO patients reported to the ELSO registry since 1986 is 74%.[1]

The data for neonatal cardiac ECMO are somewhat different, as annual case volume has been generally increasing over the past 25 years, while survival has remained at 40%–45% without a clear trend over that time period. Of the infants who die on ECMO, about half die from severe bleeding complications. Another risk factor for mortality is a birth weight less than 2 kg. A retrospective study reviewed 300 newborns supported with ECMO, and the infants who weighed less than 2.5 kg, although meeting the criteria of 2 kg, had a relative mortality risk of 3.45% compared to ECMO neonates whose birth weight exceeded 2.5 kg.[34]

Feeding and growth sequelae

Following successful decannulation from ECMO, an important determinant of readiness for discharge from the neonatal intensive care unit (NICU) is successful enteral feeding. Feeding problems have been reported in as many as one third of ECMO-treated infants and vary in presentation.[32–34] Feeding difficulties are less often a complication of ECMO and more often related to the infant's underlying disease.

Problems with feeding that present soon after completion of the ECMO course include interference from tachypnea, generalized CNS depression, poor hunger drive, pain related to endotracheal intubation, poor oral–motor coordination in an infant who has never been nipple fed, and vagal neuropraxia from manipulation or compression of the vagus nerve during the cannulation procedure.[37,38] While this last effect, specifically recurrent laryngeal nerve injury, is a well-described complication of surgery on the aortic arch and ligation of the patent ductus arteriosus, it is not observed to a significant degree among infants who have undergone ECMO cannulation. ECMO support in and of itself generally does not cause major long-term feeding problems. The feeding problems that are observed after an ECMO course are more related, rather, to the pre-ECMO diagnosis. For example, infants with CDH have a higher incidence of feeding difficulty than infants with MAS and respiratory distress syndrome (RDS).[35–37] CDH patients have associated foregut dysmotility that leads to significant reflux, delayed gastric emptying, and feeding difficulties. Respiratory compromise and severe chronic lung disease also interfere with sucking and swallowing. These babies may require prolonged nasogastric feeding or even a gastrostomy, fundoplication, and pyloroplasty to maintain adequate growth.

Although normal somatic growth is most commonly reported, ECMO-supported children are more likely to experience problems with growth than normal controls. Head circumference below the fifth percentile occurs at a higher rate (10%) in post-ECMO children. Furthermore, poor head growth is associated with a major handicapping condition with a risk greater than 75% at 5 years of age.[38] Growth problems are most commonly associated with those ECMO patients who are afflicted by CDH or residual chronic lung disease.[39]

Respiratory sequelae

Significant respiratory problems are reported in ECMO survivors during the first 2 years of life, with a high rate of rehospitalizations for pulmonary conditions.[40,41]

Approximately 15% of infants supported with ECMO require oxygen at 28 days. By the age of 5 years, ECMO patients were twice as likely to have a reported case of pneumonia as control children (25% versus 13%). Approximately half of the ECMO children with pneumonia were hospitalized compared to none of the control cases. Half of the cases of pneumonia in ECMO children occurred before 1 year of life compared to none in the control group. In addition, more than half of the ECMO rehospitalizations for pneumonia occurred within the first 6 months of life.

Among ECMO-treated neonates, the primary diagnosis of CDH, in particular, has been found to be associated with chronic lung disease as defined by the need for bronchodilators, diuretics, or supplemental oxygen for the management of pulmonary symptoms. Specifically, the use of supplemental oxygen at discharge from the hospital has been reported in 22%–80% of CDH patients.[39,42-44] Ventilator management that employs high airway pressures and oxygen concentration, as well as preexisting lung injury prior to initiating ECMO, leads to the development of BPD in these children. Persistent oxygen requirements may be due to pulmonary hypertension.

The age at the time of ECMO, which frequently correlates with the duration of mechanical ventilation prior to ECMO, is another factor associated with need for supplemental oxygen beyond 28 days of life.[8] Neonates with severe respiratory failure had an 11.5-fold increased risk of BPD if ECMO was initiated later than 96 hours of age. In addition, ECMO-treated infants with birth weights of 2–2.5 kg have a greater risk for chronic lung disease than do larger infants.[34]

Neurodevelopmental sequelae

Perhaps the most serious of post-ECMO morbidities is sensorineural handicap. Robust data on long-term neurologic outcome for newborns treated with ECMO are lacking. Reports of neurodevelopmental outcome after 1 year of age have been published from multiple institutions. Among 540 ECMO survivors from 12 institutions, the total rate of sensorineural handicap (cerebral palsy, blindness, hearing impairment) is 6% on average, ranging from 2% to 18%.[38,45-57] Significant developmental delay among ECMO survivors is 9% on average, ranging from 0% to 21%. This is comparable to other critically ill neonates. For example, newborns with extremely low birth weight (<750 g) have a 15% rate of major sensorineural handicap, with 21% testing in the mentally retarded range.[58] Additionally, newborns with PPHN not supported with ECMO have an average sensorineural handicap rate of 23% (0%–37% range) among 162 survivors from eight institutions.[59-66]

At 5 years of age, 50% of children supported with ECMO as neonates had a normal neurologic outcome as defined by lack of a developmental delay, epilepsy, or cerebral palsy.[67] The remaining children had varying degrees of disability, mostly of low severity. These authors also found that low gestational age and low birth weight were significantly associated with a negative neurologic outcome. This further supports the notion that preexisting factors, as well as ECMO support itself, contribute to negative neurologic outcomes.

The underlying diagnosis requiring ECMO support is related to risk of subsequent cognitive impairment. At an average age of 31 months at follow-up, children with CDH supported by ECMO were more likely to have an abnormal cognitive status than non-CDH ECMO survivors. Male gender and limited maternal education were other risk factors for abnormal cognitive development.[55]

Auditory deficits are reported in more than 25% of ECMO-supported neonates at the time of discharge.[68] The majority of these are mild–moderate in severity, as measured by brainstem auditory evoked response testing, and some may resolve over time. These auditory deficits may also be caused by furosemide or gentamicin ototoxicity. As a result, hearing screening is recommended at the time of NICU discharge. Examining data for 313 ECMO children from five centers shows an overall rate of 9% (range 4%–21%).[38,50,52,54] This rate is not higher than that reported for infants with PPHN who were not treated with ECMO (23%, range 0%–37%).[59-62]

Visual deficits observed among ECMO-treated neonates are usually due to the underlying retinal immaturity of premature patients. Visual deficits are rarely seen in ECMO-treated neonates weighing more than 2 kg. Concern for retinopathy of prematurity due to the hyperoxic condition of ECMO has proven to be unfounded. Haney et al.[69] reported ocular findings in 16 of 85 neonatal ECMO patients. These findings included vascular immaturity, vitreous and retinal hemorrhage, and optic nerve atrophy.[69] Not all infants were examined in this study, however, and there may have been additional complications. Long-term sequelae were not reported, and non-ECMO controls were not tested. In a study of 86 newborns supported with ECMO at the Children's Hospital of Los Angeles, examined (on average)

3 weeks after decannulation, Gonzalez et al.[70] found that 73 (85%) had normal exams, and they concluded that routine ophthalmologic screening after ECMO may not be needed.

Seizures, both clinical and electroencephalographic, are widely reported among ECMO-treated neonates, with an incidence ranging from 20% to 70%.[71-74] However, the timing and type of seizure activity vary. In a group of 5-year-old ECMO survivors, only 2% had a diagnosis of epilepsy. Seizures in the neonate are associated with neurologic disease and poorer long-term outcome, including cerebral palsy and epilepsy.[75] According to one study, the handicap rate following neonatal seizures is 8%.[76] A predictive association between abnormal EEG and developmental status has been found: 18% of infants having normal EEGs go on to have developmental delays, while delays are observed in 35% of infants with one abnormal EEG and 58% of ECMO-treated infants with two or more abnormal EEGs.[72]

Neuromotor deficits observed in ECMO survivors range from mild hypotonia, gross motor delay, and asymmetry to isolated cases of spastic quadriparesis. Although moderate hypotonia is not uncommon at discharge, it generally improves over the next 4–6 months. It should be noted that these neuromotor findings are also seen in normal control children.[41] The incidence of severe non-ambulatory cerebral palsy is less than 5%.[38,45,50] These cases are generally accompanied by cognitive disability, demonstrating a global insult to the brain. Mild cerebral palsy is seen in up to 20% of children supported with ECMO in the newborn period.

Survivors of neonatal ECMO, as a group, most commonly function within the normal range.[38,45,47,50-57,77] The rate of major handicap appears to be stable across studies with an average of 11% (range 2%–18%).

By hospital discharge, at approximately 1 month of life, ECMO-treated infants still exhibit signs of general CNS depression including lethargy, hypotonia, and weak primitive reflexes, these being indicators of moderate hypoxic–ischemic insult. By 4 months of age, ECMO-treated infants typically function within the normal range defined by Bayley mental and motor scales. Residual hypotonia or mild asymmetry persists in about 25% of ECMO patients. Mild motor delay usually accompanies the hypotonia. Significant neurological abnormalities and motor deficits (more than two standard deviations below norm) are found in approximately 10%–15% of ECMO survivors. By 3 years of age, the rate of handicap appears to be stable, but more subtle abnormalities manifest at this age, such as learning disability, particularly with language and perceptual functioning.[78-80] By age 5, a diagnosis of mental retardation (IQ < 70, delay in social adaptive functioning) becomes more certain. In one 5-year group, 11% of individuals studied were diagnosed as mentally retarded, most in the mild range with IQs of 50–70.

For ECMO children who had carotid artery cannulation and ligation, controversy remains over reconstruction of the artery. Baumgart et al. reported experience of 84 ECMO children who had carotid ligation and 41 who had right common carotid artery reconstruction.[81,82] Failure of the reanastomosis, defined by >50% occlusion or no flow, occurred in 25% of procedures. No significant differences were reported for occurrence of grades 3 and 4 hemorrhages, but more patients in the carotid repair group had moderate to severe abnormalities on EEG (60% of the reanastomosed group, compared to 35% of the nonreconstructed group). Despite this, no differences were reported in the proportion of significant neurodevelopmental delays. An additional report of neonates with CDH supported by ECMO showed a 72% incidence of occlusion or high-grade stenosis of the repaired right common carotid artery as measured by MRI at 2 years of age.[83] A more recent study reports a higher patency rate of 84% when measured by ultrasound at a median interval of 63 days following decannulation.[84] Neither study demonstrated a significant difference in neuroimaging results or neurologic outcome associated with carotid repair versus ligation.

SUMMARY

Since the first use of ECMO in neonates in 1974, much has been learned about the treatment of infants with cardiac and respiratory disease. New medications and advances in mechanical ventilatory support have been developed, which may have helped numerous babies survive and avoid ECMO cannulation, and in fact the use of ECMO for respiratory indications has been declining, from a high of 1,516 cases in 1992 to only 627 cases in 2015 (there has been an opposite trend for neonatal cardiac ECMO).[1] Qureshi et al.[85] note other interesting trends, specifically that CDH has supplanted MAS as the commonest indication for neonatal respiratory ECMO. This shift has accompanied a decreasing survival from respiratory ECMO; in 2015, survival fell to a historic low of 63%. Improved treatment for meconium aspiration has resulted in a proportional decrease in cannulations among the group with the best survival, and hence reduced overall survival. Survival to hospital discharge of infants with CDH who require ECMO support remains poor at 51%.[1]

Technological advances and improvements in ECMO circuit components continue to be made, and indications for ECMO support continue to be expanded and refined. Whereas historically many centers would not offer ECMO to infants for whom CPR was in progress, this is no longer the case. In fact, cannulation in the setting of cardiac arrest refractory to CPR (termed ECPR) is being performed with increasing frequency. In 2015, 1,254 cases of ECPR were reported to the ELSO registry, with rates of survival to decannulation and to hospital discharge of 64% and 41%, respectively. Notably, these results do not differ substantially from survival data for ECMO done for cardiac indications (not in the setting of cardiac arrest). ECMO continues to play a role in the treatment of a variety of neonatal respiratory diseases in addition to meconium aspiration and CDH. Among these diseases are persistent pulmonary hypertension of the newborn, sepsis, and pneumonia.

Challenges remain in achieving improved survival in diseases like CDH and sepsis, where survival remains poor despite the use of ECMO as a bridge to recovery. Challenges also exist in refinement of inclusion and exclusion criteria that maximize survival rates but avoid ECMO in infants with irreversible disease, high risk of ECMO-related morbidity, or very low likelihood of survival. Exclusion criteria include early gestational age, low birth weight, coagulopathy, ICH, lethal congenital anomalies, severe brain injury, and irreversible lung disease.

In summary, indications for ECMO support have evolved over the past decade, with increased use of ECMO in the setting of cardiac arrest refractory to CPR, a decrease in use for respiratory indications, and an increase in use for cardiac support. ECMO has moved into more widespread use, as indicated by the steady increase in ECMO centers over the past 10 years. It remains an important therapeutic and life-sustaining tool in the treatment of any hypoxic or hypotensive infant who has a reversible pulmonary or cardiac condition, who is physically large enough for cannulation, and who has failed maximal medical therapy. Meticulous attention and thorough documentation of each ECMO patient through the international ELSO registry will lead to continued improvement in safety, efficacy, and appropriateness of this important technology.

REFERENCES

1. Extracorporeal Life Support Organization. ECLS Registry Report: International Summary. 2016: January.
2. Cilley RE, Zwischenberger JB, Andrews AF et al. Intracranial hemorrhage during extracorporeal membrane oxygenation in neonates. *Pediatrics* 1986; 78:699–704.
3. Ballabh P. Intraventricular hemorrhage in premature infants: Mechanism of disease. *Pediatr Res* 2010; 67(1):1–8.
4. Hardart GE, Hardart KM, Arnold JM. Intracranial hemorrhage in premature neonates treated with extracorporeal membrane oxygenation correlates with conceptional age. *J Pediatr* 2004; 145:184–9.
5. Sell LL, Cullen ML, Whittlesey GC et al. Hemorrhage complications during extracorporeal membrane oxygenation: Prevention and treatment. *J Pediatr Surg* 1986; 21:1087–91.
6. Allmen D, Babcock D, Matsumoto J et al. The predictive value of head ultrasound in the ECMO candidate. *J Pediatr Surg* 1992; 27:36–9.
7. Northway WH, Rosan RC, Porter DY. Pulmonary disease following respiratory therapy of hyaline-membrane disease. *N Engl J Med* 1967; 276:357–8.
8. Kornhauser MS, Cullen JA, Baumgart S et al. Risk factors for bronchopulmonary dysplasia after extracorporeal membrane oxygenation. *Arch Pediatr Adolesc Med* 1994; 148:820–5.

9. Miana LA, Canêo LF, Tanamati C et al. Post-cardiotomy ECMO in pediatric and congenital heart surgery: Impact of team training and equipment in the results. *Revista Brasileira de Cirurgia Cardiovascular: órgão oficial da Sociedade Brasileira de Cirurgia Cardiovascular* 2015; 30(4):409–16.
10. Gamillscheg A, Zobel G, Spuller E et al. Aortic coarctation associated with alveolar capillary dysplasia and misalignment of the pulmonary veins. *Pediatr Cardiol* 2008; 29:191–4.
11. Kane TD, Greenberg JM, Bove KE, Warner BW. Alveolar capillary dysplasia with misalignment of the pulmonary veins: A rare but fatal cause of neonatal respiratory failure. *Pediatr Surg Int* 1998; 14:89–91.
12. Wung JT, James LS, Kilchevsky E, James E. Management of infants with severe respiratory failure and persistence of the fetal circulation, without hyperventilation. *Pediatrics* 1985; 76:488–94.
13. Krummel TM, Greenfield LJ, Kirkpatrick BV et al. Alveolar-arterial oxygen gradients versus the neonatal pulmonary insufficiency index for prediction of mortality in ECMO candidates. *J Pediatr Surg* 1984; 19:380–4.
14. Beck R, Anderson KD, Pearson GD et al. Criteria for extracorporeal membrane oxygenation in a population of infants with persistent pulmonary hypertension of the newborn. *J Pediatr Surg* 1986; 21:297–302.
15. Marsh TD, Wilkerson SA, Cook LN. Extracorporeal membrane oxygenation selection criteria: Partial pressure of arterial oxygen versus alveolar-arterial oxygen gradient. *Pediatrics* 1988; 82:162–6.
16. Ortiz RM, Cilley RE, Bartlett RH. Extracorporeal membrane oxygenation in pediatric respiratory failure. *Pediatr Clin North Am* 1987; 34:39–46.
17. Speggiorin S, Robinson SG, Harvey C, Westrope C, Faulkner GM, Kirkland P, Peek GJ. Experience with the Avalon bicaval double lumen veno-venous cannula for neonatal respiratory ECMO. *Perfusion* 2015; 30:250–4.
18. Blijdrop K, Cransberg K, Wildschut ED et al. Haemofiltration in newborns treated with extracorporeal membrane oxygenation: A case-comparison study. *Crit Care* 2009; 13:R48.
19. Murray D, Boylan G, Ali I, Ryan C, Murphy B, Connolly S. Defining the gap between electrographic seizure burden, clinical expression and staff recognition of neonatal seizures. *Arch Dis Child* 2008; 93:187–91.
20. Jaksic T, Hull MA, Modi BP et al. and the American Society for Parenteral and Enteral Nutrition (A.S.P.E.N.) Board of Directors. A.S.P.E.N. clinical guidelines: Nutrition support of neonates supported with extracorporeal membrane oxygenation. *J Parenter Enteral Nutr* 2010; 34:247–53.
21. Bartlett RH, Andrews AF, Toomasian JM et al. Extracorporeal membrane oxygenation for newborn respiratory failure: 45 cases. *Surgery* 1982; 92:425–33.

22. Hanekamp MN, Spoel M, Sharman-Koendjbiharie I. Routine enteral nutrition in neonates on extracorporeal membrane oxygenation. *Pediatr Crit Care Med* 2005; 6:275–9.

23. Raithel SC, Pennington DG, Boegner E et al. Extracorporeal membrane oxygenation in children after cardiac surgery. *Circulation* 1992; 86:II305–10.

24. Zwiers AJM, de Wildt SN, Hop WCJ et al. Acute kidney injury is a frequent complication in critically ill neonates receiving extracorporeal membrane oxygenation: A 14-year cohort study. *Crit Care* 2013; 17:R151.

25. Bucher BT, Guth RM, Saito JM, Najaf T, Warner BW. Impact of hospital volume on in-hospital mortality of infants undergoing repair of congenital diaphragmatic hernia. *Ann Surg* 2010; 252(4):635–41.

26. Sakai H, Tamura M, Hosokawa Y et al. Effect of surgical repair on respiratory mechanics in congenital diaphragmatic hernia. *J Pediatr* 1987; 111:432–8.

27. Cartlidge PHT, Mann NP, Kapila L. Preoperative stabilization in congenital diaphragmatic hernia. *Arch Dis Child* 1986; 61:1226–8.

28. Breaux CW Jr, Rouse TM, Cain WS, Georgenson KE. Improvement in survival of patients with congenital diaphragmatic hernia utilizing a strategy of delayed repair after medical and/or extracorporeal membrane oxygenation stabilization. *J Pediatr Surg* 1991; 26:333–8.

29. West KW, Bengston K, Rescorla FJ et al. Delayed surgical repair and ECMO improves survival in congenital diaphragmatic hernia. *Ann Surg* 1992; 216:454–62.

30. Nakayama DK, Motoyama EK, Tagge EM. Effect of preoperative stabilization on respiratory system compliance and outcome in newborn infants with congenital diaphragmatic hernia. *J Pediatr* 1991; 118:793–9.

31. Wung JT, Sahni R, Moffitt ST et al. Congenital diaphragmatic hernia: Survival treated with very delayed surgery, spontaneous respiration, and no chest tube. *J Pediatr Surg* 1995; 30:406–9.

32. Lally KP, Paranka MS, Roden J et al. Congenital diaphragmatic hernia: Stabilization and repair on ECMO. *Ann Surg* 1992; 216:569–73.

33. Does extracorporeal membrane oxygenation improve survival in neonates with congenital diaphragmatic hernia? The Congenital Diaphragmatic Hernia Study Group. *J Pediatr Surg* 1999; 34:720–34:724.

34. Revenis M, Glass P, Short BL. Mortality and morbidity rates among lower birth weight infants (2000–2500 grams) treated with extracorporeal membrane oxygenation. *J Pediatr* 1992; 121:452–8.

35. Grimm P. Feeding difficulties in infants treated with ECMO. 1993, CNMC ECMO Symposium 25.

36. Nield T, Hallaway M, Fodera C et al. Outcome in problem feeders post ECMO. 1990, CNMC ECMO Symposium 79.

37. Tarby T, Waggoner J. Are the common neurologic problems following ECMO related to jugular bulb thrombosis? 1994, CNMC ECMO Symposium 100.

38. Glass P, Wagner A, Papero P et al. Neurodevelopmental status at age five years of neonates treated with extracorporeal membrane oxygenation. *J Pediatr* 1995; 127:447–57.

39. Rajasingham S, Reed V, Glass P et al. Congenital diaphragmatic hernia—Outcome post-ECMO at 5 years. 1994, CNMC ECMO Symposium 35.

40. Gershan L, Gershan W, Day S. Airway anomalies after ECMO: Bronchoscopic findings. 1992, CNMC ECMO Symposium 65.

41. Wagner A, Glass P, Papero P et al. Neuropsychological outcome of neonatal ECMO survivors at age 5. 1994, CNMC ECMO Symposium 31.

42. D'Agostino J, Bernbaum J, Gerdes M et al. Outcome for infants with congenital diaphragmatic hernia requiring extracorporeal membrane oxygenation: The first year. *J Pediatr Surg* 1995; 30:10–5.

43. Van Meurs K, Robbins S, Reed V et al. Congenital diaphragmatic hernia: Long-term outcome in neonates treated with extracorporeal membrane oxygenation. *J Pediatr* 1993; 122:893–9.

44. Atkinson J, Poon M. ECMO and the management of congenital diaphragmatic hernia with large diaphragmatic defects requiring a prosthetic patch. *J Pediatr Surg* 1992; 27:754–6.

45. Adolph V, Ekelund C, Smith C et al. Developmental outcome of neonates treated with ECMO. *J Pediatr Surg* 1990; 25:43–6.

46. Andrews A, Nixon C, Cilley R et al. One-to-three year outcome for 14 neonatal survivors of extracorporeal membrane oxygenation. *Pediatrics* 1986; 78:692–8.

47. Flusser H, Dodge N, Engle W et al. Neurodevelopmental outcome and respiratory morbidity for ECMO survivors at 1 year of age. *J Perinatol* 1993; 13:266–71.

48. Glass P, Miller M, Short BL. Morbidity for survivors of extracorporeal membrane oxygenation: Neurodevelopmental outcome at 12 years of age. *Pediatrics* 1989; 83:72–8.

49. Griffin M, Minifee P, Landry S et al. Neurodevelopmental outcome in neonates after ECMO: Cranial magnetic resonance imaging and ultrasonography correlation. *J Pediatr Surg* 1992; 27:33–5.

50. Hofkosh D, Thompson A, Nozza R et al. Ten years of ECMO: Neurodevelopmental outcome. *Pediatrics* 1991; 87:549–55.

51. Krummel T, Greenfield L, Kirkpatrick B et al. The early evaluation of survivors after ECMO for neonatal pulmonary failure. *J Pediatr Surg* 1984; 19:585–90.

52. Schumacher R, Palmer T, Roloff D et al. Follow-up of infants treated with ECMO for newborn respiratory failure. *Pediatrics* 1991; 87:451–7.

53. Towne B, Lott I, Hicks D, Healey T. Long-term follow-up of infants and children treated with ECMO: A preliminary report. *J Pediatr Surg* 1985; 20:410–14.

54. Wildin S, Landry S, Zwischenberger J. Prospective, controlled study of developmental outcome in survivors of ECMO: The first 24 months. *Pediatrics* 1994; 93:404–8.

55. Stolar CJ, Crisafi MA, Driscoll YT. Neurocognitive outcome for neonates treated with extracorporeal membrane oxygenation: Are infants with congenital diaphragmatic hernia different? *J Pediatr Surg* 1995; 30:366–72.

56. Davis D, Wilkerson S, Stewart D. Neurodevelopmental follow-up of ECMO survivors at 7 years. 1995 CNMC ECMO Symposium 34.

57. Stanley C, Brodsky K, McKee L et al. Developmental profile of ECMO survivors at early school age and relationship to neonatal EEG status. 1995 CNMC ECMO Symposium 33.

58. Hack M, Taylor H, Klein N et al. School-age outcomes in children with birth weights under 750 g. *N Engl J Med* 1994; 331:753–9.

59. Walton J, Hendricks-Munoz K. Profile and stability of sensorineural hearing loss in persistent pulmonary hypertension of the newborn. *J Speech Lang Hear Res* 1991; 34:1362–70.

60. Naulty C, Weiss I, Herer G. Progressive sensorineural hearing loss in survivors of persistent fetal circulation. *Ear Hear* 1986; 7:74–7.

61. Leavitt A, Watchko J, Bennett F, Folson R. Neurodevelopmental outcome following persistent pulmonary hypertension of the neonate. *J Perinatol* 1987; 7:88–291.

62. Sell EJ, Gaines JA, Gluckman C, Williams E. Persistent fetal circulation: Neurodevelopmental outcome. *Am J Dis Child* 1985; 139:25–8.

63. Marron M, Crisafi M, Driscoll J et al. Hearing and neurodevelopmental outcome in survivors of persistent pulmonary hypertension of the newborn. *Pediatrics* 1992; 90:392–6.

64. Bifano E, Pfannenstiel A. Duration of hyperventilation and outcome in infants with persistent pulmonary hypertension. *Pediatrics* 1988; 81:657–61.

65. Ferrara B, Johnson D, Chang P, Thompson T. Efficacy and neurologic outcome of profound hypocapneic alkalosis for the treatment of persistent pulmonary hypertension in infancy. *Pediatrics* 1984; 105:457–61.

66. Bernbaum J, Russell P, Sheridan P et al. Long-term follow-up of newborns with persistent pulmonary hypertension. *Crit Care Med* 1984; 12:579–83.

67. Waitzer E, Riley SP, Perreault T, Shevell MI. Neurologic outcome at school entry for newborns treated with extracorporeal membrane oxygenation for noncardiac indications. *J Child Neurol* 2009; 24:801–6.

68. Desai S, Stanley C, Graziani L et al. Brainstem auditory evoked potential screening (BAEP) unreliable for detecting sensorineural hearing loss in ECMO survivors: A comparison of neonatal BAEP and follow-up behavioral audiometry. 1994, CNMC ECMO Symposium 62.

69. Haney B, Thibeault D, Sward-Comunelli S et al. Ocular findings in infants treated with ECMO. 1994, CNMC ECMO Symposium 63.

70. Gonzalez VH, Ober RR, Borchert MS, Bui KC, Raymos AD, Stout AU. Ocular findings in neonates after extracorporeal membrane oxygenation. *Retina* 1993; 13:202–7.

71. Hahn J, Baucher Y, Bejar R, Coen R. Electroencephalographic and neuroimaging findings in neonates undergoing extracorporeal membrane oxygenation. *Neuropediatrics* 1993; 24:19–24.

72. Graziani L, Streletz L, Baumgart S et al. Predictive value of neonatal electroencephalograms before and during extracorporeal membrane oxygenation. *J Pediatr* 1994; 125:969–75.

73. Campbell L, Bunyapen C, Gangarosa M et al. The significance of seizures associated with ECMO. 1991, CNMC ECMO Symposium 26.

74. Kumar P, Bedard M, Delaney-Black V, Shankaran S. Post-ECMO electroencephalogram (EEG) as a predictor of neurological outcome. 1994, CNMC ECMO Symposium 65.

75. Scher M, Kosaburo A, Beggerly M, Hamid M, Steppe D, Painter M. Electrographic seizures in preterm and full-term neonates: Clinical correlates, associated brain lesions, and risk for neurologic sequelae. *Pediatrics* 1993; 91:128–34.

76. Ittman P, Schumacher R, Vanderkerhove J. Outcome in newborns following pre-ECMO CPR. 1993, CNMC ECMO Symposium 30.

77. Khambekar K, Nichani S, Luyt DK et al. Developmental outcome in newborn infants treated for acute respiratory failure with extracorporeal membrane oxygenation: Present experience. *Arch Dis Child Fetal Neonatal Ed* 2006; 91:F21–5.

78. Stewart D, Davis D, Reese A, Wilkerson S. Neurodevelopmental outcome of extracorporeal life support (ECLS) patients using the Stanford Binet IV. 1993, CNMC ECMO Symposium 24.

79. Mendoza J, Wilkerson S, Reese A, Vogel R. Outcome of neonates treated with ECMO: Longitudinal follow-up from 1 to 3 years of age. 1991, CNMC ECMO Symposium 29.

80. Wilkerson S, Stewart D, Cook L. Developmental outcome of ECMO patients over a four year span. 1990, CNMC ECMO Symposium 23.

81. Baumgart S, Graziani L, Streletz L et al. Right common carotid artery reconstruction following ECMO: Structural and vascular imaging electroencephalography and neurodevelopmental correlates to recovery. 1993, CNMC ECMO Symposium 27.

82. Stanley C, Merton D, Desai S et al. Four year follow-up Doppler ultrasound studies in children who

received right common carotid artery (RCCA) reconstruction following neonatal ECMO. 1995, CNMC ECMO Symposium 104.

83. Beusing KA, Killian AK, Schaible T, Loff S, Sumargo S, Neff KW. Extracorporeal membrane oxygenation in infants with congenital diaphragmatic hernia: Follow-up MRI evaluating carotid artery reocclusion and neurologic outcome. *Am J Roentgenol* 2007; 188:1636–42.

84. Duggan EM, Maitre N, Zhai A et al. Neonatal carotid repair at ECMO decannulation: Patency rates and early neurologic outcomes. *J Pediatr Surg* 2015; 50(1):64–8.

85. Qureshi, FG. Jackson HT, Brown J et al. The changing population of the United States and use of extracorporeal membrane oxygenation. *J Surg Res* 2013; 184(1):572–6.

45

Bronchoscopy in the newborn

MIRA SADADCHARAM, ROHIT UMESH VERMA, AND JOHN D. RUSSELL

INTRODUCTION

The infant larynx presents some different aspects compared to the adult. Its location is higher in the neck, the cricoid cartilage being located approximately at the fourth cervical vertebra. With the growth of the child, the cricoid cartilage will gradually descend to the level of the seventh cervical vertebra, which is the location in adulthood. The size of the larynx in the newborn is about 1/3 of that in the adult. Their structures such as the vocal process of arytenoid, cuneiform cartilage, the arytenoids, and the soft tissue that makes up the supraglottic larynx are also bigger. The epiglottis is proportionally more posterior and narrower and more tubular or omega-shaped (Figure 45.1).

Bronchoscopy in the newborn is an important diagnostic and therapeutic tool.[1] The small size of the pediatric airway, anatomic differences in the pediatric larynx, as well as the distinct subset of pathologies unique to the pediatric population are all factors to be cognizant of when performing endoscopic examination in a child. Diagnosis of congenital laryngotracheal malformations and management of airway complications secondary to prolonged intubation are the two commonest indications for pediatric bronchoscopy.[2] The first pediatric bronchoscopy was performed by Killian in 1895.[3] At that time, the procedure was associated with a high complication rate due to poor visibility through small-diameter bronchoscopes, lack of a satisfactory light source, and difficulty maintaining ventilation during the procedure. Modern Hopkins lens systems, intense yet "cold" light sources, together with modern anesthetic techniques have facilitated safer examination of the airway in the newborn.[4,5] Pediatric flexible bronchoscopy was initiated in the mid-1970s, after Ikeda introduced the flexible bronchofiberscope in 1968. Since then, newer and smaller instruments and the addition of suction channels have enabled the endoscopist to examine the airway without significantly distorting the anatomy or normal physiology. Currently, flexible bronchoscopy has largely superseded rigid bronchoscopy for diagnostic purposes in the lower airway.[6,7] The development of the pediatric fiber-optic nasendoscope, while not permitting a view of the trachea or bronchi, has dramatically changed airway endoscopy in the newborn. Infants with stridor who are otherwise well can have their larynx and upper airway examined at the bedside or the outpatient clinic. If a diagnosis of laryngomalacia is made and no suspicious features are noted in the clinical history, laryngoscopy and bronchoscopy under general anesthesia may not be required. However, the airway control and therapeutic ability of rigid bronchoscopy have not been replaced, and it remains an important and potentially lifesaving procedure.

ANESTHESIA FOR PEDIATRIC BRONCHOSCOPY

Anesthesia for diagnostic/therapeutic procedures on the airway has always been challenging. Success is dependent upon careful planning and constant communication between the endoscopist and anesthetist throughout the procedure. Preoperative evaluation consists of a detailed clinical history and physical examination. As a general rule, children are recommended to fast for 6 hours if fed on formula, 4 hours if breast-fed, and 2 hours after the ingestion of clear fluids. Anesthetic technique is dependent upon the child's physical status, the presence of chemical/physical trauma to the airway, and the presence/absence of coexisting lower respiratory tract infections with consequent increased risk of bronchospasm, secretions, edema, hypoxia, and acidosis. In addition, the needs of the endoscopist in performing diagnostic/therapeutic interventions, e.g., bronchoalveolar lavage (BAL), and foreign body retrieval will need to be taken into consideration to ensure the safety of the child and minimize the risk of complications. In many instances, the perioperative use of bronchodilators and/or anticholinergic drugs may improve oxygen saturations and alveolar ventilation while attenuating the vagal responses of bradycardia and bronchoconstriction during airway manipulation.

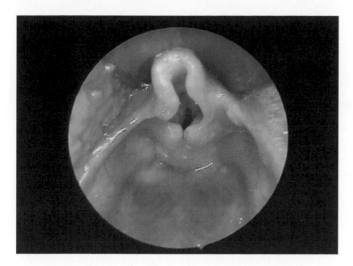

Figure 45.1 Tubular or omega-shaped epiglottis of children. The normal glottis of the infant has a very small opening, about 7 mm in anteroposterior dimension and 4 mm in the posterior transverse dimension. Following Poisseuille's law, we know that resistance to airflow is inversely proportional to the fourth power of the radius. As such, halving the radius increases resistance 16 fold.

With the exception of remifentanil, which is rapidly metabolized in neonates, as a general rule, the smaller the child, the more incomplete their metabolism, specifically in relation to drugs. The reduced intracellular calcium stores and lower myocardial mass in neonates and small children render this population susceptible to the cardiodepressant effects of anesthesia. Moreover, neonates in general and preterm neonates in particular are prone to postanesthesia apnea.

RIGID BRONCHOSCOPY

Indications for rigid bronchoscopy

Rigid bronchoscopy can be performed for both diagnostic and therapeutic purposes (Table 45.1). The commonest causes of stridor and airway obstruction in a neonate are laryngomalacia, subglottic stenosis (both congenital and acquired), and vocal cord paralysis.[8,9] Less common causes include laryngeal clefts, hemangiomas, and papillomas. Rigid bronchoscopy is the diagnostic procedure of choice in the management of airway obstruction. Most neonates with stridor will have laryngomalacia and can be diagnosed with fiber-optic laryngoscopy in an outpatient setting. However, there are three clinical situations where neonates with stridor warrant rigid bronchoscopy: (1) the neonate with severe stridor and significant airway obstruction, who will require urgent bronchoscopy and airway support; (2) the neonate with initially stable but deteriorating stridor; and (3) the neonate with mild or moderate stridor but with poor weight gain or difficulty in feeding, apnea, or cyanotic episodes. Adjuvant investigations may suggest a particular diagnosis, e.g., a vascular ring on barium swallow. However, endoscopy is needed to confirm this diagnosis. In neonates with recurrent aspiration, rigid

Table 45.1 Indications for rigid bronchoscopy

Persistent unexplained cough or wheeze
Unexplained dyspnea or stridor
Suspected congenital airway anomalies, e.g., subglottic stenosis
Foreign body removal
Hemoptysis
Recurrent lower respiratory chest infections
Persistent abnormalities on chest radiograph
Diagnostic BAL
Lung abscess
Thoracic trauma
To remove benign tumors (recurrent respiratory papillomatosis)
Endoscopic management of strictures, webs, granulation tissue
Open airway surgery

bronchoscopy is necessary to rule out a laryngotracheal cleft. Even if pathology is found in the larynx, it is important to complete a systematic assessment as about 70% neonates undergoing rigid bronchoscopy have more than one airway pathology.[4]

Instrumentation

A systematic assessment of the neonatal airway should be performed, which incorporates laryngoscopy, tracheoscopy, and bronchoscopy. A wide range of equipment of varying sizes is required including laryngoscopes, bronchoscopes, telescopes, and telescopic forceps. The senior author's preference is for Karl Storz telescopes and the Benjamin–Lindholm laryngoscope. Suspension of the laryngoscope on a Mayo stand is essential for therapeutic procedures and freeing the surgeon's second hand (Figure 45.1). The components of a modern bronchoscope are (Figure 45.2)

1. A closed gas system allowing connection to an anesthetic circuit
2. A rigid Hopkins rod telescope to allow distal illumination and vision
3. A side channel for the passage of suction catheters or flexible forceps

The bronchoscopes range in size from 2.5 (outside diameter 4.0 mm) to 6.0 (outside diameter 8.2 mm). Sizes 2.5–3.0 are the most appropriate for neonates (Table 45.2).

Technique of rigid laryngobronchoscopy

Rigid laryngobronchoscopy requires general anesthesia. Modern techniques are versatile and controlled, allowing an unhurried and complete examination.[8,9] A full range of neonatal and pediatric laryngoscopes, bronchoscopes, and telescopes are essential. Modern 1 chip and 3 chip cameras allow magnification and excellent resolution of the image on screen of these tiny airways.

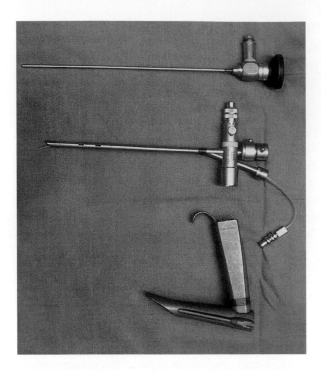

Figure 45.2 Equipment for rigid laryngobronchoscopy: 0° telescope (top); 2.5 mm ventilating bronchoscope (middle); Benjamin–Lindholm laryngoscope (bottom).

Table 45.2 Size of rigid bronchoscopes according to age

Patient age (mean)	Size	Outside diameter (mm)
Premature infant	2.5	3.7
Term newborn (birth to 3 months)	3	4.8
6 months (3–18 months)	3.5	5.7
18 months (1–3 years)	3.7	6.3
3 years (1.5–5 years)	4	6.7
5 years (3–10 years)	5	7.8
10 years (>10 years to adolescent)	6	8.2

A spontaneous respiration technique is the anesthetic method of choice and has superseded transglottic jet ventilation. However, this technique is challenging to the anesthesiologist requiring a balance as the patient must spontaneously breathe, while sedate enough to not develop laryngospasm or bronchospasm when instrumentation is introduced. Sevoflurane is, in most anesthesiologists' opinion, the anesthetic of choice. It allows a deep plane of anesthesia without causing respiratory arrest. The procedure should proceed in a systematic manner as outlined next.[10]

The neonate is anesthetized with a mixture of sevoflurane and oxygen via a facemask. The patient's chest is not covered with drapes so that respiration can be assessed. The surgeon sits at the head of the bed with the anesthetic machine positioned to the side in such a way that both the surgeon and the anesthesiologist should be able to read the patient's vital

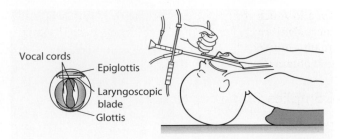

Figure 45.3 Under direct visualization of the larynx, the bronchoscope is introduced into the trachea.

signs including oxygen saturation. The camera system's monitor should be positioned over the far end of the bed. The larynx is then briefly visualized using the laryngoscope and topical 4% lidocaine (0.5–2 mg/kg) applied (to prevent laryngospasm). An appropriately sized nasopharyngeal airway is inserted, and the anesthetic agent is then provided via this route. Atropine may also be administered to prevent bradycardia and to dry up the secretions during the assessment. A baby Lindholm laryngoscope is then inserted, by placing its tip in the vallecula, exposing the whole larynx. The scope is suspended on a Mayo table to avoid compression of the baby's chest or held with the nondominant hand. The larynx is now examined using a 4 mm 0° Hopkins rod laryngeal telescope. Pathological conditions looked for in the larynx include (1) laryngeal webs, (2) laryngeal cysts, (3) subglottic stenosis, and (4) hemangiomas. The mobility of the arytenoids is then assessed using a blunt laryngeal probe, which also allows palpation for small laryngeal clefts. Once the larynx has been thoroughly examined, the telescope is passed into the subglottis and trachea. This allows a complete atraumatic inspection, easily passing to the carina. In order to examine the bronchi in detail, one has to remove the laryngoscope and introduce an appropriately sized bronchoscope (Figure 45.3). Turning the baby's head to the left allows entry through the right main bronchus, and turning the head to the right allows entry into the left mainstem bronchus. On both the left and right sides, access to the upper lobe bronchus is the most challenging and may be aided by various dynamic maneuvers including flexing the infant's chin onto the shoulder and external pressure on the chest. The final part of the assessment is to examine the trachea and vocal cords as the baby is lightening up from the anesthetic. This is the only time when tracheobronchomalacia and vocal cord paralysis can be observed.

Advantages of rigid bronchoscopy

The major advantage of rigid airway assessment is the excellent control of ventilation provided. This is of particular importance with the soft and collapsible neonatal airway. The rigid bronchoscope can also accommodate instruments, allowing therapeutic interventions to be performed endoscopically. Rigid bronchoscopy allows the lower airways to be inspected safely and in great detail while maintaining control over ventilation. Flexible bronchoscopy does not allow such control and in a small neonate or infant will cause significant, if not total, airway obstruction. The image quality obtained by the rigid telescope is also superior to that obtained with the flexible fiber-optic bundles.

Complications of rigid bronchoscopy

Despite the relative safety of modern rigid bronchoscopy, complications still occur with a reported complication rate of 2%–4%. Safety is affected by the anesthetic technique (including intraoperative monitoring), the interventions performed during the endoscopy, availability of equipment, the expertise of the staff, and the condition of the patient.[5] Complications reported include laryngospasm, vocal cord trauma, subglottic edema, pneumothorax, pneumonia, hoarseness, hemorrhage, cardiac arrhythmia, and death. In Hoeve et al.'s series in 1993, a diagnosis of tetralogy of Fallot, undertaking biopsy or drainage, foreign body extraction, and tracheal stenosis were the main risk factors for complications. Interestingly, fewer complications occurred in the age group <3 months.[11]

FLEXIBLE BRONCHOSCOPY

Flexible bronchoscopy was first performed in the 1970s, and since then, newer and smaller scopes have enabled visualization of the airway of premature infants and neonates.[12] The advantages of flexible airway bronchoscopy are that examination of the distal lobar bronchi is less challenging than rigid bronchoscopy, it can be performed as a day-case procedure, and it requires little preparation except for no oral intake 4–6 hours preoperatively. Provided flexible bronchoscopy is performed by an experienced operator in a controlled setting, the procedure is very safe. Vauthy[6] reports over 10,000 flexible bronchoscopies with no mortality.

Indications for flexible bronchoscopy

Flexible bronchoscopy may be performed for diagnostic reasons in the neonate with mild stridor, unexplained wheezing, hemoptysis, chronic cough, persistent atelectasis, and persistent pulmonary infiltrates (Table 45.3).

Table 45.3 Indications for flexible bronchoscopy

Diagnostic	Therapeutic
Unexplained stridor	To aid intubation
Unexplained wheezing	Therapeutic BAL
Hemoptysis	Brush biopsies
Unexplained cough	Removal of airway secretions
Persistent atelectasis	Diagnose and monitor after lung transplantation
Recurrent or persistent pulmonary infiltrates	Transbronchial biopsy

Flexible bronchoscopy is also increasingly performed in the neonatal intensive care unit (NICU).[13–15] Flexible bronchoscopy in the NICU can be performed via the existing endotracheal tube or tracheostomy (thus maintaining the airway) and negates the need to transfer the patient to the operating room. The bronchoscope can be used to check the position of the endotracheal tube. Sudden respiratory deterioration in the ICU can be due to severe mucous plugging, atelectasis, granuloma formation, tracheitis, or tracheobronchomalacia. In these patients, flexible bronchoscopy may be both diagnostic and therapeutic, allowing careful direction of suction catheters to improve pulmonary toilet. Full-term infants tolerate flexible bronchoscopy with a 3.4 mm scope, which has suction channels for insufflation of oxygen, suction and bronchial brushings, or BAL. BAL aids the diagnosis of infection, gastroesophageal reflux (detecting lipid-laden alveolar macrophages), and the removal of mucous plugs.[16,17]

Technique of flexible bronchoscopy

Pediatric flexible bronchoscopy can be performed directly through the nose or mouth, via a face mask or laryngeal mask airway, as well as through an endotracheal tube.[15] It is the author's experience that the vast majority of patients require general anesthesia for flexible bronchoscopy. The neonate is placed on the table with the assistant providing oxygen via a mask. The average diagnostic procedure lasts approximately 30 seconds and should be digitally recorded, so that the procedure can be reviewed. If performed as a day-case postprocedure, the patient should be clinically observed for 1.5 hours and allowed to eat prior to discharge.

Common pitfalls for the unwary flexible bronchoscopist

CONCURRENT LESIONS

Children frequently have multiple airway abnormalities, and these can often be missed due to the speed of the flexible assessment.

DIFFICULT NASAL PASSAGE

Nasal septal deviations or turbinate hypertrophy can lead to difficulty passing the flexible scopes. The use of a topical vasoconstrictor enables the nose to be entered in most cases. Wood et al. in 1990 encountered only three patients in whom the transnasal passage of the flexible bronchoscope was not possible.[20]

PHARYNGEAL HYPOTONIA

Patients with tracheostomies or who have reduced muscle tone because of neurologic disease often have pharyngeal hypotonia leading to an increase in the amount of secretions in the larynx, making visualization difficult.

Complications of flexible bronchoscopy

Complications of flexible bronchoscopy are generally minor and are reported to occur in 2%–8% of the cases.[18–21] Reported complications include laryngospasm, pneumothorax, epistaxis, bradycardia, and hemorrhage. Generally, high-risk patients are more likely to undergo rigid bronchoscopy as obstruction of a large proportion of the airway can lead to hypoxemia. It is also difficult to remove foreign bodies with a flexible scope. The relative contraindications to flexible bronchoscopy are (1) hypoxemia, (2) respiratory distress, (3) hemorrhagic diathesis, (4) cardiac arrhythmia, and (5) a foreign body. All these problems increase the risk of complications with flexible bronchoscopy.

BAL in children

Since the advent of flexible bronchoscopy in the 1980s, bronchoscopy has been increasingly used as a diagnostic tool for several pediatric pathologies.[22,23] The technique of BAL has helped determine the diagnosis in a number of respiratory conditions including persistent/recurrent lower respiratory tract infections, interstitial pulmonary infiltrates, severe refractory lower respiratory tract infections in the setting of the ICU, and pulmonary infiltrates in immunocompromised children.[24–29] Within this context, BAL is a safe, fast procedure. It is particularly useful in children in whom it is often difficult to obtain a sputum sample. Microbiologic assessment of BAL fluid may aide in identifying a causative pathogen. Even if the BAL sample is small, molecular biology techniques frequently allow for amplification and identification.[30] In addition, diagnoses of alveolar proteinosis, hemosiderosis, and recurrent pulmonary aspiration (based on the presence of lipid-laden macrophages) can also be made on the basis of BAL, potentially obviating the need for open/transbronchial biopsy. Furthermore, BAL may be used in a therapeutic capacity, e.g., in the treatment of alveolar proteinosis and for removal of inspissated secretions in children with cystic fibrosis and foreign body removal.[31,32]

CONCLUSION

Modern rigid and flexible bronchoscopy in the newborn carried out by trained personnel is a safe, relatively atraumatic procedure with a low rate of serious complications. This is due to the advances in anesthesia, pharmacology, instrumentation, and camera technologies. Rigid and flexible bronchoscopy should be viewed as complimentary and not competing mutually exclusive techniques. Both procedures should be in the armamentarium of the pediatric airway surgeon. There are advantages and disadvantages to each technique. It is to the neonate's advantage to have both types of endoscopes available so the procedure with the highest benefit-to-risk ratio can be employed.

REFERENCES

1. Lockhart CH, Elliot JL. Potential hazards of paediatric rigid bronchoscopy. *J Pediatr Surg* 1984 June; 19(3): 239–42.
2. Lindahl H, Rintala R, Malinen L, Leijala M, Sairanen H. Bronchoscopy during the first month of life. *J Pediatr Surg* 1992 May; 27(5): 548–50.
3. Clerf LH. Historical aspects of foreign bodies in the air and food passages. *Ann Otol Rhinol Laryngol* 1952 March; 61(1): 5–17.
4. Ungkanont K, Friedman EM, Sulek M. A retrospective analysis of airway endoscopy in patients less than 1-month old. *Laryngoscope* 1998 November; 108(11 Pt 1): 1724–8.
5. Holinger LD. Diagnostic endoscopy of the paediatric airway. *Laryngoscope* 1989 March; 99(3): 346–8.
6. Vauthy PA. Evaluation of the paediatric airway by flexible endoscopy. In: Cotton RT (ed). *Practical Paediatric Otolaryngology*. Philadelphia: Lipincott-Raven, 1999: 477–90.
7. Wood RE. The emerging role of flexible bronchoscopy in pediatrics. *Clin Chest Med* 2001; 22: 311–7.
8. Holinger LD. Etiology of stridor in the neonate, infant and child. *Ann Otol Rhinol Laryngol* 1980 September–October; 89(5 Pt 1): 397–400.
9. Boudewyns A, Claes J, Van de Heyning P. Clinical practice: An approach to stridor in infants and children. *Eur J Pediatr* 2010; 169: 135–41.
10. Benjamin B. Technique of laryngoscopy. *Int J Pediatr Otorhinolaryngol* 1987 October; 13(3): 299–313.
11. Farrell PT. Rigid bronchoscopy for foreign body removal: Anaesthesia and ventilation. *Paediatr Anaesth* 2004 January; 14(1): 84–9.
12. Hoeve LJ, Rombout J, Meursing AE. Complications of rigid laryngo-bronchoscopy in children. *Int J Pediatr Otorhinolaryngol* 1993 February; 26(1): 47–56.
13. Wood RE, Fink RJ. Applications of flexible fibreoptic bronchoscopes in infants and children. *Chest* 1978 May; 73(5 Suppl): 737–40.
14. Wood RE. Evaluation of the upper airway in children. *Curr Opin Pediatr* 2008; 20: 266–71.
15. Cakir E, Ersu RH, Uyan ZS, Oktem, S, Karadag B, Yapar O. Flexible bronchoscopy as a valuable tool in the evaluation of persistent wheezing in children. *Int J Pediatric Otorhinol* 2009; 73: 1666–8.
16. Myer CM 3rd, Thompson RF. Flexible fibreoptic bronchoscopy in the neonatal intensive care unit. *Int J Pediatr Otorhinolaryngol* 1988 May; 15(2): 143–7.
17. Furuya ME, Moreno-Cordova V, Ramirez-Figueroa JL, Vargas MH, Ramon-Garcia G, Ramirez-San Juan DH. Cutoff value of lipid-laden alveolar macrophages for diagnosing aspiration in infants and children. *Pediatr Pulmonol* 2007 May; 42(5): 452–7.

18. Midulla F, de Blic J, Barbato A et al. Flexible endoscopy of paediatric airways. *Eur Respir J* 2003 October; 22(4): 698–708.
19. Niggemann B, Haack M, Machotta A. How to enter the paediatric airway for bronchoscopy. *Pediatr Int* 2004 April; 46(2): 117–21.
20. Wood RE. Pitfalls in the use of the flexible bronchoscope in paediatric patients. *Chest* 1990 January; 97(1): 199–203.
21. De Blic J, Marchac V, Scheinmnann P. Complications of flexible bronchoscopy in children: Prospective study of 1.328 procedures. *Eur Respir J* 2002; 20: 1271–6.
22. Weinberger M, Abu-Hasan M. Pseudo-asthma: When cough, wheezing, and dyspnea are not asthma. *Pediatrics* 2007; 120: 855–64.
23. Cakir E, Uyan Z, Oktem S, Karakoc F, Ersu R, Karadag B. Flexible bronchoscopy for diagnosis and follow up of childhood endobronchial tuberculosis. *Pediatr Infect Dis* 2008; 27: 783–7.
24. Fiadjoe J, Stricker P. Pediatric difficult airway management: Current devices and techniques. *Anesthesiol Clin* 2009; 27: 185–95.
25. Godfrey S. Pulmonary hemorrhage/hemoptysis in children. *Pediatr Pulmonol* 2004; 37: 476–84.
26. Woods RK, Sharp RJ, Holcomb GW, Synder CL, Lofland GK, Ashcraft KW. Vascular anomalies and tracheoesophageal compression: A single institutions 25-year experience. *Ann Thorac Surg* 2001; 72: 434–8.
27. Efrati O, Sadeh-Gornik U, Modan-Moses D, Barak A, Szeinberg A, Vardi A. Flexible bronchoscopy and bronchoalveolar lavage in pediatric patients with lung disease. *Pediatr Crit Care Med* 2009; 10: 80–4.
28. Priftis KS, Anthracopoulos MB, Mermiri D, Papadopulou A, Xepapadaki P, Tsakanika C Bronchial hyperresponsiveness, atopy and bronchoalveolar lavage eosinophils in persistent middle lobe syndrome. *Pediatr Pulmonol* 2006; 41: 805–11.
29. Saito J, Harris WT, Gelfonf J, Noah TL, Leigh MW, Johnson R. Physiologic, bronchoscopic and bronchoalveolar lavage fluid findings in young children with recurrent wheeze and cough. *Pediatr Pulmonol* 2006; 41: 709–19.
30. Tessier V, Chadelat K, Baculard A, Housset B, Clement A. A controlled study of differential cytology and cytokine expression profiles by alveolar cells in pediatric sarcoidosis. *Chest* 1996; 109: 1430–8.
31. Yang LF, Xu YC, Wang YS, Wang CF, Zhu GH, Bao XE. Airway foreign body removal by flexible bronchoscopy: Experience with 1027 children during 2000–2008. *World J Pediatr* 2009; 5: 191–5.
32. Rignini CA, Morel N, Karkas A, Reyt E, Ferreti K, Pin I. What is the diagnostic value of flexible bronchoscopy in the initial investigation of children with suspected foreign body aspiration? *Int J Pediatr Otorhinolaryngol* 2007; 71: 1383–90.

PART 4

Esophagus

Esophageal atresia and tracheo-esophageal fistula

PAUL D. LOSTY

To anastomose the ends of an infant's esophagus, the surgeon must be as delicate and precise as a skilled watchmaker. No other operation offers a greater opportunity for pure technical artistry.

Willis Potts
1950[1]

INTRODUCTION

Surgery for esophageal atresia (EA) is widely regarded as one of the greatest milestones in newborn surgery. Significant advances have now led to greater than 95% survival for EA babies managed in the modern era with much attention now focusing on morbidity, health outcome(s), and quality of life (QoL) in adult survivors. Classical operation with muscle sparing thoracotomy, axillary skin crease incision, and minimally invasive surgery provide a selection of strategies for the pediatric surgeon and enthusiast. Controversy dominates best practice with regard expert management of pure (long-gap) EA without fistula, medical and surgical treatment of gastroesophageal reflux (GER) disease, therapies for anastomotic stricture, and tracheomalacia. Embryology and molecular genetic studies have yielded fascinating insight into the etiology of EA and tracheoesophageal fistula (TEF), with many important contributions emerging from animal models sharing striking similarity to the human phenotype.[2,3]

HISTORY

The history of EA–TEF is well described in the literature.[2,3] First survivors were not recorded until 1939 with Leven and Ladd achieving success with staged esophageal repair. Cameron Haight (an American surgeon working in Ann Arbor, Michigan) is credited with the first successful primary repair and survival of a 12-day-old female newborn. UK success then followed with Franklin (1947) at the Hammersmith Hospital, London; Denis Browne (1948) at the Great Ormond Street Hospital for Sick Children, London; and Peter Paul Rickham (1949) at Alder Hey Children's Hospital, Liverpool. By the 1980s, pediatric surgery units in the developed world were achieving outcomes approaching 85%–90% survival with mortality falling to less than 10%, defining the modern era of care.[2]

CLASSIFICATION

In 1929, Vogt[4] first proposed an anatomical classification of EA and TEF based on radiological and postmortem findings. A variety of surgical classifications were thereafter suggested as operative treatment became more successful, the most frequently deployed system being that attributed to Gross[5]. The most detailed classification, however, is credited to Kluth[6] and incorporates all described anatomical variants of EA and TEF. From a practical viewpoint, a working classification based on the frequency of each anomaly is of greatest value to the neonatal surgeon (Figure 46.1).

PROGNOSIS

Waterston et al.'s[7] landmark paper describing the influence of pulmonary disease, birth weight, and associated congenital

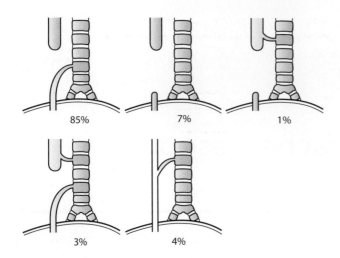

Figure 46.1 Classification and frequency of EA and TEF. EA and distal TEF—85%; isolated EA—7%; H-type TEF—4%; EA with proximal and distal fistulas—3%; EA and proximal fistula—1%.

Table 46.1 Spitz prognostic classification scoring system—survival related to birth weight and congenital heart disease (CHD)

Group		Survival
I	Birth weight ≥1500 g without major CHD	97%
II	Birth weight <1500 g or major CHD	59%
III	Birth weight <1500 g and major CHD	22%

anomalies on outcome of newborns with EA–TEF provided an important contribution for development of prognostic scoring systems. Advances in neonatal intensive care have now rendered the Waterston classification outdated. Spitz et al.[8] provided a new risk grading system based on birth weight and presence or absence of congenital heart disease that is now widely accepted as applicable to the modern era (Table 46.1). A Montreal classification system places greater emphasis on preoperative ventilator dependence and associated major anomalies as survival determinants.[9] Many studies record the negative influence of respiratory distress syndrome and pneumonia on outcome(s) and the burden of aspiration events contributing to morbidity and late death following operative repair.[10,11] Variant anatomy also features as risk factor(s) for determining favorable outcome(s). Babies with "long gap" or "pure" EA without fistula experience a high morbidity from anastomotic leak, stricture, fundoplication rate(s), "failure"/"redo" operations, and esophageal replacement.[10–12]

EPIDEMIOLOGY

In the Liverpool and Mersey region, the incidence of EA and TEF is 1 in 3300 live births.[13] The reported rates vary widely across the world from 1 in 2440 in Finland[14] to 1 in 4500 in Australia[15] and the United States.[16] Sex ratio has been quoted as equal by many authors, but some publications allude to a male preponderance.[17] EA and TEF are more common in twin pregnancies. Exposure to teratogenic drugs during pregnancy has been implicated; these include thalidomide, progesterone, and estrogens.[18]

GENETICS

Sporadic reports of familial cases of EA–TEF suggest a polygenic hereditary etiology. The best estimate of risk of recurrence for parents of a single affected child is 0.5%–2.0%, rising to 20% if another sibling is born with EA. The vertical transmission risk is 3%–4%.[19] A 10% incidence of nonspecific chromosomal abnormalities (translocations, deletions, and duplications) is recorded. Edwards syndrome (trisomy 18) and Down's (trisomy 21) are associated with the EA and TEF phenotype. Recognition of a syndrome suggestive of a major chromosomal abnormality in EA and TEF should prompt urgent involvement of a clinical geneticist before corrective surgery is undertaken. EA–TEF has also been described in association with Feingold syndrome (autosomal dominant), Holt–Oram syndrome, DiGeorge sequence, polysplenia, and in babies with Pierre Robin anomaly.[19]

ANIMAL MODELS

Significant contributions to understanding the embryology and genetic control of foregut development have evolved from laboratory research involving animal models of EA and TEF. The Adriamycin rodent model was developed by Diez-Pardo et al.[20] in Madrid. Timed pregnant rodents administered with Adriamycin (doxorubicin) in the prenatal period on gestational days 8 and 9 yield offspring with an EA–TEF variant phenotype.[20] Pups also have associated VACTERL spectrum anomalies—vertebral, anorectal, cardiac, tracheoesophageal, radial/renal, and limb defects.[21] A murine model of the VACTERL syndrome has also been generated in mice with targeted deletions of the transcription factors Gli-2 and Gli-3 for the Sonic hedgehog (Shh) gene—pivotally linked with axial organogenesis. Gli-2–/–Gli-3–/– double mutants demonstrate the full phenotypic spectrum of VACTERL syndrome, thus confirming a crucial role for Shh in genetic control of foregut development.[21,22]

EMBRYOLOGY

There is no unifying embryological theory that successfully explains all the anatomical variants of EA and TEF. The complete pathology has been demonstrated in the 5-week-old human embryo; therefore, causative factors must operate before this. In the developing embryo, the ventral aspect of the primitive foregut is destined to become the tracheobronchial tree. A median laryngotracheal groove develops in the ventral aspect of the foregut of the 23-day-old embryo. As the groove elongates with the growing esophagus, it is postulated that lateral epithelial ridges fuse to bring about foregut septation. While explaining the possible origins of tracheoesophageal cleft and H-type variant EA fistula, caudocranial separation of the ventral trachea from the dorsal esophagus by a mesenchymal tracheoesophageal septum clearly cannot adequately explain all variants of EA–TEF.

The findings of both an increased number of tracheal rings and a longer trachea in the Adriamycin rodent model of EA–TEF suggest localized abnormal proliferation and elongation of the ventral respiratory component of the common foregut tube. The preferential incorporation of tissue into the trachea may also result in esophageal discontinuity. The association of 13 pairs of ribs with long-gap TEF has also been postulated to strengthen the argument that abnormal forces, in this case hypersomatization, result in a relative deficiency of tissue, which is then preferentially absorbed into tracheal development at the expense of the esophagus.[23]

Further work in the Adriamycin model has also shown that the notochord is implicated with signaling activity to determine the fate(s) of neighboring cell populations. Shh protein, which is expressed in the notochordal tissue, is believed to be pivotal in this dynamic process.[24] Shh stimulates cell proliferation and inhibits apoptosis via intermediary HOX gene expression. Shh binds to the cell surface protein "Patched" (Ptc), which is upregulated by Shh, and thus limits the inductive capabilities of Shh. Ventral misplacement of the notochord may also result in an abnormal diffusion gradient for Shh and a localized imbalance of proliferation and apoptosis in the primitive foregut.

ASSOCIATED ANOMALIES

Associated anomalies are seen in over 50% of newborns presenting with EA and TEF.[2,25,26] Although some of these are relatively insignificant, a high proportion are life-threatening contributing directly to the morbidity and mortality of this condition. The assessment of the newborn with EA–TEF should be prioritized with some urgency to address social, ethical, and surgical strategies relating to the coexistent anomalies. The incidence of such anomalies appears to be highest in babies with pure EA without fistula and infants with orofacial cleft defects.[27] Patients born with EA–TEF have a higher incidence of prematurity than that seen in the normal healthy population. Congenital heart disease (27%) is the commonest comorbid condition and has the greatest impact on survival. Aortic arch anomalies have been shown to occur frequently with "long-gap" EA–TEF variants. Other malformations include urogenital (18%), skeletal (12%), anorectal (12%), and gastrointestinal defects (9%), most notably duodenal atresia. The spectrum of associated anomalies encountered in 581 EA patients treated at Alder Hey Children's Hospital over four decades is shown in Table 46.2.

Several phenotype variants have been described with EA–TEF babies. The VATER association,[27–28] now better referred to as the VACTERL sequence, is defined by the

Table 46.2 Abnormalities associated with esophageal atresia and TOF (Liverpool series 1953–1997)

Type	1953–1997 (581 cases)
Cardiac	154 (27%)
Urogenital	105 (18%)
Skeletal	71 (12%)
Vertebral	64 (11%)
Anorectal	67 (12%)
Gastrointestinal	53 (9%)
Palate/laryngotracheal	44 (8%)
VACTERL	25 (19%)

presence of three or more anomalies. In a study from Alder Hey Children's Hospital, Liverpool, VACTERL associations were recorded in 19% of cases.[26] CHARGE association refers to coloboma, heart disease, atresia choanae, retarded development, genital hypoplasia, and ear deformities with deafness. EA–TEF is also apparent in the SCHISIS sequence—exomphalos, neural tube defects, cleft lip palate, and genital hypoplasia.[29–31]

Interestingly, babies with EA and TEF have a higher than expected incidence of hypertrophic pyloric stenosis.[32] The almost universal association of GER with EA may lead to delay in diagnosis if gastric outlet obstruction is not suspected from pyloric stenosis. Tracheomalacia of variable severity is present in EA cases, although the full spectrum of associated tracheobronchial and pulmonary abnormalities deserves further closer scrutiny. Significant anatomical tracheobronchial variant anomalies can be seen in 47% of infants undergoing bronchoscopy.[33] Pulmonary agenesis, foregut duplication cysts, congenital cystic adenomatoid malformations, and sequestered lobe have all been described in association with EA and TEF. Other rare foregut pathology such as laryngotracheoesophageal cleft and congenital esophageal stenosis may coexist with EA and TEF.

ANTENATAL PRESENTATION

Fetal diagnosis is now possible in cases of EA and TEF.[34] This may be clearly advantageous, as delivery can be planned at or near a specialist center with full neonatal surgical capability. Counselling is essential by a multidisciplinary team (obstetrician, pediatric surgeon, neonatologist), and a careful search screen for associated chromosomal or cardiac anomalies is important. The identification of a chromosomal abnormality may have potential implications for termination of pregnancy. Antenatal diagnosis of EA should theoretically reduce the likelihood of inadvertent newborn feeding and aspiration pneumonitis. Despite potential advantages of antenatal diagnosis, it is noteworthy that fetal ultrasonography selects an "at-risk" group of infants with a significantly worse prognosis.[35,37] Perinatal mortality (excluding termination of pregnancy) in a study from Newcastle, UK was reportedly

21%.[35] The classical sonographic features of EA and TEF in the fetus are absence of the stomach bubble and associated polyhydramnios.[36] Prenatal detection rates vary widely in fetal medicine centers (9%–24%), and there also appears to be a high rate of false-positive scans. Approximately 50% of all suspected cases on fetal ultrasound scanning are later proven not to have EA after birth.[35]

CLINICAL PRESENTATION AND DIAGNOSIS

Newborns with EA have difficulty clearing saliva. Episodes of coughing, choking, and transient cyanosis may be observed shortly after delivery. These may go unnoticed, and early attempts to feed the infant result in immediate respiratory distress. Diagnosis is readily confirmed by the failure of passage of a firm nasogastric tube. A characteristic resistance is felt at the blind-ending upper esophageal pouch, and the tube cannot be introduced into the stomach. A plain x-ray, which should include the chest and abdomen, demonstrates the nasogastric tube coiled in the upper pouch. An associated TEF is confirmed by the presence of gas-filled intestinal loops below the diaphragm (Figure 46.2). In isolated or pure EA, a featureless gasless abdominal x-ray is observed (Figure 46.3). The presence of a double bubble on the abdominal plain film is highly suggestive of associated duodenal atresia (Figure 46.4). A careful and thorough search for associated abnormalities is mandatory, specifically checking for imperforate anus also. The cardiovascular system should be examined thoroughly to exclude

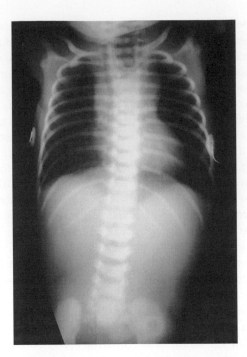

Figure 46.3 Case of "pure" EA without fistula. The nasogastric tube is lying coiled in the upper esophageal pouch. Absence of air-filled abdominal intestinal loops suggests that there is no distal esophageal fistula.

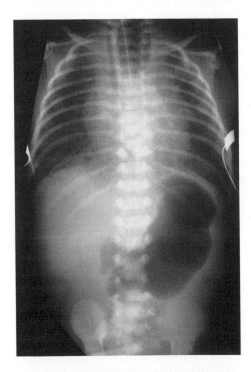

Figure 46.4 EA and TEF with duodenal atresia. Nasogastric tube coiled in upper pouch. "Double-bubble" appearance confirms duodenal atresia.

a major congenital heart defect whose treatment may take higher priority over correction of the EA defect.

Having established the diagnosis, intravenous fluids are commenced and a Replogle sump suction catheter is introduced into the upper esophageal pouch to allow continuous

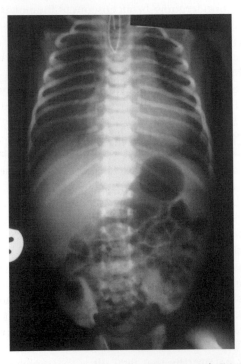

Figure 46.2 Chest x-ray film of a neonate with EA and TEF. Note the nasogastric tube coiled in the blind-ending upper esophagus. Air outlining intestinal loops below the diaphragm confirms the existence of a distal TEF.

aspiration of salivary secretions.[38] Alternatively, the upper pouch and oropharynx should be cleared of secretions by frequent intermittent suction. The infant is nursed in the supine or lateral position. Arrangements should be made for early transfer of the newborn to a specialist neonatal surgical unit. Surgery is ideally performed within the first 24 hours following birth in an otherwise healthy baby, as pneumonitis is an ever-present risk from aspiration of saliva and reflux of gastric contents through the lower pouch TEF.

Following admission to the newborn surgical unit, the infant should be fully reexamined and radiology reviewed. The x-ray study may be repeated with gentle downward firm pressure on the Replogle tube. On rare occasions, a fine nasogastric tube may coil in an otherwise normal patent esophagus, and the successful passage of a Replogle tube into the stomach prevents erroneous diagnosis and an unnecessary surgical operation. When EA is diagnosed in a newborn, an estimation of the length of the blind upper esophageal pouch on plain film radiology can give the surgeon useful clue(s) as to the ease or difficulty of a primary anastomosis. Echocardiography should be performed prior to surgery as this will alert the surgeon and the anesthetist to an underlying cardiac defect that may adversely influence prognosis, and may importantly dictate the operative approach by identifying the side of the aortic arch. Blood should be taken for cross-match and a hematological and biochemical profile arranged preoperatively. Broad-spectrum antibiotics should be administered and intravenous fluids continued. Other investigations, notably whole-spine x-rays and renal and cranial ultrasonography, can be deferred until after surgery. Contrast studies of the upper pouch to identify a rare upper pouch fistula have been superseded by preoperative bronchoscopy.

SURGICAL MANAGEMENT

Surgery for EA is now usually performed as an elective procedure.[39] Emergent operation rarely benefits the baby unless the surgeon is confronted with a "high-risk" ventilated newborn with severe respiratory distress and massive gastric distension with impending perforation, where urgent transpleural fistula ligation is lifesaving (see later). It is common practice for most surgical units to advocate bronchoscopy after induction of general anesthesia when planning elective repair of EA and TEF. We now deploy flexible miniature bronchoscopy with instruments of 2.2 mm caliber (Olympus) that can be steered through the endotracheal tube. Bronchoscopy allows precise confirmation of diagnosis and, in most cases, will demonstrate a common variant fistula just proximal to the carina. Occasionally, the fistula may be seen arising at the level of the carina or from one of the main bronchi. A careful and thorough search should be made to exclude an associated upper pouch fistula. The larynx should also be examined to exclude a laryngotracheoesophageal cleft.

Following bronchoscopy, the infant is positioned for operation. In the classical operation, a right thoracotomy is planned with the baby in a lateral position, with the right arm raised across the head so that the scapula can be easily manipulated (Figure 46.5). The surgeon may find a working headlamp and optical loupe magnification greatly facilitate the operation. A curved skin crease incision is made 1 cm below the angle of the scapula, with a muscle sparing thoracotomy. Bianchi et al.[40] have described an axillary skin crease incision, which gives excellent cosmesis, which we increasingly deploy at Alder Hey (Figure 46.6). A retractor is used to lift the scapula off the chest wall, and the ribs are counted downward from the second interspace. The thorax is then carefully entered through the fourth interspace with bipolar diathermy to separate the intercostal muscles to the level of the parietal pleura. The pleura is then gently freed from the ribs to commence the extrapleural dissection and locate the TEF. This procedure is usually started with moist pledgets and, having developed the plane, may be continued by inserting a moistened gauze swab into the extrapleural space, sweeping the pleura away from the chest wall superiorly and inferiorly. Exposure is improved by introducing a Finochettio retractor for rib retraction. Great care is required with the dissection as it is particularly easy to create a pleural tear in the anterior aspect of the incision. If a significant pleural tear occurs during the dissection, it is probably wise to convert to a transpleural approach. The practical advantages of the extrapleural over the transpleural approach include the possibility of avoiding chest drain insertion and, in the event of an anastomotic leak, the potential containment of any leak/soiling within the extrapleural space. The extrapleural exposure is completed by retracting the posterior mediastinal pleura forward with a malleable retractor until the azygos vein is clearly visualized as it enters the superior vena cava in the depths of the wound.

The azygos vein is mobilized and controlled with vascular sloops. The author advocates temporary occlusion of the vein before ligation, as venous return to the heart may rarely be critically dependent on the azygos system. Provided this maneuver does not affect cardiac output, the azygos vein may be safely ligated and divided as it enters the superior vena cava. Alternatively, some surgeons elect to preserve the azygos vein.[41] Once divided, the site of the TEF communication between the trachea and the distal esophagus is usually apparent. Having confidently identified the distal esophagus, a vascular sloop is carefully passed around it. Traction on the sloop controls the fistula and enables its junction with the trachea to be located precisely. Although it is possible to suture ligate the fistula, the author prefers to divide the fistula in stages and apply interrupted 5-0 or 6-0 monofilament prolene sutures to the tracheal component of the fistula. The distal esophagus is secured with a stay suture. The integrity of the TEF repair is evaluated by instilling saline into the thoracic cavity and requesting the anesthetist to exert positive airway pressure to ensure that no air bubbles leak from the suture line. Rarely difficulty may be

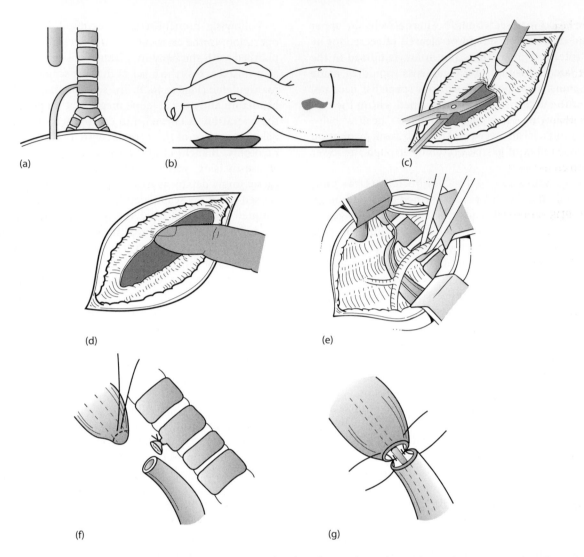

(a)

(b)

(c)

(d)

(e)

(f)

(g)

Figure 46.5 **(a)** Most frequent tracheoesophageal anomaly. **(b)** Infant in lateral position prior to operation. Location of skin incision indicated. **(c)** Exposure of intercostal space with muscle dissection. **(d)** Commencement of gentle stripping of parietal pleura from chest wall to develop extrapleural space. **(e)** Operative field when pleura and lung have been retracted medially. The azygos vein is easily seen. The other structures, i.e., the blind proximal esophageal pouch and the fistulous distal esophagus, with vagal fibers lying on its surface exposed. **(f)** Fistula ligated and divided flush with trachea. **(g)** Lateral and posterior sutures and transanastomotic tube in place.

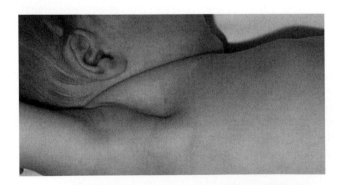

Figure 46.6 Axillary skin incision after EA–TEF repair.

encountered in locating the distal esophagus, and it is quite possible to mobilize the descending aorta in the erroneous impression that it is the esophagus. The surgeon should recognize the distal esophagus by following the vagus nerve as it courses distally, and by observing its rhythmic distension in time with ventilation.

Attention is then focused on the upper pouch—a bulbous structure—which is identified by requesting the anesthetist to push firmly on the Replogle tube. The upper pouch should be secured with a transfixion suture driven through the Replogle tube, which can then be used for traction during mobilization of the upper pouch. Bipolar diathermy is ideal for the mobilization, which should proceed to the thoracic inlet unless the gap separating the esophageal segments is short. Dissection of the plane between the upper pouch and trachea often requires great care to avoid injury to the trachea. An upper pouch fistula may be identified at this stage and should be repaired with a 5-0 or 6-0 series of interrupted nonabsorbable prolene sutures. The esophageal defect is then closed with 5-0 or 6-0 interrupted absorbable polydioxanone (PDS) sutures. Following adequate mobilization of the upper pouch, it is usually then possible to judge whether a primary anastomosis will be feasible. In most cases of EA with distal TEF, a primary anastomosis is achieved, although occasionally considerable tension is required to complete the repair.

The upper pouch is opened at its most distal extremity. The posterior wall of the anastomosis is commenced by placing two 5-0 or 6-0 PDS sutures through all layers of the lateral margins of the distal esophagus, taking great care to avoid excessive tissue handling and trauma with fine forceps. Sutures are completed by including all layers of the corresponding aspect of the upper pouch taking mucosa so that the knot comes to lie on the inside. Additional posterior wall sutures are inserted. All sutures are individually tied, drawing the esophageal ends together, commencing first with the laterally placed sutures. Having completed the posterior wall of the anastomosis, a 6–8 Fr. fine bore nasogastric tube (TAT tube) is passed by the anesthetist through the infant's nostril to the suture line, where it is grasped by the operating surgeon and carefully positioned distally along the lower esophagus into the stomach. The anterior layer of the anastomosis is completed by placing sutures with knots lying on the outside. When the gap defect length is proven to be wide, primary anastomosis may be facilitated by creating a Livaditis (1969) myotomy on the upper pouch or with an esophageal flap as described by Gough. Anastomosis created under tension requires a chest drain. For straightforward extrapleural primary EA–TEF repair, a chest drain may be unnecessary.[42] Ribs are loosely approximated with absorbable pericostal sutures, and closure of the chest wall/skin is then performed. A chest drain (if present) should be attached to underwater drainage. The baby is transferred to the intensive care unit for ventilatory support and postoperative monitoring. Should additional surgical pathology be present, such as duodenal atresia or imperforate anus, these should be dealt with accordingly under the same anesthetic in the stable infant.

Long-gap EA with distal TEF

The surgeon will encounter situation(s) where the gap between the upper pouch and the distal esophagus is clearly too wide to permit a primary anastomosis after division of the fistula with full mobilization of both the proximal and distal esophagus. Under such circumstances, it is probably wise to proceed to cervical esophagostomy as a "spit stoma" and feeding gastrostomy, accepting the need for esophageal replacement surgery at a later date.[7]

Right-sided aortic arch

Opinion is divided among pediatric surgeons regarding the optimal surgical strategy for management of patients with EA–TEF when a right-sided aortic arch (RAA) is

encountered. The incidence of RAA in association with EA is 1.8%–2.5%.[43,44] Chest x-ray may provide some clues. Preoperative echocardiography is at best 20% accurate in identifying this anomaly.[43,44] If the surgeon's suspicion remains high, magnetic resonance imaging should be arranged for definitive diagnosis. If a right-sided arch is identified from preoperative studies, experience from specialist centers advocates left thoracotomy. More commonly, the surgeon will encounter the anomaly unexpectedly in the course of an EA–TEF operation. The presence of a right-sided arch does not preclude a successful anastomosis in this situation, but the procedure is significantly more challenging as is evidenced by the 42% leak rate reported from Great Ormond Street Children's Hospital, London.[45] A trial dissection, including repair of the fistula, via right thoracotomy is appropriate, with completion of the esophageal anastomosis if this seems technically feasible.[46] Where significant difficulty is encountered with the dissection in preparation for the esophageal anastomosis, left thoracotomy is advisable following the division of the fistula through the right or left chest as circumstances dictate. The second thoracotomy may be performed immediately or delayed, depending on the stability of the infant and the experience of the surgeon.

PREMATURE INFANT WITH RDS

In premature very low birth weight (VLBW) babies with lung immaturity, emergency surgery is undertaken when adequate ventilation is compromised by the TEF with abdominal distension and diaphragmatic splinting. The surgical priority here is urgent ligation of the fistula deploying a transpleural thoracotomy to locate the TEF. Should the infant's condition stabilize sufficiently after TEF repair, primary anastomosis of the esophagus may then be appropriate. Otherwise, delayed repair of the esophagus is undertaken when the baby is physiologically stable at a later date. Sudden collapse with stomach wall perforation is equally also a "high-risk" event in fragile VLBW babies. In such situations, emergent ligation of the fistula is lifesaving. Needle paracentesis to relieve tension pneumoperitoneum with laparotomy, repair of the gut perforation, and feeding gastrostomy should follow.[47,48]

POSTOPERATIVE CARE

The infant should be nursed in the intensive care unit following repair of EA–TEF. Weaning from ventilation need not be unduly prolonged in the stable infant with a satisfactory anastomosis. Where the anastomosis is under considerable tension, elective paralysis and ventilation for a period of 3–5 days is practised.[49] It must be conceded, however, that there is no evidence base to support the claim that this technique favorably influences anastomotic healing.[50] There are some experimental data indicating that the level of tension in the anastomosis correlates with the severity of GER.[51] It is the current authors' practice to commence all patients on H_2-antagonists (e.g., ranitidine) as prophylaxis against anastomotic stricturing potentiated by GER. A contrast esophagogram is optional at the discretion of the surgeon after 5–7 days to evaluate the anastomosis, although major anastomotic leaks are clinically evident before this time. Minor "radiological" leaks are often seen on postoperative contrast studies. These are of no clinical significance and do not preclude the infant from being offered feeds.[52] In most cases, TAT tube feeding can be commenced after 48 hours and slowly increased as tolerated by the infant.

SURGICAL MANAGEMENT OF ISOLATED ("PURE") EA

The diagnosis of isolated EA without fistula is confirmed by the inability to pass a nasogastric tube with a featureless "gasless abdomen" on plain film radiology (Figure 46.3). The absence of intestinal gas below the diaphragm, however, does not always completely exclude the presence of a distal fistula, as a small proportion of babies may have a thin fibrotic connection between the lower pouch and the trachea, which does not readily permit the passage of air.[48]

Surgical management of these newborns is equally challenging and controversial. Many pediatric surgeons consider delayed primary anastomosis of the native esophagus the optimum approach. This strategy demands meticulous nursing care with regular suctioning of the bind ending upper esophageal pouch, chest physiotherapy, and careful attention to nutrition by supervised gastrostomy feeding. A prolonged period of hospitalization (6–12 weeks) is required to achieve this objective. Delayed primary esophageal anastomosis is also associated with its own attendant morbidity with further ongoing care required to manage esophageal strictures and significant GER.[53,54] The desire to preserve the infant's esophagus must be counterbalanced by the humility of knowing when to accept defeat and to abandon the esophagus in favor of a replacement procedure. A feeding gastrostomy is created by minilaparotomy with attention taken to avoid injury to the small stomach of these vulnerable babies with placement of the G-tube.[55] We do not advocate assessment of "gap length" at the time of this operation, deferring to a later session when the baby is more stable.

After a period of approximately 3 weeks, the extent of the gap defect can be assessed by fluoroscopy (Figure 46.7). A radiopaque tube is advanced into the upper pouch and either (1) contrast is instilled via the gastrostomy or (2) a metal sound is introduced through the gastrostomy site directed toward the hiatus and distal esophageal stump. This procedure can be repeated at 2–3 weekly intervals to assess whether the ends of the esophagus are sufficiently close to schedule delayed primary anastomosis.[56] Flexible endoscopy (under general anesthesia) can also be performed after several weeks when the G-tube tract site is mature by steering the "baby scope" to locate the blind esophageal stump. Images taken "on table" likewise provide an accurate gap length assessment with a radiopaque tube placed in the upper pouch. A distance of less than two vertebral bodies separating upper and lower pouches is ideal. However, in

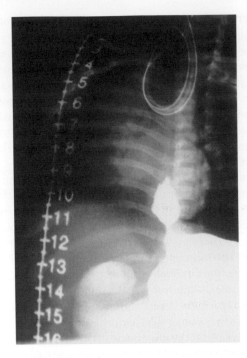

Figure 46.7 Gap assessment in a case of pure EA. The scale bar represents gap length (cm).

practical terms, there is little to be gained by the surgeon when delaying restorative surgery beyond 12 weeks of age.

The operation of delayed primary anastomosis essentially involves the same meticulous approach by the surgeon. It is to be expected that the anastomosis may be created under considerable tension. The upper pouch should be fully mobilized to the thoracic inlet. The distal esophagus is frequently a primitive stump and not readily identified at thoracotomy without the use of special aids. The surgeon can readily facilitate the location of the distal esophageal stump by passing a flexible endoscope via the G-tube tract site toward the esophageal hiatus. A brightly illuminated stump is easily identified in the depths of the thoracotomy wound. A stay suture (5-0 or 6-0 prolene) should be secured on the distal esophageal segment to aid its mobilization and dissection. Some surgeons still prefer passing metal bougies to identify the distal esophagus. The distal esophagus may be dissected to the diaphragmatic hiatus to help reduce tension on the anastomosis. A Livaditis myotomy or upper pouch flap may also be helpful.[57–61] The author prefers to perform a Livaditis myotomy over the inflated balloon of a Foley catheter passed by the anesthetist per orally to the upper pouch. Extra length can also be obtained by proceeding to laparotomy and creating a myotomy on the lesser curve as described by Scharli or a Collis gastroplasty.[57–61] If a primary anastomosis is still not possible using these techniques, the options are then to proceed cervical esophagostomy and schedule an esophageal replacement procedure when the infant is 18 months or older. A decision to convert to an immediate replacement of the esophagus is equally feasible provided that the surgeon and the team are sufficiently skilled. However, caution should be exercised when offering replacement to very young infants as risks of recurrent pulmonary aspiration are not insignificant in this age group before walking and upright posture is established. Options for esophageal replacement include gastric transposition, reverse gastric tube, colon replacement, and jejunal interposition.[2,64] Gastric transposition and colon graft interposition are currently the most popular operations.

Delays in restoring esophageal continuity have significant drawbacks. Firstly, there is the ever-present risk of aspiration pneumonitis, and secondly, the inability to feed the infant via the normal oral route. Although the child's nutritional needs are met by gastrostomy feeding, the inability to establish oral feeds may lead to long-term feeding and speech problems. Spitz has recommended formally assessing the length of the gap when the gastrostomy is initially performed. A gap length >6 vertebral bodies (6 cm) would prompt him to abandon the esophagus and perform a cervical esophagostomy.[64] This approach of early cervical esophagostomy and delayed esophageal replacement permits early sham feeding, which theoretically promotes neuronal maturation and development of the learning skills needed for feeding and later speech acquisition.

A number of other innovative approaches to the operative treatment of long-gap EA have been described. True primary repair has been performed with reported gap lengths exceeding 5 cm. The hypothesis tested by Foker et al.[65] was that a well-constructed esophageal anastomosis can withstand considerable tension. The value-added technique for esophageal reconstruction (VATER) operation involves mobilizing the gastric fundus and performing a limited Thal fundoplication. At thoracotomy, the proximal stomach is drawn into the chest, and a primary esophageal anastomosis is performed.[66] Staged neonatal colon esophagoplasty has also been described, which involves the isolation of a short length of transverse colon based on the ascending branch of the left colic vessels at the time of open gastrostomy.[67] The conduit is positioned transhiatally in the posterior mediastinum to be retrieved at thoracotomy several days later when continuity is restored.

Several well-established operations are available to restore gastrointestinal continuity in long-gap EA, where the infant's own esophagus has been abandoned.[64] Colon replacement was originally popularized by Waterston. The colon conduit may be isoperistaltic (left colon based on the left colic vessels) or anteperistaltic (right colon based on the ileocolic vessels). The colon is best routed via the posterior mediastinum (via the hiatus) or through right or left chest cavities to the neck. Cervical esophago-colon anastomosis is prone to leakage. Colon grafts also tend to dilate, and kinking is not uncommon due to tortuosity. Respiratory problems are seen due to recurrent aspiration as the new food pipe created with colon is "nonrefluxing."

The stomach may be used to create an esophageal substitute graft. A gastric tube esophagoplasty can be fashioned from the greater curvature of the stomach, based on the left gastroepiploic (anteperistaltic) or right gastroepiploic arcades (isoperistaltic), preferentially using the posterior mediastinum as a route to the neck anastomosis.[68] The long suture line of the tube created and the greater curve suture line are susceptible to bleeding and leaking. Reflux is a problem and can predispose to anastomotic stricture formation. However, dilatation and kinking are not encountered with the graft. GER may be controlled by performing a posterior partial wrap fundoplication.

Gastric transposition has been advocated by Spitz and has the merit of simplicity.[64,69] The vascular supply is based on the right gastric and right gastroepiploic vessels, which allows full mobilization of the greater and lesser curvatures. After pyloroplasty, the stomach is passed through the mediastinum via the diaphragmatic hiatus and the esophagogastric anastomosis completed in the neck. Leakage from the anastomosis is reported in some 12% of cases and strictures requiring periodic dilatation in a similar percentage of patients.[69]

Jejunal orthotopic interposition grafting reemerged as a useful technique for esophageal replacement following encouraging case series reports from the Netherlands by Klaus Bax and colleagues almost a decade ago.[70] Jejunal grafts do not dilate excessively and retain good peristalsis, which may explain why GER does not appear problematic for some of the patients.[70,71] Use of jejunal substitutes has declined with gastric transposition and colon grafts being by far the choice of many surgeons worldwide today.

H-TYPE TEF

H-type TEF comprises 4% of all EA–TEF variants.[2] It is perhaps more accurately termed N-type fistula as the track runs obliquely from trachea to esophagus. Infants with H-type TEF usually present within the first month after birth, with a characteristic history of choking with feeds and cyanotic spells. Gross abdominal distension mimicking intestinal obstruction is an occasional presenting feature, which we have encountered as the belly "accumulates wind" from the fistula communication. Older children may have frequent chest infections with recurrent right upper lobe pneumonia(s) due to chronic aspiration.

Diagnosis may be readily established by a dynamic prone video esophagogram (Figure 46.8). In this study, contrast is injected through a nasogastric tube, which is slowly withdrawn from the esophagus. However, H-type fistula(e) may be missed in approximately 50% of contrast studies. Where suspicion remains, bronchoscopy should be scheduled. At bronchoscopy, a size 4 Fr. ureteric catheter is passed through the fistula into the esophagus to facilitate identification during subsequent neck dissection. A nasogastric tube is passed into the stomach, and broad-spectrum antibiotics commenced. A right transverse skin crease incision is marked a finger's breadth above the clavicle, before positioning the neck in extension with a sandbag placed under the shoulders. The sternomastoid is retracted laterally and, if necessary, its sternal head divided. The carotid sheath is mobilized after division of the middle thyroid vein. The ipsilateral recurrent laryngeal nerve should be identified and carefully preserved.

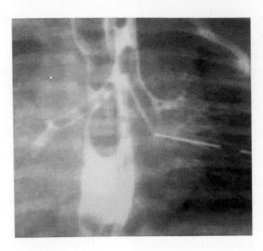

Figure 46.8 Tube esophagogram study showing H-TEF.

Intraoperatively, we have found that flexible bronchoscopy with a 2.2 mm caliber instrument (Olympus) can aid precise identification by brightly illuminating the site of the fistula tract (Figure 46.9).[72] The esophagus is carefully dissected at this point and slung with vascular sloops both above and below the fistula. Caution should be taken with dissection as the contralateral recurrent nerve is also vulnerable to injury at this point. Traction on the esophagus enables the fistula to be secured with stay sutures. After withdrawing the ureteric catheter (and 2.2 mm bronchoscope if deployed), the fistula is divided and the tracheal component repaired with 5-0 or 6-0 interrupted nonabsorbable prolene sutures. The esophagus is closed with 5-0 or 6-0 PDS sutures. Some surgeons recommend tissue interposition between esophageal and tracheal suture lines to prevent recurrent fistula.

The infant should remain intubated and ventilated in the early postoperative period, as tracheal edema can result in

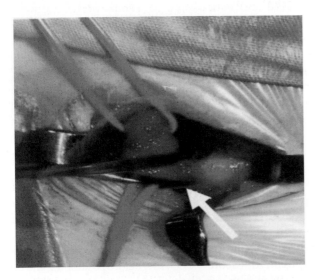

Figure 46.9 Operative photograph showing a 2.2 mm flexible bronchoscope brightly illuminating an H fistula tract—(fistula marked with arrow). Sloops secure the mobilized esophagus exposing the dissection plane between trachea and esophagus with H fistula.

progressive stridor.[73] The vocal cords should be checked on extubation, given the significant risk of recurrent nerve palsy. Nasogastric tube feeding may commence after 48 hours, and oral feeds may be slowly introduced thereafter.

The Nd:YAG laser has also been successfully used to treat congenital H-type TEF. Repeated short-duration pulses of laser light are used to coagulate the fistula.[74] Despite some success with this approach, the technique has not gained widespread acceptance, and open repair remains the gold standard.

EA–TEF—COMPLICATIONS AND SPECIAL CONSIDERATIONS

Anastomotic leak

The incidence of anastomotic leak following repair of EA and TEF ranges from 11% to 21%.[48,75] This is usually manifested by pneumothorax and salivary drainage from the chest drain. It is rare for the anastomosis to be completely disrupted. Provided that a transanastomotic tube is in place, it is usually possible to control the leak with an adequately sized chest drain. With adequate drainage, broad-spectrum antibiotics, and total parenteral nutrition, the esophagus will usually heal, although a prolonged period with a chest tube may be necessary. Some surgeons have used hyoscine patches in an attempt to "dry up" the salivary leak. Others advocate early re-exploration (<48 hours), with direct repair of the esophagus if possible, and the establishment of satisfactory drainage where a major leak is suspected.[13,75,76] When conservative management fails with uncontrolled sepsis, the establishment of a cervical esophagostomy and a feeding gastrostomy are essential. The child is committed to esophageal replacement at a later date. A clinical anastomotic leak predisposes to the development of an esophageal stricture.[77] While this association may seem logical, others contest such a correlation.[75]

Gastroesophageal reflux

GER disease occurs in 40%–50% of children following repair of EA–TEF. GER may cause failure to thrive, can predispose to recurrent aspiration episodes, and may lead to esophagitis and stricture formation.[2] Management of symptomatic GER initially requires aggressive medical therapy. Postural therapy and close attention to feeding regimes, with calorie supplementation, may prove effective management strategies. Feed thickeners (e.g., Carobel), antacid preparations (e.g., Gaviscon), H_2-antagonists (e.g., ranitidine), proton pump inhibitors (e.g., omeprazole), and prokinetic agents (e.g., domperidone) may be used in various combinations if vomiting is significant.

GER may contribute to recurrent aspiration episodes, with frequent symptoms of respiratory distress including tachypnea, apneic episodes, cyanosis, and x-ray evidence of patchy pneumonic changes. The differential diagnosis in this clinical setting also includes swallowing incoordination and respiratory distress from significant tracheomalacia.

It is not uncommon to see infants in whom all of these factors are operating to a variable degree. It is important not to overlook the possibility of a recurrent TEF as a cause of repeated episodes of respiratory distress, although the history of choking and cyanotic episodes during feeding is usually much more evident in infants with a recurrent fistula. The selective use of esophageal pH monitoring, contrast meal, bronchoscopy, and assessment of swallowing by video fluoroscopy may assist in evaluating the contribution of GER and other allied pathologies to respiratory symptoms. Failure to control GER despite full medical therapy is an indication for fundoplication.

Fundoplication rates following surgery for EA vary widely between surgery centers (6%–45%), reflecting the varied enthusiasm for antireflux operations in the clinical setting of GER and esophageal dysmotility.[2,78] There are several reasons for caution when considering fundoplication in EA patients. Dysphagia may be aggravated as a consequence of underlying foregut dysmotility. Fundoplication following EA repair has a higher failure rate (15%–38%) than is generally observed in otherwise normal patients with isolated GER.[79] Some authors recommend a partial wrap (Thal) fundoplication because of the lower incidence of postoperative dysphagia.[78] Despite such concerns, many pediatric surgeons prefer a short (1.5–2.0 cm) 360° floppy Nissen wrap for its proven effectiveness in reducing GER.[79] The high failure rate of fundoplication and the significant complications associated with surgical treatment of GER demand vigilant follow-up in this group of patients.

Anastomotic stricture

Reported definitions of esophageal stricture following repair of EA lack consistency. The incidence of symptomatic strictures requiring dilatation varies from 37% to 55%.[52,77] Some degree of anastomotic narrowing is invariably seen in all postoperative imaging studies, but this is rarely of a sufficient degree to cause symptoms in the early period after operation. Parents should be advised to report symptoms of prolonged feeding, incomplete feeding, or associated respiratory difficulty to clinicians. Contrast studies may be arranged. Such symptoms prompt us to arrange surveillance endoscopy to assess the caliber of the esophageal anastomosis. Balloon dilatation is our preferred method of treating symptomatic strictures. The radial dilating forces generated during balloon dilatation are considered to be less traumatic than the longitudinal shearing forces caused by conventional bougienage.[80,81] Balloon dilatation is performed under fluoroscopic control by passing a guide wire through the stricture, over which a balloon dilator of appropriate size is introduced. Its position is confirmed by partially filling the balloon with contrast medium, so that "waisting" due to the stricture is centrally located (Figure 46.10). The balloon is then maximally inflated using dilute contrast medium to dilate the stricture. A contrast esophagogram is performed after removing the balloon to ensure that there has been no injury perforation. Some surgeons deploy steroid injections

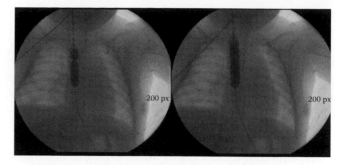

Figure 46.10 Balloon dilatation of an esophageal anastomotic stricture—"wasting" appearance shows the region of stricture.

or mitomycin C to manage stricture(s). A tailored program of surveillance endoscopy/dilatations may therefore be scheduled for some patients. If a stricture requires repeated dilatations, GER should be fully investigated by a combination of an upper GI contrast study, pH study, and endoscopy. Recalcitrant esophageal anastomotic strictures may require resection and fundoplication.

Tracheomalacia

Tracheomalacia is present to a variable degree in all patients with EA. It is thought to be responsible for the characteristically loud "barking" TEF cough.[2] Infants with tracheomalacia demonstrate expiratory stridor, which may result in episodes of desaturation, apnea, cyanosis, and bradycardia (often associated with feeding), and life-threatening so-called "dying episodes." Severe tracheomalacia may be evident in the early postoperative period, when it proves difficult to wean the infant from the ventilator.

Indications of the severity of tracheomalacia include ventilator dependency, respiratory distress characterized by stridor and chronic carbon dioxide retention, and "dying episodes." Full investigation for severe GER and recurrent TEF (see later) is advisable alongside evaluation of tracheomalacia, as aspiration secondary to GER and a recurrent fistula can mimic these symptoms. The extent of tracheomalacia is assessed by bronchoscopy under conditions of spontaneous respiration. The lumen of the trachea is significantly compressed anteroposteriorly and assumes a scabbard-like appearance during expiration due to tracheal cartilage deficiency. A further contribution is often made by the upper esophagus, which may bulge posteriorly into the airway. Tracheobronchomalacia can extend beyond the carina into the main stem bronchi.

As tracheomalacia can be self-limiting, surgical intervention is reserved for patients with life-threatening symptoms.[2] Treatment options include continuous positive airway pressure (CPAP), aortopexy, tracheostomy, and, more recently, tracheal stenting.[82,83] CPAP is a useful temporizing measure but may be required for several weeks. Aortopexy is traditionally performed by anterior left thoracotomy through the third interspace. The left lobe of the thymus is excised to gain access to the root of the aorta taking care not to damage the phrenic nerve. Plegetted sutures incorporating reinforcing Dacron squares are placed through the adventitia of the aortic root and the ascending aorta. The sutures are passed through the periosteum of the manubrium and tied, hitching the aorta forward, thereby relieving compressive forces on the trachea. Although this operation cannot resolve distal tracheobronchomalacia, it often provides immediate dramatic symptomatic relief. Failure of aortopexy may be an indication for tracheostomy, although some authors advocate tracheal stenting in this situation.[2,82,83]

Recurrent TEF

Recurrent TEF is estimated to occur in 5%–15% of cases.[84] A recurrent TEF may result from an anastomotic leak, but the possibility of a missed upper pouch fistula should always be considered. Symptoms include recurrent chest infections and choking attacks during feeding. A high index of suspicion is required if the diagnosis is not to be overlooked. Chest x-ray may sometimes reveal an air esophogram. The initial investigation of choice is prone video esophagography. If this study fails to demonstrate a fistula and the diagnosis remains strongly suspected, combined esophagoscopy and bronchoscopy should be performed. Rigid bronchoscopy is performed initially, and the site of the original fistula is carefully examined. The fistula is gently probed with a ureteric catheter, and methylene blue is carefully instilled into the fistula pit. Synchronous flexible esophagoscopy is performed to see if blue dye can be seen entering the esophagus. Should this fail to demonstrate the fistula, an "air/water test" is a useful supplementary investigation. The esophagus is filled with water and positive pressure ventilation applied to the bronchoscope. Occasionally, bubbles of air can be seen emanating from the fistulous opening into the esophagus.

Several strategies have been described to deal with the recurrent TEF. The traditional approach is formal repair via right thoracotomy. At bronchoscopy, an attempt should be made to pass a fine ureteric catheter through the fistula into the distal esophagus. A flexible miniature bronchoscope (2.2 mm, Olympus) may be useful to navigate, cannulate, and brightly illuminate the fistula tract. The fistula is repaired using a similar strategy to that deployed for the H-type variant, i.e., isolation/slooping the esophagus repairing the fistula as described earlier. Tissue interposition between suture lines is sometimes advisable in an attempt to reduce the chances of further fistula formation. A 10%–22% risk of refistulation has been reported.[84] Other approaches described to treat recurrent TEF include diathermy fulguration of the fistula tract.[85] This technique has been refined using the Nd:YAG laser to obliterate the epithelial communication. Sclerosing agents, histoacryl, and fibrin glue(s) have all been injected subepithelially to occlude fistulae. A recent review of endoscopic therapies reported an overall success rate of 55% with several sessions required to effect cure. A study from Oxford, however, concluded that formal surgical re-exploration remained the treatment of choice, except in high-risk patients.[86]

EA–TEF ADVANCES

Developments in minimally invasive surgery have now extended to the EA and TEF newborn population. In 2002, Rothenberg[87] reported the technical feasibility of endoscopic repair in a personal series of eight newborns with EA–TEF ranging in weight from 2.1 to 3.4 kg. This study followed the first pioneering operation of EA in a 2-month-old infant in 1998. Collaboration from members of the International Pediatric Endoscopic Surgery Group (IPEG) led to a 2005 multi-institutional analysis of thoracoscopic repair from centers located in the United States, Europe, and Hong Kong.[88] One hundred and four babies with common variant EA and TEF (excluding H-type and long gap without fistula) were included. Of these, there were five (4.8%) conversions to open thoracotomy and a staged repair in one baby due to unforeseen long-gap EA–TEF. Twelve infants (11.5%) developed early leaks and strictures, and 32% required esophageal dilatation(s). Survival in this selected population was 97% with three deaths recorded of which one was directly related to the EA–TEF repair on the 20th postoperative day. Additional operations were required for associated anomalies. These included duodenal atresia repair, imperforate anus surgery, aortopexy, and cardiac procedures. Twenty-five babies (24%) also underwent laparoscopic fundoplication for GER. In 2009, MacKinlay[89] (Edinburgh) reported good outcomes in a study of 26 infants—88% survival, 27% leak rate—all minor not requiring operation and 35% acquired strictures needing dilatation(s). Long-term benefits cited from minimally invasive surgery include a reduction in musculoskeletal morbidity notably winged scapula and unsightly skin scarring. For pediatric surgery centers currently not offering MIS repair, the axillary skin crease incision popularized by Bianchi provides an excellent alternative with good aesthetic outcome and comparable reductions in skeletal morbidity with all the benefits of classical open repair techniques.[40] Surgeon preference for MIS EA–TEF vs. open operation remains widely debated.

QoL AND LONG-TERM OUTCOME

The excellent survival of EA–TEF babies born in the modern era has prompted detailed analysis of morbidity with emphasis on long-term outcomes.[2,90] Several studies have examined respiratory function in EA children.[91-94] Symptoms of asthma and bronchitis are frequent, especially in a young child, and may persist into adolescence. Almost half of all children require future hospitalization due to ongoing respiratory morbidity. In a large Melbourne series comprising 334 EA children, episodes of pneumonia were seen in 31% of children under the age of 5 years, compared with 5% of those over 15 years.[91] The prevalence of annual attacks of bronchitis in these two age groups was 74% and 41%, respectively, with asthmatic symptoms reported in 40% of patients from each age range.[91] Spirometry studies have demonstrated both obstructive and restrictive abnormalities in over half the patients, and a similar proportion had a maximal working capacity below the normal range.[92] Tracheobronchial inflammation and airway narrowing have been demonstrated by bronchoscopy in one-third of patients, with histological evidence of inflammation in a further third.[93] It is plausible that abnormalities of bronchial anatomy, which are common in EA–TEF, may contribute to respiratory morbidity. Clinical assessment by a respiratory physician with use of prescribed inhalers to manage reactive airway disease and antibiotics/physiotherapy for chest infections is recommended. The contribution of aspiration episodes, whether due to esophageal dysmotility or GER, to respiratory symptoms should be actively investigated. Recognition of the long-term respiratory morbidity associated with EA patients prompted the establishment of a specialist EA–TEF clinic at Alder Hey Children's Hospital, Liverpool almost 20 years ago staffed by pediatric surgeons, respiratory physicians, physiotherapists, and dieticians. This multidisciplinary team approach ensures that vigilant health surveillance is focused on all aspects of the child's welfare including the smooth transition to adult medical/surgical services.[94,95]

Esophageal dysmotility is also a significant factor in long-term patient morbidity.[96] It is clearly implicated in many cases of food bolus impaction when endoscopy reveals no significant anastomotic narrowing. Less severe symptoms of dysphagia have been reported in up to 20% of adolescents[96] and 48% of adults on long-term follow-up. Esophageal manometry and fluoroscopy studies will demonstrate degrees of dysmotility in nearly all patients.[92] The dysmotility associated with EA may reflect intrinsic innervation abnormalities of the esophagus.[97] This may further contribute to respiratory morbidity through repeated "silent" aspiration episodes.

GER may persist into adult life. Symptoms of heartburn and acid brash range from 18% to 50% in long-term follow-up studies.[92,93] Clinical symptoms may underestimate the true incidence of GER as demonstrated by esophageal pH monitoring. An 8% incidence of Barrett's esophagus has been reported.[98,99] The relative risks of esophageal cancer developing in the lifetime of a patient are uncertain, though five cases have been recorded in the world literature.[100,101] These findings further highlight the importance of comprehensive long-term adult follow-up.[95,102]

Various QoL scoring systems have been deployed to evaluate adult populations treated for EA and TEF. Using the Spitzer index and a gastrointestinal QoL index, it has been shown that adults having primary anastomosis as newborns enjoyed an unimpaired QoL. QoL metrics were also more favorable in patients who had native esophageal repair compared to colonic interposition.[90] Psychosocial studies show more learning, emotional, and behavioral difficulties in EA adults than the healthy general population.

Cognitive performance(s) were also significantly impaired in a high-risk patient group characterized by associated major congenital anomalies and/or the requirement for prolonged ventilation in the neonatal period.[93, 103]

An energetic support group (TOFS)—a UK-based charity was founded in 1982 for the benefit of children and parents. The organization with over 1000 members (http://www.tofs.org.uk) provides a useful networking group for families together with a valuable handbook—*The TOF Child*.[104] With regular annual conferences attended by health care professionals and families, opportunities therefore exist for knowledge exchange and practical advice. TOFS UK also raises valuable funds for research.[2] Similar support networks exist in other European countries, e.g., KEKS, Germany.

REFERENCES

1. Potts WJ—Quoted by Cloud DT. Anastomotic technique in esophageal atresia. *J Pediatr Surg* 1968; 3:561–4.
2. Goyal A, Jones MO, Couriel JM, Losty PD. Oesophageal atresia and tracheo-oesophageal fistula. *Arch Dis Child Fetal Neonatal E* 2006; 91:F381–4.
3. Myers NA. The history of oesophageal atresia and tracheo-oesophageal fistula: 1670–1984. In: Rickham PP (ed). *Progress in Pediatric Surgery*, 20th edn. Heidelberg: Springer-Verlag, 1986:106–57.
4. Vogt EC. Congenital esophageal atresia. *Am J Roent* 1929; 22:463–5.
5. Gross RE. Atresia of the oesophagus. In: Gross RE (ed). *Surgery of Infancy and Childhood*, 1st edn. Philadelphia: W.B. Saunders, 1953.
6. Kluth D. Atlas of esophageal atresia. *J Pediatr Surg* 1976; 11:901–19.
7. Waterston DJ, Carter RE, Aberdeen E. Oesophageal atresia: Tracheo-oesophageal fistula. *Lancet* 1962; 1:819–22.
8. Spitz L, Kiely EM, Morecroft JA, Drake DP. Oesophageal atresia: At risk groups for the 1990's. *J Pediatr Surg* 1994; 29:723–5.
9. Teich S, Barton DP, Ginn-Pease ME, King DR. Prognostic classification for esophageal atresia and tracheo-esophageal fistula: Waterston versus Montreal. *J Pediatr Surg* 1997; 32:1075–80.
10. Yagyu M, Gitter H, Richter B, Booss D. Esophageal atresia in Bremen, Germany—evaluation of preoperative risk classification in esophageal atresia. *J Pediatr Surg* 2000; 35:584–7.
11. Choudhury SR, Ashcraft KW, Sharp RJ et al. Survival of patients with esophageal atresia: Influence of birth weight, cardiac anomaly, and late respiratory complications. *J Pediatr Surg* 1999; 34:70–4.
12. Holland AJ, Ron O, Pierro A, Drake D, Curry JI, Kiely EM, Spitz L. Surgical outcomes of esophageal atresia without fistula for 24 years at a single institution. *J Pediatr Surg* 2009; 10:1928–32.

13. Cudmore RE. Oesophageal atresia and tracheo-oesophageal fistula. In: Lister J, Irving IM (eds). *Neonatal Surgery*, 3rd edn. London: Butterworths, 1990:231–58.

14. Kyyronen P, Hemminki K. Gastro-intestinal atresia in Finland in 1970–79, indicating time-place clustering. *J Epidemiol Community Health* 1988; 42:257–65.

15. Myers NA. Oesophageal atresia: Epitome of modern surgery. *Ann R Coll Surg Eng* 1974; 54:227–87.

16. Haight C. Some observations on esophageal atresias and tracheoesophageal fistulas of congenital origin. *J Thorac Surg* 1957; 34:141–72.

17. Harris J, Kallen B, Robert E. Descriptive epidemiology of alimentary tract atresia. *Teratology* 1995; 52:15–29.

18. Harmon CM, Coran AG. Congenital anomalies of the esophagus. In: O'Neill JA Jr et al. (eds). *Pediatric Surgery*, 5th edn. St Louis: Mosby, 1998:941–67.

19. Pletcher BA, Friedes JS, Breg WR, Touloukian RJ. Familial occurrence of esophageal atresia with and without tracheoesophageal fistula: Report of two unusual kindreds. *Am J Med Genet* 1991; 39:380–4.

20. Diez-Pardo JA, Baoquan Q, Navarro C, Tovar JA. A new rodent experimental model of esophageal atresia and tracheoesophageal fistula: Preliminary report. *J Pediatr Surg* 1996; 31:498–502.

21. Kim PCW, Mo R, Hui C. Murine models of VACTERL syndrome: Role of sonic hedgehog signaling pathway. *J Pediatr Surg* 2001; 36:381–4.

22. Motoyama J, Lui J, Mo R et al. Essential function of Gli2 and Gli3 in the formation of lung, trachea and oesophagus. *Nat Genet* 1998; 20:54–7.

23. Xia H, Otten C, Migliazza L et al. Tracheobronchial malformations in experimental oesophageal atresia. *J Pediatr Surg* 1999; 34:536–9.

24. Litingtung Y, Lei L, Westphal H, Chiang C. Sonic hedgehog is essential to foregut development. *Nat Genet* 1998; 20:58–61.

25. Canty TG Jr, Boyle EM Jr, Linden B et al. Aortic arch anomalies associated with long gap esophageal atresia and tracheoesophageal fistula. *J Pediatr Surg* 1997; 32:1587–91.

26. Driver CP, Shankar KR, Jones MO et al. Phenotypic presentation and outcome of oesophageal atresia in the era of the Spitz classification. *J Pediatr Surg* 2001; 36:1419–21.

27. Quan L, Smith DW. The Vater association. *Birth Def* 1972; 8:75–8.

28. Nora AH, Nora JJ. A syndrome of multiple congenital anomalies associated with teratogenic exposure: The VACTERL syndrome. *Arch Environ Health* 1975; 30:17–21.

29. Lillquist K, Warburg M, Andersen SR. Colobomata of the iris, ciliary body and choroid in an infant with oesophagotracheal fistula and congenital heart defects. An unknown malformation complex. *Acta Paediat Scand* 1980; 69:427–30.

30. Kutiyanawala M, Wyse RKH, Brereton RJ et al. CHARGE and esophageal atresia. *J Pediatr Surg* 1992; 27:558–60.

31. Chittmittrapap S, Spitz L, Kiely EM, Brereton RJ. Oesophageal atresia and associated anomalies. *Arch Dis Child* 1989; 64:364–8.

32. Franken EA Jr, Saldino RM. Hypertrophic pyloric stenosis complicating esophageal atresia with tracheoesophageal fistula. *Am J Surg* 1969; 117:647–9.

33. Usui N, Kamata S, Ishikawa S et al. Anomalies of the tracheobronchial tree in patients with esophageal atresia. *J Pediatr Surg* 1996; 31:258–62.

34. Farrant P. The antenatal diagnosis of oesophageal atresia by ultrasound. *Br J Radiol* 1980; 53:1202–3.

35. Sparey C, Jawaheer G, Barrett AM, Robson SC. Esophageal atresia in the Northern Region Congenital Anomaly Survey, 1985–1997: Prenatal diagnosis and outcome. *Am J Obstet Gynecol* 2000; 182:427–31.

36. Stringer MD, McKenna KM, Goldstein RB et al. Prenatal diagnosis of esophageal atresia. *J Pediatr Surg* 1995; 30:1258–63.

37. Mullassery D, Llewellyn RS, Almond SL, Jesudason EC, Losty PD. Oesophageal atresia with cleft lip and palate: A marker for associated lethal anomalies. *Pediatr Surg Int* 2008; 24:815–7.

38. Replogle RL. Esophageal atresia: Plastic sump catheter for drainage of the proximal pouch. *Surgery* 1963; 54:296–7.

39. Sayari AJ, Tashiro J, Wang B, Perez EA, Lasko DS, Sola JE. Weekday vs weekend repair of esophageal atresia and tracheoesophageal fistula. *J Pediatr Surg* Feb 11, 2016 [epub ahead of print].

40. Bianchi A, Sowande O, Alizai NK, Rampersad B. Aesthetics and lateral thoracotomy in the neonate. *J Pediatr Surg* 1998; 33:1798–800.

41. Sharma S, Sinha SK, Rawat JD, Wakhlu A, Kureel SN, Tandon R. Azygos vein preservation in primary repair of esophageal atresia with tracheoesophageal fistula. *Pediatr Surg Int* 2007; 23:1215–8.

42. Kay S, Shaw K. Revisiting the role of routine retropleural drainage after repair of esophageal atresia with distal tracheoesophageal fistula. *J Pediatr Surg* 1999; 34:1082–5.

43. Parolini F, Armellini A, Boroni G, Bagolan P, Alberti D. The management of newborns with esophageal atresia and right aortic arch—A systematic review or still unsolved problem. *J Pediatr Surg* 2016; 51:304–9.

44. Bowkett B, Beasley SW, Myers NA. The frequency, significance, and management of a right aortic arch in association with esophageal atresia. *Pediatr Surg Int* 1999; 15:28–31.

45. Babu R, Pierro A, Spitz L et al. The management of oesophageal atresia in neonates with right-sided aortic arch. *J Pediatr Surg* 2000; 35:56–8.

46. Bicakci U, Tander B, Ariturk E, Rizalar R, Ayyildiz SH, Bernay F. The right-sided aortic arch in children with esophageal atresia and tracheo-esophageal fistula: A repair through the right thoracotomy. *Pediatr Surg Int* 2009; 25:423–5.

47. Maoate K, Myers NA, Beasley SW. Gastric perforation in infants with oesophageal atresia and distal tracheo-oesophageal fistula. *Pediatr Surg Int* 1999; 15:24–7.

48. Spitz L. Esophageal atresia: Lessons I have learned in a 40-year experience. *J Pediatr Surg* 2006; 41:1635–40.

49. Mackinlay GA, Burtles R. Oesophageal atresia: Paralysis and ventilation in management of the wide gap. *Pediatr Surg Int* 1987; 2:10–2.

50. Beasley SW. Does postoperative ventilation have an effect on the integrity of the anastomosis in repaired oesophageal atresia? *J Paediatr Child Health* 1999; 35:120–2.

51. Guo W, Fonkalsrud EW, Swaniker F, Kodner A. Relationship of esophageal anastomotic tension to the development of gastroesophageal reflux. *J Pediatr Surg* 1997; 32:1337–40.

52. Nambirajan L, Rintala RJ, Losty PD et al. The value of early postoperative oesophagography following repair of oesophageal atresia. *Pediatr Surg Int* 1998; 13:76–8.

53. Davison P, Poenaru D, Kamal I. Esophageal atresia: Primary repair of a long gap variant involving distal pouch mobilization. *J Pediatr Surg* 1999; 34:1881–3.

54. Lindahl H, Rintala R. Long-term complications of isolated esophageal atresia treated with esophageal anastomosis. *J Pediatr Surg* 1995; 30:1222–3.

55. Kimble RM, Harding JE, Kolbe A. The vulnerable stomach in babies born with pure oesophageal atresia. *Pediatr Surg Int* 1999; 15:467–9.

56. Rossi C, Domini M, Aquino A et al. A simple and safe method to visualize the inferior pouch in esophageal atresia without fistula. *Pediatr Surg Int* 1998; 13:535–6.

57. Livaditis A. End-end anastomosis in esophageal atresia. A clinical and experimental study. *Scand J Thorac Cardiovasc Surg* 1969; 2:7.

58. Gough M. Esophageal atresia—Use of an anterior flap in the difficult anastomosis. *J Pediatr Surg* 1980; 15:310–1.

59. Lessin MS, Wesselhoeft CW, Luks FI, DeLuca FG. Primary repair of long-gap esophageal atresia by mobilization of the distal esophagus. *Eur J Pediatr Surg* 1999; 9:369–72.

60. Davenport M, Bianchi A. Early experience with oesophageal flap oesophagoplasty for repair of oesophageal atresia. *Pediatr Surg Int* 1990; 5:332–5.

61. Sri Paran T, Decaluwe D, Corbally M, Puri P. Long-term results of delayed primary anastomosis for pure oesophageal atresia: A 27 year follow up. *Pediatr Surg Int* 2007; 23:647–51.

62. Scharli AF. Esophageal reconstruction in very long atresias by elongation of the lesser curvature. *Pediatr Surg Int* 1992; 7:101–5.

63. Evans M. Application of Collis gastroplasty to the management of esophageal atresia. *J Pediatr Surg* 1995; 30:1232–5.

64. Spitz L, Ruangtrakool R. Esophageal substitution. *Semin Pediatr Surg* 1998; 7:130–3.

65. Foker JE, Linden BC, Boyle EM Jr, Marquardt C. Development of a true primary repair for the full spectrum of esophageal atresia. *Ann Surg* 1997; 226:533–43.

66. Varjavandi V, Shi E. Early primary repair of long gap esophageal atresia: The VATER operation. *J Pediatr Surg* 2000; 35:1830–2.

67. Lipshutz GS, Albanese CT, Jennings RW et al. A strategy for primary reconstruction of long gap esophageal atresia using neonatal colon esophagoplasty: A case report. *J Pediatr Surg* 1999; 34:75–8.

68. Anderson KD, Randolph JG. The gastric tube for esophageal replacement in infants and children. *J Thorac Cardiovasc Surg* 1973; 66:333–42.

69. Spitz L. Esophageal atresia: Past, present, and future. *J Pediatr Surg* 1996; 31:19–25.

70. Bax NM, van de Zee DC. Jejunal pedicle grafts for reconstruction of the esophagus in children. *J Pediatr Surg* 2007; 42:363–9.

71. Bax NM. Jejunum for bridging long-gap esophageal atresia. *Semin Pediatr Surg* 2009; 18:34–9.

72. Goyal A, Potter F, Losty PD. Transillumination of H-type tracheoesophageal fistula using flexible miniature bronchoscopy: An innovative technique for operative localisation. *J Pediatr Surg* 2005; 40:e1–3.

73. Crabbe DC, Kiely EM, Drake DP, Spitz L. Management of isolated congenital tracheoesophageal fistula. *Eur J Pediatr Surg* 1996; 6:67–9.

74. Schmittenbecher PP, Mantel K, Hofmann U, Berlein HP. Treatment of congenital tracheoesophageal fistula by endoscopic laser coagulation: Preliminary report of three cases. *J Pediatr Surg* 1992; 27:26–8.

75. Auldist AW, Beasley SW. Esophageal complications. In: Beasley et al. (eds). *Oesophageal Atresia*, 1st edn. London: Chapman & Hall, 1991:305–22.

76. Chavin K, Field G, Chandler J et al. Save the child's esophagus: Management of major disruption after repair of esophageal atresia. *J Pediatr Surg* 1996; 31:48–52.

77. Chittmittrapap S, Spitz L, Kiely EM et al. Anastomotic stricture following repair of esophageal atresia. *J Pediatr Surg* 1990; 25:508–11.

78. Snyder CL, Ramachandran V, Kennedy AP et al. Efficacy of partial wrap fundoplication for gastroesophageal reflux after repair of esophageal atresia. *J Pediatr Surg* 1997; 32:1089–92.

79. Bergmeijer JHLJ, Tibboel D, Hazebroek FWJ. Nissen fundoplication in the management of gastro-esophageal reflux after repair of esophageal atresia. *J Pediatr Surg* 2000; 35:573–6.
80. Sandgren K, Malmfors G. Balloon dilatation of oesophageal strictures in children. *Eur J Pediatr Surg* 1998; 8:9–11.
81. Ratio A, Cresner R, Smith R, Jones MO, Losty PD. Fluoroscopic balloon dilatation for anastomotic strictures in patients with esophageal atresia—A fifteen year single center UK experience. *J Pediatr Surg* 2016; 51(9):1426–8.
82. Filler RM, Forte V, Fraga JC, Matute J. The use of expandable metallic airway stents for tracheobronchial obstruction in children. *J Pediatr Surg* 1995; 30:1050–6.
83. Corbett HJ, Mann KS, Mitra I, Jesudason EC, Losty PD, Clarke RW. Tracheostomy—A 10 year experience from a UK pediatric surgical center. *J Pediatr Surg* 2007; 42:1251–4.
84. Bruch SW, Hirschl RB, Coran AG. The diagnosis and management of recurrent tracheoesophageal fistulas. *J Pediatr Surg* 2010; 45:337–40.
85. Willetts IE, Dudley NE, Tam PKH. Endoscopic treatment of recurrent tracheo-oesophageal fistulae: Long-term results. *Pediatr Surg Int* 1998; 13:256–8.
86. Rangecroft L, Bush GH, Irving IM. Endoscopic diathermy of recurrent tracheo-esophageal fistula. *J Pediatr Surg* 1984; 19:41–3.
87. Rothenberg SS. Thoracoscopic repair of tracheo-esophageal fistula in newborns. *J Pediatr Surg* 2002; 37:869–72.
88. Holcomb GW 3rd, Rotheberg SS, Bax KM et al. Thoracoscopic repair of esophageal atresia and tracheoesophageal fistula: A multi-institutional analysis. *Ann Surg* 2005; 242:422–30.
89. MacKinlay GA. Esophageal atresia surgery in the 21st century. *Semin Pediatr Surg* 2009; 18:20–2.
90. Ure BM, Slaney E, Eypasch EP et al. Quality of life more than 20 years after repair of esophageal atresia. *J Pediatr Surg* 1998; 33:511–15.
91. Chetcuti P, Phelan PD. Respiratory morbidity after repair of oesophageal atresia and tracheo-oesophageal fistula. *Arch Dis Child* 1993; 68:167–70.
92. Montgomery M, Frenckner B, Freyschuss U, Mortensson W. Esophageal atresia: Long-term-follow-up of respiratory function, maximal working capacity, and esophageal function. *Pediatr Surg Int* 1995; 10:519–52.
93. Somppi E, Tammela O, Ruuska T et al. Outcome of patients operated on for oesophageal atresia: 30 years experience. *J Pediatr Surg* 1998; 33:1341–6.
94. de Jong EM, de Haan MA, Gischler SJ et al. A prospective comparative evaluation of persistent respiratory morbidity in esophageal atresia and congenital diaphragmatic hernia survivors. *J Pediatr Surg* 2009; 44:1683–90.
95. Sampat K, Losty PD. Transitional care and paediatric surgery. *Br J Surg* 2016; 103:163–4.
96. Romeo C, Bonanno N, Baldari S et al. Gastric motility disorders in patients operated on for esophageal atresia and tracheoesophageal fistula: Long-term evaluation. *J Pediatr Surg* 2000; 35:740–4.
97. Nakazato Y, Landing BH, Wells TR. Abnormal Auerbach plexus in the esophagus and stomach of patients with esophageal atresia and tracheo-esophageal fistula. *J Pediatr Surg* 1986; 11:831–7.
98. Lindahl H, Rintala R, Sariola H. Chronic esophagitis and gastric metaplasia are frequent late complications of esophageal atresia. *J Pediatr Surg* 1993; 28:1178–80.
99. Schneider A, Gottrand F, Bellaiche M et al. Prevalence of Barrett esophagus in adolescents and young adults with esophageal atresia. *Ann Surg* 2016; 264(6):1004–8 [epub ahead of print].
100. Adzick NS, Fisher JH, Winter HS, Sandler RH, Hendren WH. Esophageal adenocarcinoma 20 years after esophageal atresia repair. *J Pediatr Surg* 1989; 24:741–4.
101. Sistonen SJ, Koivusalo A, Lindahl H, Pukkala E, Rintala RJ, Pakarinen MP. Cancer after repair of esophageal atresia: Population-based long-term follow up. *J Pediatr Surg* 2008; 43:602–5.
102. Koivusalo AI, Parkarinen MP, Lindahl HG, Rintala RJ. Endoscopic surveillance after repair of oesophageal atresia—Longitudinal study in 209 patients. *J Pediatr Gastroenterol Nutr* 2016; 62(4):562–6 [epub ahead of print].
103. Bouman NH, Koot HM, Hazebroek FWJ. Long-term physical, psychological, and social functioning of children with esophageal atresia. *J Pediatr Surg* 1999; 34:399–404.
104. Martin V. *The TOF Child*. TOFS, Nottingham, Blueprint Group (UK) Limited, 1999.

47

Congenital esophageal stenosis

MASAKI NIO, MOTOSHI WADA, AND HIDEYUKI SASAKI

INTRODUCTION

Congenital esophageal stenosis (CES) is a rare condition. Gross[1] reviewed 38 cases of CES from the records of the Boston Children's Hospital in 1953 and reported that repeated dilatation provided complete relief in most cases; however, he later stated that CES cases who do not respond after six attempts of dilatation should be strongly considered for surgical resection or revision of the strictured area. Since then, a number of treatment modalities have been devised, but there is no consensus regarding which treatment option is the best. Although the efficacy of conservative treatments varies on a case-by-case basis, surgical treatment, which is expected to provide prompt relief of symptoms, carries certain risks of postoperative complications, including leaks, stricture, and gastroesophageal reflux (GER). Surgeons should consider differential diagnoses and understand the pathological basis of CES to be able to employ the most appropriate treatment strategy.

PATHOLOGY

CES is defined as an intrinsic stenosis of the esophagus, caused by congenital malformation of the esophageal wall. There are three pathological types of CES, namely, CES with tracheobronchial remnants in the esophageal wall,[2-16] fibromuscular thickening of the esophageal wall,[11,17-21] and membranous mucosal diaphragm or web.[8,11,22-30]

Stenosis due to tracheobronchial remnants is the most common form of CES; this condition is localized in the distal esophagus.[12] Fibromuscular thickening is observed in the middle or lower portions of the esophagus,[11,21] and membranous webs are observed in the upper or middle portions of the esophagus.[11,26-30] The stenotic area in cases with tracheobronchial remnants is usually localized, and the area of the fibromuscular stenosis varies from one to several centimeters in length, with circular thickening of the esophageal wall. In cases of membranous web, single webs have been observed in children,[26,28,30] whereas multiple webs, referred to as multiple trachea-like rings, have been observed in young adults.[31-33]

In CES with tracheobronchial remnants (mature or immature cartilages), seromucous tracheobronchial glands and ciliated epithelium have been usually observed during microscopic examination of the stenotic esophageal wall (Figure 47.1).[5,11,34] On the other hand, in fibromuscular stenosis, circumferential proliferation of smooth muscle fibers with moderate fibrosis has been observed (Figure 47.2).[11,21,34] Singaram et al.[35] reported a significant reduction of myenteric nitrinergic neurons and fibers in the muscle layer of two young adults diagnosed with the fibromuscular variant of CES. Lack of submucosa,[27] loose vascular connective tissue, and diffuse lymphocyte infiltration[26] have been microscopically observed in specimens of membranous web.

EPIDEMIOLOGY/ETIOLOGY

CES occurs in 1 in 25,000–50,000 live births.[11,36] Although the reason is unknown, the incidence of CES is higher in Japan than elsewhere.[8,37] There is no sex-associated predisposition.

CES caused by tracheobronchial remnants and fibromuscular thickening is thought to be a developmental disorder that arises during the first fetal month. The condition likely occurs during the formation and separation of the primitive foregut into the trachea and esophagus by the end of the first fetal month. The membranous mucosal diaphragm or web is believed to be a result of incomplete reformation of the esophageal lumen upon recanalization of the esophagus between the sixth and eighth week of gestation.

The incidence of anomalies associated with CES is reported to be 17%–33%[11,37]; among these, esophageal atresia/tracheoesophageal fistula (EA/TEF) is the most common,[9-11,18,19,24,37-43] and 3.6%–14% of EA/TEF cases are associated with CES.[41,44-47] Surgeons should be aware of the high incidence of association of EA/TEF with distal CES. Moreover, cardiac anomalies,[11,24] intestinal atresia,[11,23] anorectal malformation,[10,37] and chromosomal anomalies[7,11,21,23] may also be associated with CES.

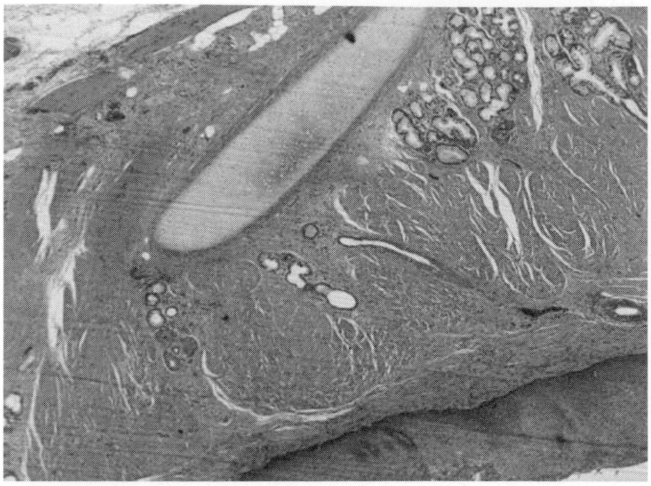

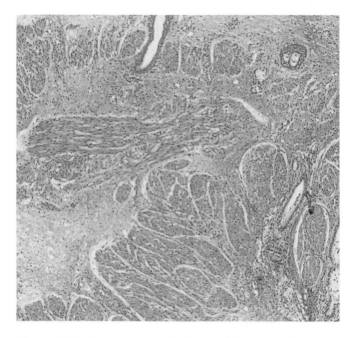

Figure 47.1 CES with tracheobronchial remnants. Mature or immature cartilages, the seromucous tracheobronchial glands and ciliated epithelium are usually seen in CES with tracheobronchial remnants.

Figure 47.2 Fibromuscular thickening of the esophageal wall. Circumferential proliferation of smooth muscle fibers with moderate fibrosis is seen in fibromuscular stenosis.

SYMPTOMS

Symptoms of CES include vomiting or regurgitation, dysphagia, recurrent respiratory tract infections, and growth retardation. Although the etiology of CES usually has congenital origins, symptoms rarely develop in newborns.[25] Characteristically, the onset of regurgitation coincides with the introduction of semisolid and solid foods around 6 months of age in patients with tracheobronchial remnants.[34] In some patients, a foreign body in the esophagus might be the first symptom observed.[36] When esophageal peristalsis is preserved, the presentation of CES might be delayed until adulthood.[48]

Patients with CES associated with EA/TEF are sometimes diagnosed at the time of surgical repair or during the postoperative course of EA/TEF before presenting any symptoms of CES.

DIAGNOSIS

Difficulties in determining the differential diagnoses of CES and being able to distinguish CES from achalasia, from secondary esophageal stenosis, and particularly, from a stricture due to reflux esophagitis[36] have resulted in various clinical problems during treatment of CES. First, achalasia, inflammatory esophagitis, and stenosis caused by a tumor or extrinsic compression of the esophagus should be excluded. The location of the stenosis varies with the type of pathology, as mentioned in the earlier section.

Patients who develop symptoms such as vomiting and dysphagia should undergo a barium swallow test to obtain an esophagogram. Esophagograms of stenoses exhibit tapered or abrupt narrowing of the esophagus with varying degrees of dilatation of the suprastenotic portion (Figure 47.3). Most of the stenoses due to tracheobronchial remnants are visible on esophagograms as abrupt esophageal narrowing, whereas fibromuscular stenoses usually exhibit tapered esophageal narrowing.[41,43] Following surgery of EA/TEF, an esophagogram should be evaluated with great care, as it is easy to overlook a narrowing at the mid-distal esophagus. To evaluate the exact site and extent of the stenosis, fluorography using a balloon catheter can be used. The balloon catheter is inserted through the esophagus, and the location and shape of the inflated balloon provide a clear image of the esophageal stenosis (Figure 47.4).

Esophageal endoscopy (i.e., esophagoscopy), manometry, and pH monitoring are helpful tools for obtaining differential diagnoses when trying to distinguish CES from achalasia and secondary esophageal stricture due to GER. Esophagoscopy can directly evaluate the stenotic area and the site of the gastroesophageal junction, as well as the presence and severity of esophagitis. The mucosa distal to the stenosis is normal in CES. In addition to esophagoscopy, endoscopic ultrasonography has recently been employed to evaluate the fine structure of CES. It is also useful for determining a treatment strategy, which may be either balloon dilatation or surgical treatment.[42,49,50] According to a systematic review by Terui et al.[51] endoscopic dilatation is recommended as the primary therapy for CES, except for patients with tracheobronchial remnants.

In CES cases, preoperative esophageal manometry demonstrates a normal pattern of the lower esophageal sphincter and a small high-pressure zone in the resting pressure profile, which corresponds to the stenotic area of the esophagus. Impaired esophageal motility is commonly observed in CES patients.[52,53] Further, pH monitoring can reveal a significant positive reflux, which is not observed in patients with CES, unlike in patients with GER.

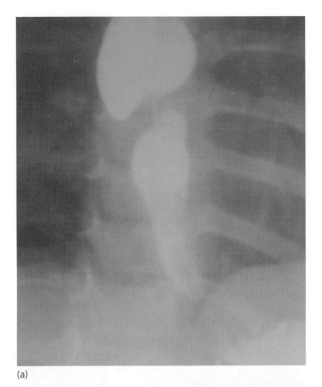

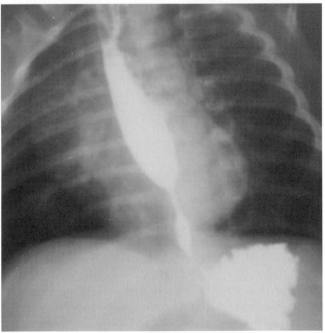

Figure 47.3 Esophagograms of CES. An abrupt (a) or tapered narrowing (b) of the esophagus evident on an esophagogram.

CES associated with EA/TEF is often overlooked at the time of the initial esophageal surgical repair and is typically only diagnosed later. Ibrahim et al.[54] reported taking a surgical specimen routinely for histopathological studies from the tip of the lower esophageal pouch during primary repair of EA/TEF.

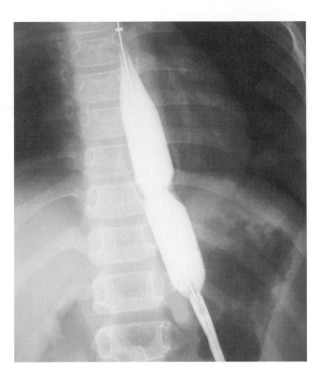

Figure 47.4 Fluorography using a balloon catheter. A low-compliance balloon catheter (RigiflexTM II, Boston Scientific Ltd, UK) is placed at the stenosis and gradually inflated, and then the location and the length of the stenosis are clearly visible.

TREATMENT

The principal aims of CES treatment include the alleviation of symptoms and maintenance of the antireflux mechanism of the gastroesophageal junction. This condition can be treated either conservatively (by nonsurgical methods) or by surgical intervention. Nonsurgical methods include balloon dilatation and endoscopic treatment.

Nonsurgical treatment

Balloon dilatation is the first choice of treatment for CES. This method should be employed in patients with tapered esophageal narrowing and abrupt esophageal narrowing when a balloon catheter can be passed safely through the stenotic area. Low-compliance balloon catheters are commonly used.[43] The effect of balloon dilatation varies with the type of pathology, and patients with membranous web of the esophagus and some cases of fibromuscular stenosis can be treated by suitable dilatation.[11,26,28,29]

It is thought that the efficacy of balloon dilatation in CES with tracheobronchial remnants is limited.[51] However, it is difficult to precisely assess the efficacy of balloon dilatation among the different types of CES pathology. This is because the histological findings of the stenotic lesions of the patients who respond positively to dilation remain unconfirmed. Currently, the responsiveness of patients with CES with tracheobronchial remnants to dilatation is uncertain. Recently, a case of successful treatment of membranous web with the use of endoscopic instruments (electrocauterization, high-frequency-wave snare/cutter) was reported.[55,56]

Surgery

When patients fail to respond to repeated (four to six times) attempts of bougienage, surgical intervention should be considered. Surgical resection of the stenosis followed by end-to-end esophageal anastomosis is a general surgical treatment, typically used in cases with tracheobronchial remnants[6,8,10–16,37,40–43] and some cases with fibromuscular thickening.[21,34]

Most cases of CES can be operated upon using the thoracic approach. However, when the stenosis is located in the abdominal esophagus, laparotomy is utilized. In a few cases of CES, complete resections of the stenotic segment using the thoracoscopic[57,58] or laparoscopic approach[59] have been reported.

In the thoracic approach, right thoracotomy is employed for stenosis in the middle esophagus, and left thoracotomy is employed for stenosis in the lower part of the esophagus. After exposing the esophagus, a balloon catheter is inserted from the mouth to locate the stenotic segment. The catheter is then inflated and pulled up to confirm the lower margin of the stenosis. Following the cut in the distal end of the stenosis, a sterile balloon catheter is passed through the stenotic area from the oral stump of the esophagus. The upper margin of the stenosis is determined by pulling down the catheter (Figure 47.5).[43]

The stenotic area is completely removed, and end-to-end anastomosis is achieved using single- or double-layer interrupted sutures of absorbable material. Surgeons should ensure that the phrenic and vagal nerves are not damaged during the surgery.

Other options for surgical treatment include simple excision of cartilaginous remnants, longitudinal myotomy, circular myectomy, and esophageal replacement. Among these procedures, simple excision of the cartilaginous remnants and subsequent repair of the esophageal wall have been reported.[5,11,43] However, these methods are rarely employed because they fail to provide sufficient relief from symptoms in most cases of CES with tracheobronchial remnants.

Longitudinal myotomy, which is more often used for esophageal achalasia than for CES, has been employed for fibromuscular stenosis. However, postoperative dilatation is frequently required, and its efficacy remains unconfirmed. Moreover, development of esophageal perforation after myotomy has been reported.[42]

Circular myectomy for CES with tracheobronchial remnants has been described,[60,61] and it might be employed for fibromuscular stenosis as well. During this surgical procedure, the lower margin of the stenotic segment is delineated while pulling up a balloon catheter inserted through the mouth. This is similar to the technique followed during resection of the stenotic portion. The upper margin is determined by pushing down the balloon catheter inserted through the mouth or by pulling down the balloon catheter inserted through a small incision at the esophageal mucosa

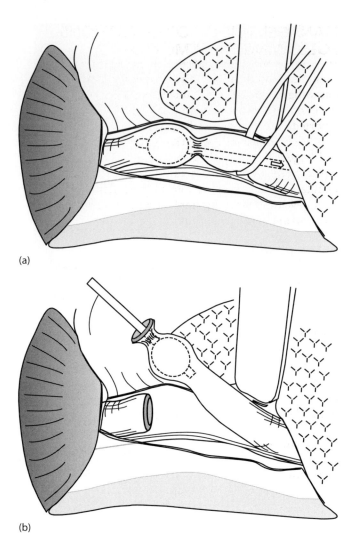

(a)

(b)

Figure 47.5 Intraoperative procedure by use of a Foley catheter to determine the distal **(a)** and proximal sites **(b)** of stenosis.

into the esophageal lumen. The muscular layer is incised up to the submucosal layer at the lower and upper margins. Subsequently, the abnormal muscular layer is dissected circumferentially using surgical scissors or cauterization. Circular myectomy is expected to prevent postoperative leakage and re-stenosis of the esophageal anastomosis.[60,61]

Among various methods of surgical treatment for CES, segmental resection with end-to-end anastomosis of the esophagus is currently the standard procedure, and circular myectomy is a promising alternative. Both procedures pose a substantial risk of developing GER, particularly when anastomosis is performed under tension. When the stenosis is situated close to the gastroesophageal junction and the surgery is performed through laparotomy, an antireflux procedure might be employed as well to prevent postoperative reflux.[43] If the vagal nerve is accidently severed, a pyloroplasty is performed.

Patients with extensive CES, necessitating the resection of >3 cm of the esophagus, might require esophageal replacement using the colon, jejunum, or a gastric tube.

MANAGEMENT OF COMPLICATIONS FOLLOWING TREATMENT

Complications, including iatrogenic esophageal perforation following bougienage[10,42,57] and leakage following segmental resection and reconstruction of the esophagus,[11] have been reported. The rate of esophageal perforation upon dilatation has been reported as 9.1%–44%.[41,43,46,51,62] Perforations and large leakages might require surgical drainage and/or repair, but minor leakages can be treated successfully by maintaining the patient on total parenteral nutrition. When GER develops following simple resection or circular myectomy, an antireflux procedure is required.

PROGNOSIS

Favorable results have been reported following appropriate treatment. Amae et al.[43] reported the treatment outcome of 14 patients with CES, of whom 11 and 3 patients became asymptomatic following surgery and dilatation, respectively. On the other hand, according to a recent report of 61 cases of CES by Michaud et al.,[63] dysphagia occurred frequently, regardless of therapeutic option, and it remained in 36% of the patients at the time of follow-up. Close, long-term follow-up is highly recommended.

REFERENCES

1. Gross RE. *The Surgery of Infancy and Childhood.* WB Saunders & Co., Philadelphia, 1953.
2. Frey EK, Duschl L. Der Kardiospasmus. *Erge Chirurg Orthopaed* 1936; 29: 637–716.
3. Bergmann M, Charnas RM. Tracheobronchial rests in the esophagus. *J Thorac Surg* 1958; 35: 97–104.
4. Kumar R. A case of congenital oesophageal stricture due to a cartilaginous ring. *Br J Surg* 1962; 69: 533–4.
5. Pauline E, Roselli A, Aprigliano F. Congenital esophageal stricture due to tracheobronchial remnants. *Surgery* 1963; 53: 547–50.
6. Ishida M, Tsuchida Y, Saito S et al. Congenital esophageal stenosis due to tracheobronchial remnants. *J Pediatr Surg* 1969; 4: 339–45.
7. Rose JS, Kassner EG, Jurgens KH et al. Congenital esophageal strictures due to cartilaginous rings. *Br J Radiol* 1975; 48: 16–8.
8. Ohkawa H, Takahashi H, Hoshino Y et al. Lower esophageal stenosis in association with tracheobronchial remnants. *J Pediatr Surg* 1975; 10: 453–7.
9. Ibrahim NBN, Sandry RJ. Congenital esophageal stenosis caused by tracheobronchial structures in the esophageal wall. *Thorax* 1981; 36: 465–8.
10. Deiraniya AK. Congenital oesophageal stenosis due to tracheobronchial remnants. *Thorax* 1974; 29: 720–5.
11. Fekete CN, Backer AD, Jacob SL. Congenital esophageal stenosis. A review of 20 cases. *Pediatr Surg Int* 1987; 2: 86–92.
12. Sneed WF, LaGarde MS, Kogutt MS et al. Esophageal stenosis due to cartilaginous tracheobronchial remnants. *J Pediatr Surg* 1979; 14: 786–8.
13. Spitz L. Congenital esophageal stenosis distal to associated esophageal atresia. *J Pediatr Surg* 1973; 8: 973–4.
14. Briceno LI, Grases PJ, Gallego S. Tracheobronchial and pancreatic remnants causing esophageal stenosis. *J Pediatr Surg* 1981; 16: 731–2.
15. Tubino P, Marouelli LF, Alves E et al. Choristoma: Esophageal stenosis, due to tracheobronchial remnants. *Z Kinderchir* 1982; 35: 14–7.
16. Shoshany G, Bar-Maor JA. Congenital stenosis of the esophagus due to tracheobronchial remnants: A missed diagnosis. *J Pediatr Gastroenterol Nutr* 1986; 5: 977–9.
17. Bonilla KB, Bower WF. Congenital esophageal stenosis; pathologic studies following resection. *Am J Surg* 1959; 97: 772–6.
18. Mahour GH, Jounston PW, Gwinn JL et al. Congenital esophageal stenosis distal to esophageal atresia. *Surgery* 1971; 69: 936–9.
19. Tuqan NA. Annular stricture of the esophagus distal to congenital tracheoesophageal fistula. *Surgery* 1962; 52: 394–5.
20. Vidne B, Levy MJ. Use of pericardium for esophagoplasty in congenital stenosis. *Surgery* 1970; 68: 389–92.
21. Todani T, Watanabe Y, Mizuguchi T et al. Congenital oesophageal stenosis due to fibromuscular thickening. *Z Kinderchir* 1984; 39: 11–4.
22. Beatty CC. Congenital stenosis of the esophagus. *Br J Child Dis* 1928; 25: 237–70.
23. Huchzermeyer H, Burdeiski M, Hruby M. Endoscopic therapy of a congenital oesophageal stricture. *Endoscopy* 1979; 11: 259–62.
24. Overton RC, Creech O. Unusual esophageal atresia with distant membranous obstruction of the esophagus. *J Thorac Surg* 1953; 35: 674–7.
25. Schwaetz SI. Congenital membranous obstruction of esophagus. *Arch Surg* 1962; 85: 480–2.
26. Grabowski ST, Andrews DA. Upper esophageal stenosis: Two case reports. *J Pediatr Surg* 1996; 31: 1438–9.
27. Takayanagi K, Ii K, Komi N. Congenital esophageal stenosis with lack of the submucosa. *J Pediatr Surg* 1975; 10: 425–6.
28. Sarihan H, Abes M. Congenital esophageal stenosis. *J Cardiovasc Surg* 1997; 38: 421–3.
29. Komuro H, Makino S, Tsuchiya I et al. Cervical esophageal web in a 13-year-old with growth failure. *Pediatr Int* 1999; 41: 568–70.
30. Roy GT, Cohen RC, Willeams SJ. Endoscopic laser division of an esophageal web in a child. *J Pediatr Surg* 1996; 31: 439–40.
31. Younes Z, Johnson DA. Congenital esophageal stenosis: Clinical and endoscopic features in adults. *Dig Dis* 1999; 17: 172–7.

32. Katzka DA, Levine MS, Ginsberg GG et al. Congenital esophageal stenosis in adults. *Am J Gastroenterol* 2000; 95: 32–6.

33. Pokieser P, Schima W, Schober E et al. Congenital esophageal stenosis in a 21-year-old man: Clinical and radiographic findings. *Am J Gastroenterol* 1998; 170: 147–8.

34. Murphy SG, Yazbeck S, Russo P. Isolated congenital esophageal stenosis. *J Pediatr Surg* 1995; 30: 1238–41.

35. Singaram C, Sweet MA, Gaumnitz EA. Peptidergic and nitrinergic denervation in congenital esophageal stenosis. *Gastroenterology* 1995; 109: 275–81.

36. Bluestone CD, Kerry R, Sieber WK. Congenital esophageal stenosis. *Laryngoscope* 1969; 79: 1095–103.

37. Nishina T, Tsuchida Y, Saito S. Congenital esophageal stenosis due to tracheobronchial remnants and its associated anomalies. *J Pediatr Surg* 1981; 16: 190–3.

38. Sheridan J, Hyde I. Oesophageal stenosis distal to oesophageal atresia. *Clin Radiol* 1990; 42: 274–6.

39. Yeung CK, Spitz L, Brereton RJ et al. Congenital esophageal stenosis due to tracheobronchial remnants: A rare but important association with esophageal atresia. *J Pediatr Surg* 1992; 27: 852–5.

40. Neilson IR, Croitoru DP, Guttman FK et al. Distal congenital esophageal stenosis associated with esophageal atresia. *J Pediatr Surg* 1991; 26: 478–81.

41. Kawahara H, Imura K, Yagi M et al. Clinical characteristics of congenital esophageal stenosis distal to associated esophageal atresia. *Surgery* 2001; 129: 29–38.

42. Takamizawa S, Tsugawa C, Mouri N et al. Congenital esophageal stenosis: Therapeutic strategy based on etiology. *J Pediatr Surg* 2002; 37: 197–201.

43. Amae S, Nio M, Kamiyama T et al. Clinical characteristics and management of congenital esophageal stenosis: A report on 14 cases. *J Pediatr Surg* 2003; 38: 565–70.

44. Yoo HJ, Kim WS, Cheon JE et al. Congenital esophageal stenosis associated with esophageal atresia/tracheoesophageal fistula: Clinical and radiologic features. *Pediatr Radiol* 2010; 40: 1353–9.

45. McCann F, Michaud L, Aspirot A et al. Congenital esophageal stenosis associated with esophageal atresia. *Dis Esophagus* 2015; 28: 211–5.

46. Newman B, Bender TM. Esophageal atresia/tracheoesophageal fistula and associated congenital esophageal stenosis. *Pediatr Radiol* 1997; 27: 530–4.

47. Vasudevan SA, Kerendi F, Lee H et al. Management of congenital esophageal stenosis. *J Pediatr Surg* 2002; 37: 1024–6.

48. McNally PR, Collier EH 3rd, Lopiano MC et al. Congenital esophageal stenosis. A rare cause of food impaction in the adult. *Dig Dis Sci* 1990; 35: 263–6.

49. Kouchi K, Yoshida H, Matsunaga T et al. Endosonographic evaluation in two children with esophageal stenosis. *J Pediatr Surg* 2002; 37: 934–6.

50. Usui N, Kamata S, Kawahara H et al. Usefulness of endoscopic ultrasonography in the diagnosis of congenital esophageal stenosis. *J Pediatr Surg* 2002; 37: 1744–6.

51. Terui K, Saito T, Mitsunaga T et al. Endoscopic management for congenital esophageal stenosis: A systematic review. *World J Gastrointest Endosc* 2015; 7: 183–91.

52. Liu Q, Yao LP, Xie HH et al. High-resolution manometry and endoscopic ultrasonography are important for diagnosing congenital esophageal stenosis. *J Dig Dis* 2015; 16: 479–82.

53. Kawahara H, Oue T, Okuyama H et al. Esophageal motor function in congenital esophageal stenosis. *J Pediatr Surg* 2003; 38: 1716–9.

54. Ibrahim AH, Al Malki TA, Hamza AF, Congenital esophageal stenosis associated with esophageal atresia: New concepts. *Pediatr Surg Int* 2007; 23: 533–7.

55. Nose S, Kubota A, Kawahara H et al. Endoscopic membranectomy with a high-frequency-wave snare/cutter for membranous stenosis in the upper gastrointestinal tract. *J Pediatr Surg* 2005; 40: 1486–8.

56. Chao HC, Chen SY, Kong MS. Successful treatment of congenital esophageal web by endoscopic electrocauterization and balloon dilatation. *J Pediatr Surg* 2008; 43: e13–5.

57. Martinez-Ferro M, Rubio M, Piaggio L et al. Thoracoscopic approach for congenital esophageal stenosis. *J Pediatr Surg* 2006; 41: E5–7.

58. van Poll D, van der Zee DC. Thoracoscopic treatment of congenital esophageal stenosis in combination with H-type tracheoesophageal fistula. *J Pediatr Surg* 2012; 47: 1611–3.

59. Deshpande AV, Shun A. Laparoscopic treatment of esophageal stenosis due to tracheobronchial remnant in a child. *J Laparoendosc Adv Surg Tech A* 2009; 19: 107–9.

60. Maeda K, Hisamatsu C, Hasegawa T et al. Circular myectomy for the treatment of congenital esophageal stenosis owing to tracheobronchial remnant. *J Pediatr Surg* 2004; 39: 1765–8.

61. Saito T, Ise K, Kawahara Y et al. Congenital esophageal stenosis because of tracheobronchial remnant and treated by circular myectomy: A case report. *J Pediatr Surg* 2008; 43: 583–5.

62. Romeo E, Foschia F, de Angelis P et al. Endoscopic management of congenital esophageal stenosis. *J Pediatr Surg* 2011; 46: 838–41.

63. Michaud L, Coutenier F, Podevin G et al. Characteristics and management of congenital esophageal stenosis: Findings from a multicenter study. *Orphanet J Rare Dis* 2013; 8: 186.

48

Esophageal duplication cysts

DAKSHESH H. PARIKH AND MICHAEL SINGH

INTRODUCTION

Esophageal duplications and bronchogenic cysts are part of the spectrum of foregut malformations as both seem to have their origin from the primitive foregut.[1] Foregut duplication cysts in children account for up to one-third of mediastinal cysts and are one of the main differential diagnoses for posterior mediastinal tumors. In the literature, approximately 21% of gastrointestinal duplications are reported to be of esophageal origin.[2,3]

Esophageal duplication cysts are seen in close proximity to the native esophagus. There may be associated duplications elsewhere in the gastrointestinal tract. Some of the esophageal duplications can be thoracoabdominal in nature.[4,5] In contrast, bronchogenic cysts are more frequent and are closely associated with the tracheobronchial tree or within the lung parenchyma. Unlike bronchogenic cysts, esophageal duplication cysts are commonly associated with vertebral anomalies. In the presence of a vertebral anomaly, rarely, an intraspinal communication can be identified. This variant is called a neuroenteric cyst.[6]

ETIOLOGY

Esophageal duplications are thought to be a result of an aberrant dorsal foregut development during the fourth to eighth week of gestation. One of the embryological theories implicates inappropriate canalization or failure of connection of the vacuoles as canalization of the gastrointestinal tract occurs to form a lumen. The other theory proposes a diverticulum occurring during the development of the gastrointestinal tract that may result in duplication with or without connection with the intestinal lumen. Both these theories fail to explain the various types of duplications occurring in the gastrointestinal tract. The split notochord theory, in contrast, can explain the association of vertebral anomalies with mediastinal duplications. The notochord is formed by the ingrowth of the mesodermal cells and separates from the endoderm. In the event of adhesion with the endodermal lining, it is drawn inside the spinal canal, not allowing the spinal canal to close ventrally. It is possible that both ends of this connecting tract may remain open or closed on either side. The cephalic end may represent a fibrous cord, connect to the cysts on either side, or disappear altogether as seen in most instances.[1]

PATHOLOGY

Esophageal duplications are described as cystic, tubular, or neuroenteric in nature. Over 60% of esophageal duplication cysts are mainly associated with the lower esophageal, and the rest are identified within the upper and middle thirds of the esophagus. They generally have a thin wall of muscle coat and are in close proximity to the native esophagus or can be within the esophageal wall. Rarely, some of the esophageal duplications can be simple epithelial-lined cysts. The cysts can contain either a clear mucoid, brown, or blood-stained serous fluid. The majority do not communicate with the spinal canal or have an associated vertebral anomaly. Duplication cysts can have a wide variety of mucosal linings: squamous, gastric, pseudostratified, cuboidal, columnar, ciliated respiratory tract lining, or pancreatic cells.[4,5] A mixed epithelial lining within the cyst is commonly reported.[3,7,8] The symptomatic duplication may therefore bleed within the cyst or cause pressure symptoms onto the surrounding structures such as the trachea, esophagus, or result in formation of a fistula.

PRESENTATION

The majority of esophageal duplication cysts present in early childhood, of which some are antenatally detected (Figure 48.1a). In our experience of the antenatally detected cystic thoracic lesions, approximately 5% of cases are subsequently diagnosed as foregut duplications. The majority of antenatally detected cases are asymptomatic at birth.

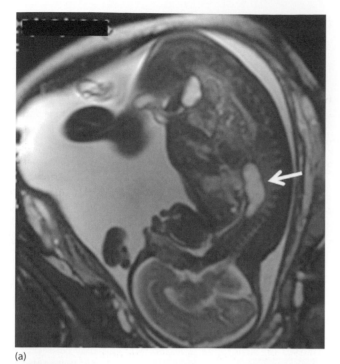

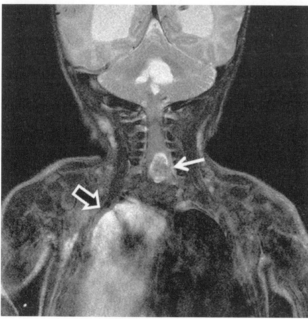

Figure 48.1 **(a)** Fetal MRI confirming antenatal ultrasound findings of foregut duplication cyst with intraspinal extension. **(b)** Postnatal MRI showing a large tubular esophageal duplication cyst (hollow arrow) with a cervical intraspinal component (white arrow).

Patients can present in infancy with acute respiratory distress, stridor, dysphagia, meningitis, and the sudden appearance of a cervical mass (Figure 48.2a,b). Sudden death has been reported in some untreated cases, where the most plausible explanation would be the rupture of the cyst into the tracheobronchial tree.[8,9]

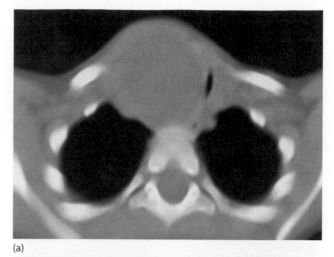

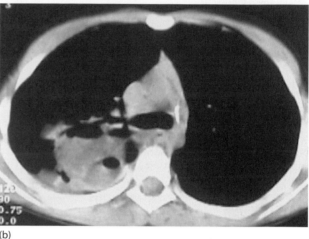

Figure 48.2 **(a)** CT scan demonstrating a large cervical esophageal duplication with tracheal compression and deviation, in a patient with acute stridor and sudden appearance of a cervical mass. **(b)** CT scan showing an infected duplication cyst with a fistula into the right-upper-lobe bronchus. This patient had recurrent pneumonia and developed a right-upper-lobe lung abscess seen on chest x-ray.

Occasionally, duplications may be an incidental finding on chest x-ray (Figure 48.3). The symptoms in older children are generally related to pressure on the surrounding structures. Esophageal compression causes dysphagia (Figure 48.4b). Tracheal compression results in stridor or respiratory compromise (Figure 48.2a). These cysts may ulcerate, bleed, and rupture into the esophagus or tracheobronchial tree, causing recurrent pneumonia, pain, hemoptysis, and lung abscess (Figure 48.2b).[3,7,8] Both squamous cell carcinoma and adenocarcinoma in esophageal duplication cysts have been reported in adults.[10,11]

A high preoperative mortality (10%) has been reported in a large retrospective study.[8] The reported deaths are a consequence of exsanguinating bleeding into the esophagus, respiratory compromise, or septic complications.[8]

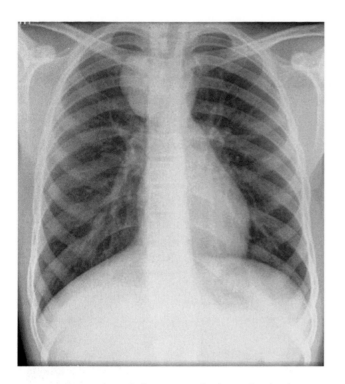

Figure 48.3 Incidental chest x-ray finding of a duplication cyst in a previously asymptomatic patient. This x-ray was done for blunt chest trauma. Subsequent investigation confirmed this to be an esophageal duplication.

DIAGNOSIS

All antenatally diagnosed thoracic cystic lesions must be investigated postnatally with a contrast-enhanced computed tomography (CT) scan. A foregut duplication on CT scan is located in the posterior mediastinum in contact with the esophagus or trachea. Typically, it is described as a low-attenuation, homogenous cystic mass with a smooth border (Figures 48.4c and 48.5d).[12]

Plain x-ray may reveal a paravertebral, smooth round shadow. In symptomatic cases, there may be a deviated or compressed trachea (Figures 48.2a and 48.4c). The plain radiograph is also useful in demonstrating associated vertebral anomalies (Figure 48.5a).

In children presenting with dysphagia, a contrast swallow will demonstrate a smooth shadow compressing the esophageal tract (Figure 48.4b). In the acute onset of stridor, a CT scan will show a cystic mass causing tracheal compression (Figure 48.2a). The lower esophageal duplication cysts are likely to remain asymptomatic and can present in adulthood either on an incidental x-ray or with symptoms such as chest pain, dysphagia, or hematemesis (Figure 48.5b). A magnetic resonance imaging (MRI) scan should be considered in the presence of vertebral anomalies for the diagnosis of an intraspinal component (Figures 48.1b and 48.5c). Upper gastrointestinal endoscopy and esophageal ultrasonography add little to the diagnosis of the esophageal cyst.

MANAGEMENT

Esophageal duplications warrant complete excision as incomplete excision inevitably results in a recurrence.[8] Antenatally diagnosed cases after investigations should be electively excised, preferably with the thoracoscopic approach. In most instances, symptomatic cases are suitable for thoracoscopic resection with the exception of infected cases with fistulation (Figure 48.2b). Thoracoscopic excision is being increasingly used for the surgical management of esophageal duplication cysts.[13–15] The thoracoscopic approach has been shown to have lower opioid requirements and shorter duration of chest tube drainage and hospital stay.[14,15] Previous inadequate resection with recurrence may require an open approach for a complete resection.

Thoracoscopic resection

Central endotracheal intubation is used in most cases, with the exception of older children, where single-lung anesthesia is possible. The patient is placed in the lateral position, with the affected side uppermost. The optical port is generally inserted just anterior to the angle of the scapula in the midaxillary line. Two or three additional ports are inserted under thoracoscopic vision for the best possible triangulation and manipulation. The lung is collapsed and retracted with creation of a pneumothorax with minimal pressures (5–7 mmHg of CO_2, flow rates of 1.5–2 L/min) to expose the posterior mediastinal cyst.

The pleura at the base of the cyst is incised with either scissors or diathermy hook. Two types of duplications are encountered requiring slightly different techniques during its resection. The commonly encountered duplication has a separate muscle wall and is attached to the native esophageal tract by connective tissue. The dissection can be completed using either diathermy hook or scissors, harmonic scalpel, or LigaSure (Valley Lab, Covidien). Electrosurgical instruments should be used precisely and with caution so as to prevent inadvertent tissue injury by electrical conduction or thermal spread. The vagus and phrenic nerves and thoracic duct are at risk of injury during the resection of the thoracic inlet duplication. Esophageal duplications sharing a common muscle wall with the native esophagus are relatively rare and a technical challenge to resect thoracoscopically. A nasogastric tube or an endoscope placed in situ during resection can help avoid resection of a major portion of the wall and mucosa of the native esophagus. The cyst should be completely excised with the esophageal mucosa left intact if possible. Marsupialization should be avoided as leaving residual cyst wall tends to result in recurrence.[8] Once the cyst is removed, the defect in the esophageal musculature and mucosa can be sutured with absorbable sutures. The specimen is decompressed by aspiration and delivered by expanding one of the anterior ports.

In the presence of a thoracoabdominal duplication cyst, complete resection is achieved by an additional laparoscopic

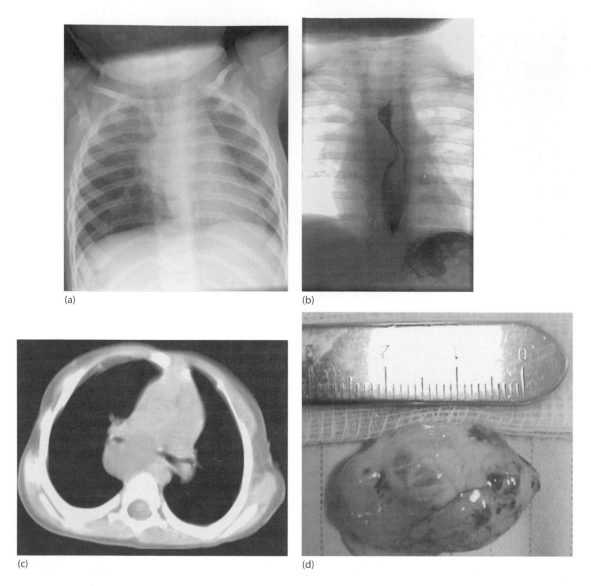

Figure 48.4 **(a)** This patient presented with recurrent chest infections. Chest x-ray shows mild emphysema of the right lung with a smooth round mediastinal mass. **(b)** A contrast swallow shows the classical smooth shadow compressing the esophageal tract. **(c)** CT scan revealed a typical low-attenuation, homogenous cystic mass with a smooth border compressing the right main bronchus. **(d)** Duplication cyst specimen following thoracoscopic excision.

approach. A separate intra-abdominal cyst can be successfully resected either in the same sitting or at a subsequent laparoscopic resection.[5]

Most esophageal duplications following resection do not require postoperative chest drains. We recommend a chest drain only if the esophageal mucosa is breached during the resection.[16] Postoperative pain is managed with oral or intravenous paracetamol and oral anti-inflammatory drugs (ibuprofen). The majority of thoracoscopically resected cases can be discharged the following day.

Thoracotomy and resection

A lateral thoracotomy through the bed of the fifth rib is recommended for an open resection. The principles of surgery are the same as for thoracoscopic resection. Adhesions,

either inflammatory or as a result of a previous operation, are the cause of complications in open operations. Bleeding and air leaks either from the lung parenchyma or from fistulation should be managed intraoperatively in order to avoid postoperative complications. The aforementioned nerves and thoracic duct are also at risk of injury as bleeding or adhesions may obscure their presence near the duplication.

Cervical and suprasternal cysts

Cervical excision can be achieved by placing the patient supine with a roll under the shoulders. Once the cyst wall is identified, the dissection is continued staying close to its surface. Electrosurgical instruments should be used precisely and with caution so as to prevent inadvertent tissue injury by electrical conduction or thermal spread. The

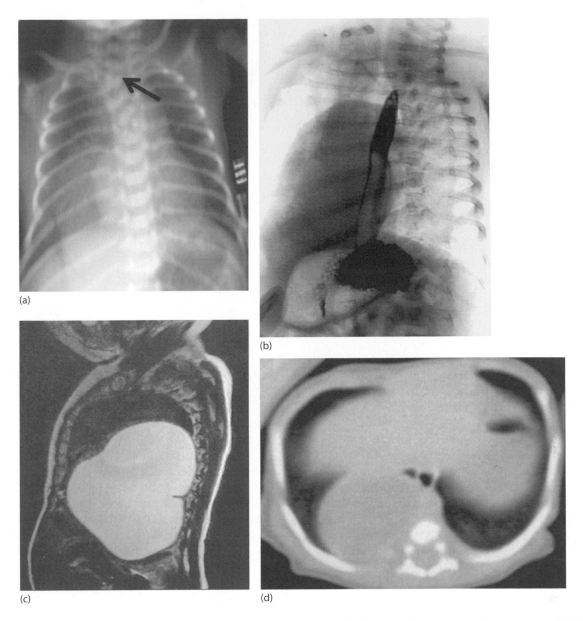

Figure 48.5 **(a)** Chest x-ray showing vertebral anomalies in an antenatally detected foregut duplication cyst. **(b)** Contrast study demonstrating a large posterior mediastinal duplication cyst. **(c)** MRI scan was done to rule out neuroenteric component in presence of vertebral anomalies. **(d)** CT scan confirmed a smooth low-attenuation posterior mediastinal duplication cyst.

recurrent laryngeal nerve is particularly at risk of injury as it can travel on the surface of the esophageal duplication.

SURGICAL COMPLICATIONS

Surgical complications are related to the site and mode of surgery. Incomplete excision is associated with recurrence and the need for further surgery.[8] Esophageal leakage is a possibility with both the open and the thoracoscopic approach. A minor leak can be managed conservatively with a period of nil by mouth with parenteral nutrition, antibiotics, and chest drainage. However, major leaks may require thoracotomy, esophageal repair, evacuation of the empyema, and chest drainage.[7,13] This group of patients is at risk of esophageal stricture long term, which may respond to dilation. Esophageal pseudodiverticulum is a long-term risk if the esophageal musculature is not approximated.[15] A persistent air leak will require thoracotomy and formal repair of the bronchus or trachea.[13] In a retrospective series, two postoperative deaths have been reported secondary to septic complications, one from an esophageal leakage and the other from cyst-related sepsis.[8]

Injury to the vagus nerve, recurrent laryngeal nerve, and phrenic nerve in the cervical and the superior mediastinal duplication can be avoided by careful dissection and staying close to the cyst wall. Judicious use of electrosurgical instruments in dissecting close to the nerves is recommended. There is a higher risk of nerve or thoracic duct injury during surgery for an infected cyst because of adhesions and bleeding.

LONG-TERM OUTCOME

All esophageal duplications should be excised because of the potential for life-threatening complications: peptic ulceration and bleeding or perforation, acute airway obstruction, recurrent infection, mediastinitis, meningitis, and the long-term risk of cancer. Thoracoscopic excision in the asymptomatic patient has a lower complication rate than surgery for a cyst-related complication. Patients who are known to have incomplete excision should be monitored for recurrence. Patients with vertebral anomalies should be monitored for scoliosis. Rarely, a motility disorder of the esophagus is noted in some cases after resection as a result of damage to the pharyngeal plexus. After resection of the cervical duplication, a pharyngeal pouch can be a long-term consequence.

REFERENCES

1. Ponski TA, Rothenberg SS. Foregut duplication cysts. In: Parikh DH, Crabb D, Aldist A, Rothenberg SS (eds). *Paediatric Thoracic Surgery*. London: Springer Verlag, 2009: 383–90.
2. Stringer MD, Spitz L, Abel R et al. Management of alimentary tract duplication in children. *Br J Surg* 1995; 82: 74–8.
3. Holcomb GW 3rd, Gheissari A, O'Neill JA Jr et al. Surgical management of alimentary tract duplications. *Ann Surg* 1989; 209: 167–74.
4. Beardmore HE, Wiglesworth FW. Vertebral anomalies and alimentary duplications; clinical and embryological aspects. *Pediatr Clin North Am* 1958; May: 457–74.
5. Cocker DM, Parikh D, Brown R. Multiple antenatally diagnosed foregut duplication cysts excised and the value of thoracoscopy in diagnosing small concurrent cysts. *Ann R Coll Surg Engl* 2006; 88: W8–10(1).
6. Bently JF, Smith JR. Developmental posterior enteric remnants and spinal malformations: The split notochord syndrome. *Arch Dis Child* 1960; 35: 76–86.
7. Carachi R, Azmy A. Foregut duplications. *Pediatr Surg Int* 2002; 18: 371–4.
8. Nobuhara KK, Gorski YC, La Quaglia MP, Shamberger RC. Bronchogenic cysts and esophageal duplications: Common origins and treatment. *J Pediatr Surg* 1997; 32: 1408–13.
9. Ravitch MM. Mediastinal cysts and tumors. In: Welch KJ, Randolph JG, Ravitch MM, O'Neill JA, Rowe MI (eds). *Pediatric Surgery*, 4rth edn. Chicago: Year Book Medical Publishers, Inc. 1986; 602–18.
10. Tapia RH, White VA. Squamous cell carcinoma arising in a duplication cyst of the esophagus. *Am J Gastroenterol* 1985; 80: 325–9.
11. Lee MY, Jensen E, Kwak S, Larson RA. Metastatic adenocarcinoma arising in a congenital foregut cyst of the esophagus: A case report with review of the literature. *Am J Clin Oncol* 1998; 21: 64–6.
12. Weiss LM, Fagelman D, Warhit JM. CT demonstration of an esophageal duplication cyst. *J Comput Assist Tomogr* 1983; 7: 716–8.
13. Michel JL, Revillon Y, Montupet P. Thoracoscopic treatment of mediastinal cysts in children. *J Pediatr Surg* 1998; 33: 1745–8.
14. Merry C, Spurbeck W, Lobe TE. Resection of foregut-derived duplications by minimal-access surgery. *Pediatr Surg Int* 1999; 15: 224–6.
15. Bratu I, Laberge JM, Flageole H, Bouchard S. Foregut duplications: Is there an advantage to thoracoscopic resection? *J Pediatr Surg* 2005; 40: 138–41.
16. Partrick D, Rothenberg SS. Thoracoscopic resection of mediastinal masses in infants and children: An evaluation of technique and results. *J Pediatr Surg* 2001; 36: 1165–7.

49

Esophageal perforation in the newborn

DAVID S. FOLEY

INTRODUCTION

Iatrogenic esophageal perforation occurs rarely in neonates and was first reported in the literature by Eklof and colleagues.[1] In the past two decades, perforation of the esophagus in extremely premature neonates has become increasingly recognized and reported. Spontaneous perforation of the esophagus (neonatal Boerhaave's syndrome) is extremely rare, and Fryfogle[2] performed the first successful repair. Despite the favorable results of nonoperative management in cases of neonatal esophageal perforation, this condition may be fatal without early diagnosis and treatment, and aggressive surgical therapy is occasionally warranted.[3–7] Surgeons must continue to play a central role in the individualization of care in these patients.

CLASSIFICATION AND ETIOLOGY

Esophageal perforation in newborns can be classified as iatrogenic or noniatrogenic. Noniatrogenic perforations are extremely rare and are usually seen in full-term infants when they occur. The most common site of perforation is the lower third of the esophagus. Etiological hypotheses for spontaneous perforation include increased intra-abdominal pressure at delivery, perinatal hypoxemia, and reflux-associated peptic esophagitis.[8]

Iatrogenic perforation of the esophagus is most commonly seen in premature, small-for-gestational-age (SGA) infants,[9] and usually occurs in the cervical esophagus or hypopharynx. Pharyngeal suctioning with a stiff catheter, traumatic laryngoscopy, esophageal intubation, and digital manipulation of the neonatal head during breech delivery have all been described as causative.[10–13]

During instrumentation, when the neck is hyperextended, perforation of the esophagus may occur at the level of the cricopharyngeus muscle, where the posterior esophageal wall is compressed by the sixth or seventh cervical vertebra. Submucosal injury by a laryngoscope blade or endotracheal tube may be the initial injury to the hypopharynx, resulting in cricopharyngeal spasm.[14] Endotracheal intubation, especially in premature, SGA neonates, may further compromise the esophageal introitus. Subsequent oropharyngeal suctioning or insertion of a nasogastric tube may extend the submucosal injury into a full-thickness perforation.

Perforation of the middle esophagus is usually associated with dilatation of a stricture, or a postoperative anastomotic leak following esophageal atresia repair.[15,16] An improperly placed chest tube may cause disruption of a fresh esophageal anastomosis or may penetrate a proximal myotomy site.[17] Chest tube–related direct pressure necrosis of an otherwise normal esophagus has been reported in a premature neonate.[18] With the increasing use of transesophageal echocardiography in the evaluation of congenital heart disease, perforations of the proximal and middle esophagus have been reported with this procedure.[19,20]

Distal esophageal perforation may be associated with dilatation of an esophageal stricture secondary to esophagitis, a technical error during antireflux surgery, or a misplaced gastrostomy balloon.[21]

DIAGNOSIS AND CLINICAL MANIFESTATIONS

Newborns with iatrogenic esophageal injury may demonstrate excessive salivation and mucoid secretions due to difficulty swallowing, and many will have overt respiratory distress. The examiner will have difficulty passing a nasogastric tube, either as the inciting event or as a result of swelling or a false tract created by prior instrumentation. In neonates, an abnormal position of the nasogastric tube on postplacement chest x-ray is commonly the first indication of esophageal perforation.[9]

In premature infants, the presence of blood-tinged oral secretions after endotracheal intubation warrants serial x-ray examinations of the chest. The proper diagnosis often will be missed in the absence of such an examination. The symptoms of perforation may not be recognized until the child develops esophageal obstruction, and may be mistaken for esophageal atresia.[9,11,13] Esophageal perforation may be differentiated from atresia of the esophagus by an asymptomatic interval after birth, a premorbid history of repeated attempts at intubation or vigorous suctioning, absence of prenatal polyhydramnios, and the position and course of the nasogastric tube on chest x-ray.[9] Some perforations of the esophagus create respiratory distress secondary to the development of hydropneumothorax. In these cases, the right pleural space is most commonly affected.[3,5,11,13] Thoracentesis or tube thoracostomy should yield serosanguinous fluid or the contents of the previous feeding. Chylopneumothorax has also been reported in association with neonatal esophageal perforation.[22]

Anteroposterior and lateral x-rays of the chest and neck should be obtained in any suspected case of perforation. The abnormalities seen in these cases depend on the site of injury. Hypopharyngeal and cervical perforations frequently demonstrate extraluminal air in the neck, without pneumomediastinum initially. Midesophageal perforations may demonstrate pneumomediastinum, pneumothorax, or hydrothorax. An unusual course of the nasogastric tube (right pleural cavity, pericardial cavity [Figure 49.1], or right side of the mediastinum) supports the diagnosis and may be confirmatory. Widening of the mediastinum and blurring of the mediastinal margin may occur secondary to the development of mediastinitis, but are later and more subtle findings. These changes should prompt esophagography. Mollit et al.[23] described three types of injuries that are seen in premature neonates: (1) a pharyngeal diverticulum created by a local cervical leak; (2) a mucosal perforation extending posteriorly in parallel to the esophagus; and (3) a free

intrapleural perforation where there is obvious leakage of air and esophageal contents into the pleural cavity.

In cases where chest x-ray demonstrates the nasogastric tube to be located in the pleural cavity or pericardium, the diagnosis of esophageal perforation can be confirmed (Figure 49.2). In this situation, precise localization of the site of perforation may be unnecessary, unless the patient's clinical condition deteriorates after removal of the nasogastric tube and tube thoracostomy drainage. If symptoms suggest esophageal obstruction, esophagography should be performed by administering a small quantity of diatrizoate meglumine (Hypaque), diatrizoate sodium (Renografin) or metrizamide into the proximal esophagus; Gastografin and barium should be avoided due to the risk of worsening mediastinitis or inducing significant pulmonary inflammation with aspiration. In cases of pharyngeal–esophageal perforation, cricopharyngeal spasm may be so severe that no contrast material will enter the native esophagus. In these cases, several clues may help to differentiate submucosal perforation or pseudodiverticular formation from congenital esophageal atresia.[24] These include the following:

- The distance between the trachea and opacified tract on lateral x-ray is greater than that of the pouch in a congenital esophageal atresia, which is closely associated with the trachea.
- The opacified tract in perforation cases is longer, narrower, and more irregular than in esophageal atresia.
- The trachea is slightly compressed on lateral x-ray by the upper pouch in esophageal atresia, but this is not so in esophageal perforation.

Esophagoscopy is usually not indicated at the time of diagnosis and may actually enlarge the perforation.

Spontaneous perforation of the neonatal esophagus usually presents with respiratory distress, which may be immediate or delayed for several hours after the event. There is a greater predilection for right-sided pneumothorax in neonatal Boerhaave's syndrome, in contrast to the left-sided

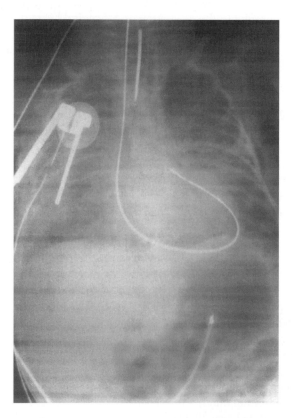

Figure 49.1 Chest x-ray shows displacement of the nasogastric tube to the pericardial sac.

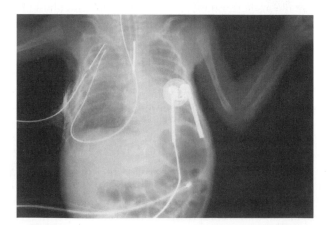

Figure 49.2 Anteroposterior view demonstrates coiled nasogastric tube in right pleural cavity and chest tube placed for tension pneumothorax.

pneumothorax typically seen in adults.[8,18] This may be explained by the close adherence of the aorta to the left side of the esophagus in neonates, which provides an additional mediastinal barrier on the left side. If the perforation remains undiagnosed, respiratory distress will worsen with subsequent feedings. Esophagography must be performed in all suspected cases of free perforation to evaluate the extent of the damage and to localize it.

MANAGEMENT

The management of neonatal esophageal perforations has favored a selective approach in recent years.[7,23–25] Esophageal perforation can be a rapidly fatal condition that requires immediate recognition and aggressive management for a successful outcome. However, the treatment of esophageal perforation must be individualized according to the site and size of injury, the systemic response of the neonate, and the time interval between the injury and initiation of treatment. Small submucosal perforations of the hypopharynx and esophagus, limited to the mediastinum and without systemic symptoms, may be managed by nonoperative methods (Figure 49.3). Identification of the exact site of perforation is not essential in these infants. If the nasogastric tube is noted in the

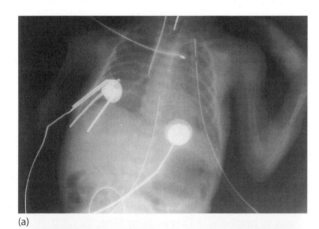

(a)

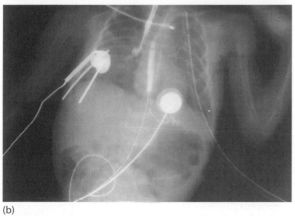

(b)

Figure 49.3 Abserrant position of nasopharyngeal tube within mediastinum **(a)**, with confirmation of contained proximal esophageal perforation on subsequent contrast evaluation **(b)**.

mediastinum or pericardial cavity, the tube can be withdrawn and a new tube placed under fluoroscopic control. A broad-spectrum antibiotic must be given for 7–14 days. Intravenous (IV) fluids and hyperalimentation should be administered, as oral feedings must be withheld. Esophagography should be performed 7–10 days after the injury. If the perforation is completely healed, oral feeding may be resumed. If the perforation has not healed during this interval, conservative treatment for another week will usually allow complete healing.

In general, routine surgical intervention does not appear to improve the rate of survival in these newborns. Tube thoracostomy should be placed when the chest x-ray indicates pneumomediastimun, pneumothorax, or hydrothorax (Figure 49.4). All newborn infants with esophageal perforation must be carefully monitored during treatment, including the use of white blood cell counts or C-reactive protein levels, platelet counts, blood gas analyses, and chest x-ray evaluation. If there is clinical deterioration or respiratory compromise, and closed-chest drainage does not handle the leak, direct repair of the perforation is indicated.

In cases where direct repair of the perforation is not technically feasible because of scarring, inflammation, and tissue friability, diverting cervical esophagostomy with closure of the perforated area and concomitant gastrostomy is indicated. If at all possible, efforts should be made to avoid future esophageal replacement. Long, linear perforations to the lower end of the esophagus require an immediate thoracotomy, debridement of the necrotic edges, and primary repair of the defect with pleural flap coverage. A gastrostomy tube may be inserted in these situations to minimize the risk of gastroesophageal reflux during healing.

If there is a delay of more than 24 hours in the diagnosis of a spontaneous perforation of the esophagus, unprotected primary repair cannot be safely accomplished. After adequate debridement, the treatment should be local esophagectomy with closure of the proximal and distal esophagus, proximal esophagostomy, and gastrostomy tube placement. Critically ill newborns should be managed with chest tube drainage, cervical esophagostomy (with or without ligation

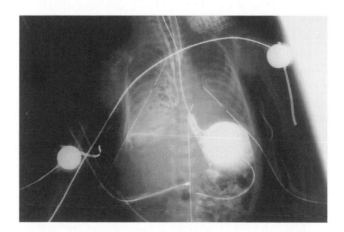

Figure 49.4 Free spillage of contrast material into right pleural cavity, indicating a free perforation in this infant. Clinical deterioration warranted direct repair.

of the cardioesophageal junction), and gastrostomy.[26] Broad-spectrum antibiotics, IV fluids, and hyperalimentation should be continued until clinical signs of sepsis improve. Gastrostomy feedings may be attempted after 48 hours. In cases where extensive debridement or resection is necessary, esophageal substitution is indicated after an interval of at least 6 months, when the mediastinal inflammation has resolved.

Perforations that occur following dilation of esophageal anastomotic strictures are usually managed nonoperatively, as long as the leak is contained or can be adequately drained by tube thoracostomy. These perforations may take some time to heal due to obstruction at the stricture site. In the last decade, endoscopic stenting has been reported as a means of containing leakage and promoting healing in these cases, although its use is limited in the neonatal population due to the size constraints of available stents.[27]

CONCLUSION

Iatrogenic perforation of the esophagus is more common than reported in the literature and may be fatal without early diagnosis. The incidence of recognized pharyngeal and esophageal perforations is low, however, considering the large number of pharyngeal instrumentations that are performed on premature infants in modern neonatal intensive care units.[23] Gentle laryngoscopy with proper visualization of the vocal cords during intubation, avoidance of protruding stylets, careful suctioning of the pharynx, and avoidance of forceful nasogastric tube placement are all essential factors in the prevention of these injuries.

It is generally accepted that most iatrogenic perforations of the esophagus in newborns are cervical and are made when inexperienced personnel attempt to intubate the trachea. With early diagnosis, most of these perforations can be managed nonoperatively with successful outcomes.[28] However, these infants should be monitored closely. If they develop systemic illness, appropriate operative intervention is often required. Early diagnosis of this condition allows for more treatment options, which include nonoperative therapy, closed-chest drainage, and primary repair. The mortality rate in neonates with esophageal perforation (4%) is significantly less than that in older children and adults (25%–50%).[6,7,29] Delayed diagnosis may result in the inability to repair the injury primarily, a significant increase in mortality, and the eventual need for esophageal replacement among survivors. Surgical consultation is warranted in all cases of esophageal perforation to allow timely and selective management, thereby limiting both mortality and long-term morbidity.

REFERENCES

1. Eklof O, Lohr G, Okmian L. Submucosal perforation of the esophagus in the neonate. *Acta Radiol* 1969; 8: 1987.
2. Fryfogle JD. Discussion of Anderson RL. Rupture of the esophagus. *J Thorac Cardiovasc Surg* 1952: 24: 369–88.
3. Michael L, Grillo HC, Malt RA. Operative and non-operative management of esophageal perforations. *Ann Surg* 1981; 194: 57.
4. Van der Zee DC, Slooff MJH, Kingma LM. Management of esophageal perforations: A tailored approach. *Neth J Surg* 1966; 38: 31.
5. Gander JW, Berdon WE, Cowles RA. Iatrogenic esophageal perforation in children. *Pediatr Surg Int* 2009; 25(5): 395–401.
6. Hesketh AJ, Behr C, Soffer S et al. Neonatal esophageal perforation: Nonoperative management. *J Surg Res* 2015; 198(1): 1–6.
7. Garey CL, Laituri CA, Kaye AJ et al. Esophageal perforation in children: A review of one institution's experience. *J Surg Res* 2010; 164(1): 13–17.
8. Aaronson IA, Cywess S, Louwh JH. Spontaneous esophageal rupture in the newborn. *J Pediatr Surg* 1975; 10: 459.
9. Ducharme JC, Bertrano R, Debie J. Perforation of the pharynx in the newborn: A condition mimicking esophageal atresia. *Med Assoc J* 1971; 104: 785.
10. Astley R, Robrts KD. Intubation perforation of the esophagus in the newborn baby. *Br J Radiol* 1970; 43: 219.
11. Su BH, Lin HY, Chiu HY et al. Esophageal perforation: A complication of nasogastric tube placement in premature neonates. *J Pediatr* 2009; 154(3): 460.
12. Lee Sb, Kuhn JP. Esophageal perforation in the neonate. *Am J Dis Child* 1976; 130: 325.
13. Wychulis AR, Fontana RS, Payne WS. Instrumental perforation of the esophagus. *Chest* 1969; 55(3): 184–9.
14. Girdany BR, Sieber W, Osman MZ. Pseudo-diverticulum of the pharynx in newborn infants. *New Engl J Med* 1969; 280: 237.
15. Sloan EI, Haight C. Congenital atresia of the esophagus in brothers. *J Thorac Surg* 1956; 32: 200.
16. Eraklis AJ, Gross RE. Esophageal atresia: Management following an anastomotic leak. *Surgery* 1966; 60: 919.
17. Johnson JF, Wright DR. Chest tube perforation of esophagus following repair of esophageal atresia. *J Pediatr Surg* 1990; 25: 1227.
18. Cairns PA, McClure BG, Halliday HL et al. Unusual site for oesophageal perforation in an extremely low birth weight infant. *Eur J Pediatr* 1999; 158: 152–3.
19. Miller JW, Hart CK, Statile CJ. Oesophageal perforation in a neonate during transesophageal echocardiography for cardiac surgery. *Cardiol Young* 2015; 25(5): 1015–8.
20. Mukerideen-Russell IA, Miller-Hance WC, Silverman NH. Unrecognized esophageal perforation in a neonate during transesophageal echocardiography. *J Am Soc Echocardiogr* 2001; 14(7): 747–9.

21. Kenigsberg, K, Levenbrown J. Esophageal perforation secondary to gastrostomy. *J Pediatr Surg* 1986; 21: 946.

22. Kairamkonda VR. A rare cause of chylopneumothorax in a preterm neonate. *Indian J Med Sci* 2007; 61(8): 476–7.

23. Mollit DC, Schullinger JW, Santulli T. Selective management of iatrogenic esophageal perforation in the newborn. *J Pediatr Surg* 1981; 16: 989.

24. Blair GK, Filler RM, Theodorescu D. Neonatal pharyngoesophageal perforation mimicking esophageal atresia: Clues to diagnosis. *J Pediatr Surg* 1987; 22: 270.

25. Johnson DE, Foker J, Munson DP et al. Management of esophageal and pharyngeal perforation in the newborn. *Pediatrics* 1982; 70: 592–9.

26. Urschel HC Jr, Razzuk MA, Wood RE et al. Improved management of esophageal perforations: Exclusion and diversion in continuity. *Ann Surg* 1974; 179: 587.

27. Rico FR, Panzer AM, Kooros K et al. Use of Polyflex Airway stent in the treatment of perforated esophageal stricture in an infant: A case report. *J Pediatr Surg* 2007; 42(7); E5–8.

28. Krasna IH, Rosenfield D, Benjamin BG et al. Esophageal perforation in the neonate: An emergency problem in the newborn nursery. *J Pediatr Surg* 1987; 227: 784.

29. Engum SA, Grosfeld JL, West KW et al. Improved survival of children with esophageal perforation. *Arch Surg* 1996; 131: 604–11.

50

Gastroesophageal reflux in the neonate and small infant

MICHAEL E. HÖLLWARTH

INTRODUCTION

Gastroesophageal reflux (GER) is a term that describes the backflow of gastric content into the esophagus, sometimes reaching even the mouth. It is a common phenomenon and occurs in otherwise normal individuals several times during the day and night, especially after ingestion of fluids, e.g., soup, tea, coffee, or milk. Therefore, reflux episodes are more common in neonates and infants as long as they are nourished mainly with milk. The typical reflux symptoms in this age group are regurgitation, spitting up, and flaccid leak-out of milk after meals and when asleep. Pathological reflux defines a situation where the reflux causes symptoms in the neonate such as failure to thrive, sleep disturbance, and obviously, pain. The aim of this chapter is to discuss the normal esophagus in newborns and its function, the typical symptoms of reflux in this age group, investigating procedures, and conservative and operative therapy.

ANATOMY

The esophagus is a muscular tubular organ responsible for the transport of food from the mouth to the stomach. The upper half is composed of striated muscles, and its lower half consists of smooth muscle. The lumen is covered by a nonkeratinized, stratified squamous epithelium. At the esophageal–gastric junction, the epithelial layer changes to a monolayer columnar epithelium, the so-called cardia epithelium.

The diaphragmatic hiatus of the esophagus is fixed by the phrenicoesophageal membrane, which is incompetent in the case of a hiatal hernia (HH). The medial wall of the esophagus directly continues into the lesser curvature of the stomach, while the lateral wall forms a kind of incisure—the so-called His angle. Within the lumen at the His angle is a mucosal fold (flutter valve), which is passively pressed against the lower esophageal sphincter (LES) when the gastric fundus is filled, thus preventing reflux (Figure 50.1).[1] The flatter the angle of His, the less developed the flutter valve, and the more readily a reflux occurs for anatomical reasons.

INNERVATION

The esophagus has a parasympathetic innervation through the vagus nerve, which runs along the esophagus. Sympathetic innervation arises from postganglionic neurons of the sympathetic chain. The myenteric plexus and the submucosal plexus contain also nonadrenergic and noncholinergic nerves, and execute the complex activity of the esophagus through a number of neurotransmitters. Most important is a central regulation by consecutively activated nuclei in the brain stem responsible for the peristalsis and relaxations of the esophageal sphincters.

THE SPHINCTERS

There are two sphincter systems at the upper and lower end of the esophagus. In adult persons, the tone is in the upper esophageal sphincter (UES), markedly higher (between 40–80 mm Hg) than in the LES (15–25 mm Hg). The UES relaxes during propulsion of food from the oral cavity but also when refluxed volume reaches the upper esophagus from below. Then refluxed material can reach the hypopharynx and eventually the oral cavity.

Reflux of the contents of the stomach into the esophagus is prevented by the LES. The pressure ranges between 15 and 25 mm Hg in adults. On manometry, the pressure zone permits easy identification of the exact position of the sphincter. The pressure transition of the LES lies exactly within the diaphragm. The upper half of the sphincter can be assigned to the chest cavity, while the lower portion of the pressure zone is assigned to the abdominal cavity (Figure 50.2).

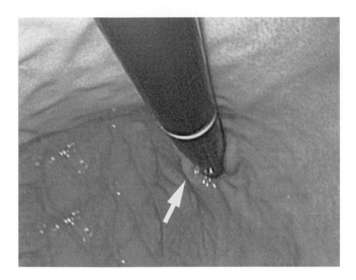

Figure 50.1 Typical mucosal flutter valve at the site of the His angle within the stomach.

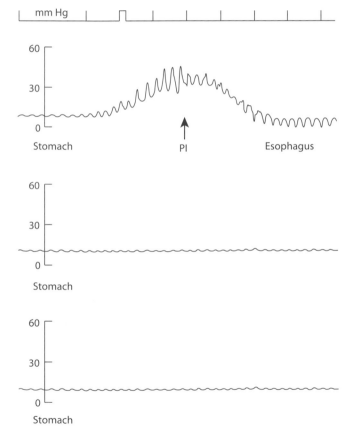

Figure 50.2 Slow pull-through manometry through the LES in a newborn child. PI indicates the pressure inversion from a typical stomach tracing to a typical esophageal tracing. Thus, the PI is located within the diaphragmatic hiatus, and one part of the LES belongs to the abdomen and the other part to the thorax. Except the sphincter, there is no intra-abdominal esophagus.

PERISTALSIS

Once food enters the esophagus, it is transported by a propulsive peristaltic wave into the stomach (primary peristalsis). With any local distension of the esophagus, as in cases of reflux, a propulsive peristaltic wave arises locally and transports the contents of the esophagus back into the stomach (secondary peristalsis). Isolated and disorderly contractions are defined as tertiary peristalsis or pathological contractions.

CAUSES OF REFLUX

One of the specific characteristics of the LES is the fact that its tonus does not only relax when food enters the esophagus through a propulsive peristaltic wave, but regular spontaneous relaxations of 5–10 seconds' duration (spontaneous transient LES relaxations [STLESRs]) occur even in the absence of any other esophageal activity in healthy individuals. Thereby, a common space is opened between the stomach and the esophagus and can be demonstrated on manometry as a sudden change of the typical esophageal tracing into an abdominal pressure curve, the *common cavity phenomenon* (CCP) (Figure 50.3). Usually, these relaxations remain unrecognized because the reflux reaches, in most events, only the lower esophagus. The volume is immediately returned to the stomach by a secondary peristalsis (volume clearance). Any drop in the pH, however, is neutralized in a stepwise manner by saliva during subsequent acts of deglutition (acid clearance). In patients with pathological reflux or reflux disease, STLESRs occur significantly more often and longer.

THE DEVELOPMENT OF THE ESOPHAGUS IN THE NEONATE AND SMALL INFANT

The best way to investigate the esophageal function in this age group is manometry combined with pH monitoring. Studies in premature infants and newborn babies have shown that the length of the LES is 10.7 mm. The tone of the LES is in these groups of babies was in the range of 18.0–23.0 mm Hg. Thus, the tone in the LES is identical with the tone in older age groups and in adults (Table 50.1).[2]

Manometric studies have shown that there is a physiologic delay in the development of propulsive esophageal peristalsis. Induced swallows in the youngest group of patients have been followed only in 59% by a propulsive peristalsis and in 41% by simultaneous contractions of the esophagus. However, already at the age of 4 weeks, nearly all investigated babies had a normal peristaltic response in 8 out of 10 induced swallows.

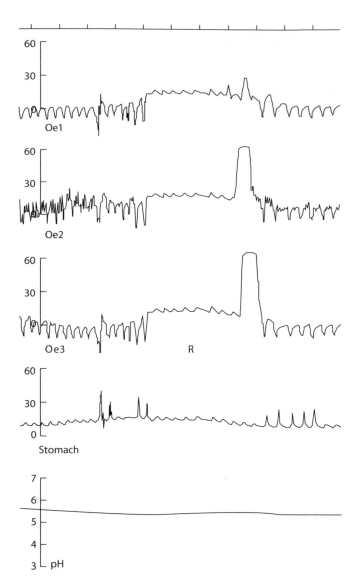

Figure 50.3 Spontaneous pressure inversion of the esophageal tracing to an abdominal tracing indicates the opening of the LES due to a transient relaxation. This is the manometric sign of reflux—the *common cavity phenomenon* (CCP). It is always terminated by a secondary propulsive peristalsis.

REFLUX IN THE NEWBORN

Mild spitting, a flaccid leak-out, or vomiting of milk as a sign of a pronounced GER is observed in approximately half of all newborns and young infants. The subsequent development shows that these symptoms become less frequent after the first 4–6 months of the infant's life and are no longer observed at 12 months in most cases. Previously, it was believed that frequent reflux in these early age groups is caused by a physiologic absence of tone in the LES. However, our former studies using adequate manometric techniques have clearly shown that the incidence of GER in newborns and infants is not caused by a low or even absent pressure of an immature LES, and not by a deficient esophageal peristalsis, but as a consequence of other factors (Table 50.1).

What is immature in this age group, and what might cause the higher incidence of reflux? Three factors have to be considered:

1. *Spontaneous LES relaxation:* We were able to show that GER in newborns and infants is caused by STLESRs. Babies with pathological reflux have significantly more frequent and more prolonged STLESRs but a normal LES tone (Table 50.2).[2,3] These findings were later confirmed by Omari et al.[4] Further investigations showed that pathological STLERs are associated with immaturity of the normal propulsive peristalsis of the esophagus. Thus, we can conclude that reflux in this age group is not caused by an absent LES tone but must be regarded as delay in the central motor coordination in the esophagus and its sphincters. The particularly high prevalence of reflux in infants with sleep apnea is an additional indication of the conclusion that immature central regulatory structures are responsible for frequent STLESRs.[5] In most cases, a spontaneous maturation of this functional instability occurs within the first year of life, and thereafter, the reflux pattern is identical with that of adults. However, it has been shown that the disappearance of the clinical signs of reflux around the age of 12 month does not necessarily mean that the

Table 50.1 Results of esophageal manometry

	n	Age (days)	LES tone (mm Hg) x̄ ± SD	LES length (mm) x̄ ± SD	PS *n* = 10
Premature infants (Gestational age [GA] 30–36)	7	7–28	23.0 ± 3.6	1.0 ± 1.1	–
Newborns	24	1–10	20.4 ± 8.0	10.7 ± 0.8	5.2*
Newborns	19	11–28	21.8 ± 10.0	11.0 ± 0.5	7.3
Infants	20	>28	18.0 ± 7.0	11.3 ± 1.1	7.9

Note: The LES pressure values in newborn babies and infants are already normal. *PS* is the response of propulsive peristaltic waves in the esophagus after 10 induced swallows. The results show that the response is significantly lower within the first 10 days of life, but thereafter, it is normal, with nearly 8 propulsive responses out of 10 induced swallows.

*$p < .05$.

Table 50.2 CCP occurs significantly more often and longer in babies with GER when compared to normal controls (However, the LES tone is not different between groups)

	Seconds	With reflux (n)	Controls (n)
CCP episodes	<7	12.4 ± 92.6[a]	3.3 ± 90.5
	7–15	9.6 ± 91.1[a]	3.4 ± 90.4
	>15	3.0 ± 90.8[a]	0.7 ± 90.2
Total CCP time (%)		2.0 ± 90.3[a]	0.5 ± 90.05
LES tone (mm Hg)		25.3 ± 92.6	30.2 ± 91.4

Note: CCP, common cavity phenomenon; GER, gastroesophageal reflux; LES, lower esophageal sphincter.

[a] $p < 0.05$.

esophageal function is normalized.[6] Despite persistent reflux, the clinical sign may be mild or even absent, but years later, sequelae of a chronic pathological reflux may become evident. Recent investigations in adults have shown that approximately half of young adults with reflux disease had marked symptoms in their childhood.[7]

2. *The His angle* is an other factor that may have a significant impact on the function of the LES and the incidence of spontaneous relaxations in this age group. In contrast to older children, the His angle in newborns and infants is not sharp but flat, and no mucosal valve can be seen during endoscopy (Figure 50.4). Any increased intragastric pressure after meals is then exerted directly toward the sphincter due to the lack of the mucosal valve mechanism.

3. Finally, it is well known that any *ingested fluid causes reflux* episodes. The largely liquid nutrition (milk) given in infancy is another factor causing frequent refluxes. The number of reflux events is significantly reduced toward the end of the first year as soon as nutrition is in larger quantities and more solid.

SYMPTOMS OF PATHOLOGICAL REFLUX IN NEWBORNS AND INFANTS

Pathological reflux in this age group may be characterized by different symptoms. The most typical reported signs are regurgitation and effortless leak-out of milk or food after meals, between meals, and when asleep. A moist pillow is another sign of reflux. Further symptoms of pathological reflux are restless sleep with sudden wake-up and crying periods. If recurrent vomiting of food is significant, the child may develop malnutrition and failure to thrive.[8–10] Rarely, one may even observe rickets despite seemingly adequate vitamin D supplementation as a consequence of the recurrent vomiting. Further suspicious symptoms are developmental disorders, recurrent respiratory tract infections due to microaspirations, greater irritability, and agitation. Quite often, reflux-related problems in feeding the baby may significantly disturb the interaction between mother and child. However, the clinical symptoms are not reliable indicators of gastroesophageal reflux disease (GERD), and show often a poor correlation with the results of 24-hour pH monitoring or histology.[11]

The most significant complication of GERD is esophagitis, which is caused by too frequent and prolonged relaxations of the LES and chronic acid exposure of the esophagus. The resulting inflammation of the mucosa may cause microbleeding and result in chronic anemia. If the inflammation spreads to deeper layers of the esophageal wall, it may eventually cause stenosis due to simultaneous formation of scars. However, in newborns and infants, as long as the babies are largely fed with milk, the acidic gastric juice is largely buffered during the first 2 hours after feeding (Figure 50.5). Thus, esophagitis is a very rare occurrence in this age group.

DIAGNOSIS OF REFLUX

There are several diagnostic tests to determine pathological reflux. However, in most cases, only a few of them are needed in the newborn age group. It depends on the underlying problem whether or not an extensive diagnosis is needed. In this section, the principal diagnostic tests to determine pathological gastroesophageal reflux will be described.

Radiological investigation of esophageal passage

The primary purpose of barium contrast radiography is to investigate the morphology and peristaltic function of the esophagus. Visualization of the gastroesophageal junction,

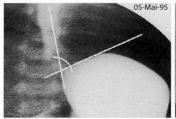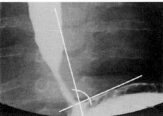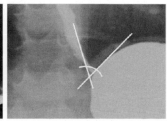

Figure 50.4 Development of the His angle: the diaphragm moves upward with age, and the His angle becomes markedly sharp-angled in this child with a primary GER problem.

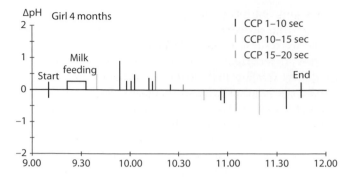

Figure 50.5 Combined manometric study and pH monitoring after a typical milk meal in a 4-month-old child. The lines indicate reflux episodes with a CCP of different duration. The result shows that refluxes are accompanied by a slight pH decrease only 1 hour after feeding.

demonstration of a gliding or fixed hiatus hernia, assessment of the angle of His, the finding of smooth or pathological pharyngoesophageal deglutition, the course of esophageal peristalsis, and any remarkable features in the epithelium as signs of inflammation constitute the most important information that needs be obtained from a radiological investigation. A further finding is evidence of aspiration of contrast medium during the investigation.

In contrast, the actual evidence of reflux is of less importance because radiological exposure time is short and the true extent of reflux may be overestimated or underestimated. Indirect signs of a pathological reflux include air reflux during the investigation and a positive water siphon test (reflux after taking a large sip of water as a reflux provocation), and the height of the reflux events must be documented.[12] This may yield an evaluation scheme that, however, should be used only if it concurs with a 24-hour pH monitoring.

Twenty-four-hour pH monitoring

This investigation is the gold standard to evaluate frequency and duration of acidic refluxes into the esophagus. The thinnest possible glass or antimony electrodes are introduced by the nasal route, and the ongoing pH values are recorded on a battery-driven recorder. Ideally multichannel probes are used, and pH values in the stomach, the lower esophagus, and the upper esophagus are registered. Thus, a pH drop in the esophagus can be correlated with the pH in the stomach, and the number of acidic refluxes that reach the upper esophagus can also be determined.

All pH drops to <4 for at least 15 seconds' duration (number of refluxes), the time required for normalization of pH and/or the increase of pH to 4 (reflux clearance), the number of refluxes with a clearance time of more than 5 minutes, and the longest reflux are evaluated. Intake of food and the time in lying or upright position are also registered. Different Institutions use different *cutoff values*, which are partly influenced by values in adults. We use the threshold values shown in Table 50.3. The low threshold value of 3% used in infants fed largely with milk takes into account the lower number of acidic refluxes during which the pH drops below 4 (Figure 50.5).

The weakness of the method is the fact that it does not demonstrate refluxes with a neutral pH or mildly alkaline refluxes with an increase in pH.

Combined multiple intraluminal impedance/pH monitoring

Combining over 24 hours the multiple intraluminal impedance (MII) technique with pH monitoring allows us to determine all refluxes and the direction of bolus movements. Thus, even neutral and alkaline refluxes can be recorded (Figure 50.6). This provides a much more informative and valuable assessment of a true reflux compared to simple pH monitoring.[13–15] The technique has been shown to be especially useful in postprandial episodes when the reflux is not acidic or only weakly so as it is in milk-fed newborns and small infants.[16] Furthermore ,it is useful to investigate the efficacy of antiacid therapy. MII can detect microaspirations of nonacid refluxes, which may play an important role in recurrent respiratory tract infection. MII recording with pH monitoring doubles the probability of documenting an association between symptoms and reflux when compared with isolated pH monitoring.[17,18] Thus, the combined MII/pH monitoring has already replaced simple pH monitoring and can be seen as the new gold standard for investigation of reflux disease.

Manometry

Manometric investigations of esophageal function were introduced as a diagnostic procedure quite early in the late 1960s, primarily to measure pressure in the LES. It was presumed at the time that low pressures are responsible for reflux. Initial manometric investigations in newborns and infants appeared to confirm this fact.[19] However, only with the introduction of low-perfusion-low-compliance pumps

Table 50.3 Cutoff values in our gastrointestinal lab

Age (years)	pH < 4 (%)	No. of refluxes	Refluxes > 5 min	Reflux number	Clearance
<1	<3%	<30	<5	<50	<1
>1	<5%	<35	<5	<50	<1

Note: The lower pH % value in children under q year of age is the result of the fact that the gastric acidity is neutralized in infants who are mainly fed with milk products (see also Figure 50.5). "Reflux Number" is "Number of refluxes" + ("Number of refluxes > 5 min" times three).

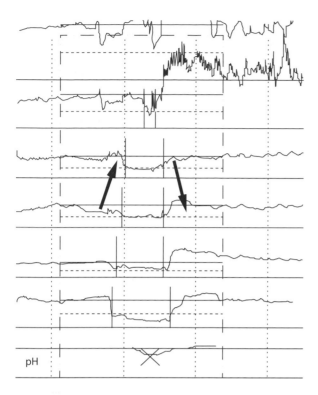

Figure 50.6 Combined impedance and pH monitoring: it shows a short reflux episode with a nonsignificant decrease of the pH in the esophagus, which would not be detected by pH monitoring alone.

did it become possible to obtain reliable pressure values and data.[2]

As mentioned earlier, our investigations performed in the 1970s showed that even at this age, normal pressure values are registered in the LES.[2] Furthermore, manometry is an excellent method to demonstrate the motor function and peristalsis of the esophagus. It shows that reflux of the contents of the stomach occurs during spontaneous transient relaxations of the LES. The manometric sign of these relaxations is the CCP, which is characterized by an increase of the esophageal pressure tracings up to abdominal pressure values and the typical reversal to abdominal pressure fluctuations with respiration (Figure 50.3). Secondary peristalsis causes the refluxed volume to be conveyed back to the stomach. Normalization of the drop in pH is achieved in a stepwise manner by swallowing saliva. In combination with simultaneous pH monitoring, the CCP also allows the investigator to analyze nonacid, neutral, or alkaline refluxes and thus draw conclusions such as those derived from impedance measurement. However, the disadvantage of manometry is that it is a motion-dependent investigation and requires a quiet child. Therefore, it is not suitable as a routine method but is indispensable for scientific questions.

Endoscopy and histology

Investigations with flexible fiber-optic endoscopes and biopsies are invasive investigations but the only way to diagnose

esophagitis. Therefore, they are a part of the standard procedure in older patients with GERD but are rarely needed as a routine procedure for reflux in newborn infants.

Briefly, the endoscope is introduced into the esophagus under visual control and is usually extended down to the duodenum. Biopsies from the duodenum and antrum of the stomach are taken routinely. The tip of the device is inverted in the stomach in order to inspect the gastroesophageal junction from below. Under normal circumstances, the esophagus encloses the device tightly, and the aforementioned flutter valve can be seen at the lateral circumference. In contrast, in a hiatus hernia, the cardia is slightly opened, and the investigator is able to see into the herniated stomach, whereas the LES encircles the device higher up.

By withdrawing the endoscope further, the gastroesophageal junction and the Z-line are inspected exactly. In normal cases, the esophageal epithelium is smooth and milky-red in color (grade 0). In the presence of esophagitis, one may find reddening, swelling (grades 1 and 2), striated erosion (grade 3), deep ulceration (grade 4), or stenosis (grade 5). Mild reddening of the mucosa at the distal esophagus is a normal condition. Grades 0–2 are largely prone to subjective assessment and often do not concur with the histological outcome. Therefore, it is essential to take several biopsy specimens, starting 1–2 cm proximal to the Z-line, upward into the upper esophagus. The quality of the biopsied material is of decisive importance for an accurate histological diagnosis. Therefore, an endoscope with the largest possible external diameter should be used to obtain the best possible material with the largest biopsy forceps. The biopsy specimens should be placed on a piece of cork, correctly oriented immediately after the specimen is taken, and then inserted in formalin. An optimal biopsy specimen should include the entire epithelium as well as the basal-cell layer. Thickening of the basal-cell layer and relative elongation of the papilla (due to a thinner epithelial zone) are signs of increased cell turnover and pathological reflux. Evidence of intraepithelial eosinophils then confirms the presence of obvious esophagitis even in the absence of corresponding symptoms. Erosions and ulcerations are, by nature, signs of severe chronic esophagitis. However, in children, this condition is not always associated with unequivocal symptoms. On the other hand, the presence of more than 20 eosinophils per high-power field is a sign of non-reflux-related allergic/atopic disease, which is also known as eosinophilic esophagitis.

Nuclear medicine investigations

Scintigraphic investigations permit the investigator to observe migration of the bolus through the esophagus, any reflux-related aspiration of nuclear medicine tracer material in the lungs, and the measurement of the time taken to empty the stomach after standardized meals. This consists of a solid and a liquid portion, e.g., an egg dish and water. ^{99m}Tc-labeled sulfur colloid is used as tracer. The act of swallowing is visualized in dynamic sequences. After setting the regions of interest (ROIs), on the one hand, refluxes are registered and on the other hand, the mean time taken to empty the stomach is measured as a time–activity curve. The disadvantage of scinitgraphic study is similar to that of barium radiography: both are short-term investigations that may overdiagnose or underdiagnose reflux numbers. However, a control scan after 24 hours may permit the investigator to document the presence of the tracer in the lung, provided aspiration has occurred in meantime.

CONSERVATIVE THERAPY OF REFLUX DISEASE

A pathological reflux may be considered to exist when the infant has a history of significant regurgitation and flaccid vomiting, suffers from recurrent respiratory tract infections and/or pain, is restless at night, or has other typical symptoms (Table 50.4).[20] As the risk of esophagitis is very low at this age, an endoscopic investigation does not need to be performed if no other indications in consequence of a congenital anomaly are present. In addition to a 24-hour pH monitoring or impedance pH monitoring, a contrast swallow of the esophagus and an ultrasound investigation of the pylorus are usually needed to exclude any pathologies that would hinder spontaneous healing of the reflux disease, such as HH, chronic organoaxial gastric volvulus, gastric stenosis, pylorus hypertrophy, or other anatomic problems.

Since esophageal dysfunction with pathological reflux matures spontaneously in 90% of otherwise normal infants, conservative measurements are the therapy of choice. Former investigations have shown that the prone position with the trunk raised most effectively prevents reflux, because the hiatus is in the highest position.[21] However, the risk of sudden infant death is markedly increased in this position because vomiting during sleep may result in an obstruction of the nose and mouth and cause prolonged apneic spells and sudden infant death syndrome (SIDS). Therefore, the prone position is acceptable if the infant is awake and observed,

Table 50.4 Symptoms that may be associated with gastroesophageal reflux

Symptoms
Recurrent regurgitation with/without vomiting
Weight loss or poor weight gain
Irritability in infants
Ruminative behavior
Wheezing
Stridor
Unexplained recurrent cough

Source: Adapted from Vandenplas Y et al., Pediatric gastroesophageal reflux clinical practice guidelines: Joint recommendations of the North American Society for Pediatric Gastroenterology, Hepatology, and Nutrition (NASPGHAN) and the European Society for Pediatric Gastroenterology, Hepatology, and Nutrition (ESPGHAN), JPGN 2009;49: 498–547.

particularly in the postprandial period. The prone position may be used in children older than 1 year whose risk of SIDS is negligible.[20] Today, the supine position with an elevated trunk or left-side positioning during sleep and elevation of the head of the bed is recommended.[22]

Frequent small-volume meals and thickening of food with rice gruel are recommended and decrease the frequency of regurgitation. There is no clear evidence from the literature that specially manufactured milk formulas are more effective in reducing reflux index scores, but they do reduce vomiting episodes, too.[20,23–25] In most cases, the symptoms abate within the next few months. Prokinetic therapy is not anymore recommended in children.[20]

As mentioned previously, the disappearance of the symptoms does not necessarily mean that there is no more reflux; it might just not reach the mouth. Therefore, at the end of the first year, a control 24-hour impedance/pH monitoring should be performed to definitively exclude persistent reflux.[26,27]

About 10% of these children still have pathological results and need further treatment and controls. In these patients addition of acid-suppressive therapy is usually indicated, e.g., proton pump inhibitors (PPIs). Experience with PPIs in 10 infants with unquietness/pain-related gastroesophageal reflux showed that the number of acidic refluxes was significantly reduced, but the total number of refluxes was unchanged.[28] PPIs only decrease the acidity of refluxate.[29] Thus, vomiting, aspiration during sleep, and chronic respiratory tract infections may still continue, despite PPI therapy. Thus, more studies are needed to determine which infants and children should be treated with PPIs.[20,30] When administering any form of antiacidic medication for the treatment of reflux, one should be aware of the fact that the production of gastric acid is largely reduced, and the consequences on the intestinal flora of infants and children have not been evaluated so far.[20]

Our experience has shown that spontaneous normalization of the esophageal function may still occur beyond the first year, up to the age of 3–4 years, and conservative treatment can be continued if the symptoms are minimal and the parents want to avoid surgery. However, after this time, a spontaneous maturation of the function cannot be expected, and surgical therapy is indicated. It has been shown that in these patients, pathological reflux patterns continue till adulthood.[7] In contrast, it has been shown that preterm birth is associated with esophagitis in childhood, but being small for gestational age is associated with esophagitis even up to adolescence.[31]

SURGICAL THERAPY

As mentioned previously, surgery of reflux is not indicated in most newborns and infants due to the spontaneous maturation of the esophageal function within the first year of life. However, there is a small group of patients in which any trials of conservative therapy are ineffective, even when treated under in-hospital supervision. Additionally, the process of spontaneous normalization of a pathological reflux cannot be expected in babies after correction of an esophageal atresia, diaphragmatic hernia, congenital HH, or even upside-down stomach, organoaxial gastric volvulus, and some other congenital anomalies. In these children, surgical procedures are indicated in order to avoid the long-term sequelae of unphysiologic neutralization of gastric acid with PPIs, which are problematic.

The strategic principles of reflux surgery consist of creating an intra-abdominal portion of the esophagus and a complete (Nissen) or partial plication (dorsal Toupet, ventral Thal) of the gastric fundus around the esophagus.[32] The standard approach today is by laparoscopy, showing a low recurrence rate (3%) during long-term follow-up.[33] Recurrence rate increases up to 12% in children with neurological impairment, esophageal atresia, or congenital diaphragmatic hernia.[34] Therefore, Hassall[35] recommends treatment with PPI as a safe alternative to surgery in many cases.

In fact, recurrent reflux has been observed with all three surgical methods (Table 50.2).[36–38] It is related to the natural agitation in this region due to the movement of the diaphragm during respiration and due to the significant shortening of the esophagus that occurs during swallowing.[39] Further risk factors for recurrence are severe rumination and regurgitation, which occur in some cerebral-handicapped children.[40] Rare complications after a Nissen procedure may occur in patients with a rather tight fundoplication and the inability to vomit, gas bloat syndrome, or dumping.

A rarely used method that might be useful in a patient with a very small stomach is the Collis gastroplasty, for which the His angle is deepened parallel to the esophagus with a stapler. The lengthened fundus is then used for a Nissen, Toupet, or Thal plication around the elongated esophagus.

The gastroesophageal dissection is an other method that is useful in rare cases of severely cerebral-handicapped infants with massive rumination and recurrent GERD.[41] The esophagus is detached from the stomach and anastomosed to a Roux-en-Y jejunal loop. Orally ingested food is thus diverted directly into the jejunum, and recurrent reflux or rumination is rendered impossible.[42]

In the last few years, a number of new technical methods have been introduced for the treatment of reflux in adults, such as creation of a mucosal fold by an intraluminal stapler, radio-wave damage of the cardia (Stretta procedure), or endoscopic submucosal injection of foreign material (Enteryx). Experiences in children are rare, and long-term results are lacking.[43–46]

SPECIAL PROBLEMS OF REFLUX IN THE NEWBORN AND INFANT

Laryngopharyngeal reflux

Chronic microaspiration of acidic reflux during the day and/or night may cause laryngeal symptoms such as hoarseness, the urge to cough, and dysphagia. Each endoscopic investigation is incomplete if the larynx is not inspected. Reddening, ulcerations, or pseudopolyps on the vocal cords are typical signs of laryngeal reflux. However, as mentioned previously, these findings are very rare in this age group as long as the babies are mainly fed with milk. As regards therapy, medication with PPIs is recommended to prevent contact of gastric acid with the laryngeal folds.

Reflux-associated infections of the respiratory tract

Aspiration of acidic or nonacidic reflux may be the cause of recurrent respiratory tract infections and pneumonia. Other causes such as cystic fibrosis, aspirated foreign bodies, H-type fistulas, or other malformations of the respiratory tract must be excluded. In cerebral-handicapped children, disruption of the pharyngoesophageal transport—disturbed swallowing—is another well-known cause of recurrent aspiration.

Diagnosis is not simple, except when the radiological investigation shows aspiration of the contrast material during reflux phases. Neither bronchoalveolar lavage nor nuclear medicine investigations are unequivocal. Twenty-four-hour combined MII/pH monitoring with several recording points along the esophagus provides indirect signs when a large number of refluxes extends into the upper esophagus.[47] If evidence of recurrent reflux-associated aspiration and chronic unexplained cough is obtained, surgery is indicated.

Reflux and apnea syndrome

Apnea and SIDS are the most common causes of death between the ages of 2–6 months. The association of reflux with apneic spells has been investigated, with unequivocal results.[48] Some studies have not proved a temporal relationship between GER and apneas.[49,50] Although an increased rate of GER was observed after feeding in preterm infants, a corresponding increase of apneic spells was not found. Our investigations with manometry and pH monitoring in infants with pathological sleep apneas have not shown that acidic refluxes are directly causing apneic spells. However, we did register a markedly delayed maturation of motor function of the esophagus in babies with sleep apnea or apparent life-threatening events (ALTEs).[5] Further studies have shown that infants investigated due to a pathologic sleep-apneic pattern frequently also have pathological reflux, whereas infants with a primary history of pathological reflux have no remarkable apneic spells.[51] These investigations support the hypothesis that infants with sleep apnea syndrome or ALTE suffer from a deeper localized underlying immaturity of regulation centers in the brain stem, while the causes for a delay in the maturation of the esophageal motor function are localized in higher brain stem regions and therefore not necessarily associated with disorders of respiratory regulation.[2]

Hiatal hernia

Any upward gliding of portions of the stomach into or above the esophageal hiatus are called hiatal hernia. A gliding HH is rare in newborns and infants, but one cannot expect a spontaneous normalization of this anatomic malformation. The previously used term *forme mineure* for minimal HH in infants is not anymore considered a pathology but is known as a normal finding of the special anatomy of the gastroesophageal junction in this age group.

Paraesophageal hernias are not-so-rare findings after fundoplication. A part of the stomach slips through the hiatus into the chest, lateral to the gastroesophageal junction. If a small postoperative paraesophageal hernia is combined with reflux or any other symptoms, surgical correction is indicated. A congenital form of paraesophageal hernia is the upside-down stomach in the newborn, which is a more or less complete displacement of the stomach into the chest while the gastroesophageal junction remains in normal position.

Esophageal atresia and diaphragmatic hernia

The lower segment of the esophagus in patients with esophageal atresia is characterized by an abnormal or absent propulsive peristalsis.[52] Due to the absent peristalsis, refluxed material remains for a prolonged time in the esophagus, and volume as well as acid clearance are significantly prolonged, especially during sleep. The long acid clearance time may cause already in this age group a chronic esophagitis. A spontaneous normalization of the pathology cannot be expected; therefore, surgical correction is usually necessary.

Children with congenital diaphragmatic hernia suffer often from a pathological reflux due to the abnormal anatomy of the gastro–esophageal–diaphragmatic anatomy.[53,54] Early fundoplication is indicated because a spontaneous normalization of the disturbed function cannot be expected.

REFLUX IN NEUROLOGICALLY IMPAIRED CHILDREN

In patients with severe neurological impairment, GERD is a common disorder that may lead to a number of complications such as esophagitis, esophageal stenosis, anemia, and/or Barrett esophagus. Although these symptoms usually become clinically evident only in later childhood, vomiting, recurrent respiratory tract infections, as well as failure to thrive are, in small babies, are strong indicators that the underlying pathology is accompanied by a significant reflux problem.[55] Manometric studies show that these children suffer not from a sphincter insufficiency but from too many spontaneous LES relaxations. These findings support again the hypothesis that pathological reflux is strongly connected with a dysfunction of the regulation centers in the brain. Whether conservative therapy including PPIs, a fundoplication (with or without a button gastrostomy), or an esophagogastric dissection is needed has to be decided on an individual basis considering the living quality and circumstances of the child.

CONCLUSION

GER is common in neonates and small infants. It is caused in most cases not by an insufficient LES but by a delay in the development of the esohageal function characterized by many spontaneous relaxations of the LES. In more than 90% of babies, a spontaneous maturation of the esophageal function can be expected till the end of the first year of life, and therefore, unspecific conservative measurements are usually sufficient. In contrast, babies with severe and recurrent complications of reflux, e.g., recurrent respiratory tract infections, and/or congenital malformations usually need surgical therapy by semicircular or complete fundoplication.

REFERENCES

1. Edwards DAW. The anti-reflux mechanism, its disorders and their consequences. *Clin Gastroenterol* 1982; 11: 479–96.
2. Höllwarth ME. Development of oesophageal motility in newborns—A manometric investigation. *Z Kinderchirurgie* 1979; 27 (3): 201–15.
3. Höllwarth ME, Uray E, Pesendorfer P. Esophageal manometry. *Ped Surg Int* 1986, 1: 177–83.
4. Omari TI, Barnett CP, Benninga MA et al. Mechanisms of gastroesophageal reflux in preterm and term infants with reflux disease. *Gut* 2002; 51: 475–9.
5. Landler U, Höllwarth ME, Uray E et al. Esophageal function in infants with sudden infant death risk. *Klin Pädiatr* 1990; 202: 37–42.
6. Pesendorfer P, Höllwarth ME, Uray, E. Long-term follow-up of infants with gastroesophageal reflux. *Klin Pädiatr* 1993; 205: 363–6.
7. El-Serag HB, Gilger M, Carter J et al. Childhood GERD is a risk factor for GERD in adolescents and young adults. *Am Gastroenterol* 2004; 99: 806–12.
8. Rudolph CD, Mazur LJ, Liptak GS et al. Guidelines for evaluation and treatment of gastroesophageal reflux in infants and children: Recommendations of the North American Society for Pediatric Gastroenterology and Nutrition. *JPGN* 2001; 32 Suppl. 2: S1–31.
9. Birch JL, Newell SJ. Gastrooesophageal reflux disease in preterm infants: Current management and diagnostic dilemmas. *Arch Dis Child Fetal Neonatal Ed* 2009; 94: F379–83.
10. Vandenplas Y, Salvatore S, Hauser, B. The diagnosis and management of gastro-oesophageal reflux in infants. *Early Hum Dev* 2005; 81: 1011–24.

11. Salvatore S, Hauser B, Vandemaele K et al. Gastroesophageal reflux disease in infants: How much is predictable with questionnaires, pH-metry, endoscopy and histology? *J Pediatr Gastroenterol Nutr* 2005; 40: 210–5.

12. Fotter R, Höllwarth ME, Uray E. Correlation between manometric and roentgenologic findings of diseases of the esophagus in infants and children. *Prog Ped Surg* 1985; 18: 14–21.

13. Vandenplas Y, Salvator S, Devreker T et al. Gastro-oesophageal reflux disease: Oesophageal impedance versus pH monitoring. *Acta Paediatr* 2007; 96: 956–62.

14. Sifrim D, Castell D, Dent J et al. Gastro-oesophageal reflux monitoring: Review and consensus report on detection and definitions of acid, non-acid, and gas reflux. *Gut* 2004; 53: 1024–31.

15. López-Alonso M, Moya MJ, Cabo JA. Twenty-four-hour esophageal impedance-pH monitoring in healthy preterm neonates: Rate and characteristics of acid, weakly acidic, and weakly alkaline gastroesophageal reflux. *Pediatrics* 2006; 118: e299–308.

16. Vandenplas Y. Challenges in the diagnosis of gastroesophageal reflux disease in infants and children. *Expert Opin Med Diagn* 2013; 7: 2–11.

17. Salvatore S, Arrigo S, Luini C et al. Esophageal impedance in children: Symptom-based results. *J Pediatr* 2010; 157: 949–54.

18. Wenzl TG, Bennigna MA, Loots CM et al. Indications, methodology, and interpretation of combined esophageal impedance-pH monitoring in children: ESPGHAN EURO-PIG Standard Protocol. *JPGN* 2012; 55: 230–4.

19. Boix-Ochoa J, Canals J. Maturation of the lower esophagus. *J Pediatr Surg* 1976; 11(5): 749–56.

20. Vandenplas Y, Rudolph CD, Di Lorenzo C et al. Pediatric gastroesophageal reflux clinical practice guidelines: Joint recommendations of the North American Society for Pediatric Gastroenterology, Hepatology, and Nutrition (NASPGHAN) and the European Society for Pediatric Gastroenterology, Hepatology, and Nutrition (ESPGHAN). *JPGN* 2009; 49: 498–547.

21. Herbst JJ. Gastroesophageal reflux and pulmonary diseases. *Pediatrics* 1981; 68(1): 132–4.

22. Corvaglia L, Rotatori R, Ferlini M et al. The effect of body positioning on gastroesophageal reflux in premature infants: Evaluation by combined impedance and pH monitoring. *J Pediatr* 2007; 151: 591–6.

23. Horvath A, Dziechciarz P, Szajewska H. The effect of thickened-feed interventions on gastroesophageal reflux in infants: Systematic review and meta-analysis of randomized, controlled trials. *Pediatrics* 2008; 112 (6): c1268–77

24. Carroll AE, Garrison MM, Christakis DA. A systematic review of nonpharmacological and nonsurgical therapies for gastroesophageal reflux in infants. *Arch Pediatr Adolesc Med* 2002; 156: 109–13.

25. Huang RC, Forges DA, Davies MW. Feed thickener for newborn infants with gastro-oesophageal reflux. *Cochrane Database Syst Rev* 2002; 3: CD003211.

26. Orenstein SR, Shalaby TM, Kelsey SF et al. Natural history of infant reflux esophagitis: Symptoms and morphometric histology during one year without pharmacotherapy. *Am J Gastroenterol* 2006; 101 (3): 628–40.

27. Gold BD. Is gastroesophageal reflux diseases really a life-long disease: Do babies who regurgitate grow up to be adults with GERD complications? *Am J Gastroenterol* 2006; 101: 641–4.

28. Catellani C, Huber-Zeiringer A, Bachmaier G et al. Proton pump inhibitors for reflux therapy in infants: Effectiveness determined by impedance pH monitoring. *Pediatr Surg Int* 2014; 30: 381–5.

29. Turk H, Hauser B, Brecelj J et al. Effect of proton pump inhibition on acid, weakly acid and weakly alkaline gastro-esophageal reflux in children. *World J Pediatr* 2013; 9: 36–41.

30. Rudolph CD. Are proton pump inhibitors indicated for the treatment of gastroesophageal reflux in infants and children? *JPGN* 2003; 37 (Suppl.): S60–4.

31. Forsell L, Cnattingius S, Bottai M et al. Risk of esophagitis among individuals born preterm and small for gestational age. *Clin Gastroenterol Hepatol* 2012; 10: 1369–75.

32. Pacilli M, Chowdhury MM, Pierro A. The surgical treatment of gastro-esophageal reflux in neonates and infants. *Semin Pediatr Surg* 2005; 14: 34–41.

33. Leung L, Wong CWY, Chung PHY et al. Laparoscopic Nissen fundoplication for gastro-esophageal reflux disease in infants. *Pediatr Surg Int* 2015; 31: 83–8.

34. Lopes-Fernandez S, Hernandez F, Hernandez-Martin S et al. Failed Nissen fundoplication in children: Causes and management. *Eur J Pediatr Surg* 2014; 24: 79–82.

35. Hassall, E. Outcomes of fundoplication: Causes for concern, newer options. *Arch Dis Child* 2005; 90: 1047–52.

36. Fonkalsrud EW, Ashcraft KW, Coran AG et al. Surgical treatment of gastroesophageal reflux in children: A combined hospital study of 7467 patients. *Pediatrics* 1998; 101 (3 Pt 1): 419–22.

37. Dall Vecchia LK, Grosfeld JL, West KW et al. Reoperation after Nissen fundoplication in children with gastroesophageal reflux: Experience with 130 patients. *Ann Surg* 1997; 226(3): 315–21.

38. Lundell L, Miettinen P, Myrvold HE et al. Comparison of outcomes twelve years after antireflux surgery or omeprazole maintenance therapy for reflux esophagitis. *Clin Gastroenterol Hepatol* 2009; 7: 1292–8.

39. Dodds WJ, Dent J, Hogan WJ et al. Mechanisms of gastroesophageal reflux in patients with reflux esophagitis. *N Engl J Med* 1982; 307: 1547–52.

40. Gössler A, Huber-Zeyringer A, Höllwarth ME. Recurrent gastroesophageal reflux in neurologically impaired patients after fundoplication. *Acta Paediatr* 2007; 96: 87–93.

41. Bianchi A. Total esophagogastric dissociation: An alternative approach. *J Pediatr Surg* 1997; 32(9): 1291–4.

42. Morabito A, Lall A, Lo Piccolo R et al. Total esophagogastric dissociation: 10 years' review. *J Pediatr Surg* 2006; 41(5): 919–22.

43. Katz PO. Gastroesophageal reflux disease: New treatments. *Rev Gastroenterol Disord* 2002; 2(2): 66–74.

44. Liu DC, Somme S, Mavrelis PG et al. Stretta as the initial antireflux procedure in children. *J Pediatr Surg* 2005; 40(1): 148–51.

45. Johnson DA. Endoscopic therapy for GERD—Baking, sewing, or stuffing: An evidence-based perspective. *Rev Gastroenterol Disord* 2003; 3(3): 142–9.

46. Johnson DA. Enteryx for gastroesophageal reflux disease. *Expert Rev Med Dev* 2005; 2(1): 19–26.

47. Blondeau K, Mertens V, Dupont L et al. The relationship between gastroesophageal reflux and cough in children with chronic unexplained cough using combined Impedance-pH–manometry recordings. *Pediatr Pulmonol* 2011; 46: 286–94.

48. Slocum C, Hibbs AM, Martin RJ et al. Infant apnea and gastroesophageal reflux: A critical review and framework for further investigation. *Curr Gastroenterol Rep* 2007; 9: 219–24.

49. Peter CS, Sprodowksi N, Bohnhorst B et al. Gastroesophageal reflux and apnea of prematurity: No temporal relationship. *Pediatrics* 2002; 109: 8–11.

50. Di Fiore JM, Arko M, Whitehouse M et al. Apnea is not prolonged by acid gastroesophageal reflux in preterm infants. *Pediatrics* 2005; 116: 1059–63.

51. Kurz R, Höllwarth ME, Fasching M et al. Combined disturbance of respiratory regulation and esophageal function in early infancy. *Prog Ped Surg* 1985; 18: 52–61.

52. Höllwarth ME. Gastroesophageal reflux disease. In: Coran AG, Adzick NS, Krummel TM, Laberge J-M, Shamberger RC, Caldamone AA (eds). *Pediatric Surgery*. Philadelphia: Elsevier/Saunders. 2012: 947–58.

53. Fasching G, Huber A, Uray E et al. Gastroesophageal reflux and diaphragmatic motility after repair of congenital diaphragmatic hernia. *Eur J Pediatr Surg* 2000; 10(6): 360–4.

54. Caruso AM, Di Pace MR, Catalano P et al. Gastroesophageal reflux in patients treated for congenital diaphragmatic hernia: Short- and long-term evaluation with multichannel intraluminal impedance. *Pediatr Surg Int* 2013; 29: 553–9.

55. Gössler A, Schalamon J, Huber-Zeyringer A et al. Gastroesophageal reflux and behavior in neurologically impaired children. *J Ped Surg* 2007; 42: 1486–90.

Gastrointestinal

51

Pyloric atresia and prepyloric antral diaphragm

ALESSIO PINI PRATO, VINCENZO JASONNI, AND GIROLAMO MATTIOLI

PYLORIC ATRESIA

Introduction

Gastric outlet obstruction in the newborn may be due to pyloric atresia (PA), antral web, or hypertrophic pyloric stenosis. The latter is most common cause of gastric outlet obstruction.

PA is a rare congenital malformation representing less than 1% of all atresias and diaphragms involving the gastrointestinal tract.[1–3] Up to 50% of these patients have associated abnormalities, of which epidermolysis bullosa (EB) is by far the most common.[1,4–6] Familial occurrence of PA has been reported.[5–7] In particular, Puri and coworkers[7] first described PA in three consecutive siblings in a family.

Etiology

Though a sure etiology is still unknown, mucosal desquamation leading to gastric outlet obstruction has been suggested to play a role, mainly in patients with associated EB.[8] Junctional epidermolysis bullosa (junctional EB) associated with pyloric atresia (EB-PA: "OMIM [Online Mendelian Inheritance in Man]" 226730) represents a rare congenital disorder also known as Carmi syndrome, named after the author who described, in 1982, the association of aplasia cutis and PA[9] and, later on, in 1998, suggested the existence of an autosomal recessive inherited disease including EB, PA, and aplasia cutis congenita,[10] in which mucocutaneous fragility is associated with congenital gastric outlet obstruction. This association is usually fatal during the first few weeks or months of life, even following surgical correction of intestinal obstruction. Mutations in the genes encoding α6β4 integrin (ITGA6 and ITGB4 genes) and plectin (PLEC gene) have been identified in a number of patients with EB-PA.[8,11–13] Regardless of whether or not it is associated with epidermolysis, several authors agreed that there is strong evidence to support an autosomal recessive model of inheritance for PA.[14,15]

Pathology

There are three main different types of pyloric obstruction: (1) type A, pyloric membrane or web; (2) type B, longitudinal segmental atresia (i.e., pylorus replaced by fibrotic tissue); and (3) type C, PA with a gap between the stomach and the duodenum (Figure 51.1). Table 51.1 shows the incidence of different types of pyloric obstruction.[2,3]

History and physical examination

Prenatal diagnosis of PA can be suspected when polyhydramnios is present and associated with a dilated stomach. Prenatal diagnosis of PA and EB can be performed in pregnancies at risk for recurrence of this syndrome. However, some sonographic signs suggest the possibility of significant cutaneous desquamation and blister formation in a fetus, especially when there is positive amniotic acetylcholinesterase coupled with elevated alphafetoprotein.[16] Since 2009, prenatal magnetic resonance imaging (MRI) has been used to confirm the diagnosis, but its utility remains unclear.[17,18]

Presentation

The newborn with complete pyloric obstruction presents shortly after birth with persistent nonbilious vomiting and epigastric distension.[19] There is no significant gender predominance, and there is a high proportion of infants with low birth weight.[5,20,21] Recently, Al-Salem and coworkers[5] reported an incidence of over 65% of prematurity in a series of 20 patients with PA.[5] Respiratory problems are common, and dyspnea, tachypnea, cyanosis, and/or excessive salivation may suggest esophageal atresia.[22] Scattered reports of the association between PA and esophageal atresia have been described.[23,24]

Delayed diagnosis of PA can determine gastric perforation, although this complication has also been reported as early as 12 hours postdelivery.[25] See Table 51.2 for clinical features.[2,3]

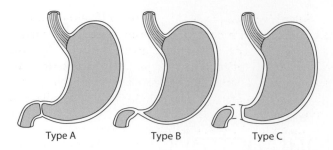

Figure 51.1 Anatomical varieties of congenital pyloric obstruction: type A—membranous pyloric obstruction; type B—longitudinal segmental atresia; type C—pyloric aplasia.

Table 51.1 Incidence of the different pyloric atresia types (n = 140)

Type of atresia	n	%
Membranous (type A)	77 cases	57
Atresia (type B)	46 cases	34
Aplasia (type C)	12 cases	9
No data	5 cases	3.5

Source: Data from Muller M et al., Pyloric atresia: Report of four cases and review of the literature, Pediatr Surg Int 1990; 5:276–9.

Diagnosis

A plain x-ray of the abdomen will usually confirm the clinical diagnosis. X-ray (Figure 51.2) will show a severely dilated stomach without air below.[26] Contrast study, although unnecessary, will confirm complete obstruction at the pyloric region. The radiological diagnosis is based on the identification of three radiological signs: the single gas bubble sign, the absence of beak sign (typical of hypertrophic pyloric stenosis), and the presence of the pyloric dimple sign on a contrast study.[27] The single gas bubble sign is not specific to the diagnosis of PA, but it is an indicator of a gastric outlet obstruction. The ultrasonographic examination can be helpful and demonstrates the absence of normal pyloric muscle and canal, which is specific for the diagnosis of this entity.[27]

Management

Depending on the type of pyloric obstruction, different operative procedures are used. The best results from operative treatment of membranous obstruction are obtained by excision of the membrane associated to pyloroplasty according to Heineke–Mikulicz or Finney.[1–4] Transgastric excision of the pyloric membrane without pyloroplasty has also been reported.[28] In case of longitudinal segmental atresia, the operative method depends on the length of the atresia. When the atresia is short, a Finney pyloroplasty can be carried out. For longer atresia, the procedure of choice is excision and end-to-end gastroduodenostomy.[4] Gastrojejunostomy is not recommended, due to the high mortality rate[4] and because of the risk of marginal ulcer and blind loop syndrome.

Table 51.2 Clinical features of pyloric atresia (n = 140 patients)

Symptoms and signs	Occurrence (%)
Bile-free vomiting	100
Single stomach bubble (one bubble) on x-ray	98
Distended epigastrium	68
Polyhydramnios	63
Birth weight <2500 g	53
Prematurity	45
Jaundice	21
Peristaltic movements in the epigastrium	18
Hemorrhagic vomiting	12

Source: Data from Muller M et al., Pyloric atresia: Report of four cases and review of the literature, Pediatr Surg Int 1990; 5:276–9.

Preoperative management

Usually, newborns are referred to the hospital and admitted within the first 48 hours of life. They are generally in good physical condition, except those with EB. Preoperative preparation should consist of gastric decompression by nasogastric tube insertion. An intravenous infusion should be started to correct dehydration, electrolyte imbalance, and metabolic alkalosis observed in most cases. A central

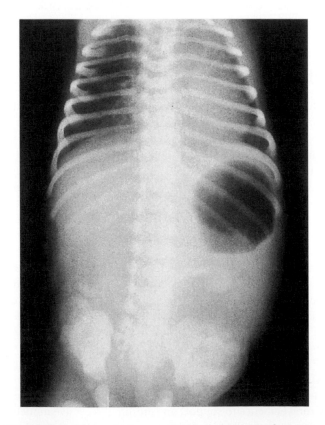

Figure 51.2 Abdominal x-ray showing absence of air beyond the stomach.

line should be inserted to administrate parenteral nutrition and long-term medical treatment specifically in those newborns with associated EB.

Operative technique

LAPAROTOMY

A transverse abdominal incision is made 2 cm above the umbilicus, starting just left of the midline and leading to the right in a skin crease for about 5 cm (Figure 51.3a). The abdominal cavity is opened in the line of the incision. Careful exploration and search of other intestinal atresias are performed at this site.[15]

IDENTIFICATION OF THE SITE OF OBSTRUCTION

During the procedure, it may become difficult to identify the exact disease; therefore, a gastrotomy can be helpful in this regard.[19] Another way to find the exact location of the web and prevent the gastrotomy can be achieved by placing a firm 12–14 Ch. nasogastric tube, to be advanced up to the region of the obstruction.[29]

PYLOROPLASTY

This procedure is indicated for membranous pyloric obstruction (type A) and short atresia (type B).[4,7,14]

After identification of the pylorus, a longitudinal incision is made with cutting diathermy or scissors, starting on the gastric side of the pylorus to the duodenum (Figure 51.3b). A blunt dissecting forceps, which is inserted into the lumen, is useful at this stage. Care must be taken that no inadvertent damage is done to the posterior wall of the stomach or duodenum. The total length of the incision should be 1.5–2 cm, extending approximated 1 cm on the gastric side and 1–1.5 cm on the duodenal side of the pylorus; it should be preformed on the midline between the greater and lesser curvatures of the stomach and superior and inferior borders of the duodenum. The greater length on the gastric side is necessary because of the thicker gastric wall in order to properly align both margins of the incision in the transverse direction. The membrane is excised circumferentially and the mucosa approximated with 5-0 absorbable sutures (Figure 51.3c). The duodenal lumen is inspected, and a catheter is pushed down to exclude further distal atresias. The longitudinal incision is then closed transversely in layers after meticulous hemostasis (Figure 51.3d).

CLOSURE OF ABDOMEN

Gastrostomy is not strictly necessary but can be considered in certain instances. In particular, it could be beneficial for

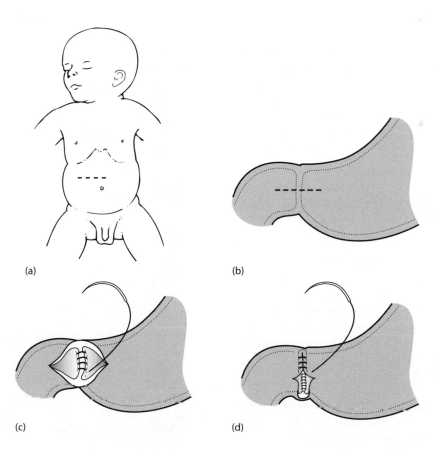

(a)

(b)

(c)

(d)

Figure 51.3 Operative technique of pyloroplasty. **(a)** Skin incision. **(b)** Pyloric longitudinal incision. **(c)** Incision of the membrane and suture. **(d)** Longitudinal incision closed transversely.

patients with EB-PA in order to avoid the need for prolonged nasogastric tube maintenance. The abdomen is closed in two layers, and the nasogastric tube is left in the stomach for decompression.

LAPAROSCOPIC APPROACH

To date, only Son and Hoan[30] have reported a complete laparoscopic treatment of a newborn with EB-PA. The authors described a successful and satisfactory outcome and suggested laparoscopy as an alternative option to the conventional laparotomic procedure. Although newborns have high sensitivity to insufflation, pneumoperitoneum is usually well tolerated provided that CO_2 pressure is maintained below 8 mmHg.[31] An advantage of laparoscopy in case of EB-PA is the reduced wall trauma and subsequent lower likelihood to develop mucocutaneous lesions related to junctional EB.

Postoperative management

Parenteral nutrition should be discontinued when the patient tolerates oral feeding well. A nasogastric tube should be kept in the site for 2–3 days to maintain gastric decompression or even longer if there are signs of delayed gastric emptying. Intravenous broad-spectrum antibiotics are administered intraoperatively and should be discontinued after 3–5 days, according to the patient's condition.

Complications

Complications are uncommon but include strictures, leakage, adhesions, infections, and bleeding as with any other abdominal surgery. Wound dehiscence and/or infection can occur, particularly in patients with EB.

Long-term results

Early diagnosis and surgical intervention with adequate neonatal supportive care significantly improve the survival of pure PA. Mortality has been associated with delayed diagnosis,[12,13] but it is mainly due to the associated malformation. Survival and long-term results are excellent in isolated forms of PA. Mortality rate ranges between 20% and 60%, and the majority of fatal cases are those with EB and/or other multiple intestinal atresia.[5,6,24,32] On the grounds of these considerations, Rosenbloom and Ranter[33] suggested a nonoperative management of PA, unless the skin disease is responsive to treatment. On the other hand, Hayashi et al.[34] reported long-term survival in four out of five patients with EB-PA. A comprehensive review from Dank and coworkers in 1999[35] reported that 51 out of 70 patients with EB-PA had been operated on worldwide, with a long-term survival of roughly 31%. Not surprisingly, survival was mainly observed in patients with mild forms of epidermolysis.

PREPYLORIC ANTRAL DIAPHRAGM

Introduction and etiology

Prepyloric antral diaphragm is a rare anomaly involving a submucosal web of gastric tissue covered by gastric mucosa and found in the distal gastric antrum. A total of about 150 cases have been reported, divided between pediatric and adult age ranges.[36] Reports have suggested both acquired and congenital forms, citing epidemiological and histological evidence.[37]

Pathology

There are three groups of patients: a neonatal group with complete or partial obstruction, a group presenting later in childhood, and a group not diagnosed until later in life.[38] Significant associated abnormalities are noted in about 30% of children with antral web, including Down syndrome, gastrointestinal issues, and cardiovascular malformations.[37,39]

History, presentation, and diagnosis

In the neonatal group, nonbilious vomiting is the predominant presenting symptom. Other symptoms include apnea, cyanosis, and no weight gain.[38] Older children complain of abdominal pain, vomiting, fullness after eating, and bloating. Prolonged retention of foreign bodies can lead to the diagnosis is older children.[40] In the elderly group, the clinical history consists of episodic cramping, epigastric pain or fullness following meals, and intermittent vomiting. There is one report describing a case diagnosed in the eighth decade of life.[41]

The diagnosis of antral web with a central aperture is with a barium meal in 90% of cases.[37] The typical appearance of a web in an infant is a thin, membranous septum, projecting into the antral lumen, perpendicular to its longitudinal axis 1–2 cm proximal to the pylorus (Figure 51.4a).

Gastroscopy has recently been noted to be of use in confirming clinical and radiological evidence of the web in

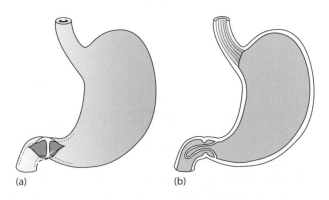

(a)   (b)

Figure 51.4 **(a)** Prepyloric antral web. **(b)** Wind-sock antral membrane protruding into the duodenum.

older infants and in children.[42] Features of the web include the following:

- A small fixed central aperture surrounded by gastric mucosa that is smooth and devoid of folds.
- No change in the opening size of the web with peristalsis.
- The gastric wall proximal and distal to the web is seen to contract normally.[43]

Management

Preoperative and postoperative management does not significantly differ from that of PA. Surgery for partially obstructing antral web consists of excision of the web, combined with pyloroplasty if the web is very close to the pylorus (same as PA). Furthermore, at operation, it is important to pass a Foley catheter distally to the stomach, and then to inflate the balloon and withdraw the catheter.[29] Wind-sock pyloric and antral membranes protruding into the duodenum have been reported (Figure 51.4b) and would be missed at laparotomy by simple inspection of the gastric lumen.[44] Other methods are reported. Most noticeably, some reports described successful endoscopic transection using a standard papillotome[45] and forceful dilatation of antral membrane without pyloroplasty.[46] Recently, Bing and coworkers reported successful laparoscopic-assisted treatment of prepyloric webs in a series of three infants who were treated by gastrostomy and resection.[47] No similar reports have been published so far.

Medical treatment has been reported with success in infants without pronounced obstruction.[48] While this concept of conservative management is supported by some surgeons, the majority of the literature preferred the surgical correction of this entity, which will reduce and prevent morbidity and unnecessary counseling in this group of babies and children.[4,36]

Complications and long-term results

Complications do not significantly differ from those of isolated PA.

REFERENCES

1. Dessanti A, Iannuccelli M, Dore A et al. Pyloric atresia: An attempt at anatomic pyloric sphincter reconstruction. *J Pediatr Surg* 2000; 35: 1372–4.
2. Muller M, Morger R, Engert J. Pyloric atresia: Report of four cases and review of the literature. *Pediatr Surg Int* 1990; 5: 276–9.
3. Dillon WP, Cilley RE. *Congenital Gastric outlet Obstruction in Ashcraft's Pediatric Surgery*, 3rd edn. Philadelphia, PA: WB Saunders Company, 2000: 394–5.
4. Hall WH, Read RC. Gastric acid secretory differences in patients with Heineke–Mikulicz and Finney pyloroplasties. *Am J Dig Dis* 1975; 20: 947–50.
5. Al-Salem AH, Abdulla MR, Kothari MR, Naga MI. Congenital pyloric atresia, presentation, management, and outcome: A report of 20 cases. *J Pediatr Surg* 2014 July; 49(7): 1078–82.
6. Al-Salem AH. Congenital pyloric atresia and associated anomalies. *Pediatr Surg Int* 2007 June; 23(6): 559–63.
7. Puri P, Guiney EJ, Carroll R. Multiple gastro-intestinal atresias in three consecutive siblings: Observations on pathogenesis. *J Pediatr Surg* 1985; 20: 22–4.
8. Mellerio JE, Pulkkimen L, McMillan JR et al. Pyloric atresia—Junctional epidermolysis bullosa syndrome: Mutations in the integrin bega4 gene (ITGB4) in two unrelated patients with mild diseases. *Br J Dermatol* 1998; 139: 862–71.
9. Carmi R, Sofer S, Karplus M, Ben-Yakar Y, Mahler D, Zirkin H, Bar-Ziv J. Aplasia cutis congenita in two sibs discordant for pyloric atresia. *Am J Med Genet* 1982; 11(3): 319–28.
10. Maman E, Maor E, Kachko L, Carmi R. Epidermolysis bullosa, pyloric atresia, aplasia cutis congenita: Histopathological delineation of an autosomal recessive disease. *Am J Med Genet* 1998; 78(2): 127–33.
11. Mencía A, García M, García E et al. Identification of two rare and novel large deletions in ITGB4 gene causing epidermolysis bullosa with pyloric atresia. *Exp Dermatol* 2016; 25(4): 269–74.
12. Dellambra E, Prislei S, Salvati AL et al. Gene correction of integrin beta 4–dependent pyloric atresia epidermolysis bullosa keratinocytes establishes a role for beta 4 tyrosines 1422 and 1440 in hemidesmosome assembly. *J Biol Chem* 2001; 44: 41336–42.
13. Nakano A, Pulkkinen L, Murrell D et al. Epidermolysis bullosas with congenital pyloric atresia: Novel mutations in the beta 4 integrin gene (ITGB4) and genotype/phenotype correlations. *Pediatr Res* 2001; 49: 618–26.
14. Bar-Maor JA, Nissan S, Nevo S. Pyloric atresia. *J Pediatr Surg* 1972; 20: 22–4.
15. El Shafie M, Stidham GL, Klippel CH et al. Pyloric atresia and epidermolysis bullosa letalis: A lethal combination in two premature newborn siblings. *J Pediatr Surg* 1979; 14: 446–9.
16. Lapinard C, Descampo P, Menegurri G et al. Prenatal diagnosis of pyloric atresia—Junctional epidermolysis bullosa syndrome in a fetus not known to be at risk. *Prenat Diagn* 2000; 20: 60–75.
17. Yu DC, Voss SD, Javid PJ, Jennings RW, Weldon CB. In utero diagnosis of congenital pyloric atresia in a single twin using MRI and ultrasound. *J Pediatr Surg* 2009 November; 44(11): e21–4.
18. Merrow AC, Frischer JS, Lucky AW. Pyloric atresia with epidermolysis bullosa: Fetal MRI diagnosis with postnatal correlation. *Pediatr Radiol* 2013; 43(12): 1656–61.

19. Ducharme JC, Benoussan AL. Pyloric atresia. *J Pediatr Surg* 1975; 10: 149–50.
20. Kume K, Ikeda K, Hayashida Y et al. Congenital pyloric atresia: A report of three cases and review of literature. *Jpn J Pediatr Surg* 1980; 16: 259–68.
21. Lloyd JR, Clatworthy HW. Hydramnios as an aid for the early diagnosis of congenital obstruction of the alimentary tract: A study of the maternal and fetal factors. *Pediatrics* 1958; 21: 903–9.
22. Campbell JE. Other conditions of the stomach. In: Welch KJ, Randolp JG, Ravitch MM et al. (eds). *Pediatric Surgery*, 4th edn. Chicago: Year Book, 1986: 821–2.
23. Friedman AP, Velcek FT, Ergin MA et al. Oesophageal atresia with pyloric atresia. *Br J Radiol* 1980; 53: 1009–11.
24. Gupta R, Soni V, Mathur P, Goyal RB. Congenital pyloric atresia and associated anomalies: A case series. *J Neonatal Surg* 2013; 2(4): 40.
25. Burnett HA, Halpert B. Perforation of the stomach of a newborn infant with pyloric atresia. *Arch Pathol* 1947; 44: 318–20.
26. Hermanowicz A, Debek W. Images in clinical medicine. Single bubble—Pyloric atresia. *N Engl J Med* 2015 August 27; 373(9): 863.
27. Grunebaum M, Kornreich L, Ziv N et al. The imaging diagnosis of pyloric atresia. *Z Kinderchir* 1985; 40: 308–11.
28. Narasimhan KL, Road KLN, Mitra SK. Membranous pyloric atresia—Local excision by a new technique. *Pediatr Surg Int* 1991; 6: 159–60.
29. Raffensperger JG. Pyloric and duodenal obstruction. In: *Swenson's Pediatric Surgery*, 5th edn. Norwalk, CT: Appleton & Lange, 1990: 509–16.
30. Son TN, Hoan VX. Laparoscopic management of pyloric atresia in a neonate with epidermolysis bullosa. *J Laparoendosc Adv Surg Tech A* 2013; 23(7): 649–50.
31. Kalfa N, Allal H, Raux O et al. Tolerance of laparoscopy and thoracoscopy in neonates. *Pediatrics* 2005 December; 116(6): e785–91.
32. Chittmittrapap S. Pyloric atresia associated with ileal and rectal atresia. *Pediatr Surg Int* 1988; 3: 426–30.
33. Rosenbloom MS, Ranter M. Congenital pyloric atresia and epidermolysis bullosa letalis in premature siblings. *J Pediatr Surg* 1987; 22: 374–6.
34. Hayashi AH, Galliana CA, Gillis DA. Congenital pyloric atresia and junctional epidermolysis bullosa: A report of long-term survival and a review of the literature. *J Pediatr Surg* 1991; 26: 1341–5.
35. Dank JP, Kim S, Parisi MA, Brown T, Smith LT, Waldhausen J, Sybert VP. Outcome after surgical repair of junctional epidermolysis bullosa-pyloric atresia syndrome: A report of 3 cases and review of the literature. *Arch Dermatol* 1999 October; 135(10): 1243–7.
36. Blazek FD, Boeckman CR. Prepyloric antral diaphragm: Delays in treatment. *J Pediatr Surg* 1987; 22: 948–9.
37. Bell MJ, Gternberg JL, Keating JP et al. Prepyloric gastric antral web: A puzzling epidemic. *J Pediatr Surg* 1978; 13: 307–13.
38. Patnaik DN, Sun S, Groff DB. Newborn gastric outlet obstruction caused by an antral web. *J Med Soc N Jers* 1976; 73: 736–7.
39. Benjamin B, Jayakumar P, Reddy LA, Abbag F. Gastric outlet obstruction caused by prepyloric web in a case of Down's syndrome. *J Pediatr Surg* 1996; 31(9): 1290–1.
40. Mandell GA, Rosenberg HK, Schnaufer L. Prolonged retention of foreign bodies in the stomach. *Pediatrics* 1977; 60(4): 460–2.
41. Rona A, Sylvestre J. Prepyloric mucosal diaphragm. *J Can Assoc Radiol* 1975; 26: 291–4.
42. Schwatx SE, Rowden DR, Dudgeon DL. Antral mucosal diaphragm. *Gastrointest Endosc* 1977; 24: 33–4.
43. Banks PA, Waye JD. The gastroscopic appearance of the antral web. *Gastrointest Endosc* 1969; 15: 228–9.
44. Haller JA Jr, Cahill JL. Combined congenital gastric and duodenal obstruction: Pitfalls in diagnosis and treatment. *Surgery* 1968; 63: 503–6.
45. Berr F, Rienmueller R, Sauerbruch T. Successful endoscopic transection of a partially obstructing antral diaphragm. *Gastroenterology* 1985; 89: 1147–51.
46. Lugo-Vincent HL. Congenital antral membrane: Prenatal diagnosis and treatment. *J Pediatr Surg* 1994; 29: 1589–90.
47. Bing L, Wei-Bing C, Shou-Qing W, Ye-Bo W. Laparoscope-assisted diagnosis and treatment of prepyloric web in children—Report of three cases. *J Pediatr Surg* 2013; 48(7): 1633–6.
48. Tunell WP, Smith EI. Antral web in infancy. *J Pediatr Surg* 1980; 15: 152–5.

52

Infantile hypertrophic pyloric stenosis

PREM PURI, BALAZS KUTASY, AND GANAPATHY LAKSHMANADASS

INTRODUCTION

Infantile hypertrophic pyloric stenosis (IHPS) is the most common condition requiring surgery in the first few months of life. It is characterized by hypertrophy of the circular muscle of the pylorus, causing pyloric channel narrowing and elongation. The incidence of IHPS varies widely with geographic location, season, and ethnic origin.[1] The incidence has been reported to be approximately 0.5–2 per 1000 live births.[2–4] A remarkable decline in the incidence of IHPS has been reported during the 1990s and early 2000s in Western countries.[2,3] Environmental changes rather than genetic ones are likely to explain this development (e.g., increased breastfeeding rate).[3,5] Boys are affected five times more often than girls, and the ratio of affected boys to girls was relatively constant throughout the past decades.[2]

ETIOLOGY

Although earlier diagnosis, advances in fluid and electrolyte therapy, and pediatric anesthesia have reduced the mortality to practically zero, the exact etiology of pyloric stenosis is unknown.[5] This condition is usually classified as a congenital disorder. It is almost unknown in stillbirths, associated anomalies are very uncommon, and the patient usually presents with vomiting after the second week of life; changes in disease incidence over the past two decades indicate that environmental factors are also important.[3,5] Rollins et al.[6] measured pyloric muscle dimensions on ultrasonography in 1400 consecutive newborn infants. Nine of these infants subsequently developed pyloric stenosis and were operated upon. Their pyloric muscle measurements at birth were all within the normal range. This study clearly showed that congenital pyloric muscular hypertrophy is not present in babies who later develop pyloric stenosis.

The occurrence of IHPS has been associated with several variables such as genetic, environmental, and mechanical factors. The pyloric sphincter, a zone of intermittently increased pressure, is able to contract tonically and phasically and produce an effect on gastric emptying. Pyloric sphincter function and motility is under a complex control system that involves the enteric nervous system, gastrointestinal (GI) hormones, and interstitial cells of Cajal (ICC); these pathways have been investigated in IHPS, and abnormalities in hormonal control, extracellular matrix (ECM), smooth muscle fibers, growth factors, and ICC have been implicated in the pathogenesis of the disease.

EXTRINSIC FACTORS

Various environmental and mechanical factors have been proposed as potential causes of IHPS. Significant correlation has been found between higher pesticide (insecticides and herbicides) use in the families' living area and the development of IHPS.[7] Maternal smoking has been shown to double the risk for IHPS.[8] The maternal age has been related with IHPS, and the following results have been found: there is a significantly increased risk for IHPS with young maternal age (<20 years), and a significantly decreased risk with maternal age 30 years and older.[9] Firstborns are at 1.8 increased risk for IHPS.[10] Very preterm birth was associated with a more than twofold increased risk for IHPS, and interestingly, premature infants with IHPS have a higher female predominance.[2,11,12] Caesarean delivery was significantly associated with an increased risk for IHPS.[2] The mechanism for how caesarean delivery could trigger the development of IHPS is unclear. Infants born by caesarean section are known to have differences in the gut flora, which may lead to IHPS.[2] Another potential link between caesarean section and IHPS could be the delayed start of breastfeeding associated with caesarean delivery.[13]

Recently, it has been demonstrated that infants who are bottle-fed has a 4.6-fold increased risk of developing IHPS compared with infants who are not bottle-fed.[3,14] Under the hypothesis that breast milk confers protection against IHPS, one suggestion has been that the presence of high levels of hormones such as vasoactive intestinal peptide in human milk favors pyloric relaxation.[14,15] Breast milk also has lower osmolarity, which could provide better gastric emptying.[14,16]

However, even within 14 days of bottle exposure, among the infants both breast- and bottle-fed, the risk is increased.[14] This observation suggests that limited exposure to bottle-feeding quickly results in a higher risk of IHPS.[14] It has been shown that formula has a higher level of whey and particularly casein proteins than breast milk, and is likely more difficult for the infants to digest causing slower gastric emptying.[14,16] Furthermore, infants fed by bottle have higher serum gastrin levels, which can be associated with pylorospasm.[3,15] Formulas have been improved over time and now approach the composition of breast milk. This could be a contributing reason for the decrease in IHPS incidence.[14]

Lund at al.[17] have found in their nationwide cohort study that macrolide (erythromycin or azithromycin) use in infants for different types of infection is associated with a strongly increased risk of IHPS, including a 30-fold increased risk with use during the first 2 weeks after birth and a lower, but significantly increased threefold risk with use on days 14 to 120. The risk of IHPS is increased more than threefold with maternal use of macrolides during the first 2 weeks after birth, but is not increased with macrolide use thereafter. They found no evidence of an association between IHPS and maternal use of macrolides during gestational weeks 0 to 27, but a possible modest association with use during weeks 28 to birth. It has been shown that both erythromycin and azithromycin are gastrin motilin receptor agonists.[18] Activation of these receptors by macrolides with consequent increased pyloric contractions has been hypothesized as a possible cause of IHPS.

A growing body of research has hinted at seasonality in IHPS epidemiology.[19] Most investigations have observed a peak summer incidence.[20–22] Others have found bimodal spring–autumn peaks[23] or winter peak,[24] or have failed to demonstrate seasonality at all.[25,26] The seasonality has raised the suspicion of an infectious etiology for IHPS.[19] In the adult patient population, resolution of pyloric stenosis after eradication of *Helicobacter pylori* has been found.[27] However, no direct link between IHPS and *H. pylori* has been discovered.[19] Any evidence of association between IHPS and common neonatal respiratory and GI viruses has also not been found.[19]

In a small number of cases, IHPS has been believed to develop as secondary effect to a primary gastric outlet obstruction by mechanical factors. Transpyloric feeding tube, an antral polyp, and a pyloric cyst have been associated with IHPS.[28]

GENETICS

As IHPS tends to run in families, genetic factors have been implicated in its etiology. IHPS is relatively rare in babies of African, Indian, and Chinese extraction.[29,30] Boys are affected five times more often than girls.[2,6] In a population-based cohort study of almost 2 million children,[31] there was a nearly 200-fold increased risk in monozygotic twins, a 20-fold increased risk among siblings. Familial aggregation of IHPS was pronounced even in more distant relatives. The aggregation was observed on both the maternal and paternal sides of the families and irrespective of sex of the cohort member and sex of relatives. Heritability was estimated to be 87%. In a follow-up study extending over 45 years, Carter and Evans[32] found that 5%–20% of the sons and 2.5%–7% of the daughters of affected patients developed IHPS. Sons and daughters of affected female patients had three to four times the incidence of IHPS than sons and daughters of affected male patients.[33] It seems that familial aggregation is primarily explained by shared genes.[31] However, the condition does not follow classic mendelian modes of inheritance.[31] A multifactorial threshold model has been discussed that suggests that IHPS is caused by polygenic inheritance of genes that are modified by sex and environmental factors.[31]

IHPS has been associated with a number of inherited genetic syndromes such as Smith–Lemli–Opitz and Cornelia de Lange, as well as chromosomal abnormalities including partial trisomy of chromosome 9, partial trisomy of chromosome 13, and partial monosomy of chromosomes 8 and 17.[34]

Although a specific gene responsible for IHPS has not yet been discovered, several susceptible loci have been identified, such as 3p25, 16p12-q13, 16q14, 11q14-q22, 11q23, and Xq23 involving NOS1, APOA1, NKX2-5, and MBNL1 genes.[35–39] In view of the implication of the enzyme neuronal nitric oxide synthase (nNOS) in the pathogenesis of IHPS, NOS1, the gene encoding nNOS on chromosome 12q, has been investigated by linkage analysis and evaluation of nNOS mRNA expression[40] and suggested as a susceptibility locus. APOA1 encodes apolipoprotein A-1, a major protein component of high-density lipoprotein (HDL) in plasma, which has been found to be associated with levels of circulating cholesterol.[37] In IHPS, lower cholesterol levels have been found at birth in infants who went on to develop IHPS compared with matched controls who did not develop the disease.[37] A number of previous findings would be consistent with low lipid levels representing an important risk factor for IHPS: The protective effect of female sex could at least partly be due to higher cholesterol levels, since it is well known that levels of LDL cholesterol and HDL cholesterol are, on average, higher in newborn girls compared to boys; IHPS risk associated with bottle-feeding could in part be caused by insufficient lipid levels since bottle-feeding is known to be associated with lower total and LDL cholesterol levels in infancy; and cholesterol has an essential role in nervous system including enteric nervous system development.[37] NKX2-5 encodes the NK2 homeobox 5 transcription factor, which has been shown to have a critical role in pyloric sphincter development.[39,41,42] It has been reported that Sox9 is critical for embryonic pyloric smooth muscle development.[41,42] Nkx2-5 and Gata3 are required for pyloric sphincter morphogenesis, and both directly or indirectly regulate Sox9.[42,43] It has been suggested that some forms of IHPS can result from overexpression of NKX2-5 at the pylorus.[42] MBNL1 is a double-stranded RNA binding protein, and it is a member of muscleblind protein family, which are important regulators of alternative splicing.[38,39] In the early postnatal period, splicing transitions from fetal to adult protein isoforms are essential for the extensive remodeling of muscle tissue that occurs as a part of normal development.[44] In studies of mouse heart and skeletal muscle development, Mbnl1 has been shown to control a set of temporally correlated splicing transitions that occur within the first 3 weeks of postnatal life.[45,46] The intriguing observation that IHPS occurs almost exclusively between 2 and 8 weeks after birth points to a possible role for misregulation of MBNL1 controlled splicing transitions in the etiology of IHPS.[38]

ABNORMALITIES OF HORMONAL CONTROL

The human pylorus is characterized by a zone of elevated pressure that relaxes with antral peristalsis, contracts in response to intraduodenal stimulation, and prevents the retrograde movement of duodenal contents into the stomach.[47] The hormonal control of the pyloric sphincter function by mediators such as gastrin, somatostatin, cholecystokinin, and secretin has been reported to be the same as in other GI sphincters.[48] Since Dodge successfully induced pyloric stenosis by prolonged perinatal maternal stimulation with pentagastrin in approximately one-half of a litter,[49] together with the finding of elevated serum gastrin levels in infants with IHPS,[50] and growing evidence of strong relation between a gastrin motilin agonist macrolide use and increased incidence of IHPS,[17] much attention has been paid to the role of gastrin in the pathogenesis of IHPS. It has been suggested that repeated hyperacid stimulation of the duodenum induced by gastrin evokes repeated pyloric sphincter contractions with work hypertrophy of the pylorus.[51] However, Janik et al.[52] failed to induce pyloric stenosis in other species by prenatal administration of pentagastrin. Some investigators found significantly high plasma gastrin levels in affected infants compared to healthy controls,[50,53] whereas others failed to confirm this finding.[54,55] Since raised serum gastrin levels return to normal following pyloromyotomy, it is believed that they are secondary to antral stasis.[54]

Prostaglandins are produced in response to acid secretion and have a role in GI motility as well as cytoprotective and trophic effects. Prostaglandins PGE2 and PGE2a in the gastric juice have been found to be elevated in IHPS as compared with controls, and based on the belief that they influence pyloric contraction, it has been suggested that these substances may be responsible for pylorospasm and pyloric hypertrophy.[56] Although the finding of elevated PGE2 in IHPS has been confirmed, evidence on prostaglandins causing relaxation of circular smooth muscle has challenged the hypothesis that prostaglandins cause pyloric hypertrophy.[57] However, prostaglandin treatment for cyanotic congenital heart disease has been shown to induce antral hyperplasia and gastric outlet obstruction that mimics IHPS.[58] Moreover, this gastric outlet obstruction can be transient and resolve spontaneously when prostaglandin treatment has been stopped.[59]

ABNORMALITIES OF PYLORIC INNERVATION

Although the smooth muscle sphincter tone is myogenic, contraction and relaxation are under neural control via activation of excitatory and inhibitory pathways, respectively. Sympathetic stimulation is believed to exert an excitatory effect on the pyloric sphincter, while parasympathetic stimulation has either an excitatory effect via cholinergic neurons or an inhibitory effect via nonadrenergic noncholinergic neurons.[60]

The innervations of the musculature regulating motility are particularly dense at the level of the smooth muscle sphincters of the GI tract.[61] Relaxation of the sphincter is accomplished by activation of inhibitory motor neurons.[62] As a defect in pyloric relaxation has been thought to be responsible for the gastric-outlet obstruction and development of pyloric muscle hypertrophy, many investigators have sought evidence for neural abnormality in specimens of IHPS that may explain the failure of pyloric muscle relaxation.[5] Earlier studies concentrated on abnormalities in the myenteric plexus[63–70] and more recent studies with advances in laboratory techniques and equipment have focused on the glial cells, the synaptic function, and the neurotransmitter status in both the myenteric plexus and pyloric muscle layers.[40,70–81]

Ganglion cells

Many investigators have reported conflicting morphologic findings as regards ganglion cells in the myenteric plexus in IHPS. A number of early authors found decreased numbers of ganglion cells, which were attributed either to degenerative changes related to vagal overstimulation[63,64,67] or to immaturity.[65,66] On the other hand, Rintoul and Kirkman[68] suggested that Dogiel type I ganglion cells (primarily motor) were selectively absent in IHPS. Belding and Kernohan[64] and Spitz and Kaufmann[69] found that the majority of myenteric ganglion cells in the hypertrophic pylorus showed degenerative changes. However, Tam[70], using immunohistochemical stains for neuron-specific enolase, stated that neurons were neither immature nor severely degenerated. Langer et al.[82] demonstrated using electron microscopy that there were fewer nerve cell bodies in the myenteric plexus in IHPS, and the total number of ganglia was lower than that in control samples.

Cholinergic and adrenergic innervations

Cholinergic nerve distribution has been studied using acetylcholinesterase (AChE) histochemical staining. Strong AChE staining was observed in the myenteric plexus and the muscle layers in controls, whereas in IHPS specimens, AChE staining was markedly decreased in the muscular layers but strong in the myenteric plexus.[74]

The studies from our laboratory have reported that adrenergic immunoreactivity is absent in the muscular layers and markedly decreased in the myenteric plexus in IHPS in comparison to controls.[5]

Nitrergic innervation

Nitric oxide (NO) is a gaseous free radical, synthesized from L-arginine in a reaction catalyzed by nNOS. NO has a well-described role as a major nonadrenergic, noncholinergic inhibitory neurotransmitter that mediates pyloric relaxation in the enteric nervous system.[83] Vanderwinden et al.[79] and Kobayashi et al.[73] have reported that enzyme NADPH diaphorase, which is identical to NO synthase,[84] is absent or markedly reduced in hypertrophic pyloric muscle, while it is preserved in the myenteric plexus in IHPS. Furthermore, a NOS gene-deleted knockout mouse model is described in which the only abnormality is a constant gastric-outlet obstruction due to pyloric hypertrophy.[85] Barbosa et al.[86] administered nitro-L-arginine methyl ester hydrochloride (L-NAME), a known NOS inhibitor, to pregnant rats and their newborns, and then noted that the L-NAME rats had a larger stomach and pyloric hypertrophy. Kusafuka and Puri[40] demonstrated low levels of nNOS mRNA in pyloric muscle of IHPS patients compared to normal controls. Since a low level of nNOS mRNA may lead to impaired local production of NO, it is suggested that the excessively contracted hypertrophied circular muscle in IHPS is a result of reduced expression of the nNOS gene at the mRNA level.[40]

More recent research showed that sphincter tone is determined by the balance between the nNOS-dependent relaxant and the Rho-associated protein kinase 2 (ROCK-2)-dependent contraction effects.[87] nNOS's NO generation potential depends on the coupled dimeric state of the enzyme.[87] When uncoupled, nNOS predominantly generates reactive oxygen species (ROS).[88] It has been shown that ROS generation promotes ROCK-2 activation.[89,90] Welsh et al.[87] have investigated nNOS and ROCK-2 expression in pyloric stenos using a hyperphenylalaninemia-1 (hph-1) newborn mouse model. These mice exhibit transient pyloric smooth muscle hypertrophy, gastric distension, and failure to gain weight that spontaneously resolves with development.[91] The hph-1 mouse has a congenital mutation in the gene coding GTPCH-1, a rate-limiting enzyme in the production of tetrahydrobiopterin (BH4), an essential nNOS cofactor.[91] BH4 deficiency results in nNOS uncoupling, leading to an increase in tissue ROS content and tissue NO deficiency.[92] Welsh et al.[87] have demonstrated that the hph-1 pyloric tissue nNOS downregulation is a secondary phenomenon and not primarily related to the gastric stasis. Both a reduction in nNOS-derived NO and ROS-induced ROCK-2 upregulation account for the newborn hph-1 mice increases in the pyloric sphincter muscle tone. The mechanism accounting for the age-dependent pyloric changes in hph-1 mice is unclear but likely related to the degree of nNOS uncoupling and tissue BH4 content. It is unclear whether BH4 deficiency plays a role in the IHPS pathogenesis. However, breast milk, as opposed to infant formulas, has a high BH4 content, and IHPS rarely occurs in infants that are exclusively breastfed.[87,93]

Synapse formation

Synapses provide the final neuronal control of the GI tract by regulating neurotransmission at the neuromuscular terminals. The reduction of synaptic vesicles and presynaptic terminals in hypertrophied pyloric muscle layers has been demonstrated.[71,77] Furthermore, a study from our laboratory reported markedly reduced neural-cell adhesion molecule (NCAM) expression on nerve fibers within circular and longitudinal muscles in patients with IHPS compared with normal pylorus.[73] NCAM plays an important role in the formation of initial contacts between nerve and muscle cells and affects tissue formation during embryogenesis.[94,95] These reports suggest that there is impairment of neurotransmission between nerves and muscle in IHPS.

Nerve-supporting cells

The nerve-supporting cells (NSCs) permit cell bodies and processes of neurons to be ordered and maintained in a proper spatial arrangement, and are essential in the maintenance of basic physiological functions of neurons.[96] The NSCs of the intrinsic enteric nervous system are often referred to as enteric glia.[5] Enteric glia have been reported to express various markers for both astrocytes and Schwann cells, such as glial fibrillary acidic protein (GFAP), a specific marker for astrocytes within the central nervous system, and S-100,[97] a marker for astrocytes and Schwann cells. A study from our laboratory demonstrated that in IHPS cases, S-100 and GFAP-immunoreactive fibers were either absent or markedly reduced within the hypertrophied circular and longitudinal muscles.[72] The absence or marked reduction of NSC in IHPS corresponds to the absence or reduction of peptidergic, nitrergic, cholinergic, and adrenergic nerve fibers, and is additional evidence that a defect of intramuscular innervation exists in IHPS.

ABNORMALITIES OF THE INTESTINAL PACEMAKER SYSTEM (ICC)

ICC are small fusiform or stellate cells with prominent nuclei and varicose processes that form networks in the GI tissues. They express C-KIT, a transmembrane protein kinase receptor, essential for their development and maintenance. Morphologic studies have suggested three major functions of ICC: (1) they are pacemaker cells in GI smooth muscle[97]; (2) they facilitate active propagation of electrical events; and (3) they mediate neurotransmission.[98,99] A number of investigators have reported a lack of ICC in hypertrophic pyloric muscle from patients with IHPS using C-KIT antibody and electron microscopy.[100,101] The lack of ICC in IHPS suggests the disruption of their network, and the interruption of the generation of slow waves may contribute to the motility disturbances of the pyloric sphincter.[100]

Carbon monoxide (CO) acts as a neurotransmitter in the GI tract and has been shown to cause smooth muscle relaxation. The main source of endogenous CO is through degradation of heme, catalyzed by heme oxygenase (HO). Heme-oxygenase-2 (HO-2), an isoform of HO, is present in the enteric neurons and in intramuscular ICC, suggesting that CO may serve as an intercellular messenger between enteric neurons, ICC, and smooth muscle cells (SMCs).[102] Our laboratory has investigated immunocolocalization of HO-2 and ICC in IHPS and reported that although intramuscular ICC were HO-2 positive in controls, HO-2 and ICC were not detected in IHPS. It is suggested that impaired intercellular communication between ICC and SMCs may contribute to motility dysfunction in infants with IHPS.[103]

ABNORMALITIES OF ECM PROTEINS

Previous studies have reported an increase in connective tissue in IHPS, particularly in the septa that run between the circular muscle bundles.[63,64] ECM proteins, particularly collagen, are important microenvironmental factors of the neuronal processing pathway in the early embryonal stage and an important matrix for cell adhesion and movement.[5] Cass and Zhang[104] reported an increase in ECM proteins such as chondroitin sulfate, fibronectin, and laminin in specimens of pyloric muscle in IHPS. Another study reported abnormal amounts of elastin fibers and elastin in the pyloric muscle in IHPS.[105] Using M-57 antibody, which can distinguish newly synthesized type I procollagen from fully processed mature collagen, it was reported that type I procollagen was markedly increased in not only the connective tissue septa between circular muscle bundles but also among the circular muscle fibers in patients with IHPS, suggesting that the hypertrophied circular muscle in IHPS is actively synthesizing collagen.[105,106] These studies suggested that increased ECM proteins may be responsible for the characteristic "firm" nature of the pyloric tumor.

Desmin is the main protein of intermediate filaments and is important for the organization and function of muscle fibers. A strong expression of desmin was observed in pyloric muscle biopsies from infants with IHPS, in contrast to absent or weak expression in tached controls. A similar pattern of strong desmin expression has been demonstrated in the fetal pylorus, suggesting that the organization of intermediate filaments in IHPS is in a fetal state of development.[107]

ABNORMALITIES OF SMCS

The ongoing contractile tone in the smooth muscle sphincters is generated by myogenic mechanisms. Langer et al.[82] found SMCs in IHPS to be morphologically normal, containing contractile filaments, intermediate filaments, dense bodies, and caveolae. They found, however, that SMCs in IHPS were frequently in a proliferative phase, with large amounts of dilated rough ER with a lower proportion of contractile filaments, and very few gap junctions exhibited between SMCs compared with control specimens. In contrast, they demonstrated significant ultrastructural abnormalities of the inhibitory enteric nervous system in IHPS.

We performed quantitative evaluation of proliferative activity in pyloric muscle in IHPS and showed that proliferative activity is markedly increased in SMCs in IHPS.[108]

Gentile et al.[109] studied cytoskeletal elements of pyloric SMCs in IHPS using immunohistochemical staining and confocal laser microscopy. Talin, a protein responsible for SMC–ECM interaction, and dystrophin, a protein with adhesion properties, were present in controls but absent in IHPS patients, suggesting that the membrane-cytoskeleton interactions and the cell-matrix communications are altered.

Romeo et al.[110] investigated dystroglycans and sarcoglycans, two proteins that, along with dystrophin, form the dystrophin–glycoprotein complex, which is important for maintaining the structural integrity and function of muscle fibers. They reported that although dystroglycans showed similar expressions in IHPS and controls, sarcoglycans were present in controls but absent in IHPS. It is suggested that lack of sarcoglycans can alter the physiology of SMCs and predispose to IHPS.

ABNORMALITIES OF GROWTH FACTORS

Growth factors are peptides that control cell proliferation and modulate cellular functions by binding to specific high-affinity cell membrane receptors. Although the mechanisms responsible for smooth muscle hypertrophy are unknown, with progress in molecular biology, there is increasing evidence to suggest that the growth of SMCs is regulated by several growth factors.[111-113] IGF-I and PDGF-BB are potent SMC mitogens in vitro and act synergistically to stimulate SMC proliferation. IGF-I mediates the growth-promoting effects of PDGF in mesenchymal cells.[114] IGF-I and PDGF have been shown to be produced by SMCs, and their effects are mediated via their receptors.[115,116] Transforming growth factor alpha (TGF-α) is a growth regulatory peptide found in a wide range of embryonic and adult tissues. It has been recognized that TGF-α has a growth-promoting effect on vascular and visceral SMCs.[117] Epidermal growth factor (EGF) is best known as a potent growth stimulator. It appears to play a critical role early in growth of cultured smooth muscle, in which its production is highest and its growth-promoting effects are greatest.[117] The studies from our laboratory have reported increased expression of IGF-I, PDGF-BB, TGF, and EGF, in hypertrophic pyloric muscle in IHPS,[5,118-120] suggesting that the increased local synthesis of peptide growth factors in SMCs may play a critical role in the development of pyloric muscle hypertrophy in IHPS.

PATHOLOGY

In IHPS, the mean appearance of the pylorus is that of an enlarged muscle mass usually measuring 2 to 2.5 cm in length and 1 to 1.5 cm in diameter. On histological examination, marked muscle hypertrophy and hypoplasia[108] primarily involving the circular layer and hypertrophy of the underlying mucosa are described.[121] Increased fibroblast, fibronectin, proteoglycan chondroitin sulfate, desmin, elastin, and collagen have been found on the immunohistochemical analysis of the hypertrophic muscle.[104,105] Abnormally contorted and thickened nerve fibers have been shown with confocal microscopy.[122] These changes are causing either partial or complete obstruction of the pyloric canal.

CLINICAL FEATURES

The usual onset of symptoms occurs between 3 and 6 weeks of age; however, it can present earlier.[123] Demian et al.[124] investigated 278 patients with IHPS, and only 16 (5.8%) were presented during the first 14 days of life. Presentation of HPS in infants older than 12 weeks of age is considered rare, and reports in the literature are few and far between.[125,126]

Vomiting is the most common presenting symptom. Initially, there is only regurgitation of feeds, but soon it is characteristically projectile and free of bile. In 17%–18% of cases, the vomitus may contain fresh or altered blood, usually attributed to irritative gastritis or esophagitis.[127] Persistent vomiting in these patients results in gastric hydrogen ion loss and subsequent hypochloremic, hypokalemic, metabolic alkalosis.[128]

Owing to inadequate fluid and calorie intake, dehydration and weight loss soon become apparent. In patients who present late, there is disappearance of subcutaneous fat and wrinkled skin. Stools become infrequent, dry, firm, and scanty. However, some infants have diarrhea (starvation diarrhea).

Jaundice occurs in about 2% of cases and has been shown to be related to decrease in glucuronyl transferase, which occurs as a consequence of starvation.[129]

Pylorospasm and gastroesophageal reflux give similar clinical findings, and it may be difficult to differentiate them from IHPS without further evaluation. Other surgical causes of nonbilious vomiting include gastric volvulus, antral web, periampullary duodenal stenosis, duplication cyst of the antropyloric lesion, and ectopic pancreatic tissue within an antropyloric muscle, which are all far less common than IHPS. Common medical causes of nonbilious vomiting are gastroenteritis, increased intracranial pressure, and metabolic disorders (Table 52.1).[34]

Associated anomalies are found in 6%–20% of patients.[130,131] These include esophageal atresia, malrotation of bowel, Hirschsprung's disease, anorectal anomalies, cleft lip and palate, and urological anomalies.

DIAGNOSIS

It should be possible to diagnose HPS on clinical features alone in 80%–90% of infants.[132–134] The important diagnostic features of pyloric stenosis are visible gastric peristalsis and a palpable pyloric tumor. Physical examination of the infant is best carried out during a test feed, which relaxes the abdominal wall and makes the detection of pyloric tumor easier. The abdomen is completely exposed and observation made for gastric peristalsis, which is often visible in this condition as a bulge appearing in the left upper quadrant and moving slowly to the right across the epigastrium. On palpation of the abdomen, an olive-shaped pyloric tumor is palpable in most cases just above the umbilicus at the lateral border of the rectus muscle below the liver edge. However, Bakal et al.[135] have shown that the frequency of development of an olive-shaped abdominal mass evident on physical examination decreased significantly over time. Early diagnosis triggers timely support and surgical intervention, and thus may prevent development of a classical clinical and laboratory findings of late-stage IHPS. The remarkable recent advances in ultrasonographic devices and techniques allow IHPS to be diagnosed earlier than formerly.[135,136]

The diagnosis by ultrasonography relies on the measurement of the pyloric diameter, pyloric length, and muscle thickness, and the hypertrophied pylorus often looks obvious at first glance: "the hot dog in a bun" appearance.[137] Of the three parameters, muscular wall thickness is considered to be the most precise on sonography. Blumhagen and Coombs[138] were the first to point out that pyloric muscle thickness of the hypoechoic ring is the most important sonographic parameter in the diagnosis of pyloric stenosis (Figure 52.1). They considered a thickness of 4 mm or more to be pathological. Other investigators believe that muscle thickness of 5 mm or more is most reliable for the diagnosis

Table 52.1 Differential diagnosis of IHPS

Surgical conditions	Medical conditions
Gastric volvolus	Pylorospasm
Antral web	Gastroesophageal reflux
Periampullary duodenal stenosis	Gastroenteritis
Duplication cyst	Increased intracranial pressure
Ectopic pancreas within the pyloric muscle	Metabolic disease

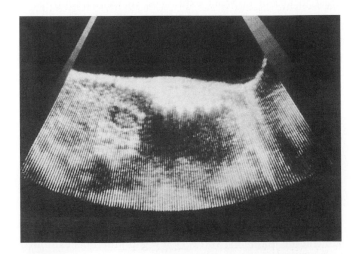

Figure 52.1 Longitudinal real-time sonogram section reveals hypoechoic ring with echogenic center typical of pyloric tumor.

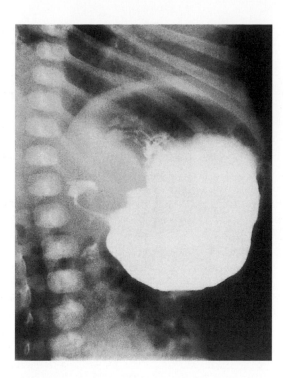

Figure 52.2 Pyloric stenosis. Severe narrowing of pyloric region giving the "string sign" in this 3-week-old infant who presented with projectile vomiting.

of pyloric stenosis.[139] False-positive results are rare, but false-negative rates range from 0% to 19% and largely depend upon the skill of the ultrasonographer.[131,139] In recent years, ultrasound has been used by surgeons to diagnose pyloric stenosis and leaving only problematic or equivocal cases for the radiologist. With this method, IHPS is diagnosed immediately from the emergency room, decreasing hospital stay.[13]

Barium meal study is still a highly sensitive examination for the diagnosis of IHPS. In patients in whom the pyloric tumor cannot be palpated and ultrasound is not definitive, usually it confirms the diagnosis and it may also detect gastroesophageal reflux or intestinal malrotation. Before barium study, the stomach should be emptied with a nasogastric tube and 30–60 mL of barium is instilled under fluoroscopic control. The characteristic radiological feature of pyloric stenosis is a narrowed elongated pyloric canal giving a "string" or "double track" sign caused by compressed invaginated folds of mucosa in the pyloric canal (Figure 52.2). However, barium meal study provides indirect information about the antropyloric canal status. Failure of the relaxation of the antropyloric lesion, known as pylorospasm, demonstrates the same findings as those of IHPS. The emptying speed of the barium meal to the distal bowel will be important to differentiate these two conditions.[140]

MANAGEMENT

Preoperative management

Estimation of serum electrolyte level, urea nitrogen level, hematocrit, and blood gases should be done to determine the state of dehydration and acid–base abnormalities. We have to keep in mind that severe metabolic alkalosis has a potential effect on central control of ventilation and respiratory drive.[141] However, several studies have shown that the classic electrolyte abnormalities of hypochloremic, hypokalemic, metabolic alkalosis are present in less than half of the patients with IHPS.[142,143] Some studies have suggested that the prevalance of electrolyte derangement in IHPS may have diminished in the past three decades.[143,144] More recent study from Tutay et al.[128] have shown that most patients with IHPS demonstrated no alkalosis and no electrolyte derangement. They suggested that this is caused by earlier diagnosis given and consequent earlier correction of dehydration and electrolytes. Anesthesia can be safely performed when serum chloride is >100 mEq/L and the serum HCO3- is <30 mEq/L.[141]

If the babies with IHPS do not show any clinical evidence of dehydration on admission, their serum electrolyte levels are usually normal. They are given their maintenance requirements of fluid as half-straight saline and are operated on as soon as feasible. If the infant is mildly dehydrated and has hypochloremic alkalosis, maintenance fluids can be given as 0.45% saline with 5% dextrose containing 10 mmol of potassium chloride per 500 mL, together with adequate volumes of isotonic saline to correct for continuing nasogastric losses. If the infant is more severely dehydrated (>5%), sodium and chloride ions must be replaced with isotonic saline to enable the kidney to excrete bicarbonate, thereby correcting the acid–base status.[30,131] The operation for IHPS is not an emergency and should never be undertaken until serum electrolyte levels have returned to normal.

A nasogastric tube is passed to keep the stomach empty. Saline irrigation through the nasogastric tube may help in removing mucus and milk curd. And if the barium meal study has been carried out prior to surgery, it may be necessary to remove the residual barium meal by gastric aspiration.

Operation

The Ramstedt's pyloromyotomy is the universally accepted operation for pyloric stenosis.

INCISION

A 3 cm transverse right upper quadrant incision provides excellent exposure and direct access to the pylorus with minimal retraction (Figure 52.3). Another incision that is commonly used is an umbilical fold incision. This technique achieves an excellent cosmetic outcome with an apparently unscarred abdomen.[145–148]

PROCEDURE

The transverse incision lateral to the rectus muscle is cut through all layers of muscle and peritoneum. The pyloric tumor is delivered by gentle traction on the stomach (Figure 52.4). The surgeon applies an index finger to the duodenal

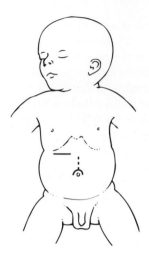

Figure 52.3 Skin incision for pyloromyotomy.

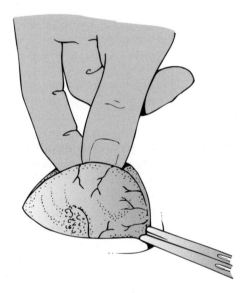

Figure 52.4 Delivery of pyloric tumor.

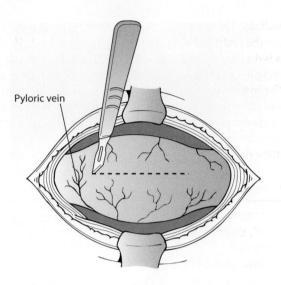

Figure 52.5 Incision through the serosa of the pyloric tumor.

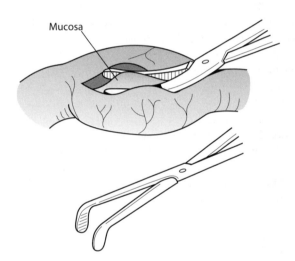

Figure 52.6 Splitting of pyloric muscle.

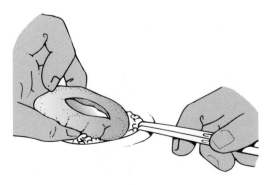

Figure 52.7 Bulging mucosa seen after complete splitting of pyloric muscle.

end of the pylorus and stabilizes the pyloric tumor. An incision is then made over the anterosuperior part of the pylorus, beginning at the clearly demarcated pyloroduodenal junction about 2 mm proximal to the pyloric vein and extending onto the gastric antrum, where muscle is thin (Figure 52.5). The pyloric muscle is then widely split down to the mucosa using mosquito forceps (Figure 52.6). Some surgeons prefer a Denis Browne pyloric spreader. When the pyloric muscle has been adequately split, the mucosa can be seen to be bulging (Figure 52.7). If mucosal injury is questionable, to test the injury, the stomach is inflated through the nasogastric tube and passage of air through the pylorus to duodenum is confirmed. Then the pylorus is dropped back into the abdomen. The peritoneum is closed with 4-0 polyglactin (Vicryl) and muscles approximated using 3-0 polyglactin (Vicryl). 5-0 Vicryl is used for subcuticular stitches.

Tan and Bianchi described the supraumbilical fold approach for pyloromyotomy. Circumumbilical incision is made through about two-thirds of the circumference of the umbilicus. The skin is undermined in a cephalad direction above the umbilical ring, and linea alba is exposed. The linea alba is divided longitudinally in the midline from the umbilical ring to as far cephalad as necessary to allow easy delivery of the pyloric tumor.[145–148] The problem with the supraumbilical incision is that it does not always allow easy access to the hypertrophic pyloric muscle. Delivery of a large pyloric tumor can be fairly difficult and time-consuming, and may damage the serosa of the stomach or duodenum by tearing.[145]

LAPAROSCOPIC PYLOROMYOTOMY

Since 1991,[149] when the first laparoscopic pyloromyotomy was reported, there have been numerous publications supporting this approach,[140,150] and recently, single incision laparoscopic pyloromyotomy also has been reported.[151] For the laparoscopic procedure, the patient is placed in the supine position at the end of the table. A 5 mm port is placed in the umbilical fold after an open technique under direct vision. Pneumoperitoneum is established with CO_2 at maximum pressure of 6–8 mmHg. Two additional access sites are placed in the left and right midclavicular line just below the costal margin under direct vision with the camera. The duodenum is grasped with atraumatic forceps just distal to the pylorus olive and stabilizes it. Endotome or diathermy hook is placed through the right incision, and the pylorus is incised in its avascular plane from the prepyloric vein well into the gastric antrum (Figure 52.8). The muscular layer is then separated with an endoscopic spreader (Figure 52.9). A satisfactory pyloromyotomy is evidenced by ballooning of the intact mucosa. The absence of mucosal perforation is checked by insufflations of air in the nasogastric tube; if none is seen, the instruments and ports are removed. The umbilical fascia is closed with 4-0 absorbable suture, and the skin of all the wound is reapproximated with 5-0 subcuticular absorbable sutures.[34]

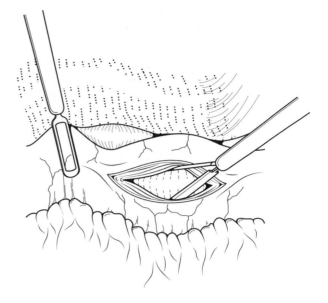

Figure 52.9 Muscular layer is separated with an endoscopic spreader.

Compared to open pyloromyotomy, laparoscopic pyloromyotomy is associated with significantly shorter postoperative recovery, decreased analgesia requirements, and superior cosmetic result in prospective, randomized controlled trials.[152–155] However, this is not much cosmetic advantage when compared with the umbilical approach. Moreover, as Hall et al.[156] have shown in their randomized controlled trials, that laparoscopy is associated with significantly higher frequency of incomplete pyloromyotomy (1.16% versus 0.29%) and a trend of higher perforation rates with laparoscopy (0.83% versus 0.29%).[157] A recent systematic review[158] has concluded that if the surgeon is able to perform both procedures, it is at the discretion of the surgeon or the center to make a well-founded decision between the two options.

Postoperative care

Maintenance i.v. fluids are continued postoperatively until the infant is feeding satisfactorily. The timing of reintroduction of feeds continues to be controversial.[159–162] Several studies have investigated postoperative feeding regimens for IHPS patients with respect to time of reintroduction of feeding and speed of advancement in an attempt to discover the safest and most cost-effective method. Some practice patterns have initiated feedings as soon as the infant awakens from anesthesia.[163] Some authors have suggested a period of withholding feedings for several hours postoperatively,[164] while others have recommended a significantly longer period of starvation up to 18 h before initiating feedings.[165] The ongoing debate arises over whether a surgeon chooses a standardized, incremental feeding regimen versus an ad libitum feeding schedule that allows the infant to decide when and how much to eat.[166] Many concerns surrounding immediate feeding regimens take into account the degree of postoperative gastroparesis.[166] Studies analyzing

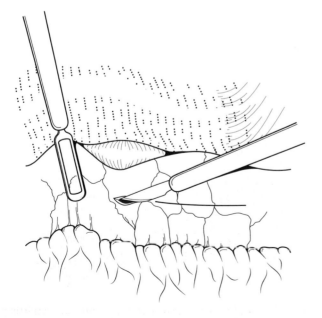

Figure 52.8 Laparoscopic incision.

radiographic and manometric functional variables suggest that gastric peristalsis completely ceases for 4–6 h postoperatively and is profoundly depressed for 12–18 h postoperatively.[167] Based on the current literature, an ad libitum feeding regimen may be superior to a variety of scheduled, incremental feeding regimens.[166] A majority of the studies found no increase in the incidence of postoperative emesis despite reaching full strength feeds more quickly, thereby decreasing time to discharge.[161,168,169] Therefore, Graham et al.[166] have recommended in their meta-analysis, based on high evidence, to delay feeds for a period of at least 4 h postoperatively, and then to initiate ad lib feedings.

COMPLICATIONS

Duodenal perforation is usually the result of excessive separation of fibers at the distal end of the pylorus. It is not serious provided that it is recognized and closed with one or two sutures. A patch of omentum should be brought up and tied over the wound.

A mucosal injury has always been a major intraoperative complication, generally occurring in less than 5% of cases.[170] Several different approaches of dealing with mucosal injury have been described: full-thickness closure, rotation of the pylorus, repyloromyotomy in a different quadrant, and simple primary mucosal repair.[170] Waldron et al.[170] have demonstrated in their recent study that most of the mucosal injuries (93%) were noticed intraoperatively. Mucosal injuries that are noticed and addressed intraoperatively resulted in few complications, regardless of the repair method. Primary mucosal repair was equivalent to full-thickness closure in terms of complications and outcomes.

The need for reoperation after pyloromyotomy because of recurrent vomiting is reported with an incidence of up to 1.6%. Other complications included hemorrhage, wound infection, wound dehiscence, and gas embolus. With improvements in techniques, the incidence of complications after pyloromyotomy is very low.

CONSERVATIVE THERAPY

The use of antimuscarinics in IHPS was first reported by Svensgaard in 1935, and until the late 1960s, IHPS was often treated medically using oral atropine sulfate.[171,172] Over the past 20 years, atropine sulfate has been used increasingly in Japan as primary therapy for IHPS.[172] As atropine sulfate is a cardioactive drug, electrocardiographic and pulse-oximetry monitoring is required during administration of the drug.[173] In Western countries, medical management of IHPS has remained a controversial issue: the success rate of medical treatment with atropine is lower (75%–88%) than that of surgery (98%), and it requires longer hospitalization because of intravenous therapy and the need to continue oral atropine after discharge, the latter requiring a lot of parental effort.[174] Additionally, due to the lower success rate, patients whose symptoms do not resolve with atropine therapy may then have to undergo surgery when their health has deteriorated

even further.[174] Surgery, on the other hand, carries the usual risks of general anesthesia, a risk of mucosal perforation, wound infection, and adhesions.[174] Mercer and Philips[174] have demonstrated in their meta-analysis that a conservative approach to the treatment of IHPS with atropine sulfate should only be considered as an alternative to surgical pyloromyotomy, where longer hospital stays and a reduced success rate are acceptable. This would apply to patients who are unsuitable or at high risk for surgery, and to areas of the world where surgery on small infants is unsafe.

REFERENCES

1. Leck I. Descriptive epidemiology of common malformations (excluding central nervous system defects). *Br Med Bull* 1976; 32:45–52.
2. Svenningsson A, Svensson T, Akre O et al. Maternal and pregnancy characteristics and risk of infantile hypertrophic pyloric stenosis. *J Pediatr Surg* 2014; 49:1226–31.
3. McAteer JP, Ledbetter DJ, Goldin AB. Role of bottle feeding in the etiology of hypertrophic pyloric stenosis. *JAMA Pediatr* 2013; 167:1143–9.
4. Vermes G, Laszlo D, Czeizel AE et al. Maternal factors in the origin of infantile hypertrophic pyloric stenosis: A population-based case-control study. *Congenit Anom* 2016; 56:65–72.
5. Ohshiro K, Puri P. Pathogenesis of infantile hypertrophic pyloric stenosis: Recent progress. *Pediatr Surg Int* 1998; 13:243–52.
6. Rollins MD, Shields MD, Quinn RJ et al. Pyloric stenosis: Congenital or acquired? *Arch Dis Child* 1989; 64:138–9.
7. Markel TA, Proctor C, Ying J et al. Environmental pesticides increase the risk of developing hypertrophic pyloric stenosis. *J Pediatr Surg* 2015; 50:1283–88.
8. Sorensen HT, Norgard B, Pedersen L et al. Maternal smoking and risk of hypertrophic infantile pyloric stenosis: 10 year population based cohort study. *BMJ* 2002; 325:1011–2.
9. Pedersen RN, Garne E, Loane M et al. Infantile hypertrophic pyloric stenosis: A comparative study of incidence and other epidemiological characteristics in seven European regions. *J Matern Fetal Neonatal Med* 2008; 21:599–604.
10. Barnhart DC. Beyond the firstborn son: Epidemiology to enlighten the pathogenesis of hypertrophic pyloric stenosis. *JAMA Pediatr* 2013; 167:1100–1, 2013.
11. Cascio S, Steven M, Livingstone H et al. Hypertrophic pyloric stenosis in premature infants: Evaluation of sonographic criteria and short-term outcomes. *Pediatr Surg Int* 2013; 29:697–702.
12. Stark CM, Rogers PL, Eberly MD et al. Association of prematurity with the development of infantile hypertrophic pyloric stenosis. *Pediatr Res* 2015; 78:218–22.

13. Boneti C, McVay MR, Kokoska ER et al. Ultrasound as a diagnostic tool used by surgeons in pyloric stenosis. *J Pediatr Surg* 2008; 43:87–91; discussion 91, 2008.

14. Krogh C, Biggar RJ, Fischer TK et al. Bottle-feeding and the risk of pyloric stenosis. *Pediatrics* 2012; 130:e943–9.

15. Pisacane A, de Luca U, Criscuolo L et al. Breast feeding and hypertrophic pyloric stenosis: Population based case-control study. *BMJ* 1996; 312:745–6.

16. Cavell B. Gastric emptying in infants fed human milk or infant formula. *Acta Paediatr Scand* 1981; 70:639–41.

17. Lund M, Pasternak B, Davidsen RB et al. Use of macrolides in mother and child and risk of infantile hypertrophic pyloric stenosis: Nationwide cohort study. *BMJ* 2014; 348:g1908.

18. Smith C, Egunsola O, Choonara I et al. Use and safety of azithromycin in neonates: A systematic review. *BMJ Open* 2015; 5:e008194.

19. Modarressi T. Question of an infectious etiology or contribution to the pathogenesis of infantile hypertrophic pyloric stenosis. *J Pediatr Gastroenterol Nutr* 2014; 58:546–8.

20. Schechter R, Torfs CP, Bateson TF. The epidemiology of infantile hypertrophic pyloric stenosis. *Paediatr Perinat Epidemiol* 1997; 11:407–27.

21. Mackay AJ, Mackellar A. Infantile hypertrophic pyloric stenosis: A review of 222 cases. *Aust N Z J Surg* 1986; 56:131–3.

22. Zamakhshary MF, Dutta S, To T et al. Seasonal variation of hypertrophic pyloric stenosis: A population-based study. *Pediatr Surg Int* 2011; 27:689–93.

23. Kwok RH, Avery G. Seasonal variation of congenital hypertrophic pyloric stenosis. *J Pediatr* 1967; 70:963–5.

24. Dodge JA. Infantile hypertrophic pyloric stenosis in Belfast, 1957–1969. *Arch Dis Child* 1975; 50:171–8.

25. Habbick BF, To T. Incidence of infantile hypertrophic pyloric stenosis in Saskatchewan, 1970-85. *CMAJ* 1989; 140:395–8.

26. Leong MM, Chen SC, Hsieh CS et al. Epidemiological features of infantile hypertrophic pyloric stenosis in Taiwanese children: A Nation-Wide Analysis of Cases during 1997–2007. *PloS One* 2011; 6:e19404.

27. de Boer WA, Driessen WM. Resolution of gastric outlet obstruction after eradication of *Helicobacter pylori*. *J Clin Gastroenterol* 1995; 21:329–30.

28. Panteli C. New insights into the pathogenesis of infantile pyloric stenosis. *Pediatr Surg Int* 2009; 25:1043–52.

29. Joseph TP NN. Congenital hypertrophic pyloric stenosis. *Ind J Surg* 1974; 36:221–3.

30. Spicer RD. Infantile hypertrophic pyloric stenosis: A review. *Br J Surg* 1982; 69:128–35.

31. Krogh C, Fischer TK, Skotte L et al. Familial aggregation and heritability of pyloric stenosis. *JAMA* 2010; 303:2393–99.

32. Carter CO, Evans KA. Inheritance of congenital pyloric stenosis. *J Med Genet* 1969; 6:233–54.

33. Finsen VR. Infantile hypertrophic pyloric stenosis—Unusual familial incidence. *Arch Dis Child* 1979; 54:720–1.

34. Fujimoto T. Infantile hypertrophic pyloric stenosis. In: Puri P, Holwarth M (eds). *Pediatric Surgery: Diagnosis and Management*. Berlin-Heidelberg: Springer-Verlag, 2009:363–8.

35. Everett KV, Capon F, Georgoula C et al. Linkage of monogenic infantile hypertrophic pyloric stenosis to chromosome 16q24. *Eur J Hum Genet* 2008; 16:1151–4.

36. Everett KV, Chioza BA, Georgoula C et al. Genome-wide high-density SNP-based linkage analysis of infantile hypertrophic pyloric stenosis identifies loci on chromosomes 11q14-q22 and Xq23. *Am J Hum Genet* 2008; 82:756–2.

37. Feenstra B, Geller F, Carstensen L et al. Plasma lipids, genetic variants near APOA1, and the risk of infantile hypertrophic pyloric stenosis. *JAMA* 2013; 310:714–21.

38. Feenstra B, Geller F, Krogh C et al. Common variants near MBNL1 and NKX2-5 are associated with infantile hypertrophic pyloric stenosis. *Nat Genet* 2012; 44:334–7.

39. Feng Z, Liang P, Li Q et al. Association between NKX2-5 rs29784 and infantile hypertrophic pyloric stenosis in Chinese Han population. *Int J Clin Exp Med* 2015; 8:2905–10.

40. Kusafuka T, Puri P. Altered mRNA expression of the neuronal nitric oxide synthase gene in Hirschsprung's disease. *J Pediatr Surg* 1997; 32:1054–8.

41. Prakash A, Udager AM, Saenz DA et al. Roles for Nkx2-5 and Gata3 in the ontogeny of the murine smooth muscle gastric ligaments. *Am J Physiol Gastrointest Liver Physiol* 2014; 307:G430–6.

42. Udager AM, Prakash A, Saenz DA et al. Proper development of the outer longitudinal smooth muscle of the mouse pylorus requires Nkx2-5 and Gata3. *Gastroenterology* 2014; 146:157–65 e110.

43. Li Y, Pan J, Wei C et al. LIM homeodomain transcription factor Isl1 directs normal pyloric development by targeting Gata3. *BMC Biol* 2014; 12:25.

44. Bland CS, Wang ET, Vu A et al. Global regulation of alternative splicing during myogenic differentiation. *Nucleic Acids Res* 2010; 38:7651–64.

45. Lin X, Miller JW, Mankodi A et al. Failure of MBNL1-dependent post-natal splicing transitions in myotonic dystrophy. *Hum Mol Genet* 2006; 15:2087–97.

46. Kalsotra A, Xiao X, Ward AJ et al. A postnatal switch of CELF and MBNL proteins reprograms alternative splicing in the developing heart. *Proc. Natl Acad Sci USA* 2008; 105:20333–8.

47. Fisher RCS. The physiologic characteristics of the human pyloric sphincter. *Gastroenterology* 1972; 64:67.

48. Knox EG, Armstrong E, Haynes R. Changing incidence of infantile hypertrophic pyloric stenosis. *Arch Dis Child* 1983; 58:582–5.

49. Dodge JA. Production of duodenal ulcers and hypertrophic pyloric stenosis by administration of pentagastrin to pregnant and newborn dogs. *Nature* 1970; 225:284–5.

50. Spitz L, Zail SS. Serum gastrin levels in congenital hypertrophic pyloric stenosis. *J Pediatr Surg* 1976; 11:33–35.

51. Fisher RS, Lipshutz W, Cohen S. The hormonal regulation of pyloric sphincter function. *J Clin Invest* 1973; 52:1289–96.

52. Janik JS, Akbar AM, Burrington JD et al. The role of gastrin in congenital hypertrophic pyloric stenosis. *J Pediatr Surg* 1978; 13:151–4.

53. Wesley JR, Fiddian-Green R, Roi LD et al. The effect of pyloromyotomy on serum and luminal gastrin in infants with hypertrophic pyloric stenosis. *J Surg Res* 1980; 28:533–8.

54. Grochowski J, Szafran H, Sztefko K et al. Blood serum immunoreactive gastrin level in infants with hypertrophic pyloric stenosis. *J Pediatr Surg* 1980; 15:279–82.

55. Hambourg MA, Mignon M, Ricour C et al. Serum gastrin levels in hypertrophic pyloric stenosis of infancy. Response to a gastrin secretion test. *Arch Dis Child* 1979; 54:208–12.

56. LaFerla G, Watson J, Fyfe AH et al. The role of prostaglandins E2 and F2 alpha in infantile hypertrophic pyloric stenosis. *J Pediatr Surg* 1986; 21:410–2.

57. Shinohara K, Shimizu T, Igarashi J et al. Correlation of prostaglandin E2 production and gastric acid secretion in infants with hypertrophic pyloric stenosis. *J Pediatr Surg* 1998; 33:1483–85.

58. Kosiak W, Swieton D, Fryze I et al. Gastric outlet obstruction due to an iatrogenic cause in a neonatal period - report of two cases. *Ultraschall Med* 30:401–3.

59. Soyer T, Yalcin S, Bozkaya D et al. Transient hypertrophic pyloric stenosis due to prostaglandin infusion. *J Perinatol* 2014; 34:800–1.

60. Saps M DLC. Gastric motility. In: Kleinman R, Goulet OG, Mieli-Vergani G, Sanderson I (eds). *Walker's Pediatric Gastrointestinal Disease*, vol 1 New York: McGraw-Hill, 2008:187–93.

61. Alumets J, Schaffalitzky de Muckadell O, Fahrenkrug J et al. A rich VIP nerve supply is characteristic of sphincters. *Nature* 1979; 280:155–6.

62. Gabella. Structure of muscle and nerves in the gastrointestinal tract. In: Johnson LR (ed). *Physiology of the Gastrointestinal Tract*. New York: Raven Press, 1994:751–93.

63. Alarotu H. The histopathologic changes in the myenteric plexus of the pylorus in hypertrophic pyloric stenosis of infants (pylorospasm). *Acta Paediatr Suppl* 1956; 45:1–131.

64. Belding HH 3rd, Kernohan JW. A morphologic study of the myenteric plexus and musculature of the pylorus with special reference to the changes in hypertrophic pyloric stenosis. *Surg Gynecol Obstet* 1953; 97:322–34.

65. Friesen SR, Boley JO, Miller DR. The myenteric plexus of the pylorus: Its early normal development and its changes in hypertrophic pyloric stenosis. *Surgery* 1956; 39:21–9.

66. Friesen SR, Pearse AG. Pathogenesis of congenital pyloric stenosis: Histochemical analyses of pyloric ganglion cells. *Surgery* 1963; 53:604–8.

67. Nielsen OS. Histological changes of the pyloric myenteric plexus in infantile pyloric stenosis; studies on surgical biopsy specimens. *Acta Paediatr* 1956; 45:636–47.

68. Rintoul JR, Kirkman NF. The myenteric plexus in infantile hypertrophic pyloric stenosis. *Arch Dis Child* 1961; 36:474–80.

69. Spitz L, Kaufmann JC. The neuropathological changes in congenital hypertrophic pyloric stenosis. *S Afr J Surg* 1975; 13:239–42.

70. Tam PK. An immunochemical study with neuron-specific-enolase and substance P of human enteric innervation—The normal developmental pattern and abnormal deviations in Hirschsprung's disease and pyloric stenosis. *J Pediatr Surg* 1986; 21:227–32.

71. Kobayashi H, Miyano T, Yamataka A et al. Use of synaptophysin polyclonal antibody for the rapid intraoperative immunohistochemical evaluation of functional bowel disorders. *J Pediatr Surg* 1997; 32:38–40.

72. Kobayashi H, O'Briain DS, Puri P. Selective reduction in intramuscular nerve supporting cells in infantile hypertrophic pyloric stenosis. *J Pediatr Surg* 1994; 29:651–4.

73. Kobayashi H, O'Briain DS, Puri P. Immunochemical characterization of neural cell adhesion molecule (NCAM), nitric oxide synthase, and neurofilament protein expression in pyloric muscle of patients with pyloric stenosis. *J Pediatr Gastroenterol Nutr* 1995; 20:319–25.

74. Kobayashi H OBD, Puri P. Defective cholinergic pyloric stenosis. *Pediatr Surg Int* 1994; 9:338–41.

75. Kobayashi H PP. Abnormal adrenergic innervation in infantile pyloric stenosis. Presented at the VII International Symposium on Pediatric Surgical Research, Heidelberg, Germany, 1994.

76. Malmfors G, Sundler F. Peptidergic innervation in infantile hypertrophic pyloric stenosis. *J Pediatr Surg* 1986; 21:303–6.

77. Okazaki T, Yamataka A, Fujiwara T et al. Abnormal distribution of synaptic vesicle proteins in infantile hypertrophic pyloric stenosis. *J Pediatr Gastroenterol Nutr* 1994; 18:254–5.

78. Shen Z SY, Wang W, Wang L. Immunohistochemical study of peptidergic nerves in infantile hypertrophic pyloric stenosis. *Pediatr Surg Int* 1990; 5:110–3.

79. Vanderwinden JM, Mailleux P, Schiffmann SN et al. Nitric oxide synthase activity in infantile hypertrophic pyloric stenosis. *N Engl J Med* 1992; 327:511–5.

80. Wattchow DA, Cass DT, Furness JB et al. Abnormalities of peptide-containing nerve fibers in infantile hypertrophic pyloric stenosis. *Gastroenterology* 1987; 92:443–8.

81. Wattchow DA, Furness JB, Costa M. Distribution and coexistence of peptides in nerve fibers of the external muscle of the human gastrointestinal tract. *Gastroenterology* 1988; 95:32–41.

82. Langer JC, Berezin I, Daniel EE. Hypertrophic pyloric stenosis: Ultrastructural abnormalities of enteric nerves and the interstitial cells of Cajal. *J Pediatr Surg* 1995; 30:1535–43.

83. Bult H, Boeckxstaens GE, Pelckmans PA et al. Nitric oxide as an inhibitory non-adrenergic non-cholinergic neurotransmitter. *Nature* 1990; 345:346–7.

84. Fatemifar G, Hoggart CJ, Paternoster L et al. Genome-wide association study of primary tooth eruption identifies pleiotropic loci associated with height and craniofacial distances. *Hum Mol Genet* 2013; 22:3807–17.

85. Huang PL, Dawson TM, Bredt DS et al. Targeted disruption of the neuronal nitric oxide synthase gene. *Cell* 1993; 75:1273–86.

86. Barbosa IM, Ferrante SM, Mandarim-De-Lacerda CA. [Role of nitric oxide synthase in the etiopathogenesis of hypertrophic pyloric stenosis in infants]. *J Pediatr (Rio J)* 2001; 77:307–12.

87. Welsh C, Shifrin Y, Pan J et al. Infantile hypertrophic pyloric stenosis (IHPS): A study of its pathophysiology utilizing the newborn hph-1 mouse model of the disease. *Am J Physiol Gastrointest Liver Physiol* 2014; 307:G1198–206.

88. Rivera LR, Poole DP, Thacker M et al. The involvement of nitric oxide synthase neurons in enteric neuropathies. *Neurogastroenterol Motil* 2100; 23:980–8.

89. Knock GA, Snetkov VA, Shaifta Y et al. Superoxide constricts rat pulmonary arteries via Rho-kinase-mediated Ca(2+) sensitization. *Free Rad Biol Med* 2009; 46:633–42.

90. Rattan S, Phillips BR, Maxwell PJt. RhoA/Rho-kinase: Pathophysiologic and therapeutic implications in gastrointestinal smooth muscle tone and relaxation. *Gastroenterology* 2010; 138:13–8 e11–3.

91. Hyland K, Gunasekara RS, Munk-Martin TL et al. The hph-1 mouse: A model for dominantly inherited GTP-cyclohydrolase deficiency. *Ann Neurol* 2003; 54 Suppl 6:S46–8.

92. Welsh C, Enomoto M, Pan J et al. Tetrahydrobiopterin deficiency induces gastroparesis in newborn mice. *Am J Physiol Gastrointest Liver Physiol* 2013; 305:G47–57.

93. Weinmann A, Post M, Pan J et al. Tetrahydrobiopterin is present in high quantity in human milk and has a vasorelaxing effect on newborn rat mesenteric arteries. *Pediatr Res* 2011; 69:325–9.

94. Figarella-Branger D, Pellissier JF, Bianco N et al. Expression of various NCAM isoforms in human embryonic muscles: Correlation with myosin heavy chain phenotypes. *J Neuropathol Exp Neurol* 1992; 51:12–23.

95. Tosney KW, Watanabe M, Landmesser L et al. The distribution of NCAM in the chick hindlimb during axon outgrowth and synaptogenesis. *Dev Biol* 1986; 114:437–52.

96. Sugimura K, Haimoto H, Nagura H et al. Immunohistochemical differential distribution of S-100 alpha and S-100 beta in the peripheral nervous system of the rat. *Muscle Nerve* 1989; 12:929–35.

97. Rollins MD, Russell K, Schall K et al. Complete VACTERL evaluation is needed in newborns with rectoperineal fistula. *J Pediatr Surg* 2014; 49:95–8; discussion 98.

98. Daniel EE, Posey-Daniel V. Neuromuscular structures in opossum esophagus: Role of interstitial cells of Cajal. *Am J Physiol* 1984; 246:G305–15.

99. Daniel EE BI. Intestinal cells of Cajal; are they major players in control of gastrointestinal motility? *J Gastointest Motil* 1992; 4:1–24.

100. Vanderwinden JM, Liu H, De Laet MH et al. Study of the interstitial cells of Cajal in infantile hypertrophic pyloric stenosis. *Gastroenterology* 1996; 111:279–88.

101. Yamataka A, Fujiwara T, Kato Y et al. Lack of intestinal pacemaker (C-KIT-positive) cells in infantile hypertrophic pyloric stenosis. *J Pediatr Surg* 1996; 31:96–8; discussion 98–9.

102. Farrugia G, Szurszewski JH. Heme oxygenase, carbon monoxide, and interstitial cells of Cajal. *Microsc Res Tech* 1999; 47:321–24.

103. Piotrowska AP, Solari V, Puri P. Distribution of heme oxygenase-2 in nerves and interstitial cells of Cajal in the normal pylorus and in infantile hypertrophic pyloric stenosis. *Arch Pathol Lab Med* 2003; 127:1182–6.

104. Cass DT ZA. Extracellular matrix changes in congenital hypertrophic pyloric stenosis. *Pediatr Surg Int* 1991; 6:190–4.

105. Oue T, Puri P. Abnormalities of elastin and elastic fibers in infantile hypertrophic pyloric stenosis. *Pediatr Surg Int* 1999; 15:540–2.

106. Miyazaki E, Yamataka T, Ohshiro K et al. Active collagen synthesis in infantile hypertrophic pyloric stenosis. *Pediatr Surg Int* 1998; 13:237–9.

107. Guarino N, Shima H, Puri P. Structural immaturity of the pylorus muscle in infantile hypertrophic pyloric stenosis. *Pediatr Surg Int* 2000; 16:282–4.

108. Oue T, Puri P. Smooth muscle cell hypertrophy versus hyperplasia in infantile hypertrophic pyloric stenosis. *Pediatr Res* 1999; 45:853–7.

109. Gentile C, Romeo C, Impellizzeri P et al. A possible role of the plasmalemmal cytoskeleton, nitric oxide synthase, and innervation in infantile hypertrophic pyloric stenosis. A confocal laser scanning microscopic study. *Pediatr Surg Int* 1998; 14:45–50.

110. Romeo C, Santoro G, Impellizzeri P et al. Sarcoglycan immunoreactivity is lacking in infantile hypertrophic pyloric stenosis. A confocal laser scanning microscopic study. *Pediatr Med Chir* 2007; 29:32–7.

111. Chen Y, Bornfeldt KE, Arner A et al. Increase in insulin-like growth factor I in hypertrophying smooth muscle. *Am J Physiol* 1994; 266:E224–9.

112. Pfeifer TL, Chegini N. Immunohistochemical localization of insulin-like growth factor (IGF-I), IGF-I receptor, and IGF binding proteins 1-4 in human fallopian tube at various reproductive stages. *Biol Reprod* 1994; 50:281–9.

113. Yamamoto M, Yamamoto K. Growth regulation in primary culture of rabbit arterial smooth muscle cells by platelet-derived growth factor, insulin-like growth factor-I, and epidermal growth factor. *Exp Cell Res* 1994; 212:62–8.

114. Clemmons DR, Van Wyk JJ. Evidence for a functional role of endogenously produced somatomedinlike peptides in the regulation of DNA synthesis in cultured human fibroblasts and porcine smooth muscle cells. *J Clin Invest* 1985; 75:1914–8.

115. Libby P, Warner SJ, Salomon RN et al. Production of platelet-derived growth factor-like mitogen by smooth-muscle cells from human atheroma. *N Engl J Med* 1988; 318:1493–8.

116. Ullrich A, Gray A, Tam AW et al. Insulin-like growth factor I receptor primary structure: Comparison with insulin receptor suggests structural determinants that define functional specificity. *EMBO J* 1986; 5:2503–12.

117. Kuemmerle JF. Autocrine regulation of growth in cultured human intestinal muscle by growth factors. *Gastroenterology* 1997; 113:817–24.

118. Ohshiro K, Puri P. Increased insulin-like growth factor and platelet-derived growth factor system in the pyloric muscle in infantile hypertrophic pyloric stenosis. *J Pediatr Surg* 1998; 33:378–81.

119. Shima H, Ohshiro K, Puri P. Increased local synthesis of epidermal growth factors in infantile hypertrophic pyloric stenosis. *Pediatr Res* 2000; 47:201–7.

120. Shima H, Puri P. Increased expression of transforming growth factor-alpha in infantile hypertrophic pyloric stenosis. *Pediatr Surg Int* 1999; 15:198–200.

121. Hernanz-Schulman M, Lowe LH, Johnson J et al. In vivo visualization of pyloric mucosal hypertrophy in infants with hypertrophic pyloric stenosis: Is there an etiologic role? *AJR Am J Roentgenol* 2001; 177:843–8.

122. Kobayashi H, Miyahara K, Yamataka A et al. Pyloric stenosis: New histopathologic perspective using confocal laser scanning. *J Pediatr Surg* 2001; 36:1277–9.

123. Tack ED, Perlman JM, Bower RJ et al. Pyloric stenosis in the sick premature infant. Clinical and radiological findings. *Am J Dis Child* 1988; 142:68–70.

124. Demian M, Nguyen S, Emil S. Early pyloric stenosis: A case control study. *Pediatr Surg Int* 2009; 25(12): 1053–7.

125. Evans AL. Hypertrophic pyloric stenosis presenting in childhood. *Postgrad Med J* 1987; 63:919.

126. Konvolinka CW, Wermuth CR. Hypertrophic pyloric stenosis in older infants. *Am J Dis Child* 1971; 122:76–7 passim.

127. Cook RCM. Hypertrophic pyloric stenosis. In: Lister J, Irving IM (eds). *Neonatal Surgery*. London: Butterwoths, 1990; 406–420.

128. Tutay GJ, Capraro G, Spirko B et al. Electrolyte profile of pediatric patients with hypertrophic pyloric stenosis. *Pediatr Emerg Care* 2013; 29:465–8.

129. Woolley MM, Felsher BF, Asch J et al. Jaundice, hypertrophic pyloric stenosis, and hepatic glucuronyl transferase. *J Pediatr Surg* 1974; 9:359–63.

130. Benson CD, Lloyd JR. Infantile pyloric stenosis. A review of 1,120 cases. *Am J Surg* 1964; 107:429–33.

131. Stringer MD, Brereton RJ. Current management of infantile hypertrophic pyloric stenosis. *Br J Hosp Med* 1990; 43:266–72.

132. Forman HP, Leonidas JC, Kronfeld GD. A rational approach to the diagnosis of hypertrophic pyloric stenosis: Do the results match the claims? *J Pediatr Surg* 1990; 25:262–6.

133. Scharli A, Sieber WK, Kiesewetter WB. Hypertrophic pyloric stenosis at the Children's Hospital of Pittsburgh from 1912 to 1967. A critical review of current problems and complications. *J Pediatr Surg* 1969; 4:108–14.

134. Zeidan B, Wyatt J, Mackersie A et al. Recent results of treatment of infantile hypertrophic pyloric stenosis. *Arch Dis Child* 1988; 63:1060–4.

135. Bakal U, Sarac M, Aydin M et al. Recent changes in the features of hypertrophic pyloric stenosis. *Pediatrics Int* 2016; 58(5):369–71.

136. Acker SN, Garcia AJ, Ross JT et al. Current trends in the diagnosis and treatment of pyloric stenosis. *Pediatr Surg Int* 2015; 31:363–6.

137. Said M, Shaul DB, Fujimoto M et al. Ultrasound measurements in hypertrophic pyloric stenosis: Don't let the numbers fool you. *Perm J* 2012; 16:25–7.

138. Blumhagen JD, Coombs JB. Ultrasound in the diagnosis of hypertrophic pyloric stenosis. *J Clin Ultrasound* 1981; 9:289–92.

139. Gribner R, Pistor G, Abou-Touk B et al. Significance of ultrasound for the diagnosis of hypertrophic pyloric stenosis. *Pediatr Surg Int* 1986; 1:130–4.

140. Fujimoto T, Lane GJ, Segawa O et al. Laparoscopic extramucosal pyloromyotomy versus open pyloromyotomy for infantile hypertrophic pyloric stenosis: Which is better? *J Pediatr Surg* 1999; 34:370–2.

141. Kamata M, Cartabuke RS, Tobias JD. Perioperative care of infants with pyloric stenosis. *Paediatr Anaesth* 2015; 25:1193–206.

142. Smith GA, Mihalov L, Shields BJ. Diagnostic aids in the differentiation of pyloric stenosis from severe gastroesophageal reflux during early infancy: The utility of serum bicarbonate and serum chloride. *Am J Emerg Med* 1999; 17:28–31.

143. Papadakis K, Chen EA, Luks FI et al. The changing presentation of pyloric stenosis. *Am J Emerg Med* 1999; 17:67–9.

144. Hulka F, Campbell TJ, Campbell JR et al. Evolution in the recognition of infantile hypertrophic pyloric stenosis. *Pediatrics* 1997; 100:E9.

145. De Caluwe D, Reding R, de Ville de Goyet J et al. Intraabdominal pyloromyotomy through the umbilical route: A technical improvement. *J Pediatr Surg* 1998; 33:1806–7.

146. Fitzgerald PG, Lau GY, Langer JC et al. Umbilical fold incision for pyloromyotomy. *J Pediatr Surg* 1990; 25:1117–8.

147. Shankar KR, Losty PD, Jones MO et al. Umbilical pyloromyotomy—An alternative to laparoscopy? *Eur J Pediatr Surg* 2001; 11:8–11.

148. Tan KC, Bianchi A. Circumumbilical incision for pyloromyotomy. *Br J Surg* 1986; 73:399.

149. Alain JL, Moulies D, Longis B et al. [Pyloric stenosis in infants. New surgical approaches]. *Ann Pediatr (Paris)* 1991; 38:630–2.

150. Downey EC Jr. Laparoscopic pyloromyotomy. *Semin Pediatr Surg* 1998; 7:220–4.

151. Muensterer OJ, Adibe OO, Harmon CM et al. Single-incision laparoscopic pyloromyotomy: Initial experience. *Surg Endosc* 2010; 24:1589–93.

152. Leclair MD, Plattner V, Mirallie E et al. Laparoscopic pyloromyotomy for hypertrophic pyloric stenosis: A prospective, randomized controlled trial. *J Pediatr Surg* 2007; 42:692–8.

153. St Peter SD, Holcomb GW, 3rd, Calkins CM et al. Open versus laparoscopic pyloromyotomy for pyloric stenosis: A prospective, randomized trial. *Ann Surg* 2006; 244:363–70.

154. Hall NJ, Pacilli M, Eaton S et al. Recovery after open versus laparoscopic pyloromyotomy for pyloric stenosis: A double-blind multicentre randomised controlled trial. *Lancet* 2009; 373:390–8.

155. Siddiqui S, Heidel RE, Angel CA et al. Pyloromyotomy: Randomized control trial of laparoscopic vs open technique. *J Pediatr Surg* 2012; 47:93–8.

156. Hall NJ, Eaton S, Seims A et al. Risk of incomplete pyloromyotomy and mucosal perforation in open and laparoscopic pyloromyotomy. *J Pediatr Surg* 2014; 49:1083–6.

157. Lawrence J. Regarding risk of incomplete pyloromyotomy and mucosal perforation in open and laparoscopic pyloromyotomy. *J Pediatr Surg* 2015; 50:497.

158. Oomen MW, Hoekstra LT, Bakx R et al. Open versus laparoscopic pyloromyotomy for hypertrophic pyloric stenosis: A systematic review and meta-analysis focusing on major complications. *Surg Endosc* 2012; 26:2104–10.

159. Foster ME, Lewis WG. Early postoperative feeding—A continuing controversy in pyloric stenosis. *J R Soc Med* 1989; 82:532–3.

160. Leahy A, Fitzgerald RJ. The influence of delayed feeding on postoperative vomiting in hypertrophic pyloric stenosis. *Br J Surg* 1982; 69:658–9.

161. Leinwand MJ, Shaul DB, Anderson KD. A standardized feeding regimen for hypertrophic pyloric stenosis decreases length of hospitalization and hospital costs. *J Pediatr Surg* 2000; 35:1063–5.

162. Wheeler RA, Najmaldin AS, Stoodley N et al. Feeding regimens after pyloromyotomy. *Br J Surg* 1990; 77:1018–9.

163. Adibe OO, Nichol PF, Lim FY et al. Ad libitum feeds after laparoscopic pyloromyotomy: A retrospective comparison with a standardized feeding regimen in 227 infants. *J Laparoendosc Adv Surg Tech Part A* 2007; 17:235–7.

164. van der Bilt JD, Kramer WL, van der Zee DC et al. Early feeding after laparoscopic pyloromyotomy: The pros and cons. *Surg Endosc* 2004; 18:746–8.

165. Turnock RR, Rangecroft L. Comparison of postpyloromyotomy feeding regimens in infantile hypertrophic pyloric stenosis. *J R Coll Surg Edinb* 1991; 36:164–5.

166. Graham KA, Laituri CA, Markel TA et al. A review of postoperative feeding regimens in infantile hypertrophic pyloric stenosis. *J Pediatr Surg* 2013; 48:2175–9.

167. Scharli AF, Leditschke JF. Gastric motility after pyloromyotomy in infants. A reappraisal of postoperative feeding. *Surgery* 1968; 64:1133–7.

168. Garza JJ, Morash D, Dzakovic A et al. Ad libitum feeding decreases hospital stay for neonates after pyloromyotomy. *J Pediatr Surg* 202; 37:493–5.

169. Adibe OO, Iqbal CW, Sharp SW et al. Protocol versus ad libitum feeds after laparoscopic pyloromyotomy: A prospective randomized trial. *J Pediatr Surg* 2014; 49:129–32; discussion 132.

170. Waldron LS, St Peter SD, Muensterer OJ. Management and outcome of mucosal injury during pyloromyotomy-an analytical survey study. *J Laparoendosc Adv Surg Tech Part A* 25:1044–6.

171. Svensgaard E. The medical treatment of congenital pyloric stenosis. *Arch Dis Child* 1935; 10:443–57.

172. Koike Y, Uchida K, Nakazawa M et al. Predictive factors of negative outcome in initial atropine therapy for infantile hypertrophic pyloric stenosis. *Pediatr Int* 2013; 55:619–23.

173. Owen RP, Almond SL, Humphrey GM. Atropine sulphate: Rescue therapy for pyloric stenosis. *BMJ Case Rep* 2012; bcr2012006489.

174. Mercer AE, Phillips R. Question 2: Can a conservative approach to the treatment of hypertrophic pyloric stenosis with atropine be considered a real alternative to surgical pyloromyotomy? *Arch Dis Child* 2013; 98:474–7.

53

Gastric volvulus

ALAN E. MORTELL AND BRENDAN R. O'CONNOR

INTRODUCTION

Gastric volvulus is a rare, potentially life-threatening condition first described by Berti in 1866.[1] A review of the world literature in 1980 identified only 51 cases in children under 12 years of age.[2] Of these, 26 (52%) were infants, and half of these were younger than 1 month of age. In a recent series, neonates have accounted for only 21% of cases of gastric volvulus.[3,4] In older children, gastric volvulus may be associated with neurodevelopmental delay and splenic abnormalities, but in neonates, there is a strong link with diaphragmatic defects. In the last three decades, numerous descriptions of acute and chronic gastric volvulus in children have been published, bringing the total number of reported cases to more than 640.[3–8]

ETIOLOGY

Gastric volvulus may be defined as an abnormal rotation of one part of the stomach around another[9]; the degree of twist varies from 180° to 360° and is associated with closed-loop obstruction and the risk of strangulation. Lesser degrees of gastric torsion are probably common, frequently asymptomatic, and not diagnostic of volvulus. Such cases may be associated with transient vomiting in infants, but spontaneous resolution is the rule.[7,10] Gastric volvulus may be either organoaxial, occurring around an axis joining the esophageal hiatus and the pyloroduodenal junction, or mesenteroaxial, around an axis joining the midpoint of the greater and lesser curves of the stomach (Figure 53.1). The majority of patients present with organoaxial volvulus (54%) compared to mesenteroaxial volvulus in 41% and combined volvulus in only approximately 2% of cases.[3] A mixed or combined picture occurs if the stomach rotates around both axes simultaneously. The usual direction of rotation is anterior; i.e., in organoaxial volvulus, the greater curve moves upward and forward above the lesser curve, causing the posterior gastric wall to face anteriorly. The gastroesophageal junction and the pylorus may both become obstructed. In anterior mesenteroaxial rotation, the antrum comes to lie anterosuperior to the fundus, and obstruction is usually in the antropyloric region.

Acute, complete volvulus is most often seen in infancy in contrast to chronic and partial varieties, which more often occur in older children and adults. More complex patterns of gastric volvulus have been described in neonates and infants with abnormal gastric bands or adhesions (see later), and in older children after gastrostomy[11,12] or Nissen fundoplication, performed either open[13–15] or laparoscopically.[16]

CLINICAL CASES

The following three cases illustrate different aspects of the presentation and management of gastric volvulus in infancy.

Case 1

A full-term male infant presented soon after birth with cyanotic attacks during feeding. A tracheoesophageal fistula was initially suspected, but a plain chest radiograph (Figure 53.2a) showed a gastric shadow lying in front of the heart, and a barium swallow (Figure 53.2b) demonstrated an organoaxial gastric volvulus within the chest. Via a left thoracotomy, the stomach was derotated and reduced into the abdomen with repair of the esophageal hiatus. A gastropexy was not performed, and subsequent progress was uneventful.

Case 2

A full-term male infant presented at 4 days of age with intermittent vomiting. This was initially attributed to a urinary infection, but the vomiting continued, and a barium meal showed that there was delayed passage of contrast into the stomach from the esophagus. When the barium was injected via a nasogastric tube, the stomach was seen to lie horizontally and to empty very slowly. At laparotomy, the pylorus was hypertrophied, and the stomach was distended. The gastrocolic omentum was deficient along most of the

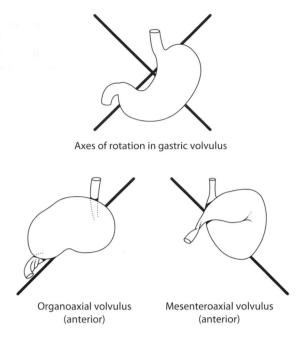

Axes of rotation in gastric volvulus

Organoaxial volvulus
(anterior)

Mesenteroaxial volvulus
(anterior)

Figure 53.1 Diagrammatic representation of the main types of gastric volvulus.

greater curve, allowing free organoaxial rotation of the stomach. A pyloromyotomy and anterior gastropexy were performed, after which the child became symptom-free.

Case 3

A female infant presented at the age of 2 months with a history of loud borborygmi, inability to bring up wind after feeding, and occasional vomiting. On examination, bowel sounds were heard in the chest. Barium meal showed an organoaxially rotated intrathoracic stomach. Via an abdominal approach, a large paraesophageal hernia was reduced, followed by a crural repair and Nissen fundoplication. The child remained asymptomatic 4 years later.

PATHOGENESIS

The stomach is relatively fixed at the esophageal hiatus and at the pyloroduodenal junction and is also stabilized by four *ligamentous* attachments—the gastrohepatic, gastrosplenic, gastrocolic, and gastrophrenic ligaments (Figure 53.3). Despite these attachments, considerable changes in shape and position of the normal stomach are possible. This is highlighted by the gastric rotation that can sometimes be observed during air insufflation of the stomach at the time of laparoscopically assisted percutaneous endoscopic gastrostomy insertion.[17] Absence or attenuation of the normal anatomical anchors results in abnormal gastric mobility, which may be encouraged still further by a coexistent diaphragmatic defect. Most cases of gastric volvulus in the newborn are secondary to diaphragmatic defects with or without deficient ligamentous attachments.[2,18–24] The contribution of the gastrocolic and gastrosplenic ligaments to

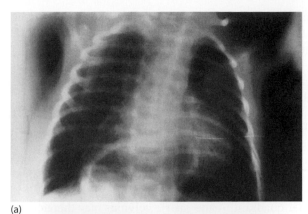

(a)

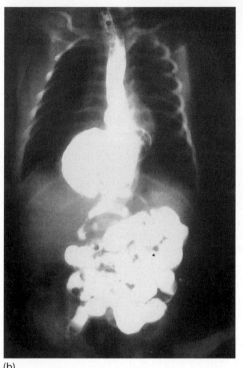

(b)

Figure 53.2 **(a)** Plain chest radiograph showing an air-filled viscus in the chest (case 1). **(b)** Barium study showing the stomach lying above the diaphragm with the greater curvature uppermost (case 1).

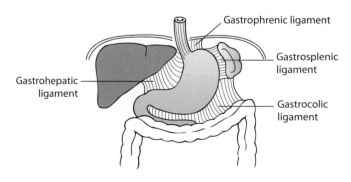

Figure 53.3 Diagrammatic view of the stabilizing gastric ligaments.

fixation of the stomach is demonstrated by the observation in the cadaver that their division allows 180° rotation of the normal stomach.[2,5,25]

Eventration or herniation of the diaphragm is present in about two-thirds of all children presenting with gastric volvulus.[3] However, this proportion is as high as 80% in some series of infants.[2,19] Diaphragmatic hernias are typically paraesophageal or posterolateral defects, but gastric volvulus within a Morgagni hernia is also possible.[3,26] The presumed mechanism of gastric volvulus in this situation is upward displacement of the transverse colon, which pulls up the greater curve of the stomach into the expanded left upper quadrant. Acute gastric volvulus may therefore present as an early complication of diaphragmatic defects.

Gastric distension may encourage the development of gastric volvulus.[25] Infantile hypertrophic pyloric stenosis may rarely be a predisposing factor, as in the second case described earlier. Two similar cases have been reported, but those infants also had diaphragmatic defects.[27,28] Air swallowing can also cause gastric distension, and intermittent gastric volvulus has been reported in an aerophagic neurologically impaired child.[23]

Other rare causes of gastric volvulus in the neonate and infant include the following: abnormal bands or adhesions producing an axis of rotation for the stomach;[6,19,29] rectal atresia with consequent overdistension of the transverse colon;[30] congenital absence or resection of the left lobe of the liver, which may promote abnormal gastric mobility;[31,32] and congenital deficiency of the gastrocolic omentum.[5,33] Asplenic syndrome (asplenia, congenital heart disease, with or without intestinal malrotation and deficiency of the gastric ligaments) is increasingly recognized as a predisposing condition.[34,35] Nakada et al.[36] reported gastric volvulus as a complication in 3 of 25 patients with asplenia, the youngest of whom was 1 month of age. Anchoring gastric ligaments were deficient in all cases. Because of the potentially fatal outcome of acute gastric volvulus in this situation, Okoye et al.[37] have recommended prophylactic gastropexy. Defective fixation and ligamentous laxity also account for the association between gastric volvulus and a wandering spleen.[38–40] Intestinal malrotation is associated with gastric volvulus, even in the absence of asplenia.[6,29,36,41]

Gastric volvulus in children may rarely arise as a postoperative complication. It has been described after Nissen fundoplication, presumably because the stomach has been extensively mobilized by division of gastrosplenic and gastrocolic attachments.[13,15,16,42] There is one recorded case of gastric volvulus developing after repair of a diaphragmatic hernia[19] and another as an iatrogenic complication of gastric transposition in infancy.[43]

CLINICAL FEATURES

The clinical features depend on the degree of rotation and obstruction. In adults and older children, the Borchardt triad is diagnostic of acute volvulus: (1) unproductive retching, (2) acute localized epigastric distension, and (3) inability

to pass a nasogastric tube.[44] These features are difficult to assess in the infant and may be absent. Persistent regurgitation and vomiting (sometimes unproductive) are common, although nonspecific, presenting symptoms in the newborn. The vomitus may or may not contain bile, depending on the degree of pyloric obstruction. Hematemesis and anemia are well described, and occasionally the vomiting is described as projectile. Failure to thrive, chest infections, and less defined respiratory complaints, such as wheeze, are sometimes evident.[41] Upper abdominal pain and distension may be noted in older infants and children. However, abdominal signs may be minimal if the stomach is intrathoracic, when respiratory distress and tachypnea are the dominant features.[2,20,22,45,46] Failure to pass a nasogastric tube may have several causes in the newborn, and the successful passage of a tube does not exclude the diagnosis.[16,19] In neonates, confusion with esophageal atresia is possible, but arrest of the nasogastric tube in the distal esophagus and radiographic abnormalities on routine films should raise suspicion and prompt investigation by contrast studies.[47] In older children, presenting symptoms may be intermittent, chronic, and also nonspecific.[16]

DIAGNOSIS

Plain abdominal and chest radiographs are essential. A distended stomach in an abnormal position should suggest the possibility of gastric volvulus. In mesenteroaxial volvulus, the stomach is spherical on the plain film taken with the patient in the supine position, and two fluid levels are often visible on the erect film—one in the fundus (the lower) and the other in the antrum (upper) (Figure 53.4a); these findings may be absent if the stomach has been decompressed by a nasogastric tube. A paucity of distal bowel gas in acute volvulus can indicate gastric outlet obstruction.[48] Contrast studies clarify the anatomy (Figure 53.4b) and the site(s) of obstruction, which is usually at the pylorus, giving a so-called beak deformity.[18] Organoaxial volvulus is more difficult to diagnose on plain films (especially if there is no associated diaphragmatic defect) and may indeed be missed during a contrast study. The distended stomach lies rather horizontally on the plain film, with a single fluid level. On contrast examination, the esophagogastric junction is lower than normal, the greater and lesser curves are inverted, and the antrum and duodenum are distorted (Figure 53.5). In the presence of a diaphragmatic defect, such as a paraesophageal hernia, the antrum may herniate into the retrocardiac position, producing a fluid level in the chest above the gastric fundus, and thus, organoaxial volvulus can also rarely give rise to two fluid levels.[49] Computed tomography (CT) has been used in cases where gastric volvulus was not diagnosed on plain films; however, it should not be necessary if an upper gastrointestinal contrast study is performed and may only serve to delay treatment.[48] A CT scan can yield further information about structural abnormalities, such as splenic position or absence.

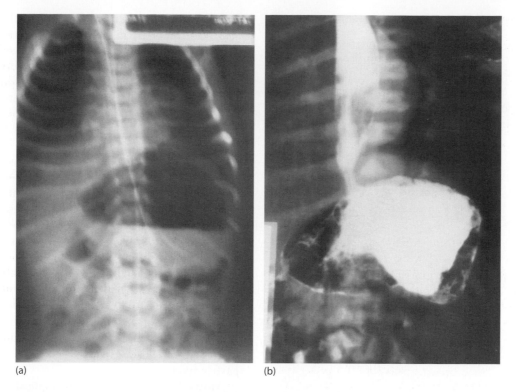

(a)   (b)

Figure 53.4 **(a)** Plain abdominal radiograph showing a distended stomach but only a single fluid level in this neonate with mesenteroaxial gastric volvulus. **(b)** Barium study confirming mesenteroaxial gastric volvulus.

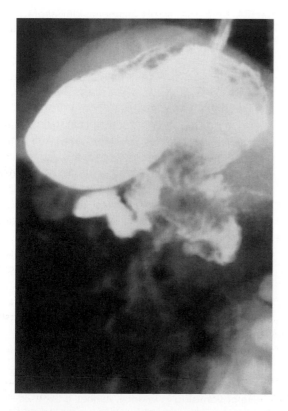

Figure 53.5 Oblique view of barium meal demonstrating an organoaxial gastric volvulus in a neonate who presented with intermittent vomiting (case 2).

TREATMENT

Acute gastric volvulus requires appropriate resuscitation and urgent surgery if ischemic necrosis and gastric perforation are to be avoided. If possible, the stomach should be decompressed preoperatively by nasogastric suction, but vigorous attempts to pass a tube must be avoided because of a risk of gastric perforation.[19] An abdominal approach is recommended, even when the stomach lies in the chest, since this allows identification of any associated gastrointestinal anomalies and accurate diaphragmatic repair if required. Occasionally, preliminary needle aspiration of the stomach may be warranted before manipulating a tensely dilated stomach and reducing the volvulus.[50] Any associated diaphragmatic defect should be repaired and the stomach fixed to the anterior abdominal wall (Table 53.1).

Gastrostomy alone may be used for gastric fixation in neonates, since it provides adequate fixation, postoperative decompression, and a route for postoperative feeding. A Stamm gastrostomy using a 10- or 12-French-gauge Malecot catheter secured by a double-purse-string absorbable suture is appropriate (Figure 53.6a). In infants with no predisposing diaphragmatic defect, an anterior gastropexy should be added (Figure 53.6b). This involves suturing the greater curve of the stomach to the parietal peritoneum of the anterior abdominal wall and the undersurface of the diaphragm by a series of nonabsorbable sutures. There are three recorded cases of recurrence following this approach.[51,52] Endoscopically assisted percutaneous anterior gastropexy has also been described as a successful

Table 53.1 Surgical options for gastric volvulus in the neonate/infant

Repair of diaphragmatic defect, division of congenital bands, etc., and anterior gastrostomy

Crural repair (if necessary) and anterior gastropexy

Crural repair and fundoplication for cases with severe gastroesophageal reflux

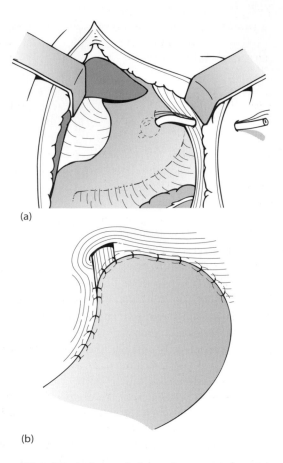

(a)

(b)

Figure 53.6 Operative techniques in neonatal gastric volvulus. **(a)** Anterior Stamm gastrostomy using a Malecot catheter. **(b)** Anterior gastropexy.

minimally invasive treatment for chronic mesenteroaxial volvulus in an older child.[53] Fundoplication may be necessary if there is evidence of gross gastroesophageal reflux, but several authors have achieved good results in such cases with a crural repair alone, and a more conservative approach is warranted provided that the tendency to volvulus is prevented.[41,42] Diaphragmatic crural repair must be performed meticulously, as there is often a common hiatus for the esophagus and aorta in these patients.[42] There is no justification for gastrectomy, gastroenterostomy, or the colonic displacement operation described by Tanner[9] in this age group.

In older children with isolated gastric volvulus, preliminary nasogastric decompression followed by a laparoscopic

anterior gastropexy is an option,[33,54] and this technique has also been reported in neonates.[55] Laparoscopic management of neonatal intrathoracic gastric volvulus due to a paraesophageal hernia has also been described, consisting of reduction of the stomach into the abdomen with resection of the hernia sac, crural repair, Nissen fundoplication, and gastrostomy.[56] In gastric volvulus due to a wandering spleen, splenopexy alone may be sufficient.[57]

COMPLICATIONS

A number of complications can result from gastric volvulus, including prolonged gastric ileus, pyloric ischemia, gastric outlet obstruction, gastric necrosis, and perforation.[6]

The mortality from gastric volvulus is difficult to assess, with recent series reporting mortality rates of 7.1% in acute gastric volvulus compared to 2.7% in chronic cases.[6] Untreated, gastric volvulus has a mortality rate of up to 80%, highlighting the importance of prompt recognition and treatment. Deaths have been reported due to missed or delayed diagnosis, with subsequent gastric necrosis and perforation, or inadequate gastric fixation.[4,8,19,21,24]

Most recent series report uncomplicated early outcomes after surgery. One long-term follow-up study of nine infants demonstrated no recurrences or late complications.[4]

REFERENCES

1. Berti A. Singalore attortigliamento dell'esofago col duodeno sequito da rapida morte. *Gazz Med Ital Prov Veneti* 1866; 9: 139.
2. Idowu J, Aitken DR, Georgeson KE. Gastric volvulus in the newborn. *Arch Surg* 1980; 115: 1046–9.
3. Cribbs RK, Gow KW, Wulkan ML. Gastric volvulus in infants and children. *Pediatrics* 2008; 122: e752–62.
4. McIntyre RC, Bensard DD, Karrer FM, Hall RJ, Lilly JR. The pediatric diaphragm in acute gastric volvulus. *J Am Coll Surg* 1994; 178: 234–8.
5. Camerton AEP, Howard ER. Gastric volvulus in childhood. *J Pediatr Surg* 1987; 22: 944–7.
6. Gerstle JT, Chiu P, Emil S. Gastric volvulus in children: Lessons learned from delayed diagnoses. *Semin Pediatr Surg* 2009; 18: 98-103.
7. Honna T, Kamii Y, Tsuchida Y. Idiopathic gastric volvulus in infancy and childhood. *J Pediatr Surg* 1990; 25: 707–10.
8. Miller DL, Pasquale MD, Seneca RP, Hodin E. Gastric volvulus in the pediatric population. *Arch Surg* 1991; 126: 1146–9.
9. Tanner NC. Chronic and recurrent volvulus of the stomach. *Am J Surg* 1968; 115: 505–15.
10. Eek S, Hagelsteen H. Torsion of the stomach as a cause of vomiting in infancy. *Lancet* 1958; i: 26–8.
11. Alawadhi A, Chou S, Soucy P. Gastric volvulus: A late complication of gastrostomy. *Can J Surg* 1991; 34: 485–6.

12. Sookpotarom P, Vejchapipat P, Chongsrisawat V et al. Gastric volvulus caused by percutaneous endoscopic gastrostomy: A case report. *J Pediatr Surg* 2005; 40: e21–3.

13. Fung KP, Rubin S, Scott RB. Gastric volvulus complicating Nissen fundoplication. *J Pediatr Surg* 1990; 25: 1242–3.

14. Trinh TD, Benson JE. Fluoroscopic diagnosis of complications after Nissen fundoplication in children. *AJR* 1997; 169: 1023–8.

15. Cameron BH, Vajarvandi V, Blair GK et al. The intermittent and variable features of gastric volvulus in childhood. *Pediatr Surg Int* 1995; 10: 26–9.

16. Kuenzler KA, Wolfson PJ, Murphy SG. Gastric volvulus after laparoscopic Nissen fundoplication with gastrostomy. *J Pediatr Surg* 2003; 38: 1241–3.

17. Croaker GD, Najmaldin AS. Laparoscopically assisted percutaneous endoscopic gastrostomy. *Pediatr Surg Int* 1997; 12: 130–1.

18. McDevitt JB. Intrathoracic volvulus of the stomach in a newborn infant. *Ir J Med Sci* 1970; 3: 131–2.

19. Cole BC, Dickinson SJ. Acute volvulus of the stomach in infants and children. *Surgery* 1971; 70:707–17.

20. Campbell JB. Neonatal gastric volvulus. *Am J Roentgenol* 1979; 132: 723–5.

21. Talukdar BC. Gastric volvulus with perforation of stomach in congenital diaphragmatic hernia in an infant. *J Indian Med Assoc* 1979; 73: 219–21.

22. Starshak RJ, Sty JR. Diaphragmatic defects with gastric volvulus in the neonate. *Wisc Med J* 1983; 82: 28–31.

23. Komuro H, Matoba K, Kaneko M. Laparoscopic gastropexy for chronic gastric volvulus complicated by pathologic aerophagia in a boy. Pediatr Int 2005; 47(6): 701–3.

24. El-Gohary MA, Etiaby A. Gastric volvulus in infants and children. *Pediatr Surg Int* 1994; 9: 486–8.

25. Dalgaard JR. Volvulus of the stomach. *Acta Chir Scand* 1952; 103: 131–53.

26. Estevao-Costa J, Soares-Oliveira M, Correia-Pinto J et al. Acute gastric volvulus secondary to a Morgagni hernia. *Pediatr Surg Int* 2000; 16: 107–8.

27. Moreno Torres E. Estenosis per hipertrofia de piloro con volvulo gastrico. *Bol Soc Valenciana Paediatr* 1968; 10: 231–2.

28. Anagnostara A, Koumanidou C, Vakaki M et al. Chronic gastric volvulus and hypertrophic pyloric stenosis in an infant. *J Clin Ultrasound* 2003; 31: 383–6.

29. Iko BO. Volvulus of the stomach: An African series and a review. *J Natl Med Assoc* 1987; 79: 171–6.

30. Mizrahi S, Vinograd I, Schiller M. Neonatal gastric volvulus secondary to rectal atresia. *Clin Pediatr* 1988; 27: 302–4.

31. Chuang JH, Hsieh CS, Hueng SC, Wan Y-L. Gastric volvulus complicating left hepatic lobectomy. *Pediatr Surg Int* 1993; 8: 255–6.

32. Koh H, Lee JS, Park YJ et al. Gastric volvulus associated with agenesis of the left lobe of the liver in a child: A case treated by laparoscopic gastropexy. *J Pediatr Surg* 2008; 43: 231–3.

33. Odaka A, Shimomura K, Fujioka M et al. Laparoscopic gastropexy for acute gastric volvulus: A case report. *J Pediatr Surg* 1999; 34: 477–8.

34. Aoyama K, Teteishi K. Gastric volvulus in three children with asplenic syndrome. *J Pediatr Surg* 1986; 21: 307–10.

35. Koga H, Yamataka A, Kobayashi H et al. Laparoscopy-assisted gastropexy for gastric volvulus in a child with situs inversus, asplenia, and major cardiac anomaly. *J Laparoendosc Adv Surg Tech A* 2007; 17: 513–6.

36. Nakada K, Kawaguchi F, Wakisaka M et al. Digestive tract disorders associated with asplenia/polysplenia syndrome. *J Pediatr Surg* 1997; 32: 91–4.

37. Okoye BO, Bailey DMC, Cusick EL, Spicer RD. Prophylactic gastropexy in the asplenia syndrome. *Pediatr Surg Int* 1997; 12: 28–9.

38. Garcia JA, Garcia-Fernandez M, Romance A, Sanchez JC. Wandering spleen and gastric volvulus. *Pediatr Radiol* 1994; 24: 535–6.

39. Liu HT, Lau KK. Wandering spleen: An unusual association with gastric volvulus. *AJR Am J Roentgenol* 2007; 188: W328–30

40. Spector JM, Chappell J. Gastric volvulus associated with wandering spleen in a child. *J Pediatr Surg* 2000; 35:641–2.

41. Samuel M, Burge DM, Griffiths DM. Gastric volvulus and associated gastro-oesophageal reflux. *Arch Dis Child* 1995; 73: 462–4.

42. Stiefel D, Willi UV, Sacher P, Schwobel MG, Stauffer UG. Pitfalls in therapy of upside-down stomach. *Eur J Pediatr Surg* 2000; 10: 162–6.

43. Chan KL, Saing H. Iatrogenic gastric volvulus during transposition for esophageal atresia: Diagnosis and treatment. *J Pediatr Surg* 1996; 31: 229–32.

44. Borchardt M. Zur Pathologie und Therapie des Magen volvulus. *Arch Klin Chir* 1904; 74: 243–60.

45. Beckmann KR, Nozicka CA. Congenital diaphragmatic hernia with gastric volvulus presenting as an acute tension gastrothorax. *Am J Emerg Med* 1999; 17: 35–7.

46. Mutabagani KH, Teich S, Long FR. Primary intrathoracic gastric volvulus in a newborn. *J Pediatr Surg* 1999; 34: 1869–71.

47. Yadav K, Myers NA. Paraesophageal hernia in the neonatal period—Another differential diagnosis of oesophageal atresia. *Pediatr Surg Int* 1997; 12: 420–1.

48. Oh SK, Han BK, Levin TL et al. Gastric volvulus in children: The twists and turns of an unusual entity. *Pediatr Radiol* 2008; 38: 297–304.

49. Scott RL, Felker R, Winer-Muram H et al. The differential retrocardiac air–fluid level: A sign of intrathoracic gastric volvulus. *J Can Assoc Radiol* 1986; 37: 119–21.

50. Asch MJ, Sherman NJ. Gastric volvulus in children: Report of two cases. *J Pediatr Surg* 1977; 12: 1059–62.

51. Stephenson RH, Hopkins WA. Volvulus of the stomach complicating eventration of the diaphragm. *Am J Gastroenterol* 1964; 41: 225–7.

52. Colijn AW, Kneepkens CM, van Amerongen AT, Ekkelkamp S. Gastric volvulus after anterior gastropexy. *J Pediatr Gastroenterol Nutr* 1993; 17: 105–7.

53. Kawai M, Hiramatsu M, Lee S-W et al. Endoscopy Assisted percutaneous anterior gastropexy for gastric volvulus: A minimally invasive technique using a special instrument. *Endoscopy* 2013; 45: E151–2.

54. Nataraja R, Mahomed A. Video demonstration of the technique of laparoscopic gastrophrenopexy for the treatment of symptomatic primary organoaxial gastric volvulus. *J Laparoendosc Adv Surg Tech A* 2010; 20(5): 507.

55. Shah A, Shah AV. Laparoscopic gastropexy in a neonate for acute gastric volvulus. *Pediatr Surg Int* 2003; 19: 217–9.

56. Bradley T, Stephenson J, Drugas G et al. Laparoscopic management of neonatal paraesophageal hernia with intrathoracic gastric volvulus. *J Pediatr Surg* 2010; 45: E21–3.

57. Zivkovic SM. Sutureless 'button and hole' splenopexy. *Pediatr Surg Int* 1998; 13: 220–2.

54

Gastric perforation

ADAM C. ALDER AND ROBERT K. MINKES

INTRODUCTION

Gastric perforation in the neonatal period is rare; however, it continues to be associated with significant morbidity and mortality. Spontaneous neonatal gastric perforation is estimated to occur in 1 in 2900 live births[1] and accounts for approximately 10%–15% of all gastrointestinal perforations in neonates and children. Gastrointestinal perforations occur more commonly in males; however, there appears to be no sex predilection for those occurring in the stomach.[2] Recent series may suggest a male predominance, but this remains inconclusive.[3] The incidence of gastrointestinal perforation is increasing in some populations; however, the relative incidence of gastric perforation is decreasing.[4] The terminology used to describe neonatal gastric perforation has been inconsistent, and its etiology remains a topic of debate. Spontaneous or idiopathic gastric perforations refer to those with no identifiable underlying cause and account for the majority of gastric perforations in most reported series.[1,5] Nevertheless, many pediatric surgeons believe that an underlying cause can be found in most cases of neonatal gastric perforation.[6]

Siebold, in 1926, is credited with the first description of a gastrointestinal perforation with no demonstrable cause, the so-called spontaneous perforation.[7] In 1929, Stern et al.[8] reported attempts at surgical repair. Agerty et al.[9] reported the first successful repair of a neonatal intestinal (ileum) perforation in 1943, and Leger et al.,[10] in 1950, described the first successful repair of a neonatal gastric perforation. Survival following a neonatal gastric perforation was rare prior to the 1960s. While mortality has improved since that time, it remains significant and ranges from 25% to over 50% in most series.[1]

ETIOLOGY

Gastric perforations in neonates can be broadly categorized as spontaneous (idiopathic), ischemic, or traumatic; however, in many instances, the etiology may be multifactorial. Ischemia, necrosis, and perforation may occur with no obvious inciting factors.[11] Table 54.1 lists several possible causes and associations with gastric perforations. Spontaneous gastric perforations most often occur on the greater curvature.[1] Neonatal gastric perforation can occur in full-term, premature, and small for gestational age neonates. Some infants appear to have been healthy and medically stable prior to the development of the perforation, whereas others have underlying medical conditions or congenital anomalies. There are reports of intrauterine gastric perforation with no known underlying cause.[12] Unrecognized overdistension or ischemic insult may result in a perforation that is thought to be spontaneous. Ischemic perforations occur in the setting of physiologic stress such as prematurity, asphyxia, sepsis, and necrotizing enterocolitis. The perforations are often associated with ulcerations and ischemic tissue. Traumatic perforation results from pneumatic distention during mask ventilation, positive pressure ventilation, or iatrogenic injury during gastric intubation. Several specific causes of neonatal gastric perforation have been reported including intestinal atresias, prenatal stress, trauma, foreign bodies or bezoars, and exposure to corticosteroids and nonsteroidal anti-inflammatory agents (Table 54.1). Several theories on the etiology of spontaneous (idiopathic) gastric perforations have been suggested, but no single theory is universally accepted. Theories include congenital absence of the gastric muscle,[13] forces exerted during vaginal delivery,[14] and pneumatic distention.[15] Studies in dogs and human neonatal cadavers suggest that rupture is caused by overdistension and is in keeping with the law of Laplace.[16] With gastric distention, the greatest wall tension is exerted on the fundus, the site of most spontaneous perforations. In addition, overdistension can cause ischemic changes, a finding present in many cases of perforation.[17]

Recent studies suggest a deficiency of the tyrosine kinase receptor C-KIT⁺ mast cells, and a lack of C-KIT⁺ interstitial cells of Cajal may contribute to idiopathic gastric perforation.[18] Mice lacking C-KIT⁺ mast cells develop spontaneous

Table 54.1 Causes and associations of neonatal gastric perforation

Idiopathic
Perinatal stress
   Hypoxia
   Asphyxia
   Prematurity[19,20]
   Anatomic defect
   Distal obstruction
      – Pyloric atresia[21]
      – Duodenal atresia[19]
      – Midgut volvulus[22]
   Tracheoesophageal fistula[23–26]
   Congenital deficiency of gastric muscle
Iatrogenic
   Nasogastric tube[27,28]
   Aggressive bag ventilation with or without tracheo-esophageal fistula[29–31]
   Cardiopulmonary resuscitation[32–35]
   Positive pressure ventilation
   Inadvertent perforation during surgery (ventriculo-peritoneal shunt)[36,37]
   Vaginal delivery[10,14]
Medication
   Indomethacin[38,39]
   Corticosteroids[40]

gastric ulceration or perforation. Pathologic specimens from nonnecrotic portions of the stomach in six spontaneous gastric perforation patients showed a decreased number in interstitial cells of Cajal.[41] In addition, postmortem examination of stomachs of neonates who died of idiopathic gastric perforation revealed a deficiency in both C-KIT⁺ mast cells and interstitial cells of Cajal when compared to controls. The authors suggest that these abnormalities could result in impaired immunity and abnormal motility predisposing to gastric perforation.[42]

CLINICAL PRESENTATION

The clinical presentation of gastric perforation is variable. The majority of cases present within the first 7 days of life; however, later presentations are reported.[2] The neonates are often premature or have a history of asphyxia or hypoxia.[19] Neonates may present with feeding intolerance or emesis that may contain blood. Many develop abrupt onset of rapidly progressive abdominal distension from pneumo- or hydroperitoneum.[43] These infants progress to respiratory distress, hemodynamic instability, and signs of shock such as hypothermia, cyanosis, poor peripheral perfusion, and low urine output. The abdomen may rapidly become tense and tender with signs of peritoneal irritation. Ventilation may be impaired or ineffective until the abdomen is decompressed. Subcutaneous emphysema in

the abdominal wall or pneumoscrotum may be appreciated.[44] Infants with posterior perforations into the lesser sac may present with a more insidious course, making the diagnosis difficult.

Infants with perforation secondary to an underlying process often have evidence of the predisposing condition such as findings of tracheoesophageal fistula, duodenal atresia or web, malrotation, gastroschisis, or diaphragmatic hernia.[19,45] In some instances, a secondary cause is found at the time of operation. In cases of iatrogenic perforation, a history of traumatic naso- or orogastric intubation, prior surgery, corticosteroid or nonsteroidal administration, and aggressive ventilation or cardiopulmonary resuscitation may be obtained.[27]

DIAGNOSIS

The diagnosis of gastric perforation is made from the clinical history, physical examination, and radiographic studies. In infants with massive pneumoperitoneum, a plain abdominal radiograph will demonstrate air under the diaphragm that extends laterally, trapping the abdominal viscera medially and producing a saddlebag appearance.[46] The stomach is not visualized by plain radiograph in 90% of the cases.[47] Other plain radiograph findings include subcutaneous emphysema, pneumoscrotum, ascites, or an oro- or nasogastric tube outside the confines of the stomach. Pneumatosis intestinalis and portal venous air are signs of necrotizing enterocolitis, which may coexist with gastric perforation. Calcification and dilated loops of bowel are common findings of more distal perforation, and a gasless abdomen is seen in cases of neonatal volvulus. A definitive diagnosis may not be made prior to laparotomy. A water-soluble contrast study will reveal extravasation from the stomach into the peritoneal cavity (Figure 54.1). Ultrasound may show ascites or fluid collections. In premature infants with known lung disease, pneumoperitoneum can result from air tracking from the mediastinum. A chest film demonstrating pneumomediastinum, an air-fluid level in the stomach, a negative peritoneal aspirate, and an intraperitoneal drain that bubbles with the ventilator cycle can help to exclude an intra-abdominal process.

DIFFERENTIAL DIAGNOSIS

The differential diagnosis is broad and includes conditions that cause sudden deterioration in the newborn and conditions that produce vomiting and abdominal distention. Conditions causing cardiovascular collapse include sepsis, pneumothorax, cardiac dysfunction, intraventricular hemorrhage, electrolyte abnormalities, hypoglycemia, necrotizing enterocolitis, perforated viscus, and malrotation with midgut volvulus. Conditions associated with vomiting and abdominal distention include Hirschsprung's disease, intestinal atresia, meconium ileus, meconium plug syndrome, imperforate anus, perforated viscus, necrotizing enterocolitis, and midgut volvulus.

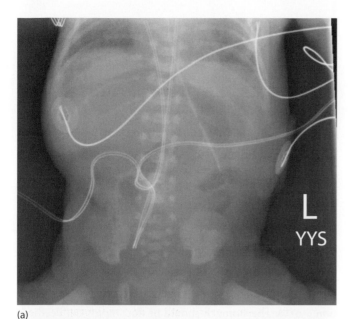

(a)

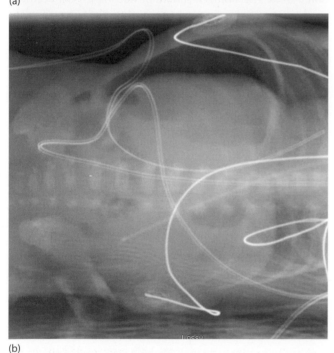

(b)

Figure 54.1 Diagnosis. Abdominal distention, pneumo-peritoneum seen on these two view films of the abdomen. **(a)** Note the lucency over the liver. **(b)** Pneumoperitoneum becomes much clearer on the lateral decubitus film. There is no evidence of lung disease and no findings suggestive of enterocolitis.

PERIOPERATIVE CARE

Infants with gastric perforation develop septic parameters and need to be resuscitated accordingly. Neonates may become unstable prior to the development of free intra-abdominal air. Infants who develop respiratory distress require intubation, and increased ventilator support is needed as the abdomen becomes more distended. Appropriate laboratory investigations include blood cultures, white blood cell count, hemoglobin, hematocrit, platelet count, electrolyte profile, and blood gas analysis. Broad-spectrum antibiotics should be initiated. Fluid boluses and blood transfusions are given to achieve hemodynamic stability and adequate urine output. An oro- or nasogastric tube should be carefully passed and placed on low intermittent suction. Once free intra-abdominal air is identified, the patient is stabilized and a laparotomy should be performed. Aspiration of the peritoneum with an i.v. cannula when an overly distended abdomen is impeding ventilation can be a lifesaving measure.[20] In select cases, peritoneal drainage has been reported with resolution of the peritonitis and healing of the perforation.[43]

SURGICAL TECHNIQUE

Historically, open exploration and repair is favored. Some reports indicate that gastrointestinal perforations have been found to be spontaneously sealed by adjacent omentum[48] or that pneumoperitoneum, possibly from gastric perforation, can be managed successfully without an operation.[49,50] These case reports often do not have a specific source for the pneumoperitoneum and make use of the non-operative management approach in high-risk patients with successful management of gastric perforation seen as a possible alternative to rather than a replacement for standard operative management. Recently, successful laparoscopic repair of neonatal gastric perforation has been reported.[51] The operative approach should be based on the abilities of the surgeon and local resources.

For an open repair, an upper abdominal transverse skin incision (Figure 54.2) is made and dissection carried through the rectus muscle until the peritoneum is entered. The umbilical vein is divided. The incision can be extended as needed. Peritoneal fluid and debris are evacuated. The abdomen is explored for the site of perforation. When a perforation of the stomach is not found, careful exploration of the gastroesophageal junction, duodenum, small bowel,

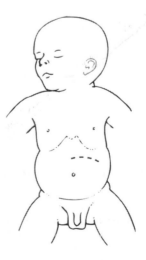

Figure 54.2 Incision. Upper abdominal transverse skin incision. The incision can be enlarged to gain access to the entire abdomen.

and colon should be performed. The lesser sac should be opened and inspected for contamination and integrity of the posterior surface of the stomach.

The most common site of a spontaneous perforation is near the greater curvature. The perforation can be small or extensive and extend high on the stomach. For isolated perforations, the devitalized edges of the perforation are debrided back to viable tissue (Figure 54.3). The defect is closed in one or two layers and may be reinforced with an omental patch (Figure 54.4). Stapled closure of a perforation as well as repair around a gastrostomy tube have also been successful. A variety of techniques have been used to manage extensive perforations or necrosis that requires subtotal or total gastrectomy. In a stable infant, subtotal gastrectomy can be performed with reconstruction with an esophago-gastric anastomosis.[52] Several techniques for reconstruction after total gastrectomy have been reported including transverse colon interposition, Roux-en-Y esophago-jejunal

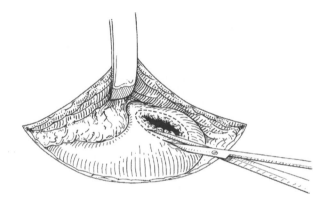

Figure 54.3 Exposure and resection. The entire perforation is exposed. A variable area of the stomach is found to be devitalized or necrotic. The edges of the perforation are resected back to bleeding viable tissue. On rare occasions, extensive resection, subtotal, or total gastrectomy are required.

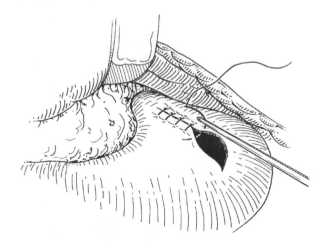

Figure 54.4 Closure. The free edges of healthy tissue are closed in one (depicted) or two layers. An omental patch may be used. Careful inspection of the posterior wall of the stomach and the entire small and large bowel should be performed to exclude additional areas of necrosis.

anastomosis, and Hunt–Lawrence pouch reconstruction.[3] Reconstruction following total gastrectomy in an unstable neonate can be delayed and performed in stages. In the initial surgery, the esophagus is closed and a feeding tube placed distally through the distal gastric remnant or separate jejunostomy. The esophagus is decompressed and the child supported with parenteral nutrition until tube feedings can be initiated through the feeding tube. Reconstruction can be considered several weeks later when the clinical condition and nutritional status have improved.

Following repair of the perforation, the abdomen is lavaged with warm saline. Peritoneal drainage is not needed for most primary repairs and has not been shown to reduce postoperative complications, but are used routinely by some surgeons. The fascia and skin are closed in standard fashions. Postoperatively, supportive and resuscitative care is continued. The child is maintained on broad spectrum antibiotics, gastric acid suppression therapy, and total parenteral nutrition (TPN). The stomach should be decompressed. Feedings are held until the infant has stabilized. Many surgeons obtain a contrast study prior to initiating enteral feeds.

Poor outcomes after gastric perforation have been associated with several clinical factors. Yang et al.[45] found that leukocytosis at admission and thrombocytopenia at 48 hours were associated with poor outcomes. Additional factors predictive of poor outcome include sepsis, metabolic acidosis, and hyponatremia.[45,53] A prompt response to identification of the perforation and appropriate supportive care for the newborn is important for the best clinical outcomes.

CONCLUSION

Gastric perforation in the newborn is a rare event, but with early recognition, appropriate care and adherence to principles of surgical management survival can be maximized. Causes of gastric perforation may be multiple including idiopathic and spontaneous perforation. Recognition of the patterns of symptoms related to gastric perforation will aid in identification of this rare clinical condition. Careful attention to preoperative preparation will aid in a successful repair. Operative principles include control of spill of the luminal contents, debridement of devitalized tissue, and closure of the defect. Postoperative care includes supportive measures, broad spectrum antibiotics, and gastric acid suppression. Nutrition plays a key role in healing with TPN until the stomach is healed. Contrast study of the stomach may be considered prior to initiation of intestinal feeds.

FUTURE DIRECTIONS

Gastric perforation remains a poorly understood and rare event in the neonatal period. Associated risk factors are poorly characterized, and future investigation may help define which patients are at the highest risk. These patients may benefit from gastric acid suppression or other trophic factors to support the stomach. Gastric perforation may be in the same spectrum as necrotizing enterocolitis or spontaneous intestinal perforation. Investigation related to improved understanding of those processes may provide improvement in the understanding of gastric perforation.

Previous studies have shown the relationship of the C-KIT⁺ mast cells and the interstitial cell of Cajal to gastric perforation. These underlying cellular and molecular deficiencies are poorly characterized and may represent future targets for therapy or possible preventive strategies.

Finally, technology has assisted in the development of minimal access techniques and minimal access instrumentation. Future instrumentation may be even smaller, and this micro access approach may allow even more technically complex procedures in the neonate. Advancements also allow endoscopic procedures in the neonate, which have been limited up to this point by the size of the endoscope and the available instrumentation. In humans and animal models, gastric perforation has been successfully approached using endoscopic clips[54] and suturing techniques.[55]

REFERENCES

1. Rosser SB, Clark CH, Elechi EN. Spontaneous neonatal gastric perforation. *J Pediatr Surg* 1982; 17(4): 390–4.
2. Bell MJ. Perforation of the gastrointestinal tract and peritonitis in the neonate. *Surg Gynecol Obstet* 1985; 160(1): 20–6.
3. Duran R, Inan M, Vatansever U, Aladag N, Acunas B. Etiology of neonatal gastric perforations: Review of 10 years' experience. *Pediatr Int* 2007; 49(5): 626–30.
4. Terui K, Iwai J, Yamada S, Takenouchi A, Nakata M, Komatsu S, Yoshida H. Etiology of neonatal gastric perforation: A review of 20 years' experience. *Pediatr Surg Int* 2012; 28(1): 9–14.
5. Kara CS, Ilce Z, Celayir S, Sarimurat N, Erdogan E, Yeker D. Neonatal gastric perforation: Review of 23 years' experience. *Surg Today* 2004; 34(3): 243–5.
6. Leone RJ Jr, Krasna IH. 'Spontaneous' neonatal gastric perforation: Is it really spontaneous? *J Pediatr Surg* 2000; 35(7): 1066–9.
7. Siebold AE. Brand in der kleinen kurvatier des magens eines atrophischen kindes. *J Geburtsch Frauenzimmer Kinderk* 1826; 5: 3–4.
8. Stern MA, Perkins E, Nessa N. Perforated gastric ulcer in a 2-day-old infant. *Lancet* 1929; 49: 492–4.
9. Agerty HA, Ziserman A, Schollenberger CL. A case of perforation of the ileum in a newborn infant with operation and recovery. *J Pediatr* 1943; 22: 233–8.
10. Leger JL, Ricard PM, Leonard C, Piette J. [Perforated gastric ulcer in a newborn with survival]. *Union Med Can* 1950; 79(11): 1277–80.
11. Pelizzo G, Dubois R, Lapillonne A, Laine X, Claris O, Bouvier R, Chappuis JP. Gastric necrosis in newborns: A report of 11 cases. *Pediatr Surg Int* 1998; 13(5–6): 346–9.
12. Woo J, Eusterbrock T, Kim S. Intrauterine gastric perforation. *Pediatr Surg Int* 2006; 22(10): 829–31.
13. Braunstein H. Congenital defect of the gastric musculature with spontaneous perforation; report of five cases. *J Pediatr* 1954; 44(1): 55–63.
14. Silbergleit A, Berkas EM. Neonatal gastric rupture. *Minn Med* 1966; 49(1): 65–8.
15. Othersen HB Jr, Gregorie HB Jr. Pneumatic rupture of the stomach in a newborn infant with esophageal atresia and tracheoesophageal fistula. *Surgery* 1963; 53: 362–7.
16. Shaw A, Blanc WA, Santulli TV, Kaiser G. Spontaneous rupture of the stomach in the newborn: A clinical and experimental study. *Surgery* 1965; 58: 561–71.
17. Touloukian RJ. Gastric ischemia: The primary factor in neonatal perforation. *Clin Pediatr (Phila)* 1973; 12(4): 219–25.
18. Ohshiro K, Yamataka A, Kobayashi H, Hirai S, Miyahara K, Sueyoshi N, Suda K, Miyano T. Idiopathic gastric perforation in neonates and abnormal distribution of intestinal pacemaker cells. *J Pediatr Surg* 2000; 35(5): 673–6.
19. Holgersen LO. The etiology of spontaneous gastric perforation of the newborn: A reevaluation. *J Pediatr Surg* 1981; 16(4 Suppl 1): 608–13.
20. Tan CE, Kiely EM, Agrawal M, Brereton RJ, Spitz L. Neonatal gastrointestinal perforation. *J Pediatr Surg* 1989; 24(9): 888–92.
21. Burnett HA, Halpert B. Perforation of the stomach of a newborn infant with pyloric atresia. *Arch Pathol (Chic)* 1947; 44(3): 318–20.
22. Miller FA. Neonatal gastrointestinal tract perforations. *J Lancet* 1957; 77(11): 439–42.
23. Reyes HM, Meller JL, Loeff D. Management of esophageal atresia and tracheoesophageal fistula. *Clin Perinatol* 1989; 16(1): 79–84.
24. Bloom BT, Delmore P, Park YI, Nelson RA. Respiratory distress syndrome and tracheoesophageal fistula: Management with high-frequency ventilation. *Crit Care Med* 1990; 18(4): 447–8.
25. Holcomb GW 3rd. Survival after gastrointestinal perforation from esophageal atresia and tracheoesophageal fistula. *J Pediatr Surg* 1993; 28(12): 1532–5.
26. Maoate K, Myers NA, Beasley SW. Gastric perforation in infants with oesophageal atresia and distal tracheo-oesophageal fistula. *Pediatr Surg Int* 1999; 15(1): 24–7.
27. Graivier L, Rundell K, McWilliams N, Carruth D. Neonatal gastric perforation and necrosis: Ninety-five percent gastrectomy and colonic interposition, with survival. *Ann Surg* 1973; 177(4): 428–31.
28. Jawad AJ, Al-Rabie A, Hadi A, Al-Sowailem A, Al-Rawaf A, Abu-Touk B, Al-Karfi T, Al-Sammarai A. Spontaneous neonatal gastric perforation. *Pediatr Surg Int* 2002; 18(5–6): 396–9.
29. Waltsad PM, Conklin W. Rupture of the normal stomach after oxygen administration. *New Engl J Med* 1961; 264: 1201–02.

30. Zamir O, Hadary A, Goldberg M, Nissan S. Spontaneous perforation of the stomach in the neonate. *Z Kinderchir* 1987; 42(1): 43–5.

31. Grosfeld JL, Molinari F, Chaet M, Engum SA, West KW, Rescorla FJ, Scherer LR 3rd. Gastrointestinal perforation and peritonitis in infants and children: Experience with 179 cases over ten years. *Surgery* 1996; 120(4): 650–5; discussion 655–6.

32. Custer JR, Polley TZ Jr, Moler F. Gastric perforation following cardiopulmonary resuscitation in a child: Report of a case and review of the literature. *Pediatr Emerg Care* 1987; 3(1): 24–7.

33. St-Vil D, LeBouthillier G, Luks FI, Bensoussan AL, Blanchard H, Youssef S. Neonatal gastrointestinal perforations. *J Pediatr Surg* 1992; 27(10): 1340–2.

34. Bush CM, Jones JS, Cohle SD, Johnson H. Pediatric injuries from cardiopulmonary resuscitation. *Ann Emerg Med* 1996; 28(1): 40–4.

35. Im SA, Lim GY, Hahn ST. Spontaneous gastric perforation in a neonate presenting with massive hydroperitoneum. *Pediatr Radiol* 2005; 35(12): 1212–4.

36. Alonso-Vanegas M, Alvarez JL, Delgado L, Mendizabal R, Jimenez JL, Sanchez-Cabrera JM. Gastric perforation due to ventriculo-peritoneal shunt. *Pediatr Neurosurg* 1994; 21(3): 192–4.

37. Christoph CL, Poole CA, Kochan PS. Operative gastric perforation: A rare complication of ventriculo-peritoneal shunt. *Pediatr Radiol* 1995; 25 Suppl 1: S173–4.

38. Gray PH, Pemberton PJ. Gastric perforation associated with indomethacin therapy in a pre-term infant. *Aust Paediatr J* 1980; 16(1): 65–6.

39. Rajadurai VS, Yu VY. Intravenous indomethacin therapy in preterm neonates with patent ductus arteriosus. *J Paediatr Child Health* 1991; 27(6): 370–5.

40. O'Neil EA, Chwals WJ, O'Shea MD, Turner CS. Dexamethasone treatment during ventilator dependency: Possible life threatening gastrointestinal complications. *Arch Dis Child* 1992; 67(1 Spec No): 10–11.

41. Jactel SN, Abramowsky CR, Schniederjan M, Durham MM, Ricketts RR, Clifton MS, Langberg KM, Elawabdeh N, Pandya S, Talebagha S, Shehata BM. Noniatrogenic neonatal gastric perforation: The role of interstitial cells of Cajal. *Fetal Pediatr Pathol* 2013; 32(6): 422–8. Epub 2013 Jun 6.

42. Yamataka A, Yamataka T, Kobayashi H, Sueyoshi N, Miyano T. Lack of C-KIT+ mast cells and the development of idiopathic gastric perforation in neonates. *J Pediatr Surg* 1999; 34(1): 34–7; discussion 37–8.

43. Aydin M, Zenciroglu A, Hakan N, Erdogan D, Okumus N, Ipek MS. Gastric perforation in an extremely low birth weight infant recovered with percutaneous peritoneal drainage. *Turk J Pediatr* 2011; 53(4): 467–70.

44. Aslan Y, Sarihan H, Dinc H, Gedik Y, Aksoy A, Dereci S. Gastric perforation presenting as bilateral scrotal pneumatoceles. *Turk J Pediatr* 1999; 41(2): 267–271.

45. Yang CY, Lien R, Fu RH, Chu SM, Hsu JF, Lai JY, Minoo P, Chiang MC. Prognostic factors and concomitant anomalies in neonatal gastric perforation. *J Pediatr Surg* 2015; 50(8): 1278–82.

46. Houck WS Jr, Griffin JA 3rd. Spontaneous linear tears of the stomach in the newborn infant. *Ann Surg* 1981; 193(6): 763–8.

47. Pochaczevsky R, Bryk D. New roentgenographic signs of neonatal gastric perforation. *Radiology* 1972; 102(1): 145–7.

48. Diesen DL, Skinner MA. Spontaneous sealing of a neonatal intestinal perforation by the omentum. *J Pediatr Surg* 2008; 43(12): 2308–10.

49. Aydin M, Deveci U, Taskin E, Bakal U, Kilic M. Percutaneous peritoneal drainage in isolated neonatal gastric perforation. *World J Gastroenterol* 2015; 21(45): 12987–8.

50. He TZ, Xu C, Ji Y, Sun XY, Liu M. Idiopathic neonatal pneumoperitoneum with favorable outcome: A case report and review. *World J Gastroenterol* 2015; 21(20): 6417–21.

51. Gluer S, Schmidt AI, Jesch NK, Ure BM. Laparoscopic repair of neonatal gastric perforation. *J Pediatr Surg* 2006; 41(1): e57–58.

52. Bilik R, Freud N, Sheinfeld T, Ben-Ari Y, Rachmel A, Ziv N, Zer M. Subtotal gastrectomy in infancy for perforating necrotizing gastritis. *J Pediatr Surg* 1990; 25(12): 1244–5.

53. Chung MT, Kuo CY, Wang JW, Hsieh WS, Huang CB, Lin JN. Gastric perforation in the neonate: Clinical analysis of 12 cases. *Zhonghua Min Guo Xiao Er Ke Yi Xue Hui Za Zhi* 1994; 35(5): 460–5.

54. Maekawa S, Nomura R, Murase T, Ann Y, Harada M. Complete closure of artificial gastric ulcer after endoscopic submucosal dissection by combined use of a single over-the-scope clip and through-the-scope clips (with videos). *Surg Endosc* 2015; 29(2): 500–4.

55. Halvax P, Diana M, Legner A, Lindner V, Liu YY, Nagao Y, Cho S, Marescaux J, Swanstrom LL. Endoluminal full-thickness suture repair of gastrotomy: A survival study. *Surg Endosc* 2015; 29(11): 3404–8.

55

Duodenal obstruction

YECHIEL SWEED AND ALON YULEVICH

INTRODUCTION

Congenital duodenal obstruction (DO) is the most common cause of intestinal obstruction in the newborn period, occurring in 1 per 5000–10,000 live births.[1,2] DO is the result of intrinsic lesion, extrinsic lesion, or a combination of both.

These pathological lesions can cause complete or incomplete obstruction. Intrinsic DO may be caused by duodenal atresia, stenosis, diaphragm, a perforated diaphragm, or a "wind-sock" web. The wind-sock web is a duodenal membrane that is ballooned distally as a result of peristalsis from above. Extrinsic DO may be caused by annular pancreas, malrotation, or preduodenal portal vein. Although the annular pancreas forms a constricting ring around the second part of the duodenum (Figure 55.1), it is not believed to be the cause of DO,[3] and there is usually an associated atresia or stenosis in patients with an annular pancreas. Similarly, preduodenal portal vein has also seldom been reported to be the cause of DO, and it is often associated with other causes of intestinal obstruction such as malrotation or duodenal atresia.[4]

Duodenal atresias have been traditionally classified by Gray and Skandalakis[5] into three types (Figure 55.2). Type I defect, the most common (Figure 55.2a), is represented by a mucosal and submucosal diaphragmatic membrane with an intact muscle wall. The opening of the bile duct at the ampulla of Vater is almost always located proximal to the duodenal web. Type II defect has a short fibrous cord that connects the two atretic ends of the duodenum (Figure 55.2b); in type III defect, there is complete separation of the atretic ends with a mesenteric defect (Figure 55.2c). The reported prevalence of type I is about 92%, type II is 1%, and type III is 7%. Duodenal stenosis is approximately half as prevalent as atresia.[6]

Figure 55.3 shows the wide spectrum of various types of DO. The proximal and distal segments of the duodenum may be separated by a gap (Figure 55.3a), be in apposition (Figure 55.3b), or be joined by a fibrous cord (Figure 55.3c). Other types include duodenal stenosis (Figure 55.3d),

complete diaphragm (Figure 55.3e), perforated diaphragm (Figure 55.3f), wind-sock web (Figure 55.3g), and annular pancreas (Figure 55.3h).

ETIOLOGY

The underlying cause of duodenal atresia remains unknown, although its pathophysiology has been well described. Frequent association of duodenal atresia or stenosis with other neonatal malformations suggests that both anomalies are due to a developmental error in the early period of gestation. Duodenal atresia differs from other atresias of the small and large bowel, which are isolated anomalies caused by mesenteric vascular accidents during later stages of development. This theory of vascular disturbance was presented by the classic study of Lauw and Barnard.[7]

No predisposing maternal risk factors are known. Although up to one-third of patients with duodenal atresia have Down syndrome (trisomy 21), it is not an independent risk factor for developing duodenal atresia. In the large California population-based registry of 2.5 million infants, the risk of duodenal atresia was found to be 265 times higher in infants with Down syndrome than in those without it, and the corresponding frequencies were 46 and 0.12 per 1000 births.[8]

Although DO is usually not regarded as a familial condition, there have been several reports of familial cases[9] and a very rare group of hereditary multiple intestinal atresias with fatal outcome.[10]

PATHOPHYSIOLOGY

Duodenal atresia, web, and stenosis usually occur in the second part of the duodenum, close to the area of intense embryological activity involved with the development of the biliary and pancreatic structures. These anomalies are believed to result from a developmental error during early fetal life.[11]

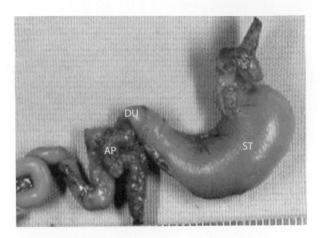

Figure 55.1 Duodenal obstruction caused by an annular pancreas associated with duodenal stenosis in a postmortem of a 14-week-old fetus with a diagnosis of Down syndrome. AP—annular, DU—duodenum, ST—stomach pancreas. (Courtesy of Prof. Bronshtein Moshe.)

Duodenal maldevelopment occurs secondary to either inadequate endodermal proliferation (gut elongation outpaces proliferation), which occurs at 5 weeks of embryonic life, or failure of the epithelial solid cord to recanalize (failure of vacuolization), which appears at 11 weeks of gestation.

Many investigators have demonstrated that the epithelium of the duodenum proliferates during 30–60 days' gestation, completely plugging the duodenal lumen. A subsequent process termed vacuolation occurs whereby the solid duodenum is recanalized. Vacuolation is believed to occur by way of apoptosis, or programmed cell death, which happens during normal development within the lumen of the duodenum. Occasionally, duodenal atresias are associated with annular pancreas. This is likely due to failure of duodenal development rather than robust and/or abnormal growth of the pancreatic buds.[12]

At the cellular level, the gastrointestinal tract develops from the embryonic gut, which is composed of an epithelium derived from endoderm, surrounded by cells of mesodermal origin. Cell signaling between these two embryonic layers appears to play a critical role in coordinating patterning and organogenesis of the duodenum. Sonic hedgehog genes encode members of the hedgehog family of cell signals. Both are expressed in gut endoderm, whereas target genes are expressed in discrete layers in the mesoderm. Mice with genetically altered sonic hedgehog signaling display duodenal stenosis, suggesting that genetic defects in the sonic hedgehog family of genes may influence the development of duodenal abnormalities.[13]

Recently, fibroblast growth factor 10 was found to be active in the duodenum at a late stage of development, and serves as a regulator in normal duodenal development. Fibroblast growth factor 10 (–/–) mutant mice demonstrated duodenal atresia with variable phenotype similar to clinical findings in humans. The phenotype occurred in an autosomal-recessive pattern with incomplete penetrance (38%).[14]

Markljung et al.[9] reported recently on a new familial case of annular pancreas and found one microduplication on chromosome 6q24 by array-based comparative genomic hybridization (CGH) shared by the affected mother and son. This microduplication may be a causative aberration or present a risk factor for the development of annular pancreas and duodenal atresia.

The obstruction of the duodenum usually occurs distal to the ampula of Vater. Preampullary obstruction is much less common, occurring in about 20% of cases. Occasionally, there may be a bifid termination of the bile duct with one limb of the duct system opening into the duodenum above the atresia and one below.[15]

ASSOCIATED MALFORMATIONS

There is a high incidence (approximately 50%) of associated anomalies in patients with intrinsic DO, especially Down syndrome, which occurs in about 30% of these patients.[16,17]

Table 55.1 presents the overall prevalence and distribution of associated anomalies of duodenal atresia. The data are the collected statistics of 1759 patients with DO from a dozen large series.[16] The associated anomalies in order of frequency are as follows: Down syndrome (28%), annular pancreas (23%), congenital heart disease (22.6%), malrotation (20%), esophageal atresia (8.5%), genitourinary malformations (8%), anorectal anomalies (4.4%), and other bowel atresias (3.5%).

Vertebral anomalies were also reported[18] in these patients. Reports of duodenal atresia have also shown a low incidence of associated epidermolysis bullosa.[19]

Other rare anomalies include De Lange syndrome,[18] chromosomal abnormalities,[16] multiple intestinal abnormalities,[19] choledochal cyst,[20] immunodeficiency,[21] and situs inversus.[22]

The complex cardiac anomalies among all other associated malformations are the major cause of morbidity and mortality in patients with duodenal atresia.[2,3,6,23] Dalla Vecchia et al.[6] attributed all the operative mortality (4%) to associated complex congenital heart anomalies in a group of 138 patients with DO in a 25-year survey. Two other important factors affecting higher morbidity and mortality of these patients are prematurity and low birth weight.[3,23,24] The mortality rate is even higher in neonates born with three or more anomalies of the VACTERL (vertebral defects, anal atresia, cardiac defects, tracheo-esophageal fistula, renal anomalies, and limb abnormalities) association, with an overall survival rate of 40%–77%.[25] Spitz and colleagues[26] and, recently, Fragoso et al.[27] reported the combination of esophageal and duodenal atresias as particularly lethal, with mortality rates ranging from 50% to 94%.

PRENATAL DIAGNOSIS/HISTORY

Maternal polyhydramnios has been reported to be present in 17%–75% of cases of duodenal atresia[24,28,29] and is the most common ultrasonographic finding in fetuses with intrinsic DO.[24] Ultrasound is usually performed for suspected fetal or maternal abnormalities when polyhydramnios or a

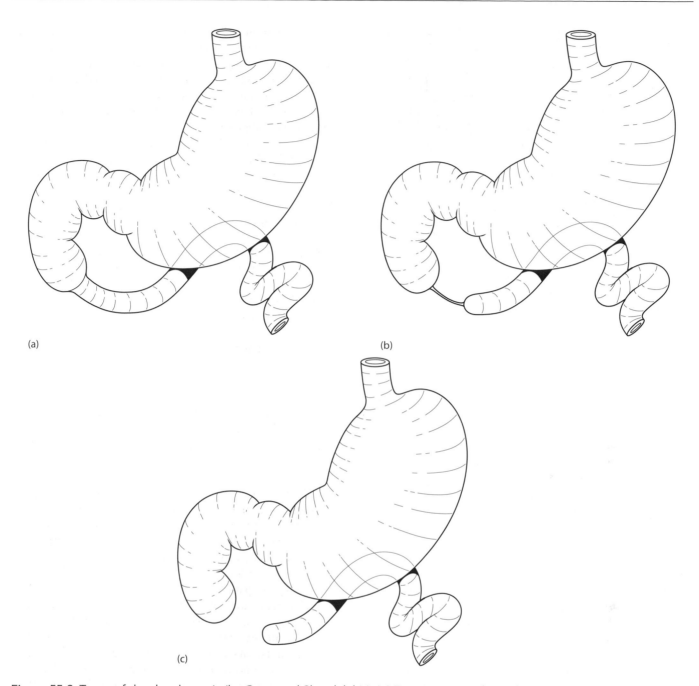

Figure 55.2 Types of duodenal atresia (by Grays and Skandalakis). **(a)** Type I—mucosal membrane with intact muscle wall. **(b)** Type II—fibrous cord connecting the two atretic ends of duodenum. **(c)** Type III—a complete separation of the atretic ends with a mesenteric defect.

large-for-date pregnancy is established. Although the majority of cases are diagnosed during the seventh or eighth month of gestation,[30] sonographic detection of duodenal atresia was reported as early as 12 gestational weeks by Tsukerman et al.[31]

There has been an increase in prenatal ultrasonographic diagnosis of duodenal atresia during the last decades, from 14% between the years 1972 and 1991[32] to a high rate of 57% for the period of 1991–1995.[29]

The prenatal sonographic diagnosis relies on the demonstration of the "double bubble" sign, which is due to simultaneous distension of the stomach and the first part of the duodenum (Figure 55.4). In many cases, this sonographic sign is observed in the second half of pregnancy probably due to hydrostatic pressure needed to dilate the duodenum and also to the degree of the DO.

Visualization of a fluid-filled double bubble (Figure 55.4) on prenatal ultrasound scan is associated with DO secondary to intrinsic lesion, extrinsic lesion, or both. This sonographic finding is known to have a low false-positive rate. Zimmer and Brohnstein[33] have reported that in a few cases, it may represent a transient finding in an otherwise healthy fetus. It is possible that intestinal peristalsis in a fetus may show transient dilatation suggesting DO.[30] On the ultrasound examination, it is also important to demonstrate

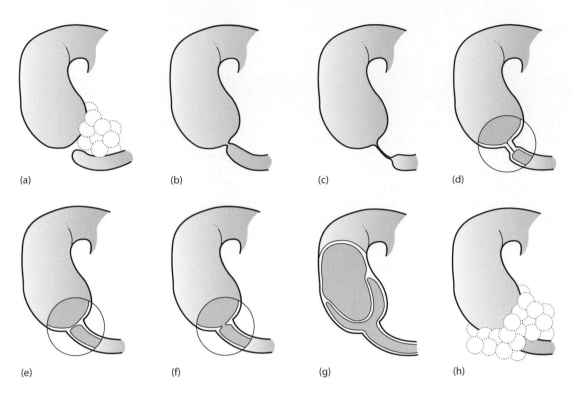

Figure 55.3 Various types of duodenal obstruction. **(a)** Blind ends separated by a gap. **(b)** Two ends in apposition. **(c)** Ends joined by a fibrous cord. **(d)** Duodenal stenosis. **(e)** Complete duodenal membrane. **(f)** Perforated diaphragm. **(g)** "Windsock" web. **(h)** Annular pancreas.

Table 55.1 The incidence of associated congenital anomalies (%) (collected statistics) (*N* =1759 patients)

Associated anomaly	%
Down syndrome	28.2
Annular pancreas	23.1
Congenital heart disease	22.6
Malrotation	19.7
Esophageal atresia and tracheo-esophageal fistula	8.5
Genitourinary	8.0
Anorectal	4.4
Other bowel atresia	3.5
Others	10.9

Source: Data from Sweed Y, Duodenal obstruction, In Puri P (ed.), *Newborn Surgery*, 3rd edn., London: Arnold, 2011: 470.

the continuity between the gastric and duodenal bubbles (Figure 55.4) to exclude other causes such as choledochal cyst, which lacks such communication,[34] or duodenal duplication.[35]

Often, other anomalies can also be diagnosed by ultrasound. Pameijer et al.[36] reported on the ultrasonic prenatal diagnosis of a fetus with combined duodenal and esophageal atresias associated with VACTERL anomalies. Prenatal ultrasonographic diagnosis of annular pancreas has also been reported showing the coincidence of the double bubble sign together with hyperechogenic bands around the duodenum (corresponding with the tissue of annular pancreas).[37]

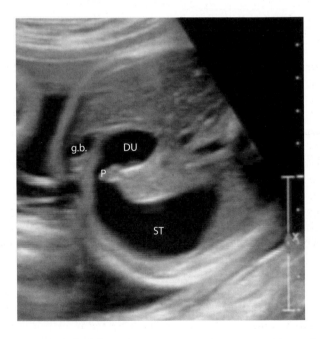

Figure 55.4 Ultrasonography (transverse view) of 24-week-gestational-age fetus showing the "double bubble" sign. DU—duodenum, g.b.—gallblader, P—pylorus, ST—stomach.

Hancock and Wiseman[24] investigated the impact of antenatal diagnosis of congenital DO in a series of 34 infants, 15 of whom were diagnosed by antenatal ultrasound. They concluded that although surgery was performed sooner, the outcome of treatment was not changed by providing an antenatal diagnosis. However, the antenatal diagnosis of DO influenced parents positively in coping with the anomaly, because it allowed them time to prepare for the medical and surgical interventions required after the birth of their infant. These authors also emphasized that a normal ultrasound in the presence of polyhydramnios does not rule out the diagnosis of DO and is an indication for repeated sonography. Cohen-Overbeek et al.[28] also reported on 91 cases diagnosed with isolated or nonisolated DO. They found that the outcomes of prenatally and postnatally diagnosed DO are not essentially different despite the fact that more prematurity and a lower birth weight were observed in the former.

The rapid advancement in imaging technology, including magnetic resonance imaging (MRI), should allow for diagnosis during the first and early second trimester, enabling abortion.[31] Alternatively, early prenatal diagnosis of DO should lead to karyotype analysis for prenatal screening for trisomy 21 and other associated anomalies.[32,38]

The prenatal diagnosis allows the mother the opportunity to receive counseling and to consider delivery at or near a tertiary care facility that is able to care for infants with gastrointestinal anomalies.[39]

CLINICAL PRESENTATION AND DIAGNOSIS

The presenting symptoms and signs are the result of high intestinal obstruction. About half of these patients are premature and low-birth-weight infants.[3,6,23] Vomiting is the most common symptom and is usually present on the first day of life. Since 80% of the obstructions are located in the postampullary region of the duodenum, vomitus in the majority of cases is bile stained. In supra-ampullary atresia, it is nonbilious. Orogastric aspiration also yields significant volumes of bile-stained gastric fluid. There is minimal or no abdominal distension because of the high level of obstruction. The infant may pass some meconium in the first 24 hours of life, and thereafter, constipation may develop. Dehydration with weight loss and electrolyte imbalance (hypokalemic/hypochloremic metabolic alkalosis) soon follows if the diagnosis is done late and if fluid and electrolyte losses have not been adequately replaced.[40]

Incomplete DO usually leads to the delayed onset of symptoms. Infants with duodenal stenosis and partial bowel obstruction may escape detection of an abnormality soon after birth and may proceed into childhood or, rarely, into adulthood before a partial obstruction is noted.[3,32]

The diagnosis of DO is confirmed on x-ray examination. An abdominal radiograph will show a dilated stomach and duodenum, giving the characteristic appearance of a double bubble sign (the stomach and the proximal duodenum are air-filled) with no gas beyond the duodenum (Figure 55.5a,b,c). In partial DO, a plain film of the abdomen will show a double bubble appearance, but there is usually some air in the distal intestine (Figure 55.6). Occasionally

in cases of duodenal atresia, air may be seen distal to the site of obstruction due to associated bile duct bifurcation.[41] Radiographic findings in patients with annular pancreas are usually indistinguishable from duodenal atresia or stenosis.

In some cases of partial DO, plain films may be normal. Upper gastrointestinal tract contrast radiography is indicated in these patients to establish the cause of incomplete DO. This may show a stenotic segment of duodenum with dilatation of the proximal segment, or a sharp termination of the dilated segment, indicating a perforated diaphragm (Figure 55.7).

Incomplete DO usually leads to delayed onset of symptoms, and the diagnosis of duodenal diaphragm with a central aperture is sometimes delayed for months or even years.[42] Mikaelsson et al.[43] reported on the late diagnosis and treatment of 8 out of 16 patients with membranous duodenal stenosis. Their patients were diagnosed and operated at 1 month to 4 years of age. Occasionally, a duodenal diaphragm may be stretched and ballooned distally, giving the wind-sock appearance on a contrast study (Figure 55.8).

The most important differential diagnosis of DO is DO caused by malrotation resulting in extrinsic compression related to Ladd bands across the duodenum, or volvulus of the midgut loop, although this is rare. Midgut volvulus may result in gangrene of the entire midgut within hours, and thus, diagnostic investigation is urgently required, though the symptoms may relent because the obstruction may be incomplete or intermittent in malrotation. Part of these extrinsic obstructions exhibit the double bubble sign with distal air on plain film, while the majority can be identified from the coil spring appearance of small bowel volvulus following barium injection. However, Samuel et al.[44] observed that volvulus neonatorum was not encountered in neonates with duodenal atresia and stenosis who had associated malrotation. They suggested that DO could perhaps be a floodgate that prevents volvulus in these children.

Preduodenal portal vein is a rare anomaly and generally asymptomatic. It is a rare cause of DO and often coexists with other anomalies resulting in bowel obstruction.[4] In most of these patients, it is impossible to diagnose preduodenal portal vein prior to surgery.

The wide variety of additional congenital anomalies, with special emphasis on cardiac malformation, often severe,[23,38] makes preoperative diagnosis imperative. Anterior–posterior and lateral chest and abdominal radiographs ascertaining visualization of the entire spine should also be performed.

Soon after the x-ray, cardiac and renal ultrasound should be carried out routinely in all these babies. A micturating cystourethrogram should be performed in those babies with abnormal urogenital ultrasound or an associated anorectal anomaly. Rectal biopsy should be taken in babies with constipation and the combination of Down syndrome and duodenal atresia, to exclude Hirschsprung disease.[45]

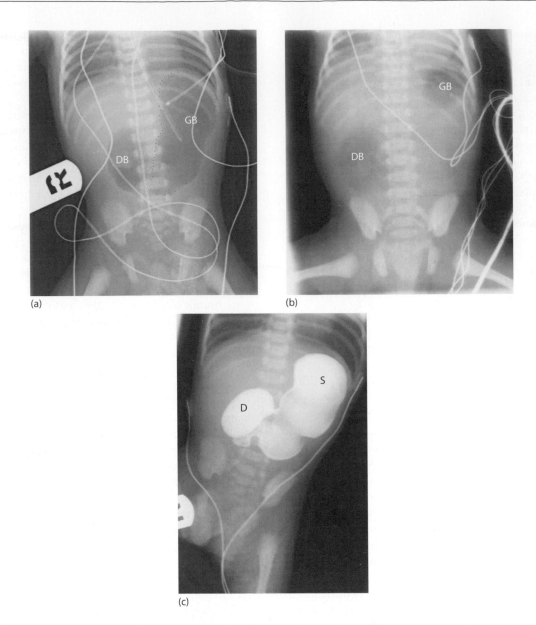

Figure 55.5 **(a)** Abdominal radiograph showing grossly distended stomach and duodenum with "double bubble" sign with no air beyond the duodenum. DB—duodenal bubble, GB—gastric bubble. **(b)** Abdominal radiograph showing the double bubble sign. In this case, the duodenal bulb is more prominent than the gastric bulb. At operation, duodenal membrane was found and excised. DB—duodenal bubble, GB—gastric bubble. **(c)** Duodenal atresia evident on upper gastrointestinal radiograph contrast study. D—duodenum, S—stomach.

PREOPERATIVE MANAGEMENT

Although duodenal atresia is a relative emergency, the patient should not be rushed to the operating room until his/her hemodynamic and fluid and electrolyte status is stable. If the clinical history and findings on physical examination indicate that the baby is in no distress, and the radiographs are consistent with the usual presentation of duodenal atresia with no air beyond the second bubble (excluding malrotation), operation should be performed on an elective basis.

An orogastric tube decompresses the stomach and intravenous fluid resuscitation can be initiated. Blood samples for electrolyte determination should be obtained, and any derangements should be corrected. Prolonged vomiting can result in a hypokalemic hypochloremic metabolic alkalosis. Passage of the orogastric tube rules out esophageal atresia, and careful inspection of anal defect variants of imperforated anus should be performed.

Care is taken to preserve body heat and avoid hypoglycemia, since many of these newborn patients are premature and small for date.[29] Very-low-birth-weight infants or those with respiratory distress syndrome and associated severe anomalies, e.g., congenital heart disease, may occasionally need special preparation such as resuscitation and ventilation.

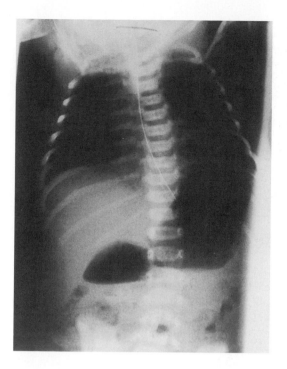

Figure 55.6 Duodenal stenosis erect abdominal x-ray demonstrating a "double bubble" sign with air beyond the duodenum.

OPERATION

Duodenoduodenostomy is the procedure of choice for patients with duodenal atresia, stenosis, and annular pancreas.[6,46]

Duodenoduodenostomy can be performed in either "diamond-shape" (proximal transverse to distal longitudinal) anastomosis as described by Kimura (Figure 55.9a,b)[47] or side-to-side fashion (Figure 55.10). The diamond-shape duodenoduodenostomy has been reported to allow earlier feeding, earlier discharge, and good long-term results.[48]

Bax et al.[49] and Rothenberg[50] reported on the first case and the first series, respectively, on the laparoscopic management of DO. They indicated that the laparoscopic approach has proven to be safe and effective and represents an alternative to the open procedure. They also emphasized that this minimally invasive surgical technique should be used only if the surgeon has appropriate instruments and suturing and laparoscopic skills (Figure 55.11).[49–51]

INCISION

The baby is placed supine on the table with a small roll under his/her upper abdomen on a warming blanket. Endotracheal anesthesia is used. The abdominal skin is prepared by cleaning with prewarmed povidone iodine.

A transverse supraumbilical abdominal incision is made 2 cm above the umbilicus starting in the midline and extending laterally into the right upper quadrant for about 5 cm. The abdominal muscles are divided transversely with cutting diathermy, and the peritoneal cavity is opened in the line of incision.

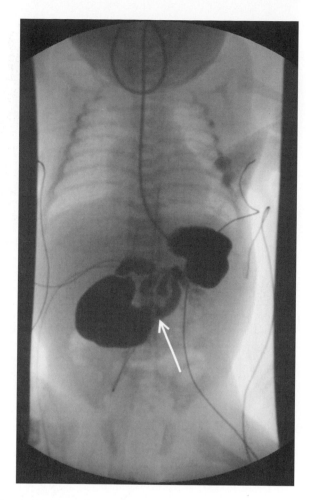

Figure 55.7 An abdominal x-ray contrast study showing marked distention of duodenum terminating abruptly with narrow caliber distally. A perforated diaphragm was found at operation.

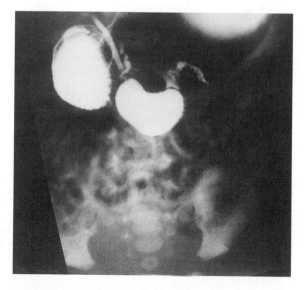

Figure 55.8 "Wind-Sock" web. Dilated duodenum demonstrated with duodenal membrane ballooned distally, giving characteristic "wind-sock" appearance. Reflux of contrast medium into pancreatic and common bile duct is seen.

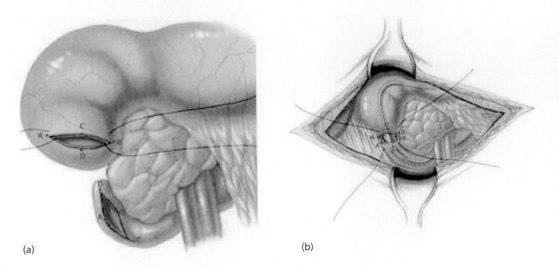

(a)   (b)

Figure 55.9 Diamond-shaped duodenoduodenostomy. **(a)** A transverse incision is made in the distal end of the proximal dilated duodenum, and a longitudinal incision is made in the smaller limb of the duodenum distal to the occlusion. **(b)** A single-layer anastomosis using interrupted 5-0 Vicryl sutures with posterior knots tied inside the posterior wall of the anastomosis and anterior knots tied outside the anterior wall is performed.

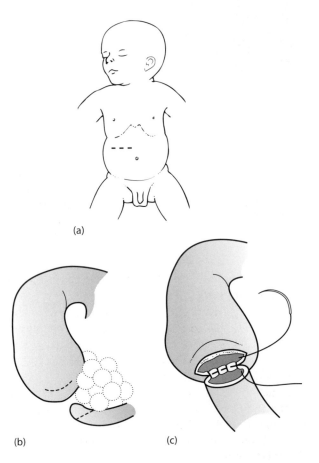

(a)

(b)   (c)

Figure 55.10 Side-to-side duodenoduodenostomy. **(a)** An upper transverse abdominal incision. **(b)** Parallel incisions of about 1 cm are made in the proximal and distal duodenum. **(c)** The anastomosis is preformed using single-layer interrupted 5-0 Vicryl sutures.

EXPLORATION AND IDENTIFICATION OF PATHOLOGY

After exposing the peritoneal cavity, the surgeon inspects the entire bowel for the presence of other bowel anomalies. There may be an associated annular pancreas, malrotation (in about one-third of the patients), or—in rare cases—preduodenal portal vein. If the colon is in normal position, malrotation is probably not a coexisting factor.

The stomach and first portion of the duodenum are usually thickened and dilated. The liver is carefully retracted superiorly. The ascending colon and the hepatic flexure of the colon are mobilized medially and downward to expose the dilated duodenum.[52]

The duodenum is then adequately mobilized and freed from its retroperitoneal attachments—Kocher maneuver. Great care must be exercised not to dissect or manipulate either segment of the duodenum medially, to avoid injury to the ampulla of Vater or the common bile duct. The tube in the stomach is then passed distally into the dilated duodenum and helps to locate the point of obstruction and determine if a wind-sock deformity is present (Figure 55.3g).

The atresia type and any pancreatic abnormality (e.g., annular pancreas) are noted. In patients with an annular pancreas, the pancreatic tissue should never be divided and should always be bypassed. The duodenum distal to the site of obstruction is small and decompressed. The requirements for distal mobilization vary according to the location of the atresia and to the gap between the two segments (Figure 55.2). If necessary, the ligament of Treitz is divided, and mobilization and displacement of the distal duodenum is performed behind the superior mesenteric vessels, thus allowing a satisfactory anastomosis to be performed without any tension.

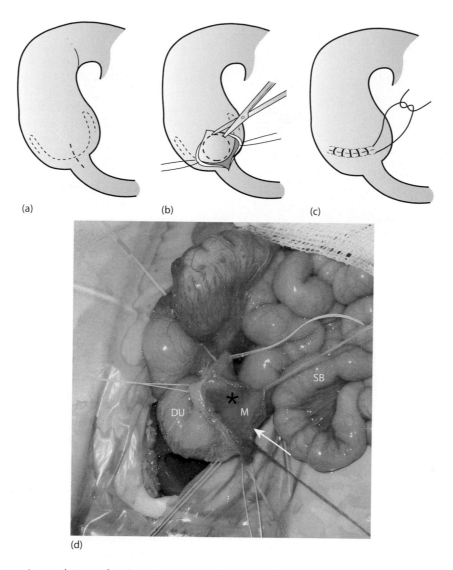

(a) (b) (c)

(d)

Figure 55.11 **(a–d)** Operative technique for duodenal web. **(a)** Longitudinal incision above the "transitional zone" of the duodenum. **(b)** Excision of the web leaving the medial third of the membrane intact. **(c)** The duodenum is closed transversely. **(d)** Intraoperative photograph of a 2-week-old infant born with duodenal web with an aperture. The papilla of Vater was identified at the proximal and medial part of the duodenal membrane (*). DU, opened duodenum; M, membrane; SB, small bowel; *, papilla of Vater.

(Continued)

DIAMOND-SHAPED DUODENODUODENOSTOMY

After abdominal exploration, the duodenum is adequately mobilized. With two traction sutures, the redundant wall of the proximal duodenum is pulled downward to overlie the proximal portion of the distal duodenal segment. A transverse incision is made in the distal end of the proximal duodenum, and a longitudinal incision is made in the smaller limb of the duodenum distal to the occlusion.

These are made in such a position as to allow good approximation of the openings without tension.

The papilla of Vater is located by observing bile flow. This is performed by gentle compression of the gallbladder.

The orientation of the sutures in the diamond-shape anastomosis and the overlapping between the proximal transverse incision and the distal longitudinal incision are shown in Figure 55.9a,b.

Additionally, an 8-French Foley catheter should be passed proximally into the stomach and distally into the jejunum and pulled back with the balloon inflated, to ensure that no additional web or wind-sock deformity is overlooked. The distal duodenum can be distended to a larger size during this maneuver, facilitating the anastomosis. Before pulling back the catheter from the distal duodenum, the surgeon should inject 30–40 mL of warm saline through the catheter to rule out distal atresias of the distal small bowel. The catheter is then removed.

A single-layer anastomosis is performed using 5-0 or 6-0 Vicryl sutures with posterior knots tied inside the posterior wall of the anastomosis and interrupted sutures with anterior knots tied outside the anterior wall. Before completion

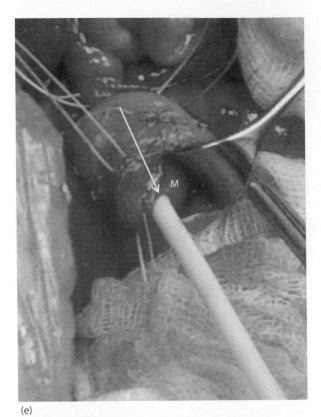

(e)

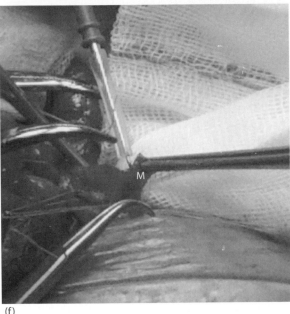

(f)

Figure 55.11 (Continued) The white arrow points to the excisional line of the membrane. **(e, f)** Intraoperative photograph of a 2-day-old infant with Down syndrome and AV canal showing: **(e)** An 8-French Foley catheter, which was introduced through an aperture of a duodenal membrane. M, membrane. The white arrow points to the aperture of the membrane. **(f)** Excision of the membrane.

of the anterior part of the anastomosis, a 5-French silicon nasojejunal transanastomotic feeding tube may be passed down into the upper jejunum for an early postoperative enteral feeding[53] using the same insertion technique as was reported for patients who underwent surgical repair for esophageal atresia and tracheoesophageal fistula.[54] Others, however, do not use the nasojejunal tube, because they suggest that it may delay the commencement of oral feeding.[48] Hall et al.[53] reported recently that a trans anastomotic tube significantly shortens time to full enteral feeds in infants with congenital DO as well as significantly reducing the need for central venous access and parenteral nutrition. Then the right colon is returned to its former position so that the mesocolon covers the anastomosis. The Ladd procedure with inversion appendectomy is performed in patients with malrotation.[32] In these patients, the cecum should be placed in the left lower quadrant to reduce the risk of midgut volvulus.

The wound is closed in layers: the peritoneum and posterior fascia, and the anterior fascia by two layers using continuous 4-0 Vicryl. The skin is closed with running intracuticular suture using 5-0 Vicryl.

SIDE-TO-SIDE DUODENODUODENOSTOMY

The dilated proximal duodenum and the distal collapsed duodenum are approximated using two stay sutures (5-0 Vicryl). Then parallel incisions about 1 cm in length are made in the proximal and distal duodenum (Figure 55.10). An 8-French Foley catheter should be inserted both to the proximal dilated duodenum and to the distal collapsed duodenum in order to rule out wind-sock membrane and distal atresias, as similarly described in the diamond-shape duodenoduodenostomy.

The posterior layer of anastomosis is completed using interrupted 5-0 Vicryl sutures.

At this stage, a transanastomotic 5-French-gauge silastic nasojejunal tube may be inserted for early enteral feeding.

The anastomosis is then completed using interrupted 5-0 Vicryl sutures for the anterior layer. The abdomen is closed in the same manner as described in the diamond-shape duodenoduodenostomy.

In premature infants some surgeons prefer to perform a gastrostomy and insert the transanastomotic silicon tube via the gastrostomy. The tip of the tube should be well down the jejunum so as to decrease the chance of it becoming displaced.

OPERATIVE TECHNIQUE FOR DUODENAL WEB

A longitudinal incision is performed above the "transitional zone" between the wide and narrow segments of the duodenum (Figure 55.11a), and the duodenum is opened. The membrane usually is located in the second part and occasionally in the third portion of the duodenum. It can be complete or have a hole. Anatomically, the ampulla of Vater may open directly into the medial part of the membrane, or posteriorly close to it; thus, the close relationship of the membrane to papilla of Vater makes its identification mandatory, before excision of the web. Excision of the web should proceed from the lateral duodenal wall, leaving the medial third of the wall intact to avoid damaging the sphincter of Oddi or the ampulla of Vater and continue leaving a circumferential rim of tissue of 1–2 mm (Figure 55.11b,d). The resection line is then oversewn using continuous sutures of Vicryl 5-0, and the duodenum is closed transversely in one layer using Vicryl 5-0 (Figure 55.11c). Because of the pitfalls in cases of the lax membrane that may bulge downward distally into the distended duodenum (the so-called wind-sock phenomenon), and in order to avoid missing the anomaly, before closure of the duodenum, the distal patency of the distal duodenum must be verified by inserting an 8-French Foley catheter through a duodenotomy (Figure 55.11e,f).

The experience with fiber-optic duodenoscopy indicates the usefulness of the technique for both the diagnosis and nonoperative management of duodenal membrane.[55] However, based on reports describing anomalous entry of the pancreatobiliary channels, the delineation of the ducts at endoscopic retrograde cholangiopancreatography (ERCP) may be necessary prior to endoscopic intervention.

Bittencourt et al.[55] reported on three female patients ages 9–12 months born with duodenal membrane who were treated successfully by two endoscopic sessions. The first and second sessions of endoscopic treatment included dilatation and resection of the membrane respectively and were carried out without complications.

Most surgeons, however, believe that a duodenotomy is preferable to the potential risk of inadvertent pancreatic or bile duct injury.

LAPAROSCOPIC MANAGEMENT OF DO

The application of minimally invasive surgical techniques (MIS) for the correction of congenital anomalies has increased significantly over the last 15 years. The ability to perform delicate dissection and intracorporeal anastomosis has broadened the scope of entities that can be approached, including neonatal DO. Although most neonatal conditions presenting with bowel obstruction present a difficult problem for laparoscopy because of the dilated bowel and limited abdominal cavity, this is not the case in duodenal atresia. The entire small and large bowel is decompressed, and there is excellent exposure of the proximal duodenum.[51,56]

For the laparoscopic approach, neonatal laparoscopic instruments (3 mm) and trocars are used. The patient is positioned supine at the end of the operating table, and the surgeon stands at the patient's feet. The abdomen is insufflated through a 5 mm umbilical port, for a 30° laparoscope, and the pneumoperitoneum is established at 6–8 mm Hg (1.5 L/minute). Then two additional trocars are inserted (Figure 55.12a). A 3 mm grasping forceps for lifting the liver can be introduced in the left upper quadrant without a trocar. A better view of the dilated duodenum can be also achieved by using a suture to lift up the falciform ligament. The suture is inserted through the abdominal wall in the right upper quadrant, lifts the ligament, and then is passed back through the abdominal wall and tied.

The first surgical step is to mobilize the colon and the duodenum. A stay suture is inserted through the abdominal wall to move the bulky part of the bulbus duodeni out of the way, allowing a view of the distal duodenum and a more convenient approach to the anastomosis. A transverse incision is made in the distal wall of the dilated duodenum (Figure 55.12b), followed by a longitudinal incision in the distal collapsed duodenum for the diamond-shaped anastomosis of Kimura (Figure 55.12c).

A diamond-shaped anastomosis is performed with either a separate running suture for the posterior and then the anterior wall, or single interrupted stitches of 5-0 Vicryl. Intracorporeal knot tying is used. The distal bowel is examined in all cases to ensure that there are no obvious secondary atresias. Once the anastomosis is completed, the ports are removed, and the sites are closed with absorbable sutures.

When a duodenal membrane is suspected, a longitudinal incision is made on the anterior wall of the duodenum, crossing from the distended duodenum to the distal collapsed duodenum (Figure 55.12d). A urinary catheter is inserted through the abdominal wall directly into the distal duodenal segment, the balloon is filled, and the catheter is gradually pulled back. A membrane with an aperture will stretch itself on top of the balloon. The membrane is incised carefully in its lateral aspect, and the longitudinal incision is closed.

The main benefits of the laparoscopic approach for treatment of duodenal atresia are the excellent visualization of the obstruction and the ease of the anastomosis. However, the possible disadvantage of this approach may be that evaluation of the distal bowel for other atretic segments is more difficult to accomplish, and if not specifically evaluated, it is feasible that a malrotation can be missed.[56] The bowel can be inspected visually for distal obstructed segments, but internal webs may be more difficult to see.

Hill et al.[56] reported recently on their results comparing 22 patients with DO treated by laparoscopy and 36 patients treated by traditional laparotomy during a 9-year period (2001–2010). They found no difference between groups in time to full feeding, postoperative length of stay, and complication rate. They found that the operative time was slightly longer in the laparoscopic group (median time 116 minutes vs. 103 minutes, respectively); however, laparoscopic management appeared to allow a shorter postoperative ventilator requirement. Six patients (26%) of the laparoscopic group were converted to open exploration because of unclear anatomy.

The experience with laparoscopic duodenoduodenostomy[57,58] demonstrates that it can be performed safely and successfully in the neonate with excellent short-term outcomes. Surgeons with experience in advanced laparoscopic techniques can learn laparoscopic duodenoduodenostomy and have good results.

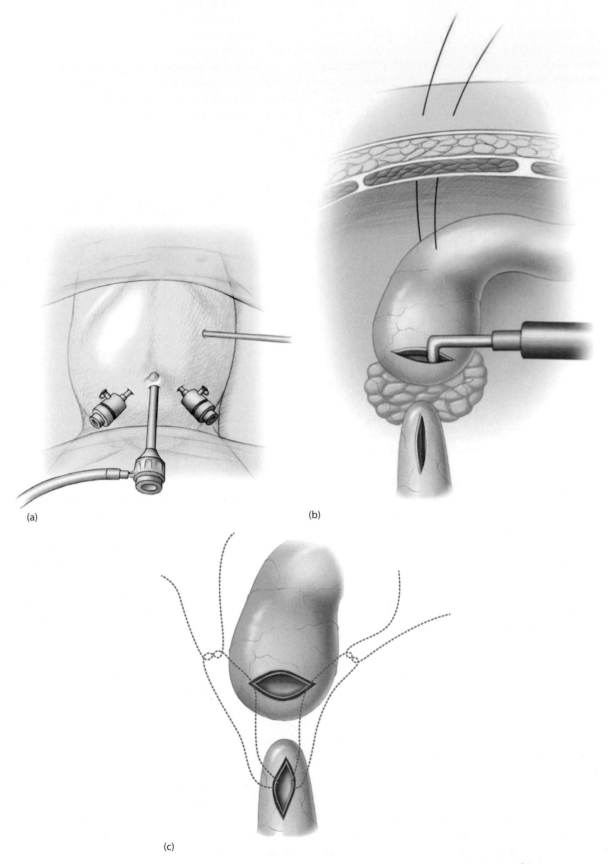

(a)

(b)

(c)

Figure 55.12 **(a)** Trocar placement and instrumentation for laparoscopic repair of duodenal atresia. **(b)** A stay suture is inserted through the abdominal wall. **(c)** A transverse incision is made in the distal wall of the dilated duodenum followed by a longitudinal incision in the distal collapsed duodenum.

(Continued)

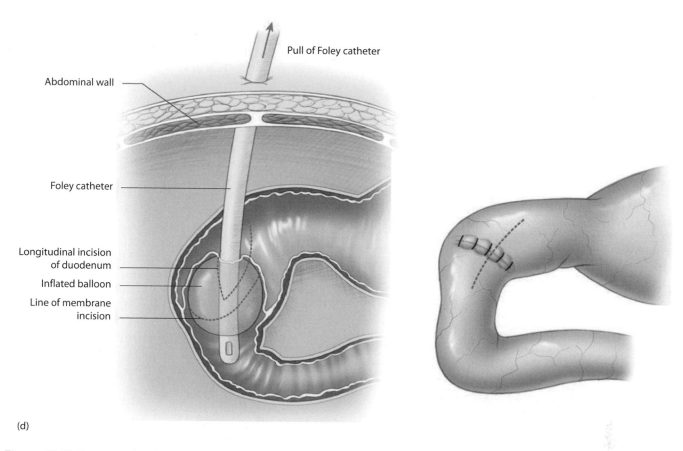

Pull of Foley catheter

Abdominal wall

Foley catheter

Longitudinal incision
of duodenum

Inflated balloon

Line of membrane
incision

(d)

Figure 55.12 (Continued) **(d)** Laparoscopic surgical treatment of duodenal membrane.

POSTOPERATIVE CARE

The baby is returned to an incubator (or radiant heat cot) at the thermoneutral temperature for its size and maturity. An intravenous infusion of the dextrose/saline is continued in the postoperative period, and further fluid and electrolyte management depends on clinical progress, loss by gastroduodenal aspiration, and serum electrolyte levels. Postoperatively, patients may have a prolonged period of bile-stained aspirate through the nasogastric tube, which is mainly due to the inability of the markedly dilated duodenum to produce effective peristalsis. Enteral feeding through the transanastomotic feeding tube is generally started within 24–48 hours postoperatively.

The commencement of oral feeding depends on the decrease of the gastric aspirate and may be delayed for several days and occasionally for 1–2 weeks or longer. Once the volume of the gastric aspirate decreases, the feeding tube is withdrawn, and the infant can be started on oral feeding.

Spigland and Yazbeck,[59] in their follow-up of 33 neonates, found that bowel transit was established for an average of 13.1 days, 7.5 days after partial web excision, 12.4 days following duodenoduodenostomy, and 15 days after duodenojejunostomy (which is rarely performed today). Spilde et al.[57] reported that the time to initial feeding was 11.3 days for patients with an open repair of DO compared to 5.4 days for those who were treated by laparoscopic approach. They also found that the average time to full oral intake was 16.9 days for the open group compared to 9 days for the laparoscopic group.

Parmentier et al.[60] reported recently that a laparoscopic approach for DO is safe and reproducible with outcomes similar to open repair even in the beginning of a learning curve for pediatric surgeons with appropriate laparoscopic skills. In their small series, laparoscopy did not appear to decrease time to full oral intake or length of stay.

MANAGEMENT OF PERSISTENT MEGADUODENUM BY DUODENOPLASTY

The deformity and dysfunction of the first part of the duodenum—the megaduodenum—are the well-known causes of morbidity,[61] and occasionally, these patients require duodenoplasty. The malfunction of the greatly dilated gut and the absence of effective peristalsis occur in the dilated duodenum proximal to the duodenal atresia. Several techniques of duodenoplasty have been described, and in all, it is of the utmost importance to visualize and identify the ampulla of Vater within the duodenal lumen prior to resection and tapering of the duodenum. Hutton and Thomas [61] have reported success by extensive tapering duodenoplasty. Adzick et al.[62] and Grosfeld and Rescorla[32] emphasized the merit of tapering duodenoplasty at the primary operation of neonates with dilated duodenum, to improve the immediate postoperative gastrointestinal function and the prevention of further development of megaduodenum. Other techniques include resection and stapling[62] and elliptical seromuscular resection.[63]

However, refashioning the anastomosis or bypass techniques usually fails.[64] Another technique of subtotal duodenal resection with reconstruction of the duodenum by the proximal jejunum as an onlay patch was demonstrated in two children. In this technique, the diseased duodenal wall is completely removed, except for the area of the ampulla of Vater, and the duodenum is reconstructed by the jejunum.[65]

OUTCOME AND LONG-TERM RESULTS

The survival of babies with DO has gradually improved over the last 40 years since the report of surgical correction of intrinsic DO by Ladd in 1932[66] (Table 55.2).[2,6,18,24,28,32,40,46,51,56,58,59] All agree that the three main factors contributing to the mortality rate in this group of patients are as follows: high incidence of associated anomalies, especially severe cardiac malformations; prematurity; and low birth weight.[2,3,32] In a recent review covering 45 years (1951–1995) of management of DO, Murshed et al.[29] found that in the first 15 years, survival reached 51%; in the next 15 years, it was 80%; and in the last 15 years, 95%.

Table 55.2 Survival rates of patients with duodenal atresia and stenosis

Reference	No. patients	% Survival
Wesley and Mahour[46]	72	74
Hancock and Wiseman[24]	34	94
Bailey et al.[18]	138	93
Grosfeld and Rescorla[32]	103	95
Dalla Vecchia et al.[6]	138	86
Cohen-Overbeek et al.[28]	91	91
Choudhry et al.[2]	65	96
Kilbride et al.[40]	51	98
Kay et al.[51,a]	17	100
Hill et al.[56,b]	58	100
Li et al.[58,c]	40	100
Parmentier et al.[60,d]	29	97

Note: Table shows gradual improvement in survival reported over the past 40 years. Most deaths are related to the associated complex cardiac malformations.

a Laparoscopic duodenoduodenostomy (years 2004–2008). N = 17 pts.
b Laparoscopic versus open repair of duodenal obstruction (years 2001–2010). Lap group: N = 22 pts, open group: N = 36 pts. One patient in the lap group who had Down syndrome, duodenal and jejunal atresias died because of sepsis 5 months after the initial operation.
c Laparoscopic duodenoduodenostomy (years 2009–2012). N = 40 pts. 20 pts with a diagnosis of congenital intestinal malrotation were operated on by laparoscopic ladd's procedure.
d Laparoscopic versus open repair of duodenal obstruction (years 2007–2010). Open group: N = 19 pts (years 2013–2014), lap group: N = 10 pts.

During the latest period, mortality was almost entirely the consequence of associated anomalies.

Dalla Vechia et al.[6] reported a relatively low rate of postoperative complications in a series of 138 infants. The early complication rate included anastomotic obstruction in 3%, congestive heart failure in 9%, prolonged adynamic ileus in 4%, pneumonia in 5%, and wound infection in 3%.

Late complications included adhesive bowel obstruction in 9%, megaduodenum and duodenal dysmotility that required tapering duodenoplasty in 4%, and gastroesophageal reflux requiring surgery in 5%.

Weber et al.[67] reported the complication rate and morbidity of three methods of technical repair in a group of 41 newborns with duodenal atresia. The three techniques were (1) side-to-side duodenoduodenostomy, (2) side-to-side duodenojejunostomy (which is rarely performed today), and (3) diamond-shaped duodenoduodenostomy. There was no difference in the complication rate, but the diamond-shape technique was found to be superior for repair, resulting in earlier feeding and discharge. Kimura et al.[48] reported on their experience with 44 patients with the diamond-shaped technique, without the use of gastrostomy or transanastomotic tube, and found a very low rate of complications and good long-term results.

Long-term results of congenital DO were reported by Kokkonen et al.[68] who studied 41 patients ages 15–35 years. They found that growth and development, including body weight, were satisfactory. Although the great majority were symptom-free, on barium meal examination, all but two had abnormal findings, including megaduodenum in nine cases. They concluded that some gastrointestinal disturbances are common, even in asymptomatic patients, and careful follow-up is important. Salonen and Makinen[69] reported previously on their experience in a small group of nine patients at age 3–21 years and found, in contrast, a normal barium meal in all groups except one. Their result was similar to the documentation by Kimura et al.[48] with the diamond-shaped technique.

Ein et al.[64] encountered five patients with late complications of duodenal atresia repair that appeared suddenly between the ages of 6 months to 24 years. The duodenal repair was functionally obstructed—caused by proximal, dilated duodenal atony. Plication of the dilated atonic proximal duodenum was curative.

Kay et al.[51] reported on their experience with 17 neonates who underwent laparoscopic duodenoduodenostomy during a 4-year period (2004–2008). There were no conversions to open procedure, no intraoperative complications, and no anastomotic leaks. Time to full feeds in this group averaged 12 days. They concluded that laparoscopic duodenoduodenostomy in the neonate can be safely and successfully performed with excellent short-term outcome. However they emphasized that the laparoscopic duodenoduodenostomy should be performed only by surgeons with adequate laparoscopic skills.

Spilde et al.[57] compared the results of open versus laparoscopic repair of congenital DO of 29 patients during the years 2003–2007. Fourteen patients underwent an open approach, and 15 patients underwent a laparoscopic operation for the repair of DO. Congenital anomalies were similar between the two groups. The diamond-shaped duodenoduodenostomy technique was performed regardless of surgical approach. Operative time was not significantly different between groups (127 minutes—laparoscopic groups, 96 minutes—open approach). The length of post-operative hospitalization, time to initial feeding, and time to full oral intake were all statistically shorter in the patients undergoing laparoscopic repair. One patient in each group developed a stenosis at the anastomosis. One patient in the open group underwent an open revision of the duodenoduodenostomy, whereas the patient in the laparoscopic group underwent a balloon dilatation of the duodenoduodenostomy via endoscopic gastroduodenoscopy.

It is important to emphasize that the most recent reports of laparoscopic approach for DO are related to the short-term follow-up. As for the long term, there are no results as yet.

Over the last few decades, advancements in neonatal intensive care, parenteral nutrition, management of associated anomalies, and improvements in operative technique including video equipment, smaller instruments, and better postoperative care have improved the outlook for patients born with duodenal atresia and stenosis. Mortality today has been reduced to 5%–10% and is now related mostly to the associated cardiac anomalies.

REFERENCES

1. Best KE, Tennant PW, Addor MC, Bianchi F, Boyd P, Calzolari E, Dias CM, Doray B et al. Epidemiology of small intestinal atresia in Europe: A register-based study. *Arch Dis Child Fetal Neonatal Ed* 2012; 97: F353–8.
2. Choudhry MS, Rahman N, Boyd P, Lakhoo K. Duodenal atresia: Associated anomalies, prenatal diagnosis and outcome. *Pediatr Surg Int* 2009; 25: 727–30.
3. Escobar MA, Ladd AP, Grosfeld JL, West KW, Rescorla FJ, Scherer LR 3rd, Engum SA, Rouse TM et al. Duodenal atresia and stenosis: Long-term follow-up over 30 years. *J Pediatr Surg* 2004; 39(6): 867–71.
4. Singal AK, Ramu C, Paul S, Matthai J. Preduodenal portal vein in association with midgut malrotation and duodenal web-triple anomaly. *J Pediatr Surg* 2009; 44(2): 5–7.
5. Gray SW, Skandalakis JE. Embryology for surgeons. In: Gray SW, Skandalakis JE (eds). *Embryology for Surgeons: The Embryology Basis for the Treatment of Congenital Defects*. Philadelphia: WB Saunders, 1972.
6. Dalla Vecchia LK, Grosfeld JL, West KW, Rescorla FJ, Scherer LR, Engum SA. Intestinal atresia and stenosis: A 25-year experience with 277 cases. *Arch Surg* 1998; 133: 490–6.
7. Lauw JH, Barnard CN. Congenital intestinal atresia: Observations on its origin. *Lancet* 1955; 2: 1065–7.
8. Torfs CP, Christianson RE. Anomalies in Down syndrome individuals in a large population-based registry. *Am J Med Genet* 1998; 77: 431–8.
9. Markljung E, Adamovic T, Ortqvist L, Wester T, Nordenskjöld A. A rare microduplication in a familial case of annular pancreas and duodenal stenosis. *J Pediatr Surg* 2012; 47: 2039–43.
10. Lambrecht W, Kluth D. Hereditary multiple atresias of the gastrointestinal tract: Report of a case and review of the literature. *J Pediatr Surg* 1998; 33: 794–7.
11. Boyden EA, Cope JG, Bill AH Jr. Anatomy and embryology of congenital intrinsic obstruction of the duodenum. *Am J Surg* 1967; 114: 190–202.
12. Sadler T. *Langman's Medical Embryology*. Lippincott Williams and Wilkins, 2003.
13. Ramalho-Santos M, Melton DA, McMahon AP. Hedgehog signals regulate multiple aspects of gastrointestinal development. *Development* 2000; 127(12): 2763–72.
14. Kanard RC, Fairbanks TJ, De Langhe SP, Sala FG, Del Moral PM, Lopez CA, Warburton D, Anderson KD et al. Fibroblast growth factor-10 serves a regulatory role in duodenal development. *J Pediatr Surg* 2005; 40: 313–6.
15. Komuro H, Ono K, Hoshino N, Urita Y, Gotoh C, Fujishiro J, Shinkai T, Ikebukuro K et al. Bile duct duplication as a cause of distal bowel gas in neonatal DO. *J Pediatr Surg* 2011; 46(12): 2301–4.
16. Sweed Y. Duodenal obstruction. In: Puri P (ed). *Newborn Surgery*, 3rd edn. Hodder & Arnold, 2011.
17. Puri P. Outlook after surgery for congenital intrinsic DO in Down syndrome. *Lancet* 1981; 2(8250): 802.
18. Bailey PV, Tracy TF Jr, Connors RH, Mooney DP, Lewis JE, Weber TR. Congenital DO; a 32 year review. *J Pediatr Surg* 1993; 28: 92–5.
19. Pulkkinen L, Kimonis VE, Xu Y, Spanou EN, McLean WH, Uitto J. Homozygous alpha6 integrin mutation in junctional epidermolysis bullosa with congenital duodenal atresia. *Hum Mol Genet* 1997; 6: 669–74.
20. Iwai A, Hamada Y, Takada K, Inagaki N, Nakatake R, Yanai H, Miki H, Araki Y et al. Choledochal cyst associated with duodenal atresia: Case report and review of the literature. *Pediatr Surg Int* 2009; 25: 995–8.
21. Moore SW, de Jongh G, Bouic P, Brown RA, Kirsten G. Immune deficiency in familial duodenal atresia. *J Pediatr Surg* 1996; 31: 1733–5.
22. Nawaz A, Matta H, Hamchou M, Jacobez A, Trad O, Al Salem AH. Situs inversus abdominus in association with congenital DO: A report of two cases and review of the literature. *Pediatr Surg Int* 2005; 21: 589–92.
23. Piper HG, Alesbury J, Waterford SD, Zurakowski D, Jaksic T. Intestinal atresia: Factors affecting clinical outcomes. *J Pediatr Surg* 2008; 43(7): 1244–8.

24. Hancock BJ, Wiseman NE. Congenital DO: Impact of an antenatal diagnosis. *J Pediatr Surg* 1989; 24: 1027–31.

25. Muraji T, Mahour GH. Surgical problems in patients with VATER-associated anomalies. *J Pediatr Surg* 1984; 19: 550–4.

26. Spitz L, Ali M, Brereton RJ. Combined esophageal and duodenal atresia: Experience of 18 patients. *J Pediatr Surg* 1981; 16: 4–7.

27. Fragoso AC, Ortiz R, Hernandez F, Olivares P, Martinez L, Tovar JA. Defective upper gastrointestinal function after repair of combined esophageal and duodenal atresia. *J Pediatr Surg* 2015; 50: 531–4.

28. Cohen-Overbeek TE, Grijseels EW, Niemeijer ND, Hop WC, Wladimiroff JW, Tibboel D. Isolated or non-isolated DO: Perinatal outcome following prenatal or postnatal diagnosis. *Ultrasound Obstet Gynecol* 2008; 32(6): 784–92.

29. Murshed R, Nicholls G, Spitz L. Intrinsic DO: Trends in management over 45 years (1951–1995) with relevance to prenatal counselling. *Br J Obstet Gynaecol* 1999; 106: 1197–9.

30. Bronshtein M, Blazer S, Zimmer EZ. The gastrointestinal tract and abdominal wall. In: Callen PW (ed). *Ultrasonography in Obstetrics and Gynecology*, 5th edn. WB Saunders, 2008.

31. Tsukerman GL, Krapiva GA, Krillova IA. First-trimester diagnosis of duodenal stenosis associated with oesophageal atresia. *Prenat Diagn* 1993; 13: 371–6.

32. Grosfeld JL, Rescorla FJ. Duodenal atresia and stenosis: Reassessment of treatment and outcome based on antenatal diagnosis, pathologic variants and long term follow up. *World J Surg* 1993; 17: 301–9.

33. Zimmer EZ, Bronshtein M. Early diagnosis of duodenal atresia and possible sonographic pitfalls. *Prenat Diagn* 1996; 16: 564–6.

34. Casaccia G, Bilancioni E, Nahom A, Trucchi A, Aite L, Marcellini M, Bagolan P. Cystic anomalies of biliary tree in the fetus: It is possible to make a more specific prenatal diagnosis? *J Pediatr Surg* 2002; 37: 1191–4.

35. Malone FD, Crombleholme TM, Nores JA, Athanassiou A, D'Alton ME. Pitfalls of the 'double bubble' sign: A case of congenital duodenal duplication. *Fetal Diagn Ther* 1997; 12: 298–300.

36. Pameijer CR, Hubbard AM, Coleman B, Flake AW. Combined pure esophageal atresia, duodenal atresia, biliary atresia and pancreatic ductal atresia: Prenatal diagnostic features and review of the literature. *J Pediatr Surg* 2000; 35: 745–7.

37. Dankovcik R, Jirasek JE, Kucera E, Feyereisl J, Radonak J, Dudas M. Prenatal diagnosis of annular pancreas: Reliability of the double bubble sign with periduodenal hyperechogenic band. *Fetal Diagn Ther* 2008; 24: 483–90.

38. Keckler SJ, St Peter SD, Spilde TL, Ostlie DJ, Snyder CL. The influence of trisomy 21 on the incidence and severity of congenital heart defects in patients with duodenal atresia. *Pediatr Surg Int* 2008; 24(8): 921–3.

39. Haeusler MC, Berghold A, Stoll C, Barisic I, Clementi M; EUROSCAN Study Group. Prenatal ultrasonographic detection of gastrointestinal obstruction: Results from 18 European congenital anomaly registries. *Prenat Diagn* 2002; 22(7): 616–23.

40. Kilbride H, Castor C, Andrews W. Congenital DO: Timing of diagnosis during the newborn period. *J Perinatol* 2010; 30(3): 197–200.

41. Knechtle SJ, Filston HC. Anomalous biliary ducts associated with duodenal atresia. *J Pediatr Surg* 1990; 25(12): 266–9.

42. Vaos G, Misiakos EP. Congenital anomalies of the gastrointestinal tract diagnosed in adulthood—Diagnosis and management. *J Gastrointest Surg* 2010; 14(5): 916–25.

43. Mikaelsson C, Arnbjörnsson E, Kullendorff CM. Membranous duodenal stenosis. *Acta Paediatr* 1997; 86(9): 953–5.

44. Samuel M, Wheeler RA, Mami AG. Does duodenal atresia and stenosis prevent midgut volvulus in malrotation? *Eur J Pediatr Surg* 1997; 7(1): 11–2.

45. Kimble RM, Harding J, Kolbe A. Additional congenital anomalies in babies with gut atresia of stenosis: When to investigate, and which investigation. *Pediatr Surg Int* 1997; 12: 565–70.

46. Wesley JR, Mahour GH. Congenital intrinsic DO: A twenty-five year review. *Surgery* 1977; 82(5): 716–20.

47. Kimura K, Tsugawa C, Ogawa K, Matsumoto Y, Yamamoto T, Asada S. Diamond-shaped anastomosis for congenital DO. *Arch Surg* 1977; 112(10): 262–3.

48. Kimura K, Mukohara N, Nishijima E, Muraji T, Tsugawa C, Matsumoto Y. Diamond-shaped anastomosis for duodenal atresia: An experience with 44 patients over 15 years. *J Pediatr Surg* 1990; 25(9): 977–9.

49. Bax NM, Ure BM, van der Zee DC, van Tuijl I. Laparoscopic duodenoduodenostomy for duodenal atresia. *Surg Endosc* 2001; 15(2): 217.

50. Rothenberg SS. Laparoscopic duodenoduodenostomy for DO in infants and children. *J Pediatr Surg* 2002; 37(7): 1088–9.

51. Kay S, Yoder S, Rothenberg S. Laparoscopic duodenoduodenostomy in the neonate. *J Pediatr Surg* 2009; 44(5): 906–8.

52. Sweed Y, DO. In: Puri P, Höllwarth M (eds). *Pediatric Surgery Atlas Series*. Springer, 2006.

53. Hall NJ, Drewett M, Wheeler RA, Griffiths DM, Kitteringham LJ, Burge DM. Trans-anastomotic tubes reduce the need for central venous access and parenteral nutrition in infants with congenital DO. *Pediatr Surg Int* 2011; 27(8): 851–5.

54. Sweed Y, Bar-Maor JA, Shoshany G. Insertion of a soft silastic nasogastric tube at operation for esophageal atresia: A new technical method. *J Pediatr Surg* 1992; 27(5): 650–1.

55. Bittencourt PF, Malheiros RS, Ferreira AR, Carvalho SD, Filho PP, Tatsuo ES, Mattos FF, Melo SO et al. Endoscopic treatment of congenital duodenal membrane. *Gastrointest Endosc* 2012; 76(6): 1273–5.

56. Hill S, Koontz CS, Langness SM, Wulkan ML. Laparoscopic versus open repair of congenital DO in infants. *J Laparoendosc Adv Surg Tech* 2011; 21(10): 961–3.

57. Spilde TL, St Peter SD, Keckler SJ, Holcomb GW 3rd, Snyder CL, Ostlie DJ. Open vs laparoscopic repair of congenital DOs: A concurrent series. *J Pediatr Surg* 2008; 43(6): 1002–5.

58. Li B, Chen WB, Zhou WY. Laparoscopic methods in the treatment of congenital duodenal obstruction for neonates. *J Laparoendosc Adv Surg Tech* A 2013; 23(10): 881–4.

59. Spigland N, Yazbeck S. Complications associated with surgical treatment of congenital intrinsic DO. *J Pediatr Surg* 1990; 25(11): 1127–30.

60. Parmentier B, Peycelon M, Muller CO, El Ghoneimi A, Bonnard A. Laparoscopic management of congenital duodenal atresia or stenosis: A single-center early experience. *J Pediatr Surg* 2015; 50(11): 1833–6.

61. Hutton KA, Thomas DF. Tapering duodenoplasty. *Pediatr Surg Int* 1988; 3: 132–4.

62. Adzick NS. Hurrison MR, deLorimier AA. Tapering duodenoplasty for megaduodenum associated with duodenal atresia. *J Pediatr Surg* 1986; 21: 311–2.

63. Kimura K, Perdzynski W, Soper RT. Elliptical seromuscular resection for tapering the proximal dilated bowel in duodenal or jejunal atresia. *J Pediatr Surg* 1996; 31: 1405–6.

64. Ein SH. Kim PC, Miller HA. The late nonfunctioning duodenal atresia repair—A second look. *J Pediatr Surg* 2000; 35: 690–1.

65. Endo M, Ukiyama E, Yokoyama J, Kitajima M. Subtotal duodenectomy with jejunal patch for megaduodenum secondary to congenital duodenal malformation. *J Pediatr Surg* 1998; 33: 1636–40.

66. Ladd WE. Congenital obstruction of the duodenum in children. *N Engl J Med* 1932; 206: 277–83.

67. Weber TR, Lewis JE, Mooney D, Connors R. Duodenal atresia: A comparison of techniques of repair. *J Pediatr Surg* 1986; 21(12): 1133–6.

68. Kokkonen ML, Kalima T, Jääskeläinen J, Louhimo I. Duodenal atresia: Late follow-up. *J Pediatr Surg* 1998; 23: 216–20.

69. Salonen IS, Makinen E. Intestinal blind pouch—And blind loop—Syndrome in children operated previously for congenital DO. *Ann Chir Gynaecol* 1976; 65: 38–45.

56

Intestinal malrotation

AUGUSTO ZANI AND AGOSTINO PIERRO

DEFINITION

Intestinal malrotation is defined as the congenital abnormal positioning of the midgut, whereby the duodenojejunal (DJ) flexure lies right of the midline and relatively close to the ileocecal valve. This makes the dorsal mesenteric root narrow and puts the bowel at risk of midgut volvulus. Intestinal malrotation is usually associated with the presence of peritoneal folds, so-called Ladd's bands, which cross from the colon and cecum to the duodenum and liver and rarely cause duodenal obstruction.

EPIDEMIOLOGY

Malrotation is estimated from autopsy studies to occur in 0.5%–1% of the population, although only 1 in 6000 live births will present with clinical symptoms. Incidence is slightly higher in males than females. Symptoms can occur at any age, but the classical teaching is that the vast majority of patients with malrotation are symptomatic in the first month of life and 90% will present before 1 year of age. However, a study on 2744 cases of intestinal rotation in children up to 17 years of age has shown that only 30% present by 1 month of age, 58% before 1 year of age, and 75% before 5 years of age. A higher incidence of malrotation is seen in patients with anterior abdominal wall defects (gastroschisis and exomphalos), congenital diaphragmatic hernia, heterotaxy syndrome, biliary atresia, intussusception (Waugh's syndrome), intestinal dysmotility syndromes, and small bowel atresia, where this is thought to be the result of an antenatal volvulus.

PATHOGENESIS

Intestinal malrotation results from an arrest of normal rotation of the embryonic gut. The intestine develops in utero through three stages that occur during the first trimester. During the first stage (5th to 10th weeks), the elongating bowel exceeds the abdominal cavity and herniates outside the abdomen. During the second stage (10th to 11th weeks), the bowel returns into the abdomen and rotates 270° counterclockwise around the superior mesenteric artery. The third stage (12th week) is characterized by the retroperitoneal fixation of the duodenum and colon. The distal duodenum comes to lie across the midline toward the left upper quadrant, attached by the ligament of Treitz at the DJ flexure to the posterior abdominal wall. The cecum passes to the right and downward and becomes fixed to the posterior abdominal wall.

CLINICAL PRESENTATION

Patients with intestinal malrotation can remain asymptomatic and be diagnosed incidentally (up to 10% of all cases). Symptomatic infants, instead, may present with signs and symptoms of acute bowel obstruction due to the development of midgut volvulus, which differ according to the age of presentation.

- In the *neonatal period,* babies present with abdominal distention and bilious vomiting. Midgut volvulus results in intestinal strangulation, passage of blood per rectum, and shock. As the strangulation progresses to gangrene, perforation, and peritonitis, the abdominal wall shows signs of edema and discoloration.
- *Older infants* and *children* present with chronic episodic obstructive symptoms, failure to thrive, malabsorption, diarrhea, and/or nonspecific colicky abdominal pain.

DIAGNOSIS

Plain abdominal radiography is usually aspecific, and can either be normal or show features of distended stomach and proximal duodenum with a distal paucity of gas.

If the physical examination and/or the abdominal radiography is indicative of volvulus with high suspicion, surgery should be expedited. Alternatively, if the patient is stable, further diagnostic imaging is recommended.

Upper gastrointestinal contrast study is the gold-standard investigation for patients presenting with signs of proximal bowel. Findings in intestinal malrotation are as follows:

- On frontal view, DJ flexure on the right of the spine and inferior to the transpyloric plane (Addison's plane).
- On lateral view, the fourth part of the duodenum lies anterior to the second part (D2), occasionally showing a corkscrew appearance.

Contrast enema has historically been used, especially to study the position of the cecal pole. However, in 15%–30% of malrotation cases, the cecum is normally located, and in many patients with normal intestinal rotation, the cecum has an abnormal location. Therefore, a contrast enema is not always helpful.

Abdominal ultrasonography that demonstrates an abnormal orientation of the mesenteric vessels can also be indicative of intestinal malrotation. In a normal situation, the superior mesenteric vein is located to the right of the superior mesenteric artery. Hence, a reversed arrangement of these vessels is suggestive of malrotation. Color Doppler ultrasonography may reveal a "whirlpool sign," which is created when the superior mesenteric vein and the mesentery wrap around the superior mesenteric artery in midgut volvulus. Ancillary ultrasonographic findings suggestive of malrotation are found when looking at the third part of the duodenum: dilatation of the proximal portion indicating obstruction and abnormal position between the superior mesenteric artery and the aorta in the retroperitoneal space are suggestive of malrotation.

Computed tomography of the abdomen is commonly used in adults as it also provides information on bowel perfusion. However, this imaging technique should not be employed in infants, children, and adolescents due to the radiation exposure risk.

TREATMENT

Management of the asymptomatic patient and timing of surgery remain controversial and are discussed in the following paragraph.

All symptomatic patients with positive investigative findings should undergo urgent laparotomy following a brief period of intensive resuscitation, with crystalloids or 5% human albumin in the form of a bolus (20 mL/kg to repeat as required) and maintenance fluids. A nasogastric tube is passed to aspirate gastric content and avoid aspiration. Blood is drawn for crossmatch, full blood count, and electrolytes. Blood for transfusion should be available at the commencement of surgery.

SURGERY

The principles of the procedure have remained almost unchanged since originally described by Ladd in 1936.

Open Ladd's procedure

The patient is positioned supine, and a right-upper-quadrant transverse incision is made. The umbilical vein is divided and ligated. The peritoneal fluid is examined. Frequently it is clear; blood-stained fluid implies bowel ischemia and volvulus; fecal staining indicates bowel perforation and should be cultured. The midgut is delivered from the wound and the base examined. Any volvulus should be derotated counterclockwise, noting the number of turns. The bowel is examined for viability, and any ischemic bowel should be wrapped in a damp swab and reexamined after 5–10 min. Nonviable bowel is resected and a primary anastomosis performed.

Ladd's bands, if present, are divided. The superior mesenteric artery is identified, and the mesenteric base is broadened as much as possible by division of the peritoneal folds. Care must be taken not to injure the superior mesenteric vessels. An appendectomy should be performed, due to the abnormal position of the appendix at the end of the surgery (left upper quadrant). However, it is still a matter of debate whether an appendectomy should be performed in neonates. Some surgeons would opt for an inversion of the appendix; others would leave the appendix untouched to prevent potential additional morbidity.

At the end of the procedure, the small bowel is placed in the right hemiabdomen and the large bowel in the left hemiabdomen. There is no need to apply any fixation sutures, as adhesions and the broad base to the mesentery developed by Ladd's procedure usually stabilize the bowel. The abdomen is closed as routine.

Midgut volvulus due to malrotation may result in loss of the small bowel. The author has reported a technique to deal with mesenteric thrombosis, which causes continuing ischemia of the intestine. This technique includes the following: (1) digital massage of the superior mesenteric vessels after derotation to restore intestinal perfusion and (2) postoperative systemic infusion of tissue-type plasminogen activator. If extensive ischemic bowel of doubtful viability is present, a second-look laparotomy is performed after 24 h in the hope of minimizing the extent of bowel resection required.

Laparoscopic Ladd's procedure

Laparoscopy can be performed for diagnosis of equivocal cases of malrotation as well as for correction of the defect. The principles of the procedure are the same as the open technique. Care must be taken to correctly identify landmarks such as the duodenum and ascending colon. To gain access to the duodenum, it is useful to raise the head of the operating table and elevate the right flank. The ascending colon falls toward the left side of the abdomen. The duodenum is exposed, and Ladd's bands are divided. After division, the bowel is examined along its length for any further causes of obstruction. Dividing the peritoneal folds broadens the root of the mesentery, and care must be taken in not injuring the superior mesenteric vein. Appendectomy is carried out either using endoloops for intracorporeal ligation or by delivering the appendix through a trocar site and excising it extra-abdominally in smaller patients.

Postoperatively, a nasogastric tube is left in situ for gastric aspirates. Intravenous fluids are continued, and gastric losses are replaced milliliter for milliliter with normal saline and potassium chloride (20 mmol/L saline). Enteral feeds are restarted when the postoperative ileus is resolved.

COMPLICATIONS

Recurrence of midgut volvulus is rare but has been reported and may be due to division of Ladd's bands without a full derotation and splaying of the mesentery. Adhesive bowel obstruction is reported in about 5% of cases. Midgut volvulus occurs in 45%–65% of children with malrotation and still carries a mortality rate of 7%–15%; necrosis of >75% of the midgut is associated with intestinal failure.

CONTROVERSIES

Management of asymptomatic patients remains controversial. It is still a matter of debate whether to look for and/or correct rotation anomalies in the following:

- Patients undergoing repair of abdominal wall defects or congenital diaphragmatic hernia. Some degree of nonrotation or malrotation is invariably encountered in these patients, and subsequent volvulus is rare.
- Asymptomatic patients with malrotation in whom the diagnosis is made incidentally during evaluation for nonspecific complaints, prior to fundoplication for gastroesophageal reflux, and in those with heterotaxy syndromes.
- Monozygotic twins with proven malrotation in the sibling.

REFERENCE

Ladd WE. Surgical diseases of the alimentary tract in infants. *N Engl J Med* 1936; 215: 705–8.

FURTHER READING

Aboagye J, Goldstein SD, Salazar JH, Papandria D, Okoye MT, Al-Omar K, Stewart D, Lukish J, Abdullah F. Age at presentation of common pediatric surgical conditions: Reexamining dogma. *J Pediatr Surg* 2014 June; 49(6): 995–9.

Bass KD, Rothenberg SS, Chang JH. Laparoscopic Ladd's procedure in infants with malrotation. *J Pediatr Surg* 1998 February; 33(2): 279–81.

Kiely EM, Pierro A, Pierce C, Cross K, De Coppi P. Clot dissolution: A novel treatment of midgut volvulus. *Pediatrics* 2012 June; 129(6): e1601–4.

Kluth D, Fiegel H. The embryology of the foregut. *Semin Pediatr Surg* 2003 February; 12(1): 3–9.

Lampl B, Levin TL, Berdon WE, Cowles RA. Malrotation and midgut volvulus: A historical review and current controversies in diagnosis and management. *Pediatr Radiol* 2009 April; 39(4): 359–66.

Millar AJ, Rode H, Cywes S. Malrotation and volvulus in infancy and childhood. *Semin Pediatr Surg* 2003 November; 12(4): 229–36.

Stanfill AB, Pearl RH, Kalvakuri K, Wallace LJ, Vegunta RK. Laparoscopic Ladd's procedure: Treatment of choice for midgut malrotation in infants and children. *J Laparoendosc Adv Surg Tech A* 2010 May; 20(4): 369–72.

Yousefzadeh DK. The position of the duodenojejunal junction: The wrong horse to bet on in diagnosing or excluding malrotation. *Pediatr Radiol* 2009 April; 39 Suppl 2: S172–7.

57

Congenital hyperinsulinism

PAUL R. V. JOHNSON

INTRODUCTION

Congenital hyperinsulinism (CHI), previously termed persistent hyperinsulinemic hyperglycemia of infancy (PHHI), is a spectrum of conditions characterized by profound hypoglycemia in the presence of inappropriately high insulin secretion.[1,2] Although rare overall, CHI is a significant cause of hypoglycaemic brain injury in the newborn[1] and subsequent mental retardation,[3] and therefore, all those involved in the medical and surgical management of neonates need to be familiar with this condition so that the diagnosis can be made promptly, and early treatment implemented. This chapter provides an overview of the etiology, clinical presentation, diagnosis, and management of CHI to facilitate this.

ETIOLOGY

Over the past decade, our understanding of the etiology of CHI has increased enormously.[4,5] This has not only led to more focused treatment for certain subforms of the condition but has also meant that genetic counseling can be offered to some families. CHI can either occur sporadically with an incidence of 1 in 40,000–50,000 or can be familial with an incidence as high as 1 in 2500. Genetically, CHI is a heterogeneous condition, and mutations of 11 different genes related to insulin secretion have now been reported.[5] Mutations can be sporadic, autosomal recessive, or autosomal dominant. The most common abnormality underlying CHI is a dysfunction of the ATP-sensitive potassium channel within the pancreatic beta cell (channelopathies).[6] This ion channel is composed of two subunits, each of which is encoded for by a different gene, namely the sulfonylurea receptor gene *SUR1* and the inward-rectifying potassium channel gene *KIR6.2*. Mutations of the SUR1 gene account for 50%–60% of CHI, whereas mutations of the KIR6.2 gene are less common and only responsible for 10%–15% of cases.[7]

The abnormal potassium channel results in the beta cell being in a constant state of depolarization, and therefore, it is constantly secreting insulin despite the cell environment being one of hypoglycemia (Figure 57.1a and b). A less common group of underlying causes of CHI are the "metabolopathies," which result from enzyme deficiencies (e.g., glutamate dehydrogenase [GDH], glucokinase [GK] or short-chain L-3-hydroxyacyl-CoA dehydrogenase [SCHAD]) or dysfunction of the insulin receptor. Finally, CHI can be associated with certain specific syndromes such as Beckwith–Wiedemann syndrome, Periman syndrome, and Sotos syndrome, each of which has associated chromosomal abnormalities.

PATHOLOGY

The original term for CHI was nesidioblastosis. This term was created by Laidlaw[8] in 1938, and described the histological finding of islet cells proliferating by budding off the pancreatic ductal tissue within pancreases of infants with severe symptoms of hypoglycemia. However, this term has since been abandoned as it was realized not only that CHI represents a spectrum of different disorders, but more specifically, that many normal neonatal pancreases also exhibit nesidioblastosis.[9]

However, the most important advance in our understanding of CHI over recent years has been the discovery that there are two distinct histopathological forms, namely, a focal form and a diffuse form. Focal CHI is characterized by a focal hyperplasia of the pancreatic beta cells and is to be distinguished from the more discrete adenoma or insulinoma seen in older children or adults. Normal islets are seen outside the focal abnormality (Figure 57.2). In the diffuse form of CHI, the islets are abnormal throughout the whole pancreas and exhibit large, pleomorphic, hyperchromatic nuclei (Figure 57.3). Distinguishing focal from diffuse CHI is important to ensure that the correct surgical treatment is undertaken.

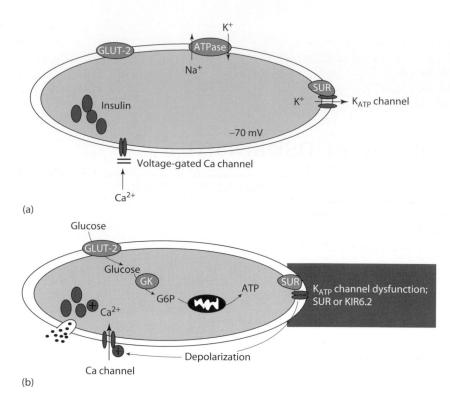

(a)

(b)

Figure 57.1 **(a)** Normal resting beta cell. At rest, the normal K_{ATP} channel is closed, which maintains the membrane potential at −70 mV. This results in the calcium channels remaining closed, preventing any calcium influx or consequent insulin release. **(b)** Congenital hyperinsulinism (CHI) beta cell. The abnormal K_{ATP} channel in the nonstimulated CHI beta cell results in the channel remaining closed even at rest. This causes depolarization of the membrane and opening of the calcium channel. The consequent calcium influx results in insulin degranulation and release.

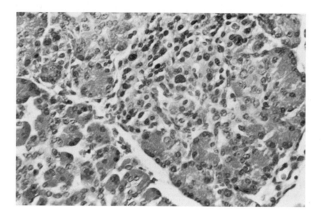

Figure 57.2 Diffuse congenital hyperinsulinism: islets have large, pleomorphic, hyperchromatic nuclei present throughout pancreas.

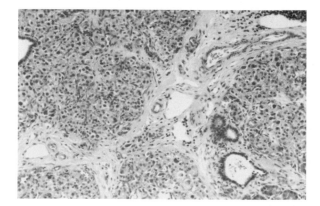

Figure 57.3 Focal congenital hyperinsulinism: nodules of adenomatous islet cell hyperplasia with normal islets outside the lesion.

CLINICAL PRESENTATION

CHI usually presents within the first few hours or days of life in both premature and term babies but can occasionally present later in infancy or childhood.[7] Babies can present with nonspecific symptoms of hypoglycemia such as poor feeding, irritability, or lethargy, or more severe symptoms such as seizures or coma. Apnea can also occur. This outlines the importance of all neonates undergoing blood glucose testing shortly after birth. Antenatal hyperinsulinism can have a profound effect on fetal development; a proportion of babies with CHI are macrosomic due to increased glycogen storage, and some have organomegaly. Some also present with mild facial abnormalities such as a high forehead, a small nasal tip, and a short columella.[10] CHI is most commonly an isolated condition but can be associated with certain specific syndromes as described earlier. CHI can sometimes be transient rather than persistent, but it is the persistent forms that are of most relevance to surgeons.

DIAGNOSIS

CHI is characterized by hyperinsulinemic, hypoketotic, hypofattyacidemic hypoglycemia.[1] The following diagnostic criteria are used: (1) laboratory blood glucose readings of <3.5 mmol/L (63 mg/dL)[11] (the diagnostic level used to be defined as 2.5–3 mmol); (2) a glucose infusion rate of >8 mg kg^{-1} min^{-1} (normal range is 4–6 mg kg^{-1} min^{-1}); (3) unsuppressed insulin concentrations of >1 mU/L; (4) a positive response to the subcutaneous or intramuscular administration of glucagon (plasma glucose concentrations increasing by 2–3 mmol/L following a 0.5 mg subcutaneous glucagon injection); and (5) negative ketone bodies in the plasma and urine.

Previously, the definitive investigation used to distinguish diffuse and focal forms of the disease was serial venous sampling of insulin. However, this procedure was invasive and time-consuming, and often resulted in inaccurate localization of focal disease. Over the last decade, the gold-standard investigation has become [18F]-DOPA positron emission tomography (PET) combined with computed tomographic (CT) angiography with 3-D reconstruction.[12,13] This test is noninvasive, is both sensitive and specific, and gives excellent localization of focal lesions. However, the [18F]-fluoro-L-DOPA isotope is only currently available in a limited number of centers.

MANAGEMENT

The main aim of management is to prevent hypoglycemic brain damage and to allow normal psychomotor development. In mild cases, it may be possible to maintain acceptable levels of blood glucose by dietary measures alone. In the majority of cases, however, intravenous administration of high concentrations of glucose are required to maintain blood glucose levels above 2.6 mmol/L. Glucose infusion rates in excess of 20 mg kg^{-1} min^{-1}, i.e., 15%–20% glucose, may be required. In these cases, it is essential to insert a central venous catheter to provide a central route for administration of high concentrations of glucose and to allow frequent monitoring of blood glucose levels.

Medical management

Diazoxide is the first-line medical treatment and is an agonist of the K_{ATP} channel. It is commenced at a dose of 5–20 mg kg^{-1} day^{-1} in three divided doses. It can be highly effective in the treatment of the transient and syndromic forms of CHI, but in the more severe neonatal forms in which a mutation of the K_{ATP} channel is present, the beta cells may be unresponsive.[7–14] Diazoxide is usually used in conjunction with chlorthiazide at a dose of 7–10 mg kg^{-1} day^{-1} in two divided doses. These two agents exert a synergistic effect on the K_{ATP} channel with diazoxide. Octreotide is a long-acting analogue of the pancreatic hormone somatostatin and is used in CHI both as a short-term measure to stabilize the baby pending definitive treatment and, sometimes,

as a long-term treatment combined with frequent feeding, for diffuse disease. Subcutaneous or intravenous glucagon is used in the acute management of hypoglycemia, often in combination with octreotide. The calcium channel blocker nifedipine has been used successfully in a small number of patients.[15] The aim of using such an agent is to reduce the calcium flux resulting from the constant depolarization of beta cells in CHI. The systemic effect of calcium blockade can be restrictive. Recently, several groups have successfully managed to treat small numbers of children with CHI with the immunosuppressive agent sirolimus (rapamycin), an inhibitor of interleukin 2 (IL-2) and other cytokines.[16]

Surgical management

Surgical treatment is indicated when an infant remains dependent on intravenous glucose administration despite maximum medical treatment. Whereas 95% pancreatectomy was, until recently, the treatment of choice for all cases of CHI that were unresponsive to medical treatment,[17] improvements in our understanding of the histopathology of CHI have enabled more limited and targeted surgical resection treatment to be used for the focal form of the disease.[18,19] Pancreatectomy can be performed using traditional open operative techniques or can be undertaken using laparoscopic techniques.[20,21] The surgical principles are the same for both techniques.

INCISION

For the open technique, a laparotomy is performed via a generous supraumbilical transverse muscle-cutting incision, extending through both rectus abdominis muscles (Figure 57.4). For the laparoscopic approach, a three-trocar technique is used with triangulation centered around the umbilicus. Within the peritoneum, a thorough search is made for sites of ectopic pancreatic tissue.

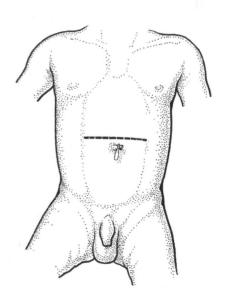

Figure 57.4 Transverse upper abdominal incision extending across both rectus abdominis muscles.

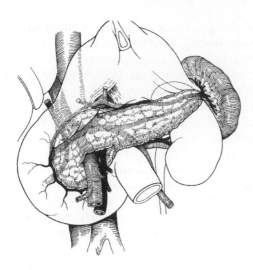

Figure 57.5 Exposure of the head, body, and tail of the pancreas by entering the lesser sac dividing the vessels in the greater omentum along the greater curvature of the stomach.

EXPOSURE

The anterior surface of the pancreas is exposed by entering the lesser peritoneal sac via the gastrocolic omentum, ligating and dividing vessels in the greater omentum along the greater curvature of the stomach (Figure 57.5). The tail of the pancreas lies in the hilum of the spleen. The hepatic flexure is reflected medially and the duodenum Kocherized to expose the head of the pancreas. The entire pancreas is carefully examined or inspected.

95% PANCREATECTOMY

In the diffuse form, the dissection of the pancreas proceeds medially from the tail toward the neck of the pancreas, which lies just to the right of the superior mesenteric vessels. It is essential for future immunologic competence to preserve the spleen whenever possible. This is accomplished by carefully exposing the short pancreatic vessels passing from the splenic vessels to the pancreas. These vessels, especially the veins, are extremely friable, but meticulous dissection will allow individual ligation, application of metal clips or electrocoagulation, and division of the vessels without traumatizing the main vessels (Figure 57.6). Should hemorrhage occur from damage to the splenic vein, direct repair should be attempted. In the event of failure to achieve hemostasis, ligation of the splenic vein with preservation of the splenic function can be expected due to collateral supply from the short gastric vessels. When the dissection has progressed to the right of the superior mesenteric vessels, attention is directed to the head of the pancreas and in particular the uncinate process (Figure 57.7).

The uncinate process is carefully dissected from behind the superior mesenteric vessels, and after positively defining the course of the common bile duct, the head of the pancreas to the left of the common duct and in the concavity of the duodenal loop is excised, leaving a sliver of pancreatic tissue on the surface of the duodenum and on the left wall of the common duct. The pancreatic duct is identified and ligated

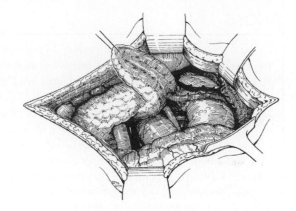

Figure 57.6 The short pancreatic vessels arising from the splenic vessels are divided, and the body and tail of the pancreas are gradually dissected toward the head.

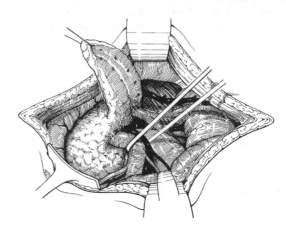

Figure 57.7 The superior mesenteric vessels are displayed and retracted toward the left, exposing the uncinate process of the pancreas.

with a nonabsorbable ligature. Hemostasis is carefully and meticulously achieved. The remaining pancreatic tissue consists of that part of the gland between the duodenum and the common bile duct and the sliver of tissue on the medial wall of the second part of the duodenum (Figure 57.8). This represents approximately 5% of the total volume of the pancreas but can vary considerably from patient to patient. A suction drain via a separate stab incision is left in the pancreatic bed.

Laparoscopic resection is performed in a similar manner, but it is easiest to perform the resection using a hook diathermy in a piecemeal manner, using a stay suture at different intervals along the pancreas as dissection proceeds from the pancreatic tail toward the head. For the transection of the pancreas itself, the harmonic scalpel ensures good hemostasis and occlusion of the pancreatic duct and cut parenchyma.

RESECTION OF FOCAL DISEASE

Exactly the same principles as described earlier apply for resection of focal disease. Based on the preoperative PET scan, the focal lesion is resected leaving the normal pancreas behind.[19] If the focal disease is within the head of the pancreas, occasionally, a major Whipple-type resection is required.

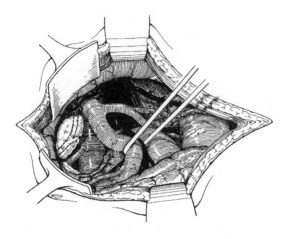

Figure 57.8 Final appearance following 95% pancreatectomy. The only remaining pancreatic tissue lies to the left of the common bile duct and a sliver in the C-curvature of the duodenum. Note splenic vessels and the completed excision of the uncinate process.

POSTOPERATIVE CARE

Postoperatively, glucose infusions and CHI medications are directed by constant monitoring of blood glucose. The infant is kept nil by mouth with a nasogastric tube in situ until the postoperative ileus has resolved.

COMPLICATIONS

Each of the medical treatments of CHI can have its side effects.[7] Long-term use of diazoxide is associated with hypertrichosis (excessive growth of hair in areas where hair does not normally grow), and this can limit its long-term use. Octreotide is associated with a wide range of side effects including gastrointestinal upset (abdominal pain, nausea, bloating, and diarrhea), and suppression of growth hormone (GH), thyroid-stimulating hormone (TSH), and adrenocorticotropic hormone (ACTH). Recurrent hypoglycemia can occur as a result of insufficient surgical resection of the diffuse form of the disease, or due to failed localization in the focal form, and should be evident within the first 72 hours after the operation. Persistent hypoglycemia may require further surgical resection. Other surgical complications include postoperative infection, bleeding, and operative trauma to the bile duct.[22] If the latter is diagnosed preoperatively, then primary repair and drainage is performed. Delayed diagnosis of bile duct injury can be treated operatively or conservatively depending on the degree of damage and the timing of presentation.

LONG-TERM RESULTS

The neurological outcome of patients with CHI depends on the age of presentation.[3] Neonates with unresponsive CHI that is unresponsive to medical treatment are at increased risk of brain injury, as are those with a delayed diagnosis and delayed implementation of treatment.[3] The

form of CHI per se does not seem to influence outcome. In patients undergoing 95% pancreatectomy, the majority will develop insulin-dependent diabetes by the second decade of life.[23,24] These patients require close monitoring of their glucose homeostasis, and a yearly glucose-tolerance test is indicated. For those that do develop diabetes, novel, minimally invasive treatments such as pancreatic islet transplantation are now achieving excellent results for reversing insulin-requiring diabetes in adults.[25] The majority of these patients will require oral pancreatic exocrine replacement. The recent emphasis on limited pancreatic resection for focal CHI means that both exocrine and endocrine insufficiency can be reduced in this group of patients. Good outcomes have been reported in this group of patients.[26]

REFERENCES

1. Arnoux J-B, de Lonlay P, Ribeiro M-J et al. Congenital hyperinsulinism. *Early Hum Dev* 2010; 86(5): 287–94.
2. Hussain K. Congenital hyperinsulinism. *Semin Fetal Neonat Med* 2005; 10: 369–76.
3. Menni F, de Lonlay P, Sevin C et al. Neurologic outcomes of 90 neonates and infants with persistent hyperinsulinaemic hypoglycaemia. *Paediatrics* 2001; 107: 476–9.
4. James C, Kapoor RR, Ismail D, Hussain K. The genetic basis of congenital hyperinsulinism. *J Med Genet* 2009; 46: 289–99.
5. Stanley CA. Perspective on the genetics and diagnosis of congenital hyperinsulinism disorders. *J Clin Endocrinol Metab* 2016 March; 101(3): 815–26.
6. Kane C, Shepherd RM, Squires PE et al. Loss of functional K_{ATP} channels in pancreatic beta-cells causes persistent hyperinsulinemic hypoglycemia of infancy. *Nat Med* 1996; (12): 1344–7.
7. Hussain K. Diagnosis and management of hyperinsulinaemic hypoglycaemia of infancy. *Hormone Res* 2008; 69: 2–13.
8. Laidlaw GF. Nesidioblastoma, the islet tumor of the pancreas. *Am J Pathol* 1938; 14: 125–34.
9. Rahler J, Guiot Y, Sempoux C. Persistent hyperinsulinaemic hypoglycaemia of infancy: A heterogeneous syndrome unrelated to nesidioblastosis. *Arch Dis Child Fetal Neonat Ed* 2002; 82(2): 108–12.
10. de Lonlay P, Cormier-Daire V, Amiel J et al. Facial appearance in persistent hyperinsulinemic hypoglycemia. *Am J Med Genet* 2002; 111: 130–3.
11. Roženková K, Güemes M, Shah P, Hussain K. The diagnosis and management of hyperinsulinaemic hypoglycaemia. *J Clin Res Pediatr Endocrinol* 2015 June; 7(2): 86–97.
12. Otonoski T, Nanto-Salonen K, Seppanen M et al. Noninvasive diagnosis of focal hyperinsulinism of infancy with [^{18}F]-DOPA positron emission tomography. *Diabetes* 2006; 55(1): 13–8.

13. Mohnike K, Blankenstein O, Christesen HT et al. Proposal for a standardized protocol for 18F-DOPA-PET (PET/CT) in congenital hyperinsulinism. *Hormone Res* 2006; 66(1): 40–2.

14. Kane C, Lindley KJ, Johnson PR et al. Therapy for persistent hyperinsulinemic hypoglycemia of infancy. Understanding the responsiveness of beta cells to diazoxide and somatostatin. *J Clin Invest* 1997; 100(7): 1888–93.

15. Lindley KJ, Dunne MJ, Kane C et al. Ionic control of beta cell function in nesidioblastosis. A possible therapeutic role for calcium channel blockade. *Arch Dis Child* 1996; 74(5): 373–8.

16. Minute M, Patti G, Tornese G, Faleschini E, Zuiani C, Ventura A. Sirolimus therapy in congenital hyperinsulinism: A successful experience beyond infancy. *Pediatrics* 2015 November; 136(5): e1373–6.

17. Gough MH. The surgical treatment of hyperinsulinism in infancy and childhood. *Br J Surg* 1984; 71(1): 75–8.

18. Nihoul-Fekete C, de Lonlay P, Jaubert F et al. The surgical management of congenital hyperinsulinaemic hypoglycaemia in infancy. *J Paediatr Surg* 2004; 39(3); 267–9.

19. Adzick NS, Thornton PS, Stanley, Kaye RD, Ruchelli E. A multidisciplinary approach to the focal form of congenital hyperinsulinism leads to successful treatment by partial pancreatectomy. *J Paediatr Surg* 2004; 39(3): 270–5.

20. Bax KN, van der Zee DC. The laparoscopic approach toward hyperinsulinism in children. *Semin Pediatr Surg* 2007; 16: 245–51.

21. Al-Shanafey S. Laparoscopic vs open pancreatectomy for persistent hyperinsulinaemic hypoglycaemia of infancy. *J Pediatr Surg* 2009; 44(5): 957–61.

22. McAndrew HF, Smith V, Spitz L. Surgical complications of pancreatectomy for persistent hyperinsulinaemic hypoglycaemia of infancy. *J Paediatr Surg* 2003; 38(1): 13–6.

23. Meissner T, Brune W, Mayatepek E. Persistent hyperinsulinaemic hypoglycaemia of infancy: Therapy, clinical outcome and mutational analysis. *Eur J Paediatr* 1997; 156: 754–7.

24. Leibowitz G, Glaser B, Higazi AA et al. Hyperinsulinaemic hypoglycaemis of infancy (nesidioblastosis) in clinical remission: High incidence of diabetes mellitus and persistent beta-cell dysfunction at long term follow up. *J Clin Endocrinol Metab* 1995; 80: 386–92.

25. Hering BJ, Clarke WR, Bridges ND, Eggerman TL, Alejandro R, Bellin MD, Chaloner K, Czarniecki CW, Goldstein JS, Hunsicker LG, Kaufman DB, Korsgren O, Larsen CP, Luo X, Markmann JF, Naji A, Oberholzer J, Posselt AM, Rickels MR, Ricordi C, Robien MA, Senior PA, Shapiro AM, Stock PG, Turgeon NA. Phase 3 trial of transplantation of human islets in type 1 diabetes complicated by severe hypoglycemia. clinical islet transplantation consortium. *Diabetes Care* 2016; 39(7): 1230–40.

26. Beltrand J, Caquard M, Arnoux JB et al. Glucose metabolism in 105 children and adolescents after pancreatectomy for congenital hyperinsulinism. *Diabetes Care* 2012; 35: 198–203.

58

Jejunoileal atresia and stenosis

ALASTAIR J. W. MILLAR, ALP NUMANOGLU, AND SHARON COX

INTRODUCTION

Jejunoileal atresia, defined as a congenital defect in continuity of the small bowel, is a common cause of intestinal obstruction in the newborn.[1-3] The incidence of jejunoileal atresia varies between 1 in 1500 and 1 in 3000 live births.[4] Jejunoileal occlusions occur more frequently than duodenal or colonic atresias.[1,5] With improved neonatal and perioperative care, safe anesthesia, refined surgical techniques, and management of short bowel syndrome, a survival rate of greater than 90% can be expected in well-resourced centers. At the Red Cross War Memorial Children's Hospital in Cape Town during the 56 years from 1959 to 2015, 363 jejunoileal atresias, 275 (76%) jejunum and 88 (24%) ileum, were seen (Table 58.1). The mortality rate was initially high, and it was only in the mid-1950s that an improved understanding of the pathogenesis and pathology of the condition led to innovative surgical techniques, which resulted in greatly improved surgical outcome.[4-6]

ETIOLOGY

In 1889, Bland Sutton postulated that atresia occurred at the site of "obliterative embryological events," and he quoted atrophy of the vitelline duct.[7] In 1900, Tandler,[8] supported by embryonal studies, suggested that intestinal atresia was related to a lack of recanalization of the solid stage of the intestine, while others have questioned these theories.[9-11] In 1952, Louw[4] published the results of an investigation of 79 patients treated at Great Ormond Street, London, and suggested that jejunoileal atresia was probably due to a vascular accident rather than the result of inadequate recanalization. At his instigation, Barnard perfected the experimental model in pregnant mongrel bitches. Mesenteric vascular insults, such as volvulus, intussusception, and interference with the blood supply to a segment of bowel, were created in the dog fetus.[12] This not only confirmed the hypothesis but led to a change in the surgical procedure for correcting atresias and stenoses of the jejunum and ileum with

a marked improvement in outcome.[13-15] Subsequently, these experimental findings were confirmed by others in several different animal models and in clinical practice.[16-20] Evidence of bowel infarction was present in 42% of 449 cases of jejunoileal atresia in a collected series, which further supported the vascular hypothesis.[21] Furthermore, the localized nature of the vascular accident occurring late in fetal life would explain the low incidence (less than 10%) of coexisting abnormalities of extra-abdominal organs.

The family history may help to identify hereditary forms and conditions that may predispose to atresia, i.e., cystic fibrosis and anomalies of intestinal rotation. The anomaly is usually not genetically determined, although affected monozygotic twins and siblings have been described.[22] A genetic basis has been established for type IIIb and IV multiple atresias.[22-27] In this situation patients typically present as premature, low-birth-weight babies and have associated malrotation and other congenital abnormalities. Sporadic jejunoileal atresia is different from the familial multiple atresias of the whole gastrointestinal tract seen in severe immune deficiency syndrome, which is an autosomal recessive condition.[28] Down syndrome is most uncommon in babies with jejunoileal atresia compared with duodenal atresias.

A classification system for familial intestinal atresia has been proposed that suggests that most cases result from disruption of a normal embryologic pathway in the development of the superior mesenteric artery and its branches.[29]

EPIDEMIOLOGY

In a 16-year study of cases documented in 20 EUROCAT registers, cases with a normal karyotype had a prevalence of 0.7 per 10,000 live births for jejunoileal atresia.[30] This is much lower than reported rates in previous studies and different geographical locations.[4] Small intestinal atresia prevalence varies in different geographical areas, but there does not seem to be any significant trend in prevalence over time. There is

Table 58.1 Jejunal atresia and stenosis: Red Cross War Memorial Children's Hospital, experience from 1959 to December 2015

Type	Jejunum	Ileum	Total	Types as % of total	% Mortality related to type
Stenosis	22	14	36	10	0
Type I	68	18	86	24	5
Type II	22	14	36	10	11
Type IIIa	28	27	55	15	15
Type IIIb	68	1	69	19	17
Type IV	67	14	81	22	12
Total	275	88	363	100	10

Note: Last 25-year survival (1990–2015) was 92% (147/160).

weak evidence of an increased risk in mothers aged less than 20 years compared with mothers aged 20–29 years.[30]

PATHOLOGY

The classification of jejunoileal atresia into three types by Bland Sutton in 1889 has stood the test of time, except for the subdivision of type III into two categories (a and b) and the addition of type IV (Figure 58.1).[7,31,32] This subdivision has allowed a better long-term prognostication. In stenosis, the proximal dilated and narrower distal bowel are in continuity with an intact mesentery, but at the point of junction, there is a short, narrow, somewhat rigid segment with a narrow but patent lumen. The small intestine is of normal length (Figure 58.2).

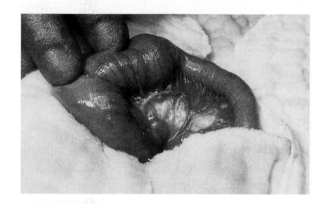

Figure 58.2 The clinical appearance of stenosis.

In atresia type I (membrane or web) (Figure 58.3a and b), the dilated proximal and collapsed bowel are in continuity, and the mesentery is intact. The intraluminal pressure in the proximal bowel produces bulging of the web into the distal intestine so that the transition from the distended to the collapsed bowel is conical in appearance—the "windsock" effect. The distal bowel is completely collapsed, and the small intestine is of normal length.

In atresia type II (blind ends joined by a fibrous band) (Figure 58.4a and b), the proximal bowel terminates in a bulbous blind end, which is grossly distended and hypertrophied for several centimeters and is often hypoperistaltic. The bowel proximal to this is usually also considerably distended and hypertrophied for a further 5–10 cm. More proximally, the bowel distension is less marked, and the bowel assumes a normal appearance. The distal collapsed bowel commences as a blind end, which is sometimes bulbous due to remains of a fetal intussusception. The two blind ends are joined by a thin fibrous band. The corresponding intestinal mesentery is normal but may occasionally be deficient, leaving a V-shaped gap. The small intestine is usually of normal length.

In atresia type IIIa (disconnected blind ends) (Figure 58.5a and b), the appearance is similar to that in type II, but the blind ends are completely separate. There is always a V-shaped gap in the mesentery, and the total bowel length is reduced.

In atresia type IIIb ("apple-peel,"[17] "Christmas tree,"[33] or "Maypole"[5] deformity), as in IIIa, the blind ends are disconnected, and the mesenteric defect is substantial

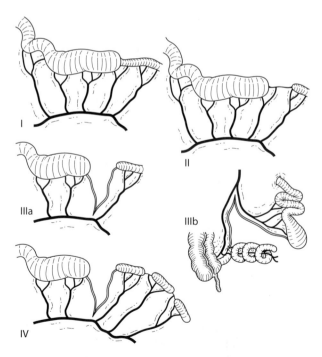

Figure 58.1 The different types of small bowel atresia according to the modified classification by Grosfeld. (From Grosfeld JL et al., Operative management of intestinal atresia and stenosis based on pathologic findings, J Pediatr Surg 1979;14(3):368–75.)

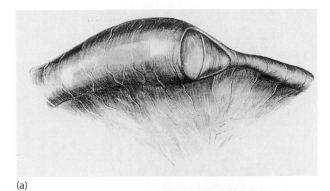

(a)

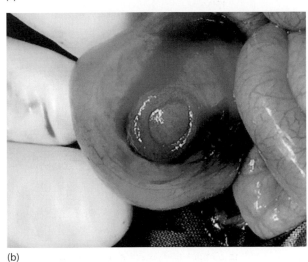

(b)

Figure 58.3 **(a)** Atresia type I. Obstruction caused by an intrinsic membrane. The proximal bowel is dilated and the distal collapsed, with intact mesentery. **(b)** Operative photograph taken from the proximal side of a type I atresia, with the bowel opened, exposing the mucosa-lined centrally placed web.

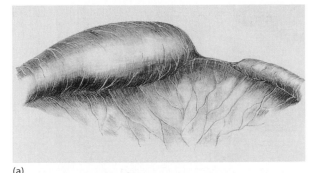

(a)

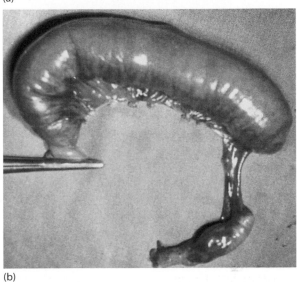

(b)

Figure 58.4 **(a)** Diagram of atresia type II. Blind ends joined by a band with an intact mesentery and normal length of bowel. **(b)** Operative photograph of a resected specimen of proximal dilated loop, band of mesentery, and 3 cm of distal collapsed bowel.

(Figure 58.6a, b, and c). This type is the consequence of an extensive infarction of the midgut secondary to a superior mesenteric artery occlusion just distal to the middle colic origin, producing a proximal jejunal atresia with loss of a varying segment of jejunum. The distal ileum remains viable, receiving an often precarious blood supply from the arterial supply to the right colon, around which the ileum is coiled. Occasionally, additional type I or type II atresias are found along the coiled length of bowel toward the distal blind end. There is always a significant reduction in intestinal length. These babies are usually born prematurely and of low birth weight. In addition, they may have associated bowel anomalies such as malrotation and may develop short bowel syndrome with increased morbidity and mortality.[21] A familial incidence has been reported by some authors.[22,34]

In atresia type IV, multiple atresias are present, which could be a combination of types I–III and often have the appearance of a string of sausages (Figure 58.7a and b). The bowel length is usually reduced. The site of the most proximal atresia determines whether it is classified as jejunal or ileal atresia.

In all types, the intestine proximal to the obstruction becomes dilated and hypertrophied. This dilated bowel frequently has a cyanosed appearance and may have some necrotic areas from either sustained intraluminal pressure or secondary volvulus. Perforation may develop antenatally, leading to meconium peritonitis, or may occur as a postnatal event, especially if diagnosis is delayed.

The peristaltic movements in the proximal segment are subnormal and ineffective, and histologic and histochemical abnormalities can be observed up to 20 cm cephalad to the atretic segment.[35,36] Recent histological and immunohistochemical studies have revealed changes in morphology and density of the enteric nervous system and interstitial cells of Cajal in the bowel both proximal and distal to the atresia.[37] In addition, pathological deterioration of the myenteric ganglia, nerve growth factor, and interstitial cells of Cajal occurs for up to 15 cm proximal and 3 cm distal to the atresia, and these changes may cause intestinal motility problems after surgical repair.[38] Macroscopically, the distal bowel is unused and wormlike in appearance but potentially normal in length and function.

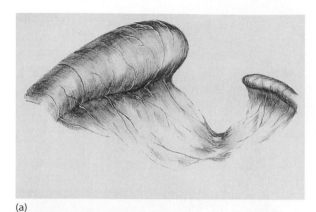

(a)

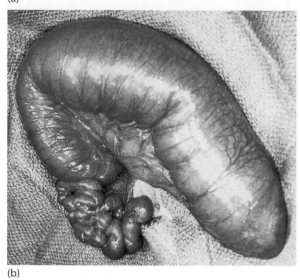

(b)

Figure 58.5 (**a** and **b**) Atresia type IIIa. Blind ends disconnected with a V-shaped defect in the mesentery. The bowel length is reduced. The grossly dilated obstructed bowel tapers proximally into intestine of normal calibre. The distal collapsed bowel illustrates how difficult it may be to assess the length of this segment.

PRENATAL DIAGNOSIS

A prenatal history of polyhydramnios is frequent. Up to 38% of patients with proximal jejunal atresia display polyhydramnios, which is less frequent in more distal cases. Many babies with intestinal atresia are diagnosed by ultrasound investigation of the fetus, which shows a dilated, echogenic, and thickened bowel loop with increased peristalsis. The distal bowel is decompressed.[39] Unfortunately, ultrasonic prenatal diagnosis has a relatively poor predictive value especially in early gestational age, and in addition, the detection is highly variable, ranging from 10% to 100%, with an overall prediction of 51% in a recent meta-analysis, jejunal atresias being detected more often than ileal atresias.[40] The use of fetal MRI scanning is increasing and may be more valuable in the prenatal diagnosis of bowel atresia.[41]

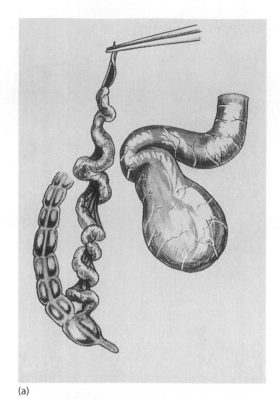

(a)

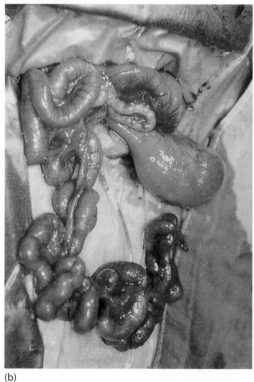

(b)

Figure 58.6 (**a** and **b**) Atresia type IIIb with a gross mesenteric defect and the coiled distal ileum with precarious collateral blood supply, producing the typical "apple-peel" appearance. Note the precarious blood supply of the terminal portion of the distal bowel and the grossly dilated proximal jejunum. There is always significant reduction in intestinal length. *(Continued)*

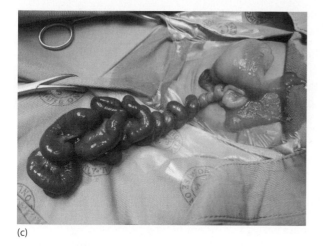

Figure 58.6 (Continued) **(c)** Type IIIb jejunal atresia with necrotic bowel at the time of initial exploration. The resulting viable bowel length may be incompatible with eventual enteral autonomy, but long-term survival may be achieved provided there is a short segment of viable terminal ileum and an intact ileocecal valve remaining.

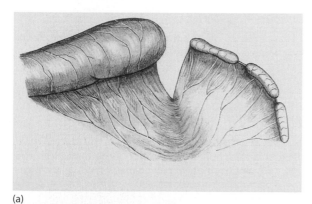

(a)

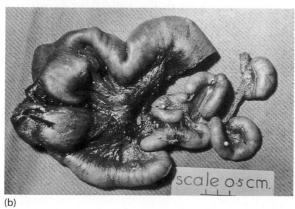

(b)

Figure 58.7 **(a)** Type IV atresia. **(b)** Operative photograph shows multiple atresias with a typical "string of sausages." The bowel length is usually reduced.

CLINICAL FEATURES

Atresia or severe stenosis of the small intestine presents clinically as neonatal intestinal obstruction with persistent bile-stained vomiting dated from the first or second day of life. In general, the higher the level of obstruction, the earlier and more forceful the vomiting, whereas in low intestinal obstruction, the vomiting may be delayed. Abdominal distension is frequently present, more so with the distal ileal intestinal atresias, where the distension is generalized, compared with the more proximal jejunal atresias, where it is confined to the upper abdomen and is relieved by nasogastric tube aspiration. In delayed diagnosis or where perforation has occurred, the distension may be severe and associated with respiratory distress. Constipation is usually not absolute, and the meconium passed varies from normal in color to the more common grey plugs of mucus. Occasionally, if ischemic bowel is present, as in type IIIb atresia, blood may be passed rectally.

Diseases that can mimic jejunoileal atresia include midgut volvulus, meconium ileus, duplication cysts, internal hernia, ileus due to sepsis, birth trauma, prematurity, and transplacental crossing of maternal medication.

Erect and supine abdominal radiographs will reveal distended small bowel loops and air–fluid levels (Figure 58.8a). The lower the obstruction, the greater the distended loops of bowel and the more fluid levels will be observed. A single large loop of bowel and air–fluid level would indicate atresia rather than other causes of neonatal intestinal obstruction. A prone lateral view is useful to distinguish between low small bowel and colonic obstruction. In some instances, the first abdominal radiograph may reveal a completely opaque abdomen due to a fluid-filled obstructed bowel. Emptying of the stomach by means of a nasogastric tube and injection of air will demonstrate the level of the obstruction. With intestinal stenosis, the calibre of the proximal obstructed intestine is greater than that of the distal gut, but because the obstruction is incomplete, the diagnosis is often delayed. When the abdominal radiograph suggests a complete obstruction, a contrast enema may be performed to exclude colonic atresia, distinguish between small and large bowel distension, determine whether the colon has the typical microcolon appearance, and locate the position of the cecum as an indication of malrotation. It also makes saline injection of the colon at surgery unnecessary, a sometimes tedious maneuver.

The classical appearance of the colon distal to jejunoileal atresia is that of an unused colon or microcolon (Figure 58.8b). When an incomplete small bowel obstruction is diagnosed, an upper gastrointestinal contrast study is indicated to demonstrate the site and nature of the obstruction. Malrotation may also be observed in 10%–30% of babies with jejunoileal atresia. Occasionally, dystrophic intraperitoneal calcification of meconium peritonitis may be seen on plain radiograph, signifying intrauterine bowel perforation. If the atresia has formed late in intrauterine life, the bowel distal to the atresia may assume the calibre of a used colon.

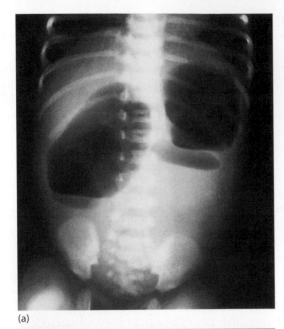

(a)

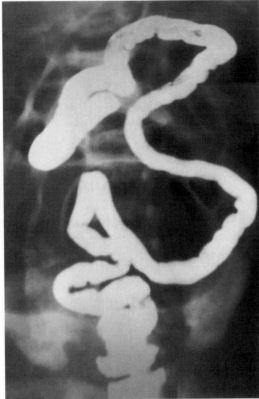

(b)

Figure 58.8 **(a)** Erect abdominal radiograph of a newborn infant showing obstructed upper small bowel loops with fluid levels. No air is visible in the distal bowel. **(b)** Contrast enema showing the unused or microcolon distal to a jejuno-ileal atresia. In addition, evidence of malrotation is present.

GUIDELINES FOR MANAGEMENT

The guidelines for management of jejunoileal atresia are as summarized in Table 58.2.

Table 58.2 Guidelines for management of jejunoileal atresia

Prenatal	Polyhydramnios, affected family: ultrasonography, MRI
Preoperative management	Gastric decompression
	Fluid management: maintenance and replacement
	Correction of electrolyte abnormalities
	Radiology: Abdominal radiograph, contrast enema
	Correction of hematological and biochemical abnormalities
	Prophylactic antibiotics
Operative management	Identify type of atresia
	Bulbous component: resect, taper, or plicate if short residual length
	Derotate and taper if high jejunal atresia
	Preserve maximal distal bowel length—measure residual bowel
	Establish patency of distal bowel with saline injection
	End-to-end single-layer interrupted anastomosis
Postoperative Management	Gastrointestinal decompression
	Antibiotics
	Parenteral nutrition
	Early graduated enteral feeds: breast, special, or polymeric feeds
	Surveillance for gastrointestinal dysfunction
Special problems	Anastomotic dysfunction
	Short bowel syndrome
	Associated congenital abnormalities

Source: Adapted from Haller JA Jr. et al., Intestinal atresia. Current concepts of pathogenesis, pathophysiology, and operative management, *Am Surg* 1983;49(7):385–91.

TREATMENT

The newborn baby tolerates operative intervention all the better after a few hours of preoperative preparation, especially if the diagnosis has been delayed. In general, this preparation should pay particular attention to hypothermia, hypoxia, hypovolemia, hypoglycemia, and hypoprothrombinemia. The operation should not be delayed unduly as there is always a danger of further infarction of the bowel, fluid and electrolyte disturbances, and increased risk of infection. In neglected cases with dehydration, more energetic therapy is required.

Sterilization of skin and draping

The use of a neonate-compatible heating mat under the baby or warm air heater is advised. The umbilical cord is cleansed with 70% alcohol and is ligated and transected at the level of the abdominal wall. The operative field is sterilized with prewarmed povidone–iodine 2% in 70% alcohol. Sterile warm Gamgee rolls or swabs are placed alongside the baby, who is then draped with towels or disposable adherent drapes. A sterile transparent adhesive drape is applied over the operative field to ensure that he/she remains dry during the operative procedure, thus preventing heat loss. Another way of keeping the neonate dry is to place adherent plastic drapes around the operative field prior to skin preparation.

Incision

An adequate incision is required. Exposure is obtained through a supraumbilical transverse incision transecting the rectus muscles 2–3 cm above the umbilicus. The ligamentum teres is subsequently divided and ligated. Alternatively, a small circumumbilical incision may be adequate.[43,44] The circumumbilical incision combines the advantages of an open approach and an abdominal scar which is aesthetically pleasing on healing.[45]

Laparoscopy has been used as an exploratory maneuver in diagnosis with exteriorization of the atretic ends of the bowel through the umbilical port site for primary anastomosis.[46,47]

Exploration

If free gas escapes on opening the peritoneum, or if there is contamination of the peritoneal cavity, a pus swab is obtained for Gram stain and culture, and the site of the perforation is sought and closed before further exploration is carried out. In the presence of peritoneal contamination, the cavity is irrigated with warm saline. The entire bowel is exteriorized to determine the site and type of obstruction and to exclude other areas of atresia or stenosis and associated lesions such as incomplete intestinal rotation or meconium ileus. The appearance of the atretic segment depends upon the type of occlusion, but in all cases, the maximal dilatation of the proximal bowel occurs at the point of obstruction; this segment is often hypoperistaltic and of questionable viability (Figure 58.9), while the bowel distal to the obstruction is collapsed, tiny, and wormlike (Figures 58.5 and 58.6).

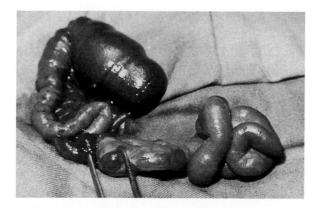

Figure 58.9 The proximal atretic bowel is grossly dilated, hypoperistaltic, and of questionable viability.

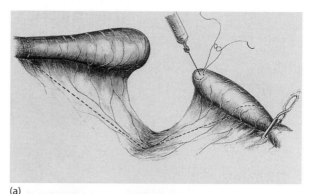

(a)

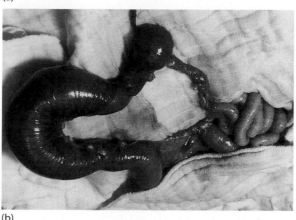

(b)

Figure 58.10 **(a)** The distal bowel is distended with saline injection proximal to the bowel clamp. The extent of the resection is indicated by the dotted lines. **(b)** The extent of resection in the clinical situation is depicted. Note that all grossly dilated bowel is to be resected.

After the location and type of lesion have been identified, the distal bowel is carefully examined to exclude other atretic segments, which are present in 10%–20% of cases. Saline is instilled into the lumen of the distal bowel to confirm patency. Malrotation is corrected if present. The total length of the small bowel is measured as this has prognostic significance and may determine the method of reconstruction. The normal length of the small bowel at full-term birth is approximately 250 cm.

After complete patency of the distal small bowel and colon has been established, the next task is to suture the disproportionate proximal and distal blind ends. This is facilitated by applying an atraumatic bowel clamp about 6–8 cm from the distal blind end and distending the intervening segment by injection with half-normal saline, taking care not to split the serosa (Figure 58.10a).

Resection

The atretic area and adjacent distended and collapsed bowel are isolated by walling off the rest of the abdominal cavity with moist packs. To ensure adequate postoperative function, the proximal distended and hypertrophied bowel should be liberally resected, even if it appears viable. If the bowel length is adequate (more than 75 cm plus ileocecal valve), the bulbous

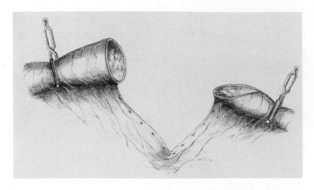

Figure 58.11 The proximal bowel has been transected at right angles and the distal obliquely with continuation of the incision along the antimesenteric border to create a "fish mouth."

hypertrophied bowel proximal to the atresia is resected to approximately normal bowel diameter; usually, a 10–15 cm section is removed. After milking the intestinal contents into the proximal bulbous end, an atraumatic bowel clamp is applied across the bowel a few centimeters proximal to the site selected for transection. The mesentery adjoining the portion to be resected is divided using bipolar diathermy or ligated up to the proposed lines of section of proximal and distal bowel (Figure 58.10a and b). The blood supply at this point should be excellent, and therefore, the bowel is divided at right angles, leaving an opening of about 1.5 cm in width. Two to three centimeters of the distal bowel is also removed. This bowel may be transected slightly obliquely, and an incision may be continued along the antimesenteric border to create a "fish mouth," which renders the opening about equal to that of the proximal bowel (Figure 58.11). Alternatively, the bowel can be transected at right angles if an end-to-end anastomosis is planned. In patients with a relatively short segment of severely dilated proximal intestine, derotation of the proximal segment, resection to the distal second part of duodenum, and establishment of continuity by end-to-end anastomosis with tapering of the duodenum is a good option. However, in patients with long segments of proximal intestine that are significantly dilated, resection of the whole involved segment may result in inadequate remaining intestinal length to allow absorption of enteric nutrients (i.e., short bowel syndrome). Therefore, these patients frequently are treated by either imbrication or tapering enteroplasty of the proximal dilated segment. In a few cases with extensive congenital short bowel, primary serial transverse enteroplasty procedure (STEP) has been attempted.[48]

Anastomosis

An inverting mattress of 5-0 or 6-0 polydioxanone sutures unites the mesenteric borders of the divided ends, and temporary stay sutures are inserted at the antimesenteric angles to facilitate accurate approximation. The *posterior* edges of the bowel are united with interrupted through-and-through 5-0 or 6-0 polydioxanone sutures tied on the mucosal aspect (Figure 58.12a). The *anterior* edges are joined by similar through-and-through sutures tied on the serosal surface (Figure 58.12b). The completed anastomosis is not strictly end to end but a modification of Denis Browne's "end-to-back" method. An alternative suture technique includes extramucosal anastomosis and the use of 5-0 or 6-0 monofilament absorbable sutures and end-to-end sutures taking larger bites on the proximal bowel. Where there is a discrepancy of less than 4:1 between the proximal and distal bowel lumens, an end-to-end extramucosal anastomosis is advised as there is thought to be an earlier return of normal peristalsis. The suture line is tested for leakage, and reinforcing sutures are inserted as required. The defect in the mesentery is repaired by approximating (and overlapping if necessary) the divided edges with interrupted sutures (Figure 58.12a and b). The intestines are returned to the peritoneal cavity. During this procedure, if the mesentery is kept in the configuration of an open fan (Figure 58.13a and b), kinking or volvulus of the bowel should be avoided.

A similar technique is used for stenosis and intraluminal membranes. Procedures such as transverse enteroplasties, excision of membranes, and bypassing techniques are not

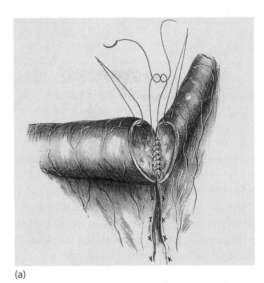

(a)

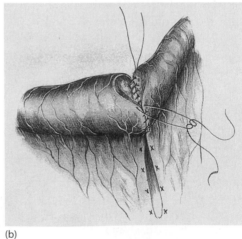

(b)

Figure 58.12 (a) Anastomosis of the posterior wall with interrupted sutures. **(b)** The anterior anastomosis.

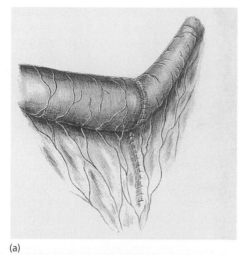

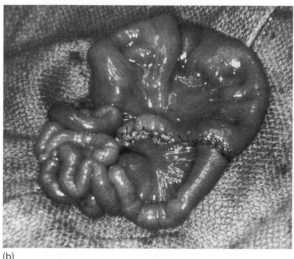

(a)

(b)

Figure 58.13 **(a)** Completed anastomosis and repair of mesenteric defect. **(b)** The clinical appearance of completed anastomosis.

recommended, because they fail to remove the abnormal segment of bowel; side-to-side anastomosis is avoided due to the risk of creating blind loops.

Gastrostomy/enteral decompression and early enteral feeding

It was customary in babies with high jejunal atresias just beyond the duodenojejunal flexure to place a transanastomotic feeding tube for early enteral feeding when parenteral feeding techniques were less sophisticated. The tube was passed into the small bowel distal to the anastomosis before completing the anterior layer of sutures and stabilized at the anastomotic site by a single tethering mucosal stitch, in order to prevent its retrograde displacement into the stomach. The transanastomotic tube was passed either via the nasogastric route or via a Stamm gastrostomy performed on the anterior wall of the stomach. More recently, the value of such transanastomotic tubes for feeding has

been questioned, and the authors have abandoned routine use of these for high jejunal and duodenal atresias.[49] Placement of a transluminal Silastic tube is, however, a useful maneuver in multiple atresias to align the atretic segments at the time of anastomosis and to provide a transluminal stent in the postoperative period. The tube can be exited via the cecum or through the colon and out the anus.[50] Nutrition is provided by the parenteral route until full enteral feeds are established.

Closure of abdominal wound

Where there has been soiling of the peritoneal cavity from a perforation, the abdominal cavity is again irrigated with saline and all macroscopic debris removed.

The abdominal wound is closed with a single continuous layer of polydioxanone 3-0 or 4-0 sutures to include all layers of the abdominal wall, excluding skin. In fat babies, the adipose layer is approximated with interrupted or continuous 4-0 absorbable sutures. The skin is approximated with continuous subcuticular 5-0 monofilament sutures.

Other surgical maneuvers

In babies in whom the initial insult has resulted in atresias with a markedly reduced length of small intestine or when large resections of multiple atretic segments are required, certain surgical techniques have been advocated in an attempt to preserve maximal intestinal length for survival and growth.[51,52] In addition, disparity in anastomotic size is reduced, and prograde duodenal function is facilitated. In high jejunal atresias, the duodenum is fully derotated and the proximal resection extended into the second part of the duodenum with antimesenteric tapering duodenoplasty or inversion plication of the proximal megaduodenum (Figures 58.14 and 58.15).[53,54] The dilated bowel is trimmed to a lumen size of a 22-French gauge catheter. An intestinal autostapling instrument may be used. Inversion plication without excision and tapering has the advantage of preserving valuable mucosa if the bowel length is short. Tapering may have an advantage over plication, as the latter has the tendency to unravel within a few months with subsequent peristaltic dysfunction, especially if the mucosal strip/excision technique has not been utilized. Following this tailoring, the anastomosis is performed as described earlier, and the bowel is returned to the abdomen in the position of nonrotation. In type IIIb, any restricting bands along the free edge of the distal narrow mesentery are released to avoid kinking and interference with the blood supply. The mesentery from any resected bowel is retained and may assist in closure of mesenteric defects. This technique is very helpful and prevents kinking or distortion of the anastomosis. Furthermore, the potential for kinking the single marginal artery and vein requires careful placement of the bowel into the peritoneal cavity at the completion of the anastomosis.

Although isolated type I atresias are best dealt with by primary resection and anastomosis, multiple diaphragms have successfully been perforated and dilated with bougies

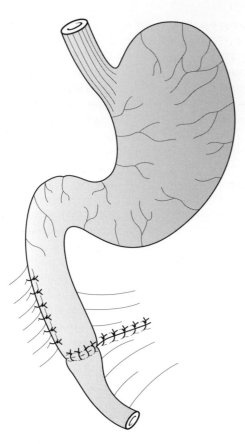

Figure 58.14 The surgical procedure for high jejunal atresia includes: derotation of the bowel, back resection into the second part of the duodenum, tapering duodenoplasty, or linear seromuscular stripping and inversion plication followed by bowel anastomosis.

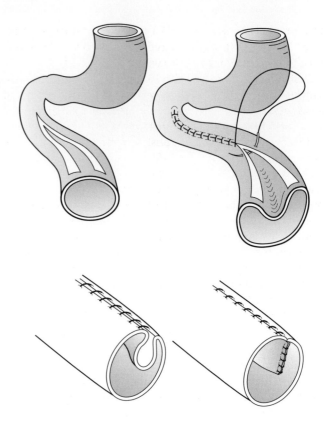

Figure 58.15 The technique of seromuscular stripping and inversion plication. This technique preserves mucosal surface for absorption and prevents unraveling of the placation.

passed along the length of the bowel. In multiple atresias, multiple resections and anastomosis may be advisable to save as much bowel length as possible. They are, however, often localized, requiring resection of all together and a single anastomosis. As mentioned previously, a Silastic tube passed through the lumen of the entire bowel facilitates these anastomotic procedures.[55]

The fashioning of stomas, e.g., Bishop–Koop,[56] Santulli and Blanc,[17] Rehbein,[57] or double barrel,[58] as practiced by some, is not routinely advocated unless there is gross intraperitoneal contamination, making a primary anastomosis unsafe. Jejunoileal atresia associated with a gastroschisis is treated by resection and primary anastomosis only if there is no evidence of edema and matting due to amniotic peritonitis. Initial reduction of the eviscerated bowel with the atresia intact and primary closure of the abdominal wall defect, if possible, is preferred. After allowing for disappearance of the edema (10–14 days), a second laparotomy is performed with resection of the atretic segment and primary anastomosis. Stomas with the potential for fluid and electrolyte loss, wound infection, and other stoma-related complications are thus avoided. There is little place for bowel lengthening procedures at the initial operation. It is advisable to delay such procedures until the neonatal bowel

has grown to its maximum potential length and maximum bowel adaptation has occurred.

POSTOPERATIVE CARE

Postoperative care is conducted according to current standards and guidelines. Nasogastric decompression is usually required until proximal gut prograde peristalsis has recovered. High jejunal atresias may require a long period of decompression. Feeding is delayed until the gastric aspirate is no longer bile stained, the abdomen is not distended, and the baby has passed meconium. In babies with a transanastomotic tube, continuous feeding is commenced 24 hours postoperatively. Graduated polymeric feeds are then commenced and increased as tolerated. Oral or gavage feeds are started with return of prograde proximal bowel function.

If at any time, there is a suspicion of a leak at the anastomosis, as suggested by clinical deterioration, abdominal distension, and vomiting, a plain radiograph of the abdomen may reveal free air in the abdomen. When more than 24 hours have elapsed since surgery, this would indicate a leak or perforation, and immediate laparotomy should be performed. Other postoperative complications observed have been ischemia leading to frank necrosis, late-onset stenosis, adhesive obstruction, and perforation of the bowel by the transanastomotic tube. Infants with human immunodeficiency virus (HIV) exposure or infection have poor healing with an increased incidence of anastomotic breakdown and wound sepsis with dehiscence.[59]

In babies in whom less than 75 cm of small bowel remains, especially if the ileocecal valve is absent, loose frequent stools and excessive water loss may become problematic. In these patients, and in every instance where normal enteral alimentation cannot be established within 5 postoperative days, parenteral feeding is indicated. Solutions containing carbohydrate, amino acid, and fat are introduced in a graduated manner over a period of 3 days. Peripheral venous push-in lines are used for short-term total parenteral nutrition (TPN), but for long-term TPN (longer than 10 days), a central Broviac® line is preferred. Once intestinal function has been reestablished, the baby is gradually weaned from a parenteral to an enteral feeding program. Careful dietary tailoring is required, as each of the patients may have different tolerance thresholds.

Predictions of the degree of intestinal dysfunction are based upon the known residual length of small intestine. Short bowel syndrome can be contemplated if more than 70% of the bowel length was lost or if the minimal bowel length left after surgery is less than 70 cm. These babies can be divided into four main functional groups: (1) those with uncorrectable intestinal insufficiency; (2) those with adequate bowel function for survival after adaptation and/ or lengthening and tailoring procedures; (3) those with adequate alimentary function for growth and development; and (4) those with normal alimentary function with a degree of intestinal reserve.

When gross intestinal insufficiency is expected, the infant is managed as short bowel syndrome.[60-62] The patient's oral intake is gradually increased in volume and energy content, while the small intestine is allowed to adapt until maximum intake tolerance is reached, which can take months to years.[63] Pharmacological control of intestinal peristaltic activity has been achieved more effectively since the introduction of loperamide hydrochloride. Vitamin B_{12} and folic acid should be administered to patients without the terminal ileum to prevent megaloblastic anemia. The long-term outcome for most of the babies is optimistic. TPN-associated complications are becoming less frequent, and parenteral nutrition (PN)-associated liver disease can be avoided in most cases, making liver and intestinal transplantation unnecessary.[64]

OUTCOMES

The first successful surgical repair of an intestinal atresia was in 1911.[6] Before 1952, the mortality rate for congenital atresias of the small intestine in Cape Town and in most other centers around the world was 90%. Between 1952 and 1955, 28% of the babies with this condition could be saved. At that stage most were treated by primary anastomosis without resection. With liberal resection of the blind ends and primary end-to-end anastomosis, the survival rate increased to 78% during 1955–58.[65,66]

Improved perioperative care and management of short bowel syndrome, both medical and surgical, has resulted in survival of nearly all cases, except those born with an ultrashort bowel incompatible with enteral autonomy (Figure 58.6c). Most patients with jejunoileal atresias have an excellent prognosis and long-term survival. Those with types III and IV atresias and resultant short bowel syndrome have more feeding problems and a higher morbidity. This increase in survival has come at the cost of a higher percentage of late complications in the surviving children.[67-69]

Associated anomalies may adversely affect outcomes. In predicting the ultimate functional outcome, the following factors must be taken into consideration: the ileum adapts to a greater degree than the jejunum, the neonatal small intestine still has a period of maturation and growth ahead of it, and the actual residual small intestinal length is difficult to determine accurately after birth particularly if the infant is born premature. The proximal obstructed bowel segment is dilated, and its functional potential may be overestimated, while that of the distal unused collapsed bowel may be underestimated. Of critical importance is an intact ileocecal valve, which allows for accelerated intestinal adaptation with shorter residual jejunoileal length. The absence of the ileocecal valve also leads to an increased intestinal content transit time, malabsorption, diarrhea, and increased bacterial contamination of the small bowel.

During the 25-year period from 1990 to 2015, 160 patients with jejunoileal atresias and stenoses were admitted to the pediatric surgical service at the Red Cross War Memorial Children's Hospital. There were 13 deaths (92% survival). Factors contributing to the mortality rate were as follows: type of atresia (type III, 32%), proximal bowel infarction with peritonitis, anastomotic leak with a missed distal atresia, atresia associated with gastroschisis, ultrashort bowel syndrome with PN-associated liver disease, sepsis, and more recently, HIV infections. Overall experience is recorded in Table 58.1.

REFERENCES

1. Grosfeld JL, Ballantine TV, Shoemaker R. Operative management of intestinal atresia and stenosis based on pathologic findings. *J Pediatr Surg* 1979; 14(3): 368–75.
2. Evans CH. Atresias of the gastrointestinal tract. *Int Abstr Surg* 1951; 92(1): 1–8.
3. Cywes S, Davies MR, Rode H. Congenital jejuno-ileal atresia and stenosis. *S Afr Med J* 1980; 57(16): 630–9.
4. Louw JH. Congenital intestinal atresia and severe stenosis in the newborn; a report on 79 consecutive cases. *S Afr J Clin Sci* 1952; 3(3): 109–29.
5. Nixon HH, Tawes R. Etiology and treatment of small intestinal atresia: Analysis of a series of 127 jejunoileal atresias and comparison with 62 duodenal atresias. *Surgery* 1971; 69(1): 41–51.
6. Fockens P. Operativ geheilter Fall von kongenitaler Dünndarmatresie. *Zentralbl Chir* 1911; 38: 532.

7. Bland-Sutton J. Imperforate ileum. *Am J Med Sci* 1889; 18: 457.

8. Tandler J. Zur Entwicklungsgeschicte des menschlichen duodenum in fruhen Embryonalstadien. *Morphol Jahrb* 1900; 29: 187.

9. Moutsouris C. The "solid stage" and congenital intestinal atresia. *J Pediatr Surg* 1966; 1(5): 446–50.

10. Lynn HB, Espinas EE. Intestinal atresia: An attempt to relate location to embryologic processes. *Arch Surg* 1959; 79: 357–61.

11. Davis DL. Congenital occlusions of the intestine. *SGO* 1922; 34: 35.

12. Louw JH, Barnard CN. Congenital intestinal atresia; observations on its origin. *Lancet* 1955; 269(6899): 1065–7.

13. Louw JH. Congenital atresia and stenosis of the small intestine. The case for resection and primary end-to-end anastomosis. *S Afr J Surg* 1966; 4(2): 57–64.

14. Lloyd DA. J.H. Louw Memorial Lecture. From puppy dogs to molecules: Small-bowel atresia and short-gut syndrome. *S Afr J Surg* 1999; 37(3): 64–8.

15. Louw JH et al. Congenital jejuno-ileal atresia: Observations on its pathogenesis and treatment. *Z Kinderchir* 1981; 33(1): 3–17.

16. Tibboel D, Molenaar JC, Van Nie CJ. New perspectives in fetal surgery: The chicken embryo. *J Pediatr Surg* 1979; 14(4): 438–40.

17. Santulli TV, Blanc WA. Congenital atresia of the intestine: Pathogenesis and treatment. *Ann Surg* 1961; 154: 939–48.

18. Nguyen DT et al. In-utero intussusception producing ileal atresia and meconium peritonitis with and without free-air—Report of 2 cases and review of the literature. *Pediatr Surg Int* 1995; 10(5–6): 406–8.

19. Koga Y et al. Intestinal atresia in fetal dogs produced by localized ligation of mesenteric vessels. *J Pediatr Surg* 1975; 10(6): 949–53.

20. Abrams JS. Experimental intestinal atresia. *Surgery* 1968; 64(1): 185–91.

21. DeLorimier AA, Fonkalsrud EW, Hays DM. Congenital atresia and stenosis of the jejunum and ileum. *Surgery* 1969; 65(5): 819–27.

22. Mishalany HG, Najjar FB. Familial jejunal atresia: Three cases in one family. *J Pediatr* 1968; 73(5): 753–5.

23. Puri P, Fujimoto T. New observations on the pathogenesis of multiple intestinal atresias. *J Pediatr Surg* 1988; 23(3): 221–5.

24. Notarangelo LD. Multiple intestinal atresia with combined immune deficiency. *Curr Opin Pediatr* 2014; 26(6): 690–6.

25. Lambrecht W, Kluth D. Hereditary multiple atresias of the gastrointestinal tract: Report of a case and review of the literature. *J Pediatr Surg* 1998; 33(5): 794–7.

26. Kimble RM, Harding JE, Kolbe A. Jejunoileal atresia—An inherited condition. *Pediatr Surg Int* 1995; 10(5–6): 400–3.

27. Guttman FM et al. Multiple atresias and a new syndrome of hereditary multiple atresias involving gastrointestinal tract from stomach to rectum. *J Pediatr Surg* 1973; 8(5): 633–40.

28. Cole C et al. Hereditary multiple intestinal atresias: 2 new cases and review of the literature. *J Pediatr Surg* 2010; 45(4): E21–4.

29. Shorter NA et al. A proposed classification system for familial intestinal atresia and its relevance to the understanding of the etiology of jejunoileal atresia. *J Pediatr Surg* 2006; 41(11): 1822–5.

30. Best KE et al. Epidemiology of small intestinal atresia in Europe: A register-based study. *Arch Dis Child Fetal Neonatal Ed* 2012; 97(5): F353–8.

31. Touloukian RJ. Intestinal atresia. *Clin Perinatol* 1978; 5(1): 3–18.

32. Martin LW, Zerella JT. Jejunoileal atresia—Proposed classification. *J Pediatr Surg* 1976; 11(3): 399–403.

33. Weitzman JJ, Vanderhoof RS. Jejunal atresia with agenesis of the dorsal mesentery. With "Christmas tree" deformity of the small intestine. *Am J Surg* 1966; 111(3): 443–9.

34. Blyth H, Dickson JA. Apple peel syndrome (congenital intestinal atresia): A family study of seven index patients. *J Med Genet* 1969; 6(3): 275–7.

35. Masumoto K et al. Abnormalities of enteric neurons, intestinal pacemaker cells, and smooth muscle in human intestinal atresia. *J Pediatr Surg* 1999; 34(10): 1463–8.

36. Doolin EJ, Ormsbee HS, Hill JL. Motility abnormality in intestinal atresia. *J Pediatr Surg* 1987; 22(4): 320–4.

37. Gfroerer S et al. Differential changes in intrinsic innervation and interstitial cells of Cajal in small bowel atresia in newborns. *World J Gastroenterol* 2010; 16(45): 5716–21.

38. Wang X et al. The clinical significance of pathological studies of congenital intestinal atresia. *J Pediatr Surg* 2013; 48(10): 2084–91.

39. Tam PK, Nicholls G. Implications of antenatal diagnosis of small-intestinal atresia in the 1990s. *Pediatr Surg Int* 1999; 15(7): 486–7.

40. Virgone C et al. Accuracy of prenatal ultrasound in detecting jejunal and ileal atresia: Systematic review and meta-analysis. *Ultrasound Obstet Gynecol*, 2015; 45(5): 523–9.

41. Veyrac C et al. MRI of fetal GI tract abnormalities. *Abdom Imaging* 2004; 29(4): 411–20.

42. Haller JA Jr et al. Intestinal atresia. Current concepts of pathogenesis, pathophysiology, and operative management. *Am Surg* 1983; 49(7): 385–91.

43. Tajiri T et al. Transumbilical approach for neonatal surgical diseases: Woundless operation. *Pediatr Surg Int* 2008; 24(10): 1123–6.

44. Banieghbal B, Beale PG. Minimal access approach to jejunal atresia. *J Pediatr Surg* 2007; 42(8): 1362–4.

45. Murphy FJ et al. Versatility of the circumumbilical incision in neonatal surgery. *Pediatr Surg Int* 2009; 25(2): 145–7.

46. Lima M et al. Evolution of the surgical management of bowel atresia in newborn: Laparoscopically assisted treatment. *Pediatr Med Chir* 2009; 31(5): 215–9.

47. Li B et al. [Application of laparoscopy in the diagnosis and treatment of neonates and infants with congenital intestinal atresia and stenosis]. *Zhonghua Wei Chang Wai Ke Za Zhi* 2014; 17(8): 816–9.

48. Wales PW, Dutta S. Serial transverse enteroplasty as primary therapy for neonates with proximal jejunal atresia. *J Pediatr Surg* 2005; 40(3): E31–4.

49. Squire R, Kiely E. Postoperative feeding in neonatal duodenal obstruction. In: *British Association of Paediatric Surgeons 38th Annual International Congress.* Budapest, Hungary, 1991.

50. Romao RL et al. Preserving bowel length with a transluminal stent in neonates with multiple intestinal anastomoses: A case series and review of the literature. *J Pediatr Surg* 2011; 46(7): 1368–72.

51. Thomas CG Jr. Jejunoplasty for the correction of jejunal atresia. *Surg Gynecol Obstet* 1969; 129(3): 545–6.

52. Millar AJW, Rode H, Cywes S. Intestinal atresia and stenosis. In: Ashcraft KW (ed). *Pediatric Surgery*, 3rd edition, WB Saunders, London 2000: 406–24.

53. Kling K et al. A novel technique for correction of intestinal atresia at the ligament of Treitz. *J Pediatr Surg* 2000; 35(2): 353–5; discussion 356.

54. Honzumi M, Okuda A, Suzuki H. Duodenal motility after tapering duodenoplasty for high jejunal and multiple intestinal atresia. *Pediatr Surg Int* 1993; 8(2): 116–8.

55. Chaet MS, Warner BW, Sheldon CA. Management of multiple jejunoileal atresias with an intraluminal SILASTIC stent. *J Pediatr Surg* 1994; 29(12): 1604–6.

56. Bishop HC, Koop CE. Management of meconium ileus; resection, Roux-en-Y anastomosis and ileostomy irrigation with pancreatic enzymes. *Ann Surg* 1957; 145(3): 410–4.

57. Rehbein F, Halsband H. The double tube technique for the treatment of meconium ileus and small bowel atresia. *J Pediatr Surg* 1968; 3: 723.

58. Rosenman JE, Kosloske AM. A reappraisal of the Mikulicz enterostomy in infants and children. *Surgery* 1982; 91(1): 34–7.

59. Karpelowsky JS et al. Outcomes of human immunodeficiency virus-infected and -exposed children undergoing surgery—A prospective study. *J Pediatr Surg* 2009; 44(4): 681–7.

60. Warner BW, Ziegler MM. Management of the short bowel syndrome in the pediatric population. *Pediatr Clin North Am* 1993; 40(6): 1335–50.

61. McMellen ME et al. Growth factors: Possible roles for clinical management of the short bowel syndrome. *Semin Pediatr Surg* 2010; 19(1): 35–43.

62. Collins JB et al. Short bowel syndrome. *Semin Pediatr Surg* 1995; 4(1): 60–72; discussion 72–3.

63. Goulet OJ et al., Neonatal short bowel syndrome. *J Pediatr* 1991; 119(1 Pt 1): 18–23.

64. Gupte GL et al. Current issues in the management of intestinal failure. *Arch Dis Child* 2006; 91(3): 259–64.

65. Smith GH, Glasson M. Intestinal atresia: Factors affecting survival. *Aust N Z J Surg* 1989; 59(2): 151–6.

66. Louw JH. Resection and end-to-end anastomosis in the management of atresia and stenosis of the small bowel. *Surgery* 1967; 62(5): 940–50.

67. Stollman TH et al. Decreased mortality but increased morbidity in neonates with jejunoileal atresia; a study of 114 cases over a 34-year period. *J Pediatr Surg* 2009; 44(1): 217–21.

68. Nusinovich Y, Revenis M, Torres C. Long-term outcomes for infants with intestinal atresia studied at Children's National Medical Center. *J Pediatr Gastroenterol Nutr* 2013; 57(3): 324–9.

69. Burjonrappa SC, Crete E, Bouchard S. Prognostic factors in jejuno-ileal atresia. *Pediatr Surg Int* 2009; 25(9): 795–8.

59

Colonic and rectal atresias

TOMAS WESTER

COLONIC ATRESIA

Introduction

Binninger was the first to describe colonic atresia in 1673.[1] The first survivor was reported in 1922, when Gaub[2] opened a diverting colostomy in a child with an atresia of the sigmoid colon. Potts[3] successfully performed a primary anastomosis in a neonate with an atresia of the transverse colon in 1947.

Atresia of the colon is a rare cause of bowel obstruction in the neonate. The incidence of colonic atresia in live births has been difficult to ascertain, but an incidence of approximately 1 in 20,000 live births has been considered to be realistic based on the experience in major pediatric surgical centers.[4] In the northwest of England, isolated colonic atresia has been reported to occur in 1 in 66,000 live births.[5] Other investigators have reported that colonic atresias account for 1.8%–10.5% of the total bowel atresias,[6,7] the incidence of which has been estimated to be 1 in 1500 to 1 in 20,000 live births.[1,8] Colonic stenosis is extremely rare.

Except for stenosis, three different types of intrinsic occlusion have been distinguished:[9,10]

1. Type I atresia or a membrane (Figure 59.1a)
2. Type II atresia with blind ends of bowel joined together by a cord-like remnant of bowel, with or without a gap in the mesentery (Figure 59.1b)
3. Type III atresia with separated blind ends of bowel and a gap in the mesentery (Figure 59.1c)

Furthermore, a hereditary form with multiple atresias of the gastrointestinal tract has been described, suggested to be of nonvascular origin.[11,12] Type III atresia appears to be the most common type proximal to the splenic flexure, whereas types I and II are more common in atresias distal to the splenic flexure.[13,14] In a literature review, it was reported that type III occurred in 60.4% of all cases.[15] Most series show an even distribution between atresias proximal and distal to the splenic flexure.[6,7,16,17]

Etiology

Colonic atresia is probably the result of intrauterine vascular insufficiency. The finding of bile, squamous epithelium, and hair in the bowel distal to the atresia supports the hypothesis that the vascular accident occurs late in development.[9] Several pathological conditions may result in compromised blood supply to the bowel, such as intussusception, volvulus, herniation, tight gastroschisis, and embolic or thrombotic events. It appears likely that focal resorption of the sterile gut occurs after ischemic necrosis. Animal experiments have been performed in which the blood supply was interrupted to different parts of the small intestine or colon, thus inducing various types of atresias. These experiments confirm the etiologic role of *in utero* vascular occlusion.[9,18,19]

Colonic atresia has been reported in monozygotic twins.[20] Benawra et al.[21] reported three cases occurring in first-degree relatives of a family. Fairbanks et al.[22] have shown that absence of fibroblast growth factor 10 (*Fgf10*) or its receptor fibroblast growth factor receptor 2b (*Fgfr2b*) results in colonic atresia in a mouse model, despite normal mesenteric vascular development. These findings suggest that genetic factors may play a role in the pathogenesis of colonic atresia.

Presentation

Neonates with colonic atresia present with symptoms of distal bowel obstruction. Abdominal distension is usually present at birth, but otherwise develops over the first 24–48 hours of life. Bile-stained vomiting is very common, but is not always an early symptom. Failure to pass meconium is the rule, and neonates that do not pass meconium within the first 24 hours of life should be considered for further investigations. On examination, the abdomen is distended and often slightly tender, sometimes with visible bowel loops. In those who have an abdominal wall defect, associated atresias should always be suspected.

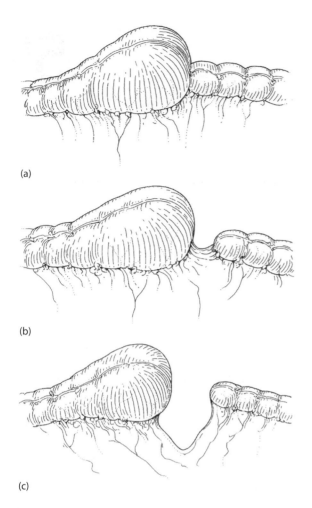

(a)

(b)

(c)

Figure 59.1 **(a)** Type 1: there is continuity of the outer layers of the bowel wall; the lumen is obstructed by a membrane covered with two layers of mucosa. **(b)** Type II: the bowel ends are connected by a fibrous band and the mesentery is intact. **(c)** Type III: a defect in the mesentery is accompanied by a gap between the bowel ends. (Reprinted from Wester T. Colonic and rectal atresias. In Puri P (ed). *Newborn Surgery*, 3rd edn. London: Hodder Arnold, 2011: 505–11, Figure 53.1. With permission.)

Colonic atresia is associated with abdominal wall defects, such as gastroschisis, cloacal exstrophy, and more rarely omphalocele, which complicates the management of these patients.[4,14] Boles et al.[14] found that 4 of their 11 patients had gastroschisis. In the series reported by Philippart,[4] 22 of 36 patients with colonic atresia had no associated anomalies, whereas 6 had cloacal exstrophy, and 3 had other abdominal wall defects; 5 of the 36 patients had jejunal atresia associated with the colonic atresia. Rarely, colonic atresia has been reported to occur concomitantly with imperforate anus.[7] Malrotation has also been reported to be a common associated anomaly.[15] One important associated anomaly is Hirschsprung's disease, which has been reported in a few cases. Although the colonic atresia was diagnosed at birth in these patients, there was a considerable delay in diagnosing the associated aganglionosis. It is therefore recommended that resected bowel is examined for Hirschsprung's disease.[23] Rectal

suction biopsies are suggested in patients that do not gain normal bowel function postoperatively.[24] Some authors recommend that rectal suction biopsies should be routinely taken in all patients with colonic atresia.[15,25] Isolated colonic atresia is sometimes associated with skeletal anomalies such as syndactyly, polydactyly, absent radius, and clubfoot.[4] Furthermore, colonic atresia has been reported in association with eye anomalies, such as exophthalmos and optic nerve hypoplasia.[13] In the series reported by Davenport et al.,[5] one patient had trisomy 18 and esophageal atresia. The fact that chromosomal abnormalities do occur in patients with colonic atresia makes it reasonable to recommend chromosomal analysis, at least in those patients who have other associated anomalies.

Diagnosis

Prenatal diagnosis of colonic atresia has been reported. However, prenatally detected colonic dilatation may also be the result of Hirschsprung's disease or anorectal malformations.[26]

Plain radiographs show a distal bowel obstruction with multiple dilated loops with air-fluid levels. A large right-sided loop, corresponding to the proximal dilated colon, has been considered characteristic in patients with colonic atresia (Figure 59.2a).[5] The level of obstruction is confirmed by a contrast enema, which reveals the distal microcolon and incomplete filling of the colon (Figure 59.2b). Pneumoperitoneum, indicating colonic perforation, is not rare and has been reported in approximately 10% of the cases.[4]

Management

PREOPERATIVE

Correction of fluid and electrolyte abnormalities is started as soon as bowel obstruction is suspected. The gastrointestinal tract is decompressed with a nasogastric tube. Prophylactic antibiotics are administered. The neonate should be in a stable condition before general anesthesia and the operation are started.

OPERATIVE

The two therapeutic options available are primary resection with anastomosis and colostomy with anastomosis at a later stage. Traditionally, many authors distinguished between the management of colonic atresia distal and proximal to the splenic flexure. Atresias proximal to the splenic flexure were treated with primary resection and anastomosis, whereas the distal atresias were treated with primary colostomy and delayed establishment of the gastrointestinal continuity.[4,7,13,17,27] More recently, it has been suggested that staged repair should be undertaken in complex cases with, for instance, questionable bowel viability, colonic perforation and peritonitis, and in patients with concomitant abdominal wall defects. On the other hand, in uncomplicated cases, resection and primary anastomosis has been proposed to be the method of choice for atresias at all levels of the colon.[28] There is no evidence that this later approach

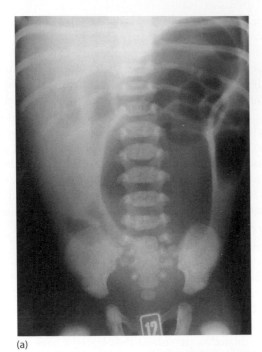

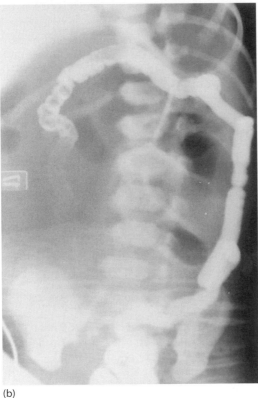

(a)

(b)

Figure 59.2 **(a)** Plain abdominal radiographs often show the hugely dilated bowel segment proximal to the atresia. **(b)** Contrast enema is diagnostic of a colonic atresia showing a microcolon and incomplete colonic filling.

increases the mortality or complication rate,[5,29] although the anastomosis may be technically difficult because of the large discrepancy between the diameters of the proximal and distal bowel.[30] England et al.[31] reported that a temporising stoma does not reduce the diameter of proximal bowel

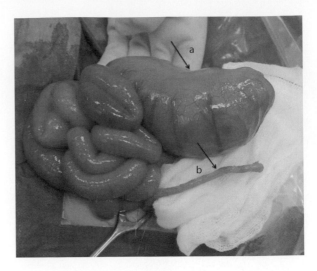

Figure 59.3 Proximal colon is hugely dilated (arrow **a**), while the distal colon is very small (arrow **b**).

and therefore recommended right hemicolectomy and primary anastomosis for proximal colonic atresia.

The abdomen is opened through a transverse incision a finger diameter above the umbilicus and to the right. The incision may be extended as required. Cautery is used to divide the muscle layers of the abdominal wall, and the umbilical vein is ligated and divided. The site and type of atresia are assessed (Figure 59.3). It is extremely important that additional atresias are excluded. The patency of the distal colon must always be tested by, for instance, injection of saline. In those with type I atresia, the bowel adjacent to the atresia is resected, and a primary anastomosis is performed. In patients with types II and III atresias, with adequate bowel length, the excessively dilated proximal bowel should also be resected (Figure 59.4a). A few centimeters of the distal narrow bowel are resected. The mesenteric vessels are divided close to the bowel wall to preserve the blood supply to the adjacent bowel. The distal bowel is incised along the antimesenteric border to achieve lumina of a similar diameter (Figure 59.4b). A single-layer anastomosis is performed using interrupted 5-0 absorbable sutures (Figure 59.5a–c). The wound is closed in layers with absorbable sutures.

POSTOPERATIVE

During the first postoperative days, parenteral nutrition is administered. Feeding can be started when the baby is well and the gastric aspirates have decreased. In cases with a primary anastomosis, it usually takes a few days before the neonate starts to pass stools. If a colostomy has been fashioned, the parents are instructed how to take care of the stoma. Usually the colostomy is closed at 2–3 months of age.

Complications and long-term results

Many factors have led to an improvement in the results of patients with colonic atresia, including early postnatal diagnosis, improved neonatal intensive care and anesthesia, and

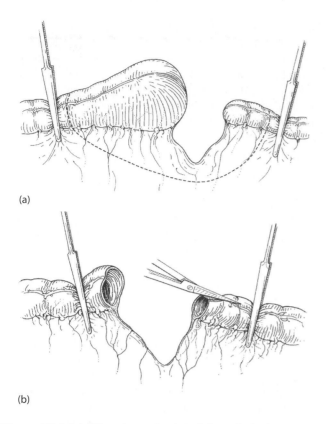

(a)

(b)

Figure 59.4 **(a)** Dilated proximal and the relatively ischemic portion of colon just distal to the atresia are resected. **(b)** Distal colon is incised along its antimesenteric border to match the luminal diameters of the two portions of bowel to be joined. (Reprinted from Wester T. Colonic and rectal atresias. In Puri P (ed). *Newborn Surgery*, 3rd edn. London: Hodder Arnold, 2011: 505–11, Figure 53.3. With permission.)

more efficient transport facilities. Today, mortality related to the colonic atresia or its treatment is rare. In the series reported by Davenport et al.,[5] no deaths occurred in the patients that underwent surgery, although one patient, who was never operated on, died of associated abnormalities.

The mortality rate in earlier series varied from 9% to 33%, in many cases as a result of associated anomalies, but also attributable to late diagnosis, nutritional deficiencies, infectious complications, and technical errors.[6,7,13,14,17] Etensel et al.[15] recently reported a lethal outcome in 27% of the cases collected for a literature review.

Powell and Raffensperger[13] reported 15 postoperative complications in 19 patients. Problems related to the colostomy were encountered in 3 of 11 patients treated with colostomy and delayed anastomosis, whereas anastomotic strictures were seen in 6 of the 19 patients. Boles et al.[14] reported significant complications in 4 of 11 cases. The use of contemporary principles of neonatal surgery has, however, reduced the morbidity rate, and Davenport et al.[5] reported recovery without complications.

RECTAL ATRESIA

Introduction

Rectal atresia is a very rare lesion, which has been reported to account for 0.3%–1.2% of all anorectal malformations.[32–34] Interestingly, a much higher incidence of 14% has been reported from Tamil Nadu in the southern part of India.[35] The reason for this high incidence has been poorly understood. However, in recent years, the incidence in Tamil Nadu has been reduced and is now similar to that in other parts of the world.

Although it has been proposed that rectal atresia should be classified as a colonic atresia,[6] it is usually considered to be part of the spectrum of anorectal malformations. Rectal atresia was classified as a type IV anomaly in the Ladd and Gross classification of anorectal anomalies.[36] In the international classification and the Wingspread classification, it was also classified as a separate type of high anomaly.[37,38] Peña's[39] classification describes rectal atresia as a separate entity, while the more recent Krickenbeck classification describes rectal atresia/stenosis among rare or regional variants of anorectal malformations.[40] Five types of rectal atresia have been distinguished: type 1 with a membrane

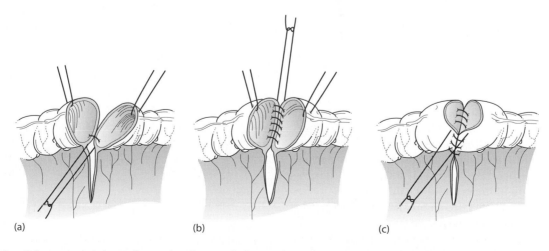

(a)

(b)

(c)

Figure 59.5 **(a–c)** Anastomosis is performed with a single layer of interrupted sutures. (Reprinted from Wester T. Colonic and rectal atresias. In Puri P (ed). *Newborn Surgery*, 3rd edn. London: Hodder Arnold, 2011: 505–11, Figure 53.4. With permission.)

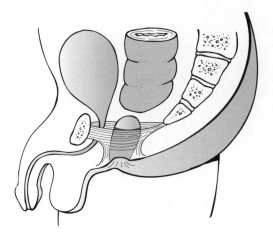

Figure 59.6 Rectal atresia. (Reprinted from Wester T. Colonic and rectal atresias. In Puri P (ed). *Newborn Surgery*, 3rd edn. London: Hodder Arnold, 2011: 505–11, Figure 53.5. With permission.)

and intact bowel wall; type 2 with blind ends separated by less than 2 cm, which is the most commonly encountered type; type 3 with a long distance between the blind ends; type 4, which is rectal stenosis; and type 5 with a urinary fistula accompanying the rectal atresia (Figure 59.6).[41]

Etiology

Magnus[42] described the autopsy findings in a female neonate with multiple atresias of the small and large bowel, including a rectal atresia. It was found that there were intact remnants of the internal sphincter, that the epithelium of the anal canal was normally developed, and that the external sphincters were normal (Figure 59.5). There was a fibromuscular band between the blind rectal pouch and the anal canal. Based on the findings in the autopsy specimen, the author suggested that rectal atresia is the result of vascular insufficiency, rather than a developmental defect. It was speculated that this could be the result of an intrauterine infection. It was also estimated that the lesion occurred between the 65 and 112 mm stages of development. Dorairajan[35] has suggested that the middle rectal artery is involved, rather than the superior rectal artery, which has been proposed by other investigators.

Presentation

Neonates with rectal atresia present with distal bowel obstruction comprising abdominal distension and failure to pass meconium. The perineum and anal canal are normal, and the diagnosis may therefore easily be delayed. The atresia is usually located 1–3 cm above the dentate line.

The incidence of associated anomalies in patients with rectal atresia has been considered to be extremely low.[43] In the series reported by Dorairajan,[35] associated anomalies were found in 2% of the 147 cases. No significant abnormalities were found in the urinary tract. Patients with rectal atresia

usually have a normal perineum and a normal sacrum. Rectal atresia occurs in patients with multiple atresias of the bowel.[42] Two of Dorairajan's[35] patients had ileal atresia, and one had multiple small bowel atresias. Patients with rectal atresia and particularly rectal stenosis may have an associated presacral mass, and it has been recommended that they should undergo MRI like other patients with anorectal malformations.

Diagnosis

The condition is diagnosed when an attempt is made to pass a thermometer or a tube to decompress the colon. After a colostomy has been opened, a contrast study with simultaneous injection of contrast material through the colostomy into the rectal pouch and the anal canal clearly outlines the anatomy of the anomaly (Figure 59.7).

Management

In the past, several different techniques, such as abdominoperineal and sacroperineal pull-through procedures, referred to by Stephens and Smith[44] and de Vries et al.[45] were used to treat rectal atresia. More recently, other methods have been described. Gauderer and Izant[46] placed a string across the membrane using fluoroscopy and progressively

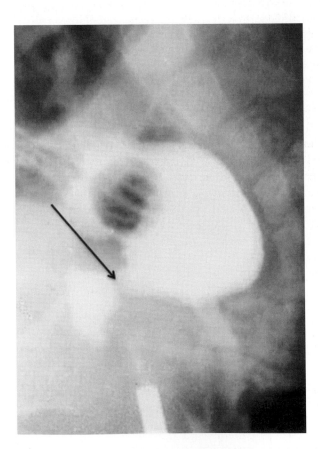

Figure 59.7 Simultaneous injection of contrast material into the upper pouch (via the sigmoid colostomy) and the anorectum clearly outlines the distance between the two pouches. The arrow shows the atresia.

dilated the rectal canal in one patient. Zia-ul-Miraj Ahmed et al.[47] used a Duhamel procedure in seven cases with rectal atresia and rectal stenosis. Dorairajan[35] fashioned a transverse colostomy in the newborn and did a definitive sacroperineal pull-through operation at approximately 1 year of age. If the blind rectal pouch ended above the pubococcygeal line, a sacro-abdomino-perineal or an abdominoperineal approach was preferred. The colostomy was closed in a third stage. Upadhyaya[41] recommended transanal end-to-end rectorectal anastomosis. One advantage of this technique is that luminal continuity is restored without injuring the functional anatomy of the region. A sigmoid colostomy is opened in the neonate, and the definitive procedure is performed at approximately 3 months of age. A Hegar dilator is advanced distally from the colostomy until it pushes the rectal pouch into the anal canal. The end of the anal canal is opened and the margins retracted with stay sutures. Then the rectal pouch is opened, and the edges of the anal canal and the rectal pouch are approximated to form an end-to-end anastomosis.[48] A similar technique, using an endoscope instead of a Hegar dilator, was recently described.[49] Transanal pull-through with mucosectomy, similar to the procedure used for Hirschsprung's disease, has been suggested also for rectal atresia.[50,51] Nguyen and Pham[52] used a combined laparoscopic and transanal approach.

Peña and DeVries[53] suggested that posterior sagittal anorectoplasty is a useful method for the repair of rectal atresia and stenosis. It is recommended that a diverting colostomy is opened in the newborn, and the definitive procedure is performed at a later stage.[39] A midline skin incision is performed, and the levator muscle and muscle complex are separated exactly at the midline to expose the bowel. The blind end of the rectum is usually separated from the anal canal with a few millimeters of fibrous tissue. The rectum has to be mobilized to allow an end-to-end anastomosis to be performed without tension. More recently, a technique sparing the anterior dentate line was introduced.[54] The wound is closed by reconstruction of the muscle structures. Daily dilatations are performed starting 2 weeks postoperatively. The colostomy is closed approximately 3 months after the operation, provided the diameter of the anastomosis is appropriate.[53]

In utero repair of rectal atresia was recently reported in a fetus that also had a sacrococcygeal teratoma.[55]

Complications and long-term results

In patients with rectal atresia, the anal canal, sacrum, and sphincteric mechanisms are virtually normal. Therefore, the prognosis with respect to functional outcome is favorable. Although the number of cases reported is very limited, the outcome in patients with rectal atresia or stenosis treated through a posterior sagittal approach is excellent. Peña[39] reported voluntary bowel movements with total continence and without soiling in a series of five cases. However, two of the five patients had constipation. The same group showed,

in a more recent series of 17 patients, that all 12 patients older than 3 years had voluntary bowel movements and were clean between bowel movements; 5 (29%) of the 17 patients had constipation that required laxatives. The authors report that complications occurred in three patients: one rectovaginal fistula and two presacral abscesses.[54] Constipation has been reported to occur frequently after other procedures were used to treat rectal atresia or stenosis as well.[47] Upadhyaya[48] reported an uneventful recovery and normal continence in two patients treated with his method. Dorairajan[35] was able to follow up 37 of 60 patients that were treated with sacroperineal pull-through operations and who had their colostomy closed. The outcome was excellent in 20% of the patients, whereas 65% had occasional soiling at night and 15% had soiling also in daytime. The mortality rate in this series was 35%.

CONCLUSION AND FUTURE DIRECTIONS

Colonic and rectal atresias are both very rare conditions. The long-term results appear to be good, although there are limited data on the outcome in adulthood in patients with colonic and rectal atresia. For colonic atresia, the surgical options are mainly resection and primary anastomosis or colostomy with delayed anastomosis. For rectal atresias, several techniques have been described. There is little evidence to show that one technique is better than the other. It is, also with multicenter studies, difficult to get a sample size that is large enough to compare the methods.

REFERENCES

1. Evans CW. Atresias of the gastrointestinal tract. *Int Abstr Surg* 1951; 92: 1–8.
2. Gaub OC. Congenital stenosis and atresia of the intestinal tract above the rectum, with a report of an operated case of atresia of the sigmoid in an infant. *Trans Am Surg Assoc* 1922; 40: 582–670.
3. Potts WJ. Congenital atresia of intestine and colon. *Surg Gynecol Obstet* 1947; 85: 14–9.
4. Philippart AI. Atresia, stenosis, and other obstructions of the colon. In: Welch KJ, Randolph JG, Ravitch MM, O'Neill JA, Rowe MI (eds). *Pediatric Surgery*, 4th edn. Chicago: Year Book Medical Publishers, 1986: 984–8.
5. Davenport M, Bianchi A, Doig CM, Gough DCS. Colonic atresia: Current results of treatment. *J R Coll Surg Edinb* 1990; 35: 25–8.
6. Freeman NV. Congenital atresia and stenosis of the colon. *Br J Surg* 1966; 53: 595–9.
7. Benson CD, Lotfi MW, Brough AJ. Congenital atresia and stenosis of the colon. *J Pediatr Surg* 1968; 3: 253–7.
8. Webb CH, Wangensteen OH. Congenital intestinal atresia. *Am J Dis Child* 1931; 41: 262–84.
9. Louw JH. Investigations into the etiology of congenital atresia of the colon. *Dis Colon Rectum* 1964; 7: 471–8.

10. Bland Sutton JD. Imperforate ileum. *Am J Med Sci* 1889; 98: 457.
11. Guttman FM, Braun P, Garance PH. Multiple atresias and a new syndrome of hereditary multiple atresias involving the gastrointestinal tract from the stomach to rectum. *J Pediatr Surg* 1973; 8: 633–4.
12. Puri P, Fujimoto T. New observations on the pathogenesis of multiple intestinal atresias. *J Pediatr Surg* 1988; 23: 221–5.
13. Powell RW, Raffensperger JG. Congenital colonic atresia. *J Pediatr Surg* 1982; 17: 166–70.
14. Boles ET, Vassy LE, Ralston M. Atresia of the colon. *J Pediatr Surg* 1976; 11: 69–75.
15. Etensel B, Temir G, Karkiner A et al. Atresia of the colon. *J Pediatr Surg* 2005; 40: 1258–68.
16. Peck DA, Lynn HB, Harris LE. Congenital atresia and stenosis of the colon. *Arch Surg* 1963; 87: 86–97.
17. Coran AG, Eraklis AJ. Atresia of the colon. *Surgery* 1969; 65: 828–31.
18. Barnard CN, Louw JH. The genesis of intestinal atresia. *Minn Med* 1956; 39: 745–8.
19. Louw JH, Barnard CN. Congenital intestinal atresia: Observations in its origin. *Lancet* 1955; 2: 1065–7.
20. Kim S, Yedlin S, Idowu O. Colonic atresia in monozygotic twins. *Am J Med Genet* 2000; 91: 204–6.
21. Benawra R, Puppala BL, Mangurten HH et al. Familial occurrence of congenital colonic atresia. *J Pediatr* 1981; 99: 435–6.
22. Fairbanks TJ, Kanard RC, Del Moral PM et al. Colonic atresia without mesenteric vascular occlusion. The role of the fibroblast growth factor 10 signalling pathway. *J Pediatr Surg* 2005; 40: 390–6.
23. Akgur FM, Olguner M, Hakguder G et al. Colonic atresia associated with Hirschsprung's disease: It is not a diagnostic challenge. *Eur J Pediatr Surg* 1998; 8: 378–9.
24. Kim PCW, Superina RA, Ein S. Colonic atresia combined with Hirschsprung's disease: A diagnostic and therapeutic challenge. *J Pediatr Surg* 1995; 30: 1216–7.
25. Lauwers P, Moens E, Wustenberghs K et al. Association of colonic atresia and Hirschsprung's disease in the newborn: Report of a new case and review of the literature. *Pediatr Surg Int* 2006; 22: 277–81.
26. Anderson N, Malpas T, Robertson R. Prenatal diagnosis of colon atresia. *Pediatr Radiol* 1993; 23: 63–4.
27. Defore WW, Garcia-Rinaldi R, Mattox KL, Harberg FJ. Surgical management of colon atresia. *Surg Gynecol Obstet* 1976; 143: 767–9.
28. Arca MJ, Oldham KT. Atresia, stenosis, and other obstructions of the colon. In: Coran AG, Adzick NS, Krummel TM, Laberge J-M, Shamberger RC, Caldamone AA (eds). *Pediatric Surgery*. Philadelphia: Elsevier Saunders, 2012: 1247–53.
29. Dassinger M, Jackson R, Smith S. Management of colonic atresia with primary resection and anastomosis. *Pediatr Surg Int* 2009; 25: 579–82.
30. Watts AC, Sabharwal AJ, MacKinlay GA et al. Congenital colonic atresia: Should primary anastomosis always be the goal? *Pediatr Surg Int* 2000; 19: 14–7.
31. England RJ, Scammel S, Murthi GV. Proximal colonic atresia: Is right hemicolectomy inevitable? *Pediatr Surg* 2011; 27: 1059–62.
32. Santulli TV, Schullinger JN, Kiesewetter WB, Bill AH. Imperforate anus: A survey from the members of the surgical section of the American Academy of Pediatrics. *J Pediatr Surg* 1971; 6: 484–7.
33. Endo M, Hayashi A, Ishihara M et al. Analysis of 1992 patients with anorectal malformations over the past two decades in Japan. *J Pediatr Surg* 1999; 34: 435–41.
34. Peña A. Posterior sagittal anorectoplasty: Results in the management of 332 cases of anorectal malformations. *Pediatr Surg Int* 1988; 3: 94–104.
35. Dorairajan T. Anorectal atresia. In: Stephens FD, Smith ED, Paul NW (eds). *Anorectal Malformations in Children*. New York: Liss, 1988: 105–10.
36. Gross RE. *The Surgery of Infancy and Childhood*. Philadelphia: W B Saunders Company, 1953: 348–68.
37. Stephens FD, Smith ED. *Anorectal Malformations in Children*. Chicago: Year Book Medical Publishers, 1971.
38. Stephens FD, Smith ED. Classification, identification, and assessment of surgical treatment of anorectal anomalies. *Pediatr Surg Int* 1986; 1: 200–5.
39. Peña A. Anorectal malformations. *Semin Pediatr Surg* 1995; 4: 35–47.
40. Holschneider A, Hutson J, Pena A et al. Preliminary report on the International conference for the development of standards for the treatment of anorectal malformations. *J Pediatr Surg* 2005; 40: 1521–6.
41. Upadhyaya P. Rectal atresia. In: Puri P (ed). *Newborn Surgery*. Oxford: Butterworth-Heinemann, 1996: 395–8.
42. Magnus RV. Rectal atresia as distinguished from rectal agenesis. *J Pediatr Surg* 1968; 3: 593–8.
43. Peña A. Anorectal anomalies. In: Puri P (ed). *Newborn Surgery*. Oxford: Butterworth-Heinemann, 1996: 379–94.
44. Stephens FD, Smith ED. Individual deformities in the male. In: *Anorectal Malformations in Children*. Chicago: Year Book Medical Publishers, 1971: 33–80.
45. de Vries PA, Dorairajan T, Guttman FM et al. Operative management of high and intermediate anomalies in males. In: Stephens FD, Smith ED, Paul NW (eds). *Anorectal Malformations in Children: Update*. New York: Liss, 1988: 317–401.
46. Gauderer MWL, Izant RJ. String placement and progressive dilatations in the management of high membranous rectal atresia. *J Pediatr Surg* 1984; 19: 600–2.

47. Zia-ul-Miraj Ahmed M, Brereton RJ, Huskinsson L. Rectal atresia and stenosis. *J Pediatr Surg* 1995; 30: 1546–50.

48. Upadhyaya P. Rectal atresia: Transanal, end-to-end, rectorectal anastomosis: A simplified, rational approach to management. *J Pediatr Surg* 1990; 25: 535–7.

49. Stenström P, Cementson Kockum C, Arnbjörnsson E. Rectal atresia-operative management with endoscopy and transanal approach: A case report. *Minim Invasive Surg* 2011; 2011: 792402. doi:10.1155/2011/792402. EPub 2011 Apr 21.

50. Luo C-C, Ming Y-C, Chu S-M et al. Individualized management of upper rectal atresia. *J Pediatr Surg* 2009; 44: 2406–9.

51. Hamzaoui M, Ghribi A, Makni W et al. Rectal and sigmoid atresia: Transanal approach. *J Pediatr Surg* 2012; 47: E41–4.

52. Nguyen TL, Pham DH. Laparoscopic and transanal approach for rectal atresia: A novel alternative. *J Pediatr Surg* 2007; 42: E25–7.

53. Peña A, DeVries PA. Posterior sagittal anorectoplasty: Important technical considerations and new applications. *J Pediatr Surg* 1982; 17: 796–811.

54. Hamrick M, Eradi B, Bischoff A et al. Rectal atresia and stenosis: Unique anorectal malformations. *J Pediatr Surg* 2012; 47: 1280–4.

55. Chiba T, Albanese CT, Jennings RW et al. In utero repair of rectal atresia after complete resection of a sacrococcygeal teratoma. *Fetal Diagn Ther* 2000; 15: 187–90.

60

Meconium ileus

GUIDO CIPRANDI AND MASSIMO RIVOSECCHI

DEFINITION

Meconium ileus is an early manifestation of cystic fibrosis (CF), due to abnormal, inspissated, and viscid mucus of intestinal origin. In children affected by this condition, the impacted meconium produces an intraluminal obstruction occurring in the midileum, leading to a progressive distension. As an ultimate evolution, different mechanical complications can be associated, including intestinal volvulus, atresia, gangrene and necrosis, perforation, peritonitis with abdominal calcifications, and finally, meconial pseudocyst. In this view, meconium diseases in infancy cannot be firmly separated into three categories, such as meconium plug syndrome, meconium ileus, and meconium peritonitis, nor can therapy of each condition.

HISTORICAL DATA

Intestinal occlusion, associated with both inspissated meconium and gross pathologic pancreatic changes, was first reported by Landsteiner[1] in 1905 and subsequently confirmed by Kornblith and Otani[2] and Fanconi et al.,[3] who correlated chronic lung disease and pancreatic insufficiency. In 1936, Fanconi et al. described this complex and lethal newborn condition as a "cystic fibrosis of the pancreas."

In the middle of the century, Bodian's[4] intuition of an abnormal sticky intestinal mucus, with a lower content of water, provided the basis for a modern treatment with intraoperative saline irrigations, thus avoiding undue small bowel resections. Mikulicz, Gross, Bishop and Koop, Santulli, and others were responsible, in those years, for different surgical techniques including distal or proximal enterostomies.[5] More recently, Noblett[6] and Shaw[7] reported relief of intestinal obstruction by irrigating with various solutions as well normal saline, 1% *N*-acetylcysteine, hyperosmolar gastrografin enema, surfactant, and DNase. With respect to different types of surgical and medical efforts, the survival rate at 1 year increased from 10% to 90%, and the operative mortality drastically decreased to 15%–23% of treated newborns.[8]

INCIDENCE

Meconium ileus accounts for 9%–33% of all neonatal intestinal obstructions (300 new cases in Italy each year) and could be defined as the third most common cause of neonatal small bowel obstruction after ileal and duodenojejunal atresia and malrotation.[9]

It is more frequently observed in predominantly white countries, where the presence of CF is higher, ranging from 1 in 1200 to 1 in 2700 live births. On the contrary, the disease is nearly absent in some Asian peoples and in black Africans. Although meconium ileus can rarely occur in otherwise normal patients, the majority of children affected by this condition have CF. The mean incidence of meconium ileus in CF is at least 18%, with no difference between sexes: when this association coexists, meconium ileus is the presenting symptom in 12% of these children.[10] In contrast to this pathology, meconium plug syndrome is more commonly seen in premature infants, is characterized by colonic obstruction, and is infrequently associated with CF.[11] Approximately half of neonates with meconium ileus present with complicated intestinal obstruction and they always require a surgical procedure. In contrast, only 6%–10% of uncomplicated forms fail nonoperative management using a water-soluble contrast enema: these patients are candidates for a temporary diversion or a major procedure.[12,13]

PATHOGENESIS

Meconium ileus is an essential expression of CF, which is the most common lethal autosomal recessive disorder in white populations, and is characterized by dysfunctional chloride ion transport across epithelial surfaces. Parents are not affected, but both are heterozygotes carrying the abnormal gene(s). The intestine, pancreas, lungs, sweat glands, liver, and salivary glands are all involved, as a result of abnormal exocrine gland activity. However, these organs will be differently affected during life, the pancreas being the first, because the progressive retention of secretions and the atrophy of the acinar cells start during fetal life; in contrast, the lungs are normal at birth, and the mucus plugging of the distal airways will be responsible for progressive pulmonary insufficiency during adolescence. Meconium ileus is a rare expression of CF in premature infants, suggesting that the intestinal abnormalities take place during the last period of the fetal life.

Although recurrent lung infections and pulmonary insufficiency are the principal causes of morbidity and death, gastrointestinal signs and symptoms commonly precede the pulmonary findings and may suggest the diagnosis in infants and young children. The gastrointestinal manifestations of CF result primarily from abnormally viscous luminal secretions within hollow viscera and the ducts of solid organs. As a result, bowel obstruction may be present at birth due to meconium plug syndrome or meconium ileus. The first biochemical studies of the altered meconium showed a lower content of carbohydrate, more proteins, and more so-called mucoproteins and albumin, which have been used as a screening test in years prior. Meconium ileus more recently appeared as a result of abnormal intestinal secretions, but not so closely related to the sweat electrolyte defect (high levels of sodium and chloride): in fact, the impermeability of CF epithelia to chloride ions is not correlated to the severity of intestinal involvement, and the pancreatic lesions plays a secondary role. Actually, the sweat test is the main laboratory test used for the diagnosis, but after the 1990s, genetic analysis commonly has been used for diagnostic as well as prognostic purposes.

From a genetic point of view, the cystic fibrosis transmembrane conductance regulator (CFTR) is the gene product defective in CF; it was first identified in 1989.

The CFTR gene is normally located in the apical membrane of the epithelial cells from the stomach to the colon: a mutation of CFTR on chromosome 7 is responsible for evidence of CF. The most common mutation is ΔF-508 and can be identified using DNA testing in affected neonates as well as in family members, possible carriers of the specific gene.

The CFTR gene codes for a 1480-amino-acid protein that acts as a chloride channel, regulated by cyclic AMP. In the small intestinal wall, the clinical expression of CF depends largely on the decreased secretion of fluid and chloride ions, the increased permeability of the paracellular space between adjacent enterocytes and the sticky mucous cover over the enterocytes. As a rule, brush border enzyme activities are normal, and there's some enhanced active transport as shown for glucose and alanine. As a result, the gastrointestinal content in children affected by meconium ileus differs mainly from the normal condition by the lower acidity in the foregut and the accretion of mucins and proteins, resulting in intestinal obstruction in the ileum but also in the colon. During growth, the small intestinal mucosa won't be functioning at maximal capacity. Better understanding of the CF gastrointestinal phenotype may contribute to improvement of the overall well-being of these first-seen newborn patients. In the recent years, the Na^+-dependent amino acid transporter called ATB(0), which has been previously localized in the 19q13.3 region, did not appear to be associated with cystic fibrosis-meconium ileus

(CF-MI) disease; however, fine chromosomal mapping of other genetic factors and loci, in human as well as animal models, such as the mouse, could be useful in determining the association with the intestinal phenotype of CF. We assume that this work will be very hard because more than 1000 mutations have been identified in the CFTR gene and the final impact of these mutations on the genotype–phenotype correlation is actually unknown. In addition, the discordant phenotype observed in CF siblings suggests that genes other than CFTR modulate the CF phenotype.[14–16]

HISTOPATHOLOGY

In meconium ileus, the intestine shows different aspects if we consider the *proximal*, the *middle*, and the *distal* ileum. In the first portion, a nearly normal evidence is present, with a progressive dilatation at the midportion borderline. In the proximal ileum, the content has a semiliquid consistency and is not yet viscous. A marked and severe dilatation of the middle ileum is ever seen: the intestine contains thick, dark green, and puttylike meconium, firmly adherent to the walls. The intestinal obstruction causing hyperperistalsis is responsible for the congestion and hypertrophy of the walls. The distal ileum is full of concretions called "rabbit pellets," gray stained and with a beaded typical appearance. This condition of the small bowel is responsible for a narrow, empty, and small colon, never used, which is called *microcolon*.[17]

When meconium ileus is complicated, more severe aspects can be seen: the dilatation is responsible for wall perforation and for secondary meconium peritonitis, with calcifications. The spontaneous healing of the ileal perforation could lead to resorption of the involved portion of bowel and finally, to an intestinal atresia. When the peristalsis is vigorous, the twisting of the ileal tract full of dense meconium may result in a massive volvulus, with a high risk of perforation. Sometimes, when the bowel perforation is massive, an intense reaction to the meconial spillage may produce a giant meconial pseudocyst. Obviously, a postnatal perforative evolution of meconium ileus is complication by bacterial peritonitis.

CLINICAL PICTURE

Polyhydramnios is the most frequent feature observed in prenatal diagnosis of complicated forms of meconium ileus. The presence of fetal hyperechogenic bowel on the ultrasound (US), associated with dilated bowel and/or ascites, could be indicative of an intestinal obstruction. A family history of CF is clearly evident in almost 25% of these patients. Meconium ileus is uncommon in premature infants (5%–12%), and associated congenital anomalies are rare.[18]

Main symptoms include abdominal distension (96%), bilious vomiting (50%), and delayed passage of meconium (36%). From a clinical point of view, it is possible to recognize two different conditions: a simple, uncomplicated, and nonsurgical type, and a complicated, severe type, with a mortality of at least 25% of all cases. In the first type

(58%), signs and symptoms of a distal ileal obstruction are seen not later than 48 hours after birth: generalized abdominal distension with dilated and visible as well as palpable loops of bowel, bilious vomiting, no stools, and narrowing of the anus and rectum, with only a dense and rubberlike gray meconium sticking to the anal wall. In the second type (42%), the neonate represents a surgical emergency that must be treated within 24 hours before birth, when the signs of hypovolemic shock or sepsis are not well established. Fetuses with complex meconium ileus are at increased risk for postnatal bowel obstruction and perforation.[19]

In this serious illness, the progressive abdominal distension may culminate in a respiratory distress. If a perforation occurs, pneumoperitoneum and sepsis are the unfavorable consequences. Infrequently, meconium in the vagina or scrotum is evidence of a fetal perforation. Sometimes, the onset is directly with a meconium peritonitis, which could involute to a giant meconial pseudocyst: when this happens, abdominal skin edema and translucency are evident and associated with a palpable right lower mass.

At present, whatever is the clinical presentation picture, the overall survival rate is at least 95%.[20]

PRENATAL US AND RADIOLOGIC PATTERN

Meconium usually fills the small bowel during the 20th week of gestation, so identification of meconium ileus before this period is rare. Prenatal US has led to confidence in the antenatal diagnosis of intestinal obstruction, allowing counseling and birth planning. In this regard, the presence of fetal hyperechogenic bowel on US, associated with dilated bowel and/or ascites, could be indicative of an intestinal obstruction. The increased echogenicity of the intestinal loops is due to a higher density of the intraluminal content (hyperdense and dry meconium). However, it is not easy to determine exactly if this feature is arising from intraluminal or extraluminal structures, and other different condition may present with similar US pattern, such as prenatal infections, neoplasm, or chromosomal trisomy. In addition, these findings may also represent transient normal variants According to final US findings in utero, patients can be classified into three types: type I (massive meconium ascites), type II (giant pseudocyst), and type III (calcification and/or small pseudocyst). This classification may be useful for perinatal management of complicated meconium ileus.[21]

The cystic or pseudocystic type of meconium peritonitis may have a potentially rapid lethal course, and the onset of fetal anemia and polyhydramnios is a bad prognostic factor. Severe evolution in hydrops and fetal distress may occur at any moment, suggesting the persistence of a leakage or rerupture of the cysts with new meconium spillage into the abdomen.

Postnatal radiological imaging does not offer further information over prenatal imaging, and surgical decision should not be influenced by the absence of abdominal free air. Urgent abdominal drainage at birth, followed by intestinal diversion of persistent intestinal perforation on the first day of life, may prevent bacterial colonization and improve prognosis.[18,22]

When meconium ileus evolves into a volvulus, the US shows enlarged hyperechogenic loops without peristalsis. Polyhydramnios is the most frequent feature observed in prenatal diagnosis of complicated forms of meconium ileus.

Obviously, if the parents are found to be carriers for a CF mutation, the correlation between US findings and meconium ileus is done.

Plain radiographs show distended and gas-filled intestinal loops. Sometimes, air–fluid levels are seen (one-third of the cases), thus mimicking an ileal atresia. Where a sharp stop image is evident, this is the exact point of the obstruction. A usual image of fine, granular soap-bubble (Singleton sign) or ground-glass appearance (Neuhauser sign) is due to a dense meconium mixed with air, typical of the distal ileum: this picture is usually located in the midabdomen or in the right iliac fossa. Nevertheless, this image has also been observed in neonates with meconium plug syndrome, Hirschsprung disease, or small bowel atresia. The meconium hyperdensity may produce various images, depending from the length or the localization of the obstructed bowel, but also on the filling (complete or partial) of the intestinal loops affected. When meconium ileus is complicated, the abdominal radiograph may show calcification as a result of meconium peritonitis due to a fetal perforation of the intestine. A double-bubble image or air–fluid levels can be seen when a secondary ileal atresia (single or double) is the final bowel remodeling after a complete volvulus associated with a severe ischemic damage. If the intestinal perforation occurs early in the antenatal period, the x-ray appearance of a round rim of calcification underlines a meconium pseudocyst. The colon is always a microcolon (unused colon) because the meconium never fills the large bowel during fetal life. So, the length is normal, but the caliber is small because of a small amount of feces (thick and dry meconium) passing through.

A water-soluble contrast enema is useful for both diagnostic and therapeutic purposes: the iso-osmolar agents facilitate evacuation of meconium without loss of large amounts of fluids and solutes.

DIAGNOSTIC CRITERIA AND DIFFERENTIAL DIAGNOSIS

The sweat test provides a quantitative estimate of sodium and chloride in a collected sample of sweat, usually from the forearm. A cholinergic drug acts by stimulating sweat production with the help of a mild electrical current applied for 3–6 minutes (pilocarpine iontophoresis technique). Concentrations of these two cations above 60 mEq/L are diagnostic if at least 100 mg of sweat is collected. However, in the early neonatal age, it is really difficult to obtain a sufficient quantity of sweat to provide an accurate analysis, and collection must be done twice or three times before being satisfactory. In borderline cases, results are not significant for CF, and further analysis is needed. Another problem is represented by the high levels of sodium and chloride in neonates who are otherwise normal. In these situations, we must wait and obtain another series of results after an interval of at least 1 month from the first test. More recently, the DNA probe analysis test for the ΔF-508 mutation and other common alleles allows for a precise diagnosis, which misses only a very small percentage of patients affected by CF. This method detects both affected children as well as heterozygote carriers.

Other causes of distal intestinal obstruction of the newborn may present with similar clinical patterns, including jejunoileal atresia, Hirschsprung disease, meconium plug syndrome, and neonatal small left colon syndrome. In particular, a congenital megacolon is suspected when the bowel contents are liquid and air–fluid levels are constantly seen in the dilated bowel.

Other conditions may mimic surgical obstruction, such as delayed peristalsis associated with prematurity (so-called functional immaturity) and adynamic ileus from sepsis. If a volvulus without malrotation or neonatal invagination is seen, the patient may undergo a sweat test to exclude CF. Although unusual, meconium ileus exists as an isolated entity, not associated with CF. These patients account for 6%–12% of the total, and the course of the illness is more often benign and without complications.[23]

MEDICAL AND SURGICAL TREATMENT

The first step of treatment includes a nasogastric tube decompression, an antibiotic prophylaxis with cephalosporin and aminoglycosides, and correction of dehydration, electrolytes, and hypothermia.

A contrast enema with water-soluble and hyperosmolar or iso-osmolar contrast is the medical treatment of choice without any mucosal damage, for uncomplicated meconium ileus. A recent study that used various enema solutions administered in a mouse model showed that surfactant and gastrografin were the most efficacious for the in vivo relief of constipation, in comparison with perflubron, Tween-80, GoLytely, DNase, N-acetylcysteine, and Viokase. Intestinal mucosal damage was absent, and viscosity was significantly reduced in vitro.[24]

Enema evacuation should be obtained under fluoroscopic control, with a gentle and progressive increase of the intraluminal pressure, thus avoiding unexpected fractures of the colon. A correct procedure prevents leakage of the contrast medium by taping the buttocks as well as catheter dislocation. If the contrast medium fails to progress into dilated small bowel loops, the presence of an acquired atresia is definite, and the radiologist must stop the examination because of a high risk of perforation. Fifty percent of neonates submitted for this procedure showed a benefit of enema alone over the next 48 hours, without any additional treatment: in some cases, a second enema may be used with

a complete evacuation of the meconium filling the ileal loops. Acetylcysteine administered by mouth is useful and helps to relieve the obstruction. Radiographs are taken at 3-, 6-, 12-, 24-, and 48-hour intervals, with the aim of evaluating progression and possible complications. At this time feeding is begun. Hypovolemic shock and early perforation are around the corner, but an appropriate and meticulous procedure can avoid these complications.

When medical treatment is unsuccessful in spite of an uncomplicated meconium ileus, surgery is mandatory, and an open evacuation, resection, and ileostomy are the different options. In a simple meconium ileus, the surgeon should perform a minimal procedure to obtain a lumen free from all kinds of rubbish, such as pellets, sticky meconium, and sometimes, small calcifications. In this case, a limited enterotomy and repeated warm saline irrigations through a smooth catheter provide the best result. In this event, meconium discharge may be manually supported, using the enterotomy placed in the dilated hypertrophic ileum. The catheter is two-way directed with care, clearing the small as well as the large bowel. At the same time as the irrigation, the surgeon controls the enema progression, and the bowel may be inspected for degree of distension, mesenteric orientation, covered perforation, gangrenous tract, and atretic single or multiple segments. The colon is inspected too, searching for possible perforation or microperforation. T-tube ileostomy could be an additional effective and safe treatment, without any additional surgery in 90% of treated patients; the T-tube should be removed within the first 8 weeks after surgery.[25,26]

At the end of this treatment, discussion is about whether to resect or not, because some authors stress the risk of a leakage at the anastomotic site: we must keep in mind that resection and termino-terminal anastomosis is possible, only if any sign of infection or sepsis is absent. Usually, a resection is done with the aim to promptly restore normal peristalsis: in these patients, the intestinal resection is limited to a huge dilation, at risk for foci of regional infection. Actually, bowel resection with primary anastomosis has been proved to be as effective and safe as stoma formation and is associated with a reduced length of initial hospital stay.[20] However, in complicated forms of meconium ileus, primary resection and anastomosis should have some advantages, such as shorter hospital stay and no later surgical procedure of stoma closure.[27,28]

An ileostomy can be performed in different ways: the simplest one is a double-barreled ileostomy (Mikulicz), with the two loops brought out side to side; this solution is quick and avoids an intra-abdominal anastomosis. However, neonates may lose a large amount of fluids and solute from this through the ileostomy, and in selected cases, as an alternative to a peripheral line, a central venous catheter is scheduled, for both nutritional and medical purposes. More and more alternatives have been described: distal ileostomy with end-to-side ileal anastomosis (Bishop–Koop) has been called "distal chimney enterostomy." The proximal chimney enterostomy is the Santulli procedure, with a proximal ileostomy with end-to-side ileal anastomosis. Complex meconium ileus or management with stomas significantly increases both length of stay and relaparotomy rate irrespective of the type of management.[29]

The enterostomy is closed between 7 and 12 days after surgery by an end-to-end anastomosis.

In a few selected cases, gastrostomy may be needed, but only when recovery of intestinal functions is expected to be delayed.

Generally, the shorter the duration of the intervention, the less extended the resection, the earlier the recovery of the peristalsis, and the less complicated and more uneventful the postoperative care.

Complications include pulmonary infections, which is the most important one, with an incidence of at least 8%–10%. Anastomotic leakage occurs for different reasons: a technical mistake, an insufficient blood supply, a distal unrecognized obstruction. Delayed recovery of peristalsis is another frequently observed complication and is due to an abnormal stretching of the intestinal walls during fetal life. Total parenteral nutrition is the support of choice, and a central venous catheter is mandatory in these situations.

PROGNOSIS

Meconium ileus may be an early indication of a more severe phenotype of CF. This is suggested by the significantly lower pulmonary function found in children with a history of meconium ileus compared to age- and sex-matched children who do not have meconium ileus.[30] The complicated form is susceptible to a higher number of long-term surgical complications, including especially small bowel obstructions and blind loop syndromes. Long-term complications in neonates affected by uncomplicated meconium ileus who were nonoperatively treated are never seen, and only mild and transient complications have been observed in newborns treated with minor surgical procedures, such as enterotomies and irrigations.

Survival of neonates with meconium ileus has improved over the last two decades because of neonatal intensive care, improved surgical technique, and medical treatment, but it has been shown that a delayed arrival at the hospital after the initial symptoms causes significant morbidity.[31] In general, an overall immediate survival of 90% is achieved using the modern protocols, and nearly all deaths are pertinent to adolescents. Only a few children die because of liver and or septic complications. Deaths are mainly due to staphylococcal or *Pseudomonas* sepsis, primary or secondary to pulmonary interstitial emphysema or to aspiration pneumonia. In a large series reported and analyzed by Fuchs,[8] only one child died because of meconium ileus itself. More recently, different studies suggest that adequate initial nutritional and medical management of meconium ileus further allows quite similar nutritional and lung wellness compared with children affected by early-discovered and symptomatic CF.[32] In conclusion, even if meconium ileus is often

associated with longer hospitalization and surgical procedures, high-risk infections, and sepsis, an early diagnosis of CF does not impair the long-term pulmonary outcome in these patients.[33]

REFERENCES

1. Landsteiner K. Darmverschluss durch eingedictes Meconium Pankreatitis. *Zentralbl Allg Pathol* 1905; 16: 903–9.
2. Kornblith BA, Otani S. Meconium ileus with congenital stenosis of the main pancreatic duct. *Am J Pathol* 1929; 5: 249–55.
3. Fanconi G, Uehlinger E, Knauer C. Das coeliakiesyndrom bei angeborener zystischer pancreasfibromatose und bronchiektasien. *Wien Med Wochenschr* 1936; 28: 753–66.
4. Bodian M. *Fibrocystic Disease of the Pancreas.* New York: Grune & Stratton, 1953.
5. Santulli TV. Meconium ileus. In: Holder TM, Ashcraft KW (eds). *Pediatric Surgery.* WB Saunders Co, Philadelphia; London; Toronto, 1980: 211–9.
6. Noblett HR. Treated of uncomplicated meconium ileus by gastrografin enema: A preliminary report. *J Pediatr Surg* 1969; 4: 190–7.
7. Shaw A. Safety of N-acetylcysteine in treatment of meconium obstruction of the newborn. *J Pediatr Surg* 1969; 4: 119–27.
8. Fuchs JR, Langer JC. Long-term outcome after neonatal meconium obstruction. *Pediatrics* 1998; 101: 4–7.
9. Kalayoglu M, Sieber WK, Rodman JB. Meconium ileus: A critical review of treatment and eventual prognosis. *J Pediatr Surg* 1971; 6: 290–300.
10. Rosenstein BJ, Langbaum TS. Incidence of meconium abnormalities in newborn infants with cystic fibrosis. *Am J Dis Child* 1980; 134: 72–83.
11. Olsen MM, Luck SR, Lloyd-Still J, Raffensperger JG. The spectrum of meconium disease in infancy. *J Pediatr Surg* 1982; 17: 479–81.
12. Caniano DA, Beaver BL. Meconium ileus: A fifteen-year experience with forty-two neonates. *Surgery* 1987; 102: 699–703.
13. Rescorla FJ, Grosfeld JL. Contemporary management of meconium ileus. *World J Surg* 1993; 17: 318–25.
14. Eggermont E. Gastrointestinal manifestations in cystic fibrosis. *Eur J Gastroenterol Hepatol* 1996; 8: 731–8.
15. Larriba S, Sumoy L, Ramos MD, Gimenez J, Estivill X, Casals T, Nunes V. ATB(0)/SLC1A5 gene. Fine localisation and exclusion of association with the intestinal phenotype of cystic fibrosis. *Eur J Hum Genet* 2001; 9: 860–6.
16. Salvatore F, Scudiero O, Castaldo G. Genotype–phenotype correlation in cystic fibrosis: The role of modifier genes. *Am J Med Genet* 2002; 111: 88–95.

17. Murshed R, Spitz L, Kiely E, Drake D. Meconium ileus: A ten-year review of thirty-six patients. *Eur J Pediatr Surg* 1997; 7: 275–7.

18. Irish MS, Ragi JM, Karamanoukian HL, Borowitz DS, Schmidt D, Glick PL. Prenatal diagnosis of the fetus with cystic fibrosis and meconium ileus. *Pediatr Surg Int* 1997; 12: 434–6.

19. Dirkes K, Crombleholme TM, Craigo SD, Latchaw LA, Jacir NN, Harris BH, D'Alton ME. The natural history of meconium peritonitis diagnosed in utero. *J Pediatr Surg* 1995; 30: 979–82.

20. Musqhtaq I, Wright VM, Drake DP, Mearns MB, Wood CB. Meconium ileus secondary to cystic fibrosis. The East London experience. *Pediatr Surg Int* 1998; 13: 365–9.

21. Kamata S, Nose K, Ishikawa S, Usui N, Sawai T, Kitayama Y, Okada A. Meconium peritonitis in utero. *Pediatr Surg Int* 2000; 16(5–6): 377–9.

22. Pelizzo G, Dell'oste C, Maso G, D'Ottavio G. Prenatal detection of the cystic form of meconium peritonitis: No issues for delayed postnatal surgery. *Pediatr Surg Int* September 2008; 24(9): 1061.

23. Kerem E, Corey M, Kerem B, Durie P, Tsui L, Levison H. Clinical and genetic comparisons of patients with cystic fibrosis, with or without meconium ileus. *J Pediatr* 1989; 114: 767–73.

24. Burke MS, Ragi JM, Karamanoukian HL, Kotter M, Brisseau GF, Borowitz DS, Ryan ME, Irish MS, Glick PL. New strategies in nonoperative management of meconium ileus. *J Pediatr Surg* 2002; 37: 760–4.

25. Steiner Z, Mogilner J, Siplovich L, Eldar S. T-tubes in the management of meconium ileus. *Pediatr Surg Int* 1997; 12: 140–1.

26. Mak GZ, Harberg FJ, Hiatt P, Deaton A, Calhoon R, Brandt ML. T-tube ileostomy for meconium ileus: Four decades of experience. *J Pediatr Surg* 2000; 35: 349–52.

27. Jawaheer J, Khalil B, Plummer T, Bianchi A, Morecroft J, Rakoczy G, Bruce J, Bowen J, Morabito A. Primary resection and anastomosis for complicated meconium ileus: A safe procedure? *Pediatr Surg Int* 2007; 23: 1091–3.

28. Jawaheer J, Khalil B, Plummer T, Bianchi A, Rakoczy G, Bowen J, Morabito A. Primary resection and anastomosis for complicated meconium ileus: A safe procedure? *Pediatr Surg Int* 2000; 16(5–6): 377–9.

29. Farrelly PJ, Charlesworth C, Lee S, Southern KW, Baillie CT. Gastrointestinal surgery in cystic fibrosis: A 20-year review. *J Pediatr Surg* February 2014; 49(2): 280–3.

30. Evans AK, Fitzgerald DA, McKay KO. The impact of meconium ileus on the clinical course of children with cystic fibrosis. *Eur Respir J* 2001; 18: 784–9.

31. Munck A, Alberti C, Colombo C, Kashirskaya N, Ellemunter H, Fotoulaki M, Houwen R, Robberecht E, Boizeau P, Wilschanski M; CF/Pancreas ESPGHAN Working Group and DIOS Study Group. International prospective study of distal intestinal obstruction syndrome in cystic fibrosis: Associated factors and outcome. *J Cyst Fibros* 2016 February; 1569–963.

32. Munck A, Gèrardin M, Alberti C, Ajzenman C, Leburgeois M, Aigrain Y, Navarro J. Clinical outcome of cystic fibrosis presenting with or without meconium ileus: A matched cohort study. *J Pediatr Surg* 2006; 41: 1556–60.

33. Kappler M, Feilcke M, Schroter C, Kraxner A, Griese M. Long-term pulmonary outcome after meconium ileus in cystic fibrosis. *Pediatr Pulmonol* 2009; 44(12): 1201–6.

61

Meconium peritonitis

JOSE L. PEIRÓ AND JOSE BOIX-OCHOA

INTRODUCTION

Meconium peritonitis (MP) is an aseptic peritonitis caused by spills of meconium in the abdominal cavity through one or several intestinal perforations that have taken place during intrauterine life. Extravasation of sterile meconium into the fetal peritoneal cavity causes an intense chemical and foreign body reaction with characteristic calcification. Often, the perforation seals before the infant is born. Gastrointestinal perforations that occur following birth, even though the gut still contains meconium, should not be included in the syndrome of "meconium peritonitis," and constitute an entirely different group of clinical problems.[1]

MP was first reported by Morgagni in 1761 in *De Sedibus et Causis Morborum*. Simpson[2] managed to find 25 cases in 1838, and it was Agerty[3] in 1943 who reported the first successful operation.

The estimated incidence of MP is currently 1:30,000.[4]

A review of the world literature up to 2015 revealed 1934 cases of MP reported, with 1167 survivors (Table 61.1). Previous collected series have made this task easier.[5,6]

In the last 20 years, continuing progress in prenatal diagnostic procedures and postnatal intensive care has decreased mortality rates below 10% in some series,[7,8] and in our last experience, the mortality rate fell to 6.6%.

The current authors' experience is based on 67 cases of pure MP who underwent surgical treatment. All of these patients presented with the classical picture of MP at laparotomy and had histological evidence of (1) meconium inclusions (Figure 61.1) or reaction to foreign bodies, and (2) visible perforation or microscopic evidence of intestinal cicatrization.

ETIOLOGY

Intrauterine intestinal perforation may result from various causes. Patients with MP are divided into those with and without associated intestinal obstruction. In the case of MP without obstruction, there is no clear-cut explanation for the perforation. Various hypotheses, such as segmental absence of the muscular coats, absence of the muscularis mucosa,[9] vascular occlusion,[10] and general hypoxia of the fetus in the perinatal period,[11] have been put forward. None of these hypotheses has been substantiated. In the current authors' research with rats, it has been clearly demonstrated that all these findings are a consequence of MP and not primary etiology.[12] In our experience, intestinal atresia, intestinal volvulus, and meconium ileus constitute 94% of etiological factors (Table 61.2). Other causes include Hirschsprung's disease, meconium plug syndrome, congenital bands, internal hernias, Meckel's diverticulum, and rectal perforation. The incidence of cystic fibrosis in infants with MP was previously reported[13] to vary between 8% and 40%.

However, in some cases, it is impossible to find its etiology, in spite of pathological changes. The tabulation of the medical and perinatal reports demonstrated that 80% of these patients had neonatal anoxia and respiratory distress.

Labor research demonstrates the consequences of the hypoxia on the splanchnic area and blood distribution in the studied animals.[14]

If these findings are correlated with the current authors' studies, as happens in isolated focal intestinal perforations in extreme prematures, it can be postulated that there is diminished blood flow to the intestine of the hypoxic infant. The mucosa, which is very sensitive to ischemia, undergoes diminished mucin production and degenerative alterations. The proteolytic enzymes can now attack the bowel wall, which is normally protected by mucin. The consequence of this is a break in the mucosal integrity followed by perforation. Sometimes the "jamming" of this reflex mechanism prevents the return to normality and can cause such severe ischemia that it leads directly to a covered perforation. The less vascularized zones, and therefore the more exposed to ischemia and perforation, are situated in the ileocecal region and splenic flexure, where the current authors have found 60% of all idiopathic lesions.

Table 61.1 Mortality rate in MP among 1934 cases reported in the world literature

Years	Total	Survivors	Mortality (%)
Before 1952	100	8	92.0
1952–1962	102	19	81.4
1963–1968	145	51	64.8
1969–1988	752	375	50.1
1989–1995	210	150	28.6
1996–2004	374	343	8.3
2004–2015	253	221	9.0
–	1934	1167	39.6

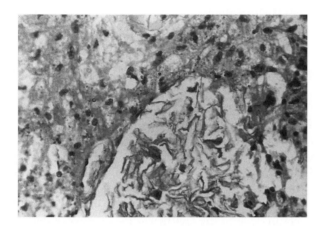

Figure 61.1 Granulomatous tissue with giant cells of foreign bodies related to meconial corpuscles.

Table 61.2 Associated congenital malformations and operative findings

Malformation	Total	Survivors	Mortality (%)
Intestinal atresia	38	34	10.5
Volvulus	12	7	41.6
Meconium ileus	11	7	36.3
Other	8	8	0

PATHOLOGY

In the current authors' experimental work[12] with rats, it has been shown that meconium gives rise to a peritoneal reaction with rapid fibroblastic proliferation enveloping the lesion. Later, foreign body granulomas and calcifications are seen. This reaction may be local or generalized, the parietal peritoneum having lost its sheen. The intestinal loops are intimately adherent structures with a fibrous tissue, which is difficult to dissect, calcifications or meconium inclusions are disseminated, and the perforation is hard to identify. When the intestinal perforation does not cicatrize and there is a fibrinous reaction instead, the consequence is the formation of a cyst, the walls of which are formed of fibrin, meconium, and intestinal loops intimately united. Such

a cyst may occupy two-thirds of the abdomen (Figure 61.2). The possibility of meconium spreading out by a hematologic or lymphatic route (via the brain or lungs) has been described.[15]

Lorimer and Ellis[16] described three major types of MP: fibroadhesive, generalized, and cystic. Two other types that have been described are the healed form of MP and microscopic MP.

The fibroadhesive type is the result of an intense fibroblastic reaction in response to the severe chemical peritonitis caused by the digestive enzymes in the meconium. This type produces obstruction by adhesive bands, and the site of perforation is usually sealed off.

The cystic type occurs when the site of perforation is not effectively sealed, and a thick-walled cyst is formed by the fixed intestinal loops.[17] This condition prevents communication of the perforation with the remainder of the viscera. Calcium deposits line the cyst wall. The formation of a pseudocyst represents an attempted intra-abdominal healing process to confine the perforation.

The generalized type usually occurs perinatally.[18,19] Calcified meconium is scattered throughout the peritoneal cavity, and the bowel loops are adherent by thin fibrinous adhesions. In the current authors' experience, this is the most frequent type (74% of all cases).

The healed form of MP, presenting as an inguinal or scrotal mass, is clinically and pathologically of special interest. These patients usually present with no relevant recent clinical history, although the majority show a unilateral hydrocele at birth. Radiological studies of the scrotum and abdomen are usually helpful in making the diagnosis by demonstrating scrotal as well as peritoneal calcifications.[20–22] This combination is pathognomonic of MP.[20,23] In some cases, the peritoneal calcifications are the only symptomatology. In cases in which the diagnosis can be established clinically, no surgical intervention is necessary and, in the majority of these cases, the nodules regress spontaneously.[23,24] Microscopic examination of the resected specimen shows a fibrosis of the serous membrane, dissociation

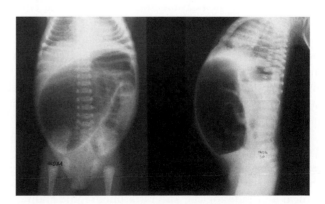

Figure 61.2 Typical roentgenogram of a giant meconium cyst. Prenatal ileal perforation was secondary to atresia of ileum.

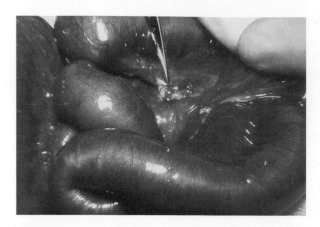

Figure 61.3 Causal finding of calcifications on an intestinal atresia without the clinical evidence and operative findings of MP. This case is not included in our material.

of the muscular layer, foci of calcification, and granulomatous lesions with foreign body giant cells.

There is another type of microscopic MP described by Tibboel et al.,[25] without clinical or therapeutic significance. In the majority of cases, it is a casual finding during laparotomy for other causes (Figure 61.3). Many patients with this "microscopic" type of MP present with atresia, and the current authors feel that such an atresia should be regarded as scarring of the site of a perforation, which must have occurred at a relatively early stage of fetal development. A careful microscopic examination of the visceral and parietal peritoneum will, however, reveal bile pigment and/or squamous cell remnants. The presence of these meconium components proves that a perforation must have occurred. The presence of collagen, calcium deposits, and giant cells surrounding meconium particles indicates that the peritoneal cavity must have contained meconium for a considerable length of time. Its etiology should be examined for intestinal perforations at an early stage of development, resulting in intestinal atresia induced by a vascular lesion. At other times, the perforation can achieve complete recovery and not lead to any significant tissue deterioration; the only remnant of this pathology is the microscopic MP as a casual finding and without clinical significance.

Interleukin 6 and interleukin 8 play important roles in the inflammatory response syndrome associated with MP, and drainage of cystic fluid did not completely suppress this inflammation. These interleukin concentrations are elevated in patient's plasma, and very high in the cyst or ascites just after birth.[26]

SYMPTOMATOLOGY AND DIAGNOSIS

The diagnosis of MP in the postnatal period is based on clinical and radiological, and ultrasonographic findings of intestinal obstruction, and occasionally one or more of the following: calcification, pneumoperitoneum, cyst formation, or ascites. The clinical symptomatology is that of any

intestinal obstruction. A typical baby with MP is born with abdominal distension, or develops it soon after birth, and this is accompanied by bile-stained vomiting and failure to pass meconium. Occasionally, severe abdominal distension may result in dystocia or respiratory distress. Sometimes, cryptorchidism is the indication that the fetal abdominal pathology has prevented the physiological descent of the testicles. Pathognomonic of this is the appearance of a scrotal edema or hydrocele with retention of the testes and intrascrotal calcification. X-ray and ultrasound[27] examinations show the intestinal ileus, the ascites when it exists, the ground-glass appearance of the abdomen due to the meconium, and rarely the presence of a pneumoperitoneum, since the quick formation of adhesions prevents the intestinal gas from escaping.

Intra-abdominal calcifications are characteristic[28,29] and can easily be seen on plain abdominal films (Figure 61.4). It is the current authors' belief that the origin of these calcifications may be the catalytic effect of the fatty meconial compounds on the precipitation of calcium salts. Proof of this is that in their investigations in laboratory animals with low serum levels of calcium, it has not been possible to reproduce calcifications. Faripor[30] is of the opinion that the pathogenesis of calcifications, after the analysis of seven cases with light microscopic observation, is undoubtedly in response to keratin debris. Keratin, however, cannot be the only source because of the presence of granulomas devoid of keratin. Due to the fact that some of these granulomas resemble gouty tophi, it may be as a result of inflammation caused by uric acid present in meconium. So early do the calcifications appear that the prenatal diagnosis of MP is easily made on sonographic exam,[31–37] finding fetal isolated intra-abdominal calcifications,[34] fetal ascites,[35] or meconium pseudocyst.[36] Diagnosis of associated pathology is

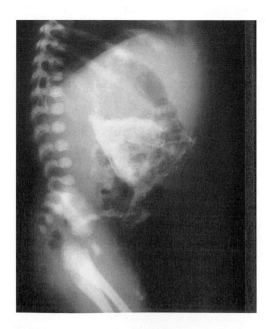

Figure 61.4 Pathognomonic abdominal calcification in a case of MP.

crucial because of its repercussions in the immediate post-operative period.[38] Finkel and Slovis indicate that the presence of intraperitoneal calcification does not exclude, but favors, a diagnosis of cystic fibrosis[39] in spite of the fact that they are scarcer than in the other types of MP. Detection of cystic fibrosis[40] is done by screening for the most common gene mutations and sweat chloride test, and also the recommended screening for congenital infections including herpes simplex virus, cytomegalovirus, parvovirus B19, and toxoplasmosis.

Newborns presenting with scrotal swelling with or without discoloration resulting from calcified meconium within the patent *processus vaginalis* have been described with increased frequency.[21,23] MP may result in a number of genital manifestations, including inguinal and scrotal or labial hydrocele containing meconium or calcifications and hard tumor-like scrotal masses.[41]

Early diagnosis is a decisive factor for the prognosis of these newborns, because bacterial colonization of the meconium starts after birth. In a study carried out by the current authors in 134 normal newborns, meconium cultures were positive in 24% at 12 hours of life and in 86% at 72 hours.[12] On the other hand, the laboratory studies carried out by the current authors already demonstrated the existence of a "meconium spreading factor," which accelerates and worsens the sepsis. Owing to this, it is not then surprising that early diagnosis is of paramount importance. In the current authors' series of 67 cases, the patients that were operated on after 36 hours of life had a mortality rate three times higher than those that were operated on during the first 24 hours of life (Table 61.3). Tibboel and Molenaar[6] reported a 91% mortality rate for patients operated on after 48 hours of life.

The natural history of MP diagnosed in utero is markedly different from that diagnosed in the newborn because some cases diagnosed prenatally normalize spontaneously during the gestational follow-up. The normal ultrasound features are polyhydramnios, fetal ascites, intra-abdominal calcifications, and dilated intestinal loops.[42]

Recently, it was reported[7] that magnetic resonance image afforded higher prenatal diagnostic accuracy of MP than ultrasonography (57.1% vs. 42%). Ultrasonography, however, is most widely used as a primary tool.

Zangheri et al.[8] proposed a prenatal classification that was divided into four grades of progressive severity, based on the number of pertinent ultrasonographic findings: grade 0, isolated intra-abdominal calcifications; grade 1, intra-abdominal calcifications and ascites, pseudocyst, or bowel dilatation; grade 2, two associated findings; and grade 3, all sonographic features. Patients with a score greater than 1 have a high probability for urgent neonatal surgery and therefore should be transferred in utero to a tertiary center with available neonatal surgery.

The cases in grade 0 that initial prenatal ultrasound findings subsequently disappeared during gestation can deliver at term without any complication at 40 weeks of gestation.

In fetuses with the described suspected intrauterine MP and pathological sonographic findings, an elective preterm delivery by cesarean section at a median gestational age of 35 weeks is recommended[43] in order to stop evolution of the disease and to operate the patient earlier. In the last years, with improvement in antenatal diagnosis, parents can decide termination of pregnancy in some cases of MP with other severe associated anomalies. Early detection is not associated with poor neonatal outcome, and selective termination is unnecessary.[44]

Dirkes et al.[13] reported that only 22% of fetuses with prenatal diagnosis of MP developed complications that required surgery, and the overall mortality rate in their series was 11%.

Meconium periorchitis is a rare disorder caused by fetal MP with subsequent spillage of meconium into the scrotal sac. The condition can be diagnosed during fetal life by ultrasonography, but usually diagnosed clinically during the first year of life, as an incidental finding of scrotal mass.[45] Surgical excision of the scrotal mass usually confirms the histological diagnosis of meconium periorchitis. Conservative treatment is also an alternative.[46]

TREATMENT

After prenatal diagnosis or suspicion, currently there is not an established prenatal therapy. There is an isolated report that used fetal abdominal injection of urinary trypsin inhibitor to reduce the meconium-induced chemical peritonitis and avoid a postnatal surgery.[47]

After a prenatal diagnosis, sometimes, fetal paracentesis could be beneficial to reduce intra-abdominal pressure, to improve mesenteric vascular supply, and to remove inflammatory debris.[48,49] Antenatal diagnosis can help us to anticipate measures at delivery and be ready for an eventual need of immediate paracentesis and cardiopulmonary resuscitation.[50] The majority of fetuses with intra-abdominal calcifications on prenatal ultrasounds do not require surgery. Associated sonographic findings, as bowel dilation or suspicion of intestinal volvulus,[51] can be used to select fetuses for delivery in tertiary neonatal surgical centers.[52]

The indication for operation in newborns with MP is a clear sign of intestinal obstruction or perforation. The diagnosis of MP without intestinal obstruction or pneumoperitoneum does not constitute an indication for operation.

Table 61.3 Time of operation related to prognosis

Time	Total	Survivors	Mortality (%)
<24 hours postnatally	25	23	8
24–36 hours	31	26	16.1
36–48 hours	6	4	33.3
>48 hours	5	1	80
	67	54	19.4

Infants with neonatal meconium calcification, meconium ascites with hydrocele, or calcified meconium found in the hernia sac do not require operation, but they have to be observed and feeding withheld for 48 hours. With absence of clinical symptoms, enteral feeding can be started with caution, gradually progressing to formula. Antibiotic coverage is desirable.

Surgical treatment

All the conditions for the preparation of the newborn for surgery, such as monitoring for vital signs and control of temperature with measures for impeding temperature loss in the operating theatre, should be adhered to. An intravenous cannula should be placed for intravenous fluid replacement. Blood should be cross-matched and prophylactic antibiotics started.

Operative treatment

Based on our experience of 67 cases with a survival rate of 92.8% in the past 20 years, the current authors act according to the following protocol:

1. If the perforation is visible, do not try to suture it. Intestinal resection and end-to-end anastomosis is performed.
2. In cases of localized or generalized peritonitis, attempt the lysis of the adhesions only to discover the perforation or to relieve obvious obstructions. Only when necessary should an attempt be made to dissect the adhesions, since fibroadhesive peritonitis disappears after 8–14 days; this has been confirmed in the current authors' patients who had the two-stage operation and investigation with laboratory animals.
3. Once the etiology has been determined (atresia, stenosis, or meconium ileus), an attempt must be made to perform an end-to-end anastomosis, according the Louw's technique,[53] if the general status of the patient and the discordance in the intestinal calibers allow it.

    Primary anastomosis can be performed for almost all patients with MP, except for nonstable extremely low birth weight infants.[54]

    The two-stage operation of Rehbein[9] (exteriorization followed by laparotomy and anastomosis) is used only if the patient's condition is very serious, or if the existing peritonitis can endanger the suture line, or when there are great differences in caliber of the two loops of bowel. The anastomosis is performed 2 weeks later, if the newborn's general status allows the second stage of the operation. During the interval between the two operations, enteral and total parenteral nutrition are indispensable for maintaining the newborn in the best condition as well as the stimulation of the distal portion with the contents of the proximal end. The two-stage operation offers a series of advantages that should always be considered by the surgeon:

- Rapid resolution of the surgical problem.
- It allows the surgeon to deal with the peritonitis, which would endanger the suture in a one-stage operation.
- It allows recovery of the general state of the patient with the increase in energy reserves by means of parenteral nutrition and antibiotic therapy.
- It gives time for the disappearance of bowel adhesions and the normalization in caliber and absorptive function of the intestinal mucosa by means of the growth stimulation offered by perfusion of the enteral diet through a soft silicone feeding tube in the distal portion.
- It allows the maturation of the neuroendocrine system.

    The two-stage operation has been associated with a lower mortality rate in the current authors' series when compared with the one-stage operation (7.2% vs 22%).

4. When faced with a meconial cyst, in view of the small number of successful cases published,[16,54] the current authors always perform decortication with great care and a two-stage operation.[55]

    Another option is cyst drainage by ultrasound-guided needle punction and later laparotomy. A drainage procedure was always accompanied by supportive treatment of decompression, broad-spectrum antibiotics, and parenteral nutrition. Tanaka et al.[56] reported two cases of cystic MP that initially underwent emergency percutaneous drainage with ultrasonic guidance under local anesthesia. They found that such procedure is safe and effective in decompression of gastrointestinal tract and prevention of bacterial infection. They recommended cyst drainage just after birth and elective surgery later based on the general condition of the baby. During the second operation, the general condition is more stable and the adhesions will be less, the identification of the bowel loops easier, and the bleeding minimal.

To summarize, the current authors are convinced that the low morbidity rate can be achieved by the adequate planning of the operation in two stages, whenever faced with the slightest doubt as to the probable success of a primary anastomosis.

With antenatal and early diagnosis, the advances in surgical techniques, and postoperative treatment, current survival of the patients with MP is nearing 100%.[57]

COMPLICATIONS

Among the postoperative complications, adhesion obstructive ileus is the most frequent. In the current authors' series of 79 patients, 8 developed adhesion ileus, 5 had anastomotic leakage, 2 had necrosis of the ileostomy stump, and 1 had an enterocutaneous fistula. There were 14 deaths in the series, 7 directly attributable to lung complications in patients with cystic fibrosis; the other 7 patients died of sepsis. Also, there are reported newborns that died from intraoperative hepatic hemorrhage, mostly in extremely low birth weight infants.[58] Gentle and delicate operative manipulation is required to reduce the mortality and morbidity in these cases.

REFERENCES

1. Cerise EJ, Whitehead W. Meconium peritonitis. *Am Surg* 1969; 35: 389.
2. Simpson JY. Peritonitis in the fetus in utero. *Edinb Med Surg J* 1838; 15: 390.
3. Agerty HA. A case of perforation of the ileum in newborn infant with operation and recovery. *J Pediatr* 1943; 22: 233.
4. Nam SH, Kim SC, Kim DY et al. Experience with meconium peritonitis. *J Pediatr Surg* 2007; 42: 1822–5.
5. Boix-Ochoa J. Meconium peritonitis. *J Pediatr Surg* 1968; 3: 715–22.
6. Tibboel D, Molenaar JC. Meconium peritonitis. A retrospective, prognostic analysis of 69 patients. *Z Kinderchir* 1984; 39: 25–8.
7. Chan KL, Tang MH, Tse HY, Tang RY, Tam PK. Meconium peritonitis: Prenatal diagnosis, postnatal management and outcome. *Prenat Diagn* 2005; 25: 676–82.
8. Zangheri G, Andreani M, Ciriello E, Urban G, Incerti M, Vergani P. Fetal intra-abdominal calcifications from meconium peritonitis: Sonographic predictors of postnatal surgery. *Prenat Diagn* 2007; 27: 960–3.
9. Rickham PP. Peritonitis of the neonatal period. *Arch Dis Child* 1955; 30: 23.
10. Vilhena-Moraes R, Cappellano G, Mattosinho Franca LC et al. Peritonite meconial. *Rev Paul Med* 1964; 65: 231.
11. Lloyd JR. The etiology of gastrointestinal perforations in the newborn. *J Pediatr Surg* 1969; 3: 77.
12. Boix-Ochoa J. Patologia quirurgica del meconio. *Med Esp* 1982; 81: 30–51.
13. Dirkes K, Crombleholme TM, Craigo SD et al. The natural history of meconium peritonitis diagnosed in utero. *J Pediatr Surg* 1995; 30: 979–82.
14. Johanssen K. Regional distribution of circulating blood during submersion asphyxia in the duck. *Acta Physiol Scand* 1964; 62: 1–3.
15. Patton WL, Lutz AM, Willmann JK et al. Systemic spread of meconium peritonitis. *Pediatr Radiol* 1998; 28: 714–6.
16. Lorimer WS, Ellis DG. Meconium peritonitis. *Surgery* 1966; 60: 470–5.
17. Kolawole TM, Bankole MA, Olurin EO, Familusi JB. Meconium peritonitis presenting as giant cysts in neonates. *Br J Radiol* 1973; 46: 964–7.
18. Fonkalstrud EW, Ellis DG, Clatworthy HW Jr. Neonatal peritonitis. *J Pediatr Surg* 1966; 1: 227–39.
19. Gugliantini P, Caione P, Rivosecchi M, Fariello G. Intestinal perforation in newborn following intrauterine meconium peritonitis. *Pediatr Radiol* 1979; 8: 113–5.
20. Cook PL. Calcified meconium in the newborn. *Clin Radiol* 1978; 29: 541–6.
21. Gunn LC, Ghionzoli OG, Gardner HG. Healed meconium peritonitis presenting as a reducible scrotal mass. *J Pediatr* 1978; 92: 847.
22. Heydenrych JJ, Marcus PB. Meconium granulomas of the tunica vaginalis. *J Urol* 1976; 115: 596–8.
23. Berdon WE, Baker DH, Becker J, De Sanctis P. Scrotal masses in healed meconium peritonitis. *N Engl J Med* 1967; 277: 585–7.
24. Heetderks DR Jr, Verbrugge GP. Healed meconium peritonitis presenting as a scrotal mass in an infant. *J Pediatr Surg* 1969; 4: 363–5.
25. Tibboel D, Gaillard JL, Molenaar JC. The 'microscopic' type of meconium peritonitis. *Z Kinderchir* 1981; 34: 9–16.
26. Kanamori Y, Terawaki K, Takayasu H et al. Interleukin 6 and interleukin 8 play important roles in systemic inflammatory response syndrome of meconium peritonitis. *Surg Today* 2012 May; 42(5): 431–4.
27. Graziani M, Bergami GL, Fasanelli S. Fibroadhesive meconium peritonitis: Ultrasonographic features. *J Pediatr Gastroenterol Nutr* 1994; 18: 241–3.
28. Smith B, Clatworthy HW. Meconium peritonitis: Prognostic significance. *Pediatrics* 1961; 27: 967.
29. Miller JP, Smith SD, Newman B, Sukarochana K. Neonatal abdominal calcification: Is it always meconium peritonitis? *J Pediatr Surg* 1988; 23: 555–6.
30. Faripor F. Origin of calcification in healed meconium peritonitis. *Med Hypoth* 1984; 14: 51–6.
31. Brugman SM, Bjelland JJ, Thomasson JE, Anderson SF, Giles HR. Sonographic findings with radiologic correlation in meconium peritonitis. *J Clin Ultrasound* 1979; 7: 305–6.
32. Bowen A, Mazer J, Zarabi M, Fujioka M. Cystic meconium peritonitis: Ultrasonographic features. *Pediatr Radiol* 1984; 14: 18–22.
33. Blumental DH, Rushovich AM, Williams RK, Rochester D. Prenatal sonographic findings of meconium peritonitis with pathologic correlation. *J Clin Ultrasound* 1982; 10: 350–2.
34. Dunne M, Haney P, Sun CCJ. Sonographic features of bowel perforation and calcific meconium peritonitis in utero. *Pediatr Radiol* 1983; 13: 231–3.
35. Garb M, Riseborough J. Meconium peritonitis presenting as fetal ascites on ultrasound. *Br J Radiol* 1980; 53: 602–4.
36. Lauer JD, Cradock TV. Meconium pseudocyst: Prenatal sonographic and antenatal radiologic correlation. *J Ultrasound Med* 1982; 1: 333–5.
37. Nancarrow PA, Mattrey FR, Edwards DK, Skram C. Fibroadhesive meconium peritonitis in utero: Sonographic diagnosis. *J Ultrasound Med* 1985; 4: 213–5.

38. Kuffer F. Die meconiumperitonitis. *Schweiz Med Wochschr* 1968; 98: 1109.

39. Finkel LI, Slovis TL. Meconium peritonitis, intraperitoneal calcifications and cystic fibrosis. *Pediatr Radiol* 1982; 12: 92–3.

40. Cassacia G, Trucchi A, Nahom A et al. The impact of cystic fibrosis on neonatal intestinal obstruction: The need for prenatal/neonatal screening. *Pediatr Surg Int* 2003; 19: 75–8.

41. Redman JF, Cottone JL Jr. Unusual sequela of meconium peritonitis in an infant: Massive contralateral extension of a hernial sac. *J Urol* 2001 January; 165(1): 228.

42. Estroff JA, Bromley B, Benacerraf BR. Fetal meconium peritonitis without sequelae. *Pediatr Radiol* 1992; 22: 277–8.

43. Saleh N, Geipel A, Gembruch U et al. Prenatal diagnosis and postnatal management of meconium peritonitis. *J Perinat Med* 2009; 37(5): 535–8.

44. Wang CN, Chang SD, Chao AS, Wang TH, Tseng LH, Chang YL. Meconium peritonitis in utero—The value of prenatal diagnosis in determining neonatal outcome. *Taiwan J Obstet Gynecol* 2008 December; 47(4): 391–6.

45. Regev RH, Markovich O, Arnon S, Bauer S, Dolfin T, Litmanovitz I. Meconium periorchitis: Intrauterine diagnosis and neonatal outcome: Case reports and review of the literature. *J Perinatol* 2009 August; 29(8): 585–7.

46. Alanbuki AH, Bandi A, Blackford N. Meconium periorchitis: A case report and literature review. *Can Urol Assoc J* 2013 July–August; 7(7–8): E495–8.

47. Izumi Y, Sato Y, Kakui K, Tatsumi K, Fujiwara H, Konishi I. Prenatal treatment of meconium peritonitis with urinary trypsin inhibitor. *Ultrasound Obstet Gynecol* 2011 March; 37(3): 366–8.

48. Shyu MK, Shih JC, Lee CN et al. Correlation of prenatal ultrasound and postnatal outcome in meconium peritonitis. *Fetal Diagn Ther* 2003; 18: 255–61.

49. Okawa T, Soeda S, Watanabe T, Sato K, Sato A. Repeated paracentesis in a fetus with meconium peritonitis with massive ascites: A case report. *Fetal Diagn Ther* 2008; 24(2): 99–102.

50. Taba R, Yamakawa M, Harada S, Yamada Y. A case of massive meconium peritonitis in utero successfully managed by planned cardiopulmonary resuscitation of the newborn. *Adv Neonat Care* 2010 December; 10(6): 307–10.

51. Sciarrone A, Teruzzi E, Pertusio A et al. Fetal midgut volvulus: Report of eight cases. *J Matern Fetal Neonat Med* 2016 April; 29(8): 1322–7.

52. Zerhouni S, Mayer C, Skarsgard ED. Can we select fetuses with intra-abdominal calcification for delivery in neonatal surgical centers? *J Pediatr Surg* 2013 May; 48(5): 946–50.

53. Louw MB. Resection and end to end anastomosis in the management of atresia and stenosis of small bowel. *Surgery* 1967; 62: 940.

54. Miyake H, Urushihara N, Fukumoto K et al. Primary anastomosis for meconium peritonitis: First choice of treatment. *J Pediatr Surg* 2011 December; 46(12): 2327–31.

55. Rao YS, Murthy TV. Giant cystic meconium peritonitis. *Indian Pediatr* 1983; 20: 773–5.

56. Tanaka K, Hashizume K, Kawarasaki H, Iwanaka T, Tsuchida Y. Elective surgery for cystic meconium peritonitis: Report of two cases. *J Pediatr Surg* 1993; 28: 960–1.

57. Al-Hindi S, Asgar M. Meconium peritonitis in neonates: Management dilemma. *Bahrain Med Bull* 2008; 30: 2.

58. Reynolds E, Douglass B, Bleacher J. Meconium peritonitis. *J Perinatol* 2000; 3: 193–5.

62

Duplications of the alimentary tract

PREM PURI, ALAN E. MORTELL, AND FARHAN TAREEN

INTRODUCTION

Duplications of the alimentary tract are rare spherical or tubular structures that can occur anywhere in the tract from mouth to anus.[1-3] Calder reported the first case of enteric duplication in 1733, and Ladd,[4] in 1937, introduced the term *alimentary tract duplication* in the hope of clarifying the nomenclature, which had previously included descriptive terms such as *enteric or enterogenous cysts*; *giant diverticula*; *ileal, jejunal, or colonic duplex*; and *unusual Meckel diverticulum*. Ladd proposed that the unifying term *alimentary tract duplications* be applied to congenital anomalies that involved the mesenteric side of the associated alimentary tract; had a smooth muscle coat; shared a common blood supply with the native bowel; and were lined by gastrointestinal (GI)-type epithelium.[4] Most duplications might indeed be called simply *enterogenous cysts*, since in only very few cases is there an actual doubling of the alimentary tract, and these are therefore deserving of the name *duplication*.

EMBRYOLOGY

Numerous theories have been developed to account for the multitude of GI tract duplications. In a comprehensive review of GI duplications, Stern and Warner[1] outlined the most widely held theories regarding GI duplication.

Embryologically, duplications have been categorized into foregut, midgut, and hindgut types.[1] Foregut duplications include the pharynx, respiratory tract, esophagus, stomach, and the first portion and proximal half of the second portion of the duodenum. Midgut duplications include the distal half of the second part of the duodenum, the jejunum, the ileum, the cecum, the appendix, the ascending colon, and the proximal two-thirds of the transverse colon. The hindgut is composed of duplications of the distal third of the transverse colon, the descending and sigmoid colon, the rectum, the anus, and components of the urological system. In one series, 39% of duplications involved the foregut, whereas 61% represented duplications of both midgut and hindgut.[5]

Partial twinning

Certain duplications appear to represent partial twinning, particularly the tubular duplications of the terminal ileum and colon.[6-10] There is a wide spectrum of abnormalities, from complete twinning of the lower trunk and extremities to mere doubling of the lumen of hindgut structures. These lesions are often associated with duplication of the lower urinary tract.[11-13] Many rare examples of abortive cephalic twinning have also been described.[14] When there is complete doubling of the colon, one or both lumens may open as a fistula into the perineum or into the genitourinary (GU) tract and may be associated with an imperforate anus. Doubling of the anus, vagina, and bladder have all been detailed and often can be associated with other severe deformities, such as double spines or two heads.

Split notochord

The most satisfactory of several theories of the origin of GI duplications is that relating to the development of the neurenteric canal. Saunders,[15] in 1943, noted that thoracic duplications are frequently associated with abnormalities of the cervical and thoracic vertebrae. These duplications may be attached to the vertebral bodies or connected to the spinal canal. These findings gave rise to the Bentley and Smith *split-notochord theory*.[16-18] The embryo initially has two layers: ectoderm and endoderm. Mesoderm forms between the two, but for a short time, these two layers remain adherent. A transient opening (the notochordal plate) appears, connecting the neural ectoderm with the intestinal endoderm. This notochordal plate normally migrates dorsally and becomes "pinched" off from the endoderm by the ingrowth of mesodermal cells from each side. If the notochordal plate fails to migrate as a result of adhesions to the endodermal lining, the spinal canal cannot close ventrally, and a tract resembling a diverticulum is established with the primitive gut. This tract may remain open, leaving a fistula between the gut and the spinal canal, or close, leaving only a fibrous tract. However, in the majority of cases, it disappears completely, leaving only the duplication of the GI tract. This theory explains the formation of thoracic and caudal duplications, which may be associated with vertebral anomalies. However, the absence of spinal defects in many alimentary tract duplications makes this theory less tenable as a unifying model of their origin.

Embryonic diverticula and recanalization defects

In a study on human (4–23 mm) and animal embryos, Lewis and Thyng[19] found tiny bands of intestinal epithelium protruding into the subepithelial connective tissue. The identification of numerous diverticula in the intestines of embryos led to the proposal of an extension of the diverticula into duplications. The frequent ileal position of these diverticula is congruous with the frequent ileal location of human GI duplications. Although this theory could explain duplications in the absence of spinal anomalies, it fails to account for the variability of the mucosal lining and specifically for the frequency of heterotopic gastric mucosa. Furthermore, the diverticula identified in this pathological series were located throughout the bowel circumference as opposed to the general locations of duplications on the mesenteric side of the intestine.

The occurrence of tubular duplications would also not be explained by this theory (Figure 62.1). Bremer[20] believed that abnormal recanalization of the intestinal lumen after the solid stage of development of the primitive gut in the sixth to seventh week of gestation resulted in duplications.[21] Such duplications, however, would not be confined to the mesenteric side of the bowel. Also opposing this theory is the finding that the solid stage of development in the human does not usually extend beyond the duodenum.[21]

In 1961, Mellish and Koop[22] proposed an environmental theory, which held that trauma or hypoxia could induce duplications and twinning in lower orders. Based on the work of Louw,[23] they concluded that vascular insufficiency could lead to the recognized GI duplications seen in humans. In addition, intrauterine vascular accidents are known precipitators of other congenital anomalies, such as GI atresias.

PATHOLOGY

Duplications are hollow structures that involve the mesenteric side of the associated GI tract.[24] They tend to share a common muscular wall and blood supply with its mature bowel, although each has its own separate lining.[25] They are usually isolated lesions and are more often cystic than tubular, with a variable size. The lesions have a muscular coat in two layers and are usually lined with epithelium similar to that found in the associated portion of the alimentary tract.[7] The duplications, however, are occasionally lined with heterotopic epithelium; the presence of colonic mucosa has been described at the base of the tongue, and sinuses lined with gastric mucosa have been found near the anus.[26] Duplications containing gastric mucosa are at risk of peptic ulceration, perforation, and hemorrhage.[27] Patches of ectopic gastric mucosa along the GI tract may represent the mildest manifestation of duplication abnormalities. Ectopic pancreatic tissue has been reported in duplications of the stomach, ileum, and colon.[28,29] The contents of a duplication vary with the type of epithelial lining of the structure, the presence or absence of a communication with the proximate part of the GI tract, and the absence or necrosis of the duplication wall. If an opening is present, the duplication contents will be similar to those of the adjacent intestinal tract. Communication between the two structures is rare, and the cysts usually contain chyle or mucus. Multiple duplications can occur in the same patient.[26,30] There is an increased incidence of other associated anomalies such as vertebral anomalies,[31] myelomeningocele,[32] imperforate anus,[33] malrotation of the bowel,[34] genital anomalies,[30] polysplenic syndrome,[35] and duodenal atresia.[36] No genetic tendency has been demonstrated.

Malignant carcinomatous changes are rare complications of intestinal duplications. Adenocarcinomas arising from small bowel as well as large bowel duplication cysts have been reported in adult life.[37–40]

INCIDENCE

Duplications of the alimentary tract are rare. Table 62.1 summarizes the larger published series of duplications. In many cases, the numbers of patients reported represent up to 40 years' work in these centers. Only a small percentage of the total cases reported actually presented in the neonatal period.[28,40–44]

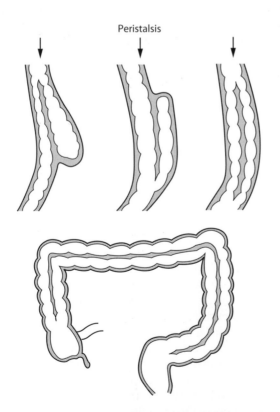

Figure 62.1 Various types of tubular duplications of the intestine.

Table 62.1 Incidence and locations of duplications

Author	Total no.	No. of neonates	Cervical	Mediastinal	Thoracoabdominal	Gastric	Duodenal	Jejunal–ileal	Colonic	Rectal
Gross[41]	68	20	1	13	3	2	4	32	9	4
Sieber[29]	25[a]	–	–	5	–	4	2	16	5	–
Grosfeld et a.[42]	20	–	–	4	–	1	–	9	4	–
Favara et al.[30]	37[b]	–	3	4	2	3	4	20	4	–
Wrenn[26]	22[c]	–	–	3	2	1	2	12	3	3
Lister[33]	32	24	–	3	–	1	–	20	5	3
Holcomb et al.[28]	96[d]	36	1	20	3	8	2	47	20	–

a One patient had two, one had three, and one had five duplications.
b One patient had three duplications.
c Two patients each had two duplications.
d Ninety-six patients had 106 atresias.

ESOPHAGEAL DUPLICATION

The esophagus is a relatively common site for foregut duplications (19%), with the majority being intramural, noncommunicating cystic structures related to the right side of the esophagus. Patients often present late in childhood as they cause relatively few symptoms; however, cervical esophageal duplications can cause significant respiratory distress requiring urgent surgery. Some lesions do not share a common wall with the esophagus and can be easily removed through open or minimally invasive techniques.[45] Plain x-rays may show an air- or fluid-filled structure adjacent to the esophagus, although this is not usually enough to confirm the diagnosis. Contrast studies can provide useful information regarding the mass effect of the lesion and whether or not their lumens communicate. Ultrasound and computed tomography (CT) are useful for establishing a diagnosis and also for ruling out multiple lesions, which can be present in 10%–20% of cases. Technetium scans (^{99m}Tc) may reveal the presence of heterotopic gastric mucosa in the case of GI bleeding.

Treatment

The surgical approach depends largely on the location of the cyst. Cervical esophageal duplications can be removed through a supraclavicular incision, with particular attention being paid to the vagus and phrenic nerves as well as the thoracic duct to avoid unnecessary damage. Intrathoracic duplications are resected through a standard posterolateral thoracotomy or a thoracoscopic approach.[46] A chest drain may be left *in situ* but is not always required.

THORACOABDOMINAL DUPLICATION

Thoracoabdominal duplications are rare, representing only 4% of all GI duplications. They often lie separate from the esophagus, more often on the right than the left side, but may be attached to other important structures, such as the aorta, azygous vein, and tracheobronchial tree. They frequently lie in the posterior mediastinum and pass through the diaphragm to communicate with the stomach, duodenum, or small bowel. The imaging studies employed are similar to those for esophageal duplications, with special attention being paid to imaging of the vertebral column/spinal cord for a possible intraspinal component. CT and/or magnetic resonance imaging (MRI) is particularly useful in this regard, especially if neurological symptoms of spinal cord compression or bony spinal abnormalities are present.

Treatment

These challenging duplications require resection of the thoracic and abdominal components through two different open procedures, or alternatively, they may be dealt with by a combined thoracolaparoscopic approach.[47]

Although the abdominal portions are often asymptomatic, the thoracic components can cause symptoms as a result of mass effect on the lungs and airway. The presence of gastric mucosa within the thoracic duplication cyst can lead to peptic ulceration and possible erosion into the lung parenchyma, presenting with hemoptysis. This complication may require a lobectomy. Once the lesion is mobilized in the thorax, it is freed from the posterior aspect of the diaphragm prior to mobilization and removal of the abdominal component.

GASTRIC DUPLICATION

The stomach is one of the less common sites of duplications, accounting for only 9% of all GI duplications. Over 60% of cases are diagnosed during the first year of life, with a significant number (40%) appearing in the neonatal period through the finding of a palpable cystic mass in the upper abdomen accompanied by vomiting and weight loss.[48,49] Rarely, they undergo peptic ulceration, and if the cyst communicates with the stomach, hematemesis and/or melena may be the presenting feature.[27] Rarely, a carcinoma may arise within a gastric duplication cyst.[50] Gastric outlet obstruction, mimicking hypertrophic pyloric stenosis, is also a common presenting feature of this duplication.[51] Gastric duplications occur twice as often in females as in males.[24] Gastric triplication, although rare, has been described in the literature.[52]

It is often difficult to make a preoperative diagnosis of gastric duplication. Plain x-rays are usually negative and therefore unhelpful. A contrast meal may show compression of the stomach, usually along the greater curvature. Contrast may delineate a connection between the stomach and duplication, but only in a small minority of cases. In these cases, contrast may be retained in the duplication long after the remainder has passed from the GI tract. Ultrasonography has been shown to be useful in the diagnosis of gastric duplications. The vast majority of gastric duplications are located in the greater curvature (Table 62.2). Occasionally, these are pedunculated,[32,53] but most are closed spherical cysts or tubular structures.

Associated anomalies occur in 3% of gastric duplications.[54] The most common is another cyst, usually of the esophagus.[55] Dual duplications of the stomach and pancreas have been reported.[56,57] These are thought to arise from an error in rotation of the ventral pancreatic anlage.

Table 62.2 Location of duplications of stomach in 87 reported cases

Location	No. of cases
Greater curvature	55
Lesser curvature	7
Anterior wall	9
Posterior wall	9
Others	7

Treatment

The management of gastric duplications is surgical because of the high incidence of complications due to obstruction, bleeding, or peritonitis. As most duplications occur in the greater curvature, a wedge of stomach is excised together with the cyst and the gap closed with a single layer of horizontal inverting mattress sutures (Figure 62.2). Partial gastrectomy should be avoided in children if possible, and if necessary, only 25%–30% of the stomach should be resected because of the associated long-term complications. When extensive resection of the adjoining stomach is impractical, as with the long tubular duplications of the greater curvature (Figure 62.3a), the main part of the duplication is excised and the mucosa stripped off (Figure 62.3b). The remaining seromuscular cuff can be sutured over the denuded area (Figure 62.3c) after checking that the common wall between the stomach and duplication has not been perforated, by insufflating the stomach with air. The use of a stapling gun to divide the common wall along the length of the greater curvature has also been described.[58]

PYLORIC DUPLICATION

True pyloric duplications are extremely rare, with very few being reported in the English literature and most of these presenting within the first week of life.[48,59–62] They simulate the symptoms and signs of hypertrophic pyloric stenosis.[63] Vomiting, weight loss, and a palpable abdominal mass are the main findings. There are certain physical features that are consistent with duplication: the mass is usually large and smooth, in contrast to the smaller and often more mobile "olive" mass in hypertrophic pyloric stenosis.[63]

Because of the nonspecific physical examination, radiographic procedures are essential for diagnosis. Plain film x-rays may show signs of gastric outlet or duodenal obstruction

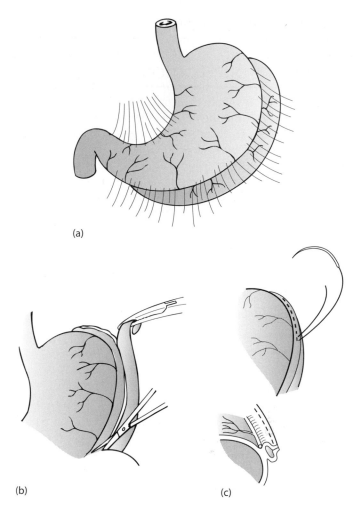

Figure 62.3 **(a)** Tubular duplication of the greater curvature of the stomach. **(b)** The mucosa is stripped from the entire length of the duplication. **(c)** The seromuscular cuff is closed over the denuded area.

with a lack of distal bowel gas,[64] or rarely, calcification within a cyst wall.[65] Ultrasonography may demonstrate an inner echogenic mucosal layer and outer hypoechoic muscular layer differentiating the duplication from a mesenteric cyst. Contrast studies may help differentiate the duplication from pyloric stenosis. If there is a clinical concern, then preoperative endoscopic retrograde cholangiopancreatography (ERCP), percutaneous transhepatic cholangiography (PTC), or magnetic resonance cholangiography/pancreatography (MRCP) should be performed to evaluate the involvement of the biliary/pancreatic ducts.

Treatment

Of the cases of pyloric duplication reported, the majority underwent simple surgical excision after opening the pyloric canal longitudinally. The pylorus was then closed transversely with no complications.[48,58,61] However, if there is a risk of damage to pancreatic or bile ducts an, acceptable

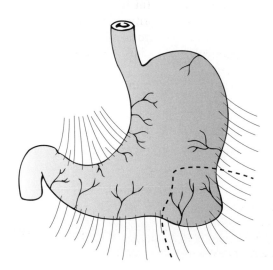

Figure 62.2 Gastric duplication located at the greater curvature. A wedge of stomach is excised together with the cyst and the gap closed with a single layer of horizontal inverted mattress sutures.

alternative is to drain the cyst into the duodenum or into a Roux limb of upper small bowel.

DUODENAL DUPLICATION

The duodenum is involved in only 4% of all duplications. They are often behind the duodenum and do not communicate with the bowel lumen.[66] Vomiting secondary to partial or complete duodenal obstruction and an upper abdominal mass are present in the majority of cases.[67] They may present with hematemesis or perforation, as gastric mucosa is present in 10%–15% of cases.[68] Alternatively, because of their location, they may present with biliary obstruction or pancreatitis. If the duplication is of sufficient size, it may appear on plain x-rays as a large opacity in the right side of the abdomen displacing the intestine (Figure 62.4a). Contrast studies will show the duodenum to be displaced upward and a beak-like projection due to compression of the duodenal lumen by the duplication (Figure 62.4b).[69] Contrast entering into the cyst confirms the presence of a luminal communication. Ultrasonography may show a cystic lesion below the liver and a classical double-layered appearance or *muscular rim* sign (Figure 62.5a).

Treatment

In view of the occasional occurrence of gastric mucosa in the duplication cyst, these lesions should, if possible, be dissected from the duodenum and excised, closing the resulting defect in the duodenum in two layers. Intraoperative

cholangiography will help determine the relationship of the cyst to the biliary and pancreatic ducts.[70]

If the lesion is extensive (Figure 62.5b), or if excision of the cyst may compromise the biliary system, then cystoduodenostomy may be performed.[71] The cyst may also be only partially excised, stripping off all the lining mucosa and leaving the part of the cyst that is adherent to the duodenum or pancreas.[70]

DUPLICATION OF THE SMALL BOWEL

Small bowel duplications constitute 45% of all alimentary tract duplications.[72] The vast majority of small bowel duplications are spherical cysts in the terminal ileum. Jejunal and ileal cysts are found on the mesenteric side of the bowel, sharing a common muscularis with the adjacent bowel. The mode of presentation depends on the site of the duplication, the mass effect of the lesion, and the presence of heterotopic gastric mucosa. They may cause obstruction by external pressure on the lumen,[73] by acting as a lead point for intussusception,[74,75] or occasionally by causing a volvulus or severe bleeding secondary to ulceration.[76]

Tubular duplications have the same features as the cystic variety, but they communicate with the normal lumen of the intestine and are more likely to contain gastric mucosa.[77] Pancreatic mucosa has also been described in these duplications. Tubular duplications can range in length from a few millimeters to the whole length of the small bowel.[78,79] The communication may be at the cephalad end, which will cause the duplication to become grossly distended with

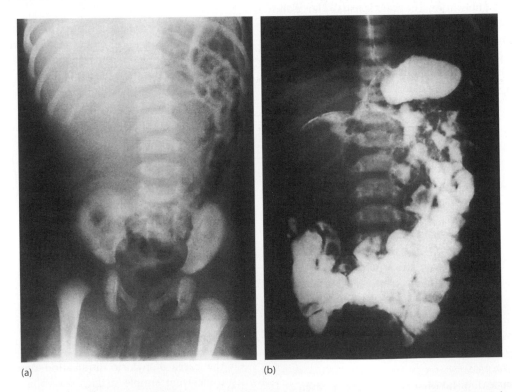

(a)   (b)

Figure 62.4 **(a)** Supine view in this 1-day-old baby showing a large soft tissue mass in the right upper and central abdomen displacing bowel loops to the left. **(b)** Barium study demonstrates beak-like projection of proximal duodenum superolaterally characteristic of duodenal duplication cyst.

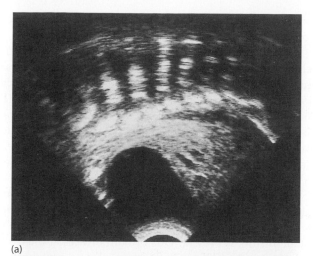

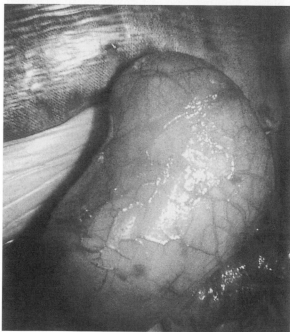

(a)

Figure 62.5 Duodenal duplication. **(a)** Ultrasound shows the cystic lesion below the liver. **(b)** Large duodenal duplication cyst.

intestinal contents, or at the caudal end, which will allow the duplication to drain freely. Communication at several different points may be present.

Hemorrhage occurs most often in tubular duplications, but perforation has been reported as well.[80,81] Plain abdominal x-rays may show nonspecific displacement of bowel gas shadows by the cyst, or signs of intestinal obstruction or perforation. Ultrasonography can help to differentiate between a mesenteric and a duplication cyst. A contrast meal may demonstrate displacement of the bowel (Figure 62.6).

Treatment

Cystic duplications are relatively straightforward to deal with. Resection of the cyst with adjacent bowel (Figure 62.7a) is performed; the two ends of the bowel are anastomosed

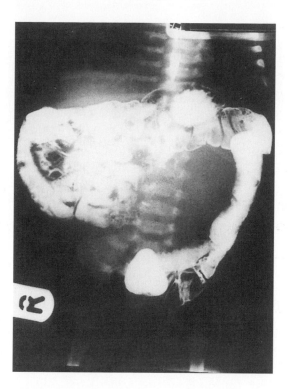

Figure 62.6 Barium study demonstrates a space-occupying lesion displacing bowel. At laparotomy, a large ileal duplication cyst was found.

with one layer of horizontal inverting mattress sutures, and the mesenteric defects are closed (Figure 62.7b).

Tubular duplications, if very short, can be resected as in a cystic lesion, but the majority involve a considerable length of small bowel, and much ingenuity and patience may be required to meet the needs of any one particular case.

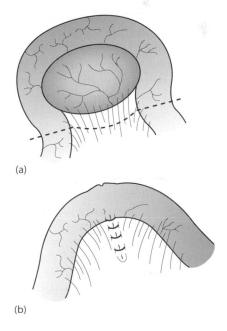

(a)

(b)

Figure 62.7 Cystic ileal duplication. **(a)** Resection of the cyst with adjacent bowel is performed. **(b)** The two ends of the bowel are anastomosed.

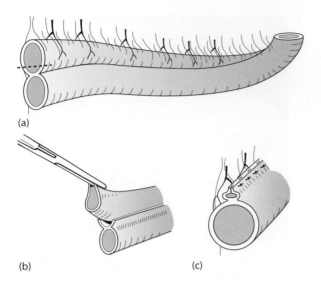

Figure 62.8 Tubular duplication of small bowel. **(a)** The main part of the tubular duplication is excised. **(b)** The mucosa is stripped from the entire length of the duplication. **(c)** The seromuscular cuff is closed over the denuded area.

Wrenn[82] suggested coring out the mucosal lining of a long tubular duplication through multiple seromuscular incisions in the wall of the duplication.

Norris et al.[83] employed a technique first described by Bianchi[84] for bowel lengthening, to separate two leashes of blood vessels passing to each side of the small intestine (Figure 62.8). Using this method, the entire mucosa and almost the entire muscle wall can be excised. The remaining cuff of muscle wall can be oversewn, preserving the blood supply to the normal bowel.

Bishop and Koop[85] described the techniques of anastomosing the distal end of the duplication to adjacent normal intestine, allowing free drainage of the contents. Malignant change in the mucosa has, however, been described as a late complication of this procedure.[86] Whichever technique is utilized, it is essential that the junction of normal and duplicated bowel is resected since heterotopic gastric mucosa is frequently present in tubular intestinal duplications.

COLONIC DUPLICATION

Colonic duplications are among the rarest reported. They are frequently diagnosed in infancy, and some reports suggest a female predilection. McPherson et al.[87] proposed a simple classification of colonic duplications: type I mesenteric cysts, type II diverticula, and the more common type III tubular colonic duplication. A number of etiological factors may be involved in the development of the "double colon." The most valid theory suggests division of the hindgut into two parts at a stage during which the anlage possesses a multiorgan developmental potential.[87,88] The hindgut anlage normally forms the distal ileum, colon, rectum, bladder, and urethra. Division of the anlage at the

same initial stage could therefore be responsible for duplication of the lower urinary tract as well.[87]

Simple cysts (type I) and diverticula (type II) occasionally result. They can be identified on plain x-rays or on contrast studies. A contrast enema may demonstrate a communication between the colon and duplications in types II and III. Associated GU and lumbosacral spinal abnormalities can also be demonstrated on the appropriate radiographic studies, particularly when dealing with type III duplications. Isotope scans are rarely of benefit with colonic duplications, as they contain only colonic mucosa.

Complete duplication of the colon is usually asymptomatic in the neonatal period unless duplication of the anus or an abnormal orifice, in addition to the normal orifice in the perineum, is present. One or both orifices at the distal end of the colon may end as rectovaginal or rectourethral fistulas.[88]

Treatment

Surgery for colonic duplication is rarely indicated in the neonatal period unless there are complications, e.g., obstruction or an associated imperforate anus. All cystic and most tubular colonic duplications can be dealt with by simple resection and anastomosis utilizing a single-layer extramucosal technique. With rare total colonic duplication, the principal aim of management is to end up with two colons draining through one anal orifice. If one part of the colon has already reached the perineum, then the other colon is divided and anatomosed to its partner. This can be achieved by using a linear stapling device. If neither colon reaches the perineum, then a formal pull-through procedure will be required. Neonatal management in any of these situations is confined to fashioning a defunctioning colostomy to drain both colons.

RECTAL DUPLICATION

Rectal duplications have now been reported in the literature, comprising only 5% of all GI duplications. More than 50% of these are examples of hindgut twinning.[89]

The embryogenesis of rectal duplication cysts is attributed to a pinching off of a diverticulum in the 20–30 mm embryo,[90] in contrast to the "caudal twinning" that occurs in the 10 mm embryo and is associated with complex hindgut anomalies.[91,92]

Rectal duplications often present in the neonatal period with a fistula or perineal mucosal swelling extending to the perianal area. Presentation of the cysts depends on the following: (1) size and their mass effect, (2) fistulas,[93] (3) infection, (4) ulceration if they contain gastric mucosa, and (5) malignancy.[94] The duplication cyst usually forms in the retrorectal space and contains colorless mucus, which can become infected. It frequently presents in 20%–45% of cases.[89,90] No cases of a fistula between the rectum and urinary tract have been described. Malignant degeneration has been reported in the rectal duplication from the fourth decade onward.[95,96]

Treatment

Treatment of the rectal duplication cyst is surgical excision or fenestration of the common wall. Depending on the anatomical variations, a transanal or transcoccygeal (Kraske) approach can be employed. For longer or more complicated cysts, a longer posterior sagittal incision will provide better exposure. As with other duplications, it is of prime importance to remove all mucosa in the duplication. The muscularis can be left *in situ*.

Associated anomalies such as presacral tumors (16%) and anorectal malformations (21%) are frequently described in the literature.[97] Management of these lesions may be difficult and often requires preoperative evaluation of both the GI and GU tracts. Continence of both systems is imperative, and therefore, treatment strategies must be individualized based on the findings of each patient.

It is clear that duplications of the GI tract represent a diverse and complex group of anomalies. Small duplications in readily accessible areas (i.e., the small intestine) may be excised with adjacent bowel. In other locations, where resection would endanger adjacent structures, simple anastomosis between the cyst and normal intestine can be performed, provided that there is no gastric mucosa in the cyst. If bleeding has been a persisting complaint, the presence of gastric mucosa can be assumed. If resection is contraindicated, the lining mucosa may be stripped from the cyst, leaving the muscle wall *in situ*.

REFERENCES

1. Stern LE, Warner BW. Gastrointestinal duplications. *Semin Pediatr Surg* 2000; 9: 135–40.
2. Chen JJ, Lee HC, Yeung CY, Chan WT, Jiang CB, Sheu JC. Meta-analysis: The clinical features of the duodenal duplication cyst. *J Pediatr Surg* 2010; 45(8): 1598–606.
3. Bhat NA, Agarwala S, Mitra DK, Bhatnagar V. Duplications of the alimentary tract in children. *Trop Gastroenterol* 2001; 22: 33–5.
4. Ladd WE. Duplications of the alimentary tract. *South Med J* 1937; 30: 363–71.
5. Ildstad ST, Tollerud DJ, Weiss RG et al. Duplications of the alimentary tract. Clinical characteristics, preferred treatment, and associated malformations. *Ann Surg* 1988; 208: 184–9.
6. Grey SW, Skandalakis JE. *Embryology for Surgeons.* Philadelphia: WB Saunders, 1972: 174.
7. Lund DP. Almentary tract duplications. In: Coran AG (ed). *Pediatric Surgery.* 7th ed. USA: Elsevier, 2012: 1155.
8. Brunschwig A, Dargeon HW, Russell WA. Duplications of the intra colon and lower ileum with termination of one colon into a vaginal anus. *Surgery* 1948; 24: 1010–2.
9. Ravitch MM. Hindgut duplications; doubling of the colon and genital urinary tracts. *Ann Surg* 1953; 137: 294–8.
10. Rowe MI, Ravitch MM, Ranniger K. Operative correction of caudal duplication (dipygus). *Surgery* 1968; 63: 840–8.
11. Smith ED. Duplication of the anus and genital tract. *Surgery* 1969; 66: 909–21.
12. Ravitch MM, Scott WW. Duplication of the entire colon bladder and urethra. *Surgery* 1953; 34: 843–58.
13. McPherson AE, Trapnell JE, Airth GR. Duplication of the colon. *Br J Surg* 1969; 56: 138–9.
14. Dykes EH, Kelleher J, Fogarty EE et al. Surgical treatment of a variant of dipygus. *Pediatr Surg Int* 1988; 3: 200–2.
15. Saunders RL. Combined anterior and posterior spina bifida in a living neonatal human female. *Anat Rec* 1943; 87: 255–75.
16. Bentley JFR, Smith JR. Developmental posterior enteric remnants and spinal malformations: The split notochord syndrome. *Arch Dis Child* 1960; 35: 76–86.
17. Mirza B, Sheikh A. Split notochord syndrome with neuroenteric fistula. *J Pediatr Neurosci* 2011 January; 6(1): 87–8.
18. Fallon M, Gordon ARC, Lendrim AC. Mediastinal cysts of foregut origin associated with vertebral anomalies. *Br J Surg* 1954; 41: 520–3.
19. Lewis FT, Thyng FW. The regular occurrence of intestinal diverticula in embryos of the pig, rabbit and man. *Am J Anat* 1970; 7: 505–19.
20. Bremer JL. Diverticula and duplications of the intestinal tract. *Arch Pathol* 1944; 38: 132–40.
21. Sandler J. Zur Entwicklung des Menschilichen duodenums in Fruhen Embryonalstadium. *Morph Jahrb* 1902; 29: 187.
22. Mellish RWP, Koop CE. Clinical manifestations of duplication of the bowel. *Pediatrics* 1961; 27: 397–407.
23. Louw JH. Congenital atresia and stenosis in the newborn. *Ann Roy Coll Surg Engl* 1959; 25: 209.
24. Ladd WE, Gross RE. Surgical treatment of duplications of the alimentary tract. *Surg Gynecol Obstet* 1940; 70: 295–307.
25. Smith JR. Accessory enteric formations: Classification and nomenclature. *Arch Dis Child* 1960; 35: 87–9.
26. Wrenn E. Alimentary tract duplications. In: Holder T, Ashcraft K (eds). *Pediatric Surgery.* Philadelphia: WB Saunders, 1992: 455–6.
27. Srikanth KP, Thapa BR, Lal SB, Menon P, Sodhi K, Vaiphei K, Rao KL. Noncommunicating gastric antral duplication cyst presenting with hematemesis due to large antral ulcer. *Trop Gastroenterol* 2015 April–June; 36(2): 134–6.
28. Holcomb GW, Gheisser A, O'Neill J et al. Surgical management of alimentary tract duplications. *Ann Surg* 1989; 209: 167–74.
29. Kobara H, Mori H, Masaki T. A gastric duplication cyst with heterotopic pancreas and ectopic submucosal gland on submucosal endoscopy. *Dig Endosc* 2015 December 22; 28(2): 223.

30. Favara BE, Franciosi RA, Akers DR. Enteric duplications: 37 cases—A vascular theory of pathogenesis. *Am J Dis Child* 1971; 122: 501–6.

31. Kremer RM, Lepoff RB, Izamt RJ. Duplication of the stomach. *J Pediatr Surg* 1970; 5: 360–4.

32. Carachi R. The split notochord syndrome: A case report on a mixed spinal enterogenous cyst in a child with spina bifida cystica. *Z Kinderchir* 1982; 35: 32–4.

33. Lister J, Zachary RB. Cystic duplication of tongue. *J Pediatr Surg* 1968; 3: 491–3.

34. Sherman NJ, Marrow D, Asch M. A triple duplication of the alimentary tract. *J Pediatr Surg* 1978; 13: 187–8.

35. Paddock RJ, Arensman RM. Polysplenic syndrome: Spectrum of gastro-intestinal anomalies. *J Pediatr Surg* 1982; 17: 563–6.

36. Soon OC, Woo HP. Duodenal duplication cyst associated with duodenal atresia. *Pediatr Surg Int* 1995; 10: 167–8.

37. Hsu H, Gueng MK, Tseng YH et al. Adenocarcinoma arising from colonic duplication cyst with metastasis to omentum: A case report. *J Clin Ultrasound* 2011; 39: 41–3.

38. Kim TH, Kim JK, Jang EH et al. Papillary adenocarcinoma arising in a tubular duplication of the jejunum. *Br J Radiol* 2010; 83: e61–4.

39. de Tullio D, Rinaldi R, Pellegrini D et al. Adenocarcinoma arising in an elderly patient's large ileal duplication. *Int J Surg Pathol* 2011; 19(5): 681–4.

40. Beltrán MA, Barría C, Contreras MA, Wilson CS, Cruces KS. Adenocarcinoma and intestinal duplication of the ileum. Report of one case. *Rev Med Chil* 2009; 137: 1341–5.

41. Gross RE. *The Surgery of Infancy and Childhood.* Philadelphia: WB Saunders, 1953: 221–45.

42. Grosfeld JL, O'Neill A, Clatworthy HW. Enteric duplications in infancy and childhood. *Ann Surg* 1970; 132: 83–6.

43. Stringer MD, Spitz L, Abel R et al. Management of alimentary tract duplications in children. *Br J Surg* 1995; 82: 74–8.

44. Iyer CP, Mahour GH. Duplications of the alimentary tract in infants and children. *Pediatr Surg* 1995; 30: 1267–70.

45. Perger L, Azzie G, Watch L, Weinsheimer R. Two cases of thoracoscopic resection of esophageal duplication in children. *J Laparoendosc Adv Surg Tech A* 2006; 16: 418–21.

46. Bratu I, Laberge JM, Flageole H, Bouchard S. Foregut duplications: Is there an advantage to thoracoscopic resection? *J Pediatr Surg* 2005; 40: 138–41.

47. Martinez-Ferro M, Laje P, Piaggio L. Combined thoraco-laparoscopy for trans-diaphragmatic thoraco-abdominal enteric duplications. *J Pediatr Surg* 2005; 40: e37–40.

48. Abrami G, Dennison WM. Duplication of the stomach. *Surgery* 1961; 49: 794–801.

49. Susan J, Pradeep JN, Tarun JJ et al. Enteric duplication in children: Experience from a tertiary center in South India. *J Indian Assoc Pediatr Surg* 2015 October–December; 20(4): 174–8.

50. Pruksapong C, Donovan RJ, Pinit A et al. Gastric duplication. *J Pediatr Surg* 1979; 14: 83–5.

51. Alschibaja T, Putram TC, Yabhin BA. Duplication of the stomach simulating hypertrophic pyloric stenosis. *Am J Dis Child* 1974; 127: 120–2.

52. Queizán A, Hernandez F, Rivas S, Herrero F. Prenatal diagnosis of gastric triplication. *Eur J Pediatr Surg* 2006; 16: 52–4.

53. Shepphard MD, Gilmour JR. Torsion of a pedunculated gastric cyst. *Br Med J* 1945; 1: 874–5.

54. Torma MJ. Of double stomachs. *Arch Surg* 1974; 109: 555–6.

55. Soundararajan S, Subramaniam TK. Gastropancreatic duplications. *Pediatr Surg Int* 1988; 4: 288–9.

56. Cloutier R. Pseudocyst of pancreas secondary to gastric duplication. *J Pediatr Surg* 1973; 8: 67.

57. Siddiqui AM, Shamberger RC, Filler RM et al. Enteric duplications of the pancreatic head: Definitive management by local resection. *J Pediatr Surg* 1998; 33: 1117–20.

58. Sammarai AI, Crankson SJ, Sadiq A. The use of mechanical sutures in the treatment of gastric duplications. *Z Kinderchir* 1989; 44: 186–7.

59. Langer JC, Superina RF, Payton D. Pyloric duplication presenting with gastric outlet obstruction in the newborn period. *Pediatr Surg Int* 1988; 4: 63–5.

60. Bamimen M, Singh MP. Pyloric duplications in a preterm neonate. *J Pediatr Surg* 1984; 19: 158–9.

61. Grosfeld JC, Boles ET, Reiner C. Duplication of the pylorus in the newborn: A rare cause of gastric outlet obstruction. *J Pediatr Surg* 1970; 5: 365–9.

62. Trainavicius K, Gurskas P, Povilavicius J. Duplication cyst of the pylorus: A case report. *J Med Case Rep* 2013; 7: 175.

63. Ramsey GS. Enterogenous cyst of the stomach simulating pyloric stenosis. *Br J Surg* 1957; 44: 632–3.

64. Tihansky DP, Sukarochana K, Hanrahan JB. Pyloroduodenal duplication cyst. *Am J Gastroenterol* 1986; 81: 189–91.

65. Sieunarine K, Manmohansingh E. Gastric duplication cyst presenting as an acute abdomen in a child. *J Pediatr Surg* 1989; 24: 1152.

66. Alfred BA, Armstrong P, Franken FA et al. Calcification associated with duodenal duplications in children. *Radiology* 1980; 134: 647–8.

67. Merrot T, Anastasescu R, Pankevych T et al. Duodenal duplications. Clinical characteristics, embryological hypotheses, histological findings, treatment. *Eur J Pediatr Surg* 2006; 16: 18–23.

68. Bower RJ, Sieber WK, Kiesewetter WB. Alimentary tract duplication in children. *Ann Surg* 1978; 188: 669–71.

69. Blake NS. Beak sign in duodenal duplication cyst. *Pediatr Radiol* 1984; 14: 232–3.

70. Byun J, Oh HM, Kim SH et al. Laparoscopic partial cystectomy with mucosal stripping of extraluminal duodenal duplication cysts. *World J Gastroenterol* 2014; 20(4): 1123–6.

71. Gardner CK, Hart J. Enterogenous cysts of the duodenum. *J Am Med Assoc* 1935; 104: 1809–12.

72. Stringer MD. Duplications of the alimentary tract. In: Spitz L, Coran AG (eds). *Operative Surgery*, 5th ed. London: Chapman & Hall, 1995: 383–95.

73. Ravitch MM. Duplications of the alimentary canal. In: Mustar WY, Ravitch MM, Snyder WH et al. (eds). *Pediatric Surgery*. Chicago: Year Book Medical Publishers, 1979: 831–40.

74. Daniss RK, Graviss ER. Jejunal intraluminal diverticular duplication with recurrent intussusception. *J Pediatr Surg* 1982; 17: 84–5.

75. Howanietz C, Lachmann D, Remes I. Volvulus as a rare complication of enterogenous cyst in newborns. *Z Kinderchir* 1969; 6: 48.

76. Wardell S, Vidican DE. Ileal duplication causing massive bleeding in a child. *J Clin Gastroenterol* 1991; 12: 681–4.

77. Lange P. Abdominal cysts and duplications. In: Mattei P. (ed). *Fundamentals of Pediatric Surgery*. Chapter 7. New York: Springer, 2011: 365–71.

78. Schwartz BC, Becker JM, Schneider KM et al. Tubular duplication with autonomous blood supply: Resection with preservation of adjacent bowel. *J Pediatr Surg* 1980; 15: 341–2.

79. Balen EM, Hernandez-Lizvain JL, Pardo F, Longo JM. Giant jejunoileal duplication: Prenatal diagnosis and complete excision without intestinal resection. *J Pediatr Surg* 1993; 28: 1586–8.

80. Doyle SG, Doig CM. Perforation of the jejunum secondary to a duplication cyst lined with ectopic gastric mucosa. *J Pediatr Surg* 1988; 23: 1025–6.

81. Dias AR, Lopes RI, do Couto RC et al. Ileal duplication causing recurrent intussusception. *J Surg Educ* 2007; 64: 51–3.

82. Wrenn E. Tubular duplication of the small intestine. *Surgery* 1962; 52: 494–8.

83. Norris R, Bereton R, Wright V et al. A new surgical approach to duplications of the intestine. *J Pediatr Surg* 1986; 21: 167–9.

84. Bianchi A. Intestinal loop lengthening—A technique for increasing small bowel length. *J Pediatr Surg* 1982; 15: 145–51.

85. Bishop HE, Koop CE. Surgical management of duplication of the alimentary tract. *Am J Surg* 1964; 107: 434–42.

86. Orr MM, Edwards AJ. Neoplastic change in duplications of the alimentary tract. *Br J Surg* 1975; 62: 269–74.

87. McPherson AG, Trapnell JE, Airth GR. Duplications of the colon. *Br J Surg* 1969; 56: 138–46.

88. Kettre JJ, Davido WT. Duplication of the large bowel. *AJR Am J Roentgenol* 1971; 113: 310–5.

89. La Quaglia MP, Fains W, Eraklis A et al. Rectal duplications. *J Pediatr Surg* 1990; 25: 980–4.

90. Ravitch MM. Hindgut duplication—Doubling of the colon and genitourinary tracts. *Ann Surg* 1953; 137: 588–601.

91. Edwards H. Congenital duplication of the intestine. *Br J Surg* 1929; 17: 7–21.

92. Van Zwalenburg RR. Double colon differentiation of cases into two groups. *AJR Am J Roentgenol* 1956; 75: 349–53.

93. Pampal A, Ozbayoglu A, Kaya et al. Rectal duplications accompanying rectovestibular fistula: Report of two cases. *Pediatr Int* 2013 August; 55(4): e86–9.

94. Kroft RO. Rectal duplications accompanying rectovestibular fistula: Report of two cases. Duplication anomalies of the rectum. *Ann Surg* 1961; 155: 230–2.

95. Ballantyne EW. Sacrococcygeal tumours. Adenocarcinoma of a cystic congenital embryonal remnant. *Arch Pathol* 1932; 14: 1–9.

96. Crowley LW, Page HG. Adenocarcinoma arising in presacral enterogenous cyst. *Arch Pathol* 1960; 69: 65–6.

96. Jasquier C, Dobremez E, Piolat C et al. Anal canal duplication in infants and children—A series of 6 cases. *Eur J Pediatr Surg* 2001; 11: 186–91.

63

Mesenteric and omental cysts

BENNO URE AND CHRISTOPH ZOELLER

INTRODUCTION

The first report on a mesenteric cyst was published by an Italian anatomist in 1507.[1] Since then, the origin and classification of mesenteric and omental cysts have been a matter of debate. Moynihan[2] attempted in 1897 a differentiation of abdominal cysts on the basis of fluid content. Serous cysts are characterized by a translucent, straw-colored fluid of low specific gravity. Their chemical composition is similar to plasma. In contrast, chylous cysts contain an opaque fluid of high specific gravity, with lipids and fat globules contributing to the fluid content. Subsequent attempts at a more appropriate classification of intra-abdominal cysts have been based on suspected etiology initially proposed by Beahrs in 1950.[3] However, the etiology of many intra-abdominal cysts is questionable, rendering classifications of this type of limited clinical usefulness. A more appropriate classification, based on histologic findings, was proposed in 1987 by Ros et al.[4] This differentiation is applicable to all operative cases and can provide the basis for a more uniform evaluation of the clinical and pathologic characteristics of these cysts (Table 63.1).

Until today, the terminology is still descriptive of anatomic location without information as to the specific histology or pathology of mesenteric, mesothelial, or omental cysts. Several authors suggested differentiating cystic lymphangiomas from mesenteric and omental cysts.[5,6] A lymphangioma wall shows endothelial cells, small lymphatic spaces, lymphoid tissue, and smooth muscle cells. Mesenteric cysts do not have lymphatic spaces and smooth muscles, and the cells of their walls are cuboidal or columnar (Table 63.2).[5] All these cystic lesions are generally of isolated pathology, with few reports of associated developmental anomalies.

The incidence of mesenteric and omental cysts is rare and has not been systematically determined in the general population. Large reviews have indicated a male predominance.[7]

SPECTRUM AND MORPHOLOGY

Lymphangiomas represent approximately 90% of the cysts encountered in the mesenterium and omentum of the neonate. They are characterized by multiple thin-walled cystic spaces with a distinct endothelial lining similar to that seen in the subcutaneous location. These lesions are presumed to be congenital, with an etiology secondary to proliferating lymphatic tissue without access to adequate drainage. Lymphangiomas appear most frequently in the mesentery of the small bowel and may be encountered in the mesocolon and omentum. Extension to the retroperitoneum has been frequently described.[7,8] Gross, solitary, multiloculated, fluid-containing cysts are encountered, which can reach an enormous size (Figure 63.1). The fluid may be serous or chylous, with chyle being characteristic of a small bowel location and the associated high lymphatic fat content. Hemorrhagic fluid is not uncommon.

Mesothelial cysts are less common but represent the majority of nonlymphangiomatous congenital cysts encountered in the omentum (Figure 63.2). They may also occur within the mesentery. Mesothelial cysts are generally unilocular, serous-containing, and lined by mesothelium. They are thought to arise from incomplete fusion of the mesothelial leaves of the omentum or mesentery.

Enteric duplication cysts are not included under the heading of mesenteric cysts but should be mentioned due to their frequent neonatal presentation, mesenteric location, and occasional similarity in appearance. Therefore, they should be included in the differential diagnosis of intra-abdominal cystic lesions in the neonate. These cysts may occur anywhere along the gastrointestinal tract as saccular or tubular unilocular lesions, usually within the mesentery adjacent to a normal intestine (Figure 63.3). Histologically, they are composed of all the layers seen in normal intestine, and they share a common blood supply with the adjacent intestine. Duplication cysts may contain mucus-producing cells.

Table 63.1 Classification of abdominal cysts[1,6,12]

Embryonic/ developmental	Enteric
	Urogenital
	Dermoid
	Embryonic defects of lymphatics (retroperitoneal, mesenteric, and omental cysts)
Traumatic/acquired	Hemorrhagic (sanguinous)
	Ruptured lacteal
	Chylous extravasation
Neoplastic	Benign (lymphangioma)
	Malignant (lymphangioendothelioma)
Infectious	Mycotic
	Parasitic
	Tuberculous
	Hydatid
	Cystic degeneration

Table 63.2 Histologic classification of mesenteric/ omental cysts[13]

Enteric cyst:	Enteric lining
	No muscle layer
Enteric duplication:	Enteric lining
	Double muscle layer with neural elements
Lymphangioma:	Endothelial lining
Mesothelial cyst:	Mesothelial lining
Pseudocyst:	No lining
(nonpancreatic)	Fibrous wall

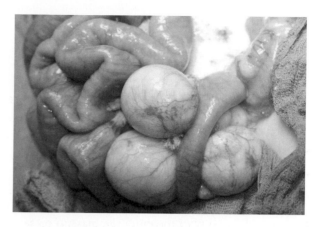

Figure 63.2 Chylous mesenteric cysts.

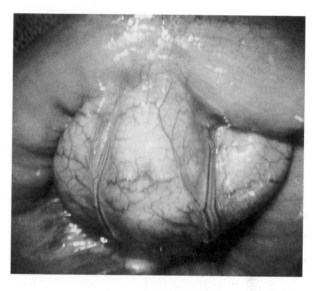

Figure 63.3 Saccular intestinal duplication simulating the appearance of a mesenteric cyst. Lesion distinguished grossly by common wall and blood supply shared with adjacent intestine.

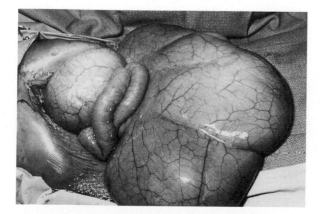

Figure 63.1 Chylous mesenteric lymphangioma.

CLINICAL CHARACTERISTICS

The cysts may be diagnosed in utero with the use of routine prenatal ultrasonography.[19] However, most series report mean ages of 3–5 years at presentation,[10–12] and the age at diagnosis has gradually decreased over the years. Omental and mesenteric cysts may be an incidental finding, but more than half of these children present with acute clinical problems.

The symptoms of mesenteric or omental cysts are related to mechanical forces due to cyst location and size. The majority of children present with abdominal complaints, such as pain, vomiting, and distension (Table 63.3). Several authors have suggested that the high incidence of symptoms in children versus adults may be related to the higher incidence of lymphangiomas in young individuals.[7,8] A palpable

Table 63.3 Clinical presentation[1–4,5,6,7,10–13,18] (281 children)

Pain	41%
Mass	35%
Obstruction	32%
Distension	25%
Miscellaneous[a]	23%

[a] Failure to thrive, nausea, gastrointestinal bleeding, diarrhea, etc.

mass is the most common physical finding, but this may be apparent in only 60% of affected children due to the flaccidity and mobility of the cyst. The mass, if present, is generally smooth, tender, and mobile in character. Of the affected children, 50% or more will present with complications. Intestinal obstruction, either partial or complete, is frequent and usually due to compression of the adjacent intestine. Volvulus can occur around the cyst and result in infarction of the bowel with perforation, peritonitis, and shock.[13] Hemorrhage within the cyst secondary to expansion or erosion may lead to rapid enlargement and pain as well as anemia.[14,15] Torsion of the cyst itself, rupture, and urinary obstruction have been reported.[14,16]

DIAGNOSIS

In most cases, a definitive preoperative diagnosis is not possible. Laboratory evaluation is pertinent only to complications that may be associated with the cyst. Sonography is the most useful diagnostic modality and represents the imaging technique of choice. The lesions appear as a well-defined, hypoechoic to anechoic smooth-walled mass, with echogenicity related to the cyst contents. In lymphangiomas, multiple thin septae may be apparent (Figure 63.4).

Computer tomography (CT) or magnetic resonance imaging (MRI) may be used in the differential diagnosis of these lesions. They frequently demonstrate a fluid-filled mass, but the thin septae, diagnostic of lymphangioma, may not be apparent. Ros et al.[4] suggested that a lymphangioma is usually a multiloculated cyst that shows no discernible wall on CT and that may have characteristics of fat. A basic radiograph of the abdomen is not routinely indicated and may demonstrate a mass, "ascites," or evidence of intestinal obstruction. Contrast radiography is rarely useful and may evidence a mass effect with varying degrees of compression of normal bowel in mesenteric cysts.

DIFFERENTIAL DIAGNOSIS

Other intra-abdominal lesions sometimes difficult to distinguish from a mesenteric or omental cyst mostly include ovarian cysts, choledochal cysts, pancreatic cysts, splenic cysts, renal cysts, hydronephrosis, cystic teratoma, dermoid cysts, hydatid cysts, and enteric duplication. The majority of these can be differentiated preoperatively by sonography and/or CT. Enteric duplication cysts have a thick wall and a

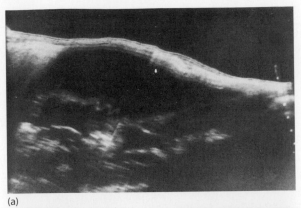

(a)

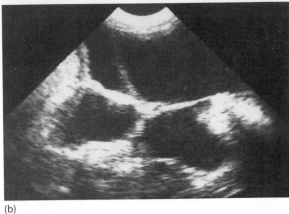

(b)

Figure 63.4 **(a)** Longitudinal and **(b)** transverse abdominal ultrasound of a child with a large omental lymphangioma demonstrating a hypoechoic, septated mass immediately beneath the anterior abdominal wall.

common muscular wall with the adjacent bowel. A mucosal line may be visible on sonography.

Large cysts may mimic ascites in the neonate. Unless the ascites is loculated, shifting will occur with movement, and the bowel will flow centrally as opposed to in the lateral dislocation associated with mesenteric or omental cysts.

Remaining lesions commonly referred to as mesenteric and/or omental cysts are nonpancreatic pseudocysts with no distinct cellular lining. They are seldom encountered in the neonate and are secondary to inflammation or trauma. Because of this etiology, the contained fluid may be hemorrhagic or purulent. A nonpancreatic pseudocyst is usually a unilocular or multilocular cyst with abundant debris sonographically and an enhancing wall on CT. An enteric duplication cyst is a unilocular cyst but also with an enhancing wall.

TREATMENT

Preoperatively, the diagnosis may be in doubt, and parents have to be informed that management may require intestinal resection. Routine mechanical bowel preparation and intraoperative bladder catheterization are not required. Routine broad-spectrum antibiotics are only administered in cases with bacterial contamination, i.e., bowel resection.

In recent years, minimally invasive techniques have been suggested for the management of cystic abdominal masses and alimentary duplications.[17,18] The initial aim of laparoscopy is to locate the cyst and to determine its nature. The patient is placed in a supine position, and the surgeon, camera assistant, and monitor are placed in line. The optimal position of the ports is determined after exploration of the abdominal cavity via the first umbilical trocar. Mesenteric and omental cysts can be resected laparoscopically, but the location and fragility of the cyst wall may interfere with the feasibility of laparoscopy. Intraoperative aspiration of the cyst and subsequent analysis prior to removal are not indicated unless there is a question of biliary or pancreatic origin. Large cysts may be punctured to reduce the size and improve exposition, but this may make dissection more difficult. Management options include enucleation or resection. If any obvious plane exists between the cyst and the adjacent bowel wall, enucleation should be undertaken. In cases requiring a limited resection of bowel, the cyst and affected loop are exteriorized via the umbilical approach, and the resection and anastomosis are performed outside the abdominal cavity. Alternatively, a transverse mini-laparotomy may be used after the optimal location has been determined by laparoscopy.

The conventional operation is performed via a supraumbilical transverse approach. Omental cysts are generally immediately apparent upon entering the peritoneal cavity. They present as large, translucent, solitary fluid-filled sacs overlying the bowel. The omentum and associated cyst is gently withdrawn from the abdomen and placed on the abdominal wall. The cyst may then be easily removed by transection at the junction with normal omentum or transverse colon (Figure 63.5). Care should be taken to ligate the numerous omental vessels at the level of the transection. Larger mesenteric cysts may also be apparent upon opening the peritoneal cavity or, if they are smaller, require exploration. Once localized, the area of involvement is mobilized

and eviscerated and the remaining bowel secured with sponges to facilitate exposure and resection (Figure 63.6).

If any obvious plane exists between the cyst and adjacent bowel wall, enucleation should be undertaken. In larger cysts, enucleation may require incision on both sides of the mesentery. Generally, a plane of loose areolar tissue is present, enabling mobilization. This may be facilitated with gentle downward traction on the cyst wall (Figure 63.7). Dissection is continued circumferentially until the cyst can be totally enucleated (Figure 63.8). Following enucleation,

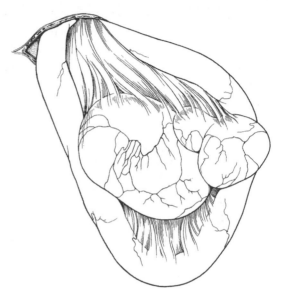

Figure 63.6 A mesenteric cyst amenable to removal without intestinal resection.

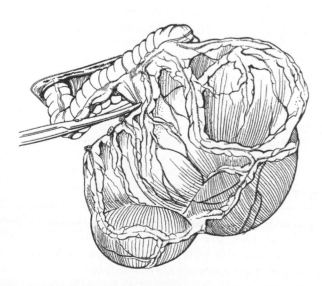

Figure 63.5 Removal of omental cyst by transection of the omentum at the transverse colon.

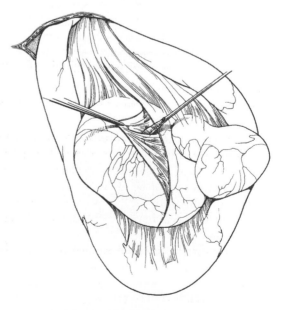

Figure 63.7 Gentle dissection of the mesenteric leaf overlying the cyst.

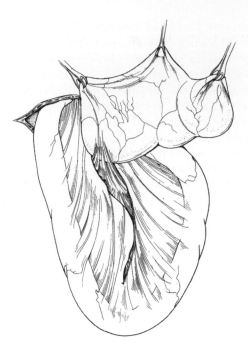

Figure 63.8 Removal of the mesenteric cyst from between the leaves of the mesentery.

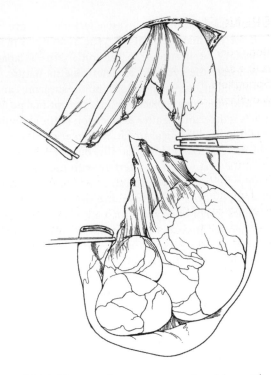

Figure 63.10 Mesenteric cyst removed en bloc with adjacent bowel.

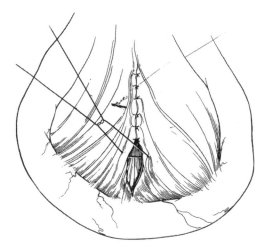

Figure 63.9 Closure of the mesenteric dissection with fine interrupted absorbable sutures.

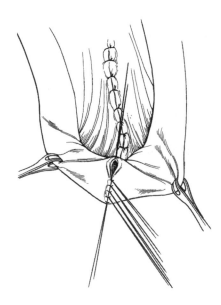

Figure 63.11 Reapproximation of the intestine with a single layer of interrupted absorbable sutures.

the mesenteric defect is closed, approximating both leaves of the mesentery (Figure 63.9).

In instances where a definite plane between the cyst and adjacent bowel cannot be identified, resection of the intestine in continuity with the cyst is required. Dissection should be planned so as to remove as little bowel as possible (Figures 63.10 and 63.11).

In patients in whom complete enucleation or resection cannot be achieved, partial excision with marsupialization and sclerotherapy are discussed. Application of agents like OK-432 remains highly controversial.[19–22]

OUTCOME

The outcome of resection or enucleation of mesenteric and omental cysts is very favorable. However, recurrence has been reported in up to 14% of patients, mostly with retroperitoneal cysts, which require re-resection.

REFERENCES

1. Benevieni A. *De abditis nonullis ac mirandis morborum e sanationum causis.* Translated by Singer CJ. Springfield, IL: Charles C. Thomas, 1954.
2. Moynihan BGA. Mesenteric cysts. *Ann Surg* 1897; 26: 1–29.
3. Beahrs OH, Judd ES, Dockerty MB. Chylous cyst of the abdomen. *Surg Clin North Am* 1950; 30: 1081–96.
4. Ros PR, Olmsted WW, Moser RP et al. Mesenteric and omental cysts—Histologic classification with imaging correlation. *Radiology* 1987; 164: 327–32.
5. Takiff H, Calabria R, Yin L et al. Mesenteric cysts and intra-abdominal cystic lymphangiomas. *Arch Surg* 1985; 120: 1266–9.
6. Losanoff JE, Richman BW, El-Sherif A et al. Mesenteric cyst lymphangioma. *J Am Coll Surg* 2003; 196: 598–611.
7. Galifer RB, Pous JG, Juskiewenski S et al. Intra-abdominal cystic lymphangiomas in childhood. *Prog Pediatr Surg* 1978; 11: 173–238.
8. Kosir MA, Sonnino RE, Gauderer MWL. Pediatric abdominal lymphangiomas: A plea for early recognition. *J Pediatr Surg* 1991; 26: 1309–13.
9. Egozi EI, Ricketts RR. Mesenteric and omental cysts in children. *Am Surg* 1997; 63: 287–90.
10. Bliss DP, Coffin CM, Bower RJ et al. Mesenteric cysts in children. *Surgery* 1994; 115: 571–7.
11. Hebra A, Brown MF, McGeehin KM et al. Mesenteric, omental, and retroperitoneal cysts in children: A clinical study of 22 cases. *South Medl J* 1993; 86: 173–6.
12. Okur H, Kuchukaydin M, Ozokutan BH. Mesenteric, omental, and retroperitoneal cysts in children. *Eur J Surg* 1997; 163: 673–7.
13. Colodny AH. Mesenteric and omental cysts. In: Welch KJ, Randolph JG, Ravitch MM et al. (eds). *Surgery.* Chicago: Yearbook Medical Publishers 1986; 921–5.
14. Gross RE. *Omental Cysts and Mesenteric Cysts. The Surgery of Infancy and Childhood.* Philadelphia: W.B. Saunders, 1953: 377–83.
15. Nam SH, Kim DY, Kim SC et al. The surgical experience for retroperitoneal, mesenteric and omental cyst in children. *J Korean Surg Soc* 2012; 83: 102–6.
16. Parrish RA, Potts JM. Torsion of omental cyst—A rare complication of ventriculoperitoneal shunt. *J Pediatr Surg* 1973; 8: 969–70.
17. Kenney B, Smith B, Bensoussan AL. Laparoscopic excision of a cystic lymphangioma. *J Laparoendosc Surg* 1996; (Suppl 1): S99–101.
18. Steyaert H, Vall J-S. Laparoscopic treatment of enteric duplications and other abdominal cystic masses. In Bax K, Georgeson KE, Rothenberg SS, Valla, J-S, Yeung CK (eds). *Endoscopic Surgery in Infants and Children.* Berlin: Springer, 2008: 321–6.
19. Luzzatto C, Lo Piccolo R, Fascetti Leon F et al. Further experience with OK-432 for lymphangiomas. *Pediatr Surg Int* 2005; 21: 969–72.
20. Luzzatto CM. OK-432 is not suitable for abdominal lymphatic malformations. *Eur J Pediatr Surg* 2011; 21: 211.
21. Ogita S, Tsuto T, Nakamura K et al. OK-432 therapy for lymphangioma in children: Why and how does it work? *J Pediatr Surg* 1996; 31: 477–80.
22. Oliveira C, Sacher P, Meuli M. Management of prenatally diagnosed abdominal lymphatic malformations. *Eur J Pediatr Surg* 2010; 20: 302–6.

64

Neonatal ascites

PREM PURI AND ELKE RUTTENSTOCK

INTRODUCTION

Ascites is defined as an abnormal accumulation of intra-peritoneal fluid in the peritoneal cavity, which consists of transudate (low protein count and low specific gravity) or exudate (high protein count and high specific gravity). The relatively rare condition of ascites in the newborn may occur due to a wide range of medical and surgical causes. The surgical conditions that most likely result in neonatal ascites are obstructive uropathy, chylous ascites, and spontaneous perforation of the extrahepatic biliary tree.

URINARY ASCITES

Urinary ascites, which occurs almost exclusively in boys, is an uncommon, life-threatening condition, which accounts for up to 30% of all cases of neonatal ascites.[1] Abdominal distension causing respiratory distress and signs of renal insufficiency are known as the most common presenting symptoms. Urinary tract obstruction from posterior urethral valves is the most common reported cause of urinary ascites, at up to 70%.[1,2] Other causes include ureteropelvic junction obstruction, ureterocele, lower ureteral atresia, bladder neck obstruction, and neuropathic bladder.[3] Ascites due to bladder rupture is also recognized, most commonly secondary to umbilical arterial catheterization causing rupture of the dome of the bladder or of a patent urachus. Predisposing factors apart from posterior urethral valves include neurogenic bladder, congenital bladder diverticulum, and detrusor areflexia. Spontaneous rupture of the bladder has also been reported as a result of profound hypoxia or morphine administration. Rarely, urinary ascites may occur in the absence of urinary tract obstruction.[4]

The ascites usually results from extravasation of urine into the peritoneal cavity due to urinary tract perforation above a point of obstruction. The perforation may occur in the bladder but most often occurs in the upper tracts.[3] In obstructive causes of extravasation, prolonged high pressure in the kidney leads to atrophy and dysplasia, which predispose to rupture of the collecting system. Urine may collect as a perinephric urinoma within the Gerota fascia encapsulating the kidney, or as urinary ascites in the peritoneal cavity.[5]

The presence of urine in the peritoneal cavity leads to an autodialysis effect, in which solutes and water follow their concentration gradients. This effect explains why ascites fluid shows sodium and potassium results not dissimilar from plasma, as well as hyponatremia and hyperkalemia. Furthermore, in all cases, one would expect higher levels of urea and creatinine with lower levels of bicarbonate in the ascites fluid than found in blood. This unique biochemical profile, in the presence of renal impairment, is peculiar to a diagnosis of urinary ascites.[6,7]

The diagnosis of urinary ascites is based on clinical assessment, together with ultrasonography and abdominal x-rays.[1,8] The typical patient with neonatal urinary ascites is a preterm male infant, who presents with gross abdominal distension, respiratory distress, and ascites at birth. Plain abdominal films will show diffuse opacity (Figure 64.1a). If the amount of intraperitoneal fluid is large, splaying of the lower rib cage and centrally located floating intestines will be demonstrated. Micturating cystourethrogram (MCUG) is necessary to diagnose posterior urethral valves, and ipsilateral vesicoureteral reflux may further elucidate the diagnosis (Figure 64.1b). Computed tomography (CT) has been recommended to reveal the underlying pathology.[9] Intravenous pyelography may show a characteristic "halo" sign produced by extravasation of contrast material into the perirenal area. Abdominal paracentesis confirms the diagnosis via elevated creatinine levels and urine in the fluid.[6,10]

The management of urinary ascites has to be prompt, with the basic aim of achieving decompression of the urinary tract. This may be accomplished by abdominal paracentesis, catheter drainage, or surgical exploration and repair of the bladder wall. One of the indications of abdominal paracentesis includes respiratory distress.[11,12] In cases of posterior urethral valves (PUV), catheter drainage by urethral route with or without vesicostomy achieves healing in most patients in 10–14 days. Catheter drainage fails in ruptures with large rents and requires surgical repair.[4]

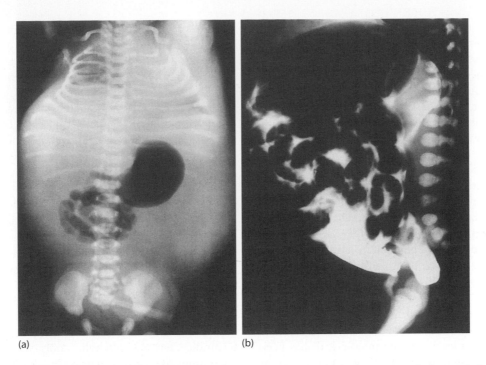

(a)   (b)

Figure 64.1 Urinary ascites. This infant had severe respiratory distress at birth due to gross abdominal distension requiring abdominal paracentesis. **(a)** Supine film immediately after removal of 650 mL of fluid shows stomach and small bowel loops floating centrally in the peritoneal fluid. Note splaying of ribs. **(b)** A micturating cystourethrogram shows leakage of contrast into the peritoneal cavity. Spontaneous perforation of the bladder was found at operation. There was no demonstrable anatomical obstruction in the urinary tract.

Long-term outcome of bladder and kidney function is reported to be surprisingly good in cases of neonatal urinary ascites secondary to severe obstructive uropathy.[3] Intrauterine pressure relief in the collecting system through urinary extravasation ("pop-off" mechanism) protects renal function, and this decompression of the urinary tract prevents severe secondary changes to bladder function.[13,14]

CHYLOUS ASCITES

Chylous ascites is a rare condition seen during the newborn period and infancy; however, it is a challenging disorder with regard to its successful treatment.[15,16] Generally, it presents with abdominal distension with or without respiratory distress and occasional signs of peritoneal irritation and malabsorption.[17] About 10% of all infants with chylous ascites have lymphedema of the limbs.[18] The most common cause of chylous ascites (45%–60% of cases) is congenital malformation of the lymphatic channels such as atresia or stenosis of the major lacteals, mesenteric cysts, and generalized lymphangiomatosis.[16,19] Other causes are obstruction of the lymphatics from external compression, as in malrotation; incarcerated hernia; intussusception; and inflammatory enlargement of lymph nodes. Furthermore, blunt abdominal trauma, child abuse, and surgical injury are reported causes of chylous ascites.[20]

Infants with chylous ascites present with abdominal distension at birth, or it may develop in the first few days of life. Ultrasonography of the abdomen is the initial step that

confirms the presence of ascites. Abdominal paracentesis is not only a diagnostic but also a therapeutic method in the management of chylous ascites.[21] Analysis of the fluid obtained by abdominal paracentesis is the most useful diagnostic method. The chyle is usually color-free; however, its appearance and composition are not constant and depend on multiple factors such as the size of fat particles, cellular content, and diet.[22] After oral feeds have been started, the chylous fluid is milky white with a high fat content. Diagnosis is confirmed by determining high protein and triglyceride content in the ascitic fluid with predominance of lymphocytes on differential count. Initial diagnostic investigations include ultrasonography and CT or magnetic resonance imaging of the abdomen to exclude conditions that necessitate immediate surgical intervention. Diagnosis of malformation of the lymphatics is suspected when everything comes out negative. Further diagnostic tests like lymphangiography and lymphoscintigraphy are imperative if surgery is decided, with the purpose of identifying the site of the leakage of chyle preoperatively.[20]

Treatment of chylous ascites is usually conservative. The majority of patients respond to abdominal paracentesis and an enteral diet containing medium-chain triglycerides (MCTs) and high protein. Dietary management is an important treatment modality in chylous ascites. An MCT-based diet is accepted as the first measure to implement for reducing the chyle production in the peritoneal fluid.[23] MCTs are not re-esterified within the intestinal cell and thus bypass the enteric lymphatics and directly enter the portal system.

It is believed that the reduction in dietary long-chain fats (long-chain triglyceride [LCT]) reduces lymphatic flow and pressure within the lymphatic system and decreases the amount of lymph leakage. For severe or complicated chylous ascites or chylous ascites that persists after a maximum of 10 weeks of diet, total parenteral nutrition (TPN) has been successfully used in treating these infants by resting the gastrointestinal tract.[24] Somatostatin analogs have been demonstrated to be effective in reducing lymphorrhea and may be proposed prior to considering the surgical approach. The exact mechanisms of somatostatin on drying lymphatic flow are not completely understood. It has been previously shown to decrease the intestinal absorption of fats, lower triglyceride concentration in the thoracic duct, and attenuate lymph flow in the major lymphatic channels.[25] Satisfactory results were achieved by the administration of the somatostatin combined with TPN.[20,26] Surgical intervention is recommended if 1–2 months of conservative approach has failed.[27] Successful surgical treatment of congenital chylous ascites by resecting the macroscopically localized anomaly or by ligation of an identifiable lymphatic leak has been described.[28] A peritoneovenous shunt, of either Leveen or Denver type, also has been reported to be successful at least temporarily, in children in whom repeated attempts of a medical or surgical approach have failed.[16,29]

BILE ASCITES

Bile ascites in infancy is a rare condition usually resulting from spontaneous perforation of bile duct (SPBD).[30–32] Most often, SPBD is seen in infants aged 2–20 weeks, but it has been reported in neonates as young as 3 days.[31,33] The site of perforation is most often the junction of the cystic duct with the common bile duct (CBD). The exact cause of SPBD is unknown. Numerous etiologies have been proposed, such as congenital mural weakness of the CBD, ischemia, stones, infection, distal bile duct stenosis, inspissated bile, and pancreatic reflux from anomalous pancreaticobiliary ductal union (APBDU).[31,32,34] In the majority of cases, there is no apparent cause for the perforation. Some authors suggest that spontaneous bile duct perforation is not merely spontaneous, but may be related to APBDU and choledochal cyst; i.e., the perforation of the bile duct and congenital choledochal cyst may be interrelated problems with a common pathogenesis.[35] Occasionally, the perforation is secondary to bile duct obstruction.[36]

Affected patients are typically previously healthy infants with unremarkable birth and perinatal histories. Signs and symptoms generally appear gradually and subacutely, but they can also present acutely with peritonitis, septic shock, or even pulmonary collapse.[33,37] The classic subacute presentation occurs in 80% of infants with fluctuating mild jaundice, normal to acholic stools, slowly progressive ascites, and abdominal distension.[38] Associated symptoms may include sepsis, lethargy, irritability, anorexia, failure to thrive, persistent emesis, fever, and dark urine.[39]

The diagnosis may not be made before surgery but should be suspected in the presence of abdominal distension, intermittent jaundice, and ascites. Abdominal x-rays will show ascites, and barium meal may demonstrate collection of fluid between the liver and stomach (Figure 64.2). If paracentesis is performed, the concentration of bilirubin in the ascetic fluid is higher than in the serum. However, paracentesis is not necessary to establish the diagnosis if a hepatobiliary

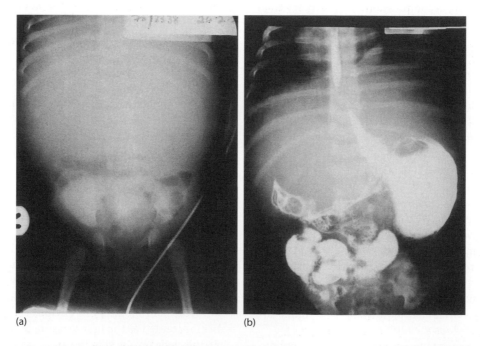

(a) (b)

Figure 64.2 Biliary ascites. **(a)** Marked abdominal distention with opacity in upper and central abdomen and downward displacement of bowel loops. **(b)** Barium study shows compression with downward displacement of stomach and duodenum. At operation, perforation of the common hepatic duct was found.

scan confirms the presence of biliary leakage.[31] Ultrasound is the imaging modality of choice in children, especially for evaluating jaundice. Free or loculated intraperitoneal fluid with normal intrahepatic and extrahepatic ducts will confirm the presence of SPBD.[40] Hepatobiliary scintigraphy is highly sensitive and specific for SPBD, and it is the preoperative test of choice when SPBD is suspected.[39,41,42] It can provide useful information about liver function, biliary patency, site of perforation based on localized accumulation of radiotracer, and any biliary leakage into the peritoneum. Magnetic resonance cholangiopancreatography (MRCP) is also useful in children, including infants.[43,44] Loculated fluid collection or pseudocyst formation can be more easily visualized on MRCP than ultrasound.

Surgical management is mandatory as soon as the diagnosis of SPBD is confirmed.[45] An intraoperative cholangiogram should be performed to delineate the location of the perforation and exclude distal obstruction. If the perforation is in the gallbladder or cystic duct, simple cholecystectomy is curative.[31] Several surgical approaches have been described, including simple drainage with or without cholecystectomy, primary repair with or without external drainage, and hepaticojejunostomy if pancreaticobiliary malformation or distal obstruction is present.[41,46,47] Most authors recommend a conservative approach of draining the abdomen to decompress the biliary tree, unless there is distal biliary tract obstruction requiring biliary–intestinal anastomosis.[48] Spontaneous closure is typical even with distal obstruction, once the biliary tree is decompressed.[37] The drains should not be removed too early, since this can lead to reaccumulation of bile in the peritoneal cavity. In situations where the surgeon encounters biliary perforation without a preoperative diagnosis, the safest policy is to drain the area and place a T-tube through the perforation. Suture repair of the bile duct or biliary reconstruction remains controversial because of the potential for stricture formation.[49] Reported complications have included portal vein thrombosis, bile leak, and cholangitis.[50] In a few cases, further surgery, including biliary revision and portosystemic shunting, was reported.[50] Overall, the prognosis is good with early recognition and surgical management.

REFERENCES

1. Hirselj DA, Zmaj PM, Firlit CF. Occult ureteropelvic junction obstruction presenting as anuria and urinary ascites in an infant with antenatal, unilateral hydronephrosis. J Pediatr Urol 2009; 5:405–7.

2. Hoffer FA, Winters WD, Retik AB et al. Urinoma drainage for neonatal respiratory insufficiency. Pediatr Radiol 1990; 20: 270–1.

3. De Vries SH, Klijn AJ, Lilien MR et al. Development of renal function after neonatal urinary ascites due to obstructive uropathy. J Urol 2002; 168: 675–8.

4. Solarin A, Gajjar P, Nourse P. Neonatal urinary ascites: A report of three cases. Case Rep Nephrol 2015; 2015: 942501.

5. Hi Sie A, Patel N, Spenceley N. Neonatal urinary ascites in renal candidal infection. J Pediatr Child Health 2006; 42: 387–8.

6. Oei J, Garvey PA, Rosenberg AR. The diagnosis and management of neonatal urinary ascites. J Paediatr Child Health 2001; 37: 513–5.

7. Clarke HS, Mills ME, Parres JA et al. The hyponatraemia of neonatal urinary ascites: Clinical observations, experimental confirmation and proposed mechanisms. J Urol 1993; 150: 778–81.

8. Ahmed S, Borghol M, Hugosson C. Urinoma and urinary ascites secondary to calyceal perforation in neonatal posterior urethral valves. Br J Urol 1997; 79: 991-2.

9. Gueroeze MK, Yildirmaz S, Dogan Y et al. A rare cause of ascites in a newborn: Posterior urethral valve. Pediatr Int 2010; 52: 154–5.

10. Sakai K, Konda R, Ota S et al. Neonatal urinary ascites caused by urinary tract obstruction: Two case reports. Int J Urol 1998; 5: 379–82.

11. Murphy D, Simmons M, Guiney EJ. Neonatal urinary ascites in the absence of urinary tract obstruction. J Pediatr Surg 1978; 13: 529–31.

12. Greenfield SP, Hensle TW, Berdon WE et al. Urinary extravasation in the newborn male with posterior urethral valves. J Pediatr Surg 1982; 17: 751–6.

13. Silveri M, Adorisio O, Pane A et al. Fetal monolateral urinoma and neonatal renal function outcome in posterior urethral valves obstruction: The pop-off mechanism. Pediatr Med Chir 2002; 24: 394–6.

14. Chun KE, Ferguson RS. Neonatal urinary ascites due to unilateral vesicoureteric junction obstruction. Pediatr Surg Int 1997; 12: 455–7.

15. Cochran WJ, Klish WJ, Curtis T et al. Chylous ascites in infants and children: A case report and literature review. J Pediatr Gastroenterol Nutr 1985; 4: 668–73.

16. Karagol BS, Zenciroglu A, Gokce S et al. Therapeutic management of neonatal chylous ascites: Report of a case and review of the literature. Acta Paediatr 2010; 19: 1–4.

17. Kuroiwa M, Toki F, Suzuki M et al. Successful laparoscopic ligation of the lymphatic trunk for refractory chylous ascites. J Pediatr Surg 2007; 42: 15–8.

18. Guttman FM, Montupet P, Bloss RS. Experience with peritovenous shunting for congenital chylous ascites in infants and children. J Pediatr Surg 1983; 17: 368–72.

19. Levine C. Primary disorder of the lymphatic vessels: A new concept. J Pediatr Surg 1989; 24: 233–40.

20. Purkait R, Saha A, Tripathy I et al. Congenital chylous ascites treated successfully with MCT-based formula and octreotide. J Indian Assoc Pediatr Surg 2014; 19(3): 175–7.

21. Campisi C, Bellini C, Eretta C et al. Diagnosis and management of primary chylous ascites. J Vasc Surg 2006; 43: 1244–8.

22. Cardenas A, Chopra S. Chylous ascites. *Am J Gastroenterol* 2002; 97: 1896–900.

23. Liao HB, Hwang RC, Chu DM et al. Neonatal chylous ascites: Report of two cases. *Acta Pediatr Sin* 1990; 31: 47–52.

24. Chye JK, Lim JT, van der Heuvel M. Neonatal chylous ascites: Report of three cases and review of the literature. *Pediatr Surg Int* 1997; 12: 296–8.

25. Collard JM, Laterre PF, Boemer F et al. Conservative treatment of postsurgical lymphatic leaks with somatostatin-14. *Chest* 2000; 117: 902–5.

26. Huang Y, Xu H. Successful treatment of neonatal idiopathic chylous ascites with total parenteral nutrition and somatostatin. *HK J Pediatr* 2008; 13: 130–4.

27. te Pas AB, vd Ven K, Stokkel MP, Walther FJ. Intractable congenital chylous ascites. *Acta Pediatr* 2004; 93: 1403–5.

28. Laterre PF, Dugernier T, Reynaert MS. Chylous ascites: Diagnosis, causes and treatment. *Acta Gastroenterol Belg* 2000; 63: 260–3.

29. Man WK, Spitz L. The management of chylous ascites in children. *J Pediatr Surg* 1985; 20: 72–5.

30. Davenport M, Betalli P, D'Antiga L et al. The spectrum of surgical jaundice in infancy. *J Pediatr Surg* 2003; 38: 1471–9.

31. Xanthakos SA, Yazigi NA, Ryckman FC et al. Spontaneous perforation of the bile duct in infancy: A rare but important cause of irritability and abdominal distension. *J Pediatr Gastroenterol Nutr* 2003; 36: 287–91.

32. Lee M-J, Kim M-J, Yonn C-S. MR cholangiopancreatography findings in children with spontaneous bile duct perforation. *Pediatr Radiol* 2010; 40: 687–92.

33. Topuzlu T, Yigit U, Bulut M. Is birth trauma responsible for idiopathic perforation of the biliary tract in infancy? *Turk J Pediatr* 1994; 36: 263–6.

34. Ando H, Ito T, Watanabe Y et al. Spontaneous perforation of choledochal cyst. *J Am Coll Surg* 1995; 181: 125–8.

35. Sai Prasad TR, Chui CH, Low Y et al. Bile duct perforation in children: Is it truly spontaneous? *Ann Acad Med Singapore* 2006; 35: 905–8.

36. Donahoe PK, Hendren WH. Bile duct perforation in a neonate with stenosis of the ampulla of Vater. *J Pediatr Surg* 1976; 1: 823–5.

37. Kanojia RP, Sinha SK, Rawat J et al. Spontaneous biliary perforation in infancy and childhood: Clues to diagnosis. *Indian J Pediatr* 2007; 74: 509–10.

38. Carubelli C, Abramo T. Abdominal distension and shock in an infant. *Am J Emerg Med* 1999; 17: 342–4.

39. Murphy JT, Koral K, Soeken T, Megison S. Complex spontaneous bile duct perforation: An alternative approach to standard porta hepatis drainage therapy. *J Pediatr Surg* 2013 April; 48(4): 893–8.

40. Tani C, Nosaka S, Masaki H et al. Spontaneous perforation of choledochal cyst: A case with unusual distribution of fluid in the retroperitoneal space. *Pediatr Radiol* 2009; 39: 629–31.

41. Saltzman DA, Snyder CL, Leonard A. Spontaneous perforation of the extrahepatic biliary tree in infancy. A case report. *Clin Pediatr* 1990; 29: 322–4.

42. Goldberg D, Rosenfeld D, Underberg-Davis S. Spontaneous biliary perforation: Biloma resembling a small bowel duplication cyst. *J Pediatr Gastroenterol Nutr* 2000; 31: 201–3.

43. Krause D, Cercueil JP, Dranssart M et al. MRI for evaluating congenital bile duct abnormalities. *J Comput Assist Tomogr* 2002; 26: 541–52.

44. Takaya J, Nakano S, Imai Y et al. Usefulness of magnetic resonance cholangiopancreatography in biliary structures in infants: A four-case report. *Eur J Pediatr* 2007; 166: 211–4.

45. Howard ER. *Spontaneous Biliary Perforation*. London: Arnold, 2002.

46. Bingol-Kologlu M, Karnak I, Ocal T et al. Idiopathic perforation of the bile duct in an infant. *J Pediatr Gastroenterol Nutr* 2000; 31: 83–5.

47. Pereira E Cotta MV, Yan J, Asaid M, Ferguson P, Clarnette T. Conservative management of spontaneous bile duct perforation in infancy: Case report and literature review. *J Pediatr Surg* 2012 September; 47(9): 1757–9.

48. Kasat LS, Borwankar SS, Jain M et al. Spontaneous perforation of the extrahepatic bile duct in an infant. *Pediatr Surg Int* 2001; 17: 463–4.

49. Suresh-Babu MV, Thomas AG, Miller V et al. Spontaneous perforation of the cystic duct. *J Pediatr Gastroenterol Nutr* 1998; 26: 461–3.

50. Chardot C, Iskandarani F, De Dreuzy O et al. Spontaneous perforation of the biliary tract in infancy: A series of 11 cases. *Eur J Pediatr Surg* 1996; 6: 341–6.

65

Necrotizing enterocolitis

STEPHANIE C. PAPILLON, SCOTT S. SHORT, AND HENRI R. FORD

INTRODUCTION

Epidemiology of necrotizing enterocolitis worldwide

Necrotizing enterocolitis (NEC) is predominantly a disease of the premature neonate. The majority of patients diagnosed with NEC are less than 32 weeks gestation. Data from population-based studies worldwide estimate the incidence of NEC to be 0.72 to 1.8 per 1000 live births.[1] The incidence is highest in extremely low birth weight infants (ELBW) weighing less than 1000 g, likely reflecting the degree of prematurity.[2-7] NEC decreases proportionally as birth weight increases, and a drastic decline occurs after 35 weeks gestation.[2,4,8]

The incidence of NEC has been increasing worldwide as a result of a steady rise in the rate of high-risk pregnancies and recent advances in neonatology that have resulted in the survival of significant numbers of ELBW infants.[9,10] Thus, the need to understand this disease has never been more imperative.

PATHOGENESIS

Risk factors

Early studies by Santulli and colleagues suggested that NEC develops in a susceptible or premature host as a result of various insults to the gastrointestinal tract inflicted by ischemia, enteral feeding, and pathogenic bacteria.[11,12] Our current understanding of the pathogenesis of NEC suggests that immaturity of the gastrointestinal tract in the preterm neonate, combined with these insults, accounts for the cascade of events that lead to NEC. The immature intestine is characterized by poor microcirculatory regulation, impaired integrity of the epithelial barrier, and various immune deficiencies, including decreased production of mucin, defensins, and secretory IgA, to name a few, which impair the host's ability to restrict the transmucosal passage of pathogenic bacteria and toxins. In addition, the dysfunctional motility and reduced digestive capacity of the premature intestine further predispose to the accumulation of toxins or noxious substances that may contribute to or exacerbate mucosal injury.[1,2] Although a normal intestinal microbiota could mitigate such mucosal injury, the premature neonate suffers from abnormal microbial colonization of the gastrointestinal tract. Thus, breakdown of the epithelial barrier is further exacerbated by loss of the vigorous and complex interaction between the mucosa and intestinal microbiota, which results in an inappropriate, exuberant inflammatory response to commensal and pathogenic bacteria. The inflammatory mediators released lead to further epithelial injury, exaggerated systemic inflammation, and the resulting adverse sequelae characteristic of NEC. The mechanisms that predispose the immature intestine to injury must be further defined in order to prevent or treat NEC in the premature neonate.[4]

Mechanisms of intestinal mucosal injury

Various studies describe some of the mechanisms by which mucosal injury occurs in NEC.[13,14] These studies have established a role for mediators such as nitric oxide, which is made in large quantities during inflammatory conditions by the inducible isoform of nitric oxide synthase (iNOS), and Toll-like receptor 4 (TLR4) in the pathogenesis of NEC. These mediators not only are elevated in neonates with NEC but also have been localized to regions of mucosal injury and have been shown to inhibit pathways necessary for restoration or repair of the damaged intestinal epithelium.[14-16] Inhibiting the activation of these mediators not only can reverse the inflammatory changes noted in the intestinal epithelium in experimental models of NEC but also can restore reparative pathways such as epithelial restitution through enterocyte migration and proliferation.[14] Interplay between these proinflammatory mediators and others such as platelet-activating factor (PAF) has been demonstrated and could represent putative pathways essential for the development of NEC.[17] Despite these observations, the sequence of events that lead to NEC has yet to be established. Nonetheless, targeted inhibition of these mediators may ultimately lead to new therapeutic approaches to prevent or attenuate NEC.

Histopathologic findings

NEC can occur anywhere along the gastrointestinal tract but most commonly affects the small intestine.[18] Morphological analysis of resected, diseased intestine and autopsy specimens has historically shaped much of our understanding of the pathogenesis of tissue injury in NEC. On gross morphology, the bowel appears distended with patchy or diffuse areas of gray to dark discoloration. Focal lesions occur as commonly as multisegmental disease.[1,19] Examination of the mucosa may reveal a hemorrhagic and friable surface. Predominant histologic findings range from acute and chronic inflammatory changes to frank necrosis or perforation. These include bowel wall edema, submucosal gas, as well as neutrophilic and lymphocytic infiltrates, which may reflect in part the acuity or chronicity of the disease (Figures 65.1 and 65.2). Subserosal or submucosal gas, a product of bacterial fermentation also known as pneumatosis intestinalis, may also be visible and lends support to the infectious nature of NEC. Rapidly progressing injury to the bowel is suggested by necrosis in the absence of inflammation, also known as coagulation necrosis, while more gradual progression is suggested by the presence of chronic inflammatory

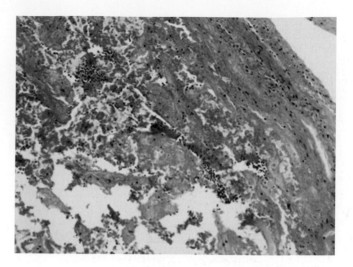

Figure 65.2 Dense lymphocytic infiltrate in the intestinal wall in NEC.

changes.[20,21] Coagulation necrosis is often, although not exclusively, the result of ischemia. Coagulation necrosis may be limited to the mucosa; however, advanced disease may ultimately result in transmural involvement and perforation. Necrosis may be accompanied by hemorrhage and intramural thrombi. Reparative changes and granulation tissue have also been observed along with active injury. These findings suggest that the acute injury characteristic of NEC probably occurred prior to the clinical manifestations that required resection of the diseased intestine.[21] Patients with transmural inflammation that do not undergo resection may subsequently develop regions of submucosal fibrosis that can manifest clinically as intestinal strictures.

RISK FACTORS FOR NEC IN THE FULL-TERM INFANT

Fewer than 10% of patients who develop NEC are full term. While the pattern of mucosal injury reflects that of preterm infants, full-term infants differ clinically from their premature counterparts and, in this population, NEC "may be initiated by different perinatal factors."[22] Most studies suggest that congenital heart disease (CHD) is the most significant predisposing risk factor for NEC in the full-term infant.[22] Infants with CHD develop intestinal ischemia due to reduced blood flow to the intestine, which may result in mucosal injury and bacterial invasion, which in turn incites the inflammatory cascade that leads to NEC.

CLINICAL FEATURES

Presentation

At initial presentation, infants who develop NEC often exhibit nonspecific systemic signs that may prompt a workup for sepsis. Symptoms specific to the gastrointestinal tract are present in over 70% of patients and include feeding

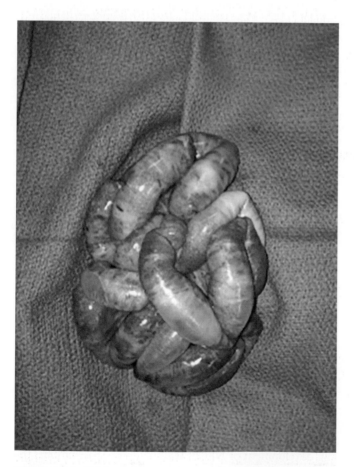

Figure 65.1 Diffuse patchy necrosis in a patient with NEC totalis. Subserosal gas can be seen.

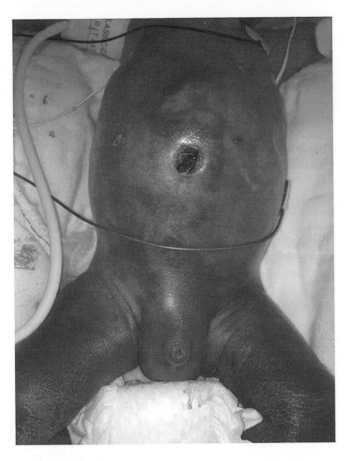

Figure 65.3 Abdominal distention and extensive abdominal wall erythema in a patient with NEC totalis.

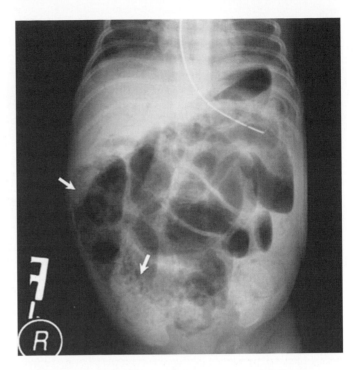

Figure 65.4 Pneumatosis intestinalis in a patient with NEC.

intolerance manifested by high gastric residuals or frank vomiting, abdominal distention, and gross or occult blood in the stool, which is seen in up to 60% of patients.[2] These symptoms may present postoperatively following the initial stages of cardiac repair for CHD in the full-term infant. As NEC progresses, patients may develop worsening abdominal distention, abdominal wall discoloration, or erythema (Figure 65.3). Within hours, patients can rapidly deteriorate and develop peritonitis with signs of cardiovascular collapse. The diagnosis is often established by radiographic imaging. Standard imaging consists of plain abdominal radiographs. Initial findings may be nonspecific such as dilated loops of intestine and a bowel gas pattern consistent with ileus. Pneumatosis intestinalis is the most common finding observed in patients with NEC (Figure 65.4).[1] Portal venous gas is another potential finding that is associated with pan-involvement and an unfavorable outcome (Figure 65.5). The NEC staging system, originally developed by Bell et al., combines the clinical symptoms with radiographic findings and has been used to classify severity of disease and guide therapy.

Laboratory findings

Laboratory data, although universally used, have not proven to be specific or reliable indicators for the diagnosis of NEC.

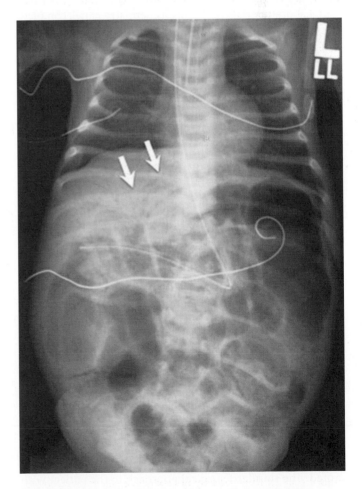

Figure 65.5 Portal venous gas in a patient with NEC.

Metabolic acidosis, leukopenia, and thrombocytopenia are common findings in patients with NEC.[1,2] Thrombocytopenia that occurs rapidly has been associated with a poor prognosis.[1,2] Studies have investigated potential indices predictive of NEC that may also serve as prognostic indicators; however, no inflammatory marker has emerged as highly sensitive and specific.[1]

ASSOCIATED COMORBIDITIES

Several retrospective studies have reported a high prevalence of NEC in patients who underwent abdominal wall closure for gastroschisis.[23–26] The patients described were often managed nonoperatively; however, recurrence was commonly observed.[23] NEC was significantly more common in patients with severe gastrointestinal dysfunction, characteristic of the premature gastrointestinal tract.

MANAGEMENT

Nonoperative

Patients with NEC are initially managed with supportive care. Upon clinical suspicion of NEC, feeds are withheld and the gastrointestinal tract is decompressed using an orogastric tube. Intravenous fluid resuscitation is initiated. Laboratory data including a chemistry panel, complete blood count with differential, blood gas, and C-reactive protein are obtained. Broad spectrum intravenous antibiotics are initiated once blood and urine are sent for culture. Close clinical observation with serial abdominal examinations as well as serial abdominal radiographs are used to monitor disease progression. Clinical improvement is expected to occur within the first 72 hours.[18] For patients who stabilize and show improvement, antibiotic therapy is continued for 1–2 weeks.

Operative indication and technique

Up to 20%–40% of patients with NEC will require surgical intervention.[1,2] Over the past decades, indications for operation have evolved as practitioners have sought to identify patients just prior to perforation; however, pneumoperitoneum remains the only consistent and definitive indication for surgical intervention. Relative indications for surgery include failure to respond to optimal medical therapy, as evidenced by worsening clinical status, abdominal wall erythema, or the presence of a persistent intestinal loop on serial abdominal radiographs. The goal of surgery is to resect gangrenous bowel while minimizing the risk of short bowel syndrome. The operation is largely determined by the extent of disease found at laparotomy. The entire length of the gastrointestinal tract is examined, and frankly necrotic bowel is resected. Where intestinal viability is questionable, a second-look laparotomy may be warranted. The standard surgical approach to the patient with NEC is resection of gangrenous or perforated bowel with

creation of a proximal ostomy. Traditionally, enterostomy creation has been accepted as the safest approach because primary anastomosis may be tenuous in a septic infant.[27] For selected stable patients with localized disease, resection with primary anastomosis may obviate the need for a second operation as well as some of the morbidity associated with ostomy creation.[2,27] In the past, multiple stoma creation had been advocated for patients with multifocal disease. However, this approach can lead to short bowel syndrome by sacrificing viable intestine; therefore, it has been abandoned.

The "clip and drop back technique," which consists of resection of all necrotic bowel leaving the remaining clipped segments within the abdominal cavity without creating ostomies or anastomoses, has been advocated for patients with extensive multifocal disease. The viable segments are then re-anastomosed at a second operation 48–72 hours later. Delayed re-exploration has been proposed in a yet more controversial technique, the "patch, drain, and wait." This approach involves irrigation of the abdominal cavity, primary approximation of intestinal perforations, placement of a Stamm gastrostomy, and insertion of two Penrose drains beneath the diaphragm that course along the lateral aspect of the peritoneal cavity and exit from the lower quadrants for continued peritoneal drainage.[28] Postoperatively, patients are kept on long-term parenteral nutrition. The drains are left in place until the drainage ceases and patients are tolerating enteral feeds. The authors advocate postponing a second operation during the 2-week period immediately postoperatively, and in cases where return of bowel function does not occur, reoperation may occur as late as 2 months.

In the 1970s, peritoneal drainage was proposed as a temporizing measure for the critically ill very low birth weight (VLBW) patient, weighing less than 1500 g, with perforated NEC. The procedure is typically performed under local anesthesia at the bedside. The major components involve copious irrigation of the abdominal cavity and placement of a Penrose drain in the lower quadrant or bilateral lower quadrants allowing for decompression and removal of fecal contamination. Peritoneal drainage is widely viewed as initial treatment, and its use as definitive treatment remains controversial. There have been two randomized controlled trials investigating the use of peritoneal drainage versus laparotomy in VLBW infants with perforated NEC to determine any survival advantage. In the first multicenter trial, 117 VLBW infants were randomized to either treatment with 55 undergoing drainage and 62 undergoing laparotomy.[29] The investigators did not observe any significant differences in 90-day mortality. Similarly, no significant differences were observed in secondary outcome measures that included total parenteral nutrition (TPN) dependency and length of hospital stay at 90 days postoperatively. In the second international multicenter randomized controlled trial,[30] 35 patients were randomized to peritoneal drainage and 34 to laparotomy. There were no significant differences in mortality or in secondary outcome measures that included length of stay and gastrointestinal and respiratory outcomes at 1 and 6 months postoperatively between the two groups. Seventy-four percent of the patients who underwent drainage subsequently required laparotomy for deteriorating clinical status. The authors concluded that peritoneal drainage is not "a safe alternative to laparotomy and is not an effective temporizing measure." While neither randomized trial detected differences in primary or secondary outcomes, each included a mixed population of patients with focal intestinal perforation and NEC, and the studies did not meet the minimum number of required participants for appropriate statistical power perhaps limiting the ability to observe differences.

OUTCOMES

Overall

NEC is associated with a high morbidity and mortality. Overall outcome is affected by the degree of prematurity and extent of disease. Over the past decades, survival for NEC has shown steady improvement. This observation has been most notable in VLBW infants and is likely related to advances in supportive care. NEC has a relatively low recurrence rate. Up to one third of patients with NEC will develop intestinal strictures. Strictures occur more frequently in patients with medically treated NEC.[2] Suspected patients should undergo contrast enema and surgical resection.

Postoperative outcomes

Postoperative complications occur in up to 40% of neonates who undergo surgical therapy for NEC. These include anastomotic leak, stoma complications such as prolapse or necrosis, and injury to the liver.[31] Other complications include intestinal strictures, sepsis, and short gut syndrome.[32,33] While mortality shows stepwise progression with decreasing gestational age, Horwitz et al.[32] found the overall number of complications to be relatively stable across all age groups.

Long-term outcomes

GASTROINTESTINAL

The most devastating complication of NEC is intestinal failure due to inadequate residual small bowel (short gut). Nearly one quarter of patients undergoing surgical resection for NEC will develop short bowel, and NEC is among the leading causes of intestinal failure in the neonatal population. Absence of the ileocecal valve does not always predict the likelihood of failure of intestinal adaptation in patients with inadequate small bowel length.[34] The patient's gestational age at the time of small bowel resection is an important prognostic indicator of the risk of intestinal failure because an increase in small bowel length typically occurs during the third trimester.[35]

Neurodevelopmental outcome

NEC has been found to be an independent risk factor for adverse neurodevelopmental outcomes. Analysis at 7 years for children included in the ORACLE Children Group, a randomized study investigating the use of broad spectrum antibiotics in preterm premature rupture of membranes, found increased risk of any functional impairment in children with a history of NEC.[36] In a multicenter retrospective study, ELBW infants who required surgery for NEC were found to have a significantly increased prevalence of neurodevelopmental and neuromotor or neurosensory deficits including cerebral palsy, blindness, and deafness.[37]

CONCLUSIONS AND FUTURE DIRECTIONS

NEC remains a vexing problem for both neonatologists and pediatric surgeons. The most devastating impact of this disease is its direct effect on patients and their families. NEC is also a major contributor to healthcare costs, and the economic burden persists beyond the initial hospitalization period. A retrospective cohort study found significantly higher healthcare costs for patients with both medical and surgical NEC compared with matched controls. These differences persisted through the first 3 years of life for patients with surgical NEC.[38] Thus, for the practitioner caring for these patients and their families, there is an urgent need to optimize current management and develop preventive strategies.

Although numerous studies have identified putative risk factors for NEC, preventive approaches are limited. Animal models have demonstrated a protective role for growth factors such as epidermal growth factor (EGF) and heparin-binding epidermal growth factor-like growth factor (HB-EGF), which can promote intestinal restitution, and for inhibitors of proinflammatory mediators. Studies in human infants have shown a beneficial role for probiotics and prebiotics in reducing the incidence of NEC and producing a fecal microbial composition that resembles that of their breastfed counterparts. However, there is insufficient evidence to recommend these interventions at this time. Restrictive feeding strategies have not shown any advantage. Corticosteroid administration has also been investigated as a therapeutic adjunct in NEC because of its ability to induce maturation of immature organs. The impact of corticosteroids on the developing intestine was first explored in the 1960s and was subsequently shown to accelerate the maturation of the mucosal barrier.[39] Randomized trials have demonstrated that steroids can reduce the number of patients who develop NEC as well as the severity of disease.[40,41] However, the direct impact of steroids on the gastrointestinal tract and their long-term effects on the developing intestine are not well defined. While antenatal steroids show benefit, use of postnatal steroids is cautioned since long-term outcomes will require further study.[42] Breast milk is the only intervention that is recommended for the preterm infant by the American Academy of Pediatrics to prevent or reduce the incidence of NEC. Clinical trials have demonstrated the ability of breast milk to reduce the incidence of NEC and its associated mortality and morbidity among preterm infants, including improved neurodevelopmental outcomes. As studies on NEC continue, identifying the child at risk, advocating for the use of breast milk, and providing aggressive care will be key in managing this perplexing problem.

REFERENCES

1. Dominguez KM, Moss RL. Necrotizing enterocolitis. In: Holcomb III GW, Murphy J, Ostlie DJ (eds). *Ashcraft's Pediatric Surgery*, 6th edn. Philadelphia, PA: Saunders, 2014: 454–73.

2. Sylvester KG, Liu GY, Albanese CT. Necrotizing enterocolitis. In: Coran AG, Adzick NS, Krummel TM, Laberge JM, Shamberger RC, Caldamone AA (eds). *Pediatric Surgery*, 7th edn. Philadelphia, PA: Mosby, 2012: 1187–207.

3. Holman RC, Stoll BJ, Curns AT, Yorita KL, Steiner CA, Schonberger LB. Necrotising enterocolitis hospitalisations among neonates in the United States. *Paediatr Perinat Epidemiol* 2006; 20(6): 498–506.

4. Llanos AR, Moss ME, Pinzon MC, Dye T, Sinkin RA, Kendig JW. Epidemiology of neonatal necrotising enterocolitis: A population-bases study. *Paediatr Perinat Epidemiol* 2002; 16(4): 342–9.

5. Sankaran K, Puckett B, Lee DS, Seshia M, Boulton J, Qiu Z et al. Variations in incidence of necrotizing enterocolitis in Canadian neonatal intensive care units. *J Pediatr Gastroenterol Nutr* 2004; 39(4): 366–72.

6. Guthrie SO, Gordon PV, Thomas V, Thorp JA, Peabody J, Clark RH. Necrotizing enterocolitis among neonates in the United States. *J Perinatol* 2003; 23(4): 278–85.

7. Christensen RD, Gordon PV, Besner. Can we cut the incidence of necrotizing enterocolitis in half-today? *Fetal Pediatr Pathol* 2010; 29(4): 185–98.

8. Hunter CJ, Podd B, Ford HR, Camerini V. Evidence vs. experience in neonatal practices in necrotizing enterocolitis. *J Perinatol* 2008; Suppl 1: S9–13.

9. Ahle M, Drott P, Anderson RE. Epidemiology and Trends of necrotizing enterocolitis in Sweden: 1987–2009. *Pediatrics* 2013; 132(2): e443–51.

10. Schlager A, Arnold M, Moore SW, Nadler EP. Necrotizing enterocolitis. In: Ameh EA, Bickler SW, Lakhoo K, Nwomeh BC, Poenaru D (eds). *Pediatric Surgery: A Comprehensive Text for Africa*. Seattle, WA: GLOBAL HELP Organization, 2012: 416–23.

11. Mizrahi A, Barlow O, Berdon W, Blanc WA, Silvermon WA. Necrotizing enterocolitis in premature infants. *J Pediatr* 1965; 66(4): 697–706.

12. Santulli TV, Schullinger JN, Heird WC, Gongaware RD, Wigger J, Barlow B et al. Acute necrotizing enterocolitis in infancy: A review of 64 cases. *Pediatrics* 1975; 55(3): 376–87.

13. Nadler EP, Dickinson E, Knisely A, Zhang XR, Boyle P, Beer-Stolz D et al. Expression of inducible nitric oxide synthase and interleukin-12 in experimental necrotizing enterocolitis. *J Surg Res* 2000; (92): 71–7.

14. Sodhi CP, Shi XH, Richardson WM, Grant ZS, Shapiro RA, Prindle T Jr et al. Toll-like receptor-4 inhibits enterocyte proliferation via impaired beta-catenin signaling in necrotizing enterocolitis. *Gastroenterology* 2010; 138(1): 185–96.

15. Ford HR. Mechanism of nitric oxide-mediated intestinal barrier failure: Insight into the pathogenesis of necrotizing enterocolitis. *J Pediatr Surg* 2006; 41(2): 294–9.

16. Afrazi A, Sodhi CP, Richardson W, Neal M, Good M, Siggers R et al. New insights into the pathogenesis and treatment of necrotizing enterocolitis: Toll-like receptors and beyond. *Pediatr Res* 2011; 63(9): 183–8.

17. Soliman A, Michelson KS, Karahashi H, Lu J, Meng FJ, Qu X et al. Platelet-activating factor induces TLR4 expression in intestinal epithelial cells: Implication for the pathogenesis of necrotizing enterocolitis. *PLoS One* 2010; 5(10): e15044.

18. Hackam DJ, Grikscheit T, Wang K, Upperman JS, Ford HR. Pediatric surgery. In: Brunicardi FC, Anderson DK, Billiar TR, Dunn DL, Hunter JG, Matthews JB et al. (eds). *Schwartz's Principles of Surgery*, 10th edn. New York: McGraw Hill: 2015.

19. Nadler EP, Upperman JS, Ford HR. Controversies in the management of necrotizing enterocolitis. *Surg Infect* 2001; 2(2): 113–9.

20. Gould SJ. The pathology of necrotizing enterocolitis. *Semin Fetal Neonat Med* 1997; 2(4): 239–44.

21. Ballance WA, Dahms BB, Shenker N, Kleigman RM. Pathology of neonatal necrotizing enterocolitis: A ten-year experience. *J Pediatr* 1990; 117(1 Pt 2): S6–13.

22. Ostlie DJ, Spilde TL, St Peter SD, Sexton N, Miller KA, Sharp RJ et al. Necrotizing enterocolitis in full-term infants. *J Pediatr Surg* 2003; 38(7): 1039–42.

23. Oldham KT, Coran AG, Drongowski RA, Baker PJ, Wesley JR, Polley TZ Jr. The development of necrotizing enterocolitis following repair of gastroschisis: A surprisingly high incidence. *J Pediatr Surg* 1988; 23(10): 945–9.

24. Amoury RA. Necrotizing enterocolitis following repair of gastroschisis. *J Pediatr Surg* 1989; 24(5): 513–4.

25. Mollitt DL, Golladay ES. Postoperative neonatal necrotizing enterocolitis. *J Pediatr Surg* 1982; 17(6): 757–63.

26. Jayanthi S, Seymour P, Puntis JW, Stringer MD. Necrotizing enterocolitis after gastroschisis repair: A preventable complication? *J Pediatr Surg* 1998; 33(5): 705–7.

27. Pierro A. The surgical management of necrotizing enterocolitis. *Early Hum Dev* 2005; 81(1): 79–85.

28. Moore TC. Successful use of the "patch, drain and wait" laparotomy approach to perforated necrotizing enterocolitis: Is hypoxia-triggered "good angiogenesis" involved? *Pediatr Surg Int* 2000; 16(5–6): 356–63.

29. Moss RL, Dimmitt RA, Barnhart DC, Sylvester KG, Brown RL, Powell DM et al. Laparotomy versus peritoneal drainage for necrotizing enterocolitis and perforation. *N Engl J Med* 2006; 354(21): 2225–34.

30. Rees CM, Eaton S, Kiely EM, Wade AM, McHugh K, Pierro A. Peritoneal drainage or laparotomy for neonatal bowel perforation? A randomized controlled trial. *Ann Surg* 2008; 248(1): 44–51.

31. Sato TT, Oldham KT. Pediatric abdomen. In: Mulholland MW, Lillemoe KD, Doherty GM, Maier RV, Simeone DM, Upchurch GR (eds). *Greenfield's Surgery Scientific Principles and Practice*, 5th edn. Philadelphia, PA: Lippincott Williams & Wilkins, 2011.

32. Horwitz JR, Lally KP, Cheu HW, Vazquez WD, Grosfeld JL, Ziegler MM. Complications after surgical interventions for necrotizing enterocolitis: A multicenter review. *J Pediatr Surg* 1995; 30(7): 994–8.

33. Blakely ML, Lally KP, McDonald S, Brown RL, Barnhart DC, Ricketts RR et al. Postoperative outcomes of extremely low birth-weight infants with necrotizing enterocolitis or isolated intestinal perforation: A prospective cohort study by the NICHD Neonatal Research Network. *Ann Surg* 2005; 241(6): 984–9.

34. Duro D, Kalish LA, Johnston P, Jaksic T, McCarthy M, Martin C et al. Risk factors of intestinal failure in infants with necrotizing enterocolitis: A Glaser Pediatric Research Network study. *J Pediatr* 2010; 157(2): 203–8.

35. Goulet O, Ruemmele F. Causes and management of intestinal failure in children. *Gastroenterology* 2006; 130(2): S16–28.

36. Pike K, Brocklehurst P, Jones D, Kenyon S, Salt A, Taylor D et al. Outcomes at 7 years for babies who developed neonatal necrotising enterocolitis: The ORACLE Children Study. Archives of disease in childhood. *Fetal Neonat Ed* 2012; 97(5): F318–22.

37. Hintz SR, Kendrick DE, Stoll BJ, Vohr BR, Fanaroff AA, Donovan EF et al. Neurodevelopmental and growth outcomes of extremely low birth weight infants after necrotizing enterocolitis. *Pediatrics* 2005; 115(3): 696–703.

38. Ganapathy V, Hay JW, Kim JH, Lee ML, Rechtman DJ. Long term healthcare costs of infants who survived neonatal necrotizing enterocolitis: A retrospective longitudinal study among infants enrolled in Texas Medicaid. *BMC Pediatr* 2013; 13 (127): 1–11.

39. Israel EJ, Schiffrin EJ, Carter EA, Freiberg E, Walker WA. Prevention of necrotizing enterocolitis in the rat with prenatal cortisone. *Gastroenterology* 1990; 99(5): 1333–8.

40. Bauer CM, Morrsion JC, Poole WK, Korones SB, Boehm JJ, Rigatto H et al. A decreased incidence of necrotizing enterocolitis after prenatal glucocorticoid therapy. *Pediatrics* 1984; 73(5): 682–8.

41. Halac E, Halac J, Begue EF, Casanas JM, Indiveri DR, Petit JF et al. Prenatal and postnatal corticosteroid therapy to prevent necrotizing enterocolitis: A controlled trial. *J Pediatr* 1990; 117(1 pt 1): 132–8.

42. Leflore JL, Salhab WA, Broyles RS, Engle WD. Association of antenatal and postnatal dexamethasone exposure with outcomes in extremely low birth weight neonates. *Pediatrics* 2002; 110(2 Pt 1): 275–9.

66

Spontaneous intestinal perforation

MARK D. STRINGER

INTRODUCTION

Spontaneous intestinal perforation (SIP) in the newborn, also known as focal, idiopathic, or isolated intestinal perforation, typically affects extremely low birth weight (ELBW; <1000 g) or very low birth weight (VLBW; <1500 g) premature babies. The perforation is most often located in the terminal ileum.[1] SIP can be difficult to distinguish from necrotizing enterocolitis (NEC), even though it is a separate clinical and pathological entity. If an infant with intestinal perforation is successfully treated by peritoneal drainage rather than primary laparotomy, the diagnosis of SIP is presumed rather than confirmed, and this has hindered interpretation of the literature. Reassuringly, however, in a large multicenter prospective study from the United States, 95% of babies undergoing laparotomy for presumed NEC or SIP were found to be correctly classified.[2]

EPIDEMIOLOGY

The incidence of SIP is approximately 1%–2% in VLBW infants[3,4] and 2%–5% in ELBW infants.[1,5,6] Boys are affected almost twice as often as girls.[4,7] The mean postconceptional age at birth of affected newborns is about 25–26 weeks, and mean birth weight about 720–820 g.[4,7] Prematurity is the single most important risk factor for SIP. Several related predisposing factors have been suggested:

Prenatal

- Chorioamnionitis—severe placental infection/inflammation and its associated treatment.[7–9] This may induce a vasculitic response in the fetus, which may in turn predispose the infant to SIP.
- Preeclampsia—identified as an independent risk factor in one retrospective study.[10]
- Maternal medication

  - Glucocorticoids. Although often stated as a risk factor, several studies have shown no association with antenatal glucocorticoids,[11,12] including one large retrospective study that included 280 babies with SIP.[13]
  - Nonsteroidal anti-inflammatory drugs have been proposed as a risk factor in one small uncontrolled study of SIP,[3] but the link remains unproven.
  - Magnesium sulfate (for fetal/neonatal neuroprotection).[14]

Postnatal

- Neonatal medication
  - Glucocorticoids. Dexamethasone given within the first week of life to prevent bronchopulmonary dysplasia in VLBW infants increases the risk of SIP,[4,12,15] but later administration of glucocorticoids does not carry this risk.[16]
  - Indomethacin. A link seems likely but the data are conflicting[4,12,13,17] and confounded by concurrent enteral feeding and glucocorticoid administration in ELBW infants. Indomethacin given for prevention of intraventricular hemorrhage does not appear to increase the risk of SIP,[18] while administration of indomethacin to treat patent ductus arteriosus does.[13]
- Hypotension requiring inotropes in the first week of life.[12]
- Delayed enteral feeding (beyond the first 3 days).[17]

PATHOLOGY AND PATHOGENESIS

The typical findings in SIP are those of a single perforation on the antimesenteric border of the terminal ileum, although perforation of the jejunum or colon has occasionally been described.[1,6,19–21] Rarely, a second perforation is present.[6,22] The rest of the bowel appears normal, and peritoneal contamination is not usually severe. Histopathologic examination shows an area of discrete ulceration and hemorrhagic necrosis, unlike the ischemic and coagulative necrosis seen in NEC.[19]

The cause of SIP is unknown, but various pathogenetic mechanisms have been implicated:

- Thinning of the muscularis propria has been observed at the site of perforation[22,23] and variably attributed to either congenital deficiency of the muscle, localized increase in intraluminal pressure, or transient focal ischemia in utero.[22,24]
- Reduced activity of nitric oxide synthase (NOS) has been implicated in an animal model after ileal perforation was produced by the administration of indomethacin or dexamethasone to NOS knockout mice.[25] Depletion of NOS is associated with disturbed intestinal motility and reduced transforming growth factor-alpha in the muscularis propria.[26]
- Upregulation of genes involved in angiogenesis, cell adhesion and chemotaxis, extracellular matrix remodeling, inflammation, and muscle contraction are reported in intestinal biopsies from infants with SIP.[27,28] Elevated serum concentrations of interleukin-6, interleukin-8, soluble type II interleukin-1 receptor, angiopoietin-2, soluble urokinase-type plasminogen activator receptor, and tumor necrosis factor-alpha are also documented.[29] Gene upregulation is more marked and diverse and serum cytokine concentrations significantly greater in infants with NEC compared to those with SIP, adding further weight to the evidence that these conditions are both pathologically and clinically distinct.

There are some reports of an association between SIP and concomitant infection with coagulase negative *Staphylococcus* or *Candida* species,[1,8,30] but this is not a consistent finding and infection with these microorganisms is not uncommon in sick premature neonates.

CLINICAL FEATURES AND DIAGNOSIS

SIP occurs predominantly in VLBW or ELBW premature babies born between 25 and 27 weeks' gestation. The key differential diagnosis is NEC with gastrointestinal perforation. It is important to try and distinguish these two conditions because they are managed differently and have a different outcome (discussed next).

Table 66.1 summarizes the features of SIP that help to differentiate it from NEC. Babies with SIP have fewer systemic and abdominal signs preceding the perforation.[28,31] Median age at perforation is usually earlier than NEC, often within the first week of life but ranging from 0 to 15 days. In SIP, there is abrupt onset of marked abdominal distension, and the abdominal wall may develop a bluish discoloration. In NEC, the abdominal wall tends to become erythematous and indurated (Figure 66.1). The bluish discoloration has been highlighted by numerous authors,[1,6,19,30] but this feature is only a pointer to SIP and does not reliably distinguish it from NEC.[2,20,32] Unlike SIP, infants with NEC may have blood in the stools.[20] Both groups of infants may develop hypotension and metabolic acidosis.[4,20]

Laboratory features in SIP may include leukocytosis and thrombocytopenia and are not helpful in the differential diagnosis with NEC.[20]

Plain abdominal radiographs in SIP show a pneumoperitoneum but without signs of pneumatosis intestinalis or portal venous gas (Figure 66.2a). The pneumoperitoneum is usually obvious on a supine abdominal radiograph, e.g., the classical football sign or Rigler's sign. If there is only a small amount of free air, then a supine cross-table lateral shoot-through view may be helpful. The radiologic signs traditionally associated with NEC, namely, pneumatosis intestinalis and portal vein gas, are highly specific but relatively insensitive (Figure 66.2b). Only rarely is pneumatosis present in SIP.[20] Thus, the presence of pneumatosis intestinalis and portal vein gas is helpful in distinguishing NEC from SIP, but their absence is not.[33] In a minority of infants with SIP, the abdominal radiograph may initially be gasless[2,19] (Figure 66.3); in such cases, the presence of

Table 66.1 Differential diagnosis of SIP and NEC

	SIP	NEC
Median age at presentation (days)	7 (0–15)	25 (8–60)
Prodrome	Few systemic or abdominal signs preceding perforation	Often systemically unwell with abdominal signs before perforation
Clinical signs	Abdominal distension Bluish discoloration	Abdominal distension Abdominal wall erythema and induration
Radiologic signs	Pneumoperitoneum Gasless abdomen	Pneumatosis intestinalis Portal vein gas Fixed dilated small bowel loops Pneumoperitoneum
Laboratory features	Leukocytosis ± thrombocytopenia	

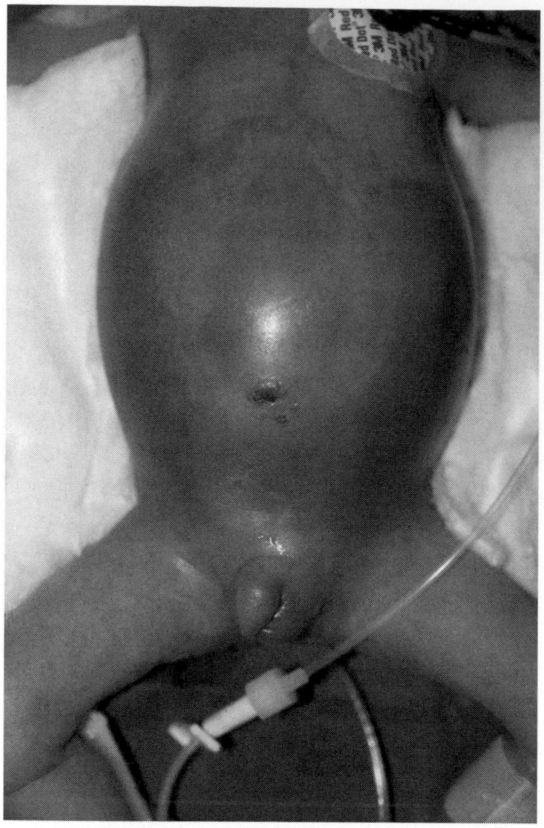

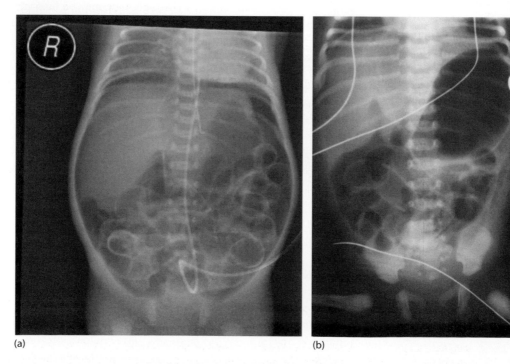

Figure 66.1 Abdominal wall discoloration in NEC. The abdominal wall is indurated and erythematous in contrast to the abdomen with SIP, which is distended and may have a bluish discoloration.

echogenic free fluid on an abdominal ultrasound scan supports the diagnosis of SIP.[32]

In summary, there are no clinical, laboratory, or radiologic features that can reliably distinguish SIP from NEC, but the earlier age of onset of the perforation and absence of pneumatosis intestinalis on the plain abdominal radiograph are features favoring the diagnosis of SIP.[2]

Other rarer differential diagnoses of SIP include (i) pneumoperitoneum secondary to pulmonary air leak, which may occur in infants who are ventilated or on continuous positive airway pressure (CPAP) and who have a pneumothorax or pneumomediastinum[34]; (ii) gastric perforation, which can affect a preterm newborn in the first week of life, although it is rare in ELBW infants[35,36] (see Chapter 54, this volume); and (iii) idiopathic pneumoperitoneum in a baby who is clinically stable and has no signs of peritoneal contamination.[37]

TREATMENT

Once SIP is suspected, enteral feeds and medications should be stopped and the stomach emptied by naso/orogastric tube. A double lumen gastric tube on low pressure suction is more effective at decompressing the gut than a standard naso/orogastric tube on free drainage and intermittent aspiration, especially if the baby is on CPAP. Other measures include intravenous fluids and broad spectrum antibiotics, analgesia, inotropes to treat hypotension that persists after fluid resuscitation, and parenteral nutrition. A prophylactic antifungal, e.g., fluconazole, is advisable.

(a)

(b)

Figure 66.2 (a) Supine abdominal radiograph of a 7-day-old 24-week-gestation female infant with SIP. There is a pneumoperitoneum with a "football" sign (note the falciform ligament) and Rigler sign (air on both sides of the intestinal wall). Radiologic features of NEC are absent. (b) Plain abdominal radiograph of an infant with intestinal perforation from NEC. Note the free air, Rigler sign, and intestinal pneumatosis, which is maximal on the infant's left side.

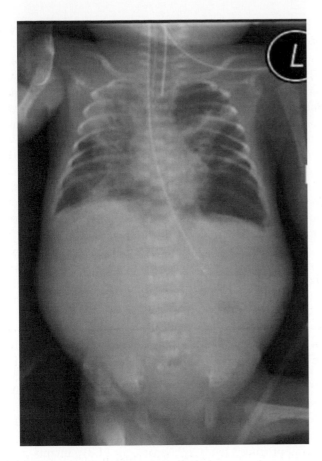

Figure 66.3 Almost completely gasless abdomen in a premature ELBW infant with chronic lung disease and SIP.

SIP is usually treated either by laparotomy and bowel resection[4,19,38] or by peritoneal drainage. Rarely, if the baby is stable, has minimal abdominal distension and no respiratory compromise, and the diagnosis of SIP is reasonably certain, the author has successfully managed the infant without any abdominal intervention. Primary peritoneal drainage (PPD) has the advantage of being performed at the cotside in the neonatal intensive care unit under local anesthesia. It avoids transfer of the baby to the operating room and the risks associated with general anesthesia and laparotomy. In many centers with modern neonatal intensive care, around 70%–80% of infants with presumed SIP treated by PPD will recover without the need for further surgical intervention[6,31,39–42] (Table 66.2). Unfortunately, there are no randomized controlled clinical trials (RCTs) comparing PPD and primary laparotomy in SIP. Such a study would be difficult to perform because in infants treated by PPD alone, the diagnosis of SIP is presumed rather than definite, and therefore some patients with SIP could, in fact, have NEC.

The reported outcomes for PPD in SIP underline the importance of attempting to distinguish SIP from intestinal perforation secondary to NEC because the utility of PPD in NEC is controversial (the evidence favoring primary laparotomy in most cases). Attempts to compare the efficacy of PPD versus primary laparotomy in premature low birth weight infants with intestinal perforation have been confounded by the inclusion of patients with either SIP or NEC. Despite this limitation, neither of the two published RCTs of PPD versus primary laparotomy in premature newborns with intestinal perforation showed a difference in mortality between the two treatment options.[43,44] However, 62% of VLBW newborns treated by PPD in the larger US study[43] avoided laparotomy (as compared to only 26% of ELBW infants in the international study[44]). Based on these two studies, a Cochrane review concluded that there was no significant benefit or harm from PPD versus laparotomy in premature VLBW newborns with intestinal perforation.[45] It should be emphasized that these studies did not differentiate patients with SIP from those with NEC. Recent retrospective reports indicate that PPD is likely to be significantly more successful in SIP than perforated NEC.[31,41]

Primary peritoneal drainage

The abdomen is prepped with antiseptic solution, and local anesthesia is injected around McBurney's point (two-thirds

Table 66.2 Recent reports of infants with (presumed) SIP managed by PPD

Author details	Study period and group[c]	No. of SIP cases	Treated by PPD alone	Subsequent "salvage" laparotomy	Survival
Cass et al.,[39] USA	1996–1999 ELBW	10	8 (80%)	2 (20%)	9 (90%)
Gollin et al.,[40] USA	1999–2002 ELBW	25	20 (80%)	5 (20%)	17(68%)
Emil et al.,[6] USA	2002–2005 ELBW	16	5 (31%)	11 (69%)	13 (81%)
Stokes et al.,[41] USA	2007–2012 VLBW	15	13 (87%)	2 (13%)	8 (53%)
Jakaitis and Bhatia,[42] USA	2003–2012 ELBW	89	67 (75%)	22[a] (25%)	71[b] (85%)
Mishra et al.,[31] New Zealand	1995–2012 <1800 g	29	22 (76%)	7 (24%)	21 (72%)

Sources: Emil S et al., *Eur J Pediatr Surg* 2008; 18: 80–5; Mishra P et al., *J Paediatr Child Health* 2016; 52: 272–7; Cass DL et al., *J Pediatr Surg* 2000; 35: 1531–6; Gollin G et al., *J Pediatr Surg* 2003; 38: 1814–7; Stokes SM et al., *Am Surg* 2014; 80: 851–4; Jakaitis BM, Bhatia AM., *J Perinatol* 2015; 35: 607–11.

[a] Four of these patients found to have NEC.
[b] Six lost to follow-up.
[c] All retrospective studies. ELBW = extremely low birth weight (<1000 g); VLBW = very low birth weight (<1500 g).

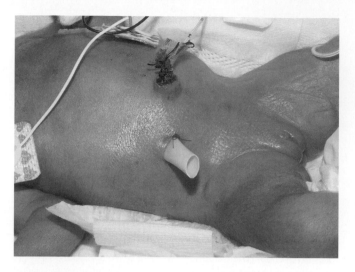

Figure 66.4 Penrose drain in the right iliac fossa of a premature infant with SIP.

of the distance along a line from the umbilicus to the anterior superior iliac spine in the right lower quadrant). A small skin incision is made, and a hemostat is used to gently dissect through the layers of the abdominal wall, taking care to avoid visceral injury. On entering the peritoneal cavity, air and a small amount of bile/meconium stained fluid are released. A culture swab is taken, and a Penrose drain is gently threaded into the peritoneal cavity using the hemostat and secured with a single skin suture. The drain should be tunneled across under the anterior abdominal wall to the left side of the abdomen (Figure 66.4). Some reports describe exiting the drain in the left iliac fossa to facilitate irrigation of the peritoneal cavity with warm saline,[6,41] but such a maneuver may risk injuring the bladder[6] and is unnecessary.

Laparotomy

Laparotomy is necessary soon after PPD if the infant fails to improve, or there is a persistent leak of air or intestinal content or evidence of uncontrolled intra-abdominal sepsis.[39,42] Exploration usually reveals an isolated bowel perforation, most often in the ileum, and the presence of otherwise healthy bowel. The short affected segment of gut is resected followed either by primary anastomosis or the creation of proximal and distal stomas. In one small uncontrolled retrospective study of 23 infants who underwent primary laparotomy for SIP, mortality and morbidity were significantly greater after primary anastomosis than after stoma formation.[38] However, these results should be interpreted cautiously as 6 of the 14 infants treated by primary anastomosis developed postoperative NEC, which was fatal in 4.

If PPD is successful, wound drainage is minimal after 5–7 days, and the drain is then gradually removed by withdrawing it by about 1 cm each day. Antibiotics are given for 7–10 days. Once the drain is out and gut function has returned (as evidenced by a soft, nondistended abdomen in a baby who is stooling and has minimal clear gastric aspirates), enteral feeding is restarted. The author has not routinely performed a gastrointestinal contrast study prior to refeeding but reserves this investigation for those babies who fail to make the expected progress with enteral feeds.

If the newborn initially responds well to PPD, a laparotomy may yet be required subsequently for several reasons: persistent drainage of enteric fluid from the drain site indicative of an enterocutaneous fistula; recurrence of the pneumoperitoneum after the drain is removed (due to recurrent SIP or NEC); or intestinal obstruction, which may develop days or weeks after the drain has been removed due to intra-abdominal adhesions or a stricture at the site of the bowel perforation.[42] The drain site itself may be complicated by development of an incisional hernia.[39,41,42]

Later complications of SIP after PPD or primary laparotomy also include NEC.[21,38] Every effort should be made to reduce the risk of this complication by giving breast milk rather than formula feed.[46,47]

OUTCOME

The outcome after SIP has progressively improved such that 70% or more of affected newborns now survive in many units, whether treated by PPD or by primary laparotomy.[2,4] However, neurodevelopmental outcomes are worse than for unaffected infants of similar gestation and weight.[7,48,49] The overall prognosis tends to be worse for ELBW infants compared to heavier babies.[4,7] Mortality after SIP is reportedly lower than after surgically treated NEC,[2,4,12] but the morbidity in both groups is high because of their profound prematurity.

REFERENCES

1. Meyer CL, Payne NR, Roback SA. Spontaneous, isolated intestinal perforations in neonates with birth weight less than 1,000 g not associated with necrotizing enterocolitis. *J Pediatr Surg* 1991; 26: 714–7.
2. Blakely ML, Lally KP, McDonald S et al. Postoperative outcomes of extremely low birth-weight infants with necrotizing enterocolitis or isolated intestinal perforation: A prospective cohort study by the NICHD Neonatal Research Network. *Ann Surg* 2005; 241: 984–94.
3. Kawase Y, Ishii T, Arai H, Uga N. Gastrointestinal perforation in very low-birthweight infants. *Pediatr Int* 2006; 48: 599–603.
4. Fisher JG, Jones BA, Gutierrez IM et al. Mortality associated with laparotomy-confirmed neonatal spontaneous intestinal perforation: A prospective 5-year multicenter analysis. *J Pediatr Surg* 2014; 49: 1215–9.
5. Blakely ML, Tyson JE, Lally KP et al. Laparotomy versus peritoneal drainage for necrotizing enterocolitis or isolated intestinal perforation in extremely low birth weight infants: Outcomes through 18 months adjusted age. *Pediatrics* 2006; 117: e680–7.

6. Emil S, Davis K, Ahmad I, Straus A. Factors associated with definitive peritoneal drainage for spontaneous intestinal perforation in extremely low birth weight neonates. *Eur J Pediatr Surg* 2008; 18: 80–5.

7. Wadhawan R, Oh W, Hintz SR et al. Neurodevelopmental outcomes of extremely low birth weight infants with spontaneous intestinal perforation or surgical necrotizing enterocolitis. *J Perinatol* 2014; 34: 64–70.

8. Ragouilliaux CJ, Keeney SE, Hawkins HK, Rowen JL. Maternal factors in extremely low birth weight infants who develop spontaneous intestinal perforation. *Pediatrics* 2007; 120: e1458–64.

9. Ducey J, Owen A, Coombs R, Cohen M. Vasculitis as part of the fetal response to acute chorioamnionitis likely plays a role in the development of necrotizing enterocolitis and spontaneous intestinal perforation in premature neonates. *Eur J Pediatr Surg* 2015; 25: 284–91.

10. Yılmaz Y, Kutman HG, Ulu HÖ et al. Preeclampsia is an independent risk factor for spontaneous intestinal perforation in very preterm infants. *J Matern Fetal Neonatal Med* 2014; 27: 1248–51.

11. Attridge JT, Clark R, Gordon PV. New insights into spontaneous intestinal perforation using a national data set (3): Antenatal steroids have no adverse association with spontaneous intestinal perforation. *J Perinatol* 2006; 26: 667–70.

12. Shah J, Singhal N, da Silva O et al. Intestinal perforation in very preterm neonates: Risk factors and outcomes. *J Perinatol* 2015; 35: 595–600.

13. Wadhawan R, Oh W, Vohr BR et al. Spontaneous intestinal perforation in extremely low birth weight infants: Association with indomethacin therapy and effects on neurodevelopmental outcomes at 18–22 months corrected age. *Arch Dis Child Fetal Neonatal Ed* 2013; 98: F127–32.

14. Rattray BN, Kraus DM, Drinker LR et al. Antenatal magnesium sulfate and spontaneous intestinal perforation in infants less than 25 weeks gestation. *J Perinatol* 2014; 34: 819–22.

15. Doyle LW, Ehrenkranz RA, Halliday HL. Early (<8 days) postnatal corticosteroids for preventing chronic lung disease in preterm infants. *Cochrane Database Syst Rev* 2014; 5: CD001146.

16. Doyle LW, Ehrenkranz RA, Halliday HL. Late (>7 days) postnatal corticosteroids for chronic lung disease in preterm infants. *Cochrane Database Syst Rev* 2014; 5: CD001145.

17. Kelleher J, Salas AA, Bhat R et al. Prophylactic indomethacin and intestinal perforation in extremely low birth weight infants. *Pediatrics* 2014; 134: e1369–77.

18. Fowlie PW, Davis PG, McGuire W. Prophylactic intravenous indomethacin for preventing mortality and morbidity in preterm infants. *Cochrane Database Syst Rev* 2010: CD000174.

19. Pumberger W, Mayr M, Kohlhauser C, Weninger M. Spontaneous localized intestinal perforation in very-low-birth-weight infants: A distinct clinical entity different from necrotizing enterocolitis. *J Am Coll Surg* 2002; 195: 796–803.

20. Hwang H, Murphy JJ, Gow KK et al. Are localized intestinal perforations distinct from necrotizing enterocolitis? *J Pediatr Surg* 2003; 38: 763–7.

21. Drewett MS, Burge DM. Recurrent neonatal gastrointestinal problems after spontaneous intestinal perforation. *Pediatr Surg Int* 2007; 23: 1081–4.

22. Kubota A, Yamanaka H, Okuyama H et al. Focal intestinal perforation in extremely-low-birth-weight neonates: Etiological consideration from histological findings. *Pediatr Surg Int* 2007; 23: 997–1000.

23. Lai S, Yu W, Wallace L et al. Intestinal muscularis propria increases in thickness with corrected gestational age and is focally attenuated in patients with isolated intestinal perforations. *J Pediatr Surg* 2014; 49: 114–9.

24. Tatekawa Y, Muraji T, Imai Y et al. The mechanism of focal intestinal perforations in neonates with low birth weight. *Pediatr Surg Int* 1999; 15: 549–52.

25. Gordon PV, Herman AC, Marcinkiewicz M et al. A neonatal mouse model of intestinal perforation: Investigating the harmful synergism between glucocorticoids and indomethacin. *J Pediatr Gastroenterol Nutr* 2007; 45: 509–19.

26. Gordon PV. Understanding intestinal vulnerability to perforation in the extremely low birth weight infant. *Pediatr Res* 2009; 65: 138–44.

27. Chan KY, Leung FW, Lam HS et al. Immunoregulatory protein profiles of necrotizing enterocolitis *versus* spontaneous intestinal perforation in preterm infants. *PLoS One* 2012; 7: e36977.

28. Chan KY, Leung KT, Tam YH et al. Genome-wide expression profiles of necrotizing enterocolitis versus spontaneous intestinal perforation in human intestinal tissues: Dysregulation of functional pathways. *Ann Surg* 2014; 260: 1128–37.

29. Bhatia AM, Stoll BJ, Cismowski MJ, Hamrick SE. Cytokine levels in the preterm infant with neonatal intestinal injury. *Am J Perinatol* 2014; 31: 489–96.

30. Adderson EE, Pappin A, Pavia AT. Spontaneous intestinal perforation in premature infants: A distinct clinical entity associated with systemic candidiasis. *J Pediatr Surg* 1998; 33: 1463–7.

31. Mishra P, Foley D, Purdie G, Pringle KC. Intestinal perforation in premature neonates: The need for subsequent laparotomy after placement of peritoneal drains. *J Paediatr Child Health* 2016; 52: 272–7.

32. Fischer A, Vachon L, Durand M, Cayabyab RG. Ultrasound to diagnose spontaneous intestinal perforation in infants weighing ⩽ 1000 g at birth. *J Perinatol* 2015; 35: 104–9.

33. Tam AL, Camberos A, Applebaum H. Surgical decision making in necrotizing enterocolitis and focal intestinal perforation: Predictive value of radiologic findings. *J Pediatr Surg* 2002; 37: 1688–91.

34. Knight PJ, Abdenour G. Pneumoperitoneum in the ventilated neonate: Respiratory or gastrointestinal origin? *J Pediatr* 1981; 98: 972–4.

35. Lin CM, Lee HC, Kao HA et al. Neonatal gastric perforation: Report of 15 cases and review of the literature. *Pediatr Neonatol* 2008; 49: 65–70.

36. Lee do K, Shim SY, Cho SJ et al. Comparison of gastric and other bowel perforations in preterm infants: A review of 20 years' experience in a single institution. *Korean J Pediatr* 2015; 58: 288–93.

37. Gupta R, Bihari Sharma S, Golash P et al. Pneumoperitoneum in the newborn: Is surgical intervention always indicated? *J Neonatal Surg* 2014; 3: 32.

38. De Haro Jorge I, Prat Ortells J, Albert Cazalla A et al. Long term outcome of preterm infants with isolated intestinal perforation: A comparison between primary anastomosis and ileostomy. *J Pediatr Surg* 2016; 51: 1251–4.

39. Cass DL, Brandt ML, Patel DL et al. Peritoneal drainage as definitive treatment for neonates with isolated intestinal perforation. *J Pediatr Surg* 2000; 35: 1531–6.

40. Gollin G, Abarbanell A, Baerg JE. Peritoneal drainage as definitive management of intestinal perforation in extremely low-birth-weight infants. *J Pediatr Surg* 2003; 38: 1814–17.

41. Stokes SM, Iocono JA, Draus JM Jr. Peritoneal drainage as the initial management of intestinal perforation in premature infants. *Am Surg* 2014; 80: 851–4.

42. Jakaitis BM, Bhatia AM. Definitive peritoneal drainage in the extremely low birth weight infant with spontaneous intestinal perforation: Predictors and hospital outcomes. *J Perinatol* 2015; 35: 607–11.

43. Moss RL, Dimmitt RA, Barnhart DC et al. Laparotomy versus peritoneal drainage for necrotizing enterocolitis and perforation. *N Engl J Med* 2006; 354: 2225–34.

44. Rees CM, Eaton S, Kiely EM et al. Peritoneal drainage or laparotomy for neonatal bowel perforation: A randomized controlled trial. *Ann Surg* 2008; 248: 44–51.

45. Rao SC, Basani L, Simmer K et al. Peritoneal drainage versus laparotomy as initial surgical treatment for perforated necrotizing enterocolitis or spontaneous intestinal perforation in preterm low birth weight infants. *Cochrane Database Syst Rev* 2011; CD006182.

46. Kantorowska A, Wei JC, Cohen RS et al. Impact of donor milk availability on breast milk use and necrotizing enterocolitis rates. *Pediatrics* 2016; 137: 1–8.

47. Colaizy TT, Bartick MC, Jegier BJ et al. Impact of optimized breastfeeding on the costs of necrotizing enterocolitis in extremely low birthweight infants. *J Pediatr* 2016; 175: 100–5.e2.

48. Roze E, Ta BD, van der Ree MH et al. Functional impairments at school age of children with necrotizing enterocolitis or spontaneous intestinal perforation. *Pediatr Res* 2011; 70: 619–25.

49. Shah TA, Meinzen-Derr J, Gratton T et al. Hospital and neurodevelopmental outcomes of extremely low-birth-weight infants with necrotizing enterocolitis and spontaneous intestinal perforation. *J Perinatol* 2012; 32: 552–8.

67

Hirschsprung's disease

PREM PURI AND CHRISTIAN TOMUSCHAT

INTRODUCTION

Hirschsprung's disease (HD) is a relatively common cause of intestinal obstruction in the newborn. It is characterized by absence of ganglionic cells in the distal bowel beginning at the internal sphincter and extending proximally for varying distances. The aganglionosis is confined to rectosigmoid in over 80% of patients. In the remaining patients, the aganglionosis extends beyond rectosigmoid involving descending colon and transverse colon, or it may involve the entire colon along with a short segment of terminal ileum. Total intestinal aganglionosis with absence of ganglion cells from the duodenum to the rectum is the rarest form of HD and is associated with high morbidity and mortality.[1-4]

The incidence of HD is estimated to be 1 in 5000 live births[5-8] (Table 67.1). Spouge and Baird[8] studied the incidence of HD in 689,118 consecutive live births in British Columbia and reported an incidence rate for this disease to be 1 in 4417 live births. Significant interracial differences in the incidence of HD have been reported: 1 in 10,000 births in Hispanic subjects, 1 in 6667 in white subjects, 1 in 4761 in black subjects, and 1 in 3571 in Asian subjects.[9] The disease is more common in boys, with a male-to-female ratio of 4:1.[5,10] The male preponderance is less evident in long-segment HD, where the male-to-female ratio is 1.5–2:1.[5-8]

ETIOLOGY

Neural crest cell migration

The enteric nervous system (ENS) is the largest and the most complex division of the peripheral nervous system. It provides the gastrointestinal tract with its unique network of innervation within its walls and functions largely independently of the central nervous system (CNS). The ENS contains more neurons than the spinal cord and is responsible for the coordination of normal bowel motility and secretory activities. Most of the neurons are located in either myenteric ganglia or submucosal ganglia and a few scattered within the mucosa. It is generally accepted that the enteric ganglion cells are derived primarily from the vagal neural crest cells.[11-14] During normal development, neuroblasts migrate from the vagal neural crest along the bowel wall in a craniocaudal direction from esophagus to anus. The embryonic neural crest arises in the neural tube, originating with the CNS, but neural crest cells detach from this tissue via reduction of cell–cell and cell–matrix adhesion. The epitheliomesenchymal transformation allows crest cells to migrate along pathways. Pathway selection is most likely achieved by balanced combinations of molecules that promote and reduce adhesion.

In the human fetus, neural crest-derived neuroblasts first appear in the developing esophagus at 5 weeks, and then migrate down to the anal canal in a craniocaudal direction during the 5th to 12th weeks of gestation. The neural crest cells first form the myenteric plexus just outside the circular muscle layer. The mesenchymally derived longitudinal muscle layer then forms, sandwiching the myenteric plexus after it has been formed in the 12th week of gestation. In addition, after the craniocaudal migration has ended, the submucous plexus is formed by the neuroblasts, which migrate from the myenteric plexus across the circular muscle layer and into the submucosa; this progresses in a craniocaudal direction during the 12th to 16th weeks of gestation.[15,16] The absence of ganglion cells in HD has been attributed to failure of migration of neural crest cells. The earlier the arrest of migration, the longer the aganglionic segment.

Several investigators have suggested that the enteric neurons follow a dual gradient of development from each end of the gut toward the middle, with vagal neural crest cells providing the main source of enteric neurons and sacral neural crest cells innervating the hindgut.[13,15,16] Whether the sacral neural crest contributes to the ENS in the human is less clear. Failure of the vagal derived neural crest cells to colonize the hindgut results in failure of ENS development in this region, suggesting that an interaction between sacral and vagal enteric neural crest cells may be necessary for sacral neural crest cell contribution to the ENS.[16]

Table 67.1 Incidence of HD

Author	Incidence	Area	
Passarge[6]		1 in 5000	Cincinnati
Orr and Scobie[5]	1 in 4500	Scotland	
Goldberg[107]		1 in 5682	Baltimore
Spouge and Baird[8]	1 in 4417	British Columbia	

Genetic factors

Genetic factors have been implicated in the etiology of HD. HD is known to occur in families. The reported incidence of familial cases varied from 3.6% to 7.8% in different series. A familial incidence of 15%–21% has been reported in total colonic aganglionosis (TCA) and 50% in the rare total intestinal aganglionosis.[17–19]

Recurrence risk to siblings is dependent upon the sex of the person affected and the extent of aganglionosis. Badner et al.[20,21] calculated the risk of HD transmission to relatives and found that the recurrence risk to siblings increases as the aganglionosis becomes more extensive (Table 67.2). The brothers of patients with rectosigmoid HD have a higher risk (4%) than sisters (1%). Much higher risks are observed in cases of long-segment HD. The brothers and sons of affected females have a 24% and 29% risk of being affected, respectively. The relationship with Down's syndrome also tends to suggest a probable genetic component in the etiology of HD. Down's syndrome is the most common chromosomal abnormality associated with aganglionosis and had been reported to occur in 4.5%–16% of all cases of HD.[22] Other chromosomal abnormalities that have been described in association with HD include interstitial deletion of distal 13q, partial deletion of 2p and reciprocal translocation, and trisomy 18 mosaic. Some of the syndromic forms of HD involve other cell types also derived from the neural crest, such as precursors of melanocytes for cranial pigment formation or in cells destined to function in the sensory components of the acoustic pathway. These include Sha–Waardenburg syndrome, Yemenite deaf–blind–hypopigmentation, piebaldism, Goldberg–Sprintzen syndrome, Smith–Lemli–Opitz syndrome, multiple endocrine neoplasia 2, and congenital central hypoventilation syndrome (Ondine's curse).[23–27]

During the past 15 years, several genes have been identified that control morphogenesis and differentiation of the ENS. These genes, when mutated or deleted, interfere with ENS development. So far, 22 genes are known to be involved in the development of HD (Table 67.3). One of these genes, the RET gene, encoding a tyrosine-kinase receptor, is the major gene causing HD.[19,28,29] Mutations in the coding region of RET are responsible for 50% of familial HD cases and 15% of sporadic ones.[19] All the genes that have been implicated in the development of HD together account for only 20% of all cases of HD.[19,27,30]

This implies that other genes are also involved in the development of HD.

PATHOPHYSIOLOGY

The pathophysiology of HD is not fully understood. It has long been recognized that obstructive symptoms in HD are secondary to the abnormal motility of the distal narrow segment, but there is still no clear explanation for the occurrence of the spastic or tonically contracted segment of bowel.[31]

Normal intestinal motility requires coordinated interaction of ENS, smooth muscle cells, and interstitial cells. Several abnormalities have been described to explain the basis for motility dysfunction in the contracted bowel in HD.

Cholinergic hyperinnervation

In association with aganglionosis, there is a marked increase in cholinergic nerve fibers in the intermuscular zone and submucosa of the aganglionic segment. These fibers appear as thick nerve trunks and correspond to extrinsic preganglionic parasympathetic nerves.[32–36] The continuous acetylcholine release from the axons of these parasympathetic nerves results in an excessive accumulation of the enzyme acetylcholinesterase (AChE) that is typically found in the lamina propria mucosae, muscularis mucosae, and circular muscle with histochemical staining technique.[37] Both the thick nerve trunks and the increased AChE activity are most pronounced in the most distal aganglionic rectum and progressively diminish proximally as normal bowel is approached.[38] The proximal extent of increased cholinergic activity does not necessarily correspond to the extent of the aganglionosis, which usually extends more proximally to a variable degree. Pharmacologic investigations of the colon in HD have demonstrated higher acetylcholine release in the aganglionic segment at rest and after stimulation compared with the proximal ganglionic bowel.[39,40] AChE concentration has also been found to be higher in the serum and erythrocytes from children suffering from HD.[41] Cholinergic nerve hyperplasia has been proposed as the cause of spasticity of the aganglionic segment since acetylcholine is the main excitatory neurotransmitter.

Adrenergic innervation

Fluorescent–histochemical studies for localization of adrenergic nerves have demonstrated that they are increased in number in the aganglionic colon of HD and have a chaotic distribution. They are also present in the circular and longitudinal muscle layers as well

Table 67.2 Recurrence risk to siblings

Relative	Recurrence risk (%)
Brothers of patients with rectosigmoid HD	?4
Sisters of patients with rectosigmoid HD	?1
Brothers of females with long-segment HD	24
Sons of females with long-segment HD	29

Table 67.3 Genes involved in the morphogenesis and differentiation of the ENS

Gene	Phenotype	Inheritance	Effects on intestinal innervation
RET	HSCR/HSCR-MEN2/FMTC	Dominant, incomplete penetrance	Absence of neuronal plexus in the small and large bowel TIA, renal agenesis
GDNF	HSCR	Dominant, low penetrance	Absence of neuronal plexus in the small and large bowel TIA, renal agenesis
EDNRB	WS4/HSCR	Recessive/dominant	Aganglionosis of the distal colon, coat spotting
SOX10	WS4/HSCR	Dominant	Aganglionosis, coat spotting
PHOX2B	CCHS/Neuroblastoma + HSCR	Dominant	TIA, no autonomic nervous system, ventilatory anomalies
NRTN	HSCR	Dominant, low penetrance	Moderate deficit of enteric neurons
PSPN	HSCR	Dominant, low penetrance	–
GFRA1	HSCR	Dominant, low penetrance	TIA, renal agenesis
EDN3	WS4/HSCR	Recessive/dominant	Aganglionosis, coat spotting
ECE1	HSCR with cardiac defects, craniofacial anomalies and autonomic dysfunction	Dominant	Aganglionosis, coat spotting, craniofacial defects
NTF3	HSCR	Dominant, low penetrance	Reduced enteric neurons
NTRK3	HSCR	Dominant, low penetrance	Reduced enteric neurons
PROKR1	HSCR	Dominant, low penetrance	–
PROKR2	HSCR	Dominant, low penetrance	Hypoplasia of the olfactory bulb and reproductive system
PROK1	HSCR	Dominant, low penetrance	–
SEMA3A	HSCR	Dominant, low penetrance	Deficit of cardiac sympathetic innervation and stellate ganglia malformation
SEMA3D	HSCR	Dominant, low penetrance	–
NRG1	HSCR	Dominant, low penetrance	Lethal from cardiac defect
NRG3	HSCR	Dominant, low penetrance	–
ZFHX1B	MWS	Dominant	Lethal at gastrulation
KIAA1279	GSS	Recessive	–
L1CAM	HSAS/MASA spectrum + HSCR	x-linked	Hydrocephalus

as in the mucosa, whereas they are almost not found in normal ganglionic colon.[42–44] However, the sensitivity of the aganglionic bowel to epinephrine is apparently not increased, despite the elevated number of adrenergic fibers.[45,46] The tissue concentration of norepinephrine is two to three times higher in the aganglionic bowel than in the normal colon; and also there is a corresponding increase in tyrosine hydroxylase, an enzyme that regulates norepinephrine biosynthesis.[43] Because adrenergic nerves normally act to relax the bowel, it is unlikely that adrenergic hyperactivity is responsible for increased tone in the aganglionic colon.[47]

Nitrergic innervation

Nitric oxide (NO) is considered to be one of the most important neurotransmitters involved in the relaxation of the smooth muscle of the gut.[48,49] It is synthesized in a reaction catalyzed by nitric oxide synthase (NOS) and depends on L-arginine and molecular oxygen as cosubstrates to form L-citrulline and NO. There are three archetypal mammalian NOS isoforms described: nNOS or neuronal NOS; iNOS, an inducible NOS isoform expressed in a variety of activated tissues; and eNOS or endothelial NOS.[50] NO binds to cytosolic guanylate cyclase and increases the production of 3'5'-cyclic guanosine monophosphate (cGMP) with subsequent relaxation of smooth muscle.[51] NOS has been shown to be colocalized with reduced nicotine adenine dinucleotide phosphate (NADPH) diaphorase, which has been demonstrated to have identical functions.[52,53] Several investigators have studied NOS distribution in the ganglionic and aganglionic bowel in patients with HD using NOS immunohistochemistry or NADPH diaphorase histochemistry.[54–59] In normal and ganglionic colon from patients with HD, there is a strong NADPH diaphorase staining of the submucous and myenteric plexuses, and a large number of positive nerve fibers in the circular and longitudinal muscle as well as in the muscularis mucosae.[51] In the aganglionic segment of HD patients, there are no ganglia and there is an absence or marked reduction of NADPH diaphorase positive nerve fibers in both muscle layers and in the muscularis mucosae. The typical hypertrophied nerve trunks appear weakly stained.[51] Kusafuka and Puri[60] examined the expression of neural NOS mRNA in the aganglionic segment from seven patients who had HD and demonstrated that NOS mRNA expression was decreased at least 1/50 to 1/100 of the level expressed in ganglionic bowel. These findings indicate that there is impaired NO synthesis in the aganglionic bowel in HD, and this deficiency could prevent smooth muscle relaxation, thereby causing the lack of peristalsis in HD. In an interesting experiment, Bealer et al.[61] compared the effect of an exogenous source of NO, S-nitroso-N-acetylpenicillamine (SNAP), on the isometric tension of smooth muscle strips from aganglionic bowel and demonstrated a 70% reduction of resting tension. These results suggest that the defective distribution of nerves containing NOS may be involved in the pathogenesis of HD.

Interstitial cells of Cajal

Abnormalities of interstitial cells of Cajal (ICCs) have been described in several disorders of human intestinal motility including HD. Vanderwinden et al.,[62] using c-kit immunohistochemistry, first described that ICCs were scarce and its network appeared disrupted in aganglionic segments of HD, whereas the distribution of ICCs in the ganglionic bowel of HD was similar to that observed in controls. Yamataka et al.[63,64] found a few c-kit positive cells in the muscle layers in HD and a moderate number around the thick nerve bundles in the space between the two muscle layers in the aganglionic bowel. Barshack et al.[65] described abnormal ICC organization in the aganglionic and ganglionic bowel of patients with HD. Horisawa et al.[66] reported no differences in c-kit immunopositive cells in aganglionic segments compared with the corresponding area of ganglionic bowel. Rolle et al.,[51] using whole-mount and frozen sections stained with c-kit immunohistochemistry preparations, showed an altered distribution of ICCs in the entire resected bowel of HD patients and not only in the aganglionic segment. Moreover, gap junctions connecting ICCs were immunolocalized by anti-Connexin 43 antibody, found to be absent from the aganglionic part of HD bowel, and highly reduced from the transitional zone.[67] A scarce, disorganized, and impaired function of ICCs in the aganglionic and ganglionic bowel of patients with HD has been suggested to contribute to the persistent dysmotility problems after properly performed pull-through operation.

Platelet-derived growth factor receptor α⁺-cells

Platelet-derived growth factor receptor α⁺-cells (PDGFRα⁺) have recently been documented in the human colon for the first time.[68] Previously known as fibroblast-like-cells, these cells are found to be distributed in a similar pattern as ICCs as well as morphologically resembling them. PDGFRα⁺ cells are found alongside ICCs, neurons, and smooth muscle cells (SMCs) and appear to have a role in neurotransmission and the modulation of smooth muscle contraction.[69] We have recently discovered a decreased expression of PDGFRα⁺ in HD colon, which suggests a role of these cells in the pathophysiology of this condition (see O'Donnell et al., article in press).

Enteroendocrine cells

Using the generic enteroendocrine cell immunohistochemical markers chromogranin A and synaptophysin, Soeda et al.[70] demonstrated that the number of enteroendocrine cells in the aganglionic colon in patients with HD was significantly increased compared with the number in the normal ganglionic segment. The increase in enteroendocrine cells in the mucosa of aganglionic colon may well influence sustained contraction of the bowel wall mainly mediated by the release of 5-hydroxytryptamine.

Smooth muscle

Smooth muscle cells are the effector cells of the bowel and, as a result of communication from the ENS, ICCs, and PDGFRα⁺, govern intestinal peristalsis. The smooth muscle cell cytoskeleton consists of proteins whose primary function is to serve as a structural framework that surrounds and supports the contractile apparatus of actin and myosin filaments in the body of the smooth muscle cell. Nemeth et al.[71] studied the distribution of cytoskeleton in the smooth muscle of HD bowel by means of immunohistochemistry and found that dystrophin, vinculin, and desmin immunoreactivity was either absent or weak in the smooth muscle of aganglionic bowel, whereas it was moderate to strong in the smooth muscle of normal bowel and ganglionic bowel from patients with HD. Neural cell adhesion molecule (NCAM) is a cell surface glycoprotein involved in cell–cell adhesion during development that has been suggested to play an important role in development and maintenance of the neuromuscular system.[72–74] NCAM is present in the innervation of normal infant bowel and, less densely, in some components of the enteric smooth muscle. Contradictory results have been published regarding the NCAM expression in the smooth muscle of aganglionic bowel. Kobayashi et al.[56] have described a lack of expression of NCAM in the muscularis propria of the aganglionic bowel compared with the ganglionic segment, whereas Romanska et al.[75] have found an increase in the NCAM expression in muscle, particularly in the muscularis mucosae. Anyhow, both authors agree that there is a strong expression of NCAM in the hypertrophic nerve trunks from the aganglionic segment.

Extracellular matrix

Although extracellular matrix (EM) abnormalities have been described mainly related to the pathogenesis of HD, they could also have an influence on its pathophysiology. The lethal spotted mouse, an animal model that develops aganglionosis in its distal bowel, displays an abnormal distribution of EM components including laminin, collagen type IV, glycosaminoglycans, and proteoglycans in the smooth muscle layer.[76,77] Parikh et al.[78] have demonstrated that the laminin concentration in aganglionic bowel was twice as high as in the normoganglionic bowel of HD and three times higher than in an age-matched control. Moreover, by means of immunohistochemistry, they found an uneven distribution of laminin and collagen type IV in the muscularis propria of aganglionic bowel, being more intensely expressed in the circular layer than in the longitudinal layer.[79] The same authors have described that EM components tenascin and fibronectin are more intensely expressed in aganglionic bowel from HD.[79] Moreover, Soret et al. demonstrate that animals with excess collagen VI develop HD-like disease due to decreased enteric neural crest-derived cell (ENCDC) migration. The inhibitory effect of collagen VI on ENCDC migration may partially explain why children with Down's syndrome have an increased risk of HD, since collagen VI genes are on chromosome 21.[80]

PATHOLOGY

The characteristic gross pathological feature in HD is dilation and hypertrophy of the proximal colon with abrupt or gradual transition to narrow distal bowel (Figure 67.1). Although the degree of dilation and hypertrophy increases with age, the cone-shaped transitional zone from dilated to narrow bowel is usually evident in the newborn.

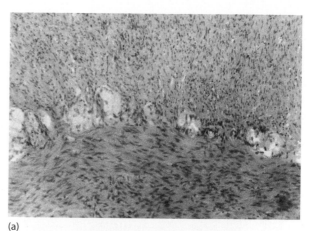

(a)

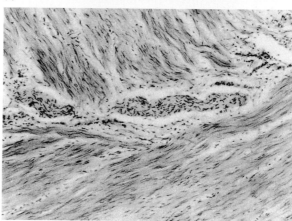

(b)

Figure 67.2 (a) Auerbach's plexus, containing ganglion cells. (b) Hypertrophied nerve trunks in rectal biopsy from a patient with HD.

Histologically, HD is characterized by the absence of ganglionic cells in the myenteric and submucous plexuses, and the presence of hypertrophied nonmyelinated nerve trunks in the space normally occupied by the ganglionic cells (Figure 67.2). The aganglionic segment of bowel is followed proximally by a hypoganglionic segment of varying length. This hypoganglionic zone is characterized by a reduced number of ganglion cells, nerve fibers in myenteric and submucous plexuses, as well as disorganized and reduced numbers of ICCs.

DIAGNOSIS

The diagnosis of HD is usually based on clinical history, radiological studies, anorectal manometry, and in particular histological examination of the rectal wall biopsy specimens.

Clinical features

Of all cases of HD, 80%–90% produce clinical symptoms and are diagnosed during the neonatal period. Delayed passage of meconium is the cardinal symptom in neonates with HD.

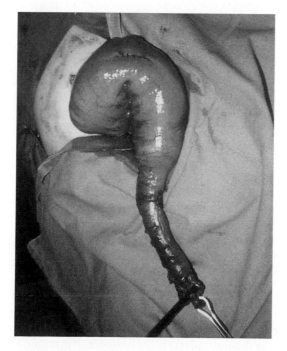

Figure 67.1 Typical gross pathology in HD, with transitional zone at rectosigmoid level.

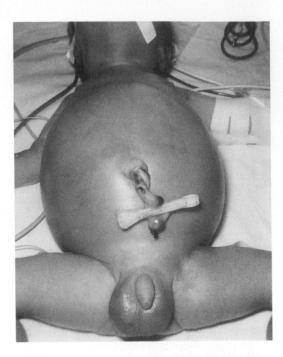

Figure 67.3 A 2-day-old infant with marked abdominal distention and failure to pass meconium. SRB confirmed HD.

Over 90% of affected patients fail to pass meconium in the first 24 hours of life. The usual presentation of HD in the neonatal period is with constipation, abdominal distension, and vomiting during the first few days of life (Figure 67.3). About one-third of the babies with HD present with diarrhea. Diarrhea in HD is always a symptom of enterocolitis, which remains the commonest cause of death. Enterocolitis may resolve with adequate therapy, or it may develop into a life-threatening condition, the toxic megacolon, characterized by the sudden onset of marked abdominal distension, bile stained vomiting, fever, and signs of dehydration, sepsis, and shock. Rectal examination or introduction of a rectal tube results in the explosive evacuation of gas and foul-smelling stools. In older children, the main symptom is persistent constipation and chronic abdominal distension.

Radiological diagnosis

Plain abdominal films in a neonate with HD will show dilated loops of bowel with fluid levels and airless pelvis. Occasionally, one may be able to see a small amount of air in the undistended rectum and dilated colon above it raising the suspicion of HD (Figure 67.4a). Plain abdominal radiographs obtained from patients with TCA may show characteristic signs of ileal obstruction with air fluid levels or simple gaseous distension of small intestinal loops.

In patients with enterocolitis complicating HD, plain abdominal radiography may show thickening of the bowel wall with mucosal irregularity or a grossly dilated colon loop, indicating toxic megacolon. Pneumoperitoneum may be found in those with perforation. Spontaneous perforation of the intestinal tract has been reported in 3% of patients with HD.[81]

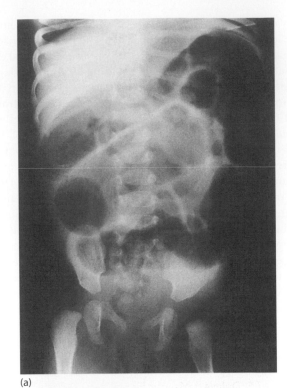

(a)

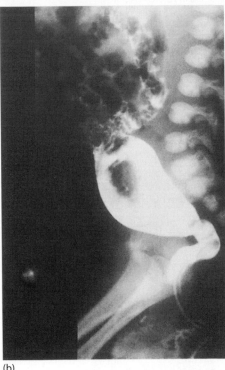

(b)

Figure 67.4 HD. **(a)** Abdominal radiograph in a 4-day-old infant showing marked dilation of large and small bowel loops. Note gas in undilated rectum. **(b)** Barium enema in this patient reveals transitional zone at sigmoid level.

Barium enema performed by an experienced radiologist using careful technique should achieve a high degree of reliability in diagnosing HD in the newborn. It is important that the infant should not have rectal washouts or even digital examinations prior to barium enema, as such interference

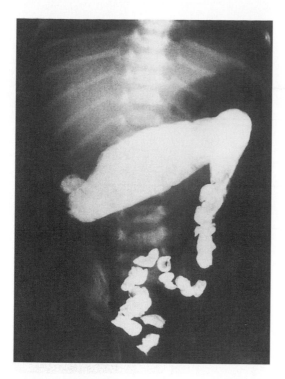

Figure 67.5 Delayed 24-hour film in lateral position showing barium retention with accentuated transition at splenic fixture in a 10-day-old baby.

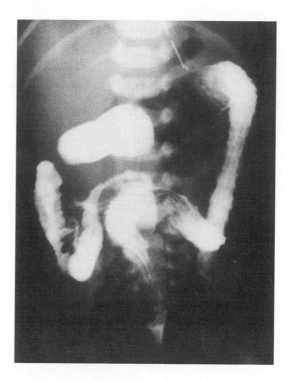

Figure 67.6 Enterocolitis complicating HD. Spasm in rectosigmoid shown in barium enema, with fine mucosal ulceration and mucosal edema giving cobblestone appearance.

may distort the transitional zone appearance and give a false-negative diagnosis. A soft rubber catheter is inserted into the lower rectum and held in position with firm strapping across the buttocks. A balloon catheter should not be used due to the risk of perforation and the possibility of distorting a transitional zone by distension. The barium should be injected slowly in small amounts under fluoroscopic control with the baby in the lateral position. A typical case of HD will demonstrate flow of barium from the undilated rectum through a cone-shaped transitional zone into dilated colon (Figure 67.4b). Some cases may show an abrupt transition between the dilated proximal colon and the distal aganglionic segment, leaving the diagnosis in little doubt.

In some cases, the findings on the barium enema are uncertain, and a delayed film at 24 hours may confirm the diagnosis by demonstrating the retained barium and often accentuating the appearance of the transitional zone (Figure 67.5). In the presence of enterocolitis complicating HD, a barium enema can demonstrate spasm, mucosal edema, and ulceration (Figure 67.6)

In TCA, the contrast enema is not pathognomic and may not provide a definitive diagnosis. The colon in TCA is of normal caliber in 25%–77% of cases.[1,82]

Anorectal manometry

In the normally innervated bowel, distension of the rectum produces relaxation of the internal sphincter rectosphincteric reflex. In normal persons, upon distending the rectal balloon with air, the rectum immediately responds with a

transient rise in pressure lasting 15–20 seconds; at the same time, the internal sphincter rhythmic activity is depressed or abolished, and its pressure falls by 15–20 cm, the duration of relaxation coinciding with the rectal wave (Figure 67.7).

In patients with HD, the rectum often shows spontaneous waves of varying amplitude and frequency in the resting phase. The internal sphincter rhythmic activity is more pronounced. On rectal distension, with an increment of air, there is complete absence of internal sphincter relaxation. Both term infants and premature babies have been shown to exhibit a well-developed recto-anal inhibitory reflex (RAIR) and anorectal pressures.[83] In the presence of a RAIR in children of under 1 year of age, HD is very unlikely. However, the specificity and positive predictive value of ARM for the diagnosis of HD are inferior to those of rectal suction biopsy. ARM may be a useful investigation in patients where a histologic specimen is inadequate and/or functional constipation is most likely diagnosed. Failure to detect the rectosphincteric reflex in premature and term infants is believed to be due to technical difficulties and not to immaturity of ganglion cells. Light sedation particularly in infants and small children may overcome technical difficulties encountered in this age group.

Rectal biopsy

The diagnosis of HD is confirmed on examination of rectal biopsy specimens. A correctly executed rectal biopsy procedure should involve sampling a segment of rectal wall 2 cm

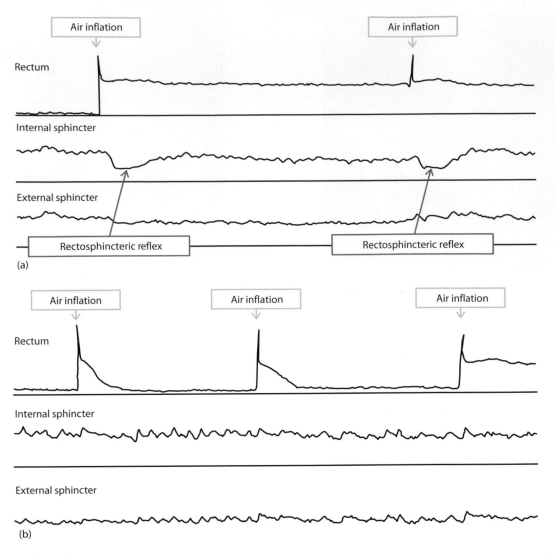

Figure 67.7 Anorectal manometry. **(a)** Normal rectosphincteric reflex on rectal balloon inflation. **(b)** Absence of rectosphincteric reflex and marked internal sphincter rhythmic activity in a patient with HD.

proximal to the dentate line along the posterior wall of the rectum. A biopsy taken too distally may collect a specimen from the physiologically aganglionic region erroneously suggesting the presence of HSCR, whereas a biopsy taken too proximally (i.e., over 4 cm) may miss very short segment of HSCR.[84]

It is also important to bear in mind that recent enemas causing mucosal edema may influence the quality of the specimens; and also a poor technique such as incorrect placement of the biopsy system, and low pressure may contribute to inadequate biopsy specimens; in addition improper techniques like incorrect placement of the biopsy system and inadequate pressure all contribute to inadequate biopsies as well.

The introduction of histochemical staining (IHC) technique for the detection of AChE activity in suction rectal biopsy (SRB) has resulted in a reliable and simple method for the diagnosis of HD.[85–87]

Full-thickness rectal biopsy is rarely indicated for the diagnosis of HD except in TCA. In normal persons, barely

detectable AChE activity is observed within the lamina propria and muscularis mucosa, and submucosal ganglion cells stain strongly for AChE. In HD, there is a marked increase in AChE activity in lamina propria and muscularis, which is evident as coarse, discrete cholinergic nerve fibers stained brown to black (Figure 67.8).

Recently, calretinin staining has been introduced in the diagnostic of HD.[65] Calretinin, a calcium-binding protein that may function as a calcium sensor/modulator, is expressed by a subset of submucosal and myenteric ganglion cells, some of which project nerve terminals into the mucosa. Aganglionic segments completely lack calretinin immunoreactivity in enteric nerves (Figure 67.9).

Kapur et al.'s findings suggest that the sensitivity and specificity of calretinin IHC are equivalent, if not superior, to rapid AChE and that calretinin IHC may be informative when inadequate tissue is available to establish an H&E diagnosis. In fact, in their comparative study, unequivocal diagnosis or exclusion of HSCR by calretinin IHC alone was more accurate than rapid AChE alone, with no major errors

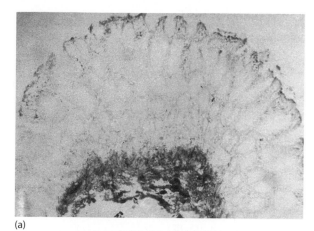

(a)

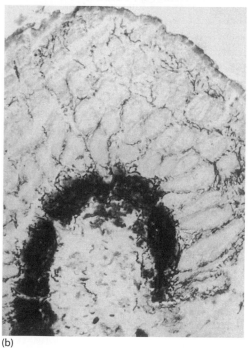

(b)

Figure 67.8 AChE staining of SRB. **(a)** Normal rectum showing minimal AChE staining in mucosa, lamina propria, and muscularis mucosae (×4). **(b)** HD characterized by marked staining of cholinesterase-positive nerves in the lamina propria and muscularis mucosae (×40).

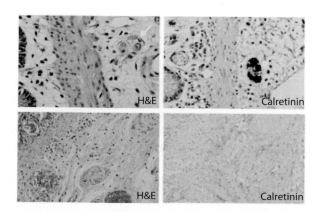

Figure 67.9 Calretinin staining of SRB.

and fewer equivocal readings.[88] Moreover, calretinin staining decreased the rate of inconclusive results and increased the likelihood of a confirmed diagnosis. On the other hand, a number of potential false-positive results described in the literature raise some concern for potential overtreatment, if calretinin is used alone.[89] However, in general, most of the results are in agreement with previous studies and argue for the addition of calretinin to the routine repertoire of stains used to diagnosis HSCR.[90]

In TCA, AChE activity in SRBs presents an atypical pattern, different from the classic one. Positive AChE fibers can be found in the lamina propria as well as the muscularis mucosae. However, cholinergic fibers present a lower density than in classical HD.

DIFFERENTIAL DIAGNOSIS

The differential diagnosis includes other causes of a lower intestinal obstruction in newborns, including intestinal atresia, meconium ileus, meconium peritonitis, meconium plug, small left colon syndrome, and imperforate anus.

Table 67.4 gives the list of common differential diagnoses. Colonic atresia gives similar plain film findings to HD but is readily excluded with barium enema showing complete mechanical obstruction. Distal small bowel atresia shows gross distension of the bowel loop immediately proximal to the obstruction with the widest fluid level in it.

In meconium ileus, the typical mottled thick meconium may be seen. Also, clear, sharp fluid levels are not a feature in erect or lateral decubitus views. However, HD can sometimes simulate meconium ileus in plain films and may give equivocal findings on Gastrografin or barium enema.

Meconium plugs obstructing the colon can present as HD with strongly suggestive history and plain films. Small left colon syndrome is associated with maternal diabetes and presents with marked distension proximal to narrowed descending colon, and simulates HD at the left colonic flexure. These two conditions usually resolve with Gastrografin enema, but a minority of these cases will actually have Hirschsprung's, which should be excluded clinically. In both of these conditions, the rectum has a greater diameter than the sigmoid colon.

Table 67.4 Differential diagnosis of HD

Neonatal bowel obstruction
Colonic atresia
Meconium ileus
Meconium plug syndrome
Small left colon syndrome
Malrotation
Low anorectal malformation
Intestinal motility disorders/pseudo-obstruction
Necrotizing enterocolitis
Medical causes: sepsis, electrolyte abnormalities, drugs, hypothyroidism, etc.

In HD, on the other hand, the rectum has a diameter smaller than the sigmoid colon. Failure to completely evacuate the barium on a 24-hour delayed film is also suggestive of HD.

MANAGEMENT

Once the diagnosis of HD has been confirmed by rectal biopsy examination, the infant should be prepared for surgery. If the newborn has enterocolitis complicating HD, correction of dehydration and electrolyte imbalance by infusion of appropriate fluids will be required, as well as antibiotics coverage. It is essential to decompress the bowel as early as possible in these babies. Deflation of the intestine may be carried out by rectal irrigations with saline via a large catheter located high in the rectum or descending colon. Some babies may require "leveling" colostomy. The level at which the colostomy is placed is determined by rapid frozen sections of seromuscular biopsies obtained from the colon during the operation. One must be assured that there are normal ganglion cells at the site of the proposed colostomy.

In recent years, the vast majority of cases of HD are diagnosed in the neonatal period. Many centers are now performing one-stage pull-through operations in the newborn with minimal morbidity rates and encouraging results. The advantages of operating on the newborn are that the colonic dilation can be quickly controlled by washouts, and at operation, the caliber of the pull-through bowel is near normal, allowing for an accurate anastomosis that minimizes leakage and cuff infection. A number of different operations have been described for the treatment of HD. The four most commonly used operations are the rectosigmoidectomy developed by Swenson and Bill, the retrorectal approach developed by Duhamel, the endorectal procedure developed by Soave, and deep anterior colorectal anastomosis developed by Rehbein.[91] The basic principle in all these procedures is to bring the ganglionic bowel down to the anus. The long-term results of any of these operations are satisfactory if they are performed correctly. Recently, a number of investigators have described and advocated a variety of one-stage pull-through procedures in the newborn using minimally invasive laparoscopic techniques. More recently, a transanal endorectal pull-through (TERPT) operation performed without opening the abdomen has been used with excellent results in rectosigmoid HD.

Transanal one-stage endorectal pull-through operation

Over 80% of patients with HD have rectosigmoid aganglionosis. A one-stage pull-through operation can be successfully performed in these patients using a transanal endorectal approach without opening the abdomen. This procedure is associated with excellent clinical results and permits early postoperative feeding, early hospital discharge, no visible scars, and low incidence of enterocolitis.[92-95] The author prefers TERPT operation in patients with classical segment rectosigmoid HD.

PREOPERATIVE MANAGEMENT

A good barium enema study is essential for this technique. A typical case of rectosigmoid HD will demonstrate flow of barium from undilated rectum through a cone-shaped transition zone into dilated sigmoid colon (Figure 67.4b). Once the diagnosis of HD is confirmed by SRB, the newborn is prepared for surgery. Rectal irrigations are carried out twice a day for 2–3 days prior to surgery. I.V. gentamicin and metronidazole are started on the morning of operation.

OPERATIVE TECHNIQUE

The patient is positioned on the operating table in the lithotomy position. The legs are strapped over sandbags. A Foley catheter is inserted into the bladder. A Denis–Browne retractor or anal retractor is placed to retract perianal skin. The rectal mucosa is circumferentially incised using the cautery with a fine tipped needle, approximately 5 mm from the dentate line, and the submucosal plane is developed. The proximal cut edge of the mucosal cuff is held with multiple fine silk sutures, which are used for traction (Figure 67.10). The endorectal dissection is then carried proximally, staying in the submucosal plane.

When the submucosal dissection has extended for about 3 cm, the rectal muscle is divided circumferentially, and the full thickness of the rectum and sigmoid colon is mobilized out through the anus. This requires division of rectal and sigmoid vessels, which can be done under direct vision using cautery.

When the transition zone is encountered, full-thickness biopsy sections are taken, and frozen section confirmation of ganglion cells is obtained. The rectal muscular cuff is split longitudinally either anteriorly or posteriorly. The colon is then divided several centimeters above the most proximal normal biopsy site, and a standard Soave–Boley anastomosis is performed (Figure 67.8). No drains are placed. The patient is started on oral feeds after 24 hours and discharged home on the third postoperative day. Digital rectal examination is performed 2 weeks after the operation. Routine rectal dilatation is not performed unless there is evidence of a stricture.

LAPAROSCOPIC-ASSISTED PULL-THROUGH

Despite the fact that many of the benefits of the pull-through procedure can be attained by transanal pull-through alone, significant advantages are realized by performing the laparoscopic dissection.[96] Prior to the irreversible step of endorectal dissection, laparoscopy allows one to verify the presence of ganglion cells in the proximal colon pedicle by seromuscular biopsy. In cases of total colon aganglionosis, a different type of pull-through operation or ostomy might be considered. In addition, laparoscopic mobilization of the intra-abdominal segment increases the mobility of the

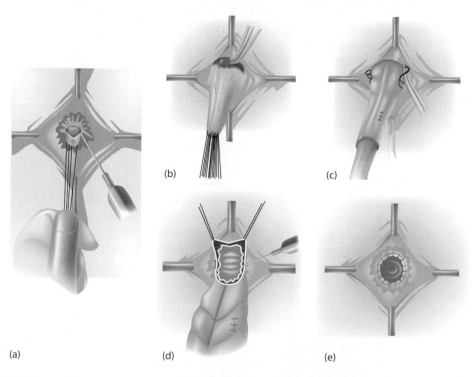

Figure 67.10 TERPT. **(a)** Rectal mucosa is circumferentially incised using the needle-tip cautery approximately 5 mm above the dentate line, and submucosa plane is developed. **(b)** When the submucosal dissection is extended proximally for about 3 cm, the muscle is divided circumferentially, and the full thickness of the rectum and sigmoid colon is mobilized out through the anus. **(c)** On reaching the transition zone, full-thickness rectal biopsies are taken for frozen section to confirm ganglion cells. **(d)** Colon is divided several centimeters above the most proximal biopsy site. **(e)** A standard Soave–Boley anastomosis is performed.

rectum and makes the endpoint of the endorectal dissection more definitive.[97]

Initially, three ports (Figure 67.11) are placed to visualize the transition zone and to perform biopsies for histologic leveling. A window is then made between the colon and superior rectal vessels, and distal dissection of the aganglionic colon is then performed circumferentially, keeping close to the colon wall, carefully preserving the mesenteric blood supply to the rectum. Blunt and sharp dissection of avascular plane posterior to the rectum follows. Anteriorly, the rectum is dissected for about 1 to 2 cm below the peritoneal reflection. It is important to avoid extensive lateral dissection, where damage to the nervi erigentes can result. Proximal mesenteric dissection of the colon pedicle with careful preservation of the marginal artery depends on the extent of the aganglionic segments; some patients require sigmoid colon mobilization or division of the lateral colonic fusion fascia up to the splenic flexure. After the endoscopic dissection of the colon and rectum has been completed, the pneumoperitoneum is released and the instruments removed, and the procedure is completed with an endorectal transanal pull-through.

Once, the anastomosis of the proximal ganglionated colon with the anorectal cuff is completed, reinsufflation for pneumoperitoneum can be performed to inspect the colon pedicle for twisting or potential internal herniation.[98]

The most frequent early complications after laparoscopically assisted endorectal pull-through (LAPT) include enterocolitis and chronic diarrhea. These problems often respond to medical management. Other less frequent problems include anastomotic leaking and bleeding, which are associated with technical error.

A recently conducted meta-analysis that included 159 patients after LAPT and 248 patients after TERPT did not find any evidence to suggest a higher rate of enterocolitis, incontinence, or constipation following TERPT compared with LAPT. Further long-term comparative studies and multicenter data pooling are needed to determine whether a laparoscopically assisted approach offers any advantages over a purely transanal approach to HD.[99]

COMPLICATIONS

Early postoperative complications that can occur after any type of pull-through operation include wound infections, anastomotic leak, anastomotic stricture, retraction or necrosis of the neorectum, intestinal adhesions, and ileus. Late complications include constipation, enterocolitis, incontinence, anastomotic problems, adhesive bowel obstruction, and urogenital complications.

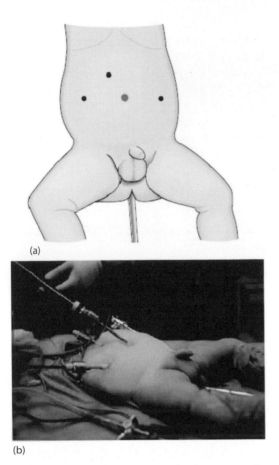

(a)

(b)

Figure 67.11 Position of trocar sites for laparoscopic pull-through. **(a)** Position of trocar port sites. **(b)** Trocars in place in an infant for the laparoscopic pull-through operation. With kind permission from Springer Science+Business Media: "Endoscopic Surgery in Children and Infants," 2008, Klaas and Georgeson.

Anastomotic leak

The most dangerous early postoperative complication following the definitive abdominoperineal pull-through procedure is leakage at the anastomotic suture line. Factors that are responsible for anastomotic leak include ischemia of the distal end of the colonic pull-through segment, tension on the anastomosis, incomplete anastomotic suture lines, and inadvertent rectal manipulation. If a leak is recognized in a patient without a colostomy, it is imperative to perform a diverting colostomy promptly, to administer intravenous antibiotics, and to irrigate the rectum with antibiotic solution a few times daily. Delay in establishing fecal diversion is likely to result in an extensive pelvic abscess, which may require laparotomy and transabdominal drainage.

Retraction of pull-through

Retraction of a portion or all of the colonic segment from the anastomosis can occur and is usually seen within 3 weeks of the operation. Evaluation under general anesthesia is generally necessary. In occasional patients, resuturing the anastomosis may be feasible transanally. For those with separation of less than 50% of the anastomosis but with adequate vascularity of

the colon, a diverting colostomy for approximately 3 months is necessary. For patients with wide separation at the anastomosis, early transabdominal reconstruction of the pull-through is recommended.

Perianal excoriation

Perianal excoriation occurs in nearly half of the patients undergoing the pull-through procedure, but generally resolves within 3 months with local therapy and resolution of diarrhea. It is helpful to begin placing a barrier cream on the perianal skin promptly after the operation and to continue after each movement for the first few weeks. Resolution of diarrhea will often hasten the clearance of perianal skin irritation.

Enterocolitis

Hirschsprung's associated enterocolitis (HAEC) is a significant complication of HD both in the pre- and postoperative periods.[81,100] HAEC can occur at any time from the neonatal period onward to adulthood and can be independent of the medical management and surgical procedure performed. The incidence of enterocolitis ranges from 20% to 58%.[81,100] Fortunately, the mortality rate has declined over the last 30 years from 30% to 1%. This decrease in mortality is related to earlier diagnosis of HD and enterocolitis, rectal decompression, appropriate vigorous resuscitation, and antibiotic therapy. It has been reported that routine postoperative rectal washouts decrease both the incidence and the severity of the episodes of enterocolitis following definitive surgery. In episodes of recurrent enterocolitis, which can develop in up to 56% of patients, anal dilatations have been recommended. However, prior to commencing a treatment regime, a contrast enema should be performed to rule out a mechanical obstruction. Patients with a normal rectal biopsy may require a sphincterotomy.

Constipation

Constipation is common after definitive repair of HD and can be due to residual aganglionosis and high anal tone. Repeated and forceful anal dilations of botulin toxin injection into the sphincter under general anesthesia may resolve the problem. In some patients, internal sphincter myectomy may be needed. In patients with scarring, stricture, or intestinal neuronal dysplasia proximal to aganglionic segment, treatment consists of treating the underlying cause.

Soiling

Soiling is fairly common after all types of pull-through operations, its precise incidence primarily dependent on how assiduously the investigator looks for it. The reported incidence of soiling ranges from 10% to 30%.[95] The attainment of normal postoperative defecation is clearly dependent on intensity of bowel training, social background, and respective intelligence of the patients. Mental handicap, including Down's syndrome, is invariably associated with long-term incontinence.[101] Those patients with preoperative enterocolitis would also seem to have a marginally higher long-term risk of incontinence. In some patients in whom soiling is intractable and a social problem, a Malone procedure may be needed to stay clean.

LONG-TERM OUTCOME

The vast majority of patients treated with any one of the standard pull-through procedures achieve satisfactory continence and function with time.[82,101–103]

FUTURE THERAPIES

Our growing understanding of what failures of normal development of ENS result in HD coupled with our progress in understanding normal gut development and motility has led to an expanding field of research into developing novel therapies for HSCR.

Stem cell transplantation using laboratory-cultured neural stem cells (NSCs) to colonize aganglionic intestine and restore intestinal motility has been proposed as a treatment for HSCR.[15]

Several potential sources of cells capable of generating enteric neurons have been investigated for ENS replenishment including CNS-derived neural stem cells (NSCs), embryonic enteric neural crest cells, postnatal ENS progenitor cells, and amnion fluid–derived stem cells.[105]

Recently, Fattahi et al. demonstrated the efficient derivation and isolation of ENS progenitors from human pluripotent stem cells, and their further differentiation into functional enteric neurons. They showed that ENS precursors derived in vitro are capable of targeted migration in the developing chick embryo and extensive colonization of the adult mouse colon.

In vivo engraftment and migration of hPSC-derived ENS precursors rescues disease-related mortality in HSCR mice (EDNRB$^{s-l/s-l}$). Finally, EDNRB-null mutant ENS precursors enable modelling of HSCR-related migration defects.[106]

Their work presents a powerful strategy to access human ENS lineages for exploring the ENS in human health and disease and for developing novel cell- and drug-based therapies for HSCR.

In conclusion, transplanted ENS may contribute to functional improvement directly by repopulating the aganglionic gut with implanted neurons and restoring neural circuits; it may also release trophic factors or neurotransmitters that can improve intestinal contractile function, and finally it can open a new field in the treatment of HD.

REFERENCES

1. Mc Laughlin D, Friedmacher F, Puri P. Total colonic aganglionosis: A systematic review and meta-analysis of long-term clinical outcome. *Pediatr Surg Int* 2012; 28:773–9.
2. Nemeth L, Yoneda A, Kader M, Devaney D, Puri P. Three-dimensional morphology of gut innervation in total intestinal aganglionosis using whole-mount preparation. *J Pediatr Surg* 2001; 36:291–5.
3. Senyüz OF, Büyükünal C, Danişmend N, Erdoğan E, Ozbay G, Söylet Y. Extensive intestinal aganglionosis. *J Pediatr Surg* 1989; 24:453–6.
4. Ziegler MM, Ross AJ, Bishop HC. Total intestinal aganglionosis: A new technique for prolonged survival. *J Pediatr Surg* 1987; 22:82–3.
5. Orr JD, Scobie WG. Presentation and incidence of Hirschsprung's disease. *Br Med J (Clin Research Ed)* 1983; 287:1671.
6. Passarge E. The genetics of Hirschsprung's disease: Evidence for heterogeneous etiology and a study of sixty-three families. *New Engl J Med* 1967; 276:138–43.
7. Passarge E. Dissecting Hirschsprung disease. *Nat Genet* 2002; 31:11–2.
8. Spouge D, Baird PA. Hirschsprung disease in a large birth cohort. *Teratology* 1985; 32:171–7.
9. Kenny SE, Tam PKH, Garcia-Barcelo M. Hirschsprung's disease. *Semin Pediatr Surg* 201; 19:194–200.
10. Sherman JO, Snyder ME, Weitzman JJ et al. A 40-year multinational retrospective study of 880 Swenson procedures. *J Pediatr Surg* 1989; 24:833–8.
11. Gershon MD. Functional anatomy of the enteric nervous system. In: *Hirschsprung's Disease and Allied Disorders*. New York: Springer, 2008:21–49.
12. Gershon MD, Chalazonitis A, Rothman TP. From neural crest to bowel: Development of the enteric nervous system. *J Neurobiol* 1993; 24:199–214.
13. Heanue TA, Pachnis V. Enteric nervous system development and Hirschsprung's disease: Advances in genetic and stem cell studies. *Nat Rev Neurosci* 2007; 8:466–79.
14. Powley TL. Vagal input to the enteric nervous system. *Gut* 2000; 47:iv30–2.
15. Wilkinson DJ, Edgar DH, Kenny SE. Future therapies for Hirschsprung's disease. *Semin Pediatr Surg* 2012; 21:364–70.
16. Burns AJ, Roberts RR, Bornstein JC, Young HM. Development of the enteric nervous system and its role in intestinal motility during fetal and early postnatal stages. *Semin Pediatr Surg* 2009; 18:196–205.
17. Angrist M, Bolk S, Thiel B et al. Mutation analysis of the RET receptor tyrosine kinase in Hirschsprung disease. *Hum Mol Genet* 1995; 4:821–30.
18. Attié T, Pelet A, Edery P et al. Diversity of RET proto-oncogene mutations in familial and sporadic Hirschsprung disease. *Hum Mol Genet* 1995; 4:1381–6.
19. Tomuschat C, Puri P. RET gene is a major risk factor for Hirschsprung's disease: A meta-analysis. *Pediatr Surg Int* 2015; 31:701–10.
20. Badner JA, Sieber WK, Garver KL, Chakravarti A. A genetic study of Hirschsprung disease. *Am J Hum Genet* 1990; 46:568–80.

21. Bergeron KF, Silversides DW, Pilon N. The developmental genetics of Hirschsprung's disease. *Clin Genet* 2013; 83:15–22.

22. Friedmacher F, Puri P. Hirschsprung's disease associated with Down syndrome: A meta-analysis of incidence, functional outcomes and mortality. *Pediatr Surg Int* 2013; 29:937–46.

23. Croaker GD, Shi E, Simpson E, Cartmill T, Cass DT. Congenital central hypoventilation syndrome and Hirschsprung's disease. *Arch Dis Child* 1998; 78:316–22.

24. Burkardt DD, Graham JM, Short SS, Frykman PK. Advances in Hirschsprung disease genetics and treatment strategies: An update for the primary care pediatrician. *Clin Pediatr (Phila)* 2014; 53:71–81.

25. Coyle D, Friedmacher F, Puri P. The association between Hirschsprung's disease and multiple endocrine neoplasia type 2a: A systematic review. *Pediatr Surg Int* 2014; 30:751–6.

26. Coyle D, Puri P. Hirschsprung's disease in children with Mowat-Wilson syndrome. *Pediatr Surg Int* 2015; 31:711–7.

27. Tam PK. Hirschsprung's disease: A bridge for science and surgery. *J Pediatr Surg* 2016; 51:18–22.

28. Edery P, Lyonnet S, Mulligan LM et al. Mutations of the RET proto-oncogene in Hirschsprung's disease. *Nature* 1994; 367:378–80.

29. Romeo G, Ronchetto P, Luo Y et al. Point mutations affecting the tyrosine kinase domain of the RET proto-oncogene in Hirschsprung's disease. *Nature* 1994; 367:377–8.

30. Moore SW. Total colonic aganglionosis and Hirschsprung's disease: A review. *Pediatr Surg Int* 2015; 31:1–9.

31. Puri P, Gosemann JH. Variants of Hirschsprung disease. *Semin Pediatr Surg* 2012; 21:310–8.

32. Kakita Y, Oshiro K, O'Briain DS, Puri P. Selective demonstration of mural nerves in ganglionic and aganglionic colon by immunohistochemistry for glucose transporter-1: Prominent extrinsic nerve pattern staining in Hirschsprung disease. *Arch Pathol Lab Med* 2000; 124:1314–9.

33. Kobayashi H, O'Briain DS, Puri P. Nerve growth factor receptor immunostaining suggests an extrinsic origin for hypertrophic nerves in Hirschsprung's disease. *Gut* 1994; 35:1605–7.

34. Payette RF, Tennyson VM, Pham TD et al. Origin and morphology of nerve fibers the aganglionic colon of the lethal spotted (ls/ls) mutant mouse. *J Comp Neurol* 1987; 257:237–52.

35. Tam PKH, Boyd GP. Origin, course, and endings of abnormal enteric nerve fibres in Hirschsprung's disease defined by whole-mount immunohistochemistry. *J Pediatr Surg* 1990; 25:457–61.

36. Watanabe Y, Ito T, Harada T, Kobayashi S, Ozaki T, Nimura Y. Spatial distribution and pattern of extrinsic nerve strands in the aganglionic segment of congenital aganglionosis: Stereoscopic analysis in spotting lethal rats. *J Pediatr Surg* 1995; 30:1471–6.

37. Tang CS-M, Tang W-K, So M-T et al. Fine mapping of the NRG1 Hirschsprung's disease locus. *PloS One* 2011; 6:e16181.

38. Weinberg AG. Hirschsprung's disease-a pathologist's view. *Perspect Pediatr Pathol* 1974; 2:207–39.

39. Frigo GM, Del Tacca M, Lecchini S, Crema A. Some observations on the intrinsic nervous mechanism in Hirschsprung's disease. *Gut* 1973; 14:35–40.

40. Vizi ES, Zseli J, Kontor E, Feher E, Verebelyi T. Characteristics of cholinergic neuroeffector transmission of ganglionic and aganglionic colon in Hirschsprung's disease. *Gut* 1990; 31:1046–50.

41. Boston VE, Cywes S, Davies MRQ. Serum and erythrocyte acetylcholinesterase activity in Hirschsprung's disease. *J Pediatr Surg* 1978; 13:407–10.

42. Garrett JR, Howard ER, Nixon HH. Autonomic nerves in rectum and colon in Hirschsprung's disease. A cholinesterase and catecholamine histochemical study. *Arch Dis Child* 1969; 44:406.

43. Nirasawa Y, Yokoyama J, Ikawa H, Morikawa Y, Katsumata K. Hirschsprung's disease: Catecholamine content, alpha-adrenoceptors, and the effect of electrical stimulation in aganglionic colon. *J Pediatr Surg* 1986; 21:136–42.

44. Touloukian RJ, Aghajanian G, Roth RH. Adrenergic hyperactivity of the aganglionic colon. *J Pediatr Surg* 1973; 8:191–5.

45. Hiramoto Y, Kiesewetter WB. The response of colonic muscle to drugs: An in vitro study of Hirschsprung's disease. *J Pediatr Surg* 1974; 9:13–20.

46. Wright PG, Shepherd JJ. Some observations on the response of normal human sigmoid colon to drugs in vitro. *Gut* 1966; 7:41–51.

47. Oldham KT, Colombani PM, Foglia RP. *Surgery of Infants and Children: Scientific Principles and Practice.* Philadelphia: Lippincott Raven Publishers, 1997.

48. Bult H, Boeckxstaens GE, Pelckmans PA, Jordaens FH, Van Maercke YM, Herman AG. Nitric oxide as an inhibitory non-adrenergic non-cholinergic neurotransmitter. *Nature* 1990; 345:346–7.

49. Rivera LR, Poole DP, Thacker M, Furness JB. The involvement of nitric oxide synthase neurons in enteric neuropathies. *Neurogastroenterol Motil* 2011; 23:980–8.

50. Michel T, Vanhoutte PM. Cellular signaling and NO production. *Pflügers Archiv-European Journal of Physiology* 2010; 459:807–16.

51. Rolle U, Nemeth L, Puri P. Nitrergic innervation of the normal gut and in motility disorders of childhood. *J Pediatr Surg* 2002; 37:551–67.

52. Dawson TM, Bredt DS, Fotuhi M, Hwang PM, Snyder SH. Nitric oxide synthase and neuronal NADPH diaphorase are identical in brain and peripheral tissues. *Proc Natl Acad Sci* 1991; 88:7797–801.

53. Hope BT, Michael GJ, Knigge KM, Vincent SR. Neuronal NADPH diaphorase is a nitric oxide synthase. *Proc Natl Acad Sci* 1991; 88:2811–4.

54. Bealer JF, Natuzzi ES, Buscher C, Flake AW. Nitric oxide synthase is deficient in the aganglionic colon of patients with Hirschsprung's disease. *Pediatrics* 1994; 93(4):647–51.

55. Guo R, Nada O, Suita S, Taguchi T, Masumoto K. The distribution and co-localization of nitric oxide synthase and vasoactive intestinal polypeptide in nerves of the colons with Hirschsprung's disease. *Virchows Arch* 1997; 430:53–61.

56. Kobayashi H, O'Briain DS, Puri P. Lack of expression of NADPH-diaphorase and neural cell adhesion molecule (NCAM) in colonic muscle of patients with Hirschsprung's disease. *J Pediatr Surg* 1994; 29:301–4.

57. Larsson LT, Shen Z, Ekblad E, Sundler F, Alm P, Andersson KE. Lack of neuronal nitric oxide synthase in nerve fibers of aganglionic intestine: A clue to Hirschsprung's disease. *J Pediatr Gastroenterol Nutr* 1995; 20:49–53.

58. Watanabe H, Ikawa H, Masuyama H, Endo M, Yokoyama J, Nakaki T. [Non-adrenergic-non-cholinergic relaxation and nitric oxide in the intestines of Hirschsprung disease]. *J Smooth Muscle Res* 1995; 31:467–70.

59. Bruder E, Meier-Ruge WA. [Twenty years diagnostic competence center for Hirschsprung's disease in Basel]. *Chirurg* 2010; 81:572–6.

60. Kusafuka T, Puri P. Altered mRNA expression of the neuronal nitric oxide synthase gene in Hirschsprung's disease. *J Pediatr Surg* 1997; 32:1054–8.

61. Bealer JF, Natuzzi ES, Flake AW, Adzick NS, Harrison MR. Effect of nitric oxide on the colonic smooth muscle of patients with Hirschsprung's disease. *J Pediatr Surg* 1994; 29:1025–9.

62. Vanderwinden JM, Rumessen JJ, Liu H, Descamps D, De Laet MH, Vanderhaeghen JJ. Interstitial cells of Cajal in human colon and in Hirschsprung's disease. *Gastroenterology* 1996; 111:901–10.

63. Yamataka A, Kato Y, Tibboel D et al. A lack of intestinal pacemaker (c-kit) in aganglionic bowel of patients with Hirschsprung's disease. *J Pediatr Surg* 1995; 30:441–4.

64. Yamataka A, Ohshiro K, Kobayashi H, Fujiwara T, Sunagawa M, Miyano T. Intestinal pacemaker C-KIT+ cells and synapses in allied Hirschsprung's disorders. *J Pediatr Surg* 1997; 32:1069–74.

65. Barshack I, Fridman E, Goldberg I, Chowers Y, Kopolovic J. The loss of calretinin expression indicates aganglionosis in Hirschsprung's disease. *J Clin Pathol* 2004; 57:712–6.

66. Horisawa M, Watanabe Y, Torihashi S. Distribution of c-Kit immunopositive cells in normal human colon and in Hirschsprung's disease. *J Pediatr Surg* 1998; 33:1209–14.

67. Nemeth L, Maddur S, Puri P. Immunolocalization of the gap junction protein Connexin43 in the interstitial cells of Cajal in the normal and Hirschsprung's disease bowel. *J Pediatr Surg* 2000; 35:823–8.

68. Kurahashi M, Nakano Y, Hennig GW, Ward SM, Sanders KM. Platelet-derived growth factor receptor α-positive cells in the tunica muscularis of human colon. *J Cell Mol Med* 2012; 16:1397–404.

69. Kurahashi M, Mutafova-Yambolieva V, Koh SD, Sanders KM. Platelet-derived growth factor receptor-α-positive cells and not smooth muscle cells mediate purinergic hyperpolarization in murine colonic muscles. *Am J Physiol Cell Physiol* 2014; 307:C561–70.

70. Soeda J, O'Briain DS, Puri P. Mucosal neuroendocrine cell abnormalities in the colon of patients with Hirschsprung's disease. *J Pediatr Surg* 1992; 27:823–7.

71. Nemeth L, Rolle U, Puri P. Altered cytoskeleton in smooth muscle of aganglionic bowel. *Arch Pathol Lab Med* 2002; 126:692–6.

72. Covault J, Sanes JR. Distribution of N-CAM in synaptic and extrasynaptic portions of developing and adult skeletal muscle. *J Cell Biol* 1986; 102:716–30.

73. Moore SE, Walsh FS. Specific regulation of N-CAM/D2-CAM cell adhesion molecule during skeletal muscle development. *EMBO J* 1985; 4:623.

74. Thiery J-P, Duband J-L, Rutishauser U, Edelman GM. Cell adhesion molecules in early chicken embryogenesis. *Proc Natl Acad Sci* 1982; 79:6737–41.

75. Romanska HM, Bishop AE, Brereton RJ, Spitz L, Polak JM. Increased expression of muscular neural cell adhesion molecule in congenital aganglionosis. *Gastroenterology* 1993; 105:1104–9.

76. Payette RF, Tennyson VM, Pomeranz HD, Pham TD, Rothman TP, Gershon MD. Accumulation of components of basal laminae: Association with the failure of neural crest cells to colonize the presumptive aganglionic bowel of lsls mutant mice. *Dev Biol* 1988; 125:341–60.

77. Tennyson VM, Payette RF, Rothman TP, Gershon MD. Distribution of hyaluronic acid and chondroitin sulfate proteoglycans in the presumptive aganglionic terminal bowel of ls/ls fetal mice: An ultrastructural analysis. *J Comp Neurol* 1990; 291:345–62.

78. Parikh DH, Tam PKH, Lloyd DA, Van Velzen D, Edgar DH. Quantitative and qualitative analysis of the extracellular matrix protein, laminin, in Hirschsprung's disease. *J Pediatr Surg* 1992; 27:991–6.

79. Parikh DH, Tam PKH, Van Velzen D, Edgar D. The extracellular matrix components, tenascin and fibronectin, in Hirschsprung's disease: An immunohistochemical study. *J Pediatr Surg* 1994; 29:1302–6.

80. Soret R, Mennetrey M, Bergeron KF et al. A collagen VI–dependent pathogenic mechanism for Hirschsprung's disease. *J Clin Investig* 2015; 125: 4483–96.

81. Murphy F, Menezes M, Puri P. Enterocolitis complicating Hirschsprung's disease. In: *Hirschsprung's Disease and Allied Disorders*. Berlin, Heidelberg: Springer, 2008:133–43.

82. Menezes M, Prato AP, Jasonni V, Puri P. Long-term clinical outcome in patients with total colonic aganglionosis: A 31-year review. *J Pediatr Surg* 2008; 43:1696–9.

83. de Lorijn F, Omari TI, Kok JH, Taminiau JAJM, Benninga MA. Maturation of the rectoanal inhibitory reflex in very premature infants. *J Pediatr* 2003; 143:630–3.

84. Muise ED, Hardee S, Morotti RA, Cowles RA. A comparison of suction and full-thickness rectal biopsy in children. *J Surg Res* 2016; 201:149–55.

85. de Arruda Lourenção PLT, Takegawa BK, Ortolan EVP, Terra SA, Rodrigues MAM. A useful panel for the diagnosis of Hirschsprung disease in rectal biopsies: Calretinin immunostaining and acetylcholinesterase histochemistry. *Ann Diagn Pathol* 2013; 17:352–6.

86. Lake BD, Puri P, Nixon HH, Claireaux AE. Hirschsprung's disease: An appraisal of histochemically demonstrated acetylcholinesterase activity in suction rectal biopsy specimens as an aid to diagnosis. *Arch Pathology Lab Med* 1978; 102:244–7.

87. Meier-Ruge W, Lutterbeck PM, Herzog B, Morger R, Moser R, Schärli A. Acetylcholinesterase activity in suction biopsies of the rectum in the diagnosis of Hirschsprung's disease. *J Pediatr Surg* 1972; 7:11–7.

88. Kapur RP, Reed RC, Finn LS, Patterson K, Johanson J, Rutledge JC. Calretinin immunohistochemistry versus acetylcholinesterase histochemistry in the evaluation of suction rectal biopsies for Hirschsprung disease. *Pediatr Dev Pathol* 2008; 12:6–15.

89. Takawira C, D'Agostini S, Shenouda S, Persad R, Sergi C. Laboratory procedures update on Hirschsprung disease. *J Pediatr Gastroenterol Nutr* 2015; 60:598–605.

90. Baker SS, Kozielski R. Calretinin and pathologic diagnosis of Hirschsprung disease: Has the time come to abandon the acetylcholinesterase stain. *J Pediatr Gastroenterol Nutr* 2014; 58:544–5.

91. Puri P. Hirschsprung's disease and variants. In: *Pediatric Surgery*. Berlin, Heidelberg: Springer, 2009:453–62.

92. De la Torre-Mondragon L, Ortega-Salgado JA. Transanal endorectal pull-through for Hirschsprung's disease. *J Pediatri Surg* 1998; 33:1283–6.

93. Kim AC, Langer JC, Pastor AC et al. Endorectal pull-through for Hirschsprung's disease—A multicenter, long-term comparison of results: Transanal vs transabdominal approach. *J Pediatr Surg* 2010; 45:1213–20.

94. Langer JC, Minkes RK, Mazziotti MV, Skinner MA, Winthrop AL. Transanal one-stage Soave procedure for infants with Hirschsprung's disease. *J Pediatr Surg* 1999; 34:148–52.

95. Ruttenstock E, Puri P. Systematic review and meta-analysis of enterocolitis after one-stage transanal pull-through procedure for Hirschsprung's disease. *Pediatr Surg Int* 2010; 26:1101–5.

96. Georgeson KE, Robertson DJ. Laparoscopic-assisted approaches for the definitive surgery for Hirschsprung's disease. *Semin Pediatr Surg* 2004; 13:256–62.

97. Georgeson KE, Fuenfer MM, Hardin WD. Primary laparoscopic pull-through for Hirschsprung's disease in infants and children. *J Pediatr Surg* 1995; 30:1017–22.

98. Georgeson KE. Laparoscopic pull-through for Hirschsprung's disease. In: *Hirschsprung's Disease and Allied Disorders*. Amsterdam: Harwood Academic Publishers, 2000; 301–10.

99. Thomson D, Allin B, Long A-M, Bradnock T, Walker G, Knight M. Laparoscopic assistance for primary transanal pull-through in Hirschsprung's disease: A systematic review and meta-analysis. *BMJ Open* 2015; 5:e006063.

100. Gosain A. Established and emerging concepts in Hirschsprung's-associated enterocolitis. *Pediatr Surg Int* 2016; 1–8.

101. Menezes M, Puri P. Long-term clinical outcome in patients with Hirschsprung's disease and associated Down's syndrome. *J Pediatr Surg* 2005; 40:810–2.

102. Granström AL, Danielson J, Husberg B, Nordenskjöld A, Wester T. Adult outcomes after surgery for Hirschsprung's disease: Evaluation of bowel function and quality of life. *J Pediatr Surg* 2015; 50:1865–9.

103. Jarvi K, Laitakari EM, Koivusalo A, Rintala RJ, Pakarinen MP. Bowel function and gastrointestinal quality of life among adults operated for Hirschsprung disease during childhood: A population-based study. *Ann Surg* 2010; 252:977–81.

104. Menezes M, Corbally M, Puri P. Long-term results of bowel function after treatment for Hirschsprung's disease: A 29-year review. *Pediatr Surg Int* 2006; 22:987–90.

105. Zhou Y, Besner G. Transplantation of amniotic fluid-derived neural stem cells as a potential novel therapy for Hirschsprung's disease. *J Pediatr Surg* 2016; 51:87–91.

106. Fattahi F, Steinbeck JA, Kriks S et al. Deriving human ENS lineages for cell therapy and drug discovery in Hirschsprung disease. *Nature* 2016; 531:105–9.

107. Goldberg EL. An epidemiological study of Hirschsprung's disease. *Int J Epidemiol* 1984; 13:479–85.

68

Anorectal anomalies

ANDREA BISCHOFF AND ALBERTO PEÑA

ANORECTAL ANOMALIES

Anorectal anomalies present with a spectrum of defects; on the "good" side of the spectrum, we see patients with minor malformations that require minimal treatment with excellent results; on the other extreme of the spectrum, we find cases with complex defects, which represent a serious technical challenge and for whom the results in terms of bowel, urinary, and sexual function are not good despite accurate anatomic reconstruction. A newborn with an anorectal malformation may represent a surgical emergency related to intestinal obstruction and (or) due to severe associated urologic, gastrointestinal, or cardiac defects, which may require aggressive and efficient management. Other patients with these defects do not represent an emergency, because they have a fistula that allows intestinal decompression and they are born without serious associated abnormalities. In these cases, the repair of the defect can become an elective procedure or, if the baby is in good condition, can be definitively managed in the newborn period.

Frequency

Anorectal malformations occur with a frequency of approximately 1 in 4000 or 5000 newborns.[1–3]

Classification

Table 68.1 shows a classification that is anatomically based, and has prognostic and therapeutic implications.[4,5]

CLINICAL FEATURES AND DIAGNOSIS

Male defects

PERINEAL FISTULA

Patients with this defect have an abnormal communication between the rectum and the perineum (Figure 68.1),

often with a "bucket-handle" malformation (Figure 68.2). The common anatomic feature is the fact that the intestinal opening is located anterior to the center of the sphincter mechanism, as demonstrated by electrical stimulation during the repair (Figure 68.3). We prefer to avoid terms such as *anterior ectopic anus*, as this opening is not really an anus as it has no pectinate line and it is not surrounded by a sphincter. We believe the term *perineal fistula* is a more accurate one. The fistula can occur anywhere along the median raphe. These defects can be treated primarily without a protective colostomy. Most of the time, the patient is able to pass small amounts of meconium through the orifice in the perineum. Sometimes it takes a few hours before the baby passes meconium. The presence of a prominent midline epithelial tag below which one can pass an instrument (bucket-handle malformation) is considered pathognomonic of this defect (Figure 68.2). Many times, one sees a midline raphe subepithelial fistula that looks like a black (meconium) or white (mucus) ribbon, which is also evidence of this type of defect (Figure 68.1). Otherwise, the patients have a perineum with signs of *good prognosis*, which include a prominent midline groove and a noticeable anal dimple. The diagnosis is made by clinical inspection, and usually, no radiologic studies are necessary. The chance of having an associated genitourinary defect is extremely low. The patient's spine should be screened for an associated, albeit rare, tethered cord.

RECTOURETHRAL BULBAR AND RECTOURETHRAL PROSTATIC FISTULAS

These two types of defects are similar from a clinical point of view. However, generally speaking, patients with rectourethral bulbar fistula are more likely to have a "good-looking" perineum (Figure 68.4); this means having a prominent midline groove and anal dimple.

In cases of prostatic fistula, the chances of having a short sacrum and a flat perineum (Figure 68.5) increase. The rectum can open into the bulbar urethra (Figure 68.6) or into the prostatic urethra (Figure 68.7). Both rectum and

Table 68.1 Classification of anorectal malformations

Male Defects

"Low" defects: perineal fistula

Rectourethral bulbar fistula

Rectourethral prostatic fistula

Rectovesical (bladder neck) fistula

Imperforate anus without fistula

Rectal atresia and stenosis

Female Defects

Low defects: perineal fistula

Vestibular fistula

Imperforate anus without fistula

Rectal atresia and stenosis

Persistent cloaca

Complex and Rare Defects

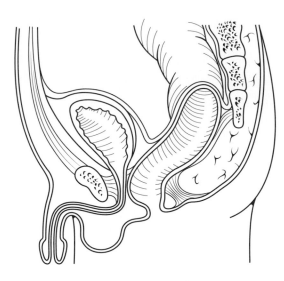

Figure 68.3 Perineal fistula—sagittal view.

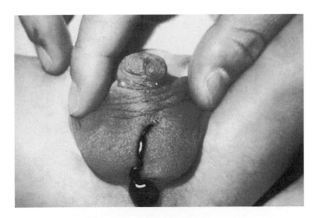

Figure 68.1 Cutaneous (subepithelial) fistula.

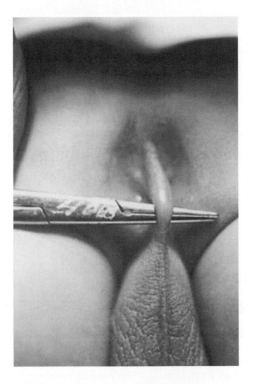

Figure 68.2 "Bucket-handle" malformation.

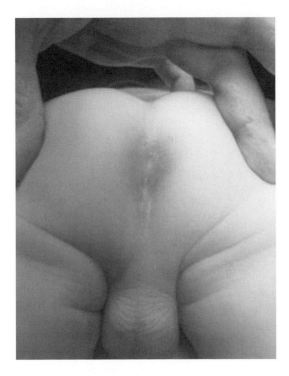

Figure 68.4 "Good-looking" perineum.

urethra have a common wall located above the fistula site, which is longer in the case of bulbar fistula and shorter in the prostatic type. The neonatal nurse may notice that the baby is passing meconium through the urethra. A cross-table lateral film, with the patient in the prone position and the pelvis elevated, is rarely necessary.[6] Figure 68.8 shows a rectum very close to the perineal skin, and Figure 68.9 shows a higher rectum. The chances of a rectourethral fistula case being associated with urological problems vary from 25% in cases of urethral bulbar fistula to 66% in cases of urethral prostatic fistula. These newborns need a diverting colostomy.

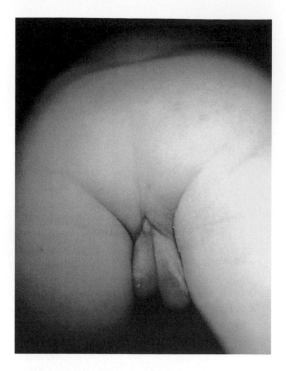

Figure 68.5 Flat bottom.

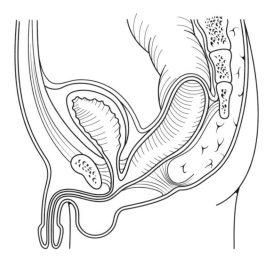

Figure 68.6 Rectourethral bulbar fistula—sagittal view.

RECTOVESICAL (BLADDER NECK) FISTULA

This defect accounts for approximately 10% of all anorectal defects in males. The rectum opens into the bladder neck in a "T" fashion (Figure 68.10). Frequently, the entire pelvis of these babies seems to be hypodeveloped. It is also common for these patients to have poor sphincter development, and the perineum looks rather flat in most patients (Figure 68.5), although some patients with these defects may have a good-looking perineum (Figure 68.4) with a midline groove and a prominent anal dimple. The frequency of associated urological anomalies in this specific defect is very high (up to 90%),[7] and therefore, a urologic workup is mandatory. A cross-table

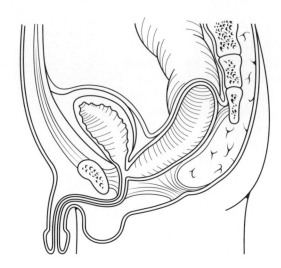

Figure 68.7 Rectourethral prostatic fistula—sagittal view.

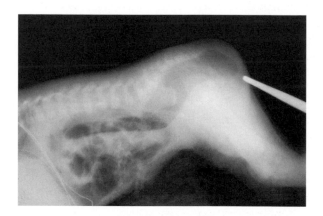

Figure 68.8 Cross-table lateral film of rectoperineal fistula, within 1–2 cm of perineal skin.

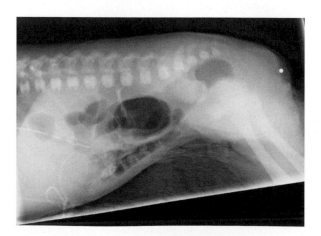

Figure 68.9 Cross-table lateral film of a rectum that is greater than 2 cm from the perineal skin representing a likely rectourethral or bladder neck fistula.

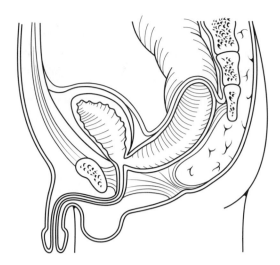

Figure 68.10 Rectovesical (bladder neck) fistula sagittal view.

lateral film, with the patient in prone position and with the pelvis elevated, shows an image consistent with air much higher than the pubococcygeus line (Figure 68.9). The neonatal nurses may note that the baby is urinating meconium. Manifestations of intestinal obstruction will become evident during the first 12–24 hours. In addition to these symptoms, the baby may show symptoms consistent with acidosis and sepsis secondary to an obstructive uropathy. These patients require a colostomy. They will require an abdominal approach (laparoscopic or laparotomy) during the definitive repair, in addition to the posterior sagittal approach.

IMPERFORATE ANUS WITHOUT FISTULA

In this type of defect, the rectum is really blind and is usually located at the level of the bulbar urethra. Even when there is no communication between rectum and urethra, the wall that separates both of them is long and has no surgical plane of separation. This defect is uncommon, but it has a good sphincter mechanism, and therefore, most of the time, the perineum is a good-looking one. The frequency of this defect is approximately 5% of male defects.[8] It is common to read reports indicating that these defects occur more often. We believe that those reports reflect diagnostic errors, consecutive to an inadequate radiologic study; a distal colostogram that is not done properly will give an incorrect assessment of "no fistula." A successful colostogram requires the injection of contrast material through the mucous fistula (distal bowel) of the colostomy, under enough hydrostatic pressure so as to demonstrate the passage of contrast material through the fistula into the urethra.[9] The rectum in all types of malformations is surrounded by voluntary muscle (Figures 68.3, 68.6, 68.7, and 68.10), and the hydrostatic pressure must be high enough to overcome the tone of the muscle that is compressing it. It is interesting to note that out of all our cases of imperforate anus with no fistula, approximately half of them have Down syndrome. The other half is predominantly made up of patients with other syndromes. Also, in all of our Down syndrome patients with imperforate anus, 95% have no fistula, clearly pointing to a genetic relationship between

the type of defect and Down syndrome.[10,11] These patients also require a newborn diverting colostomy. Chances for these patients to have an associated defect are low, except for those malformations frequently associated with Down syndrome.

RECTAL ATRESIA AND STENOSIS

This is a rare type of defect classically described as the one that is diagnosed by the nurse while passing the thermometer during the initial newborn physical examination. The reason for this is that these babies are born with a normal anal canal and have an atresia located about 1–2 cm above the anal verge. Above that, there is a dilated rectal pouch. Sometimes, the patient actually has a stenosis. The separation between the blind pouch and the anal canal may be by a very thin membrane, but more frequently, there is a thick fibrous septum 3–7 mm in length. These patients most frequently need a colostomy. The perineum looks normal. The sacrum is usually normal and the chances of associated defects are extremely low. All patients must have an anteroposterior (AP) film of the sacrum; a sacral defect is always associated with the presence of a presacral mass, which seems to occur more frequently in this malformation than in others. The presacral mass must be looked for by magnetic resonance imaging (MRI). The mass is usually a teratoma, dermoid, lipoma, anterior meningocele, or a combination of all. In addition, in cases with presacral mass, there is an associated tethered cord. These patients have all the necessary anatomical elements to become totally continent; the muscles are intact, and the anal canal has normal sensation. However, the presence of a presacral mass has a radical negative effect on the functional prognosis.

Female defects

CUTANEOUS (PERINEAL) FISTULA

This is the most benign defect seen in females, and it is equivalent to the same defect already described in males. The fistula site is located anywhere between the vestibule of the female genitalia and the center of the anal dimple (Figure 68.11). The entire fistula site is surrounded by skin,

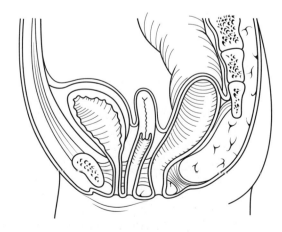

Figure 68.11 Perineal fistula in a female patient.

and therefore, it is also given the name of *cutaneous fistula*. The orifice is variable in size, and therefore, it may be sufficient for a full-bowel evacuation, or else it may require dilations to provide good bowel movements, until the main repair is done later in life. It is not uncommon to see older patients born with this malformation, which was never diagnosed. The patients suffer from severe constipation, which leads them to ask for a consultation. The defect is then diagnosed during the examination.

Our routine is to repair this malformation within the first 3 days of life, ideally when the patient is still passing meconium and before she starts being fed. Postoperatively, we keep the baby with nothing by mouth (NPO) receiving intravenous nutrition for 5 days after the repair.

These patients do not require a protective colostomy as part of their treatment. The most prominent anatomical feature in this type of defect is that the rectum and vagina are very close, although they do not share a common wall (Figure 68.11). Thus, the technical implication is that the rectum can be mobilized without risking injury to the vagina. Patients have otherwise normal sphincter mechanism and a normal sacrum. The incidence of associated defects (except for the presence of presacral mass) of the urinary tract or spine is very low.

VESTIBULAR FISTULA

This is the most frequent defect seen in females. The distal rectum opens into the vestibule, which is the space located immediately outside the hymen (Figure 68.12). The most notable anatomical feature in this defect is the presence of a very long common wall between rectum and vagina located above the fistula site (Figure 68.12). The vagina must be completely separated from the rectum in order to achieve good rectal mobilization and a tension-free repair. There is no surgical plane of separation between these two structures, and one must be carefully created. The fistula is usually represented by a short (5–15 mm) narrow rectal opening, which sometimes is not wide enough to decompress the bowel and requires dilatations if the surgeon is not proceeding with a newborn repair. Above that, one

finds a normal rectum. Sometimes, the orifice is wide enough to allow a satisfactory decompression. The opening of a colostomy is the safest way to manage these girls, but an experienced surgeon can operate on this defect primarily without a colostomy if the baby is otherwise healthy. In such a case, we would operate in the newborn period and would keep the patient NPO receiving intravenous nutrition for 7 days after surgery. The incidence of associated urogenital malformations is 30%.[7] The sacrum is usually normal. The perineum of these babies shows a prominent midline groove and a very obvious anal dimple. Once in a while in this defect, we see a "poor-looking" perineum as well as short or very abnormal sacrum.

VAGINAL FISTULA

A true vaginal fistula is a very unusual defect. Less than 1% of females have this malformation. On the other hand, vaginal fistula is presented in the traditional literature as a relatively common defect. A recent review of the authors' own experience with reoperations in female patients showed 80 female patients operated on at other institutions with a diagnosis of rectovaginal fistula. During our reoperations, we got objective evidence indicating that none of these patients actually had rectovaginal fistulas. In fact, two-thirds of them had cloacas. The original surgeons were unaware of the correct diagnosis; they repaired the rectal component of the malformation and left the patient with a persistent urogenital sinus. The remaining one-third of the patients actually had vestibular fistulas, which was evidenced by the presence of the original fistula in the vestibule.[12] The importance of this observation is not only semantic; the group of patients that were born with cloacas were mislabeled as having rectovaginal fistulas, and the patients missed a great opportunity to have their entire malformation repaired during the first operation. The results of a second procedure are never as good as the first one. Furthermore, the patients with vestibular fistula were frequently erroneously subjected to an unnecessary abdominoperineal operation (designed to repair "high" malformations), and as a result, they suffer from fecal incontinence, consecutive to the resection of the rectosigmoid, which was part of the old endorectal abdominoperineal procedures. Therefore, it is very important to increase the index of suspicion for malformations such as cloaca and vestibular fistula, and to recognize that vaginal fistulas are almost nonexistent defects.

To make the diagnosis of a real rectovaginal fistula (Figure 68.13) it is necessary to perform a meticulous inspection of the genitalia, which is sometimes not easy in the newborn period due to edema of the labia. Patients with rectovaginal fistulas would show meconium coming from inside the vagina through the hymen. These babies may have a significant incidence of associated urological defects (around 70%).[7] If the rectum is connected to the vagina very high and the urethra and vagina are normal, that could be a rare indication for a laparoscopy in a female with anorectal malformation.

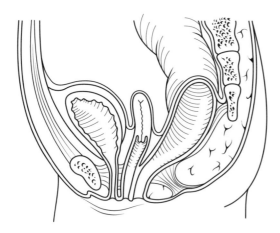

Figure 68.12 Vestibular fistula.

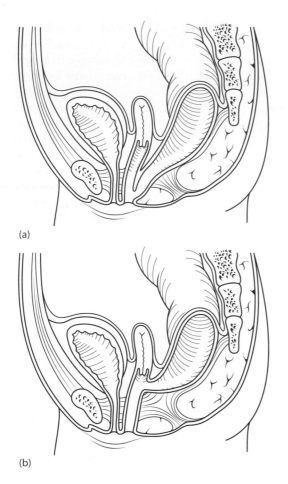

(a)

(b)

Figure 68.13 Vaginal fistula: (a) low; (b) high.

IMPERFORATE ANUS WITHOUT FISTULA

All that was written regarding this defect in males is valid regarding females, the only difference obviously being that the rectum shares a common wall with the vagina, not with the urethra.

RECTAL ATRESIA AND STENOSIS

This type of defect is identical to the one described in males, except that its frequency in females seems to be higher. The clinicians must always remember to screen for a presacral mass.

PERSISTENT CLOACA

This is the most complex anorectal malformation seen in females. It represents approximately 10% of the total number of anorectal defects. A cloaca is defined as the junction of the rectum, vagina, and urethra into a single common channel (Figure 68.14). Cloacas represent another spectrum by themselves. In other words, at one end of the spectrum one may find a rather benign, short-common-channel type of cloaca with good functional prognosis and no associated defects. At the other end of the spectrum, one can find a very complex defect with a very long common channel (3–8 cm length), with a very short vagina, severe associated obstructive uropathy, as well as very poor sacrum and poor

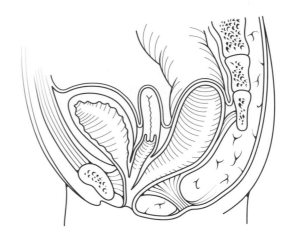

Figure 68.14 Persistent cloaca.

sphincter (Figure 68.15). The prognosis for this last type of case will be very poor for bowel and urinary control. The spectrum of cloacas includes many different types. One may see patients with a very dilated vagina, which becomes evident as a palpable abdominal mass and is called hydrocolpos. The dilated vagina usually causes urinary obstruction from compression of the ureterovesical junction at the trigone (Figure 68.16). A frequent finding is a double vagina and double uterus; in this type of case, the rectum may open at different levels in the midvaginal septum (Figure 68.17). The majority of these long-common-channel cloacas require an abdominal approach during the definitive repair, in addition to the posterior sagittal operation.[13]

The most important fact to remember in this type of defect is the high incidence of associated urinary tract obstruction (70%–90%).[7] Obstructive uropathy is the main cause of morbidity and even mortality in these patients.

The diagnosis of a cloaca is a clinical one. General practitioners, pediatricians, neonatologists, and pediatric surgeons must suspect this defect if they want to detect it and make an early diagnosis. A baby girl with an absent anus and small-looking genitalia must arouse suspicion for the presence of

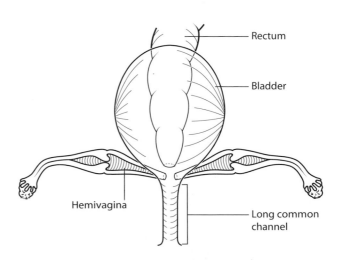

Rectum

Bladder

Hemivagina

Long common channel

Figure 68.15 High cloaca with common channel of 5 cm.

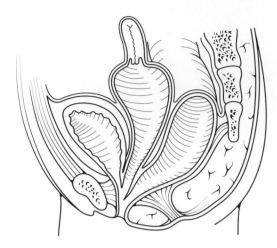

Figure 68.16 Cloaca with hydrocolpos.

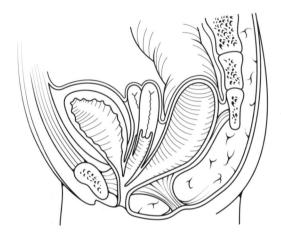

Figure 68.17 Duplicate Mullerian system.

a persistent cloaca (Figure 68.18). If one separates the labia minora, a single orifice becomes evident. These findings are pathognomonic for a cloaca. At that point, the priority in a newborn is the evaluation and treatment of the associated defects of the urinary tract. The external appearance of the perineum in these babies may vary. Sometimes, a poor-looking perineum is found, which means a flat bottom, a very poor midline groove, and almost absent anal dimple. Other times, one may find a cloaca with a good sphincter and a good sacrum. A patient with a cloaca always needs a completely diverting colostomy. If a hydrocolpos is present, the patient also needs a vaginostomy. Very rarely is a vesicostomy also needed. In addition to the mandatory urologic evaluation, in cases of cloacas, other associated malformations must be excluded, including tethered cord, cardiac defects, esophageal atresia, and spinal malformations.

In female patients, the diagnosis of the specific type of anorectal malformation is clinically obvious; a meticulous examination of the perineum and a good index of suspicion provide enough information to determine whether or not the patient has a perineal, vestibular, or vaginal fistula or a cloaca.

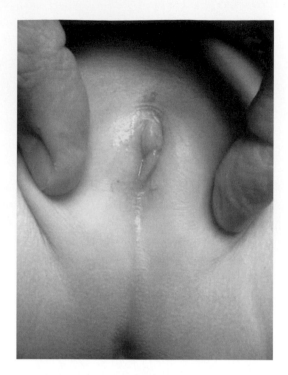

Figure 68.18 Cloaca, perineal appearance.

PREOPERATIVE CARE

Figures 68.19 and 68.20 show the decision-making algorithms for the initial management of newborns with anorectal malformations.

In approximately 90% of males, physical examination (perineal inspection) produces enough information to determine whether the patient needs a colostomy or not. The presence of a perineal subepithelial midline raphe fistula, a bucket-handle malformation, and any other type of anal orifice ectopically opening in the perineum are all considered evidence of a malformation traditionally known as "low," which can be treated during the newborn period with a simple anoplasty and without a protective colostomy. In cases of very ill babies, a series of anal dilatations may be enough to allow bowel decompression, leaving the anoplasty to be done later as an elective procedure. On the other hand, a flat bottom, or evidence of meconium in the urine, a very abnormal sacrum or spine, or other severe associated defects, is enough information to proceed with a protective colostomy. Four to eight weeks after the colostomy is done and provided the patient is growing and developing well, a radiological evaluation of the distal colon (high-pressure distal colostogram) is done to determine the specific type of malformation that the patient has and to decide the type of operation indicated; most of the time, it will consist in a posterior sagittal anorectoplasty. All these defects together represent approximately 90% of the entire group of anorectal defects in males. The remaining 10% have questionable, external, clinical evidence. In these cases, we recommend the cross-table lateral film with the patient in the prone position.[6] An intraluminal rectal bubble located above the

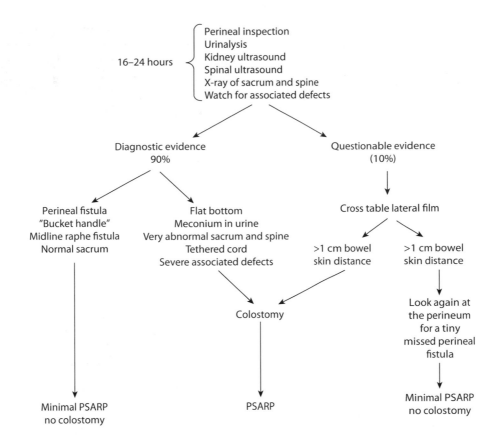

Figure 68.19 Male newborn algorithm for anorectal malformations.

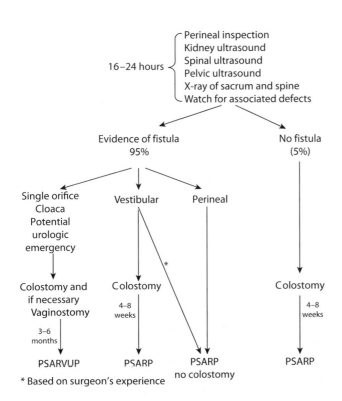

Figure 68.20 Female newborn algorithm for anorectal malformations. PSARP, posterior sagittal anorectoplasty; PSARVUP, posterior sagittal anorectovaginourethroplasty.

coccyx is considered an indication for a colostomy (Figure 68.9). If the patient does not have signs of a rectourinary fistula, most likely, the case is one of imperforate anus with no fistula. If the patient has Down syndrome,[11] it is even more likely. On the other hand, if the rectum is located below the coccyx (Figure 68.8), it means that the surgeon will be able to reach it using a posterior sagittal incision. The surgeon should inspect the perineum again and may find a tiny orifice, so narrow that it did not allow the passage of meconium in the first hours of life. The baby can then be treated with a minimal posterior sagittal anoplasty and without a colostomy.

Figure 68.20 shows the decision-making algorithm used for the initial management of newborn females with anorectal defects. The process of decision making in females is easier than in males, mainly because the vast majority of female patients have some form of fistula either to the perineum, vestibule, or genitalia, which indicates the type of defect that they have.

The presence of a cloaca (single perineal) orifice, as was previously discussed, represents an indication for an urgent urological evaluation. In addition, the patient will require a colostomy and sometimes a vaginostomy. Provided the baby is growing well, the patient may undergo the definitive repair of her defect at age 3–6 months.

In the cases in which the meconium comes from the vestibule, depending on the surgeon's experience, a primary repair or a protective colostomy can be performed. Many times, the fistula opening is big enough to decompress the bowel, and therefore, there is no need for an emergency colostomy, and the definitive repair can be delayed for several months.

The presence of a cutaneous (perineal) fistula indicates that the baby has the most benign type of anorectal defect. This can be treated with a "minimal" posterior sagittal anoplasty without a protective colostomy. If the perineal fistula is big enough to decompress the intestine, then the anoplasty can be postponed and done on an elective basis. The remaining small group of female patients that have no fistula (5%) need a colostomy followed by a PSARP 4–8 weeks later.

Every surgeon must develop his or her own learning curve in the surgical management of these defects. We like to repair perineal and vestibular fistulae in the newborn period. There are both theoretical and practical advantages in doing these repairs early in life. From the theoretical point of view, placing the rectum in its normal position early may allow the creation of new nerve synapses, which may have advantages in terms of bowel control.[14] From the practical point of view, it is much easier to dilate the anus of a small baby than trying to do it in an older patient. In addition, the babies will not remember the event.

We promote the trend to operate on newborns with anorectal malformations, primarily without a protective colostomy when feasible.[15] In addition, a single procedure is highly attractive when compared to the alternative of three operations (colostomy, main repair, and colostomy closure). However, what remains to be seen is whether or not such treatment will result in better functional results. Those who embrace the new treatment modality (primary repair) are morally obligated to report their results, including complications.

Concerning the laparoscopic approach to these malformations,[16] it must be kept in mind that, as we have described, 90% of the male cases can be repaired via the posterior sagittal route without opening the abdomen; these patients experience minimal pain, eat the same day of surgery, and could even go home the same day of the operation. Laparoscopy was created and conceived as minimally invasive surgery, to avoid the pain and potential complications inflicted by a laparotomy. Actually, there is only one particular defect in males (rectobladder neck fistula), which represents 10% of all malformations in males, that needs a laparotomy to be repaired and therefore, we feel, is ideally suited for a laparoscopic approach. For prostatic fistulas, the approach (laparoscopic or PSARP) should be based on which technique the surgeon feels most skilled at performing. For other malformations such as bulbar urethral fistula, or cases without fistula, we do not think laparoscopy is appropriate. In the female group, we believe that a laparoscopy could be indicated in patients suffering from a very unusual type of cloaca, with a rather short common channel and a rectum located very high in the pelvis; in our series, that malformation occurs only in 4% of the cloacas.

In general, babies with anorectal malformations look healthy unless they have a severe associated defect, mainly urologic, cardiac, or another, serious gastrointestinal tract malformation (esophageal atresia, duodenal atresia). The frequency of associated urologic defects in babies with anorectal malformation varies according to the statistics that one consults.[17-22] In our series, approximately half of the patients with anorectal defects had a significant associated urologic defect, and this frequency varies depending on the level of the fistula site. This, we believe, may help neonatologists and pediatricians to suspect, detect, and treat these defects early.

A constellation of associated findings (single kidney, absent sacrum, esophageal atresia, etc.) can also be detected prenatally.[23] Before the performance of the colostomy, every baby must at least have an abdominal ultrasound done to rule out the presence of obstructive uropathy.

Concerning the passage of meconium, decisions should not be made during the first 16–24 hours of life, since meconium often does not appear, either in the urine or in the perineum, until after that period of time. Abdominal distension does not become a problem during the first 16–24 hours of life. Therefore, decisions as to whether the baby should undergo primary repair or a colostomy should wait for 16–24 hours. It is after that period of time that babies with anorectal malformations will develop abdominal distention; the intraluminal pressure in the rectum will be high enough to overcome the muscle tone of the sphincter mechanism surrounding the most distal portion of the rectum. That is also the reason why diagnostic imaging studies designed to determine the position of the rectum in the pelvis should not be done before 24 hours of life. A collapsed rectum is difficult to see even using the most sophisticated imaging technology.

COLOSTOMY

At birth, once the doctor has made the diagnosis of an anorectal malformation, a nasogastric tube is placed in the stomach and intravenous fluids started. Prophylactic antibiotics are recommended. Twenty-four hours later, the surgeon must decide whether the patient needs a colostomy or a primary procedure to repair the anorectal malformation. We recommend a descending colostomy, with separated stomas: separated enough to allow the placement of a stoma bag over the proximal (functional) stoma, leaving outside the distal stoma, also called mucous fistula—all of this with the specific purpose to avoid the passing of stool from the proximal to the distal colon.

Figure 68.21a shows the type of colostomy that we recommend in the management of anorectal malformations. The advantages of this colostomy[24] over other types include the following:

- Leaves without function only a small portion of the distal intestine, allowing better water absorption.
- It is completely diverting.
- Allows for an adequate length of bowel for the pull-through. One of the most common errors in the opening of a colostomy is leaving a very short piece of distal bowel, which will eventually interfere with the pull-through of the rectum (Figure 68.21b).

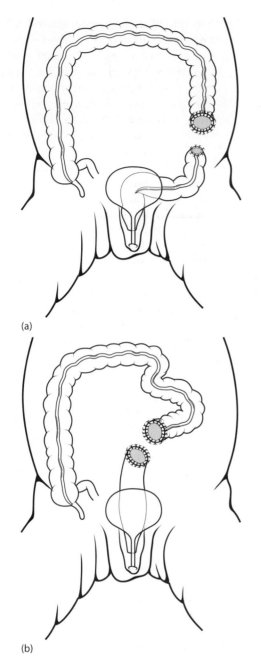

(a)

(b)

Figure 68.21 **(a)** Ideal colostomy. **(b)** Too-distal colostomy.

- Allows drainage of urine that may pass from the urinary tract back into the rectum.
- Simplifies cleaning of the distal intestine prior to the main repair. It is actually very difficult to clean the distal bowel through a transverse colostomy.
- Makes the distal colostogram easier than when dealing with a more proximal colostomy. It is very difficult to demonstrate the fistula injecting contrast material through a transverse colostomy.
- Reduces the incidence of prolapse.

Loop colostomies are problematic because they allow feces to pass into the distal stoma, provoking fecal impaction, megarectum, and urinary tract infection. Also, there is

a risk of contamination and infection of the operative field after the main repair.

Surgical technique for colostomy

The recommended incision measures approximately 6 cm, is made in the left lower quadrant, and is oblique. The proximal functional stoma is placed in the upper and lateral portion of the incision, and the mucous fistula (nonfunctional) distal stoma is intentionally created small and placed in the lower and medial portion of the incision. The distal bowel must be irrigated with saline solution during the operation, in order to remove all the meconium. In this way, the distal bowel remains completely clean and collapsed, and the patient does not need any preparation prior to the main repair.

A colostomy must be considered a serious, delicate procedure. The surgeon must carefully identify the piece of intestine that he or she is going to exteriorize to avoid serious mistakes. The most frequent errors in performing colostomies seen by the authors include the following[25]:

1. A colostomy placed too distal in the sigmoid.
2. Opening of a right upper sigmoidostomy. The surgeon thinks he or she is opening a transverse colostomy and actually grabs the sigmoid colon and exteriorizes it in the right upper quadrant. This interferes with the pull-through.
3. Retracting colostomies. In these cases, the bowel was probably handled poorly and may suffer from ischemia and retraction. In addition, most likely, the bowel was poorly fixed to the abdominal wall. To avoid this, the authors' suggestion is to fix the bowel to the peritoneum and to the anterior fascia.
4. Prolapsed colostomies. Choosing the descending colon to create the proximal, functional stoma avoids prolapse because that portion of the colon is normally attached to the posterior wall of the abdomen. The distal colostomy will never prolapse, even when it is performed in a mobile portion of the colon (sigmoid), because we specifically recommend creating a very small stoma, since it will only be used to irrigate the distal bowel and to perform a distal colostogram.

After the colostomy, once feedings are advanced, the baby can go home. If the baby is growing and developing well, 4–8 weeks later, the main repair can be performed. Prior to the final repair, it is mandatory to perform a distal colostogram in order to determine the precise type of anatomic defect that the patient has. This has important prognostic and therapeutic implications.

Distal colostogram

This is, by far, the most important diagnostic study in dealing with anorectal malformations. The study must be done under fluoroscopy. A Foley catheter is introduced into the distal stoma, the balloon is inflated, and water-soluble contrast material (never barium) is injected by hand, with a syringe, applying enough hydrostatic pressure to overcome the tone of the funnel-like muscle structure that surrounds the lowest part of the rectum. Failure to observe these principles will most likely show the dye staying above the pubococcygeus line, erroneously indicating the presence of a high defect and not showing the fistula, simply because of lack of hydrostatic pressure.[9] Figures 68.22 through 68.24 show distal colostograms in a case of rectourethral bulbar, rectoprostatic, and rectobladder (bladder neck) fistula. Having this information, the surgeon will be able to plan the surgical procedure. When dealing with a case of rectovesical (bladder neck) fistula, the surgeon will be able to predict that the prognosis in terms of bowel function is not going to be as good as in other types of defects.[5] In addition, the main repair will include a laparotomy or laparoscopy

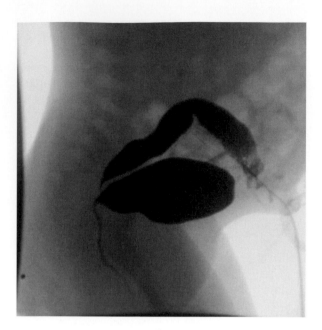

Figure 68.24 Distal colostogram in a rectovesical (bladder neck) fistula.

and will take approximately 3–4 hours. Also, a laparotomy or laparoscopy will be necessary in order to mobilize the rectum. Most importantly, the surgeon will avoid looking for the rectum through a posterior sagittal incision where it will not be found, because that would risk injury to the urinary tract, vas deferens, seminal vesicles, and ectopic ureters. The posterior sagittal approach in this case will be used only to show the trajectory of the pull-through, after its mobilization through laparoscopy or via laparotomy, and to allow tacking of the rectum to the muscle complex.

DEFINITIVE REPAIR

Minimal posterior sagittal anoplasty

This operation is done in all defects, traditionally known as low malformations, including perineal fistulas in both male and females. In cases of male newborns, it is important to place a Foley catheter in the bladder during the operation. The purpose of this is to avoid the most common accident seen during these operations, which is the urethral injury. The rectum and urethra are very close together, sharing a common wall. The operation starts by placing multiple sutures and taking the mucocutaneous junction of the fistula. This serves the purpose of exerting uniform traction, which helps in the dissection. The incision is done in the midline and posterior and around the fistula, creating what is also known as a "racket type" of incision (Figure 68.25a). The posterior sphincter mechanism is divided to identify the posterior rectal wall; the dissection then is extended to the lateral walls of the rectum. The most delicate part of the operation is the dissection of the anterior rectal wall. Special attention must be given to avoiding urethral injury. The fistula is mobilized, as well as part of the rectum,

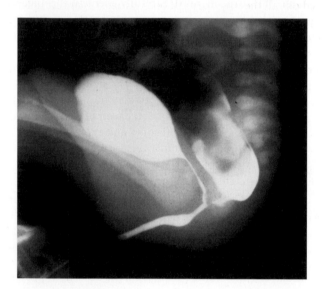

Figure 68.22 Distal colostogram in a rectourethral bulbar fistula.

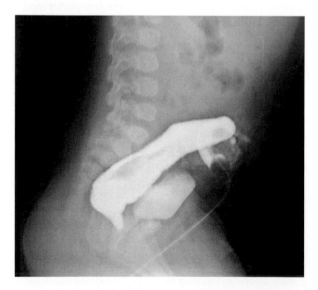

Figure 68.23 Distal colostogram in a rectourethral prostatic fistula.

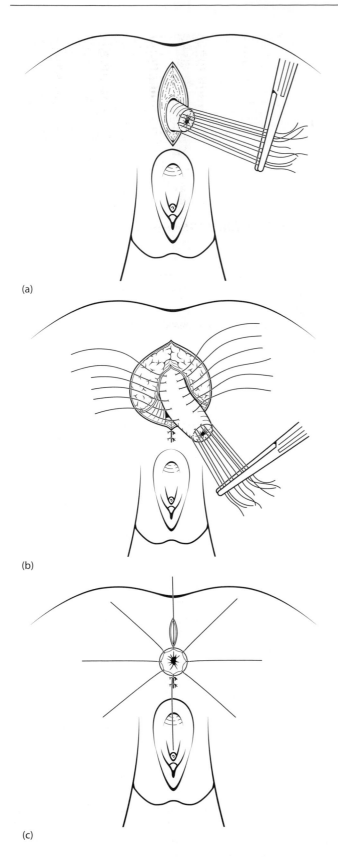

(a)

(b)

(c)

Figure 68.25 Perineal fistula repair: **(a)** incision; **(b)** reconstruction; **(c)** anoplasty.

sufficiently to be posteriorly relocated comfortably within the limits of the sphincter without tension (Figure 68.25b). The rectum is anchored to the muscle complex, and then a 16-stitch anoplasty is done, as shown in (Figure 68.25c).

Limited posterior sagittal anorectoplasty

This procedure is performed in cases of rectovestibular fistula in female newborns. The incision is very similar to the one just described, but it is extended more cephalad as far as necessary to achieve enough bowel mobilization. The main difference with the previous defect is the fact that the rectum and vagina share a rather long common wall. The most important part of the operation consists in separating the rectum and vagina by creating a plane of separation without injuring either one (Figure 68.26). The separation is carried out all the way up, until both structures are completely separated and have a full-thickness normal wall. Lack of adequate rectal mobilization is the main cause of dehiscence after this repair. The separation of the rectum from the vagina requires a meticulous and delicate technique and is performed with a needle-tip cautery, changing from cutting to coagulation where necessary to provide meticulous hemostasis. Once the rectum has been completely separated, the limits of the external sphincter are determined by electrical stimulation. This will indicate where the rectum should be located. The perineal body is then reconstructed with long-term absorbable sutures (Figure 68.27a). The rectum is anchored to the posterior edge of the muscle complex (Figure 68.27b), and then a 16-stitch anoplasty is performed in the same way as previously described (Figure 68.27c,d). If a colostomy is present, these patients can have oral feedings the same day of surgery and can go home the following day. In patients without a colostomy, our routine is to keep them NPO and on intravenous nutrition for 7–10 days. Antibiotic ointment is applied to the wound three times a day for 5 days.

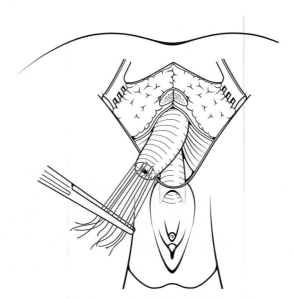

Figure 68.26 Vestibular fistula repair. Separation of rectum.

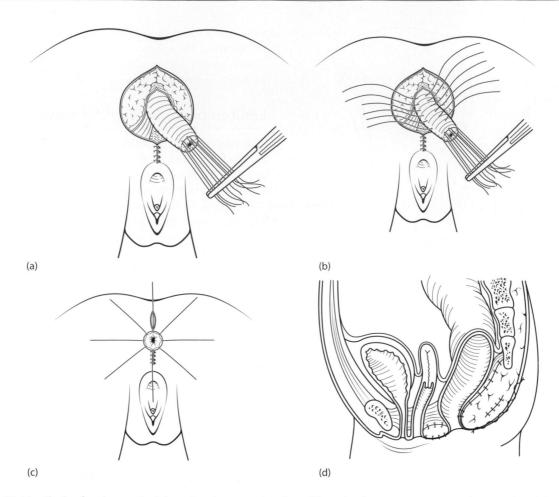

(a)

(b)

(c)

(d)

Figure 68.27 Vestibular fistula repair: **(a)** perineal reconstruction; **(b)** anchoring rectum to muscle complex; **(c)** anoplasty; **(d)** operation completed.

Posterior sagittal anorectoplasty

This technique is used for the repair of a rectourethral fistula or a rectovaginal fistula. The patient is placed as previously described in prone position, with the pelvis elevated and with a Foley catheter in the bladder. Electrical stimulation of the perineum will allow the surgeon to identify the anal dimple, which is the location of the center of the sphincter. The incision runs from the lower portion of the sacrum down and through the anal dimple, staying exactly in the midline, leaving equal amounts of sphincter muscle on both sides. After opening of the skin, one can identify the subcutaneous tissue and then the presence of parasagittal muscle fibers. The incision is deepened, and after another area of fat, the ischiorectal space, one finds the levator muscle. The levator muscle continues with the muscle complex down to the skin of the anal dimple, forming a funnel-like structure. Parasagittal fibers that run on both sides of the midline will close the lumen of the anus once this is reconstructed. Muscle complex fibers run perpendicular to the parasagittal ones and also medially. The muscle complex and parasagittal fibers cross perpendicularly, forming the posterior and anterior limits of the new anus (Figure 68.28) Under normal circumstances, in normal individuals, the

contraction of the muscle complex and levator occurs simultaneously, elevating and closing the anus. The levator muscle is divided exactly in the midline. The rectum is

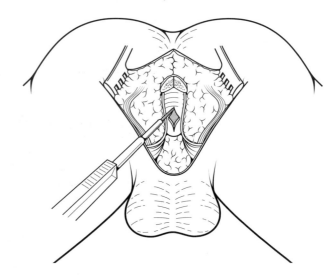

Figure 68.28 Rectourethral fistula repair. Anatomy exposed. Parasagittal fibers, muscle complex, and levator muscle have been split in the midline. The rectum is open in the midline.

then opened along its posterior wall between two traction sutures. Once the rectum is opened, one can visualize the fistula site. One must remember that the rectum and urethra share a common wall immediately above the fistula. Accordingly, a submucosal dissection must be carried out above the fistula site (Figure 68.29). After approximately 1 cm of submucosal dissection, the dissection continues taking the full thickness of rectal wall. Once the rectum has been separated from the urethra, the fistula is closed with interrupted long-term absorbable sutures. The rectum is then dissected in a circumferential manner, in order to gain enough length to reach the perineum without tension (Figure 68.30).

Tapering as shown in Figure 68.31 is rarely needed but, if necessary, must be carried out in the posterior aspect of the rectum. The bowel must then be closed in two layers of interrupted sutures. The rectum is then placed in front of the levator muscle within the limits of the sphincter mechanism and is also anchored to the posterior edge of the muscle

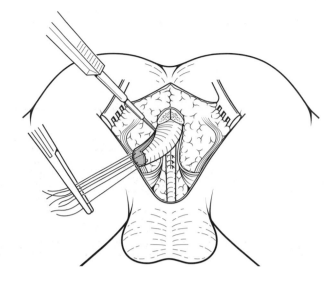

Figure 68.31 Tapering the rectum (when necessary).

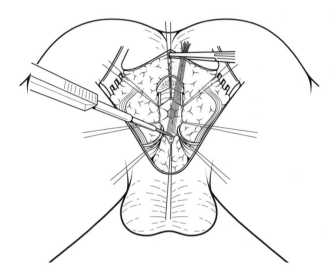

Figure 68.29 Separation of rectum from urethra.

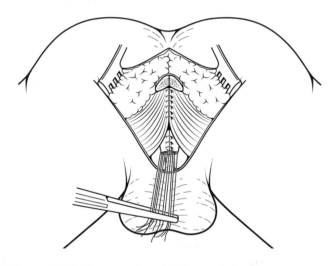

Figure 68.32 Rectum placed in front of the levator. Anchoring sutures from muscle complex to the rectum.

complex to prevent prolapse (Figure 68.32). The anoplasty is done as previously described (Figures 68.33 and 68.34).

Following the operation, the Foley catheter must remain in place for 7 days. If the catheter comes out accidentally, it is better to leave it out rather than trying to pass it back into the bladder and thus risking a urethral perforation at the urethral suture site. Most of the time, babies will be able to void with no difficulty. If this is not so, which luckily is rare, then a suprapubic cystostomy is recommended.

Posterior sagittal anorectoplasty and laparoscopy or laparotomy (bladder neck fistula)

This technique is used in cases with a very high defect, known as recto–bladder neck fistula in males. Some surgeons with experience in laparoscopy can also repair recto-prostatic fistulas with laparoscopy.

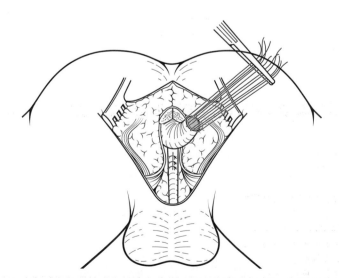

Figure 68.30 Rectum separated from urethra.

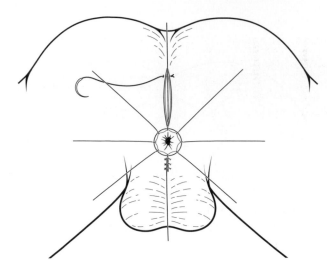

Figure 68.33 Anoplasty.

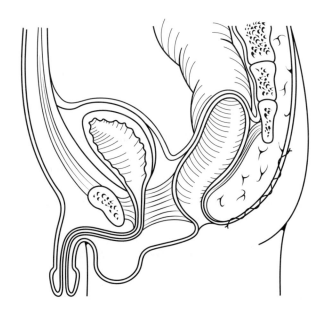

Figure 68.34 Anoplasty—operation completed.

The operation is started with the patient in the supine position. The baby is prepared with a total body preparation from nipples down. A Foley catheter is placed in the bladder. The abdomen is entered with laparoscopy, the peritoneal reflection is opened, and the sigmoid colon is dissected down to the fistula site where it is ligated and divided. The rectum in these cases opens into the bladder neck in a "T" fashion with no common wall, and therefore, the separation from the bladder is relatively easy. One must be careful to avoid damage to the vas deferens, which runs very close by. The perineal incision is the same as previously described for the posterior sagittal anoplasty but can be done in supine position with the patient's legs elevated. The sphincter mechanism is divided in the midline, and the presacral space is identified. Getting a high rectum to reach the perineum may be challenging and requires a meticulous dissection along the rectal wall, which is dependent on the rectum's

excellent intramural blood supply. A colostomy placed too distal in the sigmoid may interfere with the rectal mobilization. Also, if the distal rectum requires tapering, this may need to be done with an open abdomen. Once mobilized, the rectum is pulled through, down to the perineum. The rectum is tacked to the posterior edge of the muscle complex, and the anoplasty is done as previously described. The Foley catheter remains in the bladder for 7 days.

The posterior sagittal approach has also been used since 1982 to repair cloacas.[13] Since cloacas represent a spectrum, the operations to repair these defects may last from 3 to 14 hours and should be carried out by surgeons with significant experience. The technical maneuver that is called total urogenital mobilization has greatly facilitated the repair.[26] Using total urogenital mobilization, the rectum is separated from the vagina, and then both the urethra and vagina are mobilized together, down to the perineum. This maneuver also avoids the formation of urethrovaginal fistulas as well as vaginal stenosis. The more complex cases with common channels of 3 cm or greater require a variety of surgical maneuvers including specialized vaginal mobilizations or replacements to complete the repair.[13]

Two weeks postoperatively

After 2 weeks, the anus is calibrated, and the parents are taught to dilate, which they do twice a day, going up in size each week until the desired size is reached, at which point the colostomy can be closed. Dilations are continued thereafter with a tapering protocol.

Once the desired-size dilator goes in easily, with no pain (twice a day), the parents may start tapering the frequency of the dilatation:

- Once a day for a month
- Every other day for a month
- Every third day for a month
- Twice a week for a month
- Once a week for a month
- Once a month for 3 months

The ideal sizes of Hegar dilators are as follows:

- Number 12 for 1–4 months old
- Number 13 for 4–8 months
- Number 14 for 8–12 months old
- Number 15 for 1–3 years old
- Number 16 for 3–12 years old

Results

Each defect described here has a different prognosis. The patients with lower defects usually have excellent results, except when technical errors have been made or if they have associated sacral or spinal problems.

Table 68.2 shows the results obtained in our series. The patients with a sacral ratio (Figure 68.35) of less than 0.3

Table 68.2 Global functional results

	Voluntary bowel movement		Soiling		Totally continent[a]		Constipated	
	Pts.	%	Pts.	%	Pts.	%	Pts.	%
Perineal fistula	34/35	97%	4/33	12%	29/34	85%	19/37	51%
Rectal atresia or stenosis	8/8	100%	2/8	25%	6/8	75%	5/8	63%
Vestibular fistula	84/94	89%	34/94	36%	60/84	71%	53/93	57%
Imperforate anus without fistula	27/34	79%	15/33	45%	18/27	67%	18/35	51%
Bulbar urethra fistula	69/85	81%	45/84	54%	36/69	52%	54/85	64%
Prostatic fistula	57/86	66%	69/89	78%	17/57	30%	41/89	46%
Cloaca: short common channel	49/76	64%	52/76	68%	23/49	47%	31/77	40%
Cloaca: long common channel	17/44	39%	37/40	93%	3/17	18%	14/43	33%
Vaginal fistula	3/4	75%	3/4	75%	1/3	33%	1/4	25%
Bladder neck fistula	8/39	21%	37/39	95%	2/8	25%	7/40	18%
TOTAL	356/505	70%	298/500	60%	195/356	55%	243/511	48%

[a] Totally continent = voluntary bowel movements with no soiling.

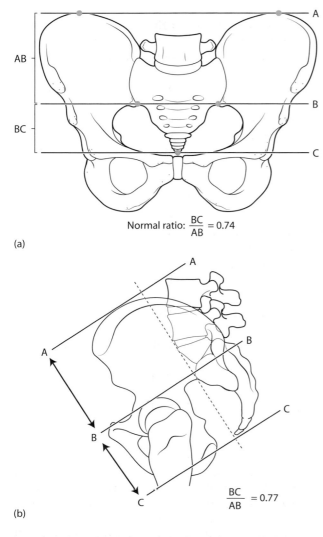

Normal ratio: $\dfrac{BC}{AB} = 0.74$

(a)

$\dfrac{BC}{AB} = 0.77$

(b)

Figure 68.35 Sacral ratios: **(a)** AP sacral view; **(b)** lateral view.

and flat perineums have fecal incontinence regardless of the type of malformation or quality of the repair. Normal sacral ratios (>.07) usually correlate with good functional prognosis.

Because persistent cloacas themselves represents another spectrum of defects, they will vary as far as potential for bowel and urinary control. The length of the common channel seems to be the most important prognostic factor for urinary control. Bowel continence seems to be influenced more by the quality of the sacrum.

BOWEL MANAGEMENT FOR FECAL INCONTINENCE

For patients suffering from fecal incontinence as a sequela of their anorectal malformations (25% of patients), we implement a bowel management program that is used after the child reaches 3 years of age.[27] The goal is to send these children to school in normal underwear. The program is implemented by trial and error, over a period of 1 week. It consists of teaching the family to clean the patient's colon once a day with an enema tailored to work for the specific child. This implementation is radiologically monitored every day during that week until the specific type of enema capable of cleaning the colon is found and the patient's underwear is kept completely clean for 24 hours.[28,29] Every year, during vacation time, the patient is subjected to a laxative test; the enemas are stopped, and the capacity of the patient to become toilet-trained without enemas is evaluated. If the patient is not ready, he or she goes back to the enema program. When the patients are old enough, sometimes they express dissatisfaction with rectal enemas; they want more privacy and do not want their parents giving them enemas. In order to further improve their quality of life, the family

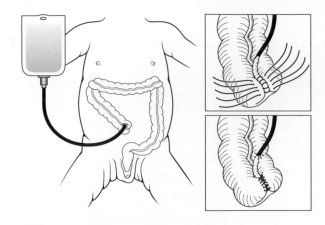

Figure 68.36 Malone appendicostomy.

is offered a procedure called *continent appendicostomy* (Malone procedure) (Figure 68.36).[30,31]

REFERENCES

1. Brenner EC. Congenital defects of the anus and rectum. *Surg Gynecol Obstet* 1915; 20: 579–88.
2. Santulli TV. Treatment of imperforate anus and associated fistulas. *Surg Gynecol Obstet* 1952; 95: 601–14.
3. Trusler GA, Wilkinson RH. Imperforate anus: A review of 147 cases. *Can J Surg* 1962; 5: 169–77.
4. Holschneider A, Hutson J, Peña A et al. Preliminary report on the international conference for the development standards for the treatment of anorectal malformations. *J Pediatr Surg* 2005; 40: 1521–6.
5. Peña A, Bischoff A. In: *Surgical Treatment of Colorectal Problems in Children*. Springer International Publishing; Switzerland, 2015. DOI 10.1007/978-3-319-14989-9.
6. Shaul DB, Harrison EA. Classification of anorectal malformations—Initial approach, diagnostic tests, and colostomy. *Semin Pediatr Surg* 1997; 6: 187–95.
7. Rich MA, Brock WA, Peña A. Spectrum of genitourinary malformations in patients with imperforate anus. *Pediatr Surg Int* 1988; 3: 110–3.
8. Peña A. Posterior sagittal anorectoplasty: Results in the management of 332 cases of anorectal malformations. *Pediatr Surg Int* 1988; 3: 94–104.
9. Gross GW, Wolfson PJ, Peña A. Augmented-pressure colostogram in imperforate anus with fistula. *Pediatr Radiol* 1991; 21: 560–2.
10. Bischoff A, Frischer J, Dickie B, Peña A. Anorectal malformation without fistula: A defect with unique characteristics. *Pediatr Surg Int* 2014; 30: 763–6.
11. Torres P, Levitt MA, Tovilla JM et al. Anorectal malformations and Down's syndrome. *Pediatr Surg* 1998; 33: 1–5.
12. Rosen NG, Hong AR, Soffer SZ et al. Rectovaginal fistula: A common diagnostic error with significant consequences in girls with anorectal malformations. *J Pediatr Surg* 2002; 37(7): 961–5.
13. Bischoff A. The surgical treatment of cloaca. *Semin Pediatr Surg* 2016; 25: 102–7.
14. Freeman NV, Burge DM, Soar IS et al. Anal evoked potentials. *Z Kinderchir* 1980; 31: 22–30.
15. Moore TC. Advantages of performing the sagittal anoplasty operation for imperforate anus at birth. *J Pediatr Surg* 1990; 25: 276.
16. Georgeson KE, Inge TH, Albanese G. Laparoscopically assisted anorectal pull-through for high imperforate anus—A new technique. *J Pediatr Surg* 2000; 35: 927–31.
17. Belman BA, King LR. Urinary tract abnormalities associated with imperforate anus. *J Urol* 1972; 108: 823–4.
18. Hoekstra WJ, Scholtmeijer RJ, Molenar JC et al. Urogenital tract abnormalities associated with congenital anorectal anomalies. *J Urol* 1983; 130: 962–3.
19. Munn R, Schillinger JF. Urologic abnormalities found with imperforate anus. *Urology* 1983; 21: 260–4.
20. Parrott TS. Urologic implications of anorectal malformations. *Urol Clin N Am* 1985; 12: 13–21.
21. Wiener ES, Kiesewetter WB. Urologic abnormalities associated with imperforate anus. *J Pediatr Surg* 1973; 8: 151–7.
22. Williams DI, Grant J. Urological complications of imperforate anus. *Br J Urol* 1969; 41: 660–5.
23. Bianchi DW, Crombleholme TM, Dalton ME. Cloacal exstrophy. In: *Fetology: Diagnosis and Management of the Fetal Patient*, 2nd edn. New York: McGraw-Hill, 2010.
24. Wilkins S, Peña A. The role of colostomy in the management of anorectal malformations. *Pediatr Surg Int* 1988; 3: 105–9.
25. Peña A, Migotto-Krieger M, Levitt MA. Colostomy in anorectal malformations: A procedure with serious but preventable complications. *J Pediatr Surg* 2006; 41(4): 748–56.
26. Peña A. Total urogenital mobilization—An easier way to repair cloacas. *J Pediatr Surg* 1997; 32(2): 263–8.
27. Bischoff A, Levitt MA, Bauer C et al. Treatment of fecal incontinence with a comprehensive bowel management program. *J Pediatr Surg* 2009; 6: 44, 1278–84.
28. Bischoff A, Levitt MA, Pena A. Bowel management for the treatment of pediatric fecal incontinence. Review article. *Pediatr Surg Int* 2009; 25: 1027–42.
29. Bischoff A, Tovilla M. A practical approach to the management of pediatric fecal incontinence. *Semin Pediatr Surg* 2010; 19: 154–9.
30. Malone PS, Ransley PC, Kiely EM. Preliminary report: The anterograde continence enema. *Lancet* 1990; 336: 1217–8.
31. Levitt MA, Soffer SZ, Peña A. Continent appendicostomy in the bowel management of fecally incontinent children. *J Pediatr Surg* 1997; 32: 163.

69

Congenital pouch colon

AMULYA K. SAXENA AND PRAVEEN MATHUR

INTRODUCTION

Congenital pouch colon (CPC) is a malformation of the colon in which the entire large bowel or segments of varying lengths of the large bowel exhibit enormous dilatations in the form of a pouch and communicate with a distal fistula to the urogenital system. CPC is a condition that comprises a high form of anorectal malformation associated with large variations in the size of the dilatations of the affected colonic segment. The scarce reporting of this condition in the 1980s precluded its inclusion in the Wingspread classification of anorectal malformations; however, with the increasing number of reports and detailed investigations of the condition, CPC has been recognized as a rare form of anorectal malformation and has been included in the Krickenbeck classification.[1]

HISTORICAL INSIGHTS

CPC is a rare congenital malformation that is almost non-existent outside the Indian subcontinent. However, this anomaly was initially recognized in England during the beginning of the twentieth century. The first description of this anomaly was documented by Spriggs[2] from a specimen carefully observed at the London Hospital Museum in 1912. He described the specimen as having an absence of half of the large bowel and rectum, where the dilatation was presumed to be the result of a congenital occlusion of the gastrointestinal tract. The next reporting of this congenital malformation was published almost half a century later in an article from Canada in 1959. In this publication, a more accurate account was provided by Trusler et al.,[3] who described more typical characteristics of this malformation, such as the pouch-like dilatation of the shortened large bowel and its association with a high form of anorectal malformation. In 1967, El-Shafie[4] described this malformation in detail as a congenital shortening of the small intestines that accompanied a cystic dilatation of the colon associated with an ectopic anus.

CPC was first reported in India in 1972, when Singh and Pathak[5] coined the term "short colon" after observing this condition in a series of six patients. The authors also speculated in this report on the possible embryogenesis of the malformation. Later on, in a successive report in 1977, a description of the anatomy of this malformation was published.[6] An important contribution to CPC was made by Chiba et al.[7] in 1976, who not only made the first attempts to classify this malformation but also reported on the management of this malformation with the technique of "colo-plasty." The term "colonic reservoir" was coined by Gopal[8] in 1978 in a report with this malformation with the distal end of the reservoir terminating into the female genitals through a rectovaginal fistula. Further efforts to describe this malformation as a "short colon malformation" associated with an atresia of the anus were made by Li in 1981.[9]

Narasimha et al.[10] in 1984 proposed the term *pouch colon syndrome* for this malformation and, after observing variations in the presentation of this malformation, presented a classification based on the length of normal colon preceding the pouch dilatation. Cloutier et al.[11] in 1987 described this malformation as a "rectal ectasia" in a newborn with a low anorectal malformation and reported an incidence of 5% of terminal bowel ectasia in their patients with low anorectal deformities. Wu et al.[12] in 1991 suggested elaborate terms to describe this malformation with acronyms such as "association of imperforate anus with short colon" (AIASC) or "association of imperforate anus with exstrophia splanchnica" (AIAES). However, Chadha et al.[13] in 1994 coined the term "congenital pouch colon," which is the nomenclature to aptly describe this anomaly.

INCIDENCE

The largest patient series of CPC are being reported exclusively from India. Smaller series of patients are being reported from neighboring countries in the Indian subcontinent such as Pakistan and Nepal but with a low incidence reported from Bangladesh.[14] Sporadic cases of CPC are being reported from the Middle East, Far East, Europe, and North America.[15-18] The incidence of CPC is the highest in the northwest regions of India and is estimated to be 5%–18% of the total number of neonates managed for anorectal malformations. Among the Indian Tertiary Care Centers reporting on large series of CPC, Udaipur in the western State of Rajasthan has reported the highest incidence of CPC in India, accounting for 37% of the high forms of anorectal malformations (which is more than double that reported in Delhi—5.2%).[19]

CPC more frequently affects the male population, with a male–female distribution of 4:1. The sex ratios of CPC reported in case reports or small series outside India predict equal gender distribution, which are not accurate since the sample size is too small to derive valid conclusions.

ETIOLOGY

The embryogenesis of CPC is not known, and the etiology is still quite elusive. The widespread use of and direct contact with pesticides in agriculture-based communities have been regarded as the possible factor in triggering of events that lead to CPC. It is also important that the effect of these factors influences the fetus after conception at a time when the hindgut is differentiating into the urinary and colonic tracts.

Various theories have been hypothesized to explain the formation of the pouch. The *chronic obstruction theory* proposed that the expansion of the large bowel was a result of chronic obstruction of the distal colon.[3] However, this theory has not been accepted since the dilated pouch does not return to assume normal proportions even after a colostomy placement to relieve the obstruction. Another hypothesis is the *interference of hindgut growth and migration theory* proposed by Dickinson.[20] In this hypothesis, it was proposed that the interference in the longitudinal growth of the hindgut (distal to the *allantois*) and failure of its migration into the pelvis following the obliteration of the inferior mesenteric artery in early embryonic life was responsible for the formation of the short colon. The *altered hindgut stimulation theory* was hypothesized by Chatterjee.[21] This theory proposed that the normal development of the cecum and the right colon was stimulated by the normal developing hindgut, and development alterations in the hindgut resulting from a primary disorder were responsible for the altered development of the cecum or the right colon. The *faulty rotation and fixation theory* proposed by Wu et al.[12] hypothesized that the faulty rotation and fixation of the large bowel was responsible for the disturbances in longitudinal growth. The *vascular insult theory* was proposed by Chadha et al.[13] in which degrees of vascular insult at the time of the partitioning of the cloaca by the urogenital septum were deemed responsible for the malformation and could explain its variations. The *vascular insult theory* was also supported by Mathur et al.[19] in explanation of double pouch formation in CPC. At present, vascular insults best explain the formation of CPC, which is evident by the abnormal vascular supply to the pouch. Also, the overwhelming vascular support provided by the superior mesenteric artery to the entire distal bowel supports this view, since the inferior mesenteric artery has been identified only in few patients with CPC during surgery.

PATHOLOGY

CPC is recognized by certain pathological characteristics that are solely found to be associated with this congenital malformation (Figure 69.1).

Gross pathology

1. The presence of anorectal malformations, which differentiates this entity from segmental dilatation of the colon.
2. Irrespective of the CPC type, there is a decrease in the length of the large bowel due to the presence of the pouch.
3. The pouch formations may differ in length and diameter and are feces or meconium impacted at the time of surgery.
4. The pouch wall is thick with a stiff consistency and is abruptly connected to the normal bowel without the presence of the transition zone.
5. There is an absence of haustrations, teniae, and appendices epiploicae in the pouch colon.
6. An abnormal vascular supply to the pouch can always be identified during surgical exploration.
7. A fistula can be identified to the urinary tract in male neonates (colovesical fistula) and to the genitourinary tract in females (colocloacal, colovaginal, or colovestibular fistula).
8. Appendiceal anomalies are present and vary from complete absence to the presence of double appendices.

Histological pathology

Histological studies of resected pouch colon demonstrate extreme variations in CPC. In most patients, acute and

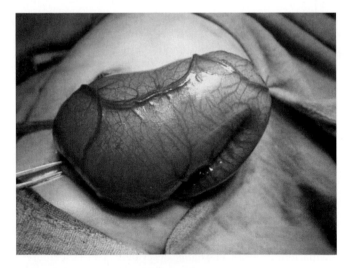

Figure 69.1 Operative view of the exteriorized grossly dilated congenital pouch colon segment visualized from a left lower quadrant "hockey-stick" incision.

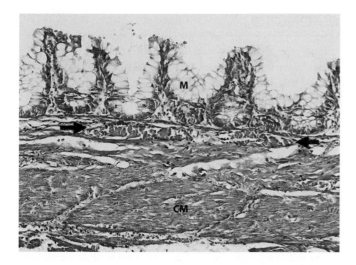

Figure 69.2 General features in the histopathology of pouch colon include inflammation of the mucosa (M) and disorganized colonic wall musculature (CM). Submucosal hemorrhage (arrows) is evident in this specimen. (Stain: Massom trichome, 20× magnification.)

chronic inflammation of the mucosal and submucosal layers is present with varying degrees of hemorrhage along with the presence of disorganized muscle layers in the colon wall (Figure 69.2). Hypotrophy of the muscle layers has been observed, which is more predominant in the outer muscle layer of the pouch.[22] Extreme variations in the muscle layer (both circular and longitudinal) have also been found, which include fibrosis, atrophy, and hypertrophy along with muscle disruption.[23] Investigations have also shown variations, from the presence of normal colon wall with normal ganglion cells in some patients to a poorly developed colon wall musculature with decreased or absent ganglion cells in others.[6,10,13,24] Interestingly, heterotrophic tissue such as gastric mucosa, small intestinal mucosa with characteristic villi, and pancreatic tissue has also been found in pouch specimens of CPC patients.[10,22]

CLASSIFICATION

CPC can present in various types, and efforts have been made to classify CPC in order to provide a basis for surgical management as well as for evaluating the outcomes.

The first efforts to classify CPC were made using a *classification based on characteristics of short colon* that grouped pouch colon into five types.[7] However, many features described in this classification did not associate with the CPC pathology. CPC was then classified by a *classification based on presence of normal colon length proximal to the pouch* into four types.[10] Although this classification had identified the major forms of CPC, it had major drawbacks since the length of the normal colon was determined using terms such as "short segment" and "significant length," and appropriate parameters or anatomic landmarks to determine the normal colon length were absent. A further classification was proposed, a *classification based on coloplasty*, which divided CPC into two types.[24] This classification was further modified into a *classification based on pull-through*, which also broadly divided CPC into two types.[25] The last two classifications considered the surgical approach with regard to coloplasty or pull-through; however, both of them offered no information about the length of the normal colon in CPC patients.

The Saxena–Mathur classification for CPC is a *classification based on anatomic morphology* and divides CPC into five types (Figure 69.3)[26]:

- *Type 1 CPC*—normal colon absent and ileum opens into pouch colon
- *Type 2 CPC*—Ileum opens into a normal cecum, which opens into pouch colon

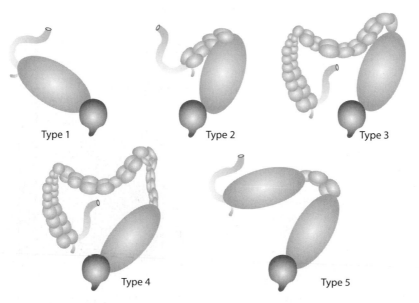

Type 1   Type 2   Type 3

Type 4   Type 5

Figure 69.3 Distribution of patients into five types of congenital pouch colon according to the Saxena–Mathur classification.

- *Type 3 CPC*—normal ascending colon and transverse colon open into pouch colon
- *Type 4 CPC*—normal colon with rectosigmoid pouch
- *Type 5 CPC*—double pouch colon with short normal interpositioned colon segment

This classification employs anatomic landmarks to determine the length of the normal colon as well as identifies the relation of the pouch to the normal colon. It also includes rare forms of CPC such as double pouch colon and offers clear guidelines toward management of CPC.

HISTORY AND PHYSICAL EXAMINATION

The presence of an anorectal malformation with gross distention of the abdomen is the hallmark of the physical examination. In male neonates, discharge of meconium (meconurea) or stool through the urethra via the colovesical fistula is evident, and these neonates are generally referred for treatment in the immediate neonatal period. However, in female patients, meconium and fecal discharge through a cloacal, uterine or vaginal fistula may delay referral in a stable neonate. Furthermore, when a colocloacal fistula (common in females with CPC) is present, it is associated with a large fistula opening that permits decompression of the pouch colon contents, the presence of which can further delay presentation in female subject for a period of several months after birth. At the time of referral, these patients with colocloacal fistulas are frequently obstipated, and physical examination shows the discharge of stools from the ectopic site.

PRESENTATION

The majority of patients with CPC present in the immediate neonatal period due to the anorectal malformation. The absence of the anal canal and excessive distention of the abdominal cavity are the two characteristic signs that raise suspicion of CPC. Although in CPC, the pouch ends through a fistula in the genitourinary tract, meconurea may be present or absent. Another common symptom in these neonates is serial episodes of bilious vomiting, which is a major symptom that leads to referrals. Delayed referrals or grossly distended pouch colon is associated with colonic perforations, which present a major challenge in the management of the newborn with septicemia and peritonitis, which further worsens the respiratory distress present due to the massive abdominal distension. Delay in diagnosis and late referrals even in the neonatal period have been largely responsible for the high mortality in CPC. Awareness of the condition and development of proper management strategies, especially through improvement in neonatal intensive care at the tertiary centers in India, have drastically reduced the mortality from 40% to the present rate of 15%.[27]

DIAGNOSIS

Plain erect abdominal radiographs performed to diagnose patients with CPC demonstrate a classical solitary, grossly dilated air fluid bowel loop that occupies more than 75% of the abdominal cavity with displacement of the small intestines (Figure 69.4). The position of the pouch and the displacement of the intestinal loops depend on CPC type.[24] Although plain abdominal radiographs can predict the CPC type, the definitive diagnosis and the CPC type can be determined only after surgical exploration.[28] False diagnosis of CPC based on plain radiographs is possible in (1) patients with significant dilatation of the sigmoid colon, (2) patients with pneumoperitonuem after perforation in anorectal malformations due to late presentation, and (3) female neonates with rectouterine fistula when severe dilatation of the meconium-filled uterus and gas exhibit the classical images of CPC radiographs.[29]

Although plain erect abdominal radiographs with the classical presentation of CPC are sufficient to establish the diagnosis, conventional invertograms used for the diagnosis in anorectal malformations are additionally performed. Prior to surgical management, further investigations such as abdominal ultrasonography, intravenous pyelography, or voiding cystouretherography and echocardiography are mandatory since a wide range of genitourinary, gastrointestinal, and other forms of associated anomalies have been found in patients with CPC (Table 69.1).

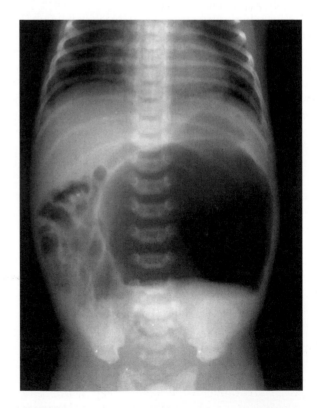

Figure 69.4 Plain abdominal erect radiograph demonstrating the classic grossly dilated pouch colon segment occupying a large area in the left abdomen, thereby displacing the small intestines toward the right abdomen.

Table 69.1 List of associated anomalies reported in congenital pouch colon patients

Genitourinary anomalies	Gastrointestinal anomalies	Other organ anomalies
Hydronephrosis	Absent appendix	Sacral agenesis
Vesicoureteral reflux	Double appendix	Congenital heart disease
Bicornuate uterus	Malrotation	Myelomeningocele
Cryptorchidism	Colon duplication	Prune belly syndrome
Hydroureteronephrosis	Meckel diverticulum	Hemivertebrae
Hypospadias	Double Meckel diverticulum	Congenital talipes equinovarus
Renal aplasia/agenesis	Esophageal atresia	Perineal teratoma
Renal dysplasia	Small intestinal duplication	Absent ribs
Double uterus	Rectal atresia	Down syndrome
Double vagina		
Septate vagina		
Ectopic kidney		
Urethra duplication (males)		
Urethral diverticula		
Bifid penis		
Megalourethra		
Urethral strictures		
Bladder exstrophy		
Duplicate bladder exstrophy		

Note: List of associated anomalies in congenital pouch colon patients distributed under genitourinary, gastrointestinal, and other organ manifestation categories.

MANAGEMENT

Preoperative management

The preoperative management is broadly dependent on the condition of the pouch (intact versus perforated). In stable neonates, preoperative management includes gastric decompression using a wide-bore nasogastric tube, intravenous fluid replacement to correct the effects of dehydration and electrolyte imbalance, and placement of a urinary bladder catheter. Antibiotic therapy is commenced and extended depending on the state of the inflammation in the pouch colon evaluated during the surgery. In neonates presenting with pouch perforations along with signs of either peritonitis or septicemia, aggressive intensive care management is necessary to stabilize the neonate for the emergency surgical procedure, which is limited to evacuation of the meconium or stool from the peritoneal cavity, placement of a ileostomy or colostomy, and closure of the perforation site. The intention in surgical management in neonates with perforations is to perform the surgery with the smallest possible incision and to complete the procedure in a short time.

Operative management

The Management algorithm of CPC is based on the type of pouch according to the Saxena–Mathur classification (Figure 69.5).[30] An abdominal incision in the lower left quadrant in shape of a hockey stick has been found to offer optimal access to inspect the malformation with the primary intention of fistula ligation irrespective of the CPC type. After the fistula has been exposed and ligated, the condition of the pouch dictates the further operative strategy. Staged procedures, employing the placement of a protective ileostomy or colostomy with ligation of the fistula in the first stage, followed by an abdominoperineal pull-through in the second stage, still offer the safest option when compared to one-stage surgery, which is associated with a higher incidence of morbidity and even mortality. The intention of surgical management in CPC is to evaluate the amount of large bowel affected and to salvage its maximum length in order to restore or partially restitute the functions of the large bowel such as absorption, transportation, and containment.

In Type 1 and Type 2 CPC, a one-stage procedure (pouch excision and pull-through) or three-stage procedure (ileostomy, pouch coloplasty with pull-through, and ileostomy closure), depending on the condition of the pouch (ischemic or healthy), can be performed. In case of severe ischemia and perforations, resection of the pouch remains the only alternative. If the pouch is resected, either a direct pull-though of the ileum or placing a protective ileostomy with delayed ileum pull-through offers the best surgical option. However, if the pouch is healthy, the surgical approach is focused on attempts to rescue and taper the pouch and to perform a pouch coloplasty through pouch tubularization. Pouch tubularization is performed after pouch mobilization and longitudinal incision on the antimesenteric side (to preserve the vascular supply) with edge reapproximation over a catheter. Although tubularized pouch coloplasty is performed in both Type 1 and Type 2 CPC, it is not uncommonly associated with increased morbidity in terms of incontinence and complications resulting from

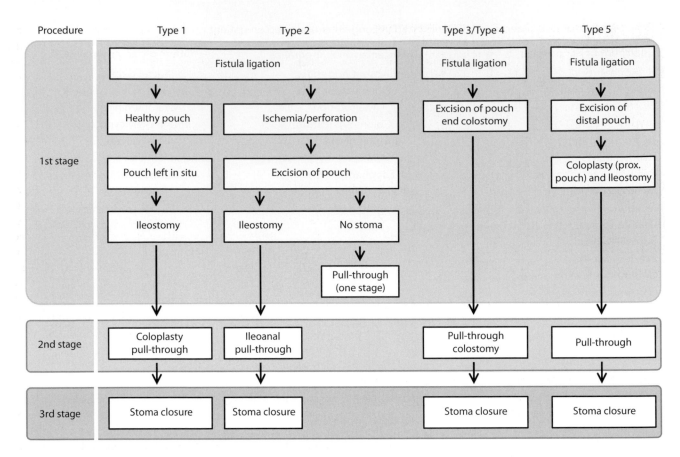

Figure 69.5 Management overview of the various types of congenital pouch colon with outline of the operative stages.

redilatation of the tubularized pouch.[31,32] Also, variations in the outcomes of surgery have been reported by various centers.[12,31,33,34] The function or the absorptive capability of the tubularized pouches is not understood; however, it is reported to be decreased since attempts to patch or augment healthy pouch colon onto normal pull-through ileum in Type 1 CPC with the intention of rescuing the absorptive surface area have been reported with success.[35]

With regard to redilatations of tubularized pouches, the technique of "window" colostomy needs to be addressed. This technique involves the placement of a stoma directly on the pouch colon, which is the most prominent part of the dilated bowel, in an attempt to provide primary decompression in a sick neonate, when extensive surgical exploration is not possible. Window colostomies are more frequently performed by surgeons not well acquainted with this malformation and are commonly associated with urinary complications when the fistula is left open. Furthermore, enormous prolapse of the pouch and failure to thrive also have been related to the placement of window colsostomies.[36] Window colostomy is also associated with mortality in patients who have been managed with this option. The option of window colostomy should not be considered in a stable infant.

The significance of the Saxena–Mathur classification in differentiating Type 1 and Type 2 CPC is to recognize the presence of the normal cecum in Type 2 CPC, which is underestimated in the classifications based on surgical approach. Various investigations and experimental studies have demonstrated the significance of the cecum and ascending colon or parts of the ascending colon in the absorption of sodium, which influences the exchange of chloride and bicarbonate in these tissues.[37,38] However, investigations need to be performed to validate these differences in patients and compare Type 1 and Type 2 CPC patients. Similarly, the absorption of potassium, which is significant in the descending colon in experimental studies,[39,40] highlights the difference between the Type 3 and Type 4 CPC since the normal functioning descending colon is only present in Type 4 CPC.

The presence of considerable lengths of normal colon in the Type 3 and Type 4 CPC enables total resection of the pouch and a staged abdominoperineal pull-through of normal colon (Figure 69.6). The approach to Type 3 and Type 4 involves the ligation of the fistula, excision of the pouch, and placement of a stoma, which is followed by a delayed abdominoperineal pull-through. Although it is debatable if a protective colostomy should be placed, or a prior high colostomy be closed during the pull-through procedure, the authors prefer the first option and place a protective colostomy during the pull-through, which is returned at a later point of time. In Type 3 and Type 4 CPC, if the high colostomy is chosen (instead of the end colostomy), appropriate placement of the colostomy is advocated since improper placement of a high colostomy may

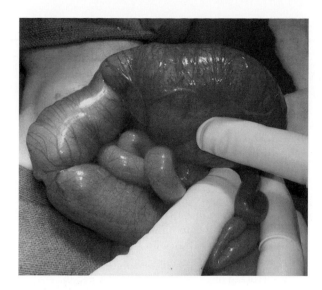

Figure 69.6 Operative view of a Type 3 CPC demonstrating the transition of normal transverse colon (left) to the pouch dilatation (right).

interfere with the pull-through procedure, especially if the length of the colon to be pulled through is too short.

Management of Type 5 CPC requires the approach of two pouch colon segments that are separated by a segment of normal colon and is best done by a three-stage procedure (Figure 69.7).[19] The first procedure involves the ligation of the fistula, excision of the distal pouch, tubularization of the proximal pouch, and the placement of a protective ileostomy. The second procedure involves the abdominoperineal pull-through keeping the protective ileostomy. In the third procedure, the protective ileostomy is returned. Another option for Type 5 CPC would be to tubularize both the proximal and the distal pouch.

Surgical management of female neonates with pouch colon is complex due to the frequent association with the cloaca as well as the associated anomalies of the genital system.[41,42] Depending on the complexity of the genital anomalies, a one-stage or three-stage approach is preferred; however, there is no consensus on the approach to date. The pouch colon has been tubularized to create a neovagina and reconstruct the anorectum with preserved vasculature also using the longitudinal incision technique.[16]

Postoperative management

The postoperative management depends on the condition of the pouch. In patients with pouch perforation, intensive care support along with parenteral nutrition is necessary until complete recovery. The use of antibiotics and the duration of treatment are also dependent on the surgical findings. In patients with protective colostomy, feeds are commenced earlier than in those who have undergone tubularization and pull-through procedures. Monitoring of bowel movements is necessary to achieve success in these patients.[43] Regular postoperative follow-up is necessary to document the bowel movements, which could range from diarrhea when the pouch is resected to obstipation, which could result in tubularized pouch redilatation and necessitate further surgical procedures.

COMPLICATIONS

Complications in the management of CPC can be divided into five distinct categories, which are related to (1) window colostomy, (2) protective colostomy, (3) tubularized pouch colon, (4) complete pouch resection, and (5) pull-through procedure. Window colostomy leads to a wide range of complications such as incomplete pouch decompression, prolapse, stoma recession, stoma stenosis, pouchitis, enterocolitis, and failure to thrive. The complications of protective colostomy or pull-through procedures are general complications associated with these procedures and are not specific to CPC. Tubularization of the pouch colon could be associated with complications of leakage along the suture line with consequent rupture. Also, redilatation after tubularized colon has been observed after long-term follow up

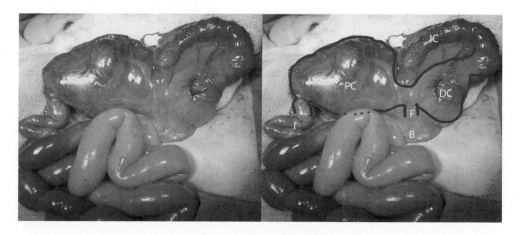

Figure 69.7 Operative view of a Type 5 CPC demonstrating the double pouch colon. (B, urinary bladder; DC, distal pouch colon; F, fistula; I, intestine; IC, intermediate colon; PC, proximal pouch colon.)

in patients with salvaged pouch colon.[32,44] Complete pouch resection is associated with the complications of recurrent watery diarrhea; excoriation around the anus, perineum, or genitals; and poor weight gain. Severe complications in neonates with pouch perforations not only are limited to the septicemia and peritonitis but also have been found to negatively influence the respiratory status as well as the anesthesia efforts intraoperatively and postoperatively, with lethal outcomes.[45]

OUTCOMES

CPC is a complex form of high anorectal malformation, and the muscle complex responsible for maintenance of continence directly influences the long-term outcomes in these patients. In types of CPC where sufficient normal bowel is present (Type 3 and Type 4 CPC), better results have been achieved in patients when the entire pouch has been resected and the normal large bowel is pulled through. This is because the pouch colon tissue investigated has demonstrated lack of normal spontaneous contractions despite maintaining acetylcholine- and histamine-induced contractility.[46] Also, fibrous tissue replaces the muscle layers of the pouch colon and affects motility adversely.[23,47] Hence, in cases of Type 1 and Type 2 CPC, the pouch colon tissue is salvaged, and a tubularized coloplasty is performed, with utilization of approximately 15 cm of tissue; this has been associated with favorable outcomes. Outcomes analyzed after tubularized coloplasty in a case report have shown normal bowel movements, adequate sensation, and a normal-sized neorectum on contrast enema.[48] Also, anorectal manometry has shown spontaneous rectal contraction and a complete rectoanal inhibitory reflex, which suggests that preservation of the native pouch colon is not contraindicated; however, this needs to be further investigated in a larger patient cohort. The defects in neuromusculature of pouch colon tissue are speculated to play a crucial role in postoperative dysmotility and redilatation of the pouch in cases when these morbidities are encountered. Therefore, the present evidence on functional outcome is variable and is probably related to the motility and histology of the retained colon.

CONCLUSION AND FUTURE DIRECTIONS

Surgical management at present focuses on the type of CPC to achieve optimal surgical results. The outcomes are variable, however, predicted with the present knowledge, based largely on the length of colon salvaged and the affected anorectal muscle complex. Future studies will be directed to investigate the etiology of CPC and details of colon histological characteristics, which are still unknown. Once the histological characteristics of the CPC are better understood, investigative studies will be necessary to correlate the histology with clinical outcomes. Greater awareness of these conditions and increased reporting in the literature will contribute toward the addition of anomalies that are associated with the spectrum of CPC.

REFERENCES

1. Holschneider A, Hutson J, Pena J et al. Preliminary report on the International conference for the development of standards for the treatment of anorectal malformations. *J Pediatr Surg* 2005; 40: 1521–6.
2. Spriggs NJ. Congenital occlusion of the gastrointestinal tract. *Guys Hosp Rep* 1912; 766: 143.
3. Trusler GA, Mestel AL, Stephens CA. Colon malformation with imperforate anus. *Surgery* 1959; 45: 328–34.
4. El-Shafie M. Congenital short intestine and cystic dilatation of the colon associated with ectopic anus. *J Pediatr Surg* 1971; 6: 76.
5. Singh S, Pathak IC. Short colon associated with imperforate anus. *Surgery* 1972; 71: 781–6.
6. Singh A, Singh R, Singh A. Short colon with anorectal malformation. *Acta Pediatr Scand* 1977; 66: 589–94.
7. Chiba T, Kasai M, Asakura Y. Two cases of coloplasty for congenital short colon. *Nippon Geva Hokan* 1976: 45: 40–4.
8. Gopal G. Congenital rectovaginal fistula with colonic reservoir. *Indian J Surg* 1978; 40: 446.
9. Li Z. Congenital atresia of the anus with short colon malformation. *Chin J Pediatr Surg* 1981; 2: 30–2.
10. Narasimha Rao KL, Yadav K, Mitra SK, Pathak IG. Congenital short colon with imperforate anus (pouch colon syndrome). *Ann Pediatr Surg* 1984; 1: 159–67.
11. Cloutier R, Archambault H, D'Amours C et al. Focal ectasia of the terminal bowel accompanying low anal deformities. *J Pediatr Surg* 1987; 22: 758–60.
12. Wu YJ, Du R, Zhang GE, Bi ZG. Association of imperforate anus with short colon: A report of eight cases. *J Pediatr Surg* 1990; 25: 282–4.
13. Chadha R, Bagga D, Malhotra CJ et al. The embryology and management of congenital pouch colon associated with anorectal agenesis. *J Pediatr Surg* 1994; 29: 439–46.
14. Gupta DK, Sharma S. Congenital pouch colon—Then and now. *J Indian Assoc Pediatr Surg* 2007; 12: 5–12.
15. Al-Salem AH. Unusual variants of congenital pouch colon with anorectal malformations. *J Pediatr Surg* 2008; 43: 2096–8.
16. Wester T, Läckgren G, Christofferson R, Rintala RJ. The congenital pouch colon can be used for vaginal reconstruction by longitudinal splitting. *J Pediatr Surg* 2006; 41: e25–8.
17. Herman TE, Coplen D, Skinner M. Congenital short colon with imperforate anus (pouch colon). Report of a case. *Pediatr Radiol* 2000; 30: 243–6.
18. Arestis NJ, Clarke C, Munro FD et al. Congenital pouch colon (CPC) associated with anorectal agenesis: A case report and review of literature. *Pediatr Dev Pathol* 2005; 8: 701–5.

19. Mathur P, Prabhu K, Jindal D. Unusual presentations of pouch colon. *J Pediatr Surg* 2002; 37: 1351–3.
20. Dickinson SJ. Agenesis of the descending colon with imperforate anus. Correlation with modern concepts of the origin of intestinal atresia. *Am J Surg* 1967; 113: 279–81.
21. Chatterjee SK. In: *Anorectal Malformations: A Surgeon's Experience.* Oxford, United Kingdom: Oxford University Press, 1991: 170–5.
22. Agarwal K, Chadha R, Ahluwalia C. The histopathology of the congenital pouch colon associated with anorectal agenesis. *Eur J Pediatr Surg* 2005; 15: 102–6.
23. Gangopadhyay AN, Patne SC, Pandey A et al. Congenital pouch colon associated with anorectal malformation—Histopathologic evaluation. *J Pediatr Surg* 2009; 44: 600–6.
24. Wakhlu AK, Wakhlu A, Pandey A et al. Congenital short colon. *World J Surg* 1996: 20107–14.
25. Gupta DK, Sharma S. Congenital pouch colon. In: Hutson J, Holschneider A (eds). *Anorectal Malformations*, 1st edn. Heidelberg: Springer, 2006: 211–22.
26. Saxena AK, Mathur P. Classification of congenital pouch colon based on anatomic morphology. *Int J Colorectal Dis* 2008; 23: 635–9.
27. Sharma S, Gupta DK, Bhatnagar V et al. Management of congenital pouch colon in association with ARM. *J Indian Assoc Pediatr Surg* 2005; 10: S22.
28. Mathur P, Saxena AK, Bajaj M et al. Role of plain abdominal radiographs in predicting type of congenital pouch colon. *Pediatr Radiol* 2010; 40: 1603–8.
29. Wakhlu AK, Tandon RK, Kalra R. Short colon with anorectal malformation. *Indian J Surg* 1982; 44: 621–9.
30. Mathur P, Saxena AK, Simlot A. Management of pouch colon based on the Saxena–Mathur classification. *J Pediatr Surg* 2009; 44: 962–6.
31. Wakhlu AK, Pandey A, Wakhlu A et al. Coloplasty for congenital short colon. *J Pediatr Surg* 1996; 31: 344–8.
32. Chadha R, Bagga D, Gupta S et al. Congenital pouch colon: Massive redilatation of the tubularized colonic pouch after pull-through surgery. *J Pediatr Surg* 2002; 37: 1376–9.
33. Wardhan H, Gangopadhyay AN, Singhal GD et al. Imperforate anus with congenital short colon (pouch colon syndrome). *Pediatr Surg Int* 1990; 5: 124–6.
34. Yadav K, Narasimharao KL. Primary pull-through as a definitive treatment of short colon associated with imperforate anus. *Aus NZJ Surg* 1983; 53: 229–30.
35. Ratan SK, Rattan KN: "Pouch colon patch graft"—An alternative treatment for congenital short colon. *Pediatr Surg Int* 2004; 20: 801–3.
36. Singhal AK, Bhatnagar V. Colostomy prolapsed and hernia following window colostomy in congenital pouch colon. *Pediatr Surg Int* 2006; 22: 459–61.
37. Hatch M, Freel RW. Electrolyte transport across the rabbit caecum in vitro. *Pflugers Arch* 1988; 411: 333–8.
38. Fromm M, Schulzke JD, Hegel U. Aldosterone low-dose, short-term action in adrenalectomized glucocorticoid-substituted rats: Na, K, Cl, HCO_3, osmolyte, and water transport in proximal and rectal colon. *Pflugers Arch* 1990; 416: 573–9.
39. Yau WM, Makhlouf GM. Comparison of transport mechanisms in isolated ascending and descending rat colon. *Am J Physiol* 1975; 228: 191–5.
40. Sweiry JH, Binder HJ. Active potassium absorption in rat distal colon. *J Physiol* 1990; 423: 155–70.
41. Chadha R, Gupta S, Mahanjan JK et al. Congenital pouch colon in females. *Pediatr Surg Int* 1999; 15: 336–42.
42. Sarin YK, Nagdeve NG, Sengar M. Congenital pouch colon in female subjects. *J Indian Assoc Pediatr Surg* 2007; 12: 17–21.
43. Gharpure V. Our experience in congenital pouch colon. *J Indian Assoc Pediatr Surg* 2007; 12: 22–4.
44. Budhiraja S, Pandit SK, Rattan KN. A report of 27 cases of congenital short colon with an imperforate anus so called "pouch colon syndrome." *Trop Doct* 1997; 2: 17–20.
45. Ghritlaharey RK, Budhwani KS, Shrivastava DK et al. Experience with 40 cases of congenital pouch colon. *J Indian Assoc Pediatr Surg* 2007; 12: 13–6.
46. Tyagi P, Mandal MS, Mandal S et al. Pouch colon associated with anorectal malformations fails to show spontaneous contractions but responds to acetylcholine and histamine in vitro. *J Pediatr Surg* 2009; 44: 2156–62.
47. Chatterjee U, Banerjee S, Basu AK et al. Congenital pouch colon: An unusual histological finding. *Pediatr Surg Int* 2009; 25: 377–80.
48. Sangkhathat S, Patrapinyokul S, Chiengkriwate P. Functional and manometric outcomes after a congenital pouch colon reconstruction: Report of a case. *J Med Assoc Thai* 2012; 95: 270–4.

70

Congenital segmental dilatation of the intestine

YOSHIAKI TAKAHASHI, YOSHINORI HAMADA, AND TOMOAKI TAGUCHI

INTRODUCTION

Congenital segmental dilatation (SD) of the intestine is a rare lesion defined as limited bowel dilatation with a 3- to 4-fold increase in size with an abrupt transition between the normal and dilated bowel and no intrinsic or extrinsic barrier distal to the dilatation. This condition is complicated by the obstruction of the intestines or chronic constipation from birth. It was first described in 1959 by Swenson and Rathauser[1] as "a new entity," which is distinct from Hirschsprung's disease in terms of the pathological finding of normal ganglion cells. Sine then, over 100 cases were reported in the world literature in 2006.[2] Thereafter, the number of case reports on patients with this condition has increased. Despite the large number of reports, the etiology of the disease remains elusive. Although the current study attempts to evaluate the roles of interstitial cells of Cajal, the enteric nervous system, and the smooth muscle in SD of the small bowel, the etiology has not been clarified.

We performed a nationwide retrospective cohort study on allied disorder of Hirschsprung's disease (ADHD) in Japan from 2000 to 2009.[3] SD was classified as an ADHD. We tried to collect all of the cases in which SD was diagnosed in Japanese authorized institutions in this period; as a result, we collected a total of 28 cases. The first and most recent retrospective cohort study of these cases was reported by Sakaguchi et al. in 2015.[4]

ETIOLOGY

The etiology of SD of the intestine remains unknown. Some of the hypotheses that have been proposed[1,5] include the following: abnormal tortuous vessels; vascular insufficiency during intussusception; disturbance during the splitting of the notochord from the endoderm; volvulus and kinking due to a long mesentery during the embryologic period; interruption of the continuity of the nerve fibers and the nerve plexus in the islands of ectopic tissue; entrapment by an omphalocele sac; and strangulation of the intestine in the umbilical ring during the early stage of development.

CLINICAL FEATURES AND DIAGNOSIS

We set the diagnostic criteria for SD based on previous reports (Table 70.1).[3]

The commonly dilated segments were the ileum (n = 14; 50%) and colon (n = 10; 35.7%) (Table 70.2).[4] Most of the described cases were discovered in neonates who presented with symptoms of intestinal obstruction in which the clinical picture was hard to differentiate from more common causes of occlusion, such as intestinal atresia, Hirschsprung's disease, meconium ileus, intestinal duplication, and midgut volvulus (Figure 70.1). Consequently, they were diagnosed with this condition when they were neonates or infants. The symptoms in children vary. The most frequent symptom beyond the infant period is gastrointestinal bleeding and anemia due to the ulceration of the dilated segment, which becomes more profuse in the presence of heterotopic gastric mucosa.[2,6-9] Rarely, the patient may present with peritonitis due to perforation of the dilated segment.[8,10] Our report showed that the onset of the disease most frequently occurred in the neonatal period (n = 18; 64.3% [including 7 cases that were prenatally diagnosed]) (Table 70.3). The common symptoms were abdominal distension and vomiting. One case had a family history of SD in cousins, and one case had a family history of severe constipation in brothers.[4]

Because the symptom is not specific and the definitive diagnosis is difficult, SD is usually diagnosed incidentally during surgery (Figure 70.2). However, the anomaly can also be suspected or diagnosed preoperatively on the basis of radiologic findings.[11,12] The classic feature of SD on plain radiographs is the marked SD of the bowel loop, with or without an air-fluid level. Contrast enema studies are often useful for confirming SD of the bowel loop.[12] In SD of the colon, the contrast enema findings are very similar to those of Hirschsprung's disease, but the two conditions can be

Table 70.1 Criteria for diagnosis of segmental dilatation of the intestine

a. Limited bowel dilatation with a three-to fourfold increase in size
b. An abrupt transition between the dilated and normal bowel
c. No intrinsic or extrinsic barrier distal to the dilatation
d. A clinical picture of intestinal occlusion or subocclusion
e. A normality of the neuronal plexus
f. Complete recovery after resection of the affected segment

Table 70.2 Location of dilatation

Ileum	14 cases (50.0%)
Colom	10 cases (35.7%)
Jejunum	3 cases (10.7%)
Duodenum	1 case (3.6%)

Table 70.3 Onset period

Neonatal	18 cases (64.3%)
Infancy	6 cases (21.4%)
Childhood	2 cases (7.1%)
Over 6 years old	2 cases (7.1%)

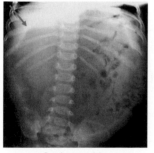
Supine position

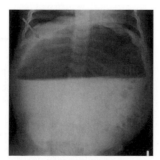
Upright position

Figure 70.1 Plain abdominal x-ray showed a dilated bowel (arrow) in the front of the abdomen. Air-fluid level was prominent in upright position.

differentiated by anorectal manometry. Additionally, histochemical studies demonstrate that there is no proliferation of the cholinergic nerve fibers of the rectal mucosa.

PATHOLOGY

The histopathological findings are the most important diagnostic criteria. The presence of ganglion cells that are normal in number and morphology is one of the criteria for the differential diagnosis. Microscopy can reveal some anomalies, essentially a hypertrophic muscular layer and a heterotopic mucosa that can include esophageal, gastric, or pancreatic tissue. Hypertrophy of the circular and longitudinal layers of the muscularis propria in the dilated segment is evident in older infants/children and is probably an acquired functional adaptation that occurs secondarily to chronic fecal distension.[13,14]

In our report, decreased numbers of ganglion cells or immature ganglion cells were found in three cases, and abnormal muscle layers were found in three cases. Ectopic pancreatic or gastric tissues were found in one case each. Immunohistological investigations showed decreasing c-kit-positive cells in the dilated segment in two of three cases.[4] Some case reports of SD detected decreasing c-kit-positive cells in the dilated segment.[15–17] In some cases, other immunohistological investigations, such as S-100 or MAP5, assisted in the diagnosis of SD.[18] Furthermore, a recent study reported the dislocation of the myenteric plexus within the circular muscle layer (Figure 70.3).[19] We experienced a similar case. Precise histological and immunohistological investigations in future cases of SD might provide more detailed information about its etiology.

TREATMENT

The treatment of SD depends on the clinical condition of the patient, the presentation, the surgeon's experience in dealing with such malformations, and the association with other malformations. The definitive surgery is resection of the involved segment and end-to-end anastomosis with/without proximal colostomy.[5,20,21] In the case of patients who are critically ill (such as patients with perforation or chromosomal abnormalities), an ileostomy can be fashioned

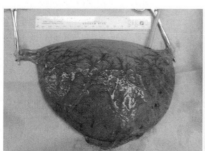
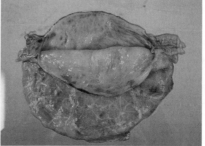

Figure 70.2 Macroscopic finding of resected dilated bowel. Both ends were normal in size.

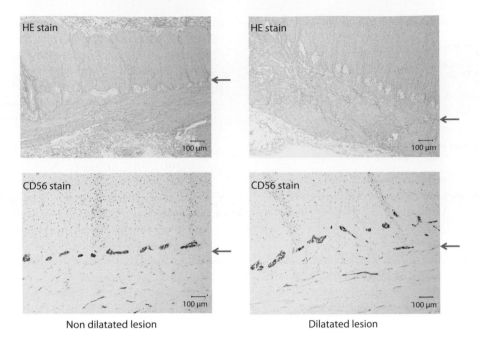

Figure 70.3 Myenteric plexus shifted to the circular muscle layer at the dilated lesion, but not at the nondilated lesion. Arrows showed intermuscular zone.

without excision of the SD.[22] In the case of associated anorectal malformations, stoma formation is always recommended for anorectoplasty in the second stage. A covering ileostomy was also fashioned due to the presence of multiple colonic anastomoses and rectal atresia.[22]

Some reports recommend the use of laparoscopic procedure in the surgical treatment of SD.[7] Laparoscopy was found to be a reliable diagnostic tool and is a minimally invasive procedure that provides safe and superior cosmetic results.[7]

PROGNOSIS

Most patients who undergo surgery for SD experience an uncomplicated postoperative course. The survival rate is excellent unless other serious complications or anomalies are present.

In Japan, SD patients respond favorably to surgical resection. One male patient who underwent ileocecal resection for cecal SD at 9 years of age died at 12 years of age from catheter-related sepsis and liver dysfunction. The patient required parenteral nutrition for 3 years after resection of the dilated bowel; thus, the case might have been complicated by chronic idiopathic intestinal pseudo-obstruction. Excluding this case, the survival rate of SD was 100%.[4]

In our experience, the initial diagnosis was SD of the transverse colon. After resection, gastric dilatation and megacolon appeared. Small intestine perforation due to abnormal dilatation arose several years later, and the final diagnosis was chronic idiopathic intestinal pseudoobstruction (CIIP). Thus, SD cases require careful follow-up. If there is a recurrence of intestinal dilation after resection, we should consider CIIP.

ACKNOWLEDGMENTS

The authors wish to acknowledge Dr. K. Ohama and Dr. N. Ishikawa for offering the data of a case. And we thank Mr. B. Quinn for an English revision.

REFERENCES

1. Swenson O, Rathauser F. Segmental dilatation of the colon. *Am J Surg* 1959; 97: 734–8.
2. Ben Brahim M, Belghith M, Mekki M et al. Segmental dilatation of the intestine. *J Pediatr Surg* 2006; 41: 1130–3.
3. Taguchi T, Ieiri S, Miyoshi K et al. The incidence and outcome of allied disorders of Hirschsprung's disease in Japan: Results from a nationwide survey. *Asian J Surg* 2015. Available online.
4. Sakaguchi T, Hamada Y, Masumoto K et al. Segmental dilatation of the intestine: Results of a nationwide survey in Japan. *Pediatr Surg Int* 2015; 31: 1073–6.
5. Balik E, Taneli C, Yazici M et al. Segmental dilatation of intestine: A case report and review of the literature. *Eur J Pediatr Surg* 1993; 3: 118–20.
6. Levent E, Dicle I, Feriha Oz et al. Segmental dilatation of the ileum accompanying hypoproteinemia. *J Pediatr Surg* 2008; 43: 15–8.
7. Porreca A, Capobianco A, Terracciano et al. Segmental dilatation of the ileum presenting with acute intestinal bleeding. *J Pediatr Surg* 2002; 37: 1506–8.
8. Kuint J, Avigad I, Husar M et al. Segmental dilatation of the ileum: An uncommon cause of neonatal intestinal obstruction. *J Pediatr Surg* 1993; 28(12): 1637–9.

9. Eradi B, Menon P, Rao KL et al. Segmental dilatation of ileum: An unusual cause of severe malnutrition. *Pediatr Surg Int* 2005; 21: 405–6.

10. Thambidorai CR, Arief H, Noor Afidah MS. Ileal perforation in segmental intestinal dilatation associated with omphalocoele. *Singapore Med J* 2009; 50: 412–4.

11. Basaran UN, Sayin C, Oner N et al. Segmental intestinal dilatation associated with omphalocele. *Pediatr Int* 2005; 47: 227–9.

12. Wasters KJ, Levine D, Lee EY et al. Segmental dilatation of the ileum. *J Ultrasound Med* 2007; 26: 1251–6.

13. Helikson MA, Schapiro MB, Garfinkel DT et al. Congenital segmental dilatation of the colon. *J Pediatr Surg* 1982; 17: 201–2.

14. Brawner J, Shafer AD. Segmental dilatation of the colon. *J Pediatr Surg* 1973; 8: 957–8.

15. Katsura S, Kudo T, Enoki T et al. Congenital segmental dilatation of the duodenum. *Surg Today* 2011; 41: 406–8.

16. Okada T, Sasaki F, Honda S et al. Disorders of interstitial cells of Cajal in a neonate with segmental dilatation of the intestine. *J Pediatr Surg* 2010; 45: 11–4.

17. Sakaguchi T, Hamada Y, Nakamura Y et al. Absence of the interstitial cells of Cajal in a neonate with segmental dilatation of ileum. *J Pediatr Surg Case Rep* 2016; 5: 19–22.

18. Cheng W, Lui VC, Chen QM et al. Enteric nervous system, interstitial cells of Cajal, and smooth muscle vacuolization in segmental dilatation of jejunum. *J Pediatr Surg* 2001; 36: 930–5.

19. Mahadevaiah SA, Panjwani P, Kini U et al. Segmental dilatation of sigmoid colon in a neonate: Atypical presentation and histology. *J Pediatr Surg* 2011; 46: 1–4.

20. Al-Salem AH, Grant C. Segmental dilatation of the colon: Report of a case and review of the literature. *Dis Colon Rectum* 1990; 33: 515–8.

21. Sarin YK, Singh VP. Congenital segmental dilatation of colon. *Indian Pediatr* 1995; 32: 116–8.

22. Mirza B, Bux N. Multiple congenital segmental dilatations of colon: A case report. *J Neonat Surg* 2012; 1: 40.

71

Intussusception

SPENCER W. BEASLEY

PRENATAL INTUSSUSCEPTION

Prenatal intussusception is a recognized cause of intestinal atresia.[1,2] The presentation is that of a bowel obstruction at birth. Preoperative evaluation usually fails to yield a definite diagnosis,[1] and the diagnosis is usually made at laparotomy.[2]

Prenatal intussusception may be associated with isolated or transient fetal ascites,[3,4] meconium peritoritis,[5] or a meconium pseudocyst.[6] Some cases are due to a Meckel's diverticulum.[7] Prenatal intussusception results in an ileal atresia following vascular impairment, necrosis, and resorption of the intussusception, irrespective of the underlying lesion causing the intussusception.[4,6,8] Sonographic findings of fetal intestinal intussusception include a "target-like" lesion (a round hyperechoic area of fetal bowel mucosa surrounded by a relatively hypoechoic ring of bowel wall), dilated bowel loops, and abdominal calcifications.[9] Sometimes, the clues to prenatal intussusception have been present on antenatal ultrasonography, so perhaps not surprisingly, the infant presents at birth with abdominal distension and features of a bowel obstruction.[10]

NEONATAL INTUSSUSCEPTION

Although intussusception is common in the first year of life, it is rare in neonates and premature infants,[3,11] accounting for fewer than 1% of cases. Extremely rarely, intussusceptions may be multiple,[11,12] which is notable because in this situation, there is generally no obvious pathological lesion at each lead point.

Generally speaking, it is reasonable to assume that when intussusception occurs in a neonate, there is a pathological lesion at the lead point, such as a duplication cyst, inverted Meckel's diverticulum, jejunal polyp,[10] or ileal polyp.[13] Even beyond the neonatal period, in any infant under 3 months of age, it is much more likely that there is a pathological lesion at the lead point than when it occurs later in the first year of life.[1,14] This is in contrast to the typical age of idiopathic intussusception (in which there is no obvious pathological lesion causing the intussusception), which is between 3 and 12 months, with a peak incidence at about 5–6 months.

The rotavirus vaccine

An early rotavirus vaccine (Rotashield) was withdrawn from the market because of its association with intussusception. Newer live, oral, attenuated rotavirus vaccines (Rota Teq and Rotarix) were believed to have no increased risk of intussusception,[15,16] but the latest data from the Centers for Disease Control and Prevention[17] suggest that 1 in 20,000–100,000 US infants who get rotavirus vaccine develop intussusception within a week of being given the vaccine. Rotarix is normally administered to infants at 6–24 weeks of age. The advantages of the vaccine still far outweigh the risks, but parents should be warned of the possibility of intussusception following vaccination, and physicians should be suspicious if symptoms consistent with intussusception occur shortly after vaccination.

CLINICAL ASSESSMENT

The key features of intussusception are those of a bowel obstruction. When intussusception occurs in premature infants or in the neonatal period, its presentation may mimic neonatal necrotizing enterocolitis: the infant develops bile-stained vomiting, increased nasogastric aspirates, blood in the stools, and intestinal dilatation—but without evidence of intramural gas (pneumatosis intestinalis) that is pathognomonic of necrotizing enterocolitis.[18] It is not surprising that diagnostic confusion with necrotizing enterocolitis can lead to delay in appropriate treatment.[19] Similarly, in the neonate, the combination of bowel obstruction and rectal bleeding may lead to confusion with malrotation and volvulus; given the rarity of the condition in this age group, the diagnosis is often made only at operation.

In the older infant, vomiting, lethargy, pallor, and colic are the most common symptoms.[20] In long-standing cases, the infant may appear shocked and septicemic, with abdominal distension. Where abdominal distension and tenderness are not pronounced, an abdominal mass may be palpable, and there may be evidence of blood mixed with the stool on rectal examination. Transanal protrusion of an intussusceptum is rare, but when it occurs, it may be confused with rectal prolapse and is associated with significant morbidity.[21]

NONOPERATIVE TREATMENT

Indication for enema

When a diagnosis of intussusception is suspected and there is no clinical evidence of necrotic bowel (i.e., peritonitis or septicemia), reduction of the intussusception by gas enema should be attempted.[22] As alternatives, hydrostatic reduction under ultrasonographic control,[23] or in institutions where gas enemas are not available, a barium enema, may be employed. Duration of symptoms, radiological evidence of small bowel obstruction,[24] and the position of the apex[25] per se are not contraindications to attempted enema reduction but can have some value in predicting the likelihood of successful reduction.

Unfortunately, a contrast enema in the neonate is diagnostic in relatively few cases, mainly because the intussusception often does not extend through the ileocecal valve, which often remains competent such that contrast cannot enter the ileum. Abdominal ultrasonography is a more reliable way to make the diagnosis (Figure 71.1) and, in many centers, is performed routinely where intussusception is suspected.[23] Routine plain radiology of the abdomen is unnecessary[26] and tends to be obtained only when the possibility of intussusception has not be considered. Ultrasonography is a more sensitive and more specific diagnostic tool.

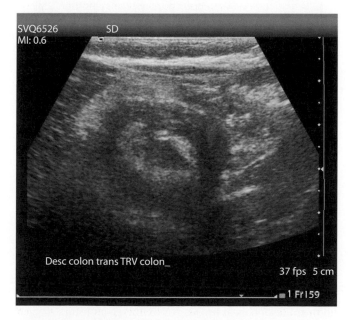

Figure 71.1 Ultrasonographic appearance of intussusception with the concentric rings of the intussusceptum within the intussuscipiens.

Preparation for gas enema

There is considerable evidence that the gas enema is more effective and safer than the barium enema for reduction of intussusception that extends beyond the ileocecal valve (Figure 71.2).[27–29] Ideally, the gas enema should be performed in a pediatric surgical institution by an experienced pediatric radiologist in the presence of a pediatric surgeon.[27] An intravenous line should be inserted and rehydration commenced before undertaking the enema. The child should be placed on a warming blanket during the procedure to prevent heat loss.

Technique of enema reduction

Gas (usually oxygen from a wall supply) is pressure-controlled and run into the colon through a Foley catheter, which has been inserted through the anal canal, as with a conventional barium enema reduction.[27] The infant lies prone with buttocks taped and squeezed tightly together by the radiologist to avoid air leakage. The upper limit of pressure can be controlled by a manometer, and the entire procedure is performed under continuous fluoroscopic control (Figure 71.3).

Cessation of gas enema

Flooding of the small bowel with gas signifies a complete reduction of the intussusception (Figure 71.4). If free intraperitoneal gas is observed, the enema should be ceased immediately. Very rarely, a tense pneumoperitoneum ensues (if there is delay in recognizing the complication) and may need decompression with an angiocath needle through the abdominal wall. Gas reduction tends to occur more rapidly than barium reduction. Both techniques have a similar recurrence rate,[30] but the perforation rate may be more common after a gas enema than a barium enema.[31,32]

Delayed gas enema after partial reduction

Where the initial attempt at reduction has been unsuccessful but there has been partial reduction, and the infant remains in good clinical condition, repetition of the gas enema after 2–3 hours is likely to be successful in about 50% of cases.[33] Where there has been further (but incomplete) reduction after the second attempt, a third attempt may be successful in around another 50%.

INDICATIONS FOR SURGERY

Clinical evidence of peritonitis or septicemia is an absolute indication for surgery, as it signifies that dead bowel is likely to be present and resection is required (Table 71.1). Other indications for surgery include failure of repeated gas enemas to reduce the intussusception or (in the case of neonates) early recurrence of intussusception after a successful enema where the presence of a pathological lesion at the lead point is likely. Occasionally, a pathological lesion at the lead

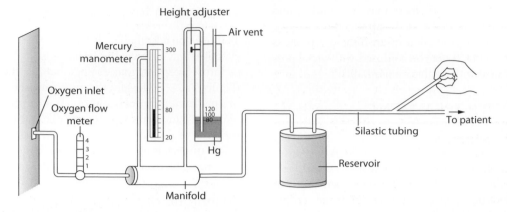

Figure 71.2 Schematic representation of the apparatus used to achieve gas (oxygen) reduction of intussusception.

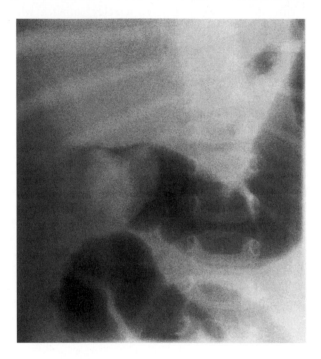

Figure 71.3 Gas reduction of intussusception: the pressure-controlled oxygen runs through the anus and outlines the intussusceptum, in this patient, encountered in the transverse colon.

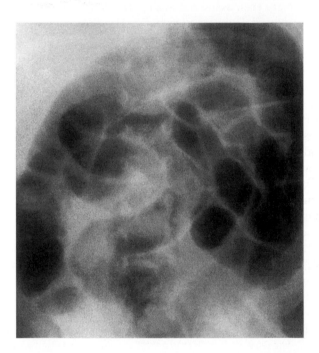

Figure 71.4 Sudden flooding of the small bowel signifies complete reduction of the intussusception.

Table 71.1 Indications for surgery

Clinical evidence for dead bowel, i.e., peritonitis, septicemia

Failure of (repeated) enema reduction

Early or multiple recurrences (relative indication)

Evidence of pathological lesion at the lead point that requires resection

point may be seen during attempted enema reduction, and typically, the intussusception cannot be reduced by enema when a pathological lesion is present. In the neonate who presents with an established bowel obstruction, the diagnosis is made when the intussusception is discovered at the time of laparotomy or laparoscopy. Surgical management involves resection of nonviable bowel and primary anastomosis. Until recent years, the mortality rate was over 20%,[11] largely because of delay in diagnosis, but it is now believed to be much lower.

Preparation for surgery

Prior to induction of general anesthesia, a nasogastric tube is inserted to empty the stomach. Prophylactic antibiotics are given intravenously at induction. The infant is paralyzed and intubated. A warming blanket must be used to prevent excessive heat loss, and temperature is monitored with a rectal or midesophageal probe. An oximeter monitors oxygen saturation. Following the procedures on the Surgical Safety Checklist ensures that every member of the team is fully informed and prepared prior to the surgery commencing.

SURGICAL TECHNIQUE

Approach

The classical approach is through a right supraumbilical transverse incision, dividing the ventral abdominal wall muscles in the line of the incision (Figure 71.5). The peritoneum is opened. This gives good exposure, irrespective of the length of intussusception. Free peritoneal fluid is aspirated, and the bowel is delivered into the wound.

Alternatively, a laparoscopic approach using a 5 mm umbilical port for the telescope and two 3 mm or 5 mm working ports is employed. The abdominal wall of the neonate is thin enough that a small incision may allow the 3 mm instruments to be introduced directly without a port. A laparoscopic approach may be difficult in the presence of marked gaseous distension of the bowel, necessitating conversion to an open approach.

Manual reduction

The intussusception is carefully reduced by manipulation of the intussusceptum within the intussuscipiens in a proximal direction (Figure 71.6). This is performed by gently squeezing the bowel between the fingers and in the cup of the hand. Time must be allowed to enable edema of the mesentery and bowel to dissipate. The intussusception is most difficult to reduce in the region of the ileocecal valve. Care must be taken to avoid splitting the serosa. A similar technique is used in the laparoscopic approach, but reduction is completely reliant on instrumental manipulation.

Check for a pathological lead point

After full reduction of the intussusception, a dimple at the lead point is a common sight and in itself does not represent a pathological lead point. Look for evidence of a duplication cyst, inverted Meckel's diverticulum, or another lesion at the lead point, because if these are present, they should be resected.

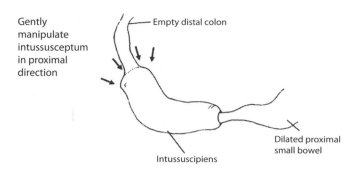

Figure 71.6 Gentle pressure on the distal limit of the intussusception coerces the intussusceptum proximally. Pulling on the bowel as it enters the intussuscipiens is not advised, as it tends to be more traumatic and less efficient at reducing the intussusception.

Technique of resection

The indicators for resection are shown in Table 71.2. The aim should be to remove as little viable bowel as possible (Figure 71.7). The small bowel mesentery is ligated and divided, and the bowel at the edges of resection is divided with scissors. An all-layers 4-0 Vicryl or similar absorbable suture is used to perform an end-to-end anastomosis. The defect in the mesentery is closed to prevent later internal herniation.

Closure

The peritoneal cavity is irrigated with warm saline. The peritoneum and posterior rectus sheath and anterior rectus sheath are closed with continuous 3-0 sutures. The skin is closed with an absorbable subcuticular suture such as a 5-0 Monocryl suture. No drainage is required. When a laparoscopic approach has been used, the 5 mm umbilical wound should be sutured, but the 3 mm working ports do not need to be closed with sutures, and the risk of incisional hernia is low.

Postoperative instructions

A nasogastric tube is usually not necessary unless there has been severe obstruction or a prolonged ileus is anticipated.

Table 71.2 Indications for resection

| Inability to reduce intussusception manually |
| Full-thickness necrosis or gangrene of the bowel |
| A pathological lesion at the lead point |

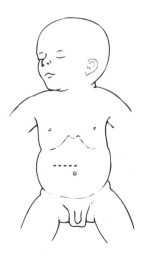

Figure 71.5 Right supraumbilical transverse incision.

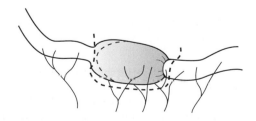

Figure 71.7 Line of resection of an irreducible intussusception.

Oral fluids are resumed when the infant appears to be hungry and the abdomen is becoming soft to palpation.

REFERENCES

1. Wang NI, Chang PY, Sheu JC et al. Prenatal and neonatal intussusception. *Pediatr Surg Int* 1998; 13(4): 232–6.
2. Huan WC, Wang CH, Yuh YS et al. A rare type of ileal atresia due to intrauterine intussusception. *Eur J Pediatr* 2007; 166(11): 1177–8.
3. Reguerre Y, de Dreuzy O, Boithias C et al. An unknown etiology of fetal ascites: Acute intestinal intussusception. *Arch Pediatr* 1997; 4(12): 1197–9.
4. Yang JI, Kim HS, Chang KH et al. Intrauterine intussusception presenting as fetal ascites at prenatal ultrasonography. *Am J Perinatol* 2004; 21(4): 241–6.
5. Lin CH, Wu SF, Lin WC et al. Meckel's diverticulum induced intrauterine intussusception associated with ileal atresia complicated by meconium peritonitis. *J Formos Med Assoc* 2007; 106(6): 495–8.
6. Gudi SN, Bhanuprakasah MR, Suneetha V, Prasanna N. Meconium pseudocysts and ileal atresia secondary to intrauterine intussusception. *J Obstet Gynaecol India* 2011; 61(5): 562–4.
7. Guandogdu HZ, Senacak ME. Intrauterine intussusception due to Meckel's diverticulum as a cause of ileal atresia: Analysis of 2 cases. *Eur J Pediatr Surg* 1996; 6(1): 52–4.
8. Chouikh T, Charieg A, Mrad C et al. Intestinal atresia caused by intrauterine intussusception: A case report and literature review. *J Pediatr Surg Case Rep* 2013; 2(4): 203–5.
9. Shimotake T, Go S, Tsuda T, Iwai N. Ultrasonographic detection of intrauterine intussusception resulting in ileal atresia complicated by meconium peritonitis. *Pediatr Surg Int* 2000; 16(1–2): 43–4.
10. Parelkar SV, Sanghvi BV, Vageriya NL et al. Neonatal jejunal polyp with jejunojejunal intussusception causing atresia: A novel case. *J Pediatr Surg* 2014; 2(2): 73–5.
11. Slam KD, Teitelbaum DH. Multiple sequential intussusceptions causing bowel obstruction in a preterm neonate. *J Pediatr Surg* July 2007; 42(7): 1279–81.
12. Bawa M, Kanojia RP, Ghai B et al. Idiopathic simultaneous intussusceptions in a neonate. *Pediatr Surg Int* May 2009; 25(5): 445–7.
13. Ong NT, Beasley SW. The lead point in intussusception. *J Pediatr Surg* 1990; 25: 640–3.
14. Blakelock RT, Beasley SW. The clinical implications of non-idiopathic intussusception. *Pediatr Surg Int* 1998; 14(3): 163–7.
15. Dennehy PH. Rotavirus vaccines: An overview. *Clin Microbiol Rev* January 2008; 21(1): 198–208.
16. Chen YE, Beasley S, Grimwood K et al. Intussusception and rotavirus associated hospitalisation in New Zealand. *Arch Dis Child* October 2005; 90(10): 1077–81.
17. Available at http://www.cdc.gov/vaccinesafety/vaccines/rotavirus-vaccine.html. Accessed December 5, 2015.
18. Mooney DP, Steinthorsson G, Shorter NA. Perinatal intussusception in premature infants. *J Pediatr Surg* 1996; 31(5): 695–7.
19. Ogundoyin OO, Ogunlana DI, Onasanya OM. Intestinal stenosis caused by perinatal intussusception in a full-term neonate. *Am J Perinatol* January 2007; 24(1): 23–5.
20. Beasley SW, Auldist AW, Stokes KB. The diagnostically difficult intussusception: Its characteristics and consequences. *Pediatr Surg Int* 1988; 3: 135–8.
21. Ameh EA, Mshelbwala PM. Transanal protrusion of intussusception in infants is associated with high morbidity and mortality. *Ann Trop Paediatr* December 2008; 28(4): 287–92.
22. Beasley SW. Can the outcome of intussusception be improved? *Aust Paediatr J* 1988; 24: 99–100.
23. Ko HS, Schenk JP, Troger J et al. Current radiological management of intussusception in children. *Eur Radiol* September 2007; 17(9): 2411–21.
24. Beasley SW, de Campo JF. Radiological evidence of small bowel obstruction in intussusception: Is it a contraindication to attempted barium reduction? *Pediatr Surg Int* 1987; 2: 291–3.
25. Ong NT, Beasley SW. Progression of intussusception. *J Pediatr Surg* 1990; 25: 644–6.
26. Robson N, Beasley SW. The role of plain abdominal radiography in the initial investigation of suspected intussusception. *J Pediatr Child Health* 2014; 50: 251–2.
27. Phelan E, de Campo JF, Maleckey G. Comparison of oxygen and barium reduction of ileocolic intussusception. *Am J Radiol* 1988; 150: 1349–52.
28. Beasley SW, Glover J. Intussusception: Prediction of outcome of gas enema. *J Pediatr Surg* 1992; 27: 474–5.
29. Guo JZ, Ma XY, Zhou QH. Results of air pressure enema reduction of intussusception: 6396 cases in 13 years. *J Pediatr Surg* 1986; 21: 1201–3.
30. Renwick AA, Beasley SW, Phelan E. Intussusception: Recurrence following gas (oxygen) enema reduction. *Pediatr Surg Int* 1992; 7: 362–3.
31. Maoate K, Beasley SW. Perforation during gas reduction of intussusception. *Pediatr Surg Int* 1998; 14: 168–70.
32. Daneman A, Alton DJ, Ein S et al. Perforation during attempted intussusception reduction in children—A comparison of perforation with barium and air. *Pediatr Radiol* 1995; 25: 81–8.
33. Saxton V, Katz M, Phelan E, Beasley SW. Intussusception: A repeat delayed gas enema increases the non-operative reduction rate. *J Pediatr Surg* 1994; 29: 1–3.

72

Inguinal hernia

THAMBIPILLAI SRI PARAN AND PREM PURI

INTRODUCTION

Inguinal hernia is one of the most common surgical conditions in infancy, with a peak incidence during the first 3 months of life. The incidence of hernia is much higher in premature infants, who are surviving in increasing numbers with improved intensive care management, and subsequently increasing the overall incidence. The diagnosis of inguinal hernia can be made without major difficulty in newborns. Early infancy carries a particularly high risk of incarceration of inguinal hernias. As a consequence, early surgical repair is advocated in a population in which there are additional surgical and anesthetic risks.

ETIOLOGY

Almost all inguinal hernias in the newborn are indirect in nature, through a patent processus vaginalis; direct inguinal hernias are exceedingly rare at this age.[1] The processus vaginalis is an outpouching of the peritoneum through the inguinal canal that is first seen during the third month of intrauterine life. In male infants, the processus accompanies the gubernaculum and the testis during their descent through the inguinal canal and reaches the scrotum by the seventh month of gestation. In the female, the processus extends along the round ligament. Obliteration of the processus vaginalis commences soon after the descent of the testis is completed and continues after birth. Most infants have a patent processus vaginalis several months after birth. Patency has been reported to be 80%–94% in the newborn period, 57% in the 4–12-month age group, and 20% in adulthood[2]; this patency is not equivalent to an inguinal hernia, and most times it has no clinical relevance.

EPIDEMIOLOGY

The incidence of congenital indirect inguinal hernia in full-term neonates is 3.5%–6.2% in males and 0.74% in females.[3,4] The incidence of inguinal hernia in preterm infants is considerably higher and ranges from 9% to 11%.[5] The incidence approaches 60% as birth weight decreases to 500–750 g.[2] Inguinal hernia is more common in males than in females. Most series report a male preponderance over females ranging from 5:1 to 10:1.[6] Of all inguinal hernias, 60% occur on the right side, 25%–30% on the left, and 10%–15% are bilateral.[2,7] Bilateral hernias are more common in premature infants and are reported to occur in 44%–55% of patients.[5,8,9] The reported risk of a metachronous contralateral hernia is 7%–10%.[10–13] There is a higher familial incidence, and inguinal hernia has been observed with increasing frequency in twins and siblings of patients.[14] There is no geographic or racial predominance reported in the literature.

ASSOCIATED CONDITIONS

There is an increased incidence of inguinal hernia in patients with the following conditions:

- Prematurity
- Undescended testis
- Ventriculoperitoneal shunts[15,16]
- Peritoneal dialysis[17,18]
- Cystic fibrosis
- Increased abdominal pressure[19] secondary to meconium ileus, necrotizing enterocolitis, chylous ascites, tight closure of gastroschisis, omphalocele
- Bladder exstrophy[20,21]
- Connective tissue disorders such as cutis laxa,[22] Ehlers–Danlos, and Marfan syndromes or Hurler–Hunter mucopolysaccharidoses[23]

CLINICAL FEATURES

Inguinal hernia can be diagnosed prenatally by ultrasonographic screening.[24] In the newborn, the presenting feature is a bulge in the groin, which increases in size with crying and which is usually noticed by the parent. This bulge may disappear spontaneously when the patient is quiet and relaxed, but sometimes it remains visible and palpable for hours causing obvious discomfort and sometimes vomiting. When the lump in the groin is reduced, it is usually possible to feel thickening of the structures of the cord due to a hernial sac. A reliable clinical history along with a palpable thickened cord is highly suggestive of inguinal hernia, and alone is sufficient to proceed to surgery, as clinical demonstration of the bulge may prove difficult at routine consultation.

In girls, the inguinal bulging is intermittently felt in the groin and is usually less obvious. Occasionally a tender, non-reducible, ovoid-shaped mass, corresponding to the ovary, sliding within the sac can be palpated; this could easily be mistaken for a swollen inguinal lymph node.

Some premature infants with previous apneic episodes have been reported to stop having them after inguinal hernia repair. The obvious interpretation is that there can be some association between both clinical conditions.[25] Although this eventuality is exceedingly rare, acute inflammation of the appendix within the hernial sac has been reported in premature and full-term newborns.[26–29]

MANAGEMENT OF INGUINAL HERNIA

The treatment of inguinal hernia is surgery and, in our opinion, there is no place for the use of trusses or other so-called conservative procedures, even in low birth weight (LBW) infants.[30] The ideal time for surgery is as soon as possible after the diagnosis has been made not only because of the high risk of incarceration[31] but also because it has been shown that comfort and weight gain of premature infants with inguinal hernias improve after repair.[32] Nowadays, most inguinal hernia operations are done as day-case procedures.[33] Premature infants and children with cardiac, respiratory, or other conditions have an increased risk of anesthetic complications and may need overnight observation for apnea. However, some authors consider it reasonably safe to operate on these patients on a day-case basis.[34,35]

ANESTHESIA

General anesthesia with endotracheal intubation is preferred in small infants. Premature infants undergoing surgery have an increased risk of life-threatening postoperative apnea.[36] The use of spinal anesthesia in LBW infants undergoing inguinal hernia repair is associated with a lower incidence of postoperative apnea.[37,38]

OPEN INGUINAL HERNIOTOMY

Inguinal herniotomy is the procedure employed in the treatment of congenital persistence processus vaginalis. The operation consists of simple ligation of the hernial sac without opening the inguinal canal.

Position: The infant is placed in the supine position on a heating blanket.

Incision: A 1.5 cm transverse inguinal skin crease incision is placed above and lateral to the pubic tubercle (Figure 72.1a).

Exposure of external ring: Hemostats are placed on subcutaneous tissue, which is cut or spread until the cord is seen to emerge from the external ring (Figure 72.1b,c).

Separation of sac: The cord is isolated over a mosquito forceps with blunt dissection around the cord. The external spermatic fascia and cremaster are separated along the length of the cord by blunt dissection. The hernial sac is seen as a glistening ivory-colored structure and is gently separated from the vas and vessels (Figure 72.1e). A hemostat is placed on the fundus of the sac, in case of incomplete hernial sacs, to aid the separation. In complete hernial sacs, it may be necessary to open the sac before the separation can be completed safely off the vas and vessels.

Herniotomy: The sac is twisted so as to reduce its content into the abdominal cavity. The spoon can be used to keep vas and vessels away from the neck of the sac. The sac is transfixed with a 4-0 absorbable suture at the level of the internal ring, which is marked by an extraperitoneal pad of fat (Figure 72.1b). The part of the sac beyond the stitch is usually excised; but there are no obvious advantages of removing the distal part of the sac after its division and transfixion, and the operation should remain as simple as possible.[39] With large preterm neonatal hernias, it may be necessary to partially tighten the deep ring around the cord structures with one or two absorbable interrupted sutures to reduce recurrence. In girls, the operation is more straightforward since there are no vas or vessels and the external ring can be closed after excising the sac. However, it is prudent to open the sac to exclude any gonadal before placing the transfixation suture.

Closure: Subcutaneous tissues are approximated using one or two 4-0 absorbable interrupted stitches (Figure 72.1g), and the skin is closed with a 5-0 absorbable continuous subcuticular suture (Figure 72.1h). A recent alternative is the use of cyano-acrylate adhesives for approximating the skin edges. A small dressing can be applied over the wound if necessary. At the end of the operation, the testis, always tractioned upward during operative maneuvers, must be routinely pulled back into the scrotum to avoid iatrogenic ascent.[40]

LAPAROSCOPIC INGUINAL HERNIA REPAIR

Laparoscopic hernia repair in infancy has gained support over the last decade. In recent years, several authors have reported that laparoscopic hernia repair in infants is feasible, safe, and effective.[41–44] Laparoscopic percutaneous techniques utilize just one port as opposed to three, and appear to work well in selected children.[45] Some authors have reported up to 20% contralateral herniotomies with the laparoscopic approach[39] and highlight the increased intervention based on appearance of patent processus, which is known not to cause any hernias in vast majority of children. Though some surgeons prefer the laparoscopic approach in

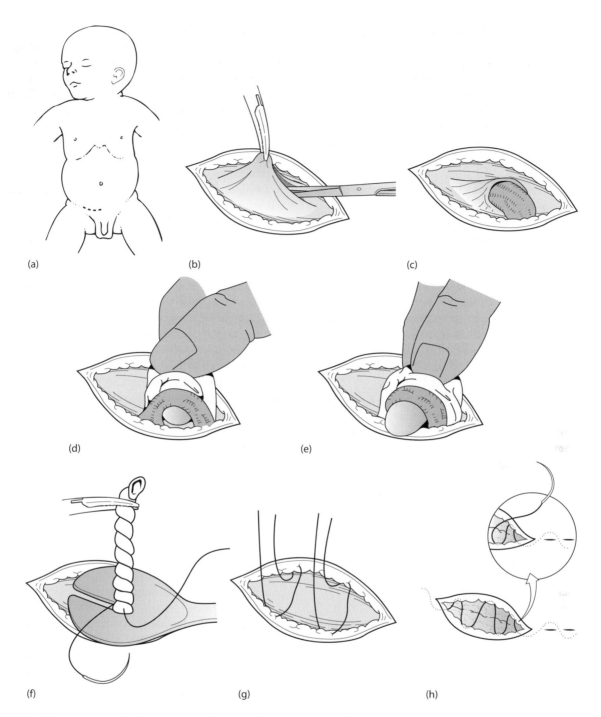

Figure 72.1 **(a)** Skin incision. **(b,c)** Exposure of external inguinal ring. **(d)** Isolation of the spermatic cord. **(e)** Separation of the hernial sac. **(f)** Transfixation of the hernial sac. **(g)** Closure of subcutaneous tissue. **(h)** Subcuticular closure of skin.

very small infants and achieve excellent results, cosmesis should not be put ahead of safety in preterm and small birth weight children.

CONTRALATERAL EXPLORATION

We don't routinely explore the contralateral side in newborns presenting with unilateral hernia. Only around 10% of these children will subsequently proceed to develop a clinically apparent inguinal hernia on the other side.[11–13]

In premature babies who have been shown to have a high incidence of bilateral hernia, which ranges from 44% to 55% according to different authors,[5,8,9] there may be a role for bilateral exploration.

IPSILATERAL ORCHIDOPEXY

Two-thirds of undescended testes detected at the time of newborn inguinal hernia repair appear to descend naturally with time.[40] If the testis remains high above the scrotal pouch after the herniotomy or if the gubernaculum has been divided in a particularly difficult neonatal hernia repair, we feel that the testis should be pexed within a scrotal pouch. Otherwise, testis can be left within the high scrotal region and observed over a period of time.

POSTOPERATIVE MANAGEMENT

Adequate postoperative analgesia is achieved by either caudal block or ilioinguinal and iliohypogastric nerve block, which is administered either before or at the end of operation. Feeding is resumed as soon as the infant is awake. Most patients can be discharged home the same day. Postoperative apnea is a well-known risk of inguinal hernia operation in premature infants.[46] Although most episodes of postoperative apnea in these babies occur in the first 4 hours following the end of the procedure,[47] they are often admitted for 24 hours for observation in order to manage this complication.[48] Postoperative apnea is inversely correlated with gestational and postconceptual ages,[49] but absolute weight at operation and previous respiratory dysfunction are apparently the best independent variables to be correlated with such risks.[50]

COMPLICATIONS OF INGUINAL HERNIOTOMY

The overall complication rates after elective hernia repair are low at about 2%,[51] while these are increased to 8%–33% for the incarcerated hernias requiring emergency operations.[5,51]

Complications of inguinal hernia repair include the following:

- *Hematoma*—Can be avoided with meticulous attention to hemostasis. It is rarely necessary to evacuate wound, cord, or scrotal hematoma.
- *Wound infection*—Low risk and should not exceed 1%.[3,47,52]
- *Gonadal complications*—Occur due to compression of the vessels by incarcerated viscera. Though large numbers of testes look nonviable in patients with incarcerated hernia, the actual incidence of testicular atrophy is low[53] and therefore, unless the testis is frankly necrotic, it should not be removed.
- *Intestinal resection*—This is necessary in about 3%–7% of patients in whom the hernia is not reduced, and it may cause some additional morbidity corresponding to resection itself and contamination of the field.[5]
- *Iatrogenic ascent of the testes*—This event is relatively rare since slightly more than 1% of patients operated upon for inguinal hernia during infancy subsequently required orchidopexy.[54] This complication is probably due to entrapment of the testis in the scar tissue or failure to pull it down into the scrotum at the end of the operation and to maintain it there.
- *Recurrence*—The acceptable recurrence rate for inguinal hernia repair is less than 1%, but when the operation is performed in the neonatal period, this complication

can occur in up to 8%.[52,55] The factors that predispose to recurrence are ventriculoperitoneal shunts, sliding hernia, incarceration, and connective tissue disorders.[56] Recurrence may be indirect or direct. Indirect recurrence is due to either failure to ligate the sac at high level, tearing of a friable sac, a slipped ligature at the neck of the sac, missed sac, or wound infection. Direct hernia may be due to inherent muscle weakness or injury to the posterior wall of the inguinal canal.
- *Mortality*—In a present-day situation, the mortality rate of inguinal hernia operation should be zero.

INCARCERATED INGUINAL HERNIA

Incarceration occurs when the protruded peritoneal contents within the hernial sac are constricted at its neck and cannot be easily reduced into the abdominal cavity. Strangulation occurs when there is vascular compromise to the contents of the sac because of prolonged and complete constriction at its neck. The contents of the hernial sac may consist of small bowel, appendix, omentum, or ovary and fallopian tube. If there is delay in treatment, incarceration rapidly progresses to strangulation and can lead to intestinal necrosis and even fecal fistula.[57]

The incidence of incarceration in neonates and young infants is reported to vary between 24% and 40%.[3,53,58] The incarceration rate is much higher in premature infants compared with full-term infants. Testicular infarction has been reported in up to 30% of infants younger than 3 months of age with incarcerated inguinal hernia,[59] and testicular atrophy following emergency operation for incarceration ranges between 10% and 15%. However, testicular volume in a group of children who had incarcerated inguinal hernia reduced by taxis during infancy and subsequently had elective herniotomy was not significantly different from age-matched controls, suggesting that this risk has been overemphasized.[53] Ovarian infarction is also possible after incarceration in females,[5] and vaginal bleeding has been reported in an infant after uterine incarceration in the hernial sac.[60] The risks of gonadal damage when the slided ovary cannot be reduced justify the fact that most surgeons advise prompt operation in these children.[33]

The risk of incarceration and clinical symptoms of partial obstruction of small bowel within the hernial sac must be balanced with the overall condition of the neonate in deciding the optimal time for surgery. Very premature infants with significant pulmonary compromise who are within a hospital environment can be safely observed till term or ready for discharge home, with intermittent reduction of hernial contents.

Diagnosis of incarcerated inguinal hernia

A newborn with incarcerated inguinal hernia usually presents with irritability, vomiting, a moderately distended abdomen, and a tender groin lump (Figure 72.2). Occasionally, the infant may pass blood per rectum. Local

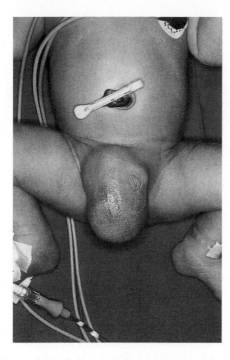

Figure 72.2 Large incarcerated right inguinal hernia in a 1-day-old infant. The hernia was reduced by taxis and herniotomy performed 2 days later.

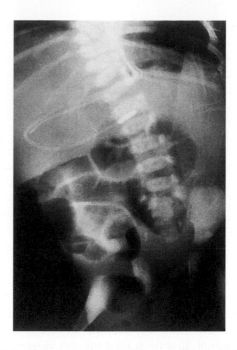

Figure 72.3 Supine abdominal film in a 10-day-old infant who presented with an irreducible lump in the right groin shows distended bowel loops extending into the right inguinal hernia.

examination reveals a tense, tender lump in the groin, the upper margin of which is usually not well defined. The ipsilateral testis may be normal or swollen and hard due to vascular compromise. Rectal examination usually is not necessary, but, if done, the contents of the hernia can be palpated at the internal ring.

The diagnosis of incarcerated inguinal hernia is usually made on clinical grounds. Abdominal radiographs may occasionally show bowel gas within the lump in the groin and confirm the diagnosis (Figure 72.3). If intestinal obstruction is present, plain abdominal films will show dilated loops of bowel with fluid levels. Ultrasonography can aid the diagnosis in some difficult cases as outlined below within the differential diagnosis.[61]

Differential diagnosis of incarcerated hernia

ENCYSTED HYDROCOELE OF THE CORD

Hydrocele of the cord or cyst of canal of Nuck is difficult to differentiate from incarcerated hernia. It may be possible to get above a hydrocoele and is nontender. Transillumination is not a reliable sign in infants, as bowel wall is very thin and is usually transilluminant. However, there will be no preceding history of reducible swelling reported by parents, and the child remains asymptomatic with no obvious signs of discomfort. Ultrasound is helpful in distinguishing this condition from an obstructed hernia.

INGUINAL LYMPHADENITIS

Usually the swelling is more laterally oriented on examination, and a thorough inspection of the area of drainage will,

at most times, reveal the source of infection. The cord and testes are found to be normal.

TORSION OF THE TESTES

In a scrotal testicular torsion, it is possible to get above the swelling. The testis is tender and slightly higher than on the other side. When there is an empty scrotum detected with a tender inguinal swelling on that side, torsion of an undescended testis must be suspected. Whether torsion of an undescended testis or an incarcerated hernia is suspected, urgent surgical exploration is necessary.

Management of incarcerated hernia

In a stable patient, there is no doubt that the preferred treatment for incarcerated hernia is reduction. This policy of nonoperative reduction is based on the following facts: the likelihood of reducing strangulated bowel in infants is extremely rare, and the complication rates are higher with emergency operations for irreducible hernia.[51]

The infant is placed in the Trendelenburg position, which helps to relieve the edema and allows mild traction of the hernial contents. Adequate sedation is given to the infant so as to relax the abdominal muscles. If the hernia is not reduced within 1 hour with these measures, an attempt is made to reduce it with gentle taxis, where constant gentle pressure is applied on the fundus of the sac in the direction of the cord. The vast majority of incarcerated hernias reduce with these nonoperative techniques. After the hernia is reduced, the infant is kept in the hospital and observed. Elective operation is carried out after 24–48 hours, when local edema has subsided.

Failure to reduce a strangulated or incarcerated inguinal hernia is an indication for emergency operation. In girls, when the ovary is not reducible, at least half of the surgeons in a recent US survey advice emergency operation.[33]

Surgery for obstructed, irreducible inguinal hernia

Infants need to be stabilized prior to surgery. Nasogastric suction and correction of fluid and electrolyte imbalance are undertaken, and antibiotics are given, but this period should be kept to a minimum. The patient is anesthetized.

SPONTANEOUS REDUCTION WITH NO ISCHEMIC BOWEL

If the hernia is spontaneously reduced after the induction of general anesthesia, the sac is opened and the peritoneal cavity is inspected as much as possible. Intestinal ischemia or necrosis will usually be accompanied with blood-stained peritoneal fluid. If there is no suspicion of bowel ischemia or only a mild suspicion exists, herniotomy is performed as described above. Usually the procedure is more difficult due to the surrounding edema and increased friability of the hernial sac. The risk of injury to vas and vessels is high, and this must be borne in mind during the dissection.

SPONTANEOUS REDUCTION WITH ISCHEMIC BOWEL

If there is any suspicion of bowel necrosis, the bowel must be inspected fully. Occasionally this may be possible through the hernial sac opening. If this cannot be achieved safely, without damage to vas or testicular vessels, then a laparotomy is warranted. This can be achieved either through a separate right iliac fossa transverse muscle cutting incision or by increasing the size of the herniotomy incision laterally, and then by retracting the skin wound superiorly to enable a muscle cutting/splitting laparotomy wound.

NO SPONTANEOUS REDUCTION WITH OR WITHOUT ISCHEMIC BOWEL

If the bowel does not reduce spontaneously when the patient is anesthetized, no attempts are made to reduce the hernia. The sac is opened and the contents are examined. If the bowel is viable, it is reduced. In case of difficulty in reducing the contents, the internal ring is either dilated or split superiorly. On the other hand, if viability of the bowel is questionable, it is delivered out and warm saline soaks are applied. The intestine is examined after 5–10 minutes. If its color returns to normal with adequate perfusion, visible peristalsis, and palpable mesenteric arterial pulsations, then the intestine is returned to the abdomen and herniotomy is completed. If the bowel is nonviable, resection and anastomosis are performed, either through the same incision or through a separate laparotomy wound as described above. Testes are put in the scrotum irrespective of whether they are normal or ischemic. Only frankly necrotic gonads may be removed. Postoperatively, if resection and anastomosis are carried out, nasogastric aspiration and intravenous fluids are continued in the infant until peristalsis returns and feeds are established. Antibiotics are continued for 5 days. The complications are as discussed above.

REFERENCES

1. Wright JE. Direct inguinal hernia in infancy and childhood. *Pediatr Surg Int* 1994; 9: 161–3.
2. Nakayama DK, Rowe MI. Inguinal hernia and the acute scrotum in infants and children. *Pediatr Rev* 1989; 11: 87–93.
3. Grosfeld JL. Current concepts in inguinal hernia in infants and children. *World J Surg* 1989; 13: 506–15.
4. Chang SJ, Chen JY, Hsu CK, Chuang FC, Yang SS. The incidence of inguinal hernia and associated risk factors of incarceration in pediatric inguinal hernia: A nation-wide longitudinal population-based study. *Hernia* 2016; 20(4): 559–63.
5. Rescorla FJ, Grosfeld JL. Inguinal hernia repair in the perinatal period and early infancy: Clinical considerations. *J Pediatr Surg* 1984; 19: 832–7.
6. Given JP, Rubin SZ. Occurrence of contralateral inguinal hernia following unilateral repair in a pediatric hospital. *J Pediatr Surg* 1989; 24: 963–5.
7. Czeizel A. Epidemiologic characteristics of congenital inguinal hernia. *Helv Paediatr Acta* 1980; 35: 57–67.
8. Harper RG, Garcia A, Sia C. Inguinal hernia: A common problem of premature infants weighing 1,000 grams or less at birth. *Pediatrics* 1975; 56: 112–5.
9. Boocock GR, Todd PJ. Inguinal hernias are common in preterm infants. *Arch Dis Child* 1985; 60: 669–670.
10. Miltenburg DM, Nuchtern JG, Jaksic T, Kozinetz CA, Brandt ML. Meta-analysis of the risk of metachronous hernia in infants and children. *Am J Surg* 1997; 174: 741–4.
11. Tuduri Limousin I, Moya Jimenez MJ, Morcillo Azcarate J, Granero Cendon R, Fernandez Pineda I, Millan Lopez A, De Agustin Asensio JC. [Incidence of metachronic contralateral inguinal hernia]. *Cir Pediatr* 2009; 22: 22–4.
12. Chertin B, De Caluwe D, Gajaharan M, Piaseczna-Piotrowska A, Puri P. Is contralateral exploration necessary in girls with unilateral inguinal hernia? *J Pediatr Surg* 2003; 38: 756–7.
13. Surana R, Puri P. Is contralateral exploration necessary in infants with unilateral inguinal hernia? *J Pediatr Surg* 1993; 28: 1026–7.
14. Czeizel A, Gardonyi J. A family study of congenital inguinal hernia. *Am J Med Genet* 1979; 4: 247–54.
15. Grosfeld JL, Cooney DR. Inguinal hernia after ventriculoperitoneal shunt for hydrocephalus. *J Pediatr Surg* 1974; 9: 311–5.

16. Moazam F, Glenn JD, Kaplan BJ, Talbert JL, Mickle JP. Inguinal hernias after ventriculoperitoneal shunt procedures in pediatric patients. *Surg Gynecol Obstet* 1984; 159: 570–2.

17. Modi KB, Grant AC, Garret A, Rodger RS. Indirect inguinal hernia in CAPD patients with polycystic kidney disease. *Adv Perit Dial* 1989; 5: 84–6.

18. Matthews DE, West KW, Rescorla FJ, Vane DW, Grosfeld JL, Wappner RS, Bergstein J, Andreoli S. Peritoneal dialysis in the first 60 days of life. *J Pediatr Surg* 1990; 25: 110–5; discussion 116.

19. Powell TG, Hallows JA, Cooke RW, Pharoah PO. Why do so many small infants develop an inguinal hernia? *Arch Dis Child* 1986; 61: 991–5.

20. Husmann DA, McLorie GA, Churchill BM, Ein SH. Inguinal pathology and its association with classical bladder exstrophy. *J Pediatr Surg* 1990; 25: 332–4.

21. Connolly JA, Peppas DS, Jeffs RD, Gearhart JP. Prevalence and repair of inguinal hernias in children with bladder exstrophy. *J Urol* 1995; 154: 1900–1.

22. Mehregan AH, Lee SC, Nabai H. Cutis laxa (generalized elastolysis). A report of four cases with autopsy findings. *J Cutan Pathol* 1978; 5: 116–26.

23. Coran AG, Eraklis AJ. Inguinal hernia in the Hurler-Hunter syndrome. *Surgery* 1967; 61: 302–4.

24. Shipp TD, Benacerraf BR. Scrotal inguinal hernia in a fetus: Sonographic diagnosis. *AJR Am J Roentgenol* 1995; 165: 1494–5.

25. Yeaton HL, Mellish RW. Resolution of prolonged neonatal apnea with hernia repair. *J Pediatr Surg* 1983; 18: 158–9.

26. Srouji MN, Buck BE. Neonatal appendicitis: Ischemic infarction in incarcerated inguinal hernia. *J Pediatr Surg* 1978; 13: 177–9.

27. Bar-Maor JA, Zeltzer M. Acute appendicitis located in a scrotal hernia of a premature infant. *J Pediatr Surg* 1978; 13: 181–2.

28. Dessanti A, Porcu, A., Scanu, A., Dettori, G. Neonatal acute appendicitis in an inguinal hernia. *Pediatr Surg Int* 1995; 10: 561–2.

29. Iuchtman M, Kirshon M, Feldman M. Neonatal pyoscrotum and perforated appendicitis. *J Perinatol* 1999; 19: 536–7.

30. Ruderman JW, Schick JB, Sherman M, Reagan Y, Hanks G, Weitzman JJ. Use of a truss to maintain inguinal hernia reduction in a very low birth weight infant. *J Perinatol* 1995; 15: 143–5.

31. Uemura S, Woodward AA, Amerena R, Drew J. Early repair of inguinal hernia in premature babies. *Pediatr Surg Int* 1999; 15: 36–9.

32. Desch LW, DeJonge MH. Weight gain: A possible factor in deciding timing for inguinal hernia repair in premature infants. *Clin Pediatr (Phila)* 1996; 35: 251–5.

33. Wiener ES, Touloukian RJ, Rodgers BM, Grosfeld JL, Smith EI, Ziegler MM, Coran AG. Hernia survey of the Section on Surgery of the American Academy of Pediatrics. *J Pediatr Surg* 1996; 31: 1166–9.

34. Lee SL, Gleason JM, Sydorak RM. A critical review of premature infants with inguinal hernias: Optimal timing of repair, incarceration risk, and postoperative apnea. *J Pediatr Surg* 2011; 46: 217–20.

35. Melone JH, Schwartz MZ, Tyson KR, Marr CC, Greenholz SK, Taub JE, Hough VJ. Outpatient inguinal herniorrhaphy in premature infants: Is it safe? *J Pediatr Surg* 1992; 27: 203–7; discussion 207–8.

36. Emberton M, Patel L, Zideman DA, Karim F, Singh MP. Early repair of inguinal hernia in preterm infants with oxygen-dependent bronchopulmonary dysplasia. *Acta Paediatr* 1996; 85: 96–9.

37. Webster AC, McKishnie JD, Kenyon CF, Marshall DG. Spinal anaesthesia for inguinal hernia repair in high-risk neonates. *Can J Anaesth* 1991; 38: 281–6.

38. Somri M, Gaitini L, Vaida S, Collins G, Sabo E, Mogilner G. Postoperative outcome in high-risk infants undergoing herniorrhaphy: Comparison between spinal and general anaesthesia. *Anaesthesia* 1998; 53: 762–6.

39. Bertozzi M, Marchesini L, Tesoro S, Appignani A. Laparoscopic herniorrhaphy in children. *Pediatr Med Chir* 2015; 37: pmc 2015 2109.

40. Meij-deVries A, van der Voort LM, Sijstermans K, Meijer RW, van der Plas EM, Hack WW. Natural course of undescended testes after inguinoscrotal surgery. *J Pediatr Surg* 2013; 48: 2540–4.

41. Shalaby R, Ismail M, Dorgham A, Hefny K, Alsaied G, Gabr K, Abdelaziz M. Laparoscopic hernia repair in infancy and childhood: Evaluation of 2 different techniques. *J Pediatr Surg* 2010; 45: 2210–6.

42. Lin CD, Tsai YC, Chang SJ, Yang SS. Surgical outcomes of mini laparoscopic herniorrhaphy in infants. *J Urol* 2011; 185: 1071–6.

43. Turial S, Enders J, Krause K, Schier F. Laparoscopic inguinal herniorrhaphy in babies weighing 5 kg or less. *Surg Endosc* 2011; 25: 72–8.

44. Alzahem A. Laparoscopic versus open inguinal herniotomy in infants and children: A meta-analysis. *Pediatr Surg Int* 2011; 27: 605–12.

45. Timberlake MD, Herbst KW, Rasmussen S, Corbett ST. Laparoscopic percutaneous inguinal hernia repair in children: Review of technique and comparison with open surgery. *J Pediatr Urol* 2015; 11:262 e261–266.

46. Warner LO, Teitelbaum DH, Caniano DA, Vanik PE, Martino JD, Servick JD. Inguinal herniorrhaphy in young infants: Perianesthetic complications and associated preanesthetic risk factors. *J Clin Anesth* 1992; 4: 455–61.

47. Audry G, Johanet S, Achrafi H, Lupold M, Gruner M. The risk of wound infection after inguinal incision in pediatric outpatient surgery. *Eur J Pediatr Surg* 1994; 4: 87–9.

48. Bell C, Dubose R, Seashore J, Touloukian R, Rosen C, Oh TH, Hughes CW, Mooney S, O'Connor TZ. Infant apnea detection after herniorrhaphy. *J Clin Anesth* 1995; 7: 219–23.

49. Cote CJ, Zaslavsky A, Downes JJ, Kurth CD, Welborn LG, Warner LO, Malviya SV. Postoperative apnea in former preterm infants after inguinal herniorrhaphy. A combined analysis. *Anesthesiology* 1995; 82: 809–22.

50. Gollin G, Bell C, Dubose R, Touloukian RJ, Seashore JH, Hughes CW, Oh TH, Fleming J, O'Connor T. Predictors of postoperative respiratory complications in premature infants after inguinal herniorrhaphy. *J Pediatr Surg* 1993; 28: 244–7.

51. Rowe MI, Clatworthy HW. Incarcerated and strangulated hernias in children. A statistical study of high-risk factors. *Arch Surg* 1970; 101: 136–9.

52. Phelps S, Agrawal M. Morbidity after neonatal inguinal herniotomy. *J Pediatr Surg* 1997; 32: 445–7.

53. Puri P, Guiney EJ, O'Donnell B. Inguinal hernia in infants: The fate of the testis following incarceration. *J Pediatr Surg* 1984; 19: 44–6.

54. Surana R, Puri P. Iatrogenic ascent of the testis: An under-recognized complication of inguinal hernia operation in children. *Br J Urol* 1994; 73: 580–1.

55. Rowe MI, Marchildon MB. Inguinal hernia and hydrocele in infants and children. *Surg Clin North Am* 1981; 61: 1137–45.

56. Grosfeld JL, Minnick K, Shedd F, West KW, Rescorla FJ, Vane DW. Inguinal hernia in children: Factors affecting recurrence in 62 cases. *J Pediatr Surg* 1991; 26: 283–7.

57. Rattan KN, Garg P. Neonatal scrotal faecal fistula. *Pediatr Surg Int* 1998; 13: 440–1.

58. Misra D, Hewitt G, Potts SR, Brown S, Boston VE. Inguinal herniotomy in young infants, with emphasis on premature neonates. *J Pediatr Surg* 1994; 29: 1496–8.

59. Schmitt M, Peiffert B, de Miscault G, Barthelme H, Poussot D, Andre M. [Complications of inguinal hernia in children]. *Chir Pediatr* 1987; 28: 193–6.

60. Zitsman JL, Cirincione E, Margossian H. Vaginal bleeding in an infant secondary to sliding inguinal hernia. *Obstet Gynecol* 1997; 89: 840–2.

61. Munden M, McEniff N, Mulvihill D. Sonographic investigation of female infants with inguinal masses. *Clin Radiol* 1995; 50: 696–8.

73

Short bowel syndrome and surgical techniques for the baby with short intestines

MICHAEL E. HÖLLWARTH

INTRODUCTION

The term *short bowel syndrome* (SBS) is defined by most authors as a state of significant maldigestion and malabsorption requiring prolonged parenteral nutrition. SBS was defined in term neonates by Rickham[1] in 1967, as an extensive resection of all but a maximum of 75 cm of the small gut. This corresponds to 30% of the total jejunoileal length in term newborns. SBS in a premature newborn corresponds, according to Touloukian, to 30% of the calculated intestinal length for the given gestational age (GA), too.[2] A more recent publication measuring bowel length *in vivo* shows that it is about 100 cm at GA of 27–29 weeks, 157 cm at 39–40 weeks, and 239 cm between 1 and 6 months.[3] The term *intestinal failure* (IF) is often used for a larger group of patients with a variety of diseases and the inability to sustain an adequate homeostasis and growth by normal enteral nutrition.[4]

Around 80% of SBS cases occur in the neonatal age group. The causes can be subdivided into prenatally acquired diseases (gastroschisis, multiple atresia, Hirschsprung disease; 17%); postnatally catastrophic events leading to a subtotal loss of small bowel, such as necrotizing enterocolitis (36%) or volvulus (19%); and other rare causes or trauma (7%). The prevalence of SBS has increased over the last decades due to the progress in intensive care medicine, allowing more babies to survive extensive loss of small bowel. A recent Italian study showed an incidence of 0.1% in all live births and 0.5% among intensive care unit (ICU) admissions.[5]

In the past, extensive loss of small bowel in newborns and babies used to be a catastrophic event nearly always followed by malnutrition and death. Reviewing the literature in 1965, Kuffer[6] found only nine surviving children with SBS. In 1972, Wilmore[7] reviewed 50 babies younger than 2 months with SBS and found that survival was possible with a 15 cm jejunoileum with the ileocecal valve, or with 38 cm

jejunoileum without the ileocecal valve. In 1985, Dorney and colleagues[8] reported that long-term nutritional support today allows survival in infants with as little as 11 cm of jejunoileum with the ileocecal valve (5% of the total), or with 25 cm of jejunoileum without the ileocecal valve (10% of the total).

Intestinal adaptation is the term that characterizes the pathophysiology that follows intensive intestinal resection, and by which more than 80% of the babies with SBS do finally reach a normal life with entirely oral nutrition.[9] Adaptation is characterized by an early increase of blood flow to the intestinal remnants[10] and by long-term stimulation of intestinal, growth which enormously enlarges the absorptive surface area.[11] The latter includes an increase of villus height, crypt depth, intestinal length, intestinal thickness, and intestinal diameter. Recent experimental studies showed that angiotensin-converting enzyme has an important function regarding the apoptosis and proliferation of enterocytes after small bowel resection.[12] Water and solute absorption is enhanced in the colon, and colonic bacteria ferment undigested carbohydrates and proteins into short-chain fatty acids, which act as important energy providers and, apparently, as additional promoters of adaptation.[13,14]

The precise mechanisms of adaptation are not clear, but intraluminal nutrients and endogenous intestinal secretions stimulate growth.[15–18] Recently, it has been shown that ω-3 fatty acids from fish oil have a beneficial effect on liver function and ameliorate parenteral nutrition–associated liver disease.[19] In general, the higher the workload required for digestion and absorption, the more potent the stimulus for adaptation. In response to the nutrients and secretions, a large number of trophic polypeptides and other mediators are secreted. Over the years, some of them have attracted attention regarding their possible clinical value in promoting adaptation in SBS patients. First, gastrin was demonstrated to exhibit trophic effects on the small bowel.[20] Gastric secretions and acid production, as well as serum gastrin levels, are initially elevated in patients with SBS. Enteroglucagon is another hormone that has been shown to stimulate the adaptive response in the intestinal tract in animal experiments and humans.[21] Since monoclonal antibodies failed to block this trophic effect, recently, precursors of enteroglucagon are considered to be responsible for the intestinal effects. Glucagon-like peptide-2 is a trophic hormone that has an important role in controlling intestinaladaptation.[22,23] Human growth hormone (GH) in combination with epidermal growth factor, or with insulin-like growth factor-1(IGF-I), has also been shown to regulate small intestinal growth and adaptation[24-27] IGF-I receptors have been identified in all segments of the gastrointestinal tract, and IGF-I stimulates DNA and RNA synthesis and cellular amino acid uptake.[28] The endogenous GH–IGF-I system is an important regulator of small intestinal growth and adaptation.[29] A number of other growth factors are widely discussed in the literature.[9]

Among the amino acids, glutamine (GL) plays an important role in the maintenance of intestinal structure and function by providing the energy required by cells with a rapid turnover, such as macrophages and enterocytes. Patients after major trauma or in chronic catabolic states benefit from GL supplementation.[30] In addition, enteral nutrition with GL has been shown to have an effect on glucose and sodium absorption in animals.[31] Ziegler et al. have shown that GH increases GL uptake after intestinal resection, supporting the evidence that GL exerts trophic effects in the small intestine and the colon of patients with SBS.[32] More research, however, is needed, since studies on GL are controversial.[25,33] Prostaglandin (Pg) E2 and polyamines have also been shown to stimulate cell proliferation in animal experiments by increasing blood flow and DNA synthesis.[34,35] Experimental evidence exists that testosterone enhances adaptation after small bowel resection in cats.[36] Recently, it has been shown that dietary supplementation with vitamin D stimulated cell proliferation and decreased cell apoptosis in a rat model of SBS.[37]

Within 1 year in more than 80% of the patients, adequate intestinal adaptation occurs, and they can be weaned off parenteral nutritional support. However, this process can cause significant embarrassment and psychological stress to the child and his/her family, as well as complications such as septicemia, cholecystitis, and chronic liver fibrosis. Therefore, the ability to reliably predict the potential of a patient to be weaned from parenteral nutrition gained significant attention. Citrulline is a free amino acid in plasma and is produced by the metabolism of GL and proline in small bowel enterocytes. It has been shown that plasma estimations of citrulline correlate well with the bowel length in children and adults, and can be used as predictors of whether weaning from parenteral nutrition will be possible or not.[38,39] The cutoff point distinguishing children who reach independence of parenteral nutrition seems to be 15 μmol/L.[40,41] Citrulline is also a potent marker of rejection after intestinal transplantation (TPX) as well as in children with graft-versus-host disease.[42]

While intestinal TPX has still limited clinical applicability with long-term survivors, ongoing interest exists in surgical methods to enhance nutrient absorption. This chapter reviews current surgical techniques for patients with SBS, with special emphasis on their clinical applicability.

SURGICAL TACTICS IN SITUATIONS REQUIRING EXTENSIVE INTESTINAL RESECTION

Malformations such as multiple intestinal atresias or gastroschisis with atresia can cause a congenital SBS in the newborn. Acquired conditions such as intestinal strangulation by midgut volvulus or necrotizing enterocolitis may require extensive intestinal resection. For patients at risk of SBS, surgery must be adapted to preserve as much small bowel as possible.

In intestinal atresias, dilated intestinal loops should be preserved instead of resected in the usual way. In volvulus, second-look procedures can help the surgeon decide which parts of the intestine are definitely lost. In extensive necrotizing enterocolitis, intestinal loops of questionable viability should be decompressed by an enterostomy, not resected. The ileum is more important than the jejunum, since it is the site of vitamin B_{12} and bile acid absorption. Also, the ileum has a much greater capacity for intestinal adaptation. When resection has been completed, the remaining jejunum and ileum should be measured from the ligament of Treitz all the way down to the ileocecal valve, with a thread laid along the antimesenteric border. Intestinal loops shrink considerably during manipulations, and the real intestinal length is difficult to measure in vivo. This may be one reason that survival does not seem strictly related to the length of the remaining bowel.

SURGICAL TECHNIQUES IN SBS PATIENTS

General agreement exists that the therapeutic priorities in patients with SBS consist of the stabilization of the patients' conditions, the evaluation of the adaptive capacities of the intestinal remnants, and the clarification of the patients' special needs. Therefore, the primary surgical aim is restoration of the bowel continuity as soon as possible in order to allow all remaining intestinal segments to take part in the adaptation process. Additional surgical strategies come into play only if

1. The absorptive area is definitely too small to allow enteral feeding
2. Dysmotility in grossly dilated loops entails stagnation of chyme
3. Intestinal transit is too fast to allow sufficient absorption of nutrients (Table 73.1)

Intestinal TPX is, of course, the most effective method to increase intestinal absorptive area immediately. Indications

Table 73.1 Surgical strategies in SBS patients

To increase passage time	To increase absorptive surface area	To improve peristalsis
Antiperistaltic segment	Serosa patching	Tapering
Colon interposition	Mucosa transplantation	Tapering and lengthening
Intestinal valves	Small bowel TPX	
Artificial invagination		

for TPX are patients after a catastrophic abdominal event with little or no small bowel remaining, and patients with SBS and irreversible liver failure due to progressive total parenteral nutrition (TPN)–associated hepatic dysfunction. Until recently, the results of intestinal TPX had been poor, mainly due to a high rejection rate. With the introduction of new immunosuppressive drugs, such as tacrolimus and OKT3 in addition to steroids, significant progress has been achieved with a 1-year transplant survival rate approaching 75% in recent series. However, 10-year results after intestinal TPX show a patient survival of around 43% and a graft survival of 23%, suggesting that a good functioning home parenteral nutrition (HPN) offers, in general, a better long-term outcome avoiding the adverse effects of immunosuppression, including lymphoproliferative diseases related to Epstein–Barr virus (EBV) infections.[43–46]

Therefore, current surgical procedures usually support only one or two of the aforementioned factors. The predominant problem in a given patient has to be evaluated carefully to choose the method most likely to enhance the absorptive capacity of the intestinal remnants. General agreement exists that most of such techniques are not indicated as a primary procedure. The priorities are as follows: (1) stabilization of the patient's condition, (2) evaluation of the adaptive capacity of the intestinal remnants, and (3) clarification of the patient's special needs.

INEFFICIENT PERISTALSIS

Tapering

In a newborn with multiple intestinal atresias resulting in SBS, bowel that is congenitally enlarged due to chronic obstruction should be preserved. However, the low contraction pressure in such bowel segments results in inefficient to-and-fro peristalsis, easily demonstrated by radiological studies. Inefficient peristalsis can lead to stasis of the chyme, symptoms of obstruction, and a contaminated bowel syndrome caused by bacterial overgrowth. Tapering of dilated loops can be accomplished by a triangular resection of an antimesenteric segment (Figure 73.1). The disadvantage of this type of tapering is that it reduces the available intestinal surface area. Thus, the technique can be recommended only for patients with sufficient intestinal length and absorptive area in whom inadequate peristalsis is the main problem.

Tapering can also be accomplished simply by turning in the redundant tissue (Figure 73.1). This technique avoids reduction of intestinal surface area and results in normal

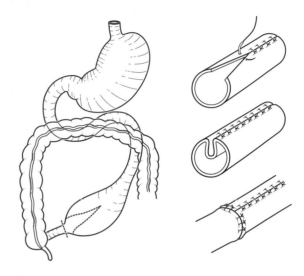

Figure 73.1 Tapering can be performed either by resection of a triangular antimesenteric segment or by turning in the redundant tissue. The latter method saves all the available resorptive surface area.

bowel function.[47,48] Whichever method is used, effective and propulsive peristalsis takes at least 3 weeks to return.

Tapering and lengthening

In 1980, Bianchi[49] reported an experimental procedure combining the tapering of dilated loops with use of the redundant tissue for lengthening the bowel. Anatomically, the mesenteric vessels from the last parallel arcade divide into anterior and posterior branches entering the bowel from either side of the midline. Especially in dilated segments, a relatively broad avascular plane in the midline can be used to separate the vascular layers. Longitudinal division of the bowel can be accomplished this way, while preserving sufficient nutrient vessels to either half of the intestine. Longitudinal closure of each intestinal segment and isoperistaltic end-to-end anastomosis doubles the intestinal length of this segment.

Bianchi[50] in his experimental reports and Boeckmann and Traylor[51] in the first clinical report used a Gastro-Intestinal-Anastomosis (GIA) stapler to divide the intestinal parts. Although the procedure using the GIA stapler is fast, it produces two rigid intestinal segments and consumes absorptive surface area. Aigrain et al.[52] recommend division with scissors and a manually sutured anastomosis. Seromuscular stitches guarantee a maximum of preserved mucosa (Figure 73.2a). Since both sections of the bowel hang on the same mesenteric segment, a helix-like

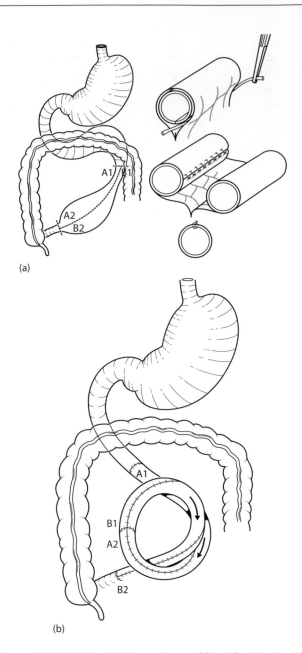

(a)

(b)

Figure 73.2 **(a)** Bianchi's tapering and lengthening is critical for the intestinal circulation. A Penrose drain facilitates the division of the segments. Seromuscular stitches save as much mucosal surface area as possible. **(b)** The helix-like arrangement of the two separated parts allows the anastomoses to be performed with minimal traction on the vessels.

isoperistaltic anastomosis is easier to perform than an anastomosis with the two segments sliding one on the other. The helix technique avoids traction on the nutrient vessels, which is critical because necrosis of the divided segments has been reported (Figure 73.2b).[53] Experimental studies in dogs showed that intestinal tapering and lengthening may impair nutritional status as well as intestinal adaptation and absorption.[54]

Bianchi's method has been used in more than 50 infants. Necrosis of half of the segments occurred in only one baby.[55] In some of these infants, the primary length

of the intestinal segments was as long as 40–80 cm, which would call into question the indication of some of these procedures. According to Bianchi's[55] own experience, the method has proved successful when performed not in the newborn or early phase of a short bowel problem but in a later stage of the disease, on so-called self-selected survivors, i.e., patients in stable general conditions and free of severe complications, such as liver failure. This statement can be confirmed by the author's experience with two SBS newborn babies with 15 cm and 20 cm small bowel remnants, no ileocecal valve, and 40% of the normal colonic length. Although Bianchi's procedure was performed completely uneventfully and nearly doubled the intestinal length, both babies suffered from a poor peristalsis and died at the age of 1 year with progressive liver failure. Thus, patients with inherent motility disorders may not be selected for this procedure.[56]

Another method of bowel tapering and elongation has been published by Kimura and Soper.[57] This procedure consists of an initial coaptation of the small bowel remnant to a host organ (liver, abdominal wall), and after collaterals have been developed, a secondary longitudinal split of the bowel is done to provide two loops, one from its antimesenteric half and the other from its mesenteric half. This procedure has been successfully used in two infants.[57,58]

A recently published procedure that can be used in cases with insufficient peristalsis due to dilated intestinal loops and also as a lengthening procedure is the so-called STEP—serial transverse enteroplasty.[59,60] The refashioning of dilated intestinal loops is achieved by serial alternating and opposite transections of one-third or half of the intestinal lumen creating a zigzag-like figure (Figure 73.3). The method has the advantage that it is technically much easier than Bianchi's procedure and the achieved lengthening is significantly longer. Long-term results show that a majority of children can be weaned off parenteral nutrition except children with motility problems.[61–63]

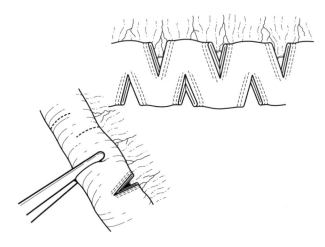

Figure 73.3 Serial transverse enteroplasty (STEP) consists of semicircular alternating incisions with the GIA stapler resulting in a zigzag-like elongation of the small bowel.

INADEQUATE INTESTINAL TRANSIT TIME

For a long time, the ileocecal valve was supposed to prolong intestinal transit time. A review from Dorney et al.[8] showed that the presence of an intact ileocecal valve is crucial to survival of newborns after extensive loss of small bowel. These findings have been confirmed by the author's experience: all babies with SBS and a preserved ileocecal valve survived, while all patients with fatal outcome did not have the valve.[64] In contrast, Coran et al.[65] and Kaufmann et al.[66] have not shown a difference in outcome of SBS patients with regard to the presence or absence of the valve. Furthermore, experimental evidence exists, that bacterial translocation in SBS rats without an ileocecal valve is significantly lower when compared with animals with a preserved ileocecal valve.[67,68] While definite evidence of a beneficial role of the ileocecal valve in SBS patients is lacking, nevertheless, the valve should be preserved whenever possible, and it probably plays a role with regard to the prolongation of the intestinal transit time.

Antiperistaltic small intestinal segment

Reversal of distal small bowel loops has been studied experimentally for years. Since the original report by Gibson and colleagues[69] of the use of reversal of small intestine in an adult, this has been, in the past, the most commonly used method for patients with SBS (Figure 73.4). The antiperistaltic small bowel segment acts as a physiological valve by causing retrograde peristalsis; therefore, it should always be located at the end of the intestinal remnants. The ideal

length of the reversed segment appears to be 10 cm in adults and 3 cm in infants. In a 3-month-old patient in the author's department, a 3 cm antiperistaltic segment (out of a total of 11 cm small bowel) was helpful for intestinal adaptation. At 4 years of age, when the child was nourished completely orally, the total radiological small bowel length had reached 1 m, with a swinging of the opaque meal at the probable location of the antiperistaltic segment.[70] The patient is today 38 years old and needs only regular supplementation of fat-soluble vitamins (A, D, E, K). A more recent report on 38 adult patients permanently depending on parenteral nutrition showed that nearly half of them could be weaned by reversal of a small bowel segment, with significant gain in absorptive bowel function.[71]

Colonic interposition

Isoperistaltic or antiperistaltic interposition of the colon has the advantage of using none of the small intestinal remnants. The method was developed by Hutcher et al.[72,73]

The isoperistaltic segment should thus be interposed proximally either between the jejunum and ileum if the jejunal segment is short and the ileal segment long, or between the duodenum and jejunum if the latter is long and the ileum short (Figure 73.5). Isoperistaltic colonic interposition slows down the rate at which nutrients are delivered to the distal intestine by slowing peristaltic activity.[74] The optimal length of an interposed colon has not been defined. Glick et al.[75] used 10–15 cm long segments in small babies, while Garcia and colleagues[76] used a 24 cm segment in a 14-month-old infant.

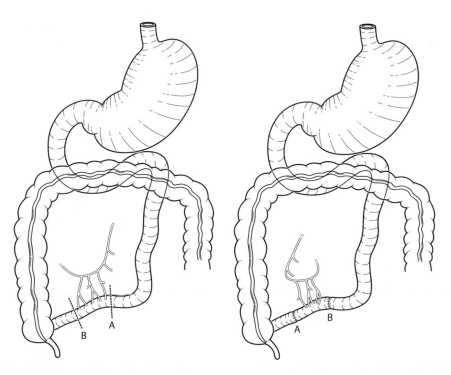

Figure 73.4 The antiperistaltic intestinal segment should be interposed close to the ileocecal valve or at the end of the small bowel. The optimal length in newborns is around 3.0 cm.

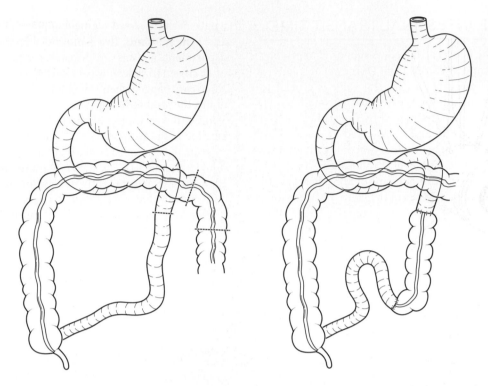

Figure 73.5 The isoperistaltic colonic interposition should be interposed proximally (while the reversed colonic interposition should be used distally). The length of an isoperistaltic interposition recommended is within 10–20 cm.

Besides the beneficial effect of slowing peristaltic activity, the interposed colonic segment increases the bowel length between the duodenum and cecum. Furthermore, colonic loops adapt to the function of the small bowel and can absorb water, electrolytes, and nutrients by active transport mechanism.[77] Experimental studies in rats have shown a significant increase in crypt depth, mucosal thickness and maltase concentration of the interposed segment.[78]

Reported clinical results show that out of seven infants with isoperistaltic interposition, four survived.[75,76] In two, the length of the intestinal remnants was not reported; in the other two, they were 39 and 63 cm. An adult patient with 5 cm of jejunum and 7 cm of ileum after a midgut volvulus could be weaned from parenteral nutrition completely after interposition of an 18-cm-long isoperistaltic colon. Recent experience in our department with proximal isoperistaltic colonic interposition and an additional distal STEP procedure in newborns with very short bowel, e.g., after gastroschisis with intrauterine volvulus and vanishing bowel, seems to be very promising.

Intestinal valves and pouches

As mentioned earlier, while the benefits of the ileocecal junction on long-term outcome of babies with SBS has been questioned, there exists a large body of evidence as to its powerful impact on intestinal transit time by slowing the passage of intraluminal nutrients into the colon. Therefore, a variety of experimental surgical procedures have been devised to slow down the intestinal transit time by creation of artificial valves.[79,80] Constriction of the bowel by sutures

and artificial sphincters,[75] mechanical or chemical denervation of segments,[81] and intussusception techniques has been studied extensively.[82,83] Clinical experience with intussuscepted valves is very limited. Waddell et al.[84] performed a reversed intussusception of the colon into the jejunum in three adults, one of whom subsequently developed an obstruction. Ricotta et al.[82] constructed a 4-cm-long nipple-like ileocecal valve (Figure 73.6) in a 15-year-old boy, which appeared to be helpful.

RESULTS

Despite the variety of surgical techniques designed to support intestinal adaptation after extensive loss of small bowel, none can be recommended unequivocally. In the past, the overwhelming majority of babies with SBS had been treated exclusively by parenteral nutritional support until intestinal adaptation allowed entirely oral nutrition. Full enteral feeding has ultimately been attained in infants with originally as little as 15 cm of the small bowel with the ileocecal valve preserved, or 25 cm of jejunoileum when it was missing.[85] Survival rates of 75%–83% are being reached in newborns, and 100% in children at or above 2 years of age.[86,87] The survival rate of surgically treated newborns with SBS born after 1985 was 96% in Goulet's clinic.[88] Survival rate of very-low-birth-weight (VLBW) infants with SBS enrolled in a national registry between 2002 and 2005 was 98% after 60 days and 79% after 180 days.[89] A further study showed that 27 out of 28 children with a bowel remnant <20 cm survived, and 48% of them have been weaned from parenteral nutrition. The successfully

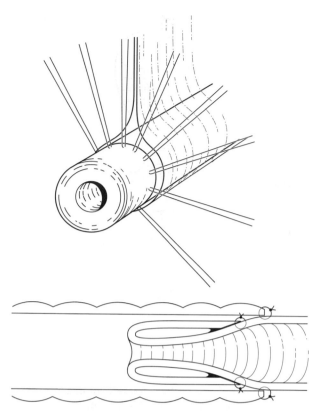

Figure 73.6 Nipple-like ileocecal valve according to Ricotta. The optimal length in newborns is not defined but will be around 1–2 cm. In a 15-year-old boy, a 4-cm-long valve worked well. Seromuscular stitches allow the precise adaptation of the mucosal layers.

rehabilitated patients were more likely to have an intact colon with the ileocecal valve.[90]

CONCLUSION

In conclusion, surgery is indicated only in selected patients either to achieve effective propulsive peristalsis or to prolong intestinal transit time. However, adjunctive surgical procedures should be postponed until the special needs of individual patients are evident. Approximately 10% will benefit from surgical interventions, either by prolongation of transit time or by remodeling parts of the intestine. Patients with total loss of small bowel or progressive liver failure may benefit from the progress made by intestinal TPX, although 5-year survival rate does not lie much above 50%.[43]

REFERENCES

1. Rickham PP. Massive small intestinal resection in newborn infants. *Ann R Coll Surg Engl* 1967; 41: 480–5.
2. Touloukian RJ, Smith GJ. Normal intestinal length in preterm infants. *J Pediatr Surg* 1983; 18: 720–3.
3. Struijs MC, Diamond IR, de Silva N et al. Establishing norms for intestinal length in children. *J Pediatr Surg* 2009; 44: 933–8.
4. D'Antiga L, Goulet O. Intestinal failure in children: The European view. *J Pediatr Gastroenterol Nutr* 2013; 56: 118–26.
5. Salvia G, Guarini A, Terrin G et al. Neonatal onset intestinal failure: An Italian multicentre study. *J Pediatr* 2008; 153: 674–6.
6. Kuffer F. Zum Problem der subtotalen Dünndarmresektion beim Säugling. *Z Kinderchir* 1965; 2: 39–55.
7. Wilmore D. Factors correlating with a successful outcome following extensive intestinal resection in newborn infants. *J Pediatr* 1973; 80: 88–95.
8. Dorney St FA, Ament ME, Berquist WE et al. Improved survival in very short small bowel of infancy with use of long term parenteral nutrition. *J Pediatr* 1985; 107: 521–5.
9. Höllwarth M. *Short Bowel Syndrome in Childhood.* E-book: http://www.morganclaypool.com. Morgan & Clydon Life Sciences, 2014.
10. Höllwarth ME, Urich-Baker MG, Kvietys PR et al. Blood flow in experimental short bowel syndrome. *Pediatr Surg Int* 1988; 4: 242–6.
11. Bristol JB, Williamson RCN. Mechanisms of intestinal adaptation. *Pediatr Surg Int* 1988; 4: 233–41.
12. Haxhija EQ, Yang H, Spencer AU et al. Modulation of mouse intestinal cell turnover in the absence of angiotensin converting enzyme. *Am J Physiol Gastrointest Liver Physiol* 2008; 295: G88–98.
13. Briet F, Flourie B, Achour L et al. Bacterial adaptation in patients with short bowel and colon in continuity. *Gastroenterology* 1995; 109: 1446–53.
14. Tappenden KA, Thomson ABR, Wild GE. Short-chain fatty acid–supplemented total parenteral nutrition enhances functional adaptation to intestinal resection in rats. *Gastroenterology* 1997; 112: 792–802.
15. Altmann GG. Influence of bile and pancreatic secretions on the size of the intestinal villi in the rat. *Am J Anat* 1971; 132: 167–78.
16. Bestermann HS, Adrian TE, Mallinson CN et al. Gut hormone release after intestinal resection. *Gut* 1982; 23: 855–61.
17. Dowling RH, Booth CC. Structural and functional changes following small bowel resection in rat. *Clin Sci (Lond)* 1967; 32: 139–149.
18. Drozdowski T, Thomson ABR. Intestinal mucosal adaptation. *World J Gastroenterol* 2006; 12: 4614–24.
19. Diamond IR, Sterescu A, Pnecharz PB, Wales PW. The rationale for the use of parenteral omega-3 lipids in children with short bowel syndrome and liver disease. *Pediatr Surg Int* 2008; 24: 773–8.
20. Johnson JR. The trophic action of gastrointestinal hormones. *Gastroenterology* 1976; 70: 278–88.
21. Bloom SR, Polak JM. The hormonal pattern of intestinal adaptation. A major role for enteroglucagon. *Scand J Gastroenterol* 1982; 74: 93–103.

22. Sigalet DL, Baeazir O, Martin GR et al. Glucagon-like Peptide-2 induces a specific pattern of adaptation in remnant jejunum. *Dig Dis Sci* 2006; 51: 1557–66.

23. Martin GR, Beck PL, Sigalet DL. Gut hormones and short bowel syndrome: The enigmatic role of glucagon-like peptide-2 in the regulation of intestinal adaptation. *World J Gastroenterology* 2006; 12: 4117–29.

24. Chow JYC, Carlstrom K, Barrett KE. Growth hormone reduces chloride secretion in human colonic epithelial cells via EGF-receptor 4 and extracellular regulated kinase. *Gastroenterology* 2003; 125: 1114–24.

25. Byrne TA, Morissey TB, Nattakorn TV et al. Growth hormone, glutamine, and a modified diet enhance nutrient absorption in patients with severe short bowel syndrome. *JPEN* 1995; 19: 296–302.

26. Ianolli P, Miller JH, Ryan CK et al. Epidermal growth factor and human growth hormone accelerate adaptation after massive enterectomy in an additive, nutrient dependent, and site-specific fashion. *Surgery* 1997; 122: 721–9.

27. Nakai K, Hamada Y, Kato Y et al. Evidence that epidermal growth factor enhances the intestinal adaptation following small bowel transplantation. *Life Sci* 2004; 75: 2091–102.

28. Clemmons DR, Underwood LE. Nutritional regulation of IGF-I and IGF binding protein. *Ann Rev Nutr* 1991; 11: 393–412.

29. Winesett DE, Ulshen DM. Hoyt EC et al. Regulation and localization of the insulin-like growth factor system in small bowel during altered nutrition status. *Am J Physiol* 1995; 268: G631–40.

30. Wilmore DW. Glutamine and the gut. *Gastroenterology* 1994; 107: 1885–901.

31. DiBaise JK, Young RJ, Vanderhoof JA. Intestinal rehabilitation and the short bowel syndrome: Part I. *Am J Gastroenterol* 2004; 99: 1386–95.

32. Ziegler TR, Mantell MP, Chow JC et al Gut adaptation and the insulin-like growth factor system: Regulation by glutamine and IGF-I administration. *Am J Physiol* 1996; 271: G866–75.

33. Cisler JJ, Buchmann AL. Intestinal adaptation in short bowel syndrome. *J Invest Med* 2005; 53: 402–13.

34. Vanderhoof JA, Park JH, Grandjean CJ Morphological and functional effects of 16,16 dimethyl-prostaglandin-E2 on mucosal adaptation after massive distal small bowel resection. *Am J Physiol* 1988; 254: G373–7.

35. Höllwarth ME, Granger DN, Ulrich-Baker MG et al. Pharmacologic enhancement of adaptive growth after extensive small bowel resection. *Pediatr Surg Int* 1988; 3: 55–61.

36. Pul M, Yilmaz N, Gürses N et al. Enhancement by testosterone of adaptive growth after small bowel resection. *Isr J Med Sci* 1991; 27: 339–42.

37. Hadjittofi CH, Coran AG, Mogilner JG et al. Dietary supplementation with vitamin D stimulates intestinal epithelial cell turnover after massive small bowel resection in rats. *Pediatr Surg Int* 2013; 29: 41–50.

38. Peterson J, Kerner JA. New advances in the management of children with intestinal failure. *JPEN* 2012; 36: S36–42.

39. Luo M, Fernández-Estívariz, C, Manatunga AK et al. Are plasma citrulline and glutamine biomarkers of intestinal absorptive function in patients with short bowel syndrome? *J Parenter Enteral Nutr* 2007; 31: 1, 1–7.

40. Crenn P, Messing B, Cynober L. Citrulline as a biomarker of intestinal failure due to enterocyte mass reduction. *Clin Nutr* 2008; 27: 328–39.

41. Fitzgibbons S, Ching YA, Valim C et al. Relationship between serum citrulline levels and progression to parenteral nutrition independence in children with short bowel syndrome. *J Pediatr Surg* 2009; 44: 928–32.

42. Merlin E, Minet-Quinard R, Pereira B et al. Non-invasive biological quantification of acute gastrointestinal graft-versus-host disease in children by plasma citrulline. *Pediatr Transplant* 2013; 17: 683–7.

43. Freeman RB, Steffick DE, Guidinger MK et al. Liver and intestinal transplantation in the United States, 1997–2006. *Am J Transplant* 2008; 8 (Part2): 958–76.

44. Jeejeebhoy KN. Editorial: Treatment of intestinal failure: Transplantation or home parenteral nutrition? *Gastroenterology* 2008; 135: 303–5.

45. Abu-Elmagd K, Costa G, Bond GJ et al. Five hundred intestinal and multivisceral transplantations at a single center. Major advances and new challenges. *Ann Surg* 2009; 250: 567–81.

46. Pironi L, Goulet O, Buchmann A et al. utcome on home parenteral nutrition for benign intestinal failure: A review of the literature and benchmarking with the European prospective survey of ESPEN. *Clin Nutr* 2012; 31: 831–45.

47. Weber TR, Vone DW, Grosfield JL. Tapering enteroplasty in infants with bowel atresia and short gut. *Arch Surg* 1982; 117: 684–8.

48. Ramanujan TM. Functional capability of blind small loops after intestinal remodelling techniques. *Aust NZJ Surg* 1986; 54: 145–50.

49. Bianchi A. Intestinal loop lengthening—A technique for increasing small intestinal length. *J Pediatr Surg* 1980; 15: 145–51.

50. Bianchi A. Intestinal lengthening: An experimental and clinical review. *J R Soc Med* 1984; 77: 35–41.

51. Boeckmann CR, Traylor R. Bowel lengthening for short gut syndrome. *J Pediatr Surg* 1981; 16: 996–7.

52. Aigrain Y, Cornet D, Cezard JP et al. Longitudinal division of small intestine: A surgical possibility for children with very short bowel syndrome. *Z Kinderchir* 1985; 40: 233–6.

53. Thompson JS, Pinch LW, Muorey N et al. Experience with intestinal lengthening for the short bowel syndrome. *J Pediatr Surg* 1991; 26: 721–4.

54. Thompson JS, Quigley EM, Adrian T. Effect of intestinal tapering and lengthening on intestinal structure and function. *Am J Surg* 1995; 169: 111–9.

55. Bianchi A. Experience with longitudinal intestinal lengthening and tailoring. *Eur J Paediatr Surg* 1999; 9: 256–9.

56. Vernon AH, Georgeson KE. Surgical options for short bowel syndrome. *Semin Pediatr Surg* 2001; 10: 91–8.

57. Kimura K, Soper RT. new bowel elongation technique for the short bowel syndrome using the isolated bowel segment Iowa models. *J Pediatr Surg* 1993; 26: 792–4.

58. Georgeson KE, Halpin D, Figueroa R et al. Sequential intestinal lengthening procedure for refractory short bowel syndrome. *J Pediatr Surg* 1994; 29: 316–21.

59. Kim HB, Fauza D, Oh J-T, Nurko S, Jaksic T. erial transverse enteroplasty (STEP): A novel bowel lengthening procedure. *J Pediatr Surg* 2003; 38: 3, 425–429.

60. Kim HB, Lee PW, Garza J, Duggan C, Fauza D, Jaksic T. Serial transverse enteroplasty for short bowel syndrome: A case report. *J Pediatr Surg* 2003; 38: 6, 881–5.

61. Javid PJ, Sanchez HE, Horslen SP et al. Intestinal lengthening and nutritional outcomes in children with short bowel syndrome. *Am J Surg* 2013; 205: 576–80.

62. Jones BA, Hull MA, Potanos KM et al. Report of 111 consecutive patients enrolled in the international serial transverse enteroplasty (STEP) data registry: A retrospective observational study. *J Am Coll Surg* 2013; 216: 438–46.

63. Mercer DF, Hobson BD, Gerhardt BK et al. Serial transverse enteroplasty allows children with short bowel to wean from parenteral nutrition. *J Pediatr* 2014; 164: 93–8.

64. Mayr J, Schober PH, Weissensteiner U et al. Morbidity and mortality of the short bowel syndrome. *Eur J Paediatr Surg* 1999; 9: 231–5.

65. Coran AG, Spivak D, Teitelbaum DH. An analysis of the morbidity and mortality of short-bowel syndrome in the pediatric age group. *Eur J Paediatr Surg* 1999; 9: 228–30.

66. Kaufman SS, Loseke CA, Lupo JV et al. Influence of bacterial overgrowth and intestinal inflammation on duration of parenteral nutrition in children with short bowel syndrome. *J Pediatr* 1997; 131: 356–61.

67. Schimpl G, Feierl G, Linni K et al. Bacterial translocation in short-bowel syndrome in rats. *Eur J Paediatr Surg* 1999; 9: 224–7.

68. Eizaguirre I, Aldazabal P, Barrena P et al. Bacterial translocation is favoured by the preservation of the ileocecal valve in experimental short bowel with total parenteral nutrition. *Eur J Paediatr Surg* 1999; 9: 220–3.

69. Gibson LD, Carter R, Hinshaw DB. Segmental reversal of small intestine after massive bowel resection. *J Am Med Assoc* 1962; 182: 952–4.

70. Kurz R, Sauer H. Treatment and metabolic findings in extreme short bowel syndrome with 11 cm jejunal remnant. *J Pediatr Surg* 1983; 18: 257–63.

71. Layec S, Beiyer L, Corcos O et al. Increased intestinal absorption by segmental reversal of the small bowel in adult patients with short bowel syndrome: A case control study. *Am J Clin Nutr* 2013; 97: 100–8.

72. Hutcher NE, Salzberg AM. re-ileal transposition of colon to prevent the development of the short bowel syndrome in puppies with 90 percent small intestine resection. *Surgery* 1971; 70: 189–97.

73. Hutcher NE, Mendez-Picon G, Salzberg AM. Prejejunal transposition of colon to prevent the development of the short bowel in puppies with 90 percent small intestine resection. *J Pediatr Surg* 1973; 8: 771–7.

74. Lloyd DA. Colonic interposition between the jejunum and ileum after massive small bowel resection in rats. *Progr Pediatr Surg* 1978; 12: 12–106.

75. Glick PL, de Lorimier AA, Adzick NS et al. olon interposition: An adjuvant operation for short gut syndrome. *J Pediatr Surg* 1984; 19: 719–25.

76. Garcia VF, Templeton JM, Eichelberger MR et al. Colon interposition for short bowel syndrome. *J Pediatr Surg* 1981; 16: 994–5.

77. Kono K, Sekikawa T, Iizuka H et al. Interposed colon between remnants of the small intestine exhibits small bowel features in a patient with short bowel syndrome. *Dig Surg* 2001; 18: 237–41.

78. King DR, Anvari M, Jamieson GG, King JM. Does the colon adopt small bowel features in a small bowel environment? *Aust N Z J* 1996; 66: 543–6.

79. Zurita M, Raurich JM, Ramirez A et al. A new neo-valve type in short bowel syndrome surgery. *Rev Esp Enfem Dig* 2004; 96: 110–8.

80. Stacchini A, Dido LJ, Primo ML et al. Artificial sphincter as a surgical treatment for experimental massive resection of small intestine. *Am J Surg* 1982; 143: 721–6.

81. Sawchuk A, Goto S, Yount J et al. Chemically induced bowel denervation improves survival in short bowel syndrome. *J Pediatr Surg* 1987; 22: 492–6.

82. Ricotta J, Zuidema GD, Gadacz TR et al. Construction of an ileocecal valve and its role in massive resection of the small intestine. *Surg Gynecol Obstet* 1981; 152: 310–4.

83. Vinograd Il, Merguerian P, Udassin R et al. An experimental model of a submucosally tunnelled valve for the replacement of the ileo-cecal valve. *J Pediatr Surg* 1984; 19: 726–31.

84. Waddell WR, Kern F, Halgrimson ChG et al. A simple jejunocolic valve. *Arch Surg* 1979; 100: 438–44.

85. Galea MH, Holliday H, Carachi R et al. Short-bowel syndrome: A collective review. Enteral and parenteral nutrition in short-bowel syndrome in children. *J Pediatr Surg* 1992; 27: 592–6.

86. Georgeson KE, Breaux CW. Outcome and intestinal adaptation in neonatal short-bowel syndrome. *J Pediatr Surg* 1992; 27: 344–50.

87. Ricour C, Duhamel JF, Arnaud-Battandier F et al. Enteral and parenteral nutrition in the short bowel syndrome in children. *World J Surg* 1985; 9: 310–5.

88. Goulet O, Baglin-Gobet S, Talbotec C. Outcome and long-term growth after extensive small bowel resection in the neonatal period: A survey of 87 children. *Eur J Pediatr Surg* 2005; 15: 95–101.

89. Cole CR, Hansen NI, Higgins RD et al. Very low birth weight preterm infants with surgical short bowel syndrome: Incidence, morbidity and mortality, and growth outcomes at 18 and 22 month. *Pediatrics* 2008; 122: e573–82.

90. Infantino BJ, Mercer DF, Hobson BD et al. Successful rehabilitation in pediatric ultra-short small bowel syndrome. *J Pediatr* 2013; 163: 1361–6.

74

Megacystis microcolon intestinal hypoperistalsis syndrome

PREM PURI AND JAN-HENDRIK GOSEMANN

INTRODUCTION

Megacystis microcolon intestinal hypoperistalsis syndrome (MMIHS) is a rare congenital and generally fatal cause of functional intestinal obstruction in the newborn. The main characteristics for this syndrome are abdominal distension caused by a massive enlarged nonobstructed urinary bladder, microcolon, and decreased or absent intestinal peristalsis.[1] MMIHS is usually associated with incomplete intestinal rotation and shortened small bowel.

PATHOGENESIS

MMIHS was first described by Berdon et al.[1] in 1976. To date, over 220 cases have been reported in the literature.[2] Although several hypotheses have been proposed to explain the pathogenetic background of MMIHS (neurogenic, myogenic, and hormonal), the etiology of this syndrome remains unclear.

In the majority of MMIHS patients, histologic studies of the myenteric and submucosal plexuses of the bowel revealed normal ganglion cells. However, in some patients, decreased amounts of ganglion cells or hyperganglionosis together with giant ganglia were found.[3,4] In 1983, Puri et al.[5] showed vacuolar degenerative changes in the smooth muscle cells (SMCs) with abundant connective tissue between muscle cells in bowel and bladder of patients with MMIHS. This leads to the suggestion that a degenerative disease of SMCs could be the cause of this syndrome. Several subsequent reports have confirmed evidence of intestinal myopathy in MMIHS.[6-8]

More recently, Piotrowska et al.[7,9] reported absence of interstitial cells of Cajal (ICCs) in bowel and urinary bladder of patients with MMIHS. ICCs are pacemaker cells, which facilitate active propagation of electrical events and neurotransmission. Their absence may result in hypoperistalsis and voiding dysfunction in MMIHS.

Furthermore, absence or marked reduction in α-smooth muscle actin and other contractile as well as cytoskeletal proteins in the smooth muscle layers of MMIHS bowel have been reported.[7,8] Contractile and cytoskeletal proteins are important structural and functional components of SMCs and play a vital role in the interaction of filaments in smooth muscle contraction.

Rolle and Puri[10] showed pathological changes within the bladder SMCs and markedly increased collagen deposits within the bladder wall of MMIHS patients, and therefore concluded that the detrusor muscle is strikingly abnormal and this is the likely cause of voiding dysfunction in the affected patients.

Other studies support the hypothesis that the absence of a functional α3 subunit of the neuronal nicotinic acetylcholine receptor (ηAChR) may be responsible for the predominant intestinal manifestation of smooth muscle myopathy, leading to manifestation of MMIHS.[11-13] This lack of functional α3 and the absence of smooth muscle actin in the circular layer of small bowel muscularis were recently suggested to be associated with a de novo deletion of the proximal long arm of chromosome 15 (15q11.2).[14]

The evaluation of the genetic background of MMIHS resulted in a number of recent publications that suggest the enteric smooth muscle actin gamma 2 (ACTG2) as the first gene to be clearly associated with MMIHS[15-17] and intestinal pseudo-obstruction. Some authors suggest to reorganize the clinical entities of MMIHS, prune belly syndrome, hollow visceral myopathy, and intestinal pseudo-obstruction into a spectrum of ACTG2-related disorders.[15] The identification of a possible genetic background might have a relevant impact on prenatal counselling in the future.

Table 74.1 Reported siblings with MMIHS

References	Gender
Berdon et al.[1]	F/F
Patel and Carty[18]	F/F
Oliveira et al.[19]	F/M
Winter and Knowles[20]	F/F
Farrell[21]	F/F
Penman and Lilford[22]	F/F
Young et al.[23]	M/M
Gakmak et al.[24]	-/-/-
Garber et al.[25]	M/M
Annerén et al.[26]	M/F
Stamm et al.[27]	F/F
Goldberg et al.[28]	F/-
Guzé et al.[29]	F/M
Bloom and Kolon[30]	F/-
Hsu et al.[31]	F/M
Köhler et al.[32]	F/M
Boissier et al.[33]	F/-
López-Muñoz et al.[34]	F/M
Lozoya Araque et al.[35]	F/-/F

Source: Data from McLaughlin D, Puri P. *Pediatr Surg Int* 2013 September; 29(9): 947–51.

Table 74.2 Prenatal ultrasound findings

Ultrasound findings	%
Enlarged bladder	88
Hydronephrosis	57
Normal amniotic fluid volume	59
Increased amniotic fluid volume	33
Decreased amniotic fluid volume	7
Dilated stomach	5

Source: Data from Puri P, Shinkai M. *Semin Pediatr Surg* 2005 February; 14(1): 58–63.

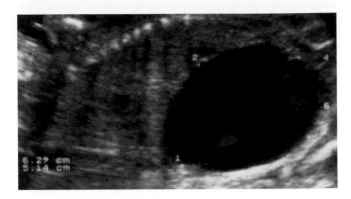

Figure 74.1 Massive enlarged fetal bladder, longitudinal view of abdominal ultrasound at 22 weeks gestation, fetus in prone position.

The occurrence of MMIHS in 15 sets of affected siblings (Table 74.1) and four further index patients with a confirmed diagnosis and a probably affected sibling as well as consanguinity in four of the confirmed sibling sets suggest an autosomal recessive pattern of inheritance.[20,26,36]

PRENATAL DIAGNOSIS

A total of 182 cases of MMIHS reported in the literature were reviewed by Puri and Shinkai.[37] The most frequent finding reported on fetal sonography (*n* = 54) associated with MMIHS was enlarged bladder (88%) together with hydronephrosis (57%). In 59% of the fetuses, normal amniotic fluid volume was detected, whereas 33% revealed increased volume and 7% had decreased volume. Only 5% showed abdominal distension caused by dilated stomach. Three cases (5%) of oligohydramnios during the second and early third trimester were reported, which may probably be related to the functional bladder obstruction (Table 74.2).

Enlarged bladder, detectable from 16 weeks of gestational age, was shown to be the earliest finding in MMIHS in serial obstetrical ultrasonography (Figure 74.1). A later finding was hydronephrosis, caused by the functional obstruction of the bladder. Usually polyhydramnios develops late, appearing during the third trimester.

Recent reports have described prenatal magnetic resonance imaging (MRI) in patients with suspected genitourinary and gastrointestinal tract abnormalities following ultrasound examination.[38–40] In contrast to sonography, MRI not only demonstrated urologic abnormalities but also

identified early stages of gastrointestinal pathology. Hence, the authors advocate MRI as an ancillary imaging technique whenever routine ultrasonography screening demonstrates genitourinary pathology with a need for further investigation.

CLINICAL PRESENTATION

Review of the current literature revealed a female-to-male ratio of 2.4:1.[2] With regard to the duration of pregnancy, 59% of the reported patients were born at term, 26% at 36–39 weeks of gestation, 12% at 32–35 weeks, and 3% at 31 weeks or less. Eight cases of dystocis delivery due to abdominal distention were reported, and caesarean section was required in four cases.[37] Nine terminations of pregnancy after the detection of MMIHS via ultrasound have been reported.[2]

In four cases, paracentesis was needed because the bladder was so distended that the baby could only be delivered vaginally after removal of 250, 500, 650, and 500 mL of urine, respectively, from fetal bladder. The mean birth weight was found normal (3000 g) for gestational age.[37]

Clinical symptoms of MMIHS are similar to other neonatal intestinal obstructions. Abdominal distension is a constant and early finding. It is a consequence of the enlarged, unobstructed urinary bladder with or without upper urinary tract dilatation. The majority of patients were not able to void spontaneously. However, a distended, nonobstructed urinary bladder could be easily relieved by catheterization.

Of 182 infants, 61 had bilious vomiting and 23 failed to pass meconium. Other symptoms included bile-stained vomiting and absent or decreased bowel sounds.[37]

RADIOLOGICAL FINDINGS

Radiological evaluation usually suggests the diagnosis of MMIHS. Plain abdominal films showed either dilated small bowel loops or a gasless abdomen with evident gastric bubble in the vast majority of 182 reviewed cases.[37] An enlarged urinary bladder was present in all patients who had cystography or ultrasonography (Figure 74.2). Vesicoureteral reflux was found in 8 patients, and in 84 patients, intravenous urography or ultrasonography detected unilateral or bilateral hydronephrosis.[3,18,37,41–43]

Barium enema showed microcolon in all 71 patients in whom this study was performed, and in 39 cases, malrotation was associated (Figure 74.3).

In patients who underwent an upper gastrointestinal series, both before and after laparotomy constantly revealed hypo- or aperistalsis in stomach, duodenum, and small bowel. Reverse peristalsis from small bowel into the stomach was observed in three cases; in two cases, hypoperistalsis was associated with gastroesophageal reflux; and in one case, the esophagus was aperistaltic.[37]

SURGICAL OR AUTOPSY FINDINGS

Surgical findings and management vary throughout the publications, and exact surgical procedures are reported inconsistently.

The most frequently reported findings at surgery or autopsy are megacystis and microcolon and are present in

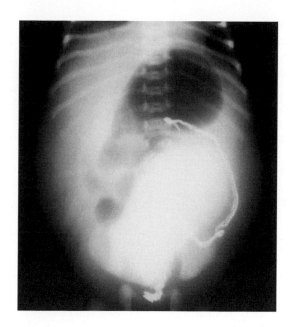

Figure 74.3 Contrast enema showing microcolon in an MMIHS patient.

all patients (Figure 74.4). Furthermore, malrotation, short bowel, and functional obstruction are frequently reported.[2] Approximately 70% of the reported patients, to date, underwent one or more surgical procedure.[37] Surgeons frequently performed gastrostomy, jejunostomy, ileostomy, cecostomy, and vesicostomy, mainly to decompress the intestinal and vesical system. However, the majority of reports state that surgical interventions did not improve enteral food intake, intestinal pseudo-obstruction, or bladder function.

Due to the various, infrequent, and fragmentary reports on surgical interventions combined with clinical outcome, no conclusion or recommendation can be made from these data. The majority of authors agree that the decision for surgical interventions should be made carefully, individualized, and restricted to supportive interventions such as enterostomy and vesicostomy.[2]

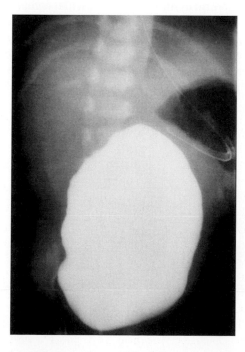

Figure 74.2 Voiding cystourethrogram showing massively enlarged bladder in an MMIHS patient.

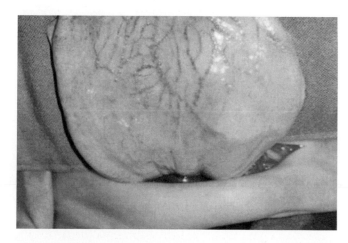

Figure 74.4 Operative photograph of a massively dilated urinary bladder in MMIHS.

HISTOLOGICAL FINDINGS

Histologic studies of the myenteric and submucosus plexuses were reported in 93 out of 182 MMIHS cases.[37] Ganglion cells were normal in appearance and number in 72 (77%). In the remaining 21 cases (23%), various neuronal abnormalities included hypoganglionosis, hyperganglionosis, and immature ganglia.[4,37,44–50] The majority of reports do not mention histologic findings in the muscle layers of bowel and bladder wall. However, some authors found significant abnormalities in SMCs, such as thinning of the longitudinal muscle, seen in light microscopy.

Vacuolar degeneration in the center of the smooth muscle of bowel (11 cases) and bladder (8 cases) was shown in electron microscopy (Figure 74.5); furthermore, connective tissue proliferation was found in the bowel (9 cases) and bladder (8 cases). In three cases, the bladder showed elastosis. Electron microscopy revealed vacuolar degeneration of smooth cells in muscle layers of bowel and bladder in addition to neuronal abnormalities in two more patients.[37]

Other investigators have reported absence or marked reduction in α-smooth muscle actin and other contractile and cytoskeletal proteins in smooth muscle layers of MMIHS bowel.[7,8]

OUTCOME

Management of patients with MMIHS is frustrating. A number of prokinetic drugs and gastrointestinal hormones have been tried without success. Surgical manipulations of the gastrointestinal tract have generally been unsuccessful. The outcome of this condition remains fatal with a survival rate of approximately 20%. Although the survival rate increased in recent years, due to inconsistent reporting, the long-term survival of patients with MMIHS remains elusive. The oldest patients alive were reported to be 19 and 24 years at the time of publication.[2,51,52]

The most frequently reported cause of death in MMIHS patients was overwhelming sepsis followed by multiple organ failure and malnutrition. Furthermore, attempts to initiate sufficient enteral feeding have been reported to result in fatal pneumonia in several cases.[2,44,53,54]

The majority of MMIHS patients are maintained by parenteral nutrition, which predisposes for fatalities such as catheter sepsis and chronic liver failure.[53,55,56] Parenteral nutrition has been further associated with dyslipidemia and consequentially parenteral nutrition-associated liver disease (PNALD). One contribution to the observed increase in survival in recent years might have been the improvements of total parenteral nutrition (TPN) products. Especially the introduction of fish oil–based lipid emulsions has been reported to improve major lipid panels and resolve cholestasis in children with PNALD.[56]

Furthermore, early referral of affected patients to tertiary care may be a significant factor that may influence the survival of MMIHS patients, since early referral to specialized centers and multidisciplinary approach have been suggested to prevent the development of PNALD and increase survival in patients with intestinal failure.[57–59]

In a recent literature, 12 cases of multivisceral transplant surgery have been described with various outcomes.[2] A 3-year survival of 50% has been reported in a series by Loinaz et al.[53] The majority received liver, pancreas, small bowel, and colon transplants. All survivors were reported to tolerate enteral feedings and showed adequate gastric emptying. In contrast, bladder function did not improve and catheterization had to be continued after transplantation.[53]

Outcome of multivisceral transplant surgery might have been improved over the last years.[60,61] However, transplant patients still face major complications such as infection/sepsis, rejection, post-transplant lymphoproliferative disease, mechanical dysfunction, and vascular complications.[62]

The decision for surgical intervention should be made carefully, individualized, and, in most cases, restricted to supportive interventions (such as feeding enterostomy and decompressing ostomy), since most explorations have not been helpful and probably are not necessary.

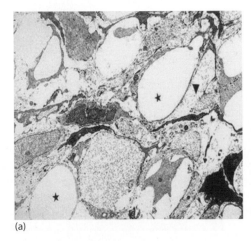
(a)

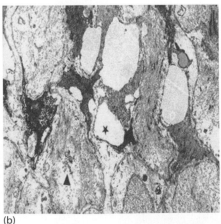
(b)

Figure 74.5 Electron microscopy: SMCs from ileum (a) and bladder (b) from a patient with MMIHS showing vacuolar degeneration (*) in the center of SMCs.

Future parenteral counselling will be based on continuously improving prenatal diagnostics and increasing knowledge on the pathogenesis of MMIHS. It is therefore crucial that the counselling physician educates the future parents to his or her best knowledge and up-to-date evidence to allow them to make a substantiated decision on the sequel of the pregnancy.

REFERENCES

1. Berdon WE, Baker DH, Blanc WA, Gay B, Santulli TV, Donovan C. Megacystis-microcolon-intestinal hypoperistalsis syndrome: A new cause of intestinal obstruction in the newborn. Report of radiologic findings in five newborn girls. *AJR Am J Roentgenol* 1976 May; 126(5): 957–64.

2. Gosemann J-H, Puri P. Megacystis microcolon intestinal hypoperistalsis syndrome: Systematic review of outcome. *Pediatr Surg Int. Springer-Verlag* 2011 October; 27(10): 1041–6.

3. Granata C, Puri P. Megacystis-microcolon-intestinal hypoperistalsis syndrome. *J Pediatr Gastroenterol Nutr* 1997 July; 25(1): 12–9.

4. Kobayashi H, O'Brian S, Puri P. *New Observation on the Pathogenesis of Megacystis Microcolon Intestinalis Hypoperistalsis Syndrome*. Presented at the American Pediatric Surgical Association Annual Meeting in Boca Raton, Florida. 1995.

5. Puri P, Lake BD, Gorman F, O'Donnell B, Nixon HH. Megacystis-microcolon-intestinal hypoperistalsis syndrome: A visceral myopathy. *J Pediatr Surg* 1983 February; 18(1): 64–9.

6. Ciftci AO, Cook RC, van Velzen D. Megacystis microcolon intestinal hypoperistalsis syndrome: Evidence of a primary myocellular defect of contractile fiber synthesis. *J Pediatr Surg* 1996 December; 31(12): 1706–11.

7. Piotrowska AP, Rolle U, Chertin B, De Caluwe D, Bianchi A, Puri P. Alterations in smooth muscle contractile and cytoskeleton proteins and interstitial cells of Cajal in megacystis microcolon intestinal hypoperistalsis syndrome. *J Pediatr Surg* 2003 May; 38(5): 749–55.

8. Rolle U, O'Briain S, Pearl RH, Puri P. Megacystis-microcolon-intestinal hypoperistalsis syndrome: Evidence of intestinal myopathy. *Pediatr Surg Int* Springer-Verlag; 2002 January; 18(1): 2–5.

9. Piaseczna Piotrowska A, Rolle U, Solari V, Puri P. Interstitial cells of Cajal in the human normal urinary bladder and in the bladder of patients with megacystis-microcolon intestinal hypoperistalsis syndrome. *BJU Int* Blackwell Science Ltd; 2004 July; 94(1): 143–6.

10. Rolle U, Puri P. Structural basis of voiding dysfunction in megacystis microcolon intestinal hypoperistalsis syndrome. *J Pediatr Urol* 2006 August; 2(4): 277–84.

11. Richardson CE, Morgan JM, Jasani B, Green JT, Rhodes J, Williams GT et al. Megacystis-microcolon-intestinal hypoperistalsis syndrome and the absence of the alpha3 nicotinic acetylcholine receptor subunit. *Gastroenterology* 2001 August; 121(2): 350–7.

12. Xu W, Gelber S, Orr-Urtreger A, Armstrong D, Lewis RA, Ou CN et al. Megacystis, mydriasis, and ion channel defect in mice lacking the alpha3 neuronal nicotinic acetylcholine receptor. *Proc Natl Acad Sci USA* Karger Publishers; 1999 May 11; 96(10): 5746–51.

13. Narayanan M, Murphy MS, Ainsworth JR, Arul GS. Mydriasis in association with MMIHS in a female infant: Evidence for involvement of the neuronal nicotinic acetylcholine receptor. *J Pediatr Surg* Elsevier; 2007 July; 42(7): 1288–90.

14. Szigeti R, Chumpitazi BP, Finegold MJ, Ranganathan S, Craigen WJ, Carter BA et al. Absent smooth muscle actin immunoreactivity of the small bowel muscularis propria circular layer in association with chromosome 15q11 deletion in megacystis-microcolon-intestinal hypoperistalsis syndrome. *Pediatr Dev Pathol* 2010 July; 13(4): 322–5.

15. Wangler MF, Gonzaga-Jauregui C, Gambin T, Penney S, Moss T, Chopra A et al. Heterozygous de novo and inherited mutations in the smooth muscle actin (ACTG2) gene underlie megacystis-microcolon-intestinal hypoperistalsis syndrome. Barsh GS (ed). *PLoS Genet. Pub Lib Sci* 2014 March; 10(3): e1004258.

16. Halim D, Hofstra RMW, Signorile L, Verdijk RM, van der Werf CS, Sribudiani Y et al. ACTG2 variants impair actin polymerization in sporadic megacystis microcolon intestinal hypoperistalsis syndrome. *Hum Mol Genet* Oxford University Press; 2015 December 8; 25(3): 571–83.

17. Tuzovic L, Tang S, Miller RS, Rohena L, Shahmirzadi L, Gonzalez K et al. New insights into the genetics of fetal megacystis: ACTG2 mutations, encoding x03B3;-2 smooth muscle actin in megacystis microcolon intestinal hypoperistalsis syndrome (Berdon syndrome). *Fetal Diagn Ther* Karger Publishers; 2015; 38(4): 296–306.

18. Patel R, Carty H. Megacystis-microcolon-intestinal hypoperistalsis syndrome: A rare cause of intestinal obstruction in the newborn. *Br J Radiol* 1980 March; 53(627): 249–52.

19. Oliveira G, Boechat MI, Ferreira MA. Megacystis-microcolon-intestinal hypoperistalsis syndrome in a newborn girl whose brother had prune belly syndrome: Common pathogenesis? *Pediatr Radiol* 1983; 13(5): 294–6.

20. Winter RM, Knowles SA. Megacystis-microcolon-intestinal hypoperistalsis syndrome: Confirmation of autosomal recessive inheritance. *J Med Genet* 1986 August; 23(4): 360–2.

21. Farrell SA. Intrauterine death in megacystis-microcolon-intestinal hypoperistalsis syndrome. *J Med Genet* 1988 May; 25(5): 350–1.

22. Penman DG, Lilford RJ. The megacystis-microcolon-intestinal hypoperistalsis syndrome: A fatal autosomal recessive condition. *J Med Genet* 1989 January; 26(1): 66–7.

23. Young ID, McKeever PA, Brown LA, Lang GD. Prenatal diagnosis of the megacystis-microcolon-intestinal hypoperistalsis syndrome. *J Med Genet* 1989 June; 26(6): 403–6.

24. Gakmak O, Pektas O, Maden HA. Megacystis-microcolon-intestinal hypoperistalsis syndrome in three siblings. Poster presentation at the Sixth International Congress of Paediatric Surgery, Istanbul, 1989.

25. Garber A, Shohat M, Sarti D. Megacystis-microcolon-intestinal hypoperistalsis syndrome in two male siblings. *Prenat Diagn* 1990 June; 10(6): 377–87.

26. Annerén G, Meurling S, Olsen L. Megacystis-microcolon-intestinal hypoperistalsis syndrome (MMIHS), an autosomal recessive disorder: Clinical reports and review of the literature. *Am J Med Genet* 1991 November 1; 41(2): 251–4.

27. Stamm E, King G, Thickman D. Megacystis-microcolon-intestinal hypoperistalsis syndrome: Prenatal identification in siblings and review of the literature. *J Ultrasound Med* 1991 October; 10(10): 599–602.

28. Goldberg M, Pruchniewski D, Beale PG, Da Fonseca JM, Davies MR. Megacystis-microcolon-intestinal hypoperistalsis syndrome. *Pediatr Surg Int* 1996 April; 11(4): 246–7.

29. Guzé CD, Hyman PE, Payne VJ. Family studies of infantile visceral myopathy: A congenital myopathic pseudo-obstruction syndrome. *Am J Med Genet* 1999 January 15; 82(2): 114–22.

30. Bloom TL, Kolon TF. Severe megacystis and bilateral hydronephrosis in a female fetus. *Urology* 2002 October; 60(4): 697.

31. Hsu CD, Craig C, Pavlik J, Ninios A. Prenatal diagnosis of megacystis-microcolon-intestinal hypoperistalsis syndrome in one fetus of a twin pregnancy. *Am J Perinatol* 2003 May; 20(4): 215–8.

32. Köhler M, Pease PW, Upadhyay V. Megacystis-microcolon-intestinal hypoperistalsis syndrome (MMIHS) in siblings: Case report and review of the literature. *Eur J Pediatr Surg* 2004 October; 14(5): 362–7.

33. Boissier K, Varlet M-N, Chauleur C, Cochin S, Clemenson A, Varlet F et al. [Early fetal megacystis at first trimester: A six-year retrospective study]. *Gynecol Obstet Fertil* 2009 February; 37(2): 115–24.

34. López-Muñoz E, Hernández-Zarco A, Polanco-Ortiz A, Villa-Morales J, Mateos-Sánchez L. Megacystis-microcolon-intestinal hypoperistalsis syndrome

(MMIHS): Report of a case with prolonged survival and literature review. *J Pediatr Urol* Elsevier; 2013 February; 9(1): e12–8.

35. Lozoya Araque T, Vila-Vives JM, Perales-Puchalt A, Soler Ferrero I, Quiroga R, Llorens-Salvador R et al. Síndrome de Berdon: Diagnóstico intrauterino y evolución posnatal. *Diagn Prenat* (Internet) 2013: 23–8.

36. McLaughlin D, Puri P. Familial megacystis microcolon intestinal hypoperistalsis syndrome: A systematic review. *Pediatr Surg Int* 2013 September; 29(9): 947–51.

37. Puri P, Shinkai M. Megacystis microcolon intestinal hypoperistalsis syndrome. *Semin Pediatr Surg* 2005 February; 14(1): 58–63.

38. Garel C, Dreux S, Philippe-Chomette P, Vuillard E, Oury JF, Muller F. Contribution of fetal magnetic resonance imaging and amniotic fluid digestive enzyme assays to the evaluation of gastrointestinal tract abnormalities. *Ultrasound Obstet Gynecol* John Wiley & Sons, Ltd; 2006 September; 28(3): 282–91.

39. Munch EM, Cisek LJJ, Roth DR. Magnetic resonance imaging for prenatal diagnosis of multisystem disease: Megacystis microcolon intestinal hypoperistalsis syndrome. *Urology* 2009 September; 74(3): 592–4.

40. Veyrac C, Couture A, Saguintaah M, Baud C. MRI of fetal GI tract abnormalities. *Abdom Imaging* 2004 July–August; 29(4): 411–20.

41. Ghavamian R, Wilcox DT, Duffy PG, Milla PJ. The urological manifestations of hollow visceral myopathy in children. *J Urol* 1997 September; 158(3 Pt 2): 1286–90.

42. Hoehn W, Thomas GG, Mearadji M. Urologic evaluation of megacystis-microcolon-intestinal hypoperistalsis syndrome. *Urology* 1981 May; 17(5): 465–6.

43. Redman JF, Jimenez JF, Golladay ES, Seibert JJ. Megacystis-microcolon-intestinal hypoperistalsis syndrome: Case report and review of the literature. *J Urol* 1984 May; 131(5): 981–3.

44. Young LW, Yunis EJ, Girdany BR, Sieber WK. Megacystis-microcolon-intestinal hypoperistalsis syndrome: Additional clinical, radiologic, surgical, and histopathologic aspects. *AJR Am J Roentgenol* 1981 October; 137(4): 749–55.

45. Vezina WC, Morin FR, Winsberg F. Megacystis-microcolon-intestinal hypoperistalsis syndrome: Antenatal ultrasound appearance. *AJR Am J Roentgenol* 1979 October; 133(4): 749–50.

46. Manco LG, Osterdahl P. The antenatal sonographic features of megacystis-microcolon-intestinal hypoperistalsis syndrome. *J Clin Ultrasound* 1984 November–December; 12(9): 595–8.

47. Kirtane J, Talwalker V, Dastur DK. Megacystis, microcolon, intestinal hypoperistalsis syndrome: Possible pathogenesis. *J Pediatr Surg* 1984 April; 19(2): 206–8.

48. Krook PM. Megacystis-microcolon-intestinal hypo-peristalsis syndrome in a male infant. *Radiology* 1980 September; 136(3): 649–50.

49. Jona JZ, Werlin SL. The megacystis microcolon intestinal hypoperistalsis syndrome: Report of a case. *J Pediatr Surg* 1981 October; 16(5): 749–51.

50. Shalev J, Itzchak Y, Avigad I, Hertz M, Straus S, Serr DM. Antenatal ultrasound appearance of megacystis microcolon intestinal hypoperistalsis syndrome. *Isr J Med Sci* 1983 January; 19(1): 76–8.

51. Talisetti A, Longacre T, Pai RK, Kerner J. Diversion colitis in a 19-year-old female with megacystis-microcolon-intestinal hypoperistalsis syndrome. *Dig Dis Sci* 2009 November; 54(11): 2338–40.

52. Trebicka J, Biecker E, Gruenhage F, Stolte M, Meier-Ruge WA, Sauerbruch T et al. Diagnosis of megacystis-microcolon intestinal hypoperistalsis syndrome with aplastic desmosis in adulthood: A case report. *Eur J Gastroenterol Hepatol* 2008 April; 20(4): 353–5.

53. Loinaz C, Rodríguez MM, Kato T, Mittal N, Romaguera RL, Bruce JH et al. Intestinal and multivisceral transplantation in children with severe gastrointestinal dysmotility. *J Pediatr Surg* Elsevier; 2005 October; 40(10): 1598–604.

54. Nazer H, Rejjal A, Abu-Osba Y, Rabeeah A, Ahmed S. Megacystis-microcolon-intestinal hypoperistalsis syndrome. *Saudi J Gastroenterol* 1995 September; 1(3): 180–3.

55. Carter BA, Karpen SJ. Intestinal failure-associated liver disease: Management and treatment strategies past, present, and future. *Semin Liver Dis* 2007 August; 27(3): 251–8.

56. Le HD, de Meijer VE, Zurakowski D, Meisel JA, Gura KM, Puder M. Parenteral fish oil as monotherapy improves lipid profiles in children with parenteral nutrition-associated liver disease. *JPEN J Parenter Enteral Nutr* 2010 September–October; 34(5): 477–84.

57. Cowles RA, Ventura KA, Martinez M, Lobritto SJ, Harren PA, Brodlie S et al. Reversal of intestinal failure-associated liver disease in infants and children on parenteral nutrition: Experience with 93 patients at a referral center for intestinal rehabilitation. *J Pediatr Surg* 2010 January; 45(1): 84–7; discussion 87–8.

58. Rhoda KM, Parekh NR, Lennon E, Shay-Downer C, Quintini C, Steiger E et al. The multidisciplinary approach to the care of patients with intestinal failure at a tertiary care facility. *Nutr Clin Pract* 2010 April; 25(2): 183–91.

59. Nucci A, Burns RC, Armah T, Lowery K, Yaworski JA, Strohm S et al. Interdisciplinary management of pediatric intestinal failure: A 10-year review of rehabilitation and transplantation. *J Gastrointest Surg* 2008 March; 12(3): 429–35; discussion 435–6.

60. Farmer DG, Venick RS, Colangelo J, Esmailian Y, Yersiz H, Duffy JP et al. Pretransplant predictors of survival after intestinal transplantation: Analysis of a single-center experience of more than 100 transplants. *Transplantation* 2010 December 27; 90(12): 1574–80.

61. Nayyar NS, McGhee W, Martin D, Sindhi R, Soltys K, Bond G et al. Intestinal transplantation in children: A review of immunotherapy regimens. *Paediatr Drugs* 2011 June 1; 13(3): 149–59.

62. Phillips GS, Bhargava P, Stanescu L, Dick AA, Parnell SE. Pediatric intestinal transplantation: Normal radiographic appearance and complications. *Pediatr Radiol* 2011 May 24: 379–88.

PART 6

Liver and biliary tract

75

Biliary atresia

MARK DAVENPORT

INTRODUCTION

There is still much to learn about biliary atresia (BA), why it happens and how it happens being good examples of areas where there is too much speculation and not enough hard evidence. What is only too obvious is that if it is untreated, it progresses to end-stage cirrhosis and is potentially fatal within the first 12–18 months. A treatment strategy has evolved, which, in the best hands, will give a 90% chance of long-term survival for all infants born with the disease, but even in these survivors, there are still significant morbidity and problems to overcome. Nonetheless, it is compatible with normal life.

HISTORY

The first documented case of BA was reported in English in 1891 by John Thompson.[1] He was a physician in Edinburgh, and his newborn patient developed jaundice, passed only white-colored stool from an early age, and ultimately died of liver failure with ascites at about 6 months. Her postmortem showed a normally formed but empty gallbladder and absence of the common hepatic duct (CHD).

Further reports followed, but no real treatment could be offered until surgeons began to operate on some of these infants. The most significant series published was that by Ladd in 1928, who reported his experience in 10 cases of surgical jaundice—some of which were BA.[2] Fairly quickly afterward, it was realized that only a small proportion (having "correctable" BA) were suitable as surgical candidates, as at exploration, a patent part of the biliary tree could be found and an hepaticojejunostomy performed. The remainder, those with "uncorrectable" BA, had an entirely solid biliary tract, certainly nothing one could anastomose to.

An alternative operation for the latter group was advocated by Morio Kasai (1922–2008), a surgeon working in Sendai, Japan.[3] He showed that a higher, more radical dissection was needed and if you removed the entire extrahepatic biliary tract, even if it looked solid, still it would contain microscopic biliary ductules, which connect to the intrahepatic biliary tract. If enough of these were uncovered, then bile flow could be restored. The reconstruction advocated was termed a *portenterostomy* to reflect this higher level of anastomosis. Once again, this proved not to be the complete answer, with unpredictable results and a significant proportion that showed no effect whatsoever.

Indeed, such was the skepticism that its value was only really recognized in North America and Europe during the 1970s. Most post-Kasai adult series as a consequence are therefore Japanese,[4] with some rare exceptions.[5] The alternative, if yet more radical, treatment for a terminally damaged liver also appeared in the 1960s—*liver transplantation*. Tom Starzl's first, albeit unsuccessful, attempt at human liver transplant occurred in 1963 in Denver, Colorado, in a 3-year-old girl with end-stage liver disease due to BA.[6] During that period, the art of immunosuppression was in its infancy, and transplant programs shut down, having failed to come to terms with consequent inevitable cellular rejection. The key discovery and clinical use of an effective immunosuppressive agent, cyclosporine, occurred in the 1980s and allowed transplant programs to flourish once more. From the 1990s, in most of the developed world, and still today, the strategy for management has been an attempt to resuscitate the native liver with a Kasai portoenterostomy, and if that fails, transplantation.[7]

ETIOLOGICAL HETEROGENEITY

BA is not one disease, certainly not one with a single cause (Figure 75.1). It seems to be a phenotype resulting from a number of different etiologies. We can define perhaps four clinically distinct groups:

1. Isolated BA
2. Biliary atresia splenic malformation (BASM) syndrome[8,9]
3. Cystic BA[10]
4. Cytomegalovirus-associated (CMV-associated) BA[11]

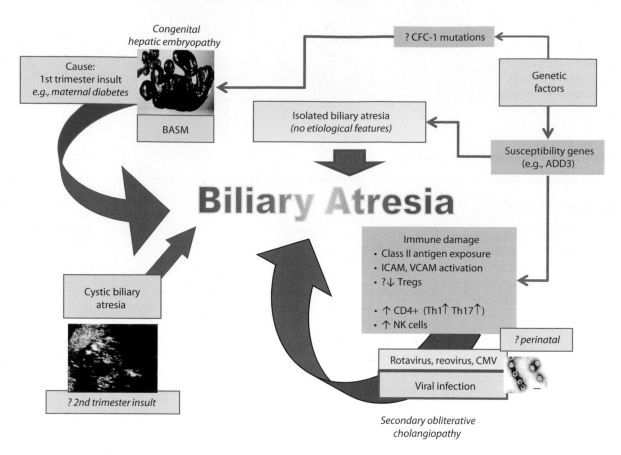

Figure 75.1 Schematic illustration of possible causes of biliary atresia: etiological heterogeneity. (Reproduced with permission from Davenport M, Biliary atresia: From Australia to the zebrafish, *J Pediatr Surg* 2016; 51:200–5.)

There are other relationships, although these are much rarer. Some cases appear to have an association with other gastrointestinal anomalies such as esophageal atresia and jejunal atresia (<2% of large series), and we have reported a small series with a defined chromosomal abnormality (e.g., cat-eye syndrome and chromosome 22 aneuploidy).[12]

We have now begun to use the term *developmental biliary atresia*[13] for those cases where there is almost unequivocal evidence for a prenatal onset and obstruction is evident by the time of birth. This would therefore include BASM (2) and cystic BA (3). By contrast, the onset of occlusion in CMV-associated BA (4) is probably perinatal with occlusion of a patent biliary system by virally mediated damage. Isolated BA (1) remains the most prevalent group, but it is more difficult to be certain of its actual etiology, because there aren't any real clues. Some of these could still be developmental in origin, and others, perinatal in timing.

BASM SYNDROME

We first reported what became known as BASM in 1993,[8] recognizing that splenic anomalies (not just polysplenia) were related in some way to BA and that there was also a peculiar but consistent association with cardiac defects, situs inversus, preduodenal portal vein, and absence of the vena cava (Table 75.1). The reasons for this are still obscure, but it has been suggested

Table 75.1 Spectrum of anomalies in biliary atresia splenic malformation syndrome

Organ system	Malformation
Splenic	Polysplenia, double spleen (95%)
	Asplenia (5%)
Situs determination	Inversus (50%)
Venous	• Preduodenal portal vein (40%)
	• Portosystemic shunt (<2%)
	Vena cava (absence) (50%)
Intestinal development	Malrotation (60%)
Cardiac	ASD, VSD, Fallot's tetralogy, etc. (~40%)
Liver	Normal, "mirror-image," or symmetrical in situs inversus
Biliary appearance	Solid and scanty gallbladder, may be absent. Gallbladder often a midline structure with solid, symmetrical proximal biliary ducts.
Pancreas	Annular (<5%)
Miscellaneous	Immotile cilia syndrome (Kartagener's syndrome)
	Sacral agenesis

that the common factor is simply an embryonic "insult" in a critical window of the developing viscera—perhaps at 30–35 days' gestation. Whether this affects single specific genes or an array of developmental genes or proteins is not known.

Furthermore, at this stage, the only biliary structure is the extrahepatic bile and emerging gallbladder. This appears at about day 20 as an outpouching from the distal foregut and develops into a funnel-shaped structure with a lumen and a gallbladder evident by day 45. It is lined by cholangiocytes derived from foregut endoderm, expressing transcription factors common to the pancreas and duodenum (e.g., PDX-1, PROX-1, HNF-6). The molecular mechanisms regulating this phase of biliary development are not well described in humans, but mice deficient in Pdx-119 or Hes1 (a Notch-dependent transcription factor), Hnf-6, Hnf-1β, or Foxf1 (a transcription factor target for Sonic Hedgehog signaling) can show altered development of the gallbladder with a normal common bile duct (CBD).[14]

The intrahepatic bile duct system develops later from around the seventh week of gestation. It is tempting, therefore, to speculate that the primary failure in BASM is that of the extrahepatic bile duct.

There are also genes that appear to be important in both bile duct development (e.g., JAG1, HNF-6[15]) and visceral and somatic symmetry (e.g., INV, CFC-1[16,17]), although most work has been done in the mouse and actual correlation with mutations in humans is not that good. A possible genetic link was reported by Davit-Spraul et al.,[18] who found an increased frequency of mutations in the CFC-1 gene (on chromosome 2) in patients with BASM, compared to controls.

A further interesting observation is that there is a definite link between maternal diabetes and BASM, in the same way that this condition can cause transposition of the great vessels, double outlet right ventricle, and sacral agenesis (although these do not form part of the usual spectrum of BASM).[8,9]

Finally, a small number of infants with BASM have immotile cilia syndrome (also known as Kartagener's syndrome), and this provides an interesting speculation as to mechanism. Certainly, dysfunctional cilia could be incriminated in the determination of visceral situs during the early days of gestation—leaving it essentially to chance. But how cilial dysfunction interacts with the developing biliary tree is not known. Normally, only rats and squirrel monkeys have ciliated intrahepatic bile ducts, although there may be chemosensory cilia on cholangiocytes in humans.

The macroscopic appearance of the biliary tree and liver is also somewhat different in BASM compared to isolated BA, with frequent absence of the CBD and a miniscule gallbladder and small proximal remnant. The liver is also usually symmetrical, whatever the nature of the abdominal situs.

PATHOLOGY OF BA

This is best described as an *occlusive pan-ductular cholangiopathy* affecting both intrahepatic and extrahepatic bile ducts.

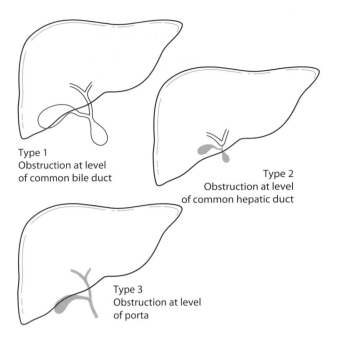

Figure 75.2 Classification of extrahepatic morphology in biliary atresia.

The commonest classification divides BA into three types based on the most proximal level of occlusion of the extrahepatic biliary tree (Figure 75.2). In types 1 and 2, there is a degree of preservation of structure in the intrahepatic bile ducts, but they are still irregular, deformed, and pruned—and do not dilate, even when obstructed. The commonest variant, type 3, occurs where there is typically a solid, dense fibroinflammatory proximal remnant at the porta hepatis. The distal duct may be atrophic, absent, or relatively well preserved—typically as a mucocele. Type 3 intrahepatic bile ducts are usually grossly abnormal with myriad small ductules coalescing at the porta hepatis. Sometimes this can be visualized radiographically as a "cloud."

Extrahepatic cyst formation may be evident and contain clear mucus or bile (depending on preservation with intrahepatic bile ductules). We prefer the name *cystic biliary atresia* for this entity, but the important thing is to distinguish it from simple obstruction in a cystic choledochal malformation.[10] The key to this is the cholangiogram, which will show a distorted, deformed nondilated intrahepatic duct system (if anything) in the former and a well-preserved and "treelike" dilated intrahepatic duct system in the latter. There should also be preservation of a decent epithelial lining in the latter on histology.

CELLULAR KINETICS AND INFLAMMATION IN BA

That BA is not simply a mechanical obstruction of the biliary tree has been obvious for some time now. There is a marked inflammatory process that is present in most types (possibly with the exception of BASM) as evidenced by an obvious mononuclear infiltrate and expression of a variety of adhesion molecules on intrahepatic biliary and vascular epithelial surfaces.[19] Whether this is a primary or secondary phenomenon (to presence of bile outside biliary canaliculi, for instance) is arguable, but there is certainly evidence to support the former as a workable hypothesis.[19,20]

The infiltrate is largely composed of CD4+ T lymphocytes (specifically Th1 and Th17)[21,22] and CD56+ natural killer (NK) cells,[19,23] which exhibit markers for proliferation (CD71+) and activation (particularly LFA-1+ but also CD25+). There is a distinct subset of CD8+ cells, but many studies suggest that these may be less important and lack various markers of activation such as perforin, granzyme B, and Fas ligand.[24]

There is abnormal expression of cell adhesion molecules (proteins involved in cell–cell binding), with both ICAM-1 and VCAM-1 (but not e-selectin) being identifiable on epithelial structures in both the liver and, to a lesser extent, the biliary remnant.[19,25]

We also identified abnormally raised levels of the soluble adhesion molecules ICAM-1 and VCAM-1 in the circulation at the time of Kasai together with rising levels of these and inflammatory cytokines (e.g., IL-2, TNFα) postoperatively.[26,27] After about 6–9 months post-Kasai, these tended to come back down to more normal values (unpublished observation).

The resident (Kupffer cells) or recruited macrophages/monocytes appear to have a crucial role in the development of fibrosis seen in established BA. This may be as both the presenters of antigenic material in the first place and later as the initiating force for fibrosis in the development of chronic liver disease. Tracy et al.[28] in 1996 first showed increases in resident macrophages (CD68+) with marked expression of the lipopolysaccharide receptor, CD14+. Increased levels of both CD68+ cells and its circulating markers (TNFα and IL-18) have been shown impair to prognosis post-Kasai.[27,29]

VIRUSES AND BA

There have been a number of studies based on serology in infants with BA that initially suggested a causal link with perinatal viral infection (originally reovirus type 3[30]) but were later disputed.[31] However, actual viral footprints within the bile ducts have been much harder to demonstrate, and a causal link is still controversial.[32,33] Rauschenfels et al.[34] from Germany looked at wedge liver biopsies obtained from 74 infants at the time of Kasai portoenterostomy (KP) for a panel of DNA and RNA hepatotropic viruses. One or, indeed, more viruses were detected in about one-third of infants, and the detection rate increased with infant age. Rauschenfels et al. suggested that this showed that viral infection was a secondary finding and unlikely to be the specific cause of BA. Zani et al.[11] from our institution showed that there are clinically distinguishing features between infants who are CMV IgM positive (about 10% of overall series) and those who are CMV IgM negative. Infants with CMV IgM associated biliary atresia tended to come to

surgery later, with worse (even if age-matched) liver biochemistry. Furthermore, histologically, the former group was characterized by a marked inflammatory infiltrate and increased fibrosis in their livers compared to the latter. The outcome following KP is also not as good as in infants with CMV IgM –ve BA (Figure 75.3). Other series, possibly where the prevalence of CMV is higher, have not shown such a marked difference.[35]

There is a mouse model of BA where just-born mice can be inoculated with rotavirus (or reovirus or CMV) and who developed jaundice with intrahepatic histology similar to that of BA.[36,37] The nature of the cholangiodestructive pathway can be examined relatively easily, and it can be shown that there is early upregulation of interferon inducers Irf7 and Irf9 genes (proinflammatory genes), with IFN-γ having greater expression at the time of bile duct obstruction.[38–40]

If not actual virally mediated damage, then it may be that we have to postulate another way of cholangiolar damage by suggesting that the virus acts as a trigger and that in some way, there is an immune-mediated destructive process.[19] One would suspect, however, that this process would continue postportoenterostomy and that no native livers would ever drain bile in the long term. There is no real observational evidence that liver loss is inevitable though.

An interesting and novel mechanism of immune damage has been recently suggested based on the observation that

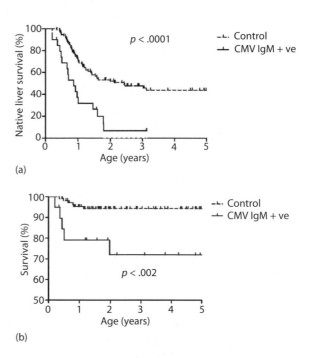

Figure 75.3 Effect of CMV IgM status on **(a)** actuarial native liver survival and **(b)** actuarial true survival. CMV IgM positive (n = 20) versus CMV IgM negative (n = 111) (dotted line). Difference between curves is significant (p < .0001 and p < .002, respectively). (Reproduced with permission from Zani A et al., Cytomegalovirus-associated biliary atresia: An aetiological and prognostic sub-group. *J Pediatr Surg* 2015; 50:1739–45.)

male BA infants have a threefold increase in maternal-origin cells in their livers.[41] These were later shown to be maternal-origin chimeric CD8+ T cells and CD45 NK cells and certainly appear capable of initiating immune cholangiolar damage.[42] This is termed *maternal microchimerism*, and it may be the reason that the destructive process is time limited.

ENVIRONMENTAL ISSUES

There have been outbreaks of BA in commercial farming. One particular famous example was reported from Burrinjuck, New South Wales, Australia, where a specific relationship with pregnant sheep grazing on land around a dam was shown. During a drought, the foreshores of the dam became exposed and colonized by a particular weed known as the red crumbweed (*Dysphania glomulifera* subsp. *glomulifera*). Almost 200 lambs subsequently born were affected by BA-like pathology.[43] In later years, whenever the exact combination of exposed foreshore, weed proliferation, and grazing pregnant livestock occurred, affected offspring were born.

This concept was further developed in the laboratory using the zebra fish model, where the genome can be manipulated and tracked as the larvae are transparent and have a fully developed biliary system by 5 days postfertilization. Potential hepatotoxic compounds derived from the various isoflavonoids found in the red crumbweed identified one, now known as *biliatresone*, which caused biliary maldevelopment[44] (Figure 75.4).

It is possible therefore that BA could arise as a result of maternal exposure to this particular toxin although not likely to be the weed itself there may be similar compounds or metabolism of non-toxic precursors such as betavulgarin which are found in more common plant foods such as sugar beet, beetroot, and chard.[45]

EPIDEMIOLOGY

Given that BA appears to be a diverse disease, it is not surprising that its epidemiology also varies. Infants with *developmental BA* have a marked female predominance not seen in the *isolated BA* group.[8,9,13] Historically, there has been a suggestion of a seasonal variation in incidence,[46,47] though when examined in large national studies, this has never been confirmed.[13,48] The implication if there were more infants with BA born during the winter months is that this might be related to the usual prevalence of viruses during this season.

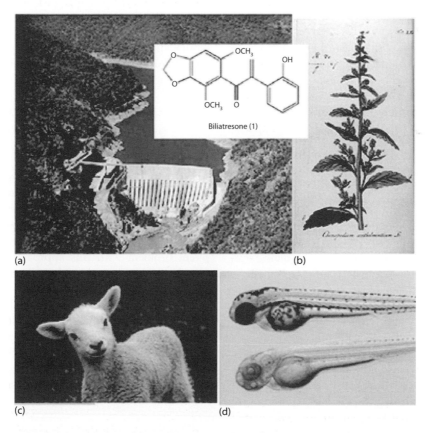

Figure 75.4 The biliatresone story: **(a)** Burunjuk Dam in Australia; **(b)** periods of drought and falling water levels allowed proliferation of the red crumbweed around the foreshore. **(c)** Pregnant ewes were allowed to graze with the following year's lambs developing biliary atresia–like pathology. **(d)** The isolated compound biliatresone was tested for its effects on developing bile ducts in zebra fish larvae. (Reproduced with permission from Davenport M, Biliary atresia: From Australia to the zebrafish, *J Pediatr Surg* 2016; 51:200–5.)

The incidence of BA varies dramatically according to geography. The highest incidences are reported from Asia, with the highest from Taiwan (1 in 5000 live births).[49] In the United Kingdom and Ireland (and much of Europe), there is an incidence of about 1 in 17,000–18,000.[13,48,50] We have reported significant regional differences within the United Kingdom, with some areas having incidences usually seen only in Asia, for instance.[13] We speculate that this may be a reflection of the current multiracial nature of the United Kingdom and, indeed, variation within the different strands of BA (e.g., developmental BA was found to be commoner in infants of Caucasian origin).

CLINICAL FEATURES

In general, infants with BA are born smaller at birth (both developmental and isolated) and fail to thrive thereafter due to fat malabsorption.[13] Antenatal detection is possible in cystic BA, and some syndromic cases may present very early because of their other malformations (e.g., malrotation, cardiac abnormities).[51]

Otherwise, the key features are conjugated jaundice together with pale, unpigmented stools and dark urine (bilirubinuria) in an otherwise healthy neonate. Liver fibrosis and cirrhosis are later developments (even in infants with intrauterine BA evident at birth),[51] and ascites and marked hepatosplenomegaly are rare features not usually seen until about 3 months.

Some infants will present with a bleeding tendency that may be catastrophic, detectable with an elevated INR or prothrombin time, and caused by fat-soluble vitamin K deficiency. This feature was particularly obvious in a recently published study in Asian-origin infants born in the United Kingdom.[52] It also tends to persist post-Kasai even if appropriately supplemented.

LABORATORY FINDINGS

Liver biochemistry will show a conjugated jaundice (variable, but rarely >250 μmol/L), modestly raised transaminases (AST > 100 IU/L), and significantly raised γ-glutamyl transpeptidase (GGT, >200 IU/L). None of this is specific.

The usual differential of a conjugated jaundice is medical and includes TORCH infections (e.g., toxoplasma, rubella, CMV, hepatitis, etc.), genetic conditions (e.g., α-1-antitrypsin deficiency, Alagille's syndrome, progressive familial intrahepatic cholestasis (PFIC) disorders, metabolic conditions (e.g., cystic fibrosis, galactosemia), and parenteral nutrition, together with something termed *neonatal hepatitis*, which is fairly nonspecific but none of the above.

The surgical differential diagnosis is less common and includes obstructed choledochal malformation, inspissated bile syndrome (usually involving the preterm), and spontaneous perforation of the bile duct.[53] The key feature in all these is that they all are able to dilate their intrahepatic bile ducts when obstructed and therefore should be distinguishable simply on ultrasound (US).

ULTRASONOGRAPHY

Ultrasound typically shows a shrunken, atrophic gallbladder with no evidence of filling between feeds. About 20% will show a "normal" gallbladder—which turns out to be a mucocele of the gallbladder in continuity with a relatively preserved CBD and, often, absence of the CHD.

Some centers appear able to actually diagnose BA, simply on US findings.[54,55] However, this is not the experience of other large institutions.[56] A specific finding is said to be the "triangular cord sign" described initially in Korean centers[54] and representing the proximal solid biliary remnant lying in front of the bifurcation of the portal vein. Accuracy rates of >80% have been reported.[55]

MISCELLANEOUS DIAGNOSTIC TECHNIQUES

In King's College Hospital, the prelaparotomy diagnosis of BA is usually made by percutaneous liver biopsy showing histological features characteristic of large duct obstruction, and this is perhaps all that is needed in >80% of cases. It is less accurate the younger the liver, though, and does require an experienced and confident liver pathologist to distinguish these very subtle features.

Other investigations have been reported but are not necessarily essential in every case. Radioisotope (technitium [Tc]-labeled iminodiacetic acid derivatives) hepatobiliary imaging has a role in some centers in showing the need for laparotomy by demonstrating absence of excretion, recognizing that severe forms of medical cholestasis also show this appearance.[57] A far simpler test is placement of a nasoduodenal tube and aspiration over 24 hours, and it is used in many Asian centers with undeniable accuracy but has never really been used in UK or North American centers.

Direct cholangiography is possible and is becoming more popular in those larger centers able to justify the small side-viewing endoscope necessary for infantile ERCPs.[58,59] Failure to cannulate the bile duct is a feature of BA but also may be the result of an inexperienced operator.[50] The current problem with this approach is that such scopes are no longer supported by their usual manufacturer, making repair and replacement difficult.

Diagnostic laparoscopy and cholangiography (± liver biopsy) is a more widely available alternative to ERCP. Direct puncture of the gallbladder is straightforward to show presence or absence of bile, and a catheter or needle can then be used to outline the biliary tree. If an atrophic gallbladder is present without a lumen, this in itself is evidence of BA and warrants further open exploration.

SURGERY—KASAI PORTOENTEROSTOMY

The preoperative management includes correcting the coagulopathy and maybe an antibacterial bowel preparation. Perioperative antibiotics should be effective against aerobic

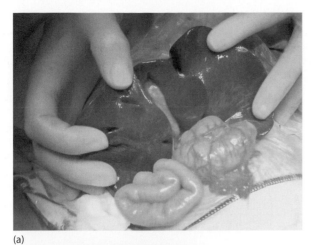

(a)

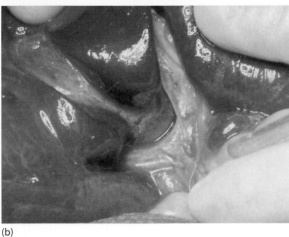

(b)

Figure 75.5 Operative appearance of liver in biliary atresia. **(a)** The liver has been mobilized and is laid out on the anterior abdominal wall. The gallbladder is collapsed and contains no bile, consistent with a type 3 BA. **(b)** The biliary remnants and gallbladder have been removed, leaving a proximal transection of the portal plate flush with liver capsule.

and anaerobic bowel flora. The various stages in this operation can be broken down into the following (Figures 75.5 and 75.6).

Cholangiogram

The diagnosis is always confirmed initially through a limited right-upper-quadrant muscle-cutting incision, allowing access to the gallbladder. To reiterate, the key observation, confirmed by needle aspiration, is presence or absence of bile. Practically, the former can only be caused by a type 1 BA, but more likely, it indicates one of the *medical* causes of a conjugated jaundice listed previously. A cholangiogram should be done to confirm. This may not be possible in some simply because the gallbladder has no lumen—but this in itself is indicative of BA. A "normal" cholangiogram for completeness should show proximal intrahepatic ducts, and sometimes, this

can be difficult, so a small vascular or bulldog clamp on the CBD should aid reflux into the more proximal ducts. Neonatal sclerosing cholangitis (a fairly controversial diagnosis) and various hypoplastic biliary syndromes (e.g., Alagille's syndrome) can then be detected.

Mobilization and eversion of liver

I believe that the most consistent and efficient dissection of the porta hepatis is facilitated by mobilization of the liver. This need not involve division of all the suspensory ligaments and can be limited to just the falciform and the left triangular and still allow the entire organ to be everted onto the anterior abdominal cavity. Care should be taken to warn the anesthetist as this maneuver kinks the cava and reduces venous return.

Portal dissection

Mobilize the gallbladder off its bed and divide the distal CBD. This allows the more proximal biliary remnant to be dissected free from the vascular elements of the porta (right hepatic artery and bifurcating portal vein). Ligate or coagulate portal lymphatics to facilitate exposure. There are always small veins passing from the superior part of the U-shaped portal vein to the portal plate—these also need careful ligation—and then the liver tissue of the caudate lobe should be seen, opposite the undersurface of segment IV. The limit of the left-sided dissection is within the recessus of Rex where the umbilical vein is in continuity with the left portal vein. If this fossa is not open, then the isthmus can be coagulated and divided. The right vascular pedicle divides into right anterior (at the base of the gallbladder bed) and posterior (lying in a small transverse depression, known as Rouviere's fossa) branches, each with an accompanying bile duct remnant. All remnant biliary tissue needs excision, and there is a definite plane of dissection from the capsule of the liver, which can be accessed using scissor dissection. Deeper dissection actually into liver parenchyma ("coring") does not seem to achieve anything useful possibly because of subsequent scarring and occlusion. Avoid coagulation on the portal plate itself and tolerate any bleeding from the edge, which will stop once the Roux loop is sutured in place.

Roux loop and portoenterostomy

A retrocolic Roux loop is constructed measuring 40 cm with the jejunojejunostomy about 10–15 cm from the ligament of Trietz (to get mobility and reduce anastomosis tension). The portoenterostomy must incorporate all the denuded portal plate and should be quite wide (at least 2 cm). I prefer an end-to-side arrangement using fine (e.g., 6/0 PDS) sutures, although other authors argue for an end-to-end arrangement.[60] A second layer can be added at the end posteriorly using adjacent periportal tissue.

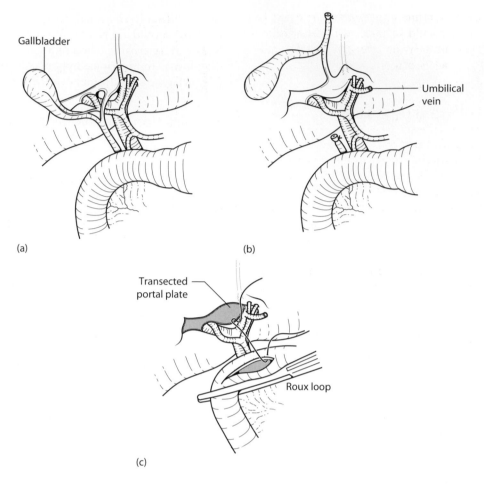

Figure 75.6 Schematic illustration of Kasai portoenterostomy. **(a)** Type 3 biliary atresia. **(b)** Mobilization of gallbladder and division of distal common bile duct. Elevation of biliary remnants and separation from vascular structures at level of porta hepatis (portal vein confluence, right and left hepatic arteries). **(c)** Transection of portal plate from "umbilical point" on left, to around right portal pedicle. Portoenterostomy with 40–45 cm retrocolic Roux loop.

Wound closure needs care as postoperative ascites can test its integrity and strength to the limit. A small drain may help to minimize ascite retention and allow the wound layers to heal. Significant bile leaks don't happen in Kasai operations—almost certainly because there's not that much bile around to leak!

CAVEATS TO SURGERY

Although visible bile-containing ducts may be evident in type 1 or 2 BA and a hepaticojejunostomy performed, it is better that further proximal tissue is resected to the level of (and therefore needing) a portoenterostomy.

Sometimes, on-table evidence of cirrhosis may seem to make a portoenterostomy futile. However, this is rarely absolutely predictable, although obviously more likely in infants of >100 days.[61] A primary transplant may be a better option, but this is arguable.

At times, it has been suggested that a frozen section of the resected portal plate is useful to determine whether ductules are large enough (Figure 75.7). In practice, the aim is to resect all visible bile duct remnants down to, but

not encroaching on, parenchyma—thus, there is nothing further to resect whatever the pathologist reports.

Portoenterostomy in BASM has a worse long-term outcome, and the outcome can be related to the age at which the surgery is performed.[8,62] The extrahepatic bile ducts

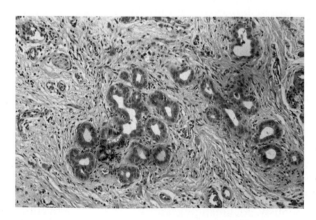

Figure 75.7 Hematoxylin and eosin microphotograph of transected biliary remnant showing multiple biliary ductules lined with relatively normal epithelium, within a fibrous stroma infiltrated by inflammatory mononuclear cells.

are rarely florid, often noninflammatory, and atrophic in appearance. Great care should be taken with the preduodenal portal vein and any aberrant arterial vessels. A malrotation may require Ladd's procedure and influence the construction of the Roux loop.

POSTOPERATIVE MANAGEMENT

Nasogastric drainage and intravenous fluids are required for 2–4 days before starting feeds. There is no clear advantage from continuing prophylactic antibiotics beyond 1 month, though it is the practice of many centers.

All infants, even those rendered anicteric, require fat-soluble vitamin supplementation (both enteral and parenteral), and levels should be monitored assiduously.[52] They should also have access to an appropriate formula milk (e.g., containing medium-chain rather than long-chain triglycerides). Failure to thrive should be aggressively attended to, with nasogastric overnight feeds if necessary. The medical management of the infant or child with serious underlying liver disease is complex, demanding, and absolutely crucial. Most centers achieve this successfully using a multidisciplinary team approach.[63]

Pharmacological improvement in bile flow is possible, by ursodeoxycholic acid, for instance, but only when a degree of flow has been established by surgery and is one of the postulated mechanisms for steroids.[63,64] There is not much evidence for other medications, although a number of Japanese and Chinese centers use the Chinese herb Inchinko-to.[65]

The use of steroids is controversial but appealing, given the possible role of inflammation in the etiology of BA. Actual evidence is somewhat contradictory. Our randomized placebo-controlled trial of oral prednisolone (2 and then 1 mg kg^{-1} day^{-1} in the first month) showed definite improvements in early clearance of jaundice but a lack of a real effect on final results and a need for transplant.[64] We then followed this using an open-label trial and a higher dose (starting at 5 mg kg^{-1} day^{-1}), which showed a statistically significant 15% increase in clearance of jaundice compared to control and placebo in those <70 days at Kasai portoenterostomy.[66] By contrast, a North American placebo-controlled trial came to a different conclusion of "no effect" despite showing the same degree of difference but with smaller numbers in the groups to be compared—hence not reaching statistical significance.[67] There is also evidence emerging to suggest that this early effect may translate to an improved native liver survival rate.[68]

OUTCOME FOLLOWING PORTOENTEROSTOMY

The actuarial 5- and 10-year survival in England and Wales for infants born this century is about 90%[7,69] (Figure 75.8). There will still be deaths: most awaiting transplantation, some as postoperative complications due to transplant, and some due to the lethal effects of other anomalies (e.g., cardiac).

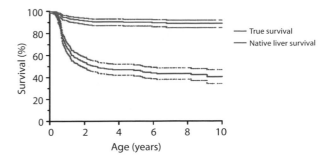

Figure 75.8 Actuarial true and native liver survival curves (median [±95% CI]) for BA (*n* = 443) in England and Wales (1999–2009). (Reproduced with permission from Davenport M et al., Biliary atresia in England and Wales: Results of centralisation and a new benchmark. *J Pediatr Surg* 2011; 46:1689–94.)

We would expect to restore enough bile flow to clear jaundice and achieve normal values for bilirubin in about 50%–60% of infants with isolated BA.[7,69] Most (>90%) of these infants can expect to survive long term with a relatively normal childhood but regular outpatient attendance to monitor progress. Their livers will however seldom be normal, however; in fact, if ever biopsied, they will be highly likely to show histological cirrhosis.[70] The 5- and 10-year native liver survival will be about 45%–50%, therefore.[7,69,70] Care should be taken in the interpretation of such figures if they are from countries with no transplant option, as their native liver survival equates to true survival.[71]

Effect of age at surgery

Cirrhosis and fibrosis are time-dependent phenomena, and it is very reasonable to surmise that the earlier in the disease the cirrhotic process is abbreviated by restoration of bile flow, the better the outcome. However, as stated earlier, BA is a heterogenous disease; especially in isolated BA, the time of onset is not known, and trying to identify a real effect of age on a large series can be difficult (Figure 75.9).[7,71–74] This hypothesis is supported by the observation that in those where there is definite evidence of intrauterine pathology (i.e., developmental BA), there is a marked relationship, while in those described as isolated (presumably much more chronologically heterogenous), this relationship is not seen (within 100 days at least).[55]

Figure 75.10 illustrates this problem. The group is as homogenous as possible, being only infants with isolated BA, and is derived from a single center with two surgeons using the same technique and outcome measured with defined end points (clearance of jaundice). Statistically, as the compendium solid black line is *virtually* flat, this implies no "cutoff" and no effect of age within pragmatic limits. There is actually a *gradual* decline, implying the truth of the original postulate (age worsens outcome) but statistically will require many more numbers to prove it.

Is there any benefit of surgery to those infants who come to surgery at >100 days? Though this is now relatively

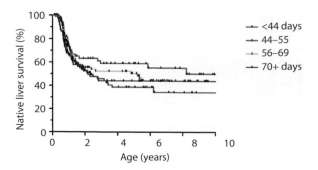

Figure 75.9 Effect of age at Kasai portoenterostomy. Infants with isolated BA (n = 318) were divided by age at surgery. No difference overall (χ = 3.3; p = .34) or for trend (χ^2 = 0.87; p = .35). Specifically, no difference between two outermost curves (χ^2 = 2.1; p = .15). (Reproduced with permission from Davenport M et al., Biliary atresia in England and Wales: Results of centralisation and a new benchmark. *J Pediatr Surg* 2011; 46:1689–94.)

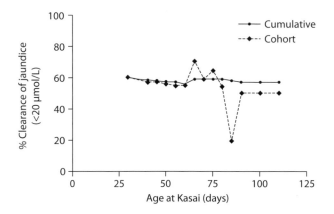

Figure 75.10 Relationship of age at surgery to clearance of jaundice in infants with isolated biliary atresia (n = 177). (Reprinted with permission from Davenport M et al., Surgical outcome in biliary atresia: Etiology affects the influence of age at surgery, *Ann Surg* 2008; 247:694–8.)

infrequent in developed countries, it still occurs. That they are much more likely to have established cirrhosis is true, and their prognosis is certainly less good. Nevertheless, a Kasai as the first step seems reasonable and has been associated with long-term jaundice-free survival in our series.[61] The alternative, of course, is a primary liver transplant.

COMPLICATIONS

Apart from end-stage liver disease in those where there is failure to restore bile flow with development of ascites, malnutrition, and deepening jaundice and that clearly can only be treated by transplantation, there are two major areas of complication.

Cholangitis

This probably occurs in relation to ascending organisms from within the Roux loop, as cholangitis is rare in those

who never show any degree of bile flow post-Kasai. It is reported in up to 50% of large series but seems only to be problematic in the first year postsurgery. It may be characterized by pyrexia, pale stools, increasing jaundice, and other signs of sepsis. Culture of organisms from blood or from liver biopsy is uncommon, and judicious use of early, broad-spectrum antibiotics is advised (e.g., ceftazidime, gentamicin etc.).

Recurrent cholangitis may occur possibly due to the formation of dilated biliary channels or cystic change within the liver acting as a nidus for infection. This should be obvious on US. Unless the cystic change is gross and the underlying liver function good, then this should probably be managed conservatively with prolonged antibiotics, often via a Hickman line. In those who do meet these criteria, it is usually possible to access the cystic change surgically and incorporate it into the preexisting Roux loop. In some cases, there is mechanical obstruction to bile drainage within the Roux loop, and this may be detectable using a radioisotope scan.[75] In older children, newer enteroscopes are now able to visualize the Roux loop directly, and this may be an alternate mode of diagnosis. Laparotomy and Roux loop exploration and revision may be indicated.

Portal hypertension

It is possible to measure portal venous pressure via the obliterated umbilical vein at the time of Kasai portoenterostomy.[76,77] This will show that most infants will have portal hypertension (PHT), but whether this persists will more likely depend upon degree of restoration of bile flow and other dynamic factors.[77] Esophagogastric varices take time to develop but will do so given sustained periods of PHT. The majority of long-term survivors will have endoscopic evidence of varices, although only a proportion will ever bleed. Our recent series review suggested that 22% will have significant varices (having bled or ≥Grade 2).[78] Surveillance endoscopy is recommended in these, although evidence is lacking for the role of prophylactic treatment (e.g., banding). Nonetheless, this is a possible option. We have also looked at a variety of scoring formulas to predict the presence of varices in this group, with the best, the varices prediction rule, to be one involving the serum albumin level and platelet count (Figure 75.11).

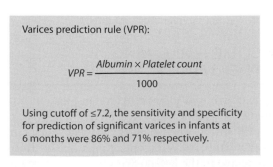

Varices prediction rule (VPR):

$$VPR = \frac{Albumin \times Platelet\ count}{1000}$$

Using cutoff of ≤7.2, the sensitivity and specificity for prediction of significant varices in infants at 6 months were 86% and 71% respectively.

Figure 75.11 Varices prediction rule.

Those who have bled will require some form of endoscopic intervention initially, either sclerotherapy or banding. The former technique is well established but not without complications such as ulceration, stenosis, and stricture formation, and currently should probably be reserved for infants and smaller children where it is not possible to actually pass the banding attachment. There will be a small proportion that have variceal bleeding of such magnitude to require immediate placement of a Sengstaken tube—this is fortunately unusual and can be lifesaving.[79] Following endoscopic control of the varices, an assessment needs to be made about the overall liver reserve. There will be some with excellent restoration of liver function and clearance of jaundice where obliteration of varices is all that is needed; there will be others (typically infants and young children <2 years) where this is simply one part of a failing system, and these need to have an expedited transplant.

ROLE OF LAPAROSCOPIC KASAI PORTOENTEROSTOMY

The tsunami of minimally invasive surgery in the 1990s swept along pediatric as well as general surgeons, and soon, more and more adventurous operations were being described through smaller multiple-port incisions—including the Kasai operation. Small series have been reported but none with good results and most with only limited outcomes.[80,81] At this present time, this operation may be the limit, and a number of enthusiasts are returning to the conventional open approach,[82] though there are still exceptions. The Japanese group led by Yamataka consciously limits the resection level at the porta hepatis, suggesting that it more closely mimics Kasai's original surgery and is certainly more easily achieved laparoscopically.[83]

The reasons for failure in other peoples' hands may be self-evident though—the dissection is unforgiving, meticulous precision is required, and therefore, even with a robot, the operations are simply not comparable. Others have suggested that it may be the effect of the paraphernalia of minimally invasive surgery. For example, Mogilner et al.[84] in an experimental model showed that the higher intra-abdominal pressures of the pneumoperitoneum may increase damage through effects on liver blood flow. A definitive answer has yet to be delivered, but in its absence, practitioners should be cautious—this surgery has a high enough "failure" rate without making it more difficult, and promises of a better cosmetic result and short hospital stays are fatuous in the context of BA. The only person benefiting is the transplant surgeon, who has a reduced amount of adhesions to deal with, and they tend to leave the biggest scars of all!

LIVER TRANSPLANTATION IN BA

This has been available in North America and Western Europe for "failed" Kasai children since the 1980s. It is still a major undertaking, with a consistent risk of postoperative mortality of 6%–15%.[85–87] The risk diminishes beyond the first year, and an actuarial plateau is then reached, although the vast majority still require oral immunosuppression. A few do develop tolerance (perhaps up to 20%) with the possibility to withdraw medication.[88] Longer-term issues such as Epstein–Barr-related posttransplant lymphoproliferative disease (PTLD) (up to 10% of some series) and chronic rejection are still a cause of morbidity and potential mortality.[89]

There are, within all countries and societies, problems coming to terms with ethical attitudes to both cadaveric and living-donor transplantation. Effective use of donor organs and, as a consequence, waiting-list death is still a major issue. There are also lingering technical issues related to size discrepancy, although organ reduction and split-liver transplants ameliorate this in the larger centers.

In conclusion, BA in many respects remains a mysterious disease with its origins cloaked and obscure; in others, though, the need for surgical intervention is straightforward, and the outcome may be somewhat capricious and unpredictable.[79] We believe that centralization of resources is one way to maximize outcome, and this appears to be the pattern now followed in the Netherlands, Denmark, Israel, and Finland. Geographic considerations clearly must play a large role in this, but surely, the time for your Kasai surgeon to be doing one or two a year should be over. Future needs will include better pharmacological options to improve bile flow post-Kasai and modify or at least abbreviate the invariable tendency to liver fibrosis (and hence PHT). This particular characteristic is a real risk to the life of a small infant on a transplant waiting list.

REFERENCES

1. Thomson J. On congenital obliteration of the bile ducts. *Edinburgh Med J* 1891; 37: 523–31.
2. Ladd WE. Congenital atresia and stenosis of the bile ducts. *J Am Med Assoc* 1928; 91: 1082–5.
3. Kasai M, Suzuki S. A new operation for "non-correctable" biliary atresia—Portoenterostomy. *Shijitsu* 1959; 13: 733–9.
4. Shinkai M, Ohhama Y, Take H et al. Long-term outcome of children with biliary atresia who were not transplanted after the Kasai operation: >20-year experience at a children's hospital. *J Pediatr Gastrol Hepatol Nutr* 2009; 48: 443–50.
5. Howard ER, MacClean G, Nio G et al. Survival patterns in biliary atresia and comparison of quality of life of long-term survivors in Japan and England. *J Pediatr Surg* 1996; 31: 1546–51.
6. Starzl TM, Marchioro TL, Von Kaulia KN et al. Homotransplantation of the liver in humans. *Surg Gynecol Obstet* 1963; 117: 659–76.
7. Davenport M, Ville de Goyet J, Stringer MD et al. Seamless management of biliary atresia. England & Wales 1999–2002. *Lancet* 2004; 363: 1354–7.
8. Davenport M, Savage M, Mowat AP, Howard ER. The biliary atresia splenic malformation syndrome. *Surgery* 1993; 113: 662–8.

9. Davenport M, Tizzard SA, Underhill J et al. The biliary atresia splenic malformation syndrome: A 28-year single-center retrospective study. *J Pediatr* 2006; 149: 393–400.

10. Caponcelli E, Knisely AS, Davenport M. Cystic biliary atresia: An etiologic and prognostic subgroup. *J Pediatr Surg* 2008; 43: 1619–24.

11. Zani A, Quaglia A, Hadžić N, Zuckerman M, Davenport M. Cytomegalovirus-associated biliary atresia: An aetiological and prognostic sub-group. *J Pediatr Surg* 2015; 50: 1739–45.

12. Allotey J, Lacaille F, Lees MM et al. Congenital bile duct anomalies (biliary atresia) and chromosome 22 aneuploidy. *J Pediatr Surg.* 2008; 43: 1736–40.

13. Livesey E, Cortina Borja M et al. Epidemiology of biliary atresia in England and Wales (1999–2006). *Arch Dis Child Fetal Neonatal Ed* 2009; 94: F451–5.

14. Kalinichenko VV, Zhou Y, Bhattacharyya D et al. Haploinsufficiency of the mouse Forkhead Box f1 gene causes defects in gall bladder development. *J Biol Chem* 2002; 277: 12369–74.

15. Kohsaka T, Yuan ZR, Guo SX et al. The significance of human jagged 1 mutations detected in severe cases of extrahepatic biliary atresia. *Hepatology* 2002; 36; 904–12.

16. Bamford RN, Roessler E, Burdine RD et al. Loss-of-function mutations in the EGF-CFC gene CFC-1 are associated with human left-right laterality defects. *Nature Genet* 2000; 26: 365–9.

17. Shimadera S, Iwai N, Deguchi E et al. The inv mouse as an experimental model of biliary atresia. *J Pediatr Surg* 2007; 42: 1555–60.

18. Davit-Spraul A, Baussan C, Hermeziu B, Bernard O, Jacquemin E. CFC1 gene involvement in biliary atresia with polysplenia syndrome. *J Pediatr Gastroenterol Nutr.* 2008; 46: 111–2.

19. Davenport M, Gonde C, Redkar R et al. Immunohistochemistry of the liver and biliary tree in extrahepatic biliary atresia. *J Pediatr Surg* 2001; 36: 1017–25.

20. Mack CL, Falta MT, Sullivan AK et al. Oligoclonal expansions of CD4+ and CD8+ T-cells in the target organ of patients with biliary atresia. *Gastroenterology* 2007; 133: 278–87.

21. Mack CL, Tucker RM, Sokol RL et al. Biliary atresia is associated with CD4+ Th1 cell-mediated portal tract inflammation. *Pediatr Res* 2004; 56: 79–87.

22. Hill R, Quaglia A, Hussain M et al. Th-17 cells infiltrate the liver in human biliary atresia and are related to surgical outcome. *J Pediatr Surg* 2015; 50: 1297–303.

23. Shivakumar P, Sabla GE, Whitington P, Chougnet CA, Bezerra JA. Neonatal NK cells target the mouse duct epithelium via Nkg2d and drive tissue-specific injury in experimental biliary atresia. *J Clin Invest* 2009; 119: 2281–90.

24. Ahmed AF, Ohtani H, Nio M et al. CD8+ T cells infiltrating into bile ducts in biliary atresia do not appear to function as cytotoxic T cells: A clinicopathological analysis. *J Pathol* 2001; 193: 383–9.

25. Dillon PW, Belchis D, Minnick K, Tracy T. Differential expression of the major histocompatibility antigens and ICAM-1 on bile duct epithelial cells in biliary atresia. *Tohoku J Exp Med* 2007; 181: 33–40.

26. Davenport M, Gonde C, Narayanaswamy B, Mieli-Vergani G, Tredger JM. Soluble adhesion molecule profiling in preoperative infants with biliary atresia. *J Pediatr Surg* 2005; 40: 1464–9.

27. Narayanaswamy B, Gonde C, Tredger JM et al. Serial circulating markers of inflammation in biliary atresia—Evolution of the post-operative inflammatory process. *Hepatology* 2007; 46: 180–7.

28. Tracy TF, Dillon P, Fox ES et al. The inflammatory response in pediatric biliary disease: Macrophage phenotype and distribution. *J Pediatr Surg* 1996; 31: 121–5.

29. Kobayashi H, Puri P, O'Briain S et al. Hepatic over-expression of MHC Class II antigens and macrophage-associated antigens (CD68) in patients with biliary atresia of poor prognosis. *J Pediatr Surg* 1997; 32; 596–3.

30. Morecki R, Glaser JH, Cho S, Balistreri WF, Horwitz MS. Biliary atresia and reovirus type 3 infection. *N Engl J Med* 1982; 307: 481–4.

31. Brown WR, Sokol RJ, Levin MR et al. Lack of correlation between infection with Reovirus type 3 and extrahepatic biliary atresia. *J Pediatr* 1988; 113: 670–6.

32. Steele MI, Marshall CM, Lloyd RE, Randolph VE. Reovirus type 3 not detected by reverse transcriptase–mediated polymerase chain reaction analysis of preserved tissue from infants with cholestatic liver disease. *Hepatology* 1995; 21: 696–702.

33. Jevon GP, Dimmick JE. Biliary atresia and cytomegalovirus infection: A DNA study. *Pediatr Dev Pathol* 1999; 2: 11–4.

34. Rauschenfels S, Krassmann M, Al-Masri AN et al. Incidence of hepatotropic viruses in biliary atresia. *Eur J Pediatr* 2009; 168: 469–76.

35. Fischler B, Rodensjo P, Nemeth A et al. Cytomegalovirus DNA detection on Guthrie cards in patients with neonatal cholestasis. *Arch Dis Child* 1999; 80: F130–4.

36. Petersen C, Grasshoff S, Luciano L. Diverse morphology of biliary atresia in an animal model. *J Hepatol* 1998; 28: 603–7.

37. Riepenhoff-Talty M, Schaekel K, Clark HF et al. Group A rotaviruses produce extrahepatic biliary obstruction in orally inoculated newborn mice. *Pediatr Res* 1993; 33: 394–9.

38. Carvalho E, Liu C, Shivakumar P et al. Analysis of the biliary transcriptome in experimental biliary atresia. *Gastroenterology* 2005; 129: 713–7.

39. Bezerra JA, Tiao G, Ryckman FC et al. Genetic induction of proinflammatory immunity in children with biliary atresia. *Lancet* 2002; 360: 1653–9.

40. Zhang DY, Sabla G, Shivakumar P et al. Coordinate expression of regulatory genes differentiates embryonic and perinatal forms of biliary atresia. *Hepatology* 2004; 39: 954–62.

41. Hayashida M, Nishimoto Y, Matsuura T et al. The evidence of maternal microchimerism in biliary atresia using fluorescent in situ hybridization. *J Pediatr Surg* 2007; 42: 2097–101.

42. Muraji T, Hosaka N, Irie N et al. Maternal microchimerism in underlying pathogenesis of biliary atresia: Quantification and phenotypes of maternal cells in the liver. *Pediatrics* 2008; 121: 517–21.

43. Harper P, Plant JW, Unger DB. Congenital biliary atresia and jaundice in lambs and calves. *Aust Vet J* 1990; 67: 18–22.

44. Lorent K, Gong W, Koo KA et al. Identification of a plant isoflavonoid that causes biliary atresia. *Sci Transl Med* 2015; 7(286): 286ra67. doi: 10.1126/sci translmed.aaa1652.

45. Davenport M. Biliary atresia: From Australia to the zebrafish. *J Pediatr Surg* 2016; 51: 200–5.

46. Yoon PW, Bresee JS, Olney RS et al. Epidemiology of biliary atresia: A population based study. *Pediatrics* 1998; 101: 729–30.

47. The NS, Honein MA, Caton AR et al. Risk factors for isolated biliary atresia, National Birth Defects Prevention Study, 1997–2002. *Am J Med Genet A* 2007; 143A: 2274–84.

48. Chardot C, Carton M, Spire-Bendelac N et al. Epidemiology of biliary atresia in France: A national study 1986–96. *J Hepatol* 1999; 31: 1006–13.

49. Hsiao CH, Chang MH, Chen HL et al. Universal screening for biliary atresia using an infant stool color card in Taiwan. *Hepatology* 2008; 47: 1233–40.

50. Serinet MO, Broué P, Jacquemin E et al. Management of patients with biliary atresia in France: Results of a decentralized policy 1986–2002. *Hepatology* 2006; 44: 75–84.

51. Makin E, Quaglia A, Kvist N et al. Congenital biliary atresia: Liver injury begins at birth. *J Pediatr Surg* 2009; 44: 630–3.

52. Ng J, Paul A, Wright N, Hadzic N, Davenport M. vitamin D levels in infants with biliary atresia: Pre and post Kasai portoenterostomy. *J Pediatr Gastroenterol Nutr.* 2016 May; 62(5): 746–50.

53. Davenport M, Betalli P, D'Antiga L et al. The spectrum of surgical jaundice in infancy. *J Pediatr Surg* 2003; 38: 1471–9.

54. Park WH, Choi SO, Lee HJ et al. A new diagnostic approach to biliary atresia with emphasis on the ultrasonographic triangular cord sign: Comparison of ultrasonography, hepatobiliary scintigraphy, and liver needle biopsy in the evaluation of infantile cholestasis. *J Pediatr Surg* 1997; 32: 1555–9.

55. Humphrey TM, Stringer MD. Biliary atresia: US diagnosis. *Radiology* 2007; 244: 845–51.

56. Jancelewicz T, Barmherzig R, Chung CT et al. A screening algorithm for the efficient exclusion of biliary atresia in infants with cholestatic jaundice. *J Pediatr Surg* 2015; 50(3): 363–70. doi: 10.1016/j .jpedsurg.2014.08.014.

57. Sevilla A, Howman-Giles R, Saleh H et al. Hepatobiliary scintigraphy with SPECT in infancy. *Clin Nucl Med* 2007; 32: 16–23.

58. Shanmugam NP, Harrison PM, Devlin J et al. Selective use of endoscopic retrograde cholangiopancreatography in the diagnosis of biliary atresia in infants younger than 100 days. *J Pediatr Gastroenterol Nutr* 2009; 49: 435–41.

59. Petersen C, Meier PN, Schneider A et al. Endoscopic retrograde cholangiopancreatography prior to explorative laparotomy avoids unnecessary surgery in patients suspected for biliary atresia. *J Hepatol* 2009; 51: 1055–60.

60. Kimura K. Biliary atresia. In: Puri P (ed). *Newborn Surgery*, 1st edn. Oxford: Butterworth-Heinemann, 1996: 423–32.

61. Davenport M, Puricelli V, Farrant P et al. The outcome of the older (>100 days) infant with biliary atresia. *J Pediatr Surg* 2004; 39: 575–81.

62. Davenport M, Caponcelli E, Livesey E, Hadzic N, Howard E. Surgical outcome in biliary atresia: Etiology affects the influence of age at surgery. *Ann Surg* 2008; 247: 694–8.

63. Thakur R, Davenport M. Improving treatment outcomes in patients with biliary atresia. *Exp Opin Orphan Drugs* 2015; 2: 12, 1267–77.

64. Davenport M, Stringer MD, Tizzard SA et al. Randomized, double-blind, placebo-controlled trial of corticosteroids after Kasai portoenterostomy for biliary atresia. *Hepatology* 2007; 46: 1821–7.

65. Iinuma Y, Kubota M, Yagi M et al. Effects of the herbal medicine Inchinko-to on liver function in postoperative patients with biliary atresia—A pilot study. *J Pediatr Surg* 2003; 38: 1607–11.

66. Davenport M, Tizzard SA, Parsons C, Hadzic N. Single surgeon, single centre: Experience with steroids in biliary atresia. *J Hepatol* 2013; 59: 1054–8.

67. Bezerra JA, Spino C, Magee JC et al. Use of corticosteroids after hepatoportoenterostomy for bile drainage in infants with biliary atresia: The START randomized clinical trial. *JAMA* 2014; 311: 1750–9.

68. Tyraskis A, Davenport M. Steroids after the Kasai procedure for biliary atresia—The effect of age at Kasai portoenterostomy. *Pediatr Surg Int* 2016; 32: 193–200.

69. Davenport M, Ong E, Sharif K et al. Biliary atresia in England and Wales: Results of centralisation and a new benchmark. *J Pediatr Surg* 2011; 46: 1689–94.

70. Hadzić N, Davenport M, Tizzard S et al. Long-term survival following Kasai portoenterostomy: Is chronic liver disease inevitable? *J Pediatr Gastroenterol Nutr* 2003; 37: 430–3.

71. Nio M, Ohi R, Miyano T et al. Five- and 10-year survival rates after surgery for biliary atresia: A report from the Japanese Biliary Atresia Registry. *J Pediatr Surg* 2003; 38: 997–1000.

72. Davenport M, Kerkar N, Mieli-Vergani G, Mowat AP, Howard ER. Biliary atresia: The King's College Hospital experience (1974–1995). *J Pediatr Surg* 1997; 32: 479–85.

73. Altman RP, Lilly JR, Greenfield et al. A multivariate risk factor analysis of the portoenterostomy (Kasai) procedure for biliary atresia: 25 years of experience from two centres. *Ann Surg* 1997; 226: 348–53.

74. Superina R, Magee JC, Brandt ML et al. The anatomic pattern of biliary atresia identified at time of Kasai hepatoportoenterostomy and early postoperative clearance of jaundice are significant predictors of transplant-free survival. *Ann Surg* 2011; 254: 577–85.

75. Houben C, Phelan S, Davenport M. Late-presenting cholangitis and Roux loop obstruction after Kasai portoenterostomy for biliary atresia. *J Pediatr Surg* 2006; 41: 1159–64.

76. Duché M, Fabre M, Kretzschmar B et al. Prognostic value of portal pressure at the time of Kasai operation in patients with biliary atresia. *J Pediatr Gastroenterol Nutr* 2006; 43: 640–5.

77. Shalaby A, Davenport M. Portal venous pressure in biliary atresia. *J Pediatr Surg* 2012; 47: 363–6.

78. Isted A, Grammatikopoulos T, Davenport M. Prediction of esophageal varices in biliary atresia: Derivation of the "varices prediction rule," a novel noninvasive predictor. *J Pediatr Surg* 2015; 50: 1734–8.

79. Jayakumar S, Patel S, Davenport M, Ade-Ajayi N. Surviving Sengstaken. *J Pediatr Surgery* 2015; 50: 1142–6.

80. Esteves E, Clemente Neto E, Ottaiano Neto M, Devanir J Jr, Esteves Pereira R. Laparoscopic Kasai portoenterostomy for biliary atresia. *Pediatr Surg Int* 2002; 18: 737–40.

81. Dutta S, Woo R, Albanese CT. Minimal access portoenterostomy: Advantages and disadvantages of standard laparoscopic and robotic techniques. *J Laparoendosc Adv Surg Tech A* 2007; 17: 258–64.

82. Wong KK, Chung PH, Chan KL, Fan ST, Tam PK. Should open Kasai portoenterostomy be performed for biliary atresia in the era of laparoscopy? *Pediatr Surg Int* 2008; 24: 931–3.

83. Wada M, Nakamura H, Koga H et al. Experience of treating biliary atresia with three types of portoenterostomy at a single institution: Extended, modified Kasai, and laparoscopic modified Kasai. *Pediatr Surg Int* 2014; 30: 863–70.

84. Mogilner J, Sukhotnik I, Brod V et al. Effect of elevated intra-abdominal pressure on portal vein and superior mesenteric artery blood flow in a rat. *Laparoendosc Adv Surg Tech A* 2009; 19 Suppl 1: S59–62.

85. Barshes NR, Lee TC, Balkrishnan R et al. Orthotopic liver transplantation for biliary atresia: The U.S. experience. *Liver Transp* 2005; 11: 1193–200.

86. Fouquet V, Alves A, Branchereau S et al. Long-term outcome of pediatric liver transplantation for biliary atresia: A 10-year follow-up in a single center. *Liver Transpl* 2008; 11: 152–60.

87. Cowles RA, Lobritto SJ, Ventura KA et al. Timing of liver transplantation in biliary atresia—Results in 71 children managed by a multidisciplinary team. *J Pediatr Surg* 2008; 43: 1605–9.

88. Lerut J, Sanchez-Fueyo A. An appraisal of tolerance in liver transplantation. *Am J Transplant* 2006; 6: 1774–80.

89. Hartley JL, Davenport M, Kelly DA. Biliary atresia. *Lancet* 2009; 374 (9702): 1704–13

76

Congenital biliary dilatation

HIROYUKI KOGA AND ATSUYUKI YAMATAKA

INTRODUCTION

Congenital biliary dilatation (CBD), or choledochal cyst, is a cystic or fusiform dilatation of the common bile duct that is uncommon in Caucasians. There is little doubt that CBD is a congenital lesion with a strong hereditary component, which may explain the higher incidence seen in Asia, and its familial occurrence in siblings and twins.[1–3] Traditionally, approximately half become symptomatic in infancy, and neonatal cases have been uncommon. However, with advances in diagnostic imaging techniques, its incidence is increasing, particularly in neonates because of an increase in prenatally diagnosed CBD.[4–12] In our series, about 20% of patients were detected either neonatally or antenatally, and interestingly, the ratio of cystic to fusiform-type CBD neonatally or antenatally is 20:1, in contrast to an overall ratio of 5:3.[13]

The treatment of CBD in early infancy has unique aspects that must be considered in relation to the risks of surgery itself and the size and physiological/immunological immaturity of the patient. Because CBD is commonly associated with pancreaticobiliary malunion (PBMU) involving concurrent anomalies of the common channel, pancreatic duct, and intrahepatic bile duct (IHBD), the importance of cholangiography both preoperatively and intraoperatively cannot be overemphasized. If these anomalies go unnoticed by surgeons, they may lead to injury during surgery and cause serious postoperative morbidity. Primary cyst excision (CE) with biliary reconstruction to avoid two-way reflux of bile and pancreatic secretions is now the standard procedure of choice.

ETIOLOGY

Various theories have been proposed for the etiology of CBD, but two factors are known to be causal—weakness of the wall of the common bile duct and obstruction distal to it. Spitz[14] stressed an obstructive factor that appears early in development based on his experimental study in sheep, in which cystic dilatation of the common bile duct could be induced by ligation of the distal end of the choledochus only in neonatal lambs and at no other stages of development. The author's animal research has confirmed this hypothesis,[15–19] and our radiologic and histologic studies on patients with CBD clearly demonstrate that distal stenosis is closely associated with cystic dilatation of the common bile duct, and that the site of stenosis is related to an abnormal choledochopancreatic ductal junction.[16,19,20] Jona et al.[21] purported that the pathogenesis of CBD-associated PBMU may be related to faulty budding of the primitive ventral pancreas. Wong and Lister[22] conducted research on human fetuses and demonstrated that the choledochopancreatic junction lies outside the duodenal wall before the eighth week of gestation, whereupon it moves inward toward the duodenal lumen, suggesting that an anomalous junction may be caused by arrest of this migration, while Tanaka[23,24] proposed that regression of the terminal choledochus and canalization of the ventral pancreatic duct (W1) caused by sinistral dislocation of the ventral pancreas are responsible for PBMU.

In recent years, cholangiography has identified anomalies of the pancreaticobiliary ductal system in association with CBD, which may allow reflux of pancreatic enzymes and subsequent dissolution of duct walls. This is known as the long common channel theory and was first proposed by Babbit in 1969.[25] Since then, numerous abnormal arrangements of the pancreaticobiliary junction associated with CBD have been reported by others based on the results of endoscopic retrograde cholangiopancreatography (ERCP), percutaneous transhepatic cholangiography, and intraoperative cholangiography. This theory is further supported by the high amylase content of fluid aspirated from dilated ducts in patients with CBD. A dilated common channel and anomalous pancreatic duct are also frequently observed, which may be responsible for the formation of protein plugs or pancreatic stones, often associated with pancreatitis. It is generally recognized that a number of patients with an anomalous long common channel and high amylase level in the gallbladder show no dilatation of the choledochus, although some had gallbladder carcinoma.[26] But, the authors' research in which choledochopancreatostomy was performed in puppies to allow regurgitation of pancreatic fluid into the common bile duct found that the chemical reaction of refluxed pancreatic fluid in the bile duct was extremely mild.[27] Interestingly, in this animal model, fusiform rather than cystic dilatation of the common bile duct was induced.

Although Babbit[25] stressed that pancreatic fluid is the most likely factor causing edema and eventual fibrosis of the distal common bile duct as well as weakness of the choledochal wall, a diagnosis of CBD can be made antenatally as early as 15–20 weeks' gestation,[9–11,28] at which time pancreatic acini are only just beginning to appear, zymogen granules are immature, and there is no evidence of secretion seen on electron microscopy.[29] Thus, the chemical reaction of pancreatic fluid on the bile duct has not been clarified in the antenatal period, and even in the neonate, the pancreas has not matured enough to produce

functional enzymes,[30] so the role of pancreatic fluid in CBD formation may be overrated.

In spite of these findings, controversy surrounds the cause of the stenosis distal to the dilated common bile duct. The authors believe that an anomalous choledochopancreatic duct junction and congenital stenosis are the basic causative factors of CBD, at least in perinatal and young infants, rather than weakness of the duct wall caused by reflux of pancreatic fluid. Both PBMU and stenosis are associated with abnormal development of the ventral pancreatic duct and biliary duct system.

CLASSIFICATION

Alonso-Lej et al.,[31] Todani et al.,[32] and Komi et al.[33] have described classifications for CBD based on anatomy and cholangiography of the hepatobiliary duct system or PBMU. Classification based on the association with PBMU is presented in Figure 76.1.

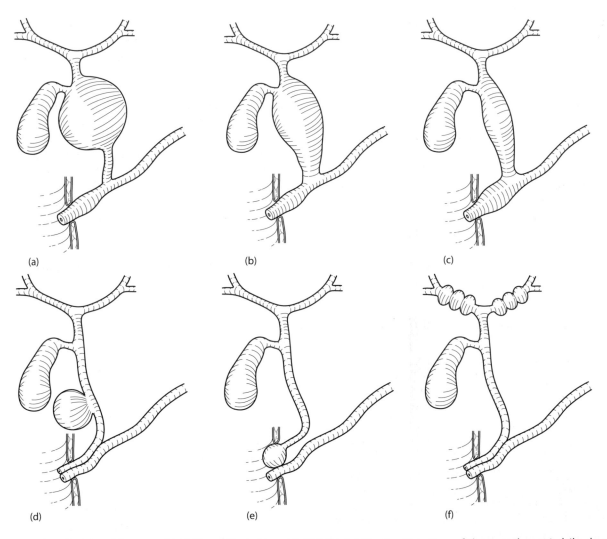

(a)

(b)

(c)

(d)

(e)

(f)

Figure 76.1 Classification of congenital biliary dilatation with PBMU. **(a)** Cystic dilatation of the extrahepatic bile duct. **(b)** Fusiform dilatation of the extrahepatic bile duct. **(c)** Forme fruste type. Without PBMU. **(d)** Cystic diverticulum of the common bile duct. **(e)** Choledochocele (diverticulum of the distal common bile duct). **(f)** Intrahepatic bile duct dilatation alone (Caroli disease). (With kind permission from Springer Science+Business Media: *Pediatric Surgery*, Puri P., Hollwarth M. (eds), Springer Surgery Atlas Series, 2006, p. 373, Miyano T., Urao M., Yamataka A., figure 34.1a–f.)

CLINICAL SIGNS AND SYMPTOMS

Clinical manifestations of CBD differ according to age. Neonates and young infants usually present with an abdominal mass, or obstructive jaundice, and acholic stools, depending on the degree of obstruction. Some present with a huge upper abdominal mass with or without jaundice. Some cases can even resemble correctable biliary atresia except that with CBD, there is a patent communication with the duodenum and a well-developed IHBD tree. In older children, the classical triad of pain, mass, and jaundice may be present. Fever and vomiting may also occur. The pattern of pain has been described as being similar to that of recurrent pancreatitis, in which a high serum amylase level is often present. However, in our series, there was no clinical evidence of pancreatitis in the neonate, and amylase levels were not found to be elevated. CBD should always be considered in the differential diagnosis of a child with abdominal signs and symptoms; the essentials of management are the same. Furthermore, we should keep in mind that there may be an association of the malignancy at the time of primary CE. The youngest case of cholangiocarcinoma associated with CBD at the time of primary CE is a 3-year-old boy.[34] Recently, we also encountered a 3 year-old boy who was found to have a carcinoma in situ in the cyst at the time of primary CE.

DIAGNOSIS

Currently, abdominal ultrasonography (US) is the best method for detecting CBD, even though it does not permit visualization of the entire duct system and is also not sensitive enough to demonstrate a non-dilated common channel and pancreatic duct. However, routine antenatal US performed mainly for dating purposes has been of increasing value for detecting fetal anomalies,[4–11,28] and the number of neonates detected as having incidental CBD has increased significantly (Figure 76.2). CBD has been detected at routine

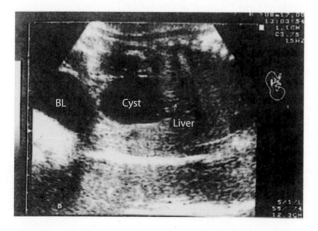

Figure 76.2 Antenatal ultrasound at 32 weeks' gestation. Sagittal view. A cystic structure is seen to be connected to the liver via a short duct (arrow). Bl: bladder. (From Miyano T., Yamataka A., in Puri P. (ed), *Newborn Surgery* (2nd ed), Edward Arnold, p. 591, figure 62.2, 2003; same figure.)

prenatal ultrasound examinations as early as 15 weeks' gestation.[9,10] Typical findings on high-resolution US are of a cyst in the porta hepatitis. These findings may be confused with duodenal atresia, biliary atresia, ovarian cysts, duplication cysts, and mesenteric cysts. Having a skilled and experienced sonologist performing the prenatal ultrasound has been critical in increasing both the sensitivity and specificity of prenatal ultrasound for CBD. Fetal magnetic resonance imaging (MRI) has additionally been performed to aid in the diagnosis. Both imaging techniques may increase the diagnostic yield in a complementary fashion.

For thorough assessment of CBD, it is important to investigate for coexisting PBMU, and anomalies of the pancreatic duct, intrahepatic ducts, and extrahepatic duct. ERCP can accurately delineate the configuration of the pancreaticobiliary duct system in detail and is unlikely to be replaced by other investigations, especially in cases where fine detail is required preoperatively. In the past, ERCP was routinely performed for the diagnosis of biliary malformations in infants and neonates in many centers in Japan, with a reasonable success rate.[35] However, it is an invasive procedure, especially in children, and therefore is unsuitable for repeated use and is contraindicated during acute pancreatitis.

The authors and others[36,37] have shown that magnetic resonance cholangiopancreatography (MRCP) can provide excellent visualization of the pancreaticobiliary ducts in patients with CBD, allowing narrowing, dilatation, and filling defects of the ducts to be detected with medium to high degrees of accuracy (Figure 76.3). Because MRCP is noninvasive, it can partially replace ERCP as a diagnostic tool for the evaluation of anatomic anomalies of the pancreaticobiliary tract, where it is available, but there are limitations of patient size, weight, and age for the use of MRCP. Another advantage of MRCP over ERCP is that the pancreatic duct can be visualized upstream to an obstruction or area of stenosis. Due to the improved quality of MRCP, ERCP, nowadays, is rarely indicated.

If preoperative imaging can allow clear visualization of the entire biliopancreatic ductal system, including the intrahepatic and extrahepatic bile ducts, and pancreatic duct in detail, intraoperative cholangiography is unnecessary; however, if sufficient information is not obtained, it must be performed. Furthermore, if the cyst is too large, intraoperative cholangiography via the gallbladder or directly via the common bile duct is useless. In such cases, intraoperative cholangiography should be performed separately for the IHBD and distal common bile duct by a selective technique during CE.

SURGERY

Choice of operative procedures

CE is currently the definitive treatment for CBD regardless of age or symptomatology because internal drainage, a commonly used treatment in the past, is associated with high morbidity and high risk for carcinoma. Basically, the only

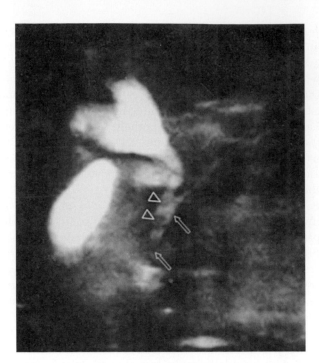

Figure 76.3 Magnetic resonance cholangiopancreatography (MRCP) in a patient with congenital biliary dilatation showing fusiform dilatation of the extrahepatic bile duct, long common channel (between arrows), protein plugs (arrowheads), and pancreatic duct. (With kind permission from Springer Science+Business Media: *Pediatric Surgery*, Puri P., Hollwarth M. (eds), 2009, p. 548, Yamataka A., Kato Y., figure 56.2.)

difference between operative procedures available is the type of biliary reconstruction performed, although the level of transection of the common hepatic duct and the level of excision of the intrapancreatic bile duct are controversial. Although most surgeons use a Roux-en-Y hepaticojejunostomy, some[38,39] recommend a wide anastomosis at the level of the hepatic hilum to allow free drainage of bile in order to prevent postoperative anastomotic stricture and stone formation. The authors[40] recommend conventional hepaticojejunostomy, while others prefer hepaticoduodenostomy. Whatever type of biliary reconstruction is used, satisfactory surgical outcome with low early morbidity is to be expected, but postoperative complications after CE, especially in the long term, generally occur more often if dilated IHBD is present. In our experience, hepaticoduodenostomy is not ideal for biliary reconstruction because of a high incidence of complications due to duodenogastric bile reflux.[40] Todani et al.[41] encountered a case of hilar bile duct carcinoma that developed 19 years after primary CE and hepaticoduodenostomy. Although Todani's team preferred hepaticoduodenostomy because they believed it was more physiologic, they have since abandoned hepaticoduodenostomy after CE and now perform hepaticojejunostomy. However, in the laparoscopic era, there are increasing reports concluding that laparoscopic CE with hepaticoduodenostomy is safe and feasible and is not inferior to hepaticojejunostomy,[42] and furthermore, that laparoscopic CE with both hepaticojejunostomy

and hepaticoduodenostomy reconstruction appears to be safe and has equivalent outcomes to open procedures in our series.[43] However, the follow-up length in these reports is short term in all. Hepaticoenterostomy (HE) at the hepatic hilum is indicated in specific cases only, such as in patients with dilated IHBD with stenosis in the common hepatic duct, or adolescent patients with severe inflammation of the common hepatic duct.

Timing of surgery

Some pediatric surgeons recommend primary CE soon after diagnosis, including prenatally diagnosed cases;[6,8,10,44–46] however, in the authors' experience,[14,47] CE need not be performed hastily if jaundice is not present. Rather, patients should be thoroughly assessed and surgery planned and performed by experienced, well-trained pediatric surgeons. In cases of bile peritonitis following perforation, severe cholangitis, poor general condition, or huge dilated CBD in neonates, external biliary drainage is recommended by either percutaneous transhepatic cholangiodrainage or direct percutaneous cyst drainage. Subsequently, delayed CE may be carried out 1–3 months later.

Neonates with CBD should receive standard medical management and nutritional support preoperatively and postoperatively; the importance of thorough preoperative assessment cannot be overemphasized. However, the timing of surgery for neonates is highly controversial despite increasing reports about the management of asymptomatic CBD detected in the antenatal or neonatal period. Diao et al.[46] mentioned that prenatally diagnosed CBD is a distinct group with a tendency of developing liver fibrosis immediately after birth and thus, early surgical intervention is warranted in the neonatal period. However, according to the authors' experience, developing liver fibrosis in CBD is extremely rare, although there have been a few cases of neonates already having liver fibrosis at the time of diagnosis; thus, the authors believe that if the neonates are asymptomatic, they, including prenatally diagnosed cases, should not be treated in the neonatal period but instead be treated around the age of 3 months, since there is an unacceptably high incidence of anastomotic leakage if treated in the neonatal period.[48] On the other hand, neonates should be treated by early surgery if they are jaundiced or have hepatic fibrosis; for example, Dewbury et al.[4] reported that a laparotomy at 10 days of age confirmed a prenatally diagnosed CBD associated with severe hepatic fibrosis, Early surgery provides the opportunity to exclude biliary atresia; prevent biliary and hepatic complications such as liver fibrosis, which can progress rapidly in cases with biliary obstruction;[4,10,45] reverse fibrosis; reduce the risk for cholangitis; prevent accumulation of biliary sludge; relieve obstructive jaundice; as well as prevent cyst perforation.[6]

Complete excision

Complete (full-thickness) excision of the cyst is much easier in neonates and young infants, because the wall of the dilated common bile duct is generally thin and there are few adhesions to surrounding structures, such as the portal vein.[49,50] Aspiration of the cyst prior to dissection makes surgery easier if the cyst is large. The cyst should be incised in the middle portion close to the duodenum, because there is often an anomalous opening of the hepatic duct, i.e., a separate opening or opening into the distal part of the cyst. The cyst is then transected after careful circumferential dissection from the hepatic artery and portal vein. Subsequently, the distal portion is dissected and excised, taking care to completely remove the dilated segment at the level of the caliber change in order to prevent malignant transformation of the remaining cyst epithelium. If the cyst has no distinct caliber change (i.e., fusiform), it should be excised just above the choledochopancreatic junction, and the stump double-sutured, ligated, and transected (Figure 76.4). If protein plugs are found in the common channel, intraoperative endoscopy should be used to wash them toward the duodenum to avoid postoperative stone formation and pancreatitis. Finally, the common hepatic duct is transected at the level of distinct caliber change to leave an adequate length for HE.

Mucosectomy/biliary reconstruction

If CE of the distal portion is difficult due to inflammation or adhesions, mucosectomy[45,47] of the distal portion of the cyst is recommended, in order to avoid damage to the pancreatic duct, hepatic artery, and portal vein, and also to prevent the residual epithelium of the distal portion of the cyst from undergoing malignant transformation (Figure 76.5). However, in neonates, infants, and small children, mucosectomy is rarely indicated because there is little inflammation around the cyst wall. Biliary reconstruction in neonates and infants is technically involved because anastomoses are often small and so should only be undertaken by experienced pediatric surgeons. Some surgeons overcome this problem by partially incising the mouth of the stoma of the anastomosis to widen it. On occasion, the authors have encountered luminal stenosis of macroscopically normal common hepatic ducts at the time of CE, which was considered to be secondary to fibrosis, probably as a consequence of inflammation associated with previous perforation.

Although an end-to-side anastomosis was initially used, the authors now prefer end-to-end anastomosis during Roux-en-Y hepaticojejunostomy, because drainage is more streamlined, with less possibility of bile stasis (Figure 76.6). With end-to-side anastomosis, there was overgrowth of the blind end, causing adhesive bowel obstruction between the blind pouch and jejunum in one case and stone formation in the blind pouch in another (Figure 76.7).[47] Bile stasis in the blind pouch can also cause stone formation in the IHBD dilatation at the porta hepatis. If end-to-side anastomosis is unavoidable, the common hepatic duct should be anastomosed as close as possible to the closed end of the blind pouch so there will be no blind pouch at the anastomosis

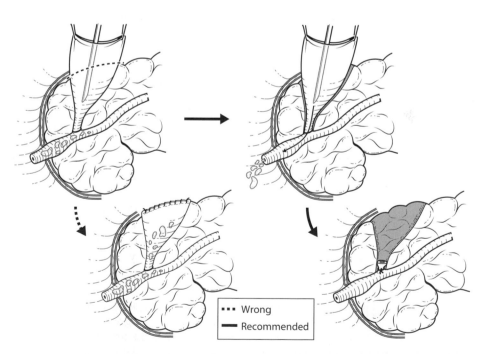

■■■ Wrong
— Recommended

Figure 76.4 Diagram of intraoperative endoscopy of the bile duct distal to a cyst with debris and protein plug. If the distal common bile duct is resected along the red line, over time, a cyst will reform around the distal duct left within the pancreas, leading to recurrent pancreatitis, stone formation, in the residual cyst, or malignant changes in the residual cyst. In contrast, if the distal duct is resected along the blue line, that is, just above the pancreaticobiliary ductal junction, cyst reformation due to residual duct within the pancreas is unlikely. (With kind permission from Springer Science+Business Media: *Pediatric Surgery*, Puri P., Hollwarth M. (eds), Springer Surgery Atlas Series, 2006, p. 381, Miyano T., Urao M., Yamataka A., figures 34.9–34.12.)

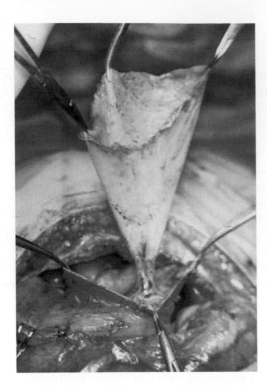

Figure 76.5 Mucosectomy of distal portion of congenital biliary dilatation. (With kind permission from Springer Science+Business Media: Pediatric Surgery, Puri P., Hollwarth M. (eds), *Springer Surgery* Atlas Series, 2006, p. 377, Miyano T., Urao M., Yamataka A., figure 34.5.)

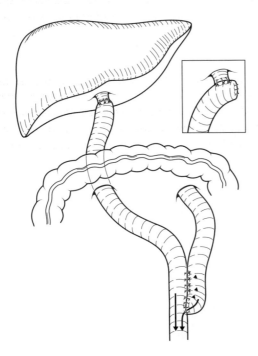

Figure 76.6 Adequate Roux-en-Y (RY) hepaticojejunostomy at the time of cyst excision. Arrowheads indicate approximated native jejunum and distal RY limb. Arrows indicate smooth flow without reflux of small bowel contents. (With kind permission from Springer Science+Business Media: *Pediatric Surgery*, Puri P., Hollwarth M. (eds), 2009, p. 548, Yamataka A., Kato Y., figure 56.12.)

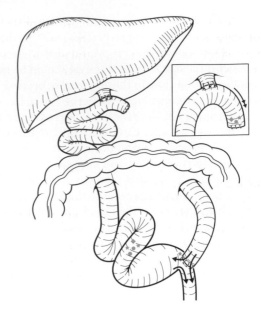

Figure 76.7 Inadequate Roux-en-Y (RY) hepaticojejunostomy (HJ) at the time of cyst excision. Note HJ far from the closed end of the blind pouch (arrowhead). Double arrows in the inset indicate elongation of the blind pouch. Arrow with an asterisk indicates reflux of jejunal contents into the RY limb through a T-shaped RY jejuno-jejunostomy. (With kind permission from Springer Science+Business Media: *Pediatric Surgery*, Puri P., Hollwarth M. (eds), 2009, p. 553, Yamataka A., Kato Y., figure 56.13.)

site; if an end-to-side anastomosis is performed far from the closed end of the blind pouch, elongation of the blind pouch will occur later in life as the child grows.

The authors have seldom performed other procedures such as HE at the hilum or valved jejunal interposition hepaticoduodenostomy to prevent reflux of digested food into the IHBD.[39] Although these procedures are appealing theoretically, there is no significant difference in morbidity. HE at the hepatic hilum is more difficult than conventional HE, particularly in neonates and infants without IHBD dilatation, and valved jejunal interposition hepaticoduodenostomy is a complicated procedure.

ASSOCIATED ANOMALIES REQUIRING TREATMENT

IBD dilatation

Recently, more attention has been paid to the treatment of IHBD anomalies such as dilatation with downstream stenosis, which is strongly associated with late postoperative complications.[32,39,51–57] In our series,[13] 8 of 21 neonatal patients (38.1%) had IHBD dilatation (in one, it was severe and was still persistent at follow-up 14 years later), which is remarkably less than the incidence in older children (53.3%).[51] IHBD dilatation can be treated by segmentectomy of the liver, intrahepatic cystoenterostomy, or balloon dilatation of the stenosis at the time of CE.[32,54,55] The authors have treated stricture of the IHBD at the hepatic hilum by intrahepatic ductoplasty and cystojejunostomy or hepatico-jejunostomy at the hepatic hilum in three cases,[51,56] creating a wide stoma by incising along the lateral wall of the hepatic ducts following excision of the narrowed segment of the common hepatic duct (Figure 76.5). By using intraoperative endoscopy, the ideal level of resection of the common hepatic duct can be safely determined without injuring the orifices of the hepatic duct or leaving a redundant duct.

Anomalies of the pancreatic duct and common channel

Anomalies of the pancreatic duct and common channel can include pathology such as stenosis of the papilla of Vater, stricture of the pancreatic ducts, protein plugs, or even a septate common channel.[33,57–59] Stone debris in the common channel and IHBD can also be responsible for postoperative abdominal pain, pancreatitis, stone formation, or jaundice and should be removed at the time of radical surgery. The authors have found intraoperative endoscopic examination of the common channel and intrahepatic duct to be of enough value to include it as a routine procedure during standard surgical treatment of CBD, because it is extremely efficient for examination and irrigation, and allows all distal pancreatic duct stone debris and stone debris in the common channel to be removed. If stenosis of the major papilla with a dilated common channel is found, a transduodenal papilloplasty or endoscopic papilloplasty should be performed.[57]

INTRAOPERATIVE ENDOSCOPY

Since 1986, the authors have routinely performed intraoperative endoscopy of the common channel, pancreatic duct, and IHBD to examine the duct system directly for stone debris and duct stenosis, and to remove stone debris by irrigation with normal saline (Figure 76.8).[51] The authors use a pediatric cystoscope or fine fiberscope with a flush channel to view the pancreatic and biliary duct systems directly at the time of CE.[56,57] In other cases, a neonatal cystoscope, a fine flexible scope (1.9–2.0 mm) with a flush channel, is required. Recently, we found there was a high incidence of IHBD debris not detected by preoperative radiographic investigations,[60] and there were some cases where IHBD debris identified on preoperative radiography was overlooked when the case was reviewed retrospectively. These facts indicate that intraoperative endoscopy is necessary at the time of CE even if preoperative radiography does not indicate the presence of IHBD debris. Another striking finding was that debris can be present in the absence of IHBD dilatation, although debris was more common when the IHBD was dilated. Thus, we believe that inspection using intraoperative endoscopy is mandatory even when there is no IHBD dilatation. In a recent review of the long-term follow-up of our intraoperative endoscopy patients, the incidence of postoperative stone formation was lower than reported in the literature,[61] evidence of the

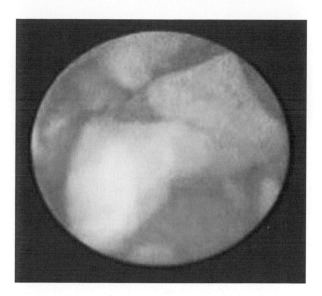

Figure 76.8 Massive debris in the common channel observed through the pediatric cystoscope.

clinical benefit of performing intraoperative endoscopy during CE.

LAPAROSCOPIC SURGERY

Recent advances in laparoscopy technology have enabled pediatric/hepatobiliary surgeons to perform minimally invasive surgery for CBD.[62] In 1995, the first laparoscopic CE in a child was reported.[63] Since then, several authors have reported the safety and feasibility of using minimally invasive techniques for advanced hepatobiliary surgery in children.[64–67] Although technically more challenging, the general concepts are the same as for open surgery. The authors' approach is to use conventionally placed trocars (right upper quadrant, left paraumbilical, left upper quadrant; scope in the umbilicus) to free the cyst and transect it at mid level. An additional 3.9 mm trocar in the left epigastrium is used for a fine ureteroscope for intralaparoscopic endoscopy, similar to intraoperative endoscopy during open CE. Under laparoscope guidance, the tip of the scope is inserted into the common channel through the distal cyst to remove any protein plugs (Figure 76.9).[68] The exact level of transection of the distal common bile duct can also be determined through intralaparoscopic endoscopy,[69] if the orifice of the pancreatic duct in the common channel is identified. After the cyst is freed, the distal part is divided as close as possible to the pancreaticobiliary junction, and the stump is ligated with an ENDOLOOP. When intralaparoscopic endoscopy cannot be performed because of a narrow opening into the intrapancreatic choledochus and common channel (common in cystic CBD), intralaparoscopic cholangiography may be performed by placing an endoscopic metal clip at the distal end of the dissected cyst to confirm the required extent of further dissection distally since the clip and the confluence between the common channel,

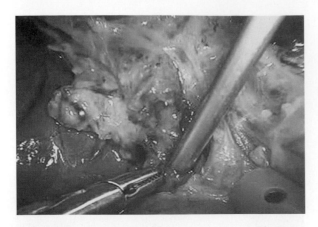

Figure 76.9 Under laparoscope guidance, the tip of the scope is inserted into the common channel through the distal cyst to remove any protein plugs.

intrapancreatic choledochus, and pancreatic duct can be visualized. If dissection is inadequate, the cyst can be further dissected distally and intralaparoscopic cholangiography repeated as previously until cyst dissection is adequate. The proximal cyst is excised leaving 5 mm of common hepatic bile duct. Another two trocars are added for the hepaticojejunostomy: lateral right subcostal, and between the lateral right subcostal and right upper quadrant trocars. Hepaticojejunostomy is performed using interrupted 5/0 or 6/0 absorbable sutures with the right upper quadrant port as a needle holder in the right hand, the 5 mm port for the scope, and the 3 mm subcostal port as a needle receiver in the left hand. Both the right and left edge sutures are exteriorized and used as traction sutures during anastomosis of the anterior wall to facilitate accuracy (Figure 76.10). From our experience, if hepaticojejunostomy is performed without extra trocars, the quality of the anastomosis deteriorates, especially when the diameter of the hepaticojejunostomy anastomosis is <9 mm.

Midterm to long-term follow-up results have been recently published,[70,71] and they found that experienced laparoscopic surgeons would appear to obtain results as good as those for open surgery. In a report comparing laparoscopic CE with open surgery in children [72–75] the operating time was found to be longer, and overall costs higher, but there was significantly less blood loss, and duration of

hospitalization was shorter. There were no significant differences for the incidence of bile leakage or wound infection rates. This would appear to suggest that in the hands of skilled laparoscopic surgeons, laparoscopic CE and Roux-en-Y reconstruction are safe and effective.[74–76] Most recently, robot-assisted laparoscopic resection of CBD has been reported.[77,78]

POSTOPERATIVE COMPLICATIONS AND MANAGEMENT

Surgical outcome is better and early morbidity lower in younger children than in older children. The authors[79] reviewed 200 children and 40 adults who underwent CE and hepaticoenterostomy (CEHE) and found that 18 out of 200 (9.0%) children developed complications post-CEHE. No stone formation was seen in the 145 children who had CEHE before the age of 5 years in our series, and there were 18 children who had 25 episodes of complications post-CEHE, including cholangitis, IHBD stone formation, pancreatitis, stone formation in the intrapancreatic terminal choledochus or pancreatic duct, and bowel obstruction. There were no complications in the 70 children who had intraoperative endoscopy in our series. Stones developed in 7 (12.7%) of 55 children who had CEHE when they were more than 5 years old. For management of complications, reoperation was required in 15 children—revision of HE in 4, percutaneous transhepatic cholangioscopic lithotomy in 1, excision of intrapancreatic terminal choledochus in 2, endoscopic sphincterotomy of the papilla of Vater in 1, pancreaticojejunostomy in 1, and laparotomy for bowel obstruction in 6.

Careful long-term follow-up is required, particularly in patients with IHBD dilatation and also dilatation of the remaining distal bile duct, pancreatic duct, and common channel, because there is a risk for chronic inflammation, stone formation, as well as the possibility of carcinoma arising at a later stage.

REFERENCES

1. Iwafuchi M, Ohsawa Y, Naito S, Naito M, Maruta Y, Saito H. Familial occurrence of congenital bile duct dilatation. *J Pediatr Surg* 1990; 25(3): 353–5.
2. Ando K, Miyano T, Fujimoto T, Ohya T, Lane G, Tawa T et al. Sibling occurrence of biliary atresia and biliary dilatation. *J Pediatr Surg* 1996; 31(9): 1302–4.
3. Lane GJ, Yamataka A, Kobayashi H, Segawa O, Miyano T. Different types of congenital biliary dilatation in dizygotic twins. *Pediatr Surg Int* 1999; 15(5–6): 403–4.
4. Dewbury KC, Aluwihare AP, Birch SJ, Freeman NV. Prenatal ultrasound demonstration of a choledochal cyst. *Br J Radiol* 1980; 53(633): 906–7.
5. Frank JL, Hill MC, Chirathivat S, Sfakianakis GN, Marchildon M. Antenatal observation of a choledochal cyst by sonography. *AJR Am J Roentgenol* 1981; 137(1): 166–8.

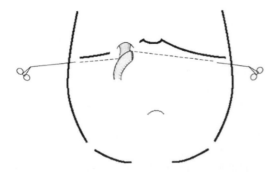

Figure 76.10 Traction sutures facilitate accurate hepaticojejunostomy.

6. Howell CG, Templeton JM, Weiner S, Glassman M, Betts JM, Witzleben CL. Antenatal diagnosis and early surgery for choledochal cyst. *J Pediatr Surg* 1983; 18(4): 387–93.

7. Wiedman MA, Tan A, Martinez CJ. Fetal sonography and neonatal scintigraphy of a choledochal cyst. *J Nucl Med* 1985; 26(8): 893–6.

8. Elrad H, Mayden KL, Ahart S, Giglia R, Gleicher N. Prenatal ultrasound diagnosis of choledochal cyst. *J Ultrasound Med* 1985; 4(10): 553–5.

9. Schroeder D, Smith L, Prain HC. Antenatal diagnosis of choledochal cyst at 15 weeks' gestation: Etiologic implications and management. *J Pediatr Surg* 1989; 24(9): 936–8.

10. Bancroft JD, Bucuvalas JC, Ryckman FC, Dudgeon DL, Saunders RC, Schwarz KB. Antenatal diagnosis of choledochal cyst. *J Pediatr Gastroenterol Nutr* 1994; 18(2): 142–5.

11. Gallivan EK, Crombleholme TM, D'Alton ME. Early prenatal diagnosis of choledochal cyst. *Prenat Diagn* 1996; 16(10): 934–7.

12. Matsumoto M, Urushihara N, Fukumoto K, Yamoto M, Miyake H, Nakajima H et al. Laparoscopic management for prenatally diagnosed choledochal cysts. *Surg Today* 2016; 46(12): 1410–14.

13. Lane G, Yamataka A, Kohno S, Fujiwara T, Fujimoto T, Sunagawa M et al. Choledochal cyst in the newborn. *Asian J Surg* 1999; 22: 310–2.

14. Spitz L. Experimental production of cystic dilatation of the common bile duct in neonatal lambs. *J Pediatr Surg* 1977; 12(1): 39–42.

15. Miyano T, Suruga K, Kimura K, Suda K. A histopathologic study of the region of the ampulla of Vater in congenital biliary atresia. *Jpn J Surg* 1980; 10(1): 34–8.

16. Suda K, Matsumoto Y, Miyano T. Narrow duct segment distal to choledochal cyst. *Am J Gastroenterol* 1991; 86(9): 1259–63.

17. Miyano T, Suruga K, Chen SC. A clinicopathologic study of choledochal cyst. *World J Surg* 1980; 4(2): 231–8.

18. Suda K, Miyano T, Konuma I, Matsumoto M. An abnormal pancreatico-choledocho-ductal junction in cases of biliary tract carcinoma. *Cancer* 1983; 52(11): 2086–8.

19. Miyano T, Takahashi A, Suruga K. Congenital stenosis associated with abnormal choledocho-pancreatico-ductal junction in concerning the pathogenesis of congenital dilatation of biliary tract. *Jpn J Pediatr Surg* 1978; 10: 539–54.

20. Miyano T, Suruga K, Suda K. Abnormal choledocho-pancreatico ductal junction related to the etiology of infantile obstructive jaundice diseases. *J Pediatr Surg* 1979; 14(1): 16–26.

21. Jona JZ, Babbitt DP, Starshak RJ, LaPorta AJ, Glicklich M, Cohen RD. Anatomic observations and etiologic and surgical considerations in choledochal cyst. *J Pediatr Surg* 1979; 14(3): 315–20.

22. Wong KC, Lister J. Human fetal development of the hepato-pancreatic duct junction—A possible explanation of congenital dilatation of the biliary tract. *J Pediatr Surg* 1981; 16(2): 139–45.

23. Tanaka T. Embryological development of the duodenal papilla, and related diseases: Primitive ampulla theory. *Am J Gastroenterol* 1993; 88(11): 1980–1.

24. Tanaka T. Pathogenesis of choledochal cyst. *Am J Gastroenterol* 1995; 90(4): 685.

25. Babbitt DP. [Congenital choledochal cysts: New etiological concept based on anomalous relationships of the common bile duct and pancreatic bulb]. *Ann Radiol* (Paris). 1969; 12(3): 231–40.

26. Tanaka K, Nishimura A, Yamada K, Ishibe R, Ishizaki N, Yoshimine M et al. Cancer of the gallbladder associated with anomalous junction of the pancreatobiliary duct system without bile duct dilatation. *Br J Surg* 1993; 80(5): 622–4.

27. Miyano T, Suruga K, Suda K. "The choledocho-pancreatic long common channel disorders" in relation to the etiology of congenital biliary dilatation and other biliary tract disease. *Ann Acad Med Singapore* 1981; 10(4): 419–26.

28. Marchildon M. Antenatal diagnosis fo choledochal cyst: The first four cases. *Pediatr Surg Int* 1988; 3: 431–6.

29. Laitio M, Lev R, Orlic D. The developing human fetal pancreas: An ultrastructural and histochemical study with special reference to exocrine cells. *J Anat* 1974; 117(Pt 3): 619–34.

30. Lebenthal E, Lee PC. Development of functional responses in human exocrine pancreas. *Pediatrics* 1980; 66(4): 556–60.

31. Alonso-Lej F, Rever WB, Jr., Pessagno DJ. Congenital choledochal cyst, with a report of 2, and an analysis of 94, cases. *Int Abstr Surg* 1959; 108(1): 1–30.

32. Todani T, Narusue M, Watanabe Y, Tabuchi K, Okajima K. Management of congenital choledochal cyst with intrahepatic involvement. *Ann Surg* 1978; 187(3): 272–80.

33. Komi N, Takehara H, Kunitomo K, Miyoshi Y, Yagi T. Does the type of anomalous arrangement of pancreaticobiliary ducts influence the surgery and prognosis of choledochal cyst? *J Pediatr Surg* 1992; 27(6): 728–31.

34 Saikusa N, Naito S, Iinuma Y, Ohtani T, Yokoyama N, Nitta, K. Invasive cholangiocarcinoma identified in congenital biliary dilatation in a 3-year-old boy. *J Pediatr Surg* 2009; 44(11): 2202–5.

35. Iinuma Y, Narisawa R, Iwafuchi M, Uchiyama M, Naito M, Yagi M et al. The role of endoscopic retrograde cholangiopancreatography in infantswith cholestasis. *J Pediatr Surg* 2000; 35(4): 545–9.

36. Yamataka A, Kuwatsuru R, Shima H, Kobayashi H, Lane G, Segawa O et al. Initial experience with non-breath-hold magnetic resonance

cholangiopancreatography: A new noninvasive technique for the diagnosis of choledochal cyst in children. *J Pediatr Surg* 1997; 32(11): 1560–2.

37. Shimizu T, Suzuki R, Yamashiro Y, Segawa O, Yamataka A, Miyano T. Progressive dilatation of the main pancreatic duct using magnetic resonance cholangiopancreatography in a boy with chronic pancreatitis. *J Pediatr Gastroenterol Nutr* 2000; 30(1): 102–4.

38. Todani T, Watanabe Y, Mizuguchi T, Fujii T, Toki A. Hepaticoduodenostomy at the hepatic hilum after excision of choledochal cyst. *Am J Surg* 1981; 142(5): 584–7.

39. Todani T, Watanabe Y, Toki A, Urushihara N, Sato Y. Reoperation for congenital choledochal cyst. *Ann Surg* 1988; 207(2): 142–7.

40. Shimotakahara A, Yamataka A, Yanai T, Kobayashi H, Okazaki T, Lane GJ et al. Roux-en-Y hepaticojejunostomy or hepaticoduodenostomy for biliary reconstruction during the surgical treatment of choledochal cyst: Which is better? *Pediatr Surg Int* 2005; 21(1): 5–7.

41. Todani T, Watanabe Y, Toki A, Hara H. Hilar duct carcinoma developed after cyst excision followed by hepatico duodenostomy In: Koyanagi Y, Aoki T (eds). *Pancreaticobiliary Maljunction*. Tokyo: Igaku tosho Shuppan, 2002: 17–21.

42. Yeung F, Chung PH, Wong KK, Tam PK. Biliary-enteric reconstruction with hepaticoduodenostomy following laparoscopic excision of choledochal cyst is associated with better postoperative outcomes: A single-centre experience. *Pediatr Surg Int* 2015; 31(2): 149–53.

43. Dalton BG, Gonzalez KW, Dehmer JJ, Andrews WS, Hendrickson RJ. Transition of techniques to treat choledochal cysts in children. *J Laparoendosc Adv Surg Tech A* 2016; 26(1): 62–5.

44. Burnweit CA, Birken GA, Heiss K. The management of choledochal cyst in the newborn. *Pediatr Surg Int* 1996; 11: 130–3.

45. Suita S, Shono K, Kinugasa Y, Kubota M, Matsuo S. Influence of age on the presentation and outcome of choledochal cyst. *J Pediatr Surg* 1999; 34(12): 1765–8.

46. Diao M, Li L, Cheng W. Timing of surgery for prenatally diagnosed asymptomatic choledochal cysts: A prospective randomized study. *J Pediatr Surg* 2012; 47(3): 506–12.

47. Miyano T, Yamataka A. Choledochal cyst. *Curr Opin Pediatr* 1997; 9: 283–8.

48. Redkar R, Davenport M, Howard ER. Antenatal diagnosis of congenital anomalies of the biliary tract. *J Pediatr Surg* 1998; 33(5): 700–4.

49. Filler RM, Stringel G. Treatment of choledochal cyst by excision. *J Pediatr Surg* 1980; 15(4): 437–42.

50. Somasundaram K, Wong TJ, Tan KC. Choledochal cyst—A review of 25 cases. *Aust N Z J Surg* 1985; 55(5): 443–6.

51. Miyano T, Yamataka A, Kato Y, Segawa O, Lane G, Takamizawa S et al. Hepaticoenterostomy after excision of choledochal cyst in children: A 30-year experience with 180 cases. *J Pediatr Surg* 1996; 31(10): 1417–21.

52. Ohi R, Yaoita S, Kamiyama T, Ibrahim M, Hayashi Y, Chiba T. Surgical treatment of congenital dilatation of the bile duct with special reference to late complications after total excisional operation. *J Pediatr Surg* 1990; 25(6): 613–7.

53. Ando H, Ito T, Kaneko K, Seo T, Ito F. Intrahepatic bile duct stenosis causing intrahepatic calculi formation following excision of a choledochal cyst. *J Am Coll Surg* 1996; 183(1): 56–60.

54. Engle J, Salmon PA. Multiple choledochal cysts. Report of a Case. *Arch Surg* 1964; 88: 345–9.

55. Tsuchida Y, Taniguchi F, Nakahara S, Uno K, Kawarasaki H, Inoue Y et al. Excision of a choledochal cyst and simultaneous hepatic lateral segmentomy. *Pediatr Surg Int* 1996; 11: 496–7.

56. Miyano T, Yamataka A, Kato Y, Kohno S, Fujiwara T. Choledochal cysts: Special emphasis on the usefulness of intraoperative endoscopy. *J Pediatr Surg* 1995; 30(3): 482–4.

57. Yamataka A, Segawa O, Kobayashi H, Kato Y, Miyano T. Intraoperative pancreatoscopy for pancreatic duct stone debris distal to the common channel in choledochal cyst. *J Pediatr Surg* 2000; 35(1): 1–4.

58. Miyano T, Suruga K, Shimomura H, Nittono H, Yamashiro Y, Matsumoto M. Choledochopancreatic elongated common channel disorders. *J Pediatr Surg* 1984; 19(2): 165–70.

59. Kaneko K, Ando H, Ito T, Watanabe Y, Seo T, Harada T et al. Protein plugs cause symptoms in patients with choledochal cysts. *Am J Gastroenterol* 1997; 92(6): 1018–21.

60. Shimotakahara A, Yamataka A, Kobayashi H, Yanai T, Lane GJ, Miyano T. Massive debris in the intrahepatic bile ducts in choledochal cyst: Possible cause of postoperative stone formation. *Pediatr Surg Int* 2004; 20(1): 67–9.

61. Takahashi T, Shimotakahara A, Okazaki T, Koga H, Miyano G, Lane GJ et al. Intraoperative endoscopy during choledochal cyst excision: Extended long-term follow-up compared with recent cases. *J Pediatr Surg* 2010; 45(2): 379–82.

62. Shimura H, Tanaka M, Shimizu S, Mizumoto K. Laparoscopic treatment of congenital choledochal cyst. *Surg Endosc* 1998; 12(10): 1268–71.

63. Farello GA, Cerofolini A, Rebonato M, Bergamaschi G, Ferrari C, Chiappetta A. Congenital choledochal cyst: Video-guided laparoscopic treatment. *Surg Laparosc Endosc* 1995; 5(5): 354–8.

64. Ure BM, Schier F, Schmidt AI, Nustede R, Petersen C, Jesch NK. Laparoscopic resection of congenital choledochal cyst, choledochojejunostomy, and

extraabdominal Roux-en-Y anastomosis. *Surg Endosc* 2005; 19(8): 1055–7.

65. Li L, Feng W, Jing-Bo F, Qi-Zhi Y, Gang L, Liu-Ming H et al. Laparoscopic-assisted total cyst excision of choledochal cyst and Roux-en-Y hepatoenterostomy. *J Pediatr Surg* 2004; 39(11): 1663–6.

66. Lee H, Hirose S, Bratton B, Farmer D. Initial experience with complex laparoscopic biliary surgery in children: Biliary atresia and choledochal cyst. *J Pediatr Surg* 2004; 39(6): 804-7; discussion 7.

67. Yeung CK, Lee KH, Tam YH. Laparoscopic excision of choledochal cyst with hepaticojejunostomy. In: Bax KMA, Georgeson KE, Rothenberg SS, Valla J, Yeung CK (eds). *Endoscopic Surgery in Infants and Children*. Berlin: Springer; 2008: 431–46.

68. Yamataka A. Removing protein plugs in the common channel during the laparoscopic excision of minimally dilated choledochal cyst: Intralaparoscopic pancreatoscopy. International pediatric endosurgery group (IPEG) annual congress; 2010.6; Hawaii 2010.

69. Koga H, Okawada M, Doi T, Miyano G, Lane GJ, Yamataka A. Refining the intraoperative measurement of the distal intrapancreatic part of a choledochal cyst during laparoscopic repair allows near total excision. *Pediatr Surg Int* 2015; 31(10): 991–4.

70. Qiao G, Li L, Li S, Tang S, Wang B, Xi H et al. Laparoscopic cyst excision and Roux-Y hepatico-jejunostomy for children with choledochal cysts in China: A multicenter study. *Surg Endosc* 2015; 29(1): 140–4.

71. Hong L, Wu Y, Yan Z, Xu M, Chu J, Chen QM. Laparoscopic surgery for choledochal cyst in children: A case review of 31 patients. *Eur J Pediatr Surg* 2008; 18(2): 67–71

72. Lee KH, Tam YH, Yeung CK, Chan KW, Sihoe JD, Cheung ST et al. Laparoscopic excision of choledochal cysts in children: An intermediate-term report. *Pediatr Surg Int* 2009; 25(4): 355–60.

73. Liem NT, Dung le A, Son TN. Laparoscopic complete cyst excision and hepaticoduodenostomy for choledochal cyst: Early results in 74 cases. *J Laparoendosc Adv Surg Tech A* 2009; 19 Suppl 1: S87–90.

74. Shen HJ, Xu M, Zhu HY, Yang C, Li F, Li KW et al. Laparoscopic versus open surgery in children with choledochal cysts: A meta-analysis. *Pediatr Surg Int* 2015; 31(6): 529–34.

75. Zhen C, Xia Z, Long L, Lishuang M, Pu Y, Wenjuan Z et al. Laparoscopic excision versus open excision for the treatment of choledochal cysts: A systematic review and meta-analysis. *Int Surg* 2015 January; 100(1): 115–22.

76. Liem NT, Pham HD, Dung le A, Son TN, Vu HM. Early and intermediate outcomes of laparoscopic surgery for choledochal cysts with 400 patients. *J Laparoendosc Adv Surg Tech A* 2012; 22(6): 599–603.

77. Alizai NK, Dawrant MJ, Najmaldin AS. Robot-assisted resection of choledochal cysts and hepaticojejunostomy in children. *Pediatr Surg Int* 2014; 30(3): 291–4.

78. Woo R, Le D, Albanese CT, Kim SS. Robot-assisted laparoscopic resection of a type I choledochal cyst in a child. *J Laparoendosc Adv Surg Tech A* 2006; 16(2): 179–83.

79. Yamataka A, Ohshiro K, Okada Y, Hosoda Y, Fujiwara T, Kohno S et al. Complications after cyst excision with hepaticoenterostomy for choledochal cysts and their surgical management in children versus adults. *J Pediatr Surg* 1997; 32(7): 1097–102.

77

Hepatic cysts and abscesses

JONATHAN P. ROACH, DAVID A. PARTRICK, AND FREDERICK M. KARRER

INTRODUCTION

Cysts and abscesses of the liver in the neonatal period are uncommon. Hepatic cysts presenting in infants are usually simple, unilocular cysts, with polycystic liver diseases presenting later in childhood or in adults. Most abscesses in infants are pyogenic, with parasitic infections occurring in older children or adults. Cross-sectional imaging studies (ultrasound, computed tomography [CT], magnetic resonance imaging) can typically make workup and localization relatively straightforward. Antenatal diagnosis of liver cysts is now more common with improving scanning technology. Treatment, however, still requires experience and judgment to prevent recurrences or complications.

SIMPLE HEPATIC CYST

Simple or solitary cysts in infants can be congenital or acquired in origin. Parasitic cysts (from hydatid disease) are rare in children and have never been reported in infancy.

Congenital cysts probably arise from defective fusion or obstruction of intrahepatic bile ducts during development, or possibly originate from peribiliary glands.[1,2] These cysts are usually single and unilocular, but septation has been reported.[3] Although one or two thin septa are regarded as normal for a simple cyst, more septae should prompt consideration of other pathologies. Simple cysts are well encapsulated with a smooth surface. There is a 2:1 female preponderance.[4] Most common in the right lobe, they abut or hang down from the liver edge.[3] The liver almost never completely covers the cyst, especially the pedunculated cysts, so the presenting portion has a bluish hue. The internal cyst wall is lined by simple cuboidal or columnar epithelium.[4] Most contain clear fluid, but it may be brownish because of remote hemorrhage. Bilious cyst fluid indicates communication with a biliary radical.

Acquired or posttraumatic cysts may result from blunt trauma or birth trauma, causing an intrahepatic hematoma. The hematoma reabsorbs, leaving behind a cyst cavity. These cysts are lined by granulation tissue and fibrosis and rarely communicate with the biliary tree.

Differential diagnosis of complex cystic structures in the liver

Cystic structures in the neonatal liver also include ciliated hepatic foregut cysts, choledochal cysts, mesenchymal hamartomas (MHs), and cystadenomas.[2,4,5,6] Simple, ciliated, and choledochal cysts usually are unilocular, whereas MH and cystadenomas are multilocular. Ciliated hepatic foregut cysts (CHFCs) are rare cystic structures in the neonatal liver thought to originate from remnants of embryonic foregut buds that are trapped in the liver during development. They are most often seen in the left lobe of the liver. Common imaging characteristics of CHFC are unilocular or bilocular, sediment-containing cysts with calcifications in the cyst wall. Fine needle aspirate of the cyst will show ciliated columnar epithelial cells in a mucoid background.[4] MH is an uncommon tumor of the liver usually presenting before 2 years of age. Characteristic findings in MH are cysts of different sizes, with a variable solid component to the mass. MH may thus be cystic, solid, or mixed in presentation. Although MH is pathologically benign, reports of malignant generation of angiosarcoma and progression to an aggressive clinical course have been described.[6] Complex cysts should be completely excised because of the reported risk of malignant degeneration of these structures.[2]

Choledochal cysts are described in a separate chapter of this textbook.

Presentation

Most congenital cysts do not have any clinical manifestations in infancy and are not diagnosed until an older age (fourth or fifth decade of life). Some are discovered prenatally or incidentally during workup of unrelated problems.[4]

When they are symptomatic in infancy, it is usually because of a visible or palpable upper abdominal mass.[5–8] They rarely cause symptoms from compression of other structures, but infants can present with abdominal distension, feeding difficulties, respiratory distress, and duodenal obstruction secondary to a large cyst.[2] Hemorrhage, secondary infection, rupture or torsion can lead to an acute abdominal condition, but such complications are extremely rare.[9]

Diagnosis

Cysts large enough to be detected on physical exam are easily distinguished from solid tumors by ultrasonography. Liver function is typically normal in spite of the impressive size of these cysts. Plain radiographs may show diaphragmatic elevation or a soft tissue mass displacing the gas pattern in the abdomen. CT is useful to identify the exact location and number of cysts. Other preoperative imaging techniques (cholangiography, angiography, nuclear scans) may provide additional information but are usually unnecessary. With improving imaging technology, many hepatic cysts are being discovered antenatally. In some series, small asymptomatic simple cysts comprised the majority of the prenatal hepatic findings, and these regressed spontaneously. Only one in seven required postnatal surgery secondary to increasing size or symptoms.[2] On prenatal ultrasound, placental pathology in conjunction with hepatic cysts has been linked to MH.[10] If such a finding is noted prenatally, early resection of the liver cyst should be considered.

Treatment

Small asymptomatic cysts (<5 cm) discovered incidentally should be left alone. Large or symptomatic cysts should be treated surgically. Percutaneous cyst aspiration may rule out biliary communication or abscess, but is not definitive therapy because of a high recurrence rate.[11,12] Complete resection is optimal and can be accomplished easily when the cyst is pedunculated.[13] Many of these may be amendable to minimally invasive surgical techniques. If complete excision cannot be accomplished by simple enucleation, formal lobectomy is not typically indicated. These are benign lesions; therefore, the risk of treatment should not exceed the risk of the disease. Under these circumstances, partial excision is preferred. By unroofing at least one-third of the cyst cavity, any serous drainage will be reabsorbed by the peritoneal cavity.[14] The edges of the cyst can be managed by oversewing with a running absorbable suture or by electrocautery. If the cyst contains bile and cholangiography confirms communication of the cyst with the biliary tree, then internal drainage via Roux-en-Y cystojejunostomy is indicated. Infected cysts should be drained externally (see below).

Prognosis

The prognosis for infants with simple hepatic cysts is excellent. Mortality and cyst recurrence should approach zero.[10,15,16,17]

POLYCYSTIC LIVER DISEASE

When liver cysts develop throughout the liver in high number, it is usually in association with an inherited polycystic disease. The two main variants of polycystic disease are autosomal dominant (adult type) and autosomal recessive (childhood type).[18] Both are associated with polycystic disease of the kidney. Autosomal dominant polycystic kidney disease (ADPKD) is the most common form (90%). Symptoms of renal involvement (pain, hypertension, renal failure, urinary tract infection) usually don't develop until adulthood. Liver cysts in autosomal dominant polycystic disease are exceptionally rare in childhood and have not been seen in infancy.

Autosomal recessive polycystic kidney disease (ARPKD) presents in childhood. There are four subgroups (perinatal, neonatal, infantile, juvenile), with varying degrees of involvement of the kidneys and liver.[19] The most severe cases present perinatally with oligohydramnios, Potter's syndrome, and pulmonary hypoplasia and usually die shortly after birth. Patients with lesser degrees of renal involvement present at an older age with renal failure and hypertension. In some children, renal involvement is minor, and they don't present until adolescence with symptoms of portal hypertension such as varicella bleeding.[20]

In all forms of ARPKD, the liver is not usually grossly cystic. The liver abnormality is termed congenital hepatic fibrosis. Microscopically, there is bile duct proliferation with irregular broad bands of fibrous tissue containing multiple microscopic cysts formed by disordered terminal bile ducts, chiefly in the portal areas. The incidence of portal hypertension in ARPKD increases with longevity and appears to be inversely related to the severity of the renal disease. Treatment for portal hypertension is not required in infancy since it takes time for esophageal varices with the tendency to bleed to develop. If portal hypertension leads to esophageal bleeding, endoscopic treatment or portosystemic shunting is preferred. Hepatic synthetic function is usually preserved and the portal hypertension may improve in adolescence as other collaterals develop. Therefore, liver transplantation is usually not needed. Rarely, fibrosis is accompanied by cystic dilation of intrahepatic biliary ducts like Carole's disease. This rare variant does not require treatment in infancy.[21]

The named subgroups of ARPKD aid discussion but are far from distinct. There is, in fact, considerable overlap among individuals and within families. In infancy, the treatment of ARPD only addresses the renal and consequent pulmonary insufficiency. No treatment is required for the hepatic lesion.

HEPATIC ABSCESSES

Incidence and etiology

The most common source of hepatic abscess in children has historically been perforated appendicitis (Figure 77.1),

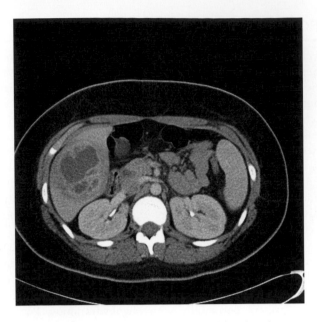

Figure 77.1 CT abdomen of a 12-year-old girl with a post-appendicitis right lobe liver abscess.

Table 77.1 Predisposing factors for neonatal hepatic abscess

Prematurity (immunocompromised)
Umbilical vein catheterization (colonizing organisms, hypertonic glucose solution, misplaced catheter)
Omphalitis
Intra-abdominal infection (necrotizing enterocolitis, bowel perforation)
Bacteremia (meningitis)

but the incidence in this population has decreased since the introduction of antibiotics. It is now more commonly seen in children with an underlying immune deficiency.[22] Although approximately 50% of children with pyogenic hepatic abscess are less than 6 years old, neonatal hepatic abscesses are rare. One study reported only 3 cases of hepatic abscesses out of 11,403 neonatal admissions.[23] Even though rare, they can definitely be lethal in this vulnerable population. In this review, only 18 neonatal cases of solitary hepatic abscess were identified in the English literature from 1900.[23] In an earlier review, 24 cases were identified historically (including cases of multiple abscesses) to which the authors added an additional 13.[24] Neonatal liver abscess seems to differ considerably from the disease in older children. The patent umbilical vein in neonates provides ready access for bacteria to the liver, and umbilical vessel catheterization is a significant predisposing factor in hepatic abscess formation.[25,26] In hospitalized infants, umbilical vein catheters allow bacteria colonizing the umbilical stump a direct route to the liver. Less common sources of liver abscesses are inoculation via the portal vein from necrotizing enterocolitis,[27] isolated bowel perforations, direct extension from surrounding structures,[25] and other intra-abdominal infections of the newborn. Bacteremia from meningitis or another septic insult can also result in hepatic abscesses via the hepatic artery.[28] Multiple pyogenic hepatic abscesses can complicate neonatal sepsis. Hepatic abscess has also been reported as a rare complication of ventriculoperitoneal shunts (six cases have been reported in the literature, primarily in older patients).[29] More recently, the majority of neonatal cases of hepatic abscess have occurred in premature neonates who are relatively immunosuppressed and have undergone umbilical vessel catheterization (Table 77.1).[21,30] There are reported associations of hepatic abscesses in infants exposed to HIV

from the mother, misplaced umbilical catheters (right-sided abscesses), or the use of hypertonic glucose solutions via an umbilical catheter.[30]

The infecting organisms in neonates are more often Gram-negative than Gram-positive. Kays[31] reviewed the infectious causes of pyogenic liver abscesses, and in 22 neonates (<1 month of age), Gram-positive aerobes accounted for only 27% of abscesses, whereas Gram-negative aerobes were responsible for 73%. Fungus was the infectious source in 5% (one patient, although an additional case has since been reported),[21] and anaerobic organisms have not been isolated from any neonatal liver abscess reported in the literature. This is in contrast to older children with hepatic abscess, where up to 50% of infecting organisms isolated are Gram-positive, 25% are Gram-negative, 10% are anaerobic, 6% are fungus, and the remainder are unknown (cryptogenic). Others have noted polymicrobial infections in up to 50% of hepatic abscesses.[32]

Presentation and diagnosis

The clinical diagnosis of neonatal hepatic abscess remains difficult. The classic findings of fever, hepatomegaly, and right-upper-quadrant pain are seldom obvious in the neonate. Signs and symptoms of sepsis may be present, but many infants are simply noted to be irritable, with only mild abdominal distention or tenderness. A rapidly enlarging and tender liver is characteristic for a hepatic abscess, but this is not commonly found on clinical examination. Fever, leukocytosis, and elevation of the sedimentation rate as well as the C-reactive protein may be present. In the majority of patients, liver function tests are normal, but direct and indirect hyperbilirubinemia, elevation of the alkaline phosphatase, elevation of serum transaminase, anemia, and hypoalbuminemia have all been reported.[20] Therefore, to make the diagnosis in neonates, a high index of suspicion is necessary in conjunction with appropriate imaging techniques.

Radiographic evaluation

Plain films may suggest the diagnosis of hepatic abscess by the presence of an elevated right hemidiaphragm and right pleural effusion. Sometimes, a gas shadow can be visualized in the liver itself corresponding to the abscess cavity. Improvements in abdominal ultrasound and CT scanning

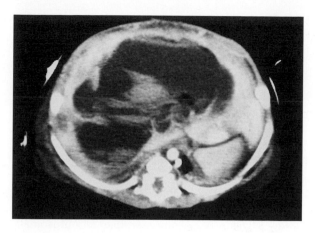

Figure 77.2 CT scan of a large hepatic abscess in a 5-day-old neonate.

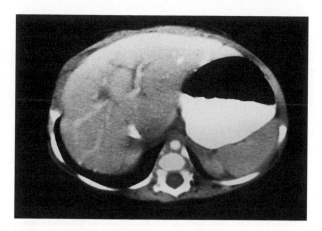

Figure 77.3 Repeat CT scan 6 weeks following open surgical drainage and intravenous antibiotic treatment demonstrating complete radiographic resolution of the hepatic abscess.

now allow for a more rapid and accurate diagnosis in neonates.[33] Ultrasound has the advantage of lower cost, no radiation exposure, relative convenience, and ease of repeating the exam (no sedation, portable).[34,35] A hepatic abscess typically shows low or variable echogenicity by ultrasound, and cystic lesions as small as 1 cm can be identified separate from liver parenchyma. A pyogenic abscess may have more irregular margins on ultrasound compared with an amoebic liver abscess, which may be round and well-defined.[36] CT scanning has demonstrated increased sensitivity compared with ultrasound, and it gives a clearer definition of the abscess.[20] The abscess margins are variably enhanced with the use of intravenous (IV) contrast. Figure 77.2 demonstrates the appearance on CT scan of a large hepatic abscess in a 5-day-old full-term baby. This neonate had an umbilical venous catheter in place with progressive hepatomegaly on physical examination. Included in the differential diagnosis of this cystic mass were hepatoblastoma, infantile hemangioendothelioma, MH, and other rare liver tumors. Any neonate with persistent fever and suggestion of upper abdominal tenderness or an enlarged liver should undergo radiographic examination, especially if risk factors are present. If the ultrasound appears normal but clinical suspicion remains high, CT scanning should be performed. Specific diagnosis requires aspiration of the lesion with Gram stain and culture, leading to subsequent identification of the infecting organism.

Treatment

Systemic antibiotic therapy remains the mainstay of therapy for neonatal hepatic abscess. Initial antibiotic treatment should be started aggressively and include broad coverage. In neonates, empiric treatment should specifically be directed against Gram-negative bacilli and *Staphylococcus aureus*, although anaerobic abscesses have been reported and specific antibiotics covering anaerobes should be considered if the patient does not respond to initial therapy. After cultures identify the infecting organism, antibiotics can be narrowed according to the reported

sensitivities. Percutaneous aspiration of smaller neonatal hepatic abscesses can be done for diagnostic purposes,[37] but larger abscesses require therapeutic drainage of the purulent fluid collection for adequate treatment.[38] Percutaneous drainage techniques have been demonstrated to be safe and efficacious in children with hepatic abscesses,[39] and recent experience in neonates has shown similar good results.[21,40] If indicated, an open abdominal exploration allows investigation and possible treatment of an intra-abdominal source of the infection. Laparoscopy may have a role in these patients in this regard. The neonate depicted in Figure 77.2 was treated aggressively with open surgical drainage and IV antibiotics (vancomycin to cover coagulase-negative staph species cultured from the abscess cavity). This aggressive treatment resulted in nearly complete resolution of the process documented by CT within 6 weeks (Figure 77.3). Investigators have variably recommended 2 to 3 weeks of drainage with a total antibiotic course of 3 to 6 weeks.

Once drained and treated with antibiotics, follow-up should include serial ultrasound examination. Most cases should have complete resolution, but chronic, partially calcified foci in the abscess site and portal vein thrombosis have been described after treatment.[40] Prevention of hepatic abscesses may not be possible in neonates given the many potential risk factors they may encounter. According to a Cochrane review,[41] there is no evidence to support the use of prophylactic antibiotics for umbilical vein catheterization to prevent sepsis or liver abscess.

AMOEBIC LIVER ABSCESS

The parasite *Entamoeba histolytica* is generally considered a possible causative organism in older children with hepatic abscess,[42,43] but it has rarely been documented to occur in newborns.[44] Hepatic abscesses due to *E. histolytica* usually follow a 1- to 2-month course of amoebic dysentery.[36] Due to nonspecific signs and symptoms, the diagnosis again rests on clinical suspicion. Serologic testing via indirect hemagglutination or complement fixation assays can be a useful diagnostic tool. Even though investigators have tried to differentiate the radiographic appearance of amoebic versus pyogenic liver abscesses,[36,45] fine needle aspiration of the abscess cavity is typically required. Return of characteristic "anchovy paste"–appearing material is suggestive of amoebic infection. Presence of trophozoites in stool and positive amoebic serology confirm the diagnosis.[36] Though surgical drainage has been described,[46] amoebic liver abscesses can often be treated successfully with metronidazole and iodoquinal over a 30-day course.[47,48]

REFERENCES

1. Moschowitz E. Non-parasitic cysts (congenital) of the liver with a study of aberrant ducts. *Am J Med Sci* 1986; 131: 674.

2. Rogers TN, Woodley H, Ramsden W et al. Solitary liver cysts in children: Not always so simple. *J Pediat Surg* 2007; 42: 333–9.

3. Saboo RM, Belsare RK, Narang R et al. Giant congenital cyst of the liver. *J Pediatr Surg* 1974; 9: 561–2.

4. Guérin F, Hadhri R, Fabre M et al. Prenatal and postnatal ciliated hepatic foregut cysts in infants. *J Pediat Surg* 2010; 45: E9–14.

5. Stringer MD, Jones MO, Woodley H et al. Ciliated hepatic foregut cyst. *J Pediatr Surg* 2006; 41: 1180–3.

6. Karpelowsky JS, Pansini A, Lazarus C et al. Difficulties in the management of mesenchymal hamartomas. *Pediatr Surg Int* 2008; 24: 1171–5.

7. Donovan MJ, Kozakewich H, Perez-Atayde A. Solitary non-parasitic cysts of the liver. *Pediatr Pathol Lab Med* 1995; 15: 419–28.

8. Avni EF, Rypens F, Donner C et al. Hepatic cysts and hyperechogenicities: Perinatal assessment and unifying theory on their origins. *Pediatr Radiol* 1994; 24: 569–72.

9. Pul N, Pul M. Congenital solitary non-parasitic cyst of the liver in infancy and childhood. *J Pediatr Gastroenterol Nutr* 1995; 21: 461–2.

10. Charlesworth P, Ade-Ajayi N, Davenport M. Natural history and long-term follow-up of antenatally detected liver cysts. *J Pediat Surg* 2007; 42: 494–9.

11. Merine D, Nussbaum AR, Sanders RC. Solitary non-parasitic hepatic cyst causing abdominal distension and respiratory distress in a newborn. *J Pediatr Surg* 1990; 25: 349–50.

12. Saini S, Mueller PR, Ferrucci JT et al. Percutaneous aspiration of hepatic cysts does not provide definitive therapy. *Am J Roentgenol* 1983; 141: 559–60.

13. Nelson J, Davidson D, McKittrick JE. Simple surgical treatment of non-parasitic hepatic cysts. *Am Surg* 1992; 58: 755–7.

14. Byrne WJ, Fonkalsrud EW. Congenital solitary non-parasitic cyst of the liver: A rare cause of a rapidly enlarging abdominal mass in infancy. *J Pediatr Surg* 1982; 17: 316–7.

15. Johnston PW. Congenital cysts of the liver in infancy and childhood. *Am J Surg* 1968; 116: 184–91.

16. Benhamou JP, Menu Y. Non-parasitic cystic disease of the liver and intrahepatic biliary tree. In: Blumgart LH (ed). *Surgery of the Liver and Biliary Tract*. Edinburgh: Churchill Livingstone, 1994; 1197–210.

17. Athey PA, Landerman JA, King DE. Massive congenital solitary non-parasitic cyst of the liver in infancy. *J Ultrasound Med* 1986; 5: 585–7.

18. Torres VE. Polycystic liver disease. *Contrib Nephrol* 1995; 115: 44–52.

19. Gang DL, Herrin JT. Infantile polycystic disease of the liver and kidneys. *Clin Nephrol* 1986; 25: 28–36.

20. Roy S, Dillon, MJ, Trompeter RS et al. Autosomal recessive polycystic kidney disease: Long-term outcome of neonatal survivors. *Pediatr Nephrol* 1997; 11: 302–6.

21. Davies CH, Stringer DA, Whyte H et al. Congenital hepatic fibrosis with saccular dilation of intrahepatic bile ducts and infantile polycystic kidneys. *Pediatr Radiol* 1986; 16: 302–9.

22. Pineiro-Carrero VM, Andres JM. Morbidity and mortality in children with pyogenic liver abscess. *Am J Dis Child* 1989; 143: 1424–7.

23. Doerr CA, Demmler GJ, Garcia-Prats JA et al. Solitary pyogenic liver abscess in neonates: Report of three cases and review of the literature. *Pediatr Infect Dis J* 1994; 13: 64–9.

24. Moss TJ, Pysher TJ. Hepatic abscess in neonates. *Am J Dis Child* 1981; 135: 726–8.

25. Simeunovic E, Arnold M, Sidler D et al. Liver abscess in neonates. *Pediatr Surg Int* 2009; 25: 153–6.

26. Brans YW, Ceballos R, Cassady G. Umbilical catheters and hepatic abscesses. *Pediatrics* 1974; 53: 264–6.

27. Lim CT, Koh MT. Neonatal liver abscess following abdominal surgery for necrotizing enterocolitis. *Pediatr Surg Int* 1994; 9: 30–1.

28. Murphy FM, Baker CJ. Solitary hepatic abscess: A delayed complication of neonatal bacteremia. *Pediatr Infect Dis J* 1988; 7: 414–6.

29. Mechaber AJ, Tuazon CU. Hepatic abscess: Rare complication of ventriculoperitoneal shunts. *Clin Infect Dis* 1997; 25: 1244–5.

30. Simeunovic E, Arnold M, Sidler D et al. Liver abscess in neonates. *Pediatr Surg Int.* 2009; 25: 153–6.

31. Kays DW. Pediatric liver cysts and abscesses. *Semin Pediatr Surg* 1992; 1: 107–14.

32. Brook I, Frazier EH. Microbiology of liver and spleen abscesses. *J Med Microbiol* 1998; 47: 1075–80.

33. Vade A, Sajous C, Anderson B et al. Neonatal hepatic abscess. *Comput Med Imaging Graph* 1998; 22: 357–9.

34. Laurin S, Kaude JV. Diagnosis of liver–spleen abscesses in children—With emphasis on ultrasound for the initial and follow-up examinations. *Pediatr Radiol* 1984; 14: 198–204.

35. Oleszczuk-Raske K, Cremin BJ, Fisher RM et al. Ultrasonic features of pyogenic and amoebic hepatic abscesses. *Pediatr Radiol* 1989; 19: 230–3.

36. Bari S, Sheikh KA, Malik AA et al. Percutaneous aspiration versus open drainage of liver abscess in children. *Pediatr Surg Int* 2007; 23: 69–74.

37. Giorgio A, Tarantino L, Mariniello N et al. Pyogenic liver abscesses: 13 years of experience in percutaneous needle aspiration with US guidance. *Radiology* 1995; 195: 122–4.

38. Wong KP. Percutaneous drainage of pyogenic liver abscesses. *World J Surg* 1990; 14: 492–7.

39. Srivastava A, Yachha SK, Arora V et al. Identification of high-risk group and therapeutic options in children with liver abscesses. *Eur J Pediatr* 2012; 171: 33–41.

40. Lee SH, Tomlinson C, Temple M et al. Image-Guided percutaneous needle aspiration or catheter drainage of neonatal liver abscesses: 14-year experience. *AJR* 2008; 190: 616–22.

41. Inglis GD, Davies MW. Prophylactic antibiotics to reduce morbidity and mortality in neonates with umbilical venous catheters. *Cochrane Database Syst Rev* 2005 October 19;(4).

42. Harrison HR, Crowe CP, Fulginiti VA. Amebic liver abscess in children: Clinical and epidemiologic features. *Pediatrics* 1979; 64: 923–8.

43. Haffar A, Boland J, Edwards MS. Amebic liver abscess in children. *Pediatr Infect Dis J* 1982; 1: 322–7.

44. Axton JH. Amoebic proctocolitis and liver abscess in a neonate. *S Afr Med J* 1972; 46: 258–9.

45. Barnes P, DeCock KM, Reynolds TN et al. A comparison of amebic and pyogenic abscess of the liver. *Medicine* 1987; 66: 472–83.

46. Short M, Desai AP. Laparoscopy and transdiaphragmatic thoracoscopy in management of ruptured amebic liver abscess. *J Laproendosc Adv Surg Tech* 2008; 18: 473–6.

47. Maltz G, Knauer CM. Amebic liver abscess: A 15-year experience. *Am J Gastroenterol* 1991; 86: 704–10.

48. Allan RJV, Katz MD, Johnson MB et al. Uncomplicated amebic liver abscess: Prospective evaluation of percutaneous therapeutic aspiration. *Radiology* 1992; 183: 827–30.

PART **7**

Anterior abdominal wall defects

78

Omphalocele and gastroschisis

STEVEN W. BRUCH AND JACOB C. LANGER

INTRODUCTION

Omphalocele (also known as exomphalos) consists of a central abdominal wall defect that permits herniation of abdominal viscera into a sac made up of a three-layered membrane consisting of peritoneum, Wharton's jelly, and amnion (Figure 78.1) that covers the viscera. Pare provided the first description of an omphalocele in 1634. Hey reported the successful treatment of an omphalocele by primary repair in 1803, and Ahlfeld described the escharotic treatment using alcohol in 1899. In 1814, Scarpa observed that omphaloceles were often associated with other congenital anomalies.

Gastroschisis is a smaller abdominal wall defect to the right of a normally positioned umbilical cord, which permits herniation of the intestine (Figure 78.2), as well as occasionally, the liver, testis, or ovary. There is never an associated sac, and other than nonrotation and intestinal atresia, there are few associated congenital anomalies. Gastroschisis was first described by Calder in 1733, and the first surgical treatment for gastroschisis was described by Fear in 1878.

The surgical repair of abdominal wall defects has evolved over many years, with advances in diagnostic ability, neonatal intensive care, and anesthetic techniques. Although Gross popularized the skin flap closure of large omphaloceles in 1948,[1] it was Olshausen who first described this technique in 1887.[2] In 1966, Izant introduced manual stretching of the abdominal wall to make more room for primary closure.[3] Schuster[4] created the first mesh silo in 1967 to temporarily house the herniated viscera until primary closure could be accomplished. Recently, a spring-loaded silo was developed that permits placement of the silo without the need for fascial sutures.[5]

Two additional advances in the medical management of infants with abdominal wall defects have had a significant impact over the past 30 years. Raffensperger and Jona[6] were the first to use postoperative paralysis and ventilator support in the neonatal intensive care unit (NICU) to hasten abdominal wall closure, either primarily or after silo placement.[6] Filler introduced the use of total parenteral nutrition (TPN) to the neonatal population, which has become a crucial component in the high survival rate of infants with abdominal wall defects.[7]

EMBRYOLOGY AND ETIOLOGY

During the sixth week of embryonic development, the intestines begin to grow rapidly and migrate out of the umbilical ring into the umbilical cord.[8] By the 10th week, the intestines return to the abdominal cavity, rotating 270° counterclockwise to attain their normal position. An omphalocele results from failure of the bowel to return to the abdomen, possibly due to delayed closure of the lateral folds with persistence of a large umbilical ring. The defect is centrally located on the abdomen, varies in size, and has a sac covering the abdominal contents that consists of peritoneum, Wharton's jelly, and amnion. Because the process of intestinal rotation normally occurs after return of the viscera to the abdomen, infants with omphalocele usually have nonrotation or malrotation. In addition to the intestine, some or all of the liver may also be present in the sac. The liver is often round and globular in appearance and central in location, and has an abnormal fixation to the diaphragm. The hepatic veins appear tortuous and wander close to the skin edge at the superior aspect of the defect. The spleen and ovaries or testes may also be found in the sac. Failure of the cephalic fold to close leads to lower sternal abnormalities and an epigastric omphalocele, which is commonly associated with cardiac defects, pericardial absence, and an anterior diaphragmatic defect, together known as the pentalogy of Cantrell. Failure of the caudal fold to close leads to a hypogastric omphalocele often associated with bladder or cloacal exstrophy.

Gastroschisis results in bowel herniation through a small defect to the right of the normally formed umbilical cord. There are several hypotheses to explain the development of the gastroschisis defect. DeVries[9] in 1980 postulated abnormal involution of the right umbilical vein, and Hoyme, 1 year later, implicated the disruption of the vitelline artery[10] as a cause of gastroschisis. These vascular etiologies are less

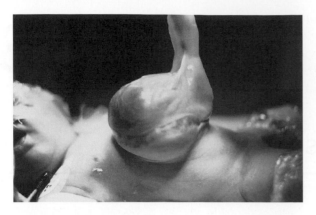

Figure 78.1 Omphalocele. The viscera (in this case liver and small bowel) are covered by a sac that is composed of peritoneum, Wharton's jelly, and amnion. The umbilical cord enters the top of the sac.

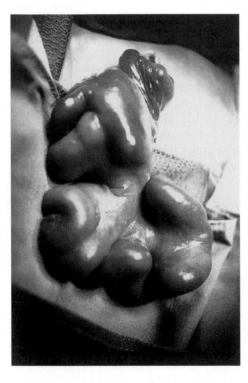

Figure 78.2 Gastroschisis. The defect is to the right of the umbilical cord, and the entire intestinal tract is exteriorized. There is no sac. The bowel wall and mesentery become thickened and foreshortened.

likely since neither the umbilical vein nor vitelline artery supplies the anterior abdominal wall. In 2007, Feldkamp et al.[11] theorized that defective closure of one or more of the embryonic body wall folds results in the gastroschisis defect. In 2009, Stevenson et al.[12] proposed that failure of the yolk sac and related vitelline structures to be incorporated into the umbilical stalk results in perforation of the abdominal wall that acts as an egress point for the intestine. More recently in 2013, Rittler proposed a defect in the umbilical ring, not the abdominal wall, with the umbilical

cord attached abnormally to the left side of the ring, leaving the right side uncovered.[13] The exact mechanism for the development of gastroschisis remains unclear. Despite this, the clinical scenario is well described. The entire intestinal tract is usually eviscerated, floating free in the amniotic cavity without an enveloping sac. The ovary, testis, and liver are less often involved. The intestines may develop a thick inflammatory peel, are foreshortened, and have a thickened mesentery—findings that correlate with functional impairment of motility and nutrient absorption. These changes result from a combination of factors, including contact with the amniotic fluid and constriction at the abdominal wall defect.

The cause of both omphalocele and gastroschisis is unknown. Omphalocele may have a genetic component, as suggested by the high incidence of structural and chromosomal anomalies, including the association with partial trisomy at chromosome 3q,[14] and by the high incidence of omphalocele in several knockout models in mice.[15] Although gastroschisis is thought not to have a genetic component to its origin, Torfs described four gene polymorphisms associated with an increased risk for gastroschisis,[16] and Kohl found a 2.4% familial recurrence rate in gastroschisis.[17]

INCIDENCE

The incidence of gastroschisis has been increasing worldwide over the past two decades. During that same time, the incidence of omphalocele has remained relatively constant, with an incidence of 1.92 per 10,000 live births in the United States.[18] The EUROCAT working group reported that the incidence of gastroschisis increased from 0.60 per 10,000 births in 1980–1984 to 2.33 per 10,000 births in 2000–2002[19] and 3.09 per 10,000 in 2011.[20] From 1987 to 2003, the overall birth prevalence for gastroschisis increased 3.2-fold in a population-based study from California.[21] The reason for this increase in gastroschisis but not in omphalocele is not well understood. Investigators have reviewed the currently available literature on nongenetic risk factors for gastroschisis including sociodemographic factors, maternal therapeutic and nontherapeutic drug exposures, chemical exposures, and other factors.[22,23] They found that the only factor definitively identified as a risk factor for gastroschisis is young maternal age. Other factors that may be associated, but require further confirmation, include ethnicity, socioeconomic status, poor nutrition,[23] cigarette smoking,[22] illicit drugs (including cocaine, methamphetamines, and marijuana),[23] certain medications (including aspirin, pseudoephedrine,[22] and selective serotonin reuptake inhibitors such as Paxil[24]), recent change in paternity, short cohabitation time,[22] gynecologic infections including *Chlamydia*,[25] and increased exposure to estrogens.[26]

ASSOCIATED ANOMALIES

As a rule, it is rare for gastroschisis to be associated with other anomalies, but it is very common for omphalocele.

A European study revealed that only 14% of infants born with omphalocele had no other anomalies. The majority of these infants, up to 88%, will have multiple associated anomalies.[27] Interestingly, small omphaloceles, less than 4 cm in diameter, have a higher incidence of multiple anomalies (55%) compared to giant omphaloceles (36%).[28] These anomalies include chromosomal abnormalities (trisomy 13, 18, and 21 being most common) in 30%–40%, cardiac abnormalities in 14%–47%, central nervous system abnormalities in 3%–33%, and associated syndromes including cloacal exstrophy, pentalogy of Cantrell, Donnai–Barrow syndrome, and Beckwith–Wiedemann syndrome in up to 12%.[27] Giant omphaloceles often develop chest wall and rib abnormalities, resulting in a narrow elongated chest with down-slanting ribs, and pulmonary hypoplasia, resulting in pulmonary insufficiency.[29] Pulmonary hypertension complicates up to 37% of giant omphaloceles, and these pulmonary issues may persist even after repair.[30] Gastroschisis, on the other hand, is usually an isolated lesion. In a review of over 3000 cases of gastroschisis, Mastroiacovo identified 14.1% of cases as nonisolated.[31] The majority of associated anomalies take the form of intestinal atresia; chromosomal abnormalities are rare. Recent Canadian Pediatric Surgery Network (CAPSNet) data broke down the anomalies associated with gastroschisis as follows: intestinal atresia 9.1%, cardiac 2.8%, genitourinary 2.4%, musculoskeletal 1.2%, and central nervous system 0.6%.[32,33] Interestingly, fetuses with gastroschisis and in utero fetal demise had a 10-fold increase in associated anomalies compared to live-born infants who survived greater than 24 hours.[33]

FUNCTION OF EXTERIORIZED VISCERA

Because of the presence of a sac in most omphaloceles, the exteriorized viscera usually function normally. In gastroschisis, the uncovered bowel is exposed to amniotic fluid, and its mesentery is subjected to varying amounts of constriction at the abdominal wall defect. Clinically, this leads to intestinal wall thickening, chronic inflammation, and often, a fibrous peel resulting in impaired motility and nutrient absorption.[34] The intestinal damage arises from exposure to fetal urine and, more importantly, meconium in the amniotic fluid, and from ischemia due to the restricted mesenteric blood flow at the gastroschisis defect.[35,36] These two insults appear to cause independent and additive damage.[37] This damage results in histologic changes in the gastroschisis bowel with increased submucosal collagen deposition and hypertrophy of the smooth muscle layer.[38] In addition, there is evidence of delayed differentiation of both smooth muscle and the Interstitial cells of Cajal in a rat model of gastroschisis.[39] The histopathologic changes along with the alteration in the intestinal nervous system lead to the impaired motility and absorption.[40] Recently, the infusion of mesenchymal stem cells into the amniotic fluid prevented the increase in bowel wall thickness usually seen in a rat gastroschisis model.[41] This may provide bowel protection for gastroschisis in the future.

PRENATAL DIAGNOSIS AND MANAGEMENT

The unique anatomic characteristics of omphalocele and gastroschisis allow them to be identified and differentiated using prenatal ultrasound. The diagnosis of omphalocele cannot be made definitively prior to the 10th gestational week, as the intestines are normally located in the umbilical cord up until that time. Although it is usually possible to sonographically differentiate omphalocele from gastroschisis, prenatal rupture of an omphalocele may make this more difficult. An abdominal wall defect is often suspected on routine screening because of elevation of the maternal serum alpha-fetoprotein (MSAFP), which is elevated in 90% of mothers carrying fetuses with omphalocele and 100% of those with gastroschisis.[42] Using a combination of maternal serum screening and ultrasound, the sensitivity and specificity for prenatal diagnosis of abdominal wall defects should approach 100%.[43]

Once an abdominal wall defect is identified, a search for additional anomalies should be carried out. If the problem is clearly gastroschisis, this can be limited to a careful anatomic ultrasound. The ultrasound exams should be repeated serially, evaluating for changes in the bowel appearance. Rare cases of vanishing gastroschisis occur where the abdominal defect closes and the extruded bowel disappears. The babies are born with an intact abdominal wall and a bowel atresia with significant loss of bowel length. Mechanistically, it is not known if the abdominal defect closes or the bowel loss occurs first, but the result is the same. For fetuses with omphalocele, both structural and chromosomal problems should be sought. Karyotype analysis by amniocentesis or chorionic villous sampling, and an anatomic ultrasound, including fetal echocardiography, should be completed. In most series, approximately two-thirds of associated abnormalities are detected prenatally in fetuses with omphalocele.[44]

Several prenatal indices may help predict neonatal outcome in fetuses with abdominal wall defects. In the case of omphalocele, the observed-to-expected fetal lung volume on magnetic resonance imaging (MRI)[45] and the ratio of omphalocele diameter to abdominal circumference ultrasound[46] have been used to predict such outcomes as primary closure within 24 hours, length of time on the ventilator, time to first and full enteral feeds, and length of neonatal stay. Investigators have studied prenatal ultrasound findings in fetuses with gastroschisis looking for signs that would predict bowel atresia and thus poorer outcomes. A recent meta-analysis revealed that intra-abdominal bowel dilation (odds ratio 5.48) and polyhydramnios (odds ratio 3.76) were risk factors for bowel atresia, whereas extra-abdominal bowel dilation and gastric dilation were not.[47]

At present, there are no intrauterine interventions indicated for fetuses with abdominal wall defects. There was interest in amnioinfusion in the past, theorizing that replacing the amniotic fluid with saline would decrease the concentration of the irritating factors in the fluid. However, amnioinfusion has not proven effective in reducing the inflammatory status of the amniotic fluid or in improving postnatal outcomes.[48] However, there continues to be controversy over the optimal timing and mode of delivery for infants with abdominal wall defects. Infants with omphalocele should be delivered at term. There is general agreement that infants with a very large omphalocele should be delivered by cesarean section to prevent injury to the exteriorized liver; however, infants with smaller defects should probably be delivered vaginally unless there are obstetric indications for cesarean section.[49] On the other hand, infants with gastroschisis may benefit from early delivery to minimize damage from exposure of the bowel to amniotic fluid, and to avoid late intrauterine fetal demise.[50] A number of investigators have reviewed this controversy, most with case series from one institution that used historical controls. There has been one randomized controlled trial with small numbers (only 20 mothers in each arm) that showed no difference in survival to hospital discharge, or any other neonatal outcome, with planned induction at 36 weeks estimated gestational age (EGA) compared with spontaneous labor.[51] Of interest, both groups had a similar gestational age at birth, suggesting that mothers carrying infants with gastroschisis tend to go into spontaneous preterm labor and deliver early. Barseghyan noted a 43% spontaneous preterm delivery rate with gastroschisis, compared to a 12.8% rate in the general US population, resulting in a mean EGA of 35 4/7 weeks.[52] In addition to this randomized controlled study, a large nationwide database is becoming mature enough to help answer this question. CAPSNet has prospectively collected data on all fetuses with the diagnosis of gastroschisis since 2005. Using these data, Al-Kaff looked at differences in neonatal outcomes depending on the planned route and timing of delivery that was made at 32 weeks EGA. He found no difference in median EGA at delivery (36 weeks) whether the labor was induced or allowed to occur spontaneously. There were also no differences in neonatal outcomes including length of stay, length of TPN required, and time to first enteral feeds. From this, he concluded that there were no major health benefits from planned early delivery.[53] Youssef, using the same database, looked at bowel damage as it relates to time of delivery. He found a 1.4% fetal loss rate, which occurred mostly early in gestation. After evaluating the gastroschisis prognostic score, which stratifies the severity of the gastroschisis bowel abnormalities at birth, and the amount of bowel matting identified at birth, he concluded that there is no indication for early delivery to prevent bowel damage.[48] Again, using the CAPSNet database and looking at the actual timing of delivery, Nasr found that infants born with gastroschisis before 36 weeks EGA had a longer time interval to full enteral feeds and more complications, while those born after 38 weeks EGA had more bowel matting. He suggested that induction of labor between 36 and 38 weeks EGA may reduce gastroschisis-related bowel morbidity while avoiding the risks related to prematurity.[54] Routine cesarean section has shown no benefit compared to vaginal delivery, so the route of delivery should be based on obstetric indications.[48]

NEWBORN MANAGEMENT

The initial treatment of a newborn with an abdominal wall defect consists of resuscitation, including evaluation of the airway and pulmonary status; this is particularly important for infants with giant omphalocele, which may be associated with pulmonary hypoplasia. Intravenous access allows volume resuscitation. In infants with gastroschisis, the bowel should be inspected to ensure that its blood supply is not compromised by twisting of the mesentery or constriction at the abdominal wall defect. If the size of the abdominal wall defect in gastroschisis is causing vascular compromise, the defect should be enlarged immediately. The bowel should be wrapped in warm saline-soaked gauze and covered with a waterproof dressing (Figure 78.3). A bowel bag or cellophane works well for this purpose. Children with gastroschisis should be transported and nursed on their right side to avoid kinking of the mesenteric vessels. In infants with omphalocele, the sac should be inspected for leaks before placing the dressing.

Newborns with abdominal wall defects should be placed in a temperature-controlled environment, as they lose a great deal of heat through the exposed bowel. Babies with gastroschisis require up to 2–3 times the amount of fluid a normal term infant would require. Despite the intact abdominal wall, babies with an omphalocele will have greater fluid and temperature losses than a normal infant, but not to the degree that is seen with gastroschisis.[28] Isotonic solutions should be used for resuscitation, and the child should be well hydrated prior to going to the operating room (OR) for repair. Once fluid resuscitation has been accomplished, parenteral nutrition, preferably through a central venous catheter, should be initiated.

All infants should be carefully examined clinically and radiologically to ensure that adequate pulmonary, cardiac, and renal function are maintained. Associated anomalies must be diligently searched for, particularly in those infants with omphalocele.

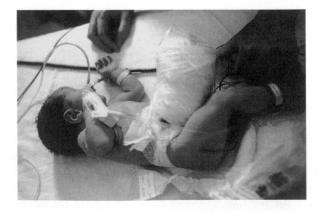

Figure 78.3 Appropriate dressing of an abdominal wall defect in the delivery room. The viscera are covered with warm saline-soaked gauze, supported on the anterior abdominal wall and covered with a waterproof dressing.

The appearance of the bowel noted in gastroschisis shortly after birth, within 6 hours, can be predictive of clinical outcome. Cowan developed the Gastroschisis Prognostic Score based on inspection of the exteriorized bowel for bowel matting (none 0, mild 1, severe 4); atresia (absent 0, suspected 1, present 2); perforation (absent 0, present 2); and necrosis (absent 0, present 4). A score of 2 or more is associated with increased complications and prolonged hospitalization, and a score of 4 or more increases the odds of mortality.[55]

SURGICAL MANAGEMENT

The goal of surgical management for abdominal wall defects is to replace the herniated viscera in the abdominal cavity and obtain fascial and skin closure with an acceptable cosmetic outcome. Various issues arise that make the closure strategy different for gastroschisis and omphalocele. The exposed bowel in gastroschisis requires an immediate intervention. Historically, primary closure was the first successful method introduce by Watkins in 1943.[56] Staged silo repair was introduced by Schuster[4] in 1967 and allowed for the survival of many more babies with gastroschisis. The

strategy at that time became an attempted primary closure, and if that was not possible, a silo was formed, and a staged reduction was performed followed by operative fascial closure (Figure 78.4). Fischer described the first preformed silo in 1995.[57] and these become popular in the late 1990s (Figure 78.5). This provided an easily placed silo that could be applied in the delivery room, the NICU, or the OR, often without the need for intubation or significant sedation. The treatment pendulum has now swung to where the majority of babies with gastroschisis are treated this way to prevent the development of abdominal compartment syndrome, which can result in ischemic or necrotic bowel, renal insufficiency, and respiratory distress.[58] Chesley reported that at his institution, their practice was to attempt primary closure and use a surgically created silo if necessary before the spring-loaded silos arrived. They achieved a 60% primary closure rate. When the spring-loaded silos became available, their primary closure rate decreased to 15%.[59] Sandler described suture-less closure for gastroschisis in 2004.[60] After intestinal reduction, the umbilical cord is used as a plug and secured in place by a clear adhesive dressing. This allows the umbilical ring to close naturally, forming

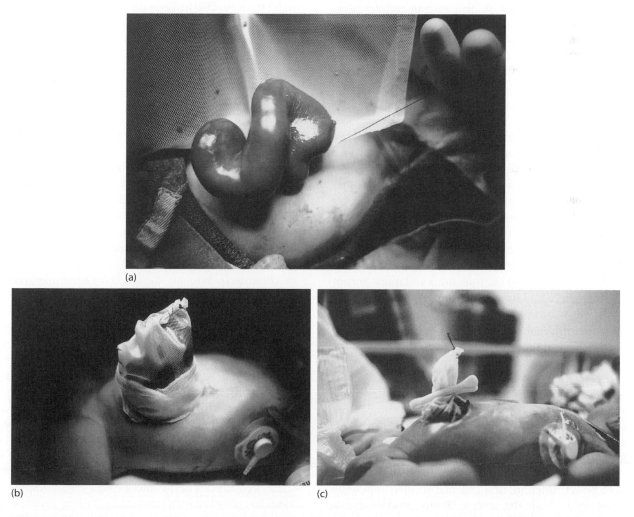

Figure 78.4 The use of a silo in a child with gastroschisis. **(a)** The silo is sewn to the abdominal wall, over the bowel. **(b)** The bowel is slowly reduced once or twice per day. **(c)** The abdominal wall is ready to be definitively closed.

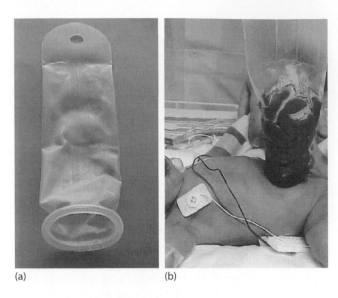

(a)   (b)

Figure 78.5 **(a)** Spring-loaded silo. **(b)** This device can be placed at the bedside without an anesthetic and permits gradual reduction of the viscera in every case, with only one trip to the operating room.

a normal-appearing umbilicus. This technique works even for the large defects resulting from a preformed silo as long as the umbilical ring is not opened,[61] which is reportedly required in 11%–44% of silo placements.[58,62] Following this, Chesley's group[59] again achieved a 60% primary closure rate. Stanger, using the CAPSNet data, reports a successful primary closure rate of 81%.[63] The majority of pediatric surgeons attempt a primary reduction with or without a suture-less closure and use a preformed silo in the event that a primary repair cannot be completed. There are, however, some proponents of an initial preformed silo placement. A randomized trial[64] and several large meta-analyses[65–67] reviewed preformed silo placement and staged closure versus primary repair in gastroschisis and found nearly all clinical outcomes equivalent. The CAPSNet data did make a distinction between successful and failed primary closure and showed that those who failed initial primary closure experienced more surgical site infections and more culture-proven bacteremia, and had a longer duration of parenteral nutrition, later initiation of enteral feeds, and more days of mechanical ventilation.[63]

The approach to the 10% of babies with bowel atresia associated with gastroschisis varies depending on the appearance of the bowel. If the atresia is identified at the time of closure and the bowel inflammation is minimal, a primary anastomosis is favored. If the bowel inflammation makes primary closure impossible, the ends should be reduced, and the abdomen closed with a plan to return in 4–6 weeks for atresia repair. On occasion, the atresia is not recognized at the time of closure. The baby will not have return of bowel function, and contrast studies from above and below will reveal the atresia. Stoma creation can be used, and on occasion, the best place to create the stoma is in the gastroschisis defect at the umbilicus.

The sac that covers the viscera in an omphalocele makes immediate surgical intervention unnecessary unless there is a hole in the sac. Historically, Hey reported the first successful primary closure of an omphalocele in 1805, and in 1948, Gross described the skin flap technique, where skin flaps but not fascia covered the bowel in giant omphaloceles.[1] The surgical strategy employed now for omphalocele is determined by the size of the defect and the physiologic status of the infant. With a small defect, a primary repair is in order. The sac is removed, and the fascia and skin are brought together. With larger defects that cannot be repaired primarily, there are several options. One is to remove the sac and place a silo, usually sewn to the fascia, as the preformed silos have a difficult time staying in the large omphalocele defects. The contents are then gradually reduced into the abdominal cavity. The silo is then removed, and the fascia and skin are closed. Occasionally, the fascia must be left open with skin closure only, or a piece of mesh can be placed either temporarily or permanently to span the fascial defect and allow skin closure. In infants with a giant omphalocele, defined as a defect greater than 5 cm in diameter with at least one-half of the liver being present in the sac, or in infants with poor physiology that would not tolerate increased intra-abdominal pressure, a second option is the "paint and wait" strategy. This involves dressing the omphalocele membrane with an antimicrobial substance, usually silver sulfadiazine, and allowing the membrane to firm up, granulate, and epithelialize, providing pseudo-skin coverage over the sac (Figure 78.6). The use of negative-pressure wound therapy applied in the first 48 hours after birth to the omphalocele sac may allow earlier epithelialization to occur. Wound healing was complete in 2 months with negative pressure compared to the 6 months often required to complete wound healing when using silver sulfadiazine.[68] The infants usually go home for a period of time and return for fascial closure later in life when their pulmonary and cardiac status has improved. On occasion, after epithelialization, there is not enough abdominal domain to allow complete reduction of the viscera in giant omphaloceles. In these situations, tissue expanders have been used to increase the space in the abdominal cavity, allowing reduction of the viscera and final closure.[69] Final closure may be obtained by bringing the fascia together primarily, using mesh, either permanent or biologic,[70] or employing a multilayered flap technique.[71]

There are a few caveats regarding these methods. When attempting primary closure or initial placement of a silo, the sac is often very adherent to the liver, so that it is often best to leave some of the sac behind on the liver to avoid significant bleeding from the attempt to separate the sac from the liver capsule. As the dissection of the sac proceeds cephalad, care should be taken not to injure the hepatic veins, which will be located just under the fascia due to the abnormal position of the liver and the inferior vena cava. The abrupt change in the position of the liver in an attempted primary closure may kink these hepatic veins or the inferior vena cava, causing cardiovascular compromise. If this occurs, the liver should be taken out of the abdomen and placed in a silo. Often, with gradual reduction in a silo, this problem will be circumvented.

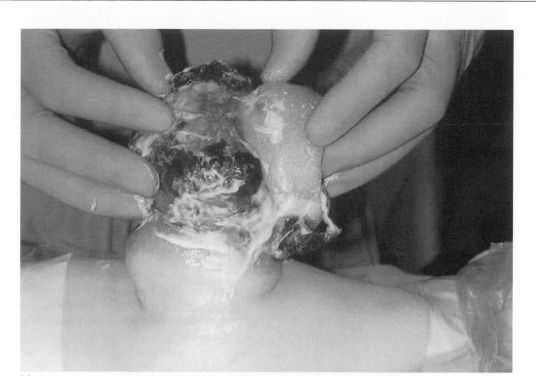

(a)

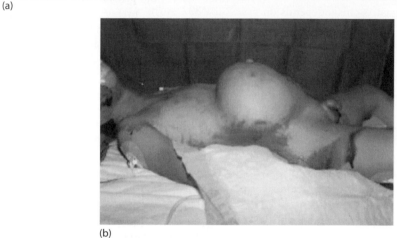

(b)

Figure 78.6 Escharotic management of a large omphalocele. **(a)** The sac is covered with silver sulfadiazine. This results in the formation of granulation tissue and ultimately in epithelialization. **(b)** The resulting ventral hernia can be repaired at any time, when the child's medical condition improves.

POSTOPERATIVE MANAGEMENT

Postoperatively, feedings are started when gastrointestinal function returns. This usually occurs more quickly in infants with omphalocele compared to gastroschisis and can take weeks to months. A review of the CAPSNet data revealed that in gastroschisis, the elapsed time from abdominal wall closure to the initiation of enteral feeds took a mean time of 17 days.[72] The abnormal intestinal motility and nutrient absorption of the exposed bowel in gastroschisis gradually improve over time but can affect the babies for up to 6–9 months. During the initial wait for bowel function to return, nasogastric decompression with parenteral nutrition sustains the infants. Feeding, or oral stimulation if feeds are not feasible, should be initiated as soon as possible to prevent oral aversion. Earlier initiation of enteral feeds predicted earlier TPN independence, a shorter length of stay, and less infectious complications in a CAPSNet review. This review also revealed a benefit to waiting at least 7 days to initiate feeds.[72] Feedings ,should be advanced cautiously in order to avoid inducing necrotizing enterocolitis which occurs in gastroschisis at a much higher frequency (up to 18.5%) than would be otherwise expected.[28]

Feeding difficulties are much less common following repair of omphalocele since the bowels have been protected by the omphalocele sac and should function normally as long as they are not compromised due to the pressure exerted by the fascial closure. However, pulmonary issues caused by pulmonary hypoplasia and pulmonary hypertension may result in prolonged mechanical ventilation following repair,

Table 78.1 Long-term quality of life

		Gastroschisis	Omphalocele
Gastrointestinal issues	Frequent	7%	10%
	Rarely or never	77%	75%
Physical limitations		9%	7%
Cosmetic results	Good or excellent	82%	73%
	Umbilical reconstruction	23%	35%
	Troubled by lack of umbilicus	24%	11%
Abdominal wall hernia		14%	20%
Delayed sitting or walking		32%	27%
Began school at usual age		77%	93%
Growth	Weight < 3rd percentile	9%	20%
	Height < 3rd percentile	14%	13%

not only in the newborn period but also following delayed repair later in childhood.

LONG-TERM OUTCOME

The outcome of infants born with gastroschisis depends on the condition of the intestine. In uncomplicated cases of gastroschisis, the overall survival is greater than 90%.[73-76] However, infants with gastroschisis that requires home TPN due to loss of bowel length or inability to tolerate enteral feeds despite normal bowel length have a 50% mortality rate in the first 2 years of life.[76] A significant number of these patients require additional surgery, usually for adhesive intestinal obstruction, and a small group of children suffer from short bowel syndrome or long-term motility disorders, which ultimately require small bowel transplantation.[77] In fact, gastroschisis is the most frequent indication for pediatric small bowel transplantation.[78] The outcome for infants with omphalocele is more dependent on the presence and severity of associated malformations. In the absence of chromosomal abnormalities, or severe pulmonary or cardiac anomalies, the majority of these children survive to live normal lives.[73,74] Henrich et al.[79] looked at several aspects of long-term quality of life in children with gastroschisis and omphalocele. These are depicted in Table 78.1. The results are similar in the two groups and reveal a satisfying overall quality of life for these children after long-term follow-up. The long-term neurodevelopmental outcomes of school-aged children and adolescents born with gastroschisis revealed overall normal intellect with a small but significant decrease in working memory index compared to normal children. There were no children with cerebral palsy or significant visual or hearing deficits noted in this group.[80]

REFERENCES

1. Gross RE. A new method for surgical treatment of large omphaloceles. *Surgery* 1948; 24: 277.
2. Olshausen RZ. Zur therapie der nadelschnurhernien. *Arch Bynak Berlin* 1887; 29: 443.
3. Izant RJ, Brown F, Rothmann BF. Current embryology and treatment of gastroschisis and omphalocele. *Arch Surg* 1966; 93: 49.
4. Schuster SR. A new method for the staged repair of large omphaloceles. *Surg Gynecol Obstet* 1967; 125: 837.
5. Minkes RK, Langer JC, Mazziotti MV et al. Routine insertion of a Silastic spring-loaded silo for infants with gastroschisis. *J Pediatr Surg* 2000; 35: 843–6.
6. Raffensperger JG, Jona JZ. Gastroschisis. *Surg Gynecol Obstet* 1974; 138: 230.
7. Filler RM, Eraklis AJ, Das JB et al. Total intravenous nutrition. An adjunct to the management of infants with ruptured omphalocele. *Am J Surg* 1971; 121: 454–9.
8. Langer JC. Normal fetal development. In: Oldham KT, Colombani PM, Foglia RP (eds). *Surgery of Infants and Children*. Philadelphia: Lippincott-Raven Publishers, 1997: 41–8.
9. deVries PA. The pathogenesis of gastroschisis and omphalocele. *J Pediatr Surg* 1980; 15: 245–51.
10. Hoyme HE, Higginbottom MC, Jones KL. The vascular pathogenesis of gastroschisis: Intrauterine interruption of the omphalomesenteric artery. *J Pediatr* 1981; 98: 228–31.
11. Feldkamp ML, Carey JC, Sadler TW. Development of gastroschisis: Review of hypothesis, a novel hypothesis, and implications for research. *Am J Med Genet A* 2007; 143: 639–52.
12. Stevenson RE, Rogers RC, Chandler JC et al. Escape of the yolk sac: A hypothesis to explain the embryogenesis of gastroschisis. *Clin Genet* 2009; 75: 326–33.
13. Rittler M, Vauthay L, Mazzitelli N. Gastroschisis is a defect of the umbilical ring: Evidence from morphological evaluation of stillborn fetuses. *Birth Defects Res* 2013; 97: 198–209.
14. Chen CP, Lin CJ, Chen YY et al. 3q26.31–q29 duplication and 9q34.3 microdeletion associated with omphalocele, ventricular septal defect, abnormal

first-trimester maternal serum screening and increased nuchal translucency: Prenatal diagnosis and aCGH characterization. *Gene* 2013; 532: 80–6.

15. Rauch F, Prud'homme J, Arabian A et al. Heart, brain, and body wall defects in mice lacking calreticulin. *Exp Cell Res* 2000; 256: 105–11.

16. Torfs CP, Christianson RE, Iovannisci DM et al. Selected gene polymorphisms and their interaction with maternal smoking as risk factors for gastroschisis. *Birth Defects Res A* 2006; 76: 723–30.

17. Kohl M, Wiesel A, Schier F. Familial recurrence of gastroschisis literature review and data from the population-based birth registry "Mainz Model." *J Pediatr Surg* 2010; 45: 1907–12.

18. Marshall J, Salemi JL, Tanner JP et al. Prevalence, correlates, and outcomes of omphalocele in the United States, 1995–2005. *Obstetr Gynecol* 2015; 126: 284–93.

19. Loane M, Dolk H, Bradbury I et al. Increasing prevalence of gastroschisis in Europe 1980–2002: A phenomenon restricted to younger mothers. *Pediatr Perinat Epi* 2007; 21: 363–9.

20. Prefumo F, Izzi C. Fetal abdominal wall defects. *Best Pract Res Clin Obstetr Gynaecol* 2014; 28: 391–402.

21. Vu LT, Nobuhara KK, Laurent C et al. Increasing prevalence of gastroschisis: Population-based study in California. *J Pediatr* 2008; 152: 807–11.

22. Rasmussen SA, Frias JL. Non-genetic risk factors for gastroschisis. *Am J Med Genet* 2008; 148c: 199–212.

23. Frolov P, Alali J, Klein MD. Clinical risk factors for gastroschisis and omphalocele in humans: A review of the literature. *Pediatr Surg Int* 2010; 26: 1135–48.

24. Reefhuis J, Devine O, Friedman JM et al. Specific SSRIs and birth defects: Bayesian analysis to interpret new data in the context of previous reports. *BMJ* 2015; 350: h3190.

25. Feldkamp ML, Enioutina EY, Gotto LD et al. *Chlamydia trachomatis* IgG3 seropositivity is associated with gastroschisis. *J Perinatol* 2015; 35: 930–4.

26. Lubinsky M. Hypothesis: Estrogen related thrombosis explains the pathogenesis and epidemiology of gastroschisis. *Am J Med Genet Part A* 2012; 158A: 808–11.

27. Gamba P, Midrio P. Abdominal wall defects: Prenatal diagnosis, newborn management, and long-term outcomes. *Semin Pediatr Surg* 2014; 23: 283–90.

28. Christison-Lagay ER, Kelleher CM, Langer JC. Neonatal abdominal wall defects. *Semin Fetal Neonat Med* 2011; 16: 164–72.

29. Panitch HB. Pulmonary complications of abdominal wall defects. *Paediatr Respir Rev* 2015; 16: 11–7.

30. Partridge EA, Hanna BD, Panitch HB et al. Pulmonary hypertension in giant omphalocele infants. *J Pediatr Surg* 2014; 49: 1767–70.

31. Mastroiacovo P, Lisi A, Castilla EE et al. Gastroschisis and associated defects: An international study. *Am J Med Genet A* 2007; 143: 660–71.

32. Alshehri A, Emil S, Laberge JM et al. Outcomes of early versus late intestinal operations in patients with gastroschisis and intestinal atresia: Results from a prospective national database. *J Pediatr Surg* 2013; 48: 2022–6.

33. Akhtar J, Skarsgard ED, The Canadian Pediatric Surgery Network (CAPSNet). Associated malformations and the "hidden mortality" of gastroschisis. *J Pediatr Surg* 2012; 47: 911–6.

34. O'Neill JA, Grosfeld JL. Intestinal malfunction after antenatal exposure of viscera. *Am J Surg* 1974; 127: 129–32.

35. Langer JC, Longaker MT, Crombleholme TM et al. Etiology of bowel damage in gastroschisis. I: Effects of amniotic fluid exposure and bowel constriction in a fetal lamb model. *J Pediatr Surg* 1989; 24: 992–7.

36. Olguner M, Akgur FM, Api A et al. The effects of intraamniotic human neonatal urine and meconium on the intestines of the chick embryo with gastroschisis. *J Pediatr Surg* 2000; 35: 458–61.

37. Phillips JD, Raval MV, Redden C et al. Gastroschisis, atresia, dysmotility: Surgical treatment strategies for a distinct clinical entity. *J Pediatr Surg* 2008; 43: 2208–12.

38. Srinathan SK, Langer JC, Blennerhassett MG et al. Etiology of intestinal damage in gastroschisis. III: Morphometric analysis of the smooth muscle and submucosa. *J Pediatr Surg* 1995; 30: 379–83.

39. Midrio P, Faussone-Pellegrini MS, Vannucchi MG et al. Gastroschisis in the rat model is associated with a delayed maturation of intestinal pacemaker cells and smooth muscle cells. *J Pediatr Surg* 2004; 39: 1541–7.

40. Dicken BJ, Sergi C, Rescorla FJ et al. Medical management of motility disorders in patients with intestinal failure: A focus on necrotizing enterocolitis, gastroschisis, and intestinal atresia. *J Pediatr Surg* 2011; 46: 1618–30.

41. Feng C, Graham CD, Connors JP et al. Transamniotic stem cell therapy (TRASCET) mitigates bowel damage in a model of gastroschisis. *J Pediatr Surg* 2016; 51: 56–61.

42. Pslomaki GE, Hill LE, Knight GJ et al. Second-trimester maternal serum alpha-fetoprotein levels in pregnancies associated with gastroschisis and omphalocele. *Obstet Gynecol* 1988; 71: 906–9.

43. Lennon CA, Gray DL. Sensitivity and specificity of ultrasound for the detection of neural tube and ventral wall defects in a high-risk population. *Obstet Gynecol* 1999; 94: 562–6.

44. Holland AJ, Ford WD, Linke RJ et al. Influence of antenatal ultrasound on the management of fetal exomphalos. *Fetal Diagn Ther* 1999; 14: 223–8.

45. Danzer E, Victoria T, Bebbington MW et al. Fetal MRI-calculated total lung volumes in the prediction of short-term outcome in giant omphalocele: Preliminary findings. *Fetal Diagn Ther* 2012; 31: 248–53.

46. Fawley JA, Peterson EL, Christensen MA et al. Can omphalocele ratio predict postnatal outcomes? *J Pediatr Surg* 2016; 51: 62–6.

47. D'Antonio F, Virgone C, Rizzo G et al. Prenatal risk factors and outcomes in gastroschisis: A meta-analysis. *Pediatrics* 2015; 136: e159–69.

48. Youssef F, Laberge JM, Baird RJ et al. The correlation between the time spent in utero and the severity of bowel matting in newborns with gastroschisis. *J Pediatr Surg* 2015; 50: 755–9.

49. How HY, Harris BJ, Pietrantoni M et al. Is vaginal delivery preferable to elective cesarean delivery in fetuses with a known ventral wall defect? *Am J Obstet Gynecol* 2000; 182: 1527–34.

50. Baud D, Lausman A, Alfaraj M et al. Expectant management compared with elective delivery at 37 weeks for gastroschisis. *Obstetr Gynecol* 2013; 121: 990–8.

51. Logghe HL, Mason GC, Stringer MD et al. A randomized controlled trial of elective preterm delivery of fetuses with gastroschisis. *J Pediatr Surg* 2005; 40: 1726–31.

52. Barseghyan K, Aghajanian P, Miller DA. The prevalence of preterm births in pregnancies complicated with fetal gastroschisis. *Arch Gynecol Obstet* 2012; 286: 889–92.

53. Al-Kaff A, MacDonald SC, Kent N et al. Delivery planning for pregnancies with gastroschisis: Findings from a prospective national registry. *Am J Obstet Gynecol* 2015; 213: 557.e1–8.

54. Nasr A, Wayne C, Bass J et al. Effect of delivery approach on outcomes in fetuses with gastroschisis. *J Pediatr Surg* 2013; 48: 2251–5.

55. Cowan KN, Puligandla PS, Laberge JM et al. The gastroschisis prognostic score: Reliable outcome prediction in gastroschisis. *J Pediatr Surg* 2012; 47: 1111–7.

56. Watkins D. Gastroschisis. *Va Med Mon* 1943; 70: 42.

57. Fischer JD, Chun K, Moores DC et al. Gastroschisis: A simple technique for staged silo closure. *J Pediatr Surg* 1995; 30: 1169–71.

58. Lobo JD, Kim AC, Davis RP et al. No free ride? The hidden costs of delayed operative management using a spring-loaded silo for gastroschisis. *J Pediatr Surg* 2010; 45: 1426–32.

59. Chesley PM, Ledbetter DJ, Meehan JJ et al. Contemporary trends in the use of primary repair for gastroschisis in surgical infants. *Am J Surg* 2015; 209: 901–6.

60. Sandler A, Lawrence J, Meehan J et al. A "plastic" sutureless abdominal wall closure in gastroschisis. *J Pediatr Surg* 2004; 39: 738–41.

61. Orion KC, Krein M, Liao J et al. Outcomes of plastic closure in gastroschisis. *Surgery* 2011; 150: 177–85.

62. Charlesworth P, Akinnola I, Hammerton C et al. Preformed silos versus traditional abdominal wall closure in gastroschisis: 163 infants at a single institution. *Eur J Ped Surg* 2014; 24: 88–93.

63. Stanger J, Mohajerani N, Skarsgard ED et al. Practice variation in gastroschisis: Factors influencing closure technique. *J Pediatr Surg* 2014; 49: 720–3.

64. Pastor A, Phillips JD, Fenton SJ et al. Routine use of a Silastic spring-loaded silo for infants with gastroschisis: A multi-center randomized controlled trial. *J Pediatr Surg* 2008; 43: 1807–12.

65. Mortellaro VE, St Peter SD, Fike FB et al. Review of the evidence on the closure of abdominal wall defects. *Pediatr Surg Int* 2011; 27: 391–7.

66. Ross AR, Eaton S, Zani A et al. The role of preformed silos in the management of infants with gastroschisis: A systematic review and meta-analysis. *Pediatr Surg Int* 2015; 31: 473–83.

67. Allin BS, Tse WH, Marven S et al. Challenges of improving the evidence base in smaller surgical specialties, as highlighted by a systematic review of gastroschisis management. *PLoS ONE* 2015; 10: e0116908.

68. Aldridge B, Ladd AP, Kepple J et al. Negative pressure wound therapy for initial management of giant omphalocele. *Am J Surg* 2016; 211: 605–9.

69. Adetayo OA, Aka AA, Ray AO. The use of intra-abdominal tissue expansion for the management of giant omphaloceles. *Ann Plastic Surg* 2012; 69: 104–8.

70. Beres A, Christison-Lagay ER, Romao RL et al. Evaluation of Surgisis for patch repair of abdominal wall defects in children. *J Pediatr Surg* 2012; 47: 917–9.

71. Kruit AS, Al-Ani SA, Jester I et al. Multilayered flap technique: A method for delayed closure of giant omphalocele. *Ann Plast Surg* 2015; Epub ahead of print.

72. Aljahdali A, Nohajerani N, Skarsgard ED et al. Effect of timing of enteral feeding on outcome in gastroschisis. *J Pediatr Surg* 2013; 48: 971–6.

73. Berseth CL, Malachowski N, Cohn RB et al. Longitudinal growth and late morbidity of survivors of gastroschisis and omphalocele. *J Pediatr Gastroent Nutr* 1982; 1: 375–9.

74. Tunell WP, Puffinbarger NK, Tuggle DW et al. Abdominal wall defects in infants: Survival and implications for adult life. *Ann Surg* 1995; 221: 525–30.

75. Davies BW, Stringer MD. The survivors of gastroschisis. *Arch Dis Child* 1997; 77: 158–60.

76. David AL, Tan A, Curry J. Gastroschisis: Sonographic diagnosis, associations, management and outcome. *Prenat Diagn* 2008; 28: 633–44.

77. Reyes J, Bueno J, Kocoshis S et al. Current status of intestinal transplantation in children. *J Pediatr Surg* 1998; 33: 243–54.

78. Wada M, Kato T, Hayashi Y et al. Intestinal transplantation for short bowel syndrome secondary to gastroschisis. *J Pediatr Surg* 2006; 41: 1841–5.

79. Henrich K, Huemmer HP, Reingruber B et al. Gastroschisis and omphalocele: Treatments and long-term outcomes. *Pediatr Surg Int* 2008; 24: 167–73.

80. Harris EL. Hart SJ, Minutillo C et al. The long-term neurodevelopmental and psychological outcomes of gastroschisis: A cohort study. *J Pediatr Surg* 2015; http://dx.doi.org/10.1016/j.jpedsurg.2015.08.062.

79

Omphalomesenteric duct remnants

KENNETH K. Y. WONG AND PAUL K. H. TAM

INTRODUCTION

The omphalomesenteric duct or the vitelline duct is a long narrow tube that joins the yolk sac to the digestive tube in the developing human embryo. This duct undergoes complete obliteration during the seventh week in most cases. However, in the rare circumstances where there is incomplete obliteration, omphalomesenteric remnants will be the result, which may be apparent in the newborn infant.[1]

ETIOLOGY

Development of the midgut in the embryo is characterized by growth and elongation of the gut at the end of the fourth week of gestation. At the apex, the intestinal loop remains connected and open to the yolk sac via the omphalomesenteric duct.[2] In some neonates, this duct persists due to incomplete obliteration and resorption (unknown cause), thus giving rise to the various anatomical anomalies as described in the next section.

PATHOLOGY

Omphalomesenteric remnants can be classified into various types according to the underlying anomaly (Figure 79.1):

1. Persistent omphalomesenteric duct (patent or obliterated)
2. Omphalomesenteric duct cyst
3. Meckel diverticulum
4. Umbilical mucosal polyp/umbilical cyst

HISTORY, PRESENTATION, AND DIAGNOSIS

Persistent omphalomesenteric duct

The persistent omphalomesenteric duct may remain patent after birth and present as an omphaloileal fistula.

The fistula may contain ectopic gastric, colonic, or pancreatic tissue. Affected neonates often present with umbilical discharge, which resembles small bowel content and can result in periumbilical excoriation. An umbilical "polyp" consisting of intestinal mucosa may also be present. The diagnosis is confirmed by passing a catheter through the fistula into the small intestine and aspirating small bowel content, or by injecting radiographic contrast medium into the fistula to perform a "fistulogram."

Rarely, the ileum may even prolapse through the omphaloileal fistula—giving rise to the so-called steer-horn abnormality (Figure 79.2), which may give rise to intestinal obstruction.

For obliterated omphalomesenteric duct, it may persist as a fibrous cord attaching the ileum to the umbilicus internally. The infant who has this anomaly is usually asymptomatic. However, there is a risk of small bowel volvulus occurring around such a band.

Omphalomesenteric duct cyst

The obliterated omphalomesenteric duct may contain one or more cysts. The clinical presentation of this is similar to obliterated duct, with a risk of small bowel volvulus. Sometimes, the cyst can become infected, and the child may present with pain and fever.

Meckel diverticulum

The most common omphalomesenteric remnant seen is the Meckel diverticulum, which is the persistence of the enteral end on the antimesenteric side of the small intestine (Figure 79.3). This anomaly occurs in around 2% of the population, with its location usually within 2 feet of the ileocecal, around 2 inches long, and usually presents below the age of 2 years ("rule of 2s"). Complications of the diverticulum include bleeding, diverticulitis, and intussusception. Asymptomatic ones are usually found incidentally at laparotomies for other conditions. A recent

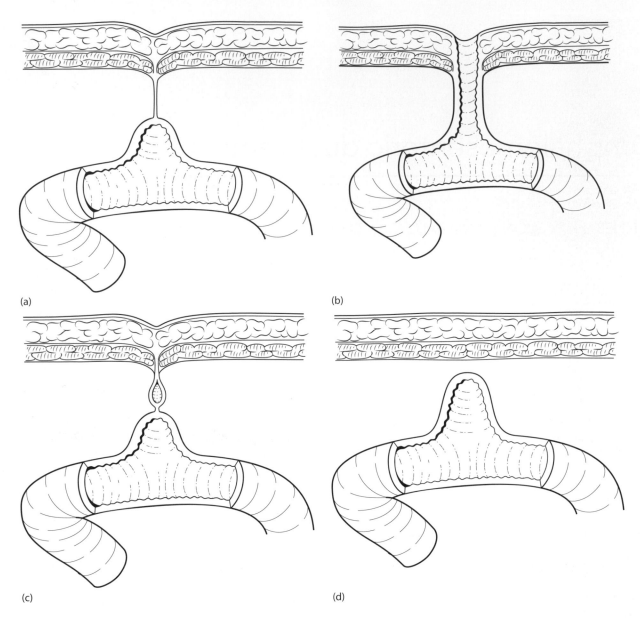

Figure 79.1 Schematic diagrams showing the various anatomical variations of omphalomesenteric remnants. **(a)** Obliterated omphalomesenteric duct. **(b)** Patent omphalomesenteric duct. **(c)** A cyst in an obliterated omphalomesenteric duct. **(d)** Meckel diverticulum.

study showed that resection of incidentally detected Meckel diverticulum had a significantly higher postoperative complication rate than leaving it in situ and that 758 resections would need to be performed to prevent 1 death from the condition. As a result, there is no evidence to support the resection of incidentally detected Meckel diverticulum.[3]

For diagnosis, the presence of ectopic gastric mucosa with the secretion of gastrin can be detected using Tc-99 radioisotope scanning (Figure 79.4), although a negative result does not exclude the presence of Meckel diverticulum (sensitivity of Tc-99 around 80%–85%).[4] In a young infant presenting with significant per rectal bleeding with hemoglobin drop, Meckel diverticulum should be one of the top diagnoses on the list.

Umbilical polyp

An umbilical polyp is a remnant of intestinal mucosa at the umbilicus. The pink, polypoid tissue produces a persistent discharge, which may be bloodstained. The other differential diagnosis is an umbilical granuloma, which should respond to simple cauterization treatment. The diagnosis of an umbilical polyp may be confirmed by biopsy to look for the presence of intestinal or gastric mucosa.

OPERATIVE MANAGEMENT

Omphalomesenteric remnants are best managed operatively,[5] and the approaches for the various anomalies are described as follows.

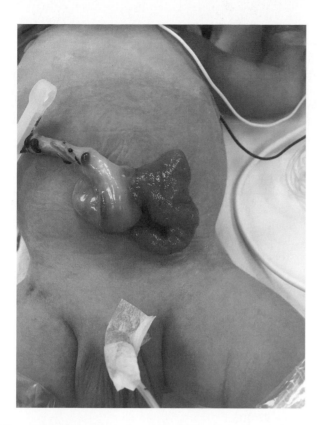

Figure 79.2 A clinical photograph showing an omphaloileal fistula giving rise to the so-called steer-horn abnormality.

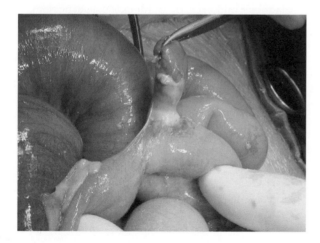

Figure 79.3 An intraoperative photograph showing Meckel diverticulum delivered out through an umbilical incision.

Excision of a patent omphalomesenteric duct

The orifice of the fistula is mobilized using a circumferential incision, preserving the surrounding umbilical skin (Figure 79.5). A separate skin-crease incision is made below the umbilicus. The superior skin flap, which includes the umbilicus, is elevated, and the fistula is brought out

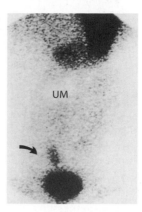

Figure 79.4 A photograph of a Tc-99 radioisotope scan taken at 20 minutes, showing the presence of gastrin-secreting mucosa in a Meckel diverticulum.

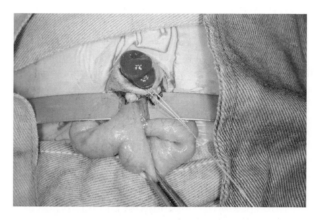

Figure 79.5 An intraoperative photograph taken after dissection of a patent omphalomesenteric duct.

through the subumbilical incision. The abdominal wall fascia is incised transversely on either side of the fistula. The umbilical vessels and the urachus are individually ligated and divided, and the peritoneal cavity is entered. The fistula is traced to its termination on the distal ileum.

The blood supply to the fistula runs across the ileum and should be ligated and divided near its origin on the mesentery. The fistula is excised with a margin of ileum using a transverse elliptical incision. The ileal defect is repaired transversely with a single interrupted layer of absorbable 4-0 sutures. The linea alba is then repaired and the subumbilical incision closed with subcuticular 5-0 suture. The circular defect in the center of the umbilicus may be left to heal by secondary intention if small, or may be loosely closed with a purse-string suture. The healed wound should resemble the umbilicus.

Meckel diverticulectomy

Symptomatic and confirmed Meckel diverticulum should be excised. For those patients who are asymptomatic, it is not essential to remove it. Nowadays, the procedure is laparoscopically assisted (where the Meckel diverticulum is brought through the subumbilical port after extension of incision to 2 cm) or even performed wholly laparoscopically in many centers. Laparoscopy is also useful in helping to diagnose symptomatic patients with negative isotope scans. The principles of laparoscopic resection remain the same as open surgery, and it is the authors' preference to resect a short segment of ileum together with the diverticulum to ensure that all abnormal mucosa is removed.[6,7] For open surgery, a 2 cm periumbilical incision is used to gain access to the peritoneal cavity. This will ensure an excellent cosmetic result postoperatively.

The Meckel diverticulum is situated on the antimesenteric border of the distal ileum and may be bound to the adjacent small bowel mesentery by a covering of peritoneum. These adhesions are divided to mobilize the diverticulum. Occasionally, the diverticulum is attached to the umbilicus, from which it must be separated. The blood vessels on the mesenteric side are ligated and divided. Ileal resection with primary end-to-end anastomosis with single-layer, interrupted absorbable 4-0 sutures is carried out. This ensures the removal of all ectopic tissue. The fascia of the subumbilical incision is closed using 3-0 absorbable sutures, and the skin is approximated with subcuticular 5-0 suture reinforced with adhesive strips.

Excision of an umbilical polyp

A circumferential incision is made around the polyp, preserving as much of the normal umbilicus as possible. The skin defect is repaired using an absorbable purse-string suture. Because of the possibility of an underlying connection to the ileum by a remnant of the omphalomesenteric duct, limited exploration of the peritoneal cavity is advisable. A subumbilical incision is made as described earlier. The abdominal wall is opened transversely and the peritoneal cavity entered. If an omphalomesenteric duct remnant is present, it is resected.

COMPLICATIONS

For conditions that involve peritoneal access (either open or laparoscopic) and intestinal resection, early postoperative complications include anastomotic leak, adhesions formation, postoperative ileus, and wound infection. These are, however, rare (<5%). Intestinal obstruction from adhesions may present as a late event.

REFERENCES

1. Mullassery D, Losty P. Omphalomesenteric remnants. In: Puri P and Höllwarth M (eds). *Pediatric Surgery: Diagnosis and Management*. Springer, New York 2009: 491–6.
2. Larsen WJ. Development of the gastrointestinal tract. In *Essentials of Human Embryology*. Churchill Livingstone, London 1998: 151–72.
3. Zani A, Eaton S, Rees CM, Pierro A. Incidentally detected Meckel diverticulum: To resect or not to resect? *Ann Surg* 2008; 247: 276–81.
4. Kiratli PO, Aksoy T, Bozkurt MF, Orhan D. Detection of ectopic gastric mucosa using 99mTc pertechnetate: Review of the literature. *Ann Nucl Med* 2009; 23: 97–105.
5. Snyder CL. Current management of umbilical abnormalities and related anomalies. *Semin Pediatr Surg* 2007; 16: 41–9.
6. Teitlebaum DH, Polley TZ, Obeid F. Laparoscopic diagnosis and excision of Meckel's diverticulum. *J Pediatr Surg* 1994; 29: 495–7.
7. Shier F. Laparoscopic treatment of Meckel's diverticulum. In: Bax KMA, Georgeson KE, Rothenberg SS, Valla JS, and Yeung CK (eds). *Endoscopic Surgery in Infants and Children*. Springer, New York 2008: 309–14.

80

Bladder exstrophy: Considerations and management of the newborn patient

PETER P. STUHLDREHER AND JOHN P. GEARHART

INTRODUCTION

In this chapter, management of the newborn with classic bladder exstrophy (CBE) is discussed based on the authors' experience and data derived from more than 1250 patients with bladder exstrophy, epispadias, and cloacal exstrophy from an institutionally approved database at the authors' institution.

The primary objectives of modern surgical management of CBE are as follows: (1) a secure abdominal wall and pelvic closure; (2) reconstruction of a functional and cosmetically acceptable penis in the male, and female external genitalia in the female; and (3) urinary continence with the preservation of renal function and volitional voiding.

Currently, several techniques exist to reconstruct the newborn with bladder exstrophy. Regardless of the technique, successful primary closure with placement of the bladder and urethra deep in the pelvis is the most important step in achieving eventual continence with an appropriately sized bladder. In the authors' experience, these objectives can best be achieved with newborn primary bladder and posterior urethral closure, early epispadias repair, and finally, bladder neck reconstruction when the bladder reaches an appropriate volume for an outlet procedure and the child desires continence. This chapter will be limited to discussion on the early management and initial primary closure of these infants.

INCIDENCE AND INHERITANCE

The incidence of bladder exstrophy has been estimated to be roughly 1 in 50,000 live births.[1-3] The male-to-female ratio has been reported to be between 1:1 and as high as 6:1 live exstrophy births.[1,2,4] We typically quote a 3:1 male-to-female ratio for our patients and their families. The risk of recurrence of bladder exstrophy in a given family is approximately 1 in 100.[4] Shapiro et al.[5] determined that the risk of bladder exstrophy in the offspring of individuals with bladder exstrophy and epispadias is 1 in 70 live births, a 500-fold greater incidence than that in the general population.[5] In reviews of exstrophy patient cohorts, three interesting trends have been found: bladder exstrophy tended to occur in infants of younger mothers, with higher risk in the Caucasian race[2] and low or high socioeconomic status[2]; an increased risk at high parity was seen for bladder exstrophy and epispadias[4]; and an increased incidence occurs with in vitro pregnancies.[6]

EMBRYOLOGY

Bladder exstrophy, cloacal exstrophy, and epispadias are variants of the exstrophy–epispadias complex. The etiology of this complex has been attributed by Muecke[7] to the failure of the cloacal membrane to be reinforced by ingrowth of the mesoderm. The cloacal membrane is a bilaminar layer situated at the caudal end of the germinal disc, which occupies the infraumbilical abdominal wall. Mesenchymal ingrowth between the ectodermal and endodermal layers of the cloacal membrane results in formation of the lower abdominal muscles and pelvic bones. After mesenchymal ingrowth occurs, downward growth of the urorectal septum divides the cloaca into a bladder anteriorly and rectum posteriorly. The paired genital tubercles migrate medially and fuse in the midline cephalad to the dorsal membrane before perforation. This process begins during the third week of gestation and continues through the sixth week of gestation. If the cloacal membrane is subject to premature rupture, its stage of development when membrane rupture occurs determines if epispadias, bladder exstrophy, or cloacal exstrophy will result.[8] Based on the timing of this disruption, the severity of the defect is determined.[9-11]

While multiple explanations have been presented, experiments in chicken embryos support the Muecke hypothesis, with experimental destruction of the cloacal membrane leading to chicks born with exstrophy.[12] Classic exstrophy accounts for 60% of patients born with this complex.[13] Of these patients, 30% are epispadias variants, and 10% are cloacal exstrophies or minor variants, such as superior vesical fissure, duplicate exstrophy, and pseudoexstrophy.

Historically, the genetics of bladder exstrophy were unknown, but recent progress using genome-wide association studies have led to a possible target gene responsible for CBE. The *ISL1* gene encodes an insulin gene enhancer protein, a LIM zinc-binding/homeobox-domain transcription factor.[14] Murine models of this gene have shown its role in multiple developing tissues.[14] The pattern of inheritance of *ISL1* is neither recessive nor purely dominant.[14] Further work into clarifying and validating *ISL1* is ongoing.

ANATOMIC CONSIDERATIONS

Exstrophy of the bladder is part of a spectrum of anomalies involving the urinary tract, genital tract, musculoskeletal system, and sometimes the intestinal tract. In CBE, most anomalies are related to birth defects of the abdominal wall, bladder, genitalia, pelvic bones, rectum, and anus (Figure 80.1).

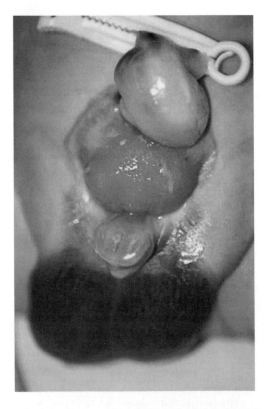

Figure 80.1 Newborn male infant with classic bladder exstrophy.

Musculoskeletal defects

Patients with CBE have a characteristic widening of the pubic symphysis caused by malrotation of the innominate bones, in relation to the sagittal plane of the body along both sacroiliac joints. In addition, they display an outward rotation or eversion of the pubic rami at their junction with the iliac bones. Using computed tomography (CT) of the pelvis with three-dimensional (3-D) reconstruction has further characterized the bony defect associated with both CBE and cloacal exstrophy.[15] Sponseller et al.[15] found that patients with CBE have a mean external rotation of the posterior aspect of the pelvis of 12° on each side, retroversion of the acetabulum, and a mean 18° of external rotation of the anterior pelvis, along with a 30% shortening of the pubic rami. The pelvic bones in children with CBE appear more like an open book or square shape compared to those of controls. These rotation deformities of the pelvic skeletal structures contribute to the short, pendular penis seen in bladder exstrophy. Additionally, this rotation also accounts for the increased distance between the hips, waddling gait, and the outward rotation of the lower limbs in these children, which in itself causes little disability and usually corrects to some degree over time.

A more recent study using 3-D CT has further increased our understanding of the pelvic anatomy in patients with bladder exstrophy.[16] The sacroiliac joints of bladder exstrophy patients are externally rotated, the pelvis is rotated inferiorly, and the pelvic volume is larger than in normal controls. One study, performed on fetal bony pelves with the exstrophy complex to determine histologic patterns and growth potential showed that despite the abnormal gross architecture, histologically, the exstrophic bone was identical to controls and completely normal; bone development was occurring at an expected rate with the potential for continued normal growth.[17]

In addition to the bony structures of the pelvis being laterally rotated, the large muscle groups constituting the pelvic floor are also flattened and laterally splayed. A fundamental tenet of bladder exstrophy repair is proper pelvic floor mobilization and placement of the vesicourethral complex deep within the pelvis. In 2001, Stec et al.[18] published the initial description using 3-D CT characterizing the pelvic floor in unclosed neonates with bladder exstrophy. This study found four primary findings that characterize the pelvic floor musculature in CBE: (1) the pelvic floor covers a twofold greater surface area in the exstrophy complex; (2) each levator ani half is outwardly rotated 38° from the midline; (3) the levator ani is 31° flatter in the exstrophy complex, thereby forming much less of a supportive sling than controls; and (4) only 32% of the puborectal sling is located anterior to the rectum for pelvic support as compared to 50% in controls. Magnetic resonance imaging (MRI) studies on the pelvic floor musculature created more advanced 3-D models of the abnormal character of the pelvic floor muscle, demonstrating one additional important caveat: the degree of pubic and bony diastasis does not account for all of the derangements in the pelvic floor anomaly in exstrophy.[19] In addition, 3-D MRI has furthered our understanding of the soft tissue anomalies in exstrophy patients. There is significant alteration of the levator ani muscle group when compared to controls. The levators are located further anterior, are flattened, and offer limited support to the pelvic organs with associated anterior placement of the anus.[20] These data of 3-D MRI also have included postoperative imaging of exstrophy repair, providing 3-D imaging that shows that closure improves the overall appearance of pelvic musculature, so that it looks much more like that of controls.[20]

Abdominal wall defects

The triangular defect caused by the premature rupture of the abnormal cloacal membrane is occupied by the exstrophied bladder and posterior urethra. The fascial defect is limited inferiorly by the intrasymphyseal band, which represents the divergent urogenital diaphragm. This band connects the bladder neck and posterior urethra to the pubic ramus on anatomical study. The anterior sheath of the rectus muscles has a fanlike extension behind the urethra and bladder neck that inserts into the intrasymphyseal band. At the upper end of the triangular fascial defect is the umbilicus. In bladder exstrophy, the distance between the umbilicus and the anus is always foreshortened. Although an umbilical hernia is usually present, it is usually of insignificant size. The umbilical hernia is repaired at the time of the abdominal wall closure. Connolly et al., in a review of 181 children with bladder exstrophy, reported inguinal hernias in 81.8% of boys and 10.5% of girls.[21]

Anorectal defects

The perineum is short and broad, with the anus situated directly behind the urogenital diaphragm, displaced anteriorly, and corresponding to the posterior limit of the triangular fascial defect. The divergent levator ani and puborectalis muscles and the distorted anatomy of the external sphincter contribute to varying degrees of anal incontinence and rectal prolapse. Anal continence is usually imperfect at an early age but typically improves. Prolapse virtually always disappears after bladder closure. If the infant develops prolapse after closure, a bladder outlet obstruction must be ruled out.

Male genital defects

The male genital defect is severe and the most troublesome aspect of the surgical reconstruction, independent of the decision about whether to treat by modern staged closure, combined closure, or some form of urinary diversion. Formerly, it was thought that the individual corpus cavernosa were of normal caliber but appeared to be shorter because of the wide separation of the crural attachments, the prominent dorsal chordee, and the shortened urethral groove. However, data by Silver et al.[22] have described the genital defect in bladder exstrophy in much greater detail. Utilizing MRI in adult men with bladder exstrophy and comparing this to age- and race-matched controls, it was found that the anterior corporal length in male patients with bladder exstrophy is almost 50% shorter and 30% wider than that in normal controls. A functional and cosmetically pleasing penis can be achieved when the dorsal chordee is released, the urethral groove lengthened, and the penis somewhat lengthened by mobilizing the crura in the midline. Potency is preserved in almost all exstrophy patients. Testis function has not been studied in a large group of postpubertal exstrophy patients, but it is generally believed that fertility is not impaired by testicular dysfunction.

Female genital defects

Reconstruction of the female genitalia presents a less complex problem than in the male (Figure 80.2). The vagina is shorter than normal, hardly greater than 6 cm in depth, but of normal caliber. The vaginal orifice is frequently stenotic and displaced anteriorly; the clitoris is bifid. The labia, mons pubis, and clitoris are divergent. The uterus enters the vagina superiorly so that the cervix is in the anterior vaginal wall. The fallopian tubes and ovaries are normal. Female patients are typically able to bear children, but given the complexity of their reconstruction, cesarean section is mandated to protect pelvic structures. Even with precautionary cesarean section, adult females are at high risk of pelvic organ prolapse. Most adolescents and young adults will undergo a vaginoplasty procedure in order to wear tampons and have intercourse.

Urinary defects

At birth, the bladder mucosa may appear to be normal; however, ectopic bowel mucosa or an isolated bowel loop may be present. More commonly, a hamartomatous polyp may also be present on the bladder surface. The size, distensibility, and neuromuscular function of the exstrophied bladder, as well as the size of the triangular fascial defect to which the bladder muscles attach, affect the decision to attempt repair. When the bladder is small, fibrosed, inelastic, and covered with polyps, functional repair may be impossible. The bladder may be invaginated or may bulge through a small fascial defect, indicating the potential for satisfactory capacity after successful initial closure, which is commonly difficult to assess on initial

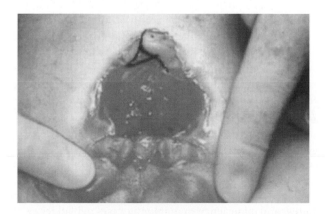

Figure 80.2 Female infant with classic bladder exstrophy.

exam. We strongly recommend examination under anesthesia to adequately diagnose true defect, as bladders that appear to be small in the nursery may have a substantial amount of bladder sequestered below the fascial defect.

The upper urinary tract is usually normal, but anomalous development does occur. Horseshoe kidney, pelvic kidney, hypoplastic kidney, solitary kidney, and dysplasia with megaureter are all encountered in these patients. The ureters have an abnormal course in their termination. The peritoneal pouch of Douglas between the bladder and the rectum is enlarged and unusually deep, forcing the ureter down laterally in its course across the true pelvis. The distal segment of ureter approaches the bladder from a point inferior and lateral to the orifice, and it enters the bladder with little or no obliquity. Due to this, the ureteral orifices are misplaced with an abnormal course of the submucosal ureters, leading, invariably, to vesicoureteral reflux,[23,24] which needs to be addressed at the time of the continence procedure.

PRENATAL DIAGNOSIS AND MANAGEMENT

It is possible to diagnose CBE prenatally with ultrasonographic findings.[25,26] The absence of a normal fluid-filled bladder on repeat examinations suggested the diagnosis, as did a mass of echogenic tissue on the lower abdominal wall.[26] In a retrospective review of 25 prenatal ultrasound examinations with the resulting birth of a newborn with CBE, several observations were made: (1) absence of bladder filling, (2) a low-set umbilicus, (3) widening of the pubic ramus, (4) diminutive genitalia, and (5) a lower abdominal mass, which increased in size as the pregnancy progressed and as the intra-abdominal viscera increased in size.[27] Surprisingly, despite very uniform ultrasound findings, even at high-volume centers, a majority of cases are diagnosed postnatally.[28] Prenatal diagnosis of bladder exstrophy allows for optimal management, including delivery in a pediatric center and appropriate prenatal counseling of the parents.

DELIVERY ROOM AND NURSERY CARE

At birth, while the bladder mucosa is usually smooth, pink, and intact, it is also sensitive and easily denuded. In the delivery room, the umbilical cord should be tied with 2-0 silk suture close to the abdominal wall so that the umbilical clamp does not traumatize the bladder mucosa and cause excoriation of the bladder surface. The bladder may be covered with a nonadherent film of plastic wrap (i.e., Saran Wrap) to prevent the mucosa from rubbing on clothes or diapers, leading to inflammation of the mucosa. In addition, each time the diaper is changed, the plastic wrap should be removed, the bladder surface irrigated with sterile saline, and a new square of plastic wrap placed.

The parents should be educated by a surgeon with a special interest and experience in managing cases of bladder exstrophy. An exstrophy support team should be available, which

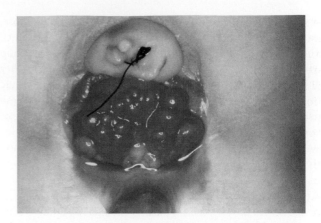

Figure 80.3 Patient with a small fibrotic bladder patch deemed too small for neonatal closure. Note the polypoid nature of the bladder mucosa.

includes a pediatric orthopedic surgeon, pediatric anesthesiologists and postoperative pain team members, social workers, nurses with special interests in bladder exstrophy, and a child psychiatrist with experience and expertise in genital anomalies. It is important to note that the need for changing the sex of rearing in CBE is not advised.

Cardiopulmonary and general physical assessment can be carried out in the first few hours of life. Ultrasound can provide evidence of renal structure, function, and drainage, even in the first few hours of life before the patient undergoes closure of the exstrophy defect, However, CBE is not heavily associated with significant renal defects. Radionucleotide imaging is reserved for a high index of suspicion for obstruction. A thorough neonatal assessment may have to be deferred until transfer of the child to a center of excellence.

Occasionally, a small fibrotic bladder template with an associated small triangular fascial defect without elasticity or contractility can be seen. When encountered, closure of these small bladders in a neonate should not be undertaken. Figure 80.3 shows a bladder that is too small for closure. Examination with the patient under anesthesia is required to assess the bladder adequately, particularly if considerable edema, excoriation, and polyp formation have developed between birth and the time of assessment. Decisions regarding the suitability of bladder closure or the need for waiting should only be made by surgeons with a great deal of experience in the bladder exstrophy condition. As illustrated by a review of our exstrophy database in 2001, it is infrequent that a bladder template is insufficient for closure.[29] After a period of time, when the bladder has grown sufficiently, closure was completed, and long-term follow-up revealed that 50% of these patients remained dry after bladder neck reconstruction and 50% required other adjunctive procedures.[29]

PRIMARY BLADDER CLOSURE

Over the past two decades, modifications in the management of functional bladder closure have contributed to a dramatic increase in the success of the treatment. The most significant changes in the management of bladder exstrophy have been as follows: (1) early bladder, posterior urethra, and abdominal wall closure; (2) the widespread use of pelvic osteotomy along with appropriate pelvic immobilization; (3) epispadias repair at 6–10 months of age; (4) reconstruction of a competent bladder neck and reimplantation of the ureters; and (5) most importantly, defining strict criteria for the selection of patients suitable for this approach.

The primary objective of functional closure is to convert the patient with bladder exstrophy into one with complete male epispadias or reconstructed female epispadias with incontinence and balanced posterior outlet resistance that preserves renal function. Typically, epispadias repair is now performed between 6 and 10 months of age in the male, after testosterone stimulation. Bladder neck reconstruction occurs when the child is 4–5 years of age, has an adequate bladder capacity and is ready to participate in a preoperative and postoperative voiding program.

Another type of staged exstrophy repair is the Kelly repair, or radical soft tissue mobilization. In this repair, the bladder and abdominal wall are closed without osteotomy after birth. Several months later, a radical soft tissue mobilization and the urogenital diaphragm and its periosteal attachments are dissected and used to allow closure of the pelvis and pelvic floor. The penis is made hypospadiac, and later, penile repair is performed. Osteotomy is never used in this repair, and thus far, continence results are modest, with up to 71% of patients achieving either complete or partial continence in the largest cohort of patients reported in the literature.[30]

This chapter will deal with the most common issue seen by the pediatric surgeon, the primary closure. Obtaining a secure primary closure is the single most important step for achieving eventual continence in exstrophy patitents.[31] It cannot be stressed enough that proper patient selection and technique selection with liberal use of osteotomy are necessary for successful closure.

Pelvic osteotomy

Pelvic osteotomies performed at the time of closure offer several advantages, including the following: (1) easy reapproximation of the symphysis with diminished tension on the abdominal wall closure eliminating the need for fascial flaps, (2) placement of the urethra deep within the pelvic ring, enhancing bladder outlet resistance, and (3) bringing the large pelvic floor muscles near the midline, where they can support the bladder neck and aid in eventual urinary control.

After pubic approximation with osteotomy, some patients show the ability to stop and start the urinary stream, experience dry intervals, and in some cases, become completely continent.[32] In a review article of a large number of patients referred to the authors' institution with failed exstrophy, a majority were referred with partial or complete dehiscence of the bladder, or major bladder prolapse, and had not undergone osteotomy at the time of initial bladder closure.[33]

Our recommendation is to perform bilateral transverse innominate and vertical iliac osteotomy when bladder closure is performed after 72 hours of age.[34] In addition, if the pelvis is not malleable or if the pubic bones are >4 cm apart at the time of initial examination under anesthesia, osteotomy should be performed, even if closed before 72 hours of age. A well-coordinated surgical and anesthesia team can perform osteotomy and proceed to bladder closure without undue loss of blood or risk of prolonged anesthesia in the child. However, one must realize that osteotomy and posterior urethral and bladder closure, along with abdominal wall closure, is a 5- to 7-hour procedure in these infants.

Combined osteotomy is performed by placing the patient in the supine position, preparing and draping the lower body below the costal margins, and placing soft absorbent gauze over the exposed bladder. The pelvis is exposed from the iliac wings inferiorly to the pectineal tubercle and posteriorly to the sacroiliac joints. The periosteum and sciatic notch are carefully elevated, and a saw is used to create the transverse innominate osteotomy, exiting anteriorly at a point halfway between the anterosuperior and anteroinferior spines (Figure 80.4). This osteotomy is created at a slightly more cranial level than that described for a Salter osteotomy, in order to allow placement of fixator pins in the distal segments.

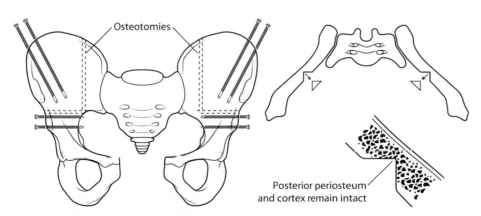

Figure 80.4 Combined transverse anterior innominate and anterior vertical iliac osteotomy with pin placement and preservation of the posterior periosteum and cortex.

In addition to the transverse osteotomy, the posterior iliac may be incised from the anterior approach in an effort to correct the deformity more completely. This is important because anatomical studies have shown that the posterior portion of the pelvis is also externally rotated in patients with exstrophy, and as patients age, they lose the elasticity of their sacroiliac ligaments. To achieve good closure, a closing wedge osteotomy is created vertically and just lateral to the sacroiliac joint. The proximal posterior iliac cortex is kept intact and used as a hinge. This combination of osteotomies easily corrects the abnormalities in both the anterior and posterior aspects of the pelvis.

Fixator pins are placed in the inferior osteotomized segment and in the wing of the ileum superiorly. The number of pins placed depends on the child's size and orthopedic surgeon discretion. Ideally, two pins are placed in either segment. Operative fluoroscopy is used to confirm pin placement. The soft tissues surrounding the osteotomy sites are closed, and the urologic procedure is then performed. At the end of the procedure, external fixators are then applied between the pins to hold the pelvis in a corrected position. Light longitudinal Buck's skin traction is used to keep the legs still. The patient remains in the supine position in traction for approximately 4 weeks to prevent dislodgement of tubes and destabilization of the pelvis. The external fixator is kept on for approximately 6 weeks until adequate callus is seen at the site of osteotomy. Postoperatively, in newborns who undergo closure without osteotomy in the first 48–72 hours of life, the baby is immobilized in modified Bryant's traction in a position in which the hips have 90° flexion. When modified Bryant's traction is used, it is employed for 4 weeks. During this time, movement control is critically important, and use of tunneled epidural catheters for pain control and use of anesthesia pain colleagues for movement control and postoperative sedation are advised.

Bladder, posterior urethral, and abdominal wall closure

The various steps in primary bladder closure are illustrated in Figure 80.5. A strip of mucosa 2 cm wide, extending from the distal trigone to below the verumontanum in the male and to the vaginal orifice in the female, is outlined for prostatic and posterior urethral reconstruction in the male and adequate urethral closure in the female. The male urethral groove length is typically adequate, and no transverse incision of the urethral plate needs to be performed for urethral lengthening. The diagrams in Figure 80.5a–c show marking of the incision with a marking pen from just above the umbilicus down around the junction of bladder and the paraexstrophy skin to the level of the urethral plate. The approximate plane is entered just above the umbilicus, and a plane is established between the rectus fascia and the bladder (Figure 80.5c,d). The umbilical vessels are doubly ligated and incised, allowing them to fall into the pelvis. The peritoneum is taken off the dome of the bladder at this point so

that the bladder can be placed deeply into the pelvis at the time of closure. Radical dissection of the peritoneal reflection from the bladder should not be done, as the vasculature to the exstrophied bladder often will occupy this space and can be inadvertently compromised. The plane is continued caudally between the bladder and the rectus fascia until the urogenital diaphragm fibers are encountered bilaterally. The pubis will be encountered at this juncture, and use of a double-pronged skin hook into the bone will accentuate the urogenital diaphragm fibers and help the surgeon radically incise these fibers between the bladder neck, posterior urethra, and pubic bone. Gentle traction on the glans of the penis at this point will show the insertion of the corporal body in the lateral inferior aspect of the pubis. These urogenital fibers are taken down sharply with electrocautery to the pelvic floor in their entirety. If this maneuver is not performed adequately, the posterior urethra and bladder will not be placed deeply into the pelvis and will compromise closure. As well, when the pubic bones are brought together, the posterior vesicourethral unit will be brought anteriorly in an unsatisfactory position for later reconstruction.

The corporal bodies are not brought together at this juncture, as later Cantwell–Ransley epispadias repair will require the urethral plate to be brought beneath the corporal bodies. If the urethral plate is left in continuity, it must be mobilized up to the level of the prostate in order to create as much additional urethral and penile length as possible. Further urethral lengthening can be performed at the time of epispadias repair, around 6 months of age.

Apparent penile lengthening is achieved by exposing the corpora cavernosa bilaterally and freeing the corpora from their attachments to the suspensory ligaments on the anterior part of the inferior pubic rami. It is important to note that there is a 50% shortage of length in the corporal bodies in exstrophy patients versus normal controls, and any penile lengthening that is obtained is more correction of chordee and changing the angulation of the penis rather than true penile lengthening.[22]

After their incision, the wide band of fibers and muscular tissue representing the urogenital diaphragm is detached subperiosteally from the pubis bilaterally (Figure 80.5e,f). Reluctance to free the bladder neck and urethral wall from the inferior ramus of the pubis moves the neobladder opening cephalad if any separation of the pubis occurs during healing. The mucosa and muscle of the bladder and the posterior urethral wall into the penis are then closed in the midline anteriorly. This orifice should accommodate a 12- to 14-French urethral catheter comfortably. The size of the opening should allow enough resistance to aid in the bladder adaptation and to prevent prolapse but not enough outlet resistance to cause upper tract changes. The posterior urethra and bladder neck are buttressed to the second layer of local tissue if possible (Figure 80.5g,h). The bladder is drained by a suprapubic nonlatex Malecot catheter for a period of 4 weeks. The urethra is not stented, in order to avoid necrosis with accumulation of secretions in the neourethra. Postoperatively, careful attention should be paid

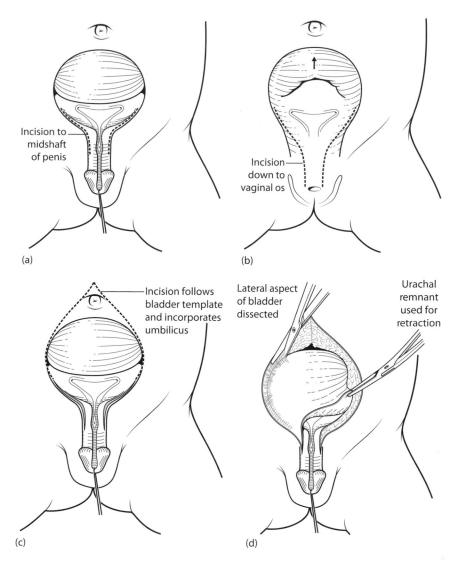

(a)

(b)

Incision to midshaft of penis

Incision down to vaginal os

(c)

(d)

Incision follows bladder template and incorporates umbilicus

Lateral aspect of bladder dissected

Urachal remnant used for retraction

Figure 80.5 **(a)** Marking of the initial incisions for a male exstrophy patient from trigone around urethral plate. **(b)** Marking of comparable incisions for closure of a female exstrophy patient down to vaginal os. **(c)** Marking of the subsequent incision around the umbilicus and bladder, joining the initial dissection. **(d)** Development of the retropubic space and division of the lateral bladder attachments.

(*Continued*)

to pooling of urine in the epispadias, as continued urine soilage can compromise repair or lead to soft tissue infection due to the immobilization of the child. Ureteral stents provide drainage for 10–14 days after closure, when swelling due to the presence of closure of a small bladder may obstruct the ureters and give rise to obstruction and transient hypertension. These stents are left in place, however, for the duration of pelvic external fixation, if used, and the duration of traction.

When the bladder and urethra have been closed and the drainage tube placed, pressure over the greater trochanters bilaterally allows the pubic bones to be approximated in the midline. Horizontal mattress sutures of number 2 nylon are placed in the pubis and tied with a knot away from the neourethra (Figure 80.5h). Oftentimes, in a good closure, the authors are able to use another stitch of

number 2 nylon at the most caudal insertion of the rectus fascia into the pubic bone. This maneuver will add to the security of the pubic closure. Research has shown that the choice of suture for pelvic closure is critically important, with nylon showing superior tensile strength compared to other choices.[35] A V-shaped flap of abdominal skin at a point corresponding to the normal position of the umbilicus is tacked down to the abdominal fascia, and the drainage tubes exit this orifice. The method described by Hanna[36] is the authors' most commonly performed procedure. Before and during the procedure, the patient is given broad-spectrum antibiotics in an attempt to convert a contaminated field into a clean surgical wound. Nonreactive sutures of polyglycolic acid (Dexon/Vicryl) and nylon are used to avoid an undesirable stitch reaction or stitch abscess.

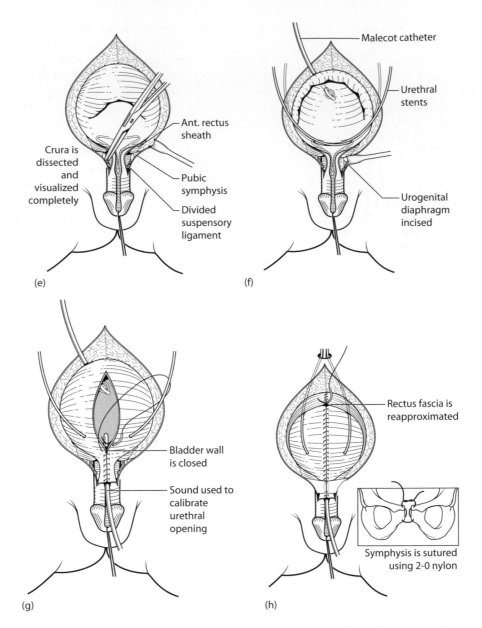

Figure 80.5 (Continued) **(e)** The urogenital diaphragm and anterior corpora are freed from the pubis in a subperiosteal plane. **(f)** Final deep incision of the remnant urogenital diaphragm fibers and insertion of a suprapubic tube. **(g)** Exit of the ureteral stents from the lateral sidewall of the bladder and the first layer of the bladder wall closure. **(h)** Closure of fascia is performed after placement of a number 2 nylon horizontal mattress suture to approximate the pubis.

Combined bladder closure and epispadias repair

The modern staged closure of bladder exstrophy has yielded consistently good cosmetic and functional results, and the utilization of osteotomy has improved the potential for successful initial closure and later continence. In an effort to decrease costs and the morbidity associated with multiple operative procedures, and possibly to effect continence, there is current interest in performing single-stage reconstruction, or combining procedures in appropriately selected patients. This technique was first described by Lattimer and Smith[1] for primary closures and Gearhart and Jeffs[37] in 1991

for failed exstrophy closures. Grady and Mitchell[38] have renewed interest in its use in newborn patients, and results have now been reported in groups of boys undergoing single-stage reconstruction (bladder closure and epispadias repair) in infancy.

The complete primary repair of bladder exstrophy is now being performed in neonates at several centers worldwide. The basics steps of the procedure have been outlined by Grady and Mitchell.[38] The initial dissection begins superiorly and is carried inferiorly to isolate the bladder template. This is carried down in a continuous fashion to then begin the penile dissection ventrally. The penile dissection will progress medially with care being taken to preserve the urethral plate for later tubularization. As previously described by Mitchell, the penis will be completely disassembled into individual corporal bodies and urethral plate with supporting spongiosum tissue.[39] Deep proximal dissection is undertaken to free the veriscourethral unit from the intersymphyseal ligaments to provide deep placement of the unit into the pelvis. Once the dissection is complete, the bladder is closed, the penis is reassembled anatomically with a hypospadiac urethra, and the abdominal wall and skin closure is completed.[38]

Long-term results of 39 children have been published that show that in experienced hands, this procedure produces comparable success rates.[40] Of children aged 4 years or older who underwent complete primary repair, 74% are continent in daytime with volitional voiding. Importantly, only 20% of boys and 43% of girls achieved primary urinary continence without the need for bladder neck reconstruction. Complication rates were comparable at 18%, with five urethrocutaneous fistulas and two patients with fascial dehiscence. However, there are published reports of significant complications from the complete primary repair. There have been multiple reports of significant penile tissue loss from complete primary repair and associated closure failures.[41-43] In a review of patients referred to our institution after complete primary repair, 13 of 55 males had major penile soft tissue loss.[44]

In the current authors' opinion, this technique should be limited to boys of older age (older than 6 months of age) because of recent experimental evidence indicating that newborn exstrophy bladders differ from bladders in older infants in the level of maturity of the muscle and connective tissue components. The senior author believes that these patients should be carefully selected, especially newborns, because of the reasons given earlier. Otherwise, boys presenting after failed initial closure and/or older than 6 months of age may be candidates for a combination of epispadias repair with bladder closure. Children should be carefully selected based on phallic size, length and depth of the urethral groove, size of the bladder template, and perivesical and urethral plate scarring in those who have undergone a prior failed closure.

CONCLUSION

The modern staged approach to treatment in patients with bladder exstrophy is able to provide a satisfactory outcome both cosmetically and functionally in most cases. This approach consists of the following: (1) initial bladder closure, (2) repair of epispadias, and (3) bladder neck reconstruction. Bladder neck reconstruction is the recommended management based on the current authors' and institutional experience with over 941 cases of the exstrophy–epispadias complex. Recent reports of a single-stage repair by other authors have proposed successful outcomes; however, follow-up is limited, and numbers of patients in these series is small. In the modern staged repair, the continence rate for males with exstrophy voiding per urethra is 80.6%, with 70% dry around the clock and 10.6% dry during the day but

damp at night.[45] In females, 74% were voiding per urethra and continent 24 hours a day, with an additional 10% being continent during the day while wet at night.[46] While recent developments in tissue engineering hold promise to improve outcomes for patients requiring genitourinary reconstruction in the future, staged functional closure remains the gold standard for patients with CBE.

REFERENCES

1. Lattimer JK, Smith MJ. Exstrophy closure: A followup on 70 cases. *J Urol* 1966; 95(3): 356–9.
2. Nelson CP, Dunn RL, Wei JT. Contemporary epidemiology of bladder exstrophy in the United States. *J Urol* 2005; 173(5): 1728–31.
3. Siffel C, Correa A, Amar E et al. Bladder exstrophy: An epidemiologic study from the International Clearinghouse for Birth Defects Surveillance and Research, and an overview of the literature. *Am J Med Genet C Semin Med Genet* 2011; 157C(4): 321–32.
4. Slaughenhoupt B. Epidemiology of bladder exstrophy and epispadias: A communication from the International Clearinghouse for Birth Defects Monitoring Systems. *Teratology* 1987; 36(2): 221–7.
5. Shapiro E, Lepor H, Jeffs RD. The inheritance of the exstrophy–epispadias complex. *J Urol* 1984; 132(2): 308–10.
6. Wood HM, Babineau D, Gearhart JP. In vitro fertilization and the cloacal/bladder exstrophy–epispadias complex: A continuing association. *J Pediatr Urol* 2007; 3(4): 305–10.
7. Muecke EC. The role of the cloacal membrane in exstrophy: The first successful experimental study. *J Urol* 1964; 92: 659–67.
8. Ambrose SS, O'Brien DP 3rd. Surgical embryology of the exstrophy–epispadias complex. *Surg Clin North Am* 1974; 54(6): 1379–90.
9. Sadler TW, Feldkamp ML. The embryology of body wall closure: Relevance to gastroschisis and other ventral body wall defects. *Am J Med Genet C Semin Med Genet* 2008; 148C(3): 180–5.
10. Ebert AK, Reutter H, Ludwig M, Rosch WH. The exstrophy–epispadias complex. *Orphanet J Rare Dis* 2009; 4: 23.
11. Yiee J, Wilcox D. Abnormalities of the fetal bladder. *Semin Fetal Neonatal Med* 2008; 13(3): 164–70.
12. Thomalla JV, Rudolph RA, Rink RC, Mitchell ME. Induction of cloacal exstrophy in the chick embryo using the CO_2 laser. *J Urol* 1985; 134(5): 991–5.
13. Marshall VF, Muecke EC. *Handbuch de Urologie.* New York: Springer-Verlag, 1968.
14. Draaken M, Knapp M, Pennimpede T et al. Genome-wide association study and meta-analysis identify ISL1 as genome-wide significant susceptibility gene for bladder exstrophy. *PLoS Genet* 2015; 11(3): e1005024.

15. Sponseller PD, Bisson LJ, Gearhart JP, Jeffs RD, Magid D, Fishman E. The anatomy of the pelvis in the exstrophy complex. *J Bone Joint Surg Am* 1995; 77(2): 177–89.

16. Stec AA, Pannu HK, Tadros YE et al. Evaluation of the bony pelvis in classic bladder exstrophy by using 3D-CT: Further insights. *Urology* 2001; 58(6): 1030–5.

17. Stec AA, Wakim A, Barbet P et al. Fetal bony pelvis in the bladder exstrophy complex: Normal potential for growth? *Urology* 2003; 62(2): 337–41.

18. Stec AA, Pannu HK, Tadros YE, Sponseller PD, Fishman EK, Gearhart JP. Pelvic floor anatomy in classic bladder exstrophy using 3-dimensional computerized tomography: Initial insights. *J Urol* 2001; 166(4): 1444–9.

19. Williams AM, Solaiyappan M, Pannu HK, Bluemke D, Shechter G, Gearhart JP. 3-dimensional magnetic resonance imaging modeling of the pelvic floor musculature in classic bladder exstrophy before pelvic osteotomy. *J Urol* 2004; 172(4 Pt 2): 1702–5.

20. Tekes A, Ertan G, Solaiyappan M et al. 2D and 3D MRI features of classic bladder exstrophy. *Clin Radiol* 2014; 69(5): e223–9.

21. Connolly JA, Peppas DS, Jeffs RD, Gearhart JP. Prevalence and repair of inguinal hernias in children with bladder exstrophy. *J Urol* 1995; 154(5): 1900–1.

22. Silver RI, Yang A, Ben-Chaim J, Jeffs RD, Gearhart JP. Penile length in adulthood after exstrophy reconstruction. *J Urol* 1997; 157(3): 999–1003.

23. Canning DA, Gearhart JP, Peppas DS, Jeffs RD. The cephalotrigonal reimplant in bladder neck reconstruction for patients with exstrophy or epispadias. *J Urol* 1993; 150(1): 156–8.

24. Mathews R, Hubbard JS, Gearhart JP. Ureteral reimplantation before bladder neck plasty in the reconstruction of bladder exstrophy: Indications and outcomes. *Urology* 2003; 61(4): 820–4.

25. Gearhart JP, Ben-Chaim J, Jeffs RD, Sanders RC. Criteria for the prenatal diagnosis of classic bladder exstrophy. *Obstet Gynecol* 1995; 85(6): 961–4.

26. Mirk M, Calisti A, Feleni A. Prenatal sonographic diagnosis of bladder exstrophy. *J Ultrasound Med* 1986; 5: 291.

27. Verco PW, Khor BH, Barbary J, Enthoven C. Ectopia vesicae in utero. *Australas Radiol* 1986; 30(2): 117–20.

28. Goyal A, Fishwick J, Hurrell R, Cervellione RM, Dickson AP. Antenatal diagnosis of bladder/cloacal exstrophy: Challenges and possible solutions. *J Pediatr Urol* 2012; 8(2): 140–4.

29. Dodson JL, Surer I, Baker LA, Jeffs RD, Gearhart JP. The newborn exstrophy bladder inadequate for primary closure: Evaluation, management and outcome. *J Urol* 2001; 165(5): 1656–9.

30. Jarzebowski AC, McMullin ND, Grover SR, Southwell BR, Hutson JM. The Kelly technique of bladder exstrophy repair: Continence, cosmesis and pelvic organ prolapse outcomes. *J Urol* 2009; 182(4 Suppl): 1802–6.

31. Chan DY, Jeffs RD, Gearhart JP. Determinants of continence in the bladder exstrophy population: Predictors of success? *Urology* 2001; 57(4): 774–7.

32. Gearhart JP, Peppas DS, Jeffs RD. The failed exstrophy closure: Strategy for management. *Br J Urol* 1993; 71(2): 217–20.

33. Sponseller PD, Gearhart JP, Jeffs RD. Anterior innominate osteotomies for failure or late closure of bladder exstrophy. *J Urol* 1991; 146(1): 137–40.

34. Gearhart JP, Forschner DC, Jeffs RD, Ben-Chaim J, Sponseller PD. A combined vertical and horizontal pelvic osteotomy approach for primary and secondary repair of bladder exstrophy. *J Urol* 1996; 155(2): 689–93.

35. Sussman JS, Sponseller PD, Gearhart JP, Valdevit AD, Kier-York J, Chao EY. A comparison of methods of repairing the symphysis pubis in bladder exstrophy by tensile testing. *Br J Urol* 1997; 79(6): 979–84.

36. Hanna MK. Reconstruction of umbilicus during functional closure of bladder exstrophy. *Urology* 1986; 27(4): 340–2.

37. Gearhart JP, Jeffs RD. Management of the failed exstrophy closure. *J Urol* 1991; 146(2 (Pt 2)): 610–2.

38. Grady RW, Mitchell ME. Complete primary repair of exstrophy. *J Urol* 1999; 162(4): 1415–20.

39. Mitchell ME, Bagli DJ. Complete penile disassembly for epispadias repair: The Mitchell technique. *J Urol* 1996; 155(1): 300–4.

40. Shnorhavorian M, Grady RW, Andersen A, Joyner BD, Mitchell ME. Long-term followup of complete primary repair of exstrophy: The Seattle experience. *J Urol* 2008; 180(4 Suppl): 1615–9; discussion 1619–20.

41. Gearhart JP, Baird AD. The failed complete repair of bladder exstrophy: Insights and outcomes. *J Urol* 2005; 174(4 Pt 2): 1669–72; discussion 1672–3.

42. Husmann DA, Gearhart JP. Loss of the penile glans and/or corpora following primary repair of bladder exstrophy using the complete penile disassembly technique. *J Urol* 2004; 172(4 Pt 2): 1696–700; discussion 1700–1.

43. Purves JT, Gearhart JP. Complications of radical soft-tissue mobilization procedure as a primary closure of exstrophy. *J Pediatr Urol* 2008; 4(1): 65–9.

44. Schaeffer AJ, Stec AA, Purves JT, Cervellione RM, Nelson CP, Gearhart JP. Complete primary repair of bladder exstrophy: A single institution referral experience. *J Urol* 2011; 186(3): 1041–6.

45. Baird AD, Nelson CP, Gearhart JP. Modern staged repair of bladder exstrophy: A contemporary series. *J Pediatr Urol* 2007; 3(4): 311–5.

46. Purves JT, Baird AD, Gearhart JP. The modern staged repair of bladder exstrophy in the female: A contemporary series. *J Pediatr Urol* 2008; 4(2): 150–3.

81

Cloacal exstrophy

ALONSO CARRASCO JR., DUNCAN T. WILCOX, AND VIJAYA M. VEMULAKONDA

INTRODUCTION

Cloacal exstrophy is an extremely rare congenital disorder first described by Littre in 1709.[1] It is the most severe form of the bladder exstrophy–epispadias complex and is characterized by findings of two exstrophy hemibladders, exstrophy hindgut, underdevelopment of hindgut, pubic diastasis, prolapsing terminal ileum, complete separation of genitalia, and omphalocele (Figure 81.1). The first successful treatment of cloacal exstrophy using a three-stage procedure was described by Rickman in 1960.[2] Since then, advances in medical and surgical care have improved survival to over 80%.[3,4] With this drastic increase in survival, the goals of care have shifted toward improvement of early diagnosis, preservation of the function of affected organs, and improvement in quality of life.

EMBRYOLOGY

The exact embryology and etiology of cloacal exstrophy are still poorly understood, but several theories have been postulated. The most commonly supported theory is the failure of mesodermal tissue migration to the lateral fold, leading to premature rupture of the cloacal membrane before the urogenital septum divides the cloaca into the anterior urogenital sinus and posterior anorectal canal.[5,6] This results in a large midline defect with exposure of both bladder and bowel elements and complete separation of the genitalia. This theory is supported by induction of cloacal exstrophy in animal models by inducing premature rupture of the cloacal membrane.[6,7] However, cases of cloacal exstrophy with intact or delayed rupture of the cloacal membrane and covered variants raise questions about this explanation.[8–11] Additionally, histopathological studies in human embryos support a much earlier defect involving the caudal eminence of the trilaminar embryo.[12,13] Other theories include insufficient cell deposition or malfunctioning of the umbilical ectodermal placode leading to impaired body wall formation.[14,15]

EPIDEMIOLOGY, GENETICS, AND ENVIRONMENTAL RISK FACTORS

Cloacal exstrophy has an overall prevalence of 1 in 200,000–300,000 live births.[16,17] Historically, there has been a male-to-female predominance of 2:1, but in recent epidemiological studies and large series, the male-to-female ratio is more evenly distributed.[16,18,19] It is often sporadic, with no genetic defect or environmental factor definitively identified as the cause of cloacal exstrophy. Small familial recurrence rate and concordance in monozygotic twins support a genetic basis in some cases.[18,20] Methylenetetrahydrofolate reductase polymorphism C677T was recently found to have a strong association with cloacal exstrophy.[21] Other gene and chromosomal abnormalities implicated include the HOX gene family, trisomy 13, trisomy 18, 9q34.1-qter deletion, del(3)(q12.2q13.2), 1p36 deletion, and mitochondrial 12SrRNA deletion.[22–27] Studies evaluating environmental factors are scarce and focused on small geographical areas or populations. Use of clomiphene citrate around time of conception was previously implicated,[28] but a prospective study later refuted this association.[29] Small case series have also suggested in vitro fertilization and smoking as potential risk factors.[18,30]

PRENATAL DIAGNOSIS

With the advent of prenatal imaging, more patients are now being diagnosed prenatally either by ultrasound or with the aid of fetal magnetic resonance imaging (MRI). Several criteria have been proposed for diagnosis. Major criteria include nonvisualization of the bladder, a large midline infraumbilical anterior wall defect or cystic anterior wall structure, omphalocele, and/or lumbosacral anomalies.[31] Other proposed minor criteria include lower extremity defects, renal anomalies, ascites, widened pubic arches, narrowed thorax, hydrocephalus, and solitary umbilical artery.[31] Additionally, the prolapsing of the terminal ileum resulting in an "elephant trunk–like"

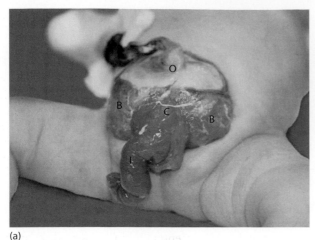

(a)

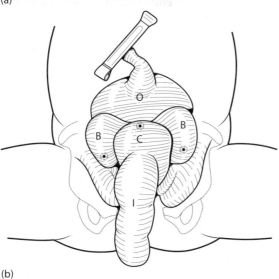

(b)

Figure 81.1 **(a)** A patient with cloacal exstrophy and **(b)** a diagram depicting the component parts of the deformity. A prolapsing terminal ileum (I) depicting the elephant trunk deformity is demonstrated with cecal place (C) between the two hemibladders (B) and omphalocele superiorly (O).

image on prenatal ultrasound has been deemed a pathognomonic finding.[32] Despite these predictive criteria, prenatal ultrasound remains a poor predictor of diagnosis, with only 25% of patients with bladder/cloacal exstrophy diagnosed by prenatal ultrasound.[33] Fetal MRI is an adjunct image modality that has been more recently used to aid in the prenatal diagnosis. Case series of this have demonstrated excellent diagnostic accuracy and the added benefit of better characterization of associated anomalies.[34–36]

Early diagnosis of cloacal exstrophy allows for early family counseling regarding extent of congenital defect, associated abnormalities, required surgical reconstruction, and long-term outcomes. Equally important, prenatal diagnosis helps with making arrangements for delivery of a patient at a center with capabilities and expertise in the postnatal management of this complex condition. It also allows for the parents to evaluate the alternative of elective termination of pregnancy, which has been reported in up to 33% of cases.[33,37]

ASSOCIATED ANOMALIES

Cloacal exstrophy often presents as part of one of three complexes: omphalocele–exstrophy–imperforate anus (OEI), omphalocele–exstrophy–imperforate anus–spinal defect (OEIS), or the exstrophy–imperforated anus–spinal defect (EIS) complex. As a result, patients should be evaluated for associated neurologic, skeletal, genitourinary, and gastrointestinal (GI) anomalies. Neurologic anomalies arise from concomitant spinal dysraphism (including tethered cord) in 64%–100% of cases.[37–41] This results in significant long-term neurologic morbidity as bladder, GI, lower extremities, and erectile function can be impaired. In addition to the bladder being affected by spinal dysraphism, there are data to support aberrant neurovascular supply to the bladder at risk for iatrogenic injury at the time of reconstruction.[42] Approximately 31% of patients with spinal dysraphism also have intracranial abnormalities such as hydrocephalus and Chiari malformation.[43] Other skeletal anomalies such as extra vertebrae, hemivertebrae, scoliosis, and kyphosis have been reported in 22%–60% of patients.[42,44] Limb deformities are also observed in 17%–26% of patients.[45]

Associated genitourinary anomalies are common. Abnormalities of the upper urinary tract have been reported in 41%–66% of patients[3,19,46,47] with renal anomalies including pelvic kidney, hydronephrosis, and renal agenesis, seen in one-third of patients.[47] In females, external and internal genitalia are affected in 73%–97% of cases.[48–50] Various degrees of duplication of Müllerian structures along with vaginal agenesis, atresia, or transverse septa are common. Ovaries are generally histologically normal.[51] The labia and clitoris are widely separated, and absence of clitoral halves may be seen. In males, the scrotum and phallic structure are similarly widely separated, and the phallic halves may be diminutive or absent (aphallia). The phallic structure can occasionally be found intravesically.[52] Cryptorchidism is common, but the testes are histologically normal.[53]

The most common GI anomalies include omphalocele, exstrophy of the cecal plate, blind-ending hindgut, and imperforate anus. Additional anomalies include short bowel syndrome, colonic duplication, duodenal web, Meckel diverticulum, malrotation, and duodenal atresia.[54] GI anomalies are associated with significant morbidity due to increase risk of nutritional malabsorption or obstruction.[38]

IMMEDIATE POSTNATAL MANAGEMENT

Cloacal exstrophy should be managed by a multidisciplinary team comprising a pediatric urologist, pediatric surgeon, neonatologist, pediatric neurosurgeon, pediatric endocrinologist, and pediatric orthopedic surgeon at a center with interest and experience in the management of this complex condition. A psychiatrist/psychologist and social worker well versed in gender assignment issues should be involved early in the process to aid with family care.[55] Upon delivery and stabilization of the neonate, all mucosal surfaces such as the exposed bladder plates, omphalocele, intestines, and myelomeningoceles should be protected. A cling-film dressing (Saran Wrap) moistened with saline can be used to cover the exposed mucosa, or a bowel bag can be use to enclose the infant's lower torso. This helps to minimize fluid losses, mucosal damage, and infection. The umbilical cord should be ligated with a nonabsorbable suture to prevent abrading the bladder plate or the hindgut with the standard umbilical clamp. Routine preoperative labs (electrolytes, hematologic, and renal function) should be drawn along with karyotyping. Preoperative imaging including renal ultrasound, chest x-ray, and spinal imaging with ultrasound or MRI should be obtained to evaluate for associated anomalies. Intravenous access should be obtained in the upper limbs to allow surgical access to the lower half of the neonate. If not done prenatally, preoperative counseling should include surgical reconstruction, gender assignment in males, anticipated needs for future surgery, and potential complications or deficits that may result in the long term.

GENDER ASSIGNMENT

Females (46XX) with cloaca exstrophy should be raised as females. Gender assignment in male (46XY) patients with cloacal exstrophy remains a complex and controversial issue. Historically, patients with insufficient phallic tissue or aphallia were reassigned and raised as female. This was accomplished by performing early orchiectomy and subsequent feminizing reconstruction. However, this practice has recently been brought into question. In a survey of pediatric urologists, two-thirds favored male gender assignment primarily based on concerns of prenatal testosterone imprinting.[53,56] In addition, studies have also demonstrated that over half of male cloacal exstrophy patients reassigned as female question their gender, exhibit stereotypical male behavior, have sexual interest in females, or declare themselves as male.[23,39,57,58] While current views are to maintain male gender, it is important that this decision be made as part of a multidisciplinary team with significant input from the family.

POSTNATAL SURGICAL MANAGEMENT

Initial surgical management should be undertaken in the newborn period (48–72 hours). Early operation minimizes bacterial colonization of exposed organs and may reduce the need for osteotomies.[39,59,60] An individualized approach to each patient usually dictates the extent of the initial surgery. The order of the repair is usually closure of the omphalocele first, followed by separation of the hemibladders from the exstrophic hindgut, tubularization of hindgut with salvage of all bowel segments including the appendix, creation of an end bowel ostomy, approximation of the hemibladders in the midline, and if feasible, closure of bladder and abdominal wall defect. If a spinal dysraphism is present, it may also be addressed at the time of initial surgery. The genitalia are managed either during initial repair or as part of a subsequent procedure. Table 81.1 outlines a typical management plan for cloacal exstrophy.

When omphalocele closure is not possible, a silo device may be required in order to minimize abdominal compartment syndrome and decrease the risk of wound dehiscence.

Table 81.1 Outline of typical management plan for cloacal exstrophy

Management phase	Patient age	Therapeutic procedures
Phase 1	Newborn	Meningocele coverage (when present)
		Closure/coverage of omphalocele
		Separation of bowel/bladder plates
		Bowel reconstruction/tubularization
		Hemibladder approximation ± closure
		Gender assignment (early orchiectomy)
		Genital reconstruction (complete or first stage)
		Pubic bone approximation (±osteotomies)
Phase 2	1–6 months	Feeding access
		Management of short bowel syndrome
Phase 3	6 months– 2 years	Bladder closure if not done
		Pubic bone approximation with osteotomies
		Genital reconstruction (complete or first stage)
Phase 4	2–18 years	Genital reconstruction (second stage or for gender reassignment)
		Bladder neck reconstruction or other continence procedure (sling, artificial urinary sphincter, etc.)
		Bladder augmentation
		Construction of catheterizable channel

A 5-French ureteral catheter should be inserted into each ureter and secured to the bladder mucosa to aid in ureteral identification during dissection and prevent postoperative obstruction. Dissection should start superiorly with ligation and division of umbilical vessels. The two hemibladders are then separated from the hindgut using diathermy, taking care to avoid the ureters. Meticulous dissection medial to the hemibladder must be performed in order to avoid iatrogenic injury of the bladder or the nerves of the corporal bodies, which travel in the midline along the posteroinferior surface of the pelvis before extending laterally.[42] If the patient has an absent hemiphallus or is aphallic, one should evaluate for potential intravesical phallic structures.[52] Preservation of all bowel segments including the appendix cannot be overemphasized due to the risk of short bowel syndrome and potential need for future urinary tract reconstruction.[39,61] It is recommended that the tubularized hindgut be turned into an end colostomy or left as a mucus fistula.[55] If possible, an ileostomy should be avoided as this can lead to fluid, electrolyte, and nutritional issues.[62,63] Bowel length should be measured and documented. The hemibladders should be approximated in the midline, thus converting the condition into a classic bladder exstrophy for subsequent staged repair.

At this point, it is usually determined if a single-stage or multistage repair is appropriate based on patient medical status, other congenital anomalies, and anatomic findings that may preclude primary single-stage repair. Studies have suggested comparable outcomes with single-stage and multistage repairs.[64,65] If the bladder plate is of adequate size and a single-stage repair is feasible, the bladder plate is dissected from its lateral attachment and lateral edges are approximated in the midline using absorbable suture. The bladder neck and proximal urethra are tubularized over an 8-French catheter either completely in girls or partially in boys (thus creating an epispadias). Ureteral stents can be brought out via the neourethra or via the anterior abdominal wall during bladder closure. The next step is genital reconstruction, which can be extremely challenging in males with cloacal exstrophy. Phallic halves are usually widely separated, asymmetric, absent, and/or rudimentary. Phallic reconstruction and epispadias repair is usually accomplished at a later time. Reconstruction during initial closure can be performed following the same principles as in classic bladder exstrophy. Current practice is to reapproximate the hemiscrota in the midline and, if necessary, perform orchiopexy. Genital reconstruction in females is usually done at the time of bladder closure. The medial aspect of the hemiclitoris may be denuded of mucosa, and the halves are brought together in the midline along with the labia minora. Müllerian structures are usually duplicated and should be joined in the midline and brought to the perineum during initial repair.

Similar to classic bladder exstrophy, placement of the bladder and proximal urethra deep in the pelvis is a key factor for success. To accomplish this, the pubic symphysis is approximated in the midline with interrupted high-tensile-strength suture. Pelvic osteotomies can be employed to improve success with closure by decreasing tension on the wound.[19,66,67] If the surgery is performed early in the neonatal period, there appears to be no difference in terms of wound dehiscence between patients with and without osteotomies.[60] The abdominal wall muscle and skin are then closed in layers with absorbable sutures.

POSTOPERATIVE MANAGEMENT

Close postoperative monitoring in the neonatal intensive care unit is necessary to ensure adequate pain control, immobilization, and nutritional support. Patients should remain immobilized for 4–6 weeks using one of a variety of described traction devices.[68–70] Avoiding abdominal distention is also important to prevent tension on the wound. Initial and aggressive use of total parental nutrition is advocated given the risk of short bowel syndrome.[71] Prophylactic antibiotics to cover for skin flora and urinary pathogens is recommended given the presence of multiple long-term indwelling catheters and associated 50%–60% risk of associated vesicoureteral reflux.[46] Serial ultrasound imaging of the kidneys is recommended to ensure adequate urinary drainage. Laboratory tests may be obtained as needed to evaluate for electrolyte disturbances and adjust nutrition supplementation.

UROLOGIC MANAGEMENT

Timing of ureteral and urethral catheter removal depends on surgeon preference and patient status. Sequential removal of stents along with upper tract monitoring with renal ultrasound is necessary to ensure adequate drainage. Once all catheters are removed, the patient should be monitored for spontaneous voiding and assessed for high postvoid residuals that may require initiation of intermittent catheterization. Bladder outcomes appear to be less favorable than those of classic bladder exstrophy, and achieving continence remains a challenge. Over 40% of patients have persistent incontinence after primary repair.[19,40,72,73] This high rate of incontinence is attributed to a smaller bladder plate and higher risk of associated neurologic condition.[40] Multiple approaches for urinary tract reconstruction to achieve continence have been described, including bladder neck reconstruction, slings, artificial urinary sphincter implantation, and bladder neck closure.[74–76] Patients often undergo multiple procedures, but a catheterizable channel and augmentation cystoplasty are necessary to achieve continence in over 50% of patients.[19,39,75,77] Patients with cloacal exstrophy should be followed closely by a pediatric urologist given the risk of bladder and upper tract deterioration associated with spinal dysraphism.

GI OUTCOMES

A considerable proportion of patients have morbidity related to the GI tract. Preservation of as much bowel as possible during initial repair is paramount as it will optimize bowel absorption by increasing transit time. It is also reported that there is potential for colonic growth with time, and any bowel segment can be of benefit during future reconstructions of the urinary tract.[39,61,78] Patients with cloacal exstrophy have traditionally been managed with diverting ostomy due to associated spinal dysmorphism, abnormal pelvic and sacral anatomy, and the absence of normal sphincter mechanisms.[78] However, several series have demonstrated good outcomes with pull-through procedures in select patients, with fecal continence in over 76% of patients using adjunct bowel management including a bulking diet, antidiarrheal medications, and enemas (antegrade or retrograde).[39,78] The ability to form solid stool and colonic length are key factors to achieving fecal continence rather than the presence of intact sphincter mechanisms.[61,63]

SEXUAL FUNCTION AND QUALITY OF LIFE

There are limited data on male patients with cloacal exstrophy with regard to sexual function and quality of life. A report of eight male patients with cloacal exstrophy demonstrated phallic inadequacy in all and erectile dysfunction in half, and only one was able to engage in vaginal intercourse.[60] While there are no reports of males with cloacal exstrophy fathering children, assisted reproductive technology can certainly be an option for these patients given normal testes.[53] Recent advancements and future developments in the field of phallic reconstruction and penile transplantation hold promise for male patients with cloacal exstrophy.[79–82] Total phallic construction using the radial artery–based forearm free flap has demonstrated excellent patient satisfaction with regard to phallic cosmesis, size, and ability to achieve sexual intercourse with the aid of a penile prosthesis.[81]

Vaginal reconstruction in female patients with cloacal exstrophy is also challenging. This is generally performed during initial repair if feasible, but oftentimes, delayed repair and additional procedures are necessary. Over 65% of patients have duplication of the vagina, uterus, or fallopian tubes due to failed fusion of the Müllerian ducts.[50,83] Pull-through vaginoplasty, flap/graft vaginoplasty, creation of neovagina using bowel, and use of the native bladder to create a neovagina have been reported.[39,61,83] There are few reports on the outcome of the uteri, but approximately half of patients require total or partial hemihysterectomy due to hydrometrocolpos, prolapse, or underdevelopment.[50] Reports on sexual function, while limited and small, demonstrate that up to half of female patients are sexually active and the majority are satisfied with their sexual life.[84,85] Successful pregnancy, although complicated and high risk, has been reported.[84,86,87] Long-term quality-of-life studies are limited in this patient population, although cases series suggest that the majority of patients are satisfied with their professional and social life.[84]

CONCLUSIONS

With advances in perinatal management and surgical reconstruction, mortality in patients with cloacal exstrophy has significantly decreased, and emphasis in care has shifted to improved diagnosis, surgical outcomes, and quality of life. Gender identity, continence, and body image can impact the quality of life of these patients, and efforts to improve in these areas are needed. Because of the rarity of this congenital condition and the lack of data, the optimal management strategy remains unclear. Treatment should be individualized to the needs of the patient and family at a center with the multidisciplinary expertise needed to adequately care for patients with this rare condition.

REFERENCES

1. Gordetsky J, Joseph DB. Cloacal exstrophy: A history of gender reassignment. *Urology* 2015 December; 86(6): 1087–9.
2. Rickham PP. Vesico-intestinal Fissure. *Arch Dis Child* 1960 February; 35(179): 97–102.
3. Hurwitz RS, Manzoni GA, Ransley PG, Stephens FD. Cloacal exstrophy: A report of 34 cases. *J Urol* 1987 October; 138(4 Pt 2): 1060–4.
4. Diamond DA, Jeffs RD. Cloacal exstrophy: A 22-year experience. *J Urol* 1985 May; 133(5): 779–82.
5. Marshall V ME. Variations in exstrophy of the bladder. *J Urol* 1962; 88: 766–96.
6. Muecke EC. The role of the cloacal membrane in exstrophy: The first successful experimental study. *J Urol* 1964 December; 92: 659–67.
7. Thomalla JV, Rudolph RA, Rink RC, Mitchell ME. Induction of cloacal exstrophy in the chick embryo using the CO_2 laser. *J Urol* 1985 November; 134(5): 991–5.
8. Langer JC, Brennan B, Lappalainen RE, Caco CC, Winthrop AL, Hollenberg RD et al. Cloacal exstrophy: Prenatal diagnosis before rupture of the cloacal membrane. *J Pediatr Surg* 1992 October; 27(10): 1352–5.
9. Bruch SW, Adzick NS, Goldstein RB, Harrison MR. Challenging the embryogenesis of cloacal exstrophy. *J Pediatr Surg* 1996 June; 31(6): 768–70.
10. Sahoo SP, Gangopadhyay AN, Sinha CK, Gupta DK, Gopal SC. Covered exstrophy: A rare variant of classical bladder exstrophy. *Scand J Urol Nephrol* 1997 February; 31(1): 103–6.
11. Borwankar SS, Kasat LS, Naregal A, Jain M, Bajaj R. Covered exstrophy: A rare variant. *Pediatr Surg Int* 1998 November; 14(1–2): 129–30.
12. van der Putte SC, Spliet WG, Nikkels PG. Common ("classical") and covered cloacal exstrophy: A histopathological study and a reconstruction of the pathogenesis. *Pediatr Dev Pathol* 2008 November–December; 11(6): 430–42.

13. Nievelstein RA, van der Werff JF, Verbeek FJ, Valk J, Vermeij-Keers C. Normal and abnormal embryonic development of the anorectum in human embryos. *Teratology* 1998 February; 57(2): 70–8.

14. Hartwig NG, Steffelaar JW, Van de Kaa C, Schueler JA, Vermeij-Keers C. Abdominal wall defect associated with persistent cloaca. The embryologic clues in autopsy. *Am J Clin Pathol* 1991 November; 96(5): 640–7.

15. Duhamel B. Embryology of exomphalos and allied malformations. *Arch Dis Child* 1963 April; 38(198): 142–7.

16. Feldkamp ML, Botto LD, Amar E, Bakker MK, Bermejo-Sanchez E, Bianca S et al. Cloacal exstrophy: An epidemiologic study from the International Clearinghouse for Birth Defects Surveillance and Research. *Am J Med Genet C Semin Med Genet* 2011 November 15; 157C(4): 333–43.

17. Cervellione RM, Mantovani A, Gearhart J, Bogaert G, Gobet R, Caione P et al. Prospective study on the incidence of bladder/cloacal exstrophy and epispadias in Europe. *J Pediatr Urol* 2015 December; 11(6): 337 e1–6.

18. Gambhir L, Holler T, Muller M, Schott G, Vogt H, Detlefsen B et al. Epidemiological survey of 214 families with bladder exstrophy–epispadias complex. *J Urol* 2008 April; 179(4): 1539–43.

19. Phillips TM, Salmasi AH, Stec A, Novak TE, Gearhart JP, Mathews RI. Urological outcomes in the omphalocele exstrophy imperforate anus spinal defects (OEIS) complex: Experience with 80 patients. *J Pediatr Urol* 2013 June; 9(3): 353–8.

20. Siebert JR, Rutledge JC, Kapur RP. Association of cloacal anomalies, caudal duplication, and twinning. *Pediatr Dev Pathol* 2005 May–June; 8(3): 339–54.

21. Raman VS, Bajpai M, Ali A. Bladder exstrophy–epispadias complex and the role of methylenetetrahydrofolate reductase C677T polymorphism: A case control study. *J Indian Assoc Pediatr Surg* 2016 January–March; 21(1): 28–32.

22. Carey JC, Greenbaum B, Hall BD. The OEIS complex (omphalocele, exstrophy, imperforate anus, spinal defects). *Birth Defects Orig Artic Ser* 1978; 14(6B): 253–63.

23. Evans JA, Chudley AE. Tibial agenesis, femoral duplication, and caudal midline anomalies. *Am J Med Genet* 1999 July 2; 85(1): 13–9.

24. Nye JS, Hayes EA, Amendola M, Vaughn D, Charrow J, McLone DG et al. Myelocystocele–cloacal exstrophy in a pedigree with a mitochondrial 12S rRNA mutation, aminoglycoside-induced deafness, pigmentary disturbances, and spinal anomalies. *Teratology* 2000 March; 61(3): 165–71.

25. Thauvin-Robinet C, Faivre L, Cusin V, Khau Van Kien P, Callier P, Parker KL et al. Cloacal exstrophy in an infant with 9q34.1-qter deletion resulting from a de novo unbalanced translocation between chromosome 9q and Yq. *Am J Med Genet A* 2004 April 30; 126A(3): 303–7.

26. Kosaki R, Fukuhara Y, Kosuga M, Okuyama T, Kawashima N, Honna T et al. OEIS complex with del(3)(q12.2q13.2). *Am J Med Genet A* 2005 June 1; 135(2): 224–6.

27. El-Hattab AW, Skorupski JC, Hsieh MH, Breman AM, Patel A, Cheung SW et al. OEIS complex associated with chromosome 1p36 deletion: A case report and review. *Am J Med Genet A* 2010 February; 152A(2): 504–11.

28. Reefhuis J, Honein MA, Schieve LA, Rasmussen SA. Use of clomiphene citrate and birth defects, National Birth Defects Prevention Study, 1997–2005. *Hum Reprod* 2011 February; 26(2): 451–7.

29. Banhidy F, Acs N, Czeizel AE. Ovarian cysts, clomiphene therapy, and the risk of neural tube defects. *Int J Gynaecol Obstet* 2008 January; 100(1): 86–8.

30. Wood HM, Trock BJ, Gearhart JP. In vitro fertilization and the cloacal–bladder exstrophy–epispadias complex: Is there an association? *J Urol* 2003 April; 169(4): 1512–5.

31. Austin PF, Homsy YL, Gearhart JP, Porter K, Guidi C, Madsen K et al. The prenatal diagnosis of cloacal exstrophy. *J Urol* 1998 September; 160(3 Pt 2): 1179–81.

32. Hamada H, Takano K, Shiina H, Sakai T, Sohda S, Kubo T. New ultrasonographic criterion for the prenatal diagnosis of cloacal exstrophy: Elephant trunk–like image. *J Urol* 1999 December; 162(6): 2123–4.

33. Goyal A, Fishwick J, Hurrell R, Cervellione RM, Dickson AP. Antenatal diagnosis of bladder/cloacal exstrophy: Challenges and possible solutions. *J Pediatr Urol* 2012 April; 8(2): 140–4.

34. Calvo-Garcia MA, Kline-Fath BM, Rubio EI, Merrow AC, Guimaraes CV, Lim FY. Fetal MRI of cloacal exstrophy. *Pediatr Radiol* 2013 March; 43(5): 593–604.

35. Yamano T, Ando K, Ishikura R, Hirota S. Serial fetal magnetic resonance imaging of cloacal exstrophy. *Jpn J Radiol* 2011 November; 29(9): 656–9.

36. Clements MB, Chalmers DJ, Meyers ML, Vemulakonda VM. Prenatal diagnosis of cloacal exstrophy: A case report and review of the literature. *Urology* 2014 May; 83(5): 1162–4.

37. Keppler-Noreuil KM. OEIS complex (omphalocele–exstrophy–imperforate anus–spinal defects): A review of 14 cases. *Am J Med Genet* 2001 April 1; 99(4): 271–9.

38. McHoney M, Ransley PG, Duffy P, Wilcox DT, Spitz L. Cloacal exstrophy: Morbidity associated with abnormalities of the gastrointestinal tract and spine. *J Pediatr Surg* 2004 August; 39(8): 1209–13.

39. Lund DP, Hendren WH. Cloacal exstrophy: A 25-year experience with 50 cases. *J Pediatr Surg* 2001 January; 36(1): 68–75.

40. Husmann DA, Vandersteen DR, McLorie GA, Churchill BM. Urinary continence after staged bladder reconstruction for cloacal exstrophy: The effect of coexisting neurological abnormalities on urinary continence. *J Urol* 1999 May; 161(5): 1598–602.

41. Dutta HK. Cloacal exstrophy: A single center experience. *J Pediatr Urol* 2014 April; 10(2): 329–35.

42. Schlegel PN, Gearhart JP. Neuroanatomy of the pelvis in an infant with cloacal exstrophy: A detailed microdissection with histology. *J Urol* 1989 March; 141(3): 583–5.

43. Suson KD, Colombani PM, Jallo GI, Gearhart JP. Intracranial anomalies and cloacal exstrophy—Is there a role for screening? *J Pediatr Surg* 2013 November; 48(11): 2256–60.

44. Greene WB, Dias LS, Lindseth RE, Torch MA. Musculoskeletal problems in association with cloacal exstrophy. *J Bone Joint Surg Am* 1991 April; 73(4): 551–60.

45. Jain M, Weaver DD. Severe lower limb defects in exstrophy of the cloaca. *Am J Med Genet A* 2004 July 30; 128A(3): 320–4.

46. Woo LL, Thomas JC, Brock JW. Cloacal exstrophy: A comprehensive review of an uncommon problem. *J Pediatr Urol* 2010 April; 6(2): 102–11.

47. Diamond DA. Management of cloacal exstrophy. *Dial Pediatr Urol* 1990; 13: 2.

48. Suson KD, Preece J, Di Carlo HN, Baradaran N, Gearhart JP. Complexities of Mullerian anatomy in 46XX cloacal exstrophy patients. *J Pediatr Adolesc Gynecol* 2016 October; 29(5): 424–8.

49. Visnesky PM, Texter JH, Galle PC, Walker GG, McRae MA. Genital outflow tract obstruction in an adolescent with cloacal exstrophy. *Obstet Gynecol* 1990 September; 76(3 Pt 2): 548–51.

50. Naiditch JA, Radhakrishnan J, Chin AC, Cheng E, Yerkes E, Reynolds M. Fate of the uterus in 46XX cloacal exstrophy patients. *J Pediatr Surg* 2013 October; 48(10): 2043–6.

51. Schober JM, Carmichael PA, Hines M, Ransley PG. The ultimate challenge of cloacal exstrophy. *J Urol* 2002 January; 167(1): 300–4.

52. Fox JA, Banihani O, Schneck FX. Is it really a hamartoma? Bringing awareness to the possibility of an intravesical phallus in the aphallic 46,xy cloacal exstrophy patient. *J Pediatr Urol* 2013 December; 9(6 Pt B): 1237–8.

53. Mathews RI, Perlman E, Marsh DW, Gearhart JP. Gonadal morphology in cloacal exstrophy: Implications in gender assignment. *BJU Int* 1999 July; 84(1): 99–100.

54. Davidoff AM, Hebra A, Balmer D, Templeton JM, Jr., Schnaufer L. Management of the gastrointestinal tract and nutrition in patients with cloacal exstrophy. *J Pediatr Surg* 1996 June; 31(6): 771–3.

55. Mathews R, Jeffs RD, Reiner WG, Docimo SG, Gearhart JP. Cloacal exstrophy—Improving the quality of life: The Johns Hopkins experience. *J Urol* 1998 December; 160(6 Pt 2): 2452–6.

56. Diamond DA, Burns JP, Mitchell C, Lamb K, Kartashov AI, Retik AB. Sex assignment for newborns with ambiguous genitalia and exposure to fetal testosterone: Attitudes and practices of pediatric urologists. *J Pediatr* 2006 April; 148(4): 445–9.

57. Reiner WG. Psychosexual development in genetic males assigned female: The cloacal exstrophy experience. *Child Adolesc Psychiatr Clin N Am* 2004 July; 13(3): 657–74, ix.

58. Zderic SA, Canning DA, Carr MC, Kodman-Jones C, Snyder HM. The CHOP experience with cloacal exstrophy and gender reassignment. *Adv Exp Med Biol* 2002; 511:135–44; discussion 44–7.

59. Howell C, Caldamone A, Snyder H, Ziegler M, Duckett J. Optimal management of cloacal exstrophy. *J Pediatr Surg* 1983 August; 18(4): 365–9.

60. Husmann DA, McLorie GA, Churchill BM. Closure of the exstrophic bladder: An evaluation of the factors leading to its success and its importance on urinary continence. *J Urol* 1989 August; 142(2 Pt 2): 522–4; discussion 42–3.

61. Soffer SZ, Rosen NG, Hong AR, Alexianu M, Pena A. Cloacal exstrophy: A unified management plan. *J Pediatr Surg* 2000 June; 35(6): 932–7.

62. Husmann DA, McLorie GA, Churchill BM, Ein SH. Management of the hindgut in cloacal exstrophy: Terminal ileostomy versus colostomy. *J Pediatr Surg* 1988 December; 23(12): 1107–13.

63. Sawaya D, Goldstein S, Seetharamaiah R, Suson K, Nabaweesi R, Colombani P et al. Gastrointestinal ramifications of the cloacal exstrophy complex: A 44-year experience. *J Pediatr Surg* 2010 January; 45(1): 171–5; discussion 5–6.

64. Thomas JC, DeMarco RT, Pope JCt, Adams MC, Brock JW 3rd. First stage approximation of the exstrophic bladder in patients with cloacal exstrophy—Should this be the initial surgical approach in all patients? *J Urol* 2007 October; 178(4 Pt 2): 1632–5; discussion 5–6.

65. Lee RS, Grady R, Joyner B, Casale P, Mitchell M. Can a complete primary repair approach be applied to cloacal exstrophy? *J Urol* 2006 December; 176(6 Pt 1): 2643–8.

66. Wild AT, Sponseller PD, Stec AA, Gearhart JP. The role of osteotomy in surgical repair of bladder exstrophy. *Semin Pediatr Surg* 2011 May; 20(2): 71–8.

67. Baka-Ostrowska M, Kowalczyk K, Felberg K, Wawer Z. Complications after primary bladder exstrophy closure—Role of pelvic osteotomy. *Cent Eur J Urol* 2013; 66(1): 104–8.

68. Wallis MC, Oottamasathien S, Wicher C, Hadley D, Snow BW, Cartwright PC. Padded self-adhesive strap immobilization following newborn bladder exstrophy closure: The Utah straps. *J Urol* 2013 December; 190(6): 2216–20.

69. Shnorhavorian M, Song K, Zamilpa I, Wiater B, Mitchell MM, Grady RW. Spica casting compared to Bryant's traction after complete primary repair of exstrophy: Safe and effective in a longitudinal cohort study. *J Urol* 2010 August; 184(2): 669–73.

70. Meldrum KK, Baird AD, Gearhart JP. Pelvic and extremity immobilization after bladder exstrophy closure: Complications and impact on success. *Urology* 2003 December; 62(6): 1109–13.

71. Hyun SJ. Cloacal exstrophy. *Neonatal Netw* 2006 March–April; 25(2): 101–15.

72. Mitchell ME, Brito CG, Rink RC. Cloacal exstrophy reconstruction for urinary continence. *J Urol* 1990 August; 144(2 Pt 2): 554–8; discussion 62–3.

73. Vliet R, Roelofs LA, Rassouli-Kirchmeier R, de Gier RP, Claahsen-van der Grinten HL, Verhaak C et al. Clinical outcome of cloacal exstrophy, current status, and a change in surgical management. *Eur J Pediatr Surg* 2015 February; 25(1): 87–93.

74. Dave S, Salle JL. Current status of bladder neck reconstruction. *Curr Opin Urol* 2008 July; 18(4): 419–24.

75. Mathews R. Achieving urinary continence in cloacal exstrophy. *Semin Pediatr Surg* 2011 May; 20(2): 126–9.

76. Hernandez-Martin S, Lopez-Pereira P, Lopez-Fernandez S, Ortiz R, Marcos M, Lobato R et al. Bladder neck closure in children: Long-term results and consequences. *Eur J Pediatr Surg* 2015 February; 25(1): 100–4.

77. Goldstein SD, Inouye BM, Reddy S, Lue K, Young EE, Abdelwahab M et al. Continence in the cloacal exstrophy patient: What does it cost? *J Pediatr Surg* 2015 December 11; 51(4): 622–5.

78. Levitt MA, Mak GZ, Falcone RA, Jr., Pena A. Cloacal exstrophy—Pull-through or permanent stoma? A review of 53 patients. *J Pediatr Surg* 2008 January; 43(1): 164–8; discussion 8–70.

79. Perovic S. Phalloplasty in children and adolescents using the extended pedicle island groin flap. *J Urol* 1995 August; 154(2 Pt 2): 848–53.

80. De Fontaine S, Lorea P, Wespes E, Schulman C, Goldschmidt D. Complete phalloplasty using the free radial forearm flap for correcting micropenis associated with vesical exstrophy. *J Urol* 2001 August; 166(2): 597–9.

81. Garaffa G, Spilotros M, Christopher NA, Ralph DJ. Total phallic reconstruction using radial artery based forearm free flap phalloplasty in patients with epispadias–exstrophy complex. *J Urol* 2014 September; 192(3): 814–20.

82. Tiftikcioglu YO, Erenoglu CM, Lineaweaver WC, Zhang F. Perioperative management of penile transplantation. *Microsurgery* 2016 February 18; 36(4): 271–5.

83. Hisamatsu E, Nakagawa Y, Sugita Y. Vaginal reconstruction in female cloacal exstrophy patients. *Urology* 2014 September; 84(3): 681–4.

84. Catti M, Paccalin C, Rudigoz RC, Mouriquand P. Quality of life for adult women born with bladder and cloacal exstrophy: A long-term follow up. *J Pediatr Urol* 2006 February; 2(1): 16–22.

85. Montagnino B, Czyzewski DI, Runyan RD, Berkman S, Roth DR, Gonzales ET, Jr. Long-term adjustment issues in patients with exstrophy. *J Urol* 1998 October; 160(4): 1471–4.

86. Dy GW, Willihnganz-Lawson KH, Shnorhavorian M, Delaney SS, Amies Oelschlager AM, Merguerian PA et al. Successful pregnancy in patients with exstrophy–epispadias complex: A University of Washington experience. *J Pediatr Urol* 2015 August; 11(4): 213 e1–6.

87. Mathews RI, Gan M, Gearhart JP. Urogynaecological and obstetric issues in women with the exstrophy–epispadias complex. *BJU Int* 2003 June; 91(9): 845–9.

82

Prune belly syndrome

SALVATORE CASCIO, HIDESHI MIYAKITA, AND PREM PURI

INTRODUCTION

Prune belly syndrome is characterized by a triad of abnormalities, including an absence or deficiency of abdominal wall musculature, cryptorchism, and anomalies of the urinary tract. The characteristic deficiency of the abdominal wall musculature was first described by Frohlich et al.[1] in 1839. Parker[2] first reported the association of the genitourinary anomalies with the deficient abdominal musculature. The term "prune belly syndrome" was coined for this complex by Osler in 1901.[3] Eagle and Barrett,[4] in 1950, further defined the triad of absent abdominal wall musculature, undescended testes, and urinary tract abnormalities. The incidence of prune belly syndrome is estimated to be 1 in 27,000 to one in 40,000 live births.[5–7] This syndrome occurs almost exclusively in boys. In females, it is extremely rare, with less than 50 cases described in the world literature.[7,8] It is also known as *pseudo–prune belly syndrome* and is characterized by hypoplastic abdominal musculature and urinary tract and genital anomalies, most commonly bicornuate uterus and vaginal atresia.[8]

ETIOLOGY

The pathogenesis of prune belly syndrome remains controversial, and many theories have been proposed to explain it.[3,4] One theory proposes that prenatal obstruction or dysfunction of the urinary tract causes urinary tract dilatation, fetal abdominal distension, and subsequent muscle wall hypoplasia and cryptorchism in males.[9–12] An embryological theory proposes that failure of primary mesodermal differentiation leads to defective muscularization of both the abdominal wall and the urinary tract.[10–12] Although both theories explain some elements of the syndrome, they fail to explain others. Reinberg et al.[8] recently suggested that the two theories should be regarded as complementary mechanisms, both operating in any given case. They theorized that teratogenic agents produce abnormal development of derivatives of the lateral plate mesoderm and abnormal epithelial–mesenchymal interactions, resulting in abnormal organ development and mechanical or functional obstruction of the urinary tract. Stephens and Gupta[13] proposed a theory of abnormal development of the intermediate mesoderm as a key factor in the pathogenesis of prune belly syndrome. This theory has two features: the first is that the terminal part of the Wolffian duct is incorporated into both the prostatic and membranous urethra, and the second is that during incorporation, the ducts including their ureteric buds overexpand. Abnormal ectasia of the terminal Wolffian duct occurring between 6 and 10 weeks' gestation may produce saccular dilatation of the prostatic urethra, prostatic hypoplasia, and the valve-like obstruction in the membranous urethra. The ectasia could explain the attenuated bladder trigone and laterally placed wide ureteric orifices. Involvement of ureteric buds may also produce irregular megaureters. Renal dysplasia can be explained as a result of primary dysplasia of the metanephros or secondary to ureteric ectopia.

The genetic basis of prune belly syndrome remains unknown. A single-gene abnormality or chromosomal defect has been suggested as the cause of this syndrome. There is an especially high incidence of prune belly syndrome associated with trisomy 21,[14] trisomy 13,[15,16] and trisomy 18.[17,18] Twelve published case reports of familial prune belly syndrome primarily affecting brothers have suggested a possible autosomal or X-linked recessive mode of inheritance.[19,20] $HNF1\beta$ is a transcription factor that regulates gene expression for normal mesodermal and endodermal development and has been proposed as a possible candidate gene for the syndrome. The most common $HNF1\beta$ phenotype is renal cysts and diabetes syndrome, also called maturity-onset diabetes of the young type 5.[21] However, a recent study has detected the V61G $HNF1\beta$ mutation only in 1 of 34 (3%) patients with prune belly syndrome.[20]

PATHOLOGY

Abdominal wall

Prune belly syndrome represents a spectrum of disease severity, ranging from those that die within the first few days of

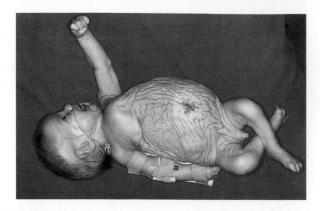

Figure 82.1 A newborn with typical features of prune belly syndrome. Note the shriveled prune-like appearance of the abdominal wall and patent urachus.

life to those that survive with relatively stable renal function in childhood. The most obvious defect in newborns with the syndrome is the shriveled prune belly–like appearance of the abdominal wall due to a deficiency in the abdominal wall musculature (Figure 82.1). The affected muscles in decreasing order of frequency are the transversus abdominis, rectus abdominis below the umbilicus, and internal oblique, external oblique, and rectus abdominis above the umbilicus.[22-24] Biopsy from the abdominal musculature shows that major functioning or recoverable muscle exists in the lateral and upper sector of the abdomen, but that little or no muscle exists in the lower central abdomen.[25] Light microscopy shows a thin mass of muscle tissue with an irregular pattern of fatty infiltration interdigitated with the muscle. Electron microscopy shows a loss of coherence and internal orientation.[26] Z-bands are shattered and disarranged, and glycogen granules are clumped in various areas. The abdominal wall defect may result in chronic constipation and respiratory infection. In addition, this defect increases the risk of postoperative pulmonary complications in patients who undergo general anesthesia. It is also impossible for the patient with a complete manifestation of the triad syndrome to raise himself/herself from the supine position to the sitting position without using the arms or rolling over and pushing up. However, the defect itself does not have prognostic significance.

Urinary tract

Abnormalities of the urinary tract are the major factors affecting the prognosis of patients with prune belly syndrome. Patients are at high risk for developing renal failure in infancy and childhood. As many as 39% of patients, typically those with impaired renal function at initial evaluation, develop chronic renal failure in childhood or adolescence, with 17% of them undergoing renal transplantation.[27]

Kidney

The kidney in prune belly syndrome has many ranges of disorders, from total agenesis (rare) or dysplasia to no significant

aberration.[28-31] Ureterohydronephrosis occurs bilaterally in 98% of patients, while renal dysplasia is detected in 35%–50% of patients and renal scarring in an additional 38%.[27,32] The degree of renal dysplasia or hydronephrosis does not appear to be related to the degree of abdominal wall deficiency.

Ureter

The ureters are characteristically markedly elongated, dilated, and tortuous. The lower end of the ureter is more severely affected than the upper one, and there are occasional saccular dilatations of the middle segment. The orifices are usually patent, and obstruction is rare. Vesicoureteral reflux is common and present in up to 78% of patients, mostly bilateral (Figure 82.2).[27] The ureteric smooth muscle is replaced by fibrous tissue in the affected areas, and there is scarcity of muscle bundles on histologic examination.[33] Ehrlich and Brown[34] studied the structure by electron microscopy and reported a marked decrease in nerve plexuses with irregularity and degeneration of nonmyelinated Schwann fibers. These findings are in keeping with the poor peristalsis of the affected ureters.

Bladder

Bladder abnormalities are common in prune belly syndrome. The typical bladder is large, irregular in shape, and thick walled. Although the bladder wall is thickened, trabeculation is rare. Histologically, the intrusion of fibrous tissue between sparse muscle layers is similar to the ureters.[35]

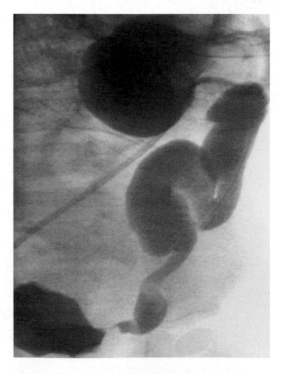

Figure 82.2 Micturating cystourethrogram showing Grade V vesicoureteral reflux into left dilated tortuous ureter.

Commonly, there is a patent urachus or urachal cyst. The trigone is surprisingly large, with very widely spaced, usually large and abnormal-appearing ureteric orifices, which can be expected to reflux. The bladder neck is often wide and ill-defined. Pelvic innervation and bladder ganglion cell distribution has been found to be normal.[28]

Urethra

A mildly dilated anterior urethra is the most common abnormality, present in 70% of patients with prune belly syndrome.[30] Both scaphoid and fusiform megalourethra have been found in association with prune belly syndrome but are rare.[36] The prostatic urethra is usually wide and elongated at the bladder neck (Figure 82.3). It tapers to a narrow point at the level of the urogenital diaphragm, even though most patients do not demonstrate true obstruction at this point.[30] Often, there is a posterior urethral diverticulum formed by a large prostatic utricle. The reduced musculature and prostatic hypoplasia cause a "functional obstruction" to bladder outflow.[3]

There are also reports of abnormalities of the penis, including ventral and dorsal chordee, hypospadias, and hypoplastic or absent corpora cavernosa.[30] Ejaculation is possible but usually is retrograde due to the open bladder neck.

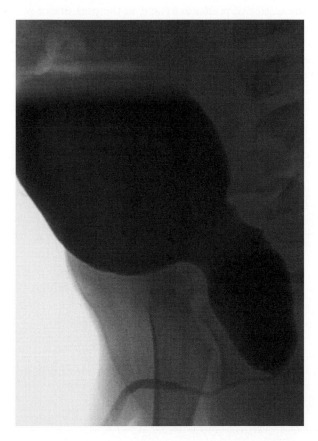

Figure 82.3 Micturating cystourethrogram showing ill-defined bladder neck with enlarged prostatic urethra. No urethral obstruction was demonstrated in the 2-week-old infant.

In females, bicornuate uterus and vaginal atresia are the most common genital anomalies encountered. Six of the seven female cases reported by Reinberg et al.[8] had vaginal atresia or uterine duplication, and these frequently coexisted in the same patient. Other urogenital anomalies include urogenital sinus and ambiguous genitalia.

Testes

Bilateral cryptorchidism is an essential characteristic of prune belly syndrome. The testes may be located anywhere from just inferior to the lower pole of the kidney to near the ureterovesical junction.[31,35] Maldescent of the testes is believed to be related to the impaired contraction of the abdominal musculature and to the mechanical obstruction caused by an enlarged bladder and dilated upper tract.[36] The gubernaculum plays an important role during testicular descent, which has been explained mainly by its action for dilatation and contraction.[37] A recent structural study of the gubernaculum testis has demonstrated a predominance of collagen type III fibers and smaller elastic fibers in fetuses with prune belly syndrome compared to a predominance of collagen type I in controls. The authors speculated that the mechanical obstruction or the altered intra-abdominal pressure hinders gubernacular remodeling.[38]

In fetuses with prune belly syndrome, testicular histology revealed reduced spermatogonia and Leydig cell hyperplasia.[39,40] Testicular biopsy samples of infant testes in prune belly syndrome demonstrate atypical germ cells with large nuclei and prominent nucleoli, and intense alkaline phosphatase staining localized to the cytoplasmic membrane.[40] The similarity of histological appearance of these testes to those in intratubular germ cell neoplasia suggests that long-term follow-up of these patients for the development of invasive germ cell tumors is important. A few cases of malignancy in the testes of patients with prune belly syndrome have been reported.[41–43]

ASSOCIATED ANOMALIES

In the last 40 years, several reports have shown a constant association between prune belly syndrome and extragenitourinary anomalies, with the most frequent being orthopedic and gastrointestinal followed by cardiopulmonary and developmental.[44]

Orthopedic comorbidities have frequently been reported in 50%–65% of patients with prune belly syndrome.[44,45] The most common abnormalities are scoliosis, talipes deformities, pectus excavatum/carinatum, developmental dysplasia of the hip, and sacral agenesis. Awareness of this association is essential either preoperatively, as pectus deformities may restrict pulmonary volumes, or intraoperatively, as developmental dysplasia of the hip may limit positioning of the patient on the operating table.

Gastrointestinal anomalies are observed in 36%–63% of patients.[44] Constipation is the most common gastrointestinal condition and may be very difficult to treat because of the lack of abdominal wall musculature. In a recent large cohort of living patients with prune belly syndrome, 58% of patients were diagnosed with constipation.[44] Due to the close anatomical and functional relationship between the gastrointestinal tract and the bladder, it is extremely important to treat the underlying constipation without delay. Malrotation of the midgut with a single mesentery and the occasional sequelae of volvulus and obstruction are found in approximately in 10% of patients.[44] Other gastrointestinal anomalies include intestinal obstruction, hepatoblastoma, gastroschisis, omphalocele, imperforate anus, Hirschsprung disease, and duodenal atresia.[44,46–49]

Cardiopulmonary anomalies have been described in 24%–49% of patients with prune belly.[44] Reactive airway disease and asthma affected nearly a quarter of patients, followed by pulmonary hypoplasia, patent ductus arteriosus, patent foramen ovale, atrial–ventricular septal defects, and pneumothorax.[44] The presence of cardiopulmonary comorbidities associated with the lack of abdominal wall musculature and limited movement of the diaphragm indicate that these patients require intraoperative antibiotics because of the increased risk of postoperative respiratory infections. In addition, micrognathia has been reported in patients with prune belly syndrome, which may result in difficulties with intubation.[50]

Neurologic anomalies have also been described in 20%–43% of patients, such as hearing loss, seizures, brain tumor, tethered cord, and spina bifida.[44]

Antenatal diagnosis

Antenatal diagnosis in the second trimester is the most common presentation of prune belly syndrome, with major renal tract abnormalities being diagnosed at as early as 13 weeks of gestation.[51] The sonographic features for the diagnosis of prune belly syndrome are bilateral hydroureter and hydronephrosis, a distended thick-walled bladder, and oligohydramnios. The differential diagnosis includes posterior urethral valves and megacystis microcolon intestinal hypoperistalsis (MMIH) syndrome. Differentiating between posterior urethral valve and prune belly syndrome could be difficult, as in posterior urethral valves, there is an isolated

dilatation of the posterior urethra in association with a thick-walled bladder, leading to a keyhole sign. Conversely, MMIH syndrome is more common in females (4:1) and has several features in common with prune belly syndrome, such as hydronephrosis, a large bladder, and laxity of the abdominal wall musculature.[52] In addition, in MMIH, there are abdominal distension, incomplete intestinal rotation, microcolon, and decreased or absent intestinal peristalsis.[52]

Unfortunately, fetal detection of prune belly syndrome has not led to an improved outcome.[53,54] Fetal vesicoamniotic shunts have been used in the hope of preventing renal parenchymal damage in children with enlarged bladder and upper renal tract dilatation.[55–57] However, studies have failed to document a beneficial effect of fetal intervention on subsequent renal function.

POSTNATAL ASSESSMENT AND INVESTIGATIONS

The prune belly appearance of the abdominal wall together with bilateral undescended testes allows easy diagnosis of this condition in a newborn. The initial postnatal course is dictated by the severity of comorbidities, which are present in up to 75% of the patients.[28] The most common is prematurity, with 43% of infants born preterm.[36] Perinatal mortality rates range between 10% and 25% and are related to the degree of prematurity and to the presence of severe cardiopulmonary abnormalities.[36] The classification proposed by Woodard and Zucker[29] is based on prenatal and postnatal findings and divide the patients into three groups (Table 82.1): Children in group 1 have poor renal function and will usually die in the immediate postnatal period due to pulmonary complications. An aggressive surgical approach in these children should be avoided. Group 2 children have mild impairment of renal function and may progress to renal failure. Group 3 consists of the majority of children with prune belly syndrome, who have normal renal function and dilated renal tracts. When antenatal oligohydramnios is present, pulmonary complications should be anticipated, and an immediate chest x-ray to exclude pneumothorax and pneumomediastinum is necessary. Initial

Table 82.1 Woodard and Zucker classification of prune belly syndrome

Category 1 (20%)	Category 2 (40%)	Category 3 (40%)
Oligohydramnios	Typical external features	External features mild or incomplete
Pulmonary hypoplasia or pneumothorax	Hydroureteronephrosis	Stable renal function
Renal dysplasia	Mild or unilateral renal dysplasia	Mild uropathy
Urethral obstruction or patent urachus	Risk of urosepsis	
Club foot	Risk of azotemia	

Source: Hassett S. et al., Prune belly syndrome, Pediatr Surg Int 2012;28:219–228.

creatinine measurements reflect maternal renal function, and repetitive sampling is necessary. The measurement of the lowest creatinine level after 5 days of life (nadir creatinine) has been demonstrated to be a valuable predictor of renal failure in boys with prune belly. None of the 35 patients reported by Noh et al.[54] with a nadir creatinine <0.7 mg/dL and without urosepsis had renal failure. Conversely, 12 of 13 children (92%) with a nadir creatinine greater than 0.7 mg/dL went into renal failure. Urine should be checked for any infection and antibiotic prophylaxis to prevent urinary tract infection (UTI) started. Renal ultrasound will provide information regarding echogenicity of the renal cortex, presence of cysts, parenchymal thickness, corticomedullary differentiation, renal tract dilatations, bladder volume, and postmicturition residue. A micturating cystourethrogram (MCUG) will provide information regarding vesicoureteral reflux and the rare presence of posterior urethral valve or megalourethra. However, contrast medium should be sparingly used in the presence of poor renal function and impaired glomerular filtration rates to avoid rapid rise in serum osmolality and subsequent intraventricular hemorrhage. Diuretic renal scintigraphy, most commonly a mercaptoacetyltriglycine (MAG-3) scan, is indicated to assess drainage, while a dimercaptosuccinic (DMSA) scan is effective in identifying renal scars or dysplasia by the presence of photopenic defects. However, both modalities may have limitations due to the inability to characterize obstruction in dilated and poorly functioning kidneys.[32] The real challenge in patients with prune belly syndrome lies in the ability to differentiate a dilated unobstructed urinary tract from an obstructed system that will benefit from surgical intervention. In patients with inconclusive drainage patterns on MAG-3 scan, the use of magnetic resonance urography (MRU) has been recommended as a reliable method of assessing renal drainage.[58] In addition, MRU allows sufficient resolution to detect renal dysplasia and loss of corticomedullary differentiation.[59] On MRU, patients with prune belly syndrome also show a wide range of abnormal calyceal morphology, from absent or decreased number of calyces to blunted or widely distorted branching.[32] The main limitation to the use of MRU in children is the requirement of deep sedation/general anesthetics, its high cost, and the use of gadolinium-based contrast, which limits use to those with normal renal function, due to the reported risk of nephrogenic systemic fibrosis.[60]

A videourodynamic (VUD) study is often performed for preoperative planning or following recurrent UTIs. The VUD findings invariably show a large capacious bladder (2.4 ± 1.4 times for estimated bladder capacity for age), normal bladder compliance, and a large postvoid residue (mean 63%).[27]

MANAGEMENT

The surgical management of the urinary tract should be tailored to suit individual cases. The initial recommended strategy is directed at bladder drainage and prevention of UTI, assuming that the renal function will stabilize and renoureteral anatomy will improve spontaneously.[31,61] This approach requires close follow-up, long-term urinary surveillance, and regular imaging. Urinary tract reconstruction should be considered in the presence of obstruction, stasis, and dilating vesicoureteral reflux associated with UTIs as these represent common risk factors for progressive renal damage. The rationale for a conservative approach is based on a few studies that have demonstrated no changes in preoperative and postoperative serum creatinine levels after early ureteric reconstruction consisting of ureteric tapering, reimplantation and reduction cystoplasty,[62] no long-term reduction in bladder capacity or improvement in voiding dynamics after reduction cystoplasty,[63] and no difference in urodynamic profiles between reconstructed and nonreconstructed patients with prune belly syndrome.[64] In addition, upper and lower urological reconstruction carries a complication rate of up to 40%, with revisional surgery often required, most likely due to the muscular deficiency present in these patients.[62,65] Multiple surgical procedures are often necessary in children with prune belly syndrome, with a mean of >2 procedures per year,[27] which include the following:

Circumcision

Circumcision is commonly recommended in children with abnormalities of the urinary tract who are at increased risk of UTI such as posterior urethral valves (>50%), vesicoureteric obstruction (46%), high-grade vesicoureteral reflux (30%), and prune belly syndrome.[66] Circumcision, by reducing the periurethral colonization of UTI-forming organisms in infants,[67] has a biologically proven protective effect, which persists into preschool children and adults, with a 90% reduction in risk of developing UTI.[66]

Orchidopexies

Bilateral intra-abdominal testes are one of the defining features of the syndrome. Current guidelines of the American Urological Association recommend, in the absence of spontaneous descent by 6 months, that orchidopexy should be performed in the first 18 months of life to preserve available fertility potential.[68] When urinary or abdominal wall reconstruction is considered in the first year of life, bilateral orchidopexies can be performed at the same time. In approximately two-thirds of boys, the testicular vessels are of adequate length to allow the testis down into the scrotum, while in the remaining one-third, it is necessary to divide either unilaterally or bilaterally the testicular vessels for a Fowler–Stephens orchidopexy,[46] with success of 80% and 85% for single- and two-stage orchidopexy, respectively.[69] The laparoscopic approach is the procedure of choice for the management of intra-abdominal testes when no other abdominal procedures are planned. Technical considerations during a laparoscopy in patients with prune belly are related to air leak due the lax abdominal wall. It is recommended to make smaller port incisions and use higher CO_2

flow rate and longer instruments.[70] Higher rates of testicular atrophy have been reported in children with prune belly syndrome, ranging from 3% for the two-stage orchidopexy[71] to 30% in children older than 2 who underwent a single-stage orchidopexy (82%) or a Fowler–Stephens orchidopexy (14%) at the same time as the urological reconstruction.[62]

Urinary tract reconstruction

Upper or lower urinary tract reconstruction is indicated in the presence of obstruction, inadequate bladder emptying, dilating vesicoureteral reflux associated with recurrent UTIs, or worsening hydronephrosis on ultrasound or differential renal function on nuclear scan. Two large contemporary series of patients with prune belly have described unilateral or bilateral ureteric reimplantation in 41%–85% of patients, formation of appendicovesicostomy in 9%–35%, reduction cystoplasty/resection of bladder dome and urachal remnant in 9%–89%, formation of vesicostomy in 11%, and urethral surgery (dilatation or urethrotomy) in 13%. Less frequently, other urological procedures may be required such as pyeloplasty, nephrectomy, ureteroureteroanastomosis, nephrostomy, and tumor resection.[27,46]

Abdominoplasty

Several techniques have been described over the years for the abdominal wall reconstruction of patients with prune belly syndrome. In 1981, Randolph et al.[25] described the only technique that utilizes a U-shaped incision between the tips of the 12 ribs and advancement of the upper abdominal layers toward the groin and pubis. The techniques described by Ehrlich in 1986, Monfort in 1991, Furness et al. in 1998, and Lesavoy in 2012 have in common a medial advancement of the lateral musculofascial layers toward the midline in a double-breasted fashion using an intraperitoneal (Ehrlich, Monfort, Lesavoy) or extraperitoneal (Furness et al.) approach.[36,72] Other differences among these techniques lie in the elliptical excision of the excessive skin and in the incision of the musculoaponeurotic fascia (MAF; midline or lateral). An innovative technique has been recently described by Denes et al.,[65] which includes an elliptical xyphopubic incision, excision of the excessive skin and subcutaneous tissue, and preservation of the umbilicus as an island attached to the MAF. A single lateral elliptical incision of the MAF is made in the most lax side of the fascia, with creation of a wider or inner flap containing the umbilicus and a shorter or outer flap. The wider inner flap is sutured over to the parietal peritoneum of the shorter flap, while the shorter outer flap is sutured over the inner to the opposite side, therefore creating a double-breasted reinforcement of the anterior abdominal wall. The umbilicus is exposed through the buttonhole incision of the outer flap and fixed to the flap.[72] This technique has a good cosmetic and functional result, requires only one incision of the MAF, and allows access to the abdominal cavity with excellent exposure of the viscera. The benefits of abdominal wall reconstruction are well established, with increased patient self-esteem;[73] improvements in continence, sensation, and urinary flow; improved postvoid residuals; and reduction in defecation time.[74] These improvements are not correlated to the genitourinary reconstruction, and the authors speculate that they may be secondary to the increased intra-abdominal pressure of the Valsalva maneuver in accordance with the Pascal principle (pressure = force/area).[74] The timing of the abdominoplasty is still a matter of debate among pediatric urologists, with some authors recommending early[46] abdominoplasty and some later.[27] It is our practice to offer abdominoplasty before starting school, between 3 and 4 years of age.

LONG-TERM OUTCOME

Long-term follow-up studies have shown that adequate bladder emptying is observed in 48%–72% of patients. In the remaining children, the bladder is managed through clean intermittent catheterization, approximately one-third through the urethra and two-thirds through a Mitrofanoff channel.[27,46] Only a minority of patients will require either Crede or Valsalva maneuvers to ensure bladder emptying.[46] Between 11% and 39% of the long-term survivors will develop chronic renal failure as a result of renal dysplasia, recurrent pyelonephritis, or obstructive nephropathy, with approximately half of them undergoing renal transplantation.[27,46] However, good bladder emptying must be achieved prior to transplantation to avoid significant risk of infection in the presence of immunosuppressant therapy.

REFERENCES

1. Frohlich F. Der Mangel der Muskon, Insbesondere der Seitenbauchmuskeln. Dissertation. Wurzburg; C.A. Zurn, 1839.
2. Parker RW. Case of an infant in whom some of the abdominal muscles were absent. *Trans Clin Soc Lond Wurzburg* 1895; 28: 201.
3. Osler W. Congenital absence of the abdominal musculature, with distended and hypertrophied urinary bladder. *Bull Johns Hopkins Hosp* 1901; 12: 331.
4. Eagle JF, Barrett GS. Congenital deficiency of abdominal musculature with associated genitourinary abnormalities. A syndrome: Report of nine cases. *Pediatrics* 1950; 6: 726.
5. Routh JC, Huang L, Retik AB. Contemporary epidemiology and characterization of newborn males with Prune Belly syndrome. *Urology* 2010; 76: 44–8.
6. Druschel CM. A descriptive study of prune-belly in New York state, 1983 to 1989. *Arch Pediatr Adolesc Med* 1995; 149: 70–6.
7. Giuliani S, Vendryes C, Malhotra A et al. Prune belly syndrome associated with cloacal anomaly, patent urachal remnant, and omphalocele in a female infant. *J Pediatr Surg* 2010; 45: E39–42.

8. Reinberg Y, Shapiro E, Manivel C et al. Prune belly syndrome in females: A triad of abdominal musculature deficiency and anomalies of the urinary and genital system. *J Pediatr* 1991; 118: 395–8.

9. Wheatley JM, Stephens FD, Hutson JM. Prune-belly syndrome: Ongoing controversies regarding pathogenesis and management. *Semin Pediatr Surg* 1996; 5(2): 95–106.

10. Popek EJ, Tyson RW, Miller GJ et al. Prostate development in prune belly syndrome (PBS) and posterior urethral valves (PUV): Etiology of PBS—Lower urinary tract obstruction or primary mesenchymal defect? *Pediatr Pathol* 1991; 11: 1–29.

11. Pagon RA, Smith DW, Shepard TH. Urethral obstruction malformation complex: A cause of abdominal muscle deficiency and the "prune belly". *J Pediatr* 1979; 94: 900–6.

12. Straub E, Spranger J. Etiology and pathogenesis of prune belly syndrome. *Kidney Int* 1981; 20: 695–9.

13. Stephens FD, Gupta D. Pathogenesis of the prune-belly syndrome. *J Urol* 1994; 152: 2328–31.

14. Amacker EA, Grass FS, Hickey DE et al. An association of prune belly anomaly with trisomy 21. *Am J Med Genet* 1986; 23: 919–23.

15. Beckmann H, Rehder H, Rauskolb R. Prune belly sequence McKeown, associated with trisomy 13. *Am J Med Genet* 1984; 19: 603–4.

16. McKeown CM, Donnai D. Prune belly in trisomy 13. *Prenat Diagn* 1986; 6: 379–81.

17. Frydmann H, Magenis RE, Mohands TK et al. Chromosome abnormalities in infants with prune belly anomaly: Associated with trisomy 18. *Am J Med Genet* 1983; 15: 145–8.

18. Hoagland MH, Frank KA, Hutchins GM. Prune belly syndrome with prostatic hypoplasia, bladder wall rupture, and massive ascites in a foetus with trisomy 18. *Arch Pathol Lab Med* 1988; 112: 1126–8.

19. Ramasamy R, Haviland M, Woodard JR, Barone JG. Patterns of inheritance in familial prune belly syndrome. *Urology* 2005; 65(6): 1227.

20. Granberg CF, Harrison SM, Dajusta D et al. Genetic basis of prune belly syndrome: Screening for HNF1β gene. *J Urol* 2012; 187: 272–8.

21. Bingham C, Hattersley AT. Renal cysts and diabetes syndrome resulting from mutations in hepatocyte nuclear factor-1 beta. *Nephrol Dial Transplant* 2004; 19: 2703.

22. Housden LG. Congenital deficiency of the abdominal muscles. *Arch Dis Child* 1934; 9: 219.

23. Lattimer JK. Congenital deficiency of the abdominal musculature and associated genito-urinary anomalies. A report of 22 cases. *J Urol* 1958; 79: 343.

24. Silverman FN, Huang N. Congenital absence of the abdominal muscles, associated with malformation of the genitourinary and alimentary tracts. *Arch Dis Child* 1950; 80: 91.

25. Randolph J, Cavett C, Eng G. Abdominal wall reconstruction in the prune belly syndrome. *J Pediatr Surg* 1981; 16: 960.

26. Mininberg DT, Montoya F, Okada K. Subcellular muscle studies in prune belly syndrome. *J Urol* 1973; 109: 524.

27. Seidel NE, Arlen AM, Smith EA et al. Clinical manifestations and management of prune-belly syndrome in a large contemporary pediatric population. *Urology* 2015; 85: 211–5.

28. Caldamone AA, Woodard JR. Prune-belly syndrome. In: Gearhart JP, Rink RC, Mouriquand PDE (eds). *Pediatric*. Philadelphia: Saunders, Elsevier, 2010: 425–36.

29. Woodard JR, Zucker I. Current management of the dilated urinary tract in prune belly syndrome. *Urol Clin N Am* 1990; 17: 407–18.

30. Kroovand RL, Al-Ansary RM, Perlmutter AD. Urethral and genital malformations in1prune belly syndrome. *J Urol* 1982; 127: 94.

31. Woodhouse CRJ, Ransly PG, Williams DJ. Prune belly syndrome report of 47 cases. *Arch Dis Child* 1982; 57: 856.

32. Garcia-Roig ML, Grattan-Smith JD, Arlen AM et al. Detailed evaluation of the upper urinary tract in patients with prune belly syndrome using magnetic resonance urography. *J Pediatr Urol* 2015; 1.e1–e7.

33. Palmer JM, Tessluk H. Ureteral pathology in the prune belly syndrome. *J Urol* 1974; 111: 701.

34. Ehrlich RM, Brown WJ. Ultrastructural anatomic obstructions of the ureter in the prune belly syndrome. *Birth Defects* 1977; 13: 101.

35. Wigger JH, Blance WA. The prune belly syndrome. *Path Ann* 1977; (Part I)12: 17.

36. Hassett S, Smith GHH, Holland AJA. Prune belly syndrome. *Pediatr Surg Int* 2012; 28: 219–28.

37. Costa WS, Sampaio FJB, Favorito LA et al. Testicular migration: Remodeling of connective tissue and muscle cells in human gubernaculum testis. *J Urol* 2002; 167: 2171.

38. Costa SF, Costa WS, Sampaio FJB et al. Structural study of gubernaculum testis in fetuses with prune belly syndrome. *J Urol* 2015; 193: 1830–6.

39. Orvis BR, Bottles K, Kogan BA. Testicular histology in fetuses with the prune belly syndrome and posterior urethral valves. *J Urol* 1988; 139: 335.

40. Massad CA, Cohen MB, Kogan BA et al. Morphology and histochemistry of infant testes in the prune belly syndrome. *J Urol* 1991; 146: 1598–600.

41. Humphrey PA, Shuch B. Seminoma in cryptorchid testis in prune belly syndrome. *J Urol* 2015: 194: 799–800.

42. Sayze R, Stephen R, Chonko AM. Prune belly syndrome and retro-peritoneal germ cell tumour. *Am J Med* 1986; 81: 895.

43. Parra RO, Cummings JM, Palmar DC. Testicular seminoma in a long term survivor of the prune belly syndrome. *Eur Urol* 1991; 19: 79–80.

44. Grimsby GM, Harrison SM, Granberg CF et al. Impact and frequency of extra-genitourinary manifestations of prune belly syndrome. *J Pediatr Urol* 2015; 11: 280.e1–e6.

45. Brinker MR, Palutsis RS, Sarwark JF. The orthopedic manifestations of prune belly syndrome (Eagle–Barrett) syndrome. *J Bone Joint Surg* 1995; 77: 251–7.

46. Lopes RI, Tavares A, Srougi M et al. 27 years of experience with the comprehensive surgical treatment of prune belly syndrome. *J Pediatr Urol* 2015; 11: 276.e1–e7.

47. Walker J, Prokurat AI, Irving IM. Prune belly syndrome associated with exomphalos and anorectal agenesis. *J Pediatr* 1987; 22: 215–7.

48. Cawthern TH, Bottene CA, Grant D. Prune belly syndrome associated with Hirschsprung's disease. *Am J Dis Child* 1979; 133: 65.

49. Willert J, Cohen H, Yu YT. Association of prune belly syndrome with gastroschisis. *Am J Dis Child* 1978; 132: 526.

50. Baris S, Karakaya D, Ustun E et al. Complicated airway management in a child with prune-belly syndrome. *Pediatr Anaesth* 2001; 11: 501–4.

51. Papantoniou N, Papoutsis D, Daskalakis G et al. Prenatal diagnosis of prune belly syndrome at 13 weeks gestation: Case report and review of literature. *J Maternal Fetal Neonat Med* 2010; 23: 1263–7.

52. Granata C, Puri P. Megacystis–microcolon–intestinal hypoperistalsis syndrome. *J Pediatr Gastroenterol Nutr* 1997; 25: 12–9.

53. Reinberg Y, Manivel JC, Pettinato G et al. Development of renal failure in children with the prune belly syndrome. *J Urol* 1991; 145: 1017–9.

54. Noh PH, Cooper CS, Winkler AC et al. Prognostic factors for long-term renal function in boys with the prune-belly syndrome. *J Urol* 1999; 162(4): 1399–401.

55. Leeners B, Sauer I, Schefels J et al. Prune-belly syndrome: Therapeutic options including in utero placement of a vesicoamniotic shunt. *J Clin Ultrasound* 2000; 28(9): 500–7.

56. Perez-Brayfield MR, Gatti J, Berkman S et al. In utero intervention in a patient with prune-belly syndrome and severe urethral hypoplasia. *Urology* 2001; 1178.

57. Galati V, Bason JH, Confer SD et al. A favourable outcome following 32 vesicocentesis and amnioinfusion procedure in a fetus with sever prune belly syndrome. *J Pediatr Urol* 2008; 4: 170–2.

58. Grattan-Smith JD, Little SB, Jones RA. MR urography evaluation of obstructive uropathy. *Pediatr Radiol* 2008; 38 (Suppl.1): S49–69.

59. McMann LP, Kirsch AJ, Scherz HC et al. Magnetic resonance urography in the evaluation of prenatally diagnosed hydronephrosis and renal dysgenesis. *J Urol* 2006; 176: 1786–92.

60. Altun E, Martin DR, Wertman R et al. Nephrogenic systemic fibrosis: Change in incidence following a switch in gadolinium agents and adoption of a gadolinium policy-report from two U.S. universities. *Radiology* 2009; 253: 689–96.

61. Tank ES, McCoy G. Limited surgical intervention in the prune belly syndrome. *J.Pediatr Surg* 1983; 18: 688–91.

62. Fallat ME, Skoog SJ, Belman AB et al. The prune belly syndrome: A comprehensive approach to management. *J Urol* 1989; 142: 802–5.

63. Bukonsky TP, Perlmutter AD. Reduction cystoplasty in the prune belly syndrome: A long term follow up. *J Urol* 1994; 152: 2113–6.

64. Kinahan TJ, Churchill BM, McLorie GA et al. The efficiency of bladder emptying in the prune belly syndrome. *J Urol* 1992; 148: 600–3.

65. Denes FT, Arap MA, Giron AM et al. Comprehensive surgical treatment of prune belly syndrome: 17 years experience with 32 patients. *Urology* 2004; 64: 789–94.

66. Bader M, McCarthy L. What is the efficacy of circumcision in boys with complex urinary tract abnormalities? *Pediatr Nephrol* 2013; 28: 2267–72.

67. Wiswell TE, Miller GM, Gelston HM et al. Effect of circumcision status on periurethral bacterial flora during the first year of life. *J Pediatr* 1988; 113: 442–6.

68. Kolon TF, Herndon CDA, Baker L et al. Evaluation and treatment of cryptorchidism: AUA guideline. *J Urol* 2014; 192: 337–45.

69. Elyas R, Guerra LA, Pike J et al. Is staging beneficial for Fowler Stephens orchidopexy? A systematic review. *J Urol* 2010; 183: 2012–8.

70. Philip J, Mullassery D, Craigie RJ et al. Laparoscopic orchidopexy in boys with prune syndrome outcome and technical considerations. *J Endourol* 2011; 25: 1115–7.

71. Patil KK, Duffy PG, Woodhouse CR et al. Long term outcome of Fowler Stephens orchidopexy in boys with prune belly syndrome. *J Urol* 2004; 171: 1666–9.

72. Dénes FT, Lopes RI, Oliveira LM et al. Modified abdominoplasty for patients with the prune belly syndrome. *Urology* 2014; 83: 451–4.

73. Arlen AM, Kirsch SS, Seidel NE et al. Health-related quality of life in children with prune belly syndrome and their caregivers. *Urology* 2016; 87: 224–7.

74. Smith CA, Smith EA, Parrott TS et al. Voiding function in patients with prune belly syndrome after Monfort abdominoplasty. *J Urol* 1998; 159: 1675–9.

83

Conjoined twins

JUAN A. TOVAR AND LEOPOLDO MARTINEZ

INTRODUCTION

Genetically identical individuals joined by a part of their anatomy and often sharing one or more organs are known as *conjoined twins*. Total prevalence of this event has been estimated at 1.47 per 100,000 live births.[1] Forty percent of all are stillborn, and a further 30% die on the first day of life. Only 18% of all conjoined twins survive longer than 24 h, and they represent one of the more difficult challenges of pediatric surgery.[2,3]

Mythologic creatures like two-faced Jano or multiple-headed Hydra were probably inspired by observation of conjoined twins.[4] Although representations of conjoined twins from ancient cultures were relatively frequent, they became popular after the original Siamese twins Chang and Eng Bunker were sent to the United States in the nineteenth century for exhibition in a circus[5]; the term *Siamese twins* was coined as a reference to them.[6] The complexity of the technical problems involved in separations of conjoined twins explains why the first attempts are relatively recent (seventeenth century).[7]

ETIOLOGY

Conjoined twinning is due to incomplete division of a primitive embryonal disk destined to produce identical twins.[1,8] These are, of course, monozygotic, monochorionic, and isosexual, and share the same genome and fingerprints.[9,10] The causes for this incomplete division are unknown, but interestingly, two-thirds of the cases are females. Two opposing theories have been suggested to explain these phenomena. Some authors support a *fusion* process because, with the exception of parapagus, all types of conjoined twins can be explained by the fusion of two separated embryos.[1,11] This fusion theory could explain some ancient experiments in amphibians, and a few modern molecular genetic observations suggest that fusion of two originally separated embryos may be the explanation for some rare cases in which there is sex discordance.[12-14]

There are supporters of a *fission* theory, claiming that conjoined twins are the result of an incomplete split of the embryonic axis.[8,15] Spencer pointed out in her monography[16] that the twins are always joined by central parts of their anatomies and that they are always homologous in the sense that they never have the head or the lower limbs on opposite sides. This seems to confirm that the mechanism is a missed cleavage of the primitive embryonal disk along the longitudinal axis.

CLASSIFICATION

The location, extent and nature of the bridge between both twins vary widely, and this complicates description of the anatomy of each set. Several classifications attempt at simplifying description. Conjoined twins are always of the same sex and are joined homologously, i.e., chest to chest, abdomen to abdomen, pelvis to pelvis.[17] They can be divided into ventrally and dorsally joined and subdivided according to the level of fusion.[16,18] We divide them by taking into account their asymmetric or symmetric nature and the level of the fusion, followed by the suffix -*pagus*.

Asymmetric twins include *fetus in fetu, acardius acephalus*, and *heteropagus* parasitic twins. The adscription of the first variety of organoid teratomata to the family of conjoined twins is only acceptable when they are "organoid" and contain a more or less rudimentary spine.[19] *Acardius acephalus* is a variety of parasitic twin devoid of heart and head that is connected by marginal placental vessels with the healthy twin (the *autositus*), who is in charge of circulation and nutrition of both.[20] *Heteropagus* twins are usually attached to the abdominal wall of an anatomically normal *autositus* twin, without or with exomphalus, as organoid parasitic masses containing various organs and limbs unable to sustain independent circulation by themselves.[21,22]

Symmetric conjoined twins may be joined by the head (*craniopagus*), the thorax (*thoracopagus*), the abdomen (*omphalopagus*), the spine (*rachiopagus*), or the caudal pole (*ischiopagus* and *pygopagus*). Occasionally, they are laterally fused along the body axis (*parapagus*).[23-25]

CLINICAL PRESENTATION

Nowadays, most conjoined twins are prenatally diagnosed by ultrasound (US) in advanced countries, preventing serious obstetric problems. Except in thoracopagus with common heart and in asymmetric twins, both fetal heart tones can be identified like in regular twins. The heads and the limbs of conjoined twins are on the same side (homologous), in contrast with regular twins, which are usually arranged in opposite directions. This allows fetal ultrasonographic diagnosis that leads to detailed US and/or magnetic resonance imaging (MRI) studies aimed at defining the anatomy of the fusion and the chances of separation.[25–27] MRI has been used more commonly in recent years to confirm the diagnosis and to define the nature of joining. Ultrafast T2 sequences eliminate the need for maternal sedation and allow precise anatomical assessment.[25] Accurate prenatal diagnosis is critical because it allows optimizing the outcome of the twins. The parents should be referred to a fetal center, and they are entitled to receive counseling by a multidisciplinary team.[2] Craniopagus and those with a sole cardiac mass or complex cardiac connections have the worst prognosis. Usually, parents are offered termination of pregnancy, an option that is chosen by 50%–70% of them when available.[28]

There are increasing risks of preterm birth, so in most cases, labor will be expected around 35 weeks of gestation. Although vaginal delivery has been reported, it is usually associated with obstetric trauma: long bone fractures, rupture of exomphalos, etc.[29–31] Most sets of twins are delivered by Cesarean section and can be taken care of by interdisciplinary teams from the beginning. The staff present at birth should be divided into two teams, one for each baby. Each person should know his or her place and role. Transfer and resuscitation of the twins require a specially designed platform than allows access from all sides.[2]

The anatomy varies widely according to the modality of joining. Thoracopagi with common hearts have almost constantly severe cardiovascular and arterial anomalies that produce early symptoms and may be rapidly lethal.[32,33] The most frequent forms, omphalopagi and thoracopagi, often have an omphalocele membrane as a part of the joining bridge (Figures 83.1 and 83.2). The livers are often fused, and the intestines are usually connected or shared. The bladder may be common and sometimes opens at the lower part of the bridge as an exstrophy (Figure 83.3). In cases joined by the rump (Figures 83.4 and 83.5), the anatomical varieties in terms of gastrointestinal (g.i.) and urogenital openings are multiple.

Serious malformations or trauma suffered by only one of the twins may create difficult clinical situations because crossed circulation creates a single internal environment, which is hard to manipulate: the healthier twin can compensate in part for the problems of the diseased one, but the latter may expose the former to disbalances, toxins, or medications.[34]

DIAGNOSIS

A comprehensive understanding of the anatomy of the organs and the distribution of their functions is necessary for planning viable separation strategies. The imaging investigation should be as extensive as possible. It aims to delineate anatomy, to assess the choice of separation, and finally, to counsel

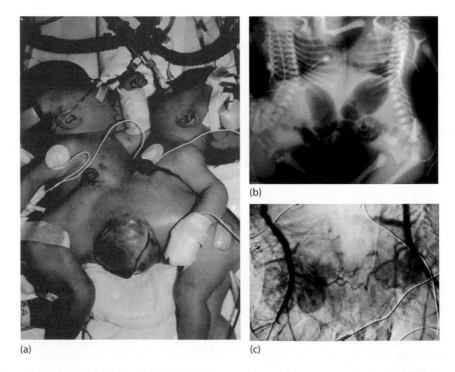

(a)

(b)

(c)

Figure 83.1 **(a)** Set of omphalopagus twins. Severe brain hemorrhage in twin on the right after vaginal delivery prompted neonatal separation. Only the twin on the left survived. Neonatal investigation demonstrated **(b)** two separated hearts and **(c)** an abdominal arterial communication between the twins.

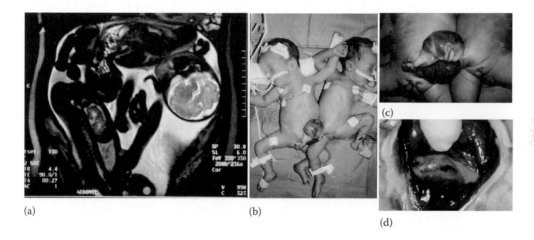

Figure 83.2 Two sets of thoracopagus twins with common heart. **(a)** Separation was undertaken only in the first set because only a narrow atrial bridge joined them; unfortunately, the twins did not survive. **(b)** Separation was considered impossible in the second set; they shared a common heart, had a gross arterial communication at abdominal level, and **(c)** the twin on the right had an hypoplastic aorta.

Figure 83.3 **(a)** Omphalopagus twins with incomplete cloacal exstrophy that was prenatally diagnosed. **(b, c)** The single bladder opened under the exomphalos. **(d)** A single colonic opening was visible in the middle of the bladder plate. Both had anorectal agenesis with one single urogenital canal and double uteruses and vaginas. Separation involved division of the colon with colostomies, and bladder closure. Later on, sagittal anorectoplasty with colonic and vaginal pull-through was performed.

parents about prognosis.[35] Plain x-rays and g.i. or urogenital tract contrast studies may depict the points of junction and other features of the corresponding organs, but due to the atypical anatomy,[36] incomplete understanding leads to unexpected surprises. Ultrasonography helps at every diagnostic step.[27,37] Angiography, which was widely used in the past for depicting the nature of the blood supply of the shared organs (Figure 83.1),[38] is being replaced by computed tomography (CT) or magnetic resonance (MR) angiography, which are now considered the best ways of depicting the vascular arrangement (Figure 85.2).[35] MRI better depicts the fused neural and meningeal tissues in craniopagus, rachiopagus, ischiopagus, pygopagus, and parapagus.[39] Both CT and MR are crucial for imaging the anatomy of conjoined hearts.[40] Helical CT reconstruction of the bony junctions may help in preparing strategies of skeletal separation (Figures 83.4 and 83.5).[41] Nuclear imaging may help to define the functional anatomy of the liver, kidney, and other organs.[42]

Hematologic and biochemical studies are often misleading due to the situation of cross-circulation. When the vascular channels are large, *parabiosis* is complete, but when only minor territories are in connection, both twins maintain some internal environmental differences that can be relevant in cases in which blood tests are necessary for diagnosis. Other tests, like electrocardiogram (ECG), are challenging when the hearts are connected.[43] Metabolic rate may show considerable differences between twins upon calorimetry.[44]

TREATMENT

Preoperative ethical issues

The principles that regulate the medical profession are particularly difficult to respect in conjoined twins, and serious ethical dilemmas are to be expected[26,45,46]:

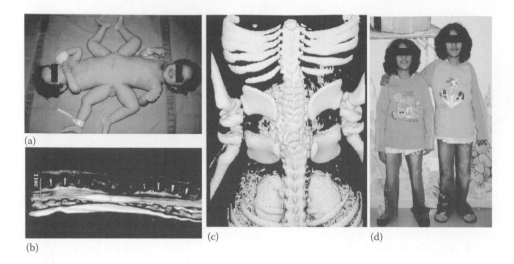

Figure 83.4 **(a)** Ischiopagus tetrapus (four legs) twins. **(b, c)** The spines and the spinal cords were joined at the caudal end as shown by helicoidal CT reconstruction. During separation, the spines were divided, the meningeal sacs were reconstructed, a quadruple iliac osteotomy was performed for joining both pubic bones in each twin, the urogenital system was reconstructed, and colostomies were fashioned. **(d)** Patients at the age of 12: they deambulate normally and enjoy relatively normal lives with permanent colostomies and intermittent bladder catheterization.

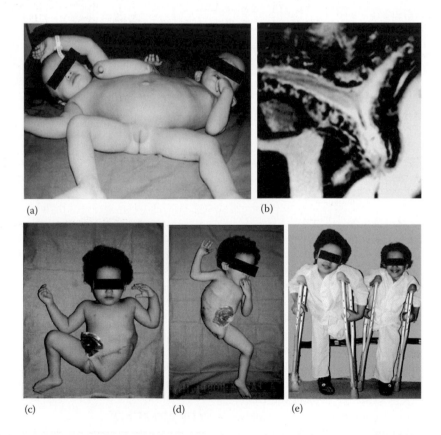

Figure 83.5 **(a)** Caudal parapagus tripus twins with an extra thoracic limb irrigated from the abdominal aorta of the twin on the left. **(b)** There was a single pelvis with two lower limbs and two spines with communicating spinal canals and joined cords. Separation involved two surgical steps. First, the spinal cords and meningeal sacs were separated and subcutaneous expanders were inserted. Secondly, the sacrum and the g.i. and g.u. tracts were divided, and the parietal defects were closed. In twin A, the skin and muscle of the additional limb were used as a vascularized flap. In twin B, a synthetic mesh was used for this purpose. Colostomies were fashioned. **(c, d, e)** Both twins are able to deambulate with braces.

The principle of *autonomy* (the decisions of the patient should be respected) is usually exerted by proxy by the parents in children, and this may be a source of conflicts among them or with doctors or the courts if unanimous decisions are not agreed upon.[47]

The principle of *justice* (similar chances for both patients) is obviously at risk when it comes to separation that may involve mutilation or sharing of organs.

The principles of *beneficiency* and *nonmaleficiency* (the benefit of the patients should be sought and no harm should be inflicted on them), which are considered as the ethical backbone of the medical decision-making process, are also difficult to apply if separation is necessary for the survival of only one twin, if distribution of organs is uneven, and if separation involves, as is usually the case, loss of some functions that might be preserved without separation.

When separation of conjoined twins is considered, the patients are usually too young to decide by themselves, the parents are heavily influenced by information delivered by doctors, and the team involved is usually so large and often ethically discordant that keeping a unified line of decision becomes difficult. Acknowledgement of a strong moral leadership after open discussion of every issue is required before providing to the parents information about the chances and the consequences of separation. In case of serious discrepancies among all participants in the process of decision, the courts might be involved.[48,49]

Furthermore, new difficulties may arise due to interference of the media, which is difficult to avoid in cases in which so many people are involved. The twins and their family should be protected from these agents, and if possible, the entire process of decision making and even the separation should be kept private.

Preoperative meetings

When separation has been decided, one or more meetings with scrub nurses, nurses, anesthesiologists, and surgeons of the required specialties (general pediatric, orthopedic, plastic, urologic, neurologic, and cardiovascular surgery) should be scheduled.[50] Technical aspects should be discussed, and the operation itself should be rehearsed because installation of the set of twins on the table, skin prep and draping, and transport of one twin with the corresponding anesthetic equipment to another table for reconstruction after separation should be carried out according to a previously established protocol. The expected order and extent of the participation of each specialist team in the separation should be scheduled as well. Everybody has to be clear on his/her exact role. The surgeon in charge of the direction of the operation acts as an orchestral conductor, and his/her coordinating activity extends well beyond the end of the separation itself. It should be kept in mind that, despite extensive previous investigation, some abnormalities will be encountered unexpectedly during operation.[51,52]

Separation

Anesthesia is a serious challenge not only because of the obvious anatomical difficulties for intubation, insertion of lines, and invasive monitoring but mainly because of the previously mentioned situation of *parabiosis* in which one single internal environment is shared to variable extents by the twins.[53] Anesthetic procedures require meticulous planning, simulation of different scenarios, and a close team work.[54] In most cases, twins require anesthesia for both diagnostic and surgical procedures prior to separation, and this should allow gaining experience before the separation.[53] Anesthesiologists should be especially aware of the difficulties of airway management, keeping intravascular volume, control of temperature, and unusual positioning of the twins. The drugs administered to one pass on into the other one, and biochemical and gas monitoring may be confusing.[55-57]

Asymmetric conjoined twins represent, in general, surgical challenges that are not unlike other ones met in this specialty. The *acardius acephalus* parasitic twin is inviable and dies upon clamping the umbilical cord of the host (autositus) twin. The *fetus in fetu* is treated as a tumor, and *heteropagus* asymmetric parasitic twins are removed with attention to preserving as much tissue as possible in order to respect the organs and allow wall reconstruction of the host.

If possible, separation should be postponed several months to allow the best possible imaging and a careful planning of surgery. Neonatal or early separation is only indicated for life-threatening reasons (for instance, one twin may be very ill or develop intestinal obstruction).[52,58,59] At this age, mortality is higher than when most anatomical and functional features of the set have been ascertained and appropriate planning has been completed. However, approximately one-third of conjoined twins require emergency procedures at birth.[52,60,61]

The separation of *craniopagus* may be extremely difficult or even impossible given the complexity of the neural, arterial, and venous connections involved. Modern imaging and sophisticated neurophysiologic monitoring are particularly useful in these cases. The final amount and nature of the brain tissue and the vascular network shared by the twins set the limits for separation.[8,62-65]

Separation of *omphalopagus* twins involves variable difficulties depending on the extent of organ sharing. These twins have, more often, fused livers and g.i. tracts. A small liver bridge without major vascular connections is relatively easy to take down, but a large mass of anatomically atypical liver with wide arterial, venous, and biliary connections[51,66,67] may be a serious undertaking. Perioperative ultrasonography and parenchyma-dividing devices used for liver resection are very useful for this purpose. The most common form of g.i. tract connection involves fusion of the small bowel from the upper jejunum down and divergence near the distal ileum. Separation consists, in most cases, of allocating half the available gut to each twin.

Additional problems may be met when atresia of one of the tracts or a common cystic dilatation of the mid bowel is present.[23,24,26,68,69]

Thoracopagus twins without connected hearts are separable, in contrast with those with a common myocardium. Only a few of them are amenable to surgery under cardiopulmonary bypass. In addition, these twins often have cardiovascular defects that may further complicate or preclude the separation. The aorta and the pulmonary arteries may be hypoplastic, and thick collaterals often largely connect the infradiaphragmatic aortas. Of those who cannot be separated, most die of the associated heart dysfunctions in the first months or years of life.[32,70]

Rachiopagus, *ischiopagus*, *pygopagus*, and *parapagus* twins share, to different extents, parts of the spine, central nervous system, and g.i. and genitourinary (g.u.) tracts, and they may represent formidable challenges. The separation of the bony parts requires highly skilled orthopedic surgeons. In some cases, the reconstruction of the pelvic rim requires bilateral iliac osteotomies and pubic fixation. In some cases, even refashioning a bony pelvis is impossible, and the subsequent prosthetic treatment is difficult.[71,72] The spine often has some malformations at other levels, and scoliosis has to be taken into account during follow-up.[73–75]

Neurosurgical separation may involve dividing a common spinal cord with reconstruction of the dural sacs on each side.[72,76] Since fusion of neural tissue is usually distal, the motor and sensitive effects tend to be limited.

The partition of a shared lower g.i. tract between both twins entails the loss of continence for one or both of them. In frontally joined twins, there is usually ileal confluence near the ileocecal valve and a single colon. The functional reconstruction of the pelvic organs is therefore rarely possible. Seldom, the rectal function can be preserved in one twin, but more often, this is impossible, and ostomies have to be fashioned at some stage. All refinements of advanced bowel management are necessary to obtain subsequent adaptation of these patients to a more or less normal life.[71,77]

The same can be said about distributing the urogenital tract structures between the twins. Keeping a bladder and urethra for one twin is rarely possible in most frontally united sets. Again, all refinements of reconstructive urology, bladder augmentation, clean intermittent catheterization, and continent urinary diversion may help to readapt these patients.[78–81] The native genital tract can be reconstructed if duplicated, but sometimes, vaginal replacement is necessary.

One of the major technical problems posed by separation of conjoined twins is the coverage of the huge parietal defects left. When only one survives, part of the wall of the other one can be used to bridge the defects, but in other cases, the skin can be expanded with subcutaneous expanders prior to separation,[82–84] and various flaps or biologic[85] or synthetic materials[86,87] may be necessary. Some authors, however, did not find any need for them to achieve a successful closure of large defects.[50,51] Since they have to be inserted in contaminated operative fields, the risks of bacterial colonization and infection are increased.

COMPLICATIONS

The nature of these risky operations involves a large number and variety of possible complications. Peroperative hemorrhage and damage to vital structures are always possible due to the often atypical anatomy. Bone division or meningeal membrane opening simultaneous to g.i. or g.u. procedures increases the risk of serious infection. Wound closure avoiding compartment syndrome may necessitate synthetic materials that are also exposed to contamination. Wound disruption and infection are therefore not rare. Finally, a wide range of complications not unlike those seen after other major operations may occur: internal hemorrhage, abscesses, vascular thrombosis, or postoperative intussusception, among others, are possible.

EARLY AND LONG-TERM RESULTS

Overall mortality in conjoined twinning is high. When diagnosis is made during early pregnancy, interruption of gestation is common practice in developed countries particularly for the forms with bad prognosis.[2,28,88,89] Fetal mortalities or stillbirths are also frequent. Obstetric mortality or severe birth trauma remains a real risk when prenatal diagnosis was missed, and this happens more often in undeveloped countries in which pregnancies are not monitored.[90] Up to 65% of the twins have associated anomalies involving various systems, the most common being cardiac defects, intestinal atresia, omphalocele, anorectal malformation, and spinal cord anomalies, that can cause demise in the first hours or days of life.[8,25] Thoracopagus twins with a common heart rarely survive because most have severe malformations. Of those sets in which separation is attempted, only a few individual twins survive.[33,91,92] However, thoracopagus without a shared heart can be successfully separated.

Most omphalopagus twins can be separated and survive if no obstetric trauma or severe associated malformation is present. In all other forms of conjoined twinning, a high proportion of the twins can be separated and survive, although with more or less extensive deficits that require follow-up for life and often additional operations.

In the long term, separation of conjoined twins rarely produces independent individuals without sequelae. Some cases of asymmetrical twins and onphalopagi may survive separation facing a normal life. Most other cases keep orthopedic or neurologic sequelae or have fecal and urinary continence problems that become predominant problems with the passage of time. Orthopedic and motor deficits may require prolonged rehabilitation and/or prosthetic appliances.[76,93] Permanent enterostomies are not rare, and the most sophisticated procedures for obtaining urinary continence or dryness are necessary.[23,75,80,81,94,95]

It is particularly discouraging that these pregnancies are often terminated in advanced medical and social environments able to provide lifelong assistance for rehabilitation and social integration, whereas twins from less privileged countries that are diagnosed at term and eventually separated lack all the necessary facilities. Reports on the long-term results usually describe sets of twins doing well with optimal social and psychological adjustments, although many of them require lifelong medical follow-up and care due to severe disabilities.[72,75,80]

Separation of conjoined twins is a major test for the quality of pediatric surgical care. Only institutions with highly sophisticated pediatric surgical specialties can undertake these operations with a reasonable chance of success. A careful study of the lessons learned from the experience of these selected centers is mandatory before any attempt at separation is undertaken.

REFERENCES

1. Mutchinick OM, Luna-Munoz L, Amar E, Bakker MK, Clementi M, Cocchi G, da Graca Dutra M, Feldkamp ML, Landau D, Leoncini E, Li Z, Lowry B, Marengo LK, Martinez-Frias ML, Mastroiacovo P, Metneki J, Morgan M, Pierini A, Rissman A, Ritvanen A, Scarano G, Siffel C, Szabova E, Arteaga-Vazquez J. Conjoined twins: A worldwide collaborative epidemiological study of the International Clearinghouse for Birth Defects Surveillance and Research. *Am J Med Genet C Semin Med Genet* 2011; 157C: 274–87.

2. O'Brien P, Nugent M, Khalil A. Prenatal diagnosis and obstetric management. *Semin Pediatr Surg* 2015; 24: 203–6.

3. Tannuri AC, Batatinha JA, Velhote MC and Tannuri U. Conjoined twins: Twenty years' experience at a reference center in Brazil. *Clinics (Sao Paulo)* 2013; 68: 371–7.

4. Dasen V. [Siamese twins in classical Antiquity: From myth to fair phenomenon]. *Rev Prat* 2002; 52: 9–12.

5. Endres L, Wilkins I. Epidemiology and biology of multiple gestations. *Clin Perinatol* 2005; 32: 301–14, v.

6. Mitchell S. Exhibiting monstrosity: Chang and Eng, the 'original' Siamese twins. *Endeavour* 2003; 27: 150–4.

7. van der Weiden RM. The first successful separation of conjoined twins (1689). *Twin Res* 2004; 7: 125–7.

8. Kaufman MH. The embryology of conjoined twins. *Childs Nerv Syst* 2004; 20: 508–25.

9. Spencer R. Theoretical and analytical embryology of conjoined twins: Part I: Embryogenesis. *Clin Anat* 2000; 13: 36–53.

10. Spencer R. Theoretical and analytical embryology of conjoined twins: Part II: Adjustments to union. *Clin Anat* 2000; 13: 97–120.

11. Spencer R. Conjoined twins: Theoretical embryologic basis. *Teratology* 1992; 45: 591–602.

12. Logrono R, Garcia-Lithgow C, Harris C, Kent M, Meisner L. Heteropagus conjoined twins due to fusion of two embryos: Report and review. *Am J Med Genet* 1997; 73: 239–43.

13. Martinez-Urrutia MJ, Lopez-Pereira P, Alvarez J, Martinez L, Lobato R, Jaureguizar E, Tovar JA. Heterozygotic twinning in a case of female vesico-urethral duplication. *J Urol* 2004; 172: 1989–90.

14. Martinez-Frias ML. Conjoined twins presenting with different sex: Description of a second case that truly represents the earliest historical evidence in humans. *Am J Med Genet A* 2009; 149A: 1595–6.

15. Weber MA, Sebire NJ. Genetics and developmental pathology of twinning. *Semin Fetal Neonatal Med* 2010; 15: 313–8.

16. Spencer R. Conjoined twins. *Developmental Malformations and Clinical Implications*. Baltimore and London: The Johns Hopkins University Press, 2003: 476 pp.

17. Spitz L. Conjoined twins. *Prenat Diagn* 2005; 25: 814–9.

18. Spencer R. Anatomic description of conjoined twins: A plea for standardized terminology. *J Pediatr Surg* 1996; 31: 941–4.

19. Spencer R. Parasitic conjoined twins: External, internal (fetuses in fetu and teratomas), and detached (acardiacs). *Clin Anat* 2001; 14: 428–44.

20. Sanjaghsaz H, Bayram MO, Qureshi F. Twin reversed arterial perfusion sequence in conjoined, acardiac, acephalic twins associated with a normal triplet. A case report. *J Reprod Med* 1998; 43: 1046–50.

21. Gupta DK, Lall A, Bajpai M. Epigastric heteropagus twins—A report of four cases. *Pediatr Surg Int* 2001; 17: 481–2.

22. Bhansali M, Sharma DB, Raina VK. Epigastric heteropagus twins: 3 case reports with review of literature. *J Pediatr Surg* 2005; 40: 1204–8.

23. Cywes S, Millar AJ, Rode H, Brown RA. Conjoined twins—The Cape Town experience. *Pediatr Surg Int* 1997; 12: 234–48.

24. Spitz L, Kiely EM. Conjoined twins. *Jama* 2003; 289: 1307–10.

25. Pierro A, Kiely EM, Spitz L. Classification and clinical evaluation. *Semin Pediatr Surg* 2015; 24: 207–11.

26. Rode H, Fieggen AG, Brown RA, Cywes S, Davies MR, Hewitson JP, Hoffman EB, Jee LD, Lawrenson J, Mann MD, Matthews LS, Millar AJ, Numanoglu A, Peter JC, Thomas J, Wainwright H. Four decades of conjoined twins at Red Cross Children's Hospital—Lessons learned. *S Afr Med J* 2006; 96: 931–40.

27. Andrews RE, McMahon CJ, Yates RW, Cullen S, de Leval MR, Kiely EM, Spitz L, Sullivan ID. Echocardiographic assessment of conjoined twins. *Heart* 2006; 92: 382–7.

28. Brizot ML, Liao AW, Lopes LM, Okumura M, Marques MS, Krebs V, Schultz R, Zugaib M. Conjoined twins pregnancies: Experience with 36 cases from a single center. *Prenat Diagn* 2011; 31: 1120–5.

29. Greening DG. Vaginal delivery of conjoined twins. *Med J Aust* 1981; 2: 356–60.

30. Mitchell T, Cheng E, Jolley J, Delaney S. Successful induction of labor of late-second-trimester conjoined twins: An alternative to hysterotomy. *Obstet Gynecol* 2014; 123: 469–72.

31. Sinha M, Gupta R, Gupta P, Tiwari A. Assisted breech vaginal delivery of dicephalus dipus dibrachius conjoined twins: A case report. *J Reprod Med* 2015; 60: 160–4.

32. Marin-Padilla M, Chin AJ, Marin-Padilla TM. Cardiovascular abnormalities in thoracopagus twins. *Teratology* 1981; 23: 101–13.

33. McMahon CJ, Spencer R. Congenital heart defects in conjoined twins: Outcome after surgical separation of thoracopagus. *Pediatr Cardiol* 2006; 27: 1–12.

34. Lai HS, Chu SH, Lee PH, Chen WJ. Unbalanced cross circulation in conjoined twins. *Surgery* 1997; 121: 591–2.

35. Watson SG, McHugh K. Conjoined twins: Radiological experience. *Semin Pediatr Surg* 2015; 24: 212–6.

36. Kingston CA, McHugh K, Kumaradevan J, Kiely EM, Spitz L. Imaging in the preoperative assessment of conjoined twins. *Radiographics* 2001; 21: 1187–208.

37. Bonilla-Musoles F, Machado LE, Osborne NG, Blanes J, Bonilla F, Jr., Raga F, Machado F. Two-dimensional and three-dimensional sonography of conjoined twins. *J Clin Ultrasound* 2002; 30: 68–75.

38. Marcinski A, Lopatec HU, Wermenski K, Wocjan J, Gajewski Z, Kaminski W, Dura W. Angiographic evaluation of conjoined twins. *Pediatr Radiol* 1978; 6: 230–2.

39. Jansen O, Mehrabi VA, Sartor K. Neuroradiological findings in adult cranially conjoined twins. Case report. *J Neurosurg* 1998; 89: 635–9.

40. McAdams RM, Milhoan KA, Hall BH, Richardson RG. Prenatal and postnatal imaging of thoracopagus conjoined twins with a shared six-chamber heart. *Pediatr Radiol* 2004; 34: 816–9.

41. Martinez L, Fernandez J, Pastor I, Garcia-Guereta L, Lassaletta L, Tovar JA. The contribution of modern imaging to planning separation strategies in conjoined twins. *Eur J Pediatr Surg* 2003; 13: 120–4.

42. Rubini G, Paradies G, Leggio A, D'Addabbo A. Scintigraphy in assessment of the feasibility of separation of a set of xipho-omphalopagous conjoined twins. *Clin Nucl Med* 1995; 20: 1074–8.

43. Izukawa T, Kidd BS, Moes CA, Tyrrell MJ, Ives EJ, Simpson JS, Shandling B. Assessment of the cardiovascular system in conjoined thoracopagus twins. *Am J Dis Child* 1978; 132: 19–24.

44. Powis M, Spitz L, Pierro A. Differential energy metabolism in conjoined twins. *J Pediatr Surg* 1999; 34: 1115–7.

45. Atkinson L. Ethics and conjoined twins. *Childs Nerv Syst* 2004; 20: 504–7.

46. Gillett G. When two are born as one: The ethics of separating conjoined twins. *J Law Med* 2009; 17: 184–9.

47. Savulescu J, Persson I. Conjoined twins: Philosophical problems and ethical challenges. *J Med Philos* 2016; 41: 41–55.

48. Davis C. The spectre of court-sanctioned sacrificial separation of teenage conjoined twins against their will. *J Law Med* 2014; 21: 973–83.

49. Spitz L. Ethics in the management of conjoined twins. *Semin Pediatr Surg* 2015; 24: 263–4.

50. Al Rabeeah A. Conjoined twins—Past, present, and future. *J Pediatr Surg* 2006; 41: 1000–4.

51. Kiely EM, Spitz L. The separation procedure. *Semin Pediatr Surg* 2015; 24: 231–6.

52. Kiely EM, Spitz L. Planning the operation. *Semin Pediatr Surg* 2015; 24: 221–3.

53. Stuart GM, Black AE, Howard RF. The anaesthetic management of conjoined twins. *Semin Pediatr Surg* 2015; 24: 224–8.

54. Simpao AF, Wong R, Ferrara TJ, Hedrick HL, Schwartz AJ, Snyder TL, Tharakan SJ, Bailey PD, Jr. From simulation to separation surgery: A tale of two twins. *Anesthesiology* 2014; 120: 110.

55. Wong TG, Ong BC, Ang C, Chee HL. Anesthetic management for a five-day separation of craniopagus twins. *Anesth Analg* 2003; 97: 999–1002, table of contents.

56. Thomas JM, Lopez JT. Conjoined twins—The anaesthetic management of 15 sets from 1991–2002. *Paediatr Anaesth* 2004; 14: 117–29.

57. Szmuk P, Rabb MF, Curry B, Smith KJ, Lantin-Hermoso MR, Ezri T. Anaesthetic management of thoracopagus twins with complex cyanotic heart disease for cardiac assessment: Special considerations related to ventilation and cross-circulation. *Br J Anaesth* 2006; 96: 341–5.

58. Spitz L, Kiely EM. Experience in the management of conjoined twins. *Br J Surg* 2002; 89: 1188–92.

59. Walton JM, Gillis DA, Giacomantonio JM, Hayashi AH, Lau HY. Emergency separation of conjoined twins. *J Pediatr Surg* 1991; 26: 1337–40.

60. Jaffray B, Russell SA, Bianchi A, Dickson AP. Necrotizing enterocolitis in omphalopagus conjoined twins. *J Pediatr Surg* 1999; 34: 1304–6.

61. Chen WJ, Chen KM, Chen MT, Liu TK, Chu SH, Tsai TC, Hwang FY. Emergency separation of omphaloischiopagus tetrapus conjoined twins in the newborn period. *J Pediatr Surg* 1989; 24: 1221–4.

62. Stone JL, Goodrich JT. The craniopagus malformation: Classification and implications for surgical separation. *Brain* 2006; 129: 1084–95.

63. Browd SR, Goodrich JT, Walker ML. Craniopagus twins. *J Neurosurg Pediatr* 2008; 1: 1–20.

64. Staffenberg DA, Goodrich JT. Separation of craniopagus conjoined twins with a staged approach. *J Craniofac Surg* 2012; 23: 2004–10.

65. Dunaway D, Jeelani NU. Staged separation of craniopagus twins. *Semin Pediatr Surg* 2015; 24: 241–8.

66. Meyers RL, Matlak ME. Biliary tract anomalies in thoraco-omphalopagus conjoined twins. *J Pediatr Surg* 2002; 37: 1716–9.

67. Al-Rabeeah A, Zamakhshary M, Al-Namshan M, Al-Jadaan S, Alshaalan H, Al-Qahtani A, Alassiri I, Kingdom of Humanity team for conjoined twins. Hepatobiliary anomalies in conjoined twins. *J Pediatr Surg* 2011; 46: 888–92.

68. el-Gohary MA. Siamese twins in the United Arab Emirates. *Pediatr Surg Int* 1998; 13: 154–7.

69. Spitz L. Surgery for conjoined twins. *Ann R Coll Surg Engl* 2003; 85: 230–5.

70. Tsang VT, Tran PK, de Leval M. Cardiothoracic surgery. *Semin Pediatr Surg* 2015; 24: 252–3.

71. Kim SS, Waldhausen JH, Weidner BC, Grady R, Mitchell M, Sawin R. Perineal reconstruction of female conjoined twins. *J Pediatr Surg* 2002; 37: 1740–3.

72. Fieggen AG, Dunn RN, Pitcher RD, Millar AJ, Rode H, Peter JC. Ischiopagus and pygopagus conjoined twins: Neurosurgical considerations. *Childs Nerv Syst* 2004; 20: 640–51.

73. Hoyle RM, Thomas CG, Jr. Twenty-three-year follow-up of separated ischiopagus tetrapus conjoined twins. *Ann Surg* 1989; 210: 673–9.

74. Spiegel DA, Ganley TJ, Akbarnia H, Drummond DS. Congenital vertebral anomalies in ischiopagus and pyopagus conjoined twins. *Clin Orthop Relat Res* 2000; 381: 137–44.

75. Votteler TP, Lipsky K. Long-term results of 10 conjoined twin separations. *J Pediatr Surg* 2005; 40: 618–29.

76. Awasthi R, Iyengar R, Rege S, Jain N. Surgical management of pygopagus conjoined twins with spinal bifida. *Eur Spine J* 2015; 24 Suppl 4: S560–3.

77. Janik JS, Hendrickson RJ, Janik JP, Bensard DD, Partrick DA, Karrer FM. Spectrum of anorectal anomalies in pygopagus twins. *J Pediatr Surg* 2003; 38: 608–12.

78. Holcomb GW 3rd, Keating MA, Hollowell JG, Murphy JP, Duckett JW. Continent urinary reconstruction in ischiopagus tripus conjoined twins. *J Urol* 1989; 141: 100–2.

79. McLorie GA, Khoury AE, Alphin T. Ischiopagus twins: An outcome analysis of urological aspects of repair in 3 sets of twins. *J Urol* 1997; 157: 650–3.

80. Lazarus J, Raad J, Rode H, Millar A. Long-term urological outcomes in six sets of conjoined twins. *J Pediatr Urol* 2011; 7: 520–5.

81. Cuckow P, Mishra P. Urological management. *Semin Pediatr Surg* 2015; 24: 237–40.

82. Shively RE, Bermant MA, Bucholz RD. Separation of craniopagus twins utilizing tissue expanders. *Plast Reconstr Surg* 1985; 76: 765–73.

83. Albert MC, Drummond DS, O'Neill J, Watts H. The orthopedic management of conjoined twins: A review of 13 cases and report of 4 cases. *J Pediatr Orthop* 1992; 12: 300–7.

84. Wirt SW, Algren CL, Wallace VR, Glass N. Separation of conjoined twins. *Aorn J* 1995; 62: 527–40, 43–5; quiz 46–50.

85. Higgins CR, Navsaria H, Stringer M, Spitz L, Leigh IM. Use of two stage keratinocyte–dermal grafting to treat the separation site in conjoined twins. *J R Soc Med* 1994; 87: 108–9.

86. Kelly DA, Rockwell WB, Siddiqi F. Pelvic and abdominal wall reconstruction using human acellular dermis in the separation of ischiopagus tripus conjoined twins. *Ann Plast Surg* 2009; 62: 417–20.

87. Dasgupta R, Wales PW, Zuker RM, Fisher DM, Langer JC. The use of Surgisis for abdominal wall reconstruction in the separation of omphalopagus conjoined twins. *Pediatr Surg Int* 2007; 23: 923–6.

88. Martinez-Frias ML, Bermejo E, Mendioroz J, Rodriguez-Pinilla E, Blanco M, Egues J, Felix V, Garcia A, Huertas H, Nieto C, Lopez JA, Lopez S, Paisan L, Rosa A, Vazquez MS. Epidemiological and clinical analysis of a consecutive series of conjoined twins in Spain. *J Pediatr Surg* 2009; 44: 811–20.

89. Pajkrt E, Jauniaux E. First-trimester diagnosis of conjoined twins. *Prenat Diagn* 2005; 25: 820–6.

90. Mackenzie TC, Crombleholme TM, Johnson MP, Schnaufer L, Flake AW, Hedrick HL, Howell LJ, Adzick NS. The natural history of prenatally diagnosed conjoined twins. *J Pediatr Surg* 2002; 37: 303–9.

91. Chiu CT, Hou SH, Lai HS, Lee PH, Lin FY, Chen WJ, Chen MT, Lin TW, Chu SH. Separation of thoracopagus conjoined twins. A case report. *J Cardiovasc Surg (Torino)* 1994; 35: 459–62.

92. Fishman SJ, Puder M, Geva T, Jenkins K, Ziegler MM, Shamberger RC. Cardiac relocation and chest wall reconstruction after separation of thoracopagus conjoined twins with a single heart. *J Pediatr Surg* 2002; 37: 515–7.

93. Jones D. Orthopedic aspects of separation. *Semin Pediatr Surg* 2015; 24: 249–51.

94. Shapiro E, Fair WR, Ternberg JL, Siegel MJ, Bell MJ, Manley CB. Ischiopagus tetrapus twins: Urological aspects of separation and 10-year followup. *J Urol* 1991; 145: 120–5.

95. Wilcox DT, Quinn FM, Spitz L, Kiely EM, Ransley PG. Urological problems in conjoined twins. *Br J Urol* 1998; 81: 905–10.

Tumors

84

Epidemiology and genetic associations of neonatal tumors

SAM W. MOORE

INTRODUCTION

Almost 50% of childhood cancer occurs under the age of 5 years[1] with clear evidence of inheritability being identified in many.

An interesting group of tumors are those occurring at birth or in the neonatal period because of the limitations of exposure to environmental factors—the so-called neonatal tumors (NNTs). NNTs include those tumors identified at birth (congenital tumors) as well as those identified during the first 28 days of life. Benign tumors and masses are not uncommon in this period, but malignant tumors, on the other hand, are uncommon, representing only 2% of childhood malignancies.[2]

It would appear necessary to define NNTs as benign or malignant. Benign tumors should probably include conditions like hamartomas, hemangiomas, lymphangiomas, and melanocytic nevi in a separate subsection. In addition, other causes of masses (e.g., abdominal masses related to the genitourinary tract, etc.) should be excluded.

Although benign tumors are not uncommon, they may be life-threatening because of their site and potential complications. They may also display variable behavior in the neonate and certain tumors [e.g., neuroblastoma, congenital fibrosarcoma (CFS)], although, having a malignant histological picture, may behave relatively benignly and even mature in the neonatal period. In addition, certain apparently benign neonatal masses (e.g., teratoma) may undergo malignant change if untreated.

Most neonatal tumors originate from mesodermal tissue with approximately 50% being present at birth (or antenatal diagnosis), with a further 20%–30% identified within the first week of life and the remainder within the rest of the neonatal period.[3]

The hypothesis that tumors (and even adult cancer) may be linked to or even initiated during fetal development[4–6] is supported by an ever-increasing number of animal experimental studies. This makes the study of NNTs particularly interesting, as a possible explanation of their early (as opposed to later) appearance may lie in the developmental processes still active in the host. However, the placenta forms a barrier to malignant cells preventing crossing from the mother to the fetus, thus protecting the fetus. Nevertheless, genetic or environmental (e.g., nutrition and exposures to environmental toxins/radiation) factors (or both) may still act as oncogenic promoters during gestation.[7]

This hypothesis is currently supported by an ever-increasing body of evidence and places the emphasis firmly on the developmental period as a focus of disease prevention and intervention. In this context, tumors occurring in the developmental and perinatal period can be regarded as a "window of opportunity" in cancer research[8,9] and may lead to the identification of potential therapeutic molecular targets.

Many of these tumors respond to therapy and have a good prognosis overall. The mortality rate for NNTs is estimated to be 6.26 per million live births.[10,11] Management of these tumors often involves the entire oncology team including neonatologists, radiologists, pediatric surgeons, pathologists, hematologists, and oncologists.

INCIDENCE OF NNTs

NNTs or perinatal tumors comprise only 2% of childhood malignancies. From an epidemiological point of view, however, there is little clarity as to the real prevalence, sites of origin, and pathological nature of NNTs, and reported series vary from unit to unit (Table 84.1), varying from 17 to 121 per million live births (Table 84.2).[12–18] Overall, the highest incidence has been reported in Japanese children and the lowest in black children in the United States.[1] The reported incidence in the United Kingdom and the United States,

Table 84.1 Published series of "neonatal" tumors since 1980

Date	Author	Country	Time span	No. of cases	Per year	Source
1978	Barson[14]	UK	N/I	270	?	Pathology review
1979	Bader	USA	1969–1971	39	13	Third National Cancer Survey
1982	Gale et al.[15]	USA (Philadelphia)	N/I	22	?	Hospital series
1985	Isaacs[19]	USA (Los Angeles)	1958–1982	110	4.4	Pathology review
1986	Las Heras[16]	USA (Los Angeles)	1964–1978	42	3	Hospital registry
1987	Campbell et al.[13]	Canada (Toronto)	1922–1982	102	1.7	Hospital series
1987	Davis et al.[17]	Scotland (Glasgow)	1955–1986	51	1.6	Hospital series
1988	Crom et al.[12]	USA (Memphis)	1962–1988	34	2.1	Hospital series
1989	Plaschkes and Dubler[20]	Switzerland (Bern)	1973–1987	39	2.6	Hospital series
1989	Mur[21]	Argentina	1967–1990	51	2.2	Hospital series
1990	Werb et al.[22]	Australia (Melbourne)	1939–1989	46	0.9	Autopsies
1992	Borch et al.[18]	Denmark (Copenhagen	1943–1985	76	1.8	National cancer registry
1992	Parkes et al.[23]	UK (Birmingham)	1960–1989	149 (+21 leuk)	5	Population-based registry
1994	Tenturier et al.[24]	France (Paris)	1975–1986	75	7.5	Hospital series
1994	Moore et al.[25]	South Africa (Cape)	1957–1991	60	1.8	Hospital series
1995	Xue[26]	USA	1956–1995	35 (<1 month)	0.9	Hospital series (35/225 < 1)
1995	Plaschkes[27]	International—SIOP	1987–1991	192	38.5	International Tumor registry
1996	Chakova and Stoyanova[28]	Bulgaria	15 years	30	2	Hospital series
1996	Zhou and Du[29]	China	N/I	15	?	Hospital autopsy series
1997	Gurney et al.[30]	USA (SEER data)	1973–1992	175 (12%)	8.76	NCI Registry
1998	Halperin[31]	USA (Durham NC)	1930–1998	23	0.33	Hospital series
2000	Rao et al.[32]	UK (Glasgow)	1955–1999	83	1.84	Hospital series
2001	Sbragia et al.[33]	USA (San Francisco)	1993–2000	64 (Antenatal)	9.1	Hospital series
2003	Hadley et al.[34]	South Africa (KZN)	1982–2002	42 malignant	4.05	Hospital series
2003	Pinter and Hock[35]	Hungary	1975–1983	+39 "benign" 142 (+ <1 year)	15.7	Hospital Series
2003	Buyukpamukcu et al.[36]	Turkey (Ankara)	1972–2000	123	2.9	Hospital series
2006	Berbel et al.[37]	Spain (Barcelona)	1990–1999	72	7.2	Hospital series
2009	Costa	Malaysia	2000–2006	28	4.6	Hospital series
2010	Bhatnagar	Portugal (Sao Jao)	1996–2006	32	3.2	Hospital series
2012		India (Mumbai)	13 years	59	4.5	Hospital series

Note: SIOP = International Society of Paediatric Oncology.

respectively, is approximately 1 in every 12500–27500 live births.[2] The Manchester Children's Registry estimated the incidence to be 121.29 per 10^6 child-years when all children under 1 year of age including those with leukemias and lymphomas are counted.[14]

One of the difficulties in assessing the true incidence of NNTs is the fairly frequent nonreporting of tumors occurring in stillborn babies and babies dying in the neonatal period.

AGE AND SEX

The majority of tumors are diagnosed when the infant is between 1 and 4 weeks of age. Fewer malignant tumors are diagnosed at birth, although benign or potentially malignant tumors are frequently encountered then.

The male-to-female ratio is equal in the majority with the exceptions of retinoblastoma (male preponderance) and teratoma (female preponderance).

Table 84.2 Incidence of NNTs—published series

Country	Author	Incidence	Source
UK	Barson[10]	70 per million live births	National Survey by Pathologists (GB)[a]
UK	Oxford Children's Cancer Group[38]	17 per million live births	Cancer Registry
UK	Manchester Children's Tumor Registry[39]	121.29 per 10^6 child-years	Tumor Registry, population based[b]
USA	Bader and Miller[40]	36.4 per 10^6 child-years	Third National Cancer Survey (USA)
Switzerland	Plaschkes and Dubler[20]	93 per million live births	Hospital activity analysis
Hungary	Pinter and Hock[35]	100.5 per million live births	Hospital activity analysis[c]
Denmark	Borch et al.[18]	23 per million live births	Danish Cancer Registry (ICD)

[a] Benign–malignant.
[b] <1 year (including neonates) includes leukemia and lymphoma.
[c] <3 months.

PRENATAL DIAGNOSIS

With the advent of routine prenatal ultrasonographic screening and the considerable recent advances in technology, many NNTs are now diagnosed antenatally. This is particularly true of patients with renal masses/tumors, mixed germ cell tumors of the sacrococcygeal region, as well as masses in other parts of the body.

The advent of neuroblastoma screening programs brought more tumors to light but did not appear to affect the overall prognosis. The reason for this is that although the histopathologic features were that of neuroblastoma, the biological characteristics of neuroblastomas detected by screening in Japan, for instance, have been shown to be mostly favorable with a few having N-myc amplification.[41] As a result, the great majority improve spontaneously and disappear, but not all, as 10%–20% have unfavorable histological features and may progress.

CLINICAL PRESENTATION

Many NNTs present with benign masses, some of which may be incidental findings or diagnosed with antenatal ultrasonography. However, the clinical behavior may vary, and 34% of the 192 patients reported by the International Society of Pediatric Oncology from 12 different centers presented with metastatic disease.[14]

PATHOLOGY

A particular problem exists in classifying NNTs in that histological features of malignancy do not always correlate with clinical behavior. As a result, there are at least four clinical groupings of NNTs[20,27]:

1. Tumors that are clearly malignant by all the usual criteria but
   a. Behave more like those occurring in older children
   b. Behave better than expected
   c. Behave worse than expected
   d. Demonstrate unpredictable or uncertain behavior

2. Tumors that show local invasiveness but have no metastatic potential
3. Benign tumors that are either
   a. Life-threatening because of size and location
   b. Have a known tendency toward malignant transformation
4. Extreme rarities, e.g., malignant carcinomas that are similar to adult-type tumors

TUMOR TYPES

True carcinoma as seen in adults remains extremely rare in childhood, making up only 1%–2% of patients.[42] Instead tumors arising from mesenchymal tissue remain the most frequent.

The distribution of the various histological types of tumors appears to be relatively constant when compared with other published series (Table 84.3). In a study of 192 cases collected from 12 different countries by the International Society of Pediatric Oncology (1987–1991), 33 different types of tumors were reported to occur within the neonatal period.[27] Teratoma is the most frequently encountered type in our own[25] as well as other large series,[23,27] and is followed by neuroblastoma, leukemia, and soft tissue tumors (STS). Certain tumors (e.g., retinoblastoma and brain tumors) vary in incidence depending on hospital referral patterns. Renal and liver tumors occurred less frequently in the neonatal period.[14] Other types of tumors tend to be rarities.

ETIOLOGY AND CARCINOGENESIS

The etiology of cancer in children is multifactorial and probably includes both genetic and environmental factors. It would appear that these tumors are initiated early in fetal development and therefore have a short window of exposure to any potential environmental interference. It therefore would appear that genetic factors predominate in their etiology and pathogenesis. This may involve a fairly straightforward genetic defect in heritable tumors, whereas a more involved multistep process is probably involved in those occurring spontaneously.

Table 84.3 International society for paediatric oncology (SIOP) tumor registry 1987–1991

Diagnosis	No. of cases
Neuroblastoma	85
Teratoma	24
Rhabdomyosarcoma	13
Retinoblastoma	10
Mesoblastic nephroma	8
Hepatoblastoma	6
Undifferentiated sarcoma	5
Histiocytosis	4
Fibromatosis	3
Hemangiopericytoma	3
Renal (unclassified)	3
Yolk sac tumor	3
Brain tumor	2
Choriocarcinoma	2
Fibrosarcoma	2
Liver tumors	2
Prospective neuroectodermal tumor (PNET)	2
Angiofibroma	2
Arterioventricular malformations	1
Embryonal tumors	1
Ependymoblastoma	1
Glioma grades III–IV	1
Infantile myofibromatosis	1
Juvenile xanthogranuloma	1
Leiomyosarcoma	1
Melanoma	1
Neurofibroma	1
Oligodendroglioma	1
Rhabdoid tumor	1
Testicular carcinoma	1
Wilms' tumor	1
Total	192

Genetic factors in NNTs

Following the first report of the Philadelphia or Ph1 chromosome,[43] in affected cells of patients with chronic myeloid leukemia, genetic mechanisms have been implicated in the etiology of many cancers, thus opening new areas for diagnosis and prognosis. Tumors are accepted as being a largely genetically based disorder at the cellular level and have been implicated in both nonhereditary and hereditary forms of malignancy in children and adults.[44] This is particularly true of NNTs where most cancer cells are monoclonal and have a high incidence of chromosomal changes and some specific genetic mutations, as well as a clear inherited predisposition to malignancy.

As such, NNTs provide a unique opportunity to study familial and genetic associations because minimal interactions between genetic and environmental factors have occurred that

soon after birth. Modern genetic surveillance techniques offer potential opportunities for prevention, in contrast to most malignancies encountered in older patients.[45]

A distinction between germline and somatic gene changes should be borne in mind, however, especially in interpreting the findings. By way of example, constitutional genetic mutations have been reported in 10–15% pediatric cancers. In neonates, these include trisomies 13, 18, and 21. In the case of trisomy 21, there is an increased association with leukemia and retroperitoneal teratoma, but other solid tumors like neuroblastoma are extremely rare.[46] In addition, the X-linked syndromes like the Klinefelter (47XXY) syndrome is associated with an increase in germ cell tumors, although once again, the prevalence of neuroblastoma is decreased.

Apart from explaining how tumors may present in the perinatal period, genetic control may also partly explain the variable behavior of certain tumors within the perinatal period.[9]

There are essentially *three groups* of genetic abnormalities involved in the epidemiology of NNTs:

1. Genes resulting in a high risk of malignancy (e.g., in retinoblastoma)
2. Genetically determined syndromes where an increased risk of malignancy exists
3. Genes that confer a higher risk by conferring an increased susceptibility to environmental factors

The frequency with which each occurs will be influenced by their incidence in the population/family at risk.

Genes resulting in a high risk of malignancy

Accumulating research over the past two decades has seen many significant advances in understanding the mechanisms of the heritability of cancer (5%–10% of all cancers). This is of particular interest in the field of NNTs.

The best example of this group is the RB1 gene, which confers a risk of retinoblastoma. Other examples include Li–Fraumeni syndrome, where there is an association of rhabdomyosarcoma (RMS), STS, breast carcinoma, adrenocortical carcinoma, brain tumors, and leukemia.

As many of the genetic mutations associated with malignancy in children appear to occur spontaneously, a double "hit"[47] or multigene etiology is a likely mechanism.

The "two-hit" or multistep model of tumor development

Whereas it is generally recognized that tumors are a genetically related disease, tumorigenesis can mostly be attributed to a multistep process, whereby each step probably correlates with one or more distinct genetic variations in the major regulatory genes.

Current understanding of this process began when Knudson,[47] in an attempt to understand the pathogenesis of neonatal retinoblastomas, proposed that the tumor resulted from a combination of a prezygotic (germinal) mutation as well as a postzygotic (somatic) event. His so-called "two-hit" theory, based on extrapolated statistical data, was later confirmed by Comings[48] who suggested that both of these events could apply to mutations of the RB1 gene.

This "two-hit" model has evolved into a widely accepted multigene or multistep model. It is particularly applicable to inherited cancer models (and possibly neonatal tumors), whereby an inherited susceptibility occurs on the basis of an identified germline mutation that results in tumor development caused by further inactivation of a second allele (often tumor suppressor genes), which gives rise to early activation of the oncogenic pathway.

This theory provides the basis for understanding the pathogenesis of a number of tumors occurring in the neonatal period and has since been validated for a number of other tumor types (e.g., retinoblastoma, Wilms' tumor [WT], neuroblastoma, and other tumors).

In sporadic tumors (as opposed to hereditary tumors) a multistep process is more likely. The initial mutational activation of an oncogene is often correlated with nonmutational inactivation of tumor suppressor genes. As this is probably an early event, it is then followed by a number of independent mutations in other genes to allow neoplastic growth.

How this applies to special circumstances such as neonatally occurring tumors outside of these known examples is still unclear. These tumors have a number of host-specific features that include the potential of spontaneous regression in some, a greater capacity for cell repair, as well as a comparatively good prognosis when compared to histologically similar tumors occurring later in childhood. It is therefore reasonable to assume that further study of the genes controlling childhood cancer and particularly cancer occurring early in life warrants further attention.

Childhood tumors arising from a developmental progenitor cell may also differ from tumors occurring in adults. Because cancer results from multiple aberrant genetic influences on the cell cycle, the cancers of childhood (as well as a number of adult cancers) may be related to prenatal development. This new paradigm of thinking has led to a concept called "the developmental basis of health and disease."

Mechanisms whereby genes may initiate malignancy include

- Oncogene activation
- Inactivation of tumor suppressor genes
- Epigenetic factors

In other words, the activation of receptors then alters gene expression and triggers signaling cascades, which then affect transcription factors.

This must take into account factors that affect gene expression in addition to genetic mutations. This process is controlled by further regulatory genes, transcription factors, and signaling proteins.

A variety of host-specific features that may influence NNTs include spontaneous regression and a greater capacity for cell repair.

The fairly good prognosis of NNTs may be reflecting the possibility that critical signaling pathways are still active in the neonatal period.

On the other hand, the malignant potential of certain tumors (e.g., sacrococcygeal teratoma) has also been shown to increase with time.

Genetically determined high-risk syndromes

The identification of a genetic association of a specific tumor may be hampered due to the fact that the precise genetic mechanisms may not be recognized by the current genetic testing methods. Etiological factors involved in the pathogenesis of certain tumors (e.g., WT) appear to be more complicated than those of others (e.g., retinoblastoma).

Increases in familial occurrence or an increased risk in monozygotic twins may be present, and an association between a specific malignancy and a set of alleles at a specific locus is thus identified. This may not be exclusive to the particular tumor under study and may be associated with the pathogenesis of other types of tumors. Examples of this are the associations between leukemia, lymphomas, central nervous system neoplasms, and STS, as well as the RB1 and WT1 genes, among others. The evaluation of clinical associations and syndromes linked to specific tumor types is therefore of considerable importance.

Mendelian single-gene-related syndromes

Syndromes arising from defects in chromosomal breakage or disorders of sexual differentiation may lead to malignancy. A number of examples of Mendelian single-gene malignancy-related syndromes are described in Table 84.4.

These may be autosomal dominant, recessive, or X-linked. In addition, certain disorders of sexual differentiation may also be associated with cancer in the pediatric age group. Autosomal dominant syndromes include familial colonic polyposis, neurofibromatosis, and the nevoid basal cell carcinoma syndrome (Gorlin syndrome), as well as the blue rubber bleb and Sotos syndromes. Skeletal abnormalities such as multiple exostoses, polyostotic fibrous dysplasia, and Maffucci syndrome are also associated with a higher incidence of tumor formation. These tumors do not normally present in the neonatal period and are added for completeness, but are extremely interesting from a genetic point of view (i.e., in tracing the affected individuals in family groups).

Autosomal recessive syndromes associated with tumors include xeroderma pigmentosum, Fanconi anemia, Bloom syndrome, and ataxia telangiectasia syndromes. Bloom syndrome includes sensitivity to ultraviolet light, growth retardation, and immunodeficiency that is related with a higher rate

Table 84.4 Inherited syndromes and childhood malignancy

Chromosome Breakage Syndromes
    Bloom syndrome
    Fanconi's anemia
    Ataxia telangiectasia
    Xeroderma pigmentosa
Neurocristopathies
Neurofibromatosis
    Tuberous sclerosis
    Turcot's syndrome
    Multiple mucosal neuroma syndrome
    Basal cell nevus syndrome
Metabolic Disorders
    Tyrosinemia (hereditary)
    Alpha-1 antitrypsin deficiency
    Glycogenolysis (type 1)
Immune Deficiency Disorders
    Sex-linked lymphoproliferative syndrome
    Wiskott–Aldrich syndrome
    Severe combined immunodeficiency
    Bruton's agammaglobulinemia

of associated malignancy occurring at an earlier age,[49] e.g., leukemias and gastrointestinal malignancies. Fanconi's anemia is also linked to leukemia and liver tumors. Tumors associated with an autosomal recessive familial inheritance as well as those associated with immunodeficient X-linked recessive syndromes occur outside of the neonatal period, suggesting some degree of an initiating environmental influence.

The Epstein–Barr virus has been suggested as a possible pathogenetic factor[50] in the X-linked lymphoproliferative syndrome. Of particular interest are the fragile chromosomal syndromes, where fragile sites associated with breakage and repair of chromosomal defects are transmitted through families. A high percentage of the inheritable and constitutive fragile sites have been mapped to genetic sites associated with human cancer.[51] These chromosomal rearrangements have been associated with malignancy in at least 6 out of the 16 inheritable fragile chromosome sites and have also been identified in other non-inherited fragile chromosome sites.[51] As a result of the chromosome fragility in these cases, deletions and chromosomal fragments may occur. Should the fragile sites break close to a proto-oncogene location, the activation of the oncogene may result in the malignant transformation of the cells. In several disorders in sexual differentiation, the incidence of gonadal tumors has been increased.

Familial associations with cancer

Although loss of a chromosome segment of a specific chromosome pair (heterozygosity) may be involved in the pathogenesis of certain tumors,[52,53] a specific chromosome from one of the parents appears to be given preference in particular situations.[54] Examples of this are the loss of a maternally derived gene on chromosome 11 in sporadic WT[55] and the successive loss of function of both alleles of RB (retinoblastoma susceptibility gene) in the development of retinoblastoma as well as certain sarcomas such as osteosarcoma.[54] Genetic processes other than chromosome anomalies may also be involved in the familial transmission of a tendency to develop certain tumors.

Large cohort studies of offspring of parents with cancer have failed to show an overall increased risk for tumors.[54] There is also little evidence to suggest that cancer treatment confers an additional risk. In a separate study of 36 survivors of 82 NNTs, the current authors found no familial increase in the incidence of malignancy, although chromosomal abnormalities were identified in three patients.[56] One patient had a chromosome 21 abnormality, one had trisomy 13, and in the other, a distinctive familial translocation pattern was located on the ninth chromosome in a girl with a neuroblastoma.[38] The lack of increase in incidence agrees with the findings of previous studies[12,39,40] where no inherited effects of childhood tumors or tumor therapy were identified in survivors of childhood neoplasms.

Other syndromes associated with an increased genetic risk of cancer

Although a family history may be observed in the group of neurocristopathies associated with neural crest abnormalities, the associated tumors appear outside the neonatal period. Examples of this are pheochromocytoma, von Recklinghausen's disease, Sturge–Wreber syndrome, tuberous sclerosis, and von Hippel–Lindau disease, as well as the MEN II tumor syndrome.

Other congenital syndromes that confer an increased risk of malignancy include the WAGR and Denys–Drash syndromes in WTs, the Beckwith–Wiedemann and Down syndromes, and neurofibromatosis (NF1 gene). There is an increased risk of leukemia and other tumors in patients with Down syndrome.[57] Leukemoid reactions may be more difficult to distinguish in the neonatal period.[58] Abnormalities of the neurofibromatosis 1 gene (NF1) have been identified in patients with von Recklinghausen's disease, and a number of different mutations on the tumor suppressor gene have been described in chromosome 17q. An additional NF2 suppressor gene has been identified on chromosome 22q, leading to tumors such as acoustic schwannomas and other neural tumors.

There is a certain amount of overlap in phenotypic expression in syndromes such as the Beckwith–Wiedemann, Denys–Drash, Simpson–Golabi–Behmel, and Perlman, as well as other overgrowth syndromes. Nephroblastomatosis may be a feature of a number of these syndromes, and long-term survey is required as these could put patients at risk for embryonic tumors.

There are additional associations between WT, aniridia, urogenital malformations and mental retardation (WAGR), and the Denys–Drash syndrome.[59] This latter syndrome includes features of disorders of sexual differentiation, nephropathy, and WT. Although initially described only in males with pseudohermaphroditism,[59,60] this syndrome has been extended to include female children with ambiguous genitalia, nephropathy, and WT.[61] An observed constant association with genetic mutations located at chromosome 11p13 (WT1 or Wilms' tumor gene) and the Denys–Drash syndrome indicates a possible molecular marker for this syndrome. The exact site of the point mutation that was identified in the majority of cases was located on the WT1 exon 9, which affects the amino acid residue 394 arginine.[61] There is also an association between other tumors such as hepatoblastoma or adrenocortical carcinoma and WT, which may coexist in 6%–10% of patients.

Genetic factors that are involved in an increased risk of tumors include tyrosinosis, the MEN II and III syndromes, congenital adrenal hyperplasia, the basal cell nevus syndrome, and the Li–Fraumeni syndrome.[62] Genetic mutations predisposing to malignant disease include the Wilms' tumor 1 gene. In this instance, an 11p13 chromosomal defect is often typical. A further example is the neurofibromatosis type 1 gene, which is common in certain tumors. Gene amplifications have been reported in certain tumors. Amplified N-myc and N-ras oncogenes have been observed in neuroblastomas. This N-myc amplification has been shown to be associated with the more severe form of the malignancy.

Association with congenital malformations

Congenital malformations are inked to tumor formation [<1 year (OR = 16.8, 95% CI: 3.1–90) vs. >1 year of age]. There is also a fairly clear relationship to congenital abnormalities, which have been reported to occur inasmuch as 15% of NNTs. In one recent study, 15 out of 72 patients with a NNT had associated congenital abnormalities.[63] The role of genetic factors in development and the link between congenital malformation and tumors (e.g., neuroblastoma[64]) are also becoming clearer.

Possible increased susceptibility to environmental toxins

In addition to genetic factors, although limited in the neonatal period, environmental exposure is also a contender for promoting oncogenesis.

Although it is true that neonates have a limited exposure to environmental toxins having just been "born," environmental influences that affect the mother may also affect the unborn baby. These include environmental exposure to ionizing radiation, drugs taken during pregnancy, infections and tumors in the mother, and congenital malformations.

As a result, events occurring during pregnancy could be of key significance in the development of NNTs. Both the environmental and genetic factors may thus influence the development of a NNT in the offspring. It is therefore conceivable that both genetic and environmental factors may

be operating (possibly in tandem) at this stage giving rise to a "unifying hypothesis" linking ontogeny to oncogenesis.

Environmental exposure may possibly influence vital signaling cascades during development. By way of example, these influences would, of necessity, have to occur during a period when normal developmentally specific mechanisms are influenced by multiple genetic and environmental factors in order to influence the epigenetic processes taking place during that period.[65] More recently, the importance of disturbances in epigenetic programming, which regulate both normal and neoplastic growth and development, are being further explored.[66,67]

The fact that NNTs have been protected from extensive environmental influences tends to mitigate against this being a major role player in their pathogenesis. However, environmental influences on epigenetic factors have already been demonstrated in patients exposed to environmental toxins in some adult tumors.[68]

It stands to reason, therefore, that a study of those genetic and environmental factors with the potential to influence this process has the potential to provide considerable information about both cancer etiology as well as the natural history of tumors, including their development and progression.

The resulting molecular epidemiological approach in investigating childhood tumors is enhanced by the current available technology, which may permit the characterization of connections between exposure and subsequent health effects in newborns by means of biomarkers (e.g., mutations in cord blood DNA).[69]

Radiation-induced tumorigenesis

One example of environmental influences is that of ionizing radiation, which has been clearly implicated in the etiology of a number of tumors in children. This may involve prenatal as well as postnatal exposure. There is a dose-related increase in tumor incidence or a tendency for tumors to occur at a younger age following prenatal or neonatal radiation exposure.[70] This is also true of internally deposited radionucleotides administered in the prenatal or neonatal periods.[71]

It is clear from experimental evidence that deletions, point mutations, translocations, and other genetic abnormalities occur as a result of ionizing radiation. As a result, a state genomic instability may occur, which may, in turn, result in malignant transformation. There does appear to be an increased susceptibility to ionizing radiation in the Li–Fraumeni syndrome mouse model (p53-deficient mice), which suggests some environmental influence in the development of tumors.[72]

Effect of drugs in pregnancy

It is becoming clearer that fetal exposure to endocrine disruptors and hormonally active substances (e.g., diethylstilboestrol) affects the prevalence of reproductive abnormalities and metabolic disorders, and thus influences cancer.[73]

Drugs may act as carcinogens or cocarcinogens in association with other agents or a particular genetic background. There is also clear evidence that tumors may arise in the children of mothers taking medication. One of the best examples of this is the fetal hydantoin syndrome.[74] There is some evidence of tumors arising from estrogens taken during pregnancy, and sacrococcygeal tumors have also been associated with maternal intake of acetazolamide.[75] This may be a greater problem than was initially thought. Satgé et al.[76] showed a history of medications being taken in 39 out of 89 (44%) neonatal tumor patients. Out of the 39 tumors, 9 were malignant, of which the main types were neuroblastomas and teratomas. Three groups of drugs were identified: IARC group 1, diethylstilboestrol and oral contraceptives; IARC group 2, possibly carcinogenic to humans; and IARC group 3, where no association has been proven. To date, the association of vitamin K with carcinogenesis remains uncertain.[77]

Environmental exposure

Results of epidemiological studies are inconsistent as far as environmental exposure is concerned, but only weak associations with risk factors such as smoking have been identified.[78] Other environmental factors such as exposure to electromagnetic radiation have proved to be difficult to determine from an epidemiological point of view.

SPECIFIC CLINICAL ASSOCIATIONS OF NNTs

Retinoblastoma

Much of the understood relationship between genetics and tumors of childhood really lies in the seminal work of Knudson[47] who in 1971 developed his "two-hit theory" of oncogenesis in retinoblastoma based on an analysis of the age of presentation of hereditary as opposed to the nonhereditary cases. His hypothesis that these tumors resulted from two separate genetic events was extended to suggest that these events could be mutations of the same RB1 gene. It has subsequently been shown that 90% of individuals with the RB1 gene mutation will develop a retinal tumor. A small number of these patients (5%) have additional associated genetic disturbances (e.g., deletions or translocations at 13q14).

To date, deregulated expression in more than 260 genes have been associated with retinoblastoma. An understanding of the function of these genes not only provides valuable insights into oncogenesis in retinoblastoma but also has yielded possible therapeutic target sites (e.g., MCM7 and WIF1) currently under investigation.[79]

Retinoblastoma remains the commonest intraocular tumor of childhood, with the average age of diagnosis being at 11–12 months of age for bilateral disease and 23 months for unilateral tumors. In cases with a strong family history

and a high index of suspicion, diagnosis may be made in the perinatal period.

The retinoblastoma protein (pRB) is part of the control of genes involved in the cell cycle and, as such, interacts with a number of transcriptional factors by modulating their activity. Therefore, deregulations and/or mutations of the retinoblastoma protein (RB/RB1) pathway have been observed in many human cancers, suggesting a fundamental role in oncogenesis. Patients with RB1 mutations carry a risk of developing other tumors such as osteogenic sarcomas, fibrosarcoma, melanoma, and even breast carcinoma in early adult life.

Neuroblastoma

Neuroblastoma is one of the most commonly occurring malignant solid tumors in childhood, which is often being advanced at diagnosis, commonly metastasizing widely to bone marrow, bone cortex, liver, lymph nodes, and lung. The tumor arises from the neural crest origin and can originate from any site along the distribution of the sympathetic chain. More than 90% are active in secreting biochemical substances, which helps in diagnosis as catecholamine metabolites may be measured in the urine.

Genetic factors play a major role in development and the link between maldevelopment and tumors. A positive association between congenital malformation and neuroblastoma has been reported in at least one recent study [odds ratio (OR) = 2.2, 95% confidence interval (95% CI): 1.1–4.5],[64] being particularly linked to those tumors presenting at <1 year of age (OR = 16.8, 95% CI: 3.1–90) as opposed to those presenting at >1 year of age.

Neuroblastoma itself may demonstrate a unique clinical behavior within the perinatal period. Although spontaneous regression is known to occur in neonates, it does not appear to be limited to fetal period or stage IVS neuroblastoma (small primary tumour, liver, skin and/or bone marrow metastases). It is noteworthy that aggressive neuroblastoma tumors are characterized by increased expression of cell cycle genes, whereas more mature forms like ganglioneuroma and ganglioneuroblastoma that mostly express genes related with neural development are associated with a more benign course.

It is also noteworthy that a few of the perinatal neuroblastoma tumors have n-myc amplification. Although its action is uncertain, other oncogenic genes alter other genes like beta-catenin, which leads to excessive cell growth (e.g., Activin-A by MYCN).

Certain tumors, although malignant in appearance, may undergo spontaneous regression, whereas others metastasize widely and aggressively. Studies have shown a favorable outcome for neuroblastoma in the majority of mass screened perinatal patients,[19,80] suggesting either a better biological profile or operative developmental signaling pathways, which still function in the perinatal period. In addition, stage IVS neuroblastomas, although widely spread [including a massively enlarged liver and extensive subcutaneous (blueberry muffin) lesions], have a relatively good clinical prognosis.

Neuroblastoma tumor cells are associated with molecular genetic features in up to 80% of cases, many of which are of biological and clinical significance as prognostic factors and are currently of value in directing treatment.

The most important of these are MYCN amplification, deletion of chromosome 1p, ploidy, additional copies of chromosome 17q, and the expression of the gene for the neurotrophin nerve growth factor gene TRKA. Multiple areas of LOH and copy number gain were seen. In many cases, the defect is found to be on chromosomes 1, 11, and 17. Gain of copy number on 17q has recently been reported in 95% of cases studied,[81] with one of the most consistent changes being a deletion on the short arm of chromosome 1 (1p36.1–1p36.3). Whereas 1p LOH is encountered in one-third of cases,[82] inactivation of the tumor suppressor gene at 11q23.3 has been found to be an even more frequently encountered element of malignant progression being identified in up to 68%.[83] LOH on both chromosomes 11q and 1p was mostly accompanied by copy number loss, indicating homozygous deletion. It is also highly associated with occurrence of chromosome 3p LOH.

Additional chromosomal abnormalities have been identified at 4p, 6q, 9q, 10q, 12q, 13q, 14q, 16q, 22p, and 22q.[84] Amplification of the n-Myc oncogene (usually found on chromosome 2) has been associated with a more advanced form of the malignancy and is a poor prognostic sign.[85] Few of the perinatal neuroblastomas have n-myc amplification, although 10%–20% have unfavorable histological features. Recent research into high-risk neuroblastoma without MYCN amplification has shown that other oncogenic genes may deregulate MYC via altered beta-catenin signaling (a transcriptional target of beta catenin), indicating some degree of interdependence with other signaling pathways.[86] Recent reports of the downregulation of Activin-A by MYCN offer an explanation for this as deprived neuroblastoma cells experience a decrease in growth-inhibitory signal transduction leading to excessive cell growth.[87] In addition, the expression of TrkA has recently been shown to inhibit angiogenesis and tumor growth in neuroblastomas, suggesting possible new treatment options.[88] It is also interesting to note that p53 gene mutations are absent in neuroblastomas,[89] although present in other tumors of childhood.

In addition, molecular genetic features have been reported in >80% neuroblastoma cases. This is particularly true of high-risk patients, in whom a number of genetic alterations exist. Examples of these include MYCN on chromosome 2, which is a poor prognostic sign. Additional high-risk sites include 1pLOH, unbalanced 11q, as well as gains of Chr 17 and 7. It has been shown that expression of neurotrophin nerve growth factor gene TRKA inhibits angiogenesis and tumor growth in neuroblastoma. Other oncogenic genes (e.g., Activin-A by MYCN) alter beta-catenin signaling, which leads to excessive cell growth.

Few perinatal neuroblastoma have n-myc amplification and have a chance to regress. This spontaneous regression, which occurs in the neonate, is not, however, limited to fetal period or stage IVS. Aggressive neuroblastoma tumors are characterized by an increased expression of cell cycle genes.

On the other hand, the more mature ganglioneuroma and ganglioneuroblastoma subtypes express genes associated with neural development.

Genomic studies of neuroblastomas have brought to light a number of possible biological mechanisms to explain the phenomenon of spontaneous regression in certain cases. Among others, these include neurotrophin deprivation, humoral or cellular immunity, loss of telomerase activity, and alterations in epigenetic regulation.[90]

TERATOMA

Germ cell tumors account for approximately 3% of pediatric malignancies worldwide and occur in gonadal (male and female) and extragonadal sites. Epidemiology should include abortions and stillbirths as the related mortality rate is high. The majority of teratomas are located in the sacrococcygeal region and gonads in childhood. Sacrococcygeal tumors are mostly benign at birth, and the majority do not develop to malignancy if adequate surgical removal is carried out before the infant is 3 months of age. After this time, the risk of malignancy increases if residual tumor is present, and older children may require chemotherapy along with delayed surgical excision.

Teratomas are thought to arise from the primordial germ cells as a result of an early event. A genetic tendency toward spontaneous gonadal teratomas is seen in a specific strain of experimental mice (strain 129).[91] An association with autosomal dominant familial recurrence has been reported, and there also appears to be a Mendelian dominant genetic predisposition to the development of a presacral mass in association with anorectal, sacral, and urogenital abnormalities.[92] Patients with an imperforate anus and a hemisacrum have a high incidence of presacral masses, which are teratomas and may occasionally be malignant.[92] Recent evidence points to an association with the long arm of chromosome 7 and Currarino's triad.[93] Mediastinal teratomas have been shown to develop in the second trimester.[94] Their sensitivity to chemotherapy and the existence of reliable tumor markers are important prognostic factors.

SOFT TISSUE TUMORS

STS are not uncommon in childhood and whereas the majority are benign lesions of connective tissue, a number of extremely aggressive tumors exist. There are arguably three separate clinical groups of STS encountered in childhood (viz., CFS, RMS, and non-rhabdomyosarcoma).[95]

Spicer[96] classified congenital fibrosarcoma separately to differentiate it from the more aggressive type of fibrosarcomas with similar histopathologic features seen in adults as they mostly have a favorable outcome and metastasize rarely. Classifying STS on prognosis and outcome, he considered that tumors of intermediate prognosis included RMS, peripheral neuroectodermal tumors (PNET), undifferentiated sarcomas, and malignant melanomas, whereas tumors with a uniformly bad prognosis included Kaposi sarcoma, malignant schwannoma, triton tumors, and juvenile hyaline fibromatosis, as well as visceral fibromatosis.

Rhabdomyosarcoma

RMS accounts for 10% of neonatal malignancies,[97] being the most common malignant STS even in the perinatal period.[21] It has a number of genetic associations that differentiate the histological subtypes and is associated with a number of genetic syndromes [viz., Beckwith–Weideman, Li–Fraumeni, and WAGR syndromes and neurofibromatosis (Type 1)]. This suggests a genetic basis for its early appearance in the neonatal period.

Associated genetic variations include loss of heterogeneity of the short arm of chromosome 11 (11p15 locus 12) in embryonal tumors, which leads to an overexpression of the insulin growth factor II (IGFII) gene. Equally, a subset of alveolar RMS has a unique chromosomal translocation between chromosomes 2 and 13, viz. (t[2;13] (q35;q14)).[98,99] This is close to the junction of the PAX3 gene, which controls neuromuscular development,[100] and the PAX/FKHR fusion gene is found in as many as 60% of alveolar RMS. A further 10% of patients with particularly poor prognosis may also carry the Ewing's sarcoma [EWS/ETS fusion genes (occasionally along with the PAX/FKHR gene)].

Numerous other genetic variations have been reported including frequent gains of chromosomes 2, 7, 8, 11, 12, 13q21, and 20, as well as losses of 1p35–36.3, 6, 9q22, 14q21–32, and 17.[101] A further loss of 1p36[102] corresponds to the locus for the paired home box PAX 7, which is characteristically altered in alveolar RMS tumors. The 1p region is interesting as it is also associated with neuroblastomas. Additional associations between mutations in the p53 tumor suppressor gene are also associated with adverse outcome.

STS and the Beckwith–Wiedemann syndrome

The Beckwith–Weideman syndrome (BWS; macrosomia, macroglossia, omphalocele, and hemihypertrophy) is associated with genetic and/or epigenetic alterations that modify imprinted gene expression on chromosome 11p15.5. There is an increased risk of soft tissue sarcomas (approx. 7.5%) especially if hemihypertrophy is present. Oncogenesis is associated with the detection of abnormal myogenic transcription factors (MyoD, Myogenin, and Myf5) and the PAX/FHKR chimeric transcription factors. Detection of other fusion genes such as EWS/WT1 in desmoplastic small round cell tumors, EWS/ATF in clear cell sarcoma, SSX/SYT in synovial cell sarcoma, or the TLS/CHOP in liposarcoma has also been described. An overexpression of MyoD in RMS is thought to inhibit the development of muscle cells and characteristically marks these tumors.[103]

The increased tumor risk in the Beckwith–Weideman overgrowth syndromes and the associated WT, hepatoblastoma, and hemihypertrophy are probably due to the complex genetic/epigenetic abnormalities of the imprinted

11p15 region.[104,105] A specific cancer risk is associated with specific areas of the gene[106] with the most common constitutional abnormalities currently appearing to be epigenetic, with aberrant methylation occurring at H19 or LIT1. As a result, untranslated RNAs are recorded on the gene at 11p15. Variations in H19DNA methylation were found to be significantly increased in at least one report [viz., 56% (9/16) vs. 17% (13/76; $p = .002$)], but not LIT1 alterations.

Ewing's family tumors

Although the cell of origin of Ewing's sarcoma is unknown, the Ewing's family of tumors most frequently has a specific translocation that results in expression of the EWS/FLI1 fusion protein responsible for malignant transformation.[107] Although a number of EWS/FLI1 downstream targets have been identified, the exact details of the oncogenic mechanism remain uncertain. It is currently thought that the FLI, ERG, FEV, ETV1, and ETV4 genes appear to be involved in chimera formation, which all upregulate EAT-2 (a previously described EWS/FLI1 target). EWS/FLI1 dysfunction appears to then result in functional activation of the retinoblastoma (pRB) family proteins, which are key mediators of the resulting probable oncogenic transformation.[108]

HEPATOBLASTOMA

Hepatoblastoma is the most common malignant liver tumor and embryonal tumor occurring particularly in the younger child and has also been associated with a low birth weight in the neonate.[109]

Although up to one-third of hepatoblastomas are associated with congenital abnormalities, the majority of cases are sporadic and the molecular pathogenesis poorly understood. Familial recurrence is extremely rare with the exception of families with adenomatous polyposis coli (FAP).[110] As a result, it is becoming clear that FAP-APC gene mutations result in transcription–activation and oncogenesis in these cases.

There is also considerable support for associations with trisomies 2, 8, and 20 in the development of HB.[111] In addition, gains on chromosomes 1q+ 2 (2q24) and 8q and 20 appear to be associated with a poor outcome. Known associations with the BWS and hemihypertrophy suggest a common genetic pathway (viz., LOH at the 11p15 site, which contains an insulin-like growth factor II and the H19 gene).

Congenital hepatoblastoma appears to have a poorer prognosis than those occurring in the older child with metastatic lesions being reported at unusual sites (viz., brain,[112] iris and choroid,[113] and placenta[114]). The latter may indicate tumor seeding during pregnancy via the fetal circulation.

An emerging association is with the CTNNB1 (beta-catenin) gene association with HB, particularly the embryonal subtype. The incidence of mutation of this gene in HB has been reported to vary widely in HB (13%–70%). Nevertheless, the SIOPEL study in 2011 found an 87% (85/98) aberrant β-catenin expression in HB specimens. Met-activated β-catenin was found in 79% of cases.[115]

WILMS' TUMOR

WT is the most common pediatric renal tumor with a peak age of incidence of 3–4 years. Although rare in the neonatal period, patients with synchronous bilateral WT, familial cases, and those with abnormalities are noted to be significantly younger. Predisposing associations with aniridia, congenital abnormalities of the genitourinary tract, and hemihypertrophy may be associated with nephroblastomatosis, which may lead to an early WT (Table 84.5). The familial associations have been shown to be part of an autosomal dominant trait and are of the order of 1% with a somewhat slight female preponderance, particularly in multicentric and bilateral tumors.

The genetic factors involved in WT are much more complex than those involved in other tumors such as retinoblastoma. Many of the genes implicated in Wilms' tumorigenesis are involved in the control of nephron progenitors or the microRNA (miRNA) processing pathway. Current research suggests important roles for miRNAs in WT etiology.[116] The familial associations have been shown to be part of an autosomal dominant trait and are of the order of 1% with a somewhat slight female preponderance, particularly in multicentric and bilateral tumors.

WT have been associated with at least two genetic variations (viz., 11p13; 11p15). Associations between WT and aniridia, urogenital malformations, and mental retardation (WAGR) and the Denys–Drash syndromes[60,61] led to the identification of a constitutional chromosomal deletion in the short arm of one copy of chromosome 11 p13 (the WT1 gene).

Table 84.5 Syndromes associated with WT

1. Aniridia (0.75%–1%)
2. Hemihypertrophy (3.3%)
3. BWS (3.7%)
4. Musculoskeletal abnormalities (2.9%)
5. Genitourinary abnormalities (5.2%)
6. Other syndromes associated with WTs

Denys–Drash syndrome
    Nephroblastoma
    Male pseudohermaphroditism
    Glomerulonephritis
    Nephrotic syndrome
    Renal failure
WAGR syndrome (11p13 deletion)
    Nephroblastoma
    Anorectal malformation
    Genitourinary anomalies
    Mental retardation
BWS
Klippel–Trelaunay syndrome
Other associated tumors
    Hepatoblastoma (6%–10% of WTs)
    Adrenocortical carcinoma

The Knudson model for WT has been validated through molecular identification of WT1 gene variation.[117,118] The WT1 gene encodes a transcription factor that appears to act both as a tumor suppressor gene[119] as well as an important regulator of renal embryological development. The deletion of this gene results in the development of a WT[120] by encoding a zinc finger transcription factor, which binds GC-rich sequences and acts as either an activator or repressor of transcription for a number of growth factors (including Igf-2)[121]. This may be a possible explanation of the mechanism of action of WT1 in the pathogenesis of WT.

The WT1 gene variations are only present in approximately 20% of WTs, suggesting further genetic associations. Despite some overlap with the WT1 gene, a combination of different genes could account for up to one-third of WTs.[122]

In addition to the WT1 gene at 11p13, there is evidence of a second WT gene at 11p15 (WT2 gene), which is associated with the BWS.

In addition, a reported high frequency of loss of heterozygosity (LOH) at 1p35–p36 (DIS247) suggests involvement in the pathogenesis of WT.[123] Further, genes (e.g., WT3 and WT4) also appear to be implicated in the oncogenesis of WTs as are gains of 1q and deletions of chromosome 22 associated with worst prognosis of WTs.

More recently, the WTX gene [Xq11.1] has been reported to be mutated in WTs. It is of interest that the 11p15 variation and the WTX genes appear to occur with similar regularity in these tumors.

Further, genetic pathways have also been reported. An association between the WNT/beta-catenin signaling pathway (the CTNNB1 gene, encoding beta-catenin) is also known.[124,125] This suggests that Wnt signaling pathway dysregulation also plays an oncogenic role in certain WTs. Further, genomic gain of the proto-oncogene transcription factor gene MYCN is associated with anaplasia and a decreased relapse-free and overall survival, independent of the histologic findings.[126] In addition, a LOH for 16q is a structural alteration identified in 20%–30% of WTs, and p53 alteration also appears to be required for the progression to the anaplastic subtype. Further, associations with p53 analogues (p73 and p63/KET) suggest that association with the p53 family may be important to cell growth and differentiation.[127] Haploinsufficiency in the PAX6 gene is also strongly associated with aniridia and may be involved.[128]

Familial WT does not, however, map to the 11th chromosome, as the known gene FWT1 is on 17q12–q21 and FWT2 on 19q13. Other susceptibility genes still remain to be identified.

OTHER TUMORS

Other genetic aberrations associated with tumors, such as the loss of heterozygosity on chromosome 5q, in identifying the gene for familial polyposis of the colon, defects in tumor-suppressive genes on 17q (p53) and 18q (DCC) in carcinoma of the colon, and translocation of the end of the long arm of chromosome 8 with chromosome 14, or an alteration in C-myc regulation or p53[129] in Burkitt's lymphoma, are interesting associations with pediatric tumors, but are not particularly associated with the neonatal period.

ANTENATALLY DIAGNOSED TUMORS

Clinical approach to antenatally diagnosed tumors

The reasons for highlighting NNTs are manifold but include the following:

1. Increased diagnosis of NNTs due to routine ultrasonography during pregnancy brings to light tumors whose natural history and optimal management are unclear.
2. Increased knowledge and understanding of pathophysiology and biological behavior of tumors may reduce unnecessary harmful forms of therapy.
3. Molecular genetics in these tumors identifies risk factors and provides models for understanding carcinogenesis in other tumors.
4. Environmental and teratogenic factors may be identified.

All evidence points toward the fact that the natural history of NNTs is different (mostly better) than that of comparable tumors in older children. The basis of this behavior is largely unknown, and hard epidemiological and etiological data in this group are lacking.

It is important that the identification of the genetic associations of these tumors continues and the cancer-producing genes to identify the genetic alleles associated with malignancy are investigated further. In addition, it is important that families with a genetic susceptibility to malignant tumors be investigated in order to identify specific genetic loci, which may or may not be related to a specific allele. Because of the rarity of these tumors, it is clear that international collaborative studies and research projects are necessary to achieve this goal.

THERAPEUTIC CONSIDERATIONS

There is also a paucity of objective information on the optimal treatment and long-term outcome of NNTs[12] and the impact of therapeutic measures to take into consideration.[13,130-132]

REFERENCES

1. Birch JM, Blair V. The epidemiology of infant cancers. *Br J Cancer* 1992; 66(Suppl XVIII): S52–4.
2. Bader JL, Miller RW. US Cancer incidence and mortality in the first year of life. *Am J Dis Child* 1979; 133: 157–9.
3. Fossati-Bellani F. Neonatal malignancies in Neonatology: A practical approach to neonatal diseases. In: Buonocore G et al. (eds). *A Practical Approach to Neonatal Diseases*. Milan: Springer-Verlag, 2012: 858–68.
4. Scotting PJ, Walker DA, Perilongo G. Childhood solid tumours: A developmental disorder. *Nat Rev Cancer* 2005; 5: 481–8.
5. Hanson MA, Gluckman PD. Developmental origins of health and disease: New insights. *Basic Clin Pharmacol Toxicol* 2008 February; 102(2): 90–3.
6. Soto AM, Maffini MV, Sonnenschein C. Neoplasia as development gone awry: The role of endocrine disruptors. *Int J Androl* 2008 April; 31(2): 288–93.
7. Grandjean P. Late insights into early origins of disease. *Basic Clin Pharmacol Toxicol* 2008 February; 102(2): 94–9.
8. Heindel JJ. Animal models for probing the developmental basis of disease and dysfunction paradigm. *Basic Clin Pharmacol Toxicol* 2008 February; 102(2): 76–81.
9. Moore SW, Satgé D, Sasco AJ, Zimmermann A, Plaschkes J. The epidemiology of neonatal tumours. Report of an international working group. *Pediatr Surg Int* 2003; 19: 509–19.
10. Anderson DH. Tumours of infancy and childhood. *Cancer* 1951; 4: 890–906.
11. Fraumeni JF Jr, Miller RW. Cancer deaths in the newborn. *Am J Dis Child* 1969 February; 117(2): 186–9.
12. Crom DB, Wilimas JA, Green AA, Pratt CB, Jenkins JJ, Behm FG. Malignancy in the neonate. *Med Pediatr Oncol* 1989; 17: 101–4.
13. Campbell AN, Chan HSL, O'Brien A, Smith CR, Becker C. Malignant tumours in the neonate. *Arch Dis Child* 1987; 62: 19–23.
14. Barson AJ. Congenital neoplasia: The society's experience. *Arch Dis Child* 1978; 53: 436.
15. Gale GB, D'Angio GJ, Uri A, ChattenJ, Koop CE. Cancer in the neonate: The experience of the childrens hospital in Philadelphia. *Pediatrics* 1982; 70: 409–13.
16. Las Heras J, Isaacs H. Congenital tumours. *Birth Defects* 1987; 23: 421–31.
17. Davis CF, Carachi R, Young DG. Neonatal tumours in Glasgow 1955–1986. *Arch Dis Child* 1988; 63: 1075–8.
18. Borch K, Jacobsen T, Olsen JH, Hirsch FR, Hertz H. Neonatal cancer in Denmark 1943–1985. *Ugeskr Laeger* 1994; 10: 156[2], 176–9.
19. Isaacs H. Perinatal (congenital and neonatal) tumours: A report of 110 cases. *Pediatr Pathol* 1985; 3: 165–216.
20. Plaschkes J, Dubler M. Neoplasmen beim neugeborenen. Medical Faculty, University of Bern, Switzerland, 1989.
21. Mur N. Neonatal malignant tumours: A retrospective experience. *Br J Cancer* 1992; 66(suppl XVIII). Paper presented at Cancer in the Very Young conference, St James University Hospital, Leeds September 1990.
22. Werb P, Scurry J, Oestoer A, Fortune-Attwood M. Survey of congenital tumours in perinatal necropsies. *Pathology* 1992; 24: 247–53.

23. Parkes SE, Muir KR, Southern L, Cameron AH, Darbyshire PJ, Stevens MCG. Neonatal tumours: A thirty year population based study. *Med Pediatr Oncol* 1994; 22: 309–17.

24. Tenturier C et al. Tumours solides malignes neonatales. Apropros de 75 cas. *Arch Fr Pediatr* 1992; 49: 187–92.

25. Moore SW, Kaschula ROC, Rode H, Millar AJW, Karabus C. The outcome of solid tumours occurring in the neonatal period. *Pediatr Surg Int* 1995; 10: 366–70.

26. Xue H, Horwitz JR, Smith MB, Lally KP, Black CT, Cangir A et al. Malignant solid tumours in Neonates: A 40 year review. *J Pediatr Surg* 1995; 30: 543–5.

27. Plaschkes J. Epidemiology of neonatal tumours. In: Puri P (ed). *Neonatal Tumours*. London: Springer-Verlag, 1996: 11–22.

28. Chakova L, Stoyanova A. Solid tumours in newborns and infants. *Folia Med (Bulgaria)* 1996; 38: 39–43.

29. Zhou X, Du X. A clinicopathological analysis of 15 cases with congenital tumours in fetus and newborn (English abstract). *Chung Hua Fu Chan Ko Tsa Chin* 1998; 33(5): 290–2.

30. Gurney JG, Ross JA, Wall DA, Bleyer WA, Severson RK, Robison LL. Infant cancer in the U.S.: Histology-specific incidence and trends, 1973 to 1992. *J Pediatr Hematol Oncol* 1997; 19(5): 428–32.

31. Halperin EC. Neonatal neoplasms. *Int J Radiat Oncol Biol Phys* 2000; 47(1): 171–8.

32. Rao S, Azmy A, Carachi R. Neonatal tumours: A single centre experience. *Pediatr Surg Int* 2002; 18: 306–9.

33. Sbragia L, Paek BW, Feldstein VA, Farrell JA, Harrison MR, Albanese CT et al. Outcome of prenatally diagnosed solid fetal tumors. *J Pediatr Surg* 2001; 36: 1244–7.

34. Hadley GP, Govender D, Landers G. Malignant solid tumours in neonates: An African perspective. *Pediatr Surg Int* 2002; 18(8): 653–7.

35. Pinter A, Hock A. Cancer in neonates and infants: National survey of 141 patients. In: Thomasson B, Holschneider AM (eds). *26th Congress of Scandinavian Association of Paediatric surgeons, Stockholm 22–24 May (Supplement)*. Stuttgart: Hippokrates Verlag, 1986: 180–4.

36. Buyukpamukcu M, Varan A, Tanyel C, Senocak ME, Gogus S, Akyuz C et al. Solid tumors in the neonatal period. *Clin Pediatr (Phila)* 2003; 42(1): 29–34.

37. Yeap BH, Zahari Z. Neonatal tumours in Malaysia: A call for heightened awareness. *Pediatr Surg Int* 2009; 26(2): 207–12.

38. Satge D, Moore SW, Stiller CA, Niggli FK, Pritchard-Jones K, Bown N et al. Abnormal constitutional karyotypes in patients with neuroblastoma: A report of four new cases and review of 47 others in the literature. *Cancer Genet Cytogenet* 2003; 147(2): 89–98.

39. Li FP, Cassady JR, Jaffe N. Risk of second tumors in survivors of childhood cancer. *Cancer* 1975 April; 35(4): 1230–5.

40. Weinberg AG, Schiller G, Windmiller J. Neonatal leukaemoid reaction: An isolated manifestation of mosaic trisomy 21. *Am J Dis Child* 1982; 136: 310–1.

41. Hachitanda Y, Ishimoto K, Hata J, Shimada H. One hundred neuroblastomas detected through a mass screening programme in Japan. *Cancer* 1994; 74: 3223–6.

42. Satgé D, Philippe E, Ruppe M et al. Les carcinomes neonatalis. Revue de la literature a propos d'un cas. *Bull Cancer* 1988; 75: 373–84.

43. Nowell PC. The minute chromosome (Phl) in chronic granulocytic leukemia. *Blut* 1962 April; 8: 65–6.

44. Nowell PC, Croce CM. Chromosomal approaches to the molecular basis of neoplasia. *Symp Fundam Cancer Res* 1986; 39: 17–29.

45. Quinn E, McGee R, Nuccio R, Pappo AS, Nichols KE. Genetic Predisposition to neonatal tumors. *Curr Pediatr Rev* 2015; 11(3): 164–78.

46. Satge D, Sasco AJ, Carlsen NL, Stiller CA, Rubie H, Hero B et al. A lack of neuroblastoma in Down syndrome: A study from 11 European countries. *Cancer Res* 1998; 58(3): 448–52.

47. Knudson AG Jr. Mutation and cancer: Statistical study of retinoblastoma. *Proc Natl Acad Sci USA* 1971; 68: 820–3.

48. Comings DE. A general theory of carcinogenesis. *Proc Natl Acad Sci USA* 1973; 70: 3324–8.

49. German J, Passarge E. Bloom's syndrome. XII. Report from the Registry for 1987. *Clin Genet* 1989 January; 35(1): 57–69.

50. Purtilo DT, Sakamoto K, Barnabei V, Seeley J, Bechtold T, Rogers G et al. Epstein–Barr virus-induced diseases in boys with the X-linked lymphoproliferative syndrome (XLP). *Am J Med* 1982; 73: 49–56.

51. Yunis E, Sieber WK, Akers DR. Does zonal aganglionosis really exist? Report of a rare variety of Hirschsprung's disease and review of the literature. *Pediatr Pathol* 1983; 1(1): 33–49.

52. Toguchida J, Ishizaki K, Sasaki MS, Nakamura Y, Ikenaga M, Kato M et al. Preferential mutation of paternally derived RB gene as the initial event in sporadic osteosarcoma. *Nature* 1989 March 9; 338(6211): 156–8.

53. Schroeder WT, Chao LY, Dao DD, Strong L, Pathak S, Riccardi V et al. Nonrandom loss of maternal chromosome 11 alleles in Wilms tumors. *Am J Hum Genet* 1987 May; 40(5): 413–20.

54. Toguchida J, Ishizaki K, Sasaki MS, Nakamura Y, Ikenaga M, Kato M et al. Preferential mutation of paternally derived RB gene as the initial event in sporadic osteosarcoma. *Nature* 1989 March 9; 338(6211): 156–8.

55. Schroeder WT, Chao LY, Dao DD, Strong L, Pathak S, Riccardi V et al. Nonrandom loss of maternal chromosome 11 alleles in Wilms tumors. *Am J Hum Genet* 1987 May; 40(5): 413–20.

56. Hawkins MM. Pregnancy outcome and offspring after childhood cancer. *BMJ* 1994; 309(6961): 1034.

57. Moore SW. Genetic and clinical associations of neonatal tumours. In: Puri P (ed). *Neonatal Tumours*. London: Springer-Verlag, 1996: 11–22.

58. Holland WW, Doll R, Carter CO. The mortality of leukaemia and other cancers among patients with Down's syndrome (Mongols) and among their parents. *Br J Cancer* 1962; 16: 177–86.

59. Li Y, Bollag G, Clark R, Stevens J, Conroy L, Fults D et al. Somatic mutations in the neurofibromatosis 1 gene in human tumors. *Cell* 1992 April 17; 69(2): 275–81.

60. Denys P, Malvaux P, Van den Berghe H, Tanghe W, Proesmans W. Association d'un syndr"me anatomopathologique de pseudohemaphroditism masculin, d'une tumeur de Wilms d'une nephropathie parenchymateuse et d'un mosaicism XX/XY. *Arch Fr Pediatr* 1967; 24: 729–39.

61. Drash A, Sherman F, Hartmann W, Blizzard RM. A syndrome of pseudohemaphroditism, Wilms tumour, hypertension and degenerative renal disease. *J Pediatr* 1970; 76: 585–93.

62. Coppes MJ, Campbell CE, Williams BRG. The role of WT1 in Wilms tumorigenesis. *FASEB J* 1993; 7: 886–95.

63. al-Sheyyab M, Muir KR, Cameron AH, Raafat F, Pincott JR, Parkes SE et al. Malignant epithelial tumours in children: Incidence and etiology. *Med Pediatr Oncol* 1993; 21(6): 421–8.

64. Berbel TO, Ortega Garcia JA, Tortajada J, Garcia CJ, Colomer J, Soldin OP et al. [Neonatal tumours and congenital malformations]. *An Pediatr (Barc)* 2008 June; 68(6): 589–95.

65. Munzer C, Menegaux F, Lacour B, Valteau-Couanet D, Michon J, Coze C et al. Birth-related characteristics, congenital malformation, maternal reproductive history and neuroblastoma: The ESCALE study (SFCE). *Int J Cancer* 2008; 122(10): 2315–21.

66. Hanson MA, Gluckman PD. Developmental origins of health and disease: New insights. *Basic Clin Pharmacol Toxicol* 2008 February; 102(2): 90–3.

67. Moore SW. Developmental genes and cancer in children. *Pediatr Blood Cancer* 2009 July; 52(7): 755–60.

68. Areci R. Mechanisms of epigenetic programming regulating normal and neoplastic growth and development. *Pediatr Blood Cancer Abstr* 2009; S.021: 707.

69. Hanson MA, Gluckman PD. Developmental origins of health and disease: New insights. *Basic Clin Pharmacol Toxicol* 2008 February; 102(2): 90–3.

70. Godschalk RW, Kleinjans JC. Characterization of the exposure-disease continuum in neonates of mothers exposed to carcinogens during pregnancy. *Basic Clin Pharmacol Toxicol* 2008 February; 102(2): 109–17.

71. Doll R, Wakeford R. Risks of childhood cancer from fetal irradiation. *Br J Radiol* 1997; 70: 130–9.

72. Sikov MR. Tumour development following internal radionuclides during the perinatal period. *IARC Sci Publ* 1989; 96: 403–19.

73. Kemp CJ, Wheldon T, Balmai A. p53-deficient mice are extremely susceptible to radiation-induced tumorigenesis. *Nat Genet* 1994 September; 8(1): 66–9.

74. Grandjean P, Bellinger D, Bergman A, Cordier S, vey-Smith G, Eskenazi B et al. The faroes statement: Human health effects of developmental exposure to chemicals in our environment. *Basic Clin Pharmacol Toxicol* 2008 February; 102(2): 73–5.

75. Sherman S, Roisen N. Fetal hydantoin syndrome and neuroblastoma. *Lancet* 1976; ii: 517.

76. Worsham F Jr, Beckman EN, Mitchell EH. Sacrococcygeal teratoma in a neonate. Association with maternal use of acetazolamide. *JAMA* 1978; 240(3): 251–2.

77. Satgé D, Sasco AJ, Little J. Antenatal therapeutic drug exposure and fetal/neonatal tumours: Review of 89 cases. *Pediatr Perinat Epidemiol* 1998; 12: 84–117.

78. Passmore SJ, Draper G, Brownbil P, Kroll M. Ecological studies of relation between hospital policies on neonatal vitamin K administration and subsequent occurrence of childhood cancer. *BMJ* 1998; 316(7126): 184–9.

79. Schuz J, Kaatch P, Kaletsch U, Meinert R, Michaelis J. Association of childhood cancer with factors related to pregnancy and birth. *Int J Epidemiol* 1999; 28(4): 631–9.

80. Yang J, Zhao JJ, Zhu Y, Xiong W, Lin JY, Ma X. Identification of candidate cancer genes involved in human retinoblastoma by data mining. *Childs Nerv Syst* 2008 March 19; 24(8): 893–900.

81. Tuchman M, Lemineieux B, Auray Blis C, Robison LL, Giguere R, McCann MT et al. Screening for neuroblastoma at 3 weeks of age: Methods and preliminary results from the Quebec neuroblastoma screening project. *Pediatrics* 1990; 86: 765–73.

82. Breit S, Ashman K, Wilting J, Rossler J, Hatzi E, Fotsis T et al. The N-myc oncogene in human neuroblastoma cells: Down-regulation of an angiogenesis inhibitor identified as activin A. *Cancer Res* 2000; 60(16): 4596–601.

83. Cowell JK, Rupniak HT. Chromosome analysis of human neuroblastoma cell line TR14 showing double minutes and an aberration involving chromosome 1. *Cancer Genet Cytogenet* 1983 July; 9(3): 273–80.

84. George RE, Attiyeh EF, Li S, Moreau LA, Neuberg D, Li C et al. Genome-wide analysis of neuroblastomas using high-density single nucleotide polymorphism arrays. *PLoS ONE* 2007; 2(2): e255.

85. Woods WG, Lemieux B, Tuchman M. Neuroblastoma represents distinct clinical-biologic entities: A review and perspective from the Quebec Neuroblastoma screening project. *Pediatrics* 1992; 89: 114–8.

86. Brodeur GM, Seeger RC, Schwab M, Varmus, HE, Bishop, JM Amplification of n-myc in untreated human neuroblastomas correlates with advanced disease state. *Science* 1984; 224: 1121–4.

87. Liu X, Mazanek P, Dam V, Wang Q, Zhao H, Guo R et al. Deregulated Wnt/beta-catenin program in high-risk neuroblastomas without MYCN amplification. *Oncogene* 2007; 27(10): 1478–88.

88. Eggert A, Grotzer MA, Ikegaki N, Liu XG, Evans AE, Brodeur GM. Expression of neurotrophin receptor TrkA inhibits angiogenesis in neuroblastoma. *Med Pediatr Oncol* 2000 December; 35(6): 569–72.

89. Vogan K, Bernstein M, Leclerc JM, Brisson L, Brossard J, Brodeur GM et al. Absence of p53 gene mutations in primary neuroblastomas. *Cancer Res* 1993; 53(21): 5269–73.

90. Brodeur GM, Bagatell R. Mechanisms of neuroblastoma regression. *Nat Rev Clin Oncol* 2014; 11(12): 704–13.

91. Illmensee K, Stevens LC. Teratomas and chimeras. *Sci Am* 1979 April; 240(4): 120–32.

92. Ashcraft KW, Holder TM. Hereditary presacral teratoma. *J Pediatr Surg* 1974 October; 9(5): 691–7.

93. Lynch SA, Bond PM, Copp AJ, Kirwan WO, Nour S, Balling R et al. A gene for autosomal dominant sacral agenesis maps to the holoprosencephaly region at 7q36. *Nat Genet* 1995; 11(1): 93–5.

94. Froberg MK, Brown RE, Maylock J, Poling E. In utero development of a mediastinal teratoma: A second-trimester event. *Prenat Diagn* 1994 September; 14(9): 884–7.

95. Dillon PW, Whalen TV, Azizkhan RG, Haase GM, Coran AG, King DR et al. Neonatal soft tissue sarcomas: The influence of pathology on treatment and survival. Children's Cancer Group Surgical Committee. *J Pediatr Surg* 1995 July; 30(7): 1038–41.

96. Spicer RD. Neonatal soft tissue tumours. *Br J Cancer Suppl* 1992 August; 18: S80–3.

97. Azizkhan RC. Neonatal tumours. In: Carachi R, Azmy A, Grosfeld JL (eds). *The Surgery of Childhood Tumours*, 1st edn. London: Arnold, 1999: 107–23.

98. Douglass EC, Valentine M, Etcubanas E, Parham D, Webber BL, Houghton PJ et al. A specific chromosomal abnormality in rhabdomyosarcoma. *Cytogenet Cell Genet* 1987; 45(3–4): 148–55.

99. Shapiro DN, Parham DM, Douglass EC, Ashmun R, Webber BL, Newton WA Jr et al. Relationship of tumor-cell ploidy to histologic subtype and treatment outcome in children and adolescents with unresectable rhabdomyosarcoma. *J Clin Oncol* 1991 January; 9(1): 159–66.

100 Barr FG. The role of chimeric paired box transcription factors in the pathogenesis of pediatric rhabdomyosarcoma. *Cancer Res* 1999; 59(7 Suppl): 1711s–5s.

101. Bridge JA, Liu J, Weibolt V, Baker KS, Perry D, Kruger R et al. Novel genomic imbalances in embryonal rhabdomyosarcoma revealed by comparative genomic hybridization and fluorescence in situ hybridization: An intergroup rhabdomyosarcoma study. *Genes Chromosomes Cancer* 2000 April; 27(4): 337–44.

102. Steenman MJ, Zijlstra N, Kruitbosch DL, Wiesmeijer C, Larizza L, Voute PA et al. Delineation and physical separation of novel translocation breakpoints on chromosome 1p in two genetically closely associated childhood tumors. *Cytogenet Cell Genet* 2000; 88(3–4): 289–95.

103. Helman LJ, Thiele CJ. New insights into the causes of cancer. *Pediatr Clin North Am* 1991 April; 38(2): 201–21.

104. Smith AC, Squire JA, Thorner P, Zielenska M, Shuman C, Grant R et al. Association of alveolar rhabdomyosarcoma with Beckwith–Wiedemann syndrome. *Pediatr Dev Pathol* 2001; 4: 550–8.

105. Weksberg R, Shuman C, Beckwith JB. Beckwith–Wiedemann syndrome. *Eur J Hum Genet* 2009; E-published June 24, 2009.

106. DeBaun MR, Niemitz EL, McNeil DE, Brandenburg SA, Lee MP, Feinberg AP. Epigenetic alterations of H19 and LIT1 distinguish patients with Beckwith–Wiedemann syndrome with cancer and birth defects. *Am J Hum Genet* 2002 March; 70(3): 604–11.

107. Jorgensen HF, Giadrossi S, Casanova M, Endoh M, Koseki H, Brockdorff N et al. Stem cells primed for action: Polycomb repressive complexes restrain the expression of lineage-specific regulators in embryonic stem cells. *Cell Cycle* 2006 July; 5(13): 1411–4.

108. Hu HM, Zielinska-Kwiatkowska A, Munro K, Wilcox J, Wu DY, Yang L et al. EWS/FLI1 suppresses retinoblastoma protein function and senescence in Ewing's sarcoma cells. *J Orthop Res* 2008; 26(6): 886–93.

109. Feusner J, Plaschkes J. Hepatoblastoma and low birth weight: A trend or chance observation? *Med Pediatr Oncol* 2002 November; 39(5): 508–9.

110. Giardiello FM, Petersen GM, Brensinger JD, Luce MC, Cayouette MC, Bacon J et al. Hepatoblastoma and APC gene mutation in familial adenomatous polyposis. *Gut* 1996 December; 39(6): 867–9.

111. Li X, Zhao X. Epigenetic regulation of mammalian stem cells. *Stem Cells Dev* 2008; 17(6): 1043–52.

112. Ammann RA, Plaschkes J, Leibundgut K. Congenital hepatoblastoma: A distinct entity? *Med Pediatr Oncol* 1999; 32(6): 466–8.

113. Endo EG, Walton DS, Albert DM. Neonatal hepatoblastoma metastatic to the choroid and iris. *Arch Ophthalmol* 1996 June; 114(6): 757–61.

114. Doss BJ, Vicari J, Jacques SM, Qureshi F. Placental involvement in congenital hepatoblastoma. *Pediatr Dev Pathol* 1998 November; 1(6): 538–42.

115. Purcell R, Childs M, Maibach R, Miles C, Turner C, Zimmermann A et al. HGF/c-Met related activation of beta-catenin in hepatoblastoma. *J Exp Clin Cancer Res* 2011; 30: 96.

116. Hohenstein P, Pritchard-Jones K, Charlton J. The yin and yang of kidney development and Wilms' tumors. *Genes Dev* 2015 March 1; 29(5): 467–82.

117. Call K, Glaser T, Ito C, Buckler A, Pelletier A, Haber D et al. Isolation and characterization of a zinc finger polypeptide gene at the human chromosome 11 Wilms tumour locus. *Cell* 1990; 60: 509–20.

118. Knudson A, Strong L. Mutation and cancer: A model for Wilms tumour of the kidney. *J Natl Cancer Inst* 1972; 48: 313–24.

119. Mulvihill JJ. Clinical ecogenetics—Cancer in families. *N Eng J Med* 2005; 312: 1569–70.

120. Orkin SH, Goldman DS, Sallan SE. Development of homozygosity for chromosome 11p markers in Wilms' tumour. Nature 1984; 309 (5964): 172–4.

121. Ruteshouser EC, Robinson SM, Huff V. Wilms tumor genetics: Mutations in WT1, WTX, and CTNNB1 account for only about one-third of tumors. *Genes Chromosomes Cancer* 2008 June; 47(6): 461–70.

122. Steinberg R, Freud E, Zer M, Ziperman I, Goshen Y, Ash S et al. High frequency of loss of heterozygosity for 1p35-p36 (D1S247) in Wilms tumor. *Cancer Genet Cytogenet* 2000 March; 117(2): 136–9.

123. Madden SL, Cook, DM, Morris, JF, Gashler, A, Sukhatme, VP, Rauscher, FJ. III. Transcriptional repression mediated by the WT1 Wilms tumor gene product Science 1991; 253(5027): 1550–3.

124. Koesters R, Niggli F, von Knebel Doeberitz M, Stallmach T. Nuclear accumulation of beta-catenin protein in Wilms' tumours. *J Pathol* 2003 January; 199(1): 68–76.

125. Maiti S, Alam R, Amos CI, Huff V. Frequent association of beta-catenin and WT1 mutations in Wilms tumors. *Cancer Res* 2000; 60(22): 6288–92.

126. Williams RD, Chagtai T, caide-German M, Apps J, Wegert J, Popov S et al. Multiple mechanisms of MYCN dysregulation in Wilms tumour. *Oncotarget* 2015 March 30; 6(9): 7232–43.

127. Scharnhorst V, Dekker P, van der Eb AJ, Jochemsen AG. Physical interaction between Wilms tumor 1 and p73 proteins modulates their functions. *J Biol Chem* 2000; 275(14): 10202–11.

128. Chao LY, Huff V, Strong LC, Saunders GF. Mutation in the PAX6 gene in twenty patients with aniridia. *Hum Mutat* 2000; 15(4): 332–9.

129. O'Connor PM, Jackman J, Jondle D, Bhatia K, Magrath I, Kohn KW. Role of the p53 tumor suppressor gene in cell cycle arrest and radiosensitivity of Burkitt's lymphoma cell lines. *Cancer Res* 1993; 53(20): 4776–80.

130. Jaffe N. Late effects of treatment (skeletal, genetic, central nervous system and oncogenic). *Pediatr Clin N Am* 1976; 23: 225–44.

131. Littman P, D'Angio GJ. Radiation therapy in the neonate. *Am J Pediatr Hematol Oncol* 1981; 3: 279–85.

132. Siegel SE, Moran RG. Problems of chemotherapy of cancer of the neonate. *Am J Hematol Oncol* 1981; 3: 287–96.

85

Hemangiomas and vascular malformations

BELINDA HSI DICKIE, ARIN K. GREENE, AND STEVEN J. FISHMAN

INTRODUCTION

Vascular anomalies are disorders of the endothelium that usually present during childhood. These lesions affect all parts of the vasculature: capillaries, veins, arteries, or lymphatics. Although nearly always benign, vascular anomalies may involve any location. In addition to disfigurement, local complications include obstruction, bleeding, infection, and pain. Systemic sequelae can include thrombocytopenia, pulmonary embolism, congestive heart failure, sepsis, and even death.

A biologic classification of vascular anomalies has clarified the difference between vascular anomalies based on physical findings, natural history, and cellular characteristics.[1] This classification has been expanded and adopted by the International Society for the Study of Vascular Anomalies (ISSVA).[2] Vascular anomalies are broadly divided into two groups: tumors and malformations (Table 85.1). Vascular tumors are characterized by endothelial cell proliferation (Figure 85.1). Vascular malformations, in contrast, arise from dysmorphogenesis and have normal endothelial cell turnover (Figure 85.2).

VASCULAR TUMORS

Infantile hemangioma (IH)

CLINICAL FEATURES

IH is a benign tumor of the endothelium that affects approximately 4%–5% of Caucasian infants.[1–4] It is more frequent in premature children and females (3:1 to 5:1).[5] IH typically is single (80%) and involves the head and neck (60%), trunk (25%), or extremity (15%).[3] The median age of appearance is 2 weeks, although 30%–50% of lesions are noted at birth as a telangiectatic stain or ecchymotic area.[6] IH grows faster than the rate of the child during the first 9 months of age (*proliferating phase*).[7] When IH involves the superficial dermis, it appears red. A deep hemangioma or lesion that does not have cutaneous involvement may not be appreciated initially, but the child may present at 3–4 months of age when it is large enough to cause a visible deformity. The overlying skin may have a bluish discoloration. By 9–12 months of age, the growth of IH plateaus to approximate that of the infant.[7] After 12 months of age, the tumor begins to shrink (*involuting phase*); the color fades and the lesion flattens. Involution stops in approximately 50% of children by 5 years of age (*involuted phase*).[6] After involution, one-half of children will have an abnormality: residual telangiectasias, scarring, fibrofatty residuum, redundant skin, or destroyed anatomical structures.

DIAGNOSIS

Ninety percent of IH is diagnosed by history and physical examination. If the history is unclear, confirmation of diagnosis can be made with Doppler ultrasound. IH appears as a soft-tissue mass with fast-flow, decreased arterial resistance, and increased venous drainage.[8] Further imaging is not usually required, but is obtained in complicated, internal IH, or part of a workup for associated syndromes. On MRI, IH is isointense on T1, is hyperintense on T2, and enhances during the proliferating phase.[9] Involuting IH has increased lobularity and adipose tissue; the number of vessels and flow is reduced.[9] Rarely, biopsy is indicated if malignancy is suspected or if the diagnosis remains unclear following imaging studies. Immunohistochemistry for GLUT1 (erythrocyte-type glucose transporter 1) is specifically expressed in proliferating IH and immunostaining and can differentiate IH from other lesions.[10]

CLINICAL CONSIDERATIONS

Head and neck memangiomas

Ten percent of proliferating IH cause significant deformity or complications, usually when located on the head or neck.[11] Ulcerated lesions may destroy the eyelid, ear, nose, or lip. IH of the scalp or eyebrow can result in alopecia.

Table 85.1 Biological classification of vascular anomalies

Tumors	Malformations	
	Slow flow	Fast flow
Infantile hemangioma (IH)	Capillary (CM)	Arteriovenous (AVM)
Congenital hemangioma (CH)	Venous (VM)	
Kaposiform hemangioendothelioma (KHE)	Lymphatic (LM)	
Pyogenic granuloma (PG)		

Periorbital hemangioma can block the visual axis or distort the cornea causing amblyopia. Subglottic hemangioma may obstruct the airway; tracheostomy rarely may be necessary. IH of the periorbital region, ear, and nose are treated more aggressively to prevent complications from mass effect or ulceration.

Multiple hemangiomas

Although 20% of infants will have more than one IH, occasionally a child will have five or more small (<5 mm), dome-like lesions termed *hemangiomatosis*.[6] These children are at increased risk for IH of internal organs. The liver is most commonly affected; the brain, gut, or lung are rarely involved. Ultrasonography (US) should be considered to rule out hepatic IH in patients with greater than five cutaneous hemangiomas, hepatomegaly, or any signs of shunting on physical examination.

Hepatic hemangiomas

The liver is the most common extracutaneous site for IH, which may be focal, multifocal, or diffuse (Figure 85.3).[12] Although most hepatic IH are nonproblematic and discovered incidentally, some tumors can cause heart failure, hepatomegaly, anemia, or hypothyroidism. Ninety percent of fast-flow hepatic lesions are hemangioma; arteriovenous malformation (AVM), hepatoblastoma, and metastatic neuroblastoma are less common and do not demonstrate significant shunting on imaging.[12] Focal hepatic IH usually are asymptomatic unless they have associated direct macrovascular shunts (hepatic artery to hepatic vein and/ or portal to hepatic vein). These direct shunts can lead to high-output cardiac failure. Focal hepatic lesions are not associated with cutaneous lesions. They are not typical IH, but rather the hepatic presentation of rapidly involuting congenital hemangioma (RICH).[13] Multifocal hepatic IH are typical IH, immunopositive for GLUT1, and may be associated with cutaneous lesions. Although usually asymptomatic, multifocal lesions also can have associated macrovascular shunts that can cause high-output cardiac failure. In either focal or multifocal variants, shunts may resolve with tumor involution, which in the multifocal type may be hastened pharmacologically. Embolization of

the shunts, although technically demanding, will quickly control cardiac failure.[14] Diffuse hepatic IH can cause massive hepatomegaly, respiratory compromise, or abdominal compartment syndrome. Infants also are at risk for hypothyroidism and subsequent irreversible brain injury because the tumor expresses a deiodinase, which inactivates thyroid hormone.[15] Patients require thyroid stimulating hormone monitoring and, if abnormal, thyroid replacement, often in massive doses, until the IH undergoes involution.

Lumbosacral hemangioma

Large, superficial, plaque-like, or reticular IH rarely may be associated with underlying spinal, urogenital, or anorectal malformations when it is located in the lumbosacral midline (tethered spinal cord, anorectal and genital malformations, renal anomalies, lipomyelomeningocele).[16,17] US is obtained to rule out associated spinal anomalies in infants less than 4 months of age. MRI is indicated in older infants or when US is equivocal. This constellation of anomalies is known as the PELVIS or SACRAL syndrome.[17,18]

PHACES association

PHACES association affects 2.3% of patients with IH and consists of a plaque-like IH in a "segmental" or trigeminal dermatomal distribution of the face with at least one of the following anomalies: posterior fossa brain malformation, hemangioma, arterial cerebrovascular anomalies, coarctation of the aorta and cardiac defects, eye/endocrine abnormalities, and sternal clefting or supraumbilical raphe.[19] Ninety percent of infants are female, and cerebrovascular anomalies are the most common associated finding (72%).[20] Because 8% of children with PHACES have a stroke in infancy, patients should have an MRI to evaluate the brain and cerebrovasculature.[21] Infants are referred for ophthalmologic, endocrine, and cardiac evaluation to rule out associated anomalies.[21]

NON-OPERATIVE MANAGEMENT

Most IH are managed by observation because 90% are small, are localized, and do not involve aesthetically or functionally important areas. During the proliferative phase, 16% of lesions will ulcerate; the lips, neck, and anogenital region are the most common areas to break down.[22] Other complications include bleeding and infection.[22] To reduce the risk of ulceration, the IH is kept moist during the proliferative phase with hydrated petroleum to minimize desiccation as well as to protect against incidental trauma. Using a petroleum gauze barrier or silicone pad dressing may further protect IH. If ulceration develops, it is managed with local wound care.

Beta-blockers

Until recently, the mainstay of treatment for IH was corticosteroids. However, in 2008, Labreze et al.[23] reported on improvement of hemangiomas in 11 patients after treatment

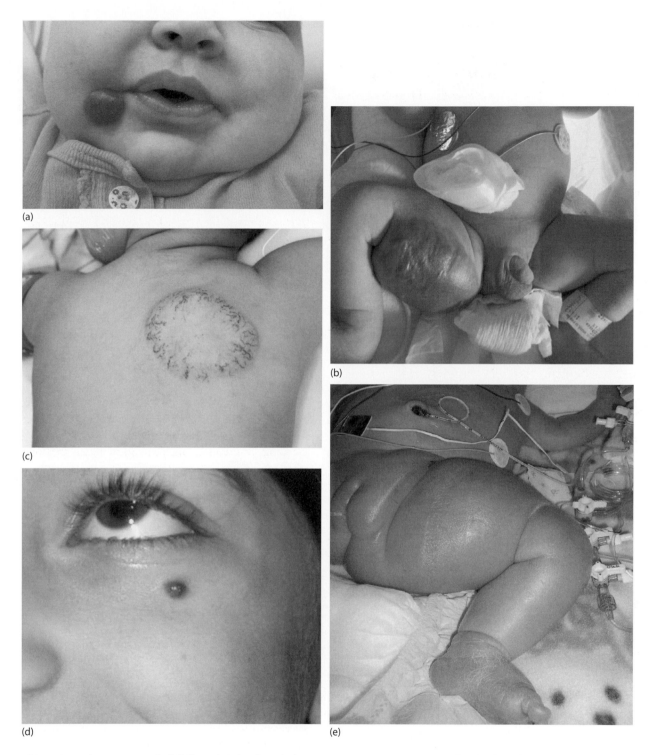

Figure 85.1 Vascular tumors of childhood. **(a)** Infantile hemangioma (IH) in a 3-month-old female. The lesion was noted 2 weeks after birth and subsequently enlarged. It was treated with corticosteroid injection. **(b)** Rapidly involuting congenital hemangioma (RICH) in a 3-week-old male. The lesion was fully grown at birth and rapidly involuted over the first year of life. **(c)** Non-involuting congenital hemangioma (NICH) in a 2.5-year-old male; the vascular mass had not changed since birth. **(d)** Pyogenic granuloma in an 8-year-old female with a 3-month history of a bleeding lesion. **(e)** Kaposiform hemangioendothelioma (KHE) in a 5-week-old neonate treated with vincristine.

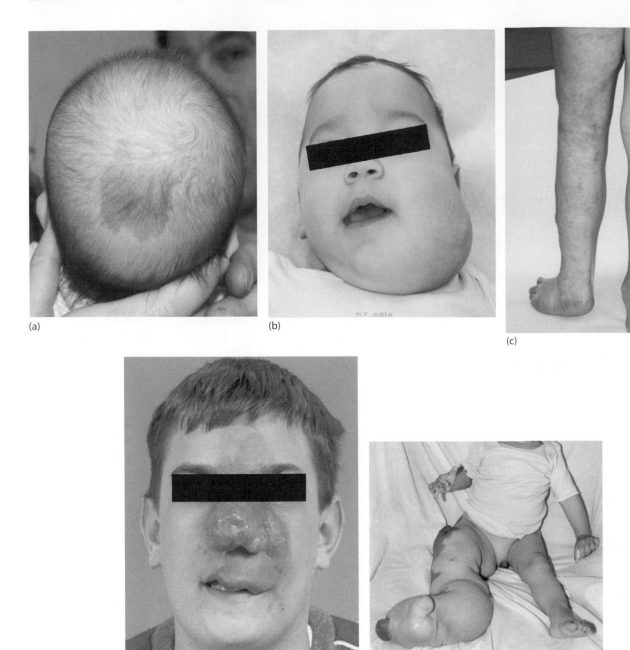

Figure 85.2 Vascular malformations of childhood. **(a)** Capillary malformation (CM) of the scalp of a 2-month-old female. **(b)** 7-month-old female with a macrocystic lymphatic malformation (LM) of the right face treated with sclerotherapy. **(c)** 7-year-old female with a diffuse venous malformation (VM) of the right lower extremity managed with compression stockings. **(d)** 16-year-old male with an arteriovenous malformation (AVM). **(e)** 1-year-old female with a combined capillary–lymphatic–venous malformation (CLVM) of the right lower extremity with overgrowth (Klippel–Trenaunay syndrome).

with propranolol. Since that time, there have been multiple published reports on the efficacy of β-blockers on the treatment of IH.[24]

Although the exact mechanism of action of β-blocker is not established, it is hypothesized that it works on vasoconstriction of the vessel, inhibition of angiogenesis, and induction of apoptosis. β-Adrenergic receptors are expressed on the IH endothelial cells, especially in proliferation.[25–28]

Systemic beta-blockers

Oral beta-blockers are usually started at a low dose and escalated. The most commonly used β-blocker is propranolol, and treatment dose is 2–3 mg/kg/day divided into two or three times a day dosing. On more complicated lesions, or diffuse or multifocal liver lesions, the dose is increased to 3 mg/kg/day. In our institution, baseline ECG is obtained and if clinically indicated, an ECHO is also done, prior to

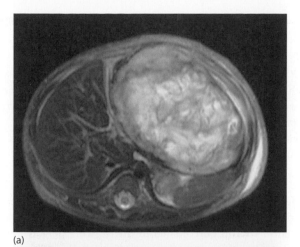

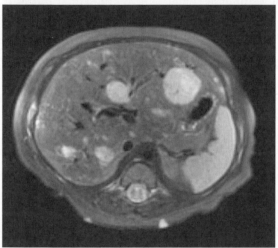

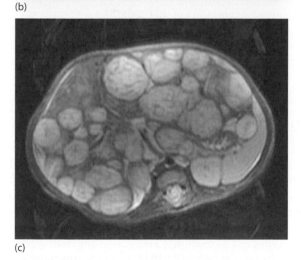

Figure 85.3 Types of hepatic hemangioma in infancy. Axial T2 MRI showing three patients with focal **(a)**, multifocal **(b)**, and diffuse **(c)** hepatic hemangiomas.

initiation of β-blockers. Infants younger than 1 month of age are monitored as inpatients on telemetry during escalation of dosage, whereas older infants are started in the outpatient setting. Heart rate, blood pressure, and blood glucose levels are monitored for 3–4 hours after the oral dose. Effect on the IH can be seen within days of initiation of the propranolol. Duration of therapy is usually determined by the response of the IH. To prevent any rebound growth, propranolol is continued until the IH is in the involutional phase.

Side effects of the β-blockers are minimal, but there are reports of hypoglycemia, diarrhea, and increased reflux.

Topical beta-blockers

For superficial hemangiomas, topical application of beta blockers can be used two to three times a day. Although there is some systemic absorption, it is not as effective on deep hemangiomas. Topical beta-blockers may result in lightening of the lesion and prevent further growth of the IH.[29]

Corticosteroids

Previously the first line of medical management of IH, corticosteroids, are now used less frequently due to the side effects. On complicated airway, periorbital, diffuse liver lesions, systemic steroids may be used in conjunction with β-blockers.

Systemic corticosteroid

Corticosteroid has been used to treat IH for over 40 years and has proven to be very safe and effective.[30–33] Overall, 84% of patients treated with different doses of corticosteroid will have (1) stabilization of growth or (2) accelerated regression.[32] Almost all patients, however, will respond to 3 mg/kg/day.[32]

Complications of systemic corticosteroid for the management of IH have been studied, and no adverse effects on neurodevelopment have been found.[33] Short-term morbidity includes cushingoid face (71%), personality change (29%), gastric irritation (21%), fungal (oral or perineal) infection (6%), myopathy (1%), decreased gain in height (35%), and decreased gain in weight (43%).[31] These findings resolve after the completion of therapy. Long-term complications of corticosteroid such as aseptic necrosis of the femoral head, diabetes, osteoporosis, long-term adrenal insufficiency, cataracts, and glaucoma have not been noted in patients treated with corticosteroid for IH.[31,34,35]

Topical corticosteroid

Topical corticosteroid has minimal efficacy, especially against IH involving the deep dermis and subcutis. Ultrapotent agents may be effective for small, superficial IH; however, their efficacy is inferior to intralesional corticosteroid. Although lightening may occur, if an underlying mass is present, it likely will not be affected.[36] Adverse effects include hypopigmentation, skin atrophy, and possible adrenal suppression.

Intralesional corticosteroid

Small, well-localized IHs that obstruct the visual axis or nasal airway, or those at risk for damaging aesthetically sensitive structures (i.e., eyelid, lip, nose), are best managed by intralesional corticosteroid. Triamcinolone (3 mg/kg) stabilizes the growth of the lesion in at least 95% of patients, and 75% of tumors will decrease in size.[37] The corticosteroid lasts 4–6 weeks, and thus, infants may require additional injections during the proliferative phase. Intralesional corticosteroid may cause subcutaneous fat atrophy. Blindness has been reported following injection of periorbital hemangioma, possibly due to embolic occlusion of the retinal artery.[38,39]

Embolic therapy

High-output congestive heart failure may be caused by macrovascular shunts seen with focal or multifocal hepatic lesions, or very rarely large nonhepatic IH. Embolization may be indicated for the initial control of heart failure, while the therapeutic effects of systemic corticosteroid are pending. Cardiac failure can recur even after initial improvement, and continued drug therapy after embolization may be indicated until the child is approximately 12 months of age when natural involution begins.

Laser therapy

Pulsed-dye laser treatment for proliferating IH is contraindicated. The laser penetrates only 0.75–1.2 mm into the dermis and thus only affects the superficial portion of the IH. Although lightening may occur, the mass of IH is not affected and accelerated involution does not occur.[40,41] Instead, patients have an increased risk of skin atrophy and hypopigmentation.[41] The thermal injury delivered by the laser to the ischemic dermis increases the risk of ulceration, pain, bleeding, and scarring.[42] The pulsed-dye laser is indicated, however, during the involuted phase to treat residual telangiectasias. Destructive laser therapy may be useful in airway hemangioma to avoid tracheostomy while awaiting successful response to pharmacotherapy.

OPERATIVE MANAGEMENT

Proliferative phase (infancy)

Operative treatment in infancy generally is not recommended. The tumor is highly vascular during this period, and the patient is at risk for blood loss, iatrogenic injury, and an inferior aesthetic outcome, compared to excising residual tissue after the tumor has regressed. Factors that lower the threshold for resection of a problematic proliferating IH include the following: (1) failure or contraindication to corticosteroid, (2) well localized in an anatomically safe area, (3) complicated reconstruction is not required, and (4) resection will be necessary in the future and the scar will be the same. Circular lesions located in visible areas, particularly the face, are best treated by circular excision and purse-string closure.[43] This technique minimizes the length of the scar as well as distortion of surrounding structures. A lenticular excision of a circular hemangioma will result in a scar as long as three times the diameter of the lesion, while a two-stage circular resection followed by lenticular excision 6–12 months later will leave a scar of approximately the same length as the diameter of the original hemangioma.[43]

Involuting phase (early childhood)

While operative management of IH generally is avoided during the proliferative phase, resection during involution is much safer because the lesion is less vascular and smaller. Because the extent of the excision and reconstruction is reduced, the aesthetic outcome is superior. Approximately 50% of IH leave behind fibrofatty tissue or damaged skin after the tumor regresses, causing a deformity.[6] Less often, children require reconstruction of damaged structures (i.e., nose, ear, lip). Staged or total excision should be considered during this period, rather than waiting for complete involution, if (1) it is clear that the patient will require resection (i.e., post-ulceration scarring, destroyed structures, expanded skin, significant fibrofatty residuum), (2) the length of the scar would be similar if the procedure was postponed to the involuted phase, or (3) the scar is in a favorable location. An advantage of operative intervention during this period, compared to late childhood, is that reconstruction is performed prior to the child's development of memory or awareness of body differences.

Involuted phase (late childhood)

Waiting until IH has fully involuted prior to resection ensures that the least amount of fibrofatty residuum and excess skin is resected, giving the smallest possible scar. Allowing full involution to occur, however, must be weighed against the psychosocial morbidity of maintaining a deformity until late childhood. Allowing full involution is advocated for lesions when it is unclear if a surgical scar would leave a worse deformity than the appearance of the residual hemangioma.

CONGENITAL HEMANGIOMA (CH)

CLINICAL FEATURES

CH is fully grown at birth and does not illustrate postnatal growth.[44-46] CH has a different appearance than IH: it is red-violaceous with coarse telangiectasias, central pallor, and a peripheral pale halo. Unlike IH, CH is more common in the extremities, has an equal sex distribution, and is almost always solitary with an average diameter of 5 cm.[44-46] Two types of CH exist: RICH and non-involuting congenital hemangioma (NICH). RICH involutes rapidly after birth and 50% of lesions have completed regression by 7 months of age.[44,46] RICH affects the head or neck (42%), limbs (52%), or trunk (6%).[44-46] RICH does not leave behind a significant adipose component, unlike IH.[46] NICH, in contrast, does not undergo involution.[42] It involves the head or neck (43%), limbs (38%), or trunk (19%).[45]

MANAGEMENT

RICH does not require operative management in infancy because it undergoes accelerated regression and is observed.

Occasionally, RICH is complicated by congestive heart failure, which is treated by beta-blockers, corticosteroid, or embolization as the lesion involutes. Since RICH undergoes such rapid natural involution, it is not clear whether the β-blockers or corticosteroid hastens involution. After regression, RICH may cause a residual deformity, usually atrophic skin and subcutaneous tissue. Operative intervention for RICH must not create a more obvious deformity than the lesion. Reconstruction with autologous grafts (fat, dermis) or acellular dermis may be indicated. NICH is rarely problematic in infancy and is observed. Because NICH is benign, asymptomatic tumors do not require excision. Symptomatic lesions in infancy are managed with embolization or resection. Resection may be indicated to improve the appearance of the affected area, as long as the surgical scar is less noticeable than the lesion. After long-term follow-up, some of these lesions are associated with pain and undergo excision at an older age. Pulse-dye laser therapy may improve the late appearance of CH by eliminating telangiectasias.

Kaposiform hemangioendothelioma

CLINICAL FEATURES

Kaposiform hemangioendothelioma (KHE) is a rare vascular neoplasm that is locally aggressive but does not metastasize.[47,48] Although one-half of lesions are present at birth, KHE may develop during infancy (58%), between age 1 and 10 years (32%), or after 11 years of age (10%).[46] KHE has an equal sex distribution, is solitary, and affects the head/neck (40%), trunk (30%), or extremity (30%).[49] The tumor is often greater than 5 cm in diameter, and thus larger than the typical IH.[48] KHE causes a visible deformity as well as pain. In addition, 50% of patients have Kassabach–Merrit phenomenon (KMP) (thrombocytopenia <25,000/mm^3, petechiae, bleeding).[47,48] KHE partially regresses after 2 years of age, although it usually persists long-term causing chronic pain and stiffness.

DIAGNOSIS

KHE is diagnosed by history and physical examination. Unlike IH, it is usually present at birth as a flat, reddish-purple, edematous lesion that does not exhibit rapid postnatal growth; it is also associated with KMP. MRI is indicated for diagnostic confirmation or to evaluate the extent of the tumor. MRI shows poorly defined margins, small vessels, and invasion of adjacent tissues.[9] KHE shows T2 hyperintensity and postgadolinium enhancement; signal voids also may be present.[9] Histologically, KHE has infiltrating sheets or nodules of endothelial cells lining capillaries.[47] Hemosiderin-filled slit-like vascular spaces with red blood cell fragments, as well as dilated lymphatics, are present.[44]

MANAGEMENT

Most lesions are large and involve multiple tissues preventing complete extirpation. Patients with KMP require systemic treatment to prevent life-threatening complications. Large, asymptomatic tumors are also managed with pharmacotherapy to minimize fibrosis and subsequent long-term pain and stiffness. KHE responds best to vincristine (90%), which is first-line therapy.[50] Recently, sirolimus, an mTOR inhibitor, has shown to be efficacious in the treatment of KHE lesions.[51] Studies comparing vincristine to sirolimus for effectiveness of treatment are ongoing. KHE does not respond as well to second-line drugs, interferon (50%) or corticosteroid (10%).[48,50] Thrombocytopenia will not be significantly improved with platelet transfusion because the platelets are trapped in the lesion. Transfusion can worsen swelling and should be avoided unless there is active bleeding or a surgical procedure is planned. By 2 years of age, the tumor often undergoes partial involution and the platelet count normalizes. Excision rarely may be indicated for symptomatic patients with well-localized lesions or who have failed chemotherapy. Resection is not required for large lesions that are not causing functional problems because KHE is benign. The risks of the resection and the resulting deformity should be weighed against the appearance of the tumor.

Pyogenic granuloma

Pyogenic granuloma (PG) has been called *lobular capillary hemangioma*.[52] PG is a solitary, red papule that grows rapidly, forming a stalk. It is small, with an average diameter of 6.5 mm; the mean age of onset is 6.7 years.[53] The male/female ratio is 2:1. PG is commonly complicated by bleeding (64.2%) and ulceration (36.3%). It primarily involves the skin (88.2%), but can involve mucous membranes as well (11.8%). PG is distributed on the head or neck (62%), trunk (19%), upper extremities (13%), or lower extremities (5%). Within the head and neck, affected sites include cheek (28.8%), oral cavity (13.5%), scalp (10.8%), forehead (9.9%), eyelids (9.0%), or lips (9.0%).[53] PG should be treated after diagnosis to prevent likely ulceration and bleeding. Numerous treatment methods have been described for PG: curettage, shave excision, laser therapy, or excision. Because the lesion can involve the reticular dermis, it may be out of the reach of the pulsed-dye laser, cautery, or shave excision. Consequently, these modalities have a recurrence rate of 43.5%.[53] Definitive treatment requires full-thickness skin excision.

VASCULAR MALFORMATIONS

Capillary malformation

CLINICAL FEATURES

Capillary malformation (CM) consists of dilated capillaries in the superficial dermis. CM is most often solitary, but can be small or extensive. It may occur in any location and over time darkens and develops fibrovascular overgrowth. It can be associated with soft tissue and skeletal hypertrophy. Sturge–Weber Syndrome consists of CM in the ophthalmic (V1) trigeminal dermatome associated with ipsilateral ocular and leptomeningeal vascular anomalies.[54] Leptomeningeal anomalies can lead to seizures, contralateral hemiplegia, and delayed motion and cognition. Patients are at risk for retinal detachment and glaucoma and should be followed by an ophthalmologist.[6]

MANAGEMENT

Pulse-dye laser (585 nm) therapy can improve the appearance of CM by lightening the color; the head and neck region has a better response compared to the extremities.[55] Outcome also is superior for smaller lesions and those treated at a younger age.[56] Fifteen percent of patients achieve at least 90% lightening, 65% improve 50%–90%, and 20% respond poorly.[57] Multiple treatments, spaced 6 weeks apart, are often required until the CM fails to improve with additional treatments. After laser treatment, CM often redarkens over time.[58] CM also can be associated with soft-tissue and skeletal overgrowth.[54] Enlargement of the maxilla or mandible can result in an occlusal cant and malocclusion. CM of the trunk or extremity may be associated with fatty overgrowth causing asymmetry. Because overgrowth may be progressive, most patients do not require contouring, usually labial, until adolescence or adulthood. Malocclusion may be corrected in adolescence with orthodontic manipulation. If orthodontics is insufficient, an orthognathic procedure is considered when the jaws are completely grown. Severe cutaneous thickening and cobblestoning can be resected and reconstructed by linear closure, skin grafts, or local flaps. Facial asymmetry caused by overgrowth of the zygoma, maxilla, or mandible can be improved by contour burring.

LYMPHATIC MALFORMATION

CLINICAL FEATURES

Lymphatic malformation (LM) results from an error in the embryonic development of the lymphatic system. LM is characterized by the size of the malformed channels: microcystic, macrocystic, or combined.[1,3] Macrocystic lesions are defined as cysts large enough to be treated by sclerotherapy.[59] Because the lymphatic and venous systems share a common embryological origin, lymphatic-venous malformation (LVM) also can occur. LM is usually noted at birth or within the first 2 years of life. It is most commonly located on the head and neck; other frequent sites include the axilla, chest, and perineum. Lesions are soft and compressible. The overlying skin may be normal, have a bluish hue, or contain pink-red vesicles.

LM typically causes a deformity and psychosocial morbidity, especially when it involves the head and neck. The two most common complications associated with LM are bleeding and infection. Intralesional bleeding occurs in up to 35% of lesions causing bluish discoloration, pain, or swelling.[60] Infection complicates as many as 71% of LMs and can progress rapidly to sepsis.[60] Cutaneous vesicles can

bleed and cause malodorous drainage as well as wounds. Swelling due to bleeding, localized infection, or systemic illness may obstruct vital structures. Two-thirds of patients with extensive cervicofacial LM require tracheostomy to maintain the airway.[60] Secondary bony overgrowth is another complication; the mandible is most commonly involved and patients can develop a malocclusion. Jaw contouring or orthognathic procedures may be required.[60] Oral lesions can cause macroglossia bleeding, pain, poor oral hygiene, and caries.[61] Thoracic or abdominal LM may lead to pleural, pericardial, or peritoneal chylous effusions. Periorbital LM leads to a permanent reduction in vision (40%), and 7% become blind in the affected eye.[62] LM may be diffuse or multifocal; patients can have splenic or osteolytic bone lesions.

DIAGNOSIS

Ninety percent of LM are diagnosed by history and physical examination.[1,3] Small, superficial lesions do not require further diagnostic workup. Large or deep lesions are evaluated by MRI to (1) confirm the diagnosis, (2) define the extent of the malformation, and (3) plan treatment. LM appears as a cystic lesion (macrocystic, microcystic, or combined) with septations of variable thickness.[63] It is hyperintense on T2-weighted sequences and does not show diffuse enhancement.[63] Although US is not as accurate as MRI, it may provide diagnostic confirmation or document intralesional bleeding. US findings for macrocystic LM include anechoic cysts with internal septations, often with debris or fluid–fluid levels.[63] Microcystic LM has ill-defined echogenic masses with diffuse involvement of adjacent tissues. Histological confirmation of LM is rarely necessary. LM shows abnormally walled vascular spaces with eosinophilic, protein-rich fluid, and collections of lymphocytes.[64] Immunostaining with the lymphatic markers D2-40 and LYVE-1 are positive.[64]

MANAGEMENT

LM is a benign condition and intervention is not mandatory; small or asymptomatic lesions may be observed. An infected LM often cannot be controlled with oral antibiotics, and intravenous antimicrobial therapy usually is required. Intervention for LM is reserved for symptomatic lesions that cause pain and significant deformity, or threaten vital structures.

Sclerotherapy

Sclerotherapy is first-line management for large or problematic macrocystic/combined LM. It involves aspiration of cysts followed by the injection of an inflammatory substance that causes scarring of the cyst walls to each other. Sclerotherapy has superior efficacy and a lower complication rate than resection.[65] Resection of macrocystic LM generally is not necessary unless (1) the lesion is symptomatic and sclerotherapy is no longer possible because all of the macrocysts have been treated, (2) resection may be curative because the lesion is small and well localized, or (3) the lesion is so massive or has a large microcystic component such that a significant mass will remain after sclerotherapy.

Several scleroscents may be used to treat LM: doxycycline, sodium tetradecyl sulfate (STS), ethanol, bleomycin, and OK-432. We prefer doxycycline because it is very effective (83% reduction in size) and safe (less than 10% risk of skin ulceration).[63,66] STS is our second-line agent. Ethanol is an effective scleroscent but has the highest complication rate. It can be used for small lesions, but large volumes should be avoided to reduce the risk of local and systemic toxicity. Ethanol can injure nerves and thus should not be used in proximity to important structures. The use of OK-432 is limited because it is not widely available in all countries.[65]

The most common complication of sclerotherapy for LM is skin ulceration (10%).[63,66] Ethanol is associated with additional systemic toxicity: CNS depression, pulmonary hypertension, hemolysis, thromboembolism, and arrhythmias.[63] Extravasation of the scleroscent into muscle can cause atrophy and contracture.[55] LM often re-expands over time; 9% recur within 3 years following OK-432 treatment, and most will re-expand with longer follow-up.[65,67] Consequently, patients often need repeat sclerotherapy over the course of their lifetime. If a problematic LM recurs and macrocysts are no longer present in the lesion, then resection is a treatment option.

Resection

Extirpation of LM can be associated with significant morbidity: major blood loss, iatrogenic injury, and deformity.[60,61,68] For example, resection of cervicofacial LM can injure the facial nerve (76%) or hypoglossal nerve (24%).[60] Excision is usually subtotal because LM involves multiple tissue planes and important structures; "recurrence" thus is common (35–64%).[67,69] Consequently, sclerotherapy is the preferred treatment for macrocystic/combined lesions. Nonproblematic microcystic lesions can be observed. Resection is reserved for (1) symptomatic microcystic LM causing bleeding, infection, obstruction/destruction of vital structures, or significant deformity; (2) symptomatic macrocystic/combined LM that no longer can be managed with sclerotherapy because all macrocysts have been treated; and (3) small, well-localized LM (microcystic or macrocystic) that may be completely excised for cure. When considering resection, the postoperative scar/deformity following removal of the LM should be weighed against the preoperative appearance of the lesion.

For diffuse malformations, staged resection of defined anatomic areas is recommended. Subtotal resections of problematic areas, such as bleeding vesicles or an overgrown lip, should be carried out rather than an attempting "complete" excision of a benign lesion, which would result in a worse deformity than the malformation itself. Macroglossia may require tongue reduction to return the tongue to the oral cavity or to correct an open-bite deformity. Bony overgrowth is corrected by osseous contouring,

and malocclusion may require orthognathic correction, usually at the time of skeletal maturity.

Bleeding or leaking cutaneous vesicles may be managed by resection if they are localized, and the wound can be closed by direct approximation of tissues. Vesicles often recur through the scar. Large areas of vesicular bleeding or drainage are best managed by sclerotherapy or carbon dioxide laser; alternatively, wide resection and skin graft coverage are required. Microcystic vesicles involving the oral cavity respond well to radiofrequency ablation.[70] Patients and families are counseled that LM can expand following any intervention, and thus additional treatments may be required in the future.

Venous malformation

CLINICAL FEATURES

Venous malformation (VM) results from an error in vascular morphogenesis; veins are dilated with thin walls and abnormal smooth muscle.[71] Consequently, lesions expand, flow stagnates, and clotting occurs. Lesions are blue, soft, and compressible; hard calcified phleboliths may be palpable. VM may range from small, localized skin lesions to diffuse malformations involving multiple tissue planes and vital structures. VM is typically sporadic and solitary in 90% of patients; 50% have a somatic mutation in the endothelial receptor TIE2.[72,73] Sporadic VM is usually greater than 5 cm (56%), single (99%), and located on the head/neck (47%), extremities (40%), or trunk (13%).[72] Almost all lesions involve the skin, mucosa, or subcutaneous tissue; 50% also affect deeper structures (i.e., muscle, bone, joints, viscera).[72]

Approximately 10% of patients with VM have multifocal, familial lesions: either glomuvenous malformation (GVM) or cutaneomucosal VM (CMVM).[72,74] GVM is an autosomal dominant condition with abnormal smooth muscle-like glomus cells along the ectatic veins. It is caused by a loss-of-function mutation in the glomulin gene.[75] Lesions are typically multiple (70%), small (two-thirds <5 cm), and located in the skin and subcutaneous tissue; deeper structures are not affected.[72] GVM involves the extremities (76%), trunk (14%), or head/neck (10%). Lesions are more painful than typical VM. CMVM are small, multifocal mucocutaneous lesions caused by a gain-of-function mutation in the TIE2 receptor.[76] The condition is autosomal dominant and less common than GVM. Lesions are small (76% <5 cm), multiple (73%), and located on the head/neck (50%), extremity (37%), or trunk (13%).[72] Blue rubber bleb nevus syndrome (BRBNS) is a rare condition with multiple, small (<2 cm) VM involving the skin, soft tissue, and gastrointestinal tract.[77] Morbidity is associated with gastrointestinal bleeding requiring chronic blood transfusions or recurrent, usually self-limited, intussusceptions.

Complications of VM include psychosocial morbidity, pain, and swelling. Head and neck VM may present with mucosal bleeding or progressive distortion leading to airway or orbital compromise. Extremity VM can cause leg-length discrepancy, hypoplasia due to disuse atrophy, pathologic fracture, hemarthrosis, and degenerative arthritis.[68] VM of muscle may result in fibrosis and subsequent pain and disability. A large VM involving the deep venous system is at risk for thrombosis and pulmonary embolism. Gastrointestinal VM can cause bleeding and chronic anemia. Stagnation within a large VM results in a localized intravascular coagulopathy (LIC) and painful phlebothromboses.

DIAGNOSIS

At least 90% of VMs are diagnosed by history and physical examination.[1,3] Dependent positioning of the anomaly can help confirm the diagnosis; VM will enlarge because of reduced venous return. Small, superficial VMs do not require further diagnostic workup. However, large or deeper lesions are evaluated by MRI to (1) confirm the diagnosis, (2) define the extent of the malformation, and (3) plan treatment. VM is hyperintense on T2-weighted sequences.[63] In contrast to LM, VM enhances with contrast, often shows phleboliths as signal voids, and is more likely to involve muscle. US may be used for some localized lesions; findings include compressible, anechoic–hypoechoic channels separated by more solid regions of variable echogenicity.[8] Phleboliths are hyperechoic with acoustic shadowing.[63] Computerized tomography (CT) is occasionally indicated to assess osseous VM. Histological diagnosis of VM is rarely necessary, but may be indicated to rule out malignancy or if imaging is equivocal.

MANAGEMENT

Patients with large extremity lesions are prescribed custom-fitted compression garments to reduce blood stagnation in the lesion and thus the risk of expansion, LIC, phlebolith formation, and pain.[78] Patients with recurrent pain secondary to phlebothrombosis may find relief from prophylactic daily aspirin (81 mg) to prevent thrombosis. Large lesions are at risk for coagulation of stagnant blood, stimulation of thrombin, and conversion of fibrinogen to fibrin. Fibrinolysis results in LIC.[78] The chronic consumptive coagulopathy can cause either thrombosis (phleboliths) or bleeding (hemarthrosis, hematoma, intraoperative blood loss).[78] Low molecular weight heparin (LMWH) is considered for patients with significant LIC or at risk for disseminated intravascular coagulation (DIC).[78] Patients with significant coagulopathy will need prophylactic treatment with LMWH prior to any significant surgical or interventional procedure. Patients who develop a serious thrombotic event require long-term anticoagulation or a vena caval filter.

Sclerotherapy

Intervention for VM is reserved for symptomatic lesions that cause pain and deformity, or threaten vital structures. First-line treatment is sclerotherapy, which is safer and more effective than resection.[59,63,79] Diffuse malformations are managed by targeting specific symptomatic areas, because the entire lesion is too extensive to treat at one time. Sclerotherapy is continued until symptoms are alleviated or when vascular spaces are no longer present to inject. Although sclerotherapy effectively reduces the size of the lesion and improves symptoms, it does not remove the malformation. Consequently, patients may continue to have a mass or visible deformity after treatment that may be improved by resection. In addition, VM usually re-expands after sclerotherapy, and thus patients often require additional sclerotherapy treatments over the course of their lifetime.

Our preferred scleroscents are STS and ethanol; STS is most commonly used.[63] Although ethanol is more effective than STS, it has a higher complication rate. Most patients, especially children, are managed under general anesthesia using US and/or fluoroscopic imaging. The most common local complication of sclerotherapy for VM is skin ulceration (10%–15%).[59,79] Extravasation of the scleroscent into muscle can cause atrophy and contracture.[59] Post-treatment swelling may necessitate close monitoring. Systemic adverse events from sclerotherapy, including hemolysis, hemoglobinuria, and DIC, are more common if large lesions are treated. Patients with low fibrinogen levels are given LMWH 14 days before and after the procedure.[78] Anticoagulation is held for 24 hours perioperatively (12 hours before and after the intervention) to prevent bleeding complications.[63,78]

Resection

Extirpation of VM can be associated with significant morbidity: major blood loss, iatrogenic injury, and deformity. In contrast to sclerotherapy, resection is not favorable because (1) the entire lesion can rarely be removed, (2) resection may cause a worse deformity than the lesion, (3) the risk of recurrence is high because channels adjacent to the visible lesion are not treated, and (4) the risk of blood loss and iatrogenic injury is greater. Resection should be considered for (1) small, well-localized lesions that can be completely removed, (2) persistent mass or deformity after completion of sclerotherapy (patent channels are not accessible for further injection), or (3) large lesions unlikely to reduce substantially with extensive sclerotherapy. When considering resection, the postoperative scar/deformity following removal of the VM should be weighed against the preoperative appearance of the lesion. Subtotal resections of problematic areas, such as an overgrown lip, should be carried out rather than attempting "complete" excision of a benign lesion, which would result in a worse deformity than the malformation itself. Patients and families are counseled that VM can expand following excision, and thus additional operative intervention may be required in the future.

Many VMs should have sclerotherapy prior to operative intervention. After adequate sclerotherapy, the VM is replaced by scar, and thus the risk of blood loss, iatrogenic injury, and recurrence is reduced. In addition, fibrosis facilitates resection and reconstruction. Very large lesions unlikely to respond to sclerotherapy should only be resected in experienced centers as massive rapid exsanguination is to be anticipated intraoperatively. Because GVM are usually small and less amenable to sclerotherapy, first-line therapy for painful lesions often is resection. Nd:YAG photocoagulation may be an adjuvant to sclerotherapy for the management of difficult airway lesions.[80] Gastrointestinal VM with chronic bleeding, anemia, and transfusion requirements are typically managed by resection. Endoscopic banding or sclerotherapy can treat solitary lesions.[81] Multifocal lesions (i.e., BRBNS) require removal of as many lesions as possible. In the gastrointestinal tract, multiple enterotomies, instead of bowel resection, is performed to preserve bowel length.[77,81] Diffuse, problematic colorectal VM may require colectomy, anorectal mucosectomy, and endorectal pull-through.[82]

Arteriovenous malformation

CLINICAL FEATURES

AVM results from an error in vascular development during embryogenesis. An absent capillary bed causes shunting of blood directly from the arterial to venous circulation, through a fistula (direct connection of an artery to a vein) or nidus (abnormal channels bridging the feeding artery to the draining veins).[71] Genetic abnormalities cause certain types of familial AVM. Hereditary hemorrhagic telangiectasia is due to mutations in endoglin and activin receptor-like kinase 1 (ALK-1), which affect transforming growth factor-beta (TGF-β) signaling.[83] Capillary malformation–AVM (CM-AVM) results from a mutation in RASA1.[84] Patients with PTEN mutations also can develop arteriovenous anomalies.[85]

The most common sites of extracranial AVM are the head and neck, followed by the limbs, trunk, and viscera.[6] Although present at birth, AVM may not become evident until childhood. Arteriovenous shunting reduces capillary oxygen delivery causing ischemia; patients are at risk for pain, ulceration, bleeding, and congestive heart failure. AVM also may cause disfigurement, destruction of tissues, and obstruction of vital structures. AVM worsens over time and can be classified according to the Schobinger staging system (Table 85.2).[86]

Table 85.2 Schobinger staging of AVM

Stage	Clinical findings
I (quiescence)	Warm, pink-blue, shunting on Doppler
II (expansion)	Enlargement, pulsation, thrill, bruit, tortuous veins
III (destruction)	Dystrophic skin changes, ulceration, bleeding, pain
IV (decompensation)	Cardiac failure

DIAGNOSIS

Most AVMs are diagnosed by history and physical examination.[1,3] If AVM is suspected, the diagnosis should be confirmed by US with color Doppler examination showing fast flow and shunting. MRI also is obtained to (1) confirm the diagnosis, (2) determine the extent of the lesion, and (3) plan treatment. MRI shows dilated feeding arteries and draining veins, enhancement, and flow voids on T2-weighted imaging.[87] If the diagnosis remains unclear after US and MRI, angiography is performed. Angiography also is indicated if embolization or resection is planned to determine the flow dynamics of the lesion. AVM shows tortuous, dilated, arteries with venous shunting and dilated draining veins on angiogram.[87] Often, a blush illustrates the nidus of the lesion. Histopathological diagnosis of AVM is rarely necessary, but may be indicated to rule out malignancy or if imaging is equivocal.

MANAGEMENT

Because AVM is often diffuse, involving multiple tissue planes and important structures, cure is rare. The goal of treatment usually is to *control* the malformation. Intervention is focused on alleviating symptoms (i.e., bleeding, pain, ulceration), preserving vital functions (i.e., vision, mastication), and improving a visible deformity. Management options include embolization, resection, or a combination. Resection offers the best chance for long-term control, but the re-expansion rate is high and extirpation may cause a worse deformity than the malformation itself.[88]

Embolization or incomplete excision of an asymptomatic lesion may stimulate it to enlarge and become problematic. Intervention is determined by (1) the size and location of the AVM, (2) the age of the patient, and (3) Schobinger stage. Although resection of an asymptomatic Stage I AVM offers the best chance for long-term control or "cure," intervention must be individualized based on the degree of deformity that would be caused by excision and reconstruction.[88] For example, a large Stage I AVM in a non-anatomically important location (i.e., trunk, proximal extremity) may be resected without consequence, before it progresses to a higher stage where resection is more difficult, and the recurrence rate is greater.[88] Similarly, a small, well-localized AVM in a more difficult location (i.e., face, hand) may be excised for possible "cure" before it expands and complete extirpation is no longer possible.

In contrast, a large, asymptomatic AVM located in an anatomically sensitive area is best observed, especially in a young child not psychologically ready for major resection and reconstruction. First, resection and reconstruction may result in a more noticeable deformity or functional problem than the malformation itself. Second, although the recurrence rate is lower when Stage I AVM is resected, it is still high, and thus, even after major resection and reconstruction, the malformation can recur. Third, some children (17.4%) do not experience significant morbidity from their lesion long term into adulthood.[88]

Intervention for Stage II AVMs is similar to Stage I lesions. However, the threshold for treatment is lower if an enlarging lesion is causing a worsening deformity or if functional problems are expected. Stage III and IV AVMs require intervention to control pain, bleeding, ulceration, or congestive heart failure.

Embolization

Embolization involves the delivery of a substance, through a catheter to the AVM, to occlude blood flow and/or fill a vascular space. Reduced arteriovenous shunting and ischemia improve symptoms and may shrink the lesion. Embolization is used either as a preoperative adjunct to resection or as monotherapy for lesions not amenable to extirpation. Because the AVM is not removed, almost all lesions eventually will expand after treatment.[71,86-89] Stage I AVM has a lower recurrence rate than higher-staged lesions. Most recurrences occur within the first year after embolization, and in an earlier era, 98.0% re-expanded within 5 years.[88] Despite the high likelihood of re-expansion, embolization can effectively palliate an AVM by reducing its size, slowing expansion, and alleviating pain and bleeding. Preoperative embolization also reduces blood loss during extirpation. In recent years, embolization from the venous outflow approach, sometimes in combination with nidus embolization from the arterial side, has offered significantly improved outcomes. Long-term outcome data are not yet available, but there is significant optimism that this approach will allow earlier and more effective embolization.

Substances used for embolization may be liquid [n-butyl cyanoacrylate (n-BCA), ethanol, Onyx (ethylene-vinyl alcohol copolymer)] or solid [polyvinyl alcohol particles (PVA), coils]. The goal of embolization is occlusion of the nidus and proximal venous outflow.[87] The embolic material is delivered to the nidus, *not* the arterial feeding vessels. Occlusion of inflow will cause collateralization and expansion of the AVM; access to the nidus also will be blocked preventing future embolization. For preoperative embolization, temporary occlusive substances (gelfoam powder, PVA, embospheres) that undergo phagocytosis are used. Permanent liquid agents capable of permeating the nidus (ethanol, n-BCA, Onyx) are used when embolization is the primary treatment. The most frequent complication of embolization is ulceration.

Resection

Resection of AVM has a lower recurrence rate than embolization and is considered for well-localized lesions or to correct focal deformities (i.e., bleeding or ulcerated areas, labial hypertrophy).[88] Wide extirpation and reconstruction of large, diffuse AVM should be exercised with caution because (1) cure is rare and the recurrence rate is high, (2) the resulting deformity is often worse than the appearance of the malformation, and (3) resection is associated with significant blood loss, iatrogenic injury, and morbidity. When excision is planned, preoperative embolization will facilitate the procedure by reducing the size of the AVM, minimizing blood loss, and creating scar tissue to aid the dissection. Multiple embolizations, spaced 6 weeks apart, may be required prior to resection. Excision should be carried out 24–72 hours after embolization, before recannalization restores blood flow to the lesion.

Surgical margins are best determined clinically, by assessing the amount of bleeding from the wound edges.[86] Most defects can be reconstructed by advancing local skin flaps. Skin grafting ulcerated areas has a high failure rate because the underlying tissue is ischemic; excision with regional flap transfer may be required. Free-flap reconstruction permits wide resection and primary closure of complicated defects, but does not improve long-term AVM control.[68,86,88-90] Despite subtotal and presumed "complete" extirpation, most AVMs treated by resection recur.[88] The majority of recurrences occur within the first year after intervention, and 86.6% re-expand within 5 years of resection.[88] Patients and families are counseled that AVM is likely to re-expand following resection, and thus, additional treatment may be required in the future.

PTEN-ASSOCIATED VASCULAR ANOMALY

The PTEN (phosphatase and tensin homologue) gene encodes a tumor suppressor lipid phosphatase.[91] Patients with PTEN mutations have PTEN hamartoma-tumor syndrome (PHTS). This autosomal dominant condition had previously been referred to as Cowden syndrome or Bannayan–Riley–Ruvalcaba syndrome (BRRS).[85,92] Males and females are equally affected, and approximately one-half (54%) of patients have a unique fast-flow vascular anomaly with arteriovenous shunting, referred to as a PTEN-associated vascular anomaly (PTEN-AVA).[85] Unlike typical AVM, PTEN-AVA may be multifocal, is associated with ectopic adipose tissue, and has disproportionate, segmental dilation of the draining veins.[85,87] Patients with PHTS have macrocephaly, and males have penile freckling.[85] Histopathology shows skeletal muscle infiltration with adipose tissue, fibrous bands, and lymphoid aggregates. In addition, tortuous arteries with transmural muscular hyperplasia and clusters of abnormal veins with variable smooth muscle are present.[85] Genetic testing is confirmative; the mutation is associated with multiple benign and malignant tumors, which require surveillance.

Combined vascular malformations

CAPILLARY MALFORMATION–ARTERIOVENOUS MALFORMATION

The prevalence of CM-AVM is estimated to be 1 in 100,000 Caucasians.[84,93] Patients have atypical CMs that are small, multifocal, round, pinkish-red, and surrounded by a pale halo (50%).[84,93] Thirty percent of individuals also have an AVM: Parkes Weber syndrome (PWS) (12%), extracerebral AVM (11%), or intracerebral AVM (7%).[93] PWS describes a diffuse AVM of an overgrown extremity with an overlying CM.[6] PWS involves the lower extremity approximately twice as often as the upper extremity.[93] CM-AVM is an autosomal dominant condition caused by a loss-of-function mutation in the *RASA1* gene.[84] A patient presenting with multiple CMs, especially with a family history of similar lesions, should be evaluated for possible AVMs on physical examination. Because 7% of patients with CM-AVM will have an intracranial fast-flow lesion, brain MRI should be considered.[74] Exploratory imaging of other anatomical areas is not necessary because extracranial AVMs have not been found to involve the viscera.[93] Although the CM is rarely problematic, associated AVMs can cause significant morbidity.

KLIPPEL–TRENAUNAY SYNDROME

Klippel–Trenaunay syndrome (KTS) is an eponym denoting a slow-flow, capillary-lymphatico-venous malformation (CLVM) in association with soft tissue and/or skeletal overgrowth.[94] KTS affects the lower extremity in 95% of patients, the upper extremity in 5% of patients, and least commonly the trunk.[94] Leg-length discrepancy is followed by plain radiographs, and MRI is used to confirm diagnosis as well as determine the extent of the anomalies. The deep venous system is commonly malformed. The marginal vein of Servelle is often located in the lateral calf and thigh and communicates with the deep venous system.[95] Complications include thrombophlebitis (20%–45%) and pulmonary embolism (4%–24%).[96] KTS of the lower extremity can involve the pelvis causing hematuria, hematochezia, constipation, and bladder outlet obstruction. Unlike some other hemihypertrophy syndromes, patients with KTS are not at increased risk for Wilms' tumor, and screening ultrasounds are unnecessary.[97] Severe enlargement of the foot requires ray, midfoot, or Syme amputation to allow the use of footwear. Management of the VM component of KTS is conservative with compressive stockings for insufficiency and aspirin to minimize phlebothrombosis. Symptomatic varicose veins may be removed or sclerosed if a functioning deep system is present. Occasionally, sclerotherapy and surgical excision are necessary for the LM component. Staged contour resection of the extremity can be performed.

CLOVEs SYNDROME

CLOVE syndrome is an overgrowth condition associated with congenital lipomatous overgrowth, vascular malformations, and epidermal nevi in a very distinct phenotype. This cohort of patients has characteristic features of truncal lipomatous overgrowth in combination with vascular anomalies, including capillary, lymphatic, venous, and arteriovenous. In addition, deformities of the extremities include wide feet and hands, macrodactyly, and a wide sandal gap. Scoliosis and renal issues are also seen, with a potential increase risk in the development of Wilms' tumors.[98] Genetic analysis of these patients demonstrates a somatic mutation in the PI3 kinase pathway.[99]

New medical treatments

In 2011, Hammill et al. published a case series of complicated vascular lesions treated with the mTOR inhibitor sirolimus. The lesions treated included KHE and complicated lymphatic or combined lymphatico-venous malformations.[51] mTOR is found in the PI3 kinase pathway, and complicated vascular lesions, especially lymphatic lesions, have been shown to have PIK3CA mutations.[100,101] There have been multiple other case series of lymphatic and complex combined vascular malformations being treated with sirolimus resulting in improved symptoms, quality of life, and bulk of the lesion. In a recent study of 53 patients with complex vascular malformations, 85% had improvement in quality of life and a partial response in the bulk of their disease (radiologically and clinically).[102]

Other pharmacologic agents that have been used to treat complex vascular lesions include propranolol and sildenafil. Similar to hemangioma treatment, propranolol is proposed to inhibit angiogenesis and induce apoptosis. Sildenafil, alternatively, is proposed to work on vascular endothelial growth factor inhibition.[103] These agents have not achieved widespread acceptance for treating vascular anomalies.

In AVMs, doxycycline has shown some promise in stabilization of the lesion. There are also reports of improved symptoms, especially pain. Doxycycline is a nonspecific matrix metalloproteinase (MMP) inhibitor, and high levels of MMP have been found in AVM tissue.[104]

REFERENCES

1. Mulliken JB, Glowacki J. Hemangiomas and vascular malformations in infants and children: A classification based on endothelial characteristics. *Plast Reconstr Surg* 1982; 69: 412.
2. Wassef M, Blei F, Adams D. Vascular anomalies classification: Recommendations from the International Society for the Study of Vascular Anomalies. *Pediatrics* 2015; 136(1): e203–14.
3. Finn MC, Glowacki J, Mulliken JB. Congenital vascular lesions: Clinical application of a new classification. *J Pediatr Surg* 1983; 18: 894–90.
4. Kilcline C, Frieden IJ. Infantile hemangiomas: How common are they? A systematic review of the medical literature. *Pediatr Dermatol* 2008; 25: 168–73.
5. Drolet BA, Swanson EA, Frieden IJ. Infantile hemangiomas: An emerging health issue linked to an increased rate of low birth weight infants. *J Pediatr* 2008; 153: 712–5.
6. Mulliken JB, Fishman SJ, Burrows PE. Vascular anomalies. *Curr Prob Surg* 2000; 37: 517–84.
7. Chang LC, Haggstrom AN, Drolet BA et al. Growth characteristics of infantile hemangiomas: Implications for management. *Pediatrics* 2008; 122: 360–7.
8. Paltiel H, Burrows PE, Kozakewich HPW et al. Soft-tissue vascular anomalies: Utility of US for diagnosis. *Radiology* 2000; 214: 747–54.

9. Burrows PE, Laor T, Paltiel H et al. Diagnostic imaging in the evaluation of vascular birthmarks. *Dermatol Clin* 1998; 16: 455–88.

10. North PE, Waner M, Mizeracki A et al. GLUT1: A newly discovered immunohistochemical marker for juvenile hemangiomas. *Hum Path* 2000; 31: 11–22.

11. Enjolras O, Gelbert F. Superficial hemangiomas: Associations and management. *Pediatr Dermatol* 1997; 14: 173–9.

12. Christison-Lagay ER, Burrows PE, Alomari A et al. Hepatic hemangiomas: Subtype classification and development of a clinical practice algorithm and registry. *J Pediatr Surg* 2007; 42: 62–7.

13. Kulungowski AM, Alomari AI, Chawla A et al. Lessons from a liver hemangioma registry: Subtype classification. *J Pediatr Surg* 2012; 47: 165–70.

14. Boon LM, Burrows PE, Paltiel HJ et al. Hepatic vascular anomalies in infancy: A twenty-seven-year experience. *J Pediatr* 1996; 129: 346–54.

15. Huang SA, Tu HM, Harney JW et al. Severe hypothyroidism caused by type 3 iodothyronine deiodinase in infantile hemangiomas. *N Engl J Med* 2000; 343: 185–9.

16. Goldberg NS, Hebert AA, Esterly NB. Sacral hemangiomas and multiple congenital anomalies. *Arch Dermatol* 1986; 122: 684–7.

17. Stockman A, Boralevi F, Taieb A et al. SACRAL syndrome: Spinal dysraphism, anogenital, cutaneous, renal and urological anomalies, associated with an angioma of lumbosacral localization. *Dermatology* 2007; 214: 40–5.

18. Girard C, Bigorre M, Guillot B et al. PELVIS syndrome. *Arch Dermatol* 2006; 142: 884–8.

19. Freiden IJ, Reese V, Cohen D. PHACE syndrome. The association of posterior fossa brain malformations, hemangiomas, arterial anomalies, coarctation of the aorta and cardiac defects and eye abnormalities. *Arch Dermatol* 1996; 132: 307–11.

20. Metry DW, Haggstrom AN, Drolet BA et al. A prospective study of PHACE syndrome in infantile hemangiomas: Demographic features, clinical findings, and complications. *Am J Med Gen* 2006; 140A: 975–86.

21. Metry DW, Garzon MC, Drolet BA et al. PHACE syndrome: Current knowledge, future directions. *Ped Derm* 2009; 26: 381–98.

22. Chamlin SL, Haggstrom AN, Drolet BA et al. Multicenter prospective study of ulcerated hemangiomas. *J Pediatr* 2007; 151: 684–9.

23. Leaute-Labreze C, Dumas de la Roque E, Hubiche T et al. Propranolol for severe hemangiomas of infancy. *N Engl J Med* 2008; 358: 2649–51.

24. Sans V, Dumas de la Roque E, Berge J et al. Propranolol for severe infantile hemangiomas: Follow-up report. *Pediatrics* 2009; 124: 423–31.

25. Storch CH, Hoeger PH. Propranolol for infantile haemangiomas: Insights into the molecular mechanisms of action. *Br J Dermatol* 2010; 163: 269–74.

26. Chisholm KM, Chang KW, Truong MT et al. beta-Adrenergic receptor expression in vascular tumors. *Mod Pathol* 2012; 25: 1446–51.

27. Stiles J, Amaya C, Pham R et al. Propranolol treatment of infantile hemangioma endothelial cells: A molecular analysis. *Exp Ther Med* 2012; 4: 594–604.

28. Sommers Smith SK, Smith DM. Beta blockade induces apoptosis in cultured capillary endothelial cells. *In Vitro Cell Dev Biol Anim* 2000; 8: 298–304.

29. Moehrle M, Leaute-Labreze C, Schmidt V et al. Topical timolol for small hemangiomas in infancy. *Pediatr Dermatol* 2013; 30: 245–9.

30. Zarem HA, Edgerton MT. Induced resolution of cavernous hemangiomas following prednisolone therapy. *Plast Reconstr Surg* 1967; 39: 76–83.

31. Boon LM, MacDonald DM, Mulliken JB. Complications of systemic corticosteroid therapy for problematic hemangiomas. *Plast Reconstr Surg* 1999; 104: 1616–23.

32. Bennett ML, Fleischer AB, Chamlin SL et al. Oral corticosteroid use is effective for cutaneous hemangiomas. *Arch Dermatol* 2001; 137: 1208–13.

33. Greene AK. Corticosteroid treatment for problematic infantile hemangioma: Evidence does not support an increased risk for cerebral palsy. *Pediatrics* 2008; 126: 1251–2.

34. George ME, Sharma V, Jacobson J et al. Adverse effects of systemic glucocorticosteroid therapy in infants with hemangiomas. *Arch Dermatol* 2004; 140: 963–9.

35. Lomenick JP, Backeljauw PF, Lucky AW. Growth, bone mineral accretion, and adrenal function in glucocorticoid-treated infants with hemangiomas—A retrospective study. *Pediatr Dermatol* 2006; 23: 169–74.

36. Garzon MC, Lucky AW, Hawrot A et al. Ultrapotent topical corticosteroid treatment of hemangiomas of infancy. *J Am Acad Dermatol* 2005; 52: 281–6.

37. Sloan GM, Renisch JF, Nichter LS et al. Intralesional corticosteroid therapy for infantile hemangiomas. *Plast Reconstr Surg* 1989; 83: 459–67.

38. Ruttum MS, Abrams GW, Harris GJ et al. Bilateral retinal embolization associated with intralesional steroid injection for capillary hemangioma of infancy. *J Pediatr Ophthalmol Strabismus* 1993; 30: 4–7.

39. Egbert JE, Schwartz GS, Walsh AW. Diagnosis and treatment of an ophthalmic artery occlusion during an intralesional injection of corticosteroid into an eyelid capillary hemangioma. *Am J Ophthalmol* 1996; 121: 638–42.

40. Scheepers JH, Quaba AA. Does the pulsed tunable dye laser have a role in the management of infantile hemangiomas: Observations based on 3 years experience. *Plast Reconstr Surg* 1995; 95: 305–12.

41. Batta K, Goodyear HM, Moss C et al. Randomized controlled study of early pulsed dye laser treatment of uncomplicated childhood haemangiomas: Results of a 1-year analysis. *Lancet* 2002; 360: 521–7.

42. Witman PM, Wagner AM, Scherer K et al. Complications following pulsed dye laser treatment of superficial hemangiomas. *Lasers Surg Med* 2006; 38: 116–23.

43. Mulliken JB, Rogers GF, Marler JJ. Circular excision of hemangioma and purse-string closure: The smallest possible scar. *Plast Reconstr Surg* 2002; 109: 1544–54.

44. Boon LM, Enjolras O, Mulliken JB. Congenital hemangioma: Evidence of accelerated involution. *J Pediatr* 1996; 128: 329–35.

45. Enjolras O, Mulliken JB, Boon LM et al. Noninvoluting congenital hemangioma: A rare cutaneous vascular anomaly. *Plast Reconstr Surg* 2001; 107: 1647–54.

46. Berenguer B, Mulliken JB, Enjolras O et al. Rapidly involuting congenital hemangioma: Clinical and histopathologic features. *Pediatr Dev Pathol* 2003; 6: 495–510.

47. Zukerberg LR, Nikoloff BJ, Weiss SW. Kaposiform hemangioendothelioma of infancy and childhood: An aggressive neoplasm associated with Kasabach–Merritt syndrome and lymphangiomatosis. *Am J Surg Pathol* 1993; 17: 321–8.

48. Mulliken JB, Anupindi S, Ezekowitz RA et al. Case 13-2004: A newborn girl with a large cutaneous lesion, thrombocytopenia, and anemia. *N Engl J Med* 2004; 350: 1764–75.

49. Lyons LL, North PE, Mac-Moune Lai F et al. Kaposiform hemangioendothelioma: A study of 33 cases emphasizing its pathologic, immunophenotypic, and biologic uniqueness from juvenile hemangioma. *Am J Surg Pathol* 2004; 28: 559–68.

50. Haisley-Royster C, Enjolras O, Frieden IJ et al. Kasabach-Merritt phenomenon: A retrospective study of treatment with vincristine. *J Pediatr Hematol Oncol* 2002; 24: 459–62.

51. Hammill AM, Wentzel MS, Gupta A et al. Sirolimus for the treatment of complicated vascular anomalies in children. *Pediatr Blood Cancer* 2011; 57: 108–24.

52. Mills SE, Cooper PH, Fechner RE. Lobular capillary hemangioma: The underlying lesion of pyogenic granuloma. *Am J Surg Pathol* 1980; 4: 470–9.

53. Patrice SJ, Wiss K, Mulliken JB. Pyogenic granuloma (lobular capillary hemangioma): A clinicopathologic study of 178 cases. *Pediatr Dermatol* 1991; 8: 267–76.

54. Greene AK, Taber SF, Ball KL et al. Sturge–Weber syndrome: Frequency and morbidity of facial overgrowth. *J Craniofac Surg* 2009; 20: 617–21.

55. Jasim ZF, Handley JM. Treatment of pulsed dye laser-resistant port wine stain birthmarks. *J Am Acad Dermatol* 2007; 57: 677–82.

56. Chapas AM, Eickhorst K, Geronemus RG. Efficacy of early treatment of facial port wine stains in newborns: A review of 49 cases. *Lasers Surg Med* 2007; 39: 563–8.

57. Astner S, Anderson RR. Treating vascular lesions. *Dermatol Ther* 2005; 18: 267–81.

58. Huikeshoven M, Koster PH, de Borgie CA et al. Redarkening of port-wine stains 10 years after pulsed-dye-laser treatment. *N Engl J Med* 2007; 356: 1235–40.

59. Burrows PE, Mason KP. Percutaneous treatment of low flow vascular malformations. *J Vasc Interv Radiol* 2004; 15: 431–45.

60. Padwa BL, Hayward PG, Ferraro NF et al. Cervicofacial lymphatic malformation: Clinical course, surgical intervention, and pathogenesis of skeletal hypertrophy. *Plast Reconstr Surg* 1995; 95: 951–60.

61. Edwards PD, Rahbar R, Ferraro NF et al. Lymphatic malformation of the lingual base and oral floor. *Plast Reconstr Surg* 2005; 115: 1906–15.

62. Greene AK, Burrows PE, Smith L et al. Periorbital lymphatic malformation: Clinical course and management in 42 patients. *Plast Reconstr Surg* 2005; 115: 22–30.

63. Choi DJ, Alomari AI, Chaudry G et al. Neurointerventional management of low-flow vascular malformations of the head and neck. *Neuroimag Clin N Am* 2009; 19: 199–218.

64. Florez-Vargas A, Vargas SO, Debelenko LV et al. Comparative analysis of D2-40 and LYVE-1 immunostaining in lymphatic malformations. *Lymphology* 2008; 41: 103–10.

65. Smith MC, Zimmerman B, Burke DK et al. Efficacy and safety of OK-432 immunotherapy of lymphatic malformations. *Laryngoscope* 2009; 119: 107–15.

66. Burrows PE, Mitri RK, Alomari A et al. Percutaneous sclerotherapy of lymphatic malformations with doxycycline. *Lymphat Res Biol* 2008; 6: 209–16.

67. Alqahtani A, Nguyen LT, Flageole H et al. 25 years' experience with lymphangiomas in children. *J Pediatr Surg* 1999; 34: 1164–8.

68. Upton J, Coombs CJ, Mulliken JB et al. Vascular malformations of the upper limb: A review of 270 patients. *J Hand Surg (Am)* 1999; 24: 1019–35.

69. Fliegelman LJ, Friedland D, Brandwein M et al. Lymphatic malformation: Predictive factors for recurrence. *Otolaryngol Head Neck Surg* 2000; 123: 706–10.

70. Grimmer JF, Mulliken JB, Burrows PE et al. Radiofrequency ablation of microcystic lymphatic malformation in the oral cavity. *Arch Otolarngol Head Neck Surg* 2006; 132: 1251–6.

71. Young AE. Pathogenesis of vascular malformations. In: Mulliken JB (ed). *Vascular Birthmarks: Hemangiomas and Malformations*. Philadelphia: Saunders, 1988: 107–13.

72. Boon LM, Mulliken JB, Enjolras O et al. Glomuvenous malformation (glomangioma) and venous malformation: Distinct clinicopathologic and genetic entities. *Arch Dermatol* 2004; 140: 971–6.

73. Limaye N, Wouters V, Uebelhoer M et al. Somatic mutations in angiopoietin receptor gene TEK cause solitary and multiple sporadic venous malformations. *Nat Gen* 2009; 41: 118–24.

74. Limaye N, Boon LM, Vikkula M. From germline towards somatic mutations in the pathophysiology of vascular anomalies. *Hum Mol Genet* 2009; 18: 65–75.

75. Brouillard P, Boon LM, Mulliken JB et al. Mutations in a novel factor, glomulin, are responsible for glomuvenous malformations ("glomangiomas"). *Am J Hum Genet* 2002; 70: 866–74.

76. Vikkula M, Boon LM, Carraway KL et al. Vascular dysmorphogenesis caused by an activating mutation in the receptor tyrosine kinase TIE2. *Cell* 1996; 87: 1181–90.

77. Fishman SJ, Smithers CJ, Folkman J et al. Blue rubber bleb nevus syndrome: Surgical eradication of gastrointestinal bleeding. *Ann Surg* 2005; 241: 523–8.

78. Adams DM, Wentzel MS. The role of the hematologist/oncologist in the care of patients with vascular anomalies. *Pediatr Clin N Am* 2008; 55: 339–55.

79. Berenguer B, Burrows PE, Zurakowski D et al. Sclerotherapy of craniofacial venous malformations: Complications and results. *Plast Reconstr Surg* 1999; 104: 1–11.

80. Ohlms LA, Forsen J, Burrows PE. Venous malformations of the pediatric airway. *Int J Pediatr Otorhinolaryngol* 1996; 37: 99–114.

81. Fishman SJ, Burrows PE, Leichtner AM et al. Gastrointestinal manifestations of vascular anomalies in childhood: Varied etiologies require multiple therapeutic modalities. *J Pediatr Surg* 1998; 33: 1163–7.

82. Fishman SJ, Shamberger RC, Fox VL et al. Endorectal pull-through abates gastrointestinal hemorrhage from colorectal venous malformations. *J Pediatr Surg* 2000; 35: 982–4.

83. Thomas B, Eyries M, Montagne K et al. Altered endothelial gene expression associated with hereditary haemorrhagic telangiectasia. *Eur J Clin Invest* 2007; 37: 580–8.

84. Eerola I, Boon LM, Mulliken JB et al. Capillary malformation-arteriovenous malformation: A new clinical and genetic disorder cased by RASA1 mutations. *Am J Hum Genet* 2003; 73: 1240–9.

85. Tan WH, Baris HN, Burrows PE et al. The spectrum of vascular anomalies in patients with PTEN mutations: Implications for diagnosis and management. *J Med Genet* 2007; 44: 594–602.

86. Kohout MP, Hansen M, Pribaz JJ et al. Arteriovenous malformations of the head and neck: Natural history and management. *Plast Reconstr Surg* 1998; 102: 643–54.

87. Wu IC, Orbach DB. Neurointerventional management of high-flow vascular malformations of the head and neck. *Neuroimag Clin N Am* 2009; 19: 219–40.

88. Liu AS, Mulliken JB, Zurakowski D et al. Extracranial arteriovenous malformations: Natural progression and recurrence after treatment. *Plast Reconstr Surg* (in press).

89. Wu JK, Bisdorff A, Gelbert F et al. Auricular arteriovenous malformation: Evaluation, management, and outcome. *Plast Reconstr Surg* 2005; 115: 985–95.

90. Hartzell LD, Stack BC Jr, Yuen J et al. Free tissue reconstruction following excision of head and neck arteriovenous malformations. *Arch Facial Plast Surg* 2009; 11: 171–7.

91. Sansal I, Sellers WR. The biology and clinical relevance of the PTEN tumor suppressor pathway. *J Clin Oncol* 2004; 22: 2954–63.

92. Eng C. PTEN: One gene, many syndromes. *Hum Mutat* 2003; 22: 183–98.

93. Revencu N, Boon LM, Mulliken JB et al. Parkes Weber syndrome, vein of galen aneurismal malformation, and other fast-flow vascular anomalies are caused by RASA1 mutations. *Hum Mutat* 2008; 29: 959–65.

94. Cohen MM. Klippel–Trenaunay syndrome. *Am J Med Genet* 2000; 93: 171–5.

95. Servelle M. Klippel and Trenaunay's syndrome: 768 operated cases. *Ann Surg* 1985; 201: 365–73.

96. Jacob AG, Driscoll DJ, Shaughnessy WJ et al. Klippel–Trenaunay syndrome: Spectrum and management. *Mayo Clin Proc* 1998; 73: 28–36.

97. Greene AK, Kieran M, Burrows PE et al. Wilms tumor screening for Klippel–Trenaunay syndrome is unnecessary. *Pediatrics* 2004; 113: E326–9.

98. Alomari, AI. Characterization of a distinct syndrome that associates truncal overgrowth, vascular, and acral anomalies: A descriptive study of 18 cases of CLOVES syndrome. *Clin Dysmorphol* 2009; 18: 1–7.

99. Kurek KC, Luks VL, Ayturk UM et al. Somatic mosaic activating mutations in PIK3CA cause CLOVES syndrome. *Am J Hum Genet* 2012; 90: 1108–15.

100. Boscolo E, Coma S, Luks VL et al. AKT hyperphosphorylation associated with PI3K mutations in lymphatic endothelial cells from a patient with lymphatic malformation. *Angiogenesis* 2015; 18: 151–62.

101. Osborn AJ, Dickie P, Neilson DE et al. Activating PIK3CA alleles and lymphangiogeneic phenotype of lymphatic endothelial cells isolated from lymphatic malformations. *Hum Mol Genet* 2015; 24: 926–38.

102. Adams DM, Trenor CC, Hammill et al. Efficacy and safety of sirolimus in the treatment of complicated vascular anomalies. *Pediatrics* 2016; 137: 1–10.

103. Bagrodia N, Defnet AM, Kandel JJ. Management of lymphatic malformations in children. *Curr Opin Pediatr* 2015; 27: 356–63.

104. Burrows PE, Mulliken JB, Fishman S et al. Pharmacological treatment of a diffuse arteriovenous malformation of the upper extremity of a child. *J Craniofac Surg* 2009; 20 (Suppl 1): 597–602.

86

Congenital nevi

LEE W. T. ALKUREISHI AND BRUCE S. BAUER

INTRODUCTION

Congenital nevi are a group of skin lesions occurring at birth or becoming apparent within the first several years of life, and are characterized by ectopic rests of dermal elements. Although most commonly melanocytic in nature, nevi may also originate from sebaceous, neural, or epidermal elements. Lesion characteristics vary according to the type of cell involved, location within the skin, and level of cell differentiation. Knowledge of the differential diagnosis and natural history of these lesions can help balance the plan of care, in order to address the potential risk of malignant degeneration while accounting for functional and aesthetic concerns encountered in the course of excision and reconstruction. This chapter outlines the presentation and management of congenital nevi, with special emphasis on congenital melanocytic nevi (CMNs).

CONGENITAL MELANOCYTIC NEVI

CMNs are the most common congenital nevi and are composed of cells of melanocytic origin that carry a varying amount of pigment. These are usually present at birth, though a small percentage may not initially be evident due to a lack of pigment production. These "tardive" CMNs are usually noted within the first 2 years of life. The presentation of CMN varies from very small, relatively insignificant nevi to giant disfiguring lesions covering large portions of the body, with significant implications in terms of the risk of melanoma, central nervous system involvement, and other associated conditions, in addition to the significant aesthetic deformity. The natural history of CMN, true melanoma risk, and optimal treatment algorithms remain controversial topics within the literature.

Epidemiology

The overall incidence of CMN is estimated to be 1%–6% of live births, with larger lesions being much less common.

Small lesions (<1.5 cm projected adult size [PAS]) are reported to occur in 1:100 births, intermediate (1.5–20 cm) lesions in 1:1,000, large (>20 cm) lesions in 1:20,000 births, and giant (>50 cm) lesions in 1:500,000.[1-3] The incidence of CMN is slightly higher in infants of Japanese and African American descent[2,4] and has a female-to-male ratio of 3:2.[5] CMNs are most commonly located on the trunk (38%), extremities (38%), head and neck, (14%) and feet and hands (10%).[6]

Etiology

Embryologically, melanocytes originate from neural crest cells as melanoblasts and migrate to the basal layer of the epidermis between the 5th and 24th week of gestation. They differentiate into dendritic melanocytes and form melanosomes, which produce pigment for transfer to keratinocytes. CMNs result from a disturbance in this migration and differentiation process, producing ectopic rests of immature cells along their course of migration.[7] As a result, nevus cells often extend deep into the subcutaneous tissues and can involve fascia, muscle, periosteum, or the leptomeninges, a condition known as neurocutaneous melanosis (NCM).

It is believed that disturbances in the melanoblast migration pathway may be related to overexpression of the proto-oncogenes *c-met* and/or *c-kit*, which produce tyrosine kinase receptors binding hepatocyte growth factor/scatter factor (HGF/SF) and stem cell factor (SCF), respectively.[8] *C-met* and *c-kit* (via the N-ras oncogene) have also been implicated in the development of rhabdomyosarcoma and melanoma in patients with large CMN (LCMN).[9,10]

Pathology

In contrast with normal melanocytes, nevus cells tend to group together in clusters and assume a rounded rather than dendritic shape. They also retain pigment within their cytoplasm instead of transferring it to the surrounding keratinocytes.[11]

Because of the higher risk of malignant transformation found in CMN compared to acquired nevi, efforts have been made to identify histologic characteristics specific to CMN. Nevus cells found within eccrine ducts, follicular epithelium, or blood vessels indicate congenital lesions; however, not all CMNs display this finding.[12] Furthermore, only congenital lesions demonstrate nevus cells within the deeper subcutaneous tissues, fascia, and/or muscle. Clinically, examination of small CMN with a dermatoscope or under loupe magnification will reveal small pigment granules at the peripheral aspect of the lesion, another specific finding to CMN.[13] Discovery of more specific markers for CMN will help to more clearly determine the true rate of melanoma associated with these lesions.

Presentation

The clinical features of CMN can differ greatly in terms of size and appearance (Figure 86.1). All CMNs are present at birth, though tardive CMN may not be visible until production of melanin increases within the first 1–2 years of life. Coloration varies from pale tan to a deep bluish black, and may be uniform or extremely variegated. The lesions are often thickened in texture with increased skin markings compared to surrounding normal skin, and may have a nodular or rugous quality. They often have hair, which can range from fine light fuzz to coarse thick follicles. When large lesions are present, they may be accompanied by smaller peripheral satellite lesions of different sizes and numbers, which may appear for the first 2–3 years of life.

In general, CMNs tend to grow in proportion with the child. The surface of CMN can become more verrucous and irregular with darkening pigmentation; however, lightening of color can also be seen in as many as 30% of patients with large and giant nevi.

Most CMNs are asymptomatic, but symptoms can include pruritus, tenderness, xerosis, and/or skin erosion or breakdown related to relative paucity of subcutaneous fat and sweat glands underlying the CMN. Skin erosion is not uncommon in the neonatal period but may also occur later. This does not necessarily indicate malignant change but warrants further investigation.

Classification

The highly variable presentation of CMN has important implications with regard to determination of malignancy risk, potential development of NCM, and treatment planning. Several authors have proposed classification schemes for CMN, the majority of which use the PAS of the nevus as the principle category.[14] The PAS can be determined by multiplying the largest diameter of the lesion in infancy by a predetermined factor, which varies by body area (Table 86.1).[16] As a general rule, a 12 cm lesion on the head or neck or 7 cm lesion on the body of an infant will grow to meet the large nevi classification (>20 cm PAS).[15] Another cited definition of large congenital nevi includes lesions >2% total body surface area.[1]

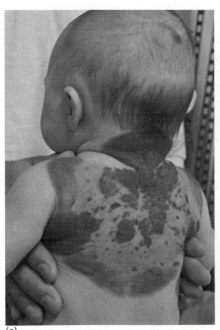
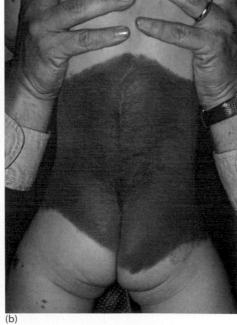
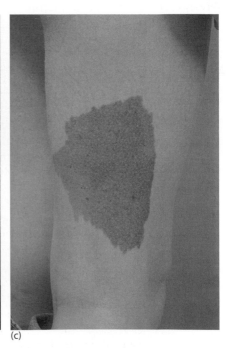

(a) (b) (c)

Figure 86.1 Variability in appearance and characteristics of congenital melanocytic nevi. **(a)** Large nevus of upper back with variable pigmentation and raised areas. **(b)** "Bathing trunk" nevus with dark pigmentation and hypertrichosis. **(c)** Medium congenital nevus of lower extremity with lighter pigmentation that is homogeneous.

Table 86.1 Estimated size of CMN in adulthood based on its diameter in infancy

CMN location on infant	CMN diameter at birth (cm)[a]	Factor[b]
Head	11.8	1.7
Hands, feet, torso, forearms, hips	7.2	2.8
Thighs	5.9	3.4
Legs	6.1	3.3

Source: Marghoob et al. Large congenital melanocytic nevi and the risk for the development of malignant melanoma. *Arch Dermatol* 1996; 132: 170–175.

Note: CMN: Congenital melanocytic nevus.

[a] Diameter in which the nevus would reach at least 20 cm in adulthood.

[b] Factor that should be multiplied by the CMN diameter in infancy to obtain its estimated size in adulthood

Comparison of study outcomes, however, has thus far been limited by inconsistent nomenclature and categorization, a finding that has become increasingly important with the development of LCMN registries pooling data from multiple institutions.[5,17] In addition to projected size, clinical features such as color variegation, localization, rugosity, hypertrichosis, and number of satellite lesions may prove equally important markers for adverse outcomes in CMN patients.[18,19] In an attempt to address these issues, Krendel and Marghoob[14] created a more inclusive classification system based on expert consensus. This classification is presented in Table 86.2.

Malignancy risk

MELANOMA

An immediate concern of the family and doctors involved with the care of these patients is the potential risk of malignancy, primarily malignant melanoma. Melanoma may arise within the nevus or in extracutaneous sites, most commonly the central nervous system. Earlier studies reporting the incidence of melanoma varied widely from 0% to 40%[1,2,20–23]; however, it is generally held that these studies may have overestimated this risk as a result of small sample sizes, selection bias, and/or overdiagnosis.[24] Nevertheless, there remains a significantly elevated risk of melanoma in CMN patients, which must be a consideration in treatment planning.

At this time, the true incidence of melanoma in CMN patients is difficult to ascertain. Heterogeneity of the patient population, lack of standardized nomenclature, and multiple treatment modalities all contribute to difficulty in determining the true natural history of CMN. However, recent literature reviews and meta-analyses have helped elucidate this to some degree.[24,25] The lifetime risk of developing melanoma, cutaneous or extracutaneous, appears likely to be less than 5% for all patients with LCMN[26] and as low as 0.7%–2% for smaller lesions.[24,25] However, it is important to note that many of the patients included in these studies have undergone partial or complete excision of their nevi, potentially underestimating the true risk of melanoma. Factors shown to be associated with an increased risk of melanoma include larger nevus size, truncal location, and the presence of multiple satellite lesions.[5,23]

The risk of melanoma arising within small CMNs before puberty is felt to be extremely unlikely.[27] However, this does not hold true for LCMN and giant CMN (GCMN). It has been reported that 50% of LCMNs that develop malignancy do so in the first 3 years of life, with 60% by childhood and 70% by puberty.[16] In a review of 289 patients with LCMN, DeDavid et al.[15] found 67 cases of melanoma, of which 34 (51%) arose within the nevus. Twenty-one cases (31.3%) developed melanoma within the CNS, and two patients (3%) developed cutaneous melanoma beyond the nevus margins. The remaining 10 patients (15%) presented with metastatic disease and an unknown primary site. It is also important to note that there has only been one reported case of melanoma developing within a satellite lesion, in a patient with CMN and neurofibromatosis type I.[5]

OTHER TUMORS ASSOCIATED WITH CMN

In addition to melanoma, patients with CMN may be at risk for the development of other tumors, both benign and malignant. These include lipomas and schwannomas, sarcomas, malignant cellular blue nevus, and undifferentiated spindle cell neoplasms.[28]

Patient evaluation

HISTORY AND PHYSICAL EXAMINATION

On initial history, any changes in the appearance of the nevus or satellite lesions should be elicited, along with any family history of melanoma. Documentation of developmental milestones and presence of any neurologic symptoms should be noted. Serial examination of the lesion(s) should be undertaken every 3–6 months, depending on the character of and variability in the lesion's appearance.

Patches of darker color or raised nodules can develop within LCMN and may represent neural nevus. This is a form of intradermal nevus, with melanocytes that appear histologically similar to Schwann cells and contain nerve organelles such as Meissner and Pacinian corpuscles. The patches may also represent local areas of proliferation that do not necessarily behave in an aggressive manner. Biopsy of any suspicious raised, ulcerating, or atypical areas can be used to exclude malignancy (Figure 86.2). Histologic findings of low mitotic rate, lack of necrosis, evidence of maturation in the cell population, and lack of high-grade nuclear atypia are clues to a benign course. The best description of these areas is melanocytic tumor of uncertain potential, and these unusual areas are best addressed earlier in the course of reconstruction.

In older children and adolescents, there can also be psychological implications associated with the diagnosis of LCMN or GCMN. In one study of 29 patients, 30% were found to have emotional, behavioral, or social problems. The reasons for this

Table 86.2 New classification of congenital melanocytic nevi

CMN parameter	Terminology	Definition
CMN project adult size	"Small CMN"	<1.5 cm
	"Medium CMN"	
	"M1"	1.5–10 cm
	"M2"	>10–20 cm
	"Large CMN"	
	"L1"	>20–30 cm
	"L2"	>30–40 cm
	"Giant CMN"	
	"G1"	>40–60 cm
	"G2"	>60 cm
	"Multiple medium CMN"	≥3 medium CMN *without a single, predominant CMN*
CMN localization[a]		
CMN of head	"Face," "scalp"	
CMN of trunk	"Neck," "shoulder," "upper back," "middle back," "lower back," "breast/chest," "abdomen," "flank," "gluteal region," "genital region"	
CMN of extremities	"Upper arm," "forearm," "hand," "thigh," "lower leg," "foot"	
No. of satellite nevi[b]	"S0"	No satellites
	"S1"	<20 satellites
	"S2"	20–50 satellites
	"S3"	>50 satellites
Additional morphological characteristics	"C0," "C1," "C2"	None, moderate, marked color heterogeneity
	"R0," "R1," "R2"	None, moderate, marked surface rugosity
	"N0," "N1," "N2"	None, scattered, extensive dermal or subcutaneous nodules
	"H0," "H1," "H2"	None, notable, marked hypertrichosis ("hairness")

Source: Krengel et al. New recommendations for the categorization of cutaneous features of congenital melanocytic nevi. *J Am Acad Dermatol* 2013; 68(3): 441–451.

Note: CMN, Congenital melanocytic nevi.

[a] One or more of this localizations should be used to describe *preponderant* area of involvement.

[b] Refers to number of satellites within first year of life; in case this number is not available, actual number should be mentioned.

are likely multifactorial, including concerns regarding malignant change, appearance of the nevus or postsurgical scarring, and anxiety related to treatment itself.[29]

NCM AND MAGNETIC RESONANCE IMAGING

The clinical presentation of NCM can range from asymptomatic to progressive, severe neurologic deterioration with developmental delay, hydrocephalus, and seizures, often with fatal outcomes. Symptoms may be caused by blockage of cerebrospinal fluid circulation by benign nevus cell proliferation, leading to hydrocephalus and increased intracranial pressure, or from malignant degeneration.

If NCM is to become symptomatic, the vast majority of cases will do so before age 3 years. The prognosis of symptomatic NCM is poor, with >90% dying within 3 years of onset of neurologic symptoms.[30] It is difficult to know the true incidence of NCM in association with LCMN, as screening of asymptomatic patients is not universally performed. However, a study of an Internet registry found NCM on magnetic resonance imaging (MRI) in approximately 5% of patients with LGCM/GCMN. Of these, only 5%–6% became symptomatic.[31] LCMN of the posterior midline and those found in association with multiple satellite nevi (greater than 20) have the highest risk of NCM and should be strongly considered for MRI screening (Figure 86.1a,b).[32]

MRI is the study of choice for detection of melanin involving the leptomeninges, which is seen as focal shortening of T1 relaxation time and, less frequently, T2 relaxation time. For increased sensitivity, the MRI should be obtained prior to age 4 months, because after that time, increasing

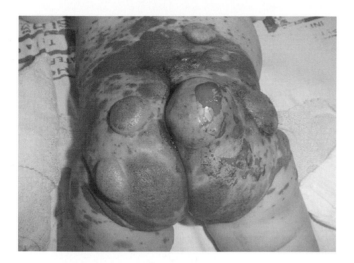

Figure 86.2 Sarcoma arising within a giant congenital melanocytic nevus at birth.

myelination of the CNS can potentially obscure visualization of nevus cells.[33]

It is important to convey that the finding of NCM on MRI does not necessarily imply the future development of neurologic symptoms. It does, however, indicate a risk for later development of benign or malignant melanotic tumors. Foster et al.[34] reported that 23% of at risk-patients had NCM on MRI imaging, with only one patient developing neurologic sequelae of hypotonia, developmental delay, and seizures during the 5-year follow-up period. More recent studies report a lower 5% incidence of NCM in patients with LCMN.[31]

In cases of symptomatic NCM, the associated poor prognosis should deter the surgeon from aggressive management of the cutaneous lesion. However, the low reported incidence of progression from asymptomatic to symptomatic NCM cautions against applying that same philosophy to this patient population. Further study will help to fully ascertain the true predicted course of disease in asymptomatic, scan-positive patients and help guide both surgical planning and the role of serial scanning. At this time, if the initial MRI is positive, we proceed with reconstruction as planned and feel that further scans are unnecessary unless neurologic symptoms develop.

Differential diagnosis

BLUE NEVI

Blue nevi are smooth, bluish-black lesions that can be present at birth but more commonly appear during childhood and puberty (Figure 86.3). They occur more frequently in females and are usually found on the head or extremities. Two variants exist: common and cellular. The common blue nevus is a relatively small (<1 cm), sharply demarcated, dome-shaped benign lesion. Histologically, it composed of intradermal and possibly subcutaneous dendritic melanocytes with normal overlying epithelium. The cellular blue

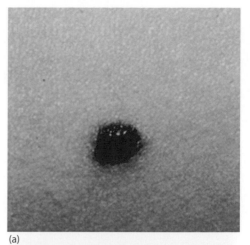

(a)

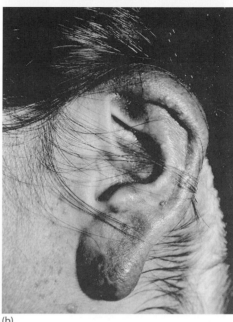

(b)

Figure 86.3 Blue nevus (a) Typical appearance. (b) Extensive blue nevus involving the external ear.

nevus is larger (1–3 cm) with less regular borders and is frequently found in the lumbosacral area. The lesion tends to be wider at the surface than at the base and is composed of spindle-shaped melanocytes in aggregates mixed within dendritic melanocytes. Unlike the common form, malignant transformation has been reported within the cellular variant, and therefore, excision is recommended.

MONGOLIAN SPOTS

Mongolian spots are blue-gray macules, usually overlying the lumbosacral area of otherwise healthy infants (Figure 86.4). They are more common in Asian and darker-skinned individuals. Mongolian spots are most often present at birth but may appear within the first weeks of life, and usually regress spontaneously by age 3–4 years of age. Lesions are made up of widely scattered dendritic melanocytes within the lower two-thirds of the dermis. No treatment of these

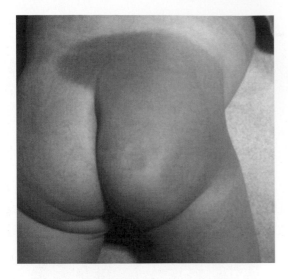

Figure 86.4 Mongolian spot of the posterior trunk.

benign lesions is necessary; however, laser can be effective for management of a persistent lesion.[35]

NEVUS OF OTA/NEVUS OF ITO

The nevus of Ota is a blue-gray facial discoloration characterized by speckled or mottled coalescing macules appearing at birth, or in childhood, in the V1/V2 distribution (Figure 86.5). Unlike Mongolian spots, these lesions do not regress and can become hyperpigmented in puberty. The lesion may extend to involve the mucosal membranes of the nose and mouth as well as sclera, conjunctiva, and retina, and ocular pathology and glaucoma have been associated. The nevus of Ota displays a female predominance and is found most commonly in Asian and Indian populations. In 10% of cases, the nevus is bilateral and associated with extensive Mongolian spots.

The nevus of Ito is a blue-gray macular lesion, similar to the nevus of Ota, that affects the shoulder area (scapula, deltoid, supraclavicular) and is sometimes associated with sensory changes. It is rarer than the nevus of Ota and more common in Asians.

Both of these lesions represent field defects of dermal melanocytosis, histologically characterized by elongated dendritic melanocytes scattered within the collagen bundles mostly in the upper third of the reticular dermis. They may contain raised areas within the lesion that are indistinguishable from blue nevus.

Although considered benign, there have been a few reported cases of malignant change, especially in areas similar to cellular blue nevus, and these may require biopsy to distinguish from melanoma.[35] Historically, cryotherapy and nonselective destruction with CO_2 laser was used with mixed aesthetic results. Current laser technology allows the surgeon to take advantage of selective photothermolysis, directing laser energy to destroy the melanocytes without damaging the surrounding tissues, with excellent cosmetic results. Multiple treatments with a Q-switched ruby laser, Q-switched alexandrite laser, or Q-switched Nd:YAG laser

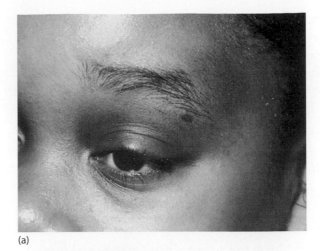

(a)

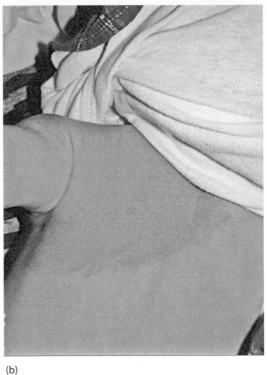

(b)

Figure 86.5 Nevus of Ota/Ito. **(a)** Nevus of Ota in its typical V1/V2 distribution. **(b)** Nevus of Ito, in typical distribution involving the shoulder, neck, and back.

are effective to fade the lesion.[35] For the nevus of Ota, an ophthalmologist should be consulted due to the risk of ocular pathology.

CAFÉ AU LAIT SPOTS

Café au lait spots are benign, sharply demarcated macules of light tan to brown regular pigmentation. They can present in normal individuals or, when multiple, can be associated with syndromes such as neurofibromatosis. Histologically, lesions are caused by increased pigment in macromelanosomes within the keratinocytes in the basal layer. Laser ablation can be used to successfully treat lesions that are of cosmetic concern, but recurrence is common.[20]

NEVUS SPILUS

Nevus spilus refers to light tan to brown macules that resemble café au lait spots, but with areas of darker speckling within them (Figure 86.6). On histology, there are both areas of increased pigment within the keratinocytes of the basal layer as well as an increased number of melanocytes. The specked areas represent a mixture of findings from freckling to CMN to blue nevi. Suspicious areas within the lesion should be excised for biopsy as the nevocellular areas do carry some malignant potential. If the entire lesion is in a cosmetically sensitive area, it can be removed surgically.

SEBACEOUS NEVI

Sebaceous nevi present at birth as a waxy, hairless, yellow-orange plaque usually on the scalp, head, or neck (Figure 86.7). Over time, they can become more nodular, verrucous, and itchy, as a child approaches puberty. Sebaceous nevi are hamartomas of sebaceous glands. They carry a 15%–20% risk of malignant transformation into basal cell carcinoma, making excision and reconstruction recommended. Sebaceous nevus syndrome is the combination of large sebaceous nevi of the scalp and face associated with developmental delay, seizures, and ophthalmologic and bony abnormalities.

Extensive linear sebaceous nevus is mostly seen in the head and neck and presents some unique challenges to the reconstructive surgeon. For the larger lesions involving the scalp and face, tissue expansion can be applied in a fashion similar to that which will be described for LCMN. Narrow linear lesions can be excised in stages, often timed so a partial excision is performed at the same time a tissue expander is placed elsewhere, and further excision is done when the expander is removed for distant flap reconstruction. Lesions on the ear are addressed with either staged excision or excision and full-thickness skin graft. Those involving the helical rim should be grafted only after full growth of the ear to avoid distortion of the cartilage. It is not uncommon to see linear nevi involving the lower lip,

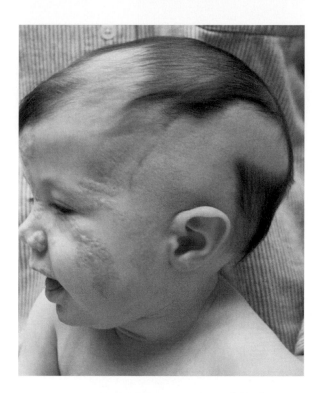

Figure 86.7 Extensive sebaceous nevus of the face and scalp.

chin, and adjacent neck. Given the linear orientation, it is important to design the reconstruction to minimize tension on the repair while breaking up the scar line to avoid scar hypertrophy and contracture. The senior author's surgical approach has been described in detail in a previous publication.[36]

SPITZ NEVI

Although not usually congenital, spitz nevi are another commonly encountered pediatric skin lesion. They present as pink, raised, firm lesions that can occasionally be pigmented (Figure 86.8). At times, they may be confused with pyogenic granulomas because of their appearance and rapid growth at onset. Originally termed *benign juvenile melanoma*, these lesions display a bizarre pathology beneath the microscope and can be confused with malignancy if the pathologist is not provided with the history of the lesion and patient's age. In fact, these lesions are benign, but do grow rapidly and tend to recur aggressively if not completely excised. Because of that, these lesions should be excised with a generous 3–4 mm border of normal tissue to decrease the chance of recurrence.

Management of CMN

The optimal management of CMN is dependent on many variables, including size and location of the lesion, malignant potential, visibility, and associated medical and psychological comorbidities. The treatment plan must therefore be tailored to the individual, with treatment

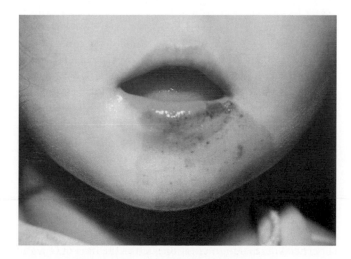

Figure 86.6 Nevus spilus of the lower lip.

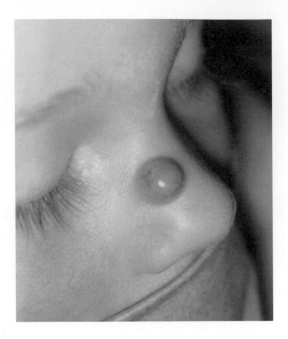

Figure 86.8 Spitz nevus.

options broadly categorized as surveillance alone, nonexcisional modalities, and excision with reconstruction.

SMALL CMN

Most CMNs fall into the small category and can usually be addressed with simple or staged excision. The low risk of melanoma before puberty in this group allows treatment to be deferred until an age at which excision can be safely performed under local anesthesia. However, if the lesion falls in a cosmetically sensitive area or is located in an area that will require general anesthesia regardless of age, consideration should be given to earlier removal to avoid potential psychological sequelae of delaying treatment. From a practical point of view, these procedures are best performed either before the patient begins toddling or just prior to school entrance in order to avoid potential complications from falls, heightened anxiety, and lack of patient cooperation found at the ages in between.

LARGE AND GIANT CONGENITAL MELANOCYTIC NEVI

Management of LCMN is a more complex, involved process that again strikes a balance between addressing the risk of malignancy and functional and aesthetic concerns, of both the lesion and subsequent reconstruction.

At this time, CMNs are not able to be diagnosed prenatally. The appearance of extensive dark, hairy lesions of the face, trunk, or extremities is, by nature, devastating for parents who have been anxiously awaiting the birth of their child. Because of this, the infant with LCMN should be referred early to a dermatologist and surgeon familiar with the management of these lesions. This allows parents to be appropriately counseled on the nature of these lesions, malignancy risk, and treatment options. If presented in a

compassionate manner, even the news of a multiple-stage reconstruction over many years can be well accepted by families. In over 30 years of experience, the senior author has developed treatment plans for the management of these lesions with the tenet that aesthetic and functional outcome are as important as removal of the nevus itself. Although the true incidence of malignant melanoma arising in untreated LCMN is unlikely to be clearly defined, these numbers encourage early removal.

Treatment for LCMN and GCMN remains controversial to some, as they feel that the risk of malignant degeneration within these lesions is too low to warrant the extensive number of surgeries and potential scar burden associated with removal. Others feel that the potential for noncutaneous melanoma to develop in nevus cells not amenable to surgical removal (such as in NCM) represents a remaining risk that negates the effectiveness of cutaneous excision for reduction of melanoma risk.[30,37,38] However, the significant deformity and associated psychological impact caused by these lesions often tip the scales toward attempted intervention. Management plans should always strive to balance removal of the nevus with a functional and aesthetic reconstruction, and lesions that cannot be effectively addressed in this manner should be considered for conservative management by serial observation by an experienced dermatologist.

DERMABRASION, CURETTAGE, AND LASER THERAPY

Nonexcisional methods of treatment for CMN have been reported as effective methods of reducing the nevus cell burden without complete removal, improving the appearance. The success of dermabrasion and curettage relies on the finding that early in infancy, the skin nevus cells lie more superficially within the upper reticular dermis and epidermis. Dermabrasion works to abrade away these surface cells, while curettage separates the cells at the natural cleavage plane between the superficial and deep dermis. Using either method, the number of nevus cells within a lesion is reduced but not eliminated. As a result, the color of the nevus may be lightened initially but can have a tendency to darken over time (Figure 86.9a,b).[39] In addition, these treatment modalities do not show any improvement in associated hypertrichosis, due to the deeper location of the hair follicles. Finally, superficial treatment modalities are theoretically less effective at reducing malignant potential compared with excision techniques due to persistence of deeper nevus cells, and resultant scarring can potentially make follow-up examination difficult. Nonetheless, good cosmesis has been reported using both methods.[40] In order to be effective, these treatments must be performed at less than 15 days of life.

Laser offers another potential treatment strategy, attractive to both the patient and the doctor as a simpler method of reducing pigmentation without scarring. Laser therapy is well suited for the treatment of lesions characterized by superficial dermal pigmentation such as the nevi of Ota and Ito, persistent Mongolian spots, café au lait macules, and

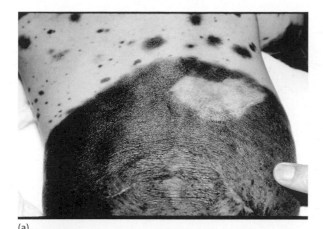

(a)

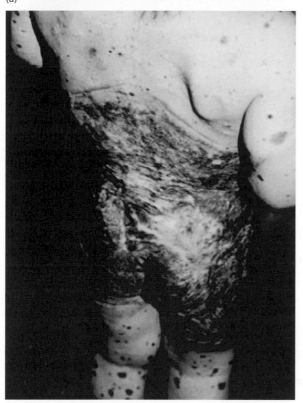

(b)

Figure 86.9 Lightening, and subsequent repigmentation, following curettage. **(a)** The pale area within the nevus was curetted immediately after birth. Seeing this result, the rest of the lesion was curetted. **(b)** As a toddler, this typical result shows recurrence of pigmentation and scarring, making clinical and histological surveillance of the lesion difficult.

some elements of nevus spilus due to their minimal thickness, location of pigment within the dermis, and low potential for malignancy. Lasers that can be used in the treatment of CMN include ruby, Q-switched, Er:YAG, and carbon dioxide, either alone or in combination with Nd:YAG or Q-switched ruby lasers.[41] Effective treatment relies on appropriate wavelength and pulse-width selection, allowing penetration of the skin and photoselective destruction of melanin while preserving the remaining elements to avoid

scarring.[35,42] Serial treatments are required, and scarring can occur with aggressive treatment or improper settings. Hypopigmentation and hyperpigmentation have also been reported, which may be temporary or permanent. Exposure to sunlight in the peritreatment period can cause significant burning, scarring, and hyperpigmentation.

Unfortunately, because CMN display nevus cells within all layers of the skin as well as within the deeper structures, it is unrealistic to think that a laser could effectively penetrate to the depths necessary to eliminate all pigment-producing nevi cells without significant secondary damage and scarring. In addition, laser treatment vaporizes the specimen, therefore eliminating histologic evaluation of the lesion to determine its nature. Finally, the impact of the exposure of nevus cells to sublethal doses of laser energy associated with laser therapy is unknown, and may not be apparent for many years into the future.[43,44]

Although dermabrasion, curettage, and laser offer relatively simple approaches to improving the appearance of CMN, they present many drawbacks. Leaving residual nevus cells within CMN imparts a continued risk of malignancy, and scarring may make monitoring the lesions more difficult posttreatment. In addition, scarring from these therapies may complicate ultimate excisional treatment options in the future. Finally, the delay of more definitive reconstruction may have its own psychological effects on a child. Although limited use of these therapies may be useful in certain areas of reconstruction (such as lightening of a thin lesion in the cosmetic and functionally sensitive eyelid area), thoughtful consideration is warranted prior to widespread implementation of these modalities in a treatment algorithm for LCMN.

SURGICAL EXCISION AND RECONSTRUCTION

The benefits of surgical excision of LCMN include complete removal of nevus cells in the involved skin and subcutaneous tissue. Although some have focused on reconstruction with skin grafts, skin substitutes, or cultured epithelium, whenever possible, the use of tissue expansion allows the most functional and aesthetic result by allowing replacement with full-thickness normal tissue. Excision of the nevus is usually carried out at the level of the deep fascia.

Goals of treatment include complete excision at an early age, minimization of scarring, and functional impact, with a low requirement for future procedures. Early excision is emphasized for four reasons. First, the greatest risk for malignancy is reported in childhood, most notably in the first 3 years of life. Second, the elasticity and healing capacity of the skin is better the younger the patient. Third, patients operated on in infancy tolerate surgery better both physically and emotionally than their older counterparts. Finally, by completing reconstruction early, the psychological impact of the lesions and surgical interventions can be reduced.

In 1988, the senior author presented a coordinated approach to the management of these lesions in 78 patients.[45] This report outlined the spectrum of treatment options

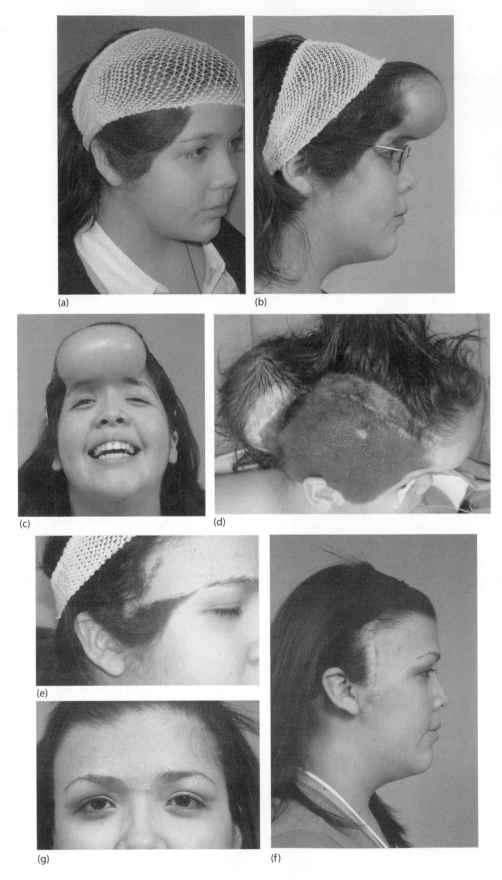

Figure 86.10 **(a)** Large CMN of scalp and forehead. **(b, c)** Lateral and frontal view after completion of forehead expansion. **(d)** At surgery with views of both forehead and occipital scalp expanders, 12 weeks after expander placement. **(e)** Result after first stage. **(f, g)** Final reconstruction of aesthetic units with scars well concealed at hairline and along the browline.

from skin graft to tissue expansion, and assessed the effectiveness of excision and reconstruction with each technique in each body region. Since then, further experience with over 300 patients has allowed further development and refinement of this approach.[46–50] Although a full discussion of the nuances of management of each type of LCMN is beyond the scope of this chapter, the following is a summary of the author's current approach.

Scalp

Scalp reconstruction is complicated by its relatively inflexible quality and the unique aesthetics of maintaining hair quality and direction. Because of this, tissue expansion remains the workhorse for scalp reconstruction following excision of LCMN. Scalp lesions are best reconstructed in stages, with placement of one or more tissue expanders in the subgaleal plane beneath adjacent normal scalp skin. Following a period of 10–12 weeks of expansion, the expanders are removed, lesions excised, and the defect closed using both advancement and transposition flaps designed to preserve hair direction and hairline.[46] Serial expansions are often necessary, and flaps should be carried out and their viability assessed before nevus excision (Figure 86.10). Safe expansion of the infant scalp can be carried out at 6 months of age, with careful attention given to the fontanel during expander placement and reconstruction. Although temporary cranial molding is common, in the authors' experience, no infants have demonstrated permanent skull deformities. Spontaneous contour correction generally occurs within 3–4 months following expander removal.

Face

LCMNs of the face present some of the greatest reconstructive challenges. By dividing the face into aesthetic units and placing expanders under adjacent normal skin in the neck and forehead, skin of excellent quality match can be used while allowing scars to lie less conspicuously at the junction of aesthetic units (Figure 86.11). When advancing tissue from the neck into the cheek area, a transposition design can help improve flap movement while aligning the scars optimally. Whether the flap is based laterally (most common) or medially, the transposition minimizes the risk of late downward drift of the flap and ectropion of the lower eyelid.[46] Lesions of the nose are best resurfaced with an expanded forehead flap carried on a superficial temporal artery pedicle when available, or with an expanded supraclavicular full-thickness skin graft. The periorbital area is also best addressed with expanded full-thickness skin grafts to allow preservation of the thin nature of the tissue while decreasing incidence of ectropion.[48] LCMN of up to 75% of the forehead can be managed with tissue expansion, often serial, and this requires careful planning to minimize distortion of the eyebrow position and maintain the normal distance from brow to hairline. Nevi extending into the temporal area must be treated by expansion of both scalp and forehead, with flaps designed to establish both normal position of the hairline and hair direction for the temporal scalp.[50]

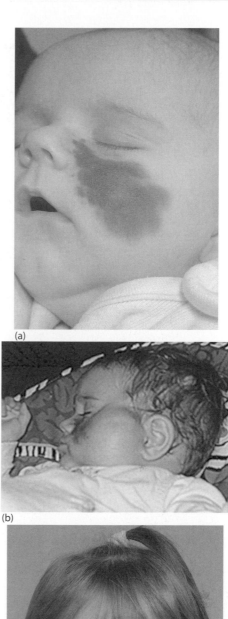
(a)

(b)

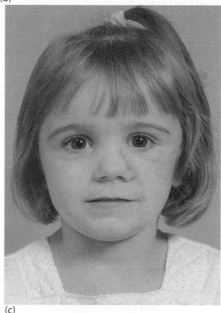
(c)

Figure 86.11 **(a)** Medium CMN involving the cheek and nasal sidewall. **(b)** Tissue expander placed in inferolateral cheek. **(c)** Result following expanded flap reconstruction. There was some later darkening pigmentation outside the margins of the original resection, best seen along the nasal sidewall.

Trunk

The frequently extensive involvement of GCMN of the trunk with relative lack of normal donor skin presents a daunting challenge to the reconstructive surgeon, leading many to resort to split-thickness skin graft–based reconstruction. The inferior functional and aesthetic results of this approach call into question whether excision should have been undertaken at all, in favor of conservative observation.

With improved expanded flap design carried out in series, or the use of expanded distant flaps with microvascular transfer, superior trunk reconstruction can be achieved.

The posterior trunk is the most common location of GCMN, often extending anteriorly in a dermatomal distribution. These lesions, including the "bathing trunk" distribution and large thoracic nevi, are best reconstructed with serial tissue expansion and subsequent transposition flap closure (Figure 86.12). Anterior trunk lesions can be

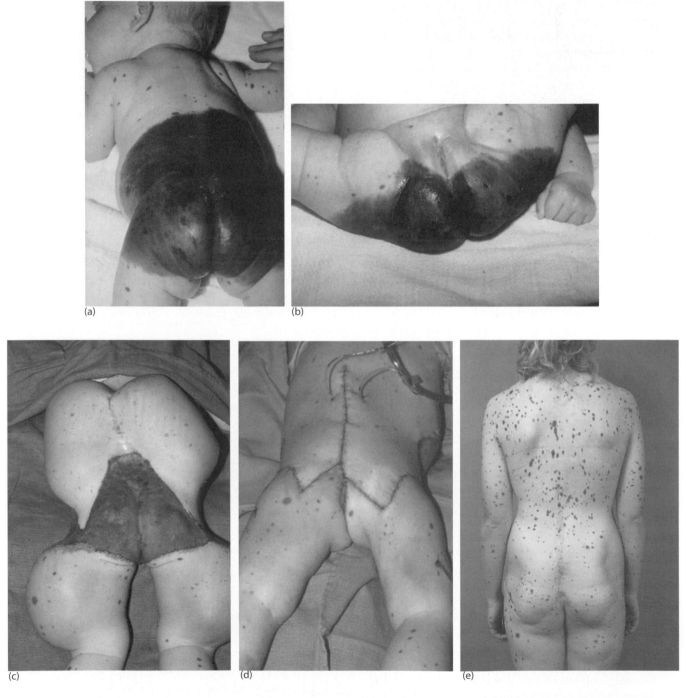

(a) (b) (c) (d) (e)

Figure 86.12 **(a, b)** Giant melanocytic nevus of the perineum and buttocks and multiple satellite nevi, both independent predictors of underlying NCM. **(c)** Serial expansion and excision techniques with transposition-designed flaps. **(d)** Total excision of the lesion was accomplished without functional disturbances, and with reasonably normal appearance. **(e)** Long-term follow-up.

treated with an abdominoplasty technique, with or without expansion depending on lesion size. When adjacent donor sites are unavailable for expansion, excision and reconstruction of shoulder, upper back, and posterior neck nevi can be accomplished using microvascular transfer of a free expanded transverse rectus abdominis musculocutaneous (TRAM) or deep inferior epigastric perforator (DIEP) flap (Figure 86.13). With increased use of expanded flaps over skin grafting for trunk reconstruction, late contour deformities seen at junction points between grafted and ungrafted areas can be significantly reduced. These modified techniques can result in aesthetic benefits far beyond what may be accomplished with alternative treatments.

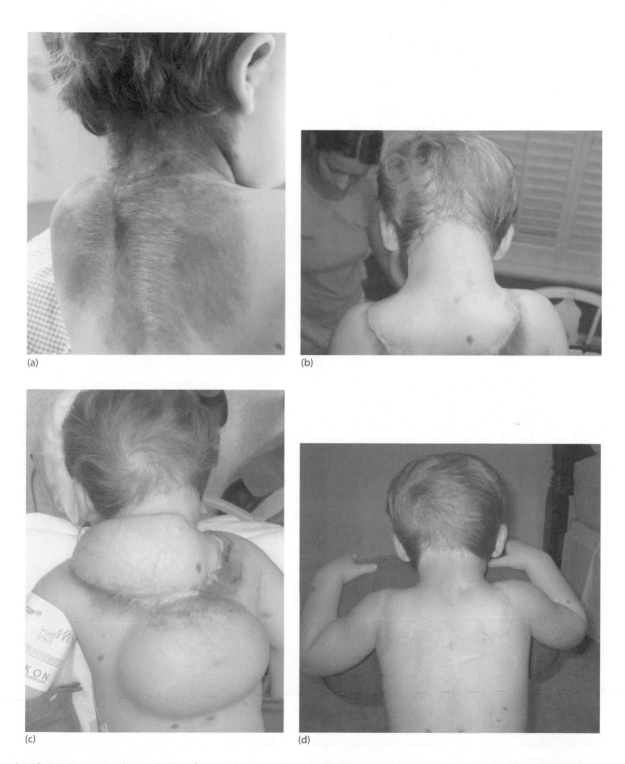

(a)

(b)

(c)

(d)

Figure 86.13 **(a)** Extensive large CMN of upper back and neck. **(b)** Reconstruction with expanded free TRAM flap. **(c)** Re-expansion of free TRAM flap. **(d)** Final result with good contour and flexibility of the shoulders and neck.

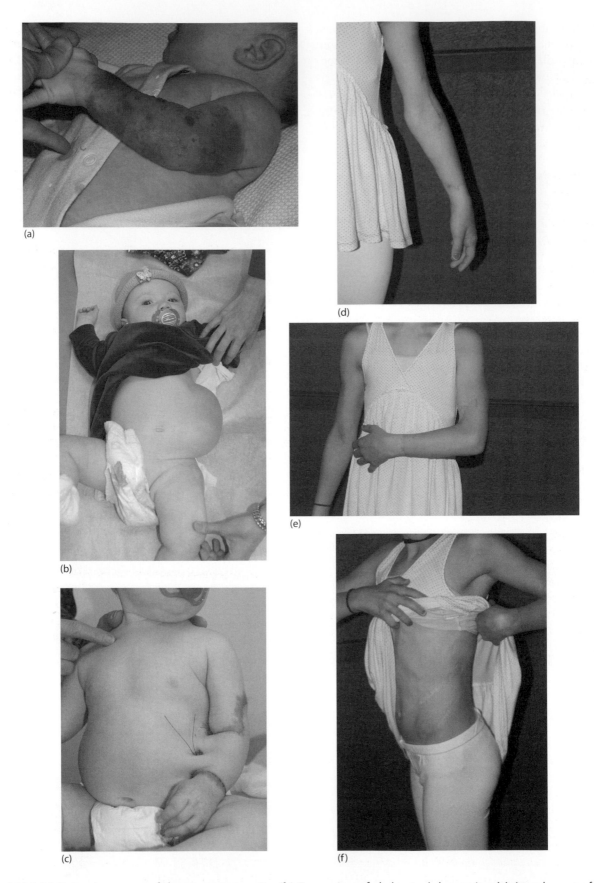

Figure 86.14 **(a)** Extensive nevus of the upper extremity. **(b)** Expansion of abdominal donor site. **(c)** Attachment of pedicled abdominal flap for circumferential arm reconstruction. **(d–f)** Final result with good contour of arm and acceptable abdominal scarring.

Extremities

LCMNs of the extremities continue to present a considerable challenge, due to the limitations of local expansion techniques in these areas and the relatively poor aesthetic outcome seen with skin grafting. The authors' prior approach utilized both split-thickness and expanded full-thickness skin grafts for most lesions, but long-term soft-tissue contour defects and pigment abnormalities in the grafted skin have led to use of alternative approaches whenever possible. In upper extremity lesions, transposition flaps from the upper back and shoulder have effectively eliminated contour defects to the proximal upper extremity. In addition, three-stage, expanded pedicled flaps from the abdomen and flank can be designed to provide complete coverage of a circumferential nevus from elbow to wrist, with excellent contour and acceptable scarring achieved at both donor and recipient sites (Figure 86.14).[49] A similar pedicled approach has been successful in providing coverage for lower leg lesions after ipsilateral thigh expansion in the young infant, when lower extremity flexibility is at its peak, with excellent results.[49] Finally, expanded free flaps offer another alternative for coverage of larger lesions of the extremities, with excellent functional and aesthetic results.

Complications

Complications of surgical excision of LCMN with expanded flap reconstruction are uncommon, despite the complex nature of these procedures. They include expander infection/exposure, partial flap necrosis, wound dehiscence, and scarring. The incidence of expander infection has been reported at 5%, which can be due to inoculation at the time of placement or during the expansion process, or by hematogenous seeding from a distant infection.[51] These infections can usually be managed conservatively with systemic antibiotics, allowing completion of expansion and successful reconstruction. A low threshold for placement on oral antibiotics during healing problems or systemic illness occurring during expansion may help minimize risk.

The expansion process effectively increases vascularity of the overlying flap through the delay phenomenon,[52] making flap ischemia rare. Preservation of the capsule and avoidance of excessive tension during closure can prevent this potentially devastating complication. Finally, meticulous closure and postoperative scar management help achieve optimal results.

CONCLUSIONS

The treatment of congenital large and giant nevi presents a continuing challenge to all individuals involved with these patients. The ability to present an organized discussion of current views on risk of malignant change to parents, older patients, referring physicians, and other allied health care workers is critical. Treatment strategies should take into consideration the varied opinions regarding malignant risk, emphasize the benefits of early excision on lowering that risk, and most importantly, provide a means of dealing with these often devastating lesions in a manner that optimizes the functional and aesthetic outcome, minimizing the need for major reconstruction in later life.

REFERENCES

1. Quaba AA, Wallace AF. The incidence of malignant melanoma (0–15 years of age) arising in "large" congenital nevocellular nevi. *Plast Reconstr Surg* 1986; 78: 174–9.
2. Alper JC, Holmes LB. The incidence and significance of birthmarks in a cohort of 4.641 newborns. *Pediatr Dermatol* 1983; 1: 58–68.
3. Illig L, Weidner F, Hundeiker ME. Congenital nevi less than or equal to 10 cm as precursors to melanoma: 52 cases, a review and a new conception. *Arch Dermatol* 1985; 121: 1274–81.
4. Hidano A, Purwoko R, Jitsukawa K. Statistical survey of skin changes in Japanese neonates. *Pediatr Dermatol* 1986; 3: 140–4.
5. Bett BJ. Large or multiple congenital melanocytic nevi: Occurrence of cutaneous melanoma in 1008 persons. *J Am Acad Dermatol* 2005; 52: 793–7.
6. Alikhan A1, Ibrahimi OA, Eisen DB. Congenital melanocytic nevi: Where are we now? Part I. Clinical presentation, epidemiology, pathogenesis, histology, malignant transformation, and neurocutaneous melanosis. *J Am Acad Dermatol* 2012 October; 67(4): 495.e1–17.
7. Cramer SF. The melanocytic differentiation pathway in congenital melanocytic nevi: Theoretical considerations. *Pediat Pathol* 1988; 8: 253–265.
8. Otsuka T, Takayama H, Sharp R et al. c-Met autocrine activation induces development of malignant melanoma and acquisition of the metastatic phenotype. *Cancer Res* 1998; 58: 5157–67.
9. Papp T, Pemsel H, Zimmermann R et al. Mutational analysis of the Nras, p53, p16INK4a, CDK4, and MC1R genes in human congenital melanocytic naevi. *J Med Genet* 1999; 36: 610–4.
10. Takayama H, Nagashima Y, Hara M et al. Immunohistochemical detection of the c-met proto-oncogene product in the congenital melanocytic nevus of an infant with neurocutaneous melanosis. *J Am Acad Derm* 2001; 44: 538–540.
11. Elder D, Elenitsas R. Benign pigmented lesions and malignant melanoma. In: Elder D (ed). *Lever's Histopathology of the Skin*, 8th edn. Philadelphia: Lippincott-Raven Publishers, 1997: 625–84.
12. Rhodes AR, Silverman RA, Harrist TJ, Melski JW. A histologic comparison of congenital and acquired nevomelanocytic nevi. *Arch Dermatol* 1986; 121: 1266–73.

13. Alper JC, Holmes LB, Mihm MC. Birthmarks with serious medical significance: Nevocellular nevi, sebaceous nevi and multiple café au lait spots. *J Pediatr* 1979; 95: 696–700.

14. Krengel S, Scope A, Dusza SW et al. New recommendations for the categorization of cutaneous features of congenital melanocytic nevi. *J Am Acad Dermatol* 2013 March; 68(3): 441–51.

15. DeDavid M, Orlow SJ, Provost N et al. A study of large congenital melanocytic nevi and associated malignant melanomas: Review of cases in the New York University Registry and the world literature. *J Am Acad Dermatol* 1997 March; 36(3 Pt 1): 409–16.

16. Marghoob AA, Schoenbach SP, Kopf AW et al. Large congenital melanocytic nevi and the risk for the development of malignant melanoma. A prospective study. *Arch Dermatol* 1996; 132: 170–5.

17. Ka VS, Dusza SW, Halpern AC, Marghoob AA. The association between large congenital melanocytic naevi and cutaneous melanoma: Preliminary findings from an Internet-based registry of 379 patients. *Melanoma Res* 2005 February; 15(1): 61–7.

18. Slutsky JB, Barr JM, Femia AN, Marghoob AA. Large congenital melanocytic nevi: Associated risks and management considerations. *Semin Cutan Med Surg* 2010 June; 29(2): 79–84.

19. Price HN, Schaffer JV. Congenital melanocytic nevi—When to worry and how to treat: Facts and controversies. *Clin Dermatol* 2010 May–June; 28(3): 293–302.

20. Kopf AW, Bart RS, Hennessey P. Congenital nevocytic nevi and malignant melanomas. *J Am Acad Dermatol* 1979; 1: 123–30.

21. Marghoob AA, Kopf AW, Bittencourt FV. Moles present at birth: Their medical significance. *Skin Cancer Found J* 1999; 36: 95–8.

22. Sandsmark M, Eskeland G, Ogaard AR et al. Treatment of large congenital naevi. *Scand J Plast Reconstr Hand Surg* 1993; 27: 223–32.

23. Bittencourt FV, Marghoob AA, Kopf AW et al. Large congenital melanocytic nevi and the risk for development of malignant melanoma and neurocutaneous melanocytosis. *Pediatrics* 2000; 106: 736–41.

24. Krengel S, Hauschild A, Schaefer T. Melanoma risk in congenital melanocytic nevi: A systematic review. *Br J Dermatol* 2006; 155: 1–8.

25. Vourc'h-Jourdain M, Martin L, Barbarot S, aRED. Large congenital melanocytic nevi: Therapeutic management and melanoma risk: A systematic review. *J Am Acad Dermatol* 2013 March; 68(3): 493-8.e1–14. Epub 2012 November 19. Review.

26. Krengel S, Marghoob AA. Current management approaches for congenital melanocytic nevi. *Dermatol Clin* 2012 July; 30(3): 377–87. Epub 2012 June 6. Review.

27. Scalzo DA, Hilda CA, Toth G et al. Childhood melanoma: A clinicopathological study of 22 cases. *Melanoma Res* 1997; 7: 63–8.

28. Hendrickson MR, Ross JC. Neoplasms arising in congenital giant nevi: Morphologic study of seven cases and a review of the literature. *Am J Surg Pathol* 1981; 5: 109–35.

29. Koot HM, DeWaard-van der Spek F, Peer CD et al. Psychosocial sequelae in 29 children with giant congenital melanocytic naevi. *Clin Exp Derm* 2000; 25: 589–93.

30. Kadonaga JN, Frieden IJ. Neurocutaneous melanosis: Definition and review of the literature. *J Am Acad Dermatol* 1991; 24: 747–55.

31. Agero AL, Benvenuto CA, Dusza SW et al. Asymptomatic neurocutaneous melanocytosis in patients with large congenital melanocytic nevi: A study of cases from an Internet-based registry. *J Am Acad Dermatol* 2005; 53: 959–65.

32. Marghoob AA, Dusza S, Oliviera S, Halpern AC. Number of satellite nevi as a correlate for neurocutaneous melanocytosis in patients with large congenital melanocytic nevi. *Arch Dermatol* 2004; 140: 171–5.

33. Barkovich AJ, Frieden IJ, Williams ML. MR of neurocutaneous melanosis. *Am J Neuroradiol* 1994; 15: 859–67.

34. Foster RD, Williams ML, Barkovich AJ et al. Giant congenital melanocytic nevi: The significance of neurocutaneous melanosis in neurologically asymptomatic children. *Plast Reconstr Surg* 2001; 107: 933–41.

35. Carpo BG, Grevelink JM, Grevelink SV. Laser treatment of pigmented lesions in children. *Semin Cutan Med Surg* 1999; 18: 233–43.

36. Margulis A, Bauer BS, Corcoran JF. Surgical management of the cutaneous manifestations of linear nevus sebaceous syndrome. *Plast Reconstr Surg* 2003; 111(3): 1043–50.

37. Kinsler VA, Birley J, Atherton DJ. Great Ormond Street Hospital for Children Registry for congenital melanocytic naevi: Prospective study 1988-2007. Part 1—Epidemiology, phenotype and outcomes. *Br J Dermatol* 2009 January; 160(1): 143–50. Epub 2008 October 22.

38. Arad E, Zuker RM. The shifting paradigm in the management of giant congenital melanocytic nevi: Review and clinical applications. *Plast Reconstr Surg* 2014 February; 133(2): 367–76. Review.

39. Magalon G, Casanova D, Bardot J, Andrac-Meyer L. Early curettage of giant congenital naevi in children. *Br J Dermatol* 1998; 138: 341–5.

40. Tromberg J, Bauer B, Benvenuto-Andrade C, Marghoob AA. Congenital melanocytic nevi needing treatment. *Dermatol Ther* 2005 March–April; 18(2): 136–50.

41. Polder KD, Landau JM, Vergilis-Kalner IJ et al. Laser eradication of pigmented lesions: A review. *Dermatol Surg* 2011 May; 37(5): 572–95.

42. Alster TS. Complete elimination of large café au lait birthmarks by the 510-nm pulsed dye laser. *Plast Reconstr Surg* 1995; 96: 1660–4.

43. Marghoob AA, Borrego JP, Halpern AC. Congenital melanocytic nevi: Treatment modalities and management options. *Semin Cutan Med Surg* 2007 December; 26(4): 231–40. Review.

44. Michel JL. Laser therapy of giant congenital melanocytic nevi. *Eur J Dermatol* 2003 January–February; 13(1): 57–64.

45. Bauer BS, Vicari FA. An approach to excision of congenital giant pigmented nevi in infancy and early childhood. *Plast Reconstr Surg* 1988; 82: 1012–21.

46. Bauer BS, Margulis A. The expanded transposition flap: Shifting paradigms based on experience gained from two decades of pediatric tissue expansion. *Plast Reconstr Surg* 2004; 114(1): 98–106.

47. Margulis A, Bauer BS, Fine NA. Large and giant congenital pigmented nevi of the upper extremity: An algorithm to surgical management. *Ann Plast Surg* 2004; 52(2): 158–67.

48. Margulis A, Adler N, Bauer BS. Congenital melanocytic nevi of the eyelids and periorbital region. *Plast Reconstr Surg* 2009 October; 124(4): 1273–83.

49. Kryger ZB, Bauer BS. Surgical management of large and giant congenital pigmented nevi of the lower extremity. *Plast Reconstr Surg* 2008; 121(5): 1674–84.

50. Unlü RE, Tekin F, Sensöz O, Bauer BS. The role of tissue expansion in the management of large congenital pigmented nevi of the forehead in the pediatric patient. *Plast Reconstr Surg* 2002; 110(4): 1191.

51. Adler N, Dorafshar AH, Bauer BS et al. Tissue expander infections in pediatric patients: Management and outcomes. *Plast Reconstr Surg* 2009; 124(2): 484–9.

52. Cherry GW, Austad E, Pasyk K et al. *Plast Reconstr Surg* 1983 November; 72(5): 680–7.

87

Lymphatic malformations

EMILY R. CHRISTISON-LAGAY AND JACOB C. LANGER

INTRODUCTION

Lymphatic malformations (LMs) constitute one subset of a larger group of so-called vascular malformations, which may affect any segment of the vascular tree, including arterial, venous, capillary, and lymphatic vessels. All vascular malformations can be considered to be the result of errors of embryonic development and can be categorized according to the particular vascular component involved as well as by physiologic flow properties. Thus, there exist slow-flow lesions (which include lymphatic, venous, and capillary malformations); fast-flow anomalies (which contain an arterial component); and complex, combined vascular malformations.

Commonly referred to as "cystic hygroma" or "lymphangioma" in the historic literature, LMs consist of a group of developmental anomalies of the lymphatic system. They are slow-flow anomalies, which range in clinical presentation from small masses to large and sometimes debilitating, disfiguring, or invasive lesions. Structurally, they may be characterized as *microcystic*, *macrocystic*, or combined lesions, and these properties have significant clinical implications for treatment. The most common presentation of a macroscopic LM is a ballottable mass beneath normal skin, although a large LM may transilluminate, causing the overlying skin to attain a blue hue. Microcystic malformations may present as vesicles that permeate the subcutaneous tissue and muscle. Dermal lymphatic involvement causes puckering, dimpling, vesiculation, or even brawny edema.[1] Approximately 40%–50% of LMs are found in the neck and shoulder; however, they may also occur in the mediastinum, retroperitoneum, groin, and other lymphatic-rich regions. Histologically, LMs are comprised of vascular spaces with a single layer of flattened epithelial cells. This chapter will provide an overview of the diagnosis and management of these often difficult lesions with emphasis on those involving the head and neck region.

EMBRYOLOGY AND ETIOLOGY

Most LMs are sporadic, but some exhibit classic Mendelian inheritance. Although our understanding of lymphatic development (and by extension, errors in lymphatic development) is less comprehensive than that of venoarterial development, recent advancements in distinguishing early lymphatic endothelial cells (LECs) from blood endothelial cells have opened the door for greater insight into observed aberrancies.

Seminal observations by Sabin[2] in the early twentieth century described the development of the lymphatic system beginning in the sixth to seventh week of embryonic life, approximately 4 weeks after the onset of vasculogenesis with the formation of five primitive "lymph sacs" originating as a set of paired sacs lateral to the jugular vein, a retroperitoneal sac at the root of the small bowel mesentery, and paired sacs posterior to the sciatic veins. It took nearly a century of investigation before this process was understood in more detail.

Migration of a specialized subset of endothelial cells from the anterior cardinal vein occurs in response to the stepwise expression of a series of transcription factors including Sox19, COUP-TPII, and Prox1.[3–5] Prox1 is considered to be a "global regulator" of lymphatic development required not only for lymphangiogenesis but also for maintenance of a lymphatic phenotype postnatally. The expression of the specific lymphatic receptor vascular endothelial growth factor receptor 3 (VEGFR3) permits separation (or budding) of the lymphatic system from the venous system.[5–8] Once the fate of LECs has been specified, migrating cells are able to respond to peripheral gradients of VEGF-C. LEC migration is a complex process that appears to depend upon relative levels of neuropilin2 and lymphatic vessel endothelial hyaluronan receptor 1 (LYVE-1). Those LECs expressing high neuropilin2 and low LYVE-1 migrate away from their precursor vein and form superficial lymphatic arbors. Conversely, those LECs expressing low levels of neuropilin2 and high LYVE-1 form a balloon-like structure adjacent to their precursor vein, eventually giving rise to larger lymphatic channels.[9,10] Complete separation of venolymphatic structures is also dependent upon the formation and signaling of platelet microthrombi. If this does not occur, the lymphatic channels end up filled with blood.[11]

Ongoing remodeling, proliferation, and maturation of LECs with lymphatic sprouting and valve development are subject to an extraordinarily precise choreography of growth factors and signaling molecules. Important regulators include VEGF and the VEGF receptor families, ephrins, angiopoietins and the Tie-2 receptor, transforming growth factor-beta (TGF-β) and its receptor, platelet-derived growth factor subunit B (PDGF-B) and its receptor, the Notch and Jagged families of membrane-associated molecules and the integrin family of cell surface receptors.[12–14]

Overexpression of the isoforms VEGF-C and VEGF-D in transgenic mice induces the formation of hyperplastic lymphatic vessels.[6] Kinase-inactivating mutations in the human *VEGFR3* gene result in Milroy disease.[15–17] Mutations in Sox18 are associated with hypotrichosis–lymphedema–telangiectasia.[9] Tie-2-deficient mouse embryos demonstrate normal initial vasculogenesis but have a disorganized vascular network lacking appropriate hierarchical organization.[18] Tie-1-deficient models demonstrate decreased endothelial cell integration leading to embryonic edema, hemorrhage, and death, and the Tie-1 receptor has recently been shown to be required for normal embryonic lymphangiogenesis.[19,20] Ang1–4, members of the angiopoietin family, likely have roles in vessel stabilization and lymphatic development.[21] Mutations in the *Fox* family of transcription factors have been associated with congenital lymphedema, and this family is thought to play a role in the formation of lymphatic valves.[22,23] Mutations or deletions in specific integrin subtypes can lead to abnormal lymphatic development.[24] Recently, integrin-α9 was found to be necessary for normal lymphatic valve morphogenesis and may be implicated as a candidate gene for primary lymphedema caused by valve defects.[25–27]

PRENATAL DIAGNOSIS

LMs are often diagnosed by prenatal ultrasound in the late first trimester.[28] The differential diagnosis of a cystic lesion in the fetus is extensive, but in experienced hands, the correct diagnosis can be made in most cases.[29] Although most LMs presenting to the pediatric surgeon have an excellent prognosis, prenatal sonography has revealed a high "hidden mortality" among fetuses with this condition.[30] Many fetuses with an LM develop hydrops fetalis or diffuse lymphangiomatosis prior to fetal demise (Figure 87.1). There is often either an associated chromosomal abnormality (e.g., Turner syndrome) or a familial syndrome associated with other structural anomalies (e.g., multiple pterygium syndrome, Robert syndrome).[31,32] Although most of these fetuses die in utero, spontaneous regression has occasionally been observed.[33–35] The natural

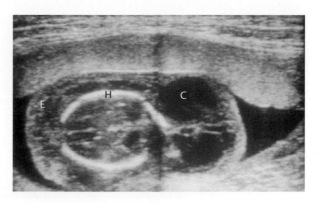

Figure 87.1 Prenatal ultrasound of a fetus with Turner syndrome and a large posterior cervical cystic hygroma. Note the diffuse subcutaneous edema (E), which is indicative of hydrops fetalis. H = fetal head, C = cystic hygroma.

history of cervical lesions detected prenatally varies according to the gestational age at which nuchal thickening appears and is further influenced by the presence or absence of hydrops or abnormal karyotyping. The cases diagnosed in the first trimester without any karyotypic abnormality usually have good prognosis with spontaneous resolution in the majority.[36–39] Conversely, those with hydrops and abnormal karyotype have a poorer outlook.[40,41] The prognosis of patients detected in the second trimester is usually poor.[42] LMs diagnosed in late gestation appear to belong to a different spectrum of disease with a much more favorable prognosis. These cases are comparatively rare and likely to represent an etiologic mechanism occurring during the latter half of pregnancy. Prenatal diagnosis should be followed by delivery and aggressive surgical management at a perinatal center.[43,44]

Occasionally, a fetus may be identified with a large anterior cervical LM that causes airway obstruction. These pose a challenge at the time of delivery and are best managed using the ex utero intrapartum (EXIT) procedure to gain access to the airway prior to dividing the umbilical cord (Figure 87.2).[45–47] In severe cases, a tracheostomy can be done, or the child can be placed on extracorporeal membrane oxygenation as part of the EXIT procedure; however, most patients with even large cervicofacial LMs can be orotracheally intubated in the delivery room.

Those LMs that are not diagnosed prenatally are generally evident at birth or before age 2 years; however, occasionally, they can manifest suddenly in older children and adults due to intralesional bleeding or infection.

CLINICAL PRESENTATION AND IMAGING

The majority of LMs occur in the head and neck, axilla, or retroperitoneum; involvement of the mediastinum, groin, extremities, or face is less common. Approximately 80% are diagnosed before the age of 5 years, and over half are present in the newborn period. Unlike infantile hemangiomas, LMs do not involute but grow proportionally with the growth of the child. LMs of the neck typically contain

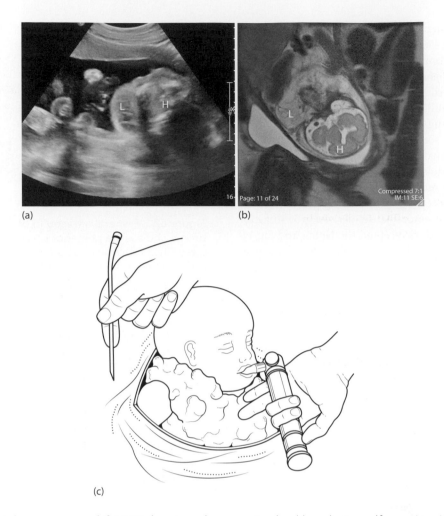

Figure 87.2 **(a)** Prenatal sonogram and **(b)** MRI showing a large pretracheal lymphatic malformation. H = fetal head, T = lymphatic malformation. **(c)** The EXIT procedure, in which intubation is accomplished prior to delivery while still on placental support.

a large macrocystic component and present as a soft, fluctuant swelling in the lateral or anterior neck. These lesions are frequently asymptomatic, and age-related growth is variable (Figure 87.3). While classically referred to as "cystic hygroma," this term is discouraged in contemporary literature as the suffix -*oma* suggests a neoplasm (which it is not) and, furthermore, the term is frequently used in the obstetrical literature to describe a posterior cervical cyst with associated lethal chromosomal abnormalities.[48] The approach to LMs depends upon anatomic location and degree of involvement of vital structures and will be discussed in greater detail in this chapter.

Head and neck

A staging system for LMs of the head and neck was proposed by de Serres et al.[49] (Table 87.1) based upon the anatomic

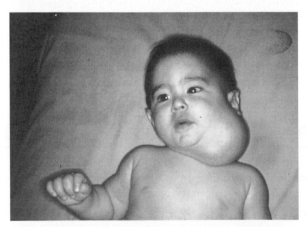

Figure 87.3 Five-month-old child with moderate-sized lymphatic malformation, which was relatively asymptomatic.

Table 87.1 De serres staging of cervicofacial lymphatic malformations

Stage	Anatomic Location
I	Unilateral infrahyoid
II	Unilateral suprahyoid
III	Unilateral infrahyoid and suprahyoid
IV	Bilateral infrahyoid
V	Bilateral infrahyoid and suprahyoid

location of the malformation. Increasing stage is correlated with increasing complexity of treatment approach, increasing complication rate, and increasing number of necessary therapeutic interventions. Since that initial description, there have been multiple refinements based upon extent of oral and pharyngeal involvement. Lesions involving the tongue are only appropriate for complete resection with organ preservation if the tongue is involved partially or superficially.

LMs in the forehead and orbit are frequently combined macrocystic and microcystic lesions and may diffusely infiltrate the intraconal and extraconal space, causing localized overgrowth and proptosis, which makes surgical excision difficult (Figure 87.4). Cervicofacial malformations can be

associated with mandibular overgrowth, causing an underbite.[50] LMs in the floor of the mouth and tongue are characterized by vesicles, intermittent swelling, and bleeding. Occasionally, huge malformations involving the floor of the mouth or the larynx will present at birth with airway obstruction. Rapid increases in size or sudden pain may be due to hemorrhage into the tumor, or to infection. Cervical malformations involving the supraglottic airway may necessitate tracheostomy.

Trunk and extremities

Diffuse thoracic lymphatic anomalies or rare abnormalities of the thoracic duct or cisterna chyli can manifest as

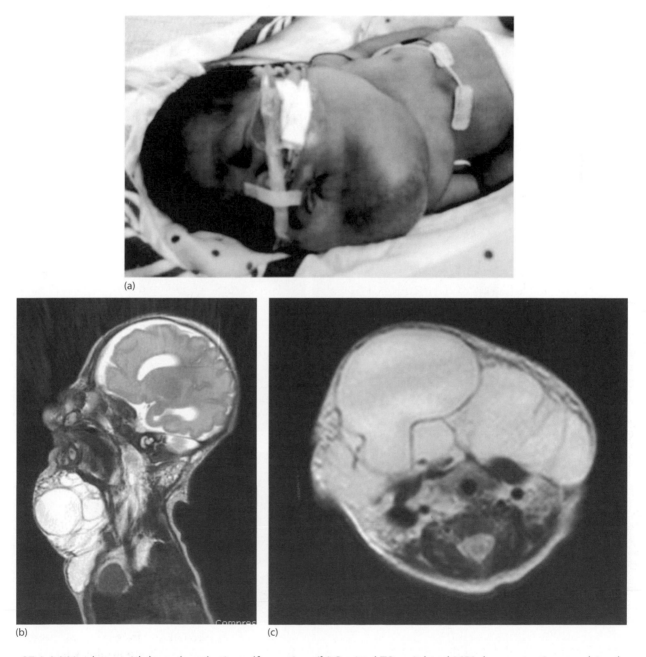

Figure 87.4 **(a)** Newborn with large lymphatic malformation. **(b)** Sagittal T2-weighted MRI demonstrating combined microcystic–macrocystic lesion. **(c)** Axial section of MRI

recurrent pleural and pericardial chylous effusion or chy-lous ascites. Anomalous lymphatics in the gastrointestinal (GI) tract can cause chylous ascites or present with a (typi-cally asymptomatic) cystic abdominal mass (Figure 87.5). Both congenital chylous ascites and chylothorax may be associated with the development of hypoalbuminemia as the result of chronic protein-losing enteropathy. LMs of the extremities may be small and localized or may involve the entire extremity in an infiltrative and debilitating fashion associated with both soft tissue and skeletal overgrowth. Pelvic malformations can be accompanied by bladder outlet obstruction, constipation, or recurrent infection.

Syndromes associated with LMs

Occasionally, LMs occur in the constellation of a well-described phenotype. The eponym *Gorham–Stout syndrome* has been applied to a phenomenon involving progressive osteolysis, caused by diffuse soft tissue and skeletal LMs. Alternative names include "disappearing bone disease" or "phantom bone disease."[51] *Klippel–Trenaunay syndrome* is a well-described combined capillary–lymphatic–venous

malformation associated with soft tissue and skeletal hypertrophy. The capillary malformations are multiple and typically arranged in a geographic pattern over the lateral side of the extremity, buttock, and/or thorax. Lymphatic hypoplasia is present in greater than 50% of patients with associated lymphedema or isolated lymphatic microcysts. *Parkes Weber syndrome* shares many similarities with Klippel-Trenaunay syndrome but should be distinguished by a component of an additional capillary–arteriovenous malformation. Lymphedema should also be included as a type of LM. Type I hereditary lymphedema (*Milroy disease*) is an autosomal dominant disorder presenting early in life with localized areas of edema. Affected areas are character-ized by absent or hypoplastic superficial lymphatics. Type II hereditary lymphedema (*Meige disease*) is a late-onset autosomal dominant disorder attributed to a mutation in the FOXC2 gene with variable penetrance and phenotype. Associated features include distichiasis (a double row of eyelashes), ptosis, cleft palate, yellow nails, and congenital heart disease.[23] The disorder is thought to arise from an impairment of lymphatic drainage, and lymphoscintigra-phy demonstrates numerous dilated lymphatic vessels.

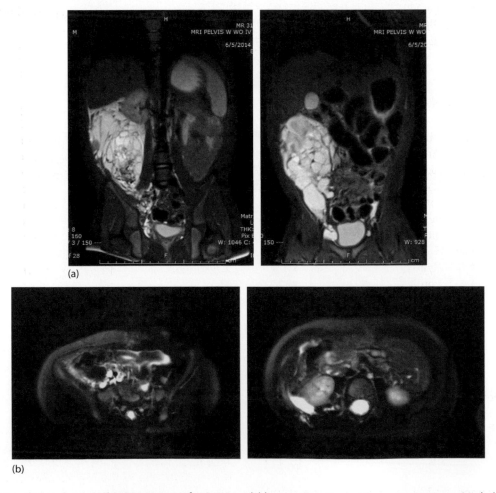

Figure 87.5 **(a)** T2-weighted coronal MRI images of a 3-year-old boy presenting with an asymptomatic abdominal LM. **(b)** Postresection MRI showing markedly reduced disease.

RADIOGRAPHIC INVESTIGATIONS

Magnetic resonance imaging (MRI) is the most useful imaging modality for LMs, aiding in the classification of macrocystic and microcystic lesions as well as defining anatomic relationships, including important neurovascular structures (e.g., brachial plexus and carotid artery).[52-55] LMs demonstrate hyperintense signal intensity in T2-weighted and turbo-Short TI Inversion Recovery (STIR) images as well as rim enhancement after contrast application. Microcystic lesions have an intermediate signal in T1 sequences and an intermediate to high signal on T2 sequences. Macrocystic lesions show low intensity in T1 and high intensity in T2. The new generation of ultrafast MRI scanners has permitted this technique to be used more frequently in small infants, and even in affected fetuses.[56,57]

Ultrasound may be a helpful adjunct in confirming the presence of macrocystic LMs, and Doppler studies may be of additional assistance in looking at flow properties.[58] Computerized tomography (CT) is extremely useful for assessing relationships to adjacent structures, especially within the mediastinum and retroperitoneum.[56,59,60]

Conventional contrast lymphangiography is rarely performed but may be of help in establishing the location of a lymphatic or chylous leak in a patient with a diffuse thoracic lymphatic anomaly.[61] Boxen et al.[62] described the use of lymphoscintigraphy to define the lymphatic supply of a large LM.

Often, a combination of techniques must be used to completely define the anatomic relationships of a large or complicated lesion.

DIFFERENTIAL DIAGNOSIS

The diagnosis of LM is usually straightforward and can be easily differentiated from lymphadenopathy, teratomas, and other solid tumors based on the clinical examination and imaging studies. Lipomas may also be confused with superficial LMs but will not have a cystic appearance on ultrasound examination. Hemangiomas may be present in the same location, but do not transilluminate and tend to collapse on compression. However, there are some patients who have features of both lymphatic and vascular malformation within the same lesion.

COMPLICATIONS

The two principal complications of LMs are intralesional bleeding and infection. Bleeding may occur spontaneously or as a consequence of trauma. It is associated with rapid, painful enlargement of the lesion with attendant ecchymosis. Analgesia and observation are generally sufficient treatment. Prophylactic antibiotics are recommended in the setting of a large bleed. Hemorrhage and infection can transform a macrocystic lesion into a microcystic and scarred lesion.

It is not uncommon for LMs to increase in size in the event of a viral or bacterial infection. This is typically self-limited and thought to be related to changes in lymphatic flow. Nonetheless, bacterial superinfection of the malformation can cause an ascending cellulitis and septicemia, and can be fatal. Additionally, an infection in a cervicofacial LM can cause obstruction of the upper airway and dysphagia. Prolonged intravenous antibiotic therapy is frequently indicated, with choice of broad-spectrum antibiotic agents directed against oral pathogens in the head and neck or enteric organisms in the trunk or perineum.

MANAGEMENT

The two principal modern strategies for treating lymphatic anomalies are sclerotherapy and surgical resection. Historically, irradiation, incision and drainage, and thermosclerosis or irritant sclerosis have all been advocated as nonsurgical treatments.[63,64] With the exception of sclerotherapy, none have demonstrated reproducible success. Sclerotherapy uses a variety of agents to induce obliteration of the lymphatic lumen by chemical destruction of the endothelium with subsequent sclerosis/fibrosis. Success parallels the degree of damage inflicted upon the endothelial and deeper muscular and connective tissue layers. In general, macrocystic LMs are more amenable to sclerotherapy than microcystic lesions because it is possible to drain the entirety of the cyst cavity and induce endothelial apposition prior to administration of a sclerosant. A number of sclerosing agents have been described including doxycycline, OK-432 (Picibanil), ethanol, sodium tetradecyl sulfate (STS), and bleomycin.[65-77] A recent meta-analysis of five retrospective series of children with macrocystic or mixed lesions of the head and neck treated with doxycycline (at a preferred concentration of 10 mg/mL) found 84.2% to be successfully treated, with 20% of those requiring only a single session.[67] Doxycycline is generally well tolerated with minimal side effects. The most commonly reported adverse reactions were cyst hemorrhage, cellulitis, pain, and transient edema. Less commonly, scarring, skin excoriation, and Horner syndrome were reported. These side effects are likely to be related to the sclerosant effect of doxycycline rather than a side effect of the medication itself and are typically self-limited.[78] OK-432, a bacterial product derived from *Streptococcus pyogenes*, induces a significant local inflammatory response and has reported durable success rates (good or excellent results) in 60%–100% of patients.[71,74] The mechanism of action of OK-432 is not completely understood but likely reflects a multitiered activation of the immunologic system including neutrophils, macrophages, natural killer (NK) cells, and T-cells.[72] Despite good success rates and infrequently reported complications, OK-432 is not available in North America but is often a first-line treatment in Europe and Japan.

Recently, several authors have supported the use of bleomycin sclerotherapy (at a concentration of 1 U/mL) in microcystic LMs. The mechanism of action that allows it to be more effective than other sclerosants on microcystic disease is not completely understood but may involve either disruption of tight junctions or induction of endothelial

(a)   (b)

Figure 87.6 **(a)** Lymphangioma circumscriptum presenting in a 4-year-old boy who had undergone resection of a lymphatic malformation at age 1. **(b)** MRI of same child demonstrating deep recurrence at same site.

mesenchymal transitsion.[75] The majority of patients exhibit either a complete (approximately 30%–40%) or partial (50%–60%) response.[75,77] Concerns about bleomycin-induced pulmonary fibrosis have not been substantiated.

Until recently, there were only anecdotal reports of medical management successfully being used as treatment for unresectable LM with no agent demonstrating consistent efficacy. Over the last several years, however, there has been considerable interest in the novel emerging role of several medications including sildenafil and propranolol. Perhaps the most excitement has been generated by sirolimus, an mTOR inhibitor, which blocks the phosphoinositide3-kinase (PI3K)/acutely transforming retrovirus (AKT) pathway of VEGF activation. A recently published Phase II study reported that 100% of patients demonstrated a partial response of large, otherwise unresectable microcystic LM to a 12-week course of sirolimus.[79] Sirolimus has also demonstrated efficacy in kaposiform lymphangiomatosis and lymphangioleiomyomatosis.[79,80]

Although safe surgical excision is possible in most small LMs, some reports in the past decade have advocated injection sclerotherapy for cases that are located in regions where resection would be too hazardous, for cases that have been incompletely resected, and for recurrent disease. Many studies suggest that in such cases, sclerotherapy and surgical therapy have similar results and the treatment selected should reflect upon the strengths and experience of the treating team.[81,82] No carefully controlled study comparing the efficacy of sclerotherapy to surgery has ever been reported. Most articles describing surgical treatment use it as the primary treatment modality, whereas sclerotherapy is described as primary therapy in most cases (approximately 70%) but as secondary therapy following surgical resection in 25%.[82] The successful surgical management of complex (often mixed or microcystic) LM is often staged. In each resection, a surgeon should focus on a defined anatomic region, attempt to limit blood loss, perform as thorough a dissection as possible and be prepared to operate as long as necessary. Even with such an intensive approach to resection, subsequent "recurrence" is as high as 40% after an incomplete excision and 17% after a macroscopically

complete excision.[83] In some patients, persistent disease at the margins can recur as vesicles along the suture line, so-called lymphangioma circumscriptum (Figure 87.6). Multiple methods have been described to treat lymphangioma circumscriptum including surgical excision, lasers, sclerotherapy, electrocoagulation therapy, and topical sirolimus.

SURGICAL MANAGEMENT

Many LMs can be resected without undue morbidity. Although pathological studies have shown that microscopic tumor is often left behind, recurrence is rare when all gross tumor is removed.[83] The following surgical principles must guide resection:

1. Adequate exposure must be obtained.
2. Meticulous dissection must be used in order to preserve vital structures, including nerves, vessels, trachea, and esophagus. We have had success with the use of a microbipolar dissection technique. This technique is of particular advantage when dissecting close to important neurovascular structures.
3. Since this is a benign disease, it is not justifiable to sacrifice a vital structure in order to completely excise the lesion.
4. Whenever possible, the lymphatic supply to the lesion should be ligated to prevent postoperative accumulation of lymph. In the head and neck region, the lymphatic supply to an LM is usually not visible, but it is possible that the microbipolar dissection technique may "weld" these channels shut.

LMs of the neck can usually be approached through a transverse cervical incision under general intratracheal anesthesia. Perioperative antibiotics should be employed. After division of the platysma muscle, the mass is carefully dissected from all surrounding structures (Figure 87.7). Large cystic malformations are usually well encapsulated, and every attempt should be made not to rupture the cysts. The fluid within the cyst aids the surgeon in defining the

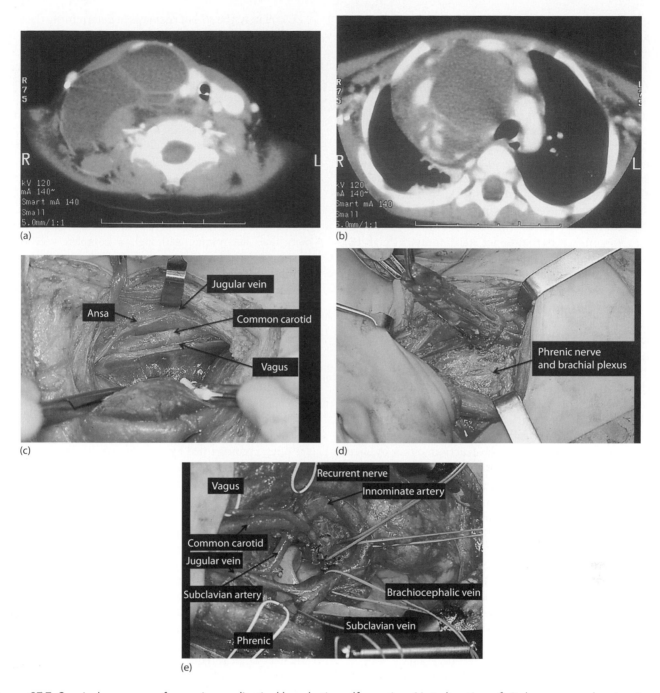

Figure 87.7 Surgical exposure of a cervicomediastinal lymphatic malformation. Note location of vital neurovascular structures, which must not be damaged during the dissection. (a and b) CT scan demonstrating the lesion. (c and d) Dissection of the cervical portion. (e) Completed mediastinal dissection after extension of the incision and sternotomy. (Courtesy of Dr. Vito Forte.)

cyst wall, and therefore in finding the correct plane in which to dissect. Particular care must be taken to avoid injury to the carotid artery and its branches, or to the internal jugular vein. Preservation of other large venous channels, if possible, may also be beneficial in promoting regional drainage. A number of nerves are often closely associated with the lesion, including the facial nerve, the spinal accessory nerve, the vagus nerve, and the brachial plexus. Once the malformation has been removed, and, if possible, the lymphatic supply to the malformation ligated,

a closed-suction drain should be left in the tumor bed to prevent early accumulation of fluid. Dietary restriction of long-chain triglycerides in the postoperative period may be of some benefit in reducing the amount of chylous lymph production.

A small number of cervical lesions extend into the axilla or the mediastinum. For axillary extension, the child should be elevated 15–20 degrees on the involved side, with the arm draped free, and both cervical and axillary crease incisions should be used. The cervical component is approached first, separating the lesion away from the brachial plexus until the cysts are seen to pass below the clavicle. The axillary portion is then dissected free. The most difficult aspect of the operation is removing the lesion from the brachial plexus behind the clavicle, where it is often densely adherent. Only careful, meticulous dissection will permit complete removal of the malformation without injury to the nerves.

Extension into the mediastinum also presents a difficult technical challenge. The best approach is one-stage resection through an "inverted hockey-stick" incision, as described by Grosfeld, whereby a transverse neck incision is extended inferiorly into a midline sternotomy.[84] Modifications of the Grosfeld approach, either by leaving a bridge of skin between the horizontal cervical and midline sternotomy incisions or by performing a partial upper sternotomy through the cervical incision, may provide a cosmetically superior result without significantly compromising exposure. These approaches provide adequate exposure to safely dissect the lesion away from the jugular, carotid, and subclavian vessels, and the aortic arch, esophagus, and pericardium, with preservation of the phrenic, vagus, and recurrent laryngeal nerves. The rare LM that is confined to the mediastinum can be approached through a lateral thoracotomy, a midline sternotomy, or a thoracoscopic approach.

Perhaps the most difficult lesions to approach surgically are the massive lesions that involve the tongue, floor of the mouth, and larynx. These lesions are usually present at birth and may result in early airway obstruction, either by sheer mass effect or as a result of hemorrhage into the tumor. In many cases, a tracheostomy is necessary, followed by multiple extensive operative procedures. Additionally, placement of a gastrostomy tube should be considered for any patient with a large cervical facial LM requiring multiple operative procedures and who may have oropharyngeal discoordination. For such lesions, combined treatment modalities including sclerotherapy (for macrocystic components), systemic therapy (sirolimus), and surgery may offer the best outcome. For prenatally diagnosed cases, access to the airway can be achieved at the time of cesarian section before clamping the umbilical cord (EXIT procedure), although emergent tracheostomy at the time of birth is rarely necessary.[45-47]

LMs involving the tongue pose a very difficult problem. As a general principle, direct surgical treatment of the tongue should be avoided if possible. Intermittent swelling of the tongue can be effectively controlled with systemic steroids. Capillary LMs involving the mucosal surface of the tongue (also known as simplex) can cause blistering, bleeding, and pain and are best handled with laser resurfacing techniques or bleomycin sclerotherapy.[77,85,86] Also, the use of laser technology for controlling airway obstruction from laryngeal or tracheal involvement has been highly successful in this group of patients. Persistent, symptomatic macroglossia involving the intrinsic muscles of the tongue may require reduction glossoplasty. LMs involving the floor of the mouth and tongue may also lead to bony malformations of the growing mandible, which may require subsequent surgical correction.[87]

Ultimately, the role of cosmesis in determining the extent of treatment is difficult to define. Severe LMs may be associated with significant social stigmatization, and this is of concern to patients and families alike.[88] However, because LM is a benign disease, gross total resection is not justified if it requires resection of vital structures. Thus, the treatment goal should be to restore function and adequate cosmesis while preserving important anatomic structures.[48]

LMs in the abdomen usually originate in the retroperitoneum or the intestinal mesentery. Choice of management depends on the type and extent of the lesion and can include surgical excision and/or sclerotherapy.[89] When surgical excision is chosen, either a laparotomy or a laparoscopic approach can be used. In either case, resection should be done using meticulous technique. Although a complete resection is sometimes possible, often some of the lesion must be left behind. Remaining cysts should be unroofed, since complications such as postoperative ascites are rarely seen. Primary intestinal lymphangiectasia presenting as a protein-losing enteropathy has been reported in case studies to be successfully treated with segmental resection of the most severely involved small bowel.[90] Occasionally, an LM will present with scrotal swelling and may be misdiagnosed and operated upon as a hydrocele. Once the diagnosis has become clear, these lesions should undergo complete resection if possible.

LMs of the extremities range from small, easily resected cysts to large, infiltrating lesions. The large malformations are often accompanied by poor lymphatic drainage, which predisposes the limb to edema, infection, and inhibition of function. Complete excision of these lesions may be impossible, and amputation may ultimately be necessary.

SURGICAL COMPLICATIONS

In the modern era, the mortality associated with surgical resection of an LM should approach zero. Early intervention before infectious complications or airway obstruction and strict adherence to the principles described here permit safe removal with little morbidity in the majority of cases. The complications of surgery include seroma, infection, and neurological sequelae such as Horner syndrome, facial nerve palsy, or spinal accessory nerve injury.

Recurrence can occur after surgical excision, especially if the first resection has been incomplete. These recurrences may represent fluid refilling cysts that had been decompressed, or may be due to filling of more distal cysts whose drainage has been interrupted by the surgical procedure. Ultrasound, CT, and MRI may all be useful for demonstrating these recurrent lesions. Options for management include further resection or injection sclerotherapy, depending on the anatomic location and the likelihood of injury to neurovascular structures.

CONCLUSION

LMs present as a clinically diverse spectrum of lesions arising at any anatomic location throughout the body. Lesions can be as simple as a single macrocyst of the neck or a complex as a microcystic cervicofacial lesion with intracerebral and mediastinal extension. For complex lesions, there is no single treatment consensus, but a treatment algorithm must be established based upon the experience and strengths of a multidisciplinary managing team. Goals and limitations of treatment should be established via thorough discussions between the patient's family and all treatment providers.

REFERENCES

1. Christison-Lagay ER, Fishman SJ. Vascular anomalies. *Surg Clin N Am* 2006; 86: 393–425, x.
2. Sabin F. The lymphatic system in human embryos with a consideration of the morphology of the system as a whole. *Am J Anat* 1909; 9.
3. Bautch VL, Caron KM. Blood and lymphatic vessel formation. *Cold Spring Harb Perspect Biol* 2015; 7: a008268.
4. Srinivasan RS, Dillard ME, Lagutin OV et al. Lineage tracing demonstrates the venous origin of the mammalian lymphatic vasculature. *Genes Dev* 2007; 21: 2422–32.
5. Yang Y, García-Verdugo JM, Soriano-Navarro M et al. Lymphatic endothelial progenitors bud from the cardinal vein and intersomitic vessels in mammalian embryos. *Blood* 2012; 120: 2340–8.
6. Jussila L, Alitalo K. Vascular growth factors and lymphangiogenesis. *Physiol Rev* 2002; 82: 673–700.
7. Karkkainen MJ, Petrova TV. Vascular endothelial growth factor receptors in the regulation of angiogenesis and lymphangiogenesis. *Oncogene* 2000; 19: 5598–605.
8. Srinivasan RS, Escobedo N, Yang Y et al. The Prox1–Vegfr3 feedback loop maintains the identity and the number of lymphatic endothelial cell progenitors. *Genes Dev* 2014; 28: 2175–87.
9. Francois M, Harvey NL, Hogan BM. The transcriptional control of lymphatic vascular development. *Physiology (Bethesda)* 2011; 26: 146–55.
10. François M, Short K, Secker GA et al. Segmental territories along the cardinal veins generate lymph sacs via a ballooning mechanism during embryonic lymphangiogenesis in mice. *Dev Biol* 2012; 364: 89–98.
11. Chen CY, Bertozzi C, Zou Z et al. Blood flow reprograms lymphatic vessels to blood vessels. *J Clin Invest* 2012; 122: 2006–17.
12. Chen H, Griffin C, Xia L, Srinivasan RS. Molecular and cellular mechanisms of lymphatic vascular maturation. *Microvasc Res* 2014; 96: 16–22.
13. Harvey NL, Oliver G. Choose your fate: Artery, vein or lymphatic vessel? *Curr Opin Genet Dev* 2004; 14: 499–505.
14. Oliver G. Lymphatic vasculature development. *Nat Rev Immunol* 2004; 4: 35–45.
15. Ferrell RE, Levinson KL, Esman JH et al. Hereditary lymphedema: Evidence for linkage and genetic heterogeneity. *Hum Mol Genet* 1998; 7: 2073–8.
16. Butler MG, Dagenais SL, Rockson SG, Glover TW. A novel VEGFR3 mutation causes Milroy disease. *Am J Med Genet A* 2007; 143A: 1212–7.
17. Mendola A, Schlögel MJ, Ghalamkarpour A et al. Mutations in the VEGFR3 signaling pathway explain 36% of familial lymphedema. *Mol Syndromol* 2013; 4: 257–66.
18. Sato TN, Tozawa Y, Deutsch U et al. Distinct roles of the receptor tyrosine kinases Tie-1 and Tie-2 in blood vessel formation. *Nature* 1995; 376: 70–4.
19. Puri MC, Rossant J, Alitalo K, Bernstein A, Partanen J. The receptor tyrosine kinase TIE is required for integrity and survival of vascular endothelial cells. *EMBO J* 1995; 14: 5884–91.
20. D'Amico G, Korhonen EA, Waltari M, Saharinen P, Laakkonen P, Alitalo K. Loss of endothelial Tie1 receptor impairs lymphatic vessel development-brief report. *Arterioscler Thromb Vasc Biol* 2010; 30: 207–9.
21. Maisonpierre PC, Suri C, Jones PF et al. Angiopoietin-2, a natural antagonist for Tie2 that disrupts in vivo angiogenesis. *Science* 1997; 277: 55–60.
22. Garabedian MJ, Wallerstein D, Medina N, Byrne J, Wallerstein RJ. Prenatal Diagnosis of Cystic Hygroma related to a Deletion of 16q24.1 with Haploinsufficiency of FOXF1 and FOXC2 Genes. *Case Rep Genet* 2012; 2012: 490408.
23. Dagenais SL, Hartsough RL, Erickson RP, Witte MH, Butler MG, Glover TW. Foxc2 is expressed in developing lymphatic vessels and other tissues associated with lymphedema–distichiasis syndrome. *Gene Expr Patterns* 2004; 4: 611–9.
24. Soldi R, Mitola S, Strasly M, Defilippi P, Tarone G, Bussolino F. Role of alphavbeta3 integrin in the activation of vascular endothelial growth factor receptor-2. *EMBO J* 1999; 18: 882–92.
25. Bazigou E, Xie S, Chen C et al. Integrin-alpha9 is required for fibronectin matrix assembly during lymphatic valve morphogenesis. *Dev Cell* 2009; 17: 175–86.
26. Bazigou E, Lyons OT, Smith A et al. Genes regulating lymphangiogenesis control venous valve formation and maintenance in mice. *J Clin Invest* 2011; 121: 2984–92.
27. Bazigou E, Wilson JT, Moore JE. Primary and secondary lymphatic valve development: Molecular, functional and mechanical insights. *Microvasc Res* 2014; 96: 38–45.
28. Gallagher PG, Mahoney MJ, Gosche JR. Cystic hygroma in the fetus and newborn. *Semin Perinatol* 1999; 23: 341–56.
29. Rempen A, Feige A. Differential diagnosis of sonographically detected tumours in the fetal cervical region. *Eur J Obstet Gynecol Reprod Biol* 1985; 20: 89–105.
30. Byrne J, Blanc WA, Warburton D, Wigger J. The significance of cystic hygroma in fetuses. *Hum Pathol* 1984; 15: 61–7.

31. Chervenak FA, Isaacson G, Blakemore KJ et al. Fetal cystic hygroma. Cause and natural history. *N Engl J Med* 1983; 309: 822–5.

32. Graham JM, Stephens TD, Shepard TH. Nuchal cystic hygroma in a fetus with presumed Roberts syndrome. *Am J Med Genet* 1983; 15: 163–7.

33. Langer JC, Fitzgerald PG, Desa D et al. Cervical cystic hygroma in the fetus: Clinical spectrum and outcome. *J Pediatr Surg* 1990; 25: 58–61; discussion -2.

34. Chodirker BN, Harman CR, Greenberg CR. Spontaneous resolution of a cystic hygroma in a fetus with Turner syndrome. *Prenat Diagn* 1988; 8: 291–6.

35. Chodirker BN, Harman CR, Greenberg CR. Survival of fetuses with abnormal karyotypes and cystic hygromas detected prenatally. *Prenat Diagn* 1990; 10: 136.

36. Nadel A, Bromley B, Benacerraf BR. Nuchal thickening or cystic hygromas in first- and early second-trimester fetuses: Prognosis and outcome. *Obstet Gynecol* 1993; 82: 43–8.

37. Johnson MP, Johnson A, Holzgreve W et al. First-trimester simple hygroma: Cause and outcome. *Am J Obstet Gynecol* 1993; 168: 156–61.

38. Shulman LP, Emerson DS, Grevengood C et al. Clinical course and outcome of fetuses with isolated cystic nuchal lesions and normal karyotypes detected in the first trimester. *Am J Obstet Gynecol* 1994; 171: 1278–81.

39. Van Vugt JM, Tinnemans BW, Van Zalen-Sprock RM. Outcome and early childhood follow-up of chromosomally normal fetuses with increased nuchal translucency at 10–14 weeks' gestation. *Ultrasound Obstet Gynecol* 1998; 11: 407–9.

40. van Vugt JM, van Zalen-Sprock RM, Kostense PJ. First-trimester nuchal translucency: A risk analysis on fetal chromosome abnormality. *Radiology* 1996; 200: 537–40.

41. Shulman LP, Emerson DS, Felker RE, Phillips OP, Simpson JL, Elias S. High frequency of cytogenetic abnormalities in fetuses with cystic hygroma diagnosed in the first trimester. *Obstet Gynecol* 1992; 80: 80–2.

42. Thomas RL. Prenatal diagnosis of giant cystic hygroma: Prognosis, counselling, and management; case presentation and review of the recent literature. *Prenat Diagn* 1992; 12: 919–23.

43. Benacerraf BR, Frigoletto FD. Prenatal sonographic diagnosis of isolated congenital cystic hygroma, unassociated with lymphedema or other morphologic abnormality. *J Ultrasound Med* 1987; 6: 63–6.

44. Goldstein I, Jakobi P, Shoshany G, Filmer S, Itskoviz I, Maor B. Late-onset isolated cystic hygroma: The obstetrical significance, management, and outcome. *Prenat Diagn* 1994; 14: 757–61.

45. Filipchuck D, Avdimiretz L. The ex utero intrapartum treatment (EXIT) procedure for fetal head and neck masses. *AORN J* 2009; 90: 661–72; quiz 73–6.

46. Lazar DA, Olutoye OO, Moise KJ et al. Ex-utero intrapartum treatment procedure for giant neck masses—Fetal and maternal outcomes. *J Pediatr Surg* 2011; 46: 817–22.

47. Liechty KW, Crombleholme TM, Flake AW et al. Intrapartum airway management for giant fetal neck masses: the EXIT (ex utero intrapartum treatment) procedure. *Am J Obstet Gynecol* 1997; 177: 870–4.

48. Elluru RG, Balakrishnan K, Padua HM. Lymphatic malformations: diagnosis and management. *Semin Pediatr Surg* 2014; 23: 178–85.

49. de Serres LM, Sie KC, Richardson MA. Lymphatic malformations of the head and neck. A proposal for staging. *Arch Otolaryngol Head Neck Surg* 1995; 121: 577–82.

50. Padwa BL, Hayward PG, Ferraro NF, Mulliken JB. Cervicofacial lymphatic malformation: Clinical course, surgical intervention, and pathogenesis of skeletal hypertrophy. *Plast Reconstr Surg* 1995; 95: 951–60.

51. Gorham LW, Stout AP. Massive osteolysis (acute spontaneous absorption of bone, phantom bone, disappearing bone); its relation to hemangiomatosis. *J Bone Joint Surg Am* 1955; 37-A: 985–1004.

52. Griauzde J, Srinivasan A. Imaging of vascular lesions of the head and neck. *Radiol Clin N Am* 2015; 53: 197–213.

53. Fung K, Poenaru D, Soboleski DA, Kamal IM. Impact of magnetic resonance imaging on the surgical management of cystic hygromas. *J Pediatr Surg* 1998; 33: 839–41.

54. Siegel MJ, Glazer HS, St Amour TE, Rosenthal DD. Lymphangiomas in children: MR imaging. *Radiology* 1989; 170: 467–70.

55. Wang H, Li S, Jiang Z. Magnetic resonance lymphangiography for the assessment of the lymphatic system in a lymphatic malformation patient undergoing sclerotherapy. *J Dermatol* 2016.

56. Cutillo DP, Swayne LC, Cucco J, Dougan H. CT and MR imaging in cystic abdominal lymphangiomatosis. *J Comput Assist Tomogr* 1989; 13: 534–6.

57. Puig S, Casati B, Staudenherz A, Paya K. Vascular low-flow malformations in children: Current concepts for classification, diagnosis and therapy. *Eur J Radiol* 2005; 53: 35–45.

58. Oates CP, Wilson AW, Ward-Booth RP, Williams ED. Combined use of Doppler and conventional ultrasound for the diagnosis of vascular and other lesions in the head and neck. *Int J Oral Maxillofac Surg* 1990; 19: 235–9.

59. Davidson AJ, Hartman DS. Lymphangioma of the retroperitoneum: CT and sonographic characteristic. *Radiology* 1990; 175: 507–10.

60. Mahboubi S, Potsic WP. Computed tomography of cervical cystic hygroma in the neck. *Int J Pediatr Otorhinolaryngol* 1989; 18: 47–51.

61. Fishman SJ, Burrows PE, Upton J, Hendren WH. Life-threatening anomalies of the thoracic duct: Anatomic delineation dictates management. *J Pediatr Surg* 2001; 36: 1269–72.

62. Boxen I, Zhang ZM, Filler RM. Lymphoscintigraphy for cystic hygroma. *J Nucl Med* 1990; 31: 516–8.

63. F. F. Radium in the treatment of multilocular lymph cysts in the neck of children. *Am J Rad* 1929; 21: 473–80.

64. G. H. Treatment of cystic hygroma of the neck by sodium morrhuate. *Br Med J* 1933; 2: 148–55.

65. Burrows PE, Mitri RK, Alomari A et al. Percutaneous sclerotherapy of lymphatic malformations with doxycycline. *Lymphat Res Biol* 2008; 6: 209–16.

66. Chaudry G, Burrows PE, Padua HM, Dillon BJ, Fishman SJ, Alomari AI. Sclerotherapy of abdominal lymphatic malformations with doxycycline. *J Vasc Interv Radiol* 2011; 22: 1431–5.

67. Cheng J. Doxycycline sclerotherapy in children with head and neck lymphatic malformations. *J Pediatr Surg* 2015; 50: 2143–6.

68. Farnoosh S, Don D, Koempel J, Panossian A, Anselmo D, Stanley P. Efficacy of doxycycline and sodium tetradecyl sulfate sclerotherapy in pediatric head and neck lymphatic malformations. *Int J Pediatr Otorhinolaryngol* 2015; 79: 883–7.

69. Chen WL, Huang ZQ, Chai Q et al. Percutaneous sclerotherapy of massive macrocystic lymphatic malformations of the face and neck using fibrin glue with OK-432 and bleomycin. *Int J Oral Maxillofac Surg* 2011; 40: 572–6.

70. Gilony D, Schwartz M, Shpitzer T, Feinmesser R, Kornreich L, Raveh E. Treatment of lymphatic malformations: A more conservative approach. *J Pediatr Surg* 2012; 47: 1837–42.

71. Ogita S, Tsuto T, Nakamura K, Deguchi E, Iwai N. OK-432 therapy in 64 patients with lymphangioma. *J Pediatr Surg* 1994; 29: 784–5.

72. Ogita S, Tsuto T, Nakamura K, Deguchi E, Tokiwa K, Iwai N. OK-432 therapy for lymphangioma in children: Why and how does it work? *J Pediatr Surg* 1996; 31: 477–80.

73. Poldervaart MT, Breugem CC, Speleman L, Pasmans S. Treatment of lymphatic malformations with OK-432 (Picibanil): Review of the literature. *J Craniofac Surg* 2009; 20: 1159–62.

74. Weitz-Tuoretmaa A, Rautio R, Valkila J, Keski-Säntti H, Keski-Nisula L, Laranne J. Efficacy of OK-432 sclerotherapy in treatment of lymphatic malformations: Long-term follow-up results. *Eur Arch Otorhinolaryngol* 2014; 271: 385–90.

75. Chaudry G, Guevara CJ, Rialon KL et al. Safety and efficacy of bleomycin sclerotherapy for microcystic lymphatic malformation. *Cardiovasc Intervent Radiol* 2014; 37: 1476–81.

76. Okada A, Kubota A, Fukuzawa M, Imura K, Kamata S. Injection of bleomycin as a primary therapy of cystic lymphangioma. *J Pediatr Surg* 1992; 27: 440–3.

77. Yang Y, Sun M, Ma Q et al. Bleomycin A5 sclerotherapy for cervicofacial lymphatic malformations. *J Vasc Surg* 2011; 53: 150–5.

78. Wang KL, Chun RH, Kerschner JE, Sulman CG. Sympathetic neuropathy and dysphagia following doxycycline sclerotherapy. *Int J Pediatr Otorhinolaryngol* 2013; 77: 1613–6.

79. Adams D, Trenor C, Hammill A, Azizkhan R. Efficacy and safety of sirolimus in the treatment of complicated vascular anomalies. *Pediatrics* 2016; 137.

80. Wang Z, Li K, Yao W, Dong K, Xiao X, Zheng S. Successful treatment of kaposiform lymphangiomatosis with sirolimus. *Pediatr Blood Cancer* 2015; 62: 1291–3.

81. Balakrishnan K, Menezes MD, Chen BS, Magit AE, Perkins JA. Primary surgery vs primary sclerotherapy for head and neck lymphatic malformations. *JAMA Otolaryngol Head Neck Surg* 2014; 140: 41–5.

82. Adams MT, Saltzman B, Perkins JA. Head and neck lymphatic malformation treatment: A systematic review. *Otolaryngol Head Neck Surg* 2012; 147: 627–39.

83. Alqahtani A, Nguyen LT, Flageole H, Shaw K, Laberge JM. 25 years' experience with lymphangiomas in children. *J Pediatr Surg* 1999; 34: 1164–8.

84. Grosfeld JL, Weber TR, Vane DW. One-stage resection for massive cervicomediastinal hygroma. *Surgery* 1982; 92: 693–9.

85. Wang LC, Krunic AL, Medenica MM, Soltani K, Busbey S. Treatment of hemorrhagic lymphatic malformation of the tongue with a pulsed-dye laser. *J Am Acad Dermatol* 2005; 52: 1088–90.

86. Wiegand S, Eivazi B, Zimmermann AP et al. Microcystic lymphatic malformations of the tongue: Diagnosis, classification, and treatment. *Arch Otolaryngol Head Neck Surg* 2009; 135: 976–83.

87. Osborne TE, Levin LS, Tilghman DM, Haller JA. Surgical correction of mandibulofacial deformities secondary to large cervical cystic hygromas. *J Oral Maxillofac Surg* 1987; 45: 1015–21.

88. Balakrishnan K, Edwards TC, Perkins JA. Functional and symptom impacts of pediatric head and neck lymphatic malformations: Developing a patient-derived instrument. *Otolaryngol Head Neck Surg* 2012; 147: 925–31.

89. Dasgupta R, Fishman SJ. Management of visceral vascular anomalies. *Semin Pediatr Surg* 2014; 23: 216–20.

90. Kim NR, Lee SK, Suh YL. Primary intestinal lymphangiectasia successfully treated by segmental resections of small bowel. *J Pediatr Surg* 2009; 44: e13–7.

88

Cervical teratomas

MICHAEL W. L. GAUDERER

INTRODUCTION

Cervical teratomas, although rare, are an important cause of neck masses in newborns and children. Because these lesions are often quite large, they can lead to precipitous airway obstruction necessitating prompt recognition and surgical intervention. Antenatal diagnosis and new techniques of multidisciplinary intrapartum management have contributed to an improved outlook for the survival of newborns at greatest risk of airway compromise.

PATHOLOGY

Teratomas are neoplastic lesions composed of tissues foreign to the anatomical site of origin, including all three germ layers. It is believed that most cervical teratomas arise from the embryonic thyroid anlage, although frequently, clear association with the gland cannot be demonstrated.[1-4] Roediger et al.[5] presented a comprehensive discussion of the histogenesis of this lesion in 1974. Although a wide variety of tissues from all three germinal layers have been found in cervical teratomas, there is a 68% incidence of neural tissue, which in many cases predominates in the solid portion of the tumor.[2-4,6] Thyroid tissue is present in 30% of specimens. The majority of cervical teratomas in the pediatric age group are benign (Figure 88.1a–c); however, malignancy with and without distant metastases has been reported.[3,7-9] Conversely, the incidence of malignancy in adults with cervical teratomas is reported to be as high as 70%.[10] Although cervical teratomas are generally located anteriorly to the major neck structures (Figure 88.2), significant distortions of normal anatomy are frequently encountered (Figure 88.3).[3,4,9,11,12] Teratomas are usually single lesions; however, they may occur in more than one site in the head and neck.[13] The presence of a teratoma arising in one fetus of a twin pregnancy has been described.[14] Associated anomalies are rare.[2-4]

INCIDENCE AND CLINICAL MANIFESTATIONS

In four large series of teratomas in infancy and childhood, the incidence of cervical location ranged from 2% to 9.3%.[15-20] Cervical teratomas are reported to occur in all races, and there is a slight female preponderance.[2-4] There is a high incidence of prematurity, polyhydramnios, and birth dystocia. Polyhydramnios is probably secondary to inability of the fetus to swallow amniotic fluid.[2] Stillbirth is usually associated with giant cervical lesions and due to a combination of compression of vital structures and congestive heart failure.[21] The most common clinical presentation, in addition to the mass, is respiratory difficulty.[1,4,12,22] Respiratory symptoms may vary from total apnea to mild dyspnea or coughing with feedings. The dyspnea may also be positional. Although airway compression may not be noted at birth, it may progress rapidly over several hours to a life-threatening obstruction. These cervical teratomas clearly represent a spectrum. Some children are referred beyond the neonatal period,[23] while in others, it only becomes manifest in adulthood.[3,10] A classification of cervical teratomas,[3] taking into consideration the age and clinical presentation (Table 88.1), clearly shows that almost half of the patients are newborns with respiratory distress (group II). Operative and nonoperative management was accompanied by a 43% mortality in this subgroup.[3] However, prenatal diagnosis, and more recently, the addition of intrapartum management, has markedly changed care and increased the survival rate, even for some of the highest-risk patients.[12,24-32]

DIAGNOSIS

Cervical teratomas can accurately be diagnosed antenatally[3,4,28] using ultrasonography,[28] which is the also the most useful immediate postnatal imaging study. Plain radiographs demonstrate calcification within the lesion in 16% of pediatric cases.[3,29] Tracheal deviation is common. Other imaging modalities such as radioisotope scans, computed axial tomography (Figure 88.3), and magnetic resonance

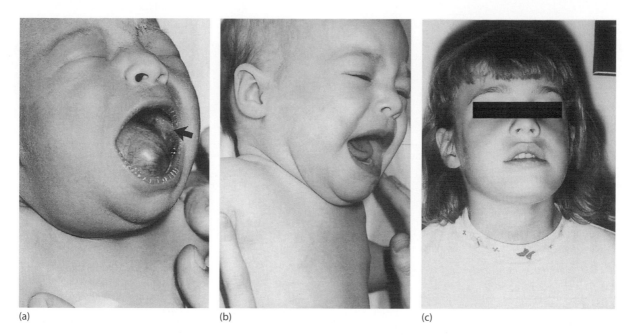

(a) (b) (c)

Figure 88.1 (a) One-day-old, full-term female newborn born with right cervical teratoma that extended into the oral floor, displacing the tongue to the left (arrow). The lesion was firm, partially cystic, and limited to the right anterior cervical triangle. She had mild respiratory distress, worsening when placed in the supine position. On the second day of life, the 6.5 × 5.5 × 4.5 cm mass was excised through a transverse cervical incision, combined with intraoral dissection. The thyroid gland was not involved. Analysis of the specimen revealed a benign cystic teratoma containing neuroglia, choroids plexus, smooth muscle, respiratory and squamous epithelium, and pancreas. Transient difficulty with oral feedings occurred in the immediate postoperative period. (b) Same child at 3 months of age. Notice the well-healed scar following the natural skin crease and the normal position of the tongue. (c) Same child at 6 years. The scar is no longer discernible. Tongue motion and dentition are normal.

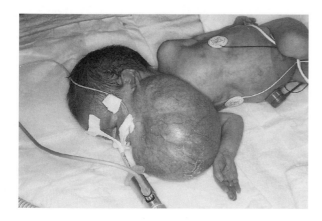

Figure 88.2 Very large cervical teratoma in a premature child.

imaging (MRI) are helpful in more complex cases but should be used with great caution because sedation for longer exposure times may be needed. MRI can be helpful in planning the operation, as it demonstrates planes of dissection and position of vital structures that have been displaced by tumor growth.[7] It is also useful in the prenatal evaluation in preparation for operating on placental support.[30–32]

DIFFERENTIAL DIAGNOSIS

Differential diagnoses should include cystic hygroma, lymphangioma, branchial cleft abnormalities, congenital

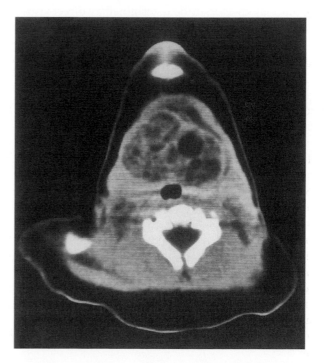

Figure 88.3 Computed tomography scan of the neck of a 5-month-old female patient. The lesion was initially thought to be a hemangiolymphangioma. Fortunately, this child had minimal or no airway compression, in spite of the location of the mass. The removed specimen was a benign teratoma containing neuroglia, choroid plexus, respiratory epithelium, pancreas, muscle, and cartilage.

Table 88.1 Classification of cervical teratomas by age and clinical presentation based on the review of 217 cases.[3]

Group	No. of cases	Total cases (%)	Malignant (%)	Mortality (%)
I Stillborn and moribund live newborn	27	12.4	2 (7.4)	100
II Newborn with respiratory distress	99	45.6	2 (2)	43.4[a]
III Newborn without respiratory distress	37	17.1	0	2.7
IV Children age 1 month to 18 years	31	14.3	0	3.2
V Adult	23	10.6	16 (69.6)	43.5[b]

Source: Jordan RB and Gauderer MWL, Cervical Teratomas: An Analysis. Literature Review and Proposed Classification. *J Pediatr Surg* 1988;23:583–91.
[a] Includes operative and nonoperative treatment.
[b] Incomplete follow up for six malignant cases.

goiter, thyroglossal duct cyst, dermoid cyst, neuroblastoma, and duplications.

MANAGEMENT

The most difficult aspect of the management of orocervical teratomas is the establishment and maintenance of an adequate airway.[3,9,12,22] Orotracheal or nasotracheal intubation requires skill and patience in these infants due to tracheal deviation and/or compression. A useful adjunct is nasotracheal intubation with the aid of a flexible fiber-optic scope. The endotracheal tube is slipped over the scope, and the endoscope is then inserted. Once the tip of the flexible scope reaches the carina, the endotracheal tube is advanced and positioned. The distance between the carina and the end of the tube can then easily be determined by direct visualization. Tracheostomy, as an emergency procedure, has obvious limitations, although it may be necessary in extreme situations.[22,26] Whenever possible, a tracheostomy should be avoided because it increases operative as well as postoperative morbidity.[3] If the teratoma is composed of one or more large cysts, emergency aspiration may be employed to reduce tumor size and alleviate pressure on the airway.

An exciting advance in the management of fetuses with giant lesions and a high probability of upper-airway compromise at or immediately after birth is the development of the *ex utero* intrapartum treatment (EXIT).[12–32] This technique permits the establishment of a secure airway while the child is on placental support. The procedure requires a multidisciplinary approach of team members from the involved specialties: obstetrics, anesthesia, pediatric surgery, and neonatology.[24–27,30–32]

The incision for cervical and orocervical teratomas should be carefully planned to allow access not only to the neck but also to the upper mediastinum or oral cavity, if needed. As opposed to lymphangiomas, teratomas usually can be dissected without great difficulty (Figure 88.4a and b). The lesion is often attached to one of the lobes of the thyroid.

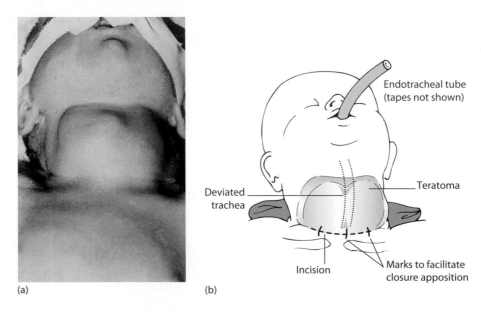

(a) (b)

Figure 88.4 Operative approach to the case in Figure 88.3. The intubated child's neck is elevated over a roll **(a)**. Wide draping with adhesive plastic sheets allows for excellent exposure and helps prevent temperature loss. The incision is drawn with a marking pen on one of the skin creases, if possible **(b)**. To facilitate proper apposition of the redundant skin following resection, multiple small crosshatches are drawn with the pen. Following the skin incision, the marks are replaced by guy sutures, which are helpful for traction on the flaps, as well as the final approximation. It must be remembered during the dissection that the trachea may not be in the center. Other vital structures may also be markedly displaced.

When dissection reaches this level, every attempt should be made to preserve the thyroid and parathyroids. Dissection around the trachea and the esophagus must be carried out with great care to avoid injury to the recurrent laryngeal nerves (Figure 88.5). Tracheal as well as esophageal deviation should be constantly kept in mind. In the small neck of the newborn, deep dissection can lead to injury to the phrenic nerves. Once the tumor is removed, a soft, fine silicone rubber drain is placed and attached to a closed drainage system. The musculoaponeurotic layers are approximated with fine synthetic absorbable sutures, and the skin is closed with subcuticular stitches. Postoperatively, vocal cord and diaphragmatic function should be assessed and recorded. Calcium levels are measured in the immediate postoperative period, and thyroid function tests are obtained after a few weeks. Careful histological examination of the entire specimen is mandatory (Figure 88.6). If the alpha-fetoprotein levels were initially elevated, follow-up determinations should be sought.

CONCLUSION

The overall prognosis for cervical teratomas is good, particularly in the newborn with little or no respiratory distress (Table 88.1).[3,4,9,17,23] If the lesion is diagnosed *in utero*, appropriate preparations can be made to assure prompt establishment of a good airway immediately at or following birth. Carefully planned excision is then possible. This should increase the survival in the newborn with significant respiratory compromise.

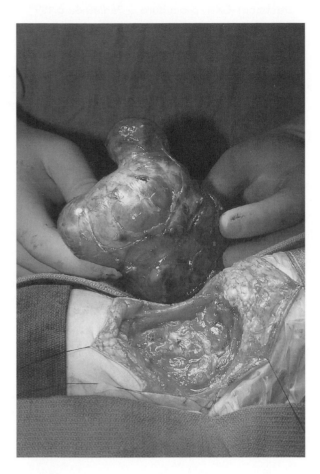

Figure 88.5 Complete excision of a large cervical teratoma. Notice the smooth surface of the removed specimen and retraction of the redundant skin flaps by the guy sutures.

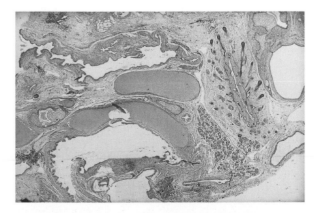

Figure 88.6 Histological section of a cervical teratoma demonstrating an array of various tissues.

REFERENCES

1. Saphir O. Teratoma of the neck. *Am J Pathol* 1929; 5: 313–22.
2. Silberman R, Mendelson IR. Teratoma of the neck. Report of two cases and review of the literature. *Arch Dis Child* 1960; 35: 159–70.
3. Jordan RB, Gauderer MWL. Cervical teratomas: An analysis. Literature review and proposed classification. *J Pediatr Surg* 1988; 23: 583–91.
4. Elmasalme F, Giacomantonio M, Clarke KD et al. Congenital cervical teratoma in neonates. Case report and review. *Eur J Pediatr Surg* 2000; 10: 252–7.
5. Roediger WE, Spitz L, Schmaman A. Histogenesis of benign cervical teratomas. *Teratology* 1974; 10: 111–18.
6. Gundry SR, Wesley JR, Klein MD et al. Cervical teratomas in the newborn. *J Pediatr Surg* 1983; 18: 382–6.
7. Touraj T, Applebaum H, Frost DB. Congenital metastatic teratoma: Diagnostic and management considerations. *J Pediatr Surg* 1989; 24: 21–3.
8. Baumann FR, Nerlich A. Metastasizing cervical teratoma of the fetus. *Pediatr Pathol* 1993; 13: 21–7.
9. Azizkhan RG, Haase GM, Applebaum H et al. Diagnosis, management, and outcome of cerviofacial teratomas in neonates: A Children's Cancer Study. *J Pediatr Surg* 1995; 30: 312–16.
10. Als C, Laeng H, Cerny T et al. Primary cervical malignant teratoma with a rib metastasis in an adult: Five-year survival after surgery and chemotherapy. A case report with a review of the literature. *Ann Oncol* 1998; 9: 1015–22.

11. Hester TO, Camnitz PS, Albernaz MS et al. Superficial carotid artery secondary to cervical teratoma. *Ear Nose Throat J* 1991; 70: 524–6.

12. Steigman SA, Nemes L, Barnewolt CE et al. Differential risk for neonatal surgical airway intervention in prenatally diagnosed neck masses. *J Pediatr Surg* 2009; 44: 76–9.

13. Dudgeon DL, Isaacs H Jr, Hays DM. Multiple teratomas of the head and neck. *J Pediatr* 1974; 85: 139–40.

14. Hitchcock A, Sears RT, O'Neill T. Immature cervical teratoma arising in one fetus of a twin pregnancy. Case report and review of the literature. *Acta Obstet Gynecol Scand* 1987; 66: 377–9.

15. Bale PM, Painter DM, Cohen D. Teratomas in childhood. *Pathology* 1975; 1: 209–18.

16. Berry CL, Keeling J, Hilton C. Teratomas in infancy and childhood: A review of 91 cases. *J Pathol* 1969; 98: 241–52.

17. Grosfeld JL, Ballantine TV, Lowe D et al. Benign and malignant teratomas in children: Analysis of 85 patients. *Surgery* 1976; 80: 297–305.

18. Tapper D, Lack EE. Teratomas in infancy and childhood. A 54 year experience at the Children's Hospital Medical Center. *Ann Surg* 1983; 198: 398–410.

19. Wakhlu A, Wakhlu AK. Head and neck teratomas in children. *Pediatr Surg Int* 2000; 16: 333–7.

20. Martino F, Avila LF, Encinas JL et al. Teratomas of the neck and mediastinum in children. *Pediatr Surg Int* 2006; 22: 627–34.

21. Grisoni ER, Gauderer MWL, Wolfson RN et al. Antenatal diagnosis of sacrococcygeal teratomas: Prognostic features. *Pediatr Surg Int* 1988; 3: 1973–5.

22. Zerella JT, Finberg FJ. Obstruction of the neonatal airway from teratomas. *Surg Gynecol Obstet* 1990; 170: 126–31.

23. Nmadu PT. Cervical teratoma in later infancy: Report of 13 cases. *Ann Trop Paediatr* 1993; 13: 95–8.

24. Mychalishka GB, Bealer JF, Graf JL et al. Operating on placental support: The ex utero intrapartum treatment (EXIT) procedure. *J Pediatr Surg* 1997; 32: 227–31.

25. Smith GM, Boyd GL, Vincent RD et al. The EXIT procedure facilitates delivery of an infant with pretracheal teratoma. *Anesthesiology* 1998; 89: 1573–75.

26. Murphy DJ, Kyle PM, Cairns P et al. Ex-utero intrapartum treatment for cervical teratoma. *Br J Obstet Gynecol* 2001; 108: 429–30.

27. Bouchard S, Johnson MP, Flake AW et al. The EXIT procedure: Experience and outcome in 31 cases. *J Pediatr Surg* 2002; 37: 418–26.

28. Patel RB, Gibson JY, D'Cruz CA et al. Sonographic diagnosis of cervical teratoma in utero. *Am J Roentgenol* 1982; 139: 1220–22.

29. Hasiotou M, Vakaki M, Pitsoulakis G et al. Congenital cervical teratomas. *Int J Pediatr Otorhinolaryngol* 2004; 68: 1133–9.

30. Hubbard AM, Crombleholme TM, Adzik NS. Prenatal MRI evaluation of giant neck masses in preparation for the fetal EXIT procedure. *Am J Perinatol* 1998; 15: 253–7.

31. Hirose S, Sydorak RM, Tsao K et al. Spectrum of intrapartum management for giant fetal cervical teratoma. *J Pediatr Surg* 2003; 38: 446–50.

32. Laje P, Johnson MP, Howell LJ et al. Ex utero intrapartum treatment in the management of giant cervical teratomas. *J Pediatr Surg* 2012; 47: 1208–16.

Sacrococcygeal teratoma

KEVIN C. PRINGLE

INTRODUCTION

A sacrococcygeal teratoma (SCT) is a neoplasm arising from the caudal end of the spine, usually protruding from the inferior end of the infant's spinal column and displacing the anus forward. These tumors have a female-to-male ratio of at least 3:1.[1-9] The incidence is approximately 1 in 40,000 live births,[10,11] although a recent article from Finland[12] found a prevalence of 1:14,900 in a study that ascertained the prevalence in the total population, including terminations of pregnancies and stillbirths. There is general agreement that SCT is the result of continued multiplication of totipotent cells from Hensen's node that fail to apoptose at the end of embryonic life.[7,13,14] This concept has received support from the work of Busch et al.,[15] who have identified histochemical markers in SCTs supporting an origin from caudal embryonic stem cells. This provides convincing evidence against the theory that these tumors arise from migrating germ cells travelling from yolk sac to gonad. Economou et al.[16] recently reported a series of experiments in mice exploring the results of injecting pluripotent cells into early embryos. They found that expression of Oct4 and Nanog in the primitive streak/tail bud after the start of somitogenesis does not result in neoplasia. Most authorities reject the concept that these are suppressed twins or parasitic fetuses. In 1976, Pantoja and Rodriguez-Ibanez[17] reviewed the conflicting theories as to the origin of these tumors. Their findings still stand. Clearly, more studies are needed to determine the genetic influences that are associated with the formation of SCTs.

A familial distribution of SCT has occasionally been reported.[18-21] Interestingly, Sonnino et al.,[19] at least, didn't recognize the similarity of their family with the triad described by Currarino et al.[21] some 8 years earlier.

PATHOLOGY

Willis[14] defines the term *teratoma* as follows: "A teratoma is a true tumour or neoplasm composed of multiple tissues

of kinds foreign to the part in which it arises." The SCT was second on Willis' list of sites where teratomata are found, but in almost all pediatric surgical series, the sacrococcygeal site is the most common site.[1-4,22] By definition, then, SCTs are composed of several types of tissue, usually derived from two or three germ layers. Robbins[23] defines a teratoma as "a tumour composed of cells representing more than one germ layer." In fact, however, in any tumor consisting of an epithelial component and a supporting stroma, at least two germ layers are represented. Most carcinomata, therefore, would meet Robbins's definition of a teratoma.

Within any one tumor, the cells can vary from totally benign (even forming well-formed teeth, hair, or other organs) to appearing frankly malignant (Figure 89.1). However, many SCTs contain malignant-looking cells (usually described as "immature"), but if they are completely excised, they do not recur. For this reason, the diagnosis of malignant SCT can only be made if there are distant metastases.[22]

The risk of malignancy depends on three factors: the site and the extent of the tumor and the age at diagnosis. Tumors diagnosed after 2 months of age have a high risk of being malignant. An exception to this statement is the relatively rare presacral "dermoid" tumors, which often present in adolescence or adult life with constipation or urinary obstruction but, if excised, completely appear to be totally benign. Altman et al.[22] classified SCTs into four groups when they reported the results of the American Academy of Pediatrics (AAP) Surgical Section survey (Figure 89.2). Type I tumors are almost exclusively exterior with a minimal pelvic component. They are rarely malignant (0% in the AAP survey). Type II tumors have a significant pelvic component. In the AAP survey, 6% of type II tumors were malignant. Type III tumors have an intrapelvic and intra-abdominal component greater than the external component. The intra-abdominal component can usually be palpated on abdominal examination. In the AAP survey, 20% of type III tumors were malignant. The type IV tumors are exclusively presacral; they had an 8% incidence of malignancy in the AAP survey.

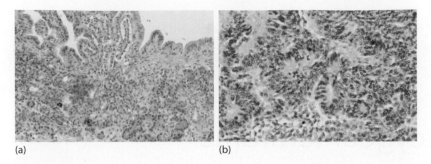

(a)   (b)

Figure 89.1 Histology of two areas of the tumor from the patient shown in Figure 89.3. **(a)** Apparently well-formed epithelium. **(b)** An area of primitive neuroglial tissue that could be diagnosed as being consistent with an aggressive neuroblastoma, were it not for the context in which it was found.

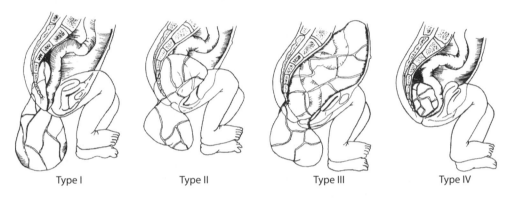

Type I   Type II   Type III   Type IV

Figure 89.2 Sacrococcygeal tumors as classified by Altman et al. (From Altman RP et al., Sacrococcygeal teratoma: American Academy of Pediatrics Surgical Section Survey—1973, *J Pediatr Surg* 1974;9:389–98.)

PRESENTATION

Before routine antenatal ultrasound examinations became widely accepted, the most common presentation was as a large sacral mass that is immediately obvious at birth.[1–5,13,24,25] The malignant tumors tend to present as a swelling of the buttock at 5–6 months of age. However, with the advent of routine antenatal ultrasound, the most common presentation is now antenatal diagnosis by ultrasonography.[24–32] Series reporting the antenatal diagnosis of SCTs have revealed that many of those fetuses diagnosed as having an SCT are likely to die before delivery.[22,26,33–35] Most of the fetuses reported to have died following antenatal diagnosis had tumors with a mass as great as or greater than the rest of the fetus. It is, therefore, entirely possible that these fetuses die of heart failure as the fetal heart is unable to pump sufficient blood to nourish both the tumor and the rest of the fetus. Certainly, in most of the antenatal series reported, fetal hydrops (nonimmune hydrops) is very common and is associated with an increased risk of fetal demise.[24,27,29,31–36] In 1990, Ikeda et al.[31] reported characteristics of 20 cases of prenatally diagnosed SCTs. Six infants delivered at a gestational age of 25–32 weeks died perinatally; 14 cases delivered after 32 weeks' gestation survived. Other articles, including three from the group in Chapel Hill (all reporting the same nine antenatally diagnosed SCTs[37–39]) also report a high mortality rate if fetal hydrops is noted or if the diagnosis is made early in gestation.[31–36] Wilson et al., from the Children's Hospital of Philadelphia, have recently emphasized the rate of growth of the tumor and the estimated fetal cardiac output as important prognostic indicators, with a growth rate >150 mL/week and a combined cardiac output >650 mL kg^{-1} min^{-1} being associated with a worse prognosis.[40] Benachi et al.[41] and Coleman et al.[42] have similarly emphasized the prognostic importance of rapid fetal growth and high vascularity. More recent studies have emphasized the importance of the tumor-to-fetal weight ratio (TFR), with a TFR >0.12 before 24 weeks' gestation indicating a poor prognosis.[43,44] Fetal echocardiographic indicators of poor prognosis have also been described.[45]

Recent improvements in magnetic resonance imaging (MRI) technology have enabled this modality to be used in the fetus without the need for fetal sedation or paralysis.[46–48] More recently, Coleman's group[49] have used MRI to define the solid tumor volume, standardized to estimated fetal weight (solid tumor volume/estimated fetal weight), as another measure of prognosis. It is becoming easier to define the anatomy of the tumor much more accurately, and it is sometimes possible to accurately determine the blood supply to the tumor in utero.

The improved diagnosis and the high mortality rate associated with fetal hydrops have provided a considerable impetus for some groups to consider fetal surgery for selected cases of antenatally diagnosed SCTs. The groups in San Francisco and at Children's Hospital of Philadelphia have had the greatest experience with this approach,[50–54] although other groups have also attempted fetal surgery[55] or percutaneous shunting or drainage to allow vaginal delivery[56,57] for these tumors. The results, so far, have been mixed.[50–57] A variety of other "minimally invasive" procedures, including radiofrequency ablation, laser ablation, and vascular embolization, have been attempted with relatively poor results in a poor-prognosis group of patients.[58,59] A detailed discussion of this aspect of the management of SCTs is beyond the scope of this chapter, but it would be fair to say that the role of fetal intervention for this tumor has still not been defined.

One further presentation (not often reported) is when the tumor becomes impacted during delivery. It either causes the death of the fetus by obstructing delivery or ruptures during delivery and the infant bleeds to death shortly after birth.[32,60–62]

CLINICAL FEATURES

Most cases presenting as neonates to pediatric surgeons will have a large skin-covered mass protruding from the coccygeal region, pushing the anus and vagina anteriorly (Figure 89.3). There may be large veins visible on the surface, and these usually drain into the surrounding structures. Large tumors may have ruptured (in which case they will bleed profusely) or may have an ulcerated area on the surface. Neonates with a tumor approaching the size of the rest of their body may be delivered prematurely and will often have some features of nonimmune hydrops.[25,27–33,35,36]

Infants presenting with malignant tumors usually present with a rapidly growing buttock mass.[63,64] In such cases, distant metastases are usually present at diagnosis. With the increasing use of antenatal ultrasound in many countries in recent times, this should become an extremely rare presentation. The management of these tumors is beyond the scope of this chapter. Recent advances in multimodal therapy of these tumors has resulted in survival rates as high as

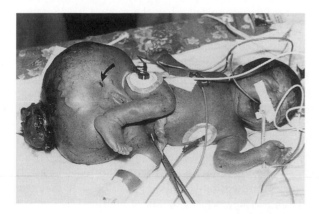

Figure 89.3 Premature infant with a large sacrococcygeal tumor that weighed almost as much as the rest of the infant. Note the displacement of the anus (arrow) and the vulva.

80%.[65,66] Children and adolescents with a benign presacral tumor usually present with constipation or urinary retention.[18,20,22,67–69] A retrorectal mass is easily recognizable on rectal examination. Again, management of these tumors is beyond the scope of this chapter.

In all cases, the tumor is firmly attached to and may be said to arise from the anterior surface of the coccyx. It may displace the coccyx posteriorly, but almost without exception, the sacrum is normal. The author has seen one infant who was delivered at 30 weeks' gestation with a large SCT associated with agenesis of the coccyx and the last two sacral vertebrae.[29] Very rarely, however, the tumor can extend superiorly. In one reported case, the tumor extended within the spinal canal as high as T4,[70] and in another case, it resulted in permanent paraplegia.[71]

In most cases, the majority of the blood supply to the tumor is derived from the median sacral artery,[5,72] and during removal, once this vessel is controlled, blood loss is usually minimal. This is not always the case, and a preliminary abdominal procedure to control the median sacral artery in very large tumors, as suggested by some authors recently,[73–75] can occasionally yield very disappointing results, with only a very small vessel being identified.[76] In an occasional case, the feeding vessels have been embolized prior to attempting resection in a premature baby.[77] In addition, on two occasions in the current author's personal series, the bulk of the venous drainage from the tumor returned through the sacral hiatus and back to the azygous system via a large network of very friable epidural veins. This resulted in a frighteningly large loss of blood when the sacrum was divided. In both cases, the initial blood loss was controlled with pressure, and the middle sacral artery was rapidly controlled, allowing the definitive control of the bleeding from the divided sacral canal with Gelfoam on one occasion and bone wax on the other. With the improvement of the resolution of modern ultrasound machines and the introduction of color flow mapping using Doppler ultrasound, it should be possible to determine whether the venous return is via the sacral hiatus. The limited experience from the current author's center suggests that this is possible. However, it should be stated that in the patients in which preoperative color flow mapping has been used over the past 5 years, no sacral flow has been noted either on ultrasound or at operation. Clearly, more experience is needed. However, the simplicity of this examination with modern ultrasound machines makes this a useful addition to preoperative workup.

Some authors have advocated laparoscopic procedures to divide the middle sacral artery.[75] This may be technically difficult if there is a large intra-abdominal component of the tumor. Another recent paper[78] has emphasized the necessity of ensuring that the vessel to be controlled is, indeed, the median sacral artery.

POSTNATAL DIAGNOSIS

The major differential diagnosis that should be considered is an anterior meningocele. This can usually be ruled out by physical examination, including rectal examination. In SCT, the rectal examination will invariably reveal a solid presacral component. If an anterior meningocele is present, this will be cystic, and an anterior sacral defect will often be palpable. Dillard et al.[4] point out the need to observe the anterior fontanel during the rectal examination. If an anterior meningocele is present, the diagnosis of Currrarino syndrome should be considered.[21,79] In anterior meningocele, pressure on the sacral mass will result in a bulging fontanel. The diagnosis can be confirmed by radiography of the lumbosacral region, which will show a characteristic defect in the sacrum in a patient with a meningomyelocele. An MRI examination will confirm the diagnosis.

Another recently described addition to the list of differential diagnoses is a sacrococcygeal chordoma.[80] Lemire et al.[81] have produced a list of 20 different lesions that can possibly enter into the differential diagnosis. Most of these are extremely rare but will usually be distinguishable from SCT on careful physical examination. An abdominal ultrasound is useful to determine the size and consistency of any pelvic or abdominal component. It may be necessary to pass a catheter into the bladder and fill the bladder with water to allow it to be used as a sonic window.

With the rapid improvements in MRI technology, it is now possible to utilize MRI in neonates with minimal sedation, although in many cases, a general anesthetic is still required for a detailed examination. Software packages allowing the use of MRI to delineate vascular anatomy are now available.[81–84] The use of gadolinium as a contrast medium has improved the delineation of the vascular anatomy. If oil is instilled into the rectum during the MRI examination while T_1-weighted images are gathered, then the oil can be used as a contrast medium during the scan,[85,86] although modern advances in MRI technology have now made this technique obsolete. MRI should clearly distinguish between SCT and anterior meningocele, and may be able to detect the occasional extension of the tumor through the sacral hiatus into the spinal canal.[70,71]

PREOPERATIVE MANAGEMENT

If the lesion is intact and the infant is stable, then there is no need for immediate resection. However, a case can be made for resecting these lesions within the first 24 hours after birth, since the gut is not usually colonized in the first 24 hours after birth. Early resection, therefore, will reduce the risk of infection if the field is contaminated by stool during the resection. Perioperative antibiotics are advisable. They should be given immediately before surgery commences and be continued for 24–48 hours postoperatively. If the infant has been fed, or is several days old, then a case can be made for a formal bowel preparation prior to the operation.

Blood should be cross-matched, and adequate intravenous access is vital. An arterial line may also be useful during the operation. It is worthwhile to obtain blood for alpha-fetoprotein (AFP) levels before surgery as a baseline, in order to confirm postoperatively that AFP levels continue to fall at a normal rate.[29,87–89] A recent paper from Italy[90] has advocated using an AFP >15,000 ng/mL as an indication for chemotherapy. In the author's opinion, this carries a significant risk of unnecessary chemotherapy. It should be noted that in very rare cases, the AFP level might not be elevated.[91]

If the tumor has ruptured, then a pressure bandage or transfixing sutures with felt pledgets,[92] may stem the blood loss for a brief time. However, there is some concern that this may "squeeze" immature cells into the venous drainage from the tumor. These cells will most likely lodge in the lungs. However, failure to slow the rate of blood loss in these infants may ensure that metastatic disease is not a problem for that infant. Obviously, emergency surgery is indicated in these circumstances.

In the past, there was often a reluctance to attempt the surgical removal of a tumor that might be as large as the rest of the baby. This is less common now, although there can be an understandable desire to let the baby grow before attempting the removal of the tumor, which will most likely be benign. This temptation should be resisted, however, as the risk of malignancy increases with age, suggesting that many of the tumors that were benign at birth become malignant after about 2 months.[3,5,7,8,13,18] If a surgeon in a peripheral hospital encounters one of these lesions, then transfer to a pediatric surgical unit is advisable, if this is possible.

OPERATION

The patient is anesthetized and intubated and a catheter placed in the bladder to measure urine output throughout the procedure, before being positioned prone with a roll under the hips. The roll is positioned so that the infant's weight is taken on the anterior superior iliac spines. It is vital that the abdomen be left hanging free to ensure that respiration is not inhibited by the baby's weight. For this reason, the baby's shoulders should be supported either by a smaller roll lying transversely across the apex of the chest at the level of the medial ends of the clavicles or by two rolls running parallel to the spine, each supporting the glenohumeral joints. The former option is illustrated in Figure 89.4. It is often useful to pack the rectum with Vaseline gauze to enable it to be readily recognized when the rectum is exposed later in the procedure. The packing also reduces the risk of stool contaminating the operative field. Many authorities state that the anus should be prepped out of the field.[13,93] This author finds that approach both inconvenient and impractical, as access to the anus is often required during the procedure. The cautery pad can usually be placed across the shoulders. A clear plastic drape may conserve body heat and assist in prevention of hypothermia. The addition of a perforated blanket through which is pumped warmed, filtered air also helps to maintain body temperature.

A chevron incision is made in the skin over the dorsum of the mass (Figure 89.5a,b), and it continues down to fascial layers. It is preferable not to dissect beyond the level of the deep fascia at this stage of the dissection. There are often several large veins in the subcutaneous tissue on either side of the midline; these should be cauterized, or if they are too

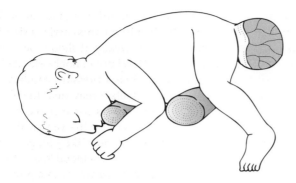

Figure 89.4 Infant with a sacrococcygeal teratoma positioned for surgical resection of the tumor. Note the large transverse roll under the pelvis and the smaller roll under the upper chest.

large for that, they may be divided between ties. The incision should be placed so as to preserve as much normal skin as possible. Excess skin can always be trimmed later if necessary. The apex of the chevron should be over the lower sacrum. In the midline, the dissection should continue directly down to the sacrococcygeal junction, or even down to the fourth or fifth sacral vertebra. The edges of the sacrum are defined, and a clamp is passed across the sacrum at the junction of the sacrum and coccyx, keeping the tips of the forceps against the ventral surface of the bone (or cartilage) to ensure that

the forceps passes between the sacrum and the underlying median sacral vessels, which are usually substantial vessels, supplying the bulk of the blood supply to the tumor. Once this maneuver is complete, the sacrum (which is usually completely, or at least largely, cartilaginous) can be divided with a scalpel and the severed section of the spine displaced slightly inferiorly to expose the median sacral vessels (Figure 89.6a,b). As mentioned earlier, this can very rarely result in catastrophic blood loss from the epidural veins, if the bulk of the venous return is passing back to the baby via the sacral hiatus. It may be necessary to divide some of the attachments of the thinned-out remnants of the levators to the edges of the lower end of the sacrum and coccyx to enable the distal portion of the sacrum and coccyx to be displaced caudally. The median sacral vessels are then ligated in continuity and divided. This early division of the median sacral vessels is essentially the same as the procedure advocated by Smith et al.[72]

This maneuver opens a plane of dissection that is outside the tumor capsule but deep to the thinned-out remnants of the levators and gluteus maximus. The levators may be so thin as to be almost invisible (Figure 89.7), but they will contract on stimulation, with either a muscle stimulator or

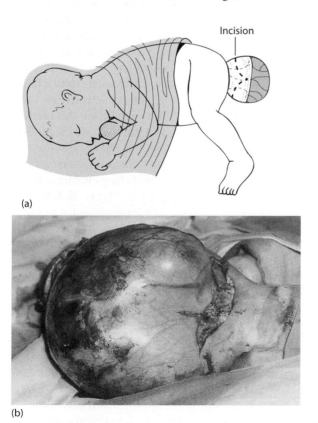

(a)

(b)

Figure 89.5 (a) Lateral view of the incision over the tumor. All normal skin that can possibly be preserved is retained, to be trimmed later if necessary. (b) Skin incision in the infant shown in Figure 89.3. Her head is to the right.

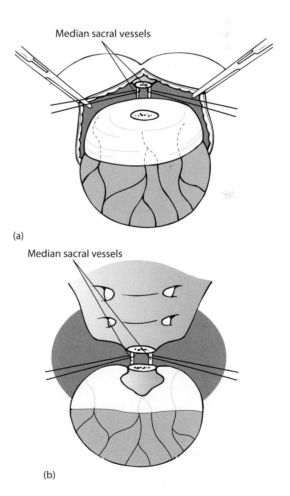

(a)

(b)

Figure 89.6 (a) Sacrum divided with the median sacral vessels slung on ties. (b) The divided fifth sacral vertebral body, showing the tumor arising from the ventral surface of the coccyx.

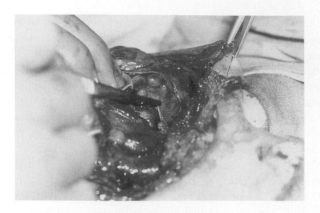

Figure 89.7 The sacrum has been divided, and the forceps demonstrates the thinned-out levators (the head is to the right).

the electrocautery. The dissection should continue laterally in this plane either side of the midline until the muscles are lost in the fascia of the tumor. At this point, they can be divided along a line parallel to the skin incision. This will allow the tumor to be further displaced in a caudal direction.

Attention is then directed to the pelvic extension of the tumor. Using blunt dissection with peanut swabs in the plane anterior to the median sacral vessels, it is usually possible to displace the pelvic component of the tumor anteriorly until its upper extent is reached. This is normally an essentially avascular plane anterior to the sacrum, although some vessels feeding into the tumor from the internal iliac vessels may be encountered laterally. These can usually be controlled with cautery or ligated if necessary. In most cases, the tumor can be dissected out from the pelvis and rolled inferiorly over the patient's legs (Figure 89.8).

This maneuver exposes the upper end of the rectum, which can be identified by the Vaseline gauze pack placed immediately before the operation is commenced or by passing a finger or a Hegar dilator through the anus. The tumor can be dissected off the rectum with a combination of sharp and blunt dissection, and rolled inferiorly until the plane of dissection moves away from the rectum and the anal canal.

At all times during this dissection, it is best to try to maintain the plane of dissection on the capsule of the tumor and to preserve all normal structures no matter how distorted and thinned-out they are. As the tumor is rolled inferiorly, it eventually becomes apparent that the plane of dissection has reached the subcutaneous tissue along the inferior surface of the tumor, posterior to the anus. Once the dissection has reached this point, the dissection can be terminated as long as the inferior skin flap that has been developed is of sufficient length to allow easy closure of the wound (Figure 89.9). The inferior skin flap can then be divided from the tumor and the tumor delivered from the field. A careful check of the tumor bed is carried out to ensure that meticulous hemostasis has been achieved. If the peritoneum has been opened during the pelvic dissection, then it is closed if possible.

Attention is then directed to reconstruction of the pelvic floor and closure of the wound. The remnants of the levator sling are identified, and the central portion is sutured to the perichondrium of the anterior surface of the sacrum using 5-0 Maxon (Cynamid Tyco Healthcare Group, Norwalk, Connecticut, USA) (a monofilament absorbable suture) (Figure 89.10a,b). This same suture is used for all subsequent muscle and fascial reconstruction. These initial fascial sutures, rather than the skin closure, should determine the siting of the anus. This aspect of the reconstruction, therefore, should be carried out with care to ensure both a functional and cosmetically pleasing result.

If a drain is to be placed, then it is placed at this stage, in the presacral space, led out through the gap in the levators, and tunneled out through the subcutaneous tissue of the buttock. A closed-suction drain is preferred. If there are remnants of the levators recognizable lateral to the midline, these are repaired with interrupted 5-0 Maxon sutures. The medial edges of the gluteus maximus are then closed in the midline over the sacrum and the lower part of the levator sling (Figure 89.11). The skin flaps are then trimmed to length. If possible, the subcutaneous tissues are closed with a running 5-0 Maxon suture, and the skin is closed

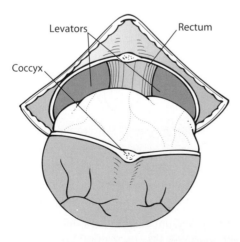

Figure 89.8 Completion of the pelvic dissection with the tumor rolled inferiorly, exposing the rectum.

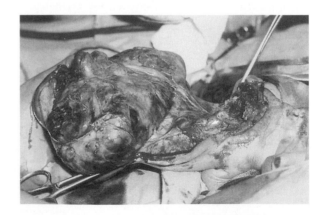

Figure 89.9 Completion of the pelvic dissection. The tumor has been dissected off the rectum (arrow), and the dissection has reached the stage where the division of the inferior skin flap can be contemplated. (Same patient as Figure 89.3; the head is to the right.)

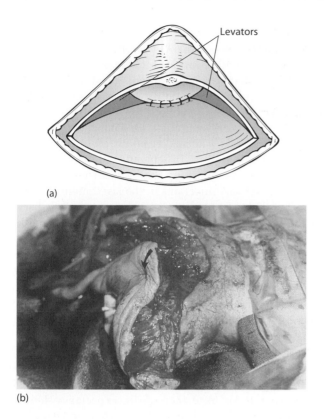

(a)

(b)

Figure 89.10 **(a)** Levators sutured to the perichondrium of the sacrum. These sutures set the anal position. **(b)** The levators have been sutured to the sacral perichondrium, resulting in the setting of the definitive anal position. (Arrow indicates the anus; same patient as in Figure 89.3; the head is to the right.)

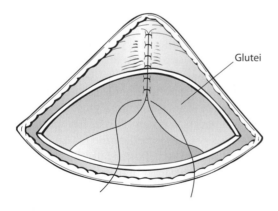

Figure 89.11 Closure of the glutei, posterior to the sacrum. This closure is continued inferior to the divided sacrum.

with a running 5-0 Maxon subcuticular suture. A Steri-Strip and collodion dressing is then applied. If it is not possible to close the subcutaneous tissue, then a subcuticular suture may not be adequate for skin closure. In this case, 5-0 nylon skin sutures are placed (Figure 89.12a,b). The rectum is repacked with Vaseline ribbon gauze at the completion of the procedure in an attempt to obliterate dead space. It is useful to attach a 2-0 silk suture to the end of this pack to aid its retrieval, should the pack become displaced higher up the rectum in the immediate postoperative period.

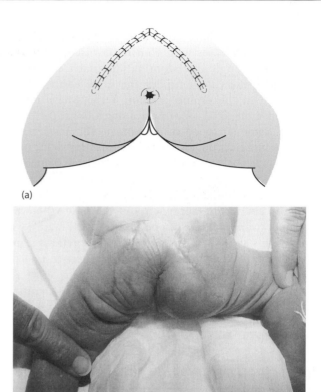

(a)

(b)

Figure 89.12 **(a)** Diagrammatic representation of the completed skin closure. **(b)** End result in the same patient illustrated in Figure 89.3.

Preliminary abdominal exploration is indicated in three circumstances:

1. If there is a large abdominal component[93,94]
2. If the tumor has been ruptured and is actively bleeding[76]
3. In the rare case when a premature baby is delivered in a hyperdynamic state and preliminary devascularization is needed to stabilize the patient before proceeding to definitive resection.[36]

In these cases, the abdomen is opened via a transverse infraumbilical incision placed just below the upper limit of any intra-abdominal mass or just below the umbilicus if there is no abdominal component. In either case, the aim is to find and ligate and then divide the median sacral vessels if at all possible. If this is not possible, then either an arterial occlusive sling[76] or a small vascular clamp is placed across the aorta below the origin of the inferior mesenteric artery. The abdomen is closed temporarily with a running 3-0 nylon mass closure and dressed with a clear plastic adhesive dressing. The patient is repositioned, and the tumor is then resected from behind as outlined previously. When the pelvic portion of the dissection is completed, the patient is repositioned in the supine position, and the clamp or aortic occlusive sling is removed before the abdomen is closed in layers with 4-0 Maxon sutures to the fascia and 5-0 Maxon subcuticular sutures to the skin. As noted previously, this procedure has been performed laparoscopically.[75,78]

Some authors[74] have advocated an abdominoperineal approach in all cases with routine devascularization of the tumor through an abdominal approach, followed by resection of the tumor (under the same aesthetic) with the patient in the supine position. Others have recently described a posterior midline approach, with the patient prone.[95] Some surgeons in Melbourne (B. Bowkett, personal communication) also advocate resection of the tumor in the supine position, with the initial incision being in the midline, extending from the sacrum down to the tumor. These authors cite the ability to devascularize the tumor from the abdominal approach and the ease with which external cardiac massage can be applied as the main advantages of this approach. The current author retains significant reservations about this approach. There is a need to control the blood supply to the tumor from above in a minority of cases, and it is felt that if there is a significant venous drainage through the epidural veins, then blood loss from this source would be extremely difficult to control with the patient in the supine position.

POSTOPERATIVE MANAGEMENT

The infant is nursed in a prone position for several days postoperatively. The urinary catheter can be removed as soon as the baby's condition is stable, and the infant can be extubated as soon as his/her respiratory condition allows. The infant can usually be fed as soon as he/she is extubated. The Vaseline pack is usually removed on the first postoperative day by pulling on the 2-0 silk suture left attached to the distal end. Any drain can usually be removed within the first few days of the procedure. A recent paper reported an unusual rare complication of a postoperative epidural hematoma that resulted in a cauda equina syndrome.[96] The patient presented 17 days after a late (11 months of age) resection of an SCT with a distended bladder, loss of rectal tone, and significant weakness of the lower limbs. After emergency surgery, the patient eventually made a full recovery.

AFP levels should be determined immediately postoperatively and on discharge. In spite of the fact that AFP is stated to have a half-life of only 3 days, the levels usually take several months to return to normal. The infant should then be followed at monthly intervals for 3 months and then at 3-month intervals for 1 year. At each visit, a rectal examination will detect any local recurrence, and an AFP level will detect any distant spread. The AFP level is often very high (of the order of 100,000 IU or more[29,87]), and even in normal babies, it may be over 100,000 IU.[87–89] These high levels usually take over a year to fall to normal adult levels. As long as the AFP level continues to fall steadily, recurrence is thought to be unlikely. However, it is important to not rely solely on the AFP levels, as in one patient in the current author's series, a very large pelvic recurrence (sufficiently large to produce urinary obstruction) occurred in the presence of a continuously falling AFP level. None of the other patients who developed recurrent tumors (including the patient who developed metastases in the inguinal lymph nodes) showed a rise in the AFP levels.

Follow-up should continue for at least 5 years, and preferably through puberty, if at all possible. It is important to obtain renal ultrasounds on an annual basis for the first few years and vital to obtain one on an urgent basis if there are any new urinary symptoms. One patient in the current author's series had a normal renal ultrasound close to her second birthday in April. In September of that year, she presented for routine follow-up with a history of having had three urinary tract infections in the last 2 months. A renal ultrasound obtained shortly after that visit revealed severe hydronephrosis bilaterally, and her serum creatinine level was significantly elevated, having been normal only a few months before. Urodynamic studies revealed that she had a hostile, high-pressure neurogenic bladder. The hydronephrosis resolved considerably with the introduction of clean intermittent catheterization, although this has placed a considerable strain on the family.

PROGNOSIS

In the absence of distant metastases at presentation, and if the excision is complete, then the life expectancy should be normal, although the appearance of the buttocks usually leaves something to be desired (Figure 89.12b).

There has been a flurry of recent papers in the literature that focus on long-term outcome. One paper[65] reported the results in a series of 23 patients followed for up to 22 years. Four patients with malignant tumors had recurrence-free intervals ranging from 9 to 14 years. They had two patients with nocturnal enuresis, one of which had perineal anesthesia. They had one child with a patulous anus and one patient with a neurogenic bladder. They emphasized the need for long-term follow-up and the need to be alert for the late appearance of urinary or fecal incontinence.

Another paper, from Liverpool, reports the results in 33 patients over 25 years treated in a single center.[97] Surprisingly, only one patient was described as having an immature teratoma, and six patients were described as having malignant tumors, two of whom died of metastatic disease. Some of the other patients in this report appear to have been diagnosed as having malignant tumors on the basis of histology and were then treated with chemotherapy on the basis of that diagnosis. In the author's series, there have been local recurrences treated only by repeat resection, without any adjuvant therapy. The only patient treated with chemotherapy was the patient who presented 2 months after resection with evidence of spread to the inguinal lymph nodes. She is a long-term survivor 18 years after a course of intensive chemotherapy.

Several other recent papers stress the need for close follow-up to detect the relatively high incidence of abnormalities of the genitourinary tract[98] and late-presenting urinary complications.[99–102]

Other papers[97,103–108] have focused on the longer-term outcomes. Overall, the quality of life in long-term survivors seems to be very good,[103,104] although some papers highlight constipation or wetting occurring with urinary and/or fecal incontinence in up to 30% of patients.[97,105,106] Another paper reports a series of 13 women who successfully delivered a baby after having an SCT excised in infancy.[107] Interestingly, the vast majority successfully delivered vaginally. One interesting case report detailed a woman who had had an SCT excised in infancy and suffered a genital prolapse in her twenties.[108]

There are mixed reports on the risk of recurrence and the incidence of malignancy. Some papers appear to rely on the histological appearance or the AFP level to diagnose malignancy.[90,109,110] The author reiterates that both recurrence and malignancy can appear in the face of a falling AFP. A paper from Japan,[110] however, does point out that malignant yolk sac tumor can appear up to 30 months after total resection in infancy, apparently arising from tumors that were entirely benign at the initial resection. Another paper[111] suggests adding CA 125 to the battery of surveillance tests. In their series of 32 patients, the CA 125 was elevated in in one-third of mature and one-third of immature recurrences.

The prognosis for patients presenting with a malignant SCT must still be guarded. Modern chemotherapy has produced a considerable improvement in survival.[62,112] The chemotherapy regimens are relatively toxic, and these patients require close monitoring during their treatment. Survival rates as high as 80% have been recorded.[62] De Corti's group[90] has recently reported survival rates of 89%. However, it appears that some of their neonatal patients were treated with chemotherapy on the basis of an AFP >15,000 ng/mL and/or histology indicating germ cell or yolk sac tumors. This may explain some of this improved result. Interestingly, although presacral tumors tend to present with malignant transformation, those found in patients with Currrarino syndrome tend to have a much better prognosis.[113]

REFERENCES

1. Bale PM, Painter DM, Cohen D. Teratomas in childhood. *Pathology* 1975; 7: 209–18.
2. Berry CL, Keeling J, Hilton C. Teratomata in infancy and childhood: A review of 91 cases. *J Pathol* 1969; 98: 241–52.
3. Billmire DF, Grosfeld JL. Teratomas in childhood: Analysis of 142 cases. *J Pediatr Surg* 1986; 21: 548–51.
4. Dillard BM, Mayer JH, McAlister WH et al. Sacrococcygeal teratoma in children. *J Pediatr Surg* 1970; 5: 53–9.
5. Donnellan WA, Swenson O. Benign and malignant sacrococcygeal teratomas. *Surgery* 1968; 64: 834–6.
6. Mahour GH, Woolley MW, Irivedi SN et al. Teratomas in infancy and childhood: Experience with 81 cases. *Surgery* 1974; 76: 309–18.
7. Vaez-Zadeh K, Sleber WK, Sherman FE et al. Sacrococcygeal teratomas in children. *J Pediatr Surg* 1972; 7: 152–6.
8. Waldhausen JA, Kilman JW, Vellios F et al. Sacrococcygeal teratoma. *Surgery* 1963; 54: 933–49.
9. Whalen TV, Mahour GH, Landing BH et al. Sacrococcygeal teratomas in infants and children. *Am J Surg* 1985; 150: 373–5.
10. Calbet JR. *Contribution a l'etude des tumeurs congénitales d'origine parasitaire de la region sacrococygiénne.* Paris: G. Steinheil, 1893.
11. McCune WS. Management of sacrococcygeal tumours. *Am Surg* 1964; 159: 911–18.
12. Pauniaho SL, Heikinheimo O, Vettenranta K et al. High prevalence of sacrococcygeal teratoma in Finland—A nationwide population-based study. *Acta Paediatr* 2013; 102: e251–6.
13. Gross RE, Clatworthy HW, Meeker IA. Sacrococcygeal teratomas in infants and children: A report of 40 cases. *Surg Gynecol Obstetr* 1951; 92: 341–54.
14. Willis RA. *The Borderland of Embryology and Pathology*, 2nd edn. London: Butterworths, 1962.
15. Busch C, Oppitz M, Wehrmann M et al. Immunohistochemical localization of nanog and Oct4 in stem cell compartments of human sacrococcygeal teratomas. *Histopathology* 2008; 52: 717–30.
16. Economou C, Tsakiridis A, Wymeersch FJ et al. Intrinsic factors and the embryonic environment influence the formation of extragonadal teratomas during gestation. *BMC Dev Biol* 2015: 15; 35.
17. Pantoja E, Rodriguez-Ibanez L. Sacrococcygeal dermoids and teratomas: Historical review. *Am J Surg* 1976; 132: 377–83.
18. Ashcraft KW, Holder TM. Hereditary presacral teratoma. *J Pediatr Surg* 1974; 9: 691–7.
19. Sonnino RE, Chou S, Guttman FM. Hereditary sacrococcygeal teratomas. *J Pediatr Surg* 1989; 24: 1074–5.
20. Bryant P, Leditschke JF, Hewett P. Hereditary presacral teratoma. *Aust N Z J Surg* 1996; 66: 418–20.
21. Currarino G, Coln D, Votteler T. Triad of anorectal, sacral, and presacral anomalies. *AJR* 1981; 137: 395–8.
22. Altman RP, Randolph JG, Lilly JR. Sacrococcygeal teratoma: American Academy of Pediatrics Surgical Section Survey—1973. *J Pediatr Surg* 1974; 9: 389–98.
23. Robbins SL. *Pathology.* In: *Neoplasia*, 3rd edn. Philadelphia: Saunders, 1967: 92.
24. Chervenak FA, Isaacson G, Touloukian R et al. Diagnosis and management of fetal teratomas. *Obstetr Gynecol* 1985; 66: 666–71.
25. Flake AW, Harrison MR, Adzick NS et al. Fetal sacrococcygeal teratoma. *J Pediatr Surg* 1986; 21: 563–6.
26. Holzgreve W, Mahony BS, Glick PL et al. Sonographic demonstration of fetal sacrococcygeal teratoma. *Prenat Diagn* 1985; 5: 245–57.
27. Holzgreve W, Miny P, Anderson R et al. Experience with 8 cases of prenatally diagnosed sacrococcygeal teratomas. *Fetal Ther* 1987; 2: 88–94.

28. Kuhlmann RS, Warsof SL, Levy DL et al. Sacrococcygeal teratoma. *Fetal Ther* 1987; 2: 95–100.

29. Pringle KC, Weiner CP, Soper RT et al. Sacrococcygeal teratoma. *Fetal Ther* 1987; 2: 80–7.

30. Sheth S, Nussbaum AR, Sanders RC et al. Prenatal diagnosis of sacrococcygeal teratoma sonographic pathologic correlation. *Radiology* 1988; 169: 131–6.

31. Ikeda H, Okumuru H, Nagashima K et al. The management of prenatally diagnosed teratoma *Pediatr Surg Int* 1990; 5: 192–4.

32. Holterman AX, Filiatrault D, Lallier M et al. The natural history of sacrococcygeal teratomas diagnosed through routine obstetric sonogram. *J Pediatr Surg* 1998; 33: 899–903.

33. Goto M, Makino Y, Tamura R et al. Sacrococcygeal teratoma with hydrops fetalis and bilateral hydronephrosis. *J Perinat Med* 2000; 28: 414–8.

34. Brace V, Grant SR, Brackley KJ et al. Prenatal diagnosis and outcome in sacrococcygeal teratomas: A review of cases between 1992 and 1998. *Prenat Diagn* 2000; 20: 51–5.

35. Tongsong T, Wanapirak C, Piyamongakol W et al. Prenatal sonographic features of sacrococcygeal teratoma. *Int J Obstetr Gynecol* 1999; 67: 95–101.

36. Robertson FM, Crombleholme TM, Frantz ID et al. Devascularisation and staged resection of giant sacrococcygeal teratoma in the premature. *J Pediatr Surg* 1995; 30: 309–11.

37. Chisholm CA, Heider AL, Kuller JA et al. Prenatal diagnosis and perinatal management of fetal sacrococcygeal teratoma. *Am J Perinatol* 1998; 15:503–5.

38. Chisholm CA, Heider AL, Kuller JA et al. Prenatal diagnosis and perinatal management of fetal sacrococcygeal teratoma. *Am J Perinatol* 1999; 16: 47–50.

39. Chisholm CA, Heider AL, Kuller JA et al. Prenatal diagnosis and perinatal management of fetal sacrococcygeal teratoma. *Am J Perinatol* 1999; 16: 89–92.

40. Wilson RD, Hedrick H, Flake AW et al. Sacrococcygeal teratomas: Prenatal surveillance, growth and pregnancy outcome. *Fetal Diagn Ther* 2009; 25: 15–20.

41. Benachi A, Durin L, Maurer SV et al. Prenatally diagnosed sacrococcygeal teratoma: A prognostic classification. *J Pediatr Surg* 2006; 41: 1517–21.

42. Coleman A, Shaaban A, Keswani S et al. Sacrococcygeal teratoma growth rate predicts adverse outcomes. *J Pediatr Surg* 2014; 49: 985–9.

43. Shue E, Bolouri M, Jelin EB et al. Tumor metrics and morphology predict poor prognosis in prenatally diagnosed sacrococcygeal teratoma: A 25-year experience at a single institution. *J Pediatr Surg* 2013; 48: 1225–31.

44. Akinkuotu AC, Coleman A, Shue E et al. Predictors of poor prognosis in prenatally diagnosed sacrococcygeal teratoma: A multiinstitutional review. *J Pediatr Surg* 2015; 50: 771–4.

45. Byrne FA, Lee H, Kipps AK et al. Echocardiographic risk stratification of fetuses with sacrococcygeal teratoma and twin-reversed arterial perfusion. *Fetal Diagn Ther* 2011; 30: 280–8.

46. Kirkinen P, Partanen K, Merikanto J et al. Ultrasonic and magnetic resonance imaging of fetal sacrococcygeal teratoma. *Acta Obstetr Gynecol Scand* 1997; 76: 917–22.

47. Okamura M, Kurauchi O, Itakura A et al. Fetal sacrococcygeal teratoma visualized by ultra-fast T_2 weighted magnetic resonance imaging. *Int J Gynaecol Obstetr* 1999; 65: 191–3.

48. Lwakatare F, Yamashita Y, Tang Y et al. Ultrafast fetal MR images of sacrococcygeal teratoma: A case report. *Comput Med Imaging Graph* 2000; 24: 49–52.

49. Coleman A, Kline-Fath B, Keswani S et al. Prenatal solid tumor volume index: Novel prenatal predictor of adverse outcome in sacrococcygeal teratoma. *J Surg Res* 2013; 184: 330–6.

50. Bullard KM, Harrison MR. Before the horse is out of the barn: Fetal surgery for hydrops. *Semin Perinatol* 1995; 19: 462–73.

51. Graf JL, Housely HT, Alabanese CT et al. A surprising histological evolution of preterm sacrococcygeal teratoma. *J Pediatr Surg* 1998; 33: 177–9.

52. Paek BW, Jennings RW, Harrison MR et al. Radiofrequency ablation of human fetal sacrococcygeal teratoma. *Am J Obstetr Gynecol* 2001; 184: 503–7.

53. Kitano Y, Flake AW, Crombleholme TM et al. Open fetal surgery for life-threatening fetal malformations. *Semin Perinatol* 1999; 23: 448–61.

54. Graf JL, Alabanese CT, Jennings RW et al. Successful fetal sacrococcygeal teratoma resection in a hydropic fetus. *J Pediatr Surg* 2000; 35: 1489–91.

55. Hecher K, Hackeloer BJ. Intrauterine endoscopic laser surgery for fetal sacrococcygeal teratoma. *Lancet* 1996; 347: 470.

56. Garcia AM, Morgan WMIII, Bruner JP. In utero decompression of a cystic grade IV sacrococcygeal teratoma. *Fetal Diagn Ther* 1998; 13: 305–8.

57. Kay S, Khalife S, Laberge JM et al. Prenatal percutaneous needle drainage of cystic sacrococcygeal teratomas. *J Pediatr Surg* 1999; 34: 1148–51.

58. Ding J, Chen Q, Stone P. Percutaneous laser photocoagulation of tumour vessels for the treatment of a rapidly growing sacrococcygeal teratoma in an extremely premature fetus. *J Maternal Fetal Neonat Med* 2010; 23: 1516–8.

59. Lee MY, Won HS, Hyun MK et al. Perinatal outcome of sacrococcygeal teratoma. *Prenat Diagn* 2011; 31: 1217–21.

60. Sarlo K. Total rupture of giant sacrococcygeal teratoma. *Kinderchirurgie* 1984; 39: 405–6.

61. Hoehn T, Krause MF, Wilhelm C et al. Fatal rupture of a sacrococcygeal teratoma during delivery. *J Perinatol* 1999; 19: 596–8.

62. Schmidt B, Haberlik A, Uray E et al. Sacrococcygeal teratoma: Clinical course and prognosis with a special view to long-term functional results. *Pediatr Surg Int* 1999; 15: 573–9.

63. Chretien PB, Milam JD, Foote FW et al. Embryonal adenocarcinomas (a type of malignant teratoma) of the sacrococcygeal region: Clinical and pathologic aspects of 21 cases. *Cancer* 1970; 26: 522–35.

64. Ein SH, Mancer K, Adeyemi SD. Malignant sacrococcygeal teratoma, endodermal sinus, yolk sac tumour—In infants and children: A 32-year review. *J Pediatr Surg* 1985; 20: 473–7.

65. Gobel U, Schneider DT, Calaminus G et al. Multimodal treatment of malignant sacrococcygeal germ cell tumors: A prospective analysis of 66 patients of the German cooperative protocols MAKEI 83/86 and 89. *J Clin Oncol* 2001; 19: 1943–50.

66. De Corti F, Sarnacki S, Patte C et al. Prognosis of malignant sacrococcygeal germ cell tumours according to their natural history and surgical management. *Surg Oncol* 2012; 21: e31–7.

67. Ghazali S. Presacral teratomas in children. *J Pediatr Surg* 1973; 8: 915–8.

68. Gwinn JL, Dockerty MB, Kennedy RLJ. Pre-sacral teratomas in infancy and childhood. *Pediatrics* 1955; 16: 239–49.

69. Swinton NW, Lehman G. Presacral tumors. *Surg Clin N Am* 1958; 38: 849–57.

70. Ribeiro PR, Guys JM, Lena G. Sacrococcygeal teratoma with an intradural and extramedullary extension in a neonate: Case report. *Neurosurgery* 1999; 44: 398–400.

71. Kunisaki SM, Maher CO, Powelson I et al. Benign sacrococcygeal teratoma with spinal canal invasion and paraplegia. *J Pediatr Surg* 2011; 46: e1–4.

72. Smith B, Passaro E, Clatworthy HW. The vascular anatomy of sacrococcygeal teratomas: Its significance in surgical management. *Pediatr Surg* 1961; 49: 534–9.

73. Angel CA, Murillo C, Mayhew J. Experience with vascular control before excision of giant, highly vascular sacrococcygeal teratomas in neonates. *J Pediatr Surg* 1998; 33: 1840–2.

74. Kamata S, Imura K, Kubota A et al. Operative management for sacrococcygeal teratoma (SCT) diagnosed in utero. *J Pediatr Surg* 2001; 36: 545–8.

75. Bax NM, van der Zee DC. Laparoscopic clipping of the median sacral artery in huge sacrococcygeal teratomas. *Surg Endosc* 1998; 12: 882–3.

76. Lindahl H. Giant sacrococcygeal teratoma: A method of simple intraoperative control of hemorrhage. *J Pediatr Surg* 1988; 23: 1068–9.

77. Lahdes-Vasama TT, Korhonen PH, Seppanen JM et al. Preoperative embolization of giant sacrococcygeal teratoma in a premature newborn. *J Pediatr Surg* 2011; 46: e5–8.

78. Solari V, Jawaid W, Jesudason EC. Enhancing safety of laparoscopic vascular control for neonatal sacrococcygeal teratoma. *J Pediatr Surg* 2011; 46: e5–7.

79. Dirix M, van Becelaere T, Berkenbosch L et al. Malignant transformation in sacrococcygeal teratoma and in presacral teratoma associated with Currarino syndrome: A comparative study. *J Pediatr Surg* 2015; 50: 462–4.

80. Cable DG, Moir C. Paediatric sacrococcygeal chordomas: A rare tumour to be differentiated from sacrococcygeal teratoma. *J Pediatr Surg* 1997; 32: 759–61.

81. Lemire RJ, Graham CB, Beckwith JB. Skin-covered sacrococcygeal masses in infants and children. *J Pediatr* 1971; 79: 948–54.

82. Davis WL, Warnock SH, Harnsberger HR et al. Intracranial MRA: Single volume vs multiple thin slab 3D time-of-flight acquisition. *J Comput Assist Tomogr* 1993; 17: 15–21.

83. Marchal G, Michiels J, Bosmans H et al. Contrast-enhanced MRA of the brain. *J Comput Assist Tomogr* 1992; 16: 25–29.

84. Ehricke H-H, Schad LR, Gadermann G et al. Use of MR angiography for stereotactic planning. *J Comput Assist Tomogr* 1992; 16: 35–40.

85. Pringle KC, Sato Y, Soper RT. Magnetic resonance imaging as an adjunct to planning an anorectal pull through. *J Pediatr Surg* 1987; 22: 571–4.

86. Sato Y, Pringle KC, Bergman RA et al. Congenital anorectal anomalies: MR imaging. *Radiology* 1988; 168: 157–62.

87. Johnston PW. The diagnostic value of alpha-fetoprotein in an infant with sacrococcygeal teratoma. *J Pediatr Surg* 1988; 23: 862–3.

88. Tsuchida Y, Endo Y, Saito S et al. Evaluation of alpha-fetoprotein in early infancy. *J Pediatr Surg* 1978; 13: 155–62.

89. Tsuchida Y, Hasegawa H. The diagnostic value of alpha-fetoprotein in infants and children with teratomas: A questionnaire survey in Japan. *J Pediatr Surg* 1983; 18: 152–5.

90. De Corti F, Sarnacki S, Patte C et al. Prognosis of malignant sacrococcygeal germ cell tumours according to their natural history and surgical management. *Surg Oncol* 2012; 21: e31–7.

91. Hung TH, Hsieh CC, Hsieh TT. Sacrococcygeal teratoma associated with a normal alpha-fetoprotein concentration. *Int J Obstetr Gynecol* 1997; 58: 321–2.

92. Smithers CJ, Javid PJ, Turner CG et al. Damage control operation for massive sacrococcygeal teratoma. *J Pediatr Surg* 2011; 46: 566–9.

93. Coran AG, Behrendt DM, Weintraub WH et al. *Surgery of the Neonate*. Boston: Little Brown, 1978: 229–32.

94. Hendren WH, Henderson BM. The surgical management of sacrococcygeal teratomas with intrapelvic extension. *Ann Surg* 1970; 171: 77–84.

95. Jan IA, Khan EA,Yasmeen N et al. Posterior sagittal approach for resection of sacrococcygeal teratomas. *Pediatr Surg Int* 2011; 27: 545–8.

96. Sears BW, Gramstad GG, Ghanayem AJ. Cauda equina syndrome in an eleven-month-old infant following sacrococcygeal teratoma tumor resection and coccyx excision: Case report. *Spine* 2010; 35: E22–4.

97. Gabra HO, Jesudason EC, McDowell, HP et al. Sacrococcygeal teratoma—A 25-year experience in a UK regional center. *J Pediatr Surg* 2006; 41: 1513–6.

98. Shalaby MS, O'Toole S, Driver C et al. Urogenital anomalies in girls with sacrococcygeal teratoma: A commonly missed association. *J Pediatr Surg* 2012; 47: 371–4.

99. Berger M, Heinrich M, Lacher M et al. Postoperative bladder and rectal function in children with sacrococcygeal teratoma. *Pediatr Blood Cancer* 2011; 56: 397–402.

100. Le LD, Alam S, Lim FY et al. Prenatal and postnatal urologic complications of sacrococcygeal teratomas. *J Pediatr Surg* 2011; 46: 1186–90.

101. Cost NG, Geller JI, Le LD et al. Urologic co-morbidities associated with sacrococcygeal teratoma and a rational plan for urologic surveillance. *Pediatr Blood Cancer* 2013; 60: 1626–9.

102. Partridge EA, Canning D, Long C et al. Urologic and anorectal complications of sacrococcygeal teratomas: Prenatal and postnatal predictors. *J Pediatr Surg* 2014; 49: 139–42; discussion 142–3.

103. Shalaby MS, Dorris L, Carachi R. The long-term psychosocial outcomes following excision of sacrococcygeal teratoma: A national study. *Arch Dis Child Fetal Neonat Ed* 2014; 99: F149–52.

104. Kremer ME, Dirix M, Koeneman MM et al. Quality of life in adulthood after resection of a sacrococcygeal teratoma in childhood: A Dutch multicentre study. *Arch Dis Child Fetal Neonat Ed* 2015; 100: F229–32.

105. Shalaby MS, Walker G, O'Toole S et al. The long-term outcome of patients diagnosed with sacrococcygeal teratoma in childhood. A study of a national cohort. *Arch Dis Child* 2014; 99: 1009–13.

106. Tailor J, Roy PG, Hitchcock R et al. Long-term functional outcome of sacrococcygeal teratoma in a UK regional center (1993 to 2006). *J Pediatr Hematol Oncol* 2009; 31: 183–6.

107. Kremer ME, Koeneman MM, Derikx JP et al. Evaluation of pregnancy and delivery in 13 women who underwent resection of a sacrococcygeal teratoma during early childhood. *BMC Pregnancy Childbirth* 2014; 14: 407.

108. Park SY, Lee JE, Lee SR. Unusual late sequela of excision surgery for sacrococcygeal teratoma: Advanced pelvic organ prolapse in a woman in her early twenties. *Eur J Obstetr Gynecol Reprod Biol* 2013; 168: 238–9.

109. Buyukpamukcu M, Varan A, Kupeli S et al. Malignant sacrococcygeal germ cell tumors in children: A 30-year experience from a single institution. *Tumori* 2013; 99; 51–6.

110. Yoshida M, Matsuoka K, Nakazawa A et al. Sacrococcygeal yolk sac tumor developing after teratoma: A clinicopathological study of pediatric sacrococcygeal germ cell tumors and a proposal of the pathogenesis of sacrococcygeal yolk sac tumors. *J Pediatr Surg* 2013; 48: 776–81.

111. Pauniaho SL, Tatti O, Lahdenne P et al. Tumor markers AFP, CA 125, and CA 19-9 in the long-term follow-up of sacrococcygeal teratomas in infancy and childhood. *Tumour Biol* 2010; 31: 261–5.

112. Marina N, Fontanesi J, Kun L et al. Treatment of childhood germ cell tumours. Review of the St Jude Experience from 1979 to 1988. *Cancer* 1992; 70: 2568–75.

113. Dirix M, van Becelaere T, Berkenbosch L et al. Malignant transformation in sacrococcygeal teratoma and in presacral teratoma associated with Currarino syndrome: A comparative study. *J Pediatr Surg* 2015; 50: 462–4.

90

Nasal tumors

UDO ROLLE

INTRODUCTION

Congenital masses of the nasal midline are very rare, occurring in 1 in every 20,000–40,000 newborns. Although benign, these masses may cause large facial deformities such as hypertelorism, cerebrospinal fluid (CSF) fistulas, cerebral herniation, visual alterations, meningitis, and cerebral abscess.[1,2]

There are various types of congenital nasal tumors. They may be classified in accordance with their embryonic origin; the most common are nasal dermal sinus, nasal glioma, and anterior encephalocele (Table 90.1).[1–5]

EMBRYOLOGY

At an early stage of development during the third and fourth weeks, there is a protrusion of the forebrain and dura through the foramen cecum into the prenasal space, which is limited by frontal and nasal bones on the anterior aspect and posteriorly by a cartilaginous capsule. During further development, the dural process is sealed, and the foramen gets obliterated. Any failure of this obliterating procedure leaves a canal, a pathway favoring the extension of the glial tissue, hence the development of encephaloceles and gliomas.[6]

An *encephalocele* is a herniation of brain tissue into the prenasal space; a *glioma* is derived from an encephalocele sequestered from the brain; for some authors, gliomas are hidden encephaloceles or sequestered encephaloceles.[7]

The frontal and nasal bones are formed by intramembranous ossification. At this stage of development, there is a gap between these bones, the fonticulus nasofrontalis, filled by a membrane; the dura and the skin are in contact without interposition of bony tissue. Part of the ectoderm may fail to separate from the dura and so remain in the depth of the nasal space. This displaced ectopic ectodermal tissue is the origin of a *dermoid cyst*. If a connection does exist with the skin, a *dermoid sinus* will result.

All these tumors or heterotopias are located in the midline (nasofrontal) or asymmetric unilateral (nasoethmoidal) position. They are present at birth. They often produce hypertelorism, telecanthus, and nasal deformity.

CONGENITAL TUMORS OF NEUROGENIC ORIGIN

Nasal glioma

Gliomas of the nose are rare, always benign heterotopias; they should not to be considered as tumors. Approximately 250 cases of nasal glioma have been described in the literature.[8] Their incidence is 1 in 250,000 births, with a male-to-female ratio of 3:1.[9,10] Nasal gliomas account for approximately 20% of all congenital nasal masses[11]; 60% of the tumors are extranasal, while 30% are intranasal and 10% both.[1,12,13] Although most gliomas are located around the midline region of the nose, there are reports with gliomas located in the scalp, cheek, soft palate, tonsils, tongue, leptomeninges, middle ear, orbit, and limbal dermoids.

A nasal glioma is a firm, gray-pink to purple, rounded or dome-shaped polypoid, noncompressible, and nonpulsatile mass of glial tissue of congenital origin that may appear in an extranasal or intranasal location at or near the root of the nose (Figure 90.1). It shows no impulse when the patient cries. The covering skin may look like a hemangioma. Gliomas are unilateral or in the midline, but are usually located at the side of the nasal bridge. The root of the nose is often enlarged; there may be an orbital hypertelorism. The diameter of the tumor varies from 1 to 3 cm. Their growth rate is usually the same as that of the surrounding tissue according to the infant's growth.

The intranasal type is located high in the nasal fossa. The septum may be displaced, and the nasal passage may be obstructed. Increased lacrimation may result from compression of the lacrimal duct. These tumors may present as early neonatal respiratory distress.[14]

Table 90.1 Differential diagnosis

Ectodermal
- Dermoid cyst
- Dermoid sinus

Neurogenic
- Meningocele
- Encephalocele
- Glioma
- Neurofibroma

Mesodermal
- Hemangioma
- Vascular malformation

Mixed origin
- Teratoma

In intra–extranasal gliomas, there is a communication between the two components of the mass, usually through a defect in the nasal bone or at the lateral margin of the nasal bone.

HISTOLOGY

A glioma consists of glial and fibrous tissue with an over-lying flattened epidermis.[12] The specimens consist of fibrillary astrocytes and fibrous connective tissue. True neurons are seen rarely.[15] It does not contain CSF-filled space communicating with the ventricular system of the brain or the subarachnoid space. In two heterotopias, cellularity in places approached that of low-grade neoplastic glioma.[16]

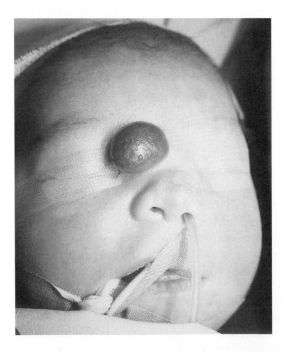

Figure 90.1   Nasal glioma in a newborn.

DIAGNOSIS—IMAGING

Preoperative imaging is essential for an appropriate surgical approach by delineating the exact site and extension of the tumor.[12,17] It is important to distinguish nasal tumors or masses from basofrontal encephaloceles to avoid inadvertent exposure of the brain during the surgical removal of mass lesions.

Computed tomography (CT) scanning is useful to visualize bony defects but is not reliable for soft-tissue contrast. Magnetic resonance imaging (MRI) is superior for imaging brain tissue; it should therefore be used preferentially for definition of the tumor mass and to disclose intracranial extension.[5,17]

TREATMENT

Though benign and relatively slow growing, these heterotopias can cause disturbances of growth and subsequent deformity by encroachment upon the bony frameworks of the nose. Furthermore, they are unsightly, and some of them, located at the root of the nose such as encephaloceles and gliomas, may interfere with vision. Hence, early surgical excision is advisable.

Complete surgical excision of nasal gliomas—with repair of any hypertelorism—is the treatment of choice. The most conservative cosmetic surgical technique should be chosen after intracranial connection has been ruled out.

TECHNIQUE

An elliptical incision is made around the base of he tumor, and the mass is removed in toto. In order to avoid recurrences, it is important to excise or coagulate the small deep stalk, which may pass upward for a short distance under the nasal bone. This tract is exposed by splaying open the nasal bones through a midline nasal incision. In the case of a high-situated intranasal glioma, an extracranial extranasal approach may be necessary to provide wide access to the nasal cavity. A lateral rhinotomy is most often used. Burckhardt and Tobon[18] described an endoscopic approach in the case of an intranasal glioma. In cases with intracranial lesion, craniotomy is mandatory.

COMPLICATIONS

Incomplete excision

Recurrences due to incomplete excision are rare (11%). In 13% of the cases, there is a connection with the intracranial nervous system by a pedicle of fibrous tissue, passing through the cribriform plate. Nasal gliomas with a cystic component seem to have a greater tendency for recurrence; the reason for this remains unclear[19] Levine et al. reported a case in which a nasal glioma masqueraded as a capillary hemangioma with subsequent inadequate treatment, which indicates the eventual need for a preoperative histologic examination in some cases.[15]

A recurrence can be avoided by a detailed evaluation of the preoperative imaging and a meticulous dissection in order to expose a stalk or a possible intracranial connection. Only a complete excision prevents recurrence.[19–21]

Dural defect

As normally there is no permeable communication with the subdural space, an accidental dural defect is theoretical. Should it occur, it must be promptly closed to prevent a CSF fistula. If such a defect is large, an epicranium graft may be needed for a safe and tight closure.

Hematoma

This can be avoided by careful hemostasis with bipolar coagulation.

Skin defect

In some cases, the skin defect is closed directly. Large defects can be covered by free-skin grafting, by glabellar skin flaps, or by tissue expansion (Figures 90.2 through 90.4).

Meningocele and encephalocele

The encephalocele is a protrusion of the brain inside a dural sac through a skull defect. The tumor contains an ependyma-lined space filled with the CSF; it communicates with the ventricular system. Encephaloceles are located at the root of the nose, midline (nasofrontal) or asymmetric lateral (nasoethmoidal); they are most frequently intranasal.[1,22] The bridge of the nose is broadened, and often hypertelorism, and nasal deformity are produced. Depending on the contents, meningoceles and encephaloceles are taut of soft, compressible, and pulsatile tumors, enlarging when the patient cries (Fürstenberg sign).

Evaluation should include a complete rhinologic and neurologic examination.[23] The dominant clinical sign of encephaloceles is an intermittent rhinoliquorrhea that can be distinguished from normal nasal secretion by the typically high glucose concentration in the liquor. The defect at the base of the skull is demonstrated by radiological examination; an intracranial lesion is best disclosed with MRI and/or CT scanning.[24] 3-D CT provides additional useful information in cases with significant bony abnormalities at little additional cost or time.[25]

TREATMENT

The treatment of choice is excision of the tumor with the herniated brain and closure of the dural defect. Usually, there are no problems for closure of the wound, the covering skin being normal. According to Macfarlane et al., primary and secondary hypertelorism regressed in most instances where patients were treated before the age of 2 years.[26] In their series of 114 patients treated in a 15-year period, in 59% of the children, the developmental outcome was normal, 18% have mild mental or physical disability, and in 23%, severe impairment occurred.

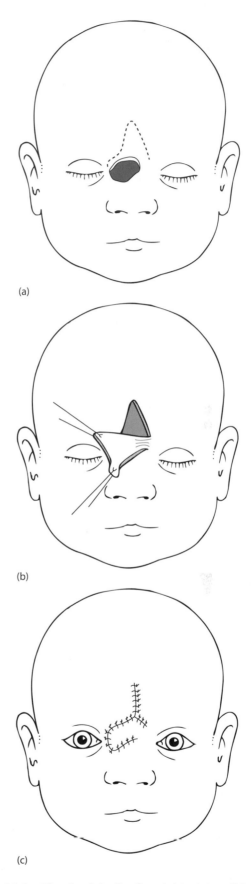

(a)

(b)

(c)

Figure 90.2   Classic glabellar flap. **(a)** Incision, **(b)** mobilization, and **(c)** result.

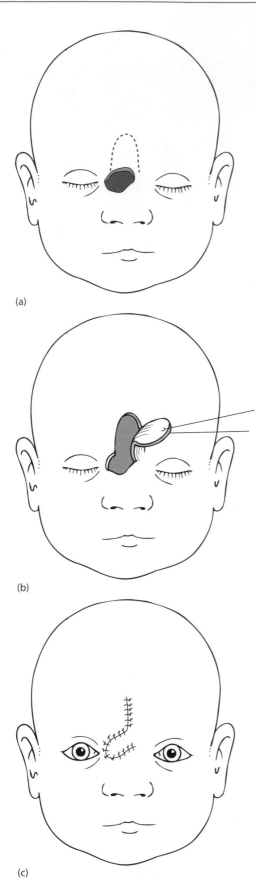

(a)

(b)

(c)

Figure 90.3 Finger flap—midline transposition flap. (a) Incision, (b) mobilization, and (c) result.

The main postoperative complication is leakage of CSF because of a large dural defect.[23,26] In the series of Macfarlane et al.,[26] it occurred in 1 patient out of 114. The dural defect must be closed tightly to prevent such a fistula. If the defect is too large for direct closure, an epicranial or a fascia lata graft may be a valid alternative.

CONGENITAL DERMOID CYSTS AND DERMOID SINUS

Congenital dermoid cysts are the most frequently found congenital nasal tumors. During early embryonic development, a portion of the dura begins to grow in close association with nasal skin. Eighty-four percent are found in the head and neck, 37% of these are located in the orbit and periorbit, and 10% are found in the midline of the nasofrontal region. External dermoid cysts present clinically as a firm, nonfluctuating, and nonpulsatile mass. The Fürstenberg sign is negative.[1] The dermoid sinus appears externally sometimes as a dimple with protruding hair; in these cases, only a thorough examination will bring up the diagnosis. The dimple usually leads to a sinus tract, which extents along the nasal septum, underneath the nasal bones, toward the base of the anterior cranial fossa; it may enter the skull (dumbbell cyst).[5] Imaging comprises CT and MRI.[27]

Nasal dermoids can be classified into superficial, intraosseous, intracranial extradural, and intracranial intradural. This classification allows precise surgical planning.[28]

Dermoid cysts and sinuses are both lined by squamous epithelium with various dermal appendages such as glands and hair follicles.

Repeated infections may form multiple sinus tracts, making complete excision difficult. Sometimes the mass of the cyst may erode nasal bones and associated sinuses. Although rare, liquorrhea may occur.

Treatment

The treatment of choice is operative removal, preferably before potentially chronic infections occur.

Technique

A midline nasal incision and excision of the mass is the best technique. The tract passing into the nasal septum must be exposed after opening the nasal bones. All epithelial elements must be removed. The stalk is carefully dissected cephalad; if it enters the skull, a craniotomy is mandatory in order to remove the intracranial part of the lesion.[29]

NASAL TERATOMA

Teratomas are rare in children. They arise from one or a combination of the three embryonic layers and could be classified as either mature, immature, or malignant. Head

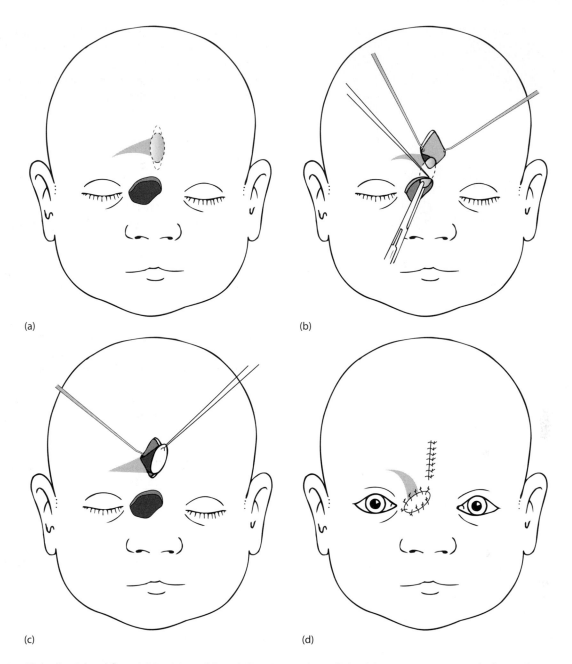

(a)

(b)

(c)

(d)

Figure 90.4   Glabellar island flap. **(a)** Incision, **(b)** mobilization with pedicle, **(c)** transposition, and **(d)** result.

and neck teratomas account for only 0.47%–6% of all teratomas; nasal teratomas are much rarer.[30]

Most nasal teratomas will be visible immediately after birth.

Diagnosis will be completed by imaging (CT, MRI).

Treatment

Complete surgical excision is the required treatment. In cases with nasopharyngeal teratomas obstructing the airway,

an ex utero intrapartum (EXIT) procedure will be required (Figure 90.5).

REFERENCES

1. Aguilar Mandret F, Oliva Izquierdo MT, Vallés Fontanet J. [Nasal glioma]. *Acta Otorrinolaringol Esp* 2004 September; 55(7): 346–50.
2. Lamesch P, Froment N, Lamesch AJ. Nasal glioma. *Pediatr Surg Int* 1988 March; 3(2): 176–80.

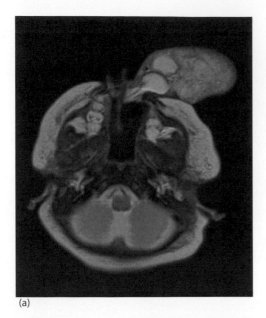

(a)

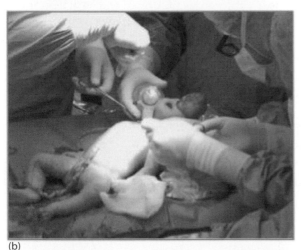

(b)

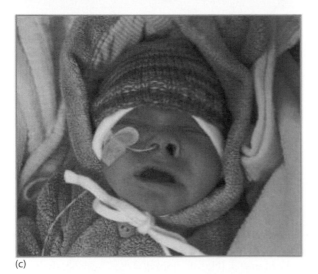

(c)

Figure 90.5   **(a)** MRI of nasal teratoma. **(b)** EXIT procedure. **(c)** Postoperative image.

3. Fitzpatrick E, Miller RH. Congenital midline nasal masses: Dermoids, gliomas, and encephaloceles. *J La State Med Soc* 1996 März; 148(3): 93–6.
4. Fairbanks D. Embryology and anatomy [Internet]. In: *Pediatric Otolaryngology*. Philadelphia: WB Saunders, 1990: 650–31. [zitiert January 25, 2010] Available from http://www.ncbi.nlm.nih.gov/sites/entrez.
5. Hedlund Congenital frontonasal masses: Developmental anatomy, malformations, and MR imaging. *Pediatr Radiol* 2006; 36: 647–62.
6. Stenberg H. Zur formalen Genese der vorderen Hirnbrücke. *Wien Med Wochenschr* 1929; 79: 463–6.
7. Tashiro Y, Sueishi K, Nakao K. Nasal glioma: An immunohistochemical and ultrastructural study. *Pathol Int* 1995 Mai; 45(5): 393–8.
8. Niedzielska G, Niedzielski A, Kotowski M. Nasal ganglioglioma—Difficulties in radiological imaging. *Int J Pediatr Otorhinolaryngol* 2008 February; 72(2): 285–7.
9. Lehner M, Rickham P. Tumours of the head and neck [Internet]. In: *Neonatal Surgery*. London: Butterworths, 1978: 91–2. [zitiert January 25, 2010] Available from http://www.ncbi.nlm.nih.gov /pubmed/19985009.
10. Whitaker SR, Sprinkle PM, Chou SM. Nasal glioma. *Arch Otolaryngol* 1981 September; 107(9): 550–4.
11. Hughes GB, Sharpino G, Hunt W, Tucker HM. Management of the congenital midline nasal mass: A review. *Head Neck Surg* 1980 February; 2(3): 222–33.
12. Arndt S, Wiech T, Mader I, Aschendorff A, Maier W. Rare extracranial localization of primary intracranial neoplasm. *Diagn Pathol* 2008; 3: 14.
13. Penner CR, Thompson L. Nasal glial heterotopia: A clinicopathologic and immunophenotypic analysis of 10 cases with a review of the literature. *Ann Diagn Pathol* 2003 December; 7(6): 354–9.
14. Puppala B, Mangurten HH, McFadden J, Lygizos N, Taxy J, Pellettiere E. Nasal glioma. Presenting as neonatal respiratory distress. Definition of the tumor mass by MRI. *Clin Pediatr (Phila)* 1990 January; 29(1): 49–52.
15. Levine MR, Kellis A, Lash R. Nasal glioma masquerading as a capillary hemangioma. *Ophthal Plast Reconstr Surg* 1993 June; 9(2): 132–4.
16. Yeoh GP, Bale PM, de Silva M. Nasal cerebral heterotopia: The so-called nasal glioma or sequestered encephalocele and its variants. *Pediatr Pathol* 1989; 9(5): 531–49.
17. Huisman TAGM, Schneider JFL, Kellenberger CJ, Martin-Fiori E, Willi UV, Holzmann D. Developmental nasal midline masses in children: Neuroradiological evaluation. *Eur Radiol* 2004 February; 14(2): 243–9.
18. Burckhardt W, Tobon D. Endoscopic approach to nasal glioma. *Otolaryngol Head Neck Surg* 1999 May; 120(5): 747–8.

19. Wilkins RB, Hofmann RJ, Byrd WA, Font RL. Heterotopic brain tissue in the orbit. *Arch Ophthalmology* 1987 March; 105(3): 390–2.
20. Newman NJ, Miller NR, Green WR. Ectopic brain in the orbit. *Ophthalmology* 1986 February; 93(2): 268–72.
21. Dasgupta NR, Bentz ML. Nasal gliomas: Identification and differentiation from hemangiomas. *J Craniofac Surg* 2003 September; 14(5): 736–8.
22. Turgut M, Ozcan OE, Benli K, Ozgen T, Gürçay O, Sağlam S, Bertan V, Erbengi A. Congenital nasal encephalocele: A review of 35 cases. *J Craniomaxillofac Surg* 1995 February; 23(1): 1–5.
23. Rahbar R, Resto VA, Robson CD, Perez-Atayde AR, Goumnerova LC, McGill TJ, Healy GB. Nasal glioma and encephalocele: Diagnosis and management. *Laryngoscope* 2003 December; 113(12): 2069–77.
24. Lusk RP, Lee PC. Magnetic resonance imaging of congenital midline nasal masses. *Otolaryngol Head Neck Surg* 1986 October; 95(3 Pt 1): 303–6.
25. Schlosser RJ, Faust RA, Phillips CD, Gross CW. Three-dimensional computed tomography of congenital nasal anomalies. *Int J Pediatr Otorhinolaryngol* 2002 September; 65(2): 125–31.
26. Macfarlane R, Rutka JT, Armstrong D, Phillips J, Posnick J, Forte V, Humphreys RP, Drake J, Hoffman HJ. Encephaloceles of the anterior cranial fossa. *Pediatr Neurosurg* 1995; 23(3): 148–58.
27. Bloom DC, Carvalho DS, Dory C, Brewster DF, Wickersham JK, Kearns DB. Imaging and surgical approach of nasal dermoids. *Int J Ped Otorhinolaryngol* 2002; 62: 111–22.
28. Hartley BEJ, Eze N, Trozzi M, Toma S, Hewitt R, Jephson C, Cochrane L, Wyatt M, Albert D. Nasal dermoids in children: A proposal for a new classification based on 103 cases at Great Ormond Street Hospital. *Int J Ped Otorhinolaryngol* 2015; 79: 18–22.
29. Hanikeri M, Waterhouse N, Kirkpatrick N, Peterson D, Macleod I. The management of midline transcranial nasal dermoid sinus cysts. *Br J Plast Surg* 2005; 58: 1043–50.
30. Alexander VRC, Manjaly JG, Pepper CM, Ifeacho SN, Hewitt RJ, Hartley BEJ. Head and neck teratomas in children—A series of 23 cases at Great Ormond Street Hospital. *Int J Ped Otorhinolaryngol* 2015; 79: 2008–14.

91

Neuroblastoma

ANDREW M. DAVIDOFF

INTRODUCTION

Cancer in the newborn is relatively rare, comprising only about 2.5% of all childhood malignancies[1]; the majority of tumors in the newborn are benign lesions. Overall, neuroblastoma is the fourth most common cancer of childhood, accounting for about 8% of all malignancies diagnosed in children younger than 15 years of age. Neonatal neuroblastoma, defined as neuroblastoma diagnosed prenatally or within 30 days after birth, accounts for approximately 5% of all cases of neuroblastoma.[2] However, neuroblastoma is second only to teratoma as the most commonly diagnosed tumor in the neonate and is, overall, the most common malignancy in the newborn, accounting for 30% of all cancers diagnosed in this age group. With the increasing use of perinatal imaging, the incidence of neonatal neuroblastoma is very likely to increase.

Neuroblastoma is a heterogeneous disease; tumors can spontaneously regress or mature without treatment, or display a very aggressive, malignant phenotype. Although the specific reasons for these differences in biologic behavior have yet to be completely elucidated, certain clinical and biologic factors have been identified that predict, to a significant degree, the tumor phenotype. Among these, patient age at diagnosis is one of the most powerful, with age less than ~1½ years conferring a favorable prognosis.[3] It follows, then, that neuroblastoma diagnosed in the newborn period is associated with a very favorable outcome. Overall, the 5-year survival for children with neuroblastoma is 79%,[4] while neonates have a 5-year survival of 85%–90%.[5,6] The challenge in managing these patients is to maintain the excellent survival rate while minimizing the toxicity of therapy.

ETIOLOGY

Neuroblastoma is an embryonal tumor that arises from neural crest cells. During normal development, neural crest cells migrate from the developing neural tube to form the sympathetic nervous system. Thus, neuroblastoma can originate anywhere along this path of migration in the neck, chest, abdomen or pelvis, including the adrenal medulla, paraspinal sympathetic ganglia, and sympathetic paraganglia, such as the organ of Zuckerkandl. Although the precise etiology of neuroblastoma is currently unknown, as with all cancer, genetic (both inherited and somatic), epigenetic, and environmental factors appear to contribute.

Inherited genetic factors

Neuroblastoma generally occurs sporadically, but familial neuroblastoma does occur in about 2% of the cases. Interestingly, however, substantial biologic and clinical heterogeneity is often observed within familial cases. The germline mutation associated with hereditary neuroblastoma has been identified—activating mutations in the tyrosine kinase domain of the anaplastic lymphoma kinase (*ALK*) oncogene on the short arm of chromosome 2 (2p23).[7] These mutations can also be somatically acquired, although the prevalence of ALK activation in sporadic neuroblastoma remains to be determined.

Somatic genetic factors

Although there is no single genetic abnormality or initiating event common to all neuroblastomas, a number of different genetic alterations have been identified that provide powerful prognostic information and play crucial roles in risk assessment and treatment planning.

DNA Content. Normal human cells contain two copies of each of 23 chromosomes; thus, a normal diploid cell has 46 chromosomes. The majority (55%) of primary neuroblastomas are triploid or *near-triploid/hyperdiploid* and contain between 58 and 80 chromosomes; the remainder (45%) are either *near-diploid* (35–57 chromosomes) or *near-tetraploid* (81–103 chromosomes).[8] The *DNA index* of a tumor is the ratio of the number of chromosomes present to a diploid number of chromosomes (i.e., 46). Therefore, diploid cells have a DNA index of 1.0, whereas near-triploid cells have a DNA index ranging from 1.26 to 1.76. Importantly, patients with near-triploid tumors typically have favorable clinical and biologic prognostic factors and excellent survival rates, as compared with those patients who have near-diploid or near-tetraploid tumors. This association is most important for infants with advanced disease[9]; the prognostic significance of tumor ploidy appears to be lost in patients older than 2 years of age.

Amplification of MYCN. Early studies of neuroblastoma cell lines showed the frequent presence of extrachromosomal double-minute chromatin bodies (DMs) and chromosomally integrated homogeneously staining regions (HSRs) characteristic of gene amplification.[10] Since that time, it has been shown that the amplified region was derived from the distal short arm of chromosome 2 (2p24) and contained the *MYCN* proto-oncogene.

Overall, approximately 25% of primary neuroblastomas have *MYCN* amplification, being present in 40% with advanced disease but only 5%–10% with low-stage disease.[11] The copy number, which can range from 5- to 500-fold amplification, is usually consistent among primary and metastatic sites and at different times during tumor evolution and treatment. This finding suggests that *MYCN* amplification is an early event in the pathogenesis of neuroblastoma. Amplification of *MYCN* is associated with advanced stages of disease, rapid tumor progression, and poor outcome; therefore, it is a powerful prognostic indicator of biologically aggressive tumor behavior.[11,12]

Chromosomal Changes. Approximately 20–35% of primary neuroblastomas exhibit 1p deletion, as determined by fluorescence in situ hybridization (FISH), with the smallest common region of loss located within region 1p36.[13] About 70% of advanced-stage neuroblastomas have 1p deletions. Molecular studies have shown that there is a strong correlation between 1p deletion and *MYCN* amplification and other high-risk features such as age older than 1 year and advanced-stage disease.[13] One study has demonstrated that 1p deletions are independently associated with a worse outcome in patients with neuroblastoma.[14] Deletion of the long arm of chromosome 11 (11q) also appears to be common in neuroblastoma, being present in about 40% of cases. Unbalanced deletion of 11q (loss with either retention or gain of 11p material) is inversely related to *MYCN* amplification[14,15] yet is strongly associated with other high-risk features. Other studies have shown that gain of genetic material on the long arm of chromosome 17 (17q) is perhaps the most common genetic abnormality in neuroblastomas, occurring in approximately 75% of primary tumors.[16] It is unclear at this time how extra copies of 17q contribute to the malignant phenotype of neuroblastoma and which genes on 17q are the critical ones. Nevertheless, gain of chromosome 17q is strongly associated with other known prognostic factors, but it may also be a powerful predictor of adverse outcome.[17]

Epigenetic factors

Epigenetic alterations are defined as those heritable changes in gene expression that do not result from direct changes in DNA sequence. Mechanisms of epigenetic regulation most commonly include DNA methylation, modification of histones, and alterations in microRNA (miRNA, a class of noncoding RNAs) expression. Each of these is likely involved in neuroblastoma pathogenesis.[18] For example, promoter methylation resulting in silencing of caspase 8, a protein involved in apoptosis, likely contributes to the pathogenesis of *MYCN*-amplified neuroblastoma.[19] Also, analyses of miRNA expression has demonstrated that many miRNAs are dysregulated in neuroblastoma,[20] where they frequently lose their function as gene silencers/tumor suppressors.

Environmental factors

In addition to genetic factors, environmental factors may have a direct impact on cell phenotype and fate by causing DNA damage that permanently alters the host genome, although few environmental factors have been convincingly linked to the development of neuroblastoma. Several case–control studies have examined the relationship between maternal and paternal occupation and exposure, and the risk of neuroblastoma in offspring.[21] Several other studies have also suggested a relationship between the use of certain medications just prior to and during pregnancy and neuroblastoma, specifically hormone use and fertility drugs, and phenylhydantoin for seizure disorders.[22] Similarly, the results for smoking, alcohol, illicit drug use, and the use of hair dye in some studies are suggestive but not conclusive.[23]

EVALUATION

Presentation

When symptomatic, children with neuroblastoma usually present with signs and symptoms that reflect the primary site and extent of disease. An abdominal mass may be detected on physical examination when the primary is adrenal or retroperitoneal. Respiratory distress may be a reflection of a thoracic tumor. Altered defecation or urination may be caused by mechanical compression by a pelvic tumor, or by spinal cord compression by a paraspinal tumor. A tumor in the neck or upper thorax can produce Horner syndrome (ptosis, miosis, and anhydrosis), enophthalmos, and heterochromia of the iris. More general signs and symptoms that reflect excessive catecholamine or vasoactive intestinal polypeptide secretion include failure to gain weight, hypertension, and diarrhea.

However, newborns with localized disease, especially those whose lesion was detected on routine perinatal imaging, are almost always asymptomatic. Paravertebral tumors presenting with spinal cord compression (a clinical emergency requiring immediate evaluation) with flaccid leg paralysis and bladder and bowel dysfunction were reported in one series in less than 20% of patients with neonatal neuroblastoma.[24] Although very uncommon, neonatal patients can also present with paraneoplastic syndromes such as opsoclonus–myoclonus–ataxia felt possibly to be secondary to a cross-reactivity of antineuroblastoma antibodies and Purkinje cells in the cerebellum. Two-thirds of these cases occur in infants with mediastinal primary tumors.[25] Although the oncologic outcome for these patients is generally very favorable, neurologic sequelae may persist.

Approximately 35% of infants with neuroblastoma will have metastatic disease at presentation, although greater than two-thirds of these will have a "special" stage of metastatic disease, which, by definition, is a localized primary tumor in patients younger than 1 year, with dissemination limited to skin, liver, or bone marrow (<10% of nucleated cells). These patients may present with "blueberry muffin" cutaneous lesions, respiratory distress secondary to massive hepatomegaly, or anemia secondary to bone marrow disease (see section "Special Considerations in Infants: Stage 4S neuroblastoma").

Laboratory findings

Lactate Dehydrogenase. Despite its lack of specificity, serum lactate dehydrogenase (LDH) can have great prognostic significance. High serum levels of LDH reflect high proliferative activity or large tumor burden, and an LDH level higher than 1500 IU/L appears to be associated with a poor prognosis.[26] Thus, LDH can be used to monitor disease activity or the response to therapy.

Ferritin. High levels of serum ferritin (>150 ng/mL) may also reflect a large tumor burden or rapid tumor progression. Elevated serum ferritin is often seen in advanced-stage neuroblastomas and indicates a poor prognosis[27]; levels often return to normal during clinical remission.

Urinary Catecholamines. Measurement of homovanillic acid (HVA) and/or vanillylmandelic acid (VMA) in the urine is a critical component of the preoperative assessment. Together with a positive bone marrow, elevated levels can be used to make the diagnosis of neuroblastoma and, if elevated at diagnosis, can be used as a marker of disease status (e.g., progression or recurrence).

Diagnostic imaging

Standard Radiographs. Chest radiography can be a useful tool for demonstrating the presence of a posterior mediastinal mass, which in an infant is usually a thoracic neuroblastoma. A Pediatric Oncology Group study demonstrated that a mediastinal mass was discovered on incidental chest radiographs in almost half of patients with thoracic neuroblastoma who had symptoms seemingly unrelated to their tumors.[28] Abdominal radiography is less often the modality by which a neuroblastoma is discovered; however, as many as half of abdominal neuroblastomas are detectable as a mass with fine calcification.

Ultrasonography. The vast majority of abdominal neuroblastomas in the newborn are diagnosed by ultrasonography, either in the prenatal period, as part of routine surveillance of the fetus, or in the postnatal period, to evaluate an abdominal mass. Although ultrasonography is the modality most often used during the initial assessment of a suspected abdominal mass, its sensitivity and accuracy are less than that of computed tomography (CT) or magnetic resonance (MR) imaging for diagnosing neuroblastoma.

Computed Tomography. CT remains a useful, commonly used modality for the evaluation of neuroblastoma. It can demonstrate calcification in almost 85% of neuroblastomas, and intraspinal extension of the tumor can be determined on contrast-enhanced CT. Overall, contrast-enhanced CT has been reported to be 82% accurate in defining neuroblastoma extent, with the accuracy increasing to nearly 97% when performed with a bone scan.[29]

Magnetic Resonance Imaging. MR imaging is becoming the most useful and most sensitive imaging modality for the diagnosis and staging of neuroblastoma. MR imaging appears to be more accurate than CT for detection of stage 4 disease: the sensitivity of MR imaging is 83%, and that of CT is 43%; and the specificity of MR imaging is 97%, and that of CT is 88%.[30] Metastases to the bone and bone marrow, in particular, are better detected by MR imaging, as is intraspinal tumor extension.[30]

Metaiodobenzylguanidine Imaging. Metaiodobenzylguanidine (MIBG) is transported to and stored in the distal storage granules of chromaffin cells in the same way as norepinephrine. MIBG has been used for scintigraphic imaging of neuroblastoma. The MIBG scintiscan is the imaging study of choice in evaluating the involvement of bone and bone marrow by neuroblastoma, having largely replaced technetium-99m methylene diphosphonate (^{99m}Tc-MDP) bone scans, as approximately 90% of neuroblastomas will take up this radiotracer.[31]

Pathology

Neuroblastoma can be distinguished histologically by the presence of neuritic processes (neuropil) and Homer Wright rosettes (neuroblasts surrounding eosinophilic neuropil). Scattered ganglion cells or immature chromaffin cells may also be seen. The appearance of the tumor cells may vary from undifferentiated cells to fully mature ganglion cells. In addition, neuroblastomas have variable degrees of Schwannian cell stroma, reactive nonneoplastic tissue recruited by the tumor cells.

In 1984, Shimada and colleagues first developed an age-linked classification system of neuroblastic tumors based on tumor morphology in which neuroblastomas were divided into two prognostic subgroups, favorable histology and unfavorable histology. The International Neuroblastoma Pathology Classification (INPC) was devised in 1999 and then modified in 2003,[32] and it is an adaptation of the original Shimada system (Table 91.1). The INPC is an age-linked classification schema that depends on the differentiation grade of the neuroblasts, the cellular turnover rate (mitosis–karyorrhexis index [MKI]), and the presence or absence of Schwannian stroma, and classifies neuroblastic tumors into three morphologic categories: neuroblastoma, ganglioneuroblastoma, and ganglioneuroma.

Table 91.1 Prognostic evaluation of neuroblastic tumors according to the international neuroblastoma pathology classification

International neuroblastoma pathology classification		Prognostic group
Neuroblastoma	Schwannian stroma-poor	
		Favorable
<1.5 years	Poorly differentiated or differentiating and low- or intermediate-MKI tumor	
1.5–5 years	Differentiating and low-MKI tumor	
		Unfavorable
<1.5 years	a. Undifferentiated tumor or b. High-MKI tumor	
1.5–5 years	a. Undifferentiated or poorly differentiated tumor or b. Intermediate- or high-MKI tumor	
≥5 years	All tumors	
Ganglioneuroblastoma, intermixed	Schwannian stroma-rich	Favorable
Ganglioneuroblastoma, nodular	Composite Schwannian stroma-rich/ stroma-dominant and stroma-poor	Unfavorable or favorable (based on nodule histology)
Ganglioneuroma	Schwannian stroma-dominant	
Maturing		Favorable
Mature		

Source: Shimada H. et al., The International Neuroblastoma Pathology Classification (the Shimada system), *Cancer,* 1999;86:364–372.
Note: MKI, mitosis–karyorrhexis index.

Neuroblastomas are, by definition, Schwannian stroma-poor (<50% of the tumor tissue) and can be subtyped as undifferentiated, poorly differentiated (<5% of tumor cells have features of differentiation), or differentiating (>5% of tumor cells show differentiation toward ganglion cells). Additional factors that contribute to the prognostic distinction of stroma-poor, neuroblastic tumors (neuroblastoma) as favorable or unfavorable subtypes include the MKI, which is defined as the number of tumor cells undergoing mitosis or karyorrhexis per 5000 neuroblastic cells (i.e., low MKI, <100 cells; intermediate, 100–200 cells; high, >200 cells) and the patient's age (<1.5 years, 1.5–5 years, >5 years). It has been hypothesized that neuroblastic cells with maturational potential require an in vivo latent period before demonstrating histologic evidence of differentiation; therefore, there is a certain allowance for mitotic and karyorrhectic activities of neuroblastic cells in tumors in infants and younger children.[33] Thus, newborns with neuroblastoma are very likely to have favorable histology disease.

Evidence for spontaneous regression of a subgroup of neuroblastoma comes from the observation that small nodules of primitive neuroblasts are routinely found in the developing adrenal gland and even during the early postnatal period. Beckwith and Perrin[34] first described these microscopic nodules that they termed "neuroblastoma in situ" in the adrenals of infants undergoing autopsy following death from non-malignancy-related causes. The incidence of this finding was more than 200-fold greater than the clinical incidence of neuroblastoma, suggesting that perhaps many neuroblastomas spontaneously regress or mature into lesions that never become clinically apparent. Even clinically apparent neuroblastoma can regress or spontaneously mature. Although initially thought to be mediated by the immune system, this may be the result of the withdrawal of neurotrophic maintenance factors such as nerve growth factor. Neuroblastoma probably represents failure of this process of regression.

Staging

International Neuroblastoma Staging System. Current staging of neuroblastoma is based on the International Neuroblastoma Staging System (INSS) (Table 91.2).[35] The INSS is a surgical–pathologic staging system that takes into account several variables, including the following: completeness of resection of primary tumor, ipsilateral and contralateral involvement of lymph nodes, and tumor location in relation to the midline. Complete evaluation for metastatic disease must also be undertaken for accurate staging, although newborns have a lower incidence of disseminated disease at presentation than children (35% vs. 60%), with bone metastases, in particular, rarely occurring in newborns.

Stage distribution varies significantly with age. Patients older than 30 days present more often with stage 4 disease (45%), whereas less than 20% of patients present with stage 1 disease. This stage distribution is notably different in neonates: more than 30% present with stage 1 disease, and only 10% present with stage 4 disease (another 25% have 4S disease). Of patients with 4S disease, more than 20% are younger than 30 days of age at diagnosis.

Table 91.2 International neuroblastoma staging system

1	Localized tumor with complete gross excision, with or without microscopic residual disease; representative ipsilateral lymph nodes negative for tumor microscopically (nodes attached to and removed with primary tumor may be positive).
2A	Localized tumor with incomplete gross excision; representative ipsilateral nonadherent lymph nodes negative for tumor microscopically.
2B	Localized tumor with or without complete gross excision, with ipsilateral nonadherent lymph nodes positive for tumor. Enlarged contralateral lymph nodes must be negative microscopically.
3	Unresectable unilateral tumor infiltrating across the midline,[a] with or without regional lymph node involvement; localized unilateral tumor with contralateral regional lymph node involvement; or midline tumor with bilateral extension by infiltration (unresectable) or by lymph node involvement.
4	Any primary tumor with dissemination to distant lymph nodes, bone marrow, bone, liver, skin, and/or other organs (except as defined for stage 4S).
4S	Localized primary tumor (as defined for stage 1, 2A, or 2B), with dissemination limited to skin, liver, and/or bone marrow[b] (limited to infants <1 year of age).

[a] The midline is defined as the vertebral column. Tumors originating on one side and crossing the midline must infiltrate to or beyond the opposite side of the vertebral column.

[b] Marrow involvement in stage 4S should be minimal, that is, <10% of total nucleated cells identified as malignant on bone marrow biopsy or on marrow aspirate. More extensive marrow involvement would be considered to be stage 4. The MIBG scan (if performed) should be negative in the marrow.

International Neuroblastoma Risk Group Staging System (INRGSS). In an effort to stage patients prior to any therapy and to avoid influences of differences in surgical approach and aggressiveness, the International Neuroblastoma Risk Group (INRG) task force developed a staging system based strictly on imaging at presentation and "image-defined risk factors" (IDRFs). This staging system was initially developed to enable comparison of risk-based clinical trials worldwide and allow for staging on the basis of tumor imaging and not the extent of surgical resection. These IDRFs (Table 91.3) were first proposed by the European International Society of Pediatric Oncology Neuroblastoma Group and generally reflect the presence of encasement of major vessels or nerves, or the infiltration of adjacent organs/structures by a locoregional tumor. Localized tumors are classified as either L1 (absence of any IDRFs) or L2 (the presence of 1 or more of 20 IDRFs). Cecchetto et al. reported in 2005 that the presence of one or more of these image-defined surgical risk factors was associated with a lower complete resection rate and a greater risk of surgery-related complications

when attempting an initial resection of a localized neuroblastoma.[36] The designation of a localized tumor as L2 at presentation is not meant to suggest that all of these tumors need to receive neoadjuvant therapy, however. Additionally, Yoneda et al.[37] recently reported that only 27% of tumors with one or more IDRFs (L2) became negative for IDRFs (L1) after neoadjuvant chemotherapy.

Stratification for risk of recurrence

As previously mentioned, one of the notable characteristics of neuroblastoma is the substantial heterogeneity of the disease. Increasing evidence indicates that the biologic and molecular features of neuroblastoma are highly predictive of clinical behavior. Current treatment is based on risk stratification that takes into account both clinical and biologic variables predictive of disease relapse. The most important clinical variables appear to be age and stage at diagnosis. The most powerful biologic factors at this time appear to be *MYCN* status,[11,12] ploidy[38] (for infants), and histopathologic classification.[39] However, additional biologic and molecular variables continue to be evaluated, and two, the allelic status at chromosomes 1p36 and 11q23 are currently being used to define the duration of therapy for certain patients. Taken together, these variables currently define the Children's Oncology Group (COG) risk stratification (Table 91.4), with children being categorized into three risk groups predictive of relapse; low, intermediate, and high risk. The probability of prolonged disease-free survival for patients in each group is >95%, >90%, and <30%, respectively. Treatment is intensified depending on the patient's increased risk of disease relapse. However, it is important to note that although low- and intermediate-risk patients account for approximately 36% and 21%, respectively, of patients of all ages, neonatal patients present with low- and intermediate-risk disease in 58% and 40% of cases, respectively; rarely do they have high-risk disease. In particular, only 3% of all patients with stage 1 or 2 neuroblastoma have *MYCN* amplification, with the incidence in newborns being even lower.[40]

MANAGEMENT

Risk-based therapy

Low-Risk Disease. The treatment for patients with low-risk disease has generally been surgical resection alone, even in the presence of microscopic residual disease (stage 1), gross residual disease (stage 2A), or gross residual disease with ipsilateral lymph node involvement (stage 2B), if the tumor is without *MYCN* amplification. Infants with stage 4S disease who are not experiencing substantial symptoms may undergo an initial biopsy and observation only, if the tumor has favorable biologic factors. Infants with a localized adrenal mass who meet certain imaging and biochemical criteria may also be observed.

Intermediate-Risk Disease. Patients receive cycles of cyclophosphamide, doxorubicin, carboplatin, and etoposide, given

Table 91.3 Objective surgical risk factors for primary resection of localized neuroblastoma

1. Neck:
   a. Tumor encasing major vessel(s) (e.g., carotid artery, vertebral artery, internal jugular vein)
   b. Tumor extending to base of skull
   c. Tumor compressing the trachea
   d. Tumor encasing the brachial plexus

2. Thorax:
   a. Tumor encasing major vessel(s) (e.g., subclavian vessels, aorta, superior vena cava)
   b. Tumor compressing the trachea or principal bronchi
   c. Lower mediastinal tumor, infiltrating the costovertebral junction between T9 and T12 (may involve the artery of Adamkiewicz supplying the lower spinal cord)

3. Abdomen:
   a. Tumor infiltrating the porta hepatis and/or the hepatoduodenal ligament
   b. Tumor encasing the origin of the celiac axis, and/or the superior mesenteric artery
   c. Tumor invading one or both renal pedicles
   d. Tumor encasing the aorta and/or vena cava
   e. Tumor encasing the iliac vessels
   f. Pelvic tumor crossing the sciatic notch

4. Dumbbell tumors with symptoms of spinal cord compression: any location

5. Infiltration of adjacent organs/structures: diaphragm, kidney, liver, duodenopancreatic block, and mesentery

Source: Cecchetto G. et al., Surgical risk factors in primary surgery for localized neuroblastoma: The LNESG1 study of the European International Society of Pediatric Oncology Neuroblastoma Group, *J Clin Oncol*, 2005;23:8483–8489.

every 3 weeks. The duration of therapy (i.e., the number of cycles) will depend upon which of three intermediate risk groups a patient is placed in, with group stratification again being based on clinical and biologic risk factors (Table 91.4). One of these biologic factors will include loss of heterozygosity (LOH—loss of one of two normally paired chromosomal regions) at chromosome 1p or 11q (unbalanced), as these events have been shown to be independently associated with decreased progression-free survival in patients with low- and intermediate-risk disease.[14]

The overall surgical goal in intermediate-risk patients is to perform the most complete tumor resection possible, consistent with preservation of full organ and neurologic function. This may necessitate leaving residual disease adherent to critical anatomic structures. It is no longer required that infants with 4S disease undergo resection of their primary tumor. In addition, if these infants are too unstable at presentation, it is no longer required that they even undergo an initial biopsy.

High-Risk Disease. This group accounts for less than 2% of neonatal neuroblastomas and comprises cases where the tumor is *MYCN* amplified. Although the incidence of high-risk neuroblastoma in neonates is much lower than that for patients older than 30 days (incidence >45%), neonates with high-risk disease have a 2-year overall survival (OS) of only 30% despite tolerating the treatment regimen.[41]

The general approach to treating patients with high-risk neuroblastoma includes intensive induction chemotherapy, myeloablative consolidation therapy with stem cell rescue, radiation therapy, and immunotherapy for minimal residual disease. The role of surgery for control of locoregional disease is controversial. Several reports have suggested that patients with INSS stage 3 or 4 disease who undergo gross total resection of their primary tumor and locoregional disease experience improved local tumor control and increased overall survival[42-44]; however, other reports have not confirmed these observations.[45,46] Despite the uncertainty of the role of surgery, the COG high-risk protocol currently recommends attempting gross total resection of the primary tumor and locoregional disease in patients with high-risk neuroblastoma.

Surgical management

Preoperative Preparation. All patients, prior to surgery, should have a complete blood count, chemistry panel (to include liver function tests if the liver is involved), and a coagulation screen. Urinary catecholamines and serum ferritin and LDH should already have been obtained as part of the initial workup. Blood pressure should be normalized with pharmacologic means if hypertension was present at presentation. Operations on neuroblastoma are often hazardous, and hemorrhage is a frequent complication; hence, packed red blood cells should be available for transfusion during or immediately after the operation.

Operative Approach (Open). Tumor size, the extent of vascular encasement, and exact tumor location should be considered in selecting the approach for a retroperitoneal neuroblastoma. Options available for the abdominal incision include a transverse incision, bilateral subcostal (Chevron) incisions, or a midline incision (Figure 91.1). A transthoracic (intercostal), transdiaphragmatic extension can be added for resection of neuroblastomas with either thoracoabdominal extension or extensive periaortic or celiac axis encasement. The tumor should be carefully exposed to determine the relation between the tumor and

Table 91.4 Children's oncology group risk stratification for children with neuroblastoma

Risk stratification	INSS stage	Age	Biology
Low			
Group 1			
	1	Any	Any
	2A/2B (>50% resected)	Any	MYCN-NA, any histology/ploidy
	4S	<365 days	MYCN-NA, FH, DI > 1
Intermediate			
Group 2			
	2A/2B (<50% resected or Bx only)	0–12 years	MYCN-NA, any histology/ploidy[a]
	3	<365 days	MYCN-NA, FH, DI > 1[a]
	3	≥365 days to 12 years	MYCN-NA, FH[a]
	4S (symptomatic)	<365 days	MYCN-NA, FH, DI > 1[a]
Group 3			
	3	<365 days	MYCN-NA, either UH or DI = 1[a]
	4	<365 days	MYCN-NA, FH, DI > 1[a]
	4S	<365 days	MYCN-NA, either UH or DI = 1[a]; or unknown biology
Group 4			
	4	<365 days	MYCN-NA, either DI = 1 or UH
	3	365 to <547 days	MYCN-NA, UH, any ploidy
	4	365 to <547 days	MYCN-NA, FH, DI > 1
High			
	2A/2B, 3, 4, 4S	Any	MYCN amplified, any histology/ploidy
	3	>547 days	MYCN-NA, UH, any ploidy
	4	365 to >547 days	MYCN-NA, UH or DI = 1
	4	>547 days	Any

Note: DI, DNA index; FH, favorable histology; MYCN-NA, MYCN not amplified; UH, unfavorable histology.

[a] If tumor contains chromosomal 1p LOH or unb11qLOH, or if data are missing, treatment assignment is upgraded to next group.

normal organs and vessels. If encasement of major vessels such as the aorta, vena cava, or their branches is found, tumor dissection must be performed to free the vessels completely. With deliberate dissection of the tumor from the mesenteric and renal vessels, injury to the liver, bowel, spleen, and kidneys can be avoided (Figure 91.2), although this frequently results in piecemeal division and excision of the tumor.[46] For a more detailed description of extensive surgical resection of neuroblastoma, see the work of Kiely.[46]

Operative Approach (Laparoscopic). Laparoscopic adrenalectomy is feasible in children and may have some benefits (less pain, shorter hospitalization, improved cosmesis) compared to open adrenalectomy. Laparoscopy may be a reasonable approach in neuroblastoma, in particular, where negative margins, piecemeal removal of the specimen, and leaving residual tumor are not usually of concern. In addition, vascular encasement, characteristic of high-risk neuroblastoma in older children, does not usually occur in newborns, making a minimally invasive approach feasible. However, an appropriate oncologic procedure, which currently still includes bilateral lymph node sampling for staging, is required. The surgeon also should consider that, as discussed previously, small adrenal masses discovered in the perinatal period and 4S neuroblastomas may not need to be removed.

Transperitoneal laparoscopic adrenalectomy is generally performed with the operative side up but in such a fashion that allows rapid transition to an open procedure, if that becomes necessary. The table is tilted into reverse Trendelenburg position and can be flexed to increase the distance between the costal margin and the iliac crest. Generally, four ports are used (Figure 91.3). Dissection is

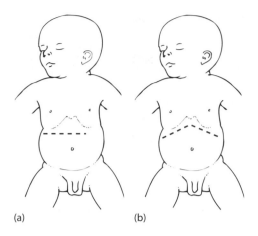

Figure 91.1 Incisions for retroperitoneal neuroblastoma resection. **(a)** Transverse abdominal incision (right-sided tumor). **(b)** Bilateral subcostal incision.

performed in much the same manner as the open procedure, with care being taken to secure the adrenal vein and to avoid the renal vessels. Bilateral retroperitoneal lymph node sampling is technically required for appropriate neuroblastoma staging although rarely done.

SPECIAL CONSIDERATIONS IN INFANTS

The best management for neuroblastoma in infants continues to be evaluated in clinical trials because of the very heterogeneous behavior of the disease and the fact that many of these tumors will follow a very benign clinical course without any therapeutic intervention, including surgery. This is an important consideration given the potential toxicities and long-term complications of adjuvant chemotherapy and radiation therapy, which include organ dysfunction and second malignancies.[47] Because extensive

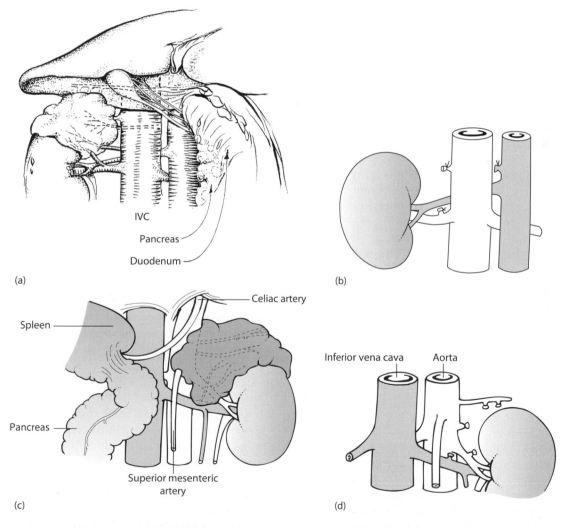

Figure 91.2 Right adrenal tumor. **(a)** The duodenum and head of the pancreas with important structures in the lesser omentum mobilized to the left. The renal vessels are dissected out, and branches to the tumor are divided. Medially, the tumor is juxtaposed to the inferior vena cava (IVC), and sharp dissection may be needed to separate it. At least one vein will need to be secured and divided. **(b)** The tumor has been removed. Left adrenal tumor. **(c)** The lienorenal ligament has been divided, allowing mobilization of the spleen and pancreas to the right. The renal vessels are visible and dissected out—branches to the tumor are divided. Next the tumor is dissected from the aorta dividing any vessels. **(d)** Tumor has been removed and the vascular supply divided.

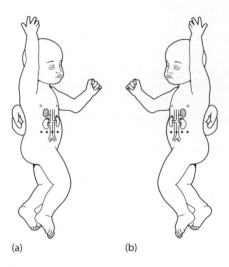

Figure 91.3 Trocar placement for laparoscopic adrenalectomy for **(a)** right-sided and **(b)** left-sided tumors.

surgery is often required, intraoperative and postoperative complications are also not uncommon.[48,49] As many as 80% of patients will experience significant blood loss during surgery. Up to 10% will suffer an injury to a major vascular structure (aorta, vena cava, or renal vessels), and injury to other viscera (bowel, liver, spleen, or kidney) occurs in approximately 5% of cases. As with all surgical procedures, there is also a risk for anesthetic complications, with infants being at higher risk. The overall mortality for young infants undergoing adrenal surgery for tumor resection may be as high as 2%.[50] Postoperative complications have a wide range. Wound complications occur in 1%–5% of cases, as does postoperative bowel obstruction. In addition, hypertension, chylous ascites, pleural effusion, infection and sepsis, diarrhea, kidney loss, and prolonged total parenteral nutrition (TPN) requirement can occur. Because of these potential therapy-related complications in neonatal patients, efforts have been directed toward reducing the treatment.

Expectant Observation of Localized Neuroblastoma. A prospective COG study, ANBL00P2, led by Nuchtern and colleagues,[51] evaluated observation alone in infants 6 months of age or younger on the date an adrenal mass was first identified that was 16 mL or less in volume if solid or 65 mL or less in volume if the mass was at least 25% cystic and did not cross the midline. Additionally, disease had to be limited to the adrenal gland as determined by adjunct imaging (e.g., MIBG, CT, or MRI scans) and bone marrow biopsy. However, parents also had the option to choose upfront surgical resection for their child. Follow-up investigations included measurement of urinary catecholamine levels and serial abdominal ultrasound studies in addition to occasional CT or MRI scans. Infants with an increase of 50% in tumor volume or an increase in catecholamine levels were referred for surgery. Of the 87 patients in this study, 83 (95.4%) were enrolled in the observation arm, of whom 56 completed the observation. A total of 20 (23.0%)

patients underwent resection: 4 immediately on enrollment into the surgery arm and 16 who were originally enrolled in the observation arm. The 3-year event-free survival for patients with small adrenal masses was 97.7%, and the 3-year OS at a median follow-up of 3.2 years was 100%. Of the 83 patients in the observation arm, 67 (81%) were spared surgery. These patients were observed without biopsy for definitive histologic diagnosis. Interestingly, however, one case has subsequently been reported detailing a patient initially observed expectantly on this protocol who, 4 years later, developed high-risk stage 4 *MYCN*-amplified neuroblastoma.[52]

Hero et al.[53] reported the German experience observing 93 infants with non-*MYCN*-amplified, localized, unresected stage 2 or 3 neuroblastoma. Forty-four (47.3%) tumors exhibited regression, 35 (37.6%) progressed locally or to stage 4S, and 4 (4.3%) progressed to stage 4, requiring high-risk therapy. Of these 35 patients, 22 received chemotherapy for tumor progression or lack of regression. Strikingly, of the 93 patients, 21 with stage 3 disease were initially observed, of whom 11 (52.4%) showed tumor regression. The entire cohort had an excellent 3-year OS of 99%. These data provide support for a trial of observation in patients with INSS stage 2 or stage 3 disease with favorable biology.

In July 2014, the COG opened a phase III study, ANBL1232 (NCT02176967), with the aim of further reducing therapy by assessing a response- and biology-based treatment approach of observation in two cohorts: infants younger than 12 months with INRG stage L1 tumors smaller than 5 cm (group A) and non-high-risk patients younger than 18 months with INRG stage L2 tumors with favorable histologic and genomic features (group B). This study will expand on ANBL00P2 findings by increasing the age cutoff for avoiding surgery from 6 months, increasing the tumor size from 3.1 cm to 5 cm, and allowing nonadrenal primaries to be observed. Patients in group A may have nonadrenal tumors confirmed by either an MIBG scan or elevated levels of catecholamine metabolites and may be observed up to 96 weeks without a biopsy. If these patients show disease progression, then surgical resection is recommended. Patients in group B must be asymptomatic and must have a diagnostic biopsy to confirm favorable biology. If these patients show a more than 25% increase in tumor volume, they will undergo two cycles of chemotherapy or surgical resection. If after initial therapy, the patients have a partial response or better, observation will be continued. Of note, this is an ongoing prospective study, so the management recommendations are not fully validated and confirmed.

Stage 4S Neuroblastoma. In 1971, D'Angio, Evans, and Koop[54] reported a number of patients with a special variant of metastatic neuroblastoma, termed IVS (now referred to as 4S [INSS] or 4M [INRGSS]). These patients were infants who typically had a single, small primary tumor but who often had extensive metastatic disease in the liver, resulting in significant hepatomegaly, skin nodules, and small amounts of disease in the bone marrow (<10% of the mononuclear cells). If there was more extensive bone marrow involvement or bone metastasis, then the disease was categorized as stage 4. They noted that these patients with 4S neuroblastoma were quite remarkable, because the large amount of disease generally underwent spontaneous regression, even without treatment, and the infants ultimately had no evidence of disease.

Gigliotti et al. reported that 45 (33.6%) of 134 neonates with neuroblastoma presented with stage 4S disease. Data from the COG suggests an incidence of 25% for neonates, which is in sharp contrast to an incidence of less than 5% in patients older than 30 days.[55] Supportive therapy only has been recommended for this stage of neuroblastoma because of the high incidence of spontaneous regression and the resultant good prognosis.[56] Most of these patients have tumor with favorable biology (single-copy *MYCN*, favorable Shimada histology, and DNA index >1); therefore, they are assigned to the low-risk classification and receive no therapy. However, despite the generally benign course of their malignancy, these infants can die of complications caused by the initial bulk of their disease. Limited chemotherapy, local irradiation, or minimal resection can be used to treat infants with life-threatening symptoms of hepatomegaly. Operative placement of a Silastic pouch as a temporary abdominal wall may be a choice for those with significant liver enlargement that causes either respiratory compromise secondary to diaphragmatic elevation or obstruction of the inferior vena cava. This procedure may help to avoid life-threatening events until shrinkage of the liver is achieved by either spontaneous regression or therapy. The rare infant with 4S disease and either unfavorable Shimada histology or a DNA index of 1 (or whose biology is not known) will be treated for intermediate-risk disease (group 3), and those with 4S disease that is *MYCN* amplified will be treated for high-risk disease.

Patients with 4S disease are also being studied prospectively on the ANBL1232 protocol. Children younger than 18 months who are asymptomatic and have tumors with favorable biology are being observed. If patients are symptomatic, then age is considered as the next criterion: patients younger than 3 months receive immediate chemotherapy (with full staging within 1 month) with plans to perform a tumor biopsy when they are stable, whereas patients 3–18 months old undergo a tumor biopsy and proceed through a response-based algorithm to determine the length of treatment. ANBL1232 will also prospectively study an objective scoring system in which values will be assigned to symptoms and laboratory results to generate a clinical score. The trial will evaluate gastrointestinal symptoms, respiratory compromise, venous return, renal compromise, and hepatic dysfunction.

Screening for Neuroblastoma. Because the two most important clinical variables for predicting outcome in patients with neuroblastoma are tumor stage and patient age at the time of diagnosis, it was hypothesized that earlier detection of neuroblastoma through mass population screening might significantly impact neuroblastoma-associated mortality. In Japan in the 1980s, mass screening of neuroblastoma was performed in infants by quantitating urinary VMA and HVA; initially, the mass screening showed very encouraging results.[57] However, subsequent population-based studies with concurrent control groups performed in Germany and North America found that although the incidence of neuroblastoma increased, the additional cases were largely early-stage, favorable biology, low-risk tumors.[47] Because the overall mortality of patients with neuroblastoma was not affected, the implication of these studies was that mass screening most likely detected tumors that would have undergone spontaneous regression and not been detected clinically. Thus, there currently appears to be no role for screening infants for neuroblastoma. A recent follow-up study by Ioka et al.[58] confirmed that the cessation of mass screening for neuroblastoma in Japan did not appear to increase mortality due to neuroblastoma or the incidence of advanced stage disease in older children.

REFERENCES

1. Isaacs HJ. Congenital and neonatal malignant tumors. A 28-year experience at Children's Hospital of Los Angeles. *Am J Pediatr Hematol Oncol* 1987; 9: 121–9.
2. Interiano RB, Davidoff AM. Current management of neonatal neuroblastoma. *Curr Pediatr Rev* 2015; 11: 179–87.
3. London WB, Castleberry RP, Matthay KK, Look AT, Seeger RC, Shimada H et al. Evidence for an age cutoff greater than 365 days for neuroblastoma risk group stratification in the Children's Oncology Group. *J Clin Oncol* 2005; 23: 6459–65.
4. Horner M, Ries L, Krapcho M, Neyman N, Aminou R, Howlader N et al. (eds). *SEER Cancer Statistics Review, 1975–2006.* Bethesda, MD: National Cancer Institute, 2009.
5. Gigliotti AR, Di CA, Sorrentino S, Parodi S, Rizzo A, Buffa P et al. Neuroblastoma in the newborn. A study of the Italian Neuroblastoma Registry. *Eur J Cancer* 2009; 45: 3220–7.
6. Zhou Y, Li K, Zheng S, Chen L. Retrospective study of neuroblastoma in Chinese neonates from 1994 to 2011: An evaluation of diagnosis, treatments, and prognosis: A 10-year restrospective study of neonatal neuroblastoma. *J Cancer Res Clin Oncol* 2014; 140: 83–7.
7. Mosse YP, Laudenslager M, Longo L, Cole KA, Wood A, Attiyeh EF et al. Identification of ALK as a major familial neuroblastoma predisposition gene. *Nature* 2008; 455: 930–5.
8. Kaneko Y, Kanda N, Maseki N, Sakurai M, Tsuchida Y, Takeda T et al. Different karyotypic patterns in early and advanced stage neuroblastomas. *Cancer Res* 1987; 47: 311–8.

9. Bowman LC, Castleberry RP, Cantor A, Joshi V, Cohn SL, Smith EI et al. Genetic staging of unresectable or metastatic neuroblastoma in infants: A Pediatric Oncology Group study. *J Natl Cancer Inst* 1997; 89: 373–80.

10. Schwab M, Alitalo K, Klempnauer KH, Varmus HE, Bishop JM, Gilbert F et al. Amplified DNA with limited homology to myc cellular oncogene is shared by human neuroblastoma cell lines and a neuroblastoma tumour. *Nature* 1983; 305: 245–8.

11. Brodeur GM, Seeger RC, Schwab M, Varmus HE, Bishop JM. Amplification of N-myc in untreated human neuroblastomas correlates with advanced disease stage. *Science* 1984; 224: 1121–4.

12. Seeger RC, Brodeur GM, Sather H, Dalton A, Siegel SE, Wong KY et al. Association of multiple copies of the N-myc oncogene with rapid progression of neuroblastomas. *N Engl J Med* 1985; 313: 1111–6.

13. Fong CT, Dracopoli NC, White PS, Merrill PT, Griffith RC, Housman DE et al. Loss of heterozygosity for the short arm of chromosome 1 in human neuroblastomas: Correlation with N-myc amplification. *Proc Natl Acad Sci U S A* 1989; 86: 3753–7.

14. Attiyeh EF, London WB, Mosse YP, Wang Q, Winter C, Khazi D et al. Chromosome 1p and 11q deletions and outcome in neuroblastoma. *N Engl J Med* 2005; 353: 2243–53.

15. Takayama H, Suzuki T, Mugishima H, Fujisawa T, Ookuni M, Schwab M et al. Deletion mapping of chromosomes 14q and 1p in human neuroblastoma. *Oncogene* 1992; 7: 1185–9.

16. Vandesompele J, Van RN, Van GM, Laureys G, Ambros P, Heimann P et al. Genetic heterogeneity of neuroblastoma studied by comparative genomic hybridization. *Genes Chromosomes Cancer* 1998; 23: 141–52.

17. Bown N, Cotterill S, Lastowska M, O'Neill S, Pearson AD, Plantaz D et al. Gain of chromosome arm 17q and adverse outcome in patients with neuroblastoma. *N Engl J Med* 1999; 340: 1954–61.

18. Domingo-Fernandez R, Watters K, Piskareva O, Stallings RL, Bray I. The role of genetic and epigenetic alterations in neuroblastoma disease pathogenesis. *Pediatr Surg Int* 2013; 29: 101–19.

19. Teitz T, Wei T, Valentine MB, Vanin EF, Grenet J, Valentine VA et al. Caspase 8 is deleted or silenced preferentially in childhood neuroblastomas with amplification of *MYCN*. *Nat Med* 2000; 6: 529–35.

20. Wei JS, Johansson P, Chen QR, Song YK, Durinck S, Wen X et al. microRNA profiling identifies cancer-specific and prognostic signatures in pediatric malignancies. *Clin Cancer Res* 2009; 15: 5560–8.

21. Bunin GR, Ward E, Kramer S, Rhee CA, Meadows AT. Neuroblastoma and parental occupation. *Am J Epidemiol* 1990; 131: 776–80.

22. Kramer S, Ward E, Meadows AT, Malone KE. Medical and drug risk factors associated with neuroblastoma: A case–control study. *J Natl Cancer Inst* 1987; 78: 797–804.

23. Bluhm EC, Daniels J, Pollock BH, Olshan AF. Maternal use of recreational drugs and neuroblastoma in offspring: A report from the Children's Oncology Group (United States). *Cancer Causes Control* 2006; 17: 663–9.

24. Moppett J, Haddadin I, Foot A. Neonatal neuroblastoma. *Arch Dis Child Fetal Neonatal Ed* 1999; 81: F134–7.

25. Rudnick E, Khakoo Y, Antunes NL, Seeger RC, Brodeur GM, Shimada H et al. Opsoclonus–myoclonus–ataxia syndrome in neuroblastoma: Clinical outcome and antineuronal antibodies—A report from the Children's Cancer Group Study. *Med Pediatr Oncol* 2001; 36: 612–22.

26. Joshi VV, Cantor AB, Brodeur GM, Look AT, Shuster JJ, Altshuler G et al. Correlation between morphologic and other prognostic markers of neuroblastoma. A study of histologic grade, DNA index, N-myc gene copy number, and lactic dehydrogenase in patients in the Pediatric Oncology Group. *Cancer* 1993; 71: 3173–81.

27. Silber JH, Evans AE, Fridman M. Models to predict outcome from childhood neuroblastoma: The role of serum ferritin and tumor histology. *Cancer Res* 1991; 51: 1426–33.

28. Adams GA, Shochat SJ, Smith EI, Shuster JJ, Joshi VV, Altshuler G et al. Thoracic neuroblastoma: A Pediatric Oncology Group study. *J Pediatr Surg* 1993; 28: 372–7.

29. Stark DD, Moss AA, Brasch RC, deLorimier AA, Albin AR, London DA et al. Neuroblastoma: Diagnostic imaging and staging. *Radiology* 1983; 148: 101–5.

30. Siegel MJ, Ishwaran H, Fletcher BD, Meyer JS, Hoffer FA, Jaramillo D et al. Staging of neuroblastoma at imaging: Report of the radiology diagnostic oncology group. *Radiology* 2002; 223: 168–75.

31. Howman-Giles R, Shaw PJ, Uren RF, Chung DK. Neuroblastoma and other neuroendocrine tumors. *Semin Nucl Med* 2007; 37: 286–302.

32. Peuchmaur M, d'Amore ES, Joshi VV, Hata J, Roald B, Dehner LP et al. Revision of the International Neuroblastoma Pathology Classification: Confirmation of favorable and unfavorable prognostic subsets in ganglioneuroblastoma, nodular. *Cancer* 2003; 98: 2274–81.

33. Shimada H, Ambros IM, Dehner LP, Hata J, Joshi VV, Roald B et al. The International Neuroblastoma Pathology Classification (the Shimada system). *Cancer* 1999; 86: 364–72.

34. Beckwith JB, Perrin E. In situ neuroblastomas: A contribution to the natural history of neural crest. *Am J Pathol* 1963; 43: 1089–104.

35. Brodeur GM, Pritchard J, Berthold F, Carlsen NL, Castel V, Castelberry RP et al. Revisions of the international criteria for neuroblastoma diagnosis, staging, and response to treatment. *J Clin Oncol* 1993; 11: 1466–77.

36. Cecchetto G, Mosseri V, De Bernardi B, Helardot P, Monclair T, Costa E et al. Surgical risk factors in primary surgery for localized neuroblastoma: The LNESG1 study of the European International Society of Pediatric Oncology Neuroblastoma Group. *J Clin Oncol* 2005; 23: 8483–9.

37. Yoneda A, Nishikawa M, Uehara S, Oue T, Usui N, Inoue M et al. Can neoadjuvant chemotherapy reduce the surgical risks for localized neuroblastoma patients with image-defined risk factors at the time of diagnosis? *Pediatr Surg Int* 2016; 32: 209–14.

38. Look AT, Hayes FA, Nitschke R, McWilliams NB, Green AA. Cellular DNA content as a predictor of response to chemotherapy in infants with unresectable neuroblastoma. *N Engl J Med* 1984; 311: 231–5.

39. Shimada H, Umehara S, Monobe Y, Hachitanda Y, Nakagawa A, Goto S et al. International neuroblastoma pathology classification for prognostic evaluation of patients with peripheral neuroblastic tumors: A report from the Children's Cancer Group. *Cancer* 2001; 92: 2451–61.

40. Bagatell R, Beck-Popovic M, London WB, Zhang Y, Pearson AD, Matthay KK et al. Significance of *MYCN* amplification in international neuroblastoma staging system stage 1 and 2 neuroblastoma: A report from the International Neuroblastoma Risk Group database. *J Clin Oncol* 2009; 27: 365–70.

41. Canete A, Gerrard M, Rubie H, Castel V, Di CA, Munzer C et al. Poor survival for infants with *MYCN*-amplified metastatic neuroblastoma despite intensified treatment: The International Society of Paediatric Oncology European Neuroblastoma Experience. *J Clin Oncol* 2009; 27: 1014–9.

42. LaQuaglia MP, Kushner BH, Su W, Heller G, Kramer K, Abramson S et al. The impact of gross total resection on local control and survival in high-risk neuroblastoma. *J Pediatr Surg* 2004; 39(3): 412–7.

43. Haase GM, O'Leary MC, Ramsay NK, Romansky SG, Stram DO, Seeger RC et al. Aggressive surgery combined with intensive chemotherapy improves survival in poor-risk neuroblastoma. *J Pediatr Surg* 1991; 26: 1119–23.

44. Grosfeld JL, Baehner RL. Neuroblastoma: An analysis of 160 cases. *World J Surg* 1980; 4: 29–37.

45. Castel V, Tovar JA, Costa E, Cuadros J, Ruiz A, Rollan V et al. The role of surgery in stage IV neuroblastoma. *J Pediatr Surg* 2002; 37: 1574–8.

46. Kiely EM. The surgical challenge of neuroblastoma. *J Pediatr Surg* 1994; 29: 128–33.

47. Laverdiere C, Liu Q, Yasui Y, Nathan PC, Gurney JG, Stovall M et al. Long-term outcomes in survivors of neuroblastoma: A report from the Childhood Cancer Survivor Study. *J Natl Cancer Inst* 2009; 101: 1131–40.

48. Azizkhan RG, Shaw A, Chandler JG. Surgical complications of neuroblastoma resection. *Surgery* 1985; 97: 514–7.

49. Kiely EM. Radical surgery for abdominal neuroblastoma. *Semin Surg Oncol* 1993; 9: 489–92.

50. Ikeda H, Suzuki N, Takahashi A, Kuroiwa M, Nagashima K, Tsuchida Y et al. Surgical treatment of neuroblastomas in infants under 12 months of age. *J Pediatr Surg* 1998; 33: 1246–50.

51. Nuchtern JG, London WB, Barnewolt CE, Naranjo A, McGrady PW, Geiger JD et al. A prospective study of expectant observation as primary therapy for neuroblastoma in young infants: A Children's Oncology Group study. *Ann Surg* 2012; 256: 573–80.

52. Salloum R, Garrison A, von AD, Sheridan R, Towbin AJ, Adams D et al. Relapsed perinatal neuroblastoma after expectant observation. *Pediatr Blood Cancer* 2015; 62: 160–2.

53. Hero B, Simon T, Spitz R, Ernestus K, Gnekow AK, Scheel-Walter HG et al. Localized infant neuroblastomas often show spontaneous regression: Results of the prospective trials NB95-S and NB97. *J Clin Oncol* 2008; 26: 1504–10.

54. D'Angio GJ, Evans AE, Koop CE. Special pattern of widespread neuroblastoma with a favourable prognosis. *Lancet* 1971; 1: 1046–9.

55. Gigliotti AR, Di CA, Sorrentino S, Parodi S, Rizzo A, Buffa P et al. Neuroblastoma in the newborn. A study of the Italian Neuroblastoma Registry. *Eur J Cancer* 2009; 45: 3220–7.

56. Nickerson HJ, Matthay KK, Seeger RC, Brodeur GM, Shimada H, Perez C et al. Favorable biology and outcome of stage IV-S neuroblastoma with supportive care or minimal therapy: A Children's Cancer Group study. *J Clin Oncol* 2000; 18: 477–86.

57. Nishihira H, Toyoda Y, Tanaka Y, Ijiri R, Aida N, Takeuchi M et al. Natural course of neuroblastoma detected by mass screening: A 5-year prospective study at a single institution. *J Clin Oncol* 2000; 18: 3012–7.

58. Ioka A, Inoue M, Yoneda A, Nakamura T, Hara J, Hashii Y et al. Effects of the cessation of mass screening for neuroblastoma at 6 months of age: A population-based study in Osaka, Japan. *J Epidemiol* 2016; 26(4): 179–84.

92

Soft-tissue sarcoma

MARTIN T. CORBALLY

INTRODUCTION

Soft-tissue sarcoma is a rare tumor in children and is considerably rarer still in the newborn period (birth to 6 weeks). Their behavior is, for the most part, benign with malignant varieties accounting for no more than 2% of all sarcomatous lesions in childhood. The very rarity of these tumors and their generally benign behavior underscore the need for a careful and balanced approach to their management. This is further emphasized by the complexity of surgery, radiotherapy, and chemotherapy in this age group, which, when weighed against the potential lifelong complications of therapy, justifies careful and measured discussion as to the most appropriate course of action.

Immature newborn metabolism, renal function, and unpredictable drug toxicity make chemotherapy complex and difficult to administer in the newborn period. In all situations where neoadjuvant or adjuvant therapy is considered appropriate, it must take into account age-dependent physiology, immature neural, and gonadal development. Certain tumors may exhibit alarming histopathological features but yet behave in a nonaggressive manner. Radical and mutilating surgery and/or toxic neoadjuvant treatment in this clinical context is clearly not indicated. However, even tumors that act in a benign manner and display no worrying histology or clinical behavior may present some cause for concern by virtue of their location such as a neck infantile fibrosarcoma (CIFS) and airway obstruction, or a perineal IFS and its potential for urinary obstruction.

From a biological perspective, it must also always be noted that certain neonatal "malignant tumors" such as neuroblastoma are subject to immunological influences that ultimately result in their spontaneous resolution. Spontaneous resolution of congenital infantile fibrosarcoma has been previously reported, and a watch-and-wait approach may be considered in some very young patients when strict observation is guaranteed. Inconsistent lack of histological correlation with clinical behavior and the known immunomodulation of some tumors therefore render the treatment options more complex and require careful discussion. Any individual center's experience of this condition may be limited and underscores the need for greater multicenter collaboration and prospective studies.

This chapter will discuss soft-tissue sarcoma in the newborn period, which strictly extends from birth to 6 weeks of age. However, most reports and series recognize the extreme rarity of this condition and usually include patients up to 2 or 3 years.

GENETICS

Although multifactorial elements are felt to contribute to the development of malignant tumors, the majority have a genetic component. Single gene mutations and more complex constitutional chromosomal anomalies favor the development of neonatal neoplasms. Some are well known, if not for the early development of neoplasia, but more for its late arrival, e.g., Down syndrome and leukemia, hepatoblastoma or rhabdomyosarcoma in Li–Fraumeni syndrome, Wilms tumor, and Denys–Drash syndrome. More recently, some reports have confirmed the association of the ETV6–NTRK3 fusion gene in more than 87% of infantile fibrosarcomas. This T chromosomal translocation is not completely specific to sarcomas, however, and has been noted in some leukemias and mesoblastic nephromas.

Soft-tissue sarcomas, however, are a heterogenous group of tumors derived from mesenchymal cells and may therefore differentiate into muscle, fibrous, and other structures. As such, they may present in many locations and with a variety of symptoms. Despite being rare, it is, however, an important diagnosis to consider in any infant presenting with an unusual mass or obstruction, or prolapse of a mass from the vagina, urethra, or other orifice.

Soft-tissue sarcomas account for approximately 10% of all neonatal tumors and only 2% of all childhood sarcomas. In general, they fall into three different groups:

1. Congenital (infantile) fibrosarcoma (CIFS)
2. Rhabdomyosarcoma (RMS)
3. Non-rhabdomyosarcoma soft-tissue sarcoma (non-RMS)

OVERVIEW OF MANAGEMENT

In general, treatment is tailored to the individual patient but should, if possible, be with a curative intent while limiting the toxicity of therapy and avoiding morbidity or mutilating surgery (Figure 92.1). Mutilating surgery is only rarely required and in exceptional and life-threatening circumstances. This is the principle mainstay of treatment. Management decisions are often complex and require discussion in a multidisciplinary forum composed of pediatric surgical oncologists, oncologists, radiotherapists, histopathologists, and nursing. While chemosensitivity and the response to radiotherapy (if utilized) vary from patient to patient, chemotherapy is modified to minimize the severity of immunosuppression and serious infection. Radiotherapy is occasionally required, but it is generally held only as a treatment of last resort with greater emphasis being placed on surgical resection where possible.

All patients need histological diagnosis either by open, tru-cut, or fine-needle aspiration cytology (FNAC). Whatever the biopsy type, it is essential that it is taken by the pediatric surgical oncologist who is ultimately responsible for the surgical care of the patient. An inappropriately sited biopsy may ultimately compromise the subsequent surgical approach and make complete tumor clearance difficult or impossible. Essentially the needle tract or open biopsy tract must be in the line of the ultimate incision for surgical clearance. The biopsy should be sufficient to allow accurate and complete diagnosis and is sent fresh to the laboratory for histology and appropriate histochemistry and biological studies. The biopsy, where possible, should minimize tumor spillage, and this may be aided by the generous use of chlorhexidine sponges, argon, or standard diathermy.

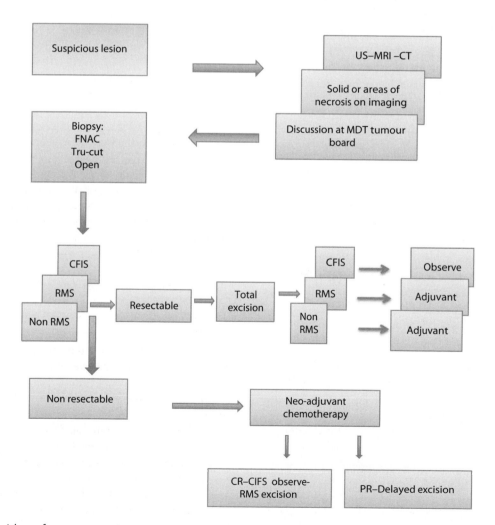

Figure 92.1 Algorithm of management.

At presentation, it is important not just to determine histology but also to accurately stage the tumor. This will include a variety of imaging, such as ultrasound, CT, and MRI. These may or may not require sedation or anesthesia to minimize movement. A PET CT may also be useful in determining stage and response to treatment and can aid the postoperative evaluation of surgical sites. In addition, a bone marrow sample is taken to determine metastatic involvement. Pleural effusions may be tapped or chest drains inserted as necessary.

Generally localized soft-tissue sarcomas are best treated by wide local excision where this does not interfere with growth or function and is not of itself mutilating. Limited surgical resection (debulking) may be the only appropriate option when complete excision is not possible or mutilating. Complete clearance can be planned after chemotherapy (see below) has reduced the tumor to a more manageable dimension.

If complete surgical excision is considered possible and nonmutilating, then representative nodal sampling should also be performed to facilitate complete surgical staging. This is also important since histological appearances may not always correlate with biological behavior. Primary excision should aim to achieve negative clear margins both clinically and histologically, and residual margins indicate the need for re-excision or adjuvant therapy in RMS but not always in CIFS. A reasonable margin of 2 cm in an en bloc excision is adequate to ensure that capsular invasion does not compromise the completeness of the surgical margin. On occasions, frozen section can help confirm negative margins or direct further excision.

CHEMOTHERAPY

The sensitivity of the young patient to the potential side effects of chemotherapy is well documented and indicates the need for treatment in a pediatric oncology center. In general, neoadjuvant therapy is indicated when the tumor is unresectable and where such an approach would interfere with function and would of itself be mutilating. Experience has shown that the majority of initially inoperable tumors are rendered operable by such therapy. Furthermore, over a third of patients treated with neoadjuvant chemotherapy for inoperable CIFS sustain a complete response with no clinical or radiological evidence of disease and do not require further surgery.

Clearly, anthracyclines and alkylating agents are associated with a significant risk of cardiac and gonadal/mutagenic complications, respectively, in the very young patient. The combination of vincristine and actinomycin D (VA regimen), while not without its own potential complications, is as effective as VAC (added cyclophosphamide), and evidence suggests that this is the safest and most effective regime in the young patient with IFS. Three-year event-free survival in the European Pediatric Soft Tissue Sarcoma Study group is currently 84%, with an overall survival of 94% over a mean follow-up of 4.7 years.

SPECIFIC TUMORS

Infantile fibrosarcoma (CIFS)

There are two main types of fibrosarcoma that share similar histological appearances but different clinical behavior: congenital and adult types (Figure 92.2).

CIFS is a well-recognized tumor with a very low tendency to metastasize. CIFS is the commonest soft-part sarcoma in children under 1 year of age and as such is regarded as of intermediate malignancy. Presentation is usually as a mass and initial rapid growth. It is more common on the extremities and in males, and is commonly an antenatal diagnosis. Although metastatic spread is uncommon, local recurrence may occur in as many as 45% following attempts at curative excision/resection. It is generally a chemosensitive tumor, but surgery remains the mainstay of treatment. The relative frequency of local recurrence and occasional advanced disease has often warranted more radical initial surgery or considerations for neoadjuvant chemotherapy. Microscopic disease after surgery does not always indicate the need for further therapy, and a watch-and-wait policy is generally the first therapeutic option.

The adult type generally occurs in older children and is indistinguishable from the CIFS type but is differentiated by its clinical behavior.

Rhabdomyosarcoma

RMS is an extremely rare tumor in the neonatal period, and of 3217 patients reported by the Intergroup Rhabdomyosarcoma Study, only 14 were in this age group. Arising from mesenchymal tissue, it has a strong tendency toward myogenesis and can spread to nodes, lung, and liver. It is associated with the Li–Fraumeni syndrome and type 1 neurofibromatosis (Figure 92.3).

There are two main histological subtypes: embryonal and alveolar with distinct clinical outcomes and chromosomal

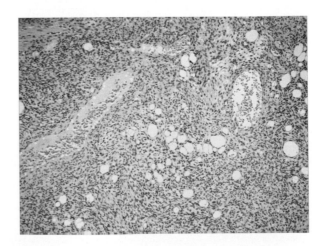

Figure 92.2 Congenital fibrosarcoma. Spindle cell proliferation infiltrating fat (adipocytes are the white blob-like cells) showing "blood lakes" characteristic of this entity.

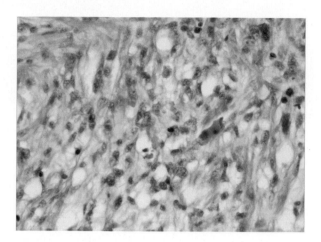

Figure 92.3 Embryonal rhabdomyosarcoma. Spindle cell sarcoma with elongated strap-like cytoplasmic processes and hyperchromatic nuclei showing considerable pleomorphism. The intensely eosinophilic cytoplasm is characteristic of skeletal muscular differentiation.

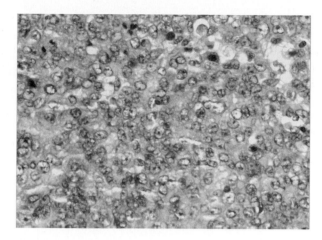

Figure 92.4 Rhabdoid sarcoma. The tumor cells are round with abundant eosinophilic cytoplasm and contain large, vesicular nuclei with prominent micronucleoli. Multiple mitotic figures are evident in the field imaged. The cytoplasm classically shows condensation of intermediate filaments, as seen here, which produces the "rhabdoid" phenotype.

translocations. Embryonal sarcoma is associated with the allelic loss of the 11p15 region and is marked histologically by degrees of myogenic differentiation that express desmin and muscle-specific actin. However, the most specific immunohistochemical markers are MyoD, Myogenin, and Vimentin.

While RMS can occur at any site, they are most common in the head and neck and genitourinary areas. Approximately 50% of RMS arises in the bladder, vagina, testicular (paratesticular), and sacrococcygeal sites, and 50% have already metastasized at presentation. Prognosis depends on histology, stage, and also site as head and neck presentations have better than 90% survival. Survival in neonates is approximately 50% with necrosis and small round cell configuration associated with a poor prognosis.

Treatment is aimed at complete surgical resection, and this may also include neoadjuvant and adjuvant chemotherapy, the latter indicated even if macroscopic clearance has been achieved. Radiotherapy is reserved for loss of local control.

Aggressive surgical management is not indicated in the presence of nonsterilized metastasis or if such an approach was extremely mutilating or associated with significant functional morbidity.

Non-rhabdomyosarcoma soft-tissue sarcoma

These comprise an extremely rare group of neonatal sarcomas such as malignant mesenchymal sarcoma, primitive sarcoma, angiosarcoma, and rhabdoid sarcoma. They tend to arise on the trunk, extremities, and head and neck area, and as such may be confused with IFS and RMS. Presenting as a painless mass, they exhibit marked clinical, histological, and biological heterogeneity (Figure 92.4).

Their management parallels that of both IFS and RMS with a need for accurate histology and planned treatment.

Wide local excision is usually sufficient as less than 10% have metastatic disease at presentation. The response to chemotherapy is less predictable, and consideration may have to be given to radiotherapy.

SUMMARY

Soft-tissue sarcoma is a rare tumor in childhood and infancy, and its management is made complex by the lack of consistency between histology and clinical behavior. Management must be tailored to the individual patient and on the basis of consensus discussion at an MDT Tumour Board. It is important to differentiate rhabdomyosarcoma from congenital infantile fibrosarcoma. In general, the aim is curative excision, but where this is not possible or considered mutilating (functionally or anatomically), then neoadjuvant chemotherapy with vincristine and actinomycin D (avoiding cyclophosphamide) is offered. Residual tumor is excised, but complete clinical and radiological remission (CIFS) can be observed without surgery. Microscopic CIFS after surgery may be observed, but RMS must be treated further. Very young patients may also be closely observed, since as many as 35% of IFS may undergo spontaneous resolution. The rarity of this tumor and the complexity of management indicate the need for multicenter prospective database and collaboration.

FURTHER READING

Blocker S, Koenig J, Ternberg, Congenital fibrosarcoma. *J Pediatric Surg* 1987; 22:665–70.

Corbally M. Soft tissue sarcoma. In: *Newborn Surgery*, 3rd edn. London: Hodder Arnold, 2013:Ch 85, 781–3.

Czernin J, Allen-Auerbach M, Schelbert HR. Improvements in cancer staging with PET/CT: Literature based evidence as of 2006. *J Nucl Med* Jan 2007; 48(1):78–88s.

Lobe TE, Wiener ES, Hays DM, Lawrence WH, Andrassy RJ, Johnston J et al. Neonatal rhabdomyosarcoma: The IRS experience. *J Pediatr Surg* 1994; 29:1167–70.

Madden NP, Spicer RD, Allibone EB, Lewis IJ. Spontaneous regression of neonatal fibrosarcoma. *Br J Cancer Suppl* 1992; 18:S72–5.

McCarville MB, Christie R, Daw NC, Spunt SL, Kaste SC. PET/CT in the evaluation of childhood sarcomas. *Am J Roentgenol* 2005; 184(4):1293–304.

Orbach D, Brennan B, De Paoli A, Gallego S, Mudry P, Francotte N et al. Conservative strategy in infantile fibrosarcoma is possible: The European paediatric soft tissue sarcoma study group experience. *Eur J Cancer* 2016; 57:1–9.

Reaman GH, Bleyer A. Infants and adolescents with cancer: Special consideration. In: Pizzo PA, Poplack DG (eds). *Principles and Practice of Paediatric Oncology*, 4th edn. Philadelphia, PA: Lippincott, 2002:409–28.

93

Hepatic tumors

BENJAMIN A. FARBER, WILLIAM J. HAMMOND, AND MICHAEL P. LA QUAGLIA

INTRODUCTION

Benign and malignant liver tumors in infants comprise 4%–5% of all neoplasms in the fetus and neonate, and are being detected perinatally with increasing frequency through ultrasound.[1,2] The spectrum of these pathological masses in newborns and infants is different from that found in older children (see Table 93.1). With advances in the understanding of the biology of these tumors over the past decades, approach to their treatment has also evolved. While most hepatic tumors are metastatic rather than primary, this chapter aims to describe the current and evolving approaches to the management of the most common benign and malignant primary liver tumors occurring in newborns (see Figure 93.1).

BENIGN LIVER TUMORS

Hepatic infantile hemangiomas

Hepatic vascular tumors are the most common benign pediatric tumor, affecting 4%–5% of white infants.[3] The true incidence is likely higher, as a large percentage of these lesions are asymptomatic and usually detected incidentally. The term hemangioma has often been indiscriminately used for vascular lesions. Generally speaking, there are two types of hemangiomas: infantile and congenital.

Infantile hemangiomas (IHs) are benign endothelial cell neoplasms characterized by proliferation of normal or abnormal blood vessels. While most infantile and congenital hemangiomas are cutaneous, liver lesions are fairly common.[4] Both visceral and cutaneous hemangiomas exhibit similar biologic behavior. Despite a landmark paper by Mulliken and Glowacki[5] that grouped vascular birthmarks into two major categories—hemangiomas and malformations—clinicians and pathologists do not agree about the descriptions of vascular lesions in the liver, using the term IH interchangeably and inclusively for true hemangiomas, arteriovenous malformations, and hemangioendothelioma.

TUMOR BIOLOGY

IHs are associated with white race, female gender, prematurity, low birth weight, and multiple gestations. The exact pathogenesis of IH remains unknown. It is thought to arise from a defect in endothelial or progenitor cells. The classification is made based on their depth of soft tissue involvement: superficial, deep, and mixed. Typically, superficial defects appear 1–4 weeks after birth, and deep lesions tend to develop between 2 and 3 months of age. There is additional differentiation for hepatic hemangiomas (HHs) and with regard to focal, multifocal, or diffuse forms of the disease. Most HHs are clinically insignificant and involute entirely without alteration of the hepatic parenchyma.

It is believed that HHs are the equivalent counterpart to rapidly involuting congenital hemangiomas (RICHs) and that they are fully formed at birth and involute faster than typical IHs. HHs can be detected on prenatal imaging, and there may be transient anemia and thrombocytopenia, but these are self-limited phenomena. They characteristically have a rapid proliferation of capillaries in the first year of life (proliferative phase), followed by a gradual, inevitable regression of the tumor over 1 to 5 years (involuting phase) and continual improvement until resolution and replacement of the tumor with fibrofatty tissue (involuted phase). Histologically, in the proliferative phase, endothelial hyperplasia with incorporation of H-thymidine and large numbers of mast cells can be observed.[6] This phase is defined by a high expression of proliferating cell nuclear antigen, type IV collagenase, and vascular endothelial growth factor (VEGF). High expression of tissue inhibitor of metalloproteinase (TIMP-1), an inhibitor of new blood vessel formation, is found exclusively in the involuting phase.[7] In contrast, vascular malformations do not express any of these biological markers or show signs of spontaneous regression and, instead, continue to grow with the child.

Glucose transporter 1 (GLUT1) immunoreactivity is found in IHs and distinguishes them from other subgroups of solitary liver hemangiomas, such as RICH, partially involuting congenital hemangiomas (PICHs), and non-involuting congenital

Table 93.1 Primary pediatric liver tumors

Age group	Malignant	Benign
Infants, toddlers	Hepatoblastoma (43%)	Hemangioma (14%)
	Rhabdoid tumors (<1%)	Mesenchymal hamartoma (6%)
	Malignant germ cell tumors (<1%)	Teratoma (<1%)
School age/adolescents	HCC and transitional cell tumors (23%)	Hepatic adenomas (2%)
	Sarcomas (7%)	Focal nodular hyperplasia (2%)

Source: Reprinted from *Semin Pediatr Surg*, 15(1), von Schweinitz D. Management of liver tumors in childhood, 17–24. Copyright 2006, with permission from Elsevier.

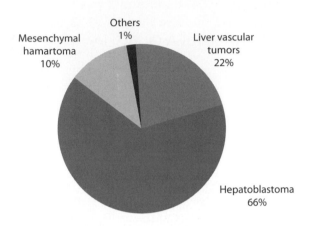

Figure 93.1 Distribution of neonatal liver tumors. (With kind permission from Springer Science+Business Media: *Semin Neonatol*, Neonatal liver tumors, 8, 2003, 403–10, von Schweinitz D.)

hemangiomas (NICHs). It is of note that vascular malformations do not express GLUT1.[8,9]

CLASSIFICATION

Hepatic IHs have been widely referred to as hemangioendotheliomas and divided into types 1 and 2. However, this term is misleading, as their behavior is different from epithelioid hemangioendotheliomas (with metastatic potential) and Kaposiform hemangioendotheliomas (KHEs; associated with the Kasabach–Merritt phenomenon [KMP][10]), both of which are true neoplasms that do not spontaneously regress.

The International Society for the Study of Vascular Anomalies (ISSVA) settled that cutaneous vascular tumors should be classified into two categories: hemangiomas (GLUT1-positive) and a heterogenous group of anomalies represented by vascular malformations (GLUT1-negative).[5,10] Drawing parallels from this, Mo et al.[9] have suggested two groups for hepatic vascular tumors: hepatic IHs (GLUT1-positive and typically multiple, but may be focal) and hepatic vascular malformations with capillary proliferation (GLUT1-negative, solitary masses).

Christison-Lagay et al.[3] and Dickie et al.[11] have proposed classifying hemangiomas based on imaging characteristics. Three types of lesions have been described: focal, multifocal, and diffuse (see Figure 93.2a–c). Focal lesions are solitary and are usually GLUT1-negative. Multifocal lesions are discrete hypodense lesions with intervening normal hepatic parenchyma. Diffuse HHs present with extensive hepatic involvement and near-total replacement of the hepatic parenchyma with innumerable lesions. Both multifocal and diffuse lesions are GLUT1-positive. Some authors have proposed that a subgroup of GLUT1-indeterminate or negative solitary hepatic vascular tumors may exhibit behavior and immunohistochemical characteristics similar to those of the RICH.[3,12,13] Table 93.2 presents the currently accepted ISSVA classification for vascular anomalies.

CLINICAL PRESENTATION

Multifocal and diffuse HHs are true IHs both by histopathology and natural history. There is a spectrum of disease with multifocal HHs randomly distributed among otherwise normal liver parenchyma and diffuse HHs exhibiting near-total liver parenchyma replacement. The diagnosis is often made while screening for visceral hemangioma based upon finding of multiple cutaneous IHs. Massive hepatomegaly from multifocal HHs can result in abdominal compartment syndrome and respiratory failure. All HHs express type III iodothyronine deiodinase and can inactivate thyroid hormone giving rise to profound hypothyroidism, resulting in exacerbation of cardiac failure and cognitive delay.

Clinical presentations of the various lesions described above overlap considerably. Infantile HHs are frequently associated with cutaneous hemangiomas, the incidence of liver lesions being higher with multiple or large skin lesions.[4] Most liver hemangiomas may be clinically silent and escape detection. Some, however, remain asymptomatic and are discovered on routine prenatal or postnatal imaging performed for unrelated reasons. The most common presenting features are an abdominal mass, hepatomegaly, and anemia. Patients with large tumors can be critically ill at presentation with congestive heart failure (CHF), inferior vena cava compression, respiratory distress, and even abdominal compartment syndrome and multiorgan failure. Hypothyroidism, which may be present due to type III iodothyronine deiodinase activity by the liver hemangioma, may contribute to the CHF. It is more common in the diffuse type, but has been noted in multifocal and large solitary hemangiomas. Screening with thyroid function tests at presentation is, therefore, advisable. Rarely, hemorrhagic shock with or without disseminated intravascular coagulation may follow a rupture of the lesion. Rupture can be precipitated by percutaneous needle biopsy.

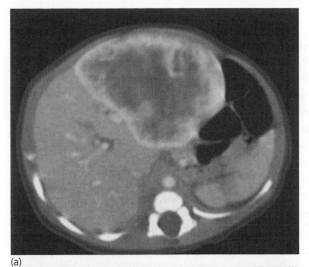

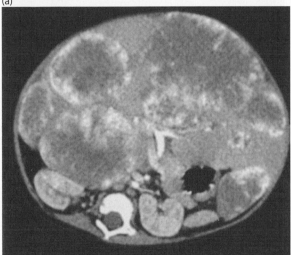

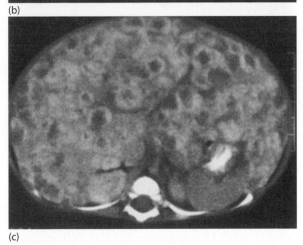

Figure 93.2 **(a)** Solitary infantile HH. **(b)** Multifocal hepatic infantile hemangioma. **(c)** Diffuse infantile HH. (Reprinted from *Surg Oncol*, 16, Meyers RL, Tumors of the liver in children, 195–203, Copyright 2007, with permission from Elsevier.)

INVESTIGATIONS

No serum marker is clinically useful for diagnosis, though elevations in alpha-fetoprotein (AFP) have been reported.[14–16]

These elevations are usually mild and call into question the importance of differentiating larger lesions from hepatoblastoma (HB).

Hepatic IHs are generally diagnosed using computed tomography (CT) and magnetic resonance imaging (MRI) with contrast enhancement. These lesions are hypodense on CT scanning with centripetal (outside-in) enhancement. On MRI, they are hypointense on T1 and hyperintense on T2-weighted sequences. Imaging criteria used in the diagnosis include nodular peripheral enhancement followed by centripetal fill-in, change to isodensity on CT, or isointensity on MRI with the blood vessels and a complete fill-in in the late phase on contrast-enhanced images.

Contrast-enhanced ultrasonography (CEUS) is being increasingly used as the first-line imaging modality in the characterization of liver lesions.[17,18] The nodular peripheral enhancement expanding centrally is also seen with CEUS. This may offer a diagnostic advantage over CT and MRI in view of the low rate of adverse reactions from the microbubble contrast, allowing for multiple injections and assessments and its use in patients with decreased renal function.[18–20]

Angiography has been declining as a diagnostic modality in vascular anomalies of the liver. Endovascular modalities are now used to outline the vasculature of tumors in a subgroup of infants who present with high-output cardiac failure for whom a high-flow shunt amenable to embolization is suspected.

Hepatic IHs must be distinguished from epithelioid hemangioendothelioma, an intermediate-grade neoplasm that has the potential to metastasize. This is a tumor seen mostly in adults and rarely in older children.[21–23] It has not been reported in newborns. It consists of multifocal and confluent masses of homogenous liver nodules with peripheral enhancement. Treatment usually involves liver resection or transplantation.

MANAGEMENT

Asymptomatic focal lesions do not need treatment and may be followed with serial ultrasound examinations until resolution. This can be every 1 to 2 months until the lesion is stable, after which scans can be performed two to three times a year until involution is demonstrated. If there are signs of asymptomatic shunts, a closer follow-up schedule can be implemented. Multifocal lesions have a similar natural history to that of focal lesions and can be similarly observed. Propranolol is the pharmacologic treatment of choice for symptomatic multifocal and diffuse HH with cardiac failure, abdominal distention, or hypothyroidism. The mechanism of propranolol is to hasten tumor involution, reducing cardiac failure and hypothyroidism. Embolization may be required for lesions with large arteriovenous shunts resulting in heart failure. Infants with HH should be followed with serial abdominal imaging until the hemangioma has involuted. If the diagnosis is unclear, a percutaneous needle biopsy may be necessary to rule out malignancy.[24] Diffuse liver lesions are the most difficult subgroup to manage. In addition to the above, an early consultation with the transplant team should be considered for patients whose disease progresses despite medical management.

Table 93.2 2014 ISSVA classification of vascular anomalies

Vascular tumors	Vascular malformations
Benign vascular tumors	*Simple vascular malformations*
Infantile hemangioma	Capillary malformations
Congenital hemangioma (RICH, NICH, and PICH)	Lymphatic malformations
Tufted angioma	Venous malformations
Spindle-cell hemangioma	Arteriovenous malformations
Epithelioid hemangioma	Arteriovenous fistula (congenital)
Pyogenic granuloma (lobular capillary hemangioma)	
Others	*Combined vascular malformations*
	Capillary–venous malformation (CVM)
Locally aggressive or borderline vascular tumors	Capillary–lymphatic malformation (CLM)
Kaposiform hemangioendothelioma	Capillary–arteriovenous malformation (CAVM)
Retiform hemangioendothelioma	Lymphatic–venous malformation (LVM)
Papillary intralymphatic angioendothelioma (PILA), Dabska tumor	Capillary–lymphatic–venous malformation (CLVM)
Composite hemangioendothelioma	Capillary–lymphatic–arteriovenous malformation (CLAVM)
Kaposi sarcoma	Capillary–venous–arteriovenous malformation (CVAVM)
Others	Capillary–lymphatic–venous–arteriovenous malformation (CLVAVM)
Malignant vascular tumors	
Angiosarcoma	
Epithelioid hemangioendothelioma	
Others	

Source: Adapted from: ISSVA Classification of Vascular Anomalies, Copyright 2014 International Society for the Study of Vascular Anomalies (http://www.issva.org). Available at https://issva.clubexpress.com/docs.ashx?id=178348. Accessed March 2016. ISSVA classification for Vascular Anomalies by International Society for the Study of Vascular Anomalies is licensed under a Creative Commons Attribution 4.0 International License.

Note: AV = arteriovenous; C = capillary; L = lymphatic; M = malformation; NICH = non-involuting congenital hemangioma; PICH = partially involuting congenital hemangioma; RICH = rapidly involuting congenital hemangioma; V = venous.

CORTICOSTEROIDS

Glucocorticoids at varying doses have been used for many decades as the first line of treatment for cutaneous hemangiomas and HHs. A possible mechanism is the negative effect of steroids on angiogenesis. Administration of 2–5 mg/kg of oral prednisolone or an intravenous equivalent is commenced for patients with hemodynamically significant shunts or signs of CHF. Response rates in the literature vary, with good responses ranging from 30% to 75% for multifocal and diffuse disease.[3,25] Steroids may also be indicated for coexisting cutaneous lesions that may threaten vision (e.g., eyelids) or be life-threatening (e.g., paratracheal or pharyngeal lesions). Lesions have been reported to stabilize between 2 and 4 months. The duration of therapy is guided by serial imaging and generally ranges from 5 to 8 months.[3,11,25]

CHEMOTHERAPEUTIC AGENTS

Interferon alpha has been used in corticosteroid unresponsive cases with promising results. In a report by Ezekowitz et al., liver hemangiomas regressed by 50% or more in 18 of 20 patients receiving interferon alpha-2a (up to 3 million units per square meter BSA) after an average of 7.8 months with no long-term adverse effects. However, its use has been guarded since 6.1% of children younger than 1 year experienced spastic diplegia and motor developmental disturbances after receiving interferon.[26,27]

Vincristine is a mitotic inhibitor that blocks the formation of tubulin microfibrils and arrests mitosis in the metaphase. It has been used in steroid-resistant, life-threatening hemangiomas at a dose of 1–2 mg/m². The high content of tubulin in the endothelial cells of hemangiomas makes this tumor particularly sensitive to vincristine.[28,29]

ENDOVASCULAR INTERVENTIONS

Use of angiography and embolization of arteriovenous shunts, though not curative, can provide major symptomatic relief from the hemodynamic effects of high-flow shunts in hemangiomas. Hemangiomas can derive collaterals from any of the hepatic, phrenic, intercostal, superior mesenteric, or adrenal arteries. It has been indicated primarily for CHF refractory to medical management, steroids, or additional chemotherapy. It has also been employed to shrink large hemangiomas symptomatic by the mass effect causing caval compression or abdominal compartment syndrome. An angiographic classification has been proposed based on the number of lesions; flow characteristics (high vs low); presence; type of shunt (arteriovenous, arterioportal, or portovenous); and major anomalies of hepatic vessels (particularly venous varices).[30] The best response to embolization is found in patients with macroscopically visible shunts on angiography associated with single or multifocal lesions. Hemangiomas with extensive portal venous supply are more difficult to treat and may require multiple embolizations.[30] There is a risk of fatal hepatic necrosis after hepatic arterial embolization. The expertise required to perform and interpret angiography in this group of infants is generally found only in highly specialized referral centers.

SURGERY

Liver resections for hemangiomas have declined with better understanding of the biologic behavior of these tumors, improvements in pharmacotherapy, advances in endovascular techniques, and better pediatric intensive care. Reports have argued for surgery to be a last recourse after pharmacotherapy for the tumor, medical management of CHF, and endovascular interventions have all failed to achieve symptomatic control and tumor regression.[11,30,31] Kassarjian et al.[30] reported a series of 15 patients managed with endovascular interventions with one death in a patient who had diffuse liver hemangioma, severe CHF, and hypothyroidism. Dickie et al.[11] reported a series of 16 patients with no mortality and only 2 patients who required surgery (a left lobectomy and an orthotopic liver transplant). In contrast, Moon et al. have employed hepatic resection as a primary treatment modality for solitary, resectable, and symptomatic lesions. They used hepatic artery embolization as a second line of treatment, with one death from postoperative hemorrhage among nine patients who underwent surgery. Surgery and open biopsy are also indicated when a distinction cannot be made between a HB and a hemangioma.[25]

LIVER TRANSPLANTATION

A small number of patients with diffuse hepatic lesions replacing most of the hepatic parenchyma develop life-threatening complications including CHF, consumptive coagulopathy, abdominal compartment syndrome, and multiorgan failure. Because these patients may be those most likely to benefit from liver transplantation, early involvement of the transplant team has been advocated if there is a poor response to initial pharmacotherapy.[3] Embolization, even in the context of diffuse lesions, has been shown to prevent transplant.[31] The outcome following transplant is varied, though some authors report good outcomes.[32-34]

FUTURE DIRECTIONS

The classification and treatment of hepatic IHs will continue to evolve. Prospective characterization of patients will further the understanding of these uncommon tumors. While there is reasonable concordance about classification of GLUT1-positive multifocal or diffuse liver lesions, there remains discord in the biologic, clinical, and radiologic characterization of certain solitary liver vascular tumors. The Children's Hospital of Boston has proposed and created an Internet-based registry for longitudinal accrual of patients with liver hemangiomas.[3]

Antiangiogenic drugs show potential in the treatment of liver hemangiomas. Bevacizumab, a recombinant monoclonal antibody against VEGF, was incidentally found to reduce the size of liver lesions significantly in a patient with colorectal adenocarcinoma initially suspected to be metastasis, but later found on biopsy to be hemangiomas.[35] A similarly dramatic response was seen in a 41-year-old patient with pulmonary epithelioid hemangioendothelioma.[36]

Mesenchymal hamartoma of the liver

Mesenchymal hamartoma of the liver (MHL) is the second most common benign liver tumor in children after hemangiomas, and typically presents as a large benign multicystic liver mass.[37] MHL has been reported in the literature to compose 6%–8% of benign pediatric liver tumors.[38-41] Median age of diagnosis is 10 months, with 80% of cases diagnosed by 2 years of age and 95% by 5 years.[40,41] Rarely, this disease can be detected in adults,[42] and the tumor is reported to have a slight male predominance.[37,40,41,43] Historically, it was described under multiple names including pseudocystic mesenchymal tumor, giant cell lymphangioma, cystic hamartoma, bile cell fibroadenoma, hamartoma, and cavernous lymphangiomatoid tumor.[44] The understanding of the biology of this tumor has evolved greatly since it was definitively described in 1956 by Edmondson.[45] Mesenchymal hamartoma must be distinguished from other congenital and infective cystic diseases, hemangiomas, and other liver tumors.

PATHOLOGY AND PATHOGENESIS

The right hepatic lobe is affected more frequently than the left (3:1), and the mass can sometimes be pedunculated.[46] A small proportion of cases may involve both lobes.[1,37] Mesenchymal hamartomas usually contain both cystic and solid components, the proportion of which varies. About 50% are multicystic, with the intervening myxoid stroma containing fibroblasts, blood vessels and lymphatics, collagen, bile ductules, and islands of hepatocytes. Less commonly, the cysts can be very small and sometimes absent, resulting in a predominantly solid tumor.[40,47] The cystic spaces are filled with a clear or mucoid liquid and may or may not be lined by epithelium, the latter seen more often in larger cysts. Tumors can be very large, up to 30 cm in diameter and weighing up to 3 kg. Over 85% of tumors in the case series reported by Kim et al.[47] were larger than 10 cm at diagnosis. Mesenchymal hamartomas are usually well circumscribed and are surrounded by a rim of compressed hepatic parenchyma but are devoid of a true capsule.[37] There have been a few reports of multifocal MHL. Small satellite lesions at the margins of the tumor have been described and may explain recurrent disease after excision of the main tumor.[48]

The pathogenesis of this tumor is not clearly defined. The three leading theories are as follows: (1) abnormal embryologic development of the mesenchyme, producing obstruction of the biliary tree as it develops, causing cystic, anaplastic, and proliferating bile ducts with most of the proliferative growth just before or after birth, since no mesenchymal mitotic activity is seen histologically[40]; (2) abnormal development of the vascular supply with ischemic necrosis and reactive cystic changes[49]; and (3) abnormal proliferation of the embryologic hepatic mesenchyme with elevated expression of fibroblast growth factor-2 (FGF-2).[50] There are associations with congenital heart disease, gut malrotation, omphalocele, myelomeningocele, Beckwith–Wiedemann syndrome, and breakpoint abnormalities on chromosome 19 (bands 19q13.3 or 19q13.4).[37,51–53]

Some have argued that MHL may be true neoplasms. The histopathologic and immunohistochemical similarities between undifferentiated embryonal sarcoma (UES) of the liver and mesenchymal hamartoma can be striking. It has been postulated that UES—with its onset in older children, benign bile ductular elements within a malignant mesenchyme, its predisposition to the right lobe, and occasional pedunculation—may be preceded by a mesenchymal hamartoma.[54,55] Several reports describe cases of UES arising within a previous MHL, two of which occurred after incomplete excision. Aneuploidy has been detected by flow cytometry in two of eight mesenchymal hamartomas in one study.[55] Cytogenetic abnormalities involving the same breakpoint on chromosome 19 (band 19q13.4) now have been reported in nine cases, three of which involved a UES originating within an MHL.[51,56–58] These karyotypic and cytogenetic abnormalities in at least some MHLs may indicate a clonal defect.

CLINICAL PRESENTATION

Mesenchymal hamartomas present most commonly as abdominal distention or an upper abdominal mass. Large tumors can cause respiratory distress or compression of the inferior vena cava with distended superficial abdominal veins or lower limb edema. Abdominal pain is unusual in children but more common in adults. Examination reveals a large, smooth, nontender mass in the upper abdomen. The tumor can be detected on prenatal ultrasound and may cause fetal hydrops, polyhydramnios, and fetal demise.[59,60] Case reports of MHL describe presentation with obstructive jaundice, vascular steal phenomenon, high-output cardiac failure, and perinatal tumor rupture in the newborn.

INVESTIGATIONS

Liver function tests are usually normal. Serum AFP concentrations may be variably elevated confounding the differential with HB. Levels return to normal after tumor removal, but may take up to a year due to liver regeneration. Thus, MHL should be distinguished from HB and may require biopsy.

A CT or ultrasound examination is diagnostic in most patients. The typical finding of a multiseptated cystic tumor with distinct margins is rarely seen in other pediatric tumors and is diagnostic of a mesenchymal hamartoma. The cystic areas appear hypodense and hypovascular on imaging. Solid areas (within mixed solid-cystic or predominantly solid tumors), septae, and peripheral areas may show heterogenous

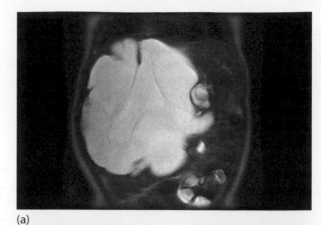

(a)

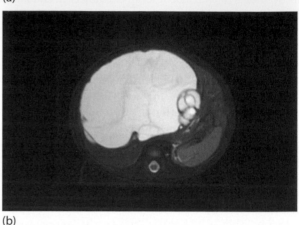

(b)

Figure 93.3 **(a)** Axial and **(b)** coronal views of the T2-weighted MRI of a large mesenchymal hamartoma showing a multiseptate cystic tumor. The patient underwent enucleation of the tumor.

enhancement after intravenous contrast on CT.[47,61] The differential diagnosis in totally solid tumors in newborns and infants should include various hepatic tumors such as HB, hepatocellular carcinoma (HCC), and hemangiomas.

On MRI, lesions typically have a low intensity on T1-weighted sequences, but have variable signal intensity on T2-weighted sequences. Where diagnosis is in doubt, the pathology is usually confirmed after resection of the tumor or by an open or percutaneous tumor biopsy (see Figure 93.3a and b).

TREATMENT

Management of MHL remains controversial. While spontaneous regression has been described, there is a lack of long-term follow-up and the safety of this approach cannot be determined. In the past, recommendations were made for nonradical resection, but there have been reports of late recurrence.[62–64] Flow cytometry studies have revealed that some MHLs are aneuploid, a finding typically observed in malignant tumors. As many controversies exist regarding the histogenetic origin of MHL and UES in addition to findings of chromosomal translocation, aneuploidy, and reports of coexistent MHL and UES, the disease is best treated by complete tumor resection, either non-anatomically with a rim of normal tissue or as an anatomic hepatic lobectomy.[37,62,65,66] While the tumors themselves are not very vascular, the surrounding compressed hepatic parenchyma can be very vascular.

In the very rare case, a liver transplantation may be an option for the recurrent or unresectable MHL. The United Network for Organ Sharing (UNOS) group reported two cases of transplants performed in children who had progressive liver failure after resection of MHL, one of whom died from postoperative bleeding. A third case was reported of a newborn girl who developed a diffuse hemangioma of the liver remnant 4 months after a resection for MHL.[23,67,68]

Kaposiform hemangioendothelioma

KHE is a relatively uncommon vascular tumor often associated with KMP. The hallmark features of KMP include an enlarging vascular lesion, microangiopathic hemolytic anemia, thrombocytopenia, and a consumptive coagulopathy that results in a life-threatening hemorrhage.[24] KHE may occur in the extremities, cervicofacial, thoracic, or retroperitoneal locations. Retroperitoneal tumors have been found to extend to involve the liver, porta hepatis, pancreas, and mesentery. Mortality may be as high as 60% for those tumors that involve the retroperitoneum.[69] In regards to nomenclature, it is generally accepted that tufted angioma and KHE exist on a spectrum and are synonymous tumors.[24]

PATHOLOGY AND PATHOGENESIS

On histology, there are sheets or lobules of spindled endothelial cells and dilated lymphatic channels that show aggressive infiltration of normal tissue. Vascular lumens are filled with erythrocytes and hemosiderin suggestive of stasis. In contrast to the endothelial cells in IH, the endothelial cells in KHE do not express GLUT-1.

CLINICAL PRESENTATION

KHEs typically present as solitary lesions at birth or early infancy with equal gender ratio. Most cases of KHE have a classic presentation of a solitary ill-defined plaque that is tense, edematous, violaceous, and warm to palpation. The lesions are often large (>5 cm) and have episodic engorgement. The associated thrombocytopenia in KMP can be profound (<50 × 10⁹/mL) as the platelets are sequestered within the tumor resulting in a platelet half-life of 1 to 24 hours. As a result, patients can be at risk of intracranial, pleural, pulmonary, peritoneal, and GI hemorrhages.[24]

INVESTIGATIONS

The imaging modality of choice for the disease is MRI with and without gadolinium. In MRI, the tumor will have enhanced T2-weighted images. Other defining characteristics include an ill-defined and infiltrative tumor penetrating multiple contiguous layers. Osteolysis may be present when KHE abuts bone. The tumor has small feeding and draining vessels relative to tumor size, and the thickening and edema of the skin will appear as stranding in the subcutaneous fat.

TREATMENT

KHE may regress with time, but a complete involution is infrequent. Areas that do undergo involution often appear as fibrotic and firm capillary malformation. The treatment for KHE with KMP is primarily medical as the tumor is often too extensive or the risk of severe bleeding is too high to be amenable for surgical resection. Successful treatment of retroperitoneal KHE with alpha-interferon has been reported, but for tumor refractory to this treatment, success has been reported with vincristine, combined with cyclophosphamide, actinomycin D, and methotrexate.[70]

In general, platelet transfusions are not advised unless there is active bleeding or in a perioperative context as the administration of platelets may actually promote tumor growth through intralesional clotting and the release of proangiogenic proteins. Heparinization is not indicated because of bleeding risk and minimal platelet effects. Should the patient develop hypofibrinogenemia (<100 mg/dL), fresh frozen plasma or cryoprecipitate can be administered.

Focal nodular hyperplasia

The diagnosis of focal nodular hyperplasia (FNH) has been reported for all ages, from newborns to the elderly. It is an infrequent diagnosis in newborns and has been reported in association with other hepatic lesions of both benign and malignant categories. FNH is a benign epithelial tumor referred to in literature under many names including benign hepatoma, solitary hyperplastic nodule, focal cirrhosis, cholangiohepatoma, and mixed adenoma.[71] Similar to other benign tumors, smaller lesions may be asymptomatic, whereas larger lesions may exert mass effect and present with symptoms such as abdominal pain. The most widely accepted theory is that FNH results from vascular abnormalities that are either acquired or congenital.[72] FNH is a well-circumscribed lobulated lesion composed of bile ducts and a central stellate scar, which contains blood vessels that supply the hyperplastic tissue. The tumor does not have a true capsule but is often surrounded by fibrous tissue. On microscopic analysis, the proliferating cells are practically identical to the surrounding hepatocytes.

FNH is suggested by ultrasound findings of a well-demarcated, homogenous mass that is hyperechoic. The mass is more appropriately imaged with CT or MR angiography. The tumors typically have normal accumulation of ⁹⁹ᵐTc sulfur colloid on liver scintigraphy. Although the central stellate scar is a characteristic finding, the radiographic appearance of FNH can be variable. Gadoxetic acid (EOVIST) enhanced MRI has emerged as an additional modality for differentiating FNH from hepatic adenoma.[73] Spontaneous regression of FNH is rare, and complete surgical resection of biopsy-proven FNH is not mandatory in an asymptomatic patient. In symptomatic patients, where biopsy is nondiagnostic, or patients in whom the diagnosis of malignancy has not been definitively ruled out, surgical excision is required.

Hepatic adenoma

Hepatic adenoma is very rare in the newborn period and can be difficult to distinguish from other more common tumors in this age range, even with multimodal imaging. One series of 17,417 perinatal autopsies found only one hepatic adenoma.[74] In a single-center series of 178 primary hepatic tumors treated over a 57-year period, two cases of hepatic adenoma were noted.[75] One case report demonstrates the detection of a hepatic adenoma in utero during routine prenatal ultrasonography.[76] The majority of neonatal hepatic adenomas occur in a sporadic manner without a known predisposing factor. Imaging typically demonstrates hepatic adenomas as a solid mass. Multimodal imaging including ultrasonography, CT, ^{99m}Tc sulfur colloid liver scintigraphy, and MRI is found to be more helpful than a single modality alone. The appearance of a hepatic adenoma can be highly variable and nonspecific. The mass is usually hypoechoic on ultrasound but may be hyperechoic; the mass is not typically cystic. On noncontrast CT, the adenoma is likely hypodense. In contrast-aided studies, the arterial phase is usually homogeneous in enhancement and the portal phase is hypodense.[76] The MRI appearance can be variable and difficult to distinguish from HCC, HB, and focal nodular hyperplasia. The common pattern observed is mild signal hypointensity in the T1-weighted images and hyperintensity in the T2-weighted images.

TREATMENT

The potential risk of life-threatening hemorrhage from a hepatic adenoma is 20%. Subsequently, complete surgical resection is recommended when technically feasible. Transarterial embolization (TAE) is preferred in instances of tumor rupture and intraperitoneal hemorrhage with hemodynamic stability.[77] TAE has also been used to electively reduce tumor mass in unruptured hepatic adenomas with up to 80% of cases showing stability, regression, or complete involution.[78,79] Additional management includes close follow-up with serial liver imaging and AFP monitoring, as it may be difficult to rule out HB. The risk of malignant transformation for a hepatic adenoma remains controversial.[75] It is recommended that hepatic adenoma be considered in the differential diagnosis even when a cystic liver mass is suggested on a fetal ultrasound. Contemporary management has included percutaneous radiofrequency ablation as an additional modality for treatment.[80]

MALIGNANT LIVER TUMORS

Hepatoblastoma

EPIDEMIOLOGY

The age-adjusted incidence for primary liver cancer for the period 2008–2012, as published by the Surveillance

Table 93.3 Age-adjusted and age-specific SEER cancer incidence rates (per million), 2008–2012

Group	Age <1 year	Age 1–4 years	Age 5–9 years
Hepatic tumors	11.1	6.7	0.7
Hepatoblastoma	11.0	6.5	–

Source: Howlader N et al., (eds). SEER Cancer Statistics Review, 1975–2012. National Cancer Institute Bethesda, MD, http://seer.cancer.gov/csr/1975_2012/. Based on November 2014 SEER data submission, posted to the SEER website in April 2015. Accessed March 25, 2016.

Epidemiology and End Result (SEER) program of the National Cancer Institute, is 11.1 per million in the <1 year age group, 6.7 per million in the 1- to 4-year-old group, and 0.7 per million among children 5–9 years old. HB comprises the overwhelming majority of malignant primary liver tumors in these age groups (Table 93.3).[81] Incidence of HB appears relatively consistent between nations with most estimates of rates among children, showing no discernible differences between continents.[82] Five percent of all cancers and more than 95% of hepatic cancers in this age group are HBs. In the Pediatric Oncology Group series, 11% of HBs occurred in the first 6 months of life. Of these, 50% were congenital, as evinced by their size at the time of diagnosis, usually at the age of 2–3 months.[83] HBs accounted for 1% of all liver and bile duct tumors diagnosed in the United States between 2008 and 2012. The incidence of HB appears to be increasing at a rate of 1.2–1.5 per million per year, likely due to the increase in survival of premature low and very low birth weight infants, a factor that has been associated with HBs.[84–87]

HISTOLOGY

HB is an embryonal tumor thought to arise from a hepatocyte precursor and usually demonstrates combinations of epithelial, mesenchymal, undifferentiated, and other histological components. HBs are broadly classified as epithelial or mixed. Epithelial HBs consist of fetal (Figure 93.4a), embryonal, macrotrabecular, small-cell undifferentiated (Figure 93.4b), and cholangioblastic types. The mixed HBs consist of stromal derivatives and teratoid types (Table 93.4).[88] Given the histologic heterogeneity of HB, biopsy samples may not always represent the entire tumor. Among all cases, 85%–90% contain both fetal and embryonal cells, and 20% may have stromal components.[83,89]

Pure fetal histology is thought to be the most favorable type, with various studies demonstrating its better prognosis with survival rates reported near 100%.[90,91] The small-cell undifferentiated type is particularly aggressive, especially when present in a significant portion of the HB (75% or so) as the sole cell type. This histology is more common in neonates and infants. AFP elevations may not be observed as seen with other histologies.[92] It has a poor prognosis due to lack of response to current therapy. The

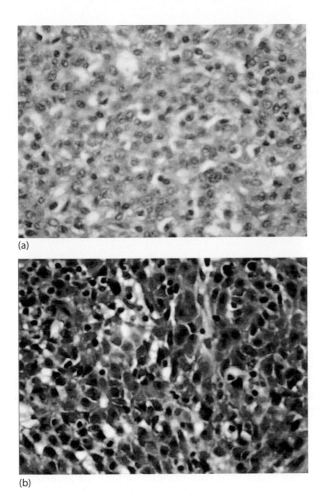

(a)

(b)

Figure 93.4 Histological subtypes of HBs. **(a)** Fetal type and **(b)** small-cell undifferentiated.

significance of smaller proportions of small cells is not yet known.

GENETIC CHANGES

Most HBs are sporadic; however, various genetic anomalies and syndromes are known to be associated with HB including low and very low birth weight, trisomy events, familial adenomatous polyposis (FAP), Gardner's syndrome, Beckwith–Weidemann syndrome, and hemihyperplasia.[93–96] The risk of HB rises 1000- to 2000-fold in children with this family history, and approximately 800-fold in those with a history of FAP.[97–101]

HB is tightly linked to excessive Wnt/β-catenin signaling. There is a high rate (50%–90%) of mutations found in *CTNNB1*, which encodes β-catenin, placing HB among the most common human tumors with constitutive activation of β-catenin/Tcf signaling.[102–104] *APC* gene (involved in degradation of β-catenin) mutations have been characterized regularly in kindred of FAP (risk of HB ~1%) but are not as commonly seen in sporadic HB. Loss-of-function somatic mutations of tumor suppressor genes *AXIN1* and *AXIN2* whose products affect the β-catenin degradation have also been reported in some HBs.[105]

Cairo et al.[106] reported two major molecular subclasses of HBs that evoke early and late phases of prenatal liver development. Using a 16-gene signature that correlated with the phase of liver development, they established a tight correlation between the stage of hepatic differentiation and clinical behavior—notably, vascular invasion, metastatic spread, and patient survival. This demonstrated strong prognostic relevance compared to clinical criteria (tumor stage and predominant histology) in multivariate analysis. Also, *Myc* overexpression has been shown to induce HB-like tumors in mice and plays a critical role in aggressive phenotype of liver tumors originating from hepatic progenitor cells.[105,106]

Other molecular mechanisms implicated in the growth of HBs include the overexpression of insulin-like growth factor-I[107,108] and downregulation of the tumor suppressor gene, *RASSF1A*, by promoter methylation.[109,110] Methylation of *RASSF1A* gene was an independent risk factor in multivariate analysis. Upregulation of the *MAPK* pathway has also been noted in aggressive HBs with a small-cell undifferentiated component.[111]

Cytogenetic analyses of HBs have shown recurring patterns of chromosomal abnormalities. The most common involve trisomies, particularly of chromosomes 2, 8, and 20, among others.[94] Numerical aberrations as well as unbalanced translocations involving the proximal region of chromosome 1q are characteristic of HB.[112] More specifically, bands 1q12-21 have been described as a location of recurring translocations in HB and were found in 20 of 55 patients in a series of HBs.[113] The *NOTCH2* gene, which encodes a transmembrane receptor critical to the development of the liver, also on chromosome 1, has been shown to have aberrant overexpression in 92% of HB cases, suggesting its role in HB pathogenesis by wrongly maintaining hepatoblast populations.[112,114]

CLINICAL FINDINGS

The majority of infants with HB present with an asymptomatic abdominal mass noticed incidentally by a relative or a pediatrician. An array of nonspecific symptoms, such as abdominal pain, pyrexia, irritability, weight loss, or gastrointestinal disturbances, may occur in a small percentage of patients, especially those with advanced disease. Clinical examination usually shows an expansile solitary mass in the liver. Thrombocytosis, with the platelet count ranging in the millions, is a well-known, albeit uncommon, feature of HB. Thrombopoietin production by the tumor has been proposed as possible cause of the thrombocytosis.[115,116] Hormone elevations that lead rarely to symptoms are due to human beta chorionic gonadotropin (β-hCG), testosterone, adrenocorticotrophic hormone, or parathormone-related peptide.[117,118]

AFP is markedly elevated in more than 90% of patients with HB, in whom it is used as a diagnostic tool and as a tumor marker to monitor therapeutic response; however, AFP elevations are not pathognomonic of disease. The half-life of AFP in the first month of life is between 5 and 6 days, increasing to approximately 42 days by 6 months of age.

Table 93.4 Classification of hepatoblastomas

Epithelial

Fetal	"Well differentiated": uniform (10–20 μm in diameter), round nuclei, cords with minimal mitotic activity (<2 per ×10/400 microscopic fields), EMH[a]
	"Crowded" or mitotically active (>2 per ×10/400 microscopic fields); conspicuous nuclei, less glycogen
	"Pleomorphic, or poorly differentiated": moderate anisonucleosis, high N/C, nucleoli
	"Anaplastic": marked nuclear enlargement and pleomorphism, hyperchromasia, abnormal mitoses
Embryonal	10–15 μm in diameter, high N/C, angulated nuclei, primitive tubules, EMH
Macrotrabecular	Epithelial HB (fetal or embryonal) growing in trabeculae of >5 cells thick (between sinusoids)
Small-cell undifferentiated	5–10 μm in diameter, no architectural pattern, minimal pale amphophilic cytoplasm, round to oval nuclei with fine chromatin and inconspicuous nucleoli, +/− mitoses; +/− INI1[b]
Cholangioblastic	Bile ducts, usually at periphery of epithelial islands, can predominate

Mixed

Stromal derivatives	Spindle cells ("blastema"), osteoid, skeletal muscle, cartilage
Teratoid	Mixed, plus primitive endoderm; neural derivative, melanin, squamous, and glandular elements

Source: Reprinted by permission from Macmillan Publishers Ltd. *Modern Pathology,* Lopez-Terrada D et al. Towards an international pediatric liver tumor consensus classification: Proceedings of the Los Angeles COG liver tumors symposium, 27:472–91, Copyright 2014.
[a] EMH = extramedullary hematopoiesis.
[b] Pure small-cell undifferentiated needs to be differentiated from MRTs (discohesive, eccentric irregular nuclei, prominent nucleoli, abundant cytoplasmic filaments including cytokeratin and vimentin, negative nuclear INI).

Levels in preterm babies (earlier than 37 weeks of gestation) are significantly higher with a negative correlation between gestational age and AFP levels.[119] AFP levels are usually less than 10 ng/mL by 1 year of age, though persistent elevations, especially in preterm babies without any known associated factors, have been observed (see Table 93.5).

Table 93.5 Average normal serum alpha-fetoprotein level in infants

Age	No. of patients analyzed	Mean ± SD (ng/mL)
Premature	11	134,734 ± 41,444
Newborn	55	48,406 ± 34,718
Newborn to 2 weeks	16	33,113 ± 32,503
2 weeks to 1 month	43	9452 ± 12,610
1 month	12	2654 ± 3080
2 months	40	323 ± 278
3 months	5	88 ± 87
4 months	31	74 ± 56
5 months	6	46.5 ± 19
6 months	9	12.5 ± 9.8
7 months	5	9.7 ± 7.1
8 months	3	8.5 ± 5.5

Source: Reprinted from Wu JT et al., *Pediatr Res* 1981; 15: 50–2. Copyright 1981 Wolters Kluwer Health. All rights reserved. Used with permission.

IMAGING

Quality imaging of patients with HB is crucial for proper staging and risk stratification so patients may receive optimal treatment. Three-phase abdominal CT (noncontrast, arterial, and venous phases) or MRI and magnetic resonance angiogram (MRA) with contrast can be performed at presentation, according to the local practice. MRI with EOVIST contrast (preferentially taken up and excreted by hepatocytes) is being used with increasing frequency.[120] A Doppler ultrasound (if an MRA has not been performed) will define any involvement of the portal or hepatic veins and inferior vena cava. It can be difficult to distinguish direct involvement of the veins from external compression.

CT of the chest (without contrast) and a anteroposterior (AP)/lateral chest x-ray should be performed on all patients with a primary liver tumor. Technetium-99m methylenediphosphonate nuclear bone scintigraphy is not routinely recommended due to the rarity of bone metastasis in HBs and is performed only if there is clinical suspicion.[121] The role of positron emission tomography (PET) is not routine in HBs. A small series showed fluoro-deoxyglucose uptake in the primary tumor, and additionally a small series evaluated PET/CT use for restaging of patients; however, larger studies need to confirm such findings and outline a role for this modality.[122,123] As resection of the primary tumor is essential for survival, liver imaging must define the segmental involvement of the liver and associated vasculature, both of which are indicators of resectability (see Figure 93.5a and b).

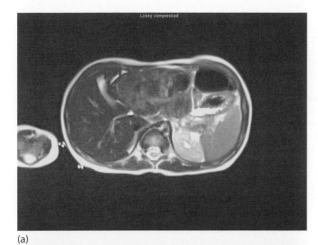

(a)

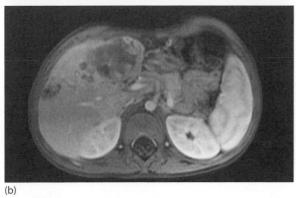

(b)

Figure 93.5 Focal and multifocal HB. **(a)** Focal HB involving the left lobe of the liver. **(b)** Multifocal HB with largest lesion involving the left lobe with multiple satellite tumors in the Segments IV, V, and VIII. This patient underwent an extended left hepatectomy.

STAGING

Two systems for staging pediatric liver tumors are used: one for treatment-naive patients and one based on postoperative extent of disease. Pretreatment staging is essential for risk stratification and outcome assessment when neoadjuvant treatments are used. However, post-operative staging systems incorporate histologic information that otherwise may not be available at time of diagnosis.[95]

The North American Children's Oncology Group (COG) employs a postoperative staging scheme (see Table 93.6). Risk stratification in the current COG HB protocol is based on the predominant tumor histology, presence of gross residual disease, distant metastasis, and the presence or absence of a low AFP (<100 ng/mL) at diagnosis (see Figure 93.6).

The Société Internationale d'Oncologie Pédiatrique/International Society of Pediatric Oncology Epithelial Liver Tumor Study Group (SIOPEL) introduced the PRETEXT (pretreatment extent of disease) system of staging liver tumors,[124,125] which defines the liver in four sections based on Couinaud's system of segmentation of the liver: (1) left lateral (Couinaud 2 and 3); (2) left medial (Couinaud 4);

Table 93.6 Children's oncology group staging system for pediatric liver tumors

Stage I	Complete gross resection at diagnosis with clear margins
Stage II	Complete gross resection at diagnosis with microscopic residual disease at the margins of resection
Stage III	Biopsy only at diagnosis; or gross total resection with nodal involvement; or preoperative tumor spill/rupture; or incomplete resection with gross residual tumor
Stage IV	Distant metastatic disease at diagnosis

Source: Reprinted from *Semin Pediatr Surg*, 21, Honeyman JN, La Quaglia MP, Malignant liver tumors, 245–54, Copyright 2012, with permission from Elsevier.

(3) right anterior (Couinaud 5 and 8); and (4) right posterior (Couinaud 6 and 7; see Figure 93.7). Risk stratification in PRETEXT is based on the number of contiguous tumor-free regions of the liver, and letters are assigned for the involvement of the caudate lobe (C); invasion of the vena cava or all three major hepatic veins (V); portal vein (P); contiguous extrahepatic growth (E); tumor rupture or hemorrhage (H); and distant metastasis (M; Table 93.7). PRETEXT stage has been shown to be an independent predictor of 5-year overall survival.[125]

The COG has used the PRETEXT staging system as an objective tool to monitor the effect of neoadjuvant chemotherapy and to determine the timing and extent of surgical resection.[126] It is hoped that this tool will allow better intergroup collaboration in the development of new therapeutic strategies for the highest-risk groups that continue to have a poor response to current treatment approaches. Recent analysis of a combined database of 1605 HB cases by the Children's Hepatic Tumors International Collaboration (CHIC) confirmed prior prognostic factors and yielded new ones for HB. Previous cooperative group studies identified variables such as PRETEXT stage, presence of metastatic disease, and very low serum AFP (<100 ng/mL) as poor prognostic factors. The CHIC group identified other variables such as spontaneous tumor rupture at enrollment, tumor multifocality, macroscopic vascular tumor invasion, contiguous extrahepatic tumor extension, older age at diagnosis, and very high (>1 million ng/mL) or borderline low AFP levels (100–999 ng/mL) as additional factors portending a poor prognosis.[87]

RISK GROUPS

The PRETEXT system established a common language for description of pediatric liver tumors and is used as the foundation for risk stratification for HB patients.[95,124] Risk group stratification allows clinicians to identify optimal treatment modalities based on their PRETEXT staging combined with histology and AFP levels. Each major study group has subtle variations on the definitions of groups between very

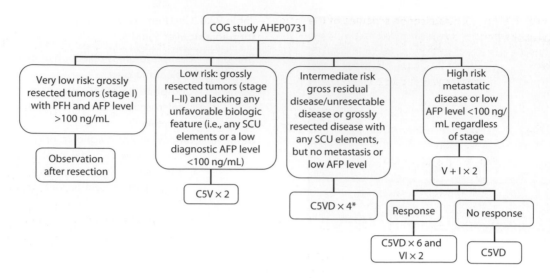

Figure 93.6 Diagram presents the patient groups and treatment algorithms for the Children's Oncology Group (COG) HB study AHEP0731 (NCT#00980460). Patient risk stratification is based on COG criteria. (Adapted from The Children's Oncology Group. Risk-based therapy in treating younger patients with newly diagnosed liver cancer [NCT00980460]. US National Library of Medicine and the National Institutes of Health; ClinicalTrials.gov. https://clinicaltrials.gov/show/NCT00980460. Accessed March 24, 2016.)

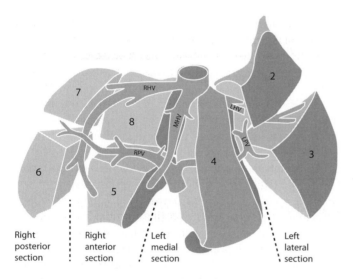

Figure 93.7 Couinaud liver segmentation and hepatic vasculature that define the surgical anatomy of the PRETEXT staging system for primary malignant liver tumors in childhood. (With kind permission from Springer Science+Business Media: *Pediatr Radiol*, PRETEXT: a revised staging system for primary malignant liver tumours of childhood developed by the SIOPEL group, 37, 2007, 123–32, Roebuck DJ et al.)

low risk, low/standard risk, intermediate risk, or high risk groups, which can be seen in Table 93.8.[120]

TREATMENT

The treatment of HBs is a success story in pediatric oncology. Overall survival has increased from 30% to 70% over the past few decades.[127] The addition of platinum-based chemotherapy to treatment regimens, along with advancements in surgical techniques, improved prognosis dramatically,

Table 93.7 SIOPEL risk stratification for hepatoblastoma

PRETEXT number	Definition
I	One section is involved and three adjoining sections are free.
II	One or two sections are involved, but two adjoining sections are free.
III	Two or three sections are involved, and no two adjoining sections are free.
IV	All four sections are involved.
High risk (HR-HB)	PRETEXT IV, additional PRETEXT criteria (V+,E+,P+,H+,M+), or AFP < 100 ng/mL
Standard risk (SR-HB)	PRETEXT I–III, V–,E–,P–,M–,H– (All other patients)

Source: With kind permission from Springer Science+Business Media: *Pediatr Radiol*, PRETEXT: A revised staging system for primary malignant liver tumours of childhood developed by the SIOPEL group, 37, 2007, Roebuck DJ et al.

Note: E = Extrahepatic disease; H = tumor rupture or intraperitoneal hemorrhage; M = distant metastases; P = portal vein involvement; V = involvement of the IVC and/or major hepatic veins.

with 5-year relative survival rates between years 2005 and 2011 reported as 86.4% for age < 1 year and 80.7% for ages 1–4 years.[81,92] Various collaborative groups have researched and developed successful treatment strategies for HBs (COG, SIOPEL, German Society for Pediatric Oncology and Hematology [GPOH], and the Japanese Study Group for Pediatric Liver Tumors [JPLT], among others).

Table 93.8 PRETEXT in risk stratification schemes of the major study groups

	COG	SIOPEL	GPOH	JPLT
Very low risk	PRETEXT I or II, pure fetal histology, and primary resection			
Low risk/ standard risk	PRETEXT I or II, any histology, primary resection	PRETEXT I, II, and III	PRETEXT I, II, and III	PRETEXT I, II, and III
Intermediate risk	PRETEXT II, III, IV unresectable at diagnosis V+, P+, E+SCU			PRETEXT IV, any PRETEXT with rupture, N1, P2, P2a, V3, and V3a multifocal
High risk	Any PRETEXT M+AFP level <100 ng/mL	Any PRETEXT V+, P+, E+, M+SCU AFP level <100 ng/mL tumor rupture	Any PRETEXT V+, P+, E+, M+multifocal	Any PRETEXT, M1, N2 AFP level <100 ng/mL

Source: Meyers RL et al., *Curr Opin Pediatrics* 2014; 26: 29–36.
Note: AFP: alpha-fetoprotein; COG: Children's Oncology Group; GPOH: German Society for Pediatric Oncology; JPLT: Japanese Study Group for Pediatric Liver Tumors; PRETEXT: pretreatment extent of disease; SIOPEL, International Society of Pediatric Oncology (SIOP) Childhood Liver Tumors Strategy Group.

Active agents against HB are cisplatin, 5-fluorouracil (5-FU), vincristine, doxorubicin, ifosfamide, and irinotecan. The standard chemotherapy regimen in SIOPEL 1 was preoperative cisplatin (PLA) and doxorubicin (DO) (PLADO) and delayed surgery.[128,129] Cisplatin monotherapy for standard risk HB (SR-HB) was evaluated against PLADO in the SIOPEL-3 trial, where it was concluded that doxorubicin could be safely omitted in these patients.[130] A review of 151 patients with high-risk HB (HR-HB) treated with alternating cycles of cisplatin and carboplatin plus doxorubicin and delayed tumor resection showed improved survival rates for this risk group.[129] The COG uses C5FV (cisplatin + 5-FU + vincristine) as the standard chemotherapy regimen for low- and intermediate-risk tumors. The addition of doxorubicin to cisplatin-based therapy offered no survival advantage for low-risk (COG stage 1 or 2) tumors and was associated with increased incidence of adverse events. However, an improved event-free survival was noted in patients receiving cisplatin–doxorubicin compared with C5FV for stage III and IV patients.[127,131] The current COG study (AHEP-0731) randomizes intermediate risk HB to cisplatin, 5-FU, vincristine, and doxorubicin against standard therapy. The use of irinotecan as window therapy for high-risk HB is also being evaluated for stage IV HB, for which outcome on current therapy continues to be dismal (see Figure 93.6).

The key difference in approach between the COG and SIOPEL is the timing of surgery and the use of neoadjuvant chemotherapy. The COG's approach has been to primarily resect tumors where possible and subsequently administer adjuvant chemotherapy for tumors with histologies other than PFH. Neoadjuvant chemotherapy after open or percutaneous needle biopsy is given to infants who present with an unresectable tumor. The SIOPEL approach has been to treat all patients diagnosed with HB (based on imaging and image-guided percutaneous needle biopsy) with neoadjuvant chemotherapy. They have argued toward less extensive surgical resections and shown operations to be easier and safer in pretreated tumors. Biopsy of the tumor, which is a prerequisite for such an approach, has also been found technically safe with a very low risk of tumor spread.[132]

The timing of surgery after induction therapy is another consideration. The current COG and SIOPEL protocols recommend an assessment for resection after two cycles of chemotherapy followed by two further cycles if the tumor is unresectable. A study found no statistically significant decline in tumor volume after the second cycle of chemotherapy.[133] These findings were similar to those of a prior study from our institution on pediatric solid tumors that included three HBs.[134] This may have implications for reduced toxicities with shorter regimens and early referral for transplant in the absence of a response.

For multifocal, PRETEXT IV tumors, liver transplant has proved to be a viable option. Six-year tumor-free survival of 82% was achieved with primary liver transplant, compared to 30% for rescue transplants due to either tumor recurrence or technical failures. Live related donor and cadaveric liver transplantation had disease-free survival of 82% and 71%, respectively. Macroscopic venous invasion, though a significant factor in overall survival, is not a contraindication to transplant, so long as the transplant can be performed without leaving gross tumor behind.[135]

The significance of pulmonary metastasis at presentation and later is currently being evaluated. The incidence of pulmonary metastatic disease can be as high as 40%. The outcome of this group of patients is markedly poorer.[136,137] The Children's Cancer Group reported long-term survival with resection of pulmonary metastasis and systemic chemotherapy where the lungs were the only site of metastatic disease and where the primary tumor had been successfully treated.[138,139] Meyers et al.'s[137] review of patients from the COG INT-0098 reported excellent outcome following pulmonary metastasectomy of lung metastasis detected at presentation (8 of 9 patients were long-term survivors), but a poorer outcome for pulmonary recurrence after chemotherapy, where 4 of 13 were long-term survivors.[137]

ADJUNCT THERAPIES

Transcatheter arterial chemoembolization (TACE), which uses a percutaneously placed intraarterial catheter, has emerged as an option in advanced, unresectable HBs (see Table 93.9). It has potential for making inoperable HBs resectable or transplantable.[140] Malogolowkin et al.[141] described the efficacy of TACE in a study including six patients with HB and found it to be well tolerated and allowed surgical resection of the primary tumor in tumors previously deemed unresectable.[141] Four series of HBs, which included 36 patients ranging from 50 days to 5 years of age, have reported a resectability rate of 88.8%.[142-145]

Further chemotherapeutic strategies for the treatment of HR-HB, especially small-cell undifferentiated HBs, which respond poorly to current chemotherapy protocols have been and continue to be investigated. A Phase II study from the COG evaluated the use of irinotecan (a topoisomerase 1 inhibitor) in children with refractory solid tumors and showed complete response in one of eight HB patients.[146] Irinotecan is currently being evaluated in HR-HB in the COG study AHEP0731, as well as a clinical trial from the National Cancer Institute (ClinicalTrials.gov Identifier:

NCT00980460), and successful treatment has been reported in case studies and small series.[147-149]

Gene-directed therapeutic strategies being investigated include Bcl-2 silencing and the targeting of *Myc* and β-catenin genes. The use of gene therapy to activate 5-fluorocytosine (an inactive prodrug) to 5-fluorouracil has been described in *in vitro* studies.[150] The neurokinin-1 receptor (NK1R), bound by the peptide substance P (SP), has been shown to induce tumor cell proliferation, angiogenesis, and migration in various cancers, and is expressed in HB cells in pre- and post-chemotherapy samples.[151] Novel studies using HB cell lines (Huh6, HepT1, HepG2) to block NK1R function with a small molecule, aprepitant, have shown growth inhibition and apoptosis by inhibition of the canonical *wnt* signaling pathway, which potentially provides another therapy to augment treatment strategies for chemoresistant cancer cells.[152] A recent study by Waters et al.[153] demonstrated that a novel rexinoid, UAB30, was able to decrease cell survival *in vitro* and decreased tumor growth in xenograft models, suggesting a possible role in the treatment of HB after further investigation.

Malignant rhabdoid tumor

Malignant rhabdoid tumors (MRTs), were initially described as the rhabdomyosarcomatoid variant of Wilms tumor,[154] although they are now known to be a distinct pathology. These tumors more commonly present as CNS or renal tumors; however, they have also been described in the liver, lungs, and soft tissues. MRTs of the liver are poorly understood extremely rare tumors with a grave prognosis. They

Table 93.9 Reports of transcatheter arterial chemoembolization in unresectable hepatoblastoma

Reference	No. of patients	Age range	No. of treatments	Resectability	Overall survival	Complications of TACE
Han et al.[142]	4	8–22 months	2	4/4 underwent hepatic resections	100%, 16–52 months follow-up	None
Li et al.[143]	16	50 days to 60 months	1–3 (cisplatin/ Adriamycin)	13/16—complete resections (incl. one OLT) 3/16—partial resection	1-year OS: 87.5% 3-year OS: 68.7% 5-year OS: 50%	None
Xuewu et al.[144]	8	2–12 months	1–3 (Adriamycin/ vincristine/ cisplatin)	6/8—complete resection; 1/8—no surgery as tumor completely regressed; 1/8—died of pneumonia before surgery	15–49 months follow-up	One case of pneumonia
Oue et al.[145]	8	4–26 months	1 (heterogenous group, 3 patients received pre- or post-TACE chemotherapy)	8/8 resected (one patient had pulmonary metastasis)	6 of 8 disease free at 46 months; 2 of 8 died of metastatic disease	Fever

have sometimes presented with an abdominal mass, distention, or fever, elevated LDH, and normal or near normal AFP levels.[155] MRTs in all sites tend to present at a young age, with one series showing 4 of 19 patients at age 3 months old or younger.[156] Differentiating the tumor from a small-cell undifferentiated type HB can be difficult, as they share clinical and histological features.[157] The tumor is very friable, can present with rupture, distant metastases, and can bleed uncontrollably following biopsy. Deletions and mutations of the tumor suppressor gene, SMARCB1 (also known as hSNF5, INI1, and BAF47), in chromosome band 22q11.2 have been demonstrated in MRTs, and the loss of SMARCB1 immunostaining may be a reliable marker of rhabdoid tumors in children.[158,159] Germline SMARCB1 mutations have been identified in up to 35% of patients. These patients have been shown to present at younger ages (~6 mo) and may carry a worse prognosis.[159]

MRTs are extremely difficult to treat with poor responses to cytotoxic chemotherapy, and reports of median survival near 15 weeks.[155,156] There are cases of long-term survival in a 13-month-old girl following right hepatectomy and multiagent chemotherapy with ifosfamide, vincristine, and actinomycin D[160]; and in a 3-year-old after combination chemotherapy with ifosfamide, carboplatin, and etoposide alternated with vincristine, doxorubicin, and cyclophosphamide as well as liver transplantation.[161]

Fibrolamellar HCC

Fibrolamellar HCC (FLHCC) is a rare primary liver tumor that typically presents in children and young adult patients with no background history of liver disease or hepatitis, and sporadic cases have been reported in infants.[162] The tumor was first described in 1956[45] as a variant of conventional HCC, but is now recognized as a unique pathologic entity. Patients typically do not have viral hepatitis or cirrhosis, and do not exhibit elevations in serum AFP. Recent advances in the tumor biology of FLHCC show a 400-kb deletion in one copy of chromosome 19 in tumor samples producing a chimeric transcript between the first exon of the heat shock protein, DNAJB1, with all but the first exon of the catalytic subunit of protein kinase A, PRKACA.[163] This chimera is a functional kinase, and few other changes are seen in the genomic DNA.[164] Total surgical resection is paramount in treatment of FLHCC, and outcomes have been reported to be more favorable for FLHCC than conventional HCC. Lymph node metastases are common, and presence of extrahepatic disease is a consistent, independent predictor of overall and recurrence-free survival.[165] Recent transcriptomic evaluation of FLHCC shows key oncologically relevant pathways to have elevated transcription levels, including EGF/ErbB and Wnt signaling pathways, which may lead to new avenues of treatment. Ongoing clinical trials are evaluating the use of an oral aurora kinase A inhibitor, the transcript of which was found to be elevated in FLHCC tumor samples (ClinicalTrials.gov identifier: NCT02234986).[166]

Germ cell tumors

While germ cell tumors in children are fairly common, their occurrence in the neonatal liver is quite rare. Large series of fetal and neonatal tumors spanning decades have documented only isolated cases in the liver. As a group, they account for around 2% of tumors in this age group.[1,167,168]

CHORIOCARCINOMA

Choriocarcinoma is a rapidly growing, hemorrhagic tumor of the trophoblastic tissues. The placenta is believed to be the site of origin, with subsequent hematogenous metastasis in the infant and/or mother. The liver is the most frequently involved site in infants. Choriocarcinoma in the neonatal period is a rare (approximately 1:40,000 pregnancies), life-threatening malignancy but one that is highly responsive to the appropriate early treatment when instituted.[169] The disease is generally recognized late in the neonate with median age of symptomatology at 1 month. Cases have been documented and treated successfully, both in the presence and absence of maternal or placental disease.[170–172] Bolze et al.[173] confirmed a case of transplacental transmission through tumor genotyping, strengthening the theorized mechanism of hematogenous spread from mother to child. The absence of placental disease can be explained by the presence of even a microscopic focus of primary disease in the placenta missed on histopathology; a placental focus of choriocarcinoma is not always present in maternal disease either.

Choriocarcinoma is detected easily in the newborn by the presence of an elevated serum β-hCG. The neonate usually presents with an abdominal mass, hepatomegaly, and anemia. This "infantile choriocarcinoma syndrome" was first described by Witzleben and Bruninga[174] in 1968 in infants aged 5 weeks to 7 months, though this can easily be applied to the newborn. The presence of choriocarcinoma in the mother who has delivered a live baby is rare and should prompt a screen for a neonatal tumor in the first month of life. Also, suspicion of choriocarcinoma in the neonate should prompt a search for the same in the mother. The tumor can metastasize rapidly to the lungs, brain, and skin, and usually is fatal within weeks owing to uncontrolled hemorrhage.[175]

If detected early, the tumor is highly chemosensitive to methotrexate and agents used for other germ cell tumors, such as etoposide, bleomycin, and cisplatin. Paclitaxel can be used as second-line chemotherapy for cisplatin unresponsive disease. Residual disease in the liver, lungs, or brain can be resected or observed as per the response monitored radiologically (CT/MRI) and biochemically (serum β-hCG). There have been an increasing number of reports of successful treatment for this disease.[171,176–181]

TERATOMAS

The few reported cases of teratomas of the liver in the newborn have been mature teratomas, though more examples of all kinds have been reported in infancy.[182–184] Interestingly, a large series of teratomas in children included two liver tumors, both of which occurred in newborns.[185] The AFP level is usually elevated regardless of the presence or absence of malignancy. Treatment usually consists of resection and chemotherapy guided by the malignant cell type. Growing teratoma syndrome is defined as an enlarging mass that consists predominately of mature teratomas with normal or falling tumor markers. While this is of concern, most series describe an older patient population.[186,187]

PRIMARY YOLK SAC TUMORS

Primary yolk sac tumors are extremely rare and highly malignant. A total of eight cases are described in the literature. The tumor is thought to develop from germ cell precursors that become arrested during embryological migration, or to arise from pluripotent embryonic cells that escaped the influences of the differentiation process during embryogenesis.[188] Yolk sac tumors can occur in a pure form or, more commonly, in combination with other germ cell tumors. Hart reported the first yolk sac tumor of the liver in an 18-month-old boy in 1975. Lesions can present as a solitary mass or as multiple masses. Serum AFP is markedly elevated, and on diagnostic imaging, there is often a finding of central necrosis or intratumoral hemorrhage. It is important to differentiate primary yolk sac tumor from HB in view of potential therapeutic implications.

PRINCIPLES OF LIVER RESECTIONS

The details of individual major hepatic resections are beyond the scope of this chapter, and the reader is referred to a text on hepatobiliary surgery.[189] However, the general principles of liver resections in neonates and infants are similar to those in adults. The potential hazards are mainly blood loss and bile leak. Eighty-five percent of the liver can be safely removed in small infants. Liver regeneration is rapid and almost complete within 3 months.[190] Central hepatectomy has also been shown to be a feasible, though technically challenging, operation in children with HBs.[191] Values on liver function tests usually return to normal within a few weeks.

Bloodless hepatic dissection is crucial in newborns for which the blood volume is no more than a few hundred milliliters. The surgical approach is based on a thorough understanding of the hepatic anatomy as described by Couinaud.[192] Skilled anesthetic management and maintenance of a low central venous pressure (CVP) in the patient minimizes blood loss. Hepatic resections in children can be carried out through a transverse or subcostal incision, and vertical extension is often unnecessary. After division of the ligamentum teres and the falciform ligament, a thorough examination of the liver is undertaken to identify the site or sites of tumor involvement. Further mobilization of the left or right lobe is undertaken with division of the respective peritoneal reflections on the diaphragm. The mobilization of the right lobe is completed once the fibrous tissue over the inferior vena cava is divided with scissors or the endoscopic gastrointestinal anastomosis vascular stapling device (Endo-GIA, United States Surgical Corporation, Norwalk, CT). The use of intraoperative ultrasound at this stage is useful in identifying the location of hepatic vessels, particularly the hepatic veins.

Next, attention is turned toward establishing inflow control and identifying and preserving the components of the biliary tree. Control of the branches of the hepatic artery and the portal vein supplying the part of the liver to be resected can be achieved individually by extrahepatic dissection or by transecting the relevant pedicle within the substance of the liver. During left hepatectomy, the left branch of the portal vein and left hepatic artery are divided within the umbilical fissure. Dissection of the extrahepatic biliary structures is not necessary and carries the risk of inadvertent bile duct injuries, especially in the presence of variant anatomy. Division of the biliary radicals can be achieved at the time of parenchymal transection by dividing them laterally within the pedicles.

Establishing control of the venous outflow is the aspect of the operation most fraught with the risk of blood loss and air embolism. This dissection is performed with the patient in 15-degree Trendelenburg position and with the anesthesiologist maintaining a CVP of less than 5 mmHg. The individual hepatic veins are carefully dissected, divided within vascular clamps, and oversewn with 3-0 polypropylene sutures. Alternatively, they can be divided using the Endo-GIA vascular stapling device.

Division of the liver parenchyma should be considered to be more akin to fine dissection than a fracture and division. This may be accomplished by a simple crushing technique. We apply intermittent inflow occlusion (Pringle maneuver) for periods up to 7 minutes with 1-minute windows when hemostasis is achieved on the cut surface. The Glisson's capsule is scored with cautery and a Kelly clamp used to fracture the liver substance. A combination of titanium hemoclips and the Endo-GIA vascular stapler is used to transect the liver substance. We employ a saline-linked radiofrequency ablation device called TissueLink (TissueLink Medical Inc, Diver, NH, USA) and the argon beam coagulator to achieve hemostasis. We do not routinely employ drainage of the abdominal cavity.[193]

CONCLUSION

The understanding of hepatic tumors in newborns and infants has evolved rapidly in the treatment of both benign and malignant disorders. Newborns and infants with these disorders present with a unique set of problems without parallel in other age groups. As many of these pathologies are so rare, international intergroup collaborations are crucial to foster continued progress and help develop novel therapeutic approaches in managing these disorders.

REFERENCES

1. Isaacs H Jr. Fetal and neonatal hepatic tumors. *J Pediatr Surg* 2007; 42(11): 1797–803.

2. Thompson PA, Chintagumpala M. Renal and hepatic tumors in the neonatal period. *Semin Fetal Neonatal Med* 2012; 17(4): 216–21.

3. Christison-Lagay ER, Burrows PE, Alomari A, Dubois J, Kozakewich HP, Lane TS et al. Hepatic hemangiomas: Subtype classification and development of a clinical practice algorithm and registry. *J Pediatr Surg* 2007; 42(1): 62–7; discussion 7–8.

4. Hughes JA, Hill V, Patel K, Syed S, Harper J, De Bruyn R. Cutaneous haemangioma: Prevalence and sonographic characteristics of associated hepatic haemangioma. *Clin Radiol* 2004; 59(3): 273–80.

5. Mulliken JB, Glowacki J. Hemangiomas and vascular malformations in infants and children: A classification based on endothelial characteristics. *Plast Reconstr Surg* 1982; 69(3): 412–22.

6. Glowacki J, Mulliken JB. Mast cells in hemangiomas and vascular malformations. *Pediatrics* 1982; 70(1): 48–51.

7. Takahashi K, Mulliken JB, Kozakewich HP, Rogers RA, Folkman J, Ezekowitz RA. Cellular markers that distinguish the phases of hemangioma during infancy and childhood. *J Clin Invest* 1994; 93(6): 2357–64.

8. North PE, Waner M, Mizeracki A, Mihm MC, Jr. GLUT1: A newly discovered immunohistochemical marker for juvenile hemangiomas. *Hum Pathol* 2000; 31(1): 11–22.

9. Mo JQ, Dimashkieh HH, Bove KE. GLUT1 endothelial reactivity distinguishes hepatic infantile hemangioma from congenital hepatic vascular malformation with associated capillary proliferation. *Hum Pathol* 2004; 35(2): 200–9.

10. Enjolras O, Mulliken JB. Vascular tumors and vascular malformations (new issues). *Adv Dermatol* 1997; 13: 375–423.

11. Dickie B, Dasgupta R, Nair R, Alonso MH, Ryckman FC, Tiao GM et al. Spectrum of hepatic hemangiomas: Management and outcome. *J Pediatr Surg* 2009; 44(1): 125–33.

12. DeAos I jC, North PE, editor. Hepatic Hemangioma: Not a singular entity. 15th International Workshop of the International Society of Vascular Anomalies; February 22, 2004; Wellington, New Zealand.

13. Paltiel HJ, Burrows PE, Kozakewich HPW. Solitary infantile liver hemangioma: A distinct clinico-pathologic entity. 15th International Workshop of the International Society of Vascular Anomalies; February 22, 2004; Wellington, New Zealand.

14. Han SJ, Tsai CC, Tsai HM, Chen YJ. Infantile hemangioendothelioma with a highly elevated serum alpha-fetoprotein level. *Hepatogastroenterology* 1998; 45(20): 459–61.

15. Seo IS, Min KW, Mirkin LD. Hepatic hemangioendothelioma of infancy associated with elevated alpha fetoprotein and catecholamine by-products. *Pediatr Pathol* 1988; 8(6): 625–31.

16. Sari N, Yalcin B, Akyuz C, Haliloglu M, Buyukpamukcu M. Infantile hepatic hemangioendothelioma with elevated serum alpha-fetoprotein. *Pediatr Hematol Oncol* 2006; 23(8): 639–47.

17. Jang HJ, Yu H, Kim TK. Contrast-enhanced ultrasound in the detection and characterization of liver tumors. *Cancer Imaging* 2009; 9: 96–103.

18. Wilson SR, Burns PN. An algorithm for the diagnosis of focal liver masses using microbubble contrast-enhanced pulse-inversion sonography. *AJR Am J Roentgenol* 2006; 186(5): 1401–12.

19. Lee JY, Choi BI, Han JK, Kim AY, Shin SH, Moon SG. Improved sonographic imaging of hepatic hemangioma with contrast-enhanced coded harmonic angiography: Comparison with MR imaging. *Ultrasound Med Biol* 2002; 28(3): 287–95.

20. Dietrich CF, Mertens JC, Braden B, Schuessler G, Ott M, Ignee A. Contrast-enhanced ultrasound of histologically proven liver hemangiomas. *Hepatology* 2007; 45(5): 1139–45.

21. Sharif K, English M, Ramani P, Alberti D, Otte JB, McKiernan P et al. Management of hepatic epithelioid haemangio-endothelioma in children: What option? *Br J Cancer* 2004; 90(8): 1498–501.

22. Makhlouf HR, Ishak KG, Goodman ZD. Epithelioid hemangioendothelioma of the liver: A clinicopathologic study of 137 cases. *Cancer* 1999; 85(3): 562–82.

23. Guiteau JJ, Cotton RT, Karpen SJ, O'Mahony CA, Goss JA. Pediatric liver transplantation for primary malignant liver tumors with a focus on hepatic epithelioid hemangioendothelioma: The UNOS experience. *Pediatr Transplant* 2010; 14(3): 326–31.

24. Foley LS, Kulungowski AM. Vascular anomalies in pediatrics. *Adv Pediatr* 2015; 62(1): 227–55.

25. Moon SB, Kwon HJ, Park KW, Yun WJ, Jung SE. Clinical experience with infantile hepatic hemangioendothelioma. *World J Surg* 2009; 33(3): 597–602.

26. Ezekowitz RA, Mulliken JB, Folkman J. Interferon alfa-2a therapy for life-threatening hemangiomas of infancy. *N Engl J Med* 1992; 326(22): 1456–63.

27. Michaud AP, Bauman NM, Burke DK, Manaligod JM, Smith RJ. Spastic diplegia and other motor disturbances in infants receiving interferon-alpha. *Laryngoscope* 2004; 114(7): 1231–6.

28. Perez Payarols J, Pardo Masferrer J, Gomez Bellvert C. Treatment of life-threatening infantile hemangiomas with vincristine. *N Engl J Med* 1995; 333(1): 69.

29. Perez J, Pardo J, Gomez C. Vincristine—An effective treatment of corticoid-resistant life-threatening infantile hemangiomas. *Acta Oncol* 2002; 41(2): 197–9.

30. Kassarjian A, Dubois J, Burrows PE. Angiographic classification of hepatic hemangiomas in infants. *Radiology* 2002; 222(3): 693–8.

31. Draper H, Diamond IR, Temple M, John P, Ng V, Fecteau A. Multimodal management of endangering hepatic hemangioma: Impact on transplant avoidance: A descriptive case series. *J Pediatr Surg* 2008; 43(1): 120–5; discussion 6.

32. Kalicinski P, Ismail H, Broniszczak D, Teisserye J, Bacewicz L, Markiewicz-Kijewska M et al. Non-resectable hepatic tumors in children—Role of liver transplantation. *Ann Transplant* 2008; 13(2): 37–41.

33. Zenzen W, Perez-Atayde AR, Elisofon SA, Kim HB, Alomari AI. Hepatic failure in a rapidly involuting congenital hemangioma of the liver: Failure of embolotherapy. *Pediatr Radiol* 2009; 39(10): 1118–23.

34. Grabhorn E, Richter A, Fischer L, Krebs-Schmitt D, Ganschow R. Neonates with severe infantile hepatic hemangioendothelioma: Limitations of liver transplantation. *Pediatr Transplant* 2009; 13(5): 560–4.

35. Mahajan D, Miller C, Hirose K, McCullough A, Yerian L. Incidental reduction in the size of liver hemangioma following use of VEGF inhibitor bevacizumab. *J Hepatol* 2008; 49(5): 867–70.

36. Belmont L, Zemoura L, Couderc LJ. Pulmonary epithelioid haemangioendothelioma and bevacizumab. *J Thorac Oncol* 2008; 3(5): 557–8.

37. Stringer MD, Alizai NK. Mesenchymal hamartoma of the liver: A systematic review. *J Pediatr Surg* 2005; 40(11): 1681–90.

38. Weinberg AG, Finegold MJ. Primary hepatic tumors of childhood. *Hum Pathol* 1983; 14(6): 512–37.

39. Stocker JT. Hepatic tumors in children. *Clin Liver Dis* 2001; 5(1): 259–81, viii–ix.

40. Stocker JT, Ishak KG. Mesenchymal hamartoma of the liver: Report of 30 cases and review of the literature. *Pediatr Pathol* 1983; 1(3): 245–67.

41. Ishak K, Stocker, JT. Benign mesenchymal tumors and pseudotumors. In: Rosai J (ed). *Atlas of Tumor Pathology*. Washington, DC: Armed Forces Institute of Pathology, 2001: 71–157.

42. Hernandez JC, Alfonso C, Gonzalez L, Samada M, Ramos L, Cepero-Valdez M et al. Solid mesenchymal hamartoma in an adult: A case report. *J Clin Pathol* 2006; 59(5): 542–5.

43. Horton KM, Bluemke DA, Hruban RH, Soyer P, Fishman EK. CT and MR imaging of benign hepatic and biliary tumors. *Radiographics* 1999; 19(2): 431–51.

44. Meyers RL. Tumors of the liver in children. *Surg Oncol* 2007; 16(3): 195–203.

45. Edmondson HA. Differential diagnosis of tumors and tumor-like lesions of liver in infancy and childhood. *AMA J Dis Child* 1956; 91(2): 168–86.

46. Chiorean L, Cui XW, Tannapfel A, Franke D, Stenzel M, Kosiak W et al. Benign liver tumors in pediatric patients—Review with emphasis on imaging features. *World J Gastroenterol* 2015; 21(28): 8541–61.

47. Kim SH, Kim WS, Cheon JE, Yoon HK, Kang GH, Kim IO et al. Radiological spectrum of hepatic mesenchymal hamartoma in children. *Korean J Radiol* 2007; 8(6): 498–505.

48. Fukahori S, Tsuru T, Tanikawa K, Akiyoshi K, Asagiri K, Tanaka Y et al. Mesenchymal hamartoma of the liver accompanied by a daughter nodule: Report of a case. *Surg Today* 2007; 37(9): 811–6.

49. Helal A, Nolan M, Bower R, Mair B, Debich-Spicer D. Pathological case of the month. Mesenchymal hamartoma of the liver. *Arch Pediatr Adolesc Med* 1995; 149(3): 315–6.

50. von Schweinitz D, Dammeier BG, Gluer S. Mesenchymal hamartoma of the liver—New insight into histogenesis. *J Pediatr Surg* 1999; 34(8): 1269–71.

51. Sharif K, Ramani P, Lochbuhler H, Grundy R, de Ville de Goyet J. Recurrent mesenchymal hamartoma associated with 19q translocation. A call for more radical surgical resection. *Eur J Pediatr Surg* 2006; 16(1): 64–7.

52. Talmon GA, Cohen SM. Mesenchymal hamartoma of the liver with an interstitial deletion involving chromosome band 19q13.4: A theory as to pathogenesis? *Arch Pathol Lab Med* 2006; 130(8): 1216–8.

53. Cajaiba MM, Sarita-Reyes C, Zambrano E, Reyes-Mugica M. Mesenchymal hamartoma of the liver associated with features of Beckwith–Wiedemann syndrome and high serum alpha-fetoprotein levels. *Pediatr Dev Pathol* 2007; 10(3): 233–8.

54. Dehner LP, Ewing SL, Sumner HW. Infantile mesenchymal hamartoma of the liver. Histologic and ultrastructural observations. *Arch Pathol* 1975; 99(7): 379–82.

55. Cozzutto C, De Bernardi B, Comelli A, Soave F. Malignant mesenchymoma of the liver in children: A clinicopathologic and ultrastructural study. *Hum Pathol* 1981; 12(5): 481–5.

56. Baboiu OE, Saal H, Collins M. Hepatic mesenchymal hamartoma: Cytogenetic analysis of a case and review of the literature. *Pediatr Dev Pathol* 2008; 11(4): 295–9.

57. Sugito K, Kawashima H, Uekusa S, Inoue M, Ikeda T, Kusafuka T. Mesenchymal hamartoma of the liver originating in the caudate lobe with t(11;19)(q13;q13.4): Report of a case. *Surg Today* 2010; 40(1): 83–7.

58. Rajaram V, Knezevich S, Bove KE, Perry A, Pfeifer JD. DNA sequence of the translocation breakpoints in undifferentiated embryonal sarcoma arising in mesenchymal hamartoma of the liver harboring the t(11;19)(q11;q13.4) translocation. *Genes Chromosomes Cancer* 2007; 46(5): 508–13.

59. Laberge JM, Patenaude Y, Desilets V, Cartier L, Khalife S, Jutras L et al. Large hepatic mesenchymal hamartoma leading to mid-trimester fetal demise. *Fetal Diagn Ther* 2005; 20(2): 141–5.

60. Bessho T, Kubota K, Komori S, Ohtsuka Y, Uneo Y, Uematsu K et al. Prenatally detected hepatic hamartoma: Another cause of non-immune hydrops. *Prenat Diagn* 1996; 16(4): 337–41.

61. Cetin M, Demirpolat G, Elmas N, Yuce G, Cetingul N, Balik E. Stromal predominant type mesenchymal hamartoma of liver: CT and MR features. *Comput Med Imaging Graph* 2002; 26(3): 167–9.

62. Meinders AJ, Simons MP, Heij HA, Aronson DC. Mesenchymal hamartoma of the liver: Failed management by marsupialization. *J Pediatr Gastroenterol Nutr* 1998; 26(3): 353–5.

63. Murray JD, Ricketts RR. Mesenchymal hamartoma of the liver. *Am Surg* 1998; 64(11): 1097–103.

64. Shuto T, Kinoshita H, Yamada C, Hirohashi K, Shiokawa C, Kubo S et al. Bilateral lobectomy excluding the caudate lobe for giant mesenchymal hamartoma of the liver. *Surgery* 1993; 113(2): 215–22.

65. Luks FI, Yazbeck S, Brandt ML, Bensoussan AL, Brochu P, Blanchard H. Benign liver tumors in children: A 25-year experience. *J Pediatr Surg* 1991; 26(11): 1326–30.

66. Virgone C, Cecchetto G, Dall'Igna P, Zanon GF, Cillo U, Alaggio R. Mesenchymal hamartoma of the liver in older children: An adult variant or a different entity? Report of a case with review of the literature. *Appl Immunohistochem Mol Morphol* 2015; 23(9): 667–73.

67. Bejarano PA, Serrano MF, Casillas J, Dehner LP, Kato T, Mitral N et al. Concurrent infantile hemangioendothelioma and mesenchymal hamartoma in a developmentally arrested liver of an infant requiring hepatic transplantation. *Pediatr Dev Pathol* 2003; 6(6): 552–7.

68. Tepetes K, Selby R, Webb M, Madariaga JR, Iwatsuki S, Starzl TE. Orthotopic liver transplantation for benign hepatic neoplasms. *Arch Surg* 1995; 130(2): 153–6.

69. Sarkar M, Mulliken JB, Kozakewich HP, Robertson RL, Burrows PE. Thrombocytopenic coagulopathy (Kasabach–Merritt phenomenon) is associated with Kaposiform hemangioendothelioma and not with common infantile hemangioma. *Plast Reconstr Surg* 1997; 100(6): 1377–86.

70. Harper L, Michel JL, Enjolras O, Raynaud-Mounet N, Riviere JP, Heigele T et al. Successful management of a retroperitoneal kaposiform hemangioendothelioma with Kasabach–Merritt phenomenon using alpha-interferon. *Eur J Pediatr Surg* 2006; 16(5): 369–72.

71. Stocker JT, Ishak KG. Focal nodular hyperplasia of the liver: A study of 21 pediatric cases. *Cancer* 1981; 48(2): 336–45.

72. Kumagai H, Masuda T, Oikawa H, Endo K, Endo M, Takano T. Focal nodular hyperplasia of the liver: Direct evidence of circulatory disturbances. *J Gastroenterol Hepatol* 2000; 15(11): 1344–7.

73. McInnes MD, Hibbert RM, Inacio JR, Schieda N. Focal nodular hyperplasia and hepatocellular adenoma: Accuracy of gadoxetic acid-enhanced MR imaging—A systematic review. *Radiology* 2015; 277(2): 413–23.

74. Werb P, Scurry J, Ostor A, Fortune D, Attwood H. Survey of congenital tumors in perinatal necropsies. *Pathology* 1992; 24(4): 247–53.

75. Lack EE, Ornvold K. Focal nodular hyperplasia and hepatic adenoma: A review of eight cases in the pediatric age group. *J Surg Oncol* 1986; 33(2): 129–35.

76. Applegate KE, Ghei M, Perez-Atayde AR. Prenatal detection of a solitary liver adenoma. *Pediatr Radiol* 1999; 29(2): 92–4.

77. Agrawal S, Agarwal S, Arnason T, Saini S, Belghiti J. Management of hepatocellular adenoma: Recent advances. *Clin Gastroenterol Hepatol* 2015; 13(7): 1221–30.

78. Erdogan D, van Delden OM, Busch OR, Gouma DJ, van Gulik TM. Selective transcatheter arterial embolization for treatment of bleeding complications or reduction of tumor mass of hepatocellular adenomas. *Cardiovasc Intervent Radiol* 2007; 30(6): 1252–8.

79. Leese T, Farges O, Bismuth H. Liver cell adenomas. A 12-year surgical experience from a specialist hepatobiliary unit. *Ann Surg* 1988; 208(5): 558–64.

80. Rocourt DV, Shiels WE, Hammond S, Besner GE. Contemporary management of benign hepatic adenoma using percutaneous radiofrequency ablation. *J Pediatr Surg* 2006; 41(6): 1149–52.

81. Howlader N NA, Krapcho M, Garshell J, Miller D, Altekruse SF, Kosary CL et al. (eds). *SEER Cancer Statistics Review, 1975–2012*. Bethesda, MD: National Cancer Institute. Available from http://seercancergov/csr/1975_2012/, based on November 2014 SEER data submission, posted to the SEER web site, April 2015.

82. Spector LG, Birch J. The epidemiology of hepatoblastoma. *Pediatr Blood Cancer* 2012; 59(5): 776–9.

83. Finegold MJ. Hepatic tumors in childhood. In: Russo P RE, Piccoli DA (eds). *Pathology of Pediatric Gastrointestinal and Liver Disease*. New York, Springer-Verlag, 2004: 300–46.

84. Spector LG, Puumala SE, Carozza SE, Chow EJ, Fox EE, Horel S et al. Cancer risk among children with very low birth weights. *Pediatrics* 2009; 124(1): 96–104.

85. Spector LG, Johnson KJ, Soler JT, Puumala SE. Perinatal risk factors for hepatoblastoma. *Br J Cancer* 2008; 98(9): 1570–3.

86. Ikeda H, Hachitanda Y, Tanimura M, Maruyama K, Koizumi T, Tsuchida Y. Development of unfavorable hepatoblastoma in children of very low birth weight: Results of a surgical and pathologic review. *Cancer* 1998; 82(9): 1789–96.

87. Czauderna P, Haeberle B, Hiyama E, Rangaswami A, Krailo M, Maibach R et al. The Children's Hepatic tumors International Collaboration (CHIC): Novel

global rare tumor database yields new prognostic factors in hepatoblastoma and becomes a research model. *Eur J Cancer* 2016; 52: 92–101.

88. Lopez-Terrada D, Alaggio R, de Davila MT, Czauderna P, Hiyama E, Katzenstein H et al. Towards an international pediatric liver tumor consensus classification: Proceedings of the Los Angeles COG liver tumors symposium. *Mod Pathol* 2014; 27(3): 472–91.

89. Hadzic N, Finegold MJ. Liver neoplasia in children. *Clin Liver Dis* 2011; 15(2): 443–62, vii–x.

90. Malogolowkin MH, Katzenstein HM, Meyers RL, Krailo MD, Rowland JM, Haas J et al. Complete surgical resection is curative for children with hepatoblastoma with pure fetal histology: A report from the Children's Oncology Group. *J Clin Oncol* 2011; 29(24): 3301–6.

91. Haas JE, Muczynski KA, Krailo M, Ablin A, Land V, Vietti TJ et al. Histopathology and prognosis in childhood hepatoblastoma and hepatocarcinoma. *Cancer* 1989; 64(5): 1082–95.

92. De Ioris M, Brugieres L, Zimmermann A, Keeling J, Brock P, Maibach R et al. Hepatoblastoma with a low serum alpha-fetoprotein level at diagnosis: The SIOPEL group experience. *Eur J Cancer* 2008; 44(4): 545–50.

93. Krush AJ, Traboulsi EI, Offerhaus JA, Maumenee IH, Yardley JH, Levin LS. Hepatoblastoma, pigmented ocular fundus lesions and jaw lesions in Gardner syndrome. *Am J Med Genet* 1988; 29(2): 323–32.

94. Finegold MJ, Lopez-Terrada DH, Bowen J, Washington MK, Qualman SJ. Protocol for the examination of specimens from pediatric patients with hepatoblastoma. *Arch Pathol Lab Med* 2007; 131(4): 520–9.

95. Honeyman JN, La Quaglia MP. Malignant liver tumors. *Semin Pediatr Surg* 2012; 21(3): 245–54.

96. Hiyama E. Pediatric hepatoblastoma: Diagnosis and treatment. *Transl Pediatr* 2014; 3(4): 293–9.

97. Hughes LJ, Michels VV. Risk of hepatoblastoma in familial adenomatous polyposis. *Am J Med Genet* 1992; 43(6): 1023–5.

98. DeBaun MR, Tucker MA. Risk of cancer during the first four years of life in children from The Beckwith–Wiedemann Syndrome Registry. *J Pediatr* 1998; 132(3 Pt 1): 398–400.

99. Kingston JE, Draper GJ, Mann JR. Hepatoblastoma and polyposis coli. *Lancet* 1982; 1(8269): 457.

100. Giardiello FM, Offerhaus GJ, Krush AJ, Booker SV, Tersmette AC, Mulder JW et al. Risk of hepatoblastoma in familial adenomatous polyposis. *J Pediatr* 1991; 119(5): 766–8.

101. Hirschman BA, Pollock BH, Tomlinson GE. The spectrum of APC mutations in children with hepatoblastoma from familial adenomatous polyposis kindreds. *J Pediatr* 2005; 147(2): 263–6.

102. Koch A, Denkhaus D, Albrecht S, Leuschner I, von Schweinitz D, Pietsch T. Childhood hepatoblastomas frequently carry a mutated degradation targeting box of the beta-catenin gene. *Cancer Res* 1999; 59(2): 269–73.

103. Taniguchi K, Roberts LR, Aderca IN, Dong X, Qian C, Murphy LM et al. Mutational spectrum of beta-catenin, AXIN1, and AXIN2 in hepatocellular carcinomas and hepatoblastomas. *Oncogene* 2002; 21(31): 4863–71.

104. Jeng YM, Wu MZ, Mao TL, Chang MH, Hsu HC. Somatic mutations of beta-catenin play a crucial role in the tumorigenesis of sporadic hepatoblastoma. *Cancer Lett* 2000; 152(1): 45–51.

105. Han ZG. Mutational landscape of hepatoblastoma goes beyond the Wnt-beta-catenin pathway. *Hepatology* 2014; 60(5): 1476–8.

106. Cairo S, Armengol C, De Reynies A, Wei Y, Thomas E, Renard CA et al. Hepatic stem-like phenotype and interplay of Wnt/beta-catenin and Myc signaling in aggressive childhood liver cancer. *Cancer Cell* 2008; 14(6): 471–84.

107. Gray SG, Eriksson T, Ekstrom C, Holm S, von Schweinitz D, Kogner P et al. Altered expression of members of the IGF-axis in hepatoblastomas. *Br J Cancer* 2000; 82(9): 1561–7.

108. Li X, Kogner P, Sandstedt B, Haas OA, Ekstrom TJ. Promoter-specific methylation and expression alterations of igf2 and h19 are involved in human hepatoblastoma. *Int J Cancer* 1998; 75(2): 176–80.

109. Sugawara W, Haruta M, Sasaki F, Watanabe N, Tsunematsu Y, Kikuta A et al. Promoter hypermethylation of the RASSF1A gene predicts the poor outcome of patients with hepatoblastoma. *Pediatr Blood Cancer* 2007; 49(3): 240–9.

110. Honda S, Haruta M, Sugawara W, Sasaki F, Ohira M, Matsunaga T et al. The methylation status of RASSF1A promoter predicts responsiveness to chemotherapy and eventual cure in hepatoblastoma patients. *Int J Cancer* 2008; 123(5): 1117–25.

111. Adesina AM, Lopez-Terrada D, Wong KK, Gunaratne P, Nguyen Y, Pulliam J et al. Gene expression profiling reveals signatures characterizing histologic subtypes of hepatoblastoma and global deregulation in cell growth and survival pathways. *Hum Pathol* 2009; 40(6): 843–53.

112. Litten JB, Chen TT, Schultz R, Herman K, Comstock J, Schiffman J et al. Activated NOTCH2 is overexpressed in hepatoblastomas: An immunohistochemical study. *Pediatr Dev Pathol* 2011; 14(5): 378–83.

113. Tomlinson GE, Douglass EC, Pollock BH, Finegold MJ, Schneider NR. Cytogenetic evaluation of a large series of hepatoblastomas: Numerical abnormalities with recurring aberrations involving 1q12-q21. *Genes Chromosomes Cancer* 2005; 44(2): 177–84.

114. Gil-Garcia B, Baladron V. The complex role of NOTCH receptors and their ligands in the development of hepatoblastoma, cholangiocarcinoma and hepatocellular carcinoma. *Biol Cell* 2016; 108(2): 29–40.

115. Hwang SJ, Luo JC, Li CP, Chu CW, Wu JC, Lai CR et al. Thrombocytosis: A paraneoplastic syndrome in patients with hepatocellular carcinoma. *World J Gastroenterol* 2004; 10(17): 2472–7.

116. Komura E, Matsumura T, Kato T, Tahara T, Tsunoda Y, Sawada T. Thrombopoietin in patients with hepatoblastoma. *Stem Cells* 1998; 16(5): 329–33.

117. Grunewald T, von Luettichau I, Welsch U, Dorr H, Hopner F, Kovacs K et al. First report of combined ectopic ACTH-syndrome and PTHrP-induced hypercalcemia due to a hepatoblastoma. *Eur J Endocrinol* 2010; 162(4): 813–8.

118. Watanabe I, Yamaguchi M, Kasai M. Histologic characteristics of gonadotropin-producing hepatoblastoma: A survey of seven cases from Japan. *J Pediatr Surg* 1987; 22(5): 406–11.

119. Blohm ME, Vesterling-Horner D, Calaminus G, Gobel U. Alpha 1-fetoprotein (AFP) reference values in infants up to 2 years of age. *Pediatr Hematol Oncol* 1998; 15(2): 135–42.

120. Meyers RL, Tiao G, de Ville de Goyet J, Superina R, Aronson DC. Hepatoblastoma state of the art: Pre-treatment extent of disease, surgical resection guidelines and the role of liver transplantation. *Curr Opin Pediatr* 2014; 26(1): 29–36.

121. McCarville MB, Kao SC. Imaging recommendations for malignant liver neoplasms in children. *Pediatr Blood Cancer* 2006; 46(1): 2–7.

122. Mody RJ, Pohlen JA, Malde S, Strouse PJ, Shulkin BL. FDG PET for the study of primary hepatic malignancies in children. *Pediatr Blood Cancer* 2006; 47(1): 51–5.

123. Cistaro A, Treglia G, Pagano M, Fania P, Bova V, Basso ME et al. A comparison between (1)(8)F-FDG PET/CT imaging and biological and radiological findings in restaging of hepatoblastoma patients. *Biomed Res Int* 2013; 2013: 709037.

124. Roebuck DJ, Aronson D, Clapuyt P, Czauderna P, de Ville de Goyet J, Gauthier F et al. 2005 PRETEXT: A revised staging system for primary malignant liver tumours of childhood developed by the SIOPEL group. *Pediatr Radiol* 2007; 37(2): 123–32; quiz 249–50.

125. Brown J, Perilongo G, Shafford E, Keeling J, Pritchard J, Brock P et al. Pretreatment prognostic factors for children with hepatoblastoma—Results from the International Society of Paediatric Oncology (SIOP) study SIOPEL 1. *Eur J Cancer* 2000; 36(11): 1418–25.

126. Meyers RL, Rowland JR, Krailo M, Chen Z, Katzenstein HM, Malogolowkin MH. Predictive power of pretreatment prognostic factors in children with hepatoblastoma: A report from the Children's Oncology Group. *Pediatr Blood Cancer* 2009; 53(6): 1016–22.

127. Ortega JA, Douglass EC, Feusner JH, Reynolds M, Quinn JJ, Finegold MJ et al. Randomized comparison of cisplatin/vincristine/fluorouracil and cisplatin/continuous infusion doxorubicin for treatment of pediatric hepatoblastoma: A report from the Children's Cancer Group and the Pediatric Oncology Group. *J Clin Oncol* 2000; 18(14): 2665–75.

128. Pritchard J, Brown J, Shafford E, Perilongo G, Brock P, Dicks-Mireaux C et al. Cisplatin, doxorubicin, and delayed surgery for childhood hepatoblastoma: A successful approach—Results of the first prospective study of the International Society of Pediatric Oncology. *J Clin Oncol* 2000; 18(22): 3819–28.

129. Zsiros J, Maibach R, Shafford E, Brugieres L, Brock P, Czauderna P et al. Successful treatment of childhood high-risk hepatoblastoma with dose-intensive multiagent chemotherapy and surgery: Final results of the SIOPEL-3HR study. *J Clin Oncol* 2010; 28(15): 2584–90.

130. Perilongo G, Maibach R, Shafford E, Brugieres L, Brock P, Morland B et al. Cisplatin versus cisplatin plus doxorubicin for standard-risk hepatoblastoma. *N Engl J Med* 2009; 361(17): 1662–70.

131. Malogolowkin MH, Katzenstein HM, Krailo M, Chen Z, Quinn JJ, Reynolds M et al. Redefining the role of doxorubicin for the treatment of children with hepatoblastoma. *J Clin Oncol* 2008; 26(14): 2379–83.

132. Schnater JM, Aronson DC, Plaschkes J, Perilongo G, Brown J, Otte JB et al. Surgical view of the treatment of patients with hepatoblastoma: Results from the first prospective trial of the International Society of Pediatric Oncology Liver Tumor Study Group. *Cancer* 2002; 94(4): 1111–20.

133. Lovvorn HN 3rd, Ayers D, Zhao Z, Hilmes M, Prasad P, Shinall MC Jr et al. Defining hepatoblastoma responsiveness to induction therapy as measured by tumor volume and serum alpha-fetoprotein kinetics. *J Pediatr Surg* 2010; 45(1): 121–8; discussion 9.

134. Medary I, Aronson D, Cheung NK, Ghavimi F, Gerald W, La Quaglia MP. Kinetics of primary tumor regression with chemotherapy: Implications for the timing of surgery. *Ann Surg Oncol* 1996; 3(6): 521–5.

135. Otte JB. Progress in the surgical treatment of malignant liver tumors in children. *Cancer Treat Rev* 2010; 36(4): 360–71.

136. Uchiyama M, Iwafuchi M, Naito M, Yagi M, Iinuma Y, Kanada S et al. A study of therapy for pediatric hepatoblastoma: Prevention and treatment of pulmonary metastasis. *Eur J Pediatr Surg* 1999; 9(3): 142–5.

137. Meyers RL, Katzenstein HM, Krailo M, McGahren ED 3rd, Malogolowkin MH. Surgical resection of pulmonary metastatic lesions in children with hepatoblastoma. *J Pediatr Surg* 2007; 42(12): 2050–6.

138. Passmore SJ, Noblett HR, Wisheart JD, Mott MG. Prolonged survival following multiple thoracotomies for metastatic hepatoblastoma. *Med Pediatr Oncol* 1995; 24(1): 58–60.

139. Feusner JH, Krailo MD, Haas JE, Campbell JR, Lloyd DA, Ablin AR. Treatment of pulmonary metastases of initial stage I hepatoblastoma in childhood. Report from the Childrens Cancer Group. *Cancer* 1993; 71(3): 859–64.

140. Hirakawa M, Nishie A, Asayama Y, Fujita N, Ishigami K, Tajiri T et al. Efficacy of preoperative transcatheter arterial chemoembolization combined with systemic chemotherapy for treatment of unresectable hepatoblastoma in children. *Jpn J Radiol* 2014; 32(9): 529–36.

141. Malogolowkin MH, Stanley P, Steele DA, Ortega JA. Feasibility and toxicity of chemoembolization for children with liver tumors. *J Clin Oncol* 2000; 18(6): 1279–84.

142. Han YM, Park HH, Lee JM, Kim JC, Hwang PH, Lee DK et al. Effectiveness of preoperative transarterial chemoembolization in presumed inoperable hepatoblastoma. *J Vasc Interv Radiol* 1999; 10(9): 1275–80.

143. Li JP, Chu JP, Yang JY, Chen W, Wang Y, Huang YH. Preoperative transcatheter selective arterial chemoembolization in treatment of unresectable hepatoblastoma in infants and children. *Cardiovasc Intervent Radiol* 2008; 31(6): 1117–23.

144. Xuewu J, Jianhong L, Xianliang H, Zhongxian C. Combined treatment of hepatoblastoma with transcatheter arterial chemoembolization and surgery. *Pediatr Hematol Oncol* 2006; 23(1): 1–9.

145. Oue T, Fukuzawa M, Kusafuka T, Kohmoto Y, Okada A, Imura K. Transcatheter arterial chemoembolization in the treatment of hepatoblastoma. *J Pediatr Surg* 1998; 33(12): 1771–5.

146. Bomgaars LR, Bernstein M, Krailo M, Kadota R, Das S, Chen Z et al. Phase II trial of irinotecan in children with refractory solid tumors: A Children's Oncology Group Study. *J Clin Oncol* 2007; 25(29): 4622–7.

147. Qayed M, Powell C, Morgan ER, Haugen M, Katzenstein HM. Irinotecan as maintenance therapy in high-risk hepatoblastoma. *Pediatr Blood Cancer* 2010; 54(5): 761–3.

148. Ijichi O, Ishikawa S, Shinkoda Y, Tanabe T, Okamoto Y, Takamatsu H et al. Response of heavily treated and relapsed hepatoblastoma in the transplanted liver to single-agent therapy with irinotecan. *Pediatr Transplant* 2006; 10(5): 635–8.

149. Palmer RD, Williams DM. Dramatic response of multiply relapsed hepatoblastoma to irinotecan (CPT-11). *Med Pediatr Oncol* 2003; 41(1): 78–80.

150. Warmann SW, Armeanu S, Heigoldt H, Ruck P, Vonthein R, Heitmann H et al. Adenovirus-mediated cytosine deaminase/5-fluorocytosine suicide gene therapy of human hepatoblastoma in vitro. *Pediatr Blood Cancer* 2009; 53(2): 145–51.

151. Berger M, Neth O, Ilmer M, Garnier A, Salinas-Martin MV, de Agustin Asencio JC et al. Hepatoblastoma cells express truncated neurokinin-1 receptor and can be growth inhibited by aprepitant in vitro and in vivo. *J Hepatol* 2014; 60(5): 985–94.

152. Ilmer M, Garnier A, Vykoukal J, Alt E, von Schweinitz D, Kappler R et al. Targeting the neurokinin-1 receptor compromises canonical Wnt signaling in hepatoblastoma. *Mol Cancer Ther* 2015; 14(12): 2712–21.

153. Waters AM, Stewart JE, Atigadda VR, Mroczek-Musulman E, Muccio DD, Grubbs CJ et al. Pre-clinical evaluation of UAB30 in pediatric renal and hepatic malignancies. *Mol Cancer Ther* 2016; 15(5): 911–921.

154. Beckwith JB, Palmer NF. Histopathology and prognosis of Wilms tumors: Results from the First National Wilms' Tumor Study. *Cancer* 1978; 41(5): 1937–48.

155. Trobaugh-Lotrario AD, Finegold MJ, Feusner JH. Rhabdoid tumors of the liver: Rare, aggressive, and poorly responsive to standard cytotoxic chemotherapy. *Pediatr Blood Cancer* 2011; 57(3): 423–8.

156. Yuri T, Danbara N, Shikata N, Fujimoto S, Nakano T, Sakaida N et al. Malignant rhabdoid tumor of the liver: Case report and literature review. *Pathol Int* 2004; 54(8): 623–9.

157. Wagner LM, Garrett JK, Ballard ET, Hill DA, Perry A, Biegel JA et al. Malignant rhabdoid tumor mimicking hepatoblastoma: A case report and literature review. *Pediatr Dev Pathol* 2007; 10(5): 409–15.

158. Versteege I, Sevenet N, Lange J, Rousseau-Merck MF, Ambros P, Handgretinger R et al. Truncating mutations of hSNF5/INI1 in aggressive paediatric cancer. *Nature* 1998; 394(6689): 203–6.

159. Hollmann TJ, Hornick JL. INI1-deficient tumors: Diagnostic features and molecular genetics. *Am J Surg Pathol* 2011; 35(10): e47–63.

160. Ravindra KV, Cullinane C, Lewis IJ, Squire BR, Stringer MD. Long-term survival after spontaneous rupture of a malignant rhabdoid tumor of the liver. *J Pediatr Surg* 2002; 37(10): 1488–90.

161. Jayaram A, Finegold MJ, Parham DM, Jasty R. Successful management of rhabdoid tumor of the liver. *J Pediatr Hematol Oncol* 2007; 29(6): 406–8.

162. Cruz O, Laguna A, Vancells M, Krauel L, Medina M, Mora J. Fibrolamellar hepatocellular carcinoma in an infant and literature review. *J Pediatr Hematol Oncol* 2008; 30(12): 968–71.

163. Honeyman JN, Simon EP, Robine N, Chiaroni-Clarke R, Darcy DG, Lim, II et al. Detection of a recurrent DNAJB1-PRKACA chimeric transcript in fibrolamellar hepatocellular carcinoma. *Science* 2014; 343(6174): 1010–4.

164. Darcy DG, Chiaroni-Clarke R, Murphy JM, Honeyman JN, Bhanot U, LaQuaglia MP et al. The genomic landscape of fibrolamellar hepatocellular carcinoma: Whole genome sequencing of ten patients. *Oncotarget* 2015; 6(2): 755–70.

165. Lim, II, Farber BA, LaQuaglia MP. Advances in fibrolamellar hepatocellular carcinoma: A review. *Eur J Pediatr Surg* 2014; 24(6): 461–6.

166. Simon EP, Freije CA, Farber BA, Lalazar G, Darcy DG, Honeyman JN et al. Transcriptomic characterization of fibrolamellar hepatocellular carcinoma. *Proc Natl Acad Sci U S A* 2015; 112(44): E5916–25.

167. Suita S, Shono K, Tajiri T, Takamatsu T, Mizote H, Nagasaki A et al. Malignant germ cell tumors: Clinical characteristics, treatment, and outcome. A report from the study group for Pediatric Solid Malignant Tumors in the Kyushu Area, Japan. *J Pediatr Surg* 2002; 37(12): 1703–6.

168. Isaacs H Jr. Perinatal (fetal and neonatal) germ cell tumors. *J Pediatr Surg* 2004; 39(7): 1003–13.

169. Yoon JM, Burns RC, Malogolowkin MH, Mascarenhas L. Treatment of infantile choriocarcinoma of the liver. *Pediatr Blood Cancer* 2007; 49(1): 99–102.

170. Moon WK, Kim WS, Kim IO, Hong JH, Yeon KM, Han MC et al. Hepatic choriocarcinoma in a neonate: MR appearance. *J Comput Assist Tomogr* 1993; 17(4): 653–5.

171. Belchis DA, Mowry J, Davis JH. Infantile choriocarcinoma. Re-examination of a potentially curable entity. *Cancer* 1993; 72(6): 2028–32.

172. Picton SV, Bose-Haider B, Lendon M, Hancock BW, Campbell RH. Simultaneous choriocarcinoma in mother and newborn infant. *Med Pediatr Oncol* 1995; 25(6): 475–8.

173. Bolze PA, Weber B, Fisher RA, Seckl MJ, Golfier F. First confirmation by genotyping of transplacental choriocarcinoma transmission. *Am J Obstet Gynecol* 2013; 209(4): e4–6.

174. Witzleben CL, Bruninga G. Infantile choriocarcinoma: A characteristic syndrome. *J Pediatr* 1968; 73(3): 374–8.

175. Johnson EJ, Crofton PM, O'Neill JM, Wilkinson AG, McKenzie KJ, Munro FD et al. Infantile choriocarcinoma treated with chemotherapy alone. *Med Pediatr Oncol* 2003; 41(6): 550–7.

176. Mailly N, Delord JP, Dubois A, Gandia P. [Metastatic placental choriocarcinoma to mother and newborn: A case report]. *J Radiol* 2008; 89(4): 517–20.

177. Fraser GC, Blair GK, Hemming A, Murphy JJ, Rogers P. The treatment of simultaneous choriocarcinoma in mother and baby. *J Pediatr Surg* 1992; 27(10): 1318–9.

178. Szavay PO, Wermes C, Fuchs J, Schrappe M, Flemming P, von Schweinitz D. Effective treatment of infantile choriocarcinoma in the liver with chemotherapy and surgical resection: A case report. *J Pediatr Surg* 2000; 35(7): 1134–5.

179. Heath JA, Tiedemann K. Successful management of neonatal choriocarcinoma. *Med Pediatr Oncol* 2001; 36(4): 497–9.

180. Blohm ME, Gobel U. Unexplained anaemia and failure to thrive as initial symptoms of infantile choriocarcinoma: A review. *Eur J Pediatr* 2004; 163(1): 1–6.

181. Blohm ME, Calaminus G, Gnekow AK, Heidemann PH, Bolkenius M, Weinel P et al. Disseminated choriocarcinoma in infancy is curable by chemotherapy and delayed tumour resection. *Eur J Cancer* 2001; 37(1): 72–8.

182. Todani T, Tabuchi K, Watanabe Y, Tsutsumi A. True hepatic teratoma with high alpha fetoprotein in serum. *J Pediatr Surg* 1977; 12(4): 591–2.

183. Kraudel K, Williams CH. Ultrasound case report of hepatic teratoma in newborn. *J Clin Ultrasound* 1984; 12(2): 98–101.

184. Witte DP, Kissane JM, Askin FB. Hepatic teratomas in children. *Pediatr Pathol* 1983; 1(1): 81–92.

185. Tapper D, Lack EE. Teratomas in infancy and childhood. A 54-year experience at the Children's Hospital Medical Center. *Ann Surg* 1983; 198(3): 398–410.

186. Spiess PE, Kassouf W, Brown GA, Kamat AM, Liu P, Gomez JA et al. Surgical management of growing teratoma syndrome: The M. D. Anderson cancer center experience. *J Urol* 2007; 177(4): 1330–4; discussion 4.

187. Jeffery GM, Theaker JM, Lee AH, Blaquiere RM, Smart CJ, Mead GM. The growing teratoma syndrome. *Br J Urol* 1991; 67(2): 195–202.

188. Littooij AS, McHugh K, McCarville MB, Sebire NJ, Bahrami A, Roebuck DJ. Yolk sac tumour: A rare cause of raised serum alpha-foetoprotein in a young child with a large liver mass. *Pediatr Radiol* 2014; 44(1): 18–22.

189. Blumgart LH. *Surgery of the Liver, Biliary Tract and Pancreas*, 4th edn. Philadelphia, PA, USA: Saunders Elsevier, 2007.

190. Wheatley JM, Rosenfield NS, Berger L, LaQuaglia MP. Liver regeneration in children after major hepatectomy for malignancy—Evaluation using a computer-aided technique of volume measurement. *J Surg Res* 1996; 61(1): 183–9.

191. Guerin F, Gauthier F, Martelli H, Fabre M, Baujard C, Franchi S et al. Outcome of central hepatectomy for hepatoblastomas. *J Pediatr Surg* 2010; 45(3): 555–63.

192. Couinaud C. [The anatomy of the liver]. *Ann Ital Chir* 1992; 63(6): 693–7.

193. Fong Y, Brennan MF, Brown K, Heffernan N, Blumgart LH. Drainage is unnecessary after elective liver resection. *Am J Surg* 1996; 171(1): 158–62.

94

Congenital mesoblastic nephroma and Wilms tumor

PHILIP J. HAMMOND AND ROBERT CARACHI

INTRODUCTION

Congenital mesoblastic nephroma (CMN), first described by Kastner in 1921,[1] is the most common renal tumor in the neonate, although rare cases present in later childhood. It is also known as a fetal renal hamartoma, mesenchymal hamartoma of infancy, or lipomyomatous hamartoma. It has an incidence of 2.8% of all renal tumors of childhood, with a mean age of presentation of 3.4 months, in contrast to an average age of 3 years in Wilms tumors.[2] It has been documented as being 22.8% of all primary tumors in children 1 year old or less.[3] A neoplasm in the kidney of a child less than 3 months old is usually a CMN. The majority of renal neoplasms originating in the fetus and found during the first weeks of life differ in structure and in biological behavior from a nephroblastoma. In contrast to cystic lesions of the kidney, solid renal neoplasms are rare in the newborn and account for only 8% of neonatal tumors. In the Children's Cancer Group (CCG) neonatal study, there were 25 neonatal renal neoplasms, of which 17 were CMN and the rest were Wilms tumors.[4] A review of neonatal Wilms tumors in the national Wilms tumor register identified 15 cases out of 6832 patients with an incidence of 0.16%, demonstrating how rare malignant renal neoplasms are in neonates. Although prenatal ultrasound is capable of detecting renal neoplasms in utero, there is no specific sonographic characteristic that can differentiate a CMN from a Wilms tumor. Both tumors present as a palpable abdominal mass in the neonate. Males outnumber females two to one with CMN, and both sexes are equally affected by Wilms tumors.

PATHOLOGY AND CYTOGENETICS

Bolande and associates,[5] in 1967, recognized CMN as a unique lesion that could be distinguished clinically and pathologically from true congenital Wilms tumor by its benign clinical behavior, a preponderance of mesenchymal derivatives, and lack of the malignant epithelial components typical of Wilms tumor. A definite infiltrative tendency distinguishes CMN from hamartomas with more limited growth potential. CMN is usually solid and unilateral and can attain a very large size like a uterine fibroid.

Histological differentiation is that of a spindle cell neoplasm with interlacing bundles of fibroblasts and myofibroblasts. Tumor types have irregular interdigitating margins in the perirenal fat, and wide margins of excision are desirable for complete removal. Incomplete removal results in tumor recurrence, which happens within a year of resection in most instances. No chemotherapy or radiotherapy is indicated here, and a wide surgical resection is the treatment of choice.[6]

Atypical and more aggressive mesoblastic nephromas tend to be soft, fleshy tumors with areas of gross hemorrhage and necrosis and are more cellular without recognizable normal glomeruli or tubules.

Another variant is congenital cystic mesoblastic nephroma (cellular variant), which can present as a unilocular hemorrhagic cyst. This can be detected antenatally and misdiagnosed as a hemorrhage into the kidney. The lining of the wall of this cyst shows a typical cellular rim comprising mitotically active small round and spindle-shaped cells, giving the diagnosis of CMN.[7] The treatment for this tumor is surgical.

Gaillard and colleagues[8] recently reported pathological and molecular characteristics of CMN in 35 cases. Based on cellular criteria, 14 were classified as classical, 4 as partly cellular, and 17 as cellular CMN. The mean ages were 24, 11, and 70 days, respectively. There were 13 intrarenal tumors (stage I), but 9 classical, 3 partly cellular, and 5 cellular CMNs extended to the perirenal fat (stage II), and 5 cellular tumors ruptured (stage III). In order to assess cellular proliferative activity, silver staining of nucleolar organizer region (Ag-NOR) proteins was performed on 19 CMNs. The number of Ag-NOR dots per cell was significantly lower in classical and partly cellular CMN than in cellular CMN,

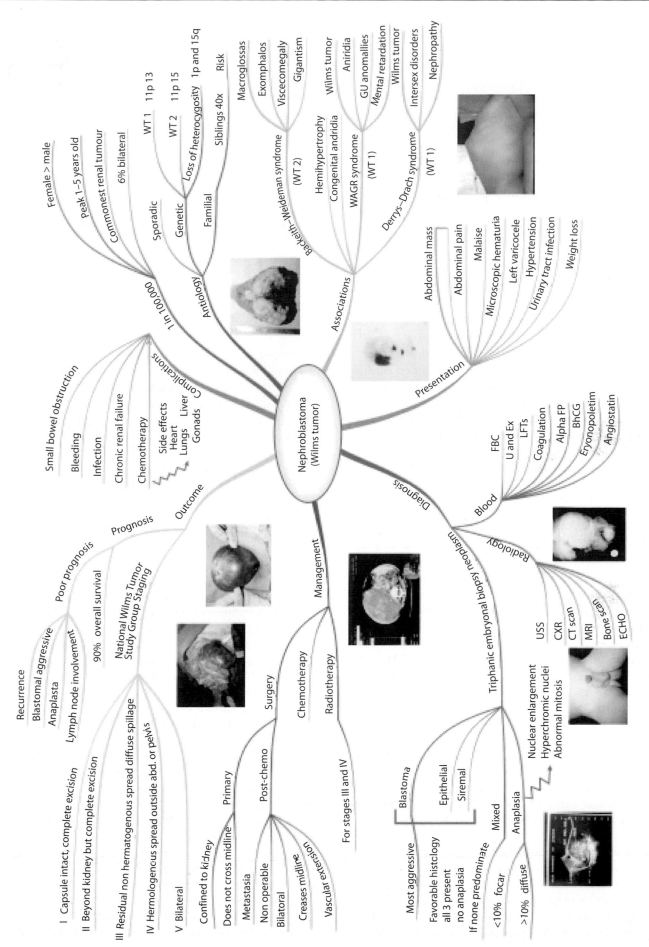

Figure 94.1 Mind map. (From *Practical Problems in Pediatric Surgery—An Atlas and Mind Maps*, Eds. R. Keilani et al., Jaypee Brothers, ISBN 978 81 8448 723 7.)

whatever the stage. Within the cellular CMNs, the mean number of Ag-NOR dots was statistically higher in the single case that recurred with fatal outcome. The number of Ag-NOR dots, DNA content measurements, the histological subclassification, and the presence or absence of tumor at the surgical margins may be useful features in selecting those patients who will benefit from further treatment after nephrectomy.

A characteristic chromosomal translocation, t(12;15)(p13;q25), has been described that results in fusion of the ETV6 (TEL) gene from 12p13 with the NRTK3 neurtrophin-3 receptor gene (TRKC) from 15q25. This results in a chimeric RNA, which is characteristic of both infantile fibrosarcoma and the cellular variant of congenital meroblastic nephroma. This suggests a close relation between these two conditions.[9]

Human epidermal growth factor receptors (HER) play a critical role in the branching morphogenesis of renal tubules. In addition, HER2 expression in Wilms tumor has been assessed, and its role in tumorgenesis has been established. Amplification and overexpression increase the metastatic potential of a tumor and promote chemoresistance.[10]

It has been reported that abnormal renin production and hypertension are common features of CMN. Several investigators have reported distinctive patterns of immunoreactive renin staining, suggesting that mesoblastic nephromas are a source of increased renin production, producing hypertension.[11,12] The most intense staining for renin was observed within areas of recognizable cortex trapped within the tumor. Renin was localized in cells in the walls of vessels running up to the glomeruli.

CLINICAL FEATURES

The newborn usually presents with a large, nontender abdominal mass. Maternal polyhydramnios and prematurity are frequently seen, although the reason for this is unclear. Male-to-female ratio ranges from 1.8:1 to 3:1.[6,12] Hypertension has been recognized as a presenting feature, and there is an association between preoperative hypertension and cardiac arrest during surgery.[6] Some patients present with hematuria. In the congenital cystic mesoblastic nephroma variant, the patient may present with a hemorrhagic problem. Recently, mind maps have been introduced to explain in a didactic fashion the clinical features, investigations, differential diagnosis, and management of CMN and Wilms tumor (Figure 94.1).

Detailed antenatal ultrasound scans may pick up a solid tumor of the kidney. Plain films of the abdomen show a large, soft-tissue abdominal mass that is rarely calcified. Sonography demonstrates the solid nature and renal origin of the mass and most commonly shows a mixed echogenic intrarenal mass (Figure 94.2a and b). CMN should easily be distinguished from more common renal masses in the newborn[13]—hydronephrosis or multicystic kidney—which are sonolucent. Magnetic resonance imaging (MRI) scans give detailed imaging of the renal tumor and its surrounding structures.

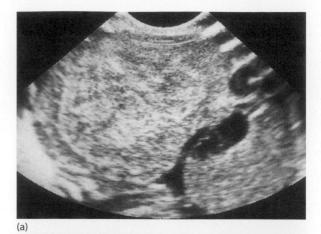
(a)

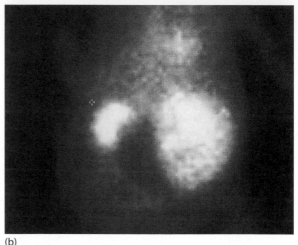
(b)

Figure 94.2 **(a)** Sonography demonstrates a mixed echogenic mass. **(b)** ^{99m}Tc-DTPA renal scintigraphy shows function within the mass in the kidney.

TREATMENT

Nephrectomy of this benign tumor is curative without the need for supplementary radiation or adjuvant chemotherapy. Even when there has been intraoperative rupture, excisional surgery is curative, and local recurrence is rare. Distant metastasis has been reported but is extremely uncommon.[14] A review of 38 patients with the cellular variant of mesoblastic nephroma showed that 7 children had recurrence and 3 died. According to them, pathologically positive surgical margins were the only statistically significant predictor of recurrent disease. Frozen section may help in obtaining tumor-free margins during surgery. Recent studies on molecular biology may shed further light on tumor behavior and add criteria for further therapy after surgery.

PREOPERATIVE PREPARATION

Blood samples are obtained for a full blood count, group, and crossmatch. Tumor markers renin, active renin, and inactive renin should also be assayed because these tumors have been documented as producing high levels of these hormones.[12] Erythropoietin levels should also be assayed. Careful monitoring and control of blood pressure is required to prevent dangerous perioperative fluctuations. A central venous cannula for intravenous infusion is inserted into the neck vein or subclavian vein as well as an arterial cannula to monitor blood pressure.

OPERATIVE TECHNIQUE

Position

The patient is placed supine with a roll under the lumbar spine to create a lordosis.

Incision

An upper transverse muscle-cutting incision from the flank across the midline provides adequate exposure (Figure 94.3a).

LAPAROTOMY AND EXPOSURE OF THE RENAL PEDICLE

The abdomen is entered, taking care not to cut into the tumor while incising the abdominal wall muscles. The small intestine is displaced toward the opposite side and covered with moist packs. The liver and the opposite kidney are inspected for the presence of any other disease. This is very rare in this condition. Free fluid is sampled and sent for cytology.

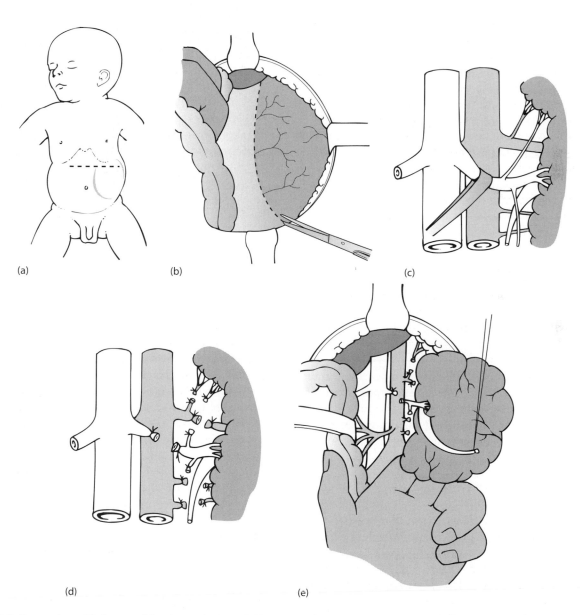

(a)   (b)   (c)

(d)   (e)

Figure 94.3 Resection of left mesoblastic nephroma: **(a)** incision; **(b)** colon retracted medially and posterior peritoneum incised; **(c)** ureter, gonadal vessels, and renal vessels identified; **(d)** ureter and gonadal vessels ligated and divided—followed by ligation and division of renal vein and artery; **(e)** tumor removed from the posterior abdominal wall using sharp and blunt dissection.

The colon overlying the tumor is retracted medially, and the posterior peritoneum lateral to the colon is incised and reflected forward to the midline (Figure 94.3b). Tumor handling should be minimized in hypertensive patients to prevent excessive release of renin. The inferior vena cava and renal veins are both palpated for the presence of tumor. The ureter is identified (Figure 94.3c), and a tape is passed around it. It is traced as far down as possible into the pelvis, ligated with 3-0 chromic catgut, and divided. Next, the gonadal vessels are ligated and divided. Before mobilization of the tumor, abdominal packs are used to isolate the operative site from the rest of the abdominal cavity. This is to prevent any dissemination of tumor if there is spillage during the time of surgery. The renal vein is doubly ligated and divided (Figure 94.3d). The renal artery is exposed and transfixed with nonabsorbable sutures. The para-aortic lymph glands, together with surrounding tissue, are dissected off the aorta and inferior vena cava and labeled carefully. The tumor is removed from the posterior abdominal wall using finger dissection (Figure 94.3e). The excised specimen should contain the kidney, Gerota fascia, fat from the lumbar fossa, and para-aortic lymph glands.

After removal of the tumor, hemostasis is obtained with diathermy coagulation or suture ligatures. No drainage is usually required.

POSTOPERATIVE CARE

Postoperative recovery following resection of mesoblastic nephroma is rapid. Nephrectomy of this benign tumor is curative. If on histology, the tumor is found to be Wilms, it should be treated in accordance with the degree of involvement as outlined in the National Wilms Tumor Study programs.

COMPLICATIONS

The main complication of CMN is rupture of the tumor during surgery. Howell and colleagues[6] reported intraoperative rupture in 20% of their cases. In practice, this is extremely rare despite intraoperative rupture; excellent subsequent relapse-free survival has been reported with this tumor.

REFERENCES

1. Kastner. Nierensarckon ber einem siebenmonatlichen. *Fotus Ztschn Path* 1921; 25: 1.
2. Crom DB, Wilimas HA, Green AA et al. Malignancy in the neonate. *Med Pediatr Oncol* 1989; 17: 101–04.
3. Campbell AN, Chan HSL, O'Brien A et al. Malignant tumours in the neonate. *Arch Dis Child* 1987; 62: 19–23.
4. Ritchey ML, Azizkhan RG, Beckwith JB et al. Neonatal Wilms' tumour. *J Pediatr Surg* 1995; 30: 856–9.
5. Bolande RP, Brough AJ, Izant RJ. Congenital mesoblastic nephroma of infancy. A report of 8 cases and the relationship to Wilms' tumour. *Pediatrics* 1967; 40: 272–8.
6. Howell CG, Otherson HB, Kiviat NE et al. Therapy and outcome in 51 children with mesoblastic nephroma. A report of the National Wilms' Tumour Study. *J Pediatr Surg* 1982; 17: 826–31.
7. Murthi S, Carachi R, Howatson A. Congenital cystic mesoblastic nephroma (cellular variant), (unilocular, haemorrhagic). Personal communication.
8. Gaillard D, Bouvier R, Sonsino E et al. Nucleolar organizer regions in congenital mesoblastic nephroma. *Pediatr Pathol* 1992; 12: 811–21.
9. Shamberger R. Renal tumors. In: Carachi R., Grosfeld JL., Azmy AF (eds). *The Surgery of Childhood Tumors*, 2nd edn. Chapter 10, pp. 171–200. Berlin: Springer.
10. Salem M, Kinoshita Y, Tajiri T et al. Association between the HER2 expression and histological differentiation in Wilms tumor. *Pediatr Surg Int* 2006; 22: 891–6.
11. Yokomori K, Hori T, Takemura T et al. Demonstration of both primary and secondary reninism in renal tumours in children. *J Pediatr Surg* 1988; 23: 403–9.
12. Malone PS, Duffy PG, Ransley PG et al. Congenital mesoblastic nephroma, renin production and hypertension. *J Pediatr Surg* 1989; 24: 599–600.
13. Kirks DR, Kaufman RA. Function with mesoblastic nephroma: Imaging–Pathologic correlation. *Pediatr Radiol* 1989; 19: 136–9.
14. Heidelberger KP, Ritchy ML, Dauser RC et al. Congenital mesoblastic nephroma metastatic to brain. *Cancer* 1993; 72: 2499–505.

95

Neonatal ovarian masses

RACHAEL L. POLIS, MARY E. FALLAT, AND CHAD WIESENAUER

INTRODUCTION

Ultrasound examination, both pre- and postnatal, has made it possible for clinicians to recognize perinatal ovarian cysts and other intra-abdominal masses for decades. True neoplasms are rare, simple ovarian cysts are common, and large or complex cysts often demand surgical attention. A variety of approaches including aspiration (both pre- and postnatal), surgical removal, or observation have been proposed and are acceptable depending on the radiographic and clinical circumstances.

ETIOLOGY

Although not fully understood, it is widely believed that ovarian cysts derive from ovarian follicles. Mature follicles can be found in up to 60% of newborn ovaries. Fetal follicle-stimulating hormone (FSH), fetal luteinizing hormone (LH), estrogens (maternal, placental and fetal), and placental human chorionic gonadotropin (HCG) all stimulate the ovarian follicle.[1-3] There is a higher incidence of larger ovarian cysts in infants born to mothers with diabetes, Rh isoimmunization, and preeclampsia due to the association with higher releases of placental chorionic gonadotropin.[4] Akin et al.[5] reviewed 20 cases of ovarian cysts diagnosed antenatally and 5 mothers had gestational diabetes, 2 had preeclampsia, 1 patient had Rh incompatibility without hydrops, and polyhydramnios was present in all cases. Follicular cysts have also been described in maternal and congenital hypothyroidism secondary to nonspecific pituitary glycoprotein hormone synthesis.[4]

At birth, HCG and estrogen levels fall precipitously, leaving only the fetal pituitary gonadotropins LH and FSH to stimulate or maintain the ovarian follicle. The newborn hypothalamus and pituitary become sensitive to negative feedback by about 4–6 months of age, decreasing secretion of LH and FSH. By this time, most if not all stimulation of the ovarian follicle halts, and fetal cysts should involute.

Simple ovarian cysts are known to resolve spontaneously in most cases by 1–6 months.[1,6-8]

An alternative theory has been proposed by Enriquez et al.[9] in which abnormal development of the primitive gonad, and not just hormonal stimulation, is the root cause of fetal cyst formation. Cyst formation becomes a consequence of germinal epithelial secretion in a dysgenetic gonad. The prevalence of ovarian cysts would argue against this being the primary mechanism.

Incidence

The normal newborn ovary will exhibit several scattered anechoic cysts from 4 to 5 mm in diameter. More than 80% of newborn ovaries will have ovarian cysts <9 mm in diameter, whereas cysts >9 mm occur in 20%–34% of ovaries.[10] There is general consensus that newborn cysts less than 2 cm in maximal diameter are considered normal and unlikely to cause problems.[1,5]

Torsion

Torsion is believed to occur when a relatively large, mobile mass twists on a long, thin pedicle. Many authors consider cysts of diameter greater than 4 or 5 cm at high risk for complications, most commonly torsion.[1,6-8,10-12] Other authors use a more conservative diameter of 2.0 cm to direct management.[13] Complex heterogeneous ovarian cysts are more likely to represent torsion of the cyst and the ovary, and autoamputation is possible.[13-15]

PATHOLOGY

Pathologic examination, possible only if surgical removal is performed, will often confirm the diagnosis of an ovarian cyst. The vast majority of cysts are of follicular origin. Torsed ovaries will have suffered a variable period of ischemia, so examination may not reveal any identifiable ovarian follicles or parenchyma. Tumors are rare in the newborn, but careful examination of the literature reveals examples. In what appears to be the most extensive review in the English language of 257 antenatally diagnosed ovarian cysts, Brandt et al.[1] reported 3 cystadenomas and 2 teratomas out of 170 surgically removed ovaries. Three other authors have reported antenatally diagnosed tumors including two germ cell tumors, one teratoma, and one serous cystadenoma.[13,16,17] There exist two reports of ovarian carcinomas found at fetal autopsy. These were bilateral ovarian cancer in a 30-week gestation fetus, and a granulosa cell carcinoma in a stillborn fetus.[18,19] Juvenile granulosa cell tumor, a tumor that may be considered malignant due to its aggressive potential, is described in children less than 7 months of age in three reports.[20–22] Finally, there exist reports of one endodermal sinus tumor and one teratoma in children under 1 year of age.[23]

HISTORY AND PHYSICAL EXAMINATION

Most newborns with ovarian cysts will have a normal physical examination at birth. Since the ovary is an intra-abdominal organ in an infant, large cysts will displace the intestinal tract and present as palpable, but generally nontender, masses. These infants rarely have signs of intestinal obstruction or hydronephrosis due to compression of the ureters if the mass reaches substantial size.[5]

PRESENTATION

Most neonatal ovarian cysts are first diagnosed at prenatal ultrasound. Their appearance is almost exclusively in the third trimester, at around 28 weeks gestational age.

DIAGNOSIS

Ultrasound is the modality of choice for both the infant and the mother, being quick, relatively inexpensive, and safe, compared to other imaging modalities. Magnetic resonance imaging has been proposed as more reliable by some authors,[24] but discounted by others,[25] based on expense and potential need for sedation. The basic criteria for ultrasound diagnosis are as follows: (1) cystic structure in the lower or lateral abdomen and (2) normal urinary and gastrointestinal tracts.[25] Differential diagnoses include urachal cyst, enteric duplication, hydrometrocolpos, choledochal cyst, renal cyst, hydronephrosis, distended bladder, meconium cyst, duodenal atresia, anterior myelomeningocele, mesenteric cyst, lymphangioma, and omental cyst, with the latter three entities being the most easily confused with ovarian cyst.[1,8,26,27]

Nussbaum et al.[28] proposed useful criteria for simple and complex ovarian cysts in 1988. Simple cysts are completely anechoic with an imperceptible cyst wall (Figure 95.1), whereas complex cysts demonstrate a fluid/debris level, have a retracting clot, are septated, or are solid (Figure 95.2). The presence of a complex heterogenous ovarian cyst with a fluid debris level can be a hallmark of ovarian torsion. Of

all "complex" cysts, Monnery-Noché et al.[13] found 89% to be torsed, with the remainder being hemorrhagic. Diagnosis or suspicion of an autoamputated ovarian cyst can be guided by the appearance of the cystic mass in different positions on postnatal ultrasound compared to prenatal ultrasound or the presence of calcifications within the cyst identified on imaging.[14]

Evolution

Prenatal and postpartum sonographic observation has allowed investigators to determine the behavior of ovarian cysts, although predictions vary by author. Anywhere from 44% to 70% of antenatally diagnosed simple cysts will convert to complex, presumably by torsion, by the time of the first postpartum ultrasound.[8,13,29–31] Five studies published between 1992 and 2008 considered simple cysts of all diameters. Some authors have correlated antenatal cyst size with risk of ovarian loss,[1,6,11] but more recent investigations have demonstrated no correlation between size and risk of ovarian loss.[13,29,30,32] The latter studies call into question the usefulness of cyst diameter in surgical decision-making.

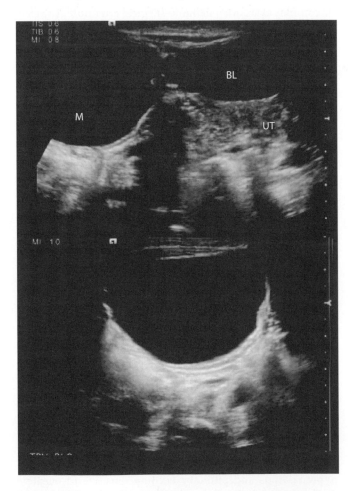

Figure 95.1   Top: Transabdominal ultrasound on day 1 of life (M = mass, BL = bladder, UT = uterus). Bottom: Same transabdominal ultrasound study with mass identified as a simple ovarian cyst measuring 4.8×3.2×4.7 cm. There is a lack of internal echoes and no perceptible cyst wall.

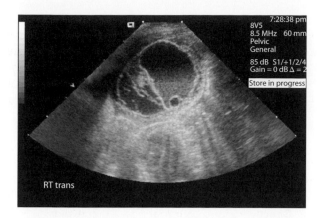

Figure 95.2 Transabdominal ultrasound of a complex ovarian cyst, 2.5 cm × 3.5 cm. Features include a relatively thick cyst wall, fluid/debris level, and multiple septations. This ovary was found to be torsed and nonviable.

Somewhat in dispute of the above prediction, simple cysts (all diameters) are also known to regress spontaneously postpartum in at least 82% of cases.[8,31] Sakala et al.[33] cite 50% resolution by 1 month, 75% by 2 months, and 90% resolution by 3 months. The remainder of these simple cysts are generally aspirated or operated upon for failure to regress in size after a period of observation.

Concerning complex cysts, three studies included 45 patients observed using serial postpartum ultrasound examinations.[8,30,31] Twenty-two followed complex cysts demonstrated regression of both the cyst and ovary at subsequent follow-up ultrasounds. Surgical removal of 15 ovaries was performed, 13 due to failed regression and 2 due to parental concern. Only eight ovaries demonstrated both cyst regression and detectable ovarian tissue.[8,30,31] Both Luzzatto et al.[8] and Foley et al.[30] noted that this occurred before 1 year of life. In cases where the complex cyst involuted and a viable ovary was not subsequently seen, it may be speculated that the gonad was torsed and necrotic and eventually resorbed spontaneously. More reports are needed to know if observation in these cases is a legitimate therapeutic option.

MANAGEMENT

The treatment of newborn ovarian cysts remains controversial. Considering only simple cysts, the majority of authors still selectively operate or aspirate (including in utero aspiration) based on a maximal diameter of 4 or 5 cm,[1,8,10,12,34–36] although other authors support close ultrasound observation for larger simple cysts with good results.[26,29,31]

As for complex cysts, a growing number of authors support ultrasound observation, with surgical treatment only if they fail to demonstrate continuous regression over time.[8,9,26,29–31,37,38] Other surgeons prefer to definitively exclude malignancy by removal of the complex ovarian cyst.[1,3,12,35] In a retrospective chart review from Papic et al.,[38] 25 asymptomatic cysts were observed including 15 complex cysts, and 6 of these had successful regression. The mean size of successfully observed complex cysts was 41 ± 16.1 mm.[38]

When failure of cyst regression occurred, the mean observation time prior to surgery was 12 weeks.[38] Complex cysts measuring ≤58 mm have been observed in the literature.[8] These complex cysts followed by ultrasonography have documented regression.[8] However, there are documented cases where no viable ovarian tissue can be identified on follow-up ultrasound imaging.[8,30,31,37] As complex cysts generally represent ovarian torsion as well, surgery would inevitably result in oophorectomy. Therefore, considering observation when ovarian regression is a possibility could preclude neonatal surgery. In a study by Papic et al.,[38] a period of observation spared about half of neonates an operation, which has relevance based on emerging data that anesthesia in the newborn period may have adverse effects on the developing brain.[39–41] See Table 95.1 for risks and benefits of early operative intervention versus observation.

Neonatal anesthesia risks

Experimental studies in animals demonstrate that exposure of the brain to a variety of anesthetic agents during developmental periods can lead to neurodegeneration or neuronal apoptosis and cause measurable functional deficits.[42–48] Flick et al.[49] concluded that exposure to multiple episodes of anesthesia, particularly during multiple surgical procedures, before the age of 2 significantly increased the risk of learning disabilities. A systematic review and meta-analysis conducted in January 2000 through February 2013 suggests a modestly elevated risk of adverse neurodevelopmental outcomes in children when exposed to anesthesia early in childhood.[40] There is a need for large, prospective observational studies and trials to investigate anesthesia effects on the developing human brain,[50] and further research is being done. It is important for clinicians to weigh the potential anesthesia risks into their management plan. Figure 95.3 outlines a surgical treatment strategy for neonatal patients with ovarian cysts modified from a study by Tajiri et al.[36]

In utero aspiration

To avoid the above-cited 44%–70% risk of in utero torsion of the simple cyst, some investigators have attempted in utero decompression.[51] Perrotin et al.[51] successfully aspirated three in utero simple cysts between 37 and 47 mm. Bagolan et al.[35] appear to have published the largest series of 14 patients without a direct technical complication in cysts measuring ≥5 cm. Of note, Bagolan et al. reported two errant prenatal diagnoses among their in utero aspirations. These masses were both hydronephrosis, and both fetuses suffered no untoward effects from these aspirations. Some would argue that these were actually technical complications.[35] Two ovaries torsed despite aspiration, making the ovarian preservation rate 86%, which is better than historic controls; however, the number of patients is small.[35] There are no recent published studies to date further investigating if in utero aspiration continues to be a viable option for management.

Table 95.1 Risks and benefits of intervention or observation

Cyst aspiration		Operative management		Observation	
Risks	Benefits	Risks	Benefits	Risks	Benefits
1. Potential of multiple aspirations if cyst recurs with associated repeated exposure to anesthesia.	1. Potential ovarian preservation.	1. Future adverse neurodevelopmental outcomes secondary to anesthesia exposure.	1. Definitive diagnosis with specimen.	1. Ovarian torsion.	1. Cyst resolves spontaneously.
2. Extended follow-up is rare and preservation of future viable ovarian tissue unknown.	2. Shorter and less invasive procedure.	2. Ovarian tissue loss due to oophorectomy.	2. Direct visualization of ovary.	2. Surgical intervention needed at a later date.	2. Avoids unnecessary surgery and exposure to anesthesia.
3. Incorrect diagnosis of an ovarian cyst with aspiration and injury to another organ system.			3. Early intervention might preclude torsion and spare ovary.	3. Patient fails to come back for follow-up. 4. No identifiable ovarian tissue on the involved side in the future.	3. Ovarian preservation.

Dera-Szymanowska et al.[52] presented a recent case report of notable recurrent complex ovarian cysts with rupture in the fetal period and recurrence of simple cysts in the neonatal period. This group suggested surgical intervention be considered postnatally and only with symptoms or in complicated cases.[52]

Postnatal aspiration

Proponents of postnatal aspiration point to maximal preservation of ovarian tissue coupled with cyst decompression to potentially prevent torsion. Also, many authors mention that the majority of operatively managed ovarian cysts involve oophorectomy, not cystectomy or fenestration, thereby removing any chance of viable ovarian tissue on the affected side. Opponents point out lack of a definitive diagnosis, i.e., risk of cancer. Kessler et al.[10] reported 17 aspirated ovarian cysts, both simple *and* complex, with a 67% ovarian preservation rate. No complications were reported, although three cysts recurred and responded to repeat aspiration. Other investigators have had similar success,[12] yet Puligandla et al. report a case whereby a proximal jejunal duplicated cyst was mistaken for ovarian pathology and aspirated. The patient was later found to have necrotic bowel secondary to a midgut volvulus, and she ultimately died.[53] Finally, Tajiri et al.[36] reported 13 cases of ultrasound-guided aspiration of cysts, one patient treated with aspiration three

times, and another undergoing the procedure twice. All 13 cases eventually had no remaining cystic lesions.[36] There was no description provided about the presence of ovarian tissue on subsequent imaging after ultrasound-guided cyst aspiration, so there may be morbidity related to the procedure itself that no one has looked for or reported.

Operative removal

The majority of large simple cysts and complex cysts are removed via laparotomy or laparoscopy. A large cyst is defined as greater than either 4 or 5 cm in maximal diameter, although at least one group operatively removed simple cysts greater than 2 cm in diameter.[13] Although the goal is always ovarian tissue preservation, more often than not, the entire ovary is removed for lack of identifiable ovarian parenchyma.[2,9,10,19,23,29,33] Fenestration of the cyst wall is an option if the cyst wall cannot safely be entirely separated from ovarian tissue. Proponents of operative removal cite this as the only method to exclude neoplasia, and also the only method that results in no chance of viable ovarian tissue on the affected side. They also cite risk of adhesive bowel obstruction as a potential complication of unremoved ovarian cysts, although this is not described even in case reports.[2,3,13]

Surgeons have come up with many creative alternatives to suprapubic laparotomy (Figure 95.4), including

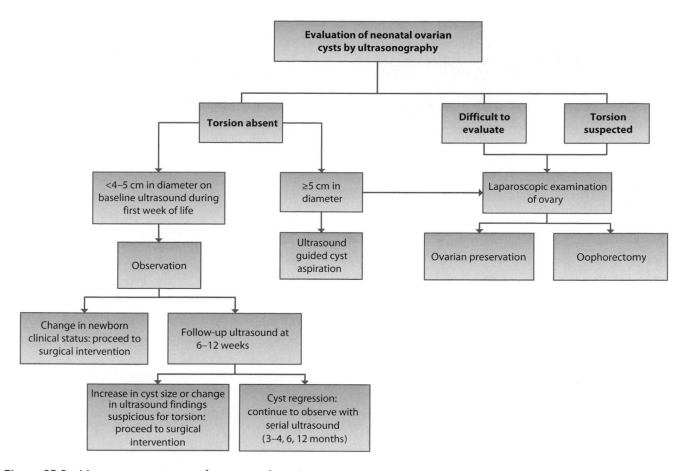

Figure 95.3   Management strategy for neonatal ovarian cysts.

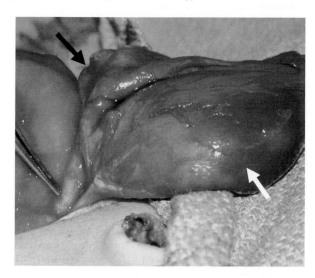

Figure 95.4   Torsed ovary with large attached cyst, exteriorized via a suprapubic transverse incision. White arrow points to cyst, black arrow points to torsed and nonviable right ovary, and forceps points to healthy uterus. Viable left ovary and tube are to the left of uterus.

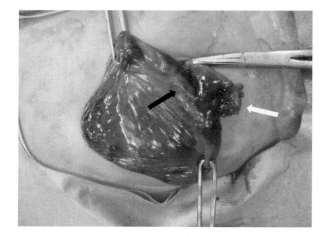

Figure 95.5   Simple ovarian cyst drained and exteriorized via umbilical incision. White arrow points to fallopian tube, black arrow to ovarian parenchyma and follicles near the blood supply of the ovary. The parenchyma is splayed out over the cyst. The cyst wall can be fenestrated or removed if it easily dissects free from the ovary.

exteriorization–aspiration, transumbilical removal (Figure 95.5), and modifications using the laparoscopic approach.[54–59] Laparoscopy is a safe and reliable treatment of ovarian cysts in the neonatal period.[59,60] If done laparoscopically, fenestration may be easier than cystectomy to avoid

removing ovarian tissue unless the ovary has torsed and is necrotic. If done open, an ovarian-sparing cystectomy can be facilitated by injecting saline in the interface between the cyst and the ovary, using a scalpel or electrocautery to begin the dissection, and then the cyst can often be peeled off the surface of the ovary using a moist

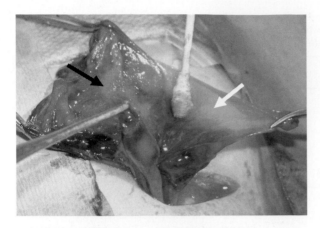

Figure 95.6 Dissection of ovarian cyst from tissue using a cotton-tipped applicator. White arrow points to cyst wall, black arrow points to ovarian parenchyma, and forceps hold fallopian tube. Despite ischemia, it is still worthwhile to spare the ovary if possible. Some tissue will atrophy, but there also may be viable ovary that will survive. It is not necessary to completely remove the cyst wall; a specimen can be sent to pathology in formalin.

cotton-tipped dissector or swab to facilitate the dissection (Figure 95.6). Subsequent bleeding at the ovarian surface can be controlled using electrocautery. It is not necessary to reapproximate ovarian tissue, but an absorbable small gauge suture should be used if this is felt necessary.

COMPLICATIONS

Complications of cyst observation include a missed malignancy, although this is very rare. As stated above, some authors believe that torsed, necrotic ovaries have the potential to cause adhesive bowel obstruction. Complications of cyst aspiration include misdiagnosis and any consequences of unintentional needle injury to another organ. Complications of operative removal include injury to viable ovarian tissue that might have been functional without intervention, and also the risk of adhesive bowel obstruction inherent to any transabdominal operation.

LONG-TERM RESULTS

Cesca et al.[37] investigated 41 neonates with congenital complex ovarian cysts managed conservatively with an average diameter of 4.16 ± 1.11 cm. Long-term follow-up was completed in 10 of the 41 patients at the mean age of 12 years, and no cyst recurrence or complications after cyst resolution were identified.[37]

No long-term studies to date have examined future fertility in the population of newborns and infants who had ovarian cysts or tumors subjected to a variety of therapeutic options.

REFERENCES

1. Brandt, Mary L., Francois I. Luks, Denis Filiatrault, Laurent Garel, Jean G. Desjardins and Sami Youssef. "Surgical indications in antenatally diagnosed ovarian cysts," *J Pediat Surg* 26 (1991): 276–282.
2. Bryant, Ann E., and Marc R. Laufer. "Fetal ovarian cysts: Incidence, diagnosis and management," *J Reprod Med* 49 (2004): 329–337.
3. Dolgin, Stephen E. "Ovarian masses in the newborn," *Seminars in Pediatric Surgery* 9 (2000): 121–127.
4. Hagen-Ansert, Sandra L. "The neonatal and pediatric pelvis," in *Textbook of Diagnostic Sonography 7th edition*, edited by Sandra L. Hagen-Ansert, 723–735. Missouri: Mosby, 2012.
5. Akin, Mustafa Ali, Leyla Aikin, Sibel Özbek, Gülay Tireli, Sultan Kavuncuoğlu, Serdar Sander, Mustafa Akçakuş, Tamer, Güneş, M. Adnan Öztürk, and Selim Kurtoğlu. "Fetal-neonatal ovarian cysts-their monitoring and management: Retrospective evaluation of 20 cases and review of the literature," *J Clin Res Ped Endo* 2 (2010): 28–33.
6. Meizner, Israel, Arie Levy, Miriam Katz, Abraham J. Maresh, and Marek Glezerman. "Fetal ovarian cysts: Prenatal ultrasonographic detection and postnatal evaluation and treatment," *Am J Obstet Gynecol* 164 (1991): 874–878.
7. Bagolan, Pietro, Massimo Rivosecchi, Claudio Giorlandino, Elena Bilancioni, Antonella Nahom, Antonio Zaccara, Alessandro Trucchi and Fabio Ferro. "Prenatal diagnosis and clinical outcome of ovarian cysts," *J Pediatr Surg* 27 (1992): 879–881.
8. Luzzatto, C., P. Midrio, T. Toffolutti, and V. Suma. "Neonatal ovarian cysts: Management and follow-up," *Pediatr Surg Int* 16 (2000): 56–59.
9. Enriquez, Goya, Carmina Durán, Nuria Torán, Joaquim Piqueras, Eduardo Gratacós, Celestino Aso, Josep Lloret, Amparo Castellote, and Javier Lucaya. "Conservative versus surgical treatment for complex neonatal ovarian cysts: Outcomes study," *AJR Am J Roentgenol* 185 (2005): 501–508.
10. Kessler, Ada, Hagith Nagar, Moshe Graif, Liat Ben-Sira, Elka Miller, Drora Fisher, and Irith Hadas-Halperin. "Percutaneous drainage as the treatment of choice for neonatal ovarian cysts," *Pediatr Radiol* 36 (2006): 954–958.
11. Giorlandino, Claudio, Elena Bilancioni, Pietro Bagolan, Ludovico Muzii, Massimo Rivosecchi, and Antonella Nahom. "Antenatal ultrasonographic diagnosis and management of fetal ovarian cysts," *Int J Gynaecol Obstet* 44 (1994): 27–31.
12. Sapin Emmanuel, Frédéric Bargy, Fanny Lewin, J.M. Baron, Catherine Adamsbaum, Jacques P. Barbet, and Pierre Helardot. "Management of ovarian cyst detected by prenatal ultrasounds," *Eur J Pediatr Surg* 4 (1994): 137–140.

13. Monnery-Noché, Marie-Emmanuelle, Frédéric Auber, Jean-Marie Jouannic, Jean-Louis Bénifla, Bruno Carbonne, Marc Dommergues, Marion Lenoir, Hubert Ducou Lepointe, Michéle Larroquet, Christine Grapin, Georges Audry, and Pierre G. Hélardot. "Fetal and neonatal ovarian cysts: Is surgery indicated?" *Prenat Diagn* 28 (2008): 15–20.

14. Ozcan, H. Nursun, Serife Balci, Saniye Ekinci, Altan Gunes, Berna Oguz, Arbay O. Ciftci, and Mithat Haliloglu. "Imaging findings of fetal-neonatal ovarian cysts complicated with ovarian torsion and autoamputation," *AJR Am J Roentgenol* 205 (2015): 185–189.

15. Amodio, John, Amer Hanano, Ernest Rudman, Francis Banfro, and Eugene Garrow. "Complex left fetal ovarian cyst with subsequent autoamputation and migration into the right lower quadrant in a neonate," *J Ultrasound Med* 29 (2010): 497–500.

16. De Backer, Antoine, Gerard C. Madern, J. Wolter Oosterhuis, Friederike G.A. Hakvoort-Cammel, and Frans W.J. Hazebroek. "Ovarian germ cell tumors in children: A clinical study of 66 patients," *Pediatr Blood Cancer* 46 (2006): 459–464.

17. Heling, K.S., R. Chaoui, F. Kirchmair, S. Stadie, and R. Bollmann. "Fetal ovarian cysts: Prenatal diagnosis, management and postnatal outcome," *Ultrasound Obstet Gynecol* 20 (2002): 47–50.

18. Ziegler, E.E. "Bilateral ovarian carcinoma in a thirty-week fetus," *Arch Pathol* 40 (1945): 279–282.

19. Marshall, John R. "Ovarian enlargements in the first year of life: Review of 45 cases," *Ann Surg* 161 (1965): 372–377.

20. Croitoru, D.P., L.E. Aaron, J.M. Laberge, I.R. Neilson, and F.M. Guttman. "Management of complex ovarian cysts presenting in the first year of life," *J Pediatr Surg* 26 (1991): 1366–1368.

21. Merras-Salmio, Laura, Kim Vettenrana, Merja Möttönen, and Markku Heikinheimo. "Ovarian granulosa cell tumors in childhood," *Pediatr Hematol Oncol* 156 (2002):145–156.

22. Schultz, Kris Ann, Susan F. Sencer, Yoav Messinger, Joseph P. Neglia, and Marie E. Steiner. "Pediatric ovarian tumors: A review of 67 cases," *Pediatr Blood Cancer* 44 (2005): 167–173.

23. Akyüz, Canan, Ali Varan, Nebil Büyükpamukçu, Tezer Kutluk, and Münevver Büyükpamukçu. "Malignant ovarian tumors in children: 22 years of experience at a single institution," *J Pediatr Hematol Oncol* 22 (2000): 422–427.

24. Kuroiwa, Minoru, Norio Suzuki, Hideaki Murai, Fumiaki Toki, Yoshiaki Tsuchida and Shin-itsu Hatakeyama. "Neonatal ovarian cysts: Management with reference to magnetic resonance imaging," *Asian J Surg* 27 (2004): 43–48.

25. Zampieri, Nicola, Franco Borruto, Carla Zamboni, and Francesco S. Camoglio. "Foetal and neonatal ovarian cysts: A 5-year experience," *Arch Gynecol Obstet* 277 (2008): 303–306.

26. Calisti, A., C. Pintus, S. Celli, C. Manzoni, I.R. Perrelli, G. Maresca, E. Saracca, L. Masini, G. Noia, and S. Candia. "Fetal ovarian cysts postnatal evolution and indications for surgical treatment," *Pediat Surg Int* 4 (1989): 341–346.

27. Lee, Hee-Jung, Seung-Ku Woo, Jung-Sik Kim, and Su-Jhi Suh. "'Daughter Cyst' sign: A sonographic finding of ovarian cyst in neonates, infants, and young children," *AJR Am J Roentgenol* 174 (2000): 1013–1015.

28. Nussbaum, Anna R., Rogers C. Sanders, David S. Hartman, David L Dudgeon, and Tim H. Parmley. "Neonatal ovarian cysts: Sonographic-pathologic correlation," *Radiology* 168 (1988): 817–821.

29. Müller-Leisse, C., U. Bick, K. Paulussen, J. Tröger, Z. Zachariou, W. Holzgreve, R. Schuhmacher, and A. Horvitz. "Ovarian cysts in the fetus and neonate—Changes in sonographic pattern in the follow-up and their management," *Pediatr Radiol* 22 (1992): 395–400.

30. Foley, P.T., W.D.A. Ford, R. McEwing, M. Furness. "Is conservative management of prenatal and neonatal ovarian cysts justifiable?" *Fetal Diagn Ther* 20 (2005): 454–458.

31. Galinier, Philippe, Luana Carfagna, Michel Juricic, Frederique Lemasson, Jacques Moscovici, Jacques Guitard, Christiane Baunin, Marcella Mendez, Audrey Cartault, Catherine Pienkowski, Sylvie Kessler, Marie-Fance Sarramon, and Philippe Vaysse. "Fetal ovarian cysts management and ovarian prognosis: A report of 82 cases," *J Pediatr Surg* 43 (2008): 2004–9.

32. Shimada, Takako, Kiyonori Miura, Hideo Gotoh, Daisuke Nakayama, and Hideaki Masuzaki. "Management of prenatal ovarian cysts," *Early Hum Dev* 84 (2008): 417–420.

33. Sakala, Elmar P., Zonia A. Leon, and Glenn A. Rouse. "Management of antenatally diagnosed fetal ovarian cysts," *Obstet Gynecol Surv* 46 (1991): 407–414.

34. Crombleholme, Timothy M., Sabrina D. Craigo, Sara Garmel, and Mary E. D'Alton. "Fetal ovarian cyst decompression to prevent torsion," *J Pediatr Surg* 32 (1997): 1447–1449.

35. Bagolan, Pietro, Claudio Giorlandino, Antonella Nahom, Elena Bilancioni, Alessandro Trucchi, Claudia Gatti, Vincenzo Aleandri, and Vincenzo Spina. "The management of fetal ovarian cysts," *J Pediatr Surg* 37 (2002): 25–30.

36. Tajiri, Tatsuro, Ryota Souzaki, Yoshiaki Kinoshita, Ryota Yosue, Kenichi Kohashi, Yoshinao Oda and Tomoaki Taguchi. "Surgical intervention strategies for pediatric ovarian tumors: Experience with 60 cases at one institution," *Pediatr Surg Int* 28 (2012): 27–31.

37. Cesca E., Paola Midrio, Rafael Boscolo-Berto, Deborah Snijders, Laura Salvador, Donato D'Antona, Giovanni Franco Zanon, and Piergiorgio Gamba.

"Conservative treatment for complex neonatal ovarian cysts: A long-term follow up analysis," *J Pediatr Surg* 48 (2013): 510–515.

38. Papic, Jonathan C., Deobrah F. Billmire, Frederick J. Rescorla, S. Maria E. Finnell, and Charles M. Leys. "Management of neonatal ovarian cysts and its effect on ovarian preservation," *J Pediatr Surg* 49 (2014): 990–994.

39. Randall P., Slavica K. Katusic, Robert C. Colligan, Robert T. Wilder, Robert G. Voigt, Michael D. Olson, Juraj Sprung, Amy L. Weaver, Darrell R. Schroeder, and David O. Warner. "Cognitive and behavioral outcomes after early exposure to anesthesia and surgery," *Pediatrics* 128 (2011):1053–1061.

40. Wang, Xin, Zheng Xu, and Chang-Hong Miao. "Current clinical evidence on the effect of general anesthesia on neurodevelopment in children: An updated systematic review with meta-regression," *PLoS One* 9 (2014): e85760. doi:10.1371/journal.pone.0085760.

41. Rappaport, Bob A., Santhanam Suresh, Sharon Hertz, Alex S. Evers, and Beverley A. Orser. "Anesthetic neurotoxicity—Clinical implications of animal models," *N Eng J Med* 372 (2015): 796–797.

42. Zhu, Changlian, Jianfeng Gao, Niklas Karlsson, Qian Li, Yu Zhang, Zhiheng Huang, Hongfu Li, H. Georg Kuhn and Klas Blomgren. "Isoflurane anesthesia induced persistent, progressive memory impairment, caused a loss of neural stem cells and reduced neurogenesis in young, but not adult, rodents," *J Cereb Blood Flow Metab* 30 (2010): 1017–1030.

43. Creeley, C., K. Dikranian, G. Dissen, L. Martin, J. Olney, and A. Brambrink. "Propofol-induced apoptosis of neurons and oligodendrocytes in fetal and neonatal rhesus macaque brain," *Br J Anaesth* 110 (2013): i29–i38.

44. Jevtovic-Todorovic, Vesna, Richard E. Hartman, Yukitoshi Izumi, Nicholas D. Benshoff, Krikor Dikranian, Charles F. Zorumski, John W. Olney, and David F. Wozniak. "Early exposure to common anesthetic agents causes widespread neurodegeneration in the developing rat brain and persistent learning deficits," *J Neurosci* 23 (2003): 876–882.

45. Stratmann, Greg, Joshua Lee, Jeffrey W. Sall, Bradley H. Lee, Rehan S. Alvi, Jennifer Shih, Allison M. Rowe, Tatiana M. Rampage, Flora L. Chang, Terri G. Alexander, David K. Lempert, Nan Lin, Kasey H. Siu, Sophie A. Elphick, Alice Wong, Caitlin I. Schnair, Alexander F. Vu, John T. Chan, Huizhen Zai, Michelle K. Wong, Amanda M. Anthony, Kyle C. Barbour, Dana Ben-Tzur, Natalie E. Kazarian, Joyce YY. Lee, Jay R. Shen, Eric Liu, Gurbir S. Behniwal, Cathy R. Lammers, Zoel Quinones, Anuj Aggarwal, Elizabeth Cedars, Andrew P. Yonelinas, and Simona Ghetti. "Effect of general anesthesia in infancy on long-term recognition memory in humans and rats," *Neuropsychopharmacology* 39 (2014): 2275–2287.

46. Brambrink, Ansgar M., Alex S. Evers, Michael S. Avidan, Nuri B. Farber, Derek J. Smith, Lauren D. Martin, Gregory A. Dissen, Catherine E. Creely, and John W. Olney. "Ketamine-induced neuroapoptosis in the fetal and neonatal rhesus macaque brain," *Anesthesiology* 116 (2012): 372–384.

47. Stratmann, Greg, Jeffrey W. Sall, Laura D.V. May, Joseph S. Bell, Kathy R. Magnusson, Vinuta Rau, Kavel H. Visrodia, Rehan S. Alvi, Ban Ku, Michael T. Lee, and Ran Dai. "Isoflurane differentially affects neurogenesis and long-term neurocognitive function in 60-day-old and 7-day-old rats," *Anesthesiology* 110 (2009): 834–848.

48. Nikizad, H. J.H. Yon, L.B. Carter, V. Jevtovic-Todorovic. "Early exposure to general anesthesia causes significant neuronal deletion in the developing rat brain," *Ann N Y Acad Sci* 1122 (2007): 69–82.

49. Flick, Randall P., Slavica K. Katusic, Robert C. Colligan, Robert T. Wilder, Robert G. Voigt, Michael D. Olson, Juraj Sprung, Amy L. Weaver, Darrell R. Schroeder, and David O. Warner. "Cognitive and Behavioral Outcomes After Early Exposure to Anesthesia and Surgery. *Pediatrics* 128 (2011): 1053–1061.

50. Davidson, Andrew J., Karin Becke, Jurgen de Graaff, Gaia Giribaldi, Walid Habre, Tom Hansen, Rodney W. Hunt, Caleb Ing, Andreas Loepke, Mary Ellen McCann, Gillian D. Ormond, Alessio Pini Prato, Ida Salvo, Lena Sun, Laszlo Vutskits, Suellen Walker, and Nicola Disma. "Anesthesia and the developing brain: A way forward for clinical research," *Paediatr Anaesth* 25 (2015): 447–452.

51. Perrotin, F., J. Potin, G. Haddad, C. Sembely-Taveau, J. Lansac, and G. Body. "Fetal ovarian cysts: A report of three cases managed by intrauterine aspiration," *Ultrasound Obstet Gynecol* 16 (2000): 655–659.

52. Dera-Szymanowska, Anna, Adam Malinger, Mateusz Madejczyk, Krzysztof Szymanowski, Gregor H. Breborowicz, and Tomasz Opal. "Recurrent fetal complex ovarian cysts with rupture followed by simple cyst in the neonatal period with no adverse sequelae," *J Matern Fetal Neonatal Med* 29 (2016): 328–330.

53. Puligandla, Pramod S., and Jean-Martin Laberge. "Lethal outcome after percutaneous aspiration of a presumed ovarian cyst in a neonate," *Semin Pediatr Surg* 18 (2009): 119–121.

54. Tseng, Daniel, Thomas J. Curran, and Mark L. Silen. "Minimally invasive management of the prenatally torsed ovarian cyst," *J Pediatr Surg* 37 (2002): 1467–1469.

55. Ferro F., B.D. Iacobelli, A. Zaccara, A. Spagnoli, A. Trucchi, and P. Bagolan. "Exteriorization-aspiration minilaparotomy for treatment of neonatal ovarian cysts," *J Pediatr and Adolesc Gynecol* 15 (2002): 205–207.

56. Lin, Jao-Lin, Zen-Fung Lee, and Yu-Tang Chang. "Transumbilical management for neonatal ovarian cysts," *J Pediatr Surg* 42 (2007): 2136–2139.
57. Schenkman, Lucy, Timothy M. Weiner, and J. Duncan Phillips. "Evolution of the surgical management of neonatal ovarian cysts: Laparoscopic-assisted transumbilical extracorporeal ovarian cystectomy," *J Laparoendosc Adv Surg Tech A* 18 (2008): 635–640.
58. Templeman, Claire L., Ann Marie J. Reynolds, S. Paige Hertweck, and Hirikati S. Nagaraj. "Laparoscopic management of neonatal ovarian cysts," *J Am Assoc Gynecol Laparosc* 7 (2000): 401–404.
59. Marinković, S. Radoica Jokić, Svetlana Bukarica, Aleksandra N. Mikić, Nada Vućković, and Jelena Antić. "Surgical treatment of neonatal ovarian cysts," *Med Pregl* 64 (2011): 408–412.
60. Pujar, Vijay C., Shirin S. Joshi, Yeshita V. Pujar, and Hema A. Dhumale. "Role of laparoscopy in the management of neonatal ovarian cysts," *N Neonatal Surg* 3 (3014): 16.

PART 9

Spina bifida and hydrocephalus

96

Spina bifida and encephalocele

JOTHY KANDASAMY, MARK A. HUGHES, AND CONOR L. MALLUCCI

INTRODUCTION

Neural tube defects (NTDs) encompass a variety of congenital anomalies ranging from anencephaly to spina bifida occulta, and arise due to defects in the morphogenesis of the neural tube. While spina bifida remains the most common congenital central nervous defect encountered in neurosurgical practice, the overall incidence of NTDs is in decline.[1-4] Multiple factors account for this change, including increased antenatal diagnosis, declining birth rates, changing social attitudes, and improved standard of living and diet. A diagnosis of spina bifida can have devastating consequences, and the "correct" management of these patients is a continued source of medical, ethical, and legal controversy. A multidisciplinary team is required, including neurosurgeons, pediatricians, neurologists, urologists, orthopedic surgeons, physiotherapists, social workers, psychologists, and nursing staff. At the center are the patient and family, with the common goal being social integration and a meaningful life.

HISTORY

Caspar Baulinin is credited with the first accurate description of spina bifida in the early seventeenth century.[5] The term *spina dorsi bifida* was coined by Nicholas Talpius (Tulp) in 1641,[6,7] and Virchow[8] introduced the term *spina bifida occulta* in 1875. The association of hydrocephalus and spina bifida was recognized by Morgagni[5] in 1761. He also described anencephaly and spina bifida as expressions of the same pathological process, and attributed bladder, rectal, and limb abnormalities to the neuronal damage in the defective spinal cord.

Aspiration of the lesion was the time-honored method of management but had catastrophic consequences. Forestus ligated the sac,[9] and sac excision was attempted by Tulp[7] with fatal results. The Clinical Society of London[9] recommended the use of a local sclerosing technique, which was initially advocated by Morton.[10] Excision of the sac was again popularized by Bayer[11] and Frazier[12] in the early twentieth century, but the mortality rate remained high. With the advent of antibiotics and introduction of cerebrospinal fluid (CSF) shunts in the 1950s, improved operative results encouraged more surgeons to introduce comprehensive, aggressive management. In 1963, Sharrard, Zachary, and Lorber[13] proposed emergency operative closure of the back lesion to decrease mortality and improve muscle function. This provided new hope for these patients, though it became evident that mortality remained high and those who survived had major disabilities. Lorber,[14] who was one of the supporters of the aggressive policy advocated by the Sheffield group, reviewed 524 cases of myelomeningocele treated actively and concluded that there were four main criteria associated with a poor prognosis: gross hydrocephalus, severe paraplegia, kyphosis, and associated gross congenital anomalies or major birth injury. He advised that patients with one or a combination of these criteria should be managed conservatively, as very few patients survived, and those that did would suffer severe mental and physically handicap. In recent years, the reliability and predictive value of these four criteria has been challenged. It has been suggested that management should be more individualized and changed whenever necessary in the best interests of the patient and family.[15-17]

INCIDENCE AND EPIDEMIOLOGY

There are geographic variations in the incidence of spina bifida and NTDs worldwide. For example, the incidence of spina bifida cystica is 0.3 per 1000 live births in Finland but 4.5 per 1000 live births in Ireland.[18] There is greater reported variation in the incidence of spina bifida occulta, which ranges between 1% and 50% depending upon the age group.[19] Caucasians are at higher risk of developing spina bifida[20] than African Caribbean people, and lower socioeconomic groups also seem to have a higher incidence of the defect.[21] Where they occur, public health initiatives promoting folate supplementation have reduced incidence of NTDs.[22] The incidence of spina bifida cystica live births is also influenced by the cultural and social norms of each society, access to antenatal diagnosis, and counseling as regards pregnancy termination and specific national legal parameters for this.

EMBRYOLOGY

NTDs result from an abnormality in the process of neurulation. The primitive streak and Hensen's nodes are present in the embryo at 2 weeks' gestation. The notochord starts extending rostrally from Hensen's node, and this induces the process of neural tube formation. Thickening of the ectoderm cephalic to Hensen's node occurs and forms the neural plate. Folding and later fusion forms the neural tube. This process continues caudally up to the somites, which start to appear from week 3. Other ectodermal tissue closes over this and buries the tube. The unfused rostral and caudal neural folds are called the anterior and posterior neuropores. These close at about 25 days and 30 days respectively, at which point the process of neurulation is complete. At this stage, there are 21–29 somites. Four somites are incorporated into the occipital bone and 20 in the cervical and thoracic vertebrae. Caudal to this, the remainder of the tube forms the caudal cell mass. During the next 4–5 weeks, canalization of this cell mass occurs, followed by regression of the most caudal part, which forms the filum terminale. The notochord separates from the neural tube dorsally and the gut ventrally, forming subchordal and epichordal spaces.

PATHOGENESIS

All developmental defects of the central nervous system are NTDs. Neurulation defects are a subgroup of NTDs. These defects can involve the following:

1. *Brain*
   Anencephaly: A result of persistence of the anterior neuropore. This allows some part of the developing brain to remain in contact with the amniotic cavity. The types are holocrine, if the defect extends to involve the foramen magnum, and mesoacrania, if the foramen is not involved.[23]
   Encephalocele: The result of defective cephalic neurulation.
2. *Spinal cord*
   Meningocele: A postneurulation defect.
   Myelomeningocele: Defective caudal neurulation results in myelomeningocele, which can occur anywhere from cervical to lumbar sites. There are various theories put forward to explain the precise mechanism of the defective neurulation. These are due to either failure of neural folds to fuse or a reopening of the normally fused neural tube. Defective neuroepithelium itself may be responsible for the failure of neural folds to fuse,[24] or the defect may lie in mesoderm, which deters the closure of neural folds. The normally fused neural tube may reopen because

of increased intraluminal pressure[25] or a primary defect in the neuroepithelium.
   Associated Arnold–Chiari malformation may be secondary to failure of ascent of the cord within the spinal column because of tethering or as a result of descent secondary to increased pressure of hydrocephalus.
3. *Brain and spinal cord*
   Craniorachischisis: Where there is failure of neural tube fusion at both brain and spinal cord level.
4. *Other defects*
   Occur secondary to various postneurulation abnormalities involving the neural tube or mesoderm, or because of persistence of totipotent cells. These lesions are diastematomyelia, complete anterior and posterior spina bifida, butterfly vertebrae, lipoma, hemangioma, dermoid cyst, and sacrococcygeal teratoma. A partial duplication and separation of the notochord can result in herniation of the endoderm of the yolk sac, called split notochord syndrome. If the hernia ruptures, it may result in ectopic bowel, sinus, or fistula.[26]

TERMINOLOGY AND CLASSIFICATION

Types of NTDs vary in severity, ranging from anencephaly to spina bifida occulta. These lesions can be classified as shown in Table 96.1. Myelomeningocele is one of the most common congenital malformations.

Spina bifida occulta

The term *spina bifida occulta* refers to spinal dysraphism not accompanied by extrusion of the contents of the vertebral column. Spina bifida occulta, without any external evidence, is rarely diagnosed in the newborn. Occasionally, it may cause neurological deficit because of a tethering of the cord. Some patients may have external evidence of spina bifida occulta, such as a small dimple, sinus, tuft of hair (Figure 96.1), or hamartomatous lesions such as hemangioma, lipoma, or nevi. Neural involvement may manifest as urinary problems, (e.g., recurrent urinary infection or enuresis), motor deficit with pedal deformity, pelvic tilt and muscle weakness, or sensory involvement in the form of trophic ulceration. All these patients warrant careful examination and investigation. Spinal x-ray will show evidence of spina bifida and other spinal abnormalities. Ultrasonography can be useful in the newborn period to diagnose diastomatomyelia.[27] The common clinically relevant lesions are lipomyelomeningocele, tethered cord, dermal sinus tract, and diastematomyelia. All of these lesions warrant craniospinal magnetic resonance imaging (MRI) and referral to a neurosurgical specialist. The increased incidence and treatment of these lesions over the last 10–20 years probably reflects more widespread availability of MRI.

Table 96.1 Classification of neural tube defects

Site	Lesion	Pathology
Craniospinal	Craniorachischisis	Involves brain and spine
Cranial	Anencephaly	Brain and skull poorly developed
	Exencephaly	Exposed brain without skin or bone cover
	Encephalocele	Brain herniation through congenital opening of skull and covered by meninges and skin
Spinal	Spina bifida cystica	Open cord defect at any point from cervical to sacral
	a. Myelomeningocele	Skin-covered sac formed of meninges—defect in
	b. Meningocele	posterior arch
	Spina bifida occulta	Absent spinous process and varying amounts of lamina (may be associated with lipomyelomeningocele, tethered cord, dermal sinus tract, diastematomyelia, hemangioma)

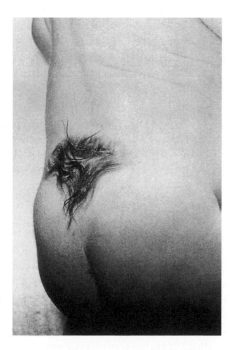

Figure 96.1 Spina bifida occulta. A large tuft of hair over the lumbosacral region in this baby was associated with spina bifida occulta and a tethered cord.

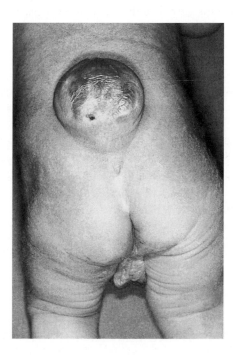

Figure 96.2 Dorsolumbar myelomeningocele. This infant had normal movement in both lower limbs.

Spina bifida cystica: meningocele

A meningocele is an epithelium-lined sac filled with CSF, which communicates with the spinal subarachnoid space. Meningocele, which comprises about 5% of all spina bifida cystica cases, is usually not associated with neurological deficit or hydrocephalus, and is most frequently observed in the lumbar region.

Spina bifida cystica: myelomeningocele

Myelomeningocele is the most common form of NTD (Figure 96.2). A neural plaque is centrally placed, around which there is a cystic lesion with attenuated meninges and skin (Figure 96.3). Although local pathological changes are obvious at the site of the lesion, additional changes may involve the whole of the nervous system and other systems, especially genitourinary and skeletal.

ETIOLOGY

The precise etiology of NTDs is not known, though genetic and environmental factors have been implicated.

Genetics

The exact mode of inheritance is unknown. Ethnic and gender variation (females are more commonly affected), and increased incidence with parental consanguinity and a

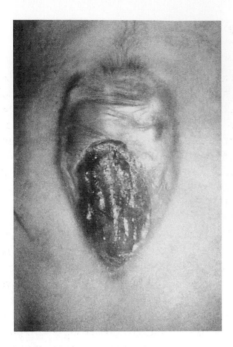

Figure 96.3 Myelomeningocele. Lesion showing neural plaque in the center covered by a thin membrane.

familial tendency, suggest a multifactorial hereditary mechanism. If there is one child with spina bifida in the family, the risk of having other children with spina bifida increases to 1 in 20–25.[28,29] This risk increases to 1 in 8–10 if there are two children with NTDs.[29] The risk of having an affected child is less if one of the parents has spina bifida (1 in 200) than if a sibling has spina bifida.[28]

Dietary factors

Substantial data have been accumulated to suggest that myelomeningocele and other neural defects can be reduced by improved maternal nutrition. Mothers of spina bifida patients were found to have an increased incidence of folate metabolism abnormalities.[30] Several studies report a beneficial role of folic acid and other vitamins.[31–34] The Medical Research Council conducted a randomized double-blind prevention trial with factorial design at 33 centers in seven countries to determine whether periconception supplementation with folic acid or a mixture of seven other vitamins (A, D, B_1, B_2, B_6, C, and nicotinamide) could prevent NTDs.[35] This study found a significant reduction in the number of children with NTDs born to high-risk mothers who had taken folic acid in the periconceptional period. Periconception use of folic acid has been recommended to all women, with or without risk. A concern that large doses of folic acid may delay the diagnosis of pernicious anemia has led to the fortification recommendations being limited to a level that may add, on average, only about 0.1 mg folic acid/day. However, others feel that a daily dose of 0.4 mg/day should be continued.[36] Studies from Canada, the United States, Australia, and China have shown a decline

in NTDs, especially in high-risk groups, with folic acid supplementation and food fortification.[3,22,37,38]

Teratogens

In utero exposure to some antiepileptic drugs increases the risk of fetal NTDs (6%–16% for sodium valproate[39,40] and 2%–6% for carbamazepine.[41,42] These are often at the severe end of the spectrum and associated with hydrocephalus.[43] Certain viruses[44] and hyperthermia have also been hypothesized to cause NTDs, and exposure to heat in the form of a hot tub, sauna, or fever in the first trimester of pregnancy has also been associated with an increased risk of NTDs.[45–47]

PRENATAL DIAGNOSIS

Prenatal diagnosis of myelomeningocele allows improved obstetric care or termination of an affected fetus.[48]

Alpha-fetoprotein in maternal serum

Alpha-fetoprotein (AFP) can be detected in maternal serum where the fetus has an open NTD. Elevated levels after 16 weeks' pregnancy are suspicious; the test is repeated a week later to confirm the presence or absence of NTDs. The sensitivity of this test is 97% for anencephaly and 72% for spina bifida.[49] This second test requires further confirmation by amniocentesis and prenatal ultrasonography after appropriate counseling.

Ultrasonography

Prenatal ultrasonography may be used as a primary screening procedure. It is a safe and effective method of antenatal screening if the ultrasonographer is experienced[50] (up to 98% specificity and 94% sensitivity).[51] Within Europe, there are formal national ultrasound screening policies for structural anomalies.[52] However, detection rates are influenced by gestational age and type of NTD. Spina bifida has a higher detection rate in the second trimester (92%–95%) compared to the first trimester (44%).[53] Three-dimensional sonography has an advantage over conventional two-dimensional ultrasound in predicting the level of lesion, and this may help to predict morbidity.[53]

Prenatal MRI

While ultrasound is the method of choice for prenatal screening, fetal MRI is a valuable second-line tool.[54] It can help to clarify unclear ultrasound findings and define the extent of confirmed lesions, thereby informing prognosis.

Amniocentesis

Many now question the use of amniocentesis in the era of high-resolution ultrasonography. In selected cases, biochemical analysis of amniotic fluid remains useful.[55] Using ultrasound guidance, amniotic fluid is obtained transabdominally at about 16 weeks' gestation. AFP and acetylcholinesterase (ACE) levels are measured. If AFP levels are ≥+3 standard deviations (SD) above normal, the risk of open NTD is 60%, rising to 86% if the levels are ≥+5SD above normal. The combined analysis of AFP and ACE in amniotic fluid increases the accuracy of diagnosis.[56]

CLINICAL MANAGEMENT

This section relates primarily to the management of myelomeningocele as this is the most common NTD that presents to pediatric neurosurgical practice.

Prenatal assessment and antenatal counseling

Once a prenatal diagnosis of myelomeningocele has been made, MRI of the fetus is performed to determine the level and extent of defect. This allows the neurosurgeon to predict the likely degree of neurological deficit and facilitates prenatal counseling. Antenatal counseling is undertaken in specialist clinics and involves fetal medicine specialists, obstetricians, neurosurgeons, and radiologists. Parents need to be given realistic expectations regarding prognosis for intellectual development, ambulation, and survival, as well as information on hydrocephalus and neurogenic bowel and bladder.

It remains controversial whether cesarean section should be carried out if a prenatal diagnosis of myelomeningocele has been made. Luthy et al.[57] reported that delivery by cesarean for a fetus with uncomplicated myelomeningocele before onset of labor may result in better motor function than vaginal delivery or cesarean section after labor has commenced. Other authors do not support this.[58] While there is no clear evidence, caesarean section facilitates a timed delivery that allows for planning of surgical closure of the myelomeningocele.[59]

In utero surgery

There is a potential role for fetal surgery for some NTDs. Techniques using endoscopy, using percutaneous fetoscopic patch coverage, and via hysterotomy have been described. The Management of Myelomeningocele Study (MOMS) was a multicenter randomized prospective trial comparing prenatal (18–25 weeks of gestation) and postnatal repair of myelomeningocele. Outcomes assessed include death, the need for ventricular shunting by 1 year of life, and neurological function at 30 months of age. The MOMS study found that prenatal surgery for myelomeningocele reduced the rate of shunting (40% compared with 82%) and improved a composite score of mental development and motor function. However, pregnancy complications were more common in the fetal surgery group, including higher risk of preterm delivery and uterine dehiscence at delivery.[60]

Postnatal assessment

LOCAL EXAMINATION

The sites affected are the lower thoracic, lumbar, sacral, cervical, and upper thoracic regions. In about 80% of infants with myelomeningocele, the defect includes the lumbar region as this is the last part of the neural tube to close. Occasionally, more than one lesion can be found,[59] and there is often concurrent kyphosis or scoliosis. Most myelomeningoceles contain an enlarged subarachnoid space ventrally, with the neural tissue displaced dorsally.

MOTOR FUNCTION

Motor function is assessed when the infant is at rest. Sharp stimulation above the level of the meningocele is administered with careful observation of voluntary movement below the affected level. Varying degrees of paralysis below the level of the lesion are common, except in rarer cervical and upper thoracic lesions, which are usually spared. The paralysis is usually flaccid, indicating a complete neural lesion. It must be borne in mind that there are some abnormal reflex activities in the lower extremities that have no bearing on volitional motor function.

SENSORY LOSS

Sensory loss is determined by pinprick test from distal to proximal, looking for an upper limb or facial response characteristic of those experiencing a pain sensation. The level at which anesthesia starts indicates the myotome level of the lesion and predicts the degree of disability.[61] Fastidious care is necessary to avoid trophic changes in anesthetic areas.

BLADDER AND BOWEL INVOLVEMENT

Over 90% of patients with myelomeningocele have some degree of neurogenic bladder. The vast majority have disturbances of detrusor and sphincter balance resulting in a large, trabeculated bladder with urinary stasis. The external anal sphincter and puborectalis are often involved, resulting in patulous anus and sometimes rectal prolapse. It is difficult to assess bladder involvement in the newborn, but steps should be taken to ensure the bladder is kept empty. There may be associated upper urinary tract abnormalities at birth.[62] All patients need careful urological and renal follow-up.

HYDROCEPHALUS

Eighty-five to ninety-five percent of patients with myelomeningocele have some degree of hydrocephalus. Assessment of the anterior fontanelle and occipitofrontal circumference is important in determining the timing of any CSF diversion procedures. In those infants with clear evidence of hydrocephalus, early CSF diversion is indicated. Delayed placement of a ventriculoperitoneal shunt is not associated with a lower infection rate compared to placement at the time of myelomeningocele closure.[63,64] Almost half of meningocele patients shunted at birth require shunt revision in the first year of life, mostly due to mechanical failure.[65] Endoscopic third ventriculostomy (ETV) has also been used in some patients, although the failure rate is high when performed as a primary procedure.[66,67] In patients presenting with shunt malfunction, secondary ETV has a better success rate and is therefore best reserved for later management.[66]

CHIARI II MALFORMATION

Chiari II malformation is invariably associated with spina bifida. MRI demonstrates cardinal findings of caudal displacement of the posterior fossa contents, an elongated brainstem, a small fourth ventricle, aqueduct stenosis, and tectal "beaking." Between 25% and 33% of patients are symptomatic from the Chiari II malformation; in the infant, this manifests as brainstem dysfunction associated with sleep apnea and lower cranial nerve palsies. Stevenson et al.[68] reported that apnea, stridor (vocal cord paresis), and swallowing difficulties in infancy were associated with a 15% mortality rate. Whether early decompression improves symptoms remains controversial as surgery-related morbidity and mortality are high in infants (up to 15%–20%).[69,70] From a practical point of view, symptomatic Chiari II is rare in infants as long as the hydrocephalus is correctly managed. Chiari II can become a secondary problem in adult life with delayed deterioration.

SKELETAL ABNORMALITIES

Clubfoot is the most common skeletal abnormality in spina bifida. Other deformities include dislocation of the hip, genu recurvatum, and kyphoscoliosis. Orthopedic assessment and specialist physiotherapy services are required to manage these problems and minimize deformity.

Investigations

A full blood count is obtained, and blood is cross-matched with maternal serum. A plain x-ray of the spine will reveal the extent of the bony abnormality and associated kyphoscoliosis. An ultrasound scan of the head and renal tract are carried out as baseline investigations. MRI of the entire craniospinal axis will determine the presence of associated congenital abnormalities.

Parental discussion

Babies born with NTDs require an ethical and humane approach to management, informed by accurate background information and full involvement of parents in the decision-making process.[15,71] The management of each child should be individualized and reviewed regularly. Despite early closure and deployment of all available therapeutic measures, there is still a significant rate of disability and mortality.[72–74] Lorber[14] previously outlined adverse criteria (including gross paraplegia, severe hydrocephalus, severe kyphosis, thoracolumbar lesions and other associated congenital anomalies; see Figure 96.4), the presence of which might prompt a conservative management strategy. These criteria are based on the belief that these patients will often

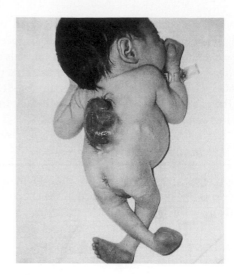

Figure 96.4 Large dorsolumbar myelomeningocele. This baby had bilateral lower limb paralysis, hydrocephalus and bilateral dysplastic kidneys. The baby was managed conservatively.

die early in infancy. These severely affected babies were often managed conservatively with demand feeding and sedation. In an era of improved antenatal diagnosis and prenatal counseling, many of the severe defects are avoided with early termination. Parents are now usually aware of the expected prognosis for intellectual development, ambulation, and survival, after antenatal counseling.

Operative treatment and technique

All actively treated spina bifida patients should undergo closure of the defect within 24–48 hours of delivery. It was previously thought that early closure resulted in improved neurological outcome,[12] but this has not been supported by more recent studies.[75,76] Early defect closure reduces the risk of infection and further damage to exposed neural tissue—the core aim is to preserve existing function. The principle of surgery is to reconstruct the defect by five-layer closure of the pia and arachnoid, lumbar fascia, subcutaneous tissue, and skin. The vascular supply to the neuroplaque is maintained, and unnecessary neural injury is avoided. The patient is placed in the prone position with a soft roll under the hips and shoulder, and with the head turned to the right through 90° (Figure 96.5a). Swabs are taken from the lesion for microbial examination and culture. An antiseptic soak is placed over the anus. The lesion is covered with a warm swab, and the surrounding skin is cleaned and draped. The skin is incised at the junction of the arachnoid membrane and skin (Figure 96.5b). The membrane between the edge of the skin defect and neural plaque is removed carefully to avoid inclusion of cysts (Figure 96.5c). The dura is freed laterally and then superiorly and inferiorly to normal intact dura (Figure 96.5d). Dura is then sutured in the midline with continuous monofilament absorbable sutures (Figure 96.5e). A suction drain may be placed extradurally, though

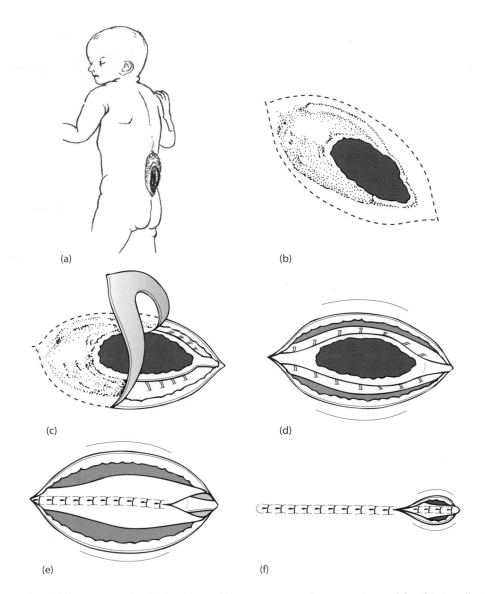

Figure 96.5 Closure of myelomeningocele. **(a)** Position of the patient on the operating table. **(b)** An elliptical incision at the junction of the arachnoid membrane and the skin. **(c)** Membrane is excised and neural plaque freed. **(d)** Dura is dissected laterally from the underlying muscle. **(e)** Dura is closed with an interrupted continuous 5-0 monofilament absorbable sutures. **(f)** Skin is closed with interrupted 5-0 nylon sutures.

this is not mandatory. The lumbodorsal fascia is incised laterally and dissected free from the posterior iliac crest. These are folded medially and sutured over the dorsal dural layer. The subcutaneous tissue is closed with absorbable interrupted sutures, and then the skin is closed with interrupted nylon stitches (Figure 96.5f). The infant is nursed in a prone position. Feeding is commenced once the bowel starts working. The wound is periodically inspected. The suction drain is removed 24–48 hours after operation.

Postoperative management and complications

Infection is common,[77] and treatment is with appropriate antibiotics and local drainage. Wound dehiscence may occur and is usually secondary to undue tension on the skin edges or skin necrosis. If infection is deep to the lumbodorsal fascia, it may cause meningitis or ventriculitis. These are vigorously treated with local dressings, systemic antibiotics, and external ventricular drainage if hydrocephalus or CSF leak occurs. With meticulous closure of the dura, CSF fistula should be rare. However, if it does occur, immediate repair is preferred rather than conservative treatment. Hydrocephalus may be present in about 15% of patients with myelomeningocele at birth, while it eventually develops in 85%. The exact reason for this is not clear; it may be aggravated by a shift in the brainstem after repair, which produces changes in the aqueduct or the Chiari malformation leading to alteration in the CSF flow dynamics. After neurosurgical closure of the defect, and shunt placement if indicated, management is continued in a multidisciplinary team context.

CLINICAL OUTCOME AND LONG-TERM MANAGEMENT

The results of myelomeningocele operations vary considerably because of differences in approach to management. Historically, in the units where a highly selective approach was taken, all conservatively managed patients died, compared with mortality of 14.3% for those actively managed.[78] Contemporary cohort studies illustrate a continuing high mortality rate in adult life. Analyzing a cohort of 117 unselectively closed spina bifida patients over a mean of 40 years showed that 40 died before the age of 5 and a further 31 died in the next 35 years (10 times average mortality).[72]

Medical problems

URINARY INCONTINENCE

Only 10% of myelomeningocele patients have a normal bladder. The remainder have a neurogenic bladder of some degree. The introduction of clean intermittent self-catheterization, pharmacological agents (e.g., anticholinergics), external devices, biofeedback, and innovative surgical procedures has allowed up to 75% of these patients to be socially continent and maintain renal function.[79] Urodynamic studies in the newborn period are useful in identifying at-risk children with high bladder pressure and detrusor instability.[80,81]

CHIARI II MALFORMATION AND HINDBRAIN DYSFUNCTION

Older children and young adults with Chiari II malformation may complain of symptoms related to foramen magnum impaction such as headache, neck pain, and upper limb sensory disturbance. Brainstem dysfunction and lower cranial nerve palsies may also be present. Surgical treatment may be indicated in symptomatic patients, once adequate CSF diversion by either shunting or ETV has been established.[82] In our own series of 21 patients with myelomeningocele surviving into adulthood, 8 patients underwent foramen magnum decompression for late deterioration, with consequent stabilization of symptoms.[83]

HYDROCEPHALUS

Shunt placement has a significant impact on the future life of the child and parents. In myelomeningocele patients, shunt malfunction and complications (e.g., infection, hemorrhage) impair cognition[84] and impact long-term survival.[73,85,86] If shunt malfunction occurs in later childhood, then ETV has a 89% success rate and should be considered before shunt revision.[82]

Lifestyle issues

Whether patients are managed conservatively or actively, quality of life is an important factor in those who survive. In the long-term follow-up study by Oakshott and Hunt,[72,73] of 117 patients treated unselectively who were followed up for 16–20 years, it was found that 41% died before 16 years of age. Of the survivors, almost 31% were mentally disabled, 48% were unable to live without help or supervision, and only about one-quarter of survivors were capable of competitive employment.[72,73]

INTELLIGENCE

Patients who have associated hydrocephalus and episodes of shunt malfunction (blockage and infection) have lower intelligence than those who only have myelomeningocele.[84] In addition, cognitive impairment can be consequent to associated structural defects, rather than repeated episodes of hydrocephalus.[87,88] Fiber tract anomalies in the limbic system have been correlated with memory deficits.[87] In a small adult cohort undergoing in-depth neuropsychological testing at our own center, visuospatial construction and memory were impaired in all myelomeningocele patients.[83] Importantly, severely physically disabled patients who have relatively mild cognitive impairment may yet be self-supporting and in competitive employment.

AMBULATION

Ambulatory potential and capacity are related to intelligence, orthopedic deformity, level of lesion, obesity, and motivation. Most of the patients with lesions below L5 are ambulators, those with lesions at L4 are functional ambulators, and those with lesions above L3 are wheelchair-bound.[89,90] The proportion of those patients who retain ambulant status into adulthood gradually decreases due to combinatorial factors including increasing weight, spinal and foot deformity, and respiratory compromise. Long-term follow-up studies have reported that only 30% of patients remain ambulant at 30 years of age.[91] A wheelchair may become a more energy-efficient means of mobility.[92]

PSYCHOSOCIAL PROBLEMS

Educational mainstreaming, special counseling, improved understanding of the patient's potential, and increased public awareness of spina bifida all contribute to a reduction in stress to patients and parents.

ENCEPHALOCELE

Encephalocele constitutes 10%–20% of all NTDs and has a prevalence of between 1 in 2000 and 1 in 5000 live births.[1,93] Encephaloceles have a higher incidence in Asian countries compared with the West.

Pathology

Encephalocele is a defect in the cranial vault, which is either oval or circular and of variable extent, ranging from a skin-covered meningocele to gross herniation of abnormal brain. These abnormalities are classified according to location as occipital, parietal, frontal, nasopharyngeal, nasal, frontoethmoid, or basal. Occipital encephalocele is the most common type in the western world, while a frontal lesion predominates in Asia.[59] The contents of the encephalocele vary according to its location and size. Brain tissue is found in 25–80% of cases, usually in occipital encephalocele. In addition to the brain tissue in the sac, the rest of the brain (especially the optic pathway) is distorted, and there may be associated microgyria, holoprosencephaly, heterotopia, agenesis, hydrocephalus, cerebellar aplasia, pyramidal tract aplasia (causing spasticity), and spinal cord distortion. Encephaloceles are commonly associated with other congenital anomalies including spina bifida, Klippel–Feil syndrome, facial cleft, and renal, cardiac, and pulmonary anomalies.

Clinical features

Most encephaloceles are obvious at birth, and some are diagnosed prenatally. The size, content, and location are variable (Figure 96.6), and there may be an overlying hamartomatous lesion. A pulsatile mass that increases in size with crying is the classical sign of an encephalocele. Anterior lesions may cause airway obstruction. Occasionally, the diagnosis may be delayed and only becomes evident when CSF leak occurs and the child presents with recurrent meningitis. A full neurological examination is necessary to determine whether any spasticity, focal motor weakness, or visual impairment exists. Physical examination will reveal any associated anomalies.

Differential diagnosis

The anterior lesion can be difficult to diagnose and may need to be differentiated from a nasal polyp, glioma, dermoid cyst, teratoma, neurofibroma, meningioma, and hamartoma.

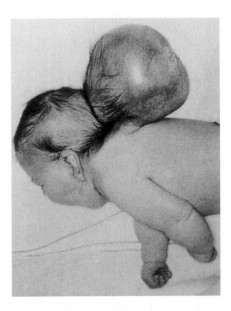

Figure 96.6 Occipital encephalocele.

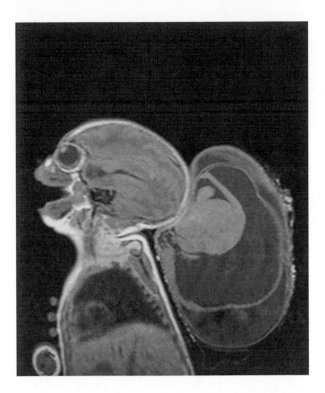

Figure 96.7 Encephalocele. Sagittal T1-weighted MRI shows a large mass arising from the occipital region.

Investigations

Craniospinal MRI should be performed on all patients with encephalocele to determine the severity and extent of the abnormality, as well as screening for associated congenital malformations (Figure 96.7). Visual evoked response will establish the presence of the occipital cortex within the sac, which may be helpful in surgical planning.

Treatment

Conservative treatment may be justified for patients with microcephaly and large amounts of brain within the encephalocele, where death is inevitable. Most patients are treated by surgical repair of the encephalocele. The aims of surgery are excision of extracranial nonfunctioning brain tissue, closure of the dura at the level of the cranium, and restoration of cranial contour with good skin coverage. Taking these steps helps to prevent infection and preserve function.

OPERATIVE TREATMENT AND TECHNIQUE

Under general anesthesia, the patient is positioned with the encephalocele uppermost. The lesion is prepped and draped while ensuring adequate support for the encephalocele. Large lesions may be aspirated to facilitate handling and dissection. A sample of CSF is sent for microbiological examination and culture. Usually, a transverse ellipse incision is made near the base of the lesion, planned to enable wound closure without tension (Figure 96.8). The incision is then deepened until the dura is seen, which is traced up to the bony defect.

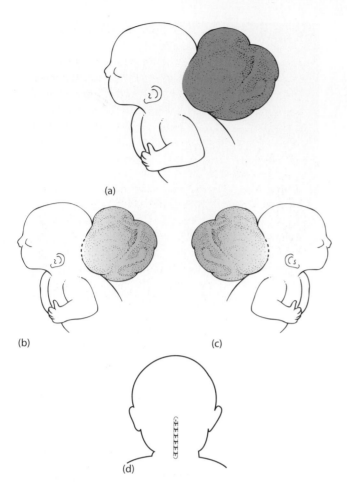

Figure 96.8 Closure of encephalocele. **(a)** Diagrammatic representation of occipital encephalocele. **(b** and **c)** Incision around the base of the encephalocele. **(d)** Skin closure.

The sac is opened where the cerebral tissue is not adherent. If the cerebral tissue is too large, or necrotic, or if no visual evoked potentials are demonstrated, it is excised. Every effort should be made to preserve brain tissue without causing an acute rise in intracranial pressure. Bony defects may sometimes need to be enlarged. While dissecting the dura and brain tissue, particular care must be taken to avoid abnormal venous sinuses and venous connections. The distal sac is then excised. The dura is closed with continuous monofilament absorbable sutures, and a dural graft may be required (pericranium is ideal). Meticulous hemostasis is achieved with the closure of all layers. A small suction drain is occasionally used. Subcutaneous tissue is approximated with fine, absorbable interrupted sutures, and the skin is closed with interrupted nylon or continuous absorbable subcuticular stitches (Figure 96.3). A dressing and bandage is applied.

POSTOPERATIVE CARE AND COMPLICATION

The infant is nursed opposite to the surgical site to minimize pressure on the wound He or she is closely observed for signs of increasing intracranial pressure or development of hydrocephalus. Meningitis is common with anterior encephalocele repair, where contamination is more likely because of proximity to the nose, mouth, and air sinuses. An intracranial approach may help to avoid this. CSF leak can occur despite meticulous dural closure. Once hydrocephalus has been excluded with a CT scan, CSF leaks are managed with additional skin sutures and a lumbar drain. If CSF leak persists, revisional surgery may be required. Most infants with encephalocele repair develop hydrocephalus requiring a CSF shunt.

RESULTS

Encephalocele carries a high rate of mortality (up to 50%).[36] These deaths may be due to cerebral anomalies, other associated congenital abnormalities, an acute rise in intracranial pressure, or complications related to management of hydrocephalus.

PROGNOSIS

Simple isolated encephalocele without associated abnormalities has a better prognosis. Larger lesions, those associated with microcephaly and hydrocephalus, and those forming part of other syndromes (e.g., trisomy 18, Meckel syndrome) have a poorer prognosis.[94,95] Anterior encephalocele has a poorer prognosis than posterior encephalocele.

REFERENCES

1. Prevalence of neural tube defects in 20 regions of Europe and the impact of prenatal diagnosis, 1980–1986. EUROCAT Working Group. *J Epidemiol Community Health* 1991; 45(1): 52–8.
2. Yen IH, Khoury MJ, Erickson JD, James LM, Waters GD, Berry RJ. The changing epidemiology of neural tube defects. United States, 1968–1989. *Am J Dis Child* 1992; 146(7): 857–61.
3. Stevenson RE, Allen WP, Pai GS, Best R, Seaver LH, Dean J et al. Decline in prevalence of neural tube defects in a high-risk region of the United States. *Pediatrics* 2000; 106(4): 677–83.
4. Kondo A, Kamihira O, Ozawa H. Neural tube defects: Prevalence, etiology and prevention. *Int J Urol* 2009; 16(1): 49–57.
5. Morgagni JB. *Je sedibus et causis morborum per indagatis.* Naples: Typographia Simoniana, 1762.
6. Doran PA, Guthkelch AN. Studies in spina bifida cystica I. General surgery and reassessment of the problem. *J Neurol Neurosurg Psychiatr* 1961; 24: 331–45.
7. Tulp N. *Observationes medicae.* Amsterdam: Elsevier, 1672.
8. Virchow R. Ein Fall von hypertrichosis circumscripta mediana kornbiniert mit spina bifida. *Ztschaz Ethnol* 1875; 7: 279.
9. Report of a committee of the society nominated to investigate spina bifida, 1882.
10. Morton J. Case of spina bifida cured by injection. *Br Med J* 1872; 1: 364.

11. Bayer C. Zur technik der operation der spina bifida and encephalocoele. *Prag Med Wochenschr* 1892; 17: 317.

12. Frazier CH. *Surgery of the Spine and Spinal Cord.* New York: Appleton & Co., 1918.

13. Sharrard WJ, Zachary RB, Lorber J. Survival and paralysis in open myelomeningocele with special reference to the time of repair of the spinal lesion. *Dev Med Child Neurol* 1967; Suppl 13: 35–50.

14. Lorber J. Results of treatment of myelomeningocele. An analysis of 524 unselected cases, with special reference to possible selection for treatment. *Dev Med Child Neurol* 1971; 13(3): 279–303.

15. Surana RH, Quinn FM, Guiney EJ, Fitzgerald RJ. Are the selection criteria for the conservative management in spina bifida still applicable? *Eur J Pediatr Surg* 1991; 1 Suppl 1: 35–7.

16. McCarthy GT. Treating children with spina bifida. *BMJ* 1991; 302(6768): 65–6.

17. Woodhouse CR. Myelomeningocele: Neglected aspects. *Pediatr Nephrol* 2008; 23(8): 1223–31.

18. Leck I. The geographical distribution of neural tube defects and oral clefts. *Br Med Bull* 1984; 40(4): 390–5.

19. Boone D, Parsons D, Lachmann SM, Sherwood T. Spina bifida occulta: Lesion or anomaly? *Clin Radiol* 1985; 36(2): 159–61.

20. Wiswell TE, Tuttle DJ, Northam RS, Simonds GR. Major congenital neurologic malformations. A 17-year survey. *Am J Dis Child* 1990; 144(1): 61–7.

21. Leck I. The etiology of human malformations: Insights from epidemiology. *Teratology* 1972; 5(3): 303–14.

22. Gong R, Wang ZP, Wang M, Gao LJ, Zhao ZT. Effects of folic acid supplementation during different pregnancy periods and relationship with the other primary prevention measures to neural tube defects. *J Matern Fetal Neonatal Med* 2016 (epub ahead of print).

23. Lemire RJ, Beckwith JB, Warkny J. *Anencephaly.* New York: Raven Press, 1978.

24. Patten BM. Overgrowth of the neural tube in young human embryos. *Anat Rec* 1952; 113(4): 381–93.

25. Gardner WJ. Rupture of the neural tube. *Arch Neurol* 1961; 4: 1–7.

26. Bentley JF, Smith JR. Developmental posterior enteric remnants and spinal malformations: The split notochord syndrome. *Arch Dis Child* 1960; 35: 76–86.

27. McConnell JR, Holder JC, Menick JR, Alexander JE. The radiology of neural tube defects. In: Keats TF, Bragg NA, Evans RG, Singleton EB, Tegtmeier CH (eds). *Diagnostic Radiology*, vol. XV, 1986: 246–76.

28. Angerpointner TA, Pockrandt L, Schroer K. Course of pregnancy, family history and genetics in children with spina bifida. *Z Kinderchir* 1990; 45(2): 72–7.

29. Carter CO. Clues to the aetiology of neural tube malformations. *Dev Med Child Neurol* 1974; 16(6 Suppl 32): 3–15.

30. Smithells RW, Chinn ER. Spina Bifida In Liverpool. *Dev Med Child Neurol* 1965; 7: 258–68.

31. Olney RS, Mulinare J. Trends in neural tube defect prevalence, folic acid fortification, and vitamin supplement use. *Semin Perinatol* 2002; 26(4): 277–85.

32. Laurence KM, James N, Miller MH, Tennant GB, Campbell H. Double-blind randomised controlled trial of folate treatment before conception to prevent recurrence of neural-tube defects. *Br Med J (Clin Res Ed)* 1981; 282(6275): 1509–11.

33. Willett WC. Folic acid and neural tube defect: Can't we come to closure? *Am J Public Health* 1992; 82(5): 666–8.

34. Folate supplements prevent recurrence of neural tube defects. *Nutr Rev* 1992; 50(1): 22–4.

35. Group MVSR. Prevention of neural tube defects: Results of the medical research council vitamin study. MRC vitamin study research group. *Lancet* 1991; 338(8760): 131–7.

36. Wald NJ, Bower C. Folic acid, pernicious anaemia, and prevention of neural tube defects. *Lancet* 1994; 343(8893): 307.

37. Bower C, D'Antoine H, Stanley FJ. Neural tube defects in Australia: Trends in encephaloceles and other neural tube defects before and after promotion of folic acid supplementation and voluntary food fortification. *Birth Defects Res A Clin Mol Teratol* 2009; 85(4): 269–73.

38. De Wals P, Tairou F, Van Allen MI, Uh SH, Lowry RB, Sibbald B et al. Reduction in neural-tube defects after folic acid fortification in Canada. *N Engl J Med* 2007; 357(2):135–42.

39. Valproate: A new cause of birth defects—Report from Italy and follow-up from France. *MMWR Morb Mortal Wkly Rep* 1983; 32(33): 438–9.

40. Valproate, spina bifida, and birth defect registries. *Lancet* 1988; 2(8625): 1404–5.

41. Rosa FW. Spina bifida in infants of women treated with carbamazepine during pregnancy. *N Engl J Med* 1991; 324(10): 674–7.

42. Pennell PB. Using current evidence in selecting antiepileptic drugs for use during pregnancy. *Epilepsy Curr* 2005; 5(2): 45–51.

43. Lindhout D, Omtzigt JG, Cornel MC. Spectrum of neural-tube defects in 34 infants prenatally exposed to antiepileptic drugs. *Neurology* 1992; 42(4 Suppl 5): 111–8.

44. Janerich DT. Influenza and neural-tube defects. *Lancet* 1971; 2(7723): 551–2.

45. Layde PM, Edmonds LD, Erickson JD. Maternal fever and neural tube defects. *Teratology* 1980; 21(1): 105–8.

46. Sandford MK, Kissling GE, Joubert PE. Neural tube defect etiology: New evidence concerning maternal hyperthermia, health and diet. *Dev Med Child Neurol* 1992; 34(8): 661–75.

47. Milunsky A, Ulcickas M, Rothman KJ, Willett W, Jick SS, Jick H. Maternal heat exposure and neural tube defects. *Jama* 1992; 268(7): 882–5.

48. White-Van Mourik MC, Connor JM, Ferguson-Smith MA. Patient care before and after termination of pregnancy for neural tube defects. *Prenat Diagn* 1990; 10(8): 497–505.

49. Wald NJ, Cuckle H, Brock JH, Peto R, Polani PE, Woodford FP. Maternal serum-alpha-fetoprotein measurement in antenatal screening for anencephaly and spina bifida in early pregnancy. Report of U.K. collaborative study on alpha-fetoprotein in relation to neural-tube defects. *Lancet* 1977; 1(8026): 1323–32.

50. Takeuchi H. [Prenatal ultrasound diagnosis of central nervous system anomalies]. *No To Hattatsu* 1991; 23(2): 183–8.

51. Romero R, Mathisen JM, Ghidini A, Sirtori M, Hobbins JC. Accuracy of ultrasound in the prenatal diagnosis of spinal anomalies. *Am J Perinatol* 1989; 6(3): 320–3.

52. Boyd PA, Devigan C, Khoshnood B, Loane M, Garne E, Dolk H. Survey of prenatal screening policies in Europe for structural malformations and chromosome anomalies, and their impact on detection and termination rates for neural tube defects and Down's syndrome. *Bjog* 2008; 115(6): 689–96.

53. Cameron M, Moran P. Prenatal screening and diagnosis of neural tube defects. *Prenat Diagn* 2009; 29(4): 402–11.

54. Herman-Sucharska I, Bekiesińska-Figatowska M, Urbanik A. Fetal central nervous system malformations on MR images. *Brain Dev* 2009; 31(3): 185–99.

55. Kooper AJ, de Bruijn D, van Ravenwaaij-Arts CM, Faas BH, Creemers JW, Thomas CM et al. Fetal anomaly scan potentially will replace routine AFAFP assays for the detection of neural tube defects. *Prenat Diagn* 2007; 27(1): 29–33.

56. Aitken DA, Morrison NM, Ferguson-Smith MA. Predictive value of amniotic acetylcholinesterase analysis in the diagnosis of fetal abnormality in 3700 pregnancies. *Prenat Diagn* 1984; 4(5): 329–40.

57. Luthy DA, Wardinsky T, Shurtleff DB, Hollenbach KA, Hickok DE, Nyberg DA et al. Cesarean section before the onset of labor and subsequent motor function in infants with meningomyelocele diagnosed antenatally. *N Engl J Med* 1991; 324(10): 662–6.

58. Sakala EP, Andree I. Optimal route of delivery for meningomyelocele. *Obstet Gynecol Surv* 1990; 45(4): 209–12.

59. Thompson DN. Postnatal management and outcome for neural tube defects including spina bifida and encephalocoeles. *Prenat Diagn* 2009; 29(4): 412–9.

60. Adzick NS, Thom EA, Spong CY, Brock JW 3rd,Burrows PK, Johnson MP, Howell LJ, Farrell JA, Dabrowiak ME, Sutton LN, Gupta N, Tulipan NB, A'Alton ME, Farmer DL; MOMS Investigators. A Randomized Trial of Prenatal versus Postnatal Repair of Myelomeningocele. *N Engl J Med* 2011; 364(11): 993–1004.

61. Sutton LN. Fetal surgery for neural tube defects. *Best Pract Res Clin Obstet Gynaecol* 2008; 22(1): 175–88.

62. Greig JD, Young DG, Azmy AF. Follow-up of spina bifida children with and without upper renal tract changes at birth. *Eur J Pediatr Surg* 1991; 1(1): 5–9.

63. Chadduck WM, Reding DL. Experience with simultaneous ventriculo-peritoneal shunt placement and myelomeningocele repair. *J Pediatr Surg* 1988; 23(10): 913–6.

64. Parent AD, McMillan T. Contemporaneous shunting with repair of myelomeningocele. *Pediatr Neurosurg* 1995; 22(3): 132–5; discussion 36.

65. Caldarelli M, Di Rocco C, La Marca F. Shunt complications in the first postoperative year in children with myelomeningocoele. *Childs Nerv Syst* 1996; 12(12): 748–54.

66. O'Brien DF, Javadpour M, Collins DR, Spennato P, Mallucci CL. Endoscopic third ventriculostomy: An outcome analysis of primary cases and procedures performed after ventriculoperitoneal shunt malfunction. *J Neurosurg* 2005; 103(5 Suppl): 393–400.

67. Fritsch MJ, Kienke S, Ankermann T, Padoin M, Mehdorn HM. Endoscopic third ventriculostomy in infants. *J Neurosurg* 2005; 56(6): 1271–8.

68. Stevenson KL. Chiari Type II malformation: Past, present, and future. *Neurosurg Focus* 2004; 16(2): E5.

69. Pollack IF, Pang D, Albright AL, Krieger D. Outcome following hindbrain decompression of symptomatic Chiari malformations in children previously treated with myelomeningocele closure and shunts. *J Neurosurg* 1992; 77(6): 881–8.

70. Vandertop WP, Asai A, Hoffman HJ, Drake JM, Humphreys RP, Rutka JT et al. Surgical decompression for symptomatic Chiari II malformation in neonates with myelomeningocele. *J Neurosurg* 1992; 77(4): 541–4.

71. Charney EB. Parental attitudes toward management of newborns with myelomeningocele. *Dev Med Child Neurol* 1990; 32(1): 14–9.

72. Oakeshott P, Hunt GM, Poulton A, Reid F. Expectation of life and unexpected death in open spina bifida: A 40-year complete, non-selective, longitudinal cohort study. *Dev Med Child Neurol* 2010; 52(8): 749–53.

73. Hunt GM, Oakeshott P. Outcome in people with open spina bifida at age 35: Prospective community based cohort study. *BMJ* 2003; 326 (7403): 1365–6.

74. Fitzgerald RJ, Healy B. The spina bifida problem. A longer term review with special reference to the quality of survival. *Ir Med J* 1974; 67(21): 565–7.

75. Charney EB, Weller SC, Sutton LN, Bruce DA, Schut LB. Management of the newborn with myelomeningocele: Time for a decision-making process. *Pediatrics* 1985; 75(1): 58–64.

76. Robards MF, Thomas GG, Rosenbloom L. Survival of infants with unoperated myeloceles. *Br Med J* 1975; 4(5987): 12–3.

77. Rickwood AMK. Infective problems encountered in neonatal closure of the neural tube defects. *Dev Med Child Neurol* 1976; 18: 164–5.

78. Lorber J, Salfield SA. Results of selective treatment of spina bifida cystica. *Arch Dis Child* 1981; 56(11): 822–30.

79. Rudy DC, Woodside JR. The incontinent myelodysplastic patient. *Urol Clin North Am* 1991; 18(2): 295–308.

80. Kasabian NG, Bauer SB, Dyro FM, Colodny AH, Mandell J, Retik AB. The prophylactic value of clean intermittent catheterization and anticholinergic medication in newborns and infants with myelodysplasia at risk of developing urinary tract deterioration. *Am J Dis Child* 1992; 146(7): 840–3.

81. Stoneking BJ, Brock JW, Pope JC, Adams MC. Early evolution of bladder emptying after myelomeningocele closure. *Urology* 2001; 58(5): 767–71.

82. Jenkinson MD, Hayhurst C, Al-Jumaily M, Kandasamy J, Clark S, Mallucci CL. The role of endoscopic third ventriculostomy in adult patients with hydrocephalus. *J Neurosurg* 2009; 110(5): 861–6.

83. Jenkinson MD, Hayhurst C, Clark S, Campbell S, Murphy P, Mallucci CL. Long-term functional and neuropsychological outcome in Chiari II malformation. *Childs Nerv Syst* 2008; 24(10): 1270.

84. Barf HA, Verhoef M, Post MW, Jennekens-Schinkel A, Gooskens RH, Mullaart RA et al. Educational career and predictors of type of education in young adults with spina bifida. *Int J Rehabil Res* 2004; 27(1): 45–52.

85. Davis BE, Daley CM, Shurtleff DB, Duguay S, Seidel K, Loeser JD et al. Long-term survival of individuals with myelomeningocele. *Pediatr Neurosurg* 2005; 41(4): 186–91.

86. Tuli S, Drake J, Lamberti-Pasculli M. Long-term outcome of hydrocephalus management in myelomeningoceles. *Childs Nerv Syst* 2003; 19(5–6): 286–91.

87. Vachha B, Adams RC, Rollins NK. Limbic tract anomalies in pediatric myelomeningocele and Chiari II malformation: Anatomic correlations with memory and learning—Initial investigation. *Radiology* 2006; 240(1): 194–202.

88. Vinck A, Maassen B, Mullaart R, Rotteveel J. Arnold–Chiari-II malformation and cognitive functioning in spina bifida. *J Neurol Neurosurg Psychiatr* 2006; 77(9): 1083–6.

89. Seitzberg A, Lind M, Biering-Sorensen F. Ambulation in adults with myelomeningocele. Is it possible to predict the level of ambulation in early life? *Childs Nerv Syst* 2008; 24(2): 231–7.

90. Asher M, Olson J. Factors affecting the ambulatory status of patients with spina bifida cystica. *J Bone Joint Surg Am* 1983; 65(3): 350–6.

91. Oakeshott P, Hunt GM. Long-term outcome in open spina bifida. *Br J Gen Pract* 2003; 53(493): 632–6.

92. Bruinings AL, van den Berg-Emons HJ, Buffart LM, van der Heijden-Maessen HC, Roebroeck ME, Stam HJ. Energy cost and physical strain of daily activities in adolescents and young adults with myelomeningocele. *Dev Med Child Neurol* 2007; 49(9): 672–7.

93. Gorlin RJ, Cohen MM, Hennekam RCM. *Syndromes of the Head and Neck*. New York: Oxford University Press, 2001.

94. Date I, Yagyu Y, Asari S, Ohmoto T. Long-term outcome in surgically treated encephalocele. *Surg Neurol* 1993; 40(2): 125–30.

95. Brown MS, Sheridan-Pereira M. Outlook for the child with a cephalocele. *Pediatrics* 1992; 90(6): 914–9.

97

Hydrocephalus

JOTHY KANDASAMY, MAGGIE K. LEE, MARK A. HUGHES, AND CONOR L. MALLUCCI

INTRODUCTION

The term *hydrocephalus* relates to the presence of an excessive amount of cerebrospinal fluid (CSF), which may cause an increase in intracranial pressure with or without abnormal enlargement of the cerebral ventricles. Hydrocephalus can result from a variety of pathological processes or insults that cause imbalance between production and absorption of CSF. Numerous classifications and categories exist with two widely used and pragmatically helpful subdivisions: obstructive (where there is macroscopic obstruction to bulk flow of CSF within the ventricles) and communicating hydrocephalus (where there is inadequate absorption of CSF from the subarachnoid space).

The estimated prevalence of congenital and infantile hydrocephalus is between 0.5 and 0.8 per 1000 births (live and still).[1-3] Until the advent of viable shunts (over 60 years ago), hydrocephalus was usually fatal. The mainstay of treatment of hydrocephalus in the infant remains CSF diversion with shunting. However, neuroendoscopic procedures (predominantly endoscopic third ventriculostomy [ETV]) are increasingly utilized in certain situations. Technological advances in neuroimaging, neuronavigation, and shunt hardware, and a better understanding of CSF dynamics is leading to a more patient-specific approach to this complex and multifactorial problem. Hydrocephalus may cause pathological changes to brain morphology, microstructure, circulation, biochemistry, metabolism, and maturation. Although treatment does not always reverse the damage, the timing of therapy is crucial in determining reversibility and outcome for the patient.

CSF CIRCULATION

The three components influencing CSF dynamics are production, circulation, and drainage. CSF is derived by adenosine triphosphate (ATP)-dependent active secretion from cerebral arterial blood across epithelial walls. The global average rate of CSF production is constant under normal and stable conditions at 0.35 mL per minute.[4,5] The current widely accepted view is that CSF circulation is via bulk flow.[6] Produced mainly in the choroid plexus of the lateral and third ventricles, CSF flows along the aqueduct of Sylvius to reach the fourth ventricle. CSF flows out of the fourth ventricle through the midline foramen of Magendie and the lateral foramina of Luschka into the subarachnoid space, comprising an interconnecting network of basal CSF cisterns. Most CSF flows around the convexities of the brain upward to the superior sagittal sinus. Some CSF flows downward toward the lumbar subarachnoid space. CSF drains into the venous compartment, predominantly via a pressure-dependent one-way pathway through arachnoid granulations in the walls of the superior sagittal sinus.[4,6]

Although our understanding of CSF dynamics is incomplete, the distinction between communicating and obstructive hydrocephalus is important (albeit sometimes knowingly inaccurate) as it informs treatment options. Obstruction of CSF flow between the third and fourth ventricles results in accumulation of CSF in the lateral and third ventricles. This may be the result of a congenital or acquired stenosis of the aqueduct, or due to a compressive mass in the posterior fossa. Endoscopic fenestration of the floor of the third ventricle (creating a new pathway for CSF to enter the subarachnoid space) can be effective in this situation. Meningitis or hemorrhage in the subarachnoid space can both impair CSF flow and also impede absorption through arachnoid granulations. In this context, third ventriculostomy is less likely to be effective, and shunting may be necessary.

CAUSES OF HYDROCEPHALUS

The numerous causes of hydrocephalus are out with the scope of this chapter. Only those most relevant to the newborn are outlined and divided into the following causative categories: obstructive hydrocephalus (radiologically visible obstructive lesion), communicating hydrocephalus (no radiologically visible obstructive lesion), external hydrocephalus, and rarely, overproduction of CSF.

Obstructive hydrocephalus

AQUEDUCT STENOSIS

This accounts for 6%–66% of cases of hydrocephalus in children. In the vast majority of cases, aqueduct stenosis is sporadic or acquired. However, rare X-linked syndromic cases have been described.[7] Aqueduct obstruction may be caused by gliosis secondary to infection or hemorrhage, or due to compression from neoplastic (e.g., tectal tumors), vascular (e.g., vein of Galen aneurysms), or congenital central nervous system (CNS) malformations (Dandy–Walker, Chiari, Spina Bifida). Magnetic resonance imaging MRI is mandatory to assess the patency of the aqueduct, which cannot be visualized adequately on computed tomography (CT).

SPINA BIFIDA AND CHIARI MALFORMATION

Approximately 95% of patients with spinal myelomeningocele have some degree of hydrocephalus, which is almost invariably associated with the Chiari II malformation.[8] The major craniocervical features of a Chiari II lesion include the following: caudal displacement of the fourth ventricle into the upper cervical canal, elongation and thinning of the upper medulla and lower pons, caudal displacement of the medulla and lower cerebellum through the foramen magnum, and various bony defects of the upper cervical vertebrae and occiput.[9] Please refer to Chapter 96, "Spina Bifida and Encephalocele."

Dandy–Walker complex and posterior fossa cysts

The *Dandy–Walker complex* refers to a rare group of malformations in which abnormal posterior fossa CSF collections show clear communication with the fourth ventricle. Dandy–Walker malformation is included in this category and typically involves cystic dilatation of the fourth ventricle, partial or complete agenesis of the cerebellar vermis, and hydrocephalus in up to 90% of cases.[10] It can be associated with other nervous or systemic abnormalities. Posterior fossa arachnoid cysts do not communicate directly with the fourth ventricle. Both third ventriculostomy and shunting are valid surgical options, and overall morbidity appears to be related to early and adequate treatment of the associated hydrocephalus.[11,12]

NEOPLASTIC LESIONS

Fortunately, brain tumors in newborns are very rare. The most common types are often of neuroectodermal origin and are more commonly supratentorial. Any neoplastic lesion can cause hydrocephalus due to obstruction of CSF pathways.

Communicating (nonobstructive) hydrocephalus

POSTHEMORRHAGIC HYDROCEPHALUS

Hemorrhage in the neonatal period is a common cause of hydrocephalus.[13,14] The premature infant born before gestation week 32 is especially vulnerable. Hemorrhage most commonly originates in the highly vascularized germinal matrix. Most studies agree that the incidence is highest in infants weighing less than 1.5 kg at birth, and up to 50% of hemorrhages occur within 8 hours of birth.[13,14] In the term neonate, the most common site of hemorrhage is the choroid plexus, but this accounts for only a small percentage of neonatal hemorrhages. Posthemorrhagic hydrocephalus (PHH) can be defined as progressive dilation of the ventricular system as a complication of neonatal intraventricular hemorrhage (IVH). Hemorrhage is postulated to provoke an inflammatory response leading to thickening of the arachnoid in the basal cisterns and temporary or permanent occlusion of the arachnoid villi.[15] PHH may contain elements of both communicating and obstructive hydrocephalus, at varying stages. The incidence of PHH after IVH of prematurity ranges from 25% to 74% and is proportionately linked to the blood load within the ventricular system.[14] The continuous improvement in perinatal care has led to increased survival rate of preterm infants and thus a greater risk of these infants developing IVH and PHH. Fernall et al. reported that an infant born very preterm has a 60 times higher risk of developing infantile hydrocephalus than an infant born at term.[16] Ultrasonography is sensitive and specific in diagnosing IVH, and some advocate routine ultrasonography in any infant born before 34 weeks' gestation and/or for those infants weighing less than 1.5 kg at birth.[17-19] Most IVHs are small and resolve spontaneously. More severe hemorrhages are associated with an increased risk of developing PHH and higher risk of mortality and neurodevelopmental impairment.

The risk of IVH in the preterm infant has been reduced significantly by measures that indirectly ameliorate fluctuation in cerebral blood flow (such as surfactant to reduce pulmonary hypertension and antenatal steroid administration).[16,20] Some advocate that premature infants should be maintained on paralytics and sedated for the first 72 hours following birth to reduce the risk of IVH.[20] Once PHH has been diagnosed, temporizing interventions can be employed. Ventricular access devices (VADs), external ventricular drains (EVDs), ventriculosubgaleal (VSG) shunts, or lumbar punctures (LPs) are potential temporizing strategies. VSG shunts may reduce the need for daily CSF aspiration compared with VADs. The routine use of serial LP is no longer recommended as a means of reducing the downstream need for a shunt.[21] Some patients are too unstable for surgery, or their hydrocephalus may resolve after degradation of the IVH. Most cases of PHH occur 3–4 weeks after IVH. Importantly, many cases are clinically silent, and early detection requires a high index of suspicion and serial radiological monitoring. Of those that develop PHH, over 50% become shunt dependent, with a high rate of neurodevelopmental disability. Medical and surgical management options will be discussed in the next sections of this chapter.

POSTINFECTIVE HYDROCEPHALUS

Intrauterine infection by cytomegalic inclusion disease, mumps, toxoplasmosis, and syphilis can cause congenital hydrocephalus. Postnatal meningitis and or ventriculitis can also lead to hydrocephalus from obstruction to arachnoid granulations and/or obstruction to CSF flow in the basal cisterns. Meningitis in the newborn may result from amniotic infection where the membranes have been ruptured for a prolonged period. In the first 2 weeks of life, the organism is usually *Escherichia coli* or other Gram-negative enteric bacilli. In the second 2-week period, Gram-positive cocci, *Listeria*, and *Pseudomonas* are more common.[22-24] Postinfective hydrocephalus (PIH) typically occurs 2–3 weeks after diagnosis of bacterial meningitis. Associated complications include abscess formation, ventriculitis and subsequent CSF loculations and intraventricular septations.[24,25] The management is difficult and frequently requires multiple shunts and revisions, with consequent poor development and high morbidity and mortality.

External hydrocephalus

This controversial entity is also linked to or referred to as *pseudohydrocephalus, benign subdural effusion, benign enlargement of the subarachnoid spaces*, and *benign pericerebral effusion*. Its etiology and pathophysiology are uncertain, but they describe abnormal collections of fluid in the subarachnoid or subdural space overlying the cerebral convexity. The condition occurs while the cranial sutures are open. Most cases do not require intervention and follow a benign course. Rarely, a subdural-peritoneal shunt is required if a patient presents with features related to mass effect and raised intracranial pressure.

Overproduction of CSF

Choroid plexus papillomas are intraventricular tumors that cause overproduction of CSF and resultant ventricular enlargement. They are most often found in the lateral ventricle and appear as homogenously enhancing lesions on MRI. Resection of the tumor may be curative if the tumor is benign.

CLINICAL FEATURES OF HYDROCEPHALUS IN THE NEWBORN

Despite a vast variation in underlying etiology, clinical presentation of hydrocephalus is remarkably consistent and relates to signs and symptoms of localized or generalized raised intracranial pressure.

An increase in head size is the major feature of hydrocephalus in the neonate, with increasing deviation of head circumference from the normal centiles for age. Incremental plotting of head circumference is essential in this regard, using a centile chart such as that produced by Gairdner and Pearson, which corrects for gestational age at birth.[26] It should be noted that there are causes for head enlargement other than hydrocephalus (e.g., a familial tendency for a large head, osteofibromatosis, macrocephaly or intracranial cysts). The head *shape* may also be abnormal.

Bulging of the anterior fontanelle with a variably open posterior fontanelle, separation of the suture lines, and dilatation of superficial scalp veins (due to venous reflux from cerebral sinuses) are classical features of raised intracranial pressure in hydrocephalus. "Setting sun sign," an upward gaze palsy, may be seen. This phenomenon consists of downward rotation of the eyeballs and retraction of the upper eyelids and may be accompanied by brow raising. Sixth-nerve palsy can occur due its sensitivity to pressure during its long intracranial course. Papilledema, decreased level of consciousness, and other focal neurological deficits can also be presenting signs. Opisthotonic posturing and bradycardic and apneic episodes are critical signs of raised intracranial pressure suggesting brain-stem compromise. This demands emergent neurosurgical assessment and treatment.

Other important, though less specific, presenting symptoms of hydrocephalus in the infant include irritability, lethargy, poor feeding, vomiting, failure to thrive, and delayed motor development. Clinical presentation may also include features specific to the underlying causative pathology.

CURRENT IMAGING AND INVESTIGATIVE TECHNIQUES FOR HYDROCEPHALUS IN THE NEWBORN

Skull x-rays are largely obsolete in the management of hydrocephalus in the newborn. Historically, widening of the sutures beyond 3 mm, with associated *lacunar* skull defects, was suggestive. Ultrasonography is exceptionally useful as a noninvasive technique (Figure 97.1).[17-19] Antenatal sonography can detect hydrocephalus in utero and is the screening procedure of choice in patients under the age of 18 months. In the newborn, the anterior fontanelle provides a window. Measurements of both the ventricle size and the cortical mantle are possible. Serial ultrasonography has not only improved the ability to detect hydrocephalus but also resulted in more prompt treatment. Ultrasound has proven especially useful in detecting IVH and associated hydrocephalus in premature infants. It is considered the initial investigation of choice for neonates with hydrocephalus (Figure 97.1) and can be performed at the bedside.[17-19] Although sensitive and specific for the detection of hydrocephalus, clarification of underlying cause usually necessitates CT or MRI.

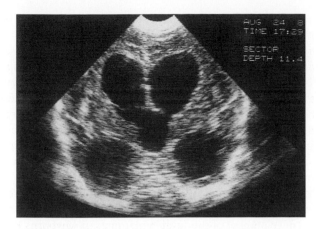

Figure 97.1 Aqueduct stenosis. Coronal section on sonography showing dilated lateral ventricles and foramina of Monro passing into a dilated third ventricle.

A complete high-resolution CT can be obtained within 2 minutes of the patient being on the CT table (Figure 97.2). MRI is the gold standard for diagnosing the *cause* of hydrocephalus and demonstrates the ventricular and CSF anatomy in exquisite detail. Pathological entities such as aqueductal stenosis, Chiari malformation, and neoplastic lesions are readily identifiable. MRI also allows detailed surgical planning when considering ETV, shunting, posterior fossa surgery, and so forth. MRI dynamic flow sequences can highlight relevant ventricular, periventricular, and other CSF flow with remarkable clarity.[27] This is particularly useful when assessing the anatomy of the third ventricle and aqueduct. Volume data sets (for both CT and MRI) allow bespoke intraoperative three-dimensional neuronavigation for shunting and neuroendoscopic procedures. MRI is increasingly used as an antenatal investigation and is valuable in both characterizing congenital malformations and detecting hemorrhage.[28]

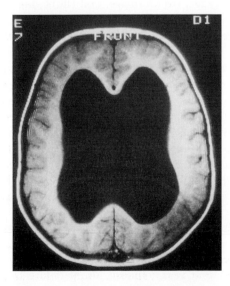

Figure 97.2 CT scan of head showing dilated lateral ventricles.

Postoperative imaging to assess ventricular size after shunting or neuroendoscopy can be performed with both CT and MRI. However, after a third ventriculostomy, phase contrast dynamic MRI sequences are required to identify CSF flow through the new stoma.[27,29] Invasive pressure measurements such as fontonometry are less often justified as they are unreliable compared with modern methods of imaging.

An antibody screen should be carried out if an intrauterine infection is suspected. CSF analysis is indicated where infection or hemorrhage is suspected. A raised protein level, or indeed bloodstained CSF, is not necessarily a contraindication to shunting but may inform the timing of shunt placement. It may be appropriate to delay surgery until the protein count and/or the blood in the CSF clears. If active infection is suspected, a temporizing EVD is preferable. Once the infection is fully treated and the CSF is sterile, a permanent shunt can be implanted.

TREATMENT OPTIONS FOR HYDROCEPHALUS IN THE NEWBORN

Nonsurgical/medical management

The complications associated with surgery in the low-birth-weight neonate, or neonates with unstable comorbidities, demand that nonsurgical means of managing hydrocephalus be considered. However, pharmacotherapeutic agents such as acetozolamide, frusemide, and steroids have not been shown to be effective in reducing the rate of shunting and are not recommended.[30,31] Although historically common practice, serial LPs are no longer recommended. Meta-analysis found no evidence of benefit but a significant risk of secondary infection.[21,32] Similarly, serial percutaneous ventricular taps have been abandoned by most tertiary neurosurgical centers due to frequent complications such *puncture porencephaly*, infection, and encephalomalacia.[33,34]

Surgical management

Surgery remains the overwhelming mainstay of treatment for hydrocephalus in the newborn. Shunting converted hydrocephalus from what was almost universally fatal to a treatable condition. The first permanent CSF diversion for hydrocephalus was performed by Mikulicz in 1893 in the form of a ventriculo–subarachnoid–subgaleal shunt.[35] Since then, virtually every anatomical cavity has been trialed as a potential reservoir or conduit for CSF drainage. This section outlines the most common surgical techniques in newborn hydrocephalus surgery.

EXTERNAL VENTRICULAR DRAINAGE

EVD is used widely in the temporary treatment of hydrocephalus. The frontal and occipital horns of the lateral ventricles are the target site, accessed via a single burr hole. CSF is drained at the desired rate into a sterile closed-circuit system. EVD is of use in the presence of active infection (where a permanent shunt system would become colonized) or when time is required to allow a transiently high CSF pressure to normalize. EVDs also provide a route for administration of intrathecal antibiotics into the infected CSF space. Similarly, EVD is useful in IVH or PHH as a temporizing measure before either persistent hydrocephalus declares itself or the blood load has reduced. In an emergent setting arising from tumor-related obstructive hydrocephalus, EVD allows decompression of the ventricular system prior to more planned definitive tumor resection. Despite the introduction of antibiotic-impregnated EVDs, these are still prone to significant infection rates, and catheters are also easily dislodged. Several studies have assessed the efficacy of intraventricular fibrinolytic therapies and CSF irrigation. With the advent of improved neuroendoscopic equipment and approaches, these techniques continue to be considered as there is some evidence that long-term outcomes may be improved in neonates with IVH-related hydrocephalus.[21,34,36,37]

SUBCUTANEOUS VAD

Here, the ventricular catheter connects to a subcutaneous reservoir under the scalp. This device may be indicated in the newborn infant whose low birth weight and/or the potential for spontaneous arrest of hydrocephalus preclude the immediate need for a permanent shunt. It is a viable option in PHH. The reservoir allows easy CSF tapping, lower infection rates compared to EVD, and access for intraventricular antibiotics. Complications and limitations include skin erosion, CSF leak, and only intermittent pressure control.

VENTRICULOPERITONEAL SHUNT

The majority of hydrocephalic newborns undergoing CSF diversion surgery will have a ventriculoperitoneal shunt (VPS). The principle of VPS remains unchanged since first described in 1908.[35] Initially, ventriculoatrial (VA), or ventriculopleural (VP) shunts were considered preferable. The peritoneum became the drainage site of choice as complications with VA shunts, such as sudden death from pulmonary embolism, endocarditis, and nephritis, were noted. Another problem in VA shunts in the neonate is the need to lengthen the lower end as the child grows and the catheter pulls up out of the atrium. This can be obviated with VPS by placing a long intraperitoneal catheter allowing scope for growth. The hardware required for a VPS includes a ventricular catheter, CSF reservoir, shunt valve, and distal peritoneal catheter. Recently, antibiotic-impregnated and antibiotic-resistant shunt tubing have been gaining popularity. Their capacity to reduce infection is currently under investigation via a large multicenter randomized controlled trial (RCT) (British Antibiotic and Silver Impregnated Catheters for VPS, http://www.basicsstudy.org.uk/index.html).[38]

The choice of shunt valve also remains a regular source of debate within the neurosurgical community. Valve types include differential pressure, flow regulating, gravity-actuated, and programmable. All valves only allow unidirectional flow of the CSF. An antisiphon device may be included in the system to prevent positional over-drainage. There are no studies that conclusively prove one valve type to be superior to another.[39-41] In practice, some factors that may influence choice include valve size/profile, cortical mantle thickness, cost, and individual surgeon experience. Some authors advocate a flow control valve for shunts in the newborn to avoid the downstream complication of slit ventricle syndrome. This is related to chronic over-drainage and seen most commonly in patients who have a shunt implanted in the first 2 years of life.[42] Overdrainage and development of subdural hematomas in newborns with large ventricles and thin cortical mantle may be avoided with high-resistance valves.[43]

Some advocate the use of a VPS in combination with a separate VAD. A VAD allows easy sampling of CSF for microbiological assessment, is a means of assessing CSF pressure, and is an easy access point for external drainage in the event of shunt blockage. Arguably, this can reduce unnecessary shunt explorations. The additional procedure of VAD insertion is not associated with increased patient morbidity.[44]

Both frameless and frame-based neuronavigation systems have been utilized to optimize the position of ventricular catheters. Recent studies have shown benefit in catheter placement accuracy, but it remains uncertain whether this translates into lower shunt revision rates in the long term.[45] With the electromagnetic (EM) frameless neuronavigation systems, there is no requirement for rigid head fixation with pins or screws. This confers a significant advantage for neonatal shunt surgery. Previous studies on endoscopic versus nonendoscopic catheter placement did not demonstrate any difference in shunt revision rates.[46]

Common complications of VPS include infection, malposition of the ventricular catheter, mechanical failure leading to blockage, overdrainage, and shunt migration. Less common complications include bowel perforation, hernia, hydrocele, appendicitis, and peritonitis. Shunt complication rates are significantly higher in the newborn, and studies have shown low birth weight to be linked to a higher incidence of shunt infection and revision rates.[47] If the CSF is sterile on insertion, the most common organisms responsible for postoperative infection are skin commensals such as *Staphylococcus epidermidis (albus)*. Where infection is proven, removal of the entire shunt system, temporary CSF diversion via an EVD, and concomitant intrathecal antibiotic administration are usually necessary. The treatment of shunt infections has been reviewed extensively by Bayston et al.[48]

Despite advances in neuronavigation and shunt hardware, shunt failure remains a considerable source of morbidity for those with hydrocephalus. Up to 40% of shunts fail in the first year.[49] Indeed, shunt failure is an almost inevitable consequence during a patient's life, with up to 80% of shunts requiring revision within 12 years.[50]

NEUROENDOSCOPY AND ETV

Advances in fiber-optic camera technology, combined with high-resolution MRI, have renewed enthusiasm for neuro-endoscopy as a therapeutic option in hydrocephalus. ETV was first performed as an open procedure by Dandy in 1922 and subsequently as an endoscopic procedure by Mixter in 1923.[34]

ETV is a minimally invasive procedure. A single parame-dian coronal burr hole allows access into the lateral ventri-cle. The ventricle is entered with a 10- or 12-French cannula, which serves as a conduit for the rigid or flexible endoscope. The endoscope is advanced toward and into the enlarged foramen of Monro and then into the third ventricle. A mid-line fenestration is formed, and dilated, in the thinned floor of the third ventricle—avoiding critical structures such as the mammillary bodies and the basilar artery. The endo-scope is then advanced through the fenestration to ensure that an effective communication into the interpeduncular and prepontine subarachnoid space has been achieved. At completion, the endoscope and cannula are removed, and no hardware is left in situ.

Circumventing the need for a shunt is an attractive surgical option. However, current evidence suggests that patient selection is crucial to success.[51] ETV in obstruc-tive hydrocephalus with maintained CSF absorption (such as in congenital aqueduct stenosis) is associated with the highest success rates. While in older children, the indica-tions for endoscopic treatment have been relatively well defined, debate continues on the utility of ETV in the first few months of life.[52–54] Various studies have reported differ-ing success rates, and there remains a lack of consensus in infants and neonates.[55]

The International Infant Hydrocephalus Study (IIHS) is an international multicenter prospective SCT of ETV versus shunting in children presenting under the age of 2 years with pure aqueduct stenosis.[56,57] The role of ETV as a secondary treatment option after initial or multiple shunt failures is gaining popularity.[58] This is relevant to the newborn with PHH or PIH who may benefit from a primary shunt (where primary ETV is ineffective) and can then be considered for a secondary ETV when presenting with a future shunt failure.

ETV may also have an important role in treatment of hydrocephalus in less economically developed countries.[59] The paucity of a follow-up in this context reinforces the advantage of a shunt-free option. PIH accounts for up to 60% of hydrocephalus cases in some developing countries.[59] In a relatively large series of patients treated in one developing country, success rates were lower in the under-1-year group compared with older children (mirroring findings in more economically developed regions). Nevertheless, ETV has enabled up to 60% shunt avoidance in developing-country infants with PIH causing acquired aqueduct stenosis.[59] The combination of ETV and choroid plexus cauterization (CPC) may also be a viable option in temporarily reducing CSF production until absorptive capacity improves. A study employing this technique in the developing world reported a success rate of over 70% in infants under 1 year old with PIH and an open aqueduct.[60]

Other applications of neuroendoscopy include aqueduc-tal stenting (for isolated fourth-ventricle enlargement), sep-tum pellucidotomies (for multiloculated hydrocephalus), cyst fenestration, and as an adjunct to shunt surgery by aid-ing shunt placement under direct endoscopic vision.

Although safe in well-trained and experienced hands, complications of neuroendoscopy can be devastating. Severe hemorrhage, cardiac arrest, cerebral infarction, diabetes insipidus, and damage to the fornices (resulting in memory deficit) have all been reported.[61] Also important is the rare but potential risk of sudden post-ETV death due to closure of the ventriculostomy.[61] Nevertheless, neuroendoscopy—together with advances in computerized neuronavigation—has an increasingly important role in the management of hydrocephalus.

FETAL SURGICAL THERAPY

Hydrocephalus is detectable in utero, raising the question of prenatal intervention. In spite of extensive experimental work, and indeed some human intervention in countries where abortions are legally banned, results on the whole have been poor.[62] The majority of patients who have under-gone fetal surgery for hydrocephalus required VPS inser-tion after birth.

However, fetal surgery in the context of myelomeningo-cele, has been shown to reduce the rate of subsequent shunt-ing. The Management of Myelomeningocele Study (MOMS) was a multicenter randomized prospective trial comparing prenatal (18–25 weeks of gestation) and postnatal repair of myelomeningocele. Outcomes assessed include death, the need for ventricular shunting by 1 year of life, and neuro-logical function at 30 months of age. MOMS found that prenatal surgery for myelomeningocele reduced the rate of shunting (40% compared with 82%) and improved a com-posite score of mental development and motor function. However, pregnancy complications were more common in the fetal surgery group, including higher risk of preterm delivery and uterine dehiscence at delivery.[63]

Shunt operation technique

VENTRICULOPERITONEAL SHUNTS

The patient is positioned while under general endotracheal anesthesia. Antibiotic prophylaxis at induction is recom-mended. The head is turned to the opposite side of intended shunt placement, with the neck extended slightly to create a straight line between the scalp and abdominal incision. The site of the burr hole and abdominal incision is to be marked prior to skin preparation and draping (Figure 97.3). Occipital burr holes are usually 3–4 cm from the midline along the lambdoid suture. Frontal burr holes are 2–3 cm along the coronal suture from the midline. It is vital to tailor the burr hole to the ventricular morphology, so as to ensure optimal ventricular catheter placement. In infants with

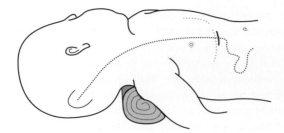

Figure 97.3 The dotted line represents the course of the ventricular catheter. The patient is positioned with a roll of Gamgee under the shoulders to straighten out the neck and allow easier passage of the cannula. The skin is marked, predisinfection, with a pen, showing the curved incision site behind the posterior parietal eminence. The transverse abdominal incision site is also marked with a dark line.

splayed sutures, access can be achieved via an opening of the sutures. The site of a burr hole is of surgeon's preference; there is little evidence showing advantages of one over the other. Occipital burr holes are more cosmetically acceptable (Figure 97.4a). After the burr hole, a durotomy is performed, and the brain pia is cauterized. Dural opening should be kept minimal to reduce the risk of CSF egress around the ventricular catheter (increasing risk of CSF leak from the wound) (Figure 97.4b).

The abdominal incision is usually performed on the same side in either an upper midline or paraumbilical site. The most important step is ensuring that the peritoneum is opened. Open technique, use of a trocar,[64] or using laparoscopic assistance have all been described.[65] The distal catheter is tunneled subcutaneously from the burr hole site to

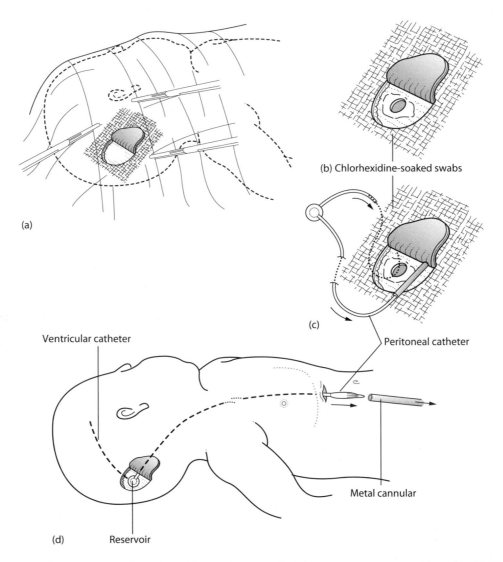

(a)

(b) Chlorhexidine-soaked swabs

(c)

Peritoneal catheter

Ventricular catheter

Metal cannular

(d)   Reservoir

Figure 97.4 (a) Wound drapes surrounding the scalp incision. Upper incision to pericranium is made. **(b)** The pericranium is diathermied and rasped peripherally and a burr hole made. **(c)** Following incision in the abdomen, a long trocar and cannula are passed percutaneously to exit at the lower incision. The long trocar is removed, allowing passage of the peritoneal catheter along the metal cannula. The trocars in some prepared shunt sets have a device for attaching the distal catheter and allowing it to be pulled through distally. **(d)** Having lightly diathermied the dura, a small hole is made in it and the ventricular catheter introduced and connected to a reservoir. With free flow from the distal end, the catheter is placed in the peritoneal cavity and the peritoneum closed snugly around it.

the abdominal opening, or vice versa. If a frontal burr hole is used, an intervening incision is made at the occiput.

The ventricular catheter is introduced mounted on a stylet. The trajectory is determined according to external landmarks or guided by neuronavigation. From an occipital burr hole, targeting the midpoint of the forehead at the hairline enables the occipital horn of the lateral ventricle to be entered. From a frontal burr hole, the target is the intersecting planes of the midpupillary line and the external auditory meatus. Intraoperative ultrasonography or image-guided stereotaxy[41] can be used for more accurate positioning of the catheter. CSF pressure can be measured once the ventricle is cannulated, and a sample of CSF taken for biochemical and microbiological examinations. The proximal catheter is connected to a reservoir and a valve system, itself connected to the tunneled distal catheter. The distal end is examined to ensure that there is free flow of CSF and then placed within the peritoneum. The peritoneum is closed followed by the rest of the abdomen in layers (Figure 97.4d).

VA SHUNTS

These may be performed in a similar fashion to VPSs except for the lower incision, which is over the right side of the neck. The objective is for the shunt tip to lie in the superior vena cava or atrium. Open access to the jugular vein can be achieved by exposing the common facial vein. This is tied proximally and held with a stay suture at the venotomy site, and the distal catheter is then fed into the superior vena cava. Throughout the procedure, the anesthetist monitors the electrocardiogram (ECG) for any cardiac alterations or rhythm changes. A purse-string suture is closed around the catheter sufficiently to prevent hemorrhage, but not so tight as to cause obstruction to the catheter. Percutaneous (Seldinger) methods can also be used to enter the jugular or subclavian veins, aided by ultrasound.[66–68] Complications include cor pulmonale, catheter emboli, and shunt nephritis.

VP SHUNTS

The proximal approach is identical to VPS placement. The pleural space can be entered safely in the fifth intercostal space along the anterior axillary line. Intercostal muscle layers are split on the upper border of the rib to avoid the neurovascular bundle. Once revealed, the parietal pleura is opened and the distal catheter gently introduced. The muscle is closed to avoid air entry into the pleural space. Intrapleural catheter placement may be aided by thoracoscopy.[65] Contraindications for this technique include previous thoracic surgery, acute or chronic pulmonary disease, and poor pulmonary function. Progressive CSF accumulation may lead to respiratory distress, and therefore, vigilance for this complication is important. This technique is rarely applicable in newborns, or indeed infants, as the pleural cavity has inadequate absorptive capacity at this age. The technique is usually reserved for older children where all other options have been exhausted.

Other sites for a distal catheter include the cerebral venous system, gallbladder, ureter, and bladder. These sites are used rarely in neonates because of their complexity and complications, leading to increased morbidity and mortality.

POSTOPERATIVE CARE

Postoperative scans are obtained and act as a reference for future surgery and shunt positioning. Continual monitoring of head circumference is required.

OUTCOMES

The outcome of hydrocephalus depends upon the underlying cause, the treatment selected (and complications thereof), the socioeconomic status of the child, and other factors beyond the scope of this chapter. The important message is that hydrocephalus is not a single disease entity and that treatment must be tailored to etiology and age. Avoidance of complications is of paramount importance and dramatically alters long-term prognosis.

REFERENCES

1. Blackburn BL, Fineman RM. Epidemiology of congenital hydrocephalus in Utah, 1940–1979: Report of an iatrogenically related "epidemic." *Am J Med Genet* 1994; 52: 123–9.
2. Fernell E, Hagberg G, Hagberg B. Infantile hydrocephalus epidemiology: An indicator of enhanced survival. *Arch Dis Child Fetal Neonatal Ed* 1994; 70: F123–8.
3. Stein S, Feldman H, Kohl S et al. The epidemiology of congenital hydrocephalus: A study in Brooklyn NY 1968–1976. *Child's Brain* 1981; 8: 253–62.
4. Kimelberg HK. Water homeostasis in the brain: Basic concepts. *Neuroscience* 2004; 129(4): 851–60.
5. Redzic ZB, Segal MB. The structure of the choroid plexus and the physiology of the choroid plexus epithelium. *Adv Drug Deliv Rev* 2004; 56(12): 1695–716.
6. Abbott NJ. Evidence for bulk flow of brain interstitial fluid: Significance for physiology and pathology. *Neurochem Int* 2004; 45(4): 545–52.
7. Halliday J, Chow CW, Wallace D, Danks DM. X-linked hydrocephalus: A survey of a 20 year period in Victoria, Australia. *J Med Genet* 1986; 23: 23–31.
8. Noetzel MJ. Myelomeningocele: Current concepts of management. *Clin Perinatol* 1989; 16: 311–29.
9. Naidich TP, McLone DG, Fulling KH. The Chiari II malformation: Part IV. The hindbrain deformity. *Neuroradiology* 1983; 25(4): 179–97.
10. Laroche JC. Malformations of the nervous system. In: Adams JH, Corsellis JAN, Duchen LW (eds). *Greenfields Neuropathology*, 4th edn. New York: Wiley, 1984: 385–450.
11. Kumar R, Jain MK, Chhabra DK. Dandy–Walker syndrome: Different modalities of treatment and outcome in 42 cases. *Child's Nerv Syst* 2001; 17: 348–52.

12. Mohanty A, Biswas A, Satish S, Praharaj SS, Sastry KV. Treatment options for Dandy–Walker malformation. *J Neurosurg* 2006 November; 105(5 Suppl): 348–56.

13. Ahmann PA, Lazzara A, Dykes FD et al. Intraventricular haemorrhage in the high risk preterm infant: Incidence and outcome. *Ann Neurol* 1980; 7: 118–24.

14. van de Bor M, Verloove-Vanhorick SP, Brand R, Keirse MJ, Ruys JH. Incidence and prediction of periventricular–intraventricular hemorrhage in very preterm infants. *J Perinat Med* 1987; 15(4): 333–9.

15. Weller RO, Shulman K. Infantile hydrocephalus: Clinical, histological, and ultrastructural study of brain damage. *J Neurosurg* 1972 March; 36(3): 255–65.

16. Fernall E, Hagberg G, Hagberg B. Infantile hydrocephalus—The impact of enhanced preterm survival. *Acta Paediatr Scand* 1990; 79: 1080–6.

17. International Society of Ultrasound in Obstetrics and Gynecology. Sonographic examination of fetal central nervous system: Guidelines for performing the "basic examination" and the "fetal neurosonogram." *Ultrasound Obstet Gynecol* 2007; 29: 109–16.

18. Quinn MW. The Doppler characteristics of hydrocephalus. MD thesis, Trinity College, Dublin University, 1991.

19. Goh D, Minns RA, Pye SD. Transcranial Doppler ultrasound as a non-invasive means of monitoring cerebrohaemodynamic change in hydrocephalus. *Eur J Paediatr Surg* 1991; 1(Suppl. I): 14–17.

20. Perlman JM, McMenamin JB, Volpe JJ. Fluctuating cerebral blood-flow velocity in respiratory-distress syndrome. Relation to the development of intraventricular hemorrhage. *N Engl J Med* 1983 July 28; 309(4): 204–9.

21. Mazzola CA, Choudhri AF, Auguste KI, Limbrick DD Jr, Rogido M, Mitchell L, Flannery AM. Pediatric hydrocephalus: Systematic literature review and evidence-based guidelines. Part 2: Management of posthemorrhagic hydrocephalus in premature infants. *J Neurosurg Pediatr* 2014; 1:8-23.

22. Sáez-Llorens X, McCracken GH Jr. Bacterial meningitis in children. *Lancet* 2003 June 21; 361(9375): 2139–48. Review.

23. Chang Chien HY, Chiu NC, Li WC et al: Characteristics of neonatal bacterial meningitis in a teaching hospital in Taiwan from 1984–1997. *J Microbiol Immunol Infect* 2000 June; 33(2): 100–4.

24. Klinger G, Chin CN, Beyene J, Perlman M. Predicting the outcome of neonatal bacterial meningitis. *Pediatrics* 2000 September; 106(3): 477–82.

25. Prats JM, López-Heredia J, Gener B, Freijo MM, Garaizar C Multilocular hydrocephalus: Ultrasound studies of origin and development. *Pediatr Neurol* 2001 February; 24(2): 149–51.

26. Zahl SM, Wester K. Routine measurement of head circumference as a tool for detecting intracranial expansion in infants: What is the gain? A nationwide survey. *Pediatrics* 2008 March; 121(3): e416–20.

27. Mallucci CI, Sgourous S. *Cerebrospinal Fluid Disorders*. Chapter 3. Informa Healthcare, 2010: 71–5.

28. Papadias A, Miller C, Martin WL, Kilby MD, Sgouros S. Comparison of prenatal and postnatal MRI findings in the evaluation of intrauterine CNS anomalies requiring postnatal neurosurgical treatment. *Childs Nerv Syst* 2008 February; 24(2): 185–92. Epub August 21, 2007.

29. O'Brien DF, Seghedoni A, Collins DR, Hayhurst C, Mallucci CL Is there an indication for ETV in young infants in aetiologies other than isolated aqueduct stenosis? *Childs Nerv Syst* 2006 December; 22(12): 1565–72. Epub September 19, 2006. Review.

30. Kennedy CR, Ayers S, Campbell MJ, Elbourne D, Hope P, Johnson A. Randomized, controlled trial of acetazolamide and furosemide in posthemorrhagic ventricular dilation in infancy: Follow-up at 1 year. *Pediatrics* 2001 September; 108(3): 597–607.

31. Diuretic therapy for newborn infants with posthemorrhagic ventricular dilatation. Whitelaw A, Kennedy CR, Brion LP. *Cochrane Database Syst Rev* 2001; (2): CD002270. Review.

32. Whitelaw A. Repeated lumbar or ventricular punctures in newborns with intraventricular hemorrhage. *Cochrane Database Syst Rev* 2001; (1): CD000216. Review. DOI:10.1002/14651858.CD000216.

33. Hudgins RJ. Posthemorrhagic hydrocephalus of infancy. *Neurosurg Clin N Am* 2001 October; 12(4): 743–51, ix. Review.

34. Shooman D, Portess H, Sparrow O. A review of the current treatments of posthaemorrhagic hydrocephalus of infants. *Cerebrospinal Fluid Res* 2009 January 30; 6: 1.

35. Lifshutz JI, Johnson WD. History of hydrocephalus and its treatments. *Neurosurg Focus* 2001 August 15; 11(2): E1.

36. Cherian S, Whitelaw A, Thoresen M, Love S. The pathogenesis of neonatal post-hemorrhagic hydrocephalus. *Brain Pathol* 2004 July; 14(3): 305–11. Review.

37. Whitelaw A, Jary S, Kmita G, Wroblewska J, Musialik-Swietlinska E, Mandera M, Hunt L, Carter M, Pople I. Randomized trial of drainage, irrigation and fibrinolytic therapy for premature infants with posthemorrhagic ventricular dilatation: Developmental outcome at 2 years. Pediatrics. 2010, 125(4):e852-8.

38. Hayhurst C, Cooke R, Williams D, Kandasamy J, O'Brien DF, Mallucci CL. The impact of antibiotic-impregnated catheters on shunt infection in children and neonates. *Childs Nerv Syst* 2008 May; 24(5): 557–62. Epub October 26, 2007.

39. Drake JM, Kestle JR, Milner R et al. Randomized trial of cerebrospinal fluid shunt valve design in pediatric hydrocephalus. *Neurosurgery* 1998 August; 43(2): 294–303; discussion 303–5.

40. Korinth MC, Gilsbach JM. What is the ideal initial valve pressure setting in neonates with ventriculo-peritoneal shunts? *Pediatr Neurosurg* 2002 April; 36(4): 169–74.

41. Baird LC, Mazzola CA, Auguste KI, Klimo P, Flannery AM.Pediatric hydrocephalus: Systematic literature review and evidence-based guidelines. Part 5: Effect of valve type on cerebrospinal fluid shunt efficacy. *Journal of Neurosurgery: Pediatrics* 2014; 14 Suppl 1, 35–43.

42. Jain H, Sgouros S, Walsh AR, Hockley AD. The treatment of infantile hydrocephalus: "Differential-pressure" or "flow-control" valves. A pilot study. *Childs Nerv Syst* 2000 April; 16(4): 242–6.

43. Rekate HL. The slit ventricle syndrome: Advances based on technology and understanding. *Pediatr Neurosurg* 2004 November–December; 40(6): 259–63.

44. Lo TY, Myles LM, Minns RA. Long-term risks and benefits of a separate CSF access device with ventriculoperitoneal shunting in childhood hydrocephalus. *Dev Med Child Neurol* 2003; 45(1): 28–33.

45. Clark S, Sangra M, Hayhurst C, Kandasamy J, Jenkinson M, Lee M, Mallucci C. The use of non-invasive electromagnetic neuronavigation for slit ventricle syndrome and complex hydrocephalus in a pediatric population. *J Neurosurg Pediatr* 2008 December; 2(6): 430–4.

46. Kestle JR, Drake JM, Cochrane DD et al. Lack of benefit of endoscopic ventriculoperitoneal shunt insertion: A multicenter randomized trial. *J Neurosurg* 2003 February; 98(2): 284–90.

47. Adams-Chapman I, Hansen NI, Stoll BJ, Higgins R. Neurodevelopmental outcome of extremely low birth weight infants with posthemorrhagic hydro-cephalus requiring shunt insertion. NICHD Research Network. *Pediatrics* 2008 May; 121(5): e1167–77. Epub April 7, 2008.

48. Bayston R. Epidemiology, diagnosis, treatment, and prevention of cerebrospinal fluid shunt infections. *Neurosurg Clin N Am* 2001 October; 12(4): 703–8, viii.

49. Drake JM, Sainte-Rose C. *The Shunt Book*. New York: Blackwell Scientific, 1995.

50. Sainte-Rose C, Piatt JH, Renier D et al. Mechanical complications in shunts. *Pediatr Neurosurg* 1991; 17: 2–9.

51. Limbrick DD Jr, Baird LC, Klimo P Jr, Riva-Cambrin J, Flannery AM; Pediatric hydrocephalus: Systematic literature review and evidence-based guidelines. Part 4: Cerebrospinal fluid shunt or endoscopic third ventriculostomy for the treatment of hydrocephalus in children. *J Neurosurg Pediatr* 2014; 14 Suppl 1: 30–4.

52. Wagner W, Koch D. Mechanisms of failure after endoscopic third ventriculostomy in young infants. *J Neurosurg* 2005 July; 103(1 Suppl): 43–9.

53. Javadpour M, Mallucci C, Brodbelt A, Golash A, May P. The impact of endoscopic third ventriculostomy on the management of newly diagnosed hydroceph-alus in infants. *Pediatr Neurosurg* 2001 September; 35(3): 131–5.

54. Buxton N, Macarthur D, Mallucci C, Punt J, Vloeberghs M. Neuroendoscopy in the premature population. *Childs Nerv Syst* 1998 November; 14(11): 649–52.

55. Zandian A, Haffner M, Johnson J, Rozzelle CJ, Tubbs RS, Loukas M. Endoscopic third ventricu-lostomy with/without choroid plexus cauterization for hydrocephalus due to hemorrhage, infection, Dandy–Walker malformation, and neural tube defect: A meta-analysis. *Childs Nerv Syst* 2014; 30(4): 571–8.

56. Kulkarni AV, Drake JM, Mallucci CL et al. Endoscopic third ventriculostomy in the treatment of childhood hydrocephalus. *J Pediatr* 2009 August; 155(2): 254–9. e1. Epub May 15, 2009.

57. Sgouros S, Kulkharni AV, Constantini S. The International Infant Hydrocephalus Study: Concept and rational. *Childs Nerv Syst* 2006 April; 22(4): 338–45. Epub October 15, 2005.

58. O'Brien DF, Javadpour M, Collins DR, Spennato P, Mallucci CL. Endoscopic third ventriculostomy: An outcome analysis of primary cases and procedures performed after ventriculoperitoneal shunt malfunc-tion. *J Neurosurg* 2005 November; 103(5 Suppl): 393–400.

59. Warf BC. Hydrocephalus in Uganda: The predomi-nance of infectious origin and primary management with endoscopic third ventriculostomy. *J Neurosurg* 2005 January; 102(1 Suppl): 1–15.

60. Warf BC. Comparison of endoscopic third ventricu-lostomy alone and combined with choroid plexus cauterization in infants younger than 1 year of age: A prospective study in 550 African children. *J Neurosurg* 2005 December; 103(6 Suppl): 475–81.

61. Javadpour M, May P, Mallucci C. Sudden death secondary to delayed closure of endoscopic third ventriculostomy. *Br J Neurosurg* 2003 June; 17(3): 266–9.

62. von Koch CS, Gupta N, Sutton LN, Sun PP. In utero surgery for hydrocephalus. *Childs Nerv Syst* 2003 August; 19(7–8): 574–86. Epub July 25, 2003. Review.

63. Adzick NS, Thom EA, Spong CY, Brock JW 3rd, Burrows PK, Johnson MP, Howell LJ, Farrell JA, Dabrowiak ME, Sutton LN, Gupta N, Tulipan NB,

A'Alton ME, Farmer DL; MOMS Investigators. A Randomized Trial of Prenatal versus Postnatal Repair of Myelomeningocele. *N Engl J Med* 2011;364(11): 993–1004.

64. Goitein D, Papasavas P, Gagné D, Ferraro D, Wilder B, Caushaj P. Single trocar laparoscopically assisted placement of central nervous system-peritoneal shunts. *J Laparoendosc Adv Surg Tech A* 2006 February; 16(1): 1–4.

65. Kurschel S, Eder HG, Schleef J. CSF shunts in children: Endoscopically-assisted placement of the distal catheter. *Childs Nerv Syst* 2005 January; 21(1): 52–5. Epub September 8, 2004.

66. Decq P, Blanquet A, Yepes C. Percutaneous jugular placement of ventriculo-atrial shunts using a split sheath. Technical note. *Acta Neurochir (Wien)* 1995; 136(1–2): 92–4.

67. Sheth SA, McGirt M, Woodworth G, Wang P, Rigamonti D. Ultrasound guidance for distal insertion of ventriculo-atrial shunt catheters: Technical note. *Neurol Res* 2009 April; 31(3): 280–2. Epub November 26, 2008.

68. Ellegaard L, Mogensen S, Juhler M. Ultrasound-guided percutaneous placement of ventriculoatrial shunts. *Childs Nerv Syst* 2007 August; 23(8): 857–62. Epub March 21, 2007.

98

Urinary tract infections

MARTIN KOYLE

INTRODUCTION

A urinary tract infection (UTI) is one of the most common bacterial infections diagnosed in childhood. This condition should be given strong consideration in the differential list when evaluating the febrile, ill neonate. The diagnosis of a UTI can lead to significant morbidity for the child, not only from the disease process itself but also from the formidable diagnostic evaluation subsequent to initial presentation. Given the premature immune system, infants, and particularly neonates, are at risk for disseminated bacteremia, which can lead to a more dangerous scenario than in older children and adults. Due to this associated danger, a thorough evaluation and prompt treatment when necessary are mandatory. In addition, the pediatric specialist needs to recognize that UTI may be a marker of a more serious, underlying urologic congenital and/or functional anomaly, which may be amenable to operative correction.

Potential urological sequelae from a UTI include renal scarring and compromised renal function, although such severe morbidity may be less likely than formerly perceived. Indeed, with the popularity of maternal fetal ultrasound (US) and antenatal detection of congenital anomalies, it is now well documented that such scarring is more often due to dysplasia. This is most obvious in the neonate with congenital vesicoureteral reflux (VUR). Regardless, it is still known that acquired renal scarring can occur in the vulnerable child, even when febrile UTI occurs and VUR is absent on radiological imaging. Current investigations are attempting to identify those specific groups at risk for renal damage. However, serious compromise of function is uncommon nowadays, especially when prompt treatment is instituted. Diagnostic tests recommended after a UTI vary, and recent guidelines have tried to help clarify the workup. Treatment, although benign and effective, has potential risks, in particular, the generation of resistant bacterial strains. Needless to say, a UTI carries with it a significant emotional and economic burden for the family of the sick child.

INCIDENCE

UTIs account for 0.7% of all pediatric office encounters and 5%–14% of pediatric emergency department (ED) visits in the United States.[6,10] Pediatric UTIs account for 1.8% of all hospitalizations in the United States, with costs for UTIs exceeding $520 million.[35] In addition, UTI has consistently been the most commonly diagnosed serious bacterial infection in the first months of life, with a prevalence varying from 1.8% to 7.5%. It is also the most consistently missed serious bacterial infection in studies attempting to define low-risk criteria for the evaluation of fever in the neonatal age group.[11] This unquestionably translates into a significant number of physician visits annually and/or extended hospitalizations of neonates, which add significantly to already escalating health care costs. It must be acknowledged that estimated costs do not include charges for subsequent evaluations, including clinic visits, follow-up studies, and time missed from work by parents.

Neonates represent a special subgroup with regard to UTI, with a male predominance of 2.5- to 6-fold, which is in striking opposition to the high prevalence rate of UTI among females in the over-6-months age group.[12] Overall, the reported incidence of neonatal UTI varies between 0.1% and 1% in the general population of healthy newborns.[2] In preterm neonates the incidence is much higher. Furthermore, this incidence is estimated at 10% in low-birth-weight infants.[10]

Reported prevalence in the preterm neonate ranges between 4% and 25%.[3] A meta-analysis of studies looking at prevalence of UTI in febrile children less than 3 months of age found that febrile female infants had a relatively high prevalence rate of UTI (5% in first 3 months). Uncircumcised males under 3 months had the highest rate at 20.1%, whereas circumcised males had the lowest rate (2.4%).[15]

ETIOLOGY

Numerous factors seem to predispose the child's urinary tract to infection. Most pathogenic bacteria that cause UTIs arise from a reservoir in the intestinal tract. *Escherichia coli* is by far the predominant bacteria to cause UTI because of the unique ability of certain serotypes to adhere to the urothelium. One way of differentiating strains of *E. coli* is based upon differences in the antigens they elaborate on their polysaccharide capsule, which surrounds the bacteria. These antigens are known as K antigens, and it has been demonstrated that certain K antigenic *E. coli* have a much higher propensity for causing UTI than other strains.

Perhaps the most significant predictor of a bacteria's uropathic potential is its ability to adhere to the epithelial membrane where they cause infection—in the urinary tract, the urothelium. Pili or fimbrae are long filamentous appendages, composed of protein, that project from the bacterial surface and allow for this adhesion to take place. In *E. coli,* type 1 pili are highly associated with bacteria that cause UTI. Type 1 pili act to bind uroplakin, a protein cap that is elaborated by the umbrella cell or urothelial cell. Another form of pili, P pili, named for its ability to bind the P antigen of blood group antigens, is highly associated with strains of *E. coli* that cause pyelonephritis. Bacterial adherence, colonization, and subsequent UTI is a complex process that involves a balance between bacterial virulence factors and a host's immune response to invasive bacterial infection and colonization. Clearly, there are specific strains of enteric bacteria that cause UTI with a much higher virulence than many of the bacteria harbored in the gut. In addition, there are also individuals who are much more prone to UTI due to the complexity of the relationship between host and bacterial factors that allow adherence to first occur. Other uncommon organisms leading to newborn UTIs include *Klebsiella, Proteus, Pseudomonas,* and *Enterobacter* (Table 98.1).

P fimbriae *E. coli* adhere to the urothelial cells and lead to a decrease in ureteral peristalsis. Bacteria secrete endotoxins that cross the ureteral mucosa and lead to paralysis of ureteral smooth muscle along with risk of ascent and reflux of bacteria. Consequently, this slows the flow in the peripheral ureters, and adherent bacteria are not washed away. Compromise of host natural immune defenses that protect the urinary tract from infection, in particular, immunologic immaturity, also predisposes pediatric patients to development of UTI. In addition, some children will have colonization of their feces by virulent bacteria.[17] This is especially true in those patients with slow stool transit times and severe constipation, a cofactor that is more common in older children in the potty-training age group.

PRESENTATION

In neonates, the most common clinical presentation varies and is less classical than in older children and adults. Symptoms such as fever, irritability, food intolerance, respiratory distress, and jaundice are common; in premature infants, symptoms encountered may be even more nondescript or non–urinary tract specific, including feeding

Table 98.1 Common uropathogens

Bacteria	Incidence
Escherichia coli	77%–93%
Klebsiella	0%–11%
Enterococcus	2%–9%
Serratia	~1%
Staphylococcus aureus	~1%
Pseudomonas aeruginosa	~1%
Enterobacter cloacae	~1%
Streptococcus	~1%
Proteus	~1%

intolerance, apnea, bradycardia, lethargy, and abdominal distention.[7] Rarely will symptoms referable to the urinary tract, such as hematuria and foul-smelling urine, be observed in the neonate. Given this diagnostic dilemma, many UTIs are either not diagnosed or diagnosed late; some are undoubtedly missed or treated as another entity. Primary care providers must have a high index of suspicion for UTI in the neonatal period to achieve an accurate diagnosis and of course obtain a properly collected urine specimen.[21]

Additional concerns of the practitioner lie in the knowledge not only that risk of serious bacterial illness is higher in young infants and neonates, but also that the clinical clues that are often used to detect serious illness are not reliable. Clinical illness indicators such as state variation and reaction to parental stimulation are not reliable predictors of serious illness. As many as 65% of neonates with a febrile illness involving a serious bacterial infections appear well on initial examination.[18]

Clinical manifestations of neonatal UTI can be similar to clinical signs of neonatal sepsis, although digestive symptoms have been reported to be more frequent in newborn infants. Elevation of body temperature and poor feeding were the most frequent clinical symptoms, in particular in infants with community-acquired infections. Children younger than 3 months with a UTI are more likely than older children to have bacteremia, sepsis, and congenital genitourinary abnormalities.[6] Bacteremia associated with UTIs is mostly observed in patients <6 months of age, particularly those <2 months of age, whose risk of bacteremia is estimated between 4.0% and 22% (Table 98.2).[1]

IMPACT OF CIRCUMCISION

As we debate the medical indications for circumcision in this country, it is well documented that newborn uncircumcised males are at higher risk for UTIs. Uncircumcised boys have an overall 12-fold increased risk of UTI compared with circumcised boys during the first 6 months of life.[14] The benefit of circumcision in terms of UTI prevention is known to extend for 6 months after birth, and possibly for as long as 1 year. After 1 year of age, there is no evidence that circumcision affects the rate of UTI in males.

Table 98.2 Prominent symptoms in neonatal nonobstructive UTI

% Symptom	Prevalence (%)
Failure to thrive/weight loss	51
Fever	41
Jaundice	12
Cyanosis	30
Vomiting	35
Diarrhea	20

Source: Modified from Phol HG, Rushton HG, Urinary Tract Infection in Children, in *The Kelalis–King–Bellman Textbook of Clinical Pediatric Urology*, Docimo SG et al., eds, Informa, UK, 2007, 103–166.

Uncircumcised boys younger than 6 months have a greater quantity of both *E. coli* and Gram-negative uropathogens in their urethras as compared with circumcised cohorts. Voiding pressures in newborn males are higher on urodynamic evaluation. Higher voiding pressures, along with a higher risk for cystitis and colonization, amount to an increased propensity for illness in these children. Total costs for treating UTI are reported to be 10-fold higher in uncircumcised than in circumcised male infants, which reflects the greater number of UTIs diagnosed in this patient group and possibly a higher number of hospital admissions.[9] Findings confirm the strong body of evidence attesting to the protective effect of newborn circumcision against UTI in the first year of life, an age when infections are most severe and likely lead to hospital admission.[9] Still, there is morbidity to this procedure, and it is estimated that the number needed to treat is approximately 111; that is, 111 boys need to undergo circumcision in order to prevent 1 UTI.[34]

BREASTFEEDING

Breastfeeding may have a protective role in preventing UTI in premature infants and should be encouraged.[7] Breastfeeding has been significantly associated with a lower risk of UTI. It has been reported to have a protective effect against many infections in the first year of life, including gastroenteritis, acute otitis media, pneumonia, bacteremia, and meningitis. The protective effect is attributed to its action on the intestinal flora, including its high concentration of IgA, which inhibits adherence of bacteria. In addition, lactoferrin prevents the growth of intestinal *E. coli*. Furthermore, the low pH of stool in breastfed babies allows for the growth of and colonization with less virulent organisms such as bifidobacteria and lactobacilli.[7]

DIAGNOSIS

Unlike older children, neonates lack diurnal temperature variation and have less normal temperature variability. During an acute infection, fever is commonly absent in neonates.[8] The general appearance and physical examination of the febrile neonate cannot be relied on to exclude a serious bacterial infection. Multicenter prospective studies of febrile infants who were 60 days of age or younger and evaluated in an emergency room for fever, circumcision status, and height of fever were associated with an increased likelihood of UTI.[11] Hyperbilirubinemia with prolonged jaundice (lasting more than 14 days) is commonly the main clinical feature at presentation, which may be the only manifestation of UTI.[2] Jaundice can be an early sign in afebrile infants, and was more common with in those neonates with nosocomial UTI. Positive urinalysis findings have been reported in approximately 56% of cases.[3]

The most common current ED practice management of even a well-appearing febrile neonate is a full sepsis evaluation, including a complete blood count (CBC), blood cultures, urinalysis and urine culture, evaluation of cerebrospinal fluid (CSF), and administration of antibiotics (ampicillin, cefotaxime, or gentamicin) with hospitalization pending culture results.[20] The initial evaluation must include a detailed history along with a thorough physical exam. Care must be taken when evaluating the newborn for abdominal masses. The back must be carefully examined for the presence of dimples or abnormalities suggestive of a spinal dysraphism. The degree of phimosis should be noted if the child is uncircumcised, and although rare, labial adhesions must be ruled out in female newborns. The presence of adhesions and recurrent UTI is an indication for intervention. In neonates, adhesions are treated surgically in order to avoid the utilization of estrogen or betamethasone ointments, which are commonly recommended in older children (older than 6 months of age).

The definitive diagnostic test of a UTI is a positive urine culture. This can be obtained through suprapubic aspiration or urethral catheterization. A false-positive culture obtained via a bag specimen may lead to inappropriate treatment, misdiagnosis, and unnecessary testing. The urinalysis, which is immediately available, is suggestive but not diagnostic. Although the presence of leukocyte esterase has a high sensitivity, it lacks in specificity; conversely, the nitrate test behaves oppositely. When combined with microscopic findings, the sensitivity approaches 100% when all three are positive, and the specificity is 100% when all three are negative.[16] The presence of any bacteria on Gram stain has a sensitivity of 93% and specificity of 95%, better than dipstick evaluation for leukocyte esterase and nitrates.[21]

There are four ways that urine can be obtained for specimen. First, a bagged specimen involves a plastic bag that is taped to the perineum and urine obtained after the child voids. This can be useful in infants, but there is a high risk of obtaining a contaminated specimen. Second is a midstream collection, which is unreliable in children, especially in young girls and uncircumcised boys in whom contamination is likely. This is useful if negative, but if positive, it is hard to tell if the collection was contaminated. Third, a catheterized specimen is more invasive and possibly traumatic in children. In the uncooperative girl, it can easily be contaminated. However, for the non-toilet-trained child, it is the most reliable and effective way to obtain a specimen. Lastly, a suprapubic bladder aspiration is the least likely to be contaminated. Again, it is invasive and rarely practiced in the current litigious environment.[21]

In neonates less than 3 months old, a catheterized urinalysis or suprapubic bladder aspiration is part of the standard workup for fever. Suprapubic aspiration, although not usually necessary, is considered the gold standard method for obtaining urine. It is performed after cleaning the suprapubic area with antiseptic solution. A 21- to 25-gauge needle is inserted one fingerbreadth above the symphysis pubis perpendicularly while aspirating until urine is obtained. Although suprapubic aspiration is popular in some EDs, it is invasive and has variable success rates for obtaining urine because of the lack of urine in the bladder. Physical examination to palpate for a full bladder is sometimes limited if the child is very upset. US, if available, may be useful to check bladder fullness before aspiration. For males with phimosis or stricture, and for girls with severe labial adhesions, suprapubic aspiration may be the only method for obtaining clean urine.[24] Although the probability of a true infection with a positive culture obtained via suprapubic aspiration is approximately 99%, this method is the most technically challenging and is associated with the lowest rate of success (23%–99%).[4]

For recovery of any organism from a suprapubic specimen, at least 50,000 colony-forming units per milliliter (CFU/mL) from a catheterized specimen or at least 100,000 CFU/mL from a clean-catch specimen is considered significant bacteriuria.[6] We should reemphasize the importance of accurate diagnosis and the appropriate collection of specimen. Results affect the child's care and can potentially subject him/her to invasive procedures, while possibly contributing to parents' undue stress. The American Association for Pediatrics (AAP) has published recommendation for diagnosis, treatment, and evaluation of initial UTI in febrile infants and young children; however, no recommendations for neonates <2 months old have been suggested.[3] Investigators have commented on the value of urine smell in the diagnosis of UTI. A study by Struthers et al. demonstrated no association between reported abnormal or different urine smell and UTI.[5]

C-reactive protein (CRP) >20 mg/L, erythrocyte sedimentation rate (ESR) >30 mm/hour, and white blood cell (WBC) count >15,000/μL are key findings in various studies on febrile infants. The diagnostic value of these for predicting serious bacterial infection in febrile infants, however, is conflicting. Lin et al.[19] showed that febrile infants with CRP >20 mg/L and ESR >30 mm/hour were at risk for UTI but that a WBC count >15,000 was not significantly associated with UTI. Although the specificity of ESR and CRP was high, their sensitivity was relatively low, demonstrating that elevated CRP and ESR are poor predictors for identifying UTI in febrile illness.

Recent guidelines have been released by the AAP on the diagnosis and management of the febrile infant. An algorithm for clinical practice can be seen in Figure 98.1.

MANAGEMENT

Developmental considerations exist that must be taken into account when treating neonates with a UTI. Glomerular filtration rate is low at birth and develops with age. This must be taken into consideration when prescribing medication and calculating fluid requirements.[10] Treatment depends on the diagnosis of either cystitis or pyelonephritis, and whether the diagnosis is simple or complicated. Simple cystitis requires a short course of oral antibiotics based of susceptibilities (3-day course). A complicated UTI will require a longer course and even parenteral antibiotic administration based on initial presentation. Pyelonephritis requires a 10- to 14-day course of parenteral medication followed by oral administration based on initial presentation. It has been established that oral and intravenous antibiotics have been equally effective in treating young children with acute pyelonephritis. It was shown that acutely, time to defervescence and return to sterile urine within 24 hours was identical, not to mention that the cost of a 10-day oral course was significantly lower, without clinical compromise, i.e., reinfection or renal scarring.[28] Studies evaluating the treatment of febrile UTIs in young children with oral versus intravenous antibiotics have demonstrated similar efficacy with the use of third-generation cephalosporins.[23]

The antibiotic repertoire available to the physician in the newborn period is significantly more limited than that available for older children. Aminoglycosides, penicillins, and cephalosporins can be utilized in the newborn period; however, their use is not without risk. Potential complications associated with their use include diarrhea, intolerance, and allergic reactions including anaphylaxis as well as nephrotoxicity if not carefully dosed and monitored. Nitrofurantoin has been linked to hemolytic anemia in the neonatal period and should not be utilized in children with glucose-6-phospate dehydrogenase deficiency, because of the risk of hemolysis. Given low tissue penetration levels attained during administration, nitrofurantoin is a poor choice for the treatment of pyelonephritis. Trimethoprim use should be avoided in patients with megaloblastic anemia and folate deficiency or in children with sodium wasting disease (i.e., posterior urethral valves [PUVs] or renal insufficiency) because of potential hyperkalemia from blocking the sodium channels present in the principal cells of the cortical collecting ducts. It can also increase serum creatinine levels by blocking the proximal tubular secretion of creatinine. Trimethoprim/sulfamethoxazole should not be used in newborn period, because of concerns for hyperbilirubinemia and

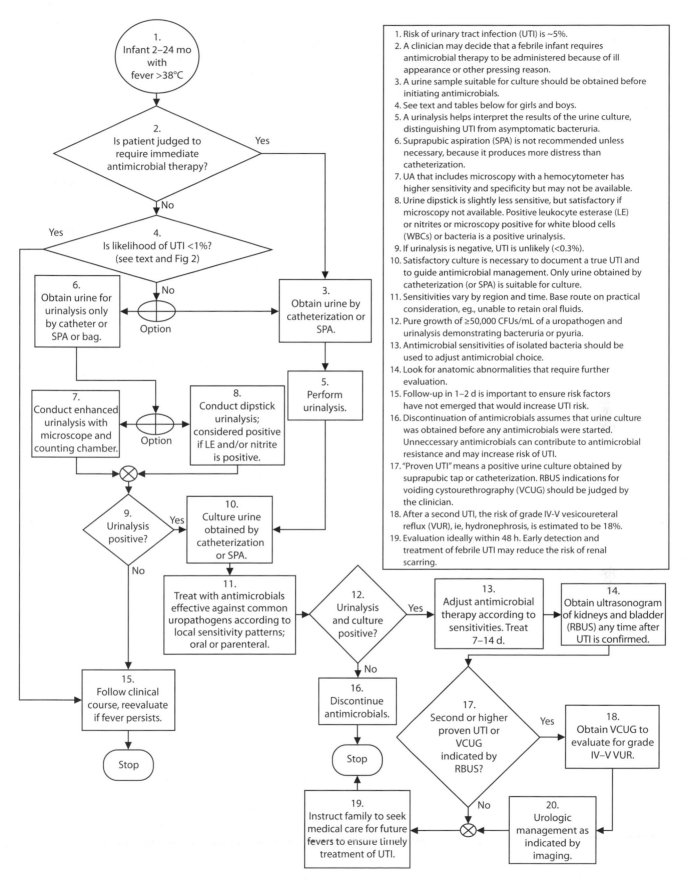

Figure 98.1 Algorithm for treating infants with unexplained fever. (From American Academy of Pediatrics, Committee on Quality Improvement, Urinary Tract Infection: Clinical Practice Guideline for the Diagnosis and Management of the Initial UTI in Febrile Infants and Children 2 to 24 Months, *Pediatrics* 2011; 128(3): 595–610.)

kernicterus. The metabolic acidosis seen in patients taking trimethoprim/sulfamethoxazole is attributed to bicarbonate loss induced by the sulfamethoxazole component through an acetazolamide-like effect on the proximal tubules.[22]

VESICOURETERAL REFLUX

Prenatal hydronephrosis is noted in 1%–5% of pregnancies. The prevalence of VUR in neonates varies from 11% to 12.5%. Considering fetal and postnatal renal pelvic anteroposterior diameter (APD) as a combined test, a value of less than 10 mm is a negative indication for a voiding cystourethrogram (VCUG). This results in increased sensitivity and diagnostic odds ratio for detecting clinically significant VUR.[33] The likelihood of significant renal abnormalities postnatally correlates with the severity of APD dilation. A meta-analysis of 17 studies reported the risk of renal abnormalities for three classifications of antenatal hydronephrosis. The probability of ureteropelvic junction obstruction increased, but there was no association of VUR with APD measurement (Tables 98.3 and 98.4).[32,37]

The incidence of VUR in children presenting with symptoms of a UTI is in the order of 30%–50%. The incidence, however, is believed to be lower in neonates. Standard of care calls for antibiotic prophylaxis in a child presenting with a febrile UTI, or recurrent nonfebrile UTIs, until VUR can be ruled out. Traditionally, recommended workup has consisted of a renal and bladder US as well as a VCUG, or a nuclear medicine cystogram, both of which are invasive studies. The false-negative rate of VCUG is estimated at 20%. A nuclear medicine cystogram involves a fraction (1%) of the radiation exposure experienced with a VCUG. Although its sensitivity is excellent, one major disadvantage is the lack of anatomic detail. It is difficult to identify Hutch diverticula, bladder trabeculation, or a dilated posterior urethra with a nuclear medicine study.

A dimercaptosuccinic acid (DMSA) scan at the time of presentation is the hallmark of the *top–down* approach.

Table 98.3 Degree of prenatal hydronephrosis and postnatal risk of renal abnormalities

Degree of hydronephrosis	Postnatal risk
Mild	11%
<7 mm in second trimester	
<9 mm in third trimester	
Moderate	45%
7–10 mm in second trimester	
9–15 mm in third trimester	
Severe	88.3%
>10 mm in second trimester	
>15 mm in third trimester	

Table 98.4 Prenatal hydronephrosis and risk of postnatal VUR

Degree of hydronephrosis	Postnatal risk
>12 mm at 20 weeks and >14 mm at 34 weeks	15%
6–8 mm during second or third trimester	5%

Source: Hothi DK, Wade AS, Gilbert R, Winyard PGT. Mild Fetal Renal Pelvis Dilatation—Much Ado About Nothing? *Clin J Am Soc Nephrol* 4: 168–177, 2009.

Some authors advocate that 50% of children will have a positive DMSA during the acute phase. Out of those children, 30%–40% will demonstrate reflux. Conversely, 90% of children with VUR will have had a positive DMSA scan. If VCUG is deferred for those children with febrile UTI and a positive acute DMSA scan, presence of hydronephrosis, or a dilated ureter, one would miss 10% of children with VUR, the majority of these being children with low-grade VUR, low risk for UTI, and late renal scarring.[27] Small studies looking into early DMSA scanning in neonates, mainly females and uncircumcised males, agree that DMSA is helpful in ruling out later development of permanent renal damage but was not predictive of the absence of dilating VUR. Therefore, if dilating VUR is to be ruled out, a VCUG needs to be performed even in the presence of a normal DMSA scan.[29] Neonatal reflux, even high grade, is more likely to resolve than VUR detected after UTI at a later age. Prospective data on the follow-up of infants with prenatal hydronephrosis diagnosed with grade III, IV, or V showed resolution rates of 53%, 28%, and 40%, respectively, at 4 years.

The goal of radiologic studies is to identify genitourinary malformations and defects that can predispose the newborn to recurrent UTI. Anatomic obstruction (PUVs, ureteropelvic junction obstruction, ureterovesical obstruction, and ureterocele) as an etiology for UTI is seen in 2%–10%.[13] Urethral obstruction during fetal development secondary to anatomic reconfiguration of the bladder neck is suggested as the cause of high-grade bilateral reflux in male neonates.[22] Hoberman et al.[30] evaluated the value of renal US after the first febrile UTI in children as young as 1 month. Their conclusion was that less than 1% of renal US after a first febrile UTI will show findings significant enough to impact management, including additional imaging studies. In their conclusion, the authors did not recommend ultrasonography after a first febrile UTI in children with an unremarkable prenatal US after 30–32 weeks of gestation. In a study of early DMSA scanning in neonates with febrile UTIs, Siomou et al.[31] found that the ability of DMSA to predict dilating VUR was low, since the majority of children with >grade III VUR had normal DMSA results. Moreover they noted that of these patients, all were noted to have a normal renal US.

AAP Imaging Guidelines

- Febrile infants with UTIs should undergo renal and bladder ultrasonography.
- VCUG should not be performed routinely after the first febrile urinary tract infection (fUTI); VCUG is indicated if renal-bladder ultrasound reveals hydronephrosis, scarring, or other findings that suggest either high-grade VUR or obstructive uropathy, as well as in other atypical or complex clinical circumstances.
- Further evaluation should be conducted if there is a recurrence of fUTI.

Source: American Academy of Pediatrics, Committee on Quality Improvement, Urinary Tract Infection: Clinical Practice Guideline for the Diagnosis and Management of the Initial UTI in Febrile Infants and Children 2 to 24 Months, *Pediatrics* 2011;128(3):595–610.

PROPHYLAXIS

The benefits from prophylactic antibiotic use have been debated, including their use in those children with VUR and those without it. Four large clinical studies have indicated no benefit of prophylaxis versus observation; however, few patients included in the studies had high-grade VUR. The Australian Prevention of Recurrent Urinary Tract Infection in Children with Vesicoureteral Reflux and Normal Renal Tracts (PRIVENT) study suggested a benefit to prophylaxis reducing incidence of UTI recurrence. Fifteen children had to be treated for 12 months to prevent a single UTI. Circumcision status, however, was not discussed in this study.[25,26] Results from the Randomized Intervention for Children with Vesicoureteral Reflux (RIVUR) trial demonstrated that prophylactic antibiotics reduced the recurrence rate of UTI (12.9% on prophylaxis vs. 23.6% on placebo), with an increase in resistance rate of 63% on prophylaxis versus 19% on placebo. While not appropriately powered to fully evaluate, there was no significant difference found in new renal scarring between placebo and prophylaxis.[36]

The use of antibiotic prophylaxis must be a partnered decision between the practitioner and the patient, considering the risks and benefits. One must remember that surveillance is not equivocal to nontreatment; however, it requires that the family be educated on signs and symptoms of a UTI and the importance of prompt evaluation and treatment (Table 98.5).

Table 98.5 Prophylactic antibiotic regimens for prevention of UTI

Antibiotic	Daily dosing
Trimethoprim	2 mg/kg
Trimethoprim sulfamethoxazole (TMP-SMX)	2 mg/kg TMP 10 mg/kg SMX
Nitrofurantoin	1–2 mg/kg
Amoxicillin	20 mg/kg
Cefixime	4 mg/kg

SURGERY

Surgical intervention in the newborn for recurrent UTI is rarely necessary. Indications for surgery include recurrent episodes of UTI and/or deteriorating renal function noted on nuclear medicine studies (Table 98.6). Infection in the face of hydronephrosis from a ureteropelvic junction obstruction mandates consideration for surgical reconstruction. Surgery can also be considered for ectopic ureteral insertion and distal ureteral obstruction with recurrent infection, with or without antibiotic prophylaxis. The size of the newborn bladder has to be taken into consideration during reconstruction, given that a ureteral reimplantation into a small newborn bladder can be technically challenging. Some authors advocate the utilization of proximal or distal diversion in order to allow the bladder time to grow and attain a larger capacity. Staged repairs can be considered especially if there is the potential need for tapering of the distal ureter during reimplantation. The presence of a ureterocele and infection calls for prompt incision followed by antibiotic prophylaxis given the high likelihood of VUR. Ureterocele puncture or incision is usually followed by reconstruction of the bladder.

Since its approval by the Federal Drug Administration, dextranomer/hyaluronic acid (Dx/HA) copolymer has revolutionized the management of VUR. Its applicability to newborns has not been well documented. However, given the low morbidity associated with this procedure, injection therapy is a viable option in the face of recurrent UTIs and low-grade VUR. It should be noted, however, that injection into a newborn bladder can be challenging, and long-term follow-up studies after injection in younger children are lacking.

UTIs in the myelodysplastic newborn warrant earlier urodynamic evaluation, the implementation of anticholinergic therapy, and clean intermittent catheterization, along with the use of prophylactic antibiotic therapy. Recurrent infections may require surgical intervention in the form of vesicostomy and, rarely, more proximal diversions such as ureterostomy or pyelostomy. Recurrent infections following ablation of PUVs and persistent hydronephrosis can also lead to diversion including the use of ureterostomy or pyelostomy to prevent recurrent infections. Prior to diversion in the PUV patient, imaging studies (such as VCUG) should be obtained confirming that the valves have been

Table 98.6 Surgical conditions leading to febrile UTI

Anatomic	Functional
Vesicoureteral reflux	Neurogenic bladder
Ureterocele	Myelomeningocele
Ureteropelvic junction obstruction	Dysfunctional voiding
Posterior urethral valves	Hinman syndrome
Obstructed megaureter/ megacalicosis	
Ureteral or renal calculi	

adequately ablated. A thorough urodynamic evaluation is also recommended. However, in the authors' opinion, the use of diversion rarely affects the clinical course of the patient and rarely seems to affect the recurrence rate.

CONCLUSION

Neonates are particularly susceptible to developing UTIs, which may be explained by the compound effect of immaturity of the local defense mechanisms (decreased uroepithelial bactericidal activity, low levels of local immunoglobulin A, decreased urinary acidification) and heavy periurethral colonization occurring in healthy neonates and gradually resolving after 6 months of age.[12] The benefit of circumcision in the prevention of early urinary tract infection is not questionable in the neonate. In the general population, the recurrence rate for UTI is very high. Within 1 year of a first infection, approximately 30% of boys and 40% of girls will develop a repeat infection. The rate will double for each subsequent episode.[13] Unfortunately, recurrence is not uncommon in the neonatal period. With the widespread use of prophylactic antibiotics, recurrence with multiresistant organisms is also a possibility. The need and extent of radiologic imaging required following a neonatal UTI are still under investigation. The usefulness of invasive, expensive studies continues to be questioned.

Pediatric UTIs constitute a significant health burden; although the actual costs are not known, it is estimated to be in the order of $180 million for inpatient costs in the United States. This fails to include the costs to society of parental productivity from lost wages, treatment, and follow-up after the infection.[21] There are a number of complex host and bacterial virulence factors that play into susceptibility of children to UTI. It is important that the clinician be familiar with the spectrum of UTI, and children at risk of UTI, so infants and children who need to be evaluated for anatomic or functional abnormalities of the urinary tract are correctly identified and managed.

REFERENCES

1. Dore-Bergeron M, Gauthier M, Chevalier I et al. Urinary tract infections in 1- to 3-month-old infants: Ambulatory treatment with intravenous antibiotics. *Pediatrics* 2009; 124: 16–21.
2. Pashapour N, Nikibahksh AA, Golmohammadlou S. Urinary tract infection in term neonates with prolonged jaundice. *Urol J* 2007; 4: 91–4.
3. Lopez Sastre JB, Aparicio AR, Coto Cotallo GD et al. Urinary tract infection in the newborn: Clinical and radio imaging studies. *Pediatr Nephrol* 2007; 22: 1735–41.
4. Chang SL, Shortliffe LD. Pediatric urinary tract infections. *Pediatr Clin N Am* 2006; 53: 379–400.
5. Struthers S, Scanlon J, Parker K et al. Parental reporting of smelly urine and urinary tract infection. *Arch Dis Child* 2003; 88: 250–2.
6. Shaikh N, Morone NE, Lopez J et al. Does This child have a urinary tract infection? *JAMA* 2007; 298(24): 2895–904.
7. Levy I, Comarsca J, Davidovits M et al. Urinary tract infection in preterm infants: the protective role of breastfeeding. *Pediatr Nephrol* 2009; 24: 527–31.
8. Phol HG, Rushton HG. Urinary tract infection in children. In: Docimo SG, Canning DA, Khoury AE (eds). *The Kelalis–King–Bellman Textbook of Clinical Pediatric Urology*. UK: Informa, 2007: 103–66.
9. Schoen EJ, Colby CJ, Ray GT. Newborn circumcision decreases incidence and costs of urinary tract infections during the first year of life. *Pediatrics* 2000; 105: 789–93.
10. Tracy MA. Pediatric genitourinary emergencies in the emergency department. *J Emerg Nurs* 2009; 35: 479–80.
11. Zorc JJ, Levine DA, Plat SL et al. Clinical and demographic factors associated with urinary tract infection in young febrile infants. *Pediatrics* 2005; 116: 644–8.
12. Cleper R, Krause I, Eisenstein B et al. Prevalence of vesicoureteral reflux in neonatal urinary tract infection. *Clin Pediatr* 2004; 43: 619–25.
13. Mingin GC, Hinds A, Nguyen HT et al. Children with a febrile urinary tract infection and a negative radiologic workup: Factors predictive of recurrence. *Urology* 2004; 63(3): 562–5.
14. Foxman B. Epidemiology of urinary tract infections: Incidence, morbidity, and economic costs. *Am J Med* 2002; 113: 5s–13s.
15. Shaikh N, Morone NE, Bost JE. Prevalence of urinary tract infection in childhood a meta-analysis. *Pediatr Infect Dis J* 2008; 27: 302–8.
16. Mesrobian HO. Urologic problems of the neonate: An update. *Clin Perinatol* 2007; 34: 667–79.
17. Rosenberg HK, Haslan H, Finkelstein MS. Work-up of urinary tract infection in infants and children. *Ultrasound Q* 2001; 17(2); 87–102.
18. Baker MD, Avner JR. The febrile infant: What's new? *Clin Ped Emerg Med* 2008; 9: 213–20.
19. Lin D, Hunag S, Lin C et al. Urinary tract infection in febrile infants younger than eight weeks of age. *Pediatrics* 2000; 105: 1–4.
20. Claudius I, Baraff LJ. Pediatric emergencies associated with fever. *Emerg Med Clin N Am* 2010; 28: 67–84.
21. Bauer R, Kogan BA. New developments in the diagnosis and management of pediatric UTIs. *Urol Clin N Am* 2008; 35: 47–58.
22. Shah G, Upandhyay J. Controversies in the diagnosis and management of urinary tract infections in children. *Pediatr Drugs* 2005; 7(6): 339–46.
23. Hoberman A, Wald ER. Urinary tract infections in young febrile children. *Pediatr Infect Dis J* 1997; 16: 11–7.

24. Santen SA, Altiery MF. Pediatric urinary tract infection. *Emerg Med Cli N Am* 2001; 19(3): 675–90.
25. Craig JC, Simpson JM, Williams GJ et al. Antibiotic prophylaxis and recurrent urinary tract infection in children. *N Engl J Med* 2009; 361: 1748–59.
26. Garin EH, Olavarria, F, Garcia V. Clinical significance of primary vesicoureteral reflux and urinary antibiotic prophylaxis after acute pyelonephritis: A multicenter, randomized, controlled study. *Pediatrics* 2006; 117: 626–32.
27. Caldamone AA, Koyle MA. Pediatric urinary tract infections and vesicoureteral reflux: What have we learned? *Afr J Urol* 2007; 13: 188–92.
28. Koyle MA. Antibiotic treatment of pyelonephritis in children: Multicentre randomised controlled non-inferiority trial. Practice Point Commentary Urology.
29. Siomou E, Griapros V, Fotopoulos A et al. Implications of 99mTC-DMSA scintigraphy performed during urinary tract infection in neonates. *Pediatrics* 2009; 124: 1–7.
30. Hoberman A, Charron M, Hickey RW et al. Imaging studies after a first febrile urinary tract infection in young children. *N Engl J Med* 2003; 348: 195–202.
31. Siomou E, Girapros V, Fotopoulous A et al. Implications of 99m Tc-DMSA scintigraphy performed during urinary tract infection in neonates. *Pediatrics* 2009; 124(3): 1–7.
32. Becker AM. Postnatal evaluation of infants with an abnormal antenatal renal sonogram. *Curr Opin Pediatr* 2009; 21: 207–13.
33. Dias CS, Bouzada MC, Pereira AK et al. Predictive factors for vesicoureteral reflux and prenatally diagnosed renal pelvic dilatation. *J Urol* 2009; 182: 2440–5.
34. Mukherjee S, Joshi A, Carroll D et al. What is the effect of circumcision on risk of urinary tract infection in boys with posterior urethral valves? *J Ped Surg* 2009; 44: 417–21.
35. Spencer JD, Schwaderer A, McHugh K et al. Pediatric urinary tract infections: An analysis of hospitalizations, charges and costs in the USA. *Pediatr Nephrol* 2010; 25: 2469–75.
36. Mattoo TK, Chesney RW, Greenfield SP et al. Renal scarring in the randomized intervention for children with vesicoureteral reflux (RIVUR) trial. *Clin J Am Soc Nephrol* 2016; 11: 54–61.
37. Hothi DK, Wade AS, Gilbert R, Winyard PGT. Mild Fetal Renal Pelvis Dilatation—Much Ado About Nothing? *Clin J Am Soc Nephrol* 4: 168–177, 2009.

99

Imaging of the renal tract in the neonate

MELANIE HIORNS AND LORENZO BIASSONI

INTRODUCTION

The widespread use of antenatal ultrasound (US) in the last 25–30 years has allowed the early identification of a number of congenital nephrourological abnormalities, which are now assessed with imaging soon after birth. In addition, a congenital nephrourological abnormality may declare itself postnatally, for example, with a urinary tract infection, anomalies in urine stream, septicemia, metabolic upset due to renal failure, or simply vomiting. Occasionally, the neonate may have hematuria due to renal vein thrombosis, especially in the case of a prolonged labor with hypoxic events. A healthy neonate may present with an abdominal mass found on routine examination or with an apparently unrelated congenital abnormality, e.g., esophageal atresia.

Once the attention of the clinical team has been focused on the genitourinary tract, the role of the radiologist is to establish whether the child has been born with a normal urinary tract and he/she is therefore suffering from an acquired condition, or whether he/she suffers from a congenital anomaly.

Usually, the questions asked by the clinical team are the following: (1) How many kidneys are present, and where are they within the abdomen? (2) Is there dilatation of the renal collecting system, and is the renal parenchyma normal or abnormal? (3) Are the bladder and the urethra normal, or is there a thick-walled bladder and/or an obstructed urethra? (4) What is the renal function, both in absolute terms and in terms of the split function of each kidney?

The radiologist has four key imaging examinations available, which can provide an answer in the vast majority of cases: abdominal US, micturating cystogram (MCUG), radioisotope examinations, and magnetic resonance imaging (MRI). Nowadays, there is absolutely no indication for intravenous urography (IVU) in the neonatal period (and almost no role in the older child), and it is considered obsolete. Computerized tomography (CT) in the neonatal period would be confined exclusively to the assessment of a renal mass if the US had not been able to provide satisfactory information and if MRI was not available. However, there are very few instances when MRI is not available locally or in a specialist center, and CT should therefore be considered a modality of last resort. MRI has an important role to play in the workup of renal tumors and in the assessment of the morphology of the urinary tract, again, if insufficient information has been obtained by US. In this instance, most newborn babies can undergo a "feed-and-wrap" technique and will not necessarily require sedation or a general anesthetic, although this will be needed in older infants or in neonates or infants needing breath-hold sequences.

COMMONLY AVAILABLE IMAGING MODALITIES

Abdominal US

The first imaging examination of the urinary tract should always be an abdominal US. With modern US equipment and well-trained personnel, it is possible to obtain anatomical detail of the entire urinary tract. The equipment is mobile, and a comprehensive US examination can be undertaken even in the ill neonate in an incubator on intensive care. The results of the US examination set the framework of the anatomical state and frequently permit the nephrourological team to begin therapy with either a short list of differential diagnoses or a presumed single diagnosis. In the majority of cases, the US examination will identify how many kidneys are present, the renal size, whether the kidneys are simplex or duplex, if the parenchyma is sonographically normal, and if there is dilation of the renal collecting systems. The bladder should be examined at the beginning of the US examination, as micturition may occur at any moment and a full bladder is useful when searching for dilated ureters behind the bladder (Figure 99.1). Bladder wall thickness is easy to identify and measure; the proximal posterior urethra may be dilated in the male with posterior urethral valves, and this can be identified during micturition if looked for. The patient needs no preparation for a

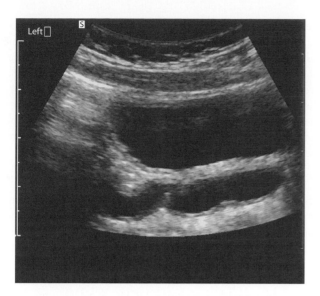

Figure 99.1 Ultrasound showing a dilated left ureter behind the bladder. In this patient, this was secondary to a vesicoureteric junction obstruction.

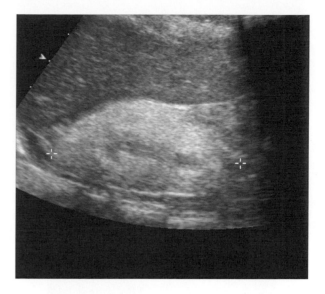

Figure 99.2 Ultrasound in a newborn male patient with primary hyperoxaluria. The kidney is echo-bright compared to the adjacent liver and has lost its corticomedullary differentiation, and in this condition, the brightness represents global nephrocalcinosis.

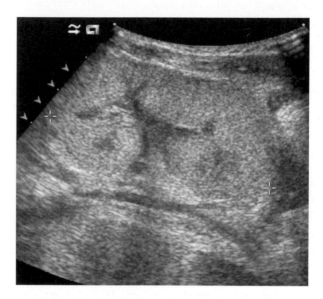

Figure 99.3 Ultrasound in a 4-week-old male patient with congenital nephrotic syndrome. The kidney is bright and enlarged, but some of the normal architecture can still be recognized.

US examination. The examination should be performed with both the standard curvilinear probe and also with a high-frequency (and thus high-resolution) linear probe. Ideally the infant should be scanned both supine and prone, although if a neonate is being ventilated, it will not be possible to obtain prone images.

The normal US appearance of the kidney in a neonate is of a slightly echo-bright cortex, when compared to the adjacent liver or spleen, with a slightly echo-poor medulla (pyramids). The difference between the cortex and the medulla is termed corticomedullary differentiation. A small kidney with loss of corticomedullary differentiation indicates an abnormal parenchyma (Figures 99.2 and 99.3). This may be due to an acute insult such as acute renal failure or renal vein thrombosis or may represent an underlying intrinsic abnormality such as renal dysplasia, which may be associated with cysts (or not) to varying degrees. The presence of dilatation of the collecting system must raise the possibility of obstruction but does not necessarily infer this. If the dilatation is bilateral, then bladder outlet pathology must be excluded. However, vesicoureteric reflux (VUR) may give a very similar appearance.

In the neonate, features on US of echogenic areas within the kidneys may suggest nephrocalcinosis (Figure 99.2), and this is the most common cause of focally echo-bright kidneys following furosemide diuretic therapy. Tamm–Horsfall proteins may give a similar appearance but are transitory.

There are two important pitfalls that must be stressed with US. The first is in the presence of a sick neonate who is either anuric or oliguric, when US may not reveal any dilation but an obstructive uropathy may still be present. In this clinical situation, a repeat US must be carried out once the infant starts to produce urine. The second pitfall is in the case of antenatally diagnosed unilateral hydronephrosis: here, the US may fail to show significant dilation during the

first 48 hours of life due to physiological dehydration, and the US should be done on the third postnatal day or later.

Micturating cystourethrogram

A micturating cystourethrogram (MCUG) gives invaluable anatomical information about the bladder, and the bladder outflow tract in the male, and if VUR is detected, then details of the ureters, pelvis, and calyces are well outlined (Figure 99.4). Contrast showing calyceal detail may suggest

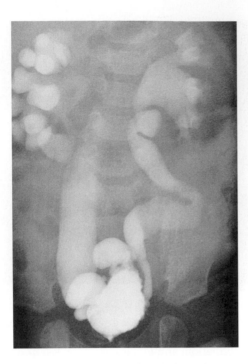

Figure 99.4 Micturating cystourethrogram in a patient with gross reflux outlining the hydroureteronephrosis and the configuration of the collecting system. There was no outflow tract obstruction in this patient (no posterior urethral valve).

renal dysplasia. The combination of US and MCUG allows adequate evaluation of all kidneys and collecting systems shortly after birth and permits appropriate management to be instituted immediately in all cases, especially if an obstructive uropathy is present, e.g., posterior urethral valves (Figure 99.5). The timing of the MCUG will depend on the clinical presentation and clinical state of the baby.

The baby will need to be catheterized, and in most patients, a 6F feeding tube can be used. It is not necessary to use a catheter with a balloon as there is no indication to inflate the balloon for this study, and indeed, inflating the balloon may/will cause bladder outlet obstruction and thus must not be done. The voiding views of the urethra in the male child should be obtained both with the tube still in and with it removed to ensure that a tiny valve leaflet is not missed as a consequence of being flattened by the presence of the catheter. Antibiotic cover should be given before and after the procedure (in accordance with local/national guidelines), and the procedure should be done under sterile conditions.

An MCUG is only rarely indicated in the immediate neonatal period, although there may be extended indications when the infant is slightly older. In the neonatal period, it is most commonly indicated with the US finding of bilateral hydronephrosis. This raises the possibility of an obstructive uropathy in the urethra (posterior urethral valve in the male infant), at the bladder base (ureterocele), or at the vesicoureteric junction (VUJ) bilaterally, or a bilateral pelviureteric junction (PUJ) obstruction. Bilateral VUR may give

identical images (Figure 99.4). In this context, an MCUG should be carried out as soon as the baby is in a good clinical state.

If an MCUG is being performed for possible posterior urethral valves and these are confirmed, then the catheter should *not* be removed; the diagnosis has been established, there is no additional information to be gained by a tube-out view, and there is a risk of a difficult recatheterization to reestablish continued bladder drainage.

The neonates with an antenatal diagnosis of hydronephrosis requiring an MCUG include all those with postnatal US confirmation of a dilated ureter, bilateral hydronephrosis, or an abnormal bladder. Unilateral hydronephrosis with a normal opposite kidney and bladder on US in a well neonate does not require an MCUG.

If the clinical question is only about the presence of VUR, and the anatomy of the urethra in a male infant has already been assessed with a previous MCUG, a radioisotope cystogram (direct isotope cystography [DIC]) will answer the question, with a negligible radiation burden (less than a chest x-ray) to the infant. This test is obtained by positioning the child on the gamma camera head and catheterizing the bladder. A minimal amount of Tc-99m pertechnetate (20 MBq is sufficient) is then instilled in the bladder via the catheter. The catheter is connected to a bag with saline; the saline is run, and the bladder is filled until the child feels the urge to void. The acquisition begins after instilling the tracer in the bladder and continues until the end of the emptying phase (or when VUR has been demonstrated). If there is VUR during the bladder-emptying phase, this will be detected with high sensitivity (Figure 99.6).

Functional imaging

Radioisotope examinations provide an in vivo evaluation of the global and regional renal cortical function, with a precise estimate of the contribution of each kidney to the total renal function. Moreover, the dynamic radionuclide shows how each kidney drains, with identification of possible holdups.

TRACERS AVAILABLE

The main tracers available are the Tc-99m dimercaptosuccinic acid (DMSA), the Tc-99m mercaptoacetyltriglicine (MAG3) and the Tc-99m diethylenetriaminepentacetic acid (DTPA). Some centers use I-123 orthoiodohippuran (OIH), but the labeling with I-123 (cyclotron produced) makes it an expensive and not readily available tracer. The DMSA is taken up by the proximal renal tubules, and once in the renal parenchyma, approximately 60% sticks within the tubules, while approximately 30%–40% of the tracer leaves the kidney with the urine. DMSA is the current gold standard for the evaluation of the differential renal function (DRF) and the evaluation of renal parenchymal integrity. The MAG3 and the OIH are secreted by the proximal tubules into the lumen and leave the kidney via the collecting ducts and the renal collecting system. The DTPA is filtered by the glomerulus and leaves the kidney via

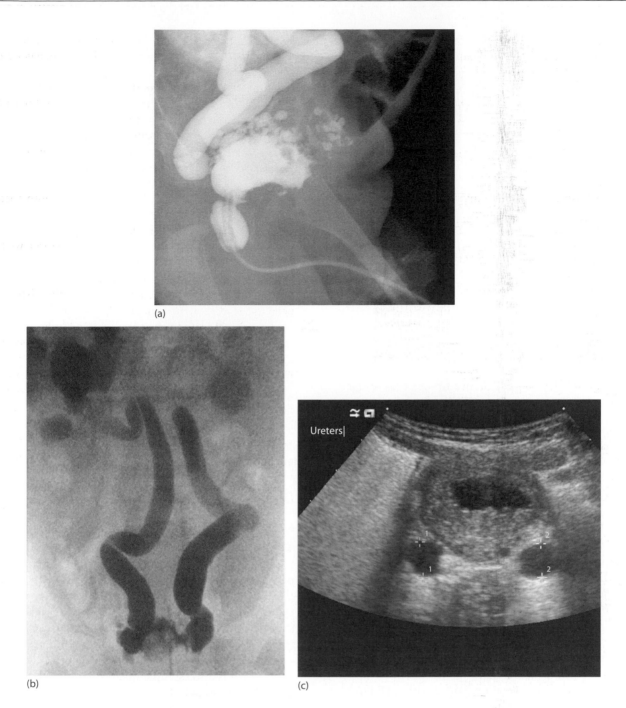

Figure 99.5 (a) Micturating cystourethrogram in a newborn male demonstrating a tight posterior urethral valve and a very trabeculated and thickened bladder wall. **(b)** A later view in the same patient showing gross reflux in both ureters to the level of the collecting systems. The bladder has preferentially refluxed contrast into the upper tracts as this presents less obstruction than overcoming the tight posterior urethral valve. **(c)** Ultrasound in the same patient showing a very thick-walled bladder and bilateral dilated ureters behind the bladder.

the collecting system. Tc-99m MAG3 has a higher extraction fraction than Tc-99m DTPA and therefore is a better tracer, especially in the neonate. The tracers used for dynamic renography can evaluate DRF almost as accurately as the DMSA. They can also provide an evaluation of renal parenchymal integrity (small scars can be missed though) and assess drainage.

Static renal scintigraphy

The DMSA scan requires the acquisition of high-quality static images in order to be clinically useful. The child has to be immobile during the acquisition process. Sedation or general anesthesia is not necessary. Good radiographic skills with distraction techniques are very important. It is

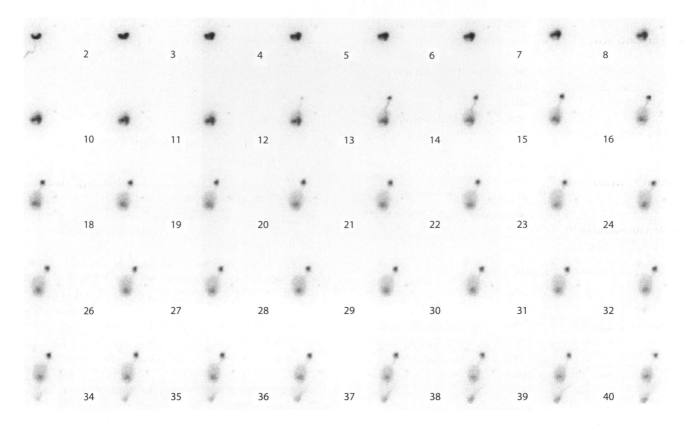

Figure 99.6 Direct isotope cystogram. Following insertion of a bladder catheter and bladder irrigation with saline, the baby feels urgency to void. Right sided vesicoureteric reflux is identified.

essential to acquire enough counts, with each image lasting, on average, between 5 and 10 minutes. A good posterior view, with a left and a right posterior oblique view, is what is needed in the vast majority of cases. The use of single photon emission computerized tomography (SPECT) is controversial. In our experience, this is almost never necessary, as we usually acquire high-quality static views, which are very informative. It is important to be aware of some normal variants: the pear-shaped kidney, the splenic impression on the lateral margin of the left kidney, the persistent fetal lobulation, and the upper or lower pole appearing hypoactive while in fact just thin. It is essential to combine the functional information gained with a DMSA scan with anatomical details, usually obtained with a US. Focal defects on DMSA are nonspecific and can be due to a wide range of conditions, including cysts, scars, calculi, tumors, foci of dysplasia, congenital abnormalities, and infarcts following arterial or venous thrombosis or congenital vascular anomalies.

In the context of urinary tract infections, an *early* DMSA scan, performed within 2–3 weeks from the infection, will inform on parenchymal inflammatory/infective involvement, which may or may not lead to permanent renal scars. A repeat DMSA scan 4–6 months after the latest infection will be able to show the presence of scars. If the clinical question is related to the presence of renal scars, then a DMSA should be done 4–6 months after the infection.

Dynamic radionuclide renography

PATIENT'S PREPARATION

The child should be appropriately hydrated. This allows normal flow of urine throughout the renal parenchyma and pelvicalyceal system. If the child is suboptimally hydrated, the tracer will progress slowly through the renal parenchyma and collecting system, thus giving a false impression of obstruction. In some centers, intravenous fluids (saline 10–15 mL/kg) are given, starting 30 minutes prior to the tracer injection. In other centers, oral hydration is preferred. It is also essential that the child is immobile during the examination: this is achieved with sandbags at both sides of the neonate and Velcro straps. If the neonate has been fed prior to the start of the examination, it is likely that he/she will fall asleep and keep still. Sedation/general anesthesia is not necessary and should not be used.

EVALUATION OF THE DRF

This is achieved by drawing regions of interest (ROIs) around each kidney at a time after tracer injection when the parenchyma-to-background ratio is optimal and no significant tracer has reached the collecting system (normally between the first and the second minute after tracer injection in the case of tracers used in dynamic renography). ROIs around each kidney, to subtract background activity, are also drawn. A precise estimate of the DRF can be challenging in the neonate, with immature kidneys and consequent reduced tracer uptake and a relatively high background activity, even more so if there is also chronic renal failure (for example, due to posterior urethral valves), because the kidneys extract the tracer with much less avidity. Another challenging clinical situation is when one of the kidneys is much bigger than the other, for example, in a neonate with prenatally diagnosed severe hydronephrosis.

In a neonate with antenatally diagnosed hydronephrosis, functional imaging is normally deferred until the child is 2 or 3 months old, with better, even if not complete, renal maturation. Occasionally, a functional study may be requested in a younger infant: the clinical question then is whether a kidney shows any significant function at all or not, leading to the consideration of a possible nephrectomy versus more conservative treatments.

EVALUATION OF DRAINAGE

Drainage can be influenced by several different factors, especially in the neonate: the function of the kidney, the hydration status, the size of the renal pelvis, the bladder status, and the effect of gravity (supine versus upright position). Therefore, an accurate evaluation of drainage has to take into account all these factors. Intravenous furosemide administration (5 mg in neonates and infants up to 6 months of age) can help to distinguish between an obstructed renal pelvis and a dilated nonobstructed one. Furosemide can be administered immediately after the radioactive tracer (F0), 15 minutes prior to tracer injection (F–15), or 20 minutes afterward (F+20). Each of these protocols causes a different diuresis during the renogram. In an attempt to avoid prolonging the renogram excessively, with likely motion artifacts as the child cannot lie still for too long, the F0 protocol is highly favored. It may happen that the neonate voids in the nappy during the dynamic renography, especially after administration of furosemide: this can be helpful as it shows the drainage pattern with an empty or almost empty bladder, and it can even demonstrate the possible presence of VUR. An image after change of position (from supine to upright) at the end of the dynamic renography is essential to differentiate an obstructed pelvis from a dilated nonobstructed one.

The use of a bladder catheter during the dynamic renography as a way of draining the bladder is controversial. This is advocated in several parts of the world, especially in North America, to eliminate the effect of a full bladder on the drainage from the upper tracts. In Europe, practitioners tend to prefer an image following change of posture and micturition. However, in the case of a neuropathic bladder, the use of a bladder catheter is strongly advised.

There are computerized methods to assess drainage. The half-time diuretic washout method calculates how long it takes to halve the counts within the renal pelvis following furosemide administration. This method is only reliable if it gives a normal value (<10 minutes half-time). If it is prolonged, it cannot differentiate between a dilated pelvis and an obstructed one, as it does not take into account the size of the renal pelvis, the bladder status, the gravity effect, and the hydration status, and therefore, in the context of

antenatally diagnosed hydronephrosis, it should not be relied upon. Methods such as the pelvic outflow efficiency (PEE) or the normalized residual activity (NORA) evaluate how much tracer has left the kidney as a percentage of what has come into the kidney (PEE), or how much tracer has remained in the kidney as a percentage of the amount that has left the kidney (NORA).

INTERPRETATION OF DRAINAGE AND DEFINITION OF OBSTRUCTION

It is important to bear in mind that slow drainage via a dilated collecting system on dynamic radionuclide renography does not necessarily mean obstruction in an asymptomatic infant with antenatally diagnosed hydronephrosis. A dilated pelvis and/or ureter can be due to a number of conditions: PUJ or VUJ anomaly with obstruction, PUJ dilatation with no obstruction, VUR, megaureter with or without VUJ dysfunction, or a complex duplex system with a dilated upper moiety. All these conditions can be associated with slow drainage on the dynamic radionuclide renography. Urinary stasis within a dilated renal pelvis/ureter does not necessarily cause suffering of the renal parenchyma. Even a stenosis at the PUJ may not cause resistance to urinary outflow that is sufficient to provoke suffering of the renal parenchyma, with a consequent drop in function. Therefore, the only definition of obstruction that has been accepted at present is "resistance to urinary outflow that, left untreated, will cause deterioration of renal function." As can be seen, unfortunately, this definition is a retrospective one. Therefore, in an asymptomatic patient who has had a single dynamic renography examination, which shows slow drainage and urinary stasis either at the PUJ or at the VUJ, obstruction cannot be reliably diagnosed, as it is not known whether this condition will cause a fall in function of that kidney or not.

MRI and CT: "cross-sectional imaging"

In the presence of a transonic/anechoic lesion on US, there is no indication for cross-sectional imaging as cystic lesions can be followed with US. Solid lesions will usually require further imaging after the initial US. The major differential diagnosis of renal tumors in the neonate is that of a mesoblastic nephroma (Figure 99.7), as Wilms tumors (Figure 99.8) are rare in the neonatal period, but still recognized. Neuroblastoma (in the adrenal) can sometimes be confused with a renal mass lesion and should also be considered. MRI is the optimal technique to assess mass lesions as it does not use radiation and has far superior inherent tissue contrast resolution compared to CT and can therefore differentiate between tissue types even if they are a similar level of density (perceived as similar "greyness") on CT. CT has good spatial resolution and is fast to acquire but carries a heavy radiation dose penalty. Furthermore, the neonate has little fat to provide contrast between adjacent structures, and CT cannot differentiate between tissues of similar density even though they may be of very different tissue types or indeed pathological. MRI can also provide exquisite depiction of the urinary tract, especially if it is dilated, as specific sequences will show water, and hence urine-containing structures, in great detail. This examination is also termed magnetic resonance urography (MRU) (Figure 99.9). It is therefore increasingly useful in supplementing the information obtained by US regarding dilatation, anatomy, and in some cases, the function of the renal tract.

The use of MRI in the neonatal age group was previously limited by the length of time to acquire various sequences (up to 10 minutes each) and, therefore, the risk of patient movement degrading the images, but the sequences are now much faster, and techniques are available to counteract the

effects of breathing and cardiac movement. MRI can be performed under general anesthetic if the feed-and-wrap technique fails.

SPECIFIC CONDITIONS IN THE NEONATAL PERIOD

Hydronephrosis

Hydronephrosis in the neonatal period is most commonly imaged subsequent to an antenatal diagnosis of renal pelvic dilatation being made at a routine antenatal US scan. It is important to clarify if the dilatation is bilateral and

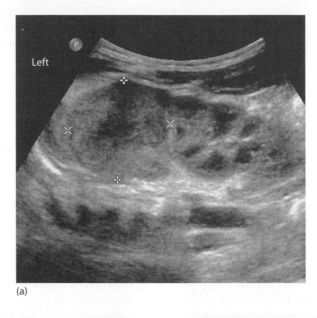

(a)

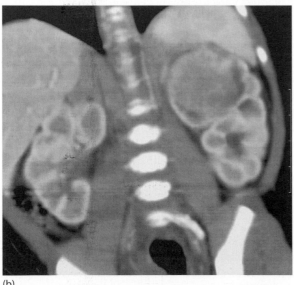

(b)

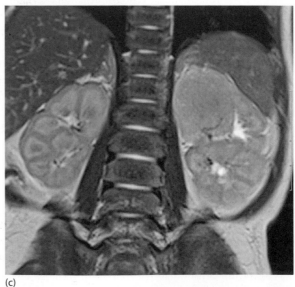

(c)

Figure 99.7 Mesoblastic nephroma in a 6-day-old male patient. **(a)** Ultrasound shows a mass at the upper pole of the left kidney. **(b)** CT scan in the same patient showing the left upper pole mass but poorly differentiating between the renal parenchyma and the collecting system. **(c)** Magnetic resonance image with T2 weighting showing the displacement of the collecting system around the mass and demonstrating the normal corticomedullary differentiation in the rest of the left kidney and in the right kidney.

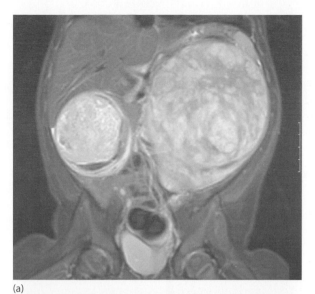

(a)

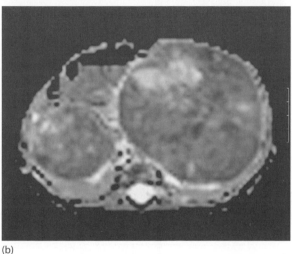

(b)

Figure 99.8 MRI in 3-month old with bilateral Wilms tumors. **(a)** Short tau inversion recovery (STIR) sequence in coronal plane showing the marked distortion of the normal anatomy due to the bulk of the tumors. **(b)** Apparent diffusion coefficient (ADC) sequence showing extensive areas of low signal (dark grey) within the tumors, which represent densely packed tumor cells. The area of high signal (white) anteriorly in the larger left-sided tumor indicates an area of necrosis.

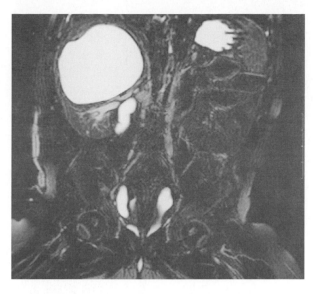

Figure 99.9 MRI in a 6-month-old female patient in whom ultrasound had been unable to differentiate between a right-sided pelviureteric junction obstruction and a dilated moiety of a duplex kidney. This heavily T2-weighted sequence shows that the right kidney is in fact duplex with a very dilated upper moiety and a small and compressed lower moiety. Incidental note was also made of a didelphus uterus in the pelvis.

how dilated the renal pelvis is. Imaging will always be by US. Bilateral pelvic dilatation (>7 mm) necessitates close inspection of the bladder (for bladder wall thickening and ureteroceles) and, in boys, will prompt MCUG to exclude posterior urethral valves. A unilateral antenatal hydronephrosis requires functional evaluation, normally with a MAG3 renography, to assess the split function of the hydronephrotic kidney and its drainage. It is important to realize that slow drainage does not necessarily mean obstruction. Follow-up of a hydronephrotic kidney is normally performed with US. Significant increase in renal pelvis dilatation on US will prompt a repeat functional study. A very

significant unilateral dilatation at diagnosis may indicate an intrinsic severe PUJ obstruction, and a functional study (often with MAG3, but also DMSA can be used—especially if the kidney is much enlarged with a very stretched renal parenchyma) will be indicated to establish if the affected kidney has any useful function. Occasionally, a PUJ anomaly may be associated with a VUJ anomaly; the MAG3 renogram may find it difficult to identify both conditions (Figure 99.10), and it is essential to interpret the findings of the isotope study in comparison with a contemporaneous US. A very enlarged and stretched kidney may still recover its function if prompt intervention is instigated. In the follow-up of an antenatally diagnosed hydronephrosis with radionuclide renography, a change in DRF of <5% is not significant. Changes between 5% and 10% have to be evaluated in context. If the child is younger than 6 months of age at the time of the first renogram (with consequent renal immaturity and poor tracer uptake on the renogram, and raised background activity) and the renal parenchyma is very stretched around a dilated renal pelvis, then the estimated value of split renal function will not be very precise. A follow-up renogram when the child is older and the kidneys are more mature, with better tracer uptake and less background activity, may show a change in split renal function between 5% and 10% in comparison to the baseline renogram but no significant change in the true function of that kidney.

A megaureter can be associated with obstruction at the distal end of the ureter and/or VUR, or may be nonobstructed and nonrefluxing. The first evaluation is with US,

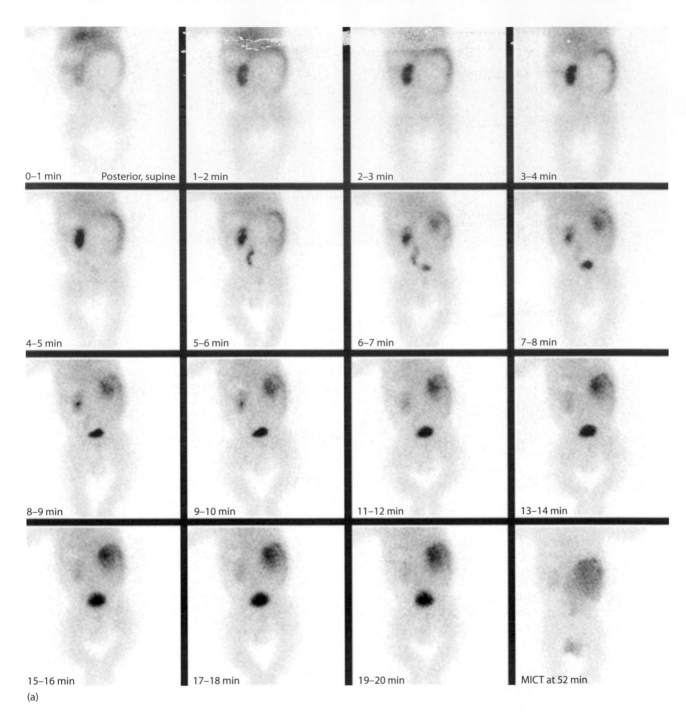

0–1 min   Posterior, supine   1–2 min   2–3 min   3–4 min

4–5 min   5–6 min   6–7 min   7–8 min

8–9 min   9–10 min   11–12 min   13–14 min

15–16 min   17–18 min   19–20 min   MICT at 52 min

(a)

Figure 99.10 **(a)** MAG3 renogram of a 6-week-old male infant with an antenatally diagnosed gross right hydronephrosis. The isotope study shows a grossly enlarged right kidney with a parenchyma severely stretched around a massively dilated collecting system, with a right renal pelvis measuring 6 cm in maximum diameter on ultrasound. Urinary stasis is seen at the level of the right PUJ, but no significant stasis is seen in the right ureter.   (*Continued*)

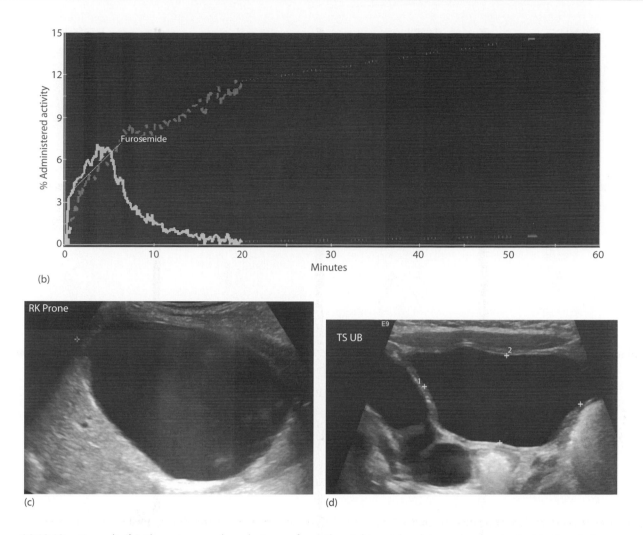

(b)

(c)

(d)

Figure 99.10 (Continued) **(b)** There is very slow drainage from the right renal pelvis as demonstrated in the drainage curve. **(c)** The ultrasound also shows marked dilatation of the renal pelvis, and these appearances combined are compatible with a right PUJ anomaly. **(d)** However, the ultrasound also shows a significantly dilated right ureter, measuring 14 mm in calibre at the distal end. Therefore, a concurrent right VUJ anomaly is also suspected. Cystoscopy confirmed a tight VUJ stenosis, which underwent balloon dilatation. A retrograde contrast study showed also a narrow right PUJ. This was corrected with a right pyeloplasty. This case highlights that a right VUJ anomaly may be missed on isotope dynamic renography, and it is essential to interpret the findings of the isotope study in comparison with a contemporaneous ultrasound.

which will show the calibre of the ureter at the proximal and at the distal ends, as well as the size of the renal pelvis. Functional imaging, often in the form of a MAG3 diuretic renography, will show the parenchymal function of the affected kidney and the level of urinary stasis (renal pelvis or ureter and where in the ureter) (Figure 99.11). It is important to realize that the radionuclide dynamic renography may fail to show significant ureteric stasis and therefore be falsely negative (Figure 99.10).

"Bright" kidneys

In an unwell neonate, US may be requested to obtain a baseline and to exclude any related renal cause for the infant's condition. On these occasions, the observation of "bright" kidneys may sometimes be made. "Bright" in this context implies that the parenchyma (both cortex and

medulla) is significantly more echo bright (i.e., hyperechoic) than the parenchyma of the adjacent liver or spleen. The kidneys may also be small, normal-sized, or large depending on the underlying cause (Figures 99.2 and 99.3). (Normal neonatal kidneys may be slightly more echogenic than the adjacent liver or spleen but not markedly so.)

The differential diagnosis of enlarged hyperechoic kidneys in the neonate includes acute tubular necrosis, renal vein thrombosis, polycystic kidney disease (autosomal dominant or autosomal recessive), autosomal dominant glomerulocystic kidneys, dysplastic kidneys (with or without an associated syndrome) (Figures 99.12a and 99.13), and rarely, an underlying metabolic disorder (Figure 99.2). In the case of renal vein thrombosis, a functional study (often DMSA) can be useful once the acute episode has resolved to assess if the kidney drained by the thrombosed vein has lost

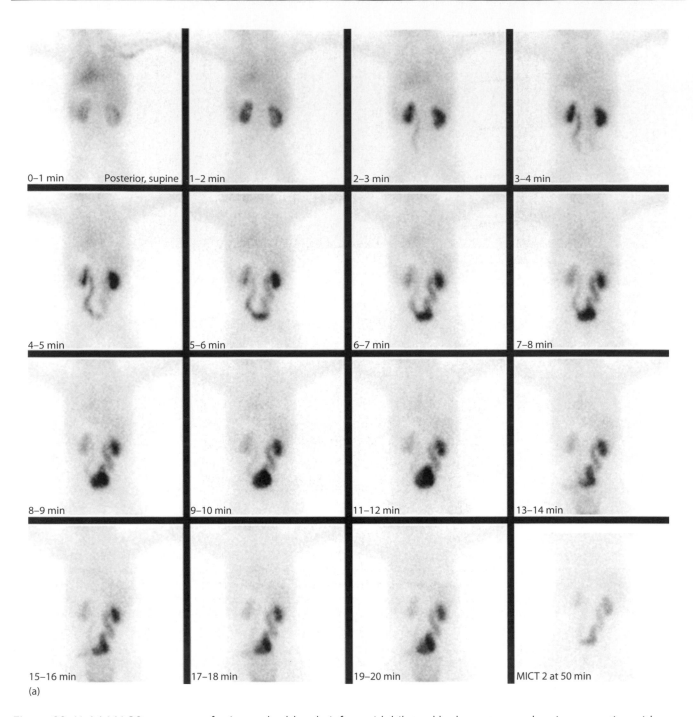

0–1 min   Posterior, supine   1–2 min   2–3 min   3–4 min

4–5 min   5–6 min   6–7 min   7–8 min

8–9 min   9–10 min   11–12 min   13–14 min

15–16 min   17–18 min   19–20 min   MICT 2 at 50 min

(a)

Figure 99. 11 **(a)** MAG3 renogram of a 4-month-old male infant with bilateral hydroureteronephrosis, presenting with urinary tract infection. Both kidneys function equally and normally.   (*Continued*)

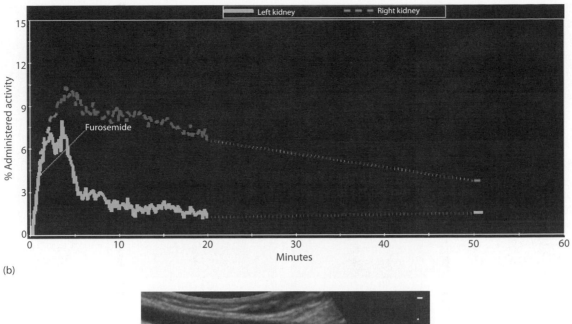

(b)

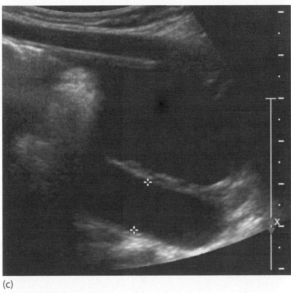

(c)

Figure 99. 11 (Continued) **(b)** The left kidney drains well via a mildly dilated ureter (5 mm on ultrasound). The right kidney shows slower drainage with significant urinary stasis in the lower third of the right ureter, even following change of posture and micturition. The ultrasound shows an 8 mm right renal pelvis. **(c)** The right ureter is dilated distally, measuring 12 mm. The imaging appearances raise the probability of a right VUJ anomaly. The baby underwent cystoscopy, which showed a tight right VUJ. This was dilated with a balloon, and a right JJ stent was placed.

significant function (Figure 99.14). A functional study may also be clinically helpful in the case of an arterial thrombosis (Figure 99.15).

Cystic kidneys

These will usually present in the neonate because the infant is in renal failure, because bilateral mass lesions can be felt in the flanks, or because the patient has a US scan for another reason. The main groups of cystic disease are listed in a previous section, "Bright Kidneys." A multicystic dysplastic kidney (MCDK) may be diagnosed antenatally but may be picked up in the neonatal period or later (Figure 99.16). Tuberous sclerosis

may also give rise to multiple cysts in the kidneys, but it would be unusual for this to present in the neonatal period (Figures 99.13 and 99.17). US will always be the first examination, and usually, no other imaging would be necessary at the neonatal stage. Functional imaging may be performed later. In the case of an MCDK, functional imaging will confirm that the kidney is nonfunctional and will look for the possible presence of slow drainage in the contralateral kidney due to ureteropelvic junction anomaly. Care must be taken not to misinterpret marked hydrophosis as an MCDK and vice versa. Differentiation is usually possible by demonstrating that the "cysts" connect to the renal pelvis and are therefore in fact dilated calyces.

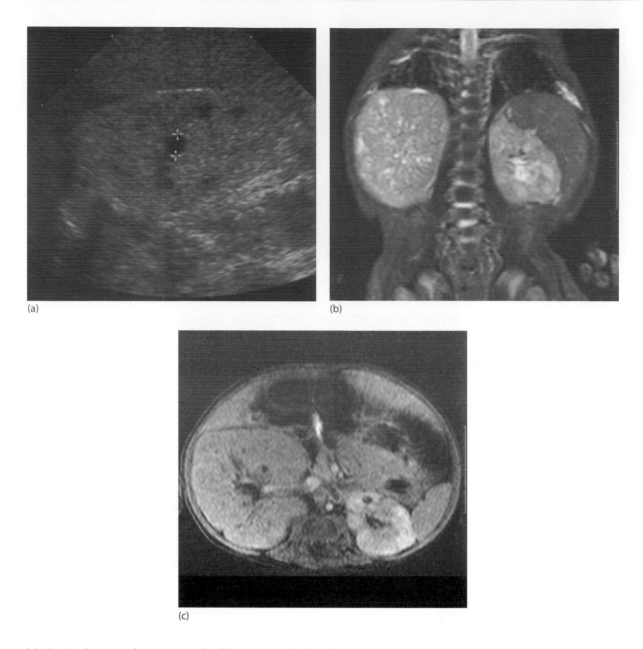

(a)

(b)

(c)

Figure 99.12 **(a)** Ultrasound in a 1-month-old patient with dysplastic kidneys. Note the small cysts in an otherwise feature-less parenchyma. **(b)** MRI in the same patient at the same time. This coronal STIR sequence shows the enlargement of the kidneys and the very abnormal renal architecture, with a typical striated appearance. **(c)** Axial T1-weighted sequence fol-lowing gadolinium demonstrating the small cysts seen on ultrasound and poor enhancement.

Tumors

Renal tumors in the neonatal period are rare, but the most likely type would be a mesoblastic nephroma. On US, this mass lesion would generally be mainly solid, if not entirely so. Usually, no further imaging is required, and surgery in the neonatal period is curative. Occasionally, the surgeon may wish for further cross-sectional imaging before oper-ating, and in this instance, MRI would be the modality of choice if it is available. There is no indication for functional imaging for the affected side, but functional imaging may be indicated to assess the function of the contralateral kid-ney before surgery.

Renal anomalies

Duplex kidneys (Figure 99.18a), cross-fused ectopic kid-neys (Figure 99.18b), horseshoe kidneys, and other anoma-lies are usually first detected by US. US will also be used for monitoring and for searching for other related anomalies, for example, spinal anomalies in patients with the VATER (Vertebral anomalies, Anal atresia, Tracheo-esophageal fis-tula and/or Esophageal atresia, Renal and radial anomalies) spectrum (Figure 99.18c). Functional imaging is essential as it informs on the function of the upper and the lower moi-eties of the duplex kidney and on the drainage (Figure 99.19). Occasionally, it can inform also on the presence of VUR

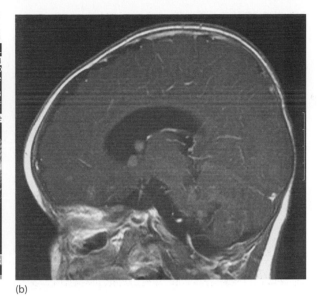

(a)

(b)

Figure 99.13 **(a)** Ultrasound in a 2-month old with large palpable kidneys showing multiple cysts. The differential is between autosomal dominant polycystic kidney disease and tuberous sclerosis. **(b)** Brain MRI in the same patient confirms the presence of tubers (shown adjacent to the lateral ventricle) and thus confirms the diagnosis of tuberous sclerosis.

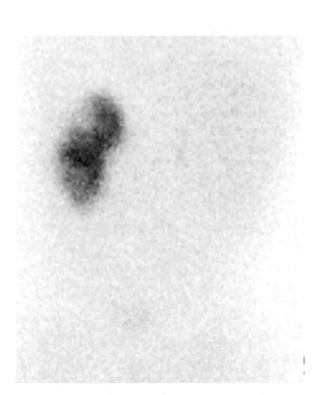

Figure 99.14 DMSA scan in a 5-month-old extremely prematurely born male infant, with a recent history of a right renal vein thrombosis. The right kidney is nonfunctional. The left kidney is damaged with focal abnormalities in the mid-upper pole laterally and at the lower pole. The ultrasound showed very dampened arterial flow to the right kidney and no detectable venous drainage.

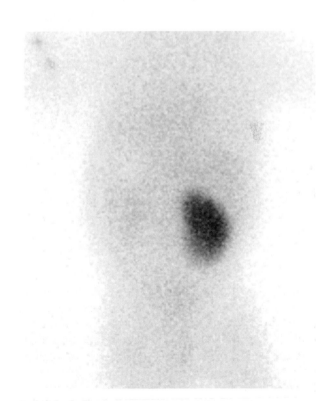

Figure 99.15 DMSA scan in a 20-day-old baby boy with extensive cerebral infarcts and significantly reduced arterial flow in the left kidney on Doppler ultrasound indicative of severe left renal artery stenosis. The left kidney is nonfunctional; the right kidney is normal.

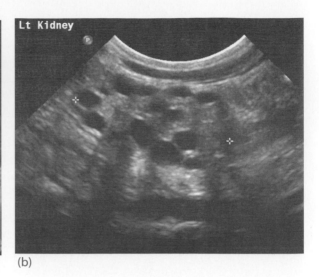

Figure 99.16 Ultrasound showing a right multicystic dysplastic kidney in a newborn patient. There are multiple non-communicating cysts in the renal parenchyma of the right kidney (a, b). The cysts may vary in size but are usually seen throughout the kidney(s), and the intervening parenchyma is echo-bright. A true MCDK has no function on DMSA.

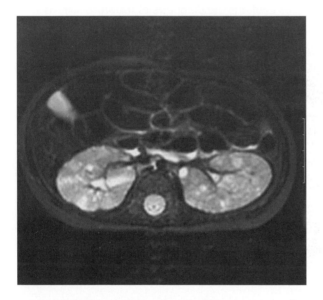

Figure 99.17 MRI in a 5-month old with tuberous sclerosis. This axial STIR sequence shows multiple cysts in both kidneys. These are easily demonstrated by ultrasound, but MRI is also performed to exclude liver or pancreatic involvement.

(Figure 99.20). MRI may be very useful in the most complicated cases, being able to demonstrate the whole of the urinary tract in any desired plane and giving some information about function and drainage. Unless there are specific complications requiring further intervention, all of the secondary imaging may be delayed till the patient is older.

Infection

Infection in the neonatal period may be acquired at the time of delivery, be secondary to an underlying urinary tract anomaly, or be a result of instrumentation/catheter placement. If imaging were required, then US would be the first modality. If the urinary tract is anatomically normal, US may not demonstrate any abnormal findings; however, echogenic debris may be seen throughout the urinary tract. If the upper tracts are involved (pyelonephritis), it may be possible to demonstrate focal areas of low echogenicity, or the kidneys may simply be enlarged. If the patient has been systemically ill (e.g., requiring intravenous antibiotics as an inpatient), the microorganism isolated is unusual (*Klebsiella*, *Pseudomonas*, *Enterococcus*), or the child has recurrent infections, functional imaging is indicated. If the clinical question is to confirm whether the child has an acute pyelonephritis with renal parenchymal inflammatory involvement and how much of the renal parenchyma has been involved, then a DMSA performed during the infection will answer the question. If the question is whether the infant has developed renal scarring as a consequence of the infection, then a DMSA scan will have to be performed between 4 and 6 months after the infection.

Renal calculi and nephrocalcinosis

Calculi are rare in the neonatal period, but nephrocalcinosis may be seen in patients with an inherited underlying metabolic abnormality such as primary hyperoxaluria (Figure 99.2). It is most commonly asymptomatic. Nephrocalcinosis is well demonstrated on US and is described as medullary, cortical, or parenchymal. Initially, there is a mild increase in echogenicity and ringing of the pyramids, which may eventually progress to filling-in of the medullae with acoustic shadowing.

Other causes of focal echogenicity mimicking nephrocalcinosis in the neonatal period include the use of furosemide (calcification seen at the tips of the pyramids, sometimes associated with stone formation) and Tamm–Horsfall

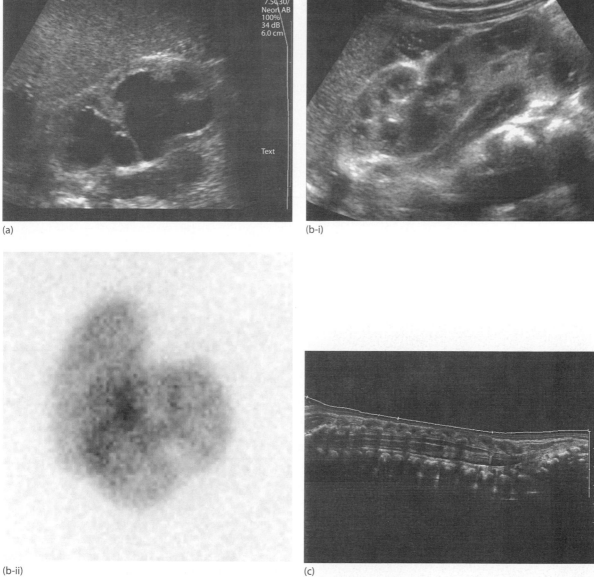

Figure 99.18 **(a)** Ultrasound of the kidney in a newborn male showing dilatation of both moieties in a duplex kidney. **(b)** Ultrasound **(i)** in a 2-month-old male infant demonstrating a crossed fused ectopic kidney and the associated DMSA **(ii)**. The two kidneys lie in the right flank and are fused obliquely. **(c)** Ultrasound of the spine was also performed in the same patient (due to other anomalies in the VATER group) and shows a normal appearance. Spine ultrasound needs to be performed in the first few weeks of life before ossification of the spine becomes established.

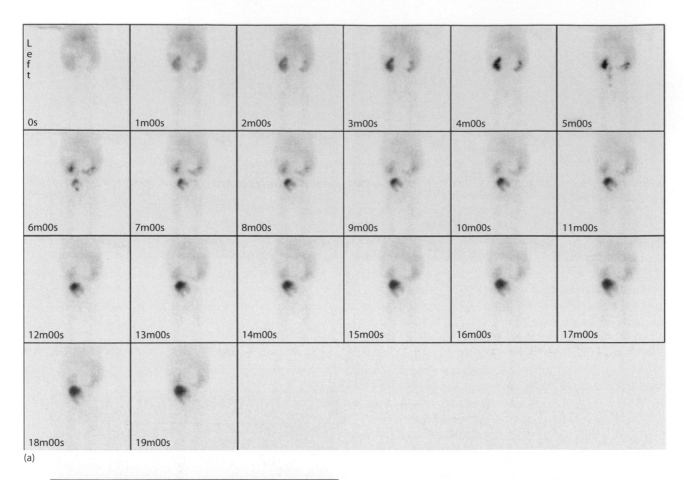

(a)

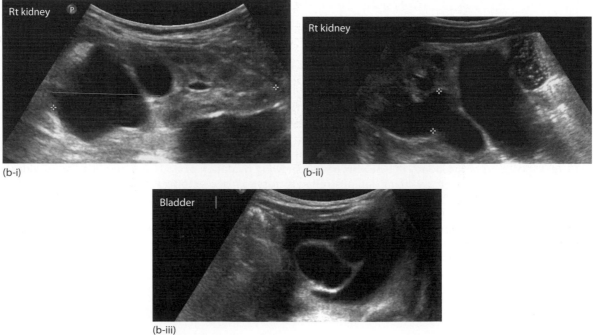

(b-i)   (b-ii)

(b-iii)

Figure 99.19 (a) MAG3 renogram of a 6-week-old female infant with a prenatal diagnosis of a right duplex kidney. This confirms a right duplex kidney with a nonfunctional upper moiety and reduced function in the lower moiety. The right kidney contributes 23% to total renal function (left kidney 77%). (b) US demonstrates dilatation of the upper moiety (i) and a tortuous dilated ureter (ii). There is a photopenic indentation in the right side of the bladder (a), in keeping with a large ureterocele as shown on US (iii).

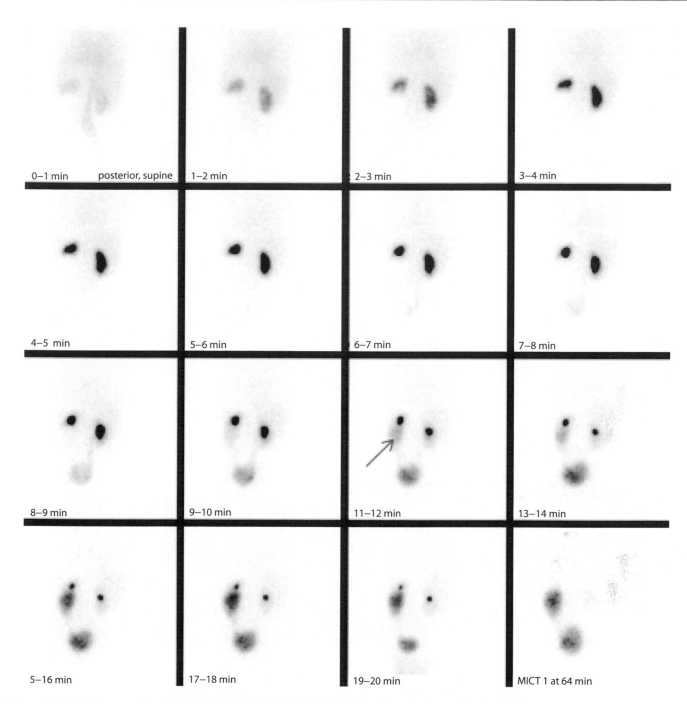

Figure 99.20 Eight-month-old baby with a left-sided duplex renal collecting system. The left lower moiety is nonfunctional. The left upper moiety shows good function. There is a clear vesicoureteric reflux in the left lower moiety during the dynamic renography, in coincidence with micturition. The right kidney is normal.

protein deposition in the medullae (which is a transitory event related to fluid regulation around the time of birth).

CONCLUSION

The US examination should always be the first imaging examination in the neonate. This may be supplemented by functional studies (DMSA or MAG3) or further anatomical studies (including MCUG and MRI [or CT]) as determined by the underlying findings on US.

FURTHER READING

Fotter R, *Paediatric Uroradiology*, 2nd edn. Berlin: Springer-Verlag, 2008. ISBN 978-3-540-33004-2.

Thomas D, Duffy P, Rickwood A (eds). *Essentials of Paediatric Urology*, 2nd edn. London: Informa Healthcare, 2008. ISBN-10: 1841846333, ISBN-13: 978-1841846330.

An excellent review on the use of functional imaging in antenatal hydronephrosis is the following:

Piepsz A. Antenatally detected hydronephrosis. *Sem Nucl Med* 2007; 37: 249–69.

Piepsz A, Ham HR. Pediatric applications of renal nuclear medicine. *Sem Nucl Med* 2006; 36: 16–35.

A comprehensive review on nuclear medicine in pediatric nephrourology is the following:

Avni FE, Garel C, Cassart M, D'Haene N, Hall M, Riccabona M. Imaging and classification of congenital cystic renal diseases. *AJR Am J Roentgenol* 2012 May; 198(5): 1004–13.

Darge K, Grattan-Smith JD, Riccabona M. Pediatric uroradiology: State of the art. *Pediatr Radiol* 2011 January; 41(1): 82–91.

Darge K, Higgins M, Hwang TJ, Delgado J, Shukla A, Bellah R. Magnetic resonance and computed tomography in pediatric urology: An imaging overview for current and future daily practice. *Radiol Clin N Am* 2013 July; 51(4): 583–98.

Dickerson EC, Dillman JR, Smith EA, DiPietro MA, Lebowitz RL, Darge K. Pediatric MR urography: Indications, techniques, and approach to review. *Radiographics* 2015 July–August; 35(4): 1208–30.

Grattan-Smith JD, Jones RA. MR urography: Technique and results for the evaluation of urinary obstruction in the pediatric population. *Magn Reson Imaging Clin N Am* 2008 November; 16(4): 643–60, viii–ix.

Jones RA, Grattan-Smith JD, Little S. Pediatric magnetic resonance urography. *J Magn Reson Imaging* 2011 March; 33(3): 510–26.

Nguyen HT, Benson CB, Bromley B, Campbell JB, Chow J, Coleman B, Cooper C, Crino J, Darge K, Herndon CD, Odibo AO, Somers MJ, Stein DR. Multidisciplinary consensus on the classification of prenatal and postnatal urinary tract dilation (UTD classification system). *J Pediatr Urol* 2014 December; 10(6): 982–98.

Renjen P, Bellah R, Hellinger JC, Darge K. Advances in uroradiologic imaging in children. *Radiol Clin N Am* 2012 March; 50(2): 207–18.

Riccabona M. Imaging of the neonatal genito-urinary tract. *Eur J Radiol* 2006 November; 60(2): 187–98.

Riccabona M. (Paediatric) magnetic resonance urography: Just fancy images or a new important diagnostic tool? *Curr Opin Urol* 2007 January; 17(1): 48–55.

Riccabona M. Basics, principles, techniques and modern methods in paediatric ultrasonography. *Eur J Radiol* 2014 September; 83(9): 1487–94.

Riccabona M. Diagnostic ultrasonography in neonates, infants and children—Why, when and how. *Eur J Radiol* 2014 September; 83(9): 1485–6.

Riccabona M. Urinary tract imaging in infancy. *Pediatr Radiol* 2009 June; 39 Suppl 3: 436–45.

100

Management of antenatal hydronephrosis

JACK S. ELDER

INTRODUCTION

An abnormality involving the genitourinary tract is detected in 1 in 50 to 1 in 100 pregnancies, depending on the sonographic criteria. The goal of management is to recognize and treat congenital anomalies that may adversely affect renal function or cause urinary tract infection (UTI) or sepsis. Many structural abnormalities of the urinary tract are characterized by hydronephrosis, which frequently is assumed to be obstructive. However, often antenatal hydronephrosis (ANH) results from non-obstructive causes, including vesicoureteral reflux (VUR), multicystic dysplastic kidney, and certain abnormalities of the ureteropelvic and ureterovesical junction.

DEVELOPMENT OF THE KIDNEY AND RENAL FUNCTION

The kidney is derived from the ureteral bud and the metanephric blastema. During the fifth week of gestation, the ureteral bud arises from the mesonephric (Wolffian) duct and penetrates the metanephric blastema, which is an area of undifferentiated mesenchyme on the nephrogenic ridge. The ureteral bud undergoes a series of approximately 15 generations of divisions, and by 20 weeks' gestation forms the entire collecting system, that is, the ureter, renal pelvis, calyces, papillary ducts, and collecting tubules. Under the inductive influence of the ureteral bud, nephron differentiation begins during the seventh week of gestation. By 20 weeks' gestation, when the collecting system is completely developed, approximately one-third of the nephrons are present. Nephrogenesis continues at a nearly exponential rate and is complete at 36 weeks' gestation. Throughout gestation, the placenta functions as the fetal hemodialyzer, and the fetal kidneys play a minor role in the maintenance of fetal salt and water homeostasis. Formation of urine begins between the fifth and ninth weeks of gestation.

The rate of urine production increases throughout gestation, and at term, volumes have been reported to be 51 mL/h.[1] The glomerular filtration rate (GFR) has been measured at 6 mL/min/1.73 m^2 at 28 weeks' gestation, increasing to 25 mL/min/1.73 m^2 at term, and thereafter triples by 3 months of age.[2] The main factors responsible for this increase in GFR after birth include an increase in the capillary surface area available for filtration, changes in intrarenal vascular resistance, and redistribution of renal blood flow to the cortical nephrons, which are much more numerous than the medullary nephrons. A congenital obstructive lesion of the urinary tract may have a deleterious effect on renal function. Severe early obstructive uropathy disrupts nephrogenesis and results in renal dysplasia.

THE FETUS WITH ANH

When a fetus is identified with a suspected urinary tract abnormality, the goals of management include determining the differential diagnosis, assessing the associated anomalies, and determining the fetal and postnatal risk of the anomaly. Hydronephrosis is recognized by demonstrating a dilated renal pelvis and calyces. The ureter and bladder may be dilated also. The likelihood of having a significant urinary tract abnormality is directly proportional to the severity of hydronephrosis.[3,4] If the renal pelvic diameter is more than 2 cm, 94% have a significant abnormality of the urinary tract requiring surgery or long-term urologic follow-up. If the fetal renal pelvic diameter is between 1.0 and 1.5 cm, 50% have an abnormality, and if the dilated renal pelvis is less than 1 cm, only 3% have a significant abnormality.[5] A renal pelvic diameter of at least 4 mm before 27 weeks' gestation and at least 7 mm after 27 weeks' gestation has been considered significant.[6] The later the sonogram is performed, the more likely an existing abnormality will be detected, because the obstructed renal pelvis gradually enlarges throughout gestation. In addition, in utero, the fetus is usually upside down in the uterus and urine is draining uphill. For example, Fugelseth et al.[7] reported that only one-third of a series of women carrying babies with a urologic anomaly had an abnormal ultrasound study at 15–21 weeks' gestation.

The differential diagnosis of ANH is provided in Table 100.1. Virtually all of these conditions can cause bilateral hydronephrosis. A distended bladder and bilateral hydronephrosis is suggestive of bladder outlet obstruction, such as posterior urethral valves (PUVs) or a large ectopic ureterocele obstructing the bladder neck, but fetuses with non-obstructive conditions, such as high-grade VUR or prune belly syndrome, also may have bilateral hydroureteronephrosis and a distended bladder. In fetuses with a urologic anomaly, associated abnormalities are common. For example, in one series of fetuses with bilateral hydronephrosis and oligohydramnios, 16 of 31 (55%) had an associated structural or chromosomal abnormality.[8] Congenital heart disease and neurologic deformities can often be detected, if they are present. In contrast, large bowel abnormalities, such as imperforate anus, are more difficult to detect by prenatal sonography, whereas recognition of small bowel anomalies, such as atresia, are usually straightforward.

The main considerations in determining fetal management include overall fetal well-being, gestational age, whether the hydronephrosis is unilateral or bilateral, and the volume of amniotic fluid. Until recently, there were no guidelines for determining how frequently to image the fetus or whether specific intervention was necessary. If hydronephrosis is unilateral, usually no specific fetal therapy is necessary. For example, if the hydronephrosis is secondary to a ureteropelvic junction (UPJ) obstruction, even if function is poor, the kidney has a significant capacity for improvement in function following neonatal pyeloplasty. Even with bilateral UPJ obstruction (characterized by bilateral hydronephrosis and a normal bladder), the amniotic fluid volume and pulmonary development typically are normal. Consequently, specific intervention, such as percutaneous drainage of the fetal kidney or early delivery to allow immediate urologic surgery, is unwarranted. These same principles apply to primary obstructive megaureter.[9]

The primary life-threatening congenital urologic anomalies include PUVs, urethral atresia, and prune belly syndrome, which are usually characterized by bilateral hydroureteronephrosis and a distended bladder that does not empty in a male fetus. Approximately one-third of infants with urethral valves eventually develop renal insufficiency or end-stage renal disease.[10] Although prune belly syndrome is considered non-obstructive, neonates with this condition frequently have renal insufficiency, in large part because of congenital renal insufficiency and also from renal deterioration in children with repeated episodes of pyelonephritis. Urethral atresia is nearly always fatal, because the kidneys are usually dysplastic. A severe adverse prognostic factor is oligohydramnios, which prevents normal pulmonary development. In fetuses with severe obstructive uropathy and renal dysplasia, neonatal demise usually results from pulmonary hypoplasia rather than chronic renal failure. Intuitively, it would seem that treatment of the obstructed fetal urinary tract by diverting the urine into the empty amniotic space might allow normal renal development to occur and restore amniotic fluid dynamics, stimulating lung development. Indeed, experimental procedures have been performed, including percutaneous placement of a vesicoamniotic shunt, creation of a fetal vesicostomy or pyelostomy, and even percutaneous urethral valve ablation through a miniscope.[11] Unfortunately, the complication rate is high, including shunt migration, urinary ascites, stimulation of preterm labor, and chorioamnionitis.[2,12] Furthermore, in most cases, irreversible renal dysplasia has already occurred, and although the procedure may be successful technically, often the baby is stillborn, dies of pulmonary hypoplasia, or is alive with end-stage renal disease.[13,14] Nevertheless, some fetuses may benefit from aggressive intervention if the kidneys do not have irreversible dysplasia. Unfavorable prognostic factors include[2,9]

- Prolonged oligohydramnios
- Renal cortical cysts
- Urinary Na >100 mEq/L, Cl >90 mEq/L, and osmolarity >210 mOsm/L
- beta2-microglobulin >6 mg/L
- Reduced lung area and thoracic or abdominal circumference

Unfavorable urinary electrolytes may reflect stale urine in the fetal urinary tract. Consequently, perinatal centers typically obtain two or three sequential samples, as subsequent samples yield fetal urine that is more reflective of true fetal renal function.[14]

GUIDELINES ON ANH

In 2010, the Society for Fetal Urology (SFU) published a consensus statement regarding the evaluation and management of ANH.[15] This document was a comprehensive attempt to provide a guide to antenatal and postnatal management of ANH, and identify areas of controversy and prioritize research endeavors. The SFU did not provide guidance on when a voiding cystourethrogram (VCUG) should be performed. With regard to antibiotic prophylaxis, the authors recommended that neonates with an increased risk of UTI (girls, uncircumcised boys, moderate to severe hydronephrosis, and familial VUR) should receive prophylaxis until the initial evaluation is completed and management is planned with the family. In 2012, the American Urological Association (AUA) was asked to establish formal guidelines for ANH, but they thought that the SFU was thorough and did not need updating. The European Society for Paediatric Urology has published recommendations on management of various congenital urinary tract malformations, but has not addressed ANH specifically.

In 2013, the Indian Society of Pediatric Nephrology published updated guidelines on ANH.[16] These recommendations were based on systematic reviews of the literature from 1990 to 2012. Level 1 recommendations included those applicable to most subjects based on consistent information.

Table 100.1 Genitourinary anomalies detectable by prenatal ultrasonography

Condition	Sex (ratio)	Frequency	Kidney(s)	Ureter(s)	Bladder	Amniotic fluid	Prognosis
Ureteropelvic junction obstruction (unilateral)	M/F (3–4:1)	1:2000	Hydronephrosis	Not seen	Normal	Normal	Good after surgical correction
Multicystic kidney (unilateral)	M/F (1:1)	1:3000	Large with cysts of variable size	Not seen	Normal	Normal	Normal
Primary obstructive megaureter	M/F (3:1)	1:10 000	Hydronephrosis	Dilated	Normal	Normal	Good after surgical correction
Ectopic ureterocele or ureter	M/F (1:6)	1:10 000	Large cyst; possible duplex kidney	Dilated	Normal or enlarged	Normal	Good after surgical correction
Posterior urethral valves	Male	1:8000	Bilateral hydronephrosis; possible cortical cysts	Dilated	Enlarged	Variable; diminished or absent in severe obstruction	Usually good after surgical correction or drainage; poor if oligo?hydramnios is present
Prune belly syndrome	Nearly always male	1:40 000	Bilateral hydronephrosis; possible cortical cysts	Dilated	Enlarged	Variable; diminished or absent if severely affected	Usually fair to good; may need surgical drainage; poor if oligohydramnios is present
Vesico-ureteral reflux	M/F (1:5)	1:100	Hydronephrosis if reflux high grade	Variable	Normal; dilated if reflux high grade	Normal	Good; may need surgical correction
Infantile polycystic kidney disease	M/F	1:6000–1:14000	Large, echogenic	Not seen	Small or not seen	Usually absent or severely diminished	Poor
Renal agenesis	M/F (2.0–2.5:1)	1:4000 (bilateral) / 1:1500 (unilateral)	Not seen	Not seen	Not seen	Severely diminished or absent	Stillbirth
			Not seen	Not seen	Normal	Normal	Normal
Hydrocolpos	Female		May have hydronephrosis	Not seen	Normal	Normal	Good after surgical correction
Ovarian cyst	Female		Normal (cyst may be confused with kidney or bladder)	Not seen	Normal	Normal	Good after surgical correction

Level 2 recommendations were those that were based on equivocal or insufficient information. Highlights of the recommendations include the following:

1. It is recommended that ANH be diagnosed and its severity graded based on anteroposterior diameter (APD) of the fetal renal pelvis (1B). ANH is present if the APD is ≥4 mm in second trimester and ≥7 mm in the third trimester.
2. Termination of pregnancy is not recommended in fetuses with unilateral or bilateral ANH, except in presence of extrarenal life threatening abnormality (1D).
3. It is recommended that all newborns with history of ANH should have postnatal ultrasound examination within the first week of life (1B). In neonates with suspected PUVs, oligohydramnios, or severe bilateral hydronephrosis, ultrasonography should be performed within 24–48 hours of birth (1C). In all other cases, the ultrasound should be performed preferably within 3–7 days, or before hospital discharge (1C).
4. It is recommended that assessment of severity of postnatal hydronephrosis be based on the classification proposed by SFU or APD of the renal pelvis (1B).
5. It is recommended that neonates with normal ultrasound examination in the first week of life should undergo a repeat study at 4–6 weeks (1C). Infants with isolated mild unilateral or bilateral hydronephrosis (APD <10 mm or SFU grade 1–2) should be followed by sequential ultrasound alone, for resolution or progression of findings (1C).
6. It is recommended that a micturating cystourethrogram (MCU) be performed in patients with unilateral or bilateral hydronephrosis with renal pelvic APD >10 mm, SFU grade 3–4, or ureteric dilatation (1B). MCU should be performed early, within 24–72 hours of life, in patients with suspected lower urinary tract obstruction (1D). In other cases, the procedure should be done at 4–6 weeks of age. MCU is recommended for infants with antenatally detected hydronephrosis who develop a UTI (1C).
7. It is recommended that infants with moderate to severe unilateral or bilateral hydronephrosis (SFU grade 3–4, APD >10 mm) who do not show VUR should undergo diuretic renography (1C). Infants with hydronephrosis and dilated ureter(s) and no evidence of VUR should undergo diuretic renography (2C). The preferred radiopharmaceuticals are ^{99m}Tc-mercaptoacetyltriglycine (^{99m}Tc-MAG3), ^{99m}Tc-ethylenedicysteine (^{99m}Tc-EC), or ^{99m}Tc-diethylenetriaminepentaacetic acid (DTPA) (2D). The differential function is estimated and renogram curve inspected for pattern of drainage. Diuretic renography should be performed after 6–8 weeks of age (2D). The procedure may be repeated after 3–6 months in infants where ultrasound shows worsening of pelvicalyceal dilatation (2D).
8. It is suggested that surgery be considered in patients with obstructed hydronephrosis, and either reduced differential renal function or its worsening on repeat evaluation (2C). It is suggested that surgery be considered in patients with bilateral hydronephrosis or hydronephrosis in a solitary kidney showing worsening dilatation and deterioration of function (2D).
9. It is recommended that parents of all infants with antenatal or postnatal hydronephrosis be counseled regarding the risk of UTIs and need for prompt management (1B). It is recommended that infants with postnatally confirmed moderate or severe hydronephrosis (SFU 3–4; renal APD >10 mm) or dilated ureter receive antibiotic prophylaxis while awaiting evaluation (1C). It is recommended that all patients detected to have VUR receive antibiotic prophylaxis through the first year of life (1B).

More recently, a multidisciplinary consensus conference involving eight societies was held and included pediatric urologists, pediatric nephrologists, pediatric radiologists, and maternal–fetal medicine specialists.[17] The purpose was to try to standardize the fetal evaluation and early postnatal management of babies with ANH. For example, several different classification schemes had been published for significant and insignificant pelvicalyceal dilation. In addition, although the SFU 4-point grading scale is used by most pediatric urologists, most pediatric radiologists classify hydronephrosis into mild, moderate, and severe.

The US parameters include anterior–posterior renal pelvic diameter (APRPD), calyceal dilation, whether it involves the major and/or minor calyces, parenchymal thickness and appearance, normal or abnormal ureter, and normal or abnormal bladder.[17] Normal values for urinary tract dilation are APRPD:

Antenatal	16–27 weeks	<4 mm
	≥28 weeks	<7 mm
Postnatal	(>48 hours)	<10 mm

Assuming there is no calyceal dilation, the kidneys have a normal appearance, and the ureter and bladder are normal, then this is considered a normal study.

The consensus group then categorized ANH into antenatal and postnatal risk groups. For antenatal, there are two risk groups: low risk and high risk. For postnatal, there are three risk groups: low risk, intermediate risk, and high risk. The panel recommended that all seven urinary tract parameters be described in a written report.

For antenatal presentation, if the APRPD is 4–7 mm at 16–27 weeks or 7–10 mm at ≥28 weeks, and there is central or no calyceal dilation, the fetus is **UTD** ["urinary tract dilation"] **A1, Low Risk**. In follow-up, for UTD A1, the panel suggested one additional antenatal US at ≥32 weeks, and after birth, a renal US at >48 hours to 1 month of age, and a second renal US 6 months later. Genetic screening is not indicated unless there are associated congenital malformations.

If the APRPD is ≥7 mm at 16–27 weeks or ≥10 mm at ≥28 weeks with any peripheral calyceal dilation or any other upper urinary tract abnormality, they are classified as **UTD A2-3** or **Increased Risk**. The assigned risk is based on the most concerning feature. For UTD A2-3, the panel recommended a follow-up US in 4–6 weeks, although with suspected PUVs or severe bilateral hydronephrosis, more frequent follow-up was recommended until delivery. Following delivery, a renal US after 48 hours but before 1 month was suggested, again with more immediate evaluation if PUV is suspected or there is significant bilateral hydronephrosis. In addition, specialist consultation with pediatric urology or nephrology was recommended.

For postnatal presentation, at >48 hours, an APRPD <10 mm is **Normal**. If the APRPD is 10–15 mm, there is central calyceal dilation, and all other parameters are normal, it is classified **UTD P1, Low Risk**. SFU hydronephrosis grades 1 and 2 correspond to UTD P1. The panel recommends a follow-up renal US in 1–6 months. A VCUG and antibiotic prophylaxis are optional, at the discretion of the clinician. A renal scan is not recommended.

If the postnatal APRPD is ≥15 mm, there is peripheral calyceal dilation, and/or abnormal ureters, it is classified **UTD P2, Intermediate Risk**. SFU hydronephrosis grade 3 corresponds to UTD P2. The panel recommends a follow-up renal US in 1–3 months. A VCUG, antibiotic prophylaxis, and a functional renal scan are optional, at the discretion of the clinician.

If the APRPD is ≥15 mm, and there is peripheral calyceal dilation, abnormal parenchymal thickness, abnormal parenchymal appearance, abnormal ureters, and/or abnormal bladder, it is classified **UTD P3, High Risk**. SFU hydronephrosis grade 4 corresponds to UTD P3. The panel recommends a follow-up renal US in 1 month. A VCUG and antibiotic prophylaxis are recommended. A functional renal scan is optional, at the discretion of the clinician (but is virtually always recommended).

This classification scheme was validated at the NIH Consensus Conference by the participants. In addition, it was evaluated in a retrospective study of 490 patients.[18] The authors found that the Urinary Tract Dilation classification appropriately identified the babies that were likely to require surgical intervention, while the SFU hydronephrosis grading system was most likely to predict likelihood of resolution of hydronephrosis.

MANAGEMENT OF THE NEWBORN WITH ANH

Management in the nursery

At birth, the abdomen is inspected to detect the presence of a mass, which most often is secondary to a multicystic dysplastic kidney or UPJ obstruction. In male newborns with PUVs, often a walnut-shaped mass, representing the bladder, is palpable just superior to the pubic symphysis. Newborns should also be evaluated for anomalies involving other organ systems, as urinary tract abnormalities often occur in babies with congenital heart disease, lung abnormalities, and anorectal malformations. Renal function should be monitored with serial serum creatinine levels, particularly in infants with bilateral hydronephrosis. At birth, the serum creatinine level is identical to the mother's, but by 1 week of age, the creatinine should decrease to 0.4 mg/dL. The exception is premature infants, in whom the creatinine may not decrease until these children reach 34–35 weeks' conceptional age because of renal immaturity before that age.

Antibiotic prophylaxis

Neonates with hydronephrosis who are at risk for UTI should be placed on antibiotic prophylaxis with either amoxicillin 50 mg daily or cephalexin 50 mg daily. At 2 months beyond term, the prophylaxis is usually changed to trimethoprim-sulfamethoxazole suspension or nitrofurantoin. In addition, circumcision should be considered in male neonates to minimize the likelihood of UTI. However, which babies are at risk and therefore who needs prophylaxis is controversial. Clearly, the risk group UTD P3, High Risk deserves prophylaxis. However, there is significant variability among pediatric urologists and nephrologists in prescribing prophylaxis for children with hydronephrosis.[19] For example, 30% of Canadian pediatric nephrologists would recommend CAP for bilateral low-grade ANH compared with 11% of pediatric urologists. With high-grade ANH, 73% of nephrologists and 38% of urologists recommended CAP. Their recommendations for VCUG also were quite variable.[19]

Early studies suggested that children with VUR, ectopic ureter and ureterocele, and PUVs benefit from prophylaxis, but that those with hydronephrosis secondary to an abnormality of the UPJ or ureterovesical junction are not at increased risk.[20] More recently, infants with high-grade hydronephrosis (OR 2.40), female gender (OR 3.16), and uncircumcised males (OR 3.63) were at highest risk, and multivariate analysis suggested that prophylaxis was not beneficial.[21] However, a subsequent prospective study from the same institution indicated that "lack of continuous antibiotic prophylaxis," hydroureteronephrosis, and VUR were significant risk factors of febrile UTI.[22] Similarly, Herz et al.[23] demonstrated in a retrospective study that the risk of febrile UTI was 7.9% in children receiving prophylaxis vs. 18.7% in those not receiving prophylaxis. In that study, children with ureteral dilation >11 mm, ureterovesical obstruction, and high-grade VUR were at greatest risk for a febrile UTI. Most agree that children with low-grade hydronephrosis do not benefit from prophylaxis.[24,25] Antibiotic resistance is a definite concern when prescribing prophylaxis unnecessarily.[26]

INITIAL RADIOLOGIC EVALUATION

Radiologic evaluation should be performed to delineate the abnormality responsible for changes on prenatal sonography. Serial renal sonograms, a VCUG, and a diuretic renogram usually provide the diagnostic information necessary to guide management, although all of these studies are unnecessary in many children.

Renal ultrasound

A renal and bladder sonogram should be obtained first. Because neonates have transient oliguria, a dilated or obstructed collecting system may appear normal for the first 24–48 hours of life (Figure 100.1). Ideally, if unilateral hydronephrosis was present prenatally, the renal sonogram should not be obtained until 72 hours to maximize its sensitivity, and unless the antenatal US showed severe unilateral or bilateral hydronephrosis, it is most appropriate to wait until 1–2 weeks of age.

Renal length, degree of caliectasis and parenchymal thickness, and presence or absence of ureteral dilation should be assessed. The severity of hydronephrosis can be graded from 1 to 4 using the SFU grading scale (Figure 100.2).[27] Inexperienced radiologists may misinterpret a normal

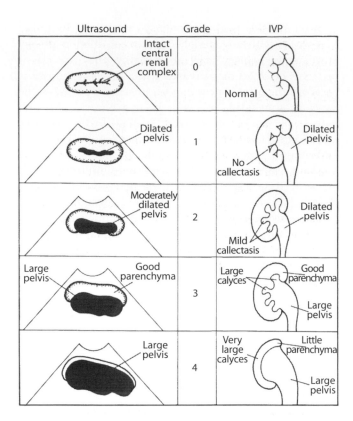

Figure 100.2 Grading system for hydronephrosis. (Reproduced with permission from the Society for Fetal Urology.)

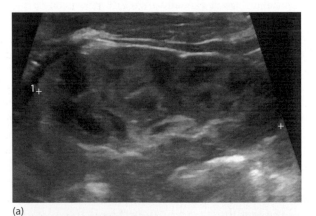

(a)

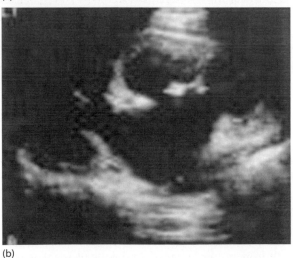

(b)

Figure 100.1 Newborn with prenatal diagnosis of left hydronephrosis. (a) Ultrasound of left kidney taken shortly after birth. Normal study. Echolucent areas in renal cortex are pyramids (normal finding). (b) Same patient. Ultrasound of left kidney at 6 weeks shows grade 4 hydronephrosis.

neonatal kidney with hypoechoic pyramids for caliectasis. Most significant urologic anomalies that require surgical correction or long-term urological follow-up are associated with grade 3 or 4 hydronephrosis.[28] More sophisticated analyses, such as the renal resistive index, as well as urinary studies have been assessed, but efforts to demonstrate obstruction have been inconsistent. The degree of pelvocaliectasis correlates closely with the likelihood that a significant urological condition is present. Lee et al.[29] performed a meta-analysis of reports of ANH and determined that the risk of finding postnatal pathology was 11.9% with mild ANH, 45.1% for moderate, and 88.3% for severe ANH. Their definitions of mild, moderate, and severe hydronephrosis depended on gestational age at the time of diagnosis. Similarly, Sidhu et al.[30] performed a meta-analysis and found that when postnatal hydronephrosis was SFU grade 1 or 2, there was stabilization or resolution of pelviectasis in 98%, whereas when there was SFU grade 3 or 4, there was stabilization or resolution in only 51%. Madden-Fuentes et al.[31] reported 416 infants with low-grade hydronephrosis. Of 398 renal units with grade 1 hydronephrosis, 96.7% resolved or remained stable; 3.3% worsened, and only one underwent ureteroneocystostomy. Of 225 units with grade 2 hydronephrosis, 98.7% resolved, improved, or remained stable, whereas 1.3% worsened, and one underwent a pyeloplasty. Only 0.7% had a febrile UTI.

The bladder should be imaged to detect a dilated posterior urethra (urethral valves), bladder wall thickening, ureteral dilation, inadequate bladder emptying, or a ureterocele. Perineal sonography may demonstrate a dilated prostatic urethra, which is consistent with PUVs.

Voiding cystourethrogram

In selected cases, a VCUG should be performed. This study may demonstrate VUR, PUVs, or a bladder diverticulum. A radiographic cystogram is preferred over a radionuclide cystogram because the latter does not provide sufficient delineation of bladder and urethral anatomy and because VUR, if present, cannot be graded. In a recent analysis by the AUA Pediatric Vesicoureteral Reflux Guidelines Committee, an overall VUR detection rate of 16.2% was found.[32] The mean incidence of VUR into a nondilated kidney was 4.1%. In cases with ANH and a normal postnatal sonogram, the incidence of VUR was 17%. The prevalence of VUR was significantly higher in girls than boys with ANH. The likelihood is highest if there is SFU grade 3 or 4 hydronephrosis or if a dilated ureter is identified. The chance of identifying VUR on a VCUG is less if there is only SFU grade 1 or 2.[33]

WHAT IF THE INITIAL SONOGRAM IS NORMAL?

A common dilemma is whether a full evaluation is necessary if the initial renal sonogram is normal. Assuming a significant degree of fetal renal pelvic dilatation (i.e., >4 mm anteroposterior pelvic diameter before 33 weeks, 7 mm diameter after 33 weeks) was present, the child may have VUR. This issue is unresolved. For example, Blane et al.[34] reported that 12% of children with grade V, 31% with grade IV, and 80% with grade III VUR had a normal renal sonogram. However, the AUA Reflux Guidelines determined that the mean incidence of VUR into a nondilated kidney was 4.1%.[32] Because VUR may cause intermittent renal pelvic dilation, theoretically babies with prenatal hydronephrosis and a normal postnatal sonogram may have VUR, and early diagnosis and medical treatment of VUR may reduce the likelihood of developing reflux nephropathy.[35] On the other hand, others have advocated performing a VCUG only if the postnatal sonogram is abnormal; however, in these reports, neonates with a normal postnatal renal sonogram were not systematically evaluated to determine the real incidence of VUR in this group. Currently, most do not recommend a VCUG unless the postnatal renal sonogram demonstrates grade 3 or 4 hydronephrosis and/or ureteral dilation.

Follow-up evaluation and treatment

If bilateral hydronephrosis or unilateral hydronephrosis in a solitary kidney is present, then close monitoring of the serum creatinine and electrolytes is necessary. If the hydronephrosis is caused by PUVs, then valve ablation should be performed before hospital discharge. If the hydronephrosis is secondary to VUR, the infant should be placed on

prophylaxis and managed, as described later in this chapter. If the hydronephrosis is grade 3 to 4 and bilateral UPJ or ureterovesical junction obstruction is suspected, prompt evaluation with diuretic renography is indicated. If unilateral hydronephrosis and a normal contralateral kidney are present, abnormalities in serum creatinine or electrolytes are uncommon. Nevertheless, these serum studies should be drawn to document that renal function is normal. Usually, follow-up functional radiographic studies can be delayed until 4–6 weeks of age, when renal function is more mature and studies of renal function and obstruction are more likely to be accurate. If the sonogram and VCUG are normal, then only a follow-up sonogram in 6–8 weeks is necessary. In general, if hydronephrosis is discovered on the initial postnatal sonogram, pediatric urologic or nephrologic consultation is advisable to direct subsequent radiologic evaluation and plan therapy.

Diuretic renogram

The diuretic renogram is used to determine whether upper urinary tract obstruction is present.[36] It is used to assess differential renal function and efficiency of drainage of the kidneys. Infants with grade 3 and 4, and occasionally grade 2, hydronephrosis should undergo this study. Mercaptoacetyltriglycine (MAG-3) is generally used and is secreted by the renal tubules. It provides excellent images with minimal background activity. During a diuretic renogram, a small dose of the radiopharmaceutical is injected intravenously. During the first 2–3 minutes, renal parenchymal uptake is analyzed and compared, allowing computation of differential renal function. Subsequently, excretion is evaluated. After 20–30 minutes, furosemide is injected intravenously, and the rapidity and pattern of drainage from the kidneys to the bladder are analyzed. If no upper urinary tract obstruction is present, then normally half of the radionuclide is cleared from the renal pelvis within 10–15 minutes, termed the t½. A t½ >20 minutes is consistent with upper urinary tract obstruction, but is not diagnostic of obstruction, because there are factors that can prolong the t½ in addition to an obstructive lesion (see below). A t½ between 15 and 20 minutes is indeterminate. The images generated usually provide an accurate assessment of the site of obstruction.

Numerous variables affect the outcome of the diuretic renogram. For example, newborn kidneys are functionally immature, and in some cases, even normal kidneys may not demonstrate normal drainage following diuretic administration. Dehydration prolongs parenchymal transit and can blunt the diuretic response. Giving an insufficient dose of furosemide may result in slow or inadequate drainage. In addition, a full bladder may impede bladder drainage. Furthermore, if VUR is present, continuous catheter drainage is mandatory to prevent the radionuclide from refluxing from the bladder into the dilated upper tract, causing a prolonged washout phase. Consequently, a urethral catheter should be inserted and bladder drainage measured.

Magnetic resonance urography

The newest study used to evaluate suspected upper urinary tract pathology is magnetic resonance urography (MRU) (Figure 100.3). The child is hydrated and given i.v. furosemide. Next, gadolinium-DTPA, which is filtered and excreted, is injected intravenously, and routine T1-weighted and fat-suppressed fast spin-echo T2-weighted imaging is performed through the kidneys, ureters, and bladder. This study provides superb images of the pathology, and methodology is being developed to allow assessment of differential renal function and drainage.[37] There is no radiation exposure, but younger children need sedation or general anesthesia. It is the procedure of choice for delineating complex genitourinary pathology (e.g., cross-fused ectopia with hydronephrosis and/or segmental multicystic kidney, cloacal anomaly).

Ancillary studies

In most cases, a renal sonogram, VCUG, and diuretic renogram provide sufficient information to establish a diagnosis and establish a plan of management. In particularly complicated cases, however, cystoscopy with retrograde pyelography, computed tomography (CT) scan, antegrade pyelography, or a Whitaker antegrade perfusion test is necessary.

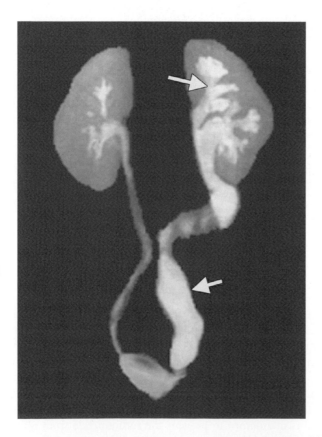

Figure 100.3 Magnetic resonance urogram in a 1-year-old demonstrating left obstructive megaureter. The right kidney is normal.

CONGENITAL ANOMALIES CAUSING ANH

UPJ obstruction or anomalous UPJ

The most common cause of severe hydronephrosis without a dilated ureter or bladder in newborn infants is UPJ obstruction, which results from an intrinsic fibrotic narrowing at the junction between the ureter and renal pelvis (Figure 100.4). At times, an accessory artery to the lower pole of the kidney also causes extrinsic obstruction, but this finding is rare in newborns with hydronephrosis; it is much more likely to occur in older children and adults. In kidneys with a UPJ obstruction, renal function may be significantly impaired from pressure atrophy.

The anomaly is corrected by performing a pyeloplasty, in which the stenotic segment is excised and the normal ureter and renal pelvis are reattached. Success rates are 91%–98%. Lesser degrees of UPJ narrowing may cause mild hydronephrosis, which is usually non-obstructive, and typically these kidneys function normally. Another cause of mild hydronephrosis is fetal folds of the upper ureter (Figure 100.5), which also are non-obstructive. The spectrum of non-obstructive UPJ abnormalities often is termed "anomalous UPJ."

Hydronephrosis in many newborns gradually diminishes or resolves over months to years. The goal of early evaluation is to determine whether a true anatomic obstruction is present that should be corrected or whether it is safe to follow the infant non-operatively. Defining what constitutes obstructive and non-obstructive hydronephrosis is a constant source of debate in pediatric urology. Cartwright et al.[38] studied 80 neonates with suspected UPJ obstruction. Of 39 with unilateral hydronephrosis and at least 35% differential renal function who were managed non-operatively, only 6 (15%) later underwent pyeloplasty, primarily because of deteriorating differential renal function on renal scintigraphy. Following pyeloplasty, the differential renal function returned to its initial level in these patients. One might question whether early pyeloplasty in these patients would have allowed renal function to improve to 50% (normal). The remaining patients managed non-operatively maintained differential function greater than 40%. Koff and Campbell[39] reported 104 consecutive neonates with unilateral hydronephrosis managed non-operatively, with follow-up as long as 5 years. In follow-up, only seven (7%) underwent pyeloplasty because of reduction in differential renal function of more than 10% or progression of hydronephrosis. Pyeloplasty returned differential renal function to prepyeloplasty levels in all cases. Of 16 patients with significantly reduced renal function on initial scan and grade 4 hydronephrosis, rapid improvement was noted on follow-up, diuretic renography in 15, and the washout curve became non-obstructive in 6. In addition, hydronephrosis disappeared in six, improved in six, remained stable in three, and deteriorated in one. The physiology of the resolution or reduction in hydronephrosis and the improvement in differential renal function in these babies is unknown. In another more recent report from the same institution, of

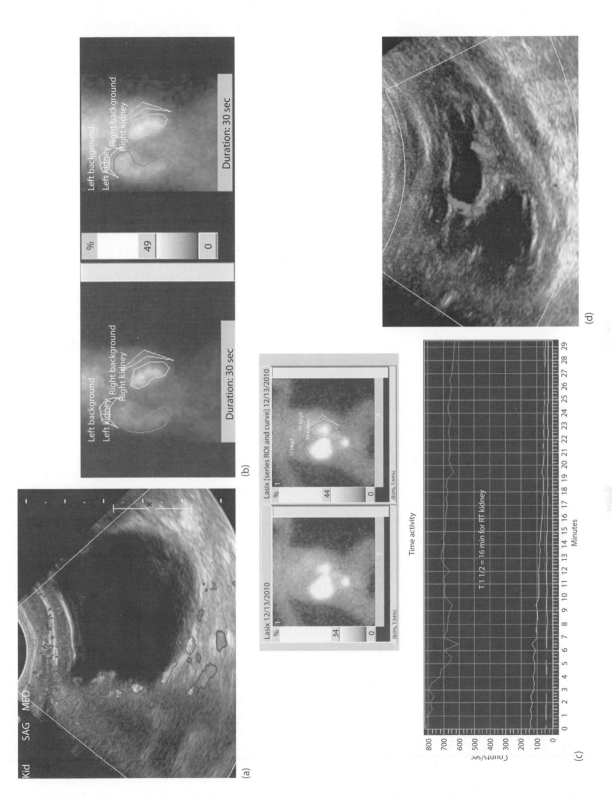

Figure 100.4 Newborn with prenatal diagnosis of left hydronephrosis. (a) Sonogram left kidney demonstrates grade 4 left hydronephrosis without a dilated ureter. The voiding cystourethrogram was normal. (b, c) MAG-3 diuretic renogram (left kidney on the left side of image) shows minimal drainage on the left side. The differential function left:right was 46:54%. Patient underwent left pyeloplasty at 2 months of age. (d) Follow-up sonogram of left kidney at 5 months of age demonstrates reduction in hydronephrosis.

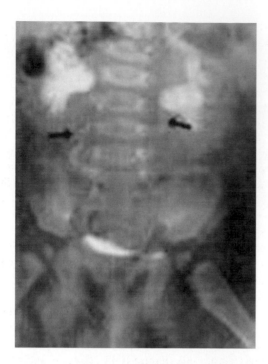

Figure 100.5 Excretory urogram in infant with bilateral grade 2 hydronephrosis shows bilateral fetal folds of upper ureters (arrows). Note sharp calyces (normal).

19 newborns with bilateral grade 3 or 4 hydronephrosis, a total of 13 kidneys were subjected to pyeloplasty.[40] Of those managed non-operatively, 21 kidneys were grade 0 to 2 and grade 3 in 2 kidneys. The mean follow-up time to achieve maximum improvement in hydronephrosis was 10 months.

Although these studies suggest that it is safe or appropriate to manage neonates with a suspected UPJ obstruction non-operatively, an infant's kidney has much greater capacity for improvement in differential renal function than an older child's. In addition, all of these studies base "differential renal function" on the uptake during the first 2–3 minutes of the study, and there is substantial variability in the way this percentage is calculated.[41] Finally, these studies have not reported the pattern of washout on diuretic renography. In a review of renal biopsies obtained at pyeloplasty at the author's previous institution, 63% showed minimal or no obstructive histologic changes; however, of those with differential function greater than 40%, 21% showed significant histopathologic changes, including reduced glomerular number, glomerular hyalinization, interstitial inflammation, and dysplastic glomeruli.[42] Of the kidneys with a differential function less than 40%, 33% showed minimal or no histologic changes. Overall, in 25% of the patients, the findings on renal biopsy did not correlate with the computed differential renal function and reflect the need for more sensitive markers of obstruction. The approach of most pediatric urologists to neonates with a suspected UPJ obstruction is as follows. The hydronephrosis is graded from 1 to 4 using the SFU grading scale and a VCUG is obtained. Nearly all infants requiring pyeloplasty have grade 3 or 4 hydronephrosis, and those with grade 1 or 2 hydronephrosis do not seem to be

at significant long-term risk. If a neonate has an abdominal mass from a hydronephrotic kidney, bilateral severe hydronephrosis, or a solitary kidney, a prompt MAG-3 diuretic renogram is obtained. If signs of obstruction are apparent, prompt pyeloplasty is performed. Otherwise, the newborn is placed on amoxicillin 50 mg daily for prophylaxis, and the diuretic renogram is obtained at 6 weeks of age. The study is not obtained right away in these cases because renal function in the newborn is immature. If diuretic renography shows at least >40% differential renal function and there is some drainage on the diuretic renogram, the child can be managed non-operatively, regardless of the drainage pattern (Figure 100.4).[43] At 2 months, prophylaxis is changed to trimethoprim sulfamethoxazole suspension 1.25 mL daily. A follow-up renal sonogram is performed 3 months later. If the hydronephrosis is unchanged from baseline, a repeat MAG-3 diuretic renogram is obtained. If there is deterioration in differential renal function or worsening of the diuretic washout curve, pyeloplasty is recommended. However, if these parameters remain stable or improved and the child does not develop a UTI, follow-up 3–6 months later with another renal sonogram or MAG-3 diuretic renogram is performed, and management is individualized. It is incumbent on clinicians caring for these infants to have a good understanding of the vagaries of the diuretic renogram and to monitor infants with a suspected UPJ obstruction closely. In addition, review of the radiologic studies (not just the radiology report) by the pediatric urologist is important.

There has been significant progress in the development of minimally invasive techniques in pediatric pyeloplasty, even in infants. Although infant pyeloplasty is performed through a small incision (lumbotomy or flank muscle-splitting) in many centers,[44] an increasing number of pediatric urologists are performing the procedure with traditional laparoscopic techniques, or the daVinci robot.[45] Success rates are being compared to series of open surgical repair; hospital stay and narcotic use are less with the minimally invasive approach. Generally, a transperitoneal approach has been used, with mobilization of the colon. However, on the left side, the pyeloplasty can be performed with a transmesenteric approach.

Multicystic dysplastic kidney

A multicystic dysplastic kidney is composed of multiple noncommunicating cysts of varying sizes with a stromal component that is composed of dysplastic elements. These kidneys do not function. Although multicystic kidney is the most common cause of an abdominal mass in neonates, the vast majority of multicystic kidneys are detected by prenatal sonography. Some clinicians incorrectly assume that multicystic kidney and polycystic kidney are synonymous terms. Polycystic kidney disease is an inherited disorder and has an "adult form" (autosomal dominant) and an "infantile form" (autosomal recessive) and affects both kidneys. In contrast, a multicystic kidney is almost always unilateral and is usually not an inherited disorder. Sonography of multicystic kidneys is often diagnostic, demonstrating multiple echolucent cysts of varying sizes with no discernible cortex (Figure 100.6). Occasionally, the cysts may resemble a severe UPJ obstruction with minimal parenchyma, termed the "hydronephrotic variant." The contralateral kidney is abnormal in 5%–10% of cases. Renal scintigraphy (MAG-3 or DMSA [dimercaptosuccinic acid] scan) shows nonfunction, but with current US techniques generally is unnecessary for confirmation.[46] On occasion, there is a segmental multicystic kidney, in which there is a complete duplication anomaly of the upper urinary tract, with the upper pole being multicystic.[47] Many also recommend obtaining a VCUG, because as many as 15% have contralateral VUR,[48] but currently it seems unnecessary unless there is contralateral hydronephrosis.[49]

The management of a multicystic kidney is becoming less controversial. If an abdominal mass that is symptomatic is present, early nephrectomy is indicated. However, left untreated, most multicystic kidneys become smaller. Potential complications include malignancy and hypertension. In a review of 26 clinical series, no cases of Wilms' tumor were reported among 1041 children, and the maximum estimated risk was 3.5 per 1000 affected children.[50] Tumors arise from the stromal, not the cystic, component of multicystic kidneys. Consequently, even if the cysts regress completely, the likelihood that the kidney could develop a neoplasm is not altered. With regard to hypertension, in a review of 29 studies, 6 cases were reported among 1115 eligible children, and the mean probability was 5.4 per 1000 affected children (95% confidence interval [CI] 1.9 to 11.7 per 1000).[51]

Generally, a follow-up sonogram is recommended at 6 months of age. If the cysts enlarge, the stromal core increases in size, or hypertension develops, laparoscopic (or possibly open) simple nephrectomy is recommended. However, further follow-up sonography is unnecessary unless there is concern regarding the contralateral kidney, because finding a Wilms' tumor incidentally would be extremely rare. Because of the occult nature of hypertension,

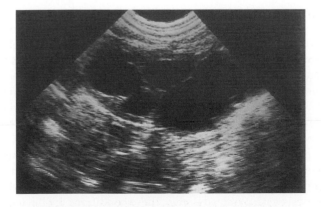

Figure 100.6 Left multicystic dysplastic kidney.

annual blood pressure measurement is recommended, and if hypertension occurs, nephrectomy should be considered.

Primary obstructive megaureter (nonrefluxing)

A megaureter refers to a wide ureter and may be (1) primary or secondary, (2) obstructive or non-obstructive, and (3) refluxing or nonrefluxing. Nonrefluxing megaureter results from an aperistaltic segment of the distal ureter that does not allow normal propulsion of urine (Figure 100.3). In this condition, sonography shows a dilated ureter and renal pelvis with variable renal parenchymal atrophy. VCUG shows no VUR in most cases. Before the antenatal sonography era, most patients with this condition presented with flank pain, flank mass, pyelonephritis, hematuria, or stone disease. Surgical correction consists of excision of the aperistaltic segment, tailoring (also known as tapering) of the ureter, and reimplantation of the ureter into the bladder. Although severe hydronephrosis may be present, often there is a tendency to gradual reduction in hydronephrosis over a period of several years (Figure 100.7). Braga et al.[52] reported that the majority of their patients demonstrated resolution of hydronephrosis in a median of 17 months, although those with a mean ureteral diameter >17 mm required surgical intervention. This group found that continuous antibiotic prophylaxis and circumcision reduced the risk of UTI. DiRenzo et al.[53] found that resolution or improvement of hydronephrosis occurs in all cases of mild postnatal dilation and 60% of those with moderate or severe upper urinary tract dilatation. The British Association of Paediatric Urologists recommends initial non-operative management of primary obstructive megaureter.[54] In follow-up, surgical intervention is recommended for UTI, pain, worsening hydronephrosis, differential renal function <40%, or a significant drop in renal function. Consequently, most of these patients may be followed non-operatively on antibiotic prophylaxis and serial monitoring of renal function and drainage.

In neonates with an antenatal diagnosis of hydroureteronephrosis, a renal sonogram and VCUG should be obtained. Early management is identical to that of neonates with suspected UPJ obstruction. If an abdominal mass, solitary kidney, or bilateral hydroureteronephrosis is present, then a MAG-3 diuretic renogram should be obtained promptly. Otherwise, the study is deferred until 6–8 weeks of age. In some centers, the diuretic-stimulated drainage from the renal pelvis and ureter are measured separately. If the differential renal function is at least 40%, the child generally is managed non-operatively, even with grade 4 hydronephrosis, and a follow-up renal sonogram or diuretic renogram is obtained every 3–6 months. These infants should receive prophylactic antibiotics while stasis is present in the upper ureter and kidney.

Early repair of megaureter has a higher complication rate than in older children. For example, Peters et al.[55] reported on megaureter repair in 42 infants operated on at

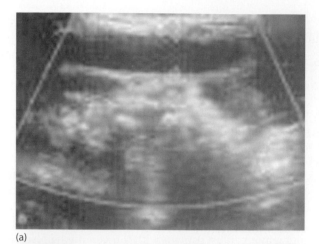

(a)

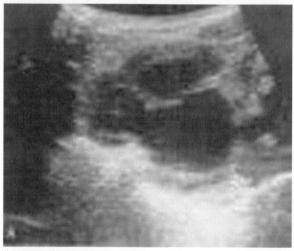

(b)

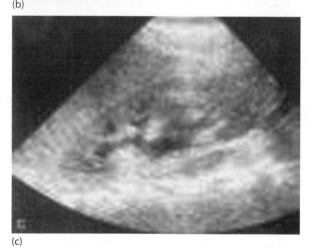

(c)

Figure 100.7 Female newborn with nonrefluxing left megaureter discovered by prenatal ultrasound. **(a, b)** Newborn ultrasound shows grade 4 hydronephrosis and dilated ureter. Diuretic renogram, 8 weeks of age, showed 50% differential renal function in left kidney. Obstructive drainage pattern was noted following administration of furosemide. Patient managed non-operatively. **(c)** Ultrasound 6 months later shows grade 1 hydronephrosis. Diuretic renogram later showed normal drainage pattern.

a mean age of 1.8 months. In that series, early complications occurred only in those less than 6 weeks of age and included transient apnea in three, UTI in one, hyponatremia in one, and meningitis in one. VUR occurred postoperatively in six infants, and none developed postoperative obstruction. The VUR resolved spontaneously between 18 and 36 months in three patients, and the remainder underwent secondary ureteroneocystostomy. Greenfield et al.[56] reported on repair of 11 megaureters in infants less than 6 months old. Of these children, two had transient ureteral obstruction immediately after stent removal and persistent grades I and II VUR in two children. In a series of older children who underwent tapered ureteral reimplantation, the success rate was 90% for obstructive megaureter.[57] The results were slightly better for intravesical compared with extravesical reimplantation.

There are three other treatment options if surgical repair seems necessary in the neonate or young infant. The first is to perform a temporary cutaneous ureterostomy, allowing the ureter to decompress over a period of 12–18 months. Subsequently, the ureterostomy can be taken down and ureteral reimplantation with or without tapering is performed. In a series of children who underwent this procedure, when undiversion and ureteral reimplantation were performed, only 5 of 23 ureters required tapering.[58] Another option is temporary refluxing ureteral reimplantation, in which the ureter is anastomosed end-to side to the bladder, and performing traditional ureteral reimplantation when the child is older.[59] The other option is to insert a double J ureteral stent through the ureterovesical junction and leave it interposed between the bladder and the kidney. Farrugia et al.[60] reported a series of 19 megaureters that were stented at a median age of 6 months, 1/3 endoscopically. Nearly 1/3 had stent-related complications, but 50% had improvement in upper tract drainage following stent removal.

In summary, if differential renal function remains normal and the child is asymptomatic, it seems safe to follow these patients with renal sonograms and diuretic renography to monitor hydronephrosis, and renal function and drainage. If renal functional deterioration, slowing of upper urinary tract drainage, or UTI occurs, ureteral reimplantation is recommended.

Ureterocele and ectopic ureter

A ureterocele is a cystic dilatation of the distal end of the ureter and is usually obstructive. In children, they usually extend through the bladder neck, termed "ectopic," but may remain entirely within the bladder, termed "intravesical" or "orthotopic." Ectopic ureteroceles and ectopic ureters occur more commonly in girls than in boys and usually are associated with the upper pole of a completely duplicated collecting system. In boys with a ureterocele, however, 40% drain a single collecting system. Prenatal sonography typically shows either hydroureteronephrosis or upper pole hydronephrosis with a dilated ureter. These conditions are bilateral in 10%–15% of patients.

Early evaluation consists of the following:

- Sonography shows a hydronephrotic upper pole connected to a dilated ureter; the ureterocele typically is visualized in the bladder (Figure 100.8a,b).
- VCUG often visualizes the ureterocele and demonstrates whether VUR is present, either into the lower pole moiety or contralateral collecting system (Figure 100.8c); an ectopic ureter that inserts into the bladder neck also typically refluxes into the upper pole obstructed ureter.
- DMSA or MAG-3 renal scan shows whether the moiety drained by the ectopic system functions; this study may be done at 1–2 weeks of age because the result does not change with functional maturity. Alternatively, a CT or MRU demonstrates the anatomy adequately, although it may not provide functional information regarding the obstructed upper pole (Figure 100.8c).

The management of neonates with a ureterocele is highly individualized.[61] The least invasive initial form of therapy is transurethral incision (TUI), which can be performed either with a 3-F Bugbee electrode or the holmium:YAG laser (Figure 100.8d,e). The ureterocele is punctured several times at its junction with the bladder mucosa. If the ureterocele is ectopic, it must be punctured both in the bladder and in the urethra. TUI provides satisfactory upper tract decompression with a single procedure in >90% of cases. However, there is a significant risk of postoperative VUR through the ureterocele into the upper pole moiety, which may require subsequent definitive treatment. If the ureterocele is orthotopic, approximately 30% show VUR following TUI, whereas if it is ectopic, 75% have VUR following TUI.[62,63] TUI is often the only procedure necessary.[64] TUI of a ureterocele draining a nonfunctioning moiety will not result in the development of any significant degree of function. In recent years, many centers have been performing minimally invasive (laparoscopic) upper pole heminephrectomy. These

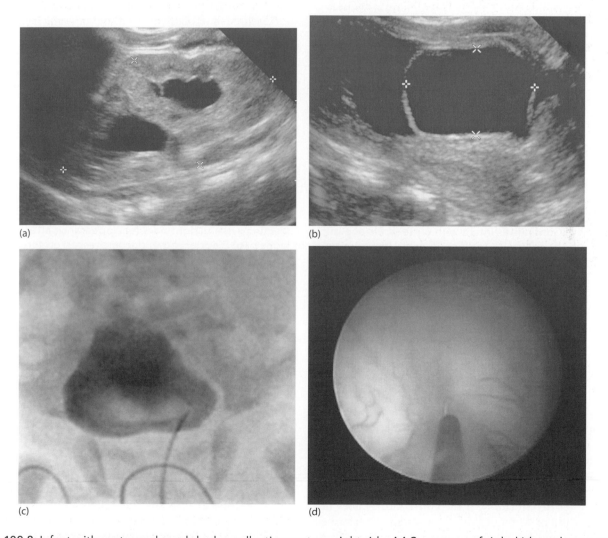

(a) (b) (c) (d)

Figure 100.8 Infant with ureterocele and duplex collecting system, right side. (a) Sonogram of right kidney demonstrating echogenic right kidney with duplex collecting system and hydronephrosis involving both upper and lower pole. (b) Ureterocele in bladder. (c) Voiding cystourethrogram shows ureterocele in bladder, and no vesicoureteral reflux. (d) Patient underwent transurethral incision; endoscopic view of ureterocele. *(Continued)*

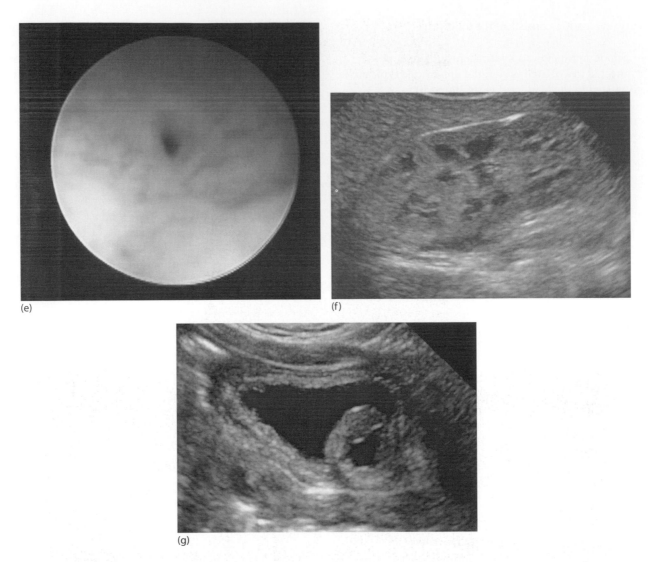

(e)

(f)

(g)

Figure 100.8 (Continued) Infant with ureterocele and duplex collecting system, right side. **(e)** Appearance after transurethral incision. **(f)** Follow-up renal sonogram shows normal right kidney. **(g)** Bladder shows decompressed ureterocele.

procedures have been performed either with a retroperitoneal[65] or transperitoneal[66] approach. One recent series with a laparoscopic retroperitoneal approach reported an overall conversion rate to open surgery of 21%, although the authors stated that they had only one conversion in their most recent 20 cases.[67] Common complications include perirenal urinoma and, in some cases, devascularization of the lower pole moiety. The latter complication is most common in infants. Another option is to perform transperitoneal laparoscopic partial nephrectomy with robotic assistance.[68] Consequently, if the hydronephrotic upper pole does not function, this author maintains the infant on antibiotic prophylaxis and laparoscopic upper pole heminephrectomy (or nephrectomy, if the entire kidney does not function) with or without robotic assistance performed electively at 6 months of age, assuming the upper pole system remains hydronephrotic. If the renal scan shows significant upper pole function, however, ureteropyelostomy or ureteroureterostomy, in which the upper pole ureter is anastomosed to the lower pole renal pelvis or ureter, is recommended. This procedure can be performed either at the level of the kidney, with removal of part of the redundant distal ureter,[69] or low, through an inguinal incision.[70] Total urinary tract reconstruction in neonates and infants is not recommended because of the high complication rate caused by the small size of the infant bladder.

Posterior urethral valves

The most common cause of severe obstructive uropathy in children is PUVs, which are tissue leaflets fanning distally from the prostatic urethra to the external urinary sphincter (Figure 100.9).[10] Typically, the leaflets are separated by a slit-like opening. Approximately one-third ultimately develop chronic renal failure or severe renal insufficiency. Prognosis is significantly better if the antenatal sonogram before 24 weeks' gestation was normal. In one study, 9 of 17 patients with PUV whose hydronephrosis was discovered before 24

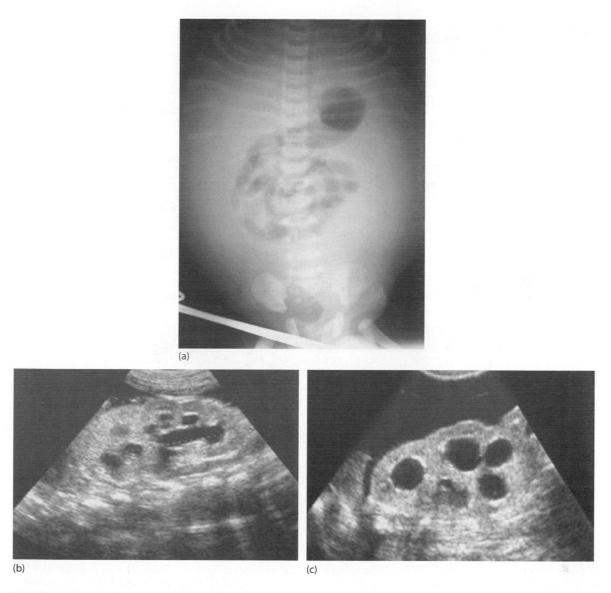

(a)

(b)

(c)

Figure 100.9 Newborn with posterior urethral valves and abdominal distension secondary to urinary ascites. **(a)** Plain film of abdomen showing ascites. **(b, c)** Renal sonogram showing bilateral hydronephrosis and urinary ascites.   (*Continued*)

weeks' gestation developed renal failure, whereas only 1 of 14 recognized after 24 weeks' gestation developed end-stage renal disease.[71] Favorable prognostic factors include a serum creatinine level of less than 0.8–1.0 mg% after bladder decompression, unilateral VUR into a nonfunctioning kidney ("VURD syndrome"), ascites, and identification of the corticomedullary junction on renal sonography. Early delivery of infants with an antenatal diagnosis of suspected PUV is not recommended, unless there is oligohydramnios. If severe bilateral renal dysplasia is present, pulmonary hypoplasia is often also present, and problems with ventilation may result. Initially, a small feeding tube should be passed into the bladder for urinary drainage until electrolyte imbalances can be corrected. A Foley catheter is not recommended because the balloon may cause significant bladder spasm and impede upper tract drainage. Care should be taken passing the catheter, as the prostatic urethra is dilated and there is bladder neck hypertrophy; the

feeding tube may coil in the prostatic urethra and not drain the bladder. In this setting, catheter irrigation typically results in fluid coming out of the urethra next to the catheter. AVCUG should be obtained to confirm the diagnosis, and a renal scan should be performed to evaluate the upper tract differential renal function.[10] In newborns, alternative treatments include transurethral endoscopic ablation of PUV, cutaneous vesicostomy, and high diversion (cutaneous pyelostomy). The ideal initial treatment is valve ablation with a small Bugbee electrode, as is used with TUI, or the holmium:YAG laser. In small neonates, the 8 or 9 Fr resectoscope may be too large for the urethra, and a temporary vesicostomy may be necessary. A vesicostomy also should be considered for those with a serum creatinine level that remains significantly elevated after bladder decompression. Cutaneous pyelostomy rarely affords better drainage compared with cutaneous vesicostomy and diverts urine away from the bladder, which may prevent normal bladder

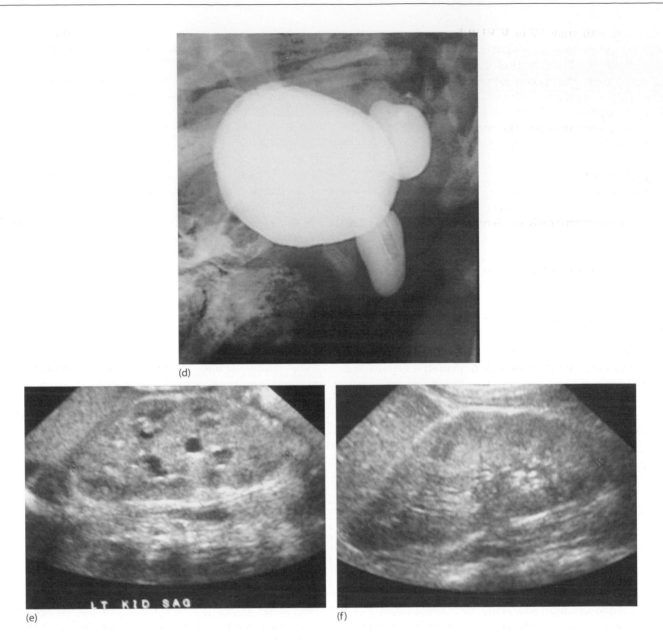

(d)

(e)

(f)

Figure 100.9 (Continued) Newborn with posterior urethral valves and abdominal distension secondary to urinary ascites. **(d)** Voiding cystourethrogram. Note dilated prostatic urethra proximal to the valve leaflets and bladder diverticulum on left side. Patient managed with upper tract drainage and transurethral incision of valve leaflets. **(e, f)** Renal sonogram, left and right kidneys at 6 months of age shows minimal hydronephrosis. At 17 years, patient had nearly normal renal appearance on ultrasound.

growth.[72] However, in selected cases, the Sober-en-T cutaneous ureterostomy is useful. In this procedure, the upper ureter is brought out to the abdomen and transected, and the distal segment is anastomosed to the renal pelvis; this option allows urine to drain both through the ureterostomy and to the bladder.[73]

Vesicoureteral reflux

Some neonates with medium- and high-grade VUR are detected following the finding of ANH. Approximately 80% of such patients are boys. In the most severe cases of massive VUR, the bladder may also become distended from aberrant

micturition into the upper urinary tract. In the AUA Reflux Guidelines analysis, reflux-related renal scarring was present in 47.9% of those with grades IV–V VUR, but only 6.2% of those with grades I–II VUR.[32] Consequently, in neonates with grades III–V VUR, a DMSA scan is recommended to determine whether reflux-related renal scarring is present. Initially, neonates with prenatally diagnosed VUR are managed medically. Most are placed on amoxicillin prophylaxis for 2 months, followed by nitrofurantoin or trimethoprim–sulfamethoxazole prophylaxis, and circumcision is recommended for male neonates to decrease the risk for UTIs.

Neonates with VUR are more likely to show spontaneous resolution than are older children. Indeed, 20%–35%

of ureters with grade IV or V VUR have reflux resolution within 2 years; however, a significant proportion develop a breakthrough UTI, and antireflux surgery is recommended in these cases. The success rate for open surgical correction of VUR in infants can be as high as in older children.[56] Another option is subureteral injection of dextranomer microspheres/hyaluronic acid into the ureterovesical junction, in which the success rate is 69% with a single injection.[74]

SUMMARY

Approximately 1%–2% of newborns have an antenatal diagnosis of hydronephrosis or significant renal pelvic dilation. Hydronephrosis is often caused by non-obstructive conditions. The likelihood of significant urologic pathology is directly related to the size of the fetal renal pelvis, and 90% with an APD >2 cm need surgical intervention or long-term urologic follow-up. Following delivery, antibiotic prophylaxis should be administered, and a renal sonogram and VCUG should be obtained. If there is grade 3 or 4 hydronephrosis, a diuretic renogram is usually also recommended. Pediatric urologic or pediatric nephrologic consultation is helpful in planning evaluation and treatment. Antenatal recognition of hydronephrosis allows postnatal diagnosis and treatment of urologic pathology, preventing complications of pyelonephritis and obstruction. In the past decade, significant progress has been made in the development of minimally invasive treatment options.

REFERENCES

1. Rabinowitz R, Peters MT, Vyas S et al. Measurement of fetal urine production in normal pregnancy by real-time ultrasonography. *Am J Obstet Gynecol* 1989; 161: 1264–6.
2. Cendron M, Elder JS. Perinatal urology. In: Gillenwater JY, Grayhack JT, Howards SS, Mitchell M (eds). *Adult and Pediatric Urology*, 4th edn. London: Lippincott Williams & Wilkins, 2002: 2041–127.
3. Stocks A, Richards D, Frentzen B et al. Correlation of prenatal renal pelvic anteroposterior diameter with outcome in infancy. *J Urol* 1996; 155: 1050–2.
4. Barker AP, Cave MM, Thomas DFM et al. Fetal pelviureteric junction obstruction: Predictors of outcome. *Br J Urol* 1995; 76: 649–52.
5. Thomas DFM, Madden NP, Irving HC et al. Mild dilatation of the fetal kidney: A follow-up study. *Br J Urol* 1994; 74: 236–9.
6. Corteville JE, Gray DL, Crane JP. Congenital hydronephrosis: Correlation of fetal ultrasonographic findings with infant outcome. *Am J Obstet Gynecol* 1991; 165: 384–8.
7. Fugelseth D, Lindemann R, Sande HA et al. Prenatal diagnosis of urinary tract anomalies: The value of two ultrasound examinations. *Acta Obst Gynecol Scand* 1994; 73: 290–3.
8. Reuss A, Wladimiroff JW, Steward PA et al. Noninvasive management of fetal obstructive uropathy. *Lancet* 1988; 2: 949.
9. Craparo FJ, Rustico M, Tassis B et al. Fetal serum beta 2-microglobulin before and after bladder shunting: A 2-step approach to evaluate fetuses with lower urinary tract obstruction. *J Urol* 2007; 178: 2576–9.
10. Elder JS, Shapiro E. Posterior urethral valves. In: Holcomb GW III, Murphy JP, Ostlie DJ (eds). *Pediatric Surgery*, 6th edn. Philadelphia, PA: Elsevier, 2014: 762–72.
11. Quintero RA, Shukla AR, Homsy YL, Bukkapatnam R. Successful in utero endoscopic ablation of posterior urethral valves: A new dimension in fetal urology. *Urology* 2000; 55: 774.
12. Elder JS, Duckett Jr JW, Snyder HW. Intervention for fetal obstructive uropathy: Has it been effective. *Lancet* 1987; 2: 1007–10.
13. Biard JM, Johnson MP, Carr MC et al. Long-term outcomes in children treated by prenatal vesicoamniotic shunting for lower urinary tract obstruction. *Obstet Gynecol* 2005; 106: 503–8.
14. Johnson MP, Corsi P, Bradfield W et al. Sequential urinalysis improves evaluation of fetal renal function in obstructive uropathy. *Am J Obstet Gynecol* 1995; 173: 59–65.
15. Nguyen HT, Herndon CD, Cooper C et al. The Society for Fetal Urology consensus statement on the evaluation and management of antenatal hydronephrosis. *J Pediatr Urol* 2010; 6: 212–31.
16. Sinha A, Bagga A, Krishna A et al. Revised guidelines on management of antenatal hydronephrosis. *Indian J Nephrol* 2013; 23: 83–97.
17. Nguyen HT, Benson CB, Bromley B et al. Multidisciplinary consensus on the classification of prenatal and postnatal urinary tract dilation (UTD classification system). *J Pediatr Urol* 2014; 10: 982–98.
18. Hodhod A, Capolicchio JP, Jednak R et al. Evaluation of urinary tract dilation classification system for grading postnatal hydronephrosis. *J Urol* 2016; 195: 725–30.
19. Braga LH, Ruzhynky V, Pemberton J et al. Evaluating practice patterns in postnatal management of antenatal hydronephrosis: A national survey of Canadian pediatric urologists and nephrologists. *Urology* 2014; 83: 909–14.
20. Roth CC, Hubanks JM, Bright BC et al. Occurrence of urinary tract infection in children with significant upper urinary tract obstruction. *Urology* 2009; 73: 74–8.
21. Zaraba P, Lorenzo AJ, Braga LH. Risk factors for febrile urinary tract infection in infants with prenatal hydronephrosis: Comprehensive single center analysis. *J Urol* 2014; 191: 1614–8.
22. Braga LH, Farrokhyar F, D'Cruz J et al. Risk factors for febrile urinary tract infection in children with prenatal hydronephrosis: A prospective study. *J Urol* 2015; 193: 1766–71.

23. Herz D, Merguerian P, McQuiston L. Continuous antibiotic prophylaxis reduces the risk of febrile UTI in children with asymptomatic antenatal hydronephrosis with either ureteral dilation, high-grade vesicoureteral reflux, or ureterovesical junction obstruction. *J Pediatr Urol* 2014; 10: 650–4.

24. Castagnetti M, Cimador M, Esposito C, Rigamonti W. Antibiotic prophylaxis in antenatal nonrefluxing hydronephrosis, megaureter and ureterocele. *Nat Rev Urol* 2012; 9: 321–9.

25. Braga LH, Mijovic H, Farrokhyar F et al. Antibiotic prophylaxis for urinary tract infections in antenatal hydronephrosis. *Pediatrics* 2013; 131: e251–61.

26. Edlin RS, Copp HL. Antibiotic resistance in pediatric urology. *Ther Adv Urol* 2014; 6: 54–61.

27. Maizels M, Reisman M, Flom LS et al. Grading nephroureteral dilatation detected in the first year of life: Correlation with obstruction. *J Urol* 1992; 148: 609–14.

28. Chertin B, Pollack A, Koulikov D et al. Conservative treatment of ureteropelvic junction obstruction in children with antenatal diagnosis of hydronephrosis: Lessons learned after 16 years of follow-up. *Eur Urol* 2006; 49: 734–48.

29. Lee RS, Cendron M, Kinnamon DD, Nguyen HT. Antenatal hydronephrosis as a predictor of postnatal outcome: A meta-analysis. *Pediatrics* 2006; 118: 586–93.

30. Sidhu G, Beyene J, Rosenblum ND. Outcome of isolated antenatal hydronephrosis: A systematic review and metaanalysis. *Pediatr Nephrol* 2006; 21: 218–24.

31. Madden-Fuentes RJ, McNamara ER, Nseyo U et al. Resolution rate of isolated low-grade hydronephrosis diagnosed within the first year of life. *J Pediatr Urol* 2014; 10: 639–44.

32. Peters CA, Skoog SJ, Arant BS Jr et al. Pediatric Vesicoureteral Reflux Guidelines Panel Summary Report. Clinical practice guidelines for the screening of siblings of children with vesicoureteral reflux (VUR) and of neonates/infants with prenatal hydronephrosis (PNH). *J Urol* 2010; 184: 1145–51.

33. Estrada CR, Peters CA, Retik AB et al. Vesicoureteral reflux and urinary tract infection in children with a history of prenatal hydronephrosis—Should voiding cystourethrography be performed in cases of postnatally persistent grade II hydronephrosis. *J Urol* 2009; 181: 801–6.

34. Blane CE, DiPietro MA, Zerin JM et al. Renal sonography is not a reliable screening examination for vesicoureteral reflux. *J Urol* 1993; 150: 752–5.

35. Elder JS. Importance of antenatal diagnosis of vesicoureteral reflux. *J Urol* 1992; 148: 1750–4.

36. Society for Fetal Urology and Pediatric Nuclear Medicine Council. The 'well tempered' diuretic renogram: A standard method to examine the asymptomatic neonate with hydronephrosis or hydroureteronephrosis. *J Nucl Med* 1992; 33: 2047–51.

37. Cerwinka WH, Damien Gratten-Smith J, Kirsch AJ. Magnetic resonance urography in pediatric urology. *J Pediatr Urol* 2009; 4: 74–82.

38. Cartwright PC, Duckett JW, Keating MA et al. Managing apparent ureteropelvic junction obstruction in the newborn. *J Urol* 1992; 148: 1224–8.

39. Koff SA, Campbell KD. The nonoperative management of unilateral neonatal hydronephrosis: Natural history of poorly functioning kidneys. *J Urol* 1994; 152: 593–5.

40. Onen A, Jayanthi VR, Koff SA. Long-term follow-up of prenatally detected severe bilateral newborn hydronephrosis initially managed nonoperatively. *J Urol* 2002; 168: 1118–20.

41. Snow BW, Gatti JM, Renschler TD et al. Variation in diethylenetriamine pentaacetic acid and mercaptoacetyltriglycine renal scans: Clinical implications of interobserver and intraobserver differences. *J Urol* 2008; 179: 1132–6.

42. Elder JS, Stansbrey R, Dahms BB et al. Renal histologic changes secondary to ureteropelvic junction obstruction. *J Urol* 1995; 154: 719–22.

43. Tekgul S, Dogan HS, Erdem E et al. Guidelines on Paediatric Urology (EAU/ESPU) 2015. Available at http://uroweb.org/wp-content/uploads/23-Paediatric-Urology_LR_full.pdf

44. Chacko JK, Koyle AM, Mingin GC et al. The minimally invasive open pyeloplasty. *J Pediatr Urol* 2006; 2: 368–72.

45. Sukumar S, Roghmann F, Elder JS et al. Correction of ureteropelvic junction obstruction in children: National trends and comparative effectiveness in operative outcomes. *J Endourol* 2014; 28: 592–8.

47. Corrales JG, Elder JS. Segmental multicystic kidney and ipsilateral duplication anomalies. *J Urol* 1996; 155: 1398–401.

48. Selzman AA, Elder JS. Contralateral vesicoureteral reflux in children with a multicystic kidney. *J Urol* 1995; 153: 1252–4.

49. Calaway AC, Whittam B, Szymanski KM et al. Multicystic dysplastic kidney: Is an initial voiding cystourethrogram necessary? *Can J Urol* 2014; 21: 7510–4.

50. Narchi H. Risk of Wilms' tumour with multicystic kidney disease: A systematic review. *Arch Dis Child* 2005; 90: 147–9.

51. Narchi H. Risk of hypertension with multicystic kidney disease: A systematic review. *Arch Dis Child* 2005; 90: 921–4.

52. Braga LH, D'Cruz J, Rickard M et al. The fate of primary nonrefluxing megaureter: A prospective outcome analysis of the rate of urinary tract infections, surgical indications and time to resolution. *J Urol* 2016; 195: 1300–5.

53. DiRenzo D, Persico A, DiNocola M et al. Conservative management of primary non-refluxing megaureter during the first year of life: A longitudinal observational study. *J Pediatr Urol* 2015; 11: 226.e1–6.

54. Farrugia MK, Hitchcock R, Radford A et al. British Association of Paediatric Urologists consensus statement on the management of the primary obstructed megaureter. *J Pediatr Urol* 2014; 10: 26–33.

55. Peters CA, Mandell J, Lebowitz RL et al. Congenital obstructed megaureters in early infancy: Diagnosis and treatment. *J Urol* 1989; 142: 641–5.

56. Greenfield SP, Griswold JJ, Wan J. Ureteral reimplantation in infants. *J Urol* 1994; 150: 1460–2.

57. DeFoor W, Minevich E, Reddy P et al. Results of tapered ureteral reimplantation for primary megaureter: Extravesical versus intravesical approach. *J Urol* 2004; 172: 1640–3.

58. Kitchens DM, DeFoor W Minevich E et al. End cutaneous ureterostomy for the management of severe hydronephrosis. *J Urol* 2007; 177: 1501–4.

59. Kaefer M, Misseri R, Frank E et al. Refluxing ureteral reimplantation: A logical method for managing neonatal UVJ obstruction. *J Pediatr Urol* 2014; 10: 824–30.

60. Farrugia MK, Steinbrecher HA, Malone PS. The utilization of stents in the management of primary obstructive megaureters requiring intervention before 1 year of age. *J Pediatr Urol* 2011; 7: 198–202.

61. Wang MH, Greenfield SP, Williot P et al. Ectopic ureteroceles in duplex systems: Long-term follow up and 'treatment-free' status. *J Pediatr Urol* 2008; 4: 183–7.

62. Coplen DE, Duckett JW. The modern approach to ureteroceles. *J Urol* 1995; 153: 166–71.

63. Smith C, Gosalbez R, Parrott TS et al. Transurethral puncture of ectopic ureteroceles in neonates and infants. *J Urol* 1994; 152: 2110–2.

64. Chertin B, de Caluwe D, Puri P. Is primary endoscopic puncture of ureterocele a long-term effective procedure? *J Pediatr Surg* 2003; 38: 116–9.

65. Mushtaq I, Haleblian G. Laparoscopic heminephrectomy in infants and children: First 54 cases. *J Pediatr Urol* 2007; 3: 100–3.

66. You D, Bang JK, Shim M et al. Analysis of the late outcome of laparoscopic heminephrectomy in children with duplex kidneys. *BJU Int* 2010; 106: 250–4.

67. Leclair MD, Vidal I, Suply E et al. Retroperitoneal laparoscopic heminephrectomy in duplex kidney in infants and children: A 15-year experience. *Eur Urol* 2009; 56: 385–9.

68. Lee RS, Sethi AS, Passerotti CC et al. Robot assisted laparoscopic partial nephrectomy: A viable and safe option in children. *J Urol* 2009; 181: 823–8.

69. Chacko JK, Koyle MA, Mingin GC et al. Ipsilateral ureteroureterostomy in the surgical management of the severely dilated ureter in ureteral duplication. *J Urol* 2007; 178: 1689–92.

70. Prieto J, Ziada A, Baker L et al. Ureteroureterostomy via inguinal incision for ectopic ureters and ureteroceles without ipsilateral lower pole reflux. *J Urol* 2009; 181: 1844–8.

71. Hutton KAR, Thomas DFM, Arthur RJ et al. Prenatally detected posterior urethral valves: Is gestational age at detection a predictor of outcome. *J Urol* 1994; 152: 698–701.

72. Podesto M, Ruarte AC, Gargiulo C et al. Bladder function associated with posterior urethral valves after primary valve ablation or proximal urinary diversion in children and adolescents. *J Urol* 2002; 168: 1830–5.

73. Ghanem MA, Nijman RJ. Long-term follow up of bilateral high (Sober) urinary diversion in patients with posterior urethral valves and its effect on bladder function. *J Urol* 2005; 173: 1721–4.

74. Puri P, Mohanan M, Menezes M et al. Endoscopic treatment of moderate and high grade vesicoureteral reflux in infants using dextranomer/hyaluronic acid. *J Urol* 2007; 178: 1714–6.

101

Multicystic dysplastic kidney

DAVID F. M. THOMAS AND AZAD S. NAJMALDIN

INTRODUCTION

It is now more than 30 years since cases of antenatally detected multicystic dysplastic kidney (MCDK) were first reported in the literature. Before then, MCDK was regarded as a rare anomaly, which generally presented as an abdominal mass in the neonatal period. Nephrectomy was the standard form of management. Over the last three decades, however, it has become apparent that MCDK is, in fact, a relatively common renal anomaly, with a prevalence in the range of 1 in 2500 to 1 in 4000.[1,2] It has also become clear that the majority of MCDKs are small and clinically undetectable and would probably have remained unrecognized throughout the individual's lifetime if they had not been detected on antenatal ultrasonography. The weight of published evidence now supports a conservative approach in the majority of cases, with nephrectomy being reserved for specific indications.

ETIOLOGY

MCDK is almost invariably associated with the presence of an atretic segment in the proximal ureter. Nevertheless, it can occasionally occur in conjunction with ureteral dilatation and an obstructive ureterocele. In both forms, the underlying mechanism is thought to be a severe obstructive insult to the developing metanephric mesenchyme at an early stage in gestation. MCDK is the most common form of cystic renal disease in children. The occurrence of bilateral MCDKs is invariably lethal and, when detected prenatally, usually leads to termination of pregnancy. Unilateral MCDK is generally a sporadic anomaly, but familial occurrence has been described, with an autosomal dominant pattern of inheritance, variable expression, and reduced penetrance.[3] MCDKs are slightly more common in boys, and the left side is affected more frequently than the right. Macroscopically, MCDKs comprise an irregular collection of tense, noncommunicating cysts of different sizes. The histological appearance is characterized by cysts lined by cuboidal or flattened tubular epithelium. Any renal parenchyma is confined to small islands or flattened plates of dysplastic tissue interposed between cysts.

The presence of a solid component of renal parenchyma effectively excludes the diagnosis of MCDK. These variants can create diagnostic confusion. Some of the reported cases of hypertension and malignancy have been incorrectly attributed to MCDKs when they have, in fact, arisen in these variants.[4]

Coexisting urological anomalies are common and include a 20% incidence of Vesico ureteric reflux (VUR) (usually low grade) and a 5% incidence of Pelvi ureteric junction (PUJ) obstruction in the contralateral kidney. Ipsilateral genital abnormalities such as Gartner duct cyst may also be present.

PRESENTATION

Patterns of presentation include the following:

1. Antenatal ultrasound detection (the majority).
2. Clinical presentation. Large multicystic kidneys generally present as a firm, "knobbly" abdominal mass, which is apparent at birth or early in the neonatal period.
3. Incidental finding during the investigation of some unrelated illness.
4. Symptomatic complications (very rare).

INVESTIGATIONS

Ultrasound

The ultrasound features that characterize MCDKs are now widely accepted and well defined in the radiological literature (Figure 101.1).[5–7] Failure to understand or apply these criteria correctly accounts for some of the purported cases of hypertension[4] and malignancy that have been incorrectly ascribed to MCDKs.

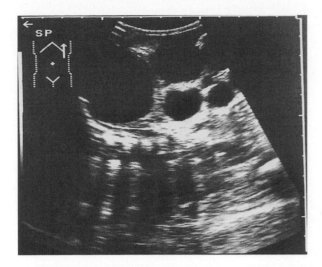

Figure 101.1 Typical ultrasonographic appearance of neonatal multicystic dysplastic kidney, i.e., noncommunicating cysts of varying size, demonstrable septa between cysts, no visible rim or cortical tissue.

The diagnostic criteria on ultrasonography comprise the following:

- Multiple oval or round cysts that do not communicate
- Presence of interfaces between the cysts
- Nonmedial location of the largest cyst (a large fluid-filled component located medially is more likely to represent the dilated pelvis of a severely hydronephrotic kidney)
- Lack of central sinus echo
- Absence of solid parenchymal tissue

When the diagnostic criteria are applied correctly, the sensitivity of ultrasonography for the diagnosis of MCDK is extremely high. Where uncertainty exists, it usually relates to severe hydronephrosis or a solid dysplastic kidney with a cystic component.

Isotope renography (nuclear medicine scan)

It has been argued that the predictive value of ultrasonography is now so high that it is no longer necessary to perform isotope renography to confirm the diagnosis.[7,8] Nevertheless, it remains standard practice in most centers to include isotope renography in the routine evaluation of MCDKs. This is intended to differentiate genuine MCDKs, which are totally nonfunctioning (0% differential function), from grossly hydronephrotic kidneys or other forms of renal dysplasia, which usually have some demonstrable function (albeit only a few percent differential function on technetium-99m dimercaptosuccinic acid [^{99m}Tc-DMSA]). In equivocal cases, nephrectomy is justified to establish a histological diagnosis and to obviate the possible risk of complications, notably hypertension.

^{99m}Tc-DMSA is the most reliable modality for demonstrating low levels of function (Figure 101.2a,b). Nevertheless, technetium-99m mercaptoacetyltriglycine (^{99m}Tc-MAG3) may be preferable if there is any suggestion of contralateral pelviureteric junction obstruction. Ideally, imaging should be deferred until after the fourth week of life.

Voiding cystourethrography

Opinion is divided on whether it is necessary to perform this invasive investigation routinely if the urinary tract

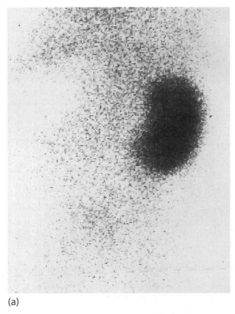

(a)

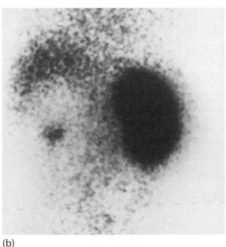

(b)

Figure 101.2 (a) ^{99m}Tc-DMSA scan demonstrating normal isotope uptake and renal morphology on the left, and no uptake or isotope in the right (multicystic) kidney. (b) A focus of poor but discernible uptake of ^{99m}Tc-DMSA in a grossly hydronephrotic right kidney. Ultrasound could not distinguish with certainty between gross hydronephrosis and multicystic kidney.

appears otherwise normal on ultrasound. The findings of several studies have endorsed the safety of omitting a routine voiding cystourethrography (VCUG) in such cases.[9,10] When VUR is present it is usually low grade and self-limiting. Children with MCDK who have not undergone a routine VCUG do not appear to be at any higher risk of urinary tract infection (UTI) or renal damage. However, if a routine VCUG is not performed, it is important that parents and general practitioners are aware that the occurrence of a documented or suspected UTI or an unexplained febrile illness should prompt further investigation to look for possible VUR.

However, VCUG is always indicated when postnatal ultrasonography reveals evidence of ipsilateral ureteric dilatation or contralateral upper tract dilatation.

NATURAL HISTORY OF PRENATALLY DETECTED MCDKS

This is characterized by a process of shrinkage (involution). MCDKs measuring less that 5–6 cm on initial assessment have a high probability of disappearing completely on ultrasound over the first 10 years of life. Those that exceed this figure on initial assessment also demonstrate considerable reduction in size but are less likely to involute completely over this timescale.[11,12] The risk of complications such as hypertension is exceedingly low regardless of initial size, and there is no evidence of any correlation between the risk of complications and initial size. Likewise, MCDKs that do not involute completely do not appear to pose a significantly greater risk than those that do. There is no evidence-based justification for advocating nephrectomy on the basis of either the initial size of the MCDK or the persistence of an MCDK on follow-up ultrasound.

Whereas MCDK is a relatively common antenatally detected anomaly, unilateral renal agenesis is rarely diagnosed *in utero*. This has been interpreted as evidence that a significant proportion of cases of apparent unilateral renal agenesis detected in adults had originated as MCDKs and then undergone complete involution. Regardless of the outcome for the MCDK, the contralateral kidney almost invariably undergoes some degree of compensatory hypertrophy.

INDICATIONS FOR SURGERY

The following are widely regarded as *definite indications for nephrectomy*:

1. *An obvious, visible and readily palpable abdominal mass.* In this situation, there is usually considerable parental anxiety. In addition, there may be apparent discomfort or other symptoms attributable to the size of the mass.
2. *Diagnostic uncertainty.* Despite the combination of ultrasound and isotope imaging, it may occasionally be impossible to distinguish with certainty between an MCDK, a poorly functioning hydronephrotic kidney,

and a rare cystic variant of renal dysplasia. The presence of demonstrable function in what otherwise appears to be an MCDK should be viewed with suspicion and represents a valid indication for nephrectomy. Isotope function equates with perfusion, and it can be reasonably argued that perfused tissue imparts a greater risk of renal hypertension. Likewise, a cystic anomaly that is also seen to contain a solid parenchymal component or that does not fulfill the other diagnostic criteria listed previously is *not* an MCDK and is, therefore, best removed.

Controversies surrounding "prophylactic" nephrectomy for asymptomatic, prenatally detected MCDKs

Although the overwhelming majority of prenatally detected MCDKs are asymptomatic and clinically undetectable, some surgeons continue to practice "prophylactic" nephrectomy. They argue that this policy is justified by published reports of complications—notably hypertension and malignant transformation.

Following the introduction of antenatal diagnosis, the assessment of risk associated with MCDKs was initially based on historical case reports. Critical analysis of the historical literature has, however, shed doubt on the accuracy of the diagnosis of MCDK in the historically reported cases. The distinguished pediatric pathologist, Beckwith, observed, "The literature concerning renal tumors in multicystic dysplastic kidney is burdened with poorly documented or unconvincing cases."[13]

It is now no longer necessary to resort to the historical literature since there is now an extensive body of literature that is devoted specifically to antenatally detected MCDKs. A detailed review is beyond the scope of this chapter, but the following summary is intended to provide readers with an evidence-based assessment of the level of risk.

Malignant transformation (Wilms tumor)

Narchi[14,15] undertook a detailed review of 26 published series totaling 1041 children with conservatively managed MCDKs. Information on duration of follow-up was available in 18 publications, and it was between 1.25 and 6.5 years, with a maximum of 23 years. No cases of Wilms tumor were identified in this literature review.

Cambio and associates[16] reviewed 105 publications on prenatally detected MCDK, to which they added unpublished data from the United States recorded in the MCDK registry on approximately 900 MCDKs.[17] From this comprehensive analysis of the literature, these authors identified 3 cases of Wilms tumor arising in a prenatally detected MCDK—none of which occurred after 4 years of age. No cases were reported to have arisen in MCDKs that had involuted. The Trent and Anglia MCDK Study Group systematically collected prospective data on 323 children with antenatally detected MCDK, with a median duration of follow-up of 10.1 years (0.3–15.4 years). No Wilms tumors were encountered in any of these patients. Similarly, no Wilms tumors occurred in 325 children with prenatally detected MCDKs managed conservatively at Great Ormond Street Hospital. Of these, 180 children with MCDKs had been followed prospectively for more than 10 years (unpublished data, Dhillon H. K., personal communication, 2009).

It could be argued that the published data might underestimate the true incidence of malignancy because not all cases have been reported in the literature. However, the risk of malignancy can also be approached from a different perspective by considering how frequently MCDKs feature in published series of Wilms tumor. This question was addressed by studying data on 7500 Wilms tumors reported to the National Wilms Tumor Study Pathology Center over an 18-year period. Of the 7500 Wilms tumors, 5 had arisen in MCDKs.[13]

On the basis of these data coupled with published data on the prevalence of MCDKs, it was calculated that individual lifetime risk of developing Wilms tumor in an MCDK was approximately 1 in 2000. If anything, this calculation overstates the risk because the overall prevalence of MCDK in the pediatric population is somewhat higher than the figure on which this calculation was based. In summary, the best available data indicate that the risk of developing a Wilms tumor in a prenatally detected MCDK is probably on the order of 1 in 5000.

The risk of hypertension has also been cited to justify the practice of prophylactic nephrectomy. There is now a growing body of evidence with which to quantify the scale of this risk. No cases of hypertension were encountered in 323 children with prenatally detected MCDK followed prospectively for a median of 10.1 years by the Trent and Anglia MCDK Study Group,[12] and no instances of hypertension were recorded in 441 children with prenatally detected MCDKs enrolled in the MCDK registry.[17]

Narchi's[14] literature review did, however, reveal a published incidence of hypertension of 0.5%. However, it is important to recognize that confirming a reliable diagnosis of hypertension in this age group can be problematic because of the difficulties inherent in obtaining accurate, reproducible blood pressure readings in fractious infants and young children.

As with malignancy, the risk of hypertension can also be viewed from a different perspective. MCDK is now known to be a relatively common anomaly with a birth incidence in the range of 1 in 2500 to 1 in 4000.[1,2] If MCDKs were resulting in hypertension on any appreciable scale, it could be expected that they would account for a sizeable proportion of children with hypertension. This is not the case. For example, in a series of 21 children with renal hypertension managed by nephrectomy at Great Ormond Street Hospital between 1968 and 2003, there was only one case of MCDK.[18]

Removing an MCDK may not entirely obviate the risk since there are well-documented cases of hypertension arising in the contralateral kidney.[19] Moreover there is also some evidence that individuals with a solitary kidney are at an increased lifetime risk of developing hypertension.

In summary, the best currently available evidence puts the risk of developing hypertension associated with a prenatally detected MCDK at less than 1% (probably significantly less).

The relative ease and safety with which MCDKs can be removed laparoscopically is sometimes cited as an argument in support of prophylactic nephrectomy. But the technical ease with which an operation can be performed can never be regarded as a legitimate indication in its own right. The overwhelming majority of children with antenatally detected MCDKs are entirely healthy and asymptomatic. There is a growing body of evidence that the scale of risk associated with an antenatally detected MCDK is exceedingly low. In these circumstances, it is important that the surgeon and parents give very careful consideration to the evidence before submitting a healthy, asymptomatic child to surgery and general anesthesia.

Timing of surgery

Large multicystic kidneys associated with a sizeable mass should be removed electively in the first few weeks of life. Smaller lesions for which surgery is nevertheless thought to be appropriate can safely be left until 6–12 months of age or later. It is important to obtain an ultrasound scan shortly before surgery to confirm that the MCDK is still visible and has not undergone involution in the period since the decision was made to operate.

SURGICAL OPTIONS

Nephrectomy for MCDK is now performed laparoscopically (conventional or robot assisted) in most western pediatric surgical centers. However, the open approach is a reasonable alternative if the surgeon lacks the necessary expertise in minimally invasive surgery or suitable pediatric equipment is not available.

Open nephrectomy

Dorsal or posterior lumbotomy has the advantages of simplicity, good cosmesis, reduced postoperative pain, and shortened hospital stay.[20,21] The major drawbacks are the limited access to the kidney afforded by this incision and difficulty in extending it if the surgeon encounters an unforeseen problem. For a small MCDK, the dorsal lumbotomy incision is ideal, and even for larger lesions, nephrectomy should not pose problems, provided that the bulk of the multicystic kidney is reduced by cyst aspiration prior to its removal.

For surgeons unfamiliar with the dorsal lumbotomy incision, the more familiar loin approach is described in detail as follows.

OPERATIVE DETAILS

Position of the patient

A full lateral position is employed (Figure 101.3). Lateral flexion of the spine is best achieved in this age group by the use of a sandbag under the contralateral loin. Once the required position has been achieved, adhesive strapping is used to maintain it. The strapping is fixed first to one side of the operating table, taken across the abdomen at the level of the iliac crests, and then is secured firmly on the other side of the table.

Incision and approach to the kidney

The twelfth rib is identified by palpation. A preoperative plain x-ray is helpful in determining the length of the twelfth rib. Care should be taken to base the incision on the twelfth rib itself (Figure 101.4a), since an inadvertent supra–eleventh rib incision may result in the pleural cavity being opened. After the skin and subcutaneous fat have been incised, cutting diathermy is used to deepen the incision to the tip of the twelfth rib. The muscles attached to the superior border of the twelfth rib (latissimus dorsi,

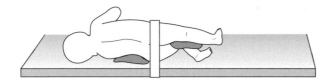

Figure 101.3 Lateral position of the patient.

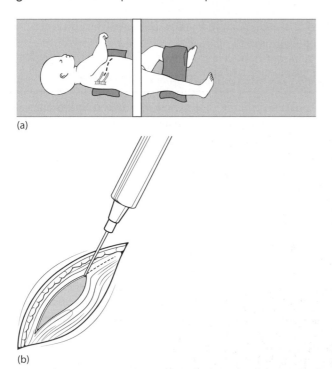

(a)

(b)

Figure 101.4 **(a)** "Supra 12" incision extending medially from the tip of the 12th rib. **(b)** Cutting diathermy used to deepen the incision through the abdominal wall muscles. Peritoneum swept anteriorly with a finger to expose the retroperitoneum.

intercostal muscles) are incised along their insertion. The rib is then deflected caudally to allow the surgeon to insert a finger to sweep the peritoneum away from the overlying abdominal wall muscles. The incision can then be extended forward in the line of the rib using the diathermy to divide the external oblique, internal oblique, and transversus abdominis muscles (Figure 101.4b). Care is needed to avoid damaging the neurovascular bundle, as this can result in a visible obvious (but usually self-limiting) postoperative weakness of the relevant segmental abdominal musculature. When the incision has been completed, a self-retaining retractor can be inserted.

Mobilization

A small MCDK may initially be difficult to identify within the retroperitoneum. If difficulty is encountered, the dissection is then extended through the retroperitoneal fat and perirenal fat—maintaining close proximity to the posterior abdominal wall to minimize the risk of damage to other viscera. More commonly, the MCDK is identified without difficulty in the renal fossa. A combination of blunt and scissor dissection is used to develop a plane between the cysts and adjacent tissues (Figure 101.5). The peritoneum is usually adherent to an extensive area of the MCDK, and care should be taken to avoid entering the peritoneal cavity. If the peritoneum is incised, the defect should be closed with a continuous absorbable suture.

Once a portion of the kidney has been exposed and mobilized in this fashion, it is helpful to aspirate the visible cysts with a syringe and needle (Figure 101.6). The decompressed cyst wall can then be grasped, e.g., with Allis Tissue Forceps, so that gentle traction can be applied to deliver the kidney out of the incision. By a combination of further dissection around the intact cysts followed by aspiration and mobilization through the incision, it is possible to remove an MCDK through a much smaller incision than would have been required if the cysts were left intact.

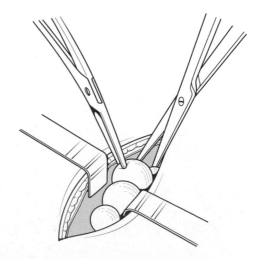

Figure 101.5 Mobilization of the kidney.

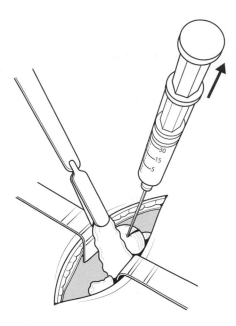

Figure 101.6 Aspiration of cysts.

Dissection of hilum

As the dissection is deepened, a malleable retractor is inserted to retract the peritoneum and expose the ureter and hilar vessels. A vascular sling or tape is placed around the ureter, and gentle traction is applied to facilitate the final dissection of the hilum (Figure 101.7). The ureter is then ligated with 4-0 absorbable suture and divided. Although it is good practice to ligate the renal arteries and veins individually (to prevent the risk of arteriovenous fistula formation), this is often impossible since the vessels are usually

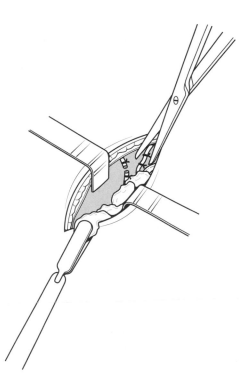

Figure 101.7 Dissection of the hilum.

small and nonpatent. The renal vessels are ligated in continuity and then divided between the ligatures.

Removal of the kidney and closure

Once the decompressed MCDK has been fully mobilized, it can be removed following division of any remaining attached tissue.

The renal bed is inspected and diathermy hemostasis performed as required. Similarly, the peritoneum should be checked and any defect closed with a continuous 4-0 absorbable suture. Drainage of the renal fossa is not necessary. This incision is closed either in two layers using a continuous absorbable suture or with a series of interrupted mass sutures encompassing the rib. The skin is then closed with a subcuticular suture of 5-0 Vicryl.

Postoperative care

Postoperative recovery is usually rapid. Feeding is reestablished within 24 hours, and the child can generally leave hospital within 1–2 days.

Laparoscopic nephrectomy

The removal of a normally sited MCDK by laparoscopic or robot-assisted nephrectomy can be performed using either a transperitoneal[22–24] or an extraperitoneal[25] approach. The transperitoneal approach is required for removal of an MCDK located in an ectopic site such as the pelvis.[26]

EQUIPMENT AND INSTRUMENTS

The following are required:

- Camera, light source, insufflator, and one or preferably two monitors with appropriate attachments.
- Diathermy unit (monopolar and bipolar) with appropriate cables and hand probes. Ultrasonic shears, LigaSure, or PlasmaKinetic coagulation devices may be used as an alternative.
- Three or four 2.5–12 mm cannulae and trocars with appropriate converters.
- A 30° or 45°, 2.5–10 mm angled telescope (0° scope may be adequate).
- An appropriate retractor may prove helpful. Often, a simple instrument such as an atraumatic grasper may be used as a retractor.
- Two atraumatic, preferably insulated, relatively fine curved or angled double-action jaw-grasping forceps (an additional forceps with ratchet can be useful).
- One insulated, curved double-action jaw scissors with appropriate diathermy lead.
- Suction/irrigation apparatus and probe.
- A single-load or multiload automatic clip applicator and clips (alternatively, suture ligatures, ultrasound shears, LigaSure, or PlasmaKinetic may be used).
- One long needle to compress cysts if necessary.
- A balloon dissector may be required for extraperitoneal approach.

The size and length of instruments depend on the size of patient, surgeon's preference, and availability of instruments. In addition to laparoscopic equipment, a set of the instruments required for open nephrectomy should always be available in case of emergency or if it becomes necessary to convert to an open approach.

PREPARATION AND POSITION OF THE PATIENT

The procedure is performed under general anesthesia with endotracheal intubation and muscle relaxants. A nasogastric tube is positioned, and a catheter should be passed to drain the bladder if it is palpable and cannot be expressed manually. The infant is placed and strapped securely in the semilateral position with soft towels under the contralateral loin/lower chest to permit lateral flexion and allow the intestine to fall medially under gravity (Figure 101.8).

TECHNIQUE FOR TRANSPERITONEAL NEPHRECTOMY

The theater layout, position of the surgeons, and placement of the cannulae are illustrated in Figure 101.8. The primary cannula is placed in the periumbilical region

using an open technique.[27] A pneumoperitoneum is created with CO_2 insufflation through the primary cannula at a flow rate of 0.2–1 L/min and pressure of 8–10 mm mercury.[28] A telescope is then placed through the cannula, and under direct vision, the working cannulae are placed in the direction of the kidney. The sites and sizes of the working "secondary" cannulae are dependent on the size of the patient, the size of the instruments to be used, and the surgeons' preference.[29] The use of two 2.5–5 mm working cannulae in addition to the primary cannula will often provide adequate access for the removal of a MCDK. An additional cannula may be placed for retraction if necessary. An incision in the peritoneum of a few centimeters in length lateral to the upper border of the colon and directly over the lower part of the kidney will allow adequate exposure.[22] Formal mobilization of the colon is not usually necessary in children. The MCDK is then mobilized by blunt and sharp dissection, with traction on the cysts when necessary to facilitate exposure (Figure 101.9). The renal vessels, which are usually attenuated, are exposed in the region of the kidney and divided between clips or ligatures. Other techniques for securing the blood vessels include unipolar or bipolar diathermy, ultrasound shears, LigaSure, or PlasmaKinetic. The ureter distal to the atretic segment is clipped or ligated and divided at a convenient level. If necessary, the bulk of the MCDK can be reduced by needle aspiration prior to removal of the specimen via the largest cannula or site of a cannula with or without 1–2 cm extension. A retrieval bag is usually difficult to accommodate in infants and is not usually necessary. A change of telescope and/or instruments from one cannula to another may serve to facilitate viewing and dissection during the procedure.[29] Postoperative drainage is not necessary. In infants, cannula sites greater than 2.5 mm are closed with absorbable sutures. The opening

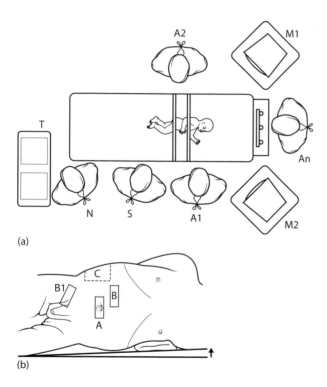

(a)

(b)

Figure 101.8 Laparoscopic transperitoneal right nephrectomy for multicystic dysplastic disease. **(a)** Theater layout. Note how the patient is fully supported and strapped in a semilateral position. A1/A2 = assistants, An = anesthetic apparatus, M1/M2 = monitors, N = scrubbed nurse, S = surgeon, T = instrument trolley. **(b)** Position of cannulae. A = periumbilical or lateral abdominal wall site for the primary cannula; B = working cannula 1; B1 = working cannula 2 in the lower abdominal skin crease, which may be extended to retrieve the specimen if necessary; C = an accessory cannula for hand instruments and/or retractor if necessary.

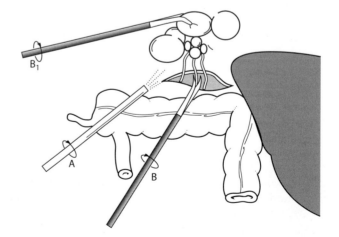

Figure 101.9 Laparoscopic transperitoneal nephrectomy. A = 2.5–10 mm angled or 0° telescope, B and B_1 = two working instruments. Note how a few-centimeters-long high paracolic peritoneal incision directly over the cystic kidney without colon mobilization allows full mobilization of the specimen and hemostasis.

in the peritoneum is covered with colon while the child is being returned to the supine position at the end of the procedure. This maneuver helps to ensure that very little, if any, raw surface is exposed that might promote adhesion formation.

In robot-assisted laparoscopic nephrectomy, position of the patient and ports and the technique are similar to that of conventional laparoscopy. However, the entire procedure can be accomplished using two instruments: an atraumatic and a PlasmaKinetic grasping forceps.[23]

POSTOPERATIVE CARE

The nasogastric tube and (if used) the urinary catheter are removed on the completion of the procedure. Local infiltration of the cannulae sites with an appropriate anesthetic agent provides generally adequate pain relief. Opiate analgesia is not usually required, but intravenous paracetamol may be administered in the early postoperative period as required. Children can usually be discharged from the hospital within 8–24 hours.

Extraperitoneal laparoscopic nephrectomy

Although challenging in infants and small children, this approach is becoming increasingly fashionable. The technique entails creating a space around the MCDK by disrupting up the loose connective tissue in the retroperitoneal plane. This is achieved either with the tip of the telescope and direct CO_2 insufflation or by the use of a balloon dissector.[25,30] This technique avoids the morbidity that may be associated with traversing the peritoneal cavity. However, it has the drawback of more restricted exposure of the kidney. In addition, it carries a risk of tearing the peritoneum, leading to an extension pneumoperitoneum and consequent difficulty in maintaining an extraperitoneal technique. The use of a single-incision retroperitoneal technique has been reported.[31] However any benefits are likely to be minimal and outweighed by the considerable technical limitations imposed by this technique. In general, the extraperitoneal approach does not appear to confer any advantage over the transperitoneal in terms of clinical outcome.[32]

FOLLOW-UP

This is determined by the nature of any coexistent abnormalities. In an otherwise normal child who has undergone nephrectomy for an MCDK, follow-up can be limited to one ultrasound scan at 6–12 months. Thereafter, it is prudent to perform an occasional precautionary ultrasound scan of the solitary remaining kidney until the child reaches an age when he or she could be expected to describe his or her symptoms in the unlikely event of development of symptomatic pathology (e.g., PUJ obstruction) in the remaining kidney. Lifelong annual blood pressure measurement is probably advisable for any individual with a solitary kidney.

REFERENCES

1. Liebeschuetz S, Thomas R. Unilateral multicystic dysplastic kidney. *Arch Dis Child* 1997 October; 77(4): 369.
2. Gordon AC, Thomas DF, Arthur RJ, Irving HC. Is Multicystic dysplastic kidney: Is nephrectomy still appropriate? *J. Urol* 1988 November; 140(5 Pt 2): 1231–4.
3. Belk RA, Thomas DF, Mueller RF, Godbole P, Markham AF, Weston MJ. A family study and the natural history of prenatally detected unilateral multicystic dysplastic kidney. *J Urol* 2002; 167: 666–9.
4. Abdulhannan P, Stahlschmidt J, Subramaniam R. Multicystic dysplastic kidney disease and hypertension: Clinical and pathological correlation. *J Pediatr Urol* 2011 October; 7(5): 566–8.
5. Stuck KJ, Koff SA, Silver TM. Ultrasonic features of multicystic dysplastic kidney: Expanded diagnostic criteria. *Radiology* 1982; 143: 217–21.
6. Sanders RC, Hartman DS. The sonographic distinction between neonatal multicystic kidney and hydronephrosis. *Radiology* 1984; 151: 621–5.
7. Whittam BM, Calaway A, Szymanski KM, Carroll AE, Misseri R, Kaefer M et al. Ultrasound diagnosis of multicystic dysplastic kidney: Is a confirmatory nuclear medicine scan necessary? *J Pediatr Urol* 2014 December; 10(6): 1059–62.
8. Hollowell JG, Kogan BA. How much imaging is necessary in patients with multicystic dysplastic kidneys? *J Urol* 2011; 186: 785–6.
9. Calaway AC, Whittam B, Szymanski KM, Misseri R, Kaefer M, Rink RC et al. Multicystic dysplastic kidney: Is an initial voiding cystourethrogram necessary? *Can J Urol* 2014 October; 21(5): 7510–4.
10. Ismaili K, Avni FE, Alexander M, Schulman C, Collier F, Hall M. Routine voiding cystourethrography is of no value in neonates with unilateral multicystic dysplastic kidney. *J Pediatr* 2005; 146: 759–63.
11. Tiryaki S, Alkac AY, Serdaroglu E, Bak M, Avanoglu A, Ulman I. Involution of multicystic dysplastic kidney: Is it predictable? *J Pediatr Urol* 2013 June; 9(3): 344–7.
12. Hayes WN, Watson AR; Trent & Anglia MCDK Study Group. Unilateral multicystic dysplastic kidney: Does initial size matter? *Pediatr Nephrol* 2012; 27: 1335–40.
13. Beckwith JB. "Wilms tumor and multicystic dysplastic kidney disease." Editorial comment, *J Urol* 1997; 158: 2259–60.
14. Narchi H. Risk of hypertension with multicystic kidney disease: A systematic review. *Arch Dis Child* 2005; 90: 921–4.
15. Narchi H. Risk of Wilms' tumour with multicystic kidney disease: A systematic review. *Arch Dis Child* 2005; 90: 147–9.
16. Cambio AJ, Evans CP, Kurzrock EA. "Non surgical management of multicystic dysplastic kidney." *BJU Int* 2008; 101: 804–8.

17. Wacksman J, Phipps L. Report of the Multicystic Kidney Registry: Preliminary findings. *J Urol* 1993; 150: 1870–2.

18. Johal NS, Kraklau D, Cuckow PM. The role of the unilateral nephrectomy in the treatment of nephronogenic hypertension in children. *BJU Int* 2005 January; 95(1): 140–2.

19. Kuwertz-Broeking E, Brinkmann OA, Von Lengerke H-J, Sciuk J, Fruend S, Bulla M et al. Unilateral multicystic kidney: Experience in children. *BJU Int* 2004; 93: 388–92.

20. Orland SN, Synder HM, Duckett JW. The dorsal lumbotomy incision in pediatric urological surgery. *J Urol* 1987; 138: 963–6.

21. Wise WR, Snow BW. The versatility of the posterior lumbotomy approach in infants. *J Urol* 1989; 141: 1148–50.

22. Najmaldin A. Transperitoneal laparoscopic nephrectomy. In: Bax NMA, Georgeson KE, Najmaldin A, Valla JS (eds). *Endoscopic Surgery in Children*. Berlin: Springer-Verlag, 1999: 371–8.

23. Najmaldin A. Paediatric telerobotic surgery: Where do we stand. *Int J Med Robotics Comput Assist Surg* 2007; 3: 183–6.

24. Ionouchene S, Mikhaylov N, Novozhilov V, Olgira O. Laparoscopic Nephrectomy: Advantages of Technique in Infants and Newborns. *J Laparo Adv Surg Tech* 2009; 19: 703–6.

25. Valla JS. Video surgery of the retroperitoneal space in children. In: Bax NMA, Georgeson KE, Najmaldin A, Valla JS (eds). *Endoscopic Surgery in Children*. Berlin: Springer-Verlag, 1999: 379–92.

26. Nishio H, Kojima Y, Mizuno K, Kamisawa H, Kohri K, Hayashi Y. Laparoscopic nephrectomy for pelvic multicystic dysplastic kidney. *Urology* 2011 August; 78(2): 434–6.

27. Humphrey GME, Najmaldin A. Modification of the Hasson technique in paediatric laparoscopy. *Br J Surg* 1994; 81:1320–3.

28. Najmaldin A. Principles of minimally invasive surgery. In Burge et al. (eds). *Paediatric Surgery*. London: Hodder Arnold, 2005; 115–9.

29. Najmaldin A. Laparoscopy—Basic technique. In: Najmaldin et al. (eds). *Operative Endoscopy and Endoscopic Surgery in Infants and Children*. London: Hodder Arnold, 2005; 179–90.

30. Najmaldin A, Guillou P (eds). *A Guide to Laparoscopic Surgery*. London: Blackwell Sciences, 1998: 56–9.

31. Cherian A, De Win G Single incision retro-peritoneoscopic paediatric nephrectomy: Early experience. *J Pediatr Urol* 2014 June; 10(3): 564–6.

32. Kim C, Mckay K, Docimo SG. Laparoscopic nephrectomy in children: Systematic review of transperitoneal and retroperitoneal approaches. *Urology* 2009; 73: 280–4.

102

Upper urinary tract obstructions

PREM PURI AND BORIS CHERTIN

INTRODUCTION

With the widespread use of maternal ultrasound, the incidence of prenatally detected hydronephrosis has increased significantly altering the practice of urology. The recent review of the trends in the prenatal sonography use and subsequent urological diagnoses in United States demonstrated significant increase in the overall ultrasound use in the last two decades. Moreover, the mean number of ultrasounds per pregnancy also increased significantly from 2.7 in 1998 to 4.2 in 2005.[1] Depending on diagnostic criteria and gestation, the prevalence of prenatally detected hydronephrosis ranges from 0.6% to 5.4%. The condition is bilateral in 17%–54%, and additional abnormalities are occasionally associated. The outcome of prenatally detected hydronephrosis depends on the underlying etiology. Although prenatally detected hydronephrosis resolves by birth or during infancy in 41%–88% patients, urological abnormalities requiring intervention are identified in 4.1%–15.4% and rates of vesicoureteric reflux (VUR) and urinary tract infections (UTIs) are several-fold higher. Pelviureteric junction (PUJ) obstruction is the most common cause of hydronephrosis detected antenatally.[2,3] The next most common cause of prenatally detected hydronephrosis is obstruction at the ureterovesical junction.[2] Management of these patients after birth remains controversial. The decision to intervene surgically in these infants has become more complex because spontaneous resolution of antenatal and neonatal upper urinary tract dilatations is being increasingly recognized.[2,4–6] The recognition and relief of significant obstruction is important to prevent irreversible damage to the kidneys.[7] Differentiating urinary tract dilatations that are significantly obstructive and require surgery from those that represent mere anatomical variants with no implications for renal function is not a simple task especially in the newborns. It has been shown that the changes in the function of the involved kidney should be used as a measure of degree of obstruction and indication for surgical intervention.[4,5,7–10]

PUJ OBSTRUCTION

The overall incidence of PUJ obstruction approximates 1 in 1500 births. The ratio of males to females is 2:1 in the neonatal period, with left-sided lesions occurring in 60%. In the newborn period, a unilateral process is most common, but bilateral PUJ obstruction was found in 10%–49% of neonates in some reported series.[7] PUJ obstruction is classified as intrinsic, extrinsic, or secondary.

Intrinsic obstruction results from failure of transmission of the peristaltic waves across the PUJ with failure of urine to be propulsed from the renal pelvis into the ureter, which results in multiple ineffective peristaltic waves that eventually causes hydronephrosis by incompletely emptying the pelvic contents.[8–11] Tainio et al.[12] have shown the abnormalities of peptidergic innervation with dense innervation of neuropeptide Y and vasoactive intestinal polypeptide, and proposed that these may have a role in intrinsic obstruction. Absence or reduction of smooth muscle with replacement by collagen fibers has been demonstrated histologically.[13,14] Some researchers proposed that downregulation of Cajal cells is responsible for the development of PUJ obstruction.[15] Extrinsic mechanical factors include aberrant renal vessels, bands, adventitial tissues, and adhesions that cause angulation, kinking, or compression of the PUJ. Extrinsic obstruction may occur alone but usually coexists with intrinsic ureteropelvic junction pathology. Secondary PUJ obstruction may develop as a consequence of severe VUR in which a tortuous ureter may kink proximately.[16] Previous reports have described VUR in 9%–15% of children who have PUJ obstruction, although the fractions that are secondary to reflux are difficult to determine.[9,16]

Prenatal diagnosis

The bladder is visualized by 14 weeks of gestation. The presence of full bladder provides evidence of renal function. The ureters are usually not seen in the absence of distal obstruction or reflux. The fetal kidney may be visualized at the same time as bladder. If not, they are always visualized by 16th week of gestation. However, it is not until 20–24 weeks of gestation, when the fetal kidney is surrounded by fat, that the internal renal structures appear distinct.[16] Renal growth can then be assessed easily.[17] Beyond 20 weeks, fetal urine production is the main source of amniotic fluid. Therefore, major abnormalities of the urinary tract may result in oligohydramnios.

Because of the distinct urine tissue interface, hydronephrosis can be detected as early as 16 weeks of gestation. An obstructive anomaly is recognized by demonstrating dilated renal calyces and pelvis. A multitude of measurement and different gestational age cutoff points have been recommended in the assessment of fetal obstructive uropathy.[18–22] Routine estimation of anteroposterior (AP) diameter of renal pelvis in fetus with hydronephrosis is considered as a useful marker for classification of renal dilatation and possible obstruction. AP renal pelvis threshold values ranged between 2.3 and 10 mm. Positive predictive values for pathological dilatation confirmed in the neonate ranged between 2.3% and >40% for AP renal measurements of 2–3 and 10 mm, respectively. A study that included more than 46,000 screening patients published the standards regarding renal pelvic measurement.[17] This study clearly demonstrated that only fetuses exhibiting third-trimester AP renal pelvis dilatations >10 mm would merit postnatal assessment. In order to standardize postnatal evolution of prenatal hydronephrosis, a grading system of postnatal hydronephrosis was implemented in 1993 by the Society for Fetal Urology (SFU).[23] In SFU system, the status of calices is paramount while the size of the pelvis is less important. In SFU grading of hydronephrosis, there is no hydronephrosis in grade 0. At grade 1, the renal pelvis is only visualized. Grade 2 of hydronephrosis is diagnosed when a few (but not all) renal calices are identified in addition to the renal pelvis. Grade 3 hydronephrosis requires that virtually all calices are depicted. Grade 4 hydronephrotic kidneys will exhibit similar calyceal status with the involved kidney exhibiting parenchymal thinning. Often this classification is applied also on prenatal hydronephrosis. We have recently published our data regarding prenatal findings with the special emphasis on the natural history of hydronephrosis during postnatal period.[7] Our data show that SFU grade of prenatal hydronephrosis is not a significant predictive factor for surgery in unilateral hydronephrosis. However, SFU grade 3–4 prenatal bilateral hydronephrosis indicates that the majority of the children will require surgical correction during postnatal period.

In case of severe prenatal bilateral hydronephrosis, severe hydroureteronephrosis or severe impairment of the solitary kidney fetal bladder aspiration for urinary proteins and electrolytes may be used in order to predict the renal injury secondary to obstructive uropathy. Fetal urinary sodium level of less than 100 mMol/L, chloride level of less than 90 mMol/L and an osmolality of less than 210 mOsm/kg are considered prognostic features for good renal function.

Clinical presentation

The clinical presentation of PUJ obstruction has dramatically changed since the advent of maternal ultrasonographic screening.[3–7] Before the routine fetal ultrasonography, the commonest presentation was with abdominal flank mass. Fifty percent abdominal masses in newborns are of renal origin with 40% being secondary to PUJ obstruction. Some patients present with UTI. Other clinical presentations include irritability, vomiting, and failure to thrive. Between 10% and 35% of PUJ obstructions are bilateral, and associated abnormalities of urinary tract are seen in about 30%.[23] PUJ problems are often associated with other congenital anomalies, including imperforated anus, contralateral dysplastic kidney, congenital heart disease, VATER syndrome, and esophageal atresia. In patients with such an established diagnosis, a renal ultrasound examination should be performed.[24] Although the majority of cases occur sporadically, familial cases have been reported. Hereditary pelviureteric obstruction, which is an autosomal dominant trait with variable penetrance, was suggested, and Izquierdo et al.[25] proposed one of the loci to short arm of chromosome 6 as responsible for the development of PUJ obstruction. Moreover, the importance of angiotensin II and its type 2 receptor (AT2) in the development of congenital urinary tract abnormalities has begun to be appreciated.[24–26] Nishimura et al.[27] reported an association of polymorphism of intron 1 of the AT2 gene (the A-1332G transition, which perturbed AT2 mRNA splicing) in patients with multicystic dysplastic kidneys and/or PUJ obstruction.

Diagnosis

With the increasing number of cases of antenatally diagnosed hydronephrosis, it is difficult to interpret the underlying pathology and its significance. Severe obstructive uropathies are detrimental to renal function. However, on the other hand, hydronephrosis without ureteral or lower tract anomaly is common. The important aspect of postnatal investigations is to identify the group of patients who will benefit from early intervention and those who need to be carefully followed up.

Ultrasound

Follow-up ultrasound examination is necessary in postnatal period in antenatally detected hydronephrosis. If the bilateral hydronephrosis is diagnosed in utero in a male infant, postnatal evaluation should be carried out within 24 hours primarily because of the possibility of posterior urethral valves. If the ultrasound scan is negative in the first 24–48 hours in any patients with unilateral or bilateral hydronephrosis, a repeat scan should be performed after 5–10 days, recognizing that neonatal physiological dehydration may mask a moderately obstructive lesion.

If hydronephrosis is confirmed on the postnatal scan, further careful scan of the kidney, ureter, bladder, and the posterior urethra in boys is essential. Ultrasonography depicts the dilated calyces as multiple intercommunicating cystic spaces of fairly uniform size that lead into a larger cystic structure at the hilum, representing the dilated renal pelvis (Figure 102.1a). Peripheral to the dilated calyces, the renal parenchyma is usually thinned with normal or increased echogenicity.

In order to standardize postnatal evolution of prenatal hydronephrosis, the aforementioned SFU grading system of postnatal hydronephrosis is utilized.

Typically, the ureter is of normal caliber and not seen.[22] But if it is dilated, the size of the ureter is also assessed ultrasonographically and graded 1–3 according to ureteral width <7, 7–10, and >10 mm, respectively.

Radionuclide scans

Diuretic renograms using 99mTc DTPA augmented with furosemide were useful in the diagnosis of urinary tract obstructions for a long time.[28,29] DTPA is completely filtered by the kidneys, with a maximum concentration of 5% being reached in 5 minutes, falling to 2% at 15 minutes. However, in the last decade, it has been reported that use of the tracers that rely on tubular extraction such as 123 I-Hippuran and 99Tc MAG3 (Figure 102.1b) may improve diagnostic accuracy.[30–32] The kidney of the young infant is immature; renal clearance, even when corrected for body surface, progressively increases until approximately 2 years of age. Therefore, the renal uptake of the tracer is particularly low in infants, and there is a high background activity. Thus, traces such as123 I-Hippuran and 99Tc MAG3 with a high

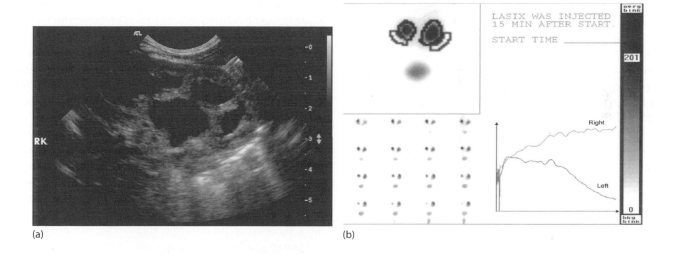

(a) (b)

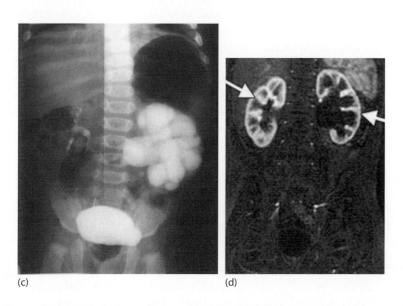

(c) (d)

Figure 102.1 **(a)** Coronal plane scan through the obstructed left kidney confirms obstruction at the level of the PUJ. **(b)** 99Tc MAG3 scan in the above patient. Clearance curve for left kidney confirming the high-grade obstruction on this side. **(c)** 20-minute full-length film from an IVU series showing left-sided high-grade PUJ obstruction in the same patient. **(d)** MRU showing PUJ obstruction in the same patient. (Lt arrow shows PUJ obstruction on the left side. Rt arrow shows normal renal pelvis.)

extraction rate provide reasonable images enabling estimation of the differential kidney function during the first few weeks of life. It is also helpful in assessing the size, shape, location, and function of the kidney. Diuretic augmented renogram is a provocative test and is intended to demonstrate or exclude obstructive hydronephrosis by stressing an upper urinary tract with a high urine flow. Obstruction usually is defined as a failure of tracer washout after diuretic stimulation. If unequivocal, it eliminates the need for further investigations. In equivocal cases, F15, in which furosemide is given 15 minutes after injection of the radionuclide trace, provides a better assessment of the drainage of the upper urinary tract. Forced hydration prior to scan increases the predictive value of nonobstructed pattern up to 94%.[31] Since glomerular filtration and glomerular blood flow are still low in the newborn, the handling of isotope is unpredictable and can be misleading. Koff et al.[32] therefore feel that the risk of making a misdiagnosis of obstruction in this age group far outweighs the potential damage to renal function that might result from delaying surgery for a few weeks until the diagnosis can be made more accurately. Therefore, the timing of the performance of radionuclide studies is of crucial importance.

In those cases where DTPA is used as an isotype, radionuclide study should be postponed until 6–8 weeks after birth allowing kidney to multiply the number of the functioning glomeruli. When 99Tc MAG3 is utilized in the diagnosis of the obstruction, the radionuclide study may be performed as early as 2 weeks of age in those cases where prompt diagnosis is required.

Diagnosis of PUJ obstruction can be made by intravenous urography. Although this investigation shows a dilated renal pelvis with clubbed calyces, it is often not helpful as the concentration of contrast is unreliable and, nowadays, it has no place in the diagnostic armamentarium (Figure 102.1c).

Recently, the value of the new tool named magnetic resonance urography (MRU) has begun to be appreciated in the diagnosis of upper tract obstructions.[33,34] The advent has facilitated the assessment of both function and morphology of the urinary tract, increasing therefore the accuracy of diagnostic workup. The advantages of this relatively new modality reside not only in the nonuse of ionizing radiation but also especially in the acquisition of images with higher contrast and spatial resolution in any orthogonal plane compared with conventional techniques. Certain pathological conditions, such as neoplasms, infections, parenchymal ischemias, and hemorrhage, as well as obstructions and anomalies, can be accurately identified. The addition of new rapid magnetic resonance imaging techniques with high temporal resolution has allowed quantification of corticomedullary perfusion along with the renal excretory function (Figure 102.1d).[34]

PRESSURE-FLOW STUDY

In the equivocal cases and in the presence of impaired function, the pressure flow study (Whitaker test) and antegrade pyelography may be necessary to confirm or exclude obstruction.[35] Whitaker test is based on the hypothesis that if the dilated upper urinary tract can transport 10 mL/min without an inordinate increase in pressure, the hydrostatic pressure under physiological conditions should not cause impairment of renal function, and the degree of obstruction, if present, is insignificant. However, it is an invasive test and is seldom required. Antegrade pyelography may be performed with ultrasound guidance in patients where diagnosis is difficult.[36] Retrograde pyelography is seldom required to determine the status of ureters. The disadvantages include difficulty in ureteral catheterization in neonates, and trauma and edema may change partial obstruction to a complete one. In patients where diagnosis is equivocal, serial examinations may be necessary.

Treatment

Considerable controversy exists regarding the management of newborn urinary tract obstructions. Some authors advocate early surgical intervention to prevent damage to maturing nephrons,[37] while others feel that early surgery carries no specific benefit.[4–7] During late prenatal and early postnatal life, there is progressive increase in the glomerular filtration rate.[5] Additionally, this transition is associated with an abrupt decline in urine output from what appears to be a quite high in utero output to a rather low early neonatal level of urine production. These physiological observations may explain the common observation of hydronephrosis detected antenatally, which on postnatal follow-up reverts to an unobstructed pattern.[1,5,10] In 1990, in a pioneering manuscript, Ransley et al.[4] reported the results of nonoperative treatment in newborns with nonrefluxing hydronephrosis and differential renal function >40%. At 6-year follow-up, only 23% needed surgical correction. The most common indication for surgery in this group of children was deterioration of renal function. Subsequently, Koff and Cambell[5] reported that out of 104 neonates with prenatally diagnosed unilateral hydronephrosis who have been followed conservatively, only 7% required pyeloplasty in long-term follow-up. Furthermore, the same group reported results of initial conservative management of children with severe unilateral hydronephrosis due to PUJ obstruction.[39] Only 22% of these children required pyeloplasty. All children who required surgery were younger than 18 months and had progressive hydronephrosis and/or reduction in renal function. Therefore, immediate postnatal surgical intervention is unnecessary in the majority of newborn children with PUJ obstruction. These babies should be followed up with serial examinations to observe anatomical and functional improvement. Surgery is undertaken in infants with deteriorating renal function.[3–5,7,38–40] We have reported our experience of over 16 years (1988–2003) with 343 children (260 males and 83 females) with antenatal diagnosis of hydronephrosis, which led to postnatal diagnosis of PUJ obstruction, who were followed conservatively. Of the 343 children, 110 had right-sided hydronephrosis and 233 had left-sided hydronephrosis. According to SFU classification, none had grade 0 of postnatal hydronephrosis, 20 had grade 1, 118 grade 2, 147 grade 3, and the remaining 58 children had grade 4 postnatal hydronephrosis. Relative renal function (RRF) on radionuclide scans revealed 235 children with RRF more than 40%, 68 with RRF between 30% and 40%, and 40 patients with RRF less than 30%. Renal function deterioration of more than 5% served as a main indication for surgery.[7] We have founded that 179 (52.2%) children required surgical correction in the course of conservative management. The average age at surgery was 10.6 months (range of 1 month to 7 years). Of those, 50% underwent surgery during the first 2 years of life, and majority of the remaining patients underwent surgery between the second and fourth years of age; only two patients required surgery later on. Univariate analysis revealed that child sex, side of hydronephrosis, and SFU grade of prenatal hydronephrosis are not significant predictive factors for surgery. However, SFU grade 3–4 of postnatal hydronephrosis and RRF less than 40% were significant independent risk factors that led to the surgical correction.

Pyeloplasty

Pathological variations in PUJ obstruction necessitate the surgeon to be conversant with the various techniques of the pyeloplasty.[41-47] The objective of the pyeloplasty is to achieve dependent, adequate calibered watertight PUJ. There are different approaches for open pyeloplasty. The classic traditional approach is an extraperitoneal one via lateral flank incision. The infant is placed on the operating table in a supine position with the affected side elevated on a roll (Figure 102.2a). Muscles are either cut or split (Figure 102.2b–d). Gerota's fascia is opened (Figure 102.2e). In the past, it was recommended to pass an appropriate-size silicone tube from opened PUJ down the ureter to the bladder in order to check for distal obstruction. However, we have abandoned this approach due to the possibility of the development of subsequent ureterovesical junction (UVJ) obstruction as a result of the injury to the fragile UVJ area from the passing catheter. The current diagnostic modalities almost certainly exclude existence of any double pathology. In those cases where suspicion to the distal to PUJ area has arisen, antegrade or retrograde study of the ureter upon or during surgery is recommended.

In some cases, the posterior lumbotomy may be applied.[41,42] The use of muscle splitting rather than muscle cutting makes it almost a minimally invasive procedure. The location of the incision just under and parallel to the 12th rib has a cosmetic advantage. The bilateral procedure is possible if indicated under the same anesthesia without changing position. This approach should not be used in older children or those who are significantly obese.

The various techniques of pyeloplasty are divided into dismembered and nondismembered pyeloplasty.

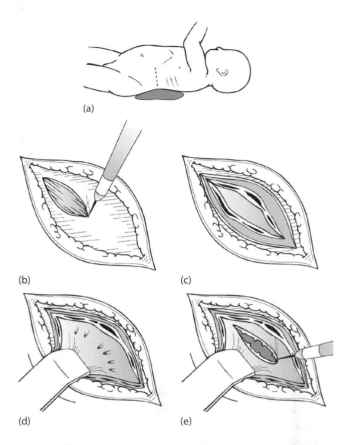

Figure 102.2 **(a)** Position of the infant on the operating table and line of skin incision. **(b)** Incision through skin and subcutaneous tissue. **(c)** Incision through external and internal oblique muscles. **(d)** Renal facia exposed. **(e)** Renal fascia has been opened.

DISMEMBERED PYELOPLASTY

Anderson–Hynes pyeloplasty

The renal pelvis, PUJ, and proximal ureter are freed of perirenal fat. Three stay sutures are placed: (1) at the superomedial aspect of the pelvis, (2) at the inferolateral aspect of the pelvis, and (3) on the ureter about 5 mm below PUJ. The ureter is divided obliquely above the ureteric stitch and the redundant pelvis trimmed (Figure 102.3a). The superior two-thirds of the pelvis is closed by using continuous 6/0 maxon stitch (Figure 102.3b). An oval-shaped anastomosis between the ureter and the lower part of the pelvis is carried out from the posterior to the anterior layer over a silastic stent using 6/0 maxon continuous stitch (Figure 102.3c and d). After the anastomosis is completed, a Redivac drain is placed. Gerota's fascia is closed with interrupted 3/0 chromic catgut sutures. Muscles are approximated in layers and skin by using subcuticular 5/0 Dexon. We have utilized a Pippi–Salle stent nephrostomy tube (Cook, USA) for dismembered pyeloplasty. In order to avoid passing of the distal end of the Pippi–Salle stent nephrostomy through the UVJ in the small children, we cut the distal tail of the tube and leave a distal end in the ureter below the anastomosis. The proximal end of the stent is positioned in the renal pelvis. The nephrostomy end is opened for the drainage for the

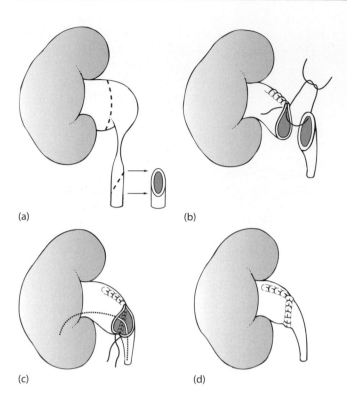

(a)

(b)

(c)

(d)

Figure 102.3 Anderson–Hynes pyeloplasty. **(a)** Vertical *en block* resection of the pelvis, PUJ, with oblique division of the ureter. **(b)** Superior part of the pelvis is closed and start of the posterior layer anastomosis between ureter and pelvis. **(c)** Posterior layer anastomosis completed and anterior layer anastomosis commenced over a stent. **(d)** Oval-shaped anastomosis completed between ureter and renal pelvis.

next 48–72 hours after surgery. After that, the nephrostomy is clamed and the patient is discharged home following removal of the drain. The tube is removed in the office usually 4 weeks after surgery.

NONDISMEMBERED PYELOPLASTY

The Y plasty (Foley)

This is based on the principle of a Y–V flap. This operation is suitable when the ureter is inserted high on the pelvis. V-shaped incision is made on the pelvis on the anterior and posterior surface. The tail of the incision is on the lateral surface of the ureter well below the obstruction. The flap of the pelvis is brought down, and posterior and anterior anastomosis of the flap and the ureter was performed using 6/0 maxon.

The spiral flap (Culp)

The spiral flap (culp) is suitable for long, dependent, stenotic ureteropelvic obstruction. The incision on the ureter must be adequate covering the stenotic area. A flap of equal length is based on a broad base (Figure 102.4a). The posterior layer of the ureter and the flap is sutured using 6/0 maxon (Figure 102.4b). The anterior layer is crossed over the stent and anastomosed using 6/0 maxon (Figure 102.4c).

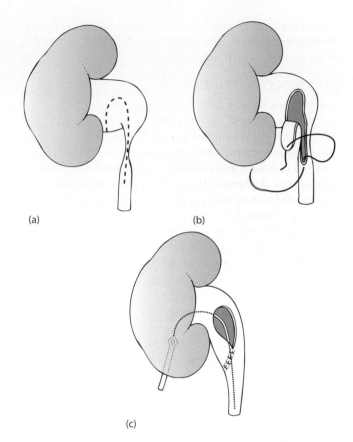

(a)

(b)

(c)

Figure 102.4 Spiral flap (culp) pyeloplasty. **(a)** Spiral fashioning of the flap. **(b)** Flap brought down and the first suture positions the rounded tip of the flap distally to the ureter. **(c)** Anterior layer closed over a stent.

The endoscopic technique has gained some popularity in the surgical treatment of PUJ obstruction.

Endopyelotomy

Endopyelotomy can be done by utilizing either percutaneous antegrade approach or endoscopic retrograde procedure.[43] Even strong and experienced surgeons do not recommend to do this procedure in neonates, infants, or young children.[44] Percutaneous endopyelotomy is performed by making an incision on the posterolateral wall using a smaller endoscope and using a 3F or 5F electrocautery probe, and followed by separating the cut edges using a balloon. A ureteral stent is placed for drainage for 6 weeks and nephrostomy tube for 3 days to 6 weeks. Kavoussi et al.[45] have shown that this procedure is also safe and effective in treating secondary PUJ obstruction.

Figenshau and Clayman[46] used a retrograde technique for old children and combined antegrade–retrograde for young children. The incision in the PUJ segment was done using an Acucise balloon with fluoroscopic control. They concluded that the technique has an 86% successful rate and should be offered to pediatric patients with PUJ obstruction. Balloon dilatation of PUJ has also been reported in infants and young children. This consists of dilatation of the PUJ segment using a dilating balloon catheter (12–24 Fr), which is positioned, confirmed, and inflated for 3 minutes under fluoroscopic control. The success rate has been reported as 63% with follow-up of up to 23 months.

LAPAROSCOPIC PYELOPLASTY

Laparoscopic Anderson–Hynes dismembered pyeloplasty has recently gained wide popularity in pediatric population.[47-49] A decade ago, Yeung et al.[48] reported the results of initial experience with retroperitoneal dismembered pyeloplasty in 13 infants and children. The authors concluded that laparoscopic Anderson–Hynes dismembered pyeloplasty is feasible and safe in infants, but stressed that the long-term results are awaited in order to prove that this method is durable in the long term in children. Since then, the visibility of the laparoscopic approach has found support in numerous publications.[49] Surgery may be performed through either retroperitoneal or transperitoneal approaches. The retroperitoneal approach is safe but technically more demanding due to the smaller operative space and additional difficulties in facilitating intracorporeal suturing. Moreover, it is more difficult to teach residents to perform laparoscopic surgery while utilizing the retroperitoneal approach. In order to facilitate laparoscopic pyeloplasty, some technical steps may be employed. Utilizing a transperitoneal approach allows increasing an operative space especially in small children. Laparoscopic pyeloplasty on the left side may be performed through the transmesenteric approach. The placement of the stay suture on the renal pelvis prior to suturing the anastomosis between renal pelvis and the ureter stabilizes the suture line and allows precise sutures placement, therefore eliminating the risk of reobstruction. Beyond the complexity imposed by the intracorporeal suturing, the presence of a ureteral stent (previously placed by cystoscopy) in front of the anastomotic site makes the suture even more difficult and time-consuming. The retrograde cystoscopic and the antegrade laparoscopic approaches are currently the two options for stent insertion during laparoscopic pyeloplasty. We have recently published our novel technique of stent placement during laparoscopic pyeloplasty. Following identification and dissection of the PUJ with the proximal part of the ureter, the ureter is dismembered just proximal to the PUJ at the level of the renal pelvis, allowing use of the excess pelvic tissue for further manipulation of the ureter. Then the abdomen is desufflated and the ureter delivered to the skin level. The externalized ureter is then spatulated and the stent inserted in an antegrade fashion to the bladder. The first stitch for further laparoscopic anastomosis is applied to the lower part of the spatulated ureteric end, and then following insufflations, the ureter is returned to the abdomen. The laparoscopic anastomosis is completed in a routine fashion.[50]

The final development in the laparoscopic reconstructive surgery in children was the employment of robot-assisted surgery. Robotic technology is changing the way surgery is performed.[51] It allows in situ surgery as well as increased magnification and dexterity for minimally invasive surgery. The development and application of pediatric robotic urology are currently manifesting themselves with rapid growth. The currently available system (DaVinci, Intuitive Surgical, Sunnyvale, CA) is a robotic manipulative device that permits a surgeon to have better control over the instruments. The impression with robot-assisted surgery is that the suturing is easier, and less operating time is required to perform laparoscopic pyeloplasty. Furthermore, it is much easier to teach a surgeon without prior laparoscopic experience to perform laparoscopic pyeloplasty while using a robot-assisted suturing technique.[52] As with laparoscopic pyeloplasty, robot-assisted pyeloplasty can be performed by a trans- or retroperitoneal approach. Suturing is done with a 6-0 monofilament absorbable suture, but one can utilize any 5-0 or 6-0 suture depending on the size of the patient. Currently, it appears that nothing larger than 6-0 for small children and infants is recommended. Robot-assisted pyeloplasty in children has been demonstrated to be feasible and to have satisfactory results. Although there are only a few published series on the long-term outcome to date, the short-term data suggest that outcomes are similar to those of open pyeloplasty in children, and it appears to be more than promising.

Recently available on the market, the da Vinci XI model allows easier docking of the system, allows more convenient manipulation in the pediatric population, and significantly decreases the operation time. However, still the high initial cost of robotic equipment and expensive maintenance of the working system cannot be ignored.

NEPHRECTOMY

Because the recovery potential of the kidney is greater in neonates, extreme conservation is justified. Salvage pyeloplasty should be considered as renal function shown on renal scintigraphy can recover.[53] At operation, an assessment should be made of the renal cortex after emptying the pelvis. Severe cystic dysplasia is an indication for nephrectomy; otherwise, every effort should be made to salvage the kidney.

BILATERAL PELVIURETERIC OBSTRUCTION

Surgical correction of the symptomatic side or the side with better function should take precedence. If a nephrectomy is considered on one side, the pyeloplasty should precede this.

Postoperative complications

Postoperative complications include infection, adhesive obstruction (transperitoneal approach), temporary obstruction at the anastomosis resulting in excessive urine leakage, and failure due to postoperative stricture at anastomotic sites. An overall reoperation rate of 8.2% was reported in the early series.[44] However, when temporally double-J stents or stent nephrostomy tube were utilized, the reoperation rate was negligible.

Follow-up and results

Follow-up ultrasound may be performed 3–6 months after operation when maximum improvement can be seen.[7] Radionuclide scans are useful to monitor the postpyeloplasty function and drainage. Pyeloplasty in the neonatal period, when indicated, gives excellent results. We have evaluated whether improved renal function after pyeloplasty for prenatal ureteropelvic junction obstruction persisted through puberty.[54] Out of more than 600 patients who underwent successful pyeloplasty and demonstrated an improvement of the renal function following surgery, 49 patients who completed puberty demonstrated that the renal function remained stable during and after puberty.

MEGAURETER

Megaureter is a ureter that is dilated out of proportion to the rest of the urinary tract and above the norms. Cussen[55] and, later, Hellstrom et al.[56] have established the normal measurement of the ureteral diameter in infants and children from 30 weeks of gestation to 12 years of age. Normal ureteral diameter in children is rarely greater than 5 mm, and ureters larger than 7 mm can be considered megaureters.

Classification

The Paediatric Urology Society in 1976[57] adopted a standard nomenclature for categorizing megaureters, which is a useful guide for management. There are three types described:

1. Refluxing ureter, which may be primary or secondary to distal obstruction or pathology
2. Obstructive ureter, which may be primary and includes intrinsic obstruction, or secondary due to distal obstruction or extrinsic causes
3. Nonrefluxing, nonobstructed ureter, which may be primary–idiopathic type or secondary to diabetes insipidus or infection

In 1980, King[58] subsequently modified this classification by adding a fourth group consisting of the refluxing, obstructed megaureters.

URETEROVESICAL JUNCTION OBSTRUCTION

The presence of an adynamic distal ureteral segment is the most common cause of a primary obstructive megaureter. The presence of narrowed terminal portion of a ureter will not convey the peristaltic wave or dilate enough to permit free passage of urine. This results in excess boluses of urine, which coalesce and cause ureteral dilatation. The contraction waves become smaller and are unable to coapt the walls of dilated ureters. This, along with infection, could damage the renal parenchyma. The proposed etiologies include the following:

1. Alteration in muscular orientation: Tanagho[59,60] noted in fetal lamb that the muscle coats of the distal ureter develop last and that late arrest in the development results in absence of longitudinally oriented musculature that conducts the peristaltic wave. This results in hypertrophy of the circular fibers causing obstruction.
2. Muscular hypoplasia with fibrosis: McLaughlin et al.[61] found that 69% of narrowed terminal ureteric segments showed muscular hypoplasia, which were separated by fibrotic sheets, thus affecting the transmission of peristalsis. This fibrotic ring prevents expansion and free urinary drainage.
3. Excessive collagen deposition resulting in a discontinuity of muscular coordination is another hypothesis.[62] Lee et al.[63] examined the histology of ureteric smooth muscle and collagen in obstruction employing computer-assisted color image analysis. They have found that the tissue matrix collagen ratios (collagen: smooth muscle) were significantly higher in patients with megaureters compared to the control.
4. Disturbance in the electric syncytium along with the nexus injury has been suggested to precede pathological innervation.[64] Dixon et al.[65] showed dense nonadrenergic innervation in a smooth muscle collar surrounding the terminal ureter in cases of an obstructed megaureter associated with ectopic ureteric insertion. Recently, it was reported that the myocyte apoptosis and decrease in the interstitial Cajal cells in the longitudinal muscular layer of the intravesical part of the ureter may lead to the development of the aperistaltic segment and subsequently to the UVJ obstruction.[66,67]

Prenatal diagnosis

Usually ureter is not seen in fetal scans. Visualization of the dilated ureter to the level of the vesicoureteric junction without abnormal bladder may suggest obstruction or reflux. However, this may be a transient phenomenon. Fetal urine flow is four to six times greater before birth than after and is due to differences in renal vascular resistance, glomerular filtration, and concentrating ability. This high outflow contributes to ureteral dilatation. Another contributing factor is increased compliance of the fetal ureter.[68]

Clinical features

The widespread use of maternal ultrasound has changed the age of presentation of congenital uropathies, including the megaureter. Currently, about half of the cases are asymptomatic and discovered on prenatal ultrasound. The commonest mode of clinical presentation is UTI.[69,70] Microscopic hematuria is frequent and may occur in the absence of infection. This is presumably caused by the disruption of mucosal vessels of the ureter secondary to ureteric distension. The primary obstructive megaureter is more common in males than females, and the left ureter is more likely to be involved than the right. Between 17% and 34% of the patients have bilateral megaureters. Contralateral renal agenesis is found in 10% of the patients.[71-76]

Diagnosis

Antenatally diagnosed ureteral dilatation needs further evaluation to confirm or exclude obstruction, reflux, or both. Clinicians are confronted with the two basic problems in assessing the dilated ureter in a neonate.[6,71,72,75–77] First, it is a real challenge to differentiate between obstructive and nonobstructive urinary tract dilatations. Second, there is no study that can determine accurately the potential of the kidney to recover after relief of obstruction.

Ultrasound

In antenatally detected cases, ultrasonography should be performed between 3 and 5 days after birth. If no dilatation is seen, repeat ultrasound should be performed after a few weeks as neonatal oliguria can mask dilatation. If dilatation persists on a repeat ultrasound, further workup can be postponed for a few weeks unless bilateral disease or a serious abnormality such as obstruction in a solitary kidney or urethral valves is suspected. Such an approach allows for the expected changes of transitional renal function in the newborn period that might otherwise cause inaccuracies with many diagnostic studies. Ultrasonography classically shows hydroureter and variable hydronephrosis, with hyperperistalsis of a lower ureter that terminates shortly above the bladder in a narrow, adynamic segment (Figure 102.5a).[77] However, the narrow segment may not always be visualized, and therefore, micturating cystourethrogram is necessary to exclude VUR.

Renal scintigraphy

Radionuclide scan is required to assess the urinary flow and stasis along with determining the differential function and the glomerular filtration rate. For the evaluation of neonatal hydronephrosis and hydroureter, MAG3 is the most frequently used (Figure 102.5b).

Intravenous urography

Intravenous urography may be necessary in equivocal cases to establish the diagnosis. It delineates the anatomy showing a dilated, obstructed ureter (Figure 102.5c). However, it is better to wait for a few weeks for renal maturation to allow concentration of contrast reliability. Occasionally, Whitaker test and antegrade pyelography may be required to establish the diagnosis.

Fung et al.[78] explored ureteral opening pressure as a novel parameter for evaluating pediatric ureterohydronephrosis. Renal pelvic pressure is assessed while simultaneously documenting the passage of contrast material from the distal ureter into the bladder. A pressure increase of 14 cm H_2O within the renal pelvis is consistent with distal ureter obstruction.

As in the diagnosis of PUJ obstruction, MRU has gained a wide popularity in the diagnosis of UVJ obstruction (Figure 102.5d).

Management

It is being increasingly recognized that many antenatal and neonatal ureteral dilatations improve with time.[5,61,70,72] Surgery is indicated in patients with progressive ureteral dilatation and deterioration in renal function. We have published our experience of over 18 years in 79 children (64 boys and 15 girls) with antenatal diagnosis of hydronephrosis, which led to postnatal diagnosis of megaureters, and tried to determine criteria for those who are at risk for surgery.[76] According to the SFU classification of hydronephrosis, 8 RU were with grade 1, 57 with grade 2, 29 with grade 3, and 11 with grade 4 of postnatal hydronephrosis. The mean ureteral diameter was 1.2 cm. RRF was more than 40% in 82 RU, between 30% and 40% in 18 RU, and less than 30% in 5 RU. Only a combination of renal function deterioration of the hydronephrotic kidney of more than 5% and worsening of hydronephrosis (considered as upgrade of SFU) served as the main indication for surgery. Twenty-five (31%) children required surgical correction. The mean age at surgery was 14.3 months (range of 3–60 months). Univariate analysis revealed that SFU grade 3–4 of postnatal hydronephrosis, RRF less than 30%, and a ureteral diameter of more than 1.33 cm were significant independent risk factors leading to reimplantation.

Operation

There are various techniques of reimplanting the ureter in a nonrefluxing manner after excision of an adynamic, narrow segment. The initial approach to the ureter can be either intravesical, extravesical, or combined.[79] The most commonly used techniques for the intravesical approach are Cohen's transtrigonal reimplantation and Politano–Leadbetter operation.

INTRAVESICAL APPROACH
Position

The patient is anesthetized and placed in supine position (Figure 102.6a).

Incision

A low transverse suprapubic skin crease incision is made (Figure 102.6a).

Exposure

The skin flaps are raised by diathermy dissection (Figure 102.6b). The rectus sheath is cut, and two recti are separated in the midline. Peritoneum is pushed upward. The bladder is opened vertically between two stay sutures. A Denis–Brown retractor is placed over the gauze inside the bladder to improve exposure. The ureter openings are inspected. A 3 or 5 Fr infant feeding tube is passed into the ureter, and a stay suture is placed around the tube. This facilitates the handling of the ureter during dissection. An incision is made circumferentially along the ureter opening, and the distal ureter is dissected from mucosa and trigonal muscle. The ureter is freed keeping away from adventitia and mesentery to avoid damage to blood supply (Figure 102.6c).

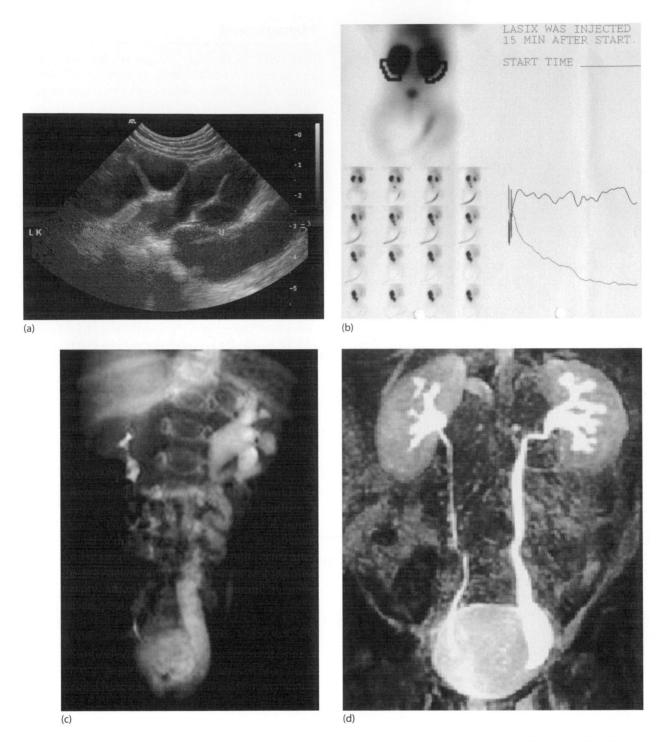

Figure 102.5 **(a)** Longitudinal scan to the left of the midline through the bladder demonstrates dilatation of the left lower ureter to the level of the vesicoureteric junction. **(b)** MAG 3 renal scan. Clearance curve for left kidney demonstrating obstructive pattern. **(c)** 30-minute full-length film from intravenous urogram series shows obstructed megaureter of the same patient. **(d)** MRU image showing obstructive left megaureter.

Bladder opening is narrowed with interrupted absorbable sutures.

COHEN'S METHOD

This method is simple and easier to perform, and is an especially useful technique in infants in whom the bladder is small. An incision is made in the mucosa above and a little lateral to the opposite ureteric orifice. A submucous tunnel is made by inserting the closed blades of scissors and performing an opening and cutting movement. The ureter is threaded through the tunnel (Figure 102.6d). The tunnel should be adequately wide for the ureter and two to three times the ureteric diameter in length to prevent reflux. The terminal narrow portion of the ureter is excised and sent for histology.

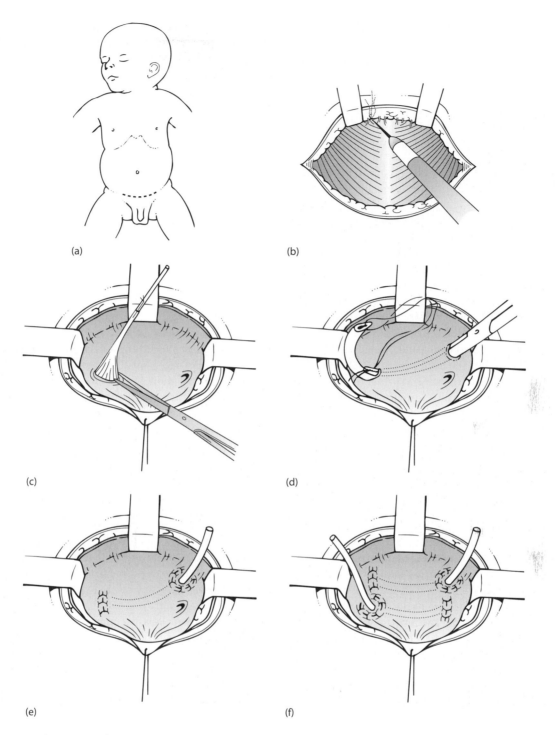

Figure 102.6 Reimplantation of ureter. **(a)** Position of patient on the operating table and line of incision. **(b)** Skin flaps being raised. **(c)** Opened bladder is retracted by Denis–Browne retractor and the stented ureter is dissected free. **(d)** Tunnel is commenced just above and lateral to the opposite ureteric orifice and continued to the original orifice. The ureter is threaded through the tunnel. **(e)** Cuff of the ureter is sutured in position. The original orifice in the bladder is closed. **(f)** In bilateral reimplantation, the second separate tunnel is parallel to the first and ends in the opposite orifice.

If the ureter is very dilated, remodeling is necessary, which may be performed by one of the following methods.

1. A nonexcisional tapering technique has the advantage of avoiding a suture line with potential urinary leakage. However, it is inappropriate for a very dilated ureter as it reduces the diameter by only 50%, and in neonates, it can become too bulky for the tunnel.

   a. Folding (Kalikinski) where a 10–12 Fr catheter is placed into the ureter and a running mattress suture placed proximally and continued distally. The lateral excluded segment is folded posteriorly and its edge fixed to the medial wall with another running suture.

b. Plication (Starr) of the ureteral wall is achieved by multiple mattress sutures in the antimesenteric border.

2. Excisional tapering technique where part of the ureteral wall is excised by using knife and scissors or Hendren clamps. The remaining ureteral strip is tubularized over 8 Fr double-J stent or feeding tube utilizing a running absorbable suture. The distal end of the ureter is closed with interrupted absorbed sutures to allow for any shortening that might be necessary. The proximal segment of the tailored ureter should stay outside the bladder after completion of the reimplantation in order to avoid a dilated obstruction of the tailored segment.

The cuff of the ureter is then sutured in position. First, a 4/0 Dexon suture is inserted laterally through the full thickness of the ureter and also through the full thickness of the bladder muscle so as to prevent the ureter from retracting. Next, the bladder and ureteral mucosa are approximated using interrupted 5/0 Dexon. The stents are placed in the ureter (Figure 102.6e). In bilateral reimplantation, the second ureter has its tunnel below and parallel to the first ending in the orifice of the opposite side (Figure 102.6b).

3. Politano–Leadbetter technique: The ureter is further freed up to the dome of the bladder. The new opening for the entrance of the ureter is made on the posterolateral aspect of the bladder. The new submucosal tunnel formed from there to the old ureteric orifice. Then the stay suture of the ureter passed and gently threaded through the new tunnel. The narrow terminal portion of the ureter is excised, the ureter is narrowed by one of the above techniques if needed, and the neo-ureter opening is fixed at the old opening with 5/0 Dexon. Stents are put in place.

A suprapubic catheter is left in the bladder and the bladder closed in two layers, the mucosa with 4/0 plain catgut and the muscles with 4/0 Dexon. A retropubic drain is brought out through a separate incision and the muscles are approximated with 3/0 Dexon. The rectus sheath is sutured with 3/0 Dexon and the skin approximated with 5/0 Dexon subcuticular stitch.

Endoscopic repair of ureter

Recent progress in endoscopic tools (such as miniscopes, balloons, and guide wires) has led to the widespread use of endoscopy for ureteral repair.[80,81] Some suggested that a simple insertion of the double-J stent into the obstructive ureter for 6 months may solve the problem.[82] Others have advocated balloon dilatation of the obstructed segment with 3.5 Fr dilating balloon, which is inflated to 12–14 atm, or until disappearance of the stenotic obstructive area.[83] This technique demonstrated 90% success rate not only in the short-term period but also in the long-term follow-up. Barat et al.[85] recently reported preliminary results with

endoureterotomy for congenital megaureters. The technique consists of incision of the obstructive segment of the ureter, which is inserted into the ureteral orifice ureteroscope. All of the layers of the ureter are incised in the long axis through the entire obstructive segment to expose the periureteral areolar tissue. A double-J stent is inserted for 3 weeks after the procedure. The risk of secondary reflux, which is a main concern after this type of procedure, has not been systematically checked. The role of endoureterotomy in the treatment of megaureters in children has not been widely established. Recently, some authors have advocated a laser incision on the obstructive segment following balloon dilatation at the same setting.[84] Although the initial results in the small group of patients were promising, long-term follow-up into adolescent period is required.

In some small children with a severe obstructive megaureter, refluxing ureteric reimplantation was suggested as a novel method to temporize an obstruction.[86] The treatment consists of anastomosing the ureter proximal to the obstruction to the dome of the bladder in a freely high-grade refluxing fashion. This technique allows time for the child to mature while accurately establishing renal function and preparing for a definitive surgical solution. We as well as others have employed end cutaneous ureterostomy in small infants, when the surgical treatment of a severe megaureter can pose formidable technical challenges, as an ideal way to release an obstruction and to allow the hydronephrosis to subside and to restore, or at least to preserve renal function while awaiting definitive ureteral reimplantation.[87]

Laparoscopic reimplantation

In recent years, laparoscopic reimplantation has gained popularity in some medical centers.[88–91] Employment of robot-assisted laparoscopic techniques in pediatric urology led to even wider application of laparoscopic reimplantation to the surgical armamentarium. Three procedures have been attempted laparoscopically: extravesical reimplantation, Gil–Vernet procedure, and the Cohen cross-trigonal reimplantation. Some difficulties were noticed with this approach such as long operative time, steep learning curve, and the technical challenges in the creation of a submucosal channel without injury to the intact bladder mucosa, and suturing aspects of the procedure. Utilization of the robot-assisted technique is supposed to overcome these difficulties. A recently published review of the national database of ureteral surgery from the United States showed that robot-assisted ureteric reimplantation still appears to be in its adoption phase and is clustered at a small number of hospitals.[91] The new da Vinci XI robot with 8-mm trocars might further optimize four-quadrant surgeries and probably will facilitate incorporeal dissection and suturing even in small infants.

POSTOPERATIVE COURSE

Patients are fasted for 24 hours in case of development of ileus. Ureteral reimplantation using the extravesical approach can be performed without stenting.[92,93] An indwelling urethral catheter is placed usually for 3–5 days to avoid urinary retention. If a double-JJ stent is used, they can be removed 7–10 days following surgery.

Complications

Complications include wound infection, vesicoureteral reflux due to short tunnel with no effective flap valve mechanism, or obstruction due to a fibrotic distal end secondary to ischemia.

Follow-up and results

Radiologic studies are used to assess initial and long-term surgical results and to monitor renal growth. These include ultrasound, intravenous urography, or radionuclide scans. The success is measured by normal urinary drainage with no reflux and control of urinary infections.

REFERENCES

1. Hsieh MH, Lai J, Saigal CS. Urological Diseases in America Project. Trends in prenatal sonography use and subsequent urologic diagnosis and abortions in the United States. *J Pediatr Urol* 2009; 5: 490–4.
2. Nguyen HT, Herndon CD, Cooper C et al. The Society for Fetal Urology consensus statement on the evaluation and management of antenatal hydronephrosis. *J Pediatr Urol* 2010; 6: 212–31.
3. Passerotti CC, Kalish LA, Chow J et al. The predictive value of the first postnatal ultrasound in children with antenatal hydronephrosis. *J Pediatr Urol* 2011; 7: 128–36.
4. Ransley PG, Dhillon HK, Gordon I et al. The postnatal management of hydronephrosis diagnosed by prenatal ultrasound. *J Urol* 1990; 144: 584–7.
5. Koff SA, Campbell K. Non-operative management of unilateral neonatal hydronephrosis. *J Urol* 1992; 148: 525–31.
6. Shukla AR, Cooper J, Patel PR et al. Prenatally detected primary megaureter: A role for extended follow up. *J Urol* 2005; 173(4): 1353–6.
7. Chertin B, Pollack A, Koulikov D et al. Conservative treatment of uretero-pelvic junction obstruction in children with antenatal diagnosis of hydronephrosis: Lessons learned after 16 years of follow up. *Eur Urol* 2006; 49(4): 734–9.
8. Peters CA. Congenital urine flow impairments of the upper urine tract: Pathophysiology and experimental studies. In: Gearhart JP, Rink RC, Mouriquand PDE (eds). *Pediatric Urology*, 2nd edn. Philadelphia: W.B. Saunders, 2009: 237–326.
9. El-Dahr SS, Lewy JE. Urinary tract obstruction and infection in the neonate. *Clin Perinatol* 1992; 19: 213–22.
10. Koff SA. Pathophysiology of ureteropelvic junction obstruction. Clinical and experimental observations. *Urol Clin N Am* 1990; 17: 263–72.
11. Weiss RM. Obstructive uropathy: Pathophysiology and diagnosis. In: Kelalis PP, King LR, Barry Belman A (eds). *Clinical Pediatric Urology*, 3rd ed. Philadelphia: W.B. Saunders Co., 1992: 664–82.
12. Tainio H, Kylmala T, Heikkinen A. Peptidergic innervation of the normal and obstructed human pyelo-ureteral junctions. *Urol Int* 1992; 48: 31–4.
13. Krueger RP, Ash JM, Silver MM et al. Primary hydronephrosis assessment of diureteric renography pelvis perfusion pressure, operative findings and renal and ureteral histology. *Urol Clin N Am* 1980; 7: 231–42.
14. Starr NT, Maizels M, Chou P et al. Microanatomy and morphometry of the hydronephrotic "obstructed" renal pelvis in asymptomatic infants. *J Urol* 1992; 148: 519–24.
15. Solari V, Piotrowska AP, Puri P. Altered expression of interstitial cells of Cajal in congenital uretero-pelvic junction obstruction. *J Urol* 2003; 170(6Pt1): 2420–2.
16. Kim YS, Do SH, Hong CH et al. Does every patient with ureteropelvic junction obstruction need voiding cystourethrography. *J Urol* 2001; 165: 2305–7.
17. Sherer DM. Is fetal hydronephrosis overdiagnosed? *Ultrasound Obstet Gynecol* 2000; 16: 601–6.
18. Harrison MR, Filly RA. The fetus with obstructive uropathy. In: Harrison MR, Gollous MS, Filly RA (eds). *Pathophysiology, Natural History, Selection and Treatment in the Unborn Patient: Prenatal diagnosis and treatment*. Philadelphia: W.B. Saunders Co., 1990: 238–402.
19. Fasolato V, Poloniato A, Bianchi C et al. Feto-neonatal ultrasonography to detect renal abnormalities: Evaluation of 1-year screening program. *Am J Perinatol* 1998; 15: 161–4.
20. Roth JA, Diamond DA. Prenatal hydronephrosis. *Curr Opin Pediatr* 2001; 13: 138–41.
21. Shokeir A, Nijman R. Antenatal hydronephrosis: Changing concepts in diagnosis and subsequent management. *BJU Int* 2000; 85: 987–94.
22. Avni FE, Cos T, Cassart M et al. Evolution of fetal ultrasonography. *Eur Radiol* 2007; 17(2): 419–31.
23. Fernloach SK, Maizels M, Conway JJ. Ultrasound grading of hydronephrosis: Introduction to the system used by the society for fetal urology. *Pediatric Radiol* 1993; 23: 278–80.
24. Woolf AA. A molecular and genetic view of human renal and urinary tract malformations. *Kidney Int* 2000; 58: 500–12.
25. Izquierdo L, Porteous M, Paramo PG, Connor JM. Evidence for genetic heterogeneity in hereditary hydronephrosis caused by pelvi-ureteric junction obstruction, with one locus assigned to chromosome 6p. *Hum Genet* 1992; 89: 557–60.

26. Pope JC, Brock JW III, Adams MC et al. Congenital anomalies of the kidney and urinary tract-role of the loss of function mutation in the pluripotent angiotensin type 2 receptor gene. *J Urol* 2001; 165: 196–202.

27. Nishimura H, Yerkes E, Hohenfellner K et al. Role of the angiotensin type 2 receptor gene in congenital anomalies of the kidney and urinary tract, CAKUT, of mice and men. *Mol Cell* 1999; 3: 1–10.

28. O'Reilly PH. Diuresis renography. Recent advances and recommended protocols. *Br J Urol* 1992; 69: 113–20.

29. Piepsz A, Blaufox MD, Gordon I et al. Consensus on renal cortical scintigraphy in children with urinary tract infection. Scientific Committee of Radionuclides in Nephrourology. *Semin Nucl Med* 1999; 2: 160–74.

30. Upsdell SM, Testa HJ, Lawson RS. The F-15, diuresis renogram in suspected obstruction of the upper urinary tract. *Br J Urol* 1992; 69: 126–31.

31. Nauta J, Pot DJ, Kooij PPM et al. Forced hydration prior to renography in children with hydronephrosis. An evaluation. *B J Urol* 1991; 68: 93–7.

32. Koff SA, McDowell GC, Byard M. Diureteric radionuclide assessment of obstruction in the infant. Guidelines for successful interpretation. *J Urol* 1988; 140: 1167–8.

33. Riccabona M, Avni FE, Blickman JG et al. Imaging recommendations in paediatric uroradiology. Minutes of the ESPR uroradiology task force session on childhood obstructive uropathy, high-grade fetal hydronephrosis, childhood haematuria, and urolithiasis in childhood. ESPR Annual Congress, Edinburgh, UK. *Pediatr Radiol* 2009; 39(8): 891–8.

34. Khrichenko D, Darge K. Functional analysis in MR urography—Made simple. *Pediatr Radiol* 2010; 40(2): 182–99.

35. Whitaker RH. Methods of assessing obstruction in dilated ureters. *Br J Urol* 1973; 45: 15–22.

36. Rohatagi M, Bajpai M, Gupta DK, Gupta AK. Role of ultrasound guided percutaneous antegrade pyelography (USPCAP) in the diagnosis of obstructive uropathy. *Indian Pediatr* 1992; 29: 425–31.

37. King LR, Coughlin PW, Bloch EC et al. The case for immediate pyeloplasty in the neonate with ureteropelvic junction obstruction. *J Urol* 1984; 132: 725–7.

38. Chevalier RL, Gomez RA, Jones CE. Developmental determinants of recovery after relief of partial ureteral obstruction. *Kidney Int* 1988; 33: 775–81.

39. Ulman I, Jayanthi VR, Koff SA. The long-term follow-up of newborns with severe unilateral hydronephrosis initially treated nonoperatively. *J Urol* 2000; 164(3 Pt2): 1101–5.

40. Thorup J, Mortensen T, Diemer H et al. The prognosis of surgically treated congenital hydronephrosis after diagnosis in utero. *J Urol* 1985; 134: 914–7.

41. Sheldon CA, Duckett JW, Snyder HM. Evolution in the management of infant pyeloplasty. *J Pediatr Surg* 1992; 27: 501–5.

42. Carr MC, El-Ghoneimi A. Anomalies and surgery of the ureteropelvic junction obstruction in children. In: Wein AJ, Kavoussi LR, Novick AC, Partin AW, Peters CA (eds). *Campbell–Walsh Urology*, 9th edn. Philadelphia: Saunders, Elsevier, 2007: 3359–82.

43. Palmer LS, Proano JM, Palmer JS. Renal pelvis cuff pyeloplasty for ureteropelvic junction obstruction for high inserting ureter: An initial experience. *J Urol* 2005; 174(3): 1088–90.

44. Motola JA, Badlani GH, Smith AD. Results of 212 consecutive endopyelotomies: An 8-year follow-up. *J Urol* 1993; 149: 453–6.

45. Kavoussi LR, Meretyk S, Dierks SM et al. Endopyelotomy for secondary uretero-pelvic junction obstruction in children. *J Urol* 1991; 145: 345–9.

46. Figenshau RS, Clayman RV. Endourologic options for management ureteropelvic junction obstruction in the pediatric patient. *Urol Clin N Am* 1998; 25: 199–209.

47. Tan HL. Laparoscopic Anderson–Hynes dismembered pyeloplasty in children using needlescopic instrumentation. *Urol Clin N Am* 2001; 28(1): 43–51.

48. Yeung CK, Tam YH, Sihoe JD et al. Retroperitoneoscopic dismembered pyeloplasty for pelvi-ureteric junction obstruction in infants and children. *BJU Int* 2001; 87(6): 509–13.

49. Seixas-Mikelus SA, Jenkins LC, Williot P, Greenfield SP. Pediatric pyeloplasty: Comparison of literature meta-analysis of laparoscopic and open techniques with open surgery at a single institution. *J Urol* 2009; 182(5): 2428–32.

50. Kocherov S, Lev G, Chertin L, Chertin B. Extracorporeal ureteric stenting for pediatric laparoscopic pyeloplasty. *Eur J Pediatr Surg* 2016; 1: 1–137.

51. Casale P. Robotic pyeloplasty in the pediatric population. *Curr Opin Urol* 2009; 19(1): 97–101.

52. O'Brien ST, Shukla AR. Transition from open to robotic-assisted pediatric pyeloplasty: A feasibility and outcome study. *J Pediatr Urol* 2014; 8(3): 276–81.

53. Bassiouny IE. Salvage pyeloplasty in non-visualising hydronephrotic kidney secondary to ureteropelvic junction obstruction. *J Urol* 1992; 148: 685–7.

54. Chertin B, Pollack A, Koulikov D et al. Does renal function remain stable after puberty in children with prenatal hydronephrosis and improved renal function after pyeloplasty? *J Urol* 2009; 182(4 Suppl): 1845–8.

55. Cussen LJ. The morphology of congenital dilatation of ureter: Intrinsic ureteral lesions. *Aust NZJ Surg* 1971; 41: 185–94.

56. Hellstrom M, Hajlmas K, Jacobsson B et al. Normal ureteral diameter in infancy and childhood. *Acta Radiol* 1985; 26: 433–5.

57. Smith ED, Cussen LJ, Glenn J et al. Report of working party to establish an international nomenclature for the large ureter. *Birth Defects* 1977; 13: 3–5.

58. King LR. Megaloureter: Definition, diagnosis and management. (Ed.) *J Urol* 1980; 123: 222–3.

59. Tanagho EA. Intrauterine fetal ureteral obstruction. *J Urol* 1973; 109: 196–203.
60. Tanagho EA, Smith DR, Guthrie TM. Pathophysiology of functional ureteral obstruction. *J Urol* 1970; 104: 73–8.
61. McLaughlin AP III, Pfister RC, Leadbetter WF et al. The pathophysiology of primary megaloureter. *J Urol* 1973; 109: 805–11.
62. Hanna MK, Jeffs RD, Sturgess JM, Barkin M. Ureteral structure and ultrastructure. Part II. Congenital uretero-pelvic junction obstruction and primary obstructive megaureter. *J Urol* 1976; 116: 725–30.
63. Lee BR, Partin AW, Epstein JI et al. A quantitative histological analysis of the dilated ureter of childhood. *J Urol* 1992; 148: 1482–6.
64. Fridrich U, Schreiber D, Gottschalk E, Dietz W. Ultrastructure of the distal ureter in congenital malformations in childhood. *Z Fur Kinderchirurgie* 1987; 42: 94–102.
65. Dixon JS, Jen PYP, Yeung CK et al. The vesico-ureteric junction in three cases of primary obstructive megaureter associated with ectopic ureteric insertion. *BJU Int* 1998; 81: 580–4.
66. Payabvash S, Kajbafzadeh AM, Tavangar SM et al. Myocyte apoptosis in primary obstructive megaureters: The role of decreased vascular and neural supply. *J Urol* 2007; 179(1): 259–64.
67. Arena E, Nicotina PA, Arena S et al. Interstitial cells of Cajal network in primary obstructive megaureter. *Pediatr Med Chir* 2007; 29(1): 28–31.
68. Seeds JW, Mittlestaedt CA, Mandell J. Prenatal and postnatal ultrasonographic diagnosis of congenital obstructive uropathies. *Urol Clin N Am* 1988; 13: 131–54.
69. Helin I, Persson P. Prenatal diagnosis of urinary tract abnormalities by ultrasound. *Pediatr* 1986; 78: 879–83.
70. Shokeir AA, Nijman RJM. Primary megaureter: Current trends in diagnosis and treatment. *BJU Int* 2000; 86: 861–8.
71. Mclellan DL, Retic AB, Bauer SB et al. Rate and predictors of spontaneous resolution of prenatally diagnosed primary nonrefluxing megaureter. *J Urol* 2002; 168: 2177–80.
72. Hanna MK, Jeffs RD. Primary obstructive megaureter in children. *Urol* 1975; 6: 419–27.
73. Retik AB, McEvoy JP, Bauer SB. Megaureters in children. *Urol* 1978; 11: 231–6.
74. Williams DI, Hulme-Moir I. Primary obstructive megaureter. *Br J Urol* 1970; 42: 140–9.
75. Keating MA, Retik AB. Management of the dilated obstructed ureter. *Urol Clin N Am* 1990; 17: 291–306.
76. Chertin B, Pollack A, Koulikov D et al. Long-term follow up of antenatal diagnosed megaureters. *J Ped Urol* 2008; 4: 188–91.
77. Wood BP, Ben-Ami T, Teele RL, Rabinowitz R. Uretero-vesical obstruction and megaloureter: Diagnosis by real time US. *Radiol* 1985; 156: 79–81.
78. Fung LCT, Churchill BM, McLorie GA et al. Ureteral opening pressure: A novel parameter for the evaluation of pediatric hydronephrosis. *J Urol* 1998; 159: 1326–30.
79. Koo HP, Bloom DA. Lower ureteral reconstruction. *Urol Clin N Am* 1999; 26(1): 167–73.
80. Desgrandchamps F. Endoscopic and surgical repair of the ureter. *Curr Opin Urol* 2001; 11: 271–4.
81. Kajbafzadeh AM, Payabvash S, Salmasi AH et al. Endoureterotomy for treatment of primary obstructive megaureter in children. *J Endourol* 2007; 21(7): 743–9.
82. Castagnetti M, Cimador M, Sergio M et al. Double J stent insertion across vesicoureteral junction is it a valuable initial approach in neonates and infants with severe primary nonrefluxing megaureter. *Urology* 2006; 68(4): 870–5.
83. Bujons A, Saldaña L, Caffaratti J et al. Can endoscopic balloon dilation for primary obstructive megaureter be effective in a long-term follow-up? *J Pediatr Urol* 2015; 11(1): 37,e1–6.
84. Christman MS, Kasturi S, Lambert SM et al. Endoscopic management and the role of double stenting for primary obstructive megaureters. *J Urol* 2012; 187(3): 1018–22.
85. Barat S, Barat M, Kirpekar D. Endoureterotomy for congenital primary obstructive megaureter: Preliminary report. *J Endourol* 2000; 14: 263–7.
86. Lee SD, Akbal C, Kaefer M. Refluxing ureteral reimplant as temporary treatment of obstructive megaureter in neonate and infant. *J Urol* 2005; 173(4): 1357–60.
87. Kitchens DM, DeFoor W, Minevich E et al. End cutaneous ureterostomy for the management of severe hydronephrosis. *J Urol* 2007; 177(4): 1501–4.
88. Canon SJ, Jayanthi VR, Patel AS. Vesicoscopic cross-trigonal ureteral reimplantation: A minimally invasive option for repair of vesicoureteral reflux. *J Urol* 2007; 178(1): 269–73.
89. Smaldone MC, Polsky E, Ricchiuti DJ et al. Advances in pediatric urologic laparoscopy. *Sci World J* 2007; 22(7): 727–41.
90. Lee RS, Sethi AS, Passerotti CC et al. Robot-assisted laparoscopic nephrectomy and contralateral ureteric reimplantation in children. *J Endourol* 2010; 24(1): 123–8.
91. Bowen DK, Faasse MA, Liu DB et al. Use of pediatric open, laparoscopic and robot-assisted laparoscopic ureteral reimplantation in the United States: 2000 to 2012. *J Urol* 2016; 196(1): 207–12.
92. Wacksman J, Gilbert A, Sheldon CA. Results of the renewed extravesical reimplant for surgical correction of vesicoureteral reflux. *J Urol* 1992; 148: 359–61.
93. Burbige KA, Miller M, Connor JP. Extravesical ureteral reimplantation: Results in 128 patients. *J Urol* 1996; 155: 1721–2.

103

Ureteral duplication anomalies

PREM PURI AND HIDESHI MIYAKITA

INTRODUCTION

Duplication of the ureter and renal pelvis is the most common upper urinary tract anomaly with a reported incidence of 0.8%[1] in the population and in 1.8%–4.2% of pyelograms.[2–5] The vast majority of these anomalies have normally developed renal moieties and cause nonfunctional problems. However, they can challenge the diagnostic acumen with a wide variety of manifestations. Complete duplex systems may be associated with vesicoureteral reflux (VUR) or may be ectopic or subtended by an ectopic ureterocele. Incomplete duplex systems are most often associated with ureteroureteral reflux or ureteropelvic junction obstruction of the lower pole of the kidney.[6,7]

EMBRYOLOGY

The ureteric bud appears at 5 weeks' gestation from the place where the Wolffian duct bends centrally and medially to the cloaca and pushes into the pelvic metanephrogenic mass and eventually forms the ureter and renal pelvis. Premature division of the ureteral bud gives rise to incomplete duplication. If two ureteral buds arise from the Wolffian duct and if both are incorporated into the urogenital sinus, then complete duplication occurs. The upper pole ureter is more closely associated with the Wolffian duct, while the lower pole ureteric bud is closest to the urogenital sinus and incorporated first. The upper pole ureter is carried medially and caudally along with the Wolffian duct. Therefore, the upper pole ureter opens more medially and inferiorly than the lower pole ureter, according to the Weigert–Mayer law.[8–10] Sometimes this upper pole ureter has an abnormally prolonged or close attachment to the Wolffian duct, which will migrate into the segment of urogenital sinus that is destined to become the urethra.

Occasionally in males, a separate opening into the urogenital sinus is not established and the bud continues to be linked to the Wolffian duct much longer, and the ureter comes to insert in the male genital tract such as in seminal vesicles, vas deferens, or even epididymis.

Stephens[11] proposed that, in females, the fused Mullerian ducts after penetrating the urogenital sinus undergo significant epithelial activity and incorporate any Wolffian duct remnants; thus, the ureteral bud along with the Wolffian duct may be carried along as part of caudal Mullerian migration, and this in turn would lead to drainage sites into the vestibule, vagina, cervix, and uterus.

CLASSIFICATION

A standard set of definitions used to describe ureteral duplications anomalies now exists. These definitions were established by the Urologic Section of the American Academy of Pediatrics Committee on Terminology, Nomenclature and Classification.[12] The following are the different types of ureteropelvic duplications, the recognition of which is important in understanding the pathophysiology, clinical manifestations, and management:

1. Incomplete ureteral duplication, where two ureters unite and enter the bladder through a common orifice.
2. Complete ureteral duplication
   a. Intravesical: Two ureters drain separately into the bladder. The upper pole opens caudal and medial to lower pole ureter and has a longer ureterovesical course and therefore less risk of reflux.
   b. Extravesical: Where the ureter opens into the urethra or genital tract.
3. Inverted Y ureteral duplication. Two distal ureters fuse to drain a single kidney; one of the limbs may be ectopic, blind-ending, or atretic.
4. Blind bifid ureter. One branch ends blindly, and this is thought to be because one ureteral bud does not join the metanephrogenic mass.
5. Ureteral triplication and even quadruplication have been reported and are due to formation and/or division into three or four buds.[13–15]

CLINICAL MANIFESTATION

Most often, ureteral duplication anomalies are discovered incidentally unassociated with any symptoms. Infants may come to medical attention because of the complications of obstruction of the upper moiety or infection. VUR is common, occurring much more frequently in the lower segment and is present in 70% of children with duplex systems who present with urinary tract infections.[1,16]

A total of 60% of duplex systems have bifid ureters, with 40% showing complete ureteral duplication. Duplication affects both sides equally, while 15% of patients have bilateral duplications. It is more common in females, who are more likely to exhibit pathological complications. The 8%–11% prevalence of duplex anomalies in females was reported,[17,18] and girls were affected about two times more often than boys.[6]

There is a familial tendency with the risk of duplication in a sibling up to one in eight and is suggestive of autosomal dominant inheritance with incomplete penetration.[4,19] A recent study reported prevalence of duplex systems in familial VUR.[20] Duplex systems were present in 39 (7.6%) of the 513 siblings with VUR. Families with exclusively boys affected with VUR had significantly higher rate (15%) of duplex systems than in families with mixed affected siblings and girls.

Ureterocele, a cystic dilatation of the terminal intramural segment of the distal ureter, is classified as either simple or ectopic.[12] The ectopic variety is symptomatic in infants far more commonly than simple ureterocele and is nearly always with an obstructed upper segment of a duplex kidney. The bulging ureterocele protrudes into the intravesical space and terminates ectopically at the bladder neck or in the urethra. Whether associated with single or duplex systems, the problems of ureterocele are much more common in girls than in boys.

Ureteral duplication can present with diverse clinical manifestations and include the following:

- Urinary tract infection, which may be due to reflux or obstruction. This can vary from overwhelming sepsis to asymptomatic bacteria.
- Epididymo-orchitis as a result of an ectopic ureter opening into the male genital tract.
- Incontinence, which is due to an ectopic ureter opening beyond the sphincter and is thus more common in females or because of infection causing urge incontinence.
- Urinary retention. A ureterocele occupying the bladder neck can cause urinary retention and overflow incontinence. Rarely, it may prolapse through the urethra (Figure 103.1).
- Abdominal mass. Hydronephrosis secondary to obstruction may present with abdominal mass.
- Failure to thrive, because of chronic persistent urinary infection.

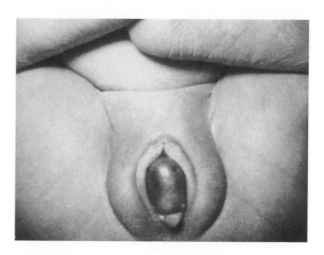

Figure 103.1 Ureterocele prolapsing through the urethra in a newborn.

Prenatal diagnosis

The kidneys can be imaged at the 12th gestational week by abdominal ultrasound. With the increased availability and use of maternal ultrasonography, the incidence of urinary tract disorders diagnosed in utero has increased considerably. Oligohydramnios or anhydramnios in the mother is usually due to diminished amniotic fluid. Because amniotic fluid after 18 weeks of gestation is voided urine, it suggests bilateral renal agenesis or outflow obstruction. In order to be certain that renal development is normal, ultrasound at or beyond 20 weeks of gestation is necessary. An obstruction anomaly is recognized by demonstrating a dilated renal pelvis, calyces, or ureter. However, it is not possible to detect an uncomplicated duplex anomaly prenatally.[21] Detection of duplex kidney in the prenatal period offers several potential benefits. For affected fetus, there is the opportunity to plan postnatal management to minimize the risk of long-term renal impairment, by early administration of antibiotics, investigation, and treatment.

Postnatal diagnosis

Ultrasonography, which does not visualize the excretory pathway, may be unable to differentiate between kidneys with and without pyeloureteral duplication, but is able to recognize thick transverse intermediate cortical mass (1 cm) in the latter group and also on the basis of the ratio between the longitudinal and transverse diameter, which is greater than in kidneys without duplication.[22] An obstructed or refluxing system and ureteroceles can be visualized on the ultrasound scans (Figure 103.2).

Micturating cystourethrograms will delineate reflux and ureteroceles. Despite its declining role in the routine evaluation of infants with UTIs, intravenous urography is a useful and easily available modality of investigation.[23] It accurately defines the anatomy, while in the nonfunctioning segment the remaining pole will exhibit the "drooping lily" sign (Figure 103.3). Radionuclide scans are useful in determining the differential function.[24] Computerized tomography and magnetic

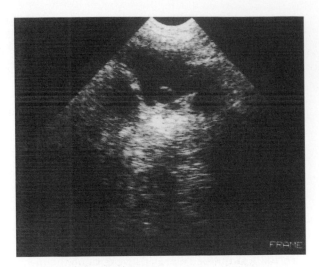

Figure 103.2 Sonographic appearance of a ureterocele within the bladder.

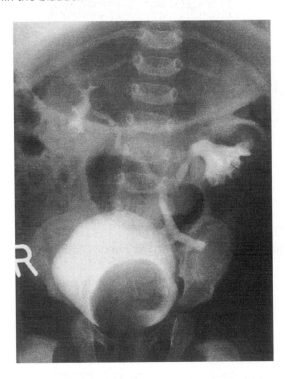

Figure 103.3 Twenty-minute film from urogram showing "drooping lily" sign on the left as a consequence of an obstructed nonfunctioning upper moiety on this side due to a large ureterocele.

resonance imaging (MRI) scans may help to define the anatomy of kidneys, and MRI is particularly useful in cases where conventional imaging fails to delineate occult dysplastic renal moieties, ectopic ureters, and ureteroceles. Diagnosis is usually confirmed by cystoscopy and endoscopic visualization of the ureteral orifices. It also helps to assess the extent of ureterocele.

MANAGEMENT

Asymptomatic uncomplicated ureteral duplications do not require active clinical management.

Vesicoureteral reflux

VUR is the most common problem associated with ureteral duplication and is more common in lower poles than in upper poles. Most of the recent reports suggest that there is no difference in the rate of spontaneous resolution of minor grades of reflux into single ureters or lower pole ureters in duplex systems.[24-27] Medical surveillance should be continued in these patients to prevent renal scarring. High-grade VUR in duplex systems is unlikely to resolve and generally considered an indication for surgical treatment.[16,25] Comparing the outcome of VUR in duplex systems with VUR in a single system, it was found that VUR in duplex systems was resolved in only 7% of refluxing units with grade III and none of those with grades IV and V at a median follow-up of 33 months.[16] The reported rates of spontaneous resolution of grades I and II reflux in duplex systems vary from 22% to 85%.[25-27]

In the newborn period, conservative antimicrobial treatment combined with full urological investigations is the management of choice. Infants with grades I–III reflux should continue on chemoprophylaxis. High grades of reflux in infants associated with ureteral duplication, breakthrough infections in spite of prophylaxis, and progressive renal scarring and poor function constitute indications for antireflux operation[28,29] or endoscopic correction.[30]

Polar nephroureterectomy is performed in patients who have one pole ureter reflux with poorly functioning segment of kidney, while nephroureterectomy may be necessary if both poles are involved. Recently, the role of laparoscopic heminephrectomy in pediatric patients has begun to be appreciated.[31-34] Both transperitoneal and retroperitoneal laparoscopic techniques have been used for heminephrectomy in infants and children. The transperitoneal approach for moiety excision is technically simple and offers the added advantage of complete ureterectomy. The retroperitoneal approach, although technically more challenging, offers the advantages of a direct access to the kidney, minimal mobilization of kidney and surrounding structures, and a decreased risk of intraperitoneal organ injury and postoperative adhesions.

In patients with lower pole reflux only in complete ureter duplication, Ahmed and Boucout[29] and Bivens and Palken[35] recommend ipsilateral ureteroureterostomy when there is no abnormality on the contralateral side, or there is history of bladder operation or abnormality thickened bladders. They propose that this operation has fewer complications and requires shorter hospitalization, no postoperative bladder catheters are required, and, as the nonrefluxing ureteral orifice and submucosal tunnel are not disturbed, there is no risk of creating reflux. This can be undertaken either by suprapubic incision or extraperitoneal iliac fossa incision. Ureteroureterostomy would be carried out for complete ureteral duplication associated with VUR, obstructing ureterocele, and ectopic ureters, as well as using laparoscopic surgery.[36,37] The significant discrepancy in ureteral size did not preclude ureteroureterostomy.

Another surgical option is reimplantation of ureters. Only a refluxing ureter may be undertaken if it can be safely separated. In patients with reflux into both ureters and those where the refluxing ureter cannot be safely separated, common sheath ureteric reimplantation is undertaken. Ellsworth et al.[38] reported 10-year experience with common sheath reimplantation in 54 refluxing units. Common sheath reimplantation yields a 98% success rate with minimal morbidity. Recently, laparoscopic extravesical transperitoneal ureteral reimplantation using the Lich–Gregoir procedure was developed in refluxing duplicated collecting systems.[39] Furthermore, robot-assisted laparoscopic surgery is spreading ureteral reimplantation as well as heminephrectomy.[40,41] All procedures were successfully completed laparoscopically, and reflux was corrected in all children.

In incompletely duplicated ureters, surgical options include reimplantation of the common distal ureter if the junction is proximal or when the junction is close to bladder excision of the common segment, with reimplantation of both ureters in the bladder or ureteroureterostomy with reimplantation of one ureter. However, if the function is poor, nephroureterectomy is necessary to avoid a diverticulum-like defect.

Minimally invasive endoscopic technique for the correction of VUR has become an established alternative to long-term antibiotic prophylaxis and surgical treatment. Endoscopic subureteric Deflux® injection is effective in treating duplex reflux of higher grades in complete and incomplete systems.[28,42,43] The technique of endoscopic injection of Deflux® is simple and straightforward. With an incomplete duplex system, the technique is the same as in a single system. All cystoscopes available for infants and children can be used for this procedure. The disposable Puri flexible catheter (STORZ) or a rigid metallic can be used for injection. A 1 ml syringe filled with Deflux® is attached to the injection catheter. Under direct vision through the cystoscope, the needle is introduced under the bladder mucosa 2–3 mm below the affected ureteral orifice at the 6 o'clock position. In children with grades IV and V reflux with wide ureteral orifices, the needle should be inserted not below but directly

in the affected ureteral orifice. The needle is advanced about 4–5 mm under the mucosa and the injection started slowly. As the Deflux® is injected, a bulge appears in the floor of the submucosal ureter. A correctly placed injection creates the appearance of a nipple on the top, which is a slit-like or inverted crescent orifice (Figures 103.4 and 103.5).

In the case of a complete ureteral duplication, the needle is introduced 2–3 mm below the lower ureteric orifice at

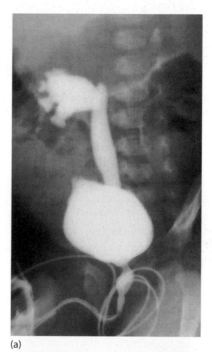

(a)

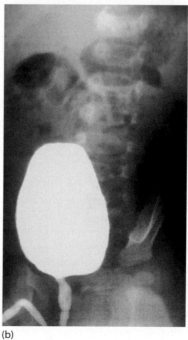

(b)

Figure 103.5 **(a)** Micturating cystogram in an 8-week-old boy shows grade IV vesicoureteric reflux into the lower moiety of the right duplex system. **(b)** Micturating cystogram in the same boy following endoscopic correction of reflux.

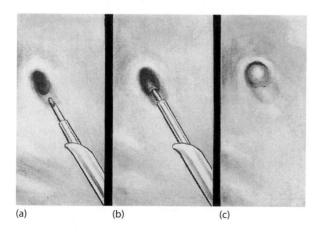

(a)　　　　(b)　　　　(c)

Figure 103.4 Technique of subureteric injection in an incomplete duplex system. **(a)** Site of placement of needle. **(b)** Injection in progress. **(c)** Slit-like orifice at the finish of injection.

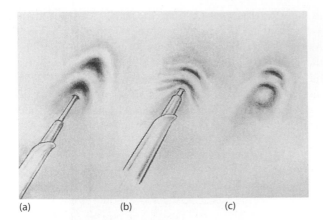

Figure 103.6 Technique of subureteric injection in a complete duplex system. **(a)** Site of placement of needle in a complete duplex system. **(b)** Injection in progress. **(c)** Slit-like orifice at the completion of injection.

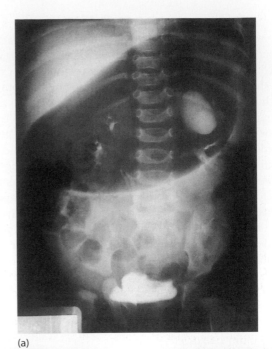

(a)

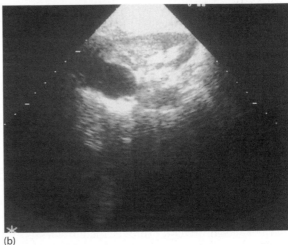

(b)

the 6 o'clock position, but the entire length of the needle (8 mm) is advanced behind the two ureters. During injection, the needle is slowly withdrawn until a "volcanic" bulge of paste is seen and the two ureteric orifices look slit-like (Figure 103.6). Patients are treated as day cases, and a voiding cystourethrogram and ultrasound are performed 6–12 weeks after discharge.

Ureteropelvic junction obstruction

In the bifid system, obstruction commonly involves the lower pole.[34–38] Upper pole ureteropelvic junction obstruction is uncommon (Figure 103.7a and b). In patients with low bifurcations and who have long ureteral segments, a standard pyeloplasty can safely be performed. If the lower pole ureteral segment is short, an end-to-end anastomosis of the lower pole pelvis to the upper pole ureter, eliminating the short lower pole ureter, may be necessary. Alternatively, the short lower pole ureter is retained and incorporated into a wider anastomosis. In patients with incomplete duplications, it is possible to widen the narrowed junction of the lower pole segment to the upper pole ureter by making a vertical incision in the anterior wall and suturing it transversely.[44] If there is nonfunction of the obstructed segment, a heminephroureterectomy to the level of the bifurcation is necessary to avoid leaving a ureteral stump into which ureteroureteral reflux can occur.[44]

The management of ureterocele is complex.[45–47] Consideration of ureterocele as intravesical or extravesical is important because the technique of surgical reconstruction can be different. If the function is good, endoscopic incision of the ureterocele may be tried. The advantage of this procedure is that this is straightforward management, especially in septic babies. The obstruction can be solved by simple puncture of ureterocele rather than endoscopic incision. The reflux rate to the ureterocele moiety following endoscopic puncture is negligible. We have used in all our babies a stylet of the 3-Fr ureteral catheter for endoscopic puncture. The puncture hole is made high enough and lateral on

Figure 103.7 **(a)** Bilateral duplex system. Urogram showing obstructed upper moiety on the left due to pelvi-ureteric junction obstruction. **(b)** Longitudinal sonographic scan through the left kidney in the coronal plane in the same patient, demonstrating pelvi–ureteric junction obstruction to upper moiety and normal lower moiety.

the ureterocele in order to avoid reobstruction and to create postpuncture flap sufficient to preserve the flap-valve antireflux mechanism. If the reflux developed after endoscopic puncture, it is usually a low grade and does not require any treatment. If the child develops breakthrough infections or high-grade reflux, endoscopic correction of reflux can be easily performed.[30]

REFERENCES

1. Privett JTJ, Jeans WD, Roylance J. The incidence and importance of renal duplication. *Clin Radiol* 1976; 27: 521–30.

2. Nordmarck B. Double formations of the pelvis of the kidney and ureters: Embryology, occurrence and clinical significance. *Ann Rad* 1948; 30: 276.

3. Nation FF. Duplication of the kidney and ureter: A statistical study of two hundred thirty new cases. *J Urol* 1944; 51: 456–65.

4. Atwell JD, Cook PL, Howell CJ. Familial incidence of bifid and double ureters. *Arch Dis Child* 1974; 49: 390–3.

5. Hartman GW, Hodson CJ. The duplex kidney and related abnormalities. *Clin Radiol* 1969; 20: 387.

6. Decter RN. Renal duplication and fusion anomalies. *Pediatr Clin N Am* 1997; 44: 1323.

7. Fernbach SK, Feinstein KA, Spencer K, Lindstrom CA. Ureteral duplication and its complications. *Radiographics* 1997; 17: 109.

8. Churchill BM, Abovea EO, McLorie GA. Ureteral duplication, ectopy and ureterocele. *Pediatr Clin N Am* 1987; 34: 1273–89.

9. Mayer R. Development of the ureter in the human embryo: A mechanistic consideration. *Anat Rec* 1946; 96: 355.

10. Weigert C. Uebeteinige bildunsfetster der Ureteren. *Virch Arch* 1877; 70: 490.

11. Stephens FO. *Congenital Malformations of the Urinary Tract*. New York: Prager, 1983: 186–363.

12. Glassberg KI, Braren V, Duckett JW. Suggested terminology for duplex systems, ectopic ureters and ureteroceles. Report of the Committee on Terminology, Nomenclature and Classification. American Academy of Pediatrics. *J Urol* 1986; 132: 1153–5.

13. Gosalbes R Jr, Gosalbes R, Piro C et al. Ureteral triplication and ureterocoele. Report of three cases and review of the literature. *J Urol* 1991; 145: 105–8.

14. Luque Mialdea R, DeThomas E, Aprojo F et al. Ureteral triplication: Double extravesical ureteral ectopic. *J Urol* 1991; 145: 109–11.

15. Soderahl DW, Shivaki LW, Sabamber DT. Bilateral ureteral quadruplication. *J Urol* 1976; 116: 255.

16. Afshar K, Papanikolaou F, Malek R et al. Vesicoureteral reflux and complete ureteral duplication, conservative or surgical management? *J Urol* 2005; 173: 1725–7.

17. Bisset GS 3rd, Strife JL. The duplex collecting system in girls with urinary tract infection: Prevalence and significance. *AJR Am J Roentgenol* 1987; 148: 497.

18. Siomou E, Papadpoulou F, Kollios KD et al. Duplex collecting system diagnosed during the first 6 tears of life after a first urinary tract infection: A study of 63 children *J Urol* 2006; 175: 678–82.

19. Whitaker J, Banks DM. A study of the inheritance of duplication of the kidneys and ureters. *J Urol* 1966; 95: 176.

20. Hunziker M, Mohanan N, Menezes M et al. Prevalence of duplex collecting systems in familial vesicoureteral reflux. *Pediatr Surg Int* 2010; 26: 115–7.

21. Bronshtein M, Yoffe N, Brandes JM et al. First and early second trimester diagnosis of fetal urinary tract anomalies using transvaginal sonography. *Prenat Diag* 1990; 10: 653–66.

22. Dalla Palma L, Bazzocchi M, Cressa C et al. Radiological anatomy of the kidney revisited. *Br J Radiol* 1990; 63: 680–90.

23. Fernbach SK, Feinstein KA, Spencer K et al. Ureteral duplication and its complications. *Radiographics* 1997; 17(1): 109–27.

24. Pattaras JG, Rushton HG, Majd M. The role of 99mtechnetium dimercapto-succinic acid renal scan in the evaluation of the occult ectopic ureters in girls with paradoxical incontinence. *J Urol* 1999; 162(3 Pt 1): 821–5.

25. Lee PH, Diamond DA, Duffy P et al. Duplex reflux: A study of 105 children. *J Urol* 1991; 146: 657–9.

26. Hausmann DA, Allen TD. Resolution of vesico-ureteral reflux in completely duplicated systems: Fact or fiction? *J Urol* 1991; 145: 1022–3.

27. Ben-Ami T, Gayer G, Hertz M et al. The natural history of reflux in the lower pole of duplicating collecting systems: A controlled study. *Pediatr Radiol* 1989; 19: 308–10.

28. Amar AD, Chabra K. Reflux in duplicated ureters. *J Pediatr Surg* 1970; 5: 419–30.

29. Ahmed S, Boucout HA. Vesicoureteral reflux in complete ureteral duplication: Surgical options. *J Urol* 1988; 140: 1092–4.

30. Puri P, Mohanan NU, Menezes M et al. Endoscopic treatment of moderate and high grade vesicoureteral reflux in infants using dextranomer/hyaluronic acid. *J Urol* 2007; 178: 1714–6.

31. Mushtaq I, Haleblian G. Laparoscopic heminephrectomy in infants and children: First 54 cases. *J Pediatr Urol* 2007; 3(2): 100–3.

32. Gao Z, Wu J, Lin C et al. Transperitoneal laparoscopic heminephrectomy in duplex kidney: Our initial experience. *Urology* 2011; 77(1): 231–6.

33. Leclair MD, Vidal I, Suply E et al. Retroperitoneal laparoscopic heminephrectomy in duplex kidney in infants and children: A 15-year experience. *Eur Urol* 2009; 56(2): 385–9.

34. Singh RR, Wagener S, Chandran H. Laparoscopic management and outcomes in non-functioning moieties of duplex kidneys in children. *J Pediatr Urol* 2010; 6(1): 66–9.

35. Bivens A, Palken M. Ureteroureterostomy for reflux in duplex systems. *J Urol* 1971; 106: 290.

36. Lashley DB, McAleer IM, Kaplan GW. Ipsilateral ureteroureterostomy for the treatment of vesicoureteral reflux or obstruction associated with complete ureteral duplication. *J Urol* 2001; 165: 552–4.

37. Corbett ST, Burris MB, Hemdon CD. Pediatric robot-assisted laparoscopic ipsilateral ureteroureterostomy in a duplicated collecting system. *J Pedatr Urol* 2013; 1239.e1–2.

38. Ellsworth PI, Lim DJ, Walker RD et al. Common sheath reimplantation yields excellent results in the treatment of vesicoureteral reflux in duplicated collecting system. *J Urol* 1996; 155(4): 1407–9.

39. Lopez M, Melo C, Francois M et al. Laparoscopic extravesical transperitoneal approach following the lich-gregoir procedure in refluxing duplicated collecting systems: Initial experience. *J Laparoendosc Adv Surg Tech A* 2011, 21: 165–9.

40. Hayashi Y, Mizuno K, Kurokawa S et al. Extravesical robot-assisted laparoscopic ureteral re-implantation for vesicoureteral reflux: Initial experience in Japan with the ureteral advancement technique. *Int J Urol* 2014; 10: 1016–21.

41. Tostivint V, Doumerc N, Roumiguie M et al. Laparoscopic robot-assisted partial nephrectomy with total uretectomy in symptomatic complete duplicated system: Advantages of transperitoneal approach. *Prog Urol* 2014; 12: 738–43.

42. Bayne AP, Roth DR. Dextranomer/Hyaluronic injection for the management of vesicoureteric reflux in complete ureteral duplication: Should age and gender be factors in decision making? *J Endourol* 2010; 24(6): 1013–6.

43. Hensle TW, Reiley EA, Ritch C et al. The clinical utility and safety of the endoscopic treatment of vesicoureteral reflux in patients with duplex ureters. *J Pediatr Urol* 2010; 6(1): 15–22.

44. Fernbach SK, Zawin JK, Lebowitz RL. Complete duplication of the ureter with uteropelvic junction obstruction of the lower pole of the kidney: Imaging findings. *Am J Roentgenol* 1995; 164: 701–4.

45. Monofort G, Guys JM, Roth CK et al. Surgical management of duplex ureters. *J Pediatr Surg* 1992; 27: 634–8.

46. Chertin B, Fridmans A, Hadas-Halpren I et al. Endoscopic puncture of ureterocele as a minimally invasive and effective long-term procedure in children. *Eur Urol* 2001; 39: 332–6.

47. Coplen DE, Barthold JS. Controversies in the management of ectopic ureteroceles. *Urology* 2000; 56: 665–8.

104

Vesicoureteral reflux

PREM PURI AND MANUELA HUNZIKER

INTRODUCTION

Primary vesicoureteral reflux (VUR)—the retrograde flow of urine from the bladder into the upper urinary tract—is the most common urological anomaly in children. It occurs in 1%–2% of the pediatric population and in 30%–50% of children who present with urinary tract infection (UTI).[1,2] The association of VUR, UTI, and renal damage is well known. Marra et al.[3] reviewed data on children with chronic renal failure who had high-grade VUR in the Italkid project, a database of Italian children with chronic renal failure, and found that those with VUR accounted for 26% of all children with chronic renal failure. Parenchymal injury in VUR occurs early, in most patients before age 3 years. Kidneys of young infants are more vulnerable to renal damage. Most renal scars are present when reflux is discovered at initial evaluation for UTI. One of the main goals of treating the child with VUR is prevention of recurring febrile UTIs and minimizing risk of renal damage and long-term renal impairment.

The hereditary and familial nature of VUR is now well recognized, and several studies have shown that siblings of children with VUR have a much higher incidence of reflux than the general pediatric population. Prevalence rates of 27%–51% in siblings of children with VUR and a 66% rate of VUR in offspring of parents with previously diagnosed reflux have been reported.[4–8] However, because VUR can resolve spontaneously with age, it is difficult to accurately determine the exact prevalence in family members. It has become evident that familial clustering of VUR must have a genetic basis, but no single major locus or gene for VUR has yet been identified, and most researchers now acknowledge that VUR is genetically heterogeneous.[9]

ETIOLOGY

Urinary tract development in the embryo begins with the formation of the ureteric bud, which is an outgrowth of the mesonephric duct. Growth of the ureteric bud is stimulated by reciprocal signaling between the bud and the metanephrogenic mesenchyme, and results in the formation of the ureter and branching to form the collecting ducts. Signaling between the bud and the mesenchyme stimulates the metanephrogenic mesenchyme to form the kidney. Apoptosis occurs in the part of the mesonephric duct between the newly developed ureter and the urogenital sinus. The free end of the developing ureter inserts into the bladder wall and forms the vesicoureteric valve.[9]

The ureterovesical junction (UVJ) acts as a valve and closes during micturation or when the bladder contracts. The UVJ is structurally and functionally adapted to allow the intermittent passage of urine and prevent the reflux of urine into the bladder. The main defect in patients with VUR is believed to involve the malformation of the UVJ, in part due to shortening of the submucosal ureteric segment due to congenital lateral ectopia of the ureteric orifice. This leads to retrograde flow of urine into the ureter or kidney. Since VUR primarily involves abnormalities of the ureter and ureteric orifice, it has been suggested that the timing and positioning of branching of the ureteric bud from the Wolffian duct may be related to VUR. Many genes are involved in the ureteric budding and subsequent urinary tract and kidney development. Primary VUR could be due to mutations in one or more developmental genes that control these processes.

Mechanism of renal scarring

The association between VUR and renal scarring is now widely recognized. Scarring is directly related to the severity of reflux. Belman and Skoog[10] assessed renal scarring in 804 refluxing units and found renal scars in 5% of those with grade I reflux, 6% of those with grade II reflux, 17% of those with grade III reflux, 25% of those with grade IV reflux, and 50% of those with grade V reflux.

The mechanism by which reflux produces renal scars is still not clear. Renal parenchymal damage can be congenital or acquired. Congenital reflux nephropathy occurs as a result of abnormal embryological development with subsequent renal dysplasia and is largely seen in male infants with high-grade VUR. Exposure to UTIs in patients with congenital renal dysplasia can lead to progression of renal parenchymal damage. Both experimental and clinical studies have shown that acquired renal scarring associated with VUR is the result of an acute inflammatory reaction caused by bacterial infection of the renal parenchyma.[11] It is well known that the risk of renal scarring after an episode of pyelonephritis is increased in children with high-grade VUR, affecting up to 89% of children with grades IV–V VUR[12] Exposure to UTIs in patients with congenital renal dysplasia can lead to progression of renal parenchymal damage. Reflux-associated nephropathy is an important cause of hypertension and end-stage renal disease.[13]

Dimercaptosuccinic acid (DMSA) scans have allowed us to follow sequentially the evolution of a scar from an area of decreased blood flow during the acute inflammatory phase to a parenchymal defect indicative of a mature scar. Yet only half of patients with acute pyelonephritis will have such a scar. What converts an acute inflammatory process into a scar in some patients and not in others is not clearly understood. Factors implicated in the formation of a mature scar include the magnitude of the pressure driving the organisms into the tissues, the intrinsic virulence of the organism itself, and the host defense mechanisms. Furthermore, some of the worst examples of renal injury associated with VUR are those that are present at birth. As renal damage at that time cannot be the consequence of infection, such injury is assumed to be developmental in origin, but the pathophysiology of this is not entirely clear.

The three mechanisms considered potential etiologies for renal scar formation are (1) reflux of infected urine with interstitial inflammation and damage; (2) sterile, usually high-grade reflux, which may damage the kidney through a mechanical or immunological mechanism; and (3) abnormal embryological development with subsequent renal dysplasia. Patients in the latter group may also have UTI in the postnatal period, resulting in extensive parenchymal damage. It is well recognized that in the first two groups of renal parenchymal damage, it is essential to discover reflux early before damage can be initiated. In the third group, it is clear that congenital damage currently cannot be prevented. However, in these patients, it is mandatory to discover reflux at the early stages to prevent exposure to UTI and avoid the possible progression of renal parenchymal damage.

DIAGNOSIS

Antenatally diagnosed reflux

Prenatal ultrasonography has resulted in a dramatic increase in the number of infants detected with significant asymptomatic uropathology, allowing treatment before the potential devastating consequences of UTI occur. An incidental anomaly is detected by antenatal ultrasonography in about 1% of studies and 20%–30% involving the urinary tract.[14] By far, the most common abnormal finding is hydronephrosis, comprising over 90% of the urological abnormalities detected. Underlying diagnoses include pelvic–ureteric junction obstruction, vesicoureteric junction obstruction, posterior urethral valves, and VUR.

Although antenatal hydronephrosis is generally considered to represent an obstructive lesion, VUR is not an uncommon cause. In children diagnosed with antenatal hydronephrosis, VUR has been reported in 10%–20%.[15] Skoog et al.[16] published guidelines for screening siblings of children with VUR and neonates/infants with prenatal hydronephrosis. They reported a prevalence of VUR of 16.2% in screened populations with prenatal hydronephrosis. Based on review of data and panel consensus, voiding cystourethrogram (VCUG) is recommended for infants with high-grade hydronephrosis, hydroureter, or abnormal bladder on ultrasound, or who develop a UTI on observation.

Natural history of prenatally diagnosed VUR

The vast majority of infants found to have VUR following detection of antenatal hydronephrosis are males. The male preponderance is reported to range from 2:1 to 5:1 in various series.[17,18] This is in total contrast to the female preponderance that has been consistently reported in later childhood. It is also important to recognize that the calculated ratio between the genders is dependent upon the method of ascertainment. UTIs are more common in females, and it is no surprise that when VUR is detected by screening children who presented with symptoms of UTI, more girls than boys are diagnosed with VUR. However, 80% of cases detected by the appearance of antenatal hydronephrosis on prenatal ultrasound are boys, and these patients often have high-grade VUR-associated renal damage.[19] In approximately two-thirds of the cases, the reflux is bilateral. VUR diagnosed prenatally tends to be of high grade.[17,18]

It also has been reported that boys are more vulnerable to UTI, especially in the first 6 months of life, where different factors play a significant role.[20] Host factors such as the inner nonkeratinized epithelium of the foreskin create a moist reservoir for uropathogens and contribute to the first contact between the host and the bacteria. Once the prepuce has been colonized, the bacteria can ascend the urinary tract, causing cystitis or pyelonephritis. Rushton and Majd[20] showed a clear predominance of males among infants less than 6 months old with febrile UTI, and a disproportionately high frequency of uncircumcised male infants. Cascio et al.[21] showed a pure growth of a uropathogen in 48% of uncircumcised infants with VUR despite the use of prophylactic antibiotics.

A meta-analysis performed by Skoog et al.[16] showed that VUR in infants diagnosed by screening after an antenatally detected hydronephrosis was significantly associated with renal damage. Renal abnormalities occurred in a mean of 6.2% versus 47.9% of those with grades I–III versus IV–V reflux.[16]

Yeung et al.[19] studied 155 infants with prenatal hydronephrosis and postnatally diagnosed VUR. They observed renal parenchymal damage in 42% of the 135 infants (101 male and 34 female) without history of UTI. Furthermore, Nguyen et al.[22] reported renal parenchymal abnormalities in 65% of predominantly male infants with sterile high-grade reflux. The resolution rate of antenatally diagnosed high-grade VUR (grade IV or V) is approximately 20% by the age of 2 years.[14] However, in approximately 25% of boys followed nonoperatively, UTIs developed by the age of 2 years, despite antimicrobial chemoprophylaxis.[14]

Early detection of febrile UTI is critical in infants, who are unable to verbally communicate lower urinary tract symptoms. Detection of VUR by screening infants in at-risk population before presentation with febrile UTI is recommendable, but its outcomes remain unknown.[16]

CLINICAL PRESENTATION

It is obviously important to diagnose VUR at the earliest possible age, preferably in infancy. There are a number of clinical presentations, which should raise the suspicion of VUR in an infant. As antenatal ultrasound becomes increasingly routine, many cases will be suspected before birth and should be investigated within the first month of life. Infants with a poor urinary stream as in posterior urethral valves or infants with spina bifida have a high incidence of VUR, while early investigations are indicated in the first-degree relatives of patients with high-grade VUR.

In most cases, VUR is discovered clinically after investigations for UTI. The incidence of VUR in infants with febrile UTI is 30%–50%, with even higher incidence in male infants. Cascio et al.[23] found VUR in 33% of the 57 neonates investigated for first hospitalized UTI. Sixteen had bilateral VUR and three unilateral, with 91% having high-grade VUR.

RADIOLOGICAL INVESTIGATIONS

Ultrasound

Sonography should be performed in any infant with suspicion of VUR. The bladder and lower ureters are assessed by real-time examination at each ureterovesical junction for dilatation, configuration, peristalsis, and continuity with the bladder base. VUR is suspected in the presence of a dilated pelvicaliceal system, upper or lower ureter, unequal renal size, or cortical loss and increased echogenicity (Figure 104.1a–d). Sonography is not sufficiently sensitive or specific for diagnosing VUR.[18,24,25] The intermittent and dynamic nature of VUR probably contributes to the insensitivity of routine renal sonography in the detection of even higher grades of reflux.

Phan et al.[15] reported a 15% prevalence of VUR in infants diagnosed with antenatal hydronephrosis, many of whom had normal postnatal ultrasound or mild postnatal pelviectasis. They concluded that a micturating cystogram is the only reliable test for detecting postnatal VUR.

Micturating cystography

VUR is a dynamic process. Bladder filling and voiding are necessary for its elucidation, which requires catheterization for adequate documentation. Micturating cystogram remains the gold standard for detecting VUR (Figure 104.2). Despite the unpleasant nature of the procedure, it has a low false-negative rate and provides accurate anatomical detail, allowing grading of the VUR (Figure 104.3a–c). It is commonly performed as a first-line investigation, together with ultrasound.

Some investigators employ nuclear cystography for diagnosing VUR. This can be either direct or indirect using technetium-labeled diaminotetra-ethyl-pentaacetic acid (DTPA). In direct nuclear cystography, DTPA is instilled into the bladder by urethral catheter or suprapubic injection, and the ureters and kidneys are observed on camera during bladder filling and voiding. In indirect nuclear cystography, DTPA is injected intravenously. After the bladder is filled, the patient is instructed to void, and the counts taken over the ureters and kidneys are used to assess the presence of VUR. Indirect nuclear cystography requires a cooperative patient and therefore is of no value in infants. The main disadvantage of nuclear cystography is that it does not give anatomical detail and VUR cannot be graded according to international classification.

According to the international classification of reflux, there are five grades of reflux:

- Grade I, ureter only
- Grade II, ureter, pelvis, and calices—no dilatation, normal caliceal fornices
- Grade III, mild dilatation and/or tortuosity of the ureter and mild dilatation of the renal pelvis—minor blunting of the fornices
- Grade IV, moderate, dilatation and/or tortuosity of the ureter and moderate dilatation of the renal pelvis and calices—complete obliteration of the sharp angle of fornices but maintenance of the papillary impressions in the majority of calices
- Grade V, gross dilatation of the renal pelvis and calices (Figure 104.4)

DMSA scan

DMSA is the most sensitive technique for detecting renal scarring. When performed in the course of acute UTI, the DMSA scan is currently the most reliable test for the diagnosis of acute pyelonephritis. Several reports have suggested that a normal[26,27] acute DMSA scan rules out the possibility of high-grade VUR. However, others have reported that acute DMSA scintigraphy has limited overall ability in revealing VUR after first febrile UTI in infants.[25,28] This was

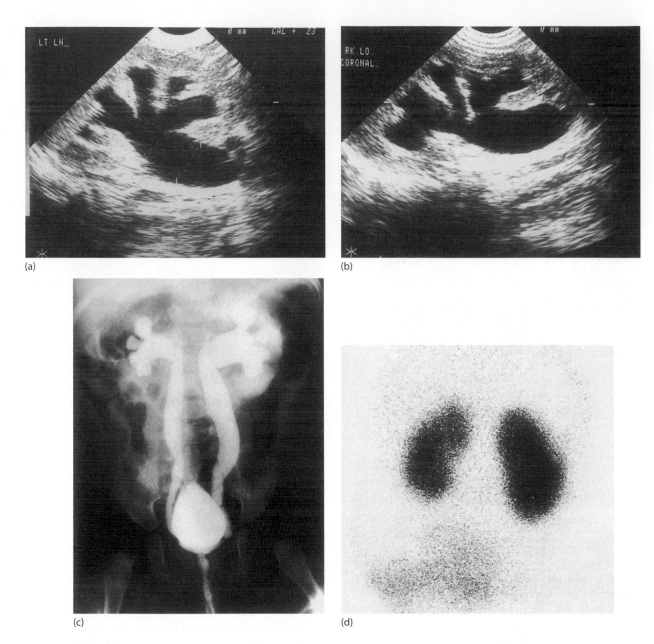

Figure 104.1 **(a, b)** Ultrasound shows bilateral hydronephrosis in a 6-week-old infant. **(c)** Micturating cystography in the same infant shows bilateral high-grade vesicoureteric reflux. Note intrarenal reflux on the left side. **(d)** DMSA scan demonstrates significant left renal scarring, particularly in upper and lower poles.

true even when the findings of the acute DMSA scan were combined with those of renal ultrasonography.

Timing of investigations

Management of VUR has changed over the last few years from only prevention of renal scarring to, in addition, improvement of quality of life and reduction of number of infections and unnecessary diagnostic tests.[29] New international guidelines are reflecting these changes in our understanding of VUR and trying to set up algorithms for clinical management.[29] However, consensus has not been reached today.[30] In the past, micturating cystourethrogram (MCUG) used to be included in all guidelines as an investigation for the assessment of

children with UTIs.[31] To date, most guidelines recommend that MCUG is not used routinely and is limited to highly selected cases, although it remains the gold standard to define VUR. The American Academy of Pediatrics (AAP) guidelines do not advocate routine MCUG after the first UTI. MCUG is indicated if renal and bladder ultrasound reveals hydronephrosis, scarring, or other pathological findings.[32] MCUG should be performed in all patients between the ages of 2 and 24 months with recurrent febrile UTI. The National Institute for Health and Clinical Excellence (NICE) guidelines do not recommend the routine use of MCUG in children with recurrent UTI; MCUG is reserved only for exceptional cases. The guidelines from the European Association of Urology (EUA) recommend a more proactive approach with early detection

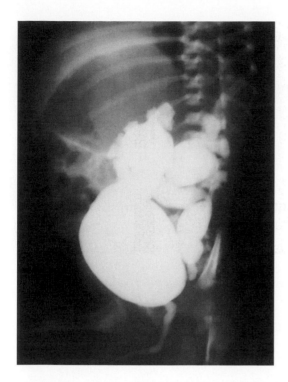

Figure 104.2 Four-week-old male infant with bilateral grade V vesicoureteric reflux. Note normal urethra and bladder wall.

of VUR using MCUG in all children younger than 2 years once a first febrile UTI is confirmed.[33] Nevertheless, most guidelines recommend the routine use of a DMSA scan for the evaluation of patients with recurrent UTIs.[30]

MANAGEMENT

The goals of treating the child with VUR are (1) to prevent recurring febrile UTIs, (2) to prevent renal injury, and (3) to minimize the morbidity of treatment and follow-up.

Management of VUR has been controversial. The various options currently available for the management of VUR are (1) long-term antibiotic prophylaxis, (2) open surgical treatment, (3) observation or intermittent therapy with management of bladder/bowel dysfunction and treatment of UTIs as they occur, and (4) minimally invasive endoscopic treatment.

Medical management

This strategy is based on three important assumptions: (1) Sterile VUR in most cases is not harmful to the kidneys and has no relevant affect on kidney function. (2) Children can outgrow VUR, at least the lower grades. (3) Continuous low-dose antibiotic prophylaxis can prevent infection for many years while VUR is still present.

The patient is required to take low-dose daily antibiotics, and annual ultrasound and VCUG are performed to assess if the reflux has resolved.

Continuing antibiotic prophylaxis is reliant on the patient's compliance and has the risk of bacterial resistance accompanied by potential breakthrough UTIs. Compliance to antibiotic therapy has been reported to be poor. Data of 11,000 children under the age of 11 years with a diagnosis of VUR were reviewed with 76% of VUR patients initiated on antibiotic prophylaxis. Only 17% of pediatric VUR patients on prophylactic antibiotics were compliant with therapy. Of patients on prophylactic therapy, 58% had a diagnosis of a UTI within 1 year of treatment.[34] Furthermore, several large, prospective, randomized controlled trials have shown little or no benefit of medical therapy in terms of reducing the incidence of febrile UTI or renal scarring.[35]

Spontaneous resolution is inversely proportional to the initial grade of reflux.[36] Resolution rates for grade I and II VUR have been reported to be between 80% and 68%, respectively. However, the resolution rate for grade III reflux was only 45% and for grade IV/V VUR only 17%.[37]

The International Reflux Study Group, at 10-year follow-up, showed that 58% of children with grade III and IV reflux randomly allocated to medical treatment still had reflux after 5 years and 27.5% after 10 years.[38]

The Randomized Intervention for Children with Vesicoureteral Reflux (RIVUR) trial, which is, to date, the largest randomized, placebo-controlled, double-blind, multicenter study, showed that there was a 50% reduction in the risk of recurrent UTI in those children on the prophylaxis. However, antimicrobial prophylaxis did not decrease the risk of renal scarring.[39,40]

Surgical treatment

OPEN ANTIREFLUX PROCEDURES

Open surgical treatment of reflux has been the gold standard. However, surgery is not without risks, and in infants, it is technically more challenging. The majority of the open antireflux procedures entail opening the bladder and performing a variety of procedures on the ureters such as transvesical reimplantation (Politano–Leadbetter technique) and transtrigonal advancement of the ureters (Cohen technique). These procedures, although effective, involve open surgery and prolonged in-hospital stay and are not free of complications, even in the best hands. Although open surgery achieves a success rate of 92%–98% in grades II–IV VUR, the American Urological Association (AUA) report on VUR reported persistence of VUR in 19.3% of ureters after reimplantation of ureters for grade V reflux.[41] The rate of obstruction after ureteral reimplantation needing reoperation reported by the AUA in 33 studies was 0.3%–9.1%.

LAPAROSCOPIC URETERAL REIMPLANTATION

In recent years, several authors have reported their experience of ureteral reimplantation with laparoscopic extravesical transperitoneal approach as well as pneumovesical approach.[42–44] This technique results in a shorter hospital stay and less postoperative discomfort compared to open operation. Furthermore, robotic-assisted laparoscopic extravesical ureteral reimplantation has shown high success rates similar to open ureteral reimplantation as well as minimal morbidity.[45–47]

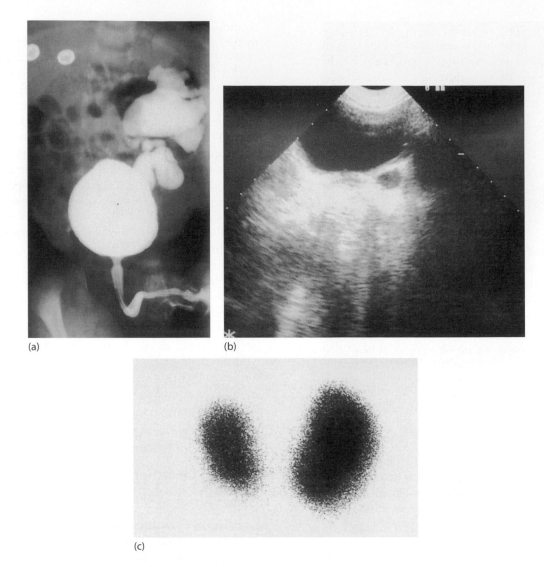

(a) (b)

(c)

Figure 104.3 **(a)** Male infant showing grade V left vesicoureteric reflux; **(b)** ultrasound in the same patient. Transverse scan through the full bladder demonstrates dilated left ureter. **(c)** DMSA scan in the same patient demonstrates small left kidney.

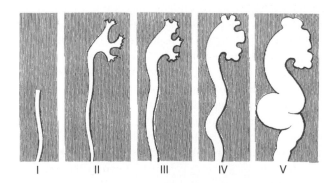

I II III IV V

Figure 104.4 International classification of vesicoureteric reflux (grades I–V).

ENDOSCOPIC TREATMENT OF VUR

The concept of endoscopic treatment was introduced by Puri and O'Donnell[48] in 1984 as a minimally invasive treatment for VUR following a successful experimental study in piglets. Minimally invasive endoscopic technique for the correction of VUR has become an established alternative to long-term antibiotic prophylaxis and open surgical treatment.

The AUA guidelines recently updated the management of primary VUR in children. They extracted data from 131 articles, and data from 17,972 patients were included in their analysis. Success rates are 98.1% for open surgical procedures and 83.0% for endoscopic therapy after one injection.[35] With the high success rate of endoscopic treatment, the AUA guidelines included endoscopic treatment in the management options for VUR.

Endoscopic treatment has several advantages over the two other options. In contrast to long-term antibiotic prophylaxis, it offers immediate cure of reflux with a high success rate, its success does not rely on patient or parent compliance, and the procedure is virtually free of adverse side effects. Long-term administration of antibiotics implies the danger of bacterial resistance with promotion of breakthrough UTIs, and antibiotics are usually needed for years. In 2001, Deflux was approved by the Food and

Drug Administration (FDA) as an acceptable tissue-augmenting substance for subureteral injection therapy for VUR. Since then, endoscopic treatment has become increasingly popular worldwide for managing VUR, and Deflux is the most widely used tissue-augmenting substance.

Recently, the Swedish Reflux Trial in Children recruited children between 1 and 2 years old with grade III–IV VUR for a prospective, open, randomized controlled multicenter study. Children were treated in 3 groups, including low-dose antibiotic prophylaxis, endoscopic therapy, and a surveillance group on antibiotics only for febrile UTI. After 2 years, endoscopic treatment results were significantly better than the spontaneous resolution rate or downgrading in the prophylaxis and surveillance groups.[49]

The technique of endoscopic injection of Deflux is simple and straightforward.[50,51] The patients should be placed in a lithotomy position. The cystoscope is passed, and the bladder wall, trigone, bladder neck, and both ureteric orifices are inspected. All cystoscopes available for infants and children can be used for this procedure. The bladder should be almost empty before proceeding with injection, since this helps to keep the ureteric orifice flat rather than away in a lateral field. The disposable Puri flexible catheter or a rigid metallic can be used for injection. A 1 mL syringe filled with Deflux is attached to the injection catheter. Under direct vision through the cystoscope, the needle is introduced under the bladder mucosa 2–3 mm below the affected ureteral orifice at 6 o'clock position (Figure 104.5). In children with grade IV and V reflux with wide ureteral orifices, the needle should be inserted not below but directly into the affected ureteral orifice. The needle is advanced about 4–5 mm under the mucosa and the injection started slowly. As the Deflux is injected, a budge appears in the floor of the submucosal ureter. Most refluxing ureters require 0.4–1.0 mL Deflux to correct reflux. A correctly placed injection creates the appearance of a nipple on the top, which is a slit-like or inverted crescent orifice. Patients are treated as day cases, and a voiding cystourethrogram and ultrasound are performed 6–12 weeks after discharge.

Between 2001 and 2010, the author treated 1551 infants and children with intermediate and high-grade VUR by endoscopic injection of Deflux. VUR was unilateral in 765 children and bilateral in 786. Renal scarring was detected in 369 (26.7%) of the 1384 patients who had a DMSA scan. Reflux grade in the 2341 ureters was grade II, III, IV, and V in 98 (4.2%), 1340 (57.3%), 818 (34.9%), and 85 (3.6%), respectively. VUR resolved after the first, second, and third endoscopic injection of dextranomer/hyaluronic acid (Dx/HA) in 2039 (87.1%), 264 (11.3%), and 38 (1.6%) ureters, respectively. Of the 1512 patients who were followed up, 69 (4.6%) developed febrile UTIs during a median follow-up of 5.6 years. None of the patients in the series needed reimplantation of ureters or developed any significant complications, confirming the efficacy and safety of this 15-minute outpatient procedure in the management of intermediate and high-grade VUR.[52]

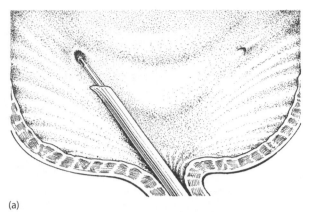

(a)

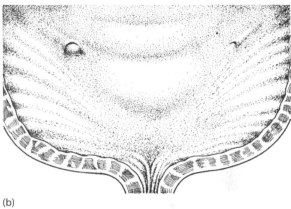

(b)

Figure 104.5 Technique of endoscopic subureteric injection: (a) site of insertion of needle; (b) appearance of ureteric orifice at completion of injection.

Endoscopic subureteral injection of Deflux is excellent first-line treatment in children, with 87% success in high-grade VUR after one injection. This 15-minute outpatient procedure is safe and simple to perform, and it can be easily repeated in failed cases.

REFERENCES

1. Smellie JM, Barratt TM, Chantler C, Gordon I, Prescod NP, Ransley PG, Woolf AS. Medical versus surgical treatment in children with severe bilateral vesicoureteric reflux and bilateral nephropathy: A randomised trial. *Lancet* 2001; 357(9265): 1329–33.

2. Hoberman A, Charron M, Hickey RW, Baskin M, Kearney DH, Wald ER. Imaging studies after a first febrile urinary tract infection in young children. *N Engl J Med* 2003; 348(3): 195–202.

3. Marra G, Oppezzo C, Ardissino G, Dacco V, Testa S, Avolio L, Taioli E, Sereni F. Severe vesicoureteral reflux and chronic renal failure: A condition peculiar to male gender? Data from the ItalKid Project. *J Pediatr* 2004; 144(5): 677–81.

4. Noe HN. The long-term results of prospective sibling reflux screening. *J Urol* 1992; 148(5 Pt 2): 1739–42.

5. Wan J, Greenfield SP, Ng M, Zerin M, Ritchey ML, Bloom D. Sibling reflux: A dual center retrospective study. *J Urol* 1996; 156(2 Pt 2): 677–9.

6. Connolly LP, Treves ST, Connolly SA, Zurakowski D, Share JC, Bar-Sever Z, Mitchell KD, Bauer SB. Vesicoureteral reflux in children: Incidence and severity in siblings. *J Urol* 1997; 157(6): 2287–90.

7. Parekh DJ, Pope JCt, Adams MC, Brock JW 3rd. Outcome of sibling vesicoureteral reflux. *J Urol* 2002; 167(1): 283–4.

8. Noe HN, Wyatt RJ, Peeden JN, Jr., Rivas ML. The transmission of vesicoureteral reflux from parent to child. *J Urol* 1992; 148(6): 1869–71.

9. Puri P, Gosemann JH, Darlow J, Barton DE. Genetics of vesicoureteral reflux. *Nat Rev Urol* 2011; 8(10): 539–52.

10. Belman AB, Skoog SJ. Nonsurgical approach to the management of vesicoureteral reflux in children. *Pediatr Infect Dis J* 1989; 8(8): 556–9.

11. Peters C, Rushton HG. Vesicoureteral reflux associated renal damage: Congenital reflux nephropathy and acquired renal scarring. *J Urol* 2010; 184(1): 265–73.

12. Swerkersson S, Jodal U, Sixt R, Stokland E, Hansson S. Relationship among vesicoureteral reflux, urinary tract infection and renal damage in children. *J Urol* 2007; 178(2): 647–51; discussion 650–1.

13. Mattoo TK. Vesicoureteral reflux and reflux nephropathy. *Adv Chronic Kidney Dis* 2011; 18(5): 348–54.

14. Elder JS. Guidelines for consideration for surgical repair of vesicoureteral reflux. *Curr Opin Urol* 2000; 10(6): 579–85.

15. Phan V, Traubici J, Hershenfield B, Stephens D, Rosenblum ND, Geary DF. Vesicoureteral reflux in infants with isolated antenatal hydronephrosis. *Pediatr Nephrol* 2003; 18(12): 1224–8.

16. Skoog SJ, Peters CA, Arant BS, Jr., Copp HL, Elder JS, Hudson RG, Khoury AE, Lorenzo AJ, Pohl HG, Shapiro E, Snodgrass WT, Diaz M. Pediatric vesicoureteral reflux guidelines panel summary report: Clinical practice guidelines for screening siblings of children with vesicoureteral reflux and neonates/infants with prenatal hydronephrosis. *J Urol* 2010; 184(3): 1145–51.

17. Steele BT, Robitaille P, DeMaria J, Grignon A. Follow-up evaluation of prenatally recognized vesicoureteric reflux. *J Pediatr* 1989; 115(1): 95–6.

18. Blane CE, DiPietro MA, Zerin JM, Sedman AB, Bloom DA. Renal sonography is not a reliable screening examination for vesicoureteral reflux. *J Urol* 1993; 150(2 Pt 2): 752–5.

19. Yeung CK, Godley ML, Dhillon HK, Gordon I, Duffy PG, Ransley PG. The characteristics of primary vesico-ureteric reflux in male and female infants with pre-natal hydronephrosis. *Br J Urol* 1997; 80(2): 319–27.

20. Rushton HG, Majd M. Pyelonephritis in male infants: How important is the foreskin? *J Urol* 1992; 148(2 Pt 2): 733–6; discussion 737–8.

21. Cascio S, Colhoun E, Puri P. Bacterial colonization of the prepuce in boys with vesicoureteral reflux who receive antibiotic prophylaxis. *J Pediatr* 2001; 139(1): 160–2.

22. Nguyen HT, Bauer SB, Peters CA, Connolly LP, Gobet R, Borer JG, Barnewolt CE, Ephraim PL, Treves ST, Retik AB. 99m Technetium dimercapto-succinic acid renal scintigraphy abnormalities in infants with sterile high grade vesicoureteral reflux. *J Urol* 2000; 164(5): 1674–8; discussion 1678–9.

23. Cascio S, Chertin B, Yoneda A, Rolle U, Kelleher J, Puri P. Acute renal damage in infants after first urinary tract infection. *Pediatr Nephrol* 2002; 17(7): 503–5.

24. Venhola M, Huttunen NP, Renko M, Pokka T, Uhari M. Practice guidelines for imaging studies in children after the first urinary tract infection. *J Urol* 2010; 184(1): 325–8.

25. Fouzas S, Krikelli E, Vassilakos P, Gkentzi D, Papanastasiou DA, Salakos C. DMSA scan for revealing vesicoureteral reflux in young children with urinary tract infection. *Pediatrics* 2010; 126(3): e513–519.

26. Tseng MH, Lin WJ, Lo WT, Wang SR, Chu ML, Wang CC. Does a normal DMSA obviate the performance of voiding cystourethrography in evaluation of young children after their first urinary tract infection? *J Pediatr* 2007; 150(1): 96–9.

27. Preda I, Jodal U, Sixt R, Stokland E, Hansson S. Normal dimercaptosuccinic acid scintigraphy makes voiding cystourethrography unnecessary after urinary tract infection. *J Pediatr* 2007; 151(6): 581–4, 584 e581.

28. Siomou E, Giapros V, Fotopoulos A, Aasioti M, Papadopoulou F, Serbis A, Siamopoulou A, Andronikou S. Implications of 99mTc-DMSA scintigraphy performed during urinary tract infection in neonates. *Pediatrics* 2009; 124(3): 881–7.

29. Springer A, Subramaniam R. Relevance of current guidelines in the management of VUR. *Eur J Pediatr* 2014; 173(7): 835–43.

30. Awais M, Rehman A, Zaman MU, Nadeem N. Recurrent urinary tract infections in young children: Role of DMSA scintigraphy in detecting vesicoureteric reflux. *Pediatr Radiol* 2015; 45(1): 62–8.

31. Tullus K. Vesicoureteric reflux in children. *Lancet* 2015; 385(9965): 371–9.

32. Subcommittee on Urinary Tract Infection SCoQI, Management, Roberts KB. Urinary tract infection: Clinical practice guideline for the diagnosis and management of the initial UTI in febrile infants and children 2 to 24 months. *Pediatrics* 2011; 128(3): 595–610.

33. Stein R, Dogan HS, Hoebeke P, Kocvara R, Nijman RJ, Radmayr C, Tekgul S, European Association of U, European Society for Pediatric U. Urinary tract infections in children: EAU/ESPU guidelines. *Eur Urol* 2015; 67(3): 546–58.

34. Hensle TW, Grogg AL, Eaddy M. Pediatric vesicoureteral reflux: Treatment patterns and outcomes. *Nat Clin Pract Urol* 2007; 4(9): 462–3.

35. Peters CA, Skoog SJ, Arant BS, Jr., Copp HL, Elder JS, Hudson RG, Khoury AE, Lorenzo AJ, Pohl HG, Shapiro E, Snodgrass WT, Diaz M. Summary of the AUA guideline on management of primary vesicoureteral reflux in children. *J Urol* 2010; 184(3): 1134–44.

36. Sung J, Skoog S. Surgical management of vesicoureteral reflux in children. *Pediatr Nephrol* 2011; doi:10.1007/s00467-011-1933-7

37. Knudson MJ, Austin JC, McMillan ZM, Hawtrey CE, Cooper CS. Predictive factors of early spontaneous resolution in children with primary vesicoureteral reflux. *J Urol* 2007; 178(4 Pt 2): 1684–8.

38. Jodal U, Smellie JM, Lax H, Hoyer PF. Ten-year results of randomized treatment of children with severe vesicoureteral reflux. Final report of the International Reflux Study in Children. *Pediatr Nephrol* 2006; 21(6): 785–92.

39. Mathews R, Mattoo TK. The role of antimicrobial prophylaxis in the management of children with vesicoureteral reflux—The RIVUR study outcomes. *Adv Chronic Kidney* Dis 2015; 22(4): 325–30. doi:10.1053/j.ackd.2015.04.002

40. Mattoo TK, Chesney RW, Greenfield SP, Hoberman A, Keren R, Mathews R, Gravens-Mueller L, Ivanova A, Carpenter MA, Moxey-Mims M, Majd M, Ziessman HA, Investigators RT. Renal scarring in the Randomized Intervention for Children with Vesicoureteral Reflux (RIVUR) Trial. *Clin J Am Soc Nephrol* 2016; 11(1): 54–61.

41. Elder JS, Peters CA, Arant BS, Jr., Ewalt DH, Hawtrey CE, Hurwitz RS, Parrott TS, Snyder HM 3rd, Weiss RA, Woolf SH, Hasselblad V. Pediatric Vesicoureteral Reflux Guidelines Panel summary report on the management of primary vesicoureteral reflux in children. *J Urol* 1997; 157(5): 1846–51.

42. Chung PH, Tang DY, Wong KK, Yip PK, Tam PK. Comparing open and pneumovesical approach for ureteric reimplantation in pediatric patients—A preliminary review. *J Pediatr Surg* 2008; 43(12): 2246–9.

43. Lopez M, Varlet F. Laparoscopic extravesical transperitoneal approach following the Lich–Gregoir technique in the treatment of vesicoureteral reflux in children. *J Pediatr Surg* 2010; 45(4): 806–10.

44. Kawauchi A, Naitoh Y, Soh J, Hirahara N, Okihara K, Miki T. Transvesical laparoscopic cross-trigonal ureteral reimplantation for correction of vesicoureteral reflux: Initial experience and comparisons between adult and pediatric cases. *J Endourol* 2009; 23(11): 1875–8.

45. Kasturi S, Sehgal SS, Christman MS, Lambert SM, Casale P. Prospective long-term analysis of nerve-sparing extravesical robotic-assisted laparoscopic ureteral reimplantation. *Urology* 2011; 79(3): 680–3.

46. Chalmers D, Herbst K, Kim C. Robotic-assisted laparoscopic extravesical ureteral reimplantation: An initial experience. *J Pediatr Urol* 2011; 8(3): 268–71.

47. Bayne AP, Shoss JM, Starke NR, Cisek LJ. Single-center experience with pediatric laparoscopic extravesical reimplantation: Safe and effective in simple and complex anatomy. *J Laparoendosc Adv Surg Tech A* 2012; 22(1): 102–6.

48. Puri P, O'Donnell B. Correction of experimentally produced vesicoureteric reflux in the piglet by intravesical injection of Teflon. *Br Med J (Clin Res Ed)* 1984; 289(6436): 5–7.

49. Holmdahl G, Brandstrom P, Lackgren G, Sillen U, Stokland E, Jodal U, Hansson S. The Swedish reflux trial in children: II. Vesicoureteral reflux outcome. *J Urol* 2010; 184(1): 280–5.

50. Dawrant MJ, Mohanan N, Puri P. Endoscopic treatment for high grade vesicoureteral reflux in infants. *J Urol* 2006; 176(4 Pt 2): 1847–50.

51. Puri P, Mohanan N, Menezes M, Colhoun E. Endoscopic treatment of moderate and high grade vesicoureteral reflux in infants using dextranomer/hyaluronic acid. *J Urol* 2007; 178(4 Pt 2): 1714–6; discussion 1717.

52. Puri P, Kutasy B, Colhoun E, Hunziker M. Single center experience with endoscopic subureteral dextranomer/hyaluronic acid injection as first line treatment in 1,551 children with intermediate and high grade vesicoureteral reflux. *J Urol* 2012; 188(4 Suppl): 1485–9.

105

Ureteroceles in the newborn

JONATHAN F. KALISVAART AND ANDREW J. KIRSCH

INTRODUCTION

Ureteroceles are congenital, cystic dilations of the terminal, intravesical portion of the ureter. The associated ureteral orifice, often extremely difficult to visualize, may be partially or totally obstructed, resulting in variability in size from small to very large. Ureteroceles can also vary in location from intravesical to ectopic. The use of fetal ultrasonography has improved the diagnosis of ureteroceles; however, they often remain difficult to diagnose and require complete postnatal evaluation when suspected.

PATHOGENESIS

The pathogenesis of the ureterocele remains unclear, although several theories have sought to explain it. Chwalla[1] and Ericsson[2] attributed the ureterocele formation to the persistence of an epithelial sheet (Chwalla's membrane) separating the lumen of the distal portion of the Wolffian duct and the urogenital sinus. Chwalla's membrane is a normal embryologic structure that disappears spontaneously approximately 2 months after conception. If it persists, it can balloon out and form the ureterocele. Stephens,[3] on the other hand, postulates that the terminal ureter becomes involved in the growth of the bladder and undergoes extensive enlargement, resulting in the formation of the ureterocele. Tanagho[4] suggests that the ureterocele forms secondary to local dilatation of the ureteral bud prior to its migration from the Wolffian duct. Tokunaka and colleagues[5] demonstrated poor muscle development in the dome of the ureterocele and suggest that ureterocele formation is based on a segmental embryonic arrest of the development of the most distal portion of the ureter. These theories regarding the pathogenesis of ureteroceles are still only speculations.

Pathological anatomy and associated pathology

Ureteroceles can be associated with the ureter draining the upper moiety of a duplex collecting system or with the ureter of a single system. Duplex-system ureteroceles occur in approximately 85% of diagnosed cases and can vary in size and position. The upper renal moiety is nonfunctional and dysplastic in over 80% of cases.[6,7] Occasionally, ureteroceles are small and well demarcated from the bladder wall, but often, they present as very large subtrigonal masses. The ureterocele may also protrude toward the contralateral ureteral orifice or the bladder neck, causing contralateral ureteral or bladder outlet obstruction. More commonly, the ipsilateral orifice of the ureter draining the lower pole is pushed upward by the distended ectopic ureterocele, shortening the intratrigonal tunnel, leading to reflux and hydronephrosis. On the contralateral side, reflux and secondary hydronephrosis can be seen, likely due to the disruption of the normal trigonal anatomy. Less commonly, reflux can be seen to occur into the ureterocele itself.

Ureteroceles are attached to single collecting systems in approximately 15% of cases, often in males.[6,7] The cystic swelling tends to be asymmetric, with the ureteral orifice located in an eccentric position. The single-system ureterocele is usually smaller in size than the ectopic ureterocele, and the size of the ureterocele is generally related to the degree of obstruction caused by the pinpoint orifice.[8]

Single-system ureteroceles rarely prolapse and cause bladder neck obstruction, and reflux is extremely uncommon. Although the ureter and pelvicalyceal structures are hydronephrotic to varying degrees, function of the renal unit is often preserved.

CLASSIFICATION

In 1954, Ericsson[2] classified ureteroceles into *orthotopic or simple* ureteroceles if the ureter forming the ureterocele ends in a normal site in the bladder or *ectopic* ureteroceles if the ureter ends in an ectopic location. However, confusingly, a simple ureterocele can also mean a ureterocele involving a single system, and an ectopic ureterocele can describe a ureterocele associated with a duplicated system. Stephens[3] classified ureteroceles based on the anatomic location and appearance of the orifice into *stenotic* (narrowed opening found in the bladder), *sphincteric* (an orifice distal to the bladder neck), *sphincterostenotic* (a narrowed opening distal to the bladder neck), and a *cecoureterocele* (intravesical orifice with a submucosal extension into the urethra). These traditional classifications, based on the location of the ureteral orifices or on the anatomical description, can be quite confusing. The modern classification system is based on the report of the Committee on Terminology, Nomenclature and Classification of the Urology Section of the American Academy of Pediatrics.[9] It subdivides ureteroceles based on the following:

1. Number of ureters that drain the kidney ipsilateral to the ureterocele
2. Location and extent of the ureterocele
3. Any additional anatomic distortions of the ureterocele resulting from eversion, prolapse, or secondary incompetence or obstruction of the other ureteral orifice or the bladder neck

Thus, a duplex-system ureterocele is when the ureterocele is attached to the upper pole ureter of a completely duplicated collecting system, and a single-system ureterocele is when the ureterocele is attached to a single ureter draining the kidney. If the ureterocele and its orifice are located entirely within the bladder, the term *intravesical* is used, and if the ureterocele and its orifice extend beyond the trigone to the bladder neck or outside of the bladder to involve the urethra, the term *ectopic* is applied. Single-system ureteroceles are generally intravesical, and ectopic ureteroceles are usually associated with the upper pole ureter of a duplex system (Figure 105.1).[10]

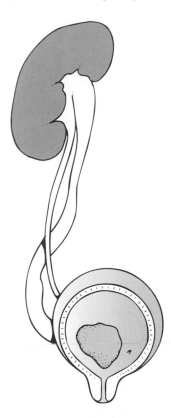

Figure 105.1 Ectopic ureterocele in relation to the upper moiety of a duplex collecting system.

INCIDENCE

The incidence of ureteroceles varies between 1:1,500 and 1:12,000 pediatric admissions, depending on the study,[11,12] and is 1:4000 autopsies.[13] Ureteroceles occur most frequently in females with a 4:1 ratio and are more common in Caucasians.[14] Duplex-system ureteroceles are four to seven times more common in females than in males,[15] and single-system ureteroceles appear to have a slightly male predilection.[10]

There does not appear to be a predilection toward laterality as both kidneys are equally affected[16] and bilateral ureteroceles are found in approximately 10% of cases.[8]

CLINICAL PRESENTATION

The clinical presentation of ureteroceles in infants and children is a febrile urinary tract infection in 39%–73.5% of the cases.[7,17–19] Sepsis, hematuria, urinary incontinence, and/or flank pain can be present. Nonspecific symptoms such as failure to thrive, irritability, urinary retention, or recurrent vomiting should also lead to further investigation of the urinary tract. In cases of severe obstruction and consequent gross megaureter and hydronephrosis, a palpable mass may be present in the abdomen or in the pelvis. Severe electrolyte disturbances, such as hyperkalemia, may occur, and in very rare cases of hyponatremia and hyperkalemia, *pseudohypoaldosteronism* should be suspected.[20]

In baby girls, the ureterocele may prolapse through the urethra and can be seen as an apparent vaginal or vulvar mass (Figure 105.2).

DIAGNOSIS

Ureteroceles can be diagnosed in the antenatal period as part of a screening ultrasound. After the 30th week of pregnancy, the ureterocele may be demonstrated in the fetal bladder (Figure 105.3). More often, however, the antenatal ultrasound performed after the 16th gestational week shows only hydronephrosis. The causative pathology of this hydronephrosis can generally only be established by immediate

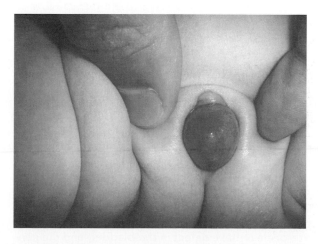

Figure 105.2 Prolapsing ureterocele in a female newborn.

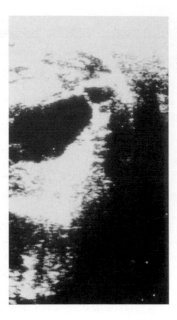

Figure 105.3 Antenatal ultrasonography. Ureterocele in the fetal bladder as seen in the 30th gestational week.

postnatal investigations. These investigations have traditionally consisted of ultrasonography, voiding cystourethrogram (VCUG), and cystoscopy. In addition, Dimercaptosuccinic acid (DMSA), Diethylenetriaminepentaacetic acid (DTPA), Mercaptoacetyltriglycine (MAG3) renal scintigraphy, or magnetic resonance urography (MRU) should be used to detect renal cortical defects, and evaluate renal function and

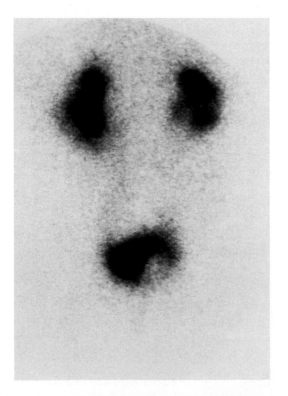

Figure 105.4 Isotope scan (DMSA) demonstrating the ureterocele (uptake defect in the bladder) and the non-function of the upper renal moiety.

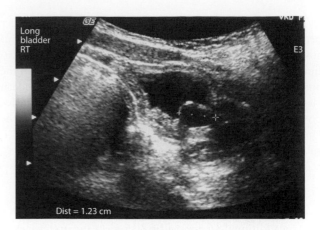

Figure 105.5 Postnatal ultrasonography. Ureterocele within the bladder.

the degree of ureteral obstruction (Figure 105.4). Although inferior in many ways, Intravenous Urogram (IVU) may be used in cases where other imaging modalities are unavailable.

Ultrasonographic findings are of a cystic mass within the bladder, often with dilatation of the associated ureter and pelvicalyceal structures (Figure 105.5). VCUG shows a filling defect within the bladder varying in size and position. The ectopic ureterocele is seen as a filling defect placed eccentrically along the bladder wall extending into the bladder neck or into the posterior urethra. The intravesical ureterocele is generally surrounded by contrast medium demonstrating most of its circumference. If the images are taken when the bladder is full, the ureterocele may evert, mimicking a bladder diverticulum (Figure 105.6).

With the VCUG, reflux into all renal units can also be assessed. Studies have estimated that 50% will have reflux into the ipsilateral lower pole, 25% into the contralateral ureter, and 10% into the ureterocele-bearing ureter.[21]

MRU has also been used to diagnose ureteroceles both in fetal life and in infants with a sensitivity of 89%–100%. The advantages of MRU include anatomic images of both the upper and lower tracts, and with the correct sequences, functional data of the upper tract can also be delineated.[22–25] This information can be useful both in decision making and in surgical planning (Figure 105.7).

Once the diagnosis is suspected based on imaging, cystoscopy can confirm the diagnosis and help with surgical planning.

TREATMENT

Ureteroceles are often complex anomalies. Although considerable controversy still exists regarding the best treatment, the final aims of the surgical management of the ureterocele are to relieve obstruction, prevent urinary infection, prevent or correct vesicoureteral reflux, and preserve renal function. The latter goal may be considered secondary as the upper pole moiety serving the ureterocele is often dysplastic with marginal function.

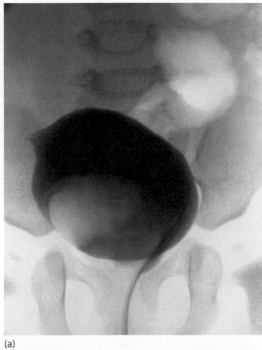

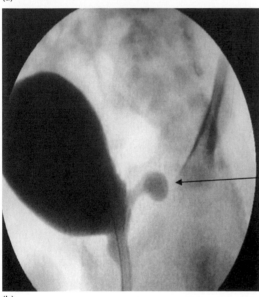

Figure 105.6 Voiding cystourethrogram (VCUG) showing **(a)** ureterocele in the bladder and **(b)** eversion of the ureterocele with filling of the bladder (arrow).

As a result of these goals, four aspects have to be taken into account in the planning of the correct surgical treatment[25]:

1. Degree of renal dysplasia and its resulting loss of renal function
2. Presence of reflux into the ureterocele-bearing ureter, the ipsilateral ureter, and/or the contralateral ureter
3. Altered trigonal anatomy as well as the weakness of the detrusor muscle backing the ureterocele

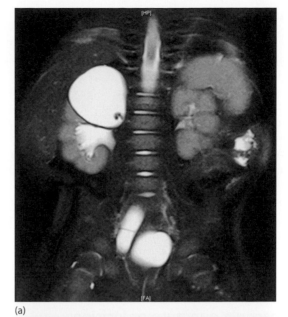

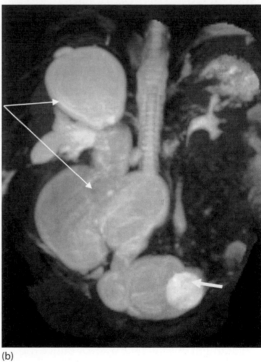

Figure 105.7 T2-weighted Magnetic resonance urography (MRU) showing **(a)** the dilated upper pole associated with the ectopic ureterocele and **(b)** the characteristic appearance of the ureterocele (thick white arrow) with the associated dilated renal upper pole and ureter (thin white arrows).

4. Degree of obstruction caused by the prolapsing or ballooning ureterocele

A standardized approach is probably impossible, and it seems reasonable to individualize the management according to the aspect of each particular case.[26]

Conservative management

Patients meeting specific criteria have been successfully managed with prophylactic antibiotics only. These criteria are as follows:

1. Either a well-functioning renal moiety associated with the ureterocele or a completely nonfunctioning renal unit associated with the ureterocele
2. No evidence of obstruction on functional renal imaging
3. No other pathology (i.e., bladder outlet obstruction)

Sixty to seventy percent of these highly selected patients managed conservatively had resolution of reflux and hydronephrosis,[27,28] showing that, in this highly selected group, surgery may be avoided. However, the long-term potential sequela of small persistent ureteroceles, such as urolithiasis and infection, have not been evaluated.

Endoscopic puncture or incision

With improvements in urologic endoscopic technology, a more conservative approach in the surgical management of the ureterocele is feasible. Several authors have demonstrated the advantages of the endoscopic incision or puncture of ureteroceles in the preservation of renal tissue,[29-32] and in the case of the septic or acutely ill child with an obstructing ureterocele, endoscopic puncture should be considered to be the first-line treatment. This procedure can be performed with the patient under general or regional anesthesia, on a same-day surgery or outpatient basis.[33] Satisfactory postoperative urinary tract decompression has been reported in 85%–100% of cases of endoscopic decompression,[33-35] and recovery of renal function following endoscopic puncture or incision has been reported.[33,34]

Several techniques of endoscopic puncture or incision of ureteroceles exist, but the most common technique consists of a small 2–3 mm incision or puncture made just above the distal junction of the ureterocele with the bladder using a Bugbee electrode[36] or a sharp electrode[29] through a pediatric cystoscope (Figure 105.8). This avoids leaving a flap of ureterocele that might obstruct the bladder outlet and works to preserve a flap valve of the collapsed ureterocele. All these techniques bear the risk of interfering with the structures of the lower pole orifice, and an attempt to visualize the lower pole orifice should be made to prevent such damage. Postincision imaging should be performed to detect reflux in all renal segments and to determine the need for further surgery. A second puncture should be considered in cases where a large ureterocele persists postoperatively and the degree of hydroureteronephrosis on ultrasound remains unchanged or worsened. In the future, even less invasive methods of puncture may be available such as pulsed focused ultrasound.[37]

Controversy still exists regarding the advantages of the endoscopic puncture or incision of ureteroceles as a

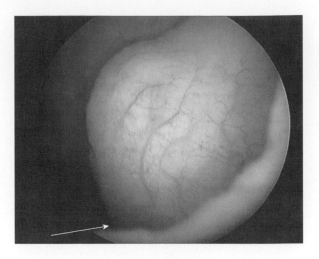

Figure 105.8 Cystoscopic view of an ureterocele. The arrow indicates the target for endoscopic puncture. (Image courtesy of Dr. Edwin Smith.)

"first-stage" treatment, principally due to the high association of postoperative reflux and secondary operations.[21,38–40,41] Surgeons in favor of the endoscopic puncture or incision first-stage treatment in neonates with ureteroceles suggest the following:

1. Approximately one-third of these patients will be definitively treated by this technique.
2. Early renal and ureteral decompression will allow improvement or stabilization of renal function, as well as a decreased risk of pyelonephritis.
3. It allows for a delay in definitive surgical correction, if necessary, and a technically easier operation after the neonatal period due to bladder growth and decreased distention of the affected ureter.[21,29,30,38,39,41–43]

A recent meta-analysis found that, among patients undergoing endoscopic puncture of their ureterocele, risk factors for repeat surgery included an ectopic versus an intravesical ureterocele (Relative Risk, 2.78), ureteroceles draining the upper pole of a duplex system versus those draining a single system (RR, 3.93), and patients with preoperative reflux versus those without reflux (RR, 1.56).[44,45] Thus, the anatomy of each individual patient needs to be taken into account prior to any attempt at endoscopic puncture as a primary treatment.

Duplex-system ureteroceles

For the treatment of duplex-system ureteroceles, four definitive surgical options are available:

1. Heminephrectomy with partial or total ureterectomy, allowing the ureterocele to collapse (upper-tract approach)
2. Excision or marsupialization of the ureterocele, reconstruction of the bladder, and reimplantation of the ureter(s) (lower-tract approach)

3. Combination of heminephrectomy and excision or marsupialization of the ureterocele (combined upper- and lower-tract approach)
4. Ureteroureterostomy (UU) to bypass the obstructed lower ureter and allow for adequate drainage of the upper pole

Ureterocele excision or marsupialization

The traditional open surgical approach involves the complete excision of the ureterocele with reconstruction of the bladder and bladder neck to create a functional bladder neck mechanism. Potential problems with this approach involve injury to adjacent structures, primarily the bladder neck; sphincteric mechanism; or creation of a vesicovaginal fistula. An alternative involves the marsupialization of the ureterocele, which leaves the floor of the ureterocele intact and adhered to the bladder mucosa. This prevents the potential injury to the surrounding structures due to the decreased dissection needed. One study has found no statistical difference between these two techniques.[46]

Procedure

Using a modified Pfannenstiel incision, the skin and the anterior rectus sheath are opened transversally. The recti are bluntly separated in the midline, and the bladder is well mobilized laterally. Over the bladder dome, the peritoneal covering has to be carefully stripped off, avoiding entry into the peritoneal cavity.

The previously filled bladder is incised longitudinally, taking care to avoid injury to the bladder neck. The lower end of the incision can be secured with a holding stitch to prevent tearing into the bladder neck or urethral sphincter and to make for easy identification when closing. The edges of the incised bladder are suspended and held open with holding sutures over the Denis-Browne ring retractor. Several sponges are placed into the superior bladder (the exact number varies depending on the size of the bladder), and the cranial blade is positioned inside the bladder dome over the sponges, pulling it upward and forward, exposing the trigonal area. The ureterocele, the orifice of the lower renal pole ureter, and the contralateral ureter are visualized (Figure 105.9). Each ureter is catheterized with an infant feeding tube or a ureteral catheter. Stay sutures are placed in the dome of the ureterocele, and the urothelium is incised in an elliptical fashion (Figure 105.10a,b).

If the ureterocele is to be completely excised, a dissection plane between the wall of the ureterocele and the urothelium and the detrusor muscle is found, and the ureterocele is dissected off the urothelium (Figure 105.10c). Once the ureterocele is freed completely, the remaining intramural ureter is mobilized as with a standard intravesical ureteral reimplantation (Figure 105.10d). If the ureterocele reaches into the bladder neck or the posterior urethra, this procedure can be extremely difficult to perform, and care has to be taken not to damage the urethral sphincter or its nerve supply. Once the ureterocele is resected, its backing detrusor muscle must be carefully reconstructed using resorbable

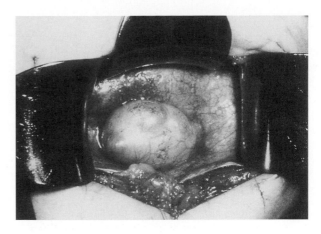

Figure 105.9 Operative treatment: intraoperative findings of a duplex-system ectopic ureterocele.

monofilament sutures (Figure 105.10e). This is to minimize diverticulum formation.[47] In girls, damage to the underlying vagina and, in boys, damage to the ipsilateral vas deferens has to be avoided during this procedure.

Alternatively, the ureterocele can be marsupialized by excision of the anterior and lateral walls of the ureterocele using cattery. This leaves the posterior wall in continuity with the detrusor muscle behind it. The edges of the ureterocele are then reapproximated to the surrounding mucosa using absorbable sutures.

At this stage, the ureters are reimplanted according to Cohen's technique,[48] creating a cross-trigonal submucosal tunnel. Stenting of the reimplanted ureter can be performed according to the surgeon's preference. We generally do not stent the ureter unless there is a specific reason to, i.e., a solitary kidney, an abnormally small ureter, etc.

The bladder is then closed in a standard two-layer technique using resorbable sutures. The bladder is drained with a transurethral catheter. The urethral catheter is generally removed between 1 and 7 days after surgery depending on surgeon preference. Prophylactic antibiotics are administered perioperatively and are continued until absence of reflux is confirmed with postoperative imaging.

Heminephroureterectomy

This procedure can be performed in the traditional open technique, laparoscopically, or using a robot-assisted technique. The laparoscopic partial (or polar) nephrectomy has had good results reported but is widely considered to be one of the hardest laparoscopic procedures to perform.[49] The robot-assisted technique removes many of the technical barriers to the laparoscopic approach. The open and robot-assisted surgical approaches will be covered here.

Procedure

The open upper pole nephrectomy is performed through a flank incision just off the tip of the 12th rib. The incision is extended to a length of 3–4 cm.

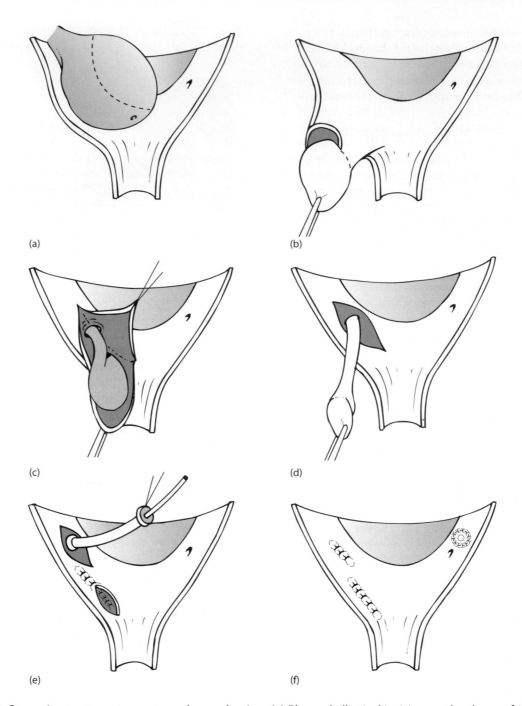

(a)

(b)

(c)

(d)

(e)

(f)

Figure 105.10 Operative treatment—ureterocele enucleation. **(a)** Planned elliptical incision on the dome of the ureterocele. **(b)** The ureterocele is held with stay sutures, and the elliptical incision is performed. **(c)** A plane between the wall of the ureterocele and the urothelium or the detrusor muscle is dissected. **(d)** The intramural ureter of the upper moiety is mobilized, taking care not to damage the lower moiety ureter. **(e)** Reconstruction of the detrusor muscle backing the ureterocele and the urothelial defect. **(f)** The lower moiety ureter is reimplanted according to Cohen's technique, creating a transverse suburothelial tunnel.

The muscle layers are incised using cautery down to the level of the retroperitoneum. The retroperitoneum is entered, and the peritoneum is gently dissected anteriorly. The wound is held open with a retractor. Gerota's fascia is exposed and opened posteriorly.

In the robot-assisted technique, an 8.5 or 12 mm robotic camera port is placed in the umbilicus, and two additional 5 or 8 mm ports are placed with one in the midline superior to the umbilicus and one in the midline or just lateral to it inferior to the umbilicus. The colon is reflected medially along the white line of Toldt to expose the ureters.[50]

In both techniques, the upper pole ureter can then be identified, generally quite easily due to its size. The upper pole ureter is dissected free from the surrounding tissue. The lower pole ureter needs to be identified and dissected free, being careful to leave a sufficient amount of periureteral tissue in place to avoid devascularization. The dilated upper pole ureter is then followed up toward the renal hilum. It is brought under the renal vessels, being careful not to injure them. There is often a separate renal artery to the upper pole segment, which needs to be identified, isolated, and ligated. Once this is accomplished, the ureter can be followed to the upper pole segment, which can be dissected free from the remainder of the renal parenchyma. There is generally a renal groove between the upper and lower pole segments, which can assist in the dissection. The different color and consistency of the dysplastic upper renal pole can be of additional help in the anatomical definition of the two segments (Figure 105.11a). Alternatively, the upper pole system can be entered and can be dissected away from the lower pole from the inside of the collecting system. Extreme care must be taken to preserve the lower renal vasculature.

It is important to remove the entire pelvicocalyceal structures of the upper renal pole and to carefully inspect the remaining kidney for opened lower pole calyces, which need to be closed meticulously with absorbable sutures.

Once hemostasis is achieved, the renal capsule is approximated and sutured with absorbable sutures (Figure 105.11b). Hemostatic agents such as Floseal, Tisseel, or Surgicel can be of additional help to control hemostasis.

Heminephrectomy is now accomplished without having interrupted the circulation to the lower moiety.

Following this procedure, the upper pole ureter is dissected toward its distal portion as far as possible. The dissection line is kept close to the diseased ureter in order not to disturb the lower pole ureter blood supply. If the ureter refluxes, it is ligated and transected, but if it is obstructed, it is transected without ligation to prevent infection.

Once the heminephroureterectomy is completed, a drain can be placed according to surgeon preference, and the muscular layers are approximated using continuous 3-0 or 4-0

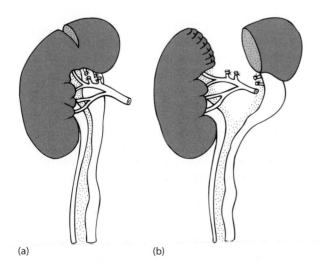

(a)　　　　　(b)

Figure 105.11 Operative treatment—heminephrectomy. **(a)** Transverse resection of the affected upper renal moiety of a duplex system. **(b)** After hemostasis, the renal parenchyma and the renal capsule are closed, often over a bolster of hemostatic material.

resorbable sutures. The subcutaneous tissues are approximated and the skin closed with a subcuticular suture.

Ureteroureterostomy

UU is increasingly being used to repair duplex systems with reasonable function of the upper pole and relatively equal calibre of ureters, although it has been shown to be effective in systems with any degree of function and ureteral size.[51] The UU enjoys the advantage of avoiding the renal vasculature and lower pole of the kidney and the potential for injury to these structures. The primary disadvantage is that the normal, lower pole ureter is involved in a surgery that has the potential to cause damage to it. The UU can be performed using a straight laparoscopic technique, but only the open and robot-assisted techniques will be described here.

Open procedure

Once under anesthesia, cystoscopy is generally performed, and a stent is placed up the normal-calibre, lower pole, "recipient" ureter. This helps with identification and to stent the ureter at the end of the case.

The skin and the anterior rectus sheath are opened transversally using a modified Pfannenstiel incision. The recti are bluntly separated in the midline, and the bladder is well mobilized laterally on the affected side. Over the bladder dome, the peritoneal covering has to be carefully stripped off, avoiding entry into the peritoneal cavity. The ureters are identified in the retroperitoneum and isolated and gently separated from one another, being careful to avoid devascularization of either ureter. The upper pole ureter ("donor" ureter) is transected as close to the bladder as possible and the stump irrigated out. If the ureter refluxes, the stump should be tied off. The recipient ureter is opened in an anteromedial ureterotomy, and the anastomosis is completed using absorbable suture. The stent can either be left in the recipient ureter or be brought across the anastomosis going from the distal recipient ureter to the proximal donor ureter. A drain is placed, and a bladder catheter is left in place, generally overnight. The stent is left in place for 4–6 weeks.

Robot-assisted laparoscopic procedure

In the robot-assisted technique, cystoscopy and stent placement are performed as in the open technique. Three ports are placed with an 8.5 or 12 mm robotic camera port placed in the umbilicus. Two additional 5 or 8 mm instrument ports are placed in the midclavicular line on either side, often 1–2 cm below the umbilicus.

The ureters are identified transperitoneally in the area of the iliac vessels. They are exposed and mobilized approximately 2–3 cm in either direction. The recipient ureter is identified (the stent can assist with this) and is mobilized away from the donor ureter, being careful not to devascularize either ureter. The donor ureter is identified and divided as far distal as possible with the stump sutured or tied off

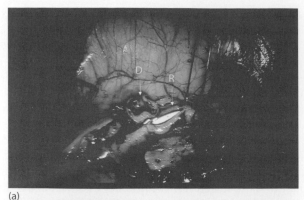

(a)

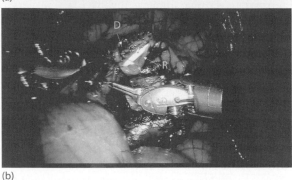

(b)

Figure 105.12 Operative treatment—ureteroureterostomy (UU). **(a)** View of the donor (D) and recipient (R) ureters prior to anastomosis. The stent is in the recipient (lower pole) ureter. (Image courtesy of Dr. Thomas Lendvay.) **(b)** View of the donor (D) and recipient (R) ureters after the back wall has been anastomosed. The stent is in the recipient (lower pole) ureter. (Image courtesy of Dr. Thomas Lendvay.)

if reflux is present (Figure 105.12a). The anastomosis of the ureters is completed in an identical fashion to the open procedure (Figure 105.12b), again with the stent either left in the recipient ureter or placed across the anastomosis.[50,52]

Percutaneous drainage

Percutaneous drainage of systems with ureteroceles is generally only indicated in cases in which the patient is acutely ill and endoscopic puncture is not an option due to small urethral size or the inability to undergo anesthesia.

SUMMARY

Ureteroceles are a fairly common urologic finding. The management of the ureterocele can be quite complex and needs to be individualized for the patient and his/her condition as well as the findings of imaging and functional studies.

REFERENCES

1. Chwalla R. The process of formation of cystic dilatations of vesical end of ureter and of diverticula at ureteral ostium. *Urol Cutan Rev* 1927; 31: 499.

2. Ericsson NO. Ectopic ureterocele in infants and children: A clinical study. *Acta Chir Scand* 1954; 197 (Suppl.): 1.

3. Stephens FD. Caecoureterocele and concepts on embryology and aetiology of ureteroceles. *Aust N Z J Surg* 1971; 40: 239–48.

4. Tanagho EA. Anatomy and management of ureteroceles. *J Urol* 1972; 107: 729–36.

5. Tokunaka S, Gotoh T, Koyanagi T, Tsuji I. Morphological study of the ureterocele: A possible clue to its embryogenesis as evidence by a locally arrested myogenesis. *J Urol* 1981; 126: 726–9.

6. Caldamone AA. Duplication anomalies of the upper tract in infants and children. *Urol Clin N Am* 1985; 12: 75–91.

7. Frey P, Cohen SJ. Ureteroceles in infancy childhood: In search of the correct surgical approach. Experience in 61 cases. *Pediatr Surg Int* 1989; 4: 175.

8. Innes Williams D. Ureteric duplications and ectopia. In: Innes Williams D, Johnston JH (eds). *Paediatric Urology*, 2nd edn. London: Butterworths, 1982: 167–87.

9. Glassberg KI, Braren V, Duckett JW, Jacobs EC, King LR, Lebowitz RL, Perlmutter AD, Stephens FD. Suggested terminology for duplex systems, ectopic ureters and ureteroceles. Report of the Committee on Terminology, Nomenclature and Classification, American Academy of Pediatrics. *J Urol* 1984; 132: 1153–4.

10. Zerin JM, Baker DR, Casale JA. Single-system ureteroceles in infants and children: Imaging features. *Pediatr Radiol* 2000; 30: 139–46.

11. Malek RS, Utz DC. Crossed, fused, renal ectopia with an ectopic ureterocele. *J Urol* 1970; 104: 665–7.

12. Genton N, Markwalder F. Ureterozele. In: Bettex M, Genton N, Stockmann M (eds). *Kinderchirurgie*, 2nd edn. Stuttgart: Thieme, 1982: 8.98–8.104.

13. Campbell M. Ureterocele: A study of 94 instances in 80 infants and children. *Surg Gynecol Obstetr* 1951; 93: 705.

14. Scherz H, Kaplan G, Packer M, Brock W. Ectopic ureteroceles: Surgical management with preservation of continence—Review of 60 cases. *J Urol* 1989; 142: 538.

15. Eklöf O, Löhr G, Ringertz H, Thomasson B. Ectopic ureterocele in the male infant. *Acta Radiol (Diagn.)* (Stockh.) 1978; 19: 145–53.

16. Brock WA, Kaplan WG. Ectopic ureteroceles in children. *J Urol* 1978; 119: 800–3.

17. Shekarriz B, Upadhyay J, Fleming P, Gonzalez R, Barthold JS. Long-term outcome based in the initial surgical approach to ureterocele. *J Urol* 1999; 162: 1072–6.

18. De Jong TP, Dik P, Klijn AJ, Uiterwaal CS, van Gool JD. Ectopic ureterocele: Results of open surgical therapy in 40 patients. *J Urol* 2000; 164: 2040–3.

19. Besson R, Tran Ngoc B, Laboure S, Debeugny P. Incidence of urinary tract infection in neonates with antenatally diagnosed ureteroceles. *Eur J Pediatr Surg* 2000; 10: 111–3.

20. Perez M, Gatti J, Smith EA, Kirsch AJ. Pseudohypoaldosteronism associated with ureterocele and upper pole moiety obstruction. *Urology* 2001; 57: 1178.

21. Cooper CS, Passerini-Glazel G, Hutcheson JC, Iafrate M, Camuffo C, Milani C, Snyder HM 3rd. Long-term follow-up of endoscopic incision of ureteroceles: Intravesical versus extravesical. *J Urol* 2000; 164: 1097–9.

22. Payabvash S, Kajbafzadeh AM, Saeedi P, Sadeghi Z, Elmi A, Mehdizadeh M. Application of magnetic resonance urography in diagnosis of congenital urogenital anomalies in children. *Pediatr Surg Int* 2008; 24: 979.

23. Adeb M, Darge K, Dillman JR, Carr M, Epelman M. Magnetic resonance urography in evaluation of duplicated renal collecting systems. *Magn Reson Imaging Clin N Am* 2013; 21: 717–30.

24. Kirsch AJ and Grattan-Smith JD. Magnetic resonance imaging of the pediatric urinary tract. In: Gearhart JP, Rink RC, Mouriquand PDE (eds). *Pediatric Urology*, 2nd edn. Amsterdam: WB Saunders, 2010: 162–71.

25. Kelalis PP. Renal pelvic and ureter. In: Kelalis PP, King LR, Belman AB (eds). *Clinical Pediatric Urology*, 2nd edn. Philadelphia: WB Saunders, 1985: 672–725.

26. Cohen SA, Juwono T, Palazzi KL, Kaplan GW, Chiang G. Examining trends in the treatment of ureterocele yields no definitive solution. *J Pediatr Urol* 2014; 11: 29.e1–e6.

27. Han M, Gibbins M, Belman A, Pohl H, Majd M, Rushton H. Indications for nonoperative management of ureteroceles. *J Urol* 2005; 174: 1652.

28. Direnna T, Leonard M. Watchful waiting for prenatally detected ureteroceles. *J Urol* 2006; 175: 1493.

29. Monfort G, Morrisson-Lacombe G, Coquet M. Endoscopic treatment of ureteroceles revisited. *J Urol* 1985; 133: 1031–3.

30. Gotoh T, Koyanagi T, Matsuno T. Surgical management of ureteroceles in children: Strategy based on the classification of ureteral hiatus and the eversion of ureteroceles. *J Pediatr Surg* 1988; 23: 159–65.

31. Di Benedetto V, Meyrat BJ, Sorrentino G, Monfort G. Management of ureteroceles detected by prenatal ultrasound. *Pediatr Surg Int* 1995; 10: 485.

32. Patil U, Mathews R. Minimal surgery with renal preservation in anomalous complete duplicated systems. *J Urol* 1995; 154: 727–8.

33. Di Benedetto V, Morrison-Lacombe G, Begnara V, Monfort G. Transurethral puncture of ureterocele associated with single collecting system in neonates. *J Pediatr Surg* 1997; 32: 1325–7.

34. Pfister C, Ravasse P, Barret E, Petit T, Mitrofanoff P. The value of endoscopic treatment for ureteroceles during the neonatal period. *J Urol* 1998; 159: 1006–9.

35. Jelloul L, Berger D, Frey P. Endoscopic management of ureteroceles in children *Eur Urol* 1997; 32: 321–6.

36. Rich MA, Keating MA, Snyder HM 3rd, Duckett JW. Low transurethral incision of single system intravesical ureteroceles in children. *J Urol* 1990; 144: 120–1.

37. Maxwell AD, His RS, Bailey MR, Casale P, Lendvay TS. Noninvasive ureterocele puncture using pulsed focused ultrasound: An in vitro study. *J Endourol* 2014; 28: 342–6.

38. Blyth B, Passerini-Glazel G, Camuffo C, Snyder HM 3rd, Duckett JW. Endoscopic incision of ureteroceles: Intravesical versus ectopic. *J Urol* 1993; 149: 556–9.

39. Smith C, Gosalbez R, Parrott TS, Woodard JR, Broecker B, Massad C. Transurethral puncture of ectopic ureteroceles in neonates and infants. *J Urol* 1994; 152: 2110–2.

40. Spencer Barthold J. Editorial: Individualized approach to the prenatally diagnosed ureterocele. *J Urol* 1998; 159: 1011–2.

41. Sander JC, Bilgutay AN, Stanasel I, Koh CJ, Janzen N, Gonzales ET, Roth DR, Seth A. Outcomes of endoscopic incision for the treatment of ureterocele in children at a single institution. *J Urol* 2015; 193: 662–7.

42. Jayanthi VR, Koff SA. Long-term outcome of transurethral puncture of ectopic ureteroceles. Initial success and late problems. *J Urol* 1999; 162: 1077–80.

43. Di Benedetto V, Monfort G. How prenatal ultrasound can change the treatment of ectopic ureterocele in neonates? *Eur J Pediatr Surg* 1997; 7: 338–40.

44. Byun E, Merguerian P. A meta-analysis of surgical practice patterns in the endoscopic management of ureteroceles. *J Urol* 2006; 176: 1871.

45. Castagnetti M, Cimador M, Sergio M, de Grazia E. Transurethral incision of duplex system ureteroceles in neonates: Does it increase the need for secondary surgery in intravesical and ectopic cases? *BJU Int* 2004; 93: 1313–7.

46. Lewis J, Cheng E, Campbell J, Kropp B, Liu D, Kropp K, Kaplan W. Complete excision or marsupialisation of ureteroceles: Does choice of surgical approach affect outcome? *J Urol* 2008; 180: 1819.

47. Gomez F, Stephens GD. Cecoureterocele: Morphology and clinical correlations. *J Urol* 1983; 129: 1017–9.

48. Cohen SJ. The Cohen technique of ureteroneocystostomy. In: Eckstein HB, Hohenfellner R, Williams DI (eds). *Surgical Pediatric Urology*. Stuttgart: Thieme, 1977: 269–74.

49. Denes F, Danilovic A, Srougi M. Outcomes of laparoscopic upper-pole nephrectomy in children with duplex systems. *J Endourol* 2007; 21: 162.

50. Timberlake MD, Corbett ST. Minimally invasive techniques for management of the ureterocele and ectopic ureter—Upper tract versus lower tract approach. *Urol Clin N Am* 2015; 42: 61–76.

51. McLeod DJ, Alpert SA, Ural Z, Jayanthi VR. Ureteroureterostomy irrespective of ureteral size of upper pole function: A single center experience. *J Pediatr Urol* 2014; 10: 616–9.

52. Leavitt DA, Rambachan A, Haberman K, DeMarco R, Shukla AR. Robot-assisted laparoscopic ipsilateral ureteroureterostomy for ectopic ureters in children: Description of technique. *J Endourol* 2012; 10: 1279–83.

106

Posterior urethral valves

PAOLO CAIONE AND MICHELE INNOCENZI

INTRODUCTION

Posterior urethral valves (PUVs) are the main cause of urethral obstruction in newborns and infants that continues to be a significant cause of morbidity and mortality in pediatric-age patients.[1,2] In males, children born with bladder obstructive uropathy and renal dysplasia represent the single largest group undergoing renal dialysis and transplantation under 5 years of age. End-stage renal disease develops in a significant proportion, varying from 30% to 42%.[1] In 2003, the ItalKid Project, which consists of a prospective population-based registry assessing the epidemiology of chronic renal failure (CRF) in pediatric age on the basis of 1197 patients recruited in 10 years, showed that renal hypodysplasia with identified congenital uropathy was the most common cause of CRF (43.6%): in this group, PUVs were second only to vesicoureteral reflux (VUR), accounting for 23.8%.[3]

HISTORICAL NOTES

Congenital obstruction of posterior the urethra has been recognized for almost 200 years, as the earliest description of this condition in infants was by an Italian anatomist, Giovanni Battista Morgagni, in 1717.[4] Langenbeck[5] described infravesical urethral obstruction in 1802 in his monograph on stone disease, and a few years later, in 1832, Velpeau[6] utilized for the first time the term *valves*. Subsequently, many reports of posterior urethral obstruction can be found in the literature. The most important contribution to define the anatomical aspects of valves was made by Hugh Hampton Young in 1919[7] and 1929.[8] Young was the first to describe clearly the features of PUV. The description included the first classification of this entity based on his initial report on 12 patients, and a review of the literature.[7] The Young classification distinguished congenital obstruction of the posterior urethra on three types of valves (Type I, Type II, Type III), which he described in detail (Figure 106.1).[9] In more recent years, some criticism arose from the analysis of Young's original work, revealing different opinions from his conclusions.[10–13] A large contribution to a better anatomical definition of PUV and urethral diaphragm was given by Hendren and more recently by P. A. Dewan and coauthors,[14,15] who identified the morphological evidence of the congenital membrane obstructing the male posterior urethra (see section titled "Classification"). Anyway, Young's classification, although not anatomically precise, is well known worldwide and still utilized currently.

EPIDEMIOLOGICAL DATA

The epidemiology of PUV is uncertain to define, as most authors believe that only those with typical appearance on voiding cystourethrograms (VCUGs) should be counted. The incidence of PUV often is reported as 1:5000 to 1:8000 infant males,[14–16] 1 child in 25,000 live births,[16] but this value seems to be underestimated.[17] The point is that the true incidence of congenital posterior urethral obstruction is difficult to ascertain.

The lesion could be more common than previously thought: this is due to the fact that the widespread use of prenatal and postnatal ultrasonography and of the VCUG during the recent few decades led to the recognition of a higher number of congenital valves, diaphragms, or strictures on the male posterior urethra, not always recognized as classic valves.

Moreover, at endoscopy or at VCUG, "mild" or "minor" forms of inframontanal *plicae* or mucosal folds, responsible for partial or little urinary outflow, are nowadays a more common observation in male children and infants, as a consequence of widespread use of cystourethroscopy. So, the full spectrum of congenital posterior obstruction is probably twice as frequent as previously thought.[18]

EMBRYOLOGY

Obstruction of the male posterior urethra is a congenital abnormality, which is considered to have no genetic basis and no pattern of inheritance. There is no agreement as regards the true embryogenesis. It has been argued that posterior valves could originate from an abnormality of development during formation of the urogenital sinus.[19] Livne et al.[20] proposed that the valves' embryogenesis arises from maldevelopment of the urethrovaginal folds, appearing at 11 weeks' gestation, from the *plicae colliculi* diverging from the distal end of the *verumontanum* (mesonephric Wolffian duct). Field and Stephens[21] believed that valves could be vestiges of the receding Wolffian ducts, which migrated posterolaterally to converge on the posterior wall of the urethra, creating the inferior urethral crests. Fusion of these folds anteriorly would explain the formation of a membranous obstruction with a posterior deficit, as described by Dewan.[15] A detailed review of the literature has recently been focused by Krishman and coauthors,[22] better elucidating the precise origins regarding the anatomy, classification, and embryology of PUV. Anyway, the embryological development of the congenital posterior urethra obstruction in male fetuses and infants remains uncertain. With the advent of more accurate imaging techniques, such as ultrasonography, VCUG, and fetal/infant magnetic resonance imaging (MRI), the obstructive membranes of the posterior male urethra are now better defined. It is hypothesized that the severity of the congenital diaphragm obstructing the urethra is variable, consistent with the differential clinical presentation of PUV. In some cases, the membrane is only partially obstructing, whereas in other situations, it may be totally obstructing, as in infants with severe renal sequelae. When a feeding tube or catheter is passed in the newborn urethra, the membrane could be ruptured ventrally, modifying the appearance into Young's classic valves.[22]

CLASSIFICATION

Young and colleagues in 1919 divided PUV into Types I, II, and III, based primarily on autopsy findings.[7] Young described Type I valves as sails or strong plicae colliculi, which extend distally from either side of the verumontanum to attach to the anterolateral walls of the urethra; Type II valves are folds that arise from the verumontanum and pass proximally toward the bladder neck, where they divide into finlike membranes; Type III valves are diaphragms with a central perforation located distal or proximal to the verumontanum, but not attached to it (Figure 106.1).

Most authors agree that Young's classification is incorrect. In particular, the existence of Type II valves has been questioned, as these plicae should be considered as normal mucosal folds.[15–17]

The Type I valves are the most commonly recognized. The clinical description of a valve with two separate leaflets is derived from autopsy specimens in which the urethra is laid open by cutting through the anterior wall. However, when viewed endoscopically, it is seen to be a single structure originating from the inferior margin of the verumontanum, the lateral folds fusing anteriorly to form a slit-like aperture. Dewan and colleagues, in accurate endoscopic studies, demonstrated that the commonly defined PUVs are represented by a single membrane with a posterior defect, distal to the verumontanum but connected to it by mucosal folds. Dewan proposed the term "congenital obstructive posterior urethral membrane" (COPUM) to define this lesion.[14,15,23]

Type III valves are considered very uncommon, and they represent a severe form of urethral obstruction.[16] In a review of cystoendoscopies of boys with urethral obstruction, Dewan described a fibrous membrane without attachment to the verumontanum, with a central defect below the verumontanum in the bulbar urethra.[14,15] These lesions are known as Cobb's collar,[24] Moormann's ring,[25] or congenital bulbar urethra stricture, but should be distinguished from the COPUM or misnamed Type III valves.[23]

In conclusion, nowadays we consider PUV as a spectrum of anatomical and pathological entities, presenting different severities of urinary outflow obstruction and having probably only two structural features:

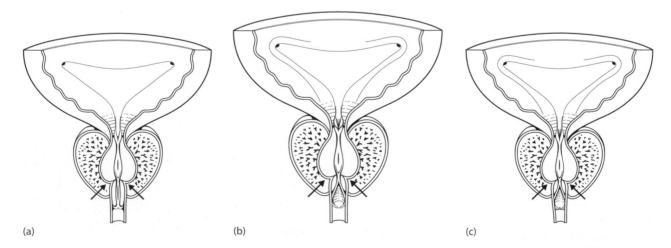

(a) (b) (c)

Figure 106.1 **(a, b, c)** Posterior urethral valves: The original classification proposed by Young in 1919 in 3 types. (From Macpherson RI et al., Posterior urethral valves: An update and review, *Radiographics* 1986; 6(5):753–791. Young HH and McKay RW, Congenital valvular obstruction of the posterior urethra, *Surg Gynecol Obstet* 1929;48:509. Waterhouse K and Hamm FC, The importance of urethral valves as a cause of vesical neck obstruction in children, *J Urol* 1962;87:404.)

1. A membrane at the level of the posterior urethra distal to the *verumontanum*, with connecting folds and a posterior defect (COPUM)
2. A fibrous membrane in the bulbar urethra with a central defect (Cobb's collar)

PATHOPHYSIOLOGY OF PUVs

Congenital posterior urethral obstruction interferes with all the lower and upper urinary tract, causing significant anatomical and functional changes. In pediatric urology, PUV could represent a severe congenital uropathy, with lifelong consequences.

Valves of the posterior urethra represent a spectrum of lesions within the male urethra, grouped under the more extensive term *COPUM*.[15] The macroscopic appearance has been described in the preceding section, "Classification." The severity of the obstruction is varying from small folds without obstruction to unyielding and hard membranes with a small deficit, causing a high degree of outlet obstruction.[26] The valves cause a mechanical and functional obstruction in the urethral conduit, leading to sequential secondary pathological changes. The heaviness of the secondary pathological changes in the upper urinary tract will depend on the degree and timing of the primary obstruction.

Proximally to the obstructive valves, high back pressure prenatally determined is responsible for significant changes in the anatomical appearance. The prostatic urethra is enlarged and elongated, and the *verumontanum* is much more evident; the posterior aspect of the bladder neck is very pronounced, as consequence of muscular hypertrophy, and it could cause impaired bladder emptying also after urethral disobstruction.

The severity of the pathological changes in the urethral and bladder structures and secondarily in the upper tract depends on the degree and timing of the primary urethral obstruction, such as variable morphological expression of the same embryological abnormality, which is considered to have onset very early during the embryological life (16th–18th week of gestational age).[22]

SECONDARY CONSEQUENCES

Secondary pathology on bladder and upper urinary tract

Not only does the posterior urethra dilate and elongate secondarily to the congenital urethral obstruction, but also, the bladder, the ureter, and the kidneys will present significant structural and functional consequences.

Bladder secondary changes

The congenital urethral obstruction is responsible for significant changes in the bladder reservoir, with consequences also in the upper urinary tract and in the renal parenchyma. These changes may persist, although the primary urethral obstruction could be fully solved. As the valve's onset is very early during the fetal life, the abnormal condition of high endoluminal pressure and overdistension of the urinary structures leads to a pathological development and dysfunctional activity of the entire urinary tract and of the renal parenchyma.[24] Experimental studies on fetal lambs demonstrated the induction of renal parenchyma dysplasia and significant histological and functional bladder changes.[27] Bladder dysfunction may present a variety of different pictures, changing throughout the years, before and after puberty.[28]

Macroscopically, the bladder wall presents trabeculations as a consequence of hypertrophy of the muscular components and of the high-pressure regimen. Histologic studies of the bladder wall have shown increased collagen and connective tissue elements within the muscular cells. The collagen/muscular ratio could be increased with reduced muscular components of the bladder wall. The overall structural and functional changes of the bladder, which persist after urethral obstruction release, were named *valve bladder syndrome*.[29]

Ureteral pathology

Dilatation of one or both ureters is often seen in newborns or infants presenting PUV. Ureteric dilatation may be due to vesicoureteric reflux, vesicoureteric junction obstruction, or inefficient ureteric drainage secondary to high vesical pressures. These changes may persist following valve removal,[30] and the ureters may remain enlarged and tortuous, with thickened and rigid walls (Figure 106.2).

Vesicoureteric reflux

Reflux is frequently associated with PUV. It has been reported in 19%–78% of children[31,32] and is thought to be due to a high-pressure regimen in the prenatally obstructed bladder (Figure 106.3). Once the urethral obstruction has been resolved, a significant proportion of patients are expected to have resolution of their reflux.[33] Thus, a conservative approach to VUR

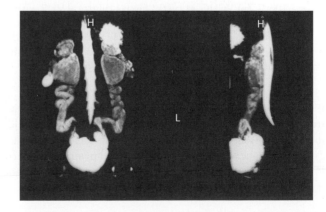

Figure 106.2 MRI of urinary tract in a boy, aged 5 years, born with PUV ablated shortly after birth: The pyelocaliceal system remains bilaterally dilated, with ureters enlarged and tortuous.

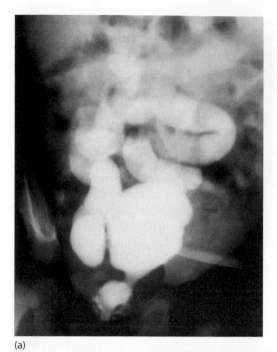

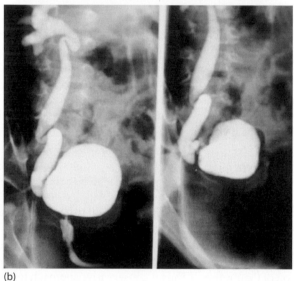

Figure 106.3 **(a)** VCUG at birth: Gross bilateral VUR with enlarged trabeculated bladder presenting congenital posterior urethra obstruction, before valve ablation. **(b)** VCUG of the same patient at 4 years of age: Normalization of the bladder and urethra outline, with persisting right VUR.

in children with previous valves or diaphragm on posterior urethra is strongly recommended in infancy and early childhood. The incidences of bilateral and unilateral reflux are almost equal; however, bilateral reflux and posterior urethral obstruction denotes a more severe disease with higher grade of renal parenchymal involvement and risk of CRF.[33]

"VURD" syndrome

John Duckett and coauthors focus on the protective factors in PUV, pointing out that unilateral reflux denotes less severe disease, although the VUR is usually high grade and ipsilateral renal parenchyma is very damaged and dysplastic.[34] In fact, in such cases, the contralateral side is protected by the "pop-off" mechanism that keeps bladder pressures low.[34,35] The kidney on the side affected with reflux is usually nonfunctioning as a result of dysplasia (Figure 106.4). VUR and renal dysplasia in posterior urethral obstruction could be a primary event due to abnormal location of the ureteric bud arising from the Wolffian duct. More probably, the pathogenesis of unilateral renal dysplasia in the "vesicoureteral reflux and dysplasia" (VURD) syndrome, unilateral VURD, is due to the high-pressure regimen of the upper urinary tract, started very early during the fetal life, with consequent impairment of the renal parenchymal maturation.[35]

Renal dysplasia and hydronephrosis

Renal damage is very frequent in PUV, and it can be attributed to a variety of reasons:

1. Primary renal dysplasia
2. Renal dysplasia induced by early intrauterine bladder outlet obstruction, VUR, or ureterovesical obstruction
3. Postnatal urinary tract infection
4. Persistent bladder dysfunction

The association between renal dysplasia and hydronephrosis can be seen as consequence of severe obstructive posterior valves or urethral diaphragm. Renal dysplasia is typically associated with abnormal histology and is not reversible. Hydronephrosis and stasis secondary to obstructive uropathy has normal renal histology and is reversible with treatment.

On the other hand, Hoover and Duckett[35] described the frequent association of posterior urethral obstruction, reflux, and renal dysplasia, suggesting a common embryological error. Henneberry[36] and Stephens proposed that renal dysplasia associated with posterior urethral obstruction is not secondary to reflux or high pressures, but is a primary embryologic malformation that is the result of an abnormal position of the primitive urethral bud.

Early bladder outlet obstruction as in PUV can also produce impaired tubular function. Pediatric nephrologists and urologists from the Great Ormond Street Children's Hospital in London observed that defective urine concentration occurs in as many as 60% of boys with urethral obstruction and is severe in 15%.[37] The resultant concentrating defect causes high urinary output and sodium loss, and the severe polyuria carries a risk of dehydration and electrolyte imbalance. Furthermore, high urine output may increase the overload of work of the lower tract and enhance the bladder dysfunction, causing incontinence and further renal damage in the attempt of obtaining dryness in toilet-trained boys and adolescents.[30] This clinical picture was named valve bladder syndrome.[38]

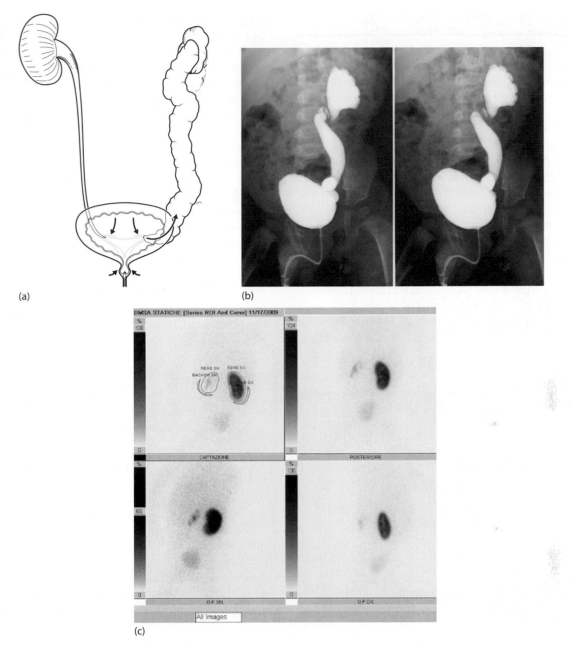

Figure 106.4 **(a)** The "VURD" syndrome (valve, unilateral reflux, dysplasia) as a protective factor for the contralateral kidney and bladder activity. **(b)** Left severe VUR in a 6-month-old infant with previously ablated PUV: Normal light kidney. **(c)** Poor-functioning left kidney at dimercaptosuccinic acid (DMSA) scan. (**[a]** From Glick PL et al., Management of the fetus with congenital hydronephrosis II: Prognostic criteria and selection for treatment, *J Pediatr Surg* 1985;20:376–387.)

These secondary consequences on the pathophysiology of the kidneys and lower urinary tract in boys with previous valves have a significant role in the management of these patients after obstruction removal.[38]

Pulmonary hypoplasia

During the pregnancy, oligohydramnios secondary to decreased fetal urine output produces an abnormally small uterine cavity. This compresses the fetus and interferes with the normal growth and expansion of the fetal thorax, resulting in pulmonary hypoplasia. The kidneys themselves have an important role in early lung growth, while the presence of amniotic fluid contributes to growth later in gestation. Amniotic fluid index (AFI) is an important marker of renal physiology during pregnancy. If severe oligohydramnios is present in early fetal life (19th–26th week gestational age), repeated maternal amnioinfusions or fetal bladder shunting may be considered, in the attempt to prevent lung maldevelopment. Preliminary hypoplasia represents the main cause of postnatal death in newborns with severe PUV or other congenital obstruction of the urethra.[39,40]

CLINICAL FEATURES

In the last three decades, advances in antenatal diagnosis have resulted in an increase in the number of babies with urinary tract obstruction being diagnosed either in utero or within the first few days of life, some of whom have posterior urethral obstruction. The ultrasonographic features of bilateral hydronephrosis in a male newborn with dilated and winding ureters, associated with an enlarged and poor-emptying bladder with thickened walls, are very suspicious for PUV or urethral diaphragm (Figure 106.5).

In the neonatal period, the baby may present with urinary tract infection, septicemia, uremia, and metabolic acidosis. Urinary symptoms may include a poor urinary stream, which can be an unreliable sign as some infants with severe obstruction have developed detrusor hypertrophy, enabling them to have a good stream. Quite often, the bladder and/or kidneys are palpable in infants with bladder outlet obstruction.[17,31]

More commonly, infants with PUV can present with chronic urinary stasis and upper tract changes, vomiting, failure, to thrive and loss of weight. Rarely, they may present with abdominal distension due to urinary ascites or peri-renal urine collection. Urinary ascites is usually a result of perforation of the kidney, and in many instances, the site of the actual leak is not obvious radiologically. The newborn may present with a severe abdominal distension due to urinary tract dilatation and/or urinary ascites (Figure 106.6). Dispnoic or polypnoic breathing is often observed, as consequence of pulmonary dysplasia, metabolic acidosis, and abdominal distension.

INVESTIGATIONS

Ultrasound scan is the first diagnostic step that often is suggested by the prenatal sonographic studies during pregnancy. The ultrasound should be performed at earliest convenience. The kidneys are scanned to determine the severity of hydronephrosis and to identify any perineal collections of urine. The dilated ureters can be traced down to the bladder. In an uncatheterized patient, a dilated posterior urethra can be demonstrated by a perineal sagittal scan.

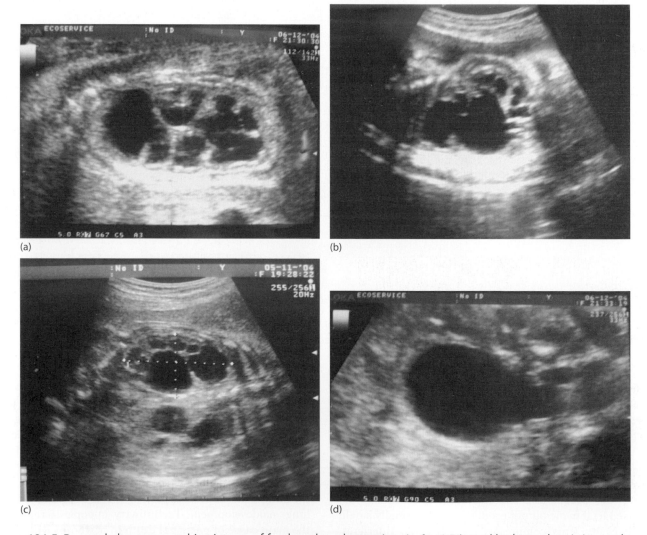

(a)

(b)

(c)

(d)

Figure 106.5 Prenatal ultrasonographic pictures of fetal urethra obstruction. **(a, b, c)** Bilateral hydronephrosis in a male newborn, with dilated ureters. **(d)** Enlarged and poorly emptying bladder, presenting thickened walls and wide bladder neck.

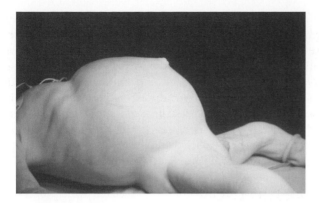

Figure 106.6 Picture of a very sick newborn with severe abdominal distension due to urinary ascites from congenital posterior urethral obstruction.

The bladder is thick-walled and with irregular edges, by the presence of pseudodiverticula (Figure 106.7).

After birth, once the infection has been brought under control, the diagnosis can be confirmed by a *micturating cystogram* (VCUG), which is the gold standard for the diagnosis of posterior urethral obstruction. The examination should be performed to record the micturition in the lateral oblique position. The following features can usually be demonstrated (Figure 106.8): trabeculated bladder walls, poor emptying, and dilatation and elongation of the posterior urethra, with prominence of the bladder neck, particularly the posterior lip. VUR may be present in many infants (Figures 106.3 and 106.4).

Intravenous pyelogram is nowadays not anymore utilized in infants and young children, as it has been replaced by ultrasound and radionuclide studies. Useful anatomical information on ureters for boys requiring upper tract surgery or bladder enlargement can be obtained by *magnetic resonance imaging* (MRI) studies (Figure 106.2).

Radionuclide studies should not be utilized in the neonatal period, but they are very useful to assess the later functional

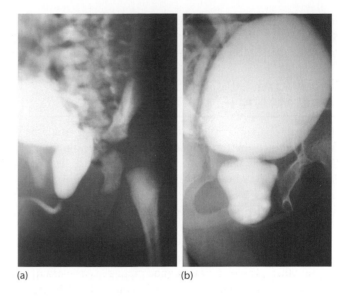

(a)   (b)

Figure 106.8 VCUG imaging in PUV. **(a)** Trabeculated bladder walls, dilatation, and elongation of the posterior urethra and sharp-cut reduced lumen of the urethra distally to the obstructing membrane. **(b)** Late presentation of PUV, with prominence of the bladder neck and wide prostatic urethra. Right VUR is present.

status of both kidneys and to guide the urologist's decision on upper tract repair and on nephrectomy (VURD syndrome). In infants in whom a postoperative ultrasound scan shows no improvement, a mercaptoacetyltriglycine (MAG3) scan may help to distinguish between persistent obstruction and cystic dysplasia. The uptake is negligible in dysplasia. A renogram should be performed to assess the differential glomerular filtration rate, and the ureterovesical or pyeloureteral junction obstruction.

Urodynamic investigations are not usually performed at neonatal age or before valve ablation, but it is essential for the outcome evaluation of bladder changes across time.[41] Urodynamic studies are necessary to investigate the functional manifestation of the valve bladder syndrome and their relationship with urinary incontinence, voiding dysfunction and upper tract persisting dilatation. From initial patterns of hypercontractility in infancy and early childhood, bladder activity may gradually change to hypocontractility in many boys, especially after puberty[41] (Figure 106.9). The overdistended bladders in adolescence may lead to decompensation and increasing postmicturition

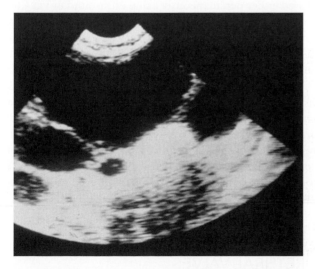

Figure 106.7 Ultrasonographic findings in an infant with PUV: Bilateral hydronephrosis, enlarged ureters with distended bladder.

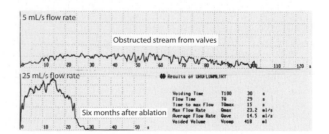

Figure 106.9 Uroflowmetry in a 4-year-old child with PUV. Reduced flow rate at presentation and normal pattern at 6 months after ablation.

residual and maximum bladder capacity. Upper tract persisting dilatation is a possible severe consequence, necessitating drug manipulation and/or intermittent catheterization.[36]

PRENATAL DIAGNOSIS AND MANAGEMENT

Urethral obstruction can be suspected in a male fetus with the introduction of screening ultrasonography and improvement of technology. A more frequent in utero diagnosis of PUV is now feasible.[42] Classic sonographic findings of PUV include a combination of megacystis, thickened bladder wall, dilated posterior urethra, with the "keyhole sign," and bilateral hydronephrosis in a male fetus (Figure 106.10). Oligohydramnios may be associated in more severe forms.[39] Even in the absence of these signs, antenatal diagnosis of urethral obstruction can be considered, especially in the presence of a constellation of findings including oligohydramnios and evidence of spontaneous urinary tract decompression (ascites, perirenal urinoma) (Figure 106.11).

Urethral obstruction in utero produces a wide variety of clinically significant effects in addition to obvious obstructive uropathy. Fetal urine is produced by the 13th gestational week, a decrease in the production of which results in an abnormally small uterine cavity. This compresses the fetus and interferes with normal growth and expansion of the fetal thorax, resulting in pulmonary hypoplasia. Bladder distension and urinary ascites expand the fetal abdomen and compromise the development of abdominal wall muscle, resulting in the prune belly appearance. In conclusion, prenatal ultrasound can accurately detect fetal lower urinary tract obstruction, with a sensitivity of 95% and a specificity of 80%.[43]

MRI may be increasingly used in the diagnosis and assessment of fetuses with lower urinary tract obstruction, enhancing the ultrasound findings.

Pulmonary and renal consequences vary in severity with the degree of urethral obstruction in utero, where high-grade

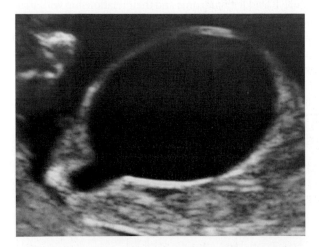

Figure 106.10 The "keyhole sign" of the fetal bladder at prenatal ultrasonography: Poorly emptying megacystis, with thickened bladder wall and dilated posterior urethra in a male fetus.

oligohydramnios and pulmonary hypoplasia develop and lead to postnatal respiratory insufficiency and death. In less severe cases, enough urine passes to give a sufficient amniotic fluid volume to allow adequate pulmonary growth.

The advantage of prenatal diagnosis is considerable. The maternal and fetal management can be planned early, which usually results in maternal transport to a tertiary center where the newborn can receive optimal treatment immediately after birth. A flowchart on the prenatal management of PUV is presented in Figure 106.12.

Fetal lower urinary tract obstruction is a condition of high mortality and morbidity, associated with progressive renal dysfunction, oligohydramnios, and secondary pulmonary hypoplasia. *Intrauterine intervention* was developed from the pioneering research of Harrison and coworkers.[37,38] The most difficult problem has been the *selection* of the fetus with obstructive uropathy who might benefit from in utero treatment. Studies of the natural history of untreated congenital hydronephrosis have shown that the fetus with mild bilateral hydronephrosis and normal amniotic fluid volume requires no in utero intervention. Also, the fetus who presents with severe oligohydramnios and severely dysplastic kidneys sonographically is unlikely to benefit from antenatal intervention. Between the two groups, cases with obstructive uropathy can be observed, where potentially fatal renal and pulmonary damage may be averted by intervention. Prognostic criteria have been developed by Glick et al. (Table 106.1).[44] Fetal urine analysis may provide improvement in prenatal determination of renal prognosis. Anyway, precise criteria to guide prenatal management remain uncertain.[45] Further predictors of renal dysplasia have been examined in fetal obstructive uropathy, such as bladder pressure and beta-2-microglobulin assessment, to achieve prenatal evaluation of fetal renal function.[45]

It is possible to decompress the obstruction in utero, through *percutaneous vesicoamniotic shunting or cystoscopic techniques.* Quintero and colleagues[46] pointed to the technique and results of the insertion of a vesicoamniotic shunt passed either percutaneously using ultrasound or via a fetoscope, allowing the bladder to decompress into the amniotic cavity. The shunts are not satisfactory for long-term fetal urinary tract decompression due to the high incidence of catheter obstruction, displacement, and risk of chorioamnionitis.[47]

In appropriately selected fetuses, prenatal intervention may improve perinatal survival, but long-term renal damage remains mostly unsolved. Randomized multicentric studies are warranted.[48] At the moment, the initial enthusiasm has been reduced by the poor ability to modify the long-term outcome for the severely affected newborns. Open decompression for fetal obstructive uropathy is still in the experimental stage, awaiting further control trials to establish its efficacy.[47,48]

POSTNATAL MANAGEMENT OF NEONATES WITH POSTERIOR URETHRAL VALVES

Infants born with posterior urethral obstruction often may have often upper tract dilatation and renal damage

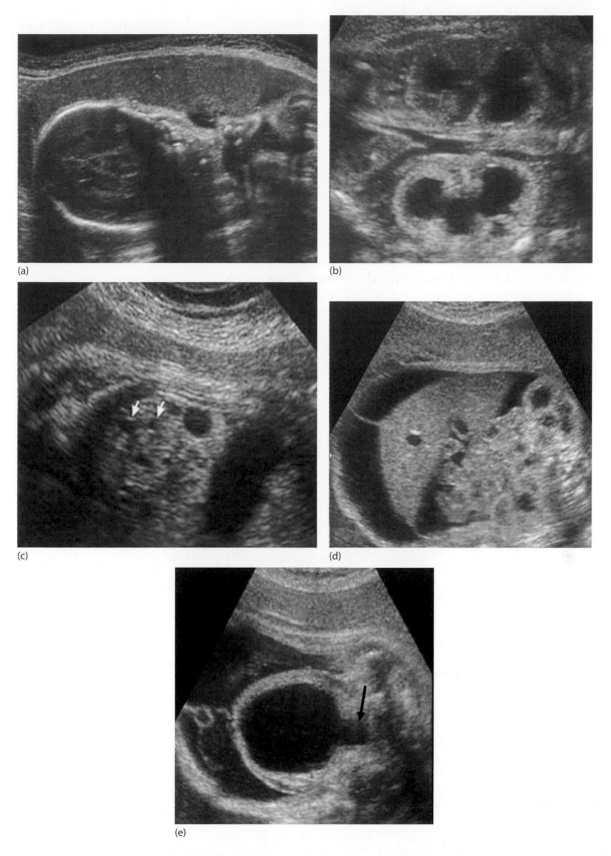

Figure 106.11 Prenatal ultrasonographic pictures. (a) Severe oligohydramnios. (b) Bilateral hydronephrosis. (c) Dysplastic kidneys. (d and e) Fetal urinary ascites with enlarged thickened bladder. The arrows indicate the exact point of the urine outflow obstruction caused by valves.

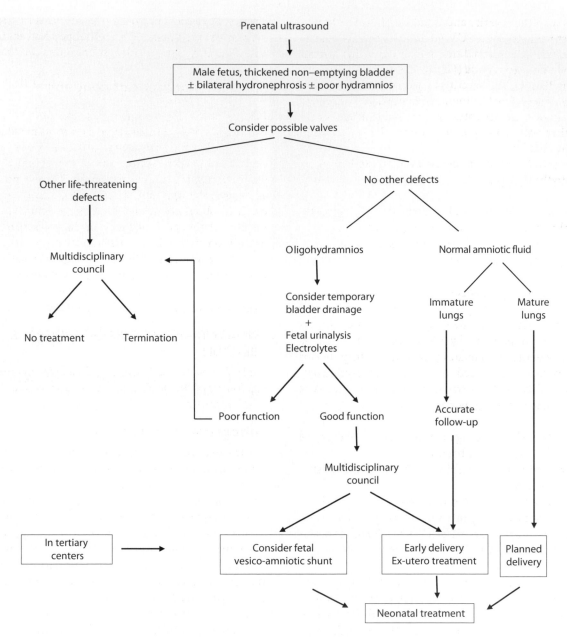

Figure 106.12 Posterior urethral valves: prenatal diagnosis and management.

Table 106.1 Favorable prognostic criteria of prenatally detected posterior urethral valves

Urinary electrolytes	=	Na^+ <100 mmol/L
	=	Cl^- <90 mmol/L
Fetal osmolarity	=	<2/0 mOsm/L
Beta-2-microglobulin	=	<5 mg/L
Renal parenchyma ultrasound	=	Preserved appearance or mild hyperecogenicity. No cortical cysts.
Amniotic fluid (AFI)	=	Normal or slightly reduced.
Diuresis	=	>2 mL/h

that varies with the severity and duration of obstruction in utero. Most neonates with PUV when first seen are acutely ill with electrolyte abnormalities, metabolic acidosis, renal insufficiency, and septicemia (Figure 106.6). They may have respiratory distress, the severity of which will depend on the degree of associated pulmonary hypoplasia. Improved management of these neonates has resulted in a better outcome for the treatment of posterior urethral obstruction in the last two decades.

The *treatment strategy* in neonates with PUV can be divided into three stages:

1. Immediate management and confirmation of diagnosis
2. Surgical treatment of the obstructing valves
3. Long-term follow-up and treatment of associated pathology and complications

Immediate management

The initial resuscitation of the sick neonate and confirmation of clinical impression by ultrasound and VCUG is mandatory. Almost all neonates presenting with posterior urethral obstruction will need intravenous rehydration and electrolyte replacement. At the same time, blood samples can be obtained for the following:

- Full blood count, including platelet count, which may be low or high in septicemic babies.
- Urea, creatinine, and electrolytes, which should be estimated as baseline values.
- Blood and urine should be sent for culture and sensitivity tests prior to starting antibiotic therapy.
- Arterial blood samples to determine the degree of acidosis, to be treated by sodium bicarbonate infusion.

Temporary vesical drainage can be achieved by passing a fine feeding tube (size 5 or 6 Fr gauge) transurethrally. Balloon catheters are not suitable for vesical drainage in posterior urethral obstruction. Recently, the use of double-J transurethral stenting has been advanced.[49] If the bladder is not emptying, a suprapubic catheter can decompress the urinary tract without interfering with the congenital urethra obstruction and its radiological study. A sample of urine obtained on catheterization should be sent for microscopy and culture.

Once urine and blood samples are obtained for culture and sensitivity tests, the baby should be treated by antibiotic therapy. An aminoglycoside or cephalosporin is suitable initially, and changes can be made once the urine and blood culture results are available. Respiratory insufficiency should be considered and treated aggressively as and when necessary, and information of the respiratory states is given by means of a chest x-ray and blood gas estimation. A multidisciplinary team in the neonatal intensive care unit is often needed.

The confirmation of diagnosis usually involves a VCUG, performed when the general condition of the patient is improved and the infection is brought under control

(Figure 106.8). However, an ultrasound scan can be done even in a sick neonate, by a sagittal perineal scan. The keyhole sign, although specific, cannot always be observed.[50]

Surgical treatment of congenital PUVs

Release of the congenital obstruction in a male newborn with PUV should be considered as early as possible, because the indwelling transurethral catheter is only very transient, for the risk of serious urinary tract infections and of defunctionalized bladder retraction. There is no consensus as regards the optimum method of treatment of posterior urethral obstruction, and its management constitutes an ongoing challenge in pediatric urology practice. The range of opinion varies from primary ablation alone to upper renal tract drainage, followed by delayed ablation. Ideally, the treatment option should be individualized, depending on the condition of the baby, the state of the upper renal tracts, and the size of the baby's genitalia.

PRIMARY TRANSURETHRAL RETROGRADE ABLATION

It can be performed under endoscopic view or blindly, depending on the preference of the surgeons and the available instrumentation.

Retrograde endoscopic ablation

It is the treatment most widely utilized, thanks to appropriate neonatal cystoscopes and resectoscopes now available, which may reduce the risk of secondary urethral damage and strictures in the newborn.[51] Fulguration can be undertaken once the infant's overall condition and renal function have stabilized. The development of smaller endoscopic equipment, as well as improved fiber optics, has permitted transurethral endoscopic incision or fulguration of posterior urethral obstruction in virtually all but the most premature patients. In most cases, primary ablation is sufficient to decompress the bladder and upper renal tracts.

Bugbee electrodes, available for use with the 8 Fr cystoscope, can be used for fulguration of PUV. One satisfactory alternative is to use a 3 Fr ureteric catheter with a metal stylet that can be used to coagulate. This can be passed through the side channel of an 8 Fr cystoscope. The obstructing membranes are incised at the 5, 7, and 12 o'clock positions. The neonatal resectoscope is commonly used in term newborns, as the caliber is 8 Fr (Figure 106.13). This instrument allows hooking of the valve leaflets and cutting them with more precision than the Bugbee catheter. It must be stressed that the valves or the congenital obstructive membrane should not be resected, but a full section of the leaflets should be undertaken at 5, 7, and 12 hours (Figure 106.14). The section is enough to release the bladder outlet obstruction and avoid the main severe complication that is postoperative urethral stricture. The reported incidence of strictures following endoscopic ablation is between 3.6% and 25%, but incidence of 0% has been reported with improved delicate maneuvers.[51]

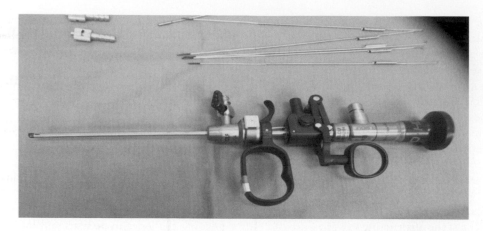

Figure 106.13 Neonatal resectoscope, suitable in newborns presenting congenital obstructing membrane or valves on posterior urethra.

Blind transurethral ablation

Especially in very small newborns or premature babies, transurethral endoscopy cannot be accomplished without the risk of urethral injury. Blind ablation of valves and urethral diaphragm was performed, utilizing different instrumentation and techniques.

1. *Fogarty balloon catheter*

    The baby is anesthetized, and a 6 Fr urethral catheter is passed transurethrally. The bladder is filled with contrast material until the posterior urethra is filled and an obstructing membrane identified. The catheter is then removed, and under fluoroscopic control, a no. 4 Fr Fogarty balloon catheter is placed into the bladder and inflated with approximately 0.75 mL of saline. With gentle withdrawal, the operator visualizes engagement at the level by the balloon. Sharp withdrawal of the catheter ruptures the valves or the membrane without injuring the sphincter.[52] Postoperative catheter drainage is recommended for 48–72 hours.

2. *Mohan's valvotome*

    This simple instrumentation may solve the problem of valve ablation in little infants. The advantages of the technique are its suitability in small neonates and the fact that it can be performed in areas of the world where pediatric endoscopic equipment is not easily available. However, a significant number of children have shown urethrorrhagia and periurethral extravasation of contrast in a postablation cystourethrogram.[53]

3. *Whitaker–Sherwood diathermy hook*

    Innes Williams successfully used a diathermy hook to ablate posterior urethral obstruction. Whitaker and Sherwood have modified the hook to its present form, which is fully insulated, except for the inside of the hook itself where the metal is bare for application of the diathermy.[54] The advantages are its small caliber, 6–7 Fr, and applicability without the need for a general anesthetic. However, the proximal end of external stricture is above the obstruction, putting the sphincter at risk.

The sterile lubricated hook is passed up the urethra, pointing to the 12 o'clock position, with the bladder full of contrast medium. The obstructive membrane is immediately engaged by rotating it to either side, and often, it will not disengage until the diathermy is applied. The obstructing membrane is destroyed with the smallest effective diathermy current at the 3 and 9 o'clock positions, and elsewhere if it can be reengaged.

With the advances in small cystoscopes, all these relatively blinded techniques are less favored in recent years.

Primary antegrade ablation

A *percutaneous antegrade ablation* technique was proposed by Zaontz,[55] combining the techniques of antegrade urethral obstruction ablation and percutaneous endoscopy. The disadvantages of urethral instrumentation are avoided, and the technique is applicable even in small premature infants.

Antegrade laser ablation has been proposed by some authors[56,57] in newborns. The Nd:YAG laser can be used via antegrade or retrograde access. The main advantage should be the limited inflammatory response of the injured tissue, with reduced risk of bleeding and of secondary stenosis.

Initial urinary diversion followed by secondary transurethral ablation

There is general agreement on some indications for temporary diversion in neonates, including prematurity, small body size, and/or small urethral caliber with massive VUR.

VESICOSTOMY

In 1974, Duckett[58] described the use of cutaneous vesicostomy as an alternative to primary ablation in a neonate. By creating a vesicostomy, urethral instrumentation is avoided, high voiding pressures causing persistent high-grade reflux are managed, and hydroureteronephrosis due to poor ureterovesical drainage is relieved. The bladder should be closed at the time of the subsequent diathermy of the urethral obstruction. However, vesicoureteric junction obstruction

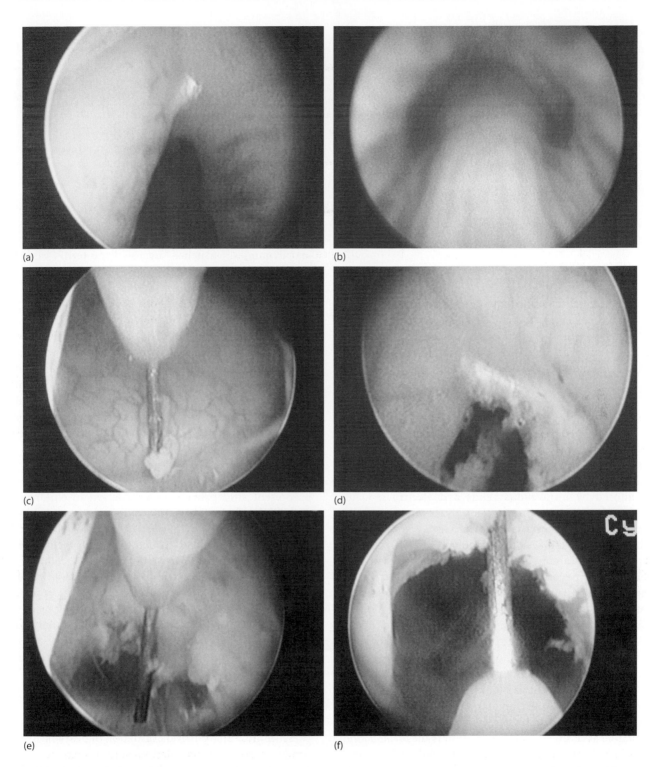

Figure 106.14 Endoscopic pictures of the section of the valve leaflets; a male newborn with PUV. **(a)** The obstructing membrane. **(b)** Dilated prostatic urethra. **(c)** Diathermic hook. **(d** and **e)** The valve flaps are hooked at 12, 5, and 7 hours. **(f)** Final appearance after PUV fulguration.

and shrinkage of a defunctionalized hypertrophied bladder may occur, if the vesicostomy is long-term.

UPPER TRACT DIVERSION

Upper tract diversion in posterior urethral obstruction is practiced in some limited indications. Primary ablation or temporary vesicostomy will be enough for hydroureteronephrosis to resolve in most cases. But for severe or late-presentation cases, and if significant dilatation of the upper tract persists, in spite of lower tract drainage and ablation, nonintubated upper tract drainage may be beneficial. However, we know that dilatation does not mean obstruction and that temporary nephrostomy diversion in the use of double-J catheters may ameliorate the hydronephrosis. In a series by Krueger and associates[59] infants treated with high-loop cutaneous ureterostomy ultimately had better outcome with regard to renal function and growth than the group managed by primary transurethral ablation of the valves. Reinberg et al.[2] demonstrated in 79% of patients who were treated initially with high diversion that mild to severe renal failure developed, versus 47% with primary ablation. Although no controlled study has been conducted, unilateral low ureterocutaneostomy could be useful in the case of VURD syndrome with refluxing ureter and nonfunctioning kidney, allowing urinary tract decompression without interfering with bladder cycling and maturation in the small infant.

TEMPORARY NEPHROSTOMY DIVERSION ON INSERTION OF DOUBLE-J STENTS

If the upper tract is needed in spite of a successful ablation, temporary nephrostomy with an insertion of double-J stents may be useful in patients with vesicoureteric junction obstruction or severely dilated upper tract. The insertion of double-J stents prevents dry bladder and keeps the bladder cycle, which is needed for normal bladder development.

Early postoperative management

The urethral catheter is left in situ after valve ablation for 48–72 hours, to allow the edema to subside and the urinary output to be measured. Accurate hydroelectrolytic balance is monitored by intravenous fluids and electrolyte solutions. Serial serum creatinine, electrolytes, and urinalysis are monitored after the patient is discharged with antibiotic prophylaxis. Postvoid residual urine volume is frequently checked by ultrasound, and sonographic appearance of kidneys and the upper tract is observed at 4–6 months' interval time. If the postvoid residual urine volume is significant (greater than 10% of expected bladder capacity), alpha-1 adrenergic blocker drug treatment can be started (terazosin 0.04–0.4 mg/kg per day), after obtaining informed consent. Blood pressure must be monitored routinely.

The first VCUG is usually performed at 3 months from valve ablation, and a "second-look" cystoscopy is indicated if residual valves or leaflets are suspected, to guarantee full urethral disobstruction. A simple measurement that allows quantitative assessment of valve ablation is the *urethral ratio* on VCUG.[60] A postfulguration urethral ratio of 2.5–3.0 represents a positive result postoperatively. Renal radionuclide scan (MAG3 or DMSA) is suggested at 6–12 months from valve ablation to check parenchymal function.

FOLLOW-UP AND TREATMENT OF LONG-TERM SEQUELAE AND COMPLICATIONS

Urethral stricture

It can be a significant complication following the transurethral approach for treatment of PUV, as a consequence of mechanical trauma on the posterior urethral wall. The stricture can happen where the lesion on the urethral wall is deeper and the *corpus spongiosum* could be injured. The incidence of urethral strictures following PUV ablation has been reduced from 25% to near 0%, but it can be avoided, utilizing small endoscopes and delicate maneuvers.[51,61]

DYSFUNCTIONAL VOIDING AND URINARY INCONTINENCE

Valve bladder syndrome

Early valve ablation allows the bladder to fill and empty with normal cycling, starting shortly after birth. The restored bladder cycling is crucial for regaining its normal function and dynamics.[62] Mitchell suggested the term "valve bladder syndrome" to denote the association of a noncompliant bladder and upper tract dilatation in boys with a history of previous PUV.[30]

At least 30% of children with previous PUV have different degrees of dysfunctional bladder. It often presents with daytime and nighttime urinary incontinence at the toilet-trained age. Initially it was thought to be secondary to external sphincter incompetence, depending on primary maldevelopment of the sphincteric urethra, rather than iatrogenic injuring of this structure during endoscopic manipulations. Further urodynamic studies showed the presence of vesical dysfunction, which does not resolve after complete urethral obstruction removal.[41]

A number of different voiding dysfunction pictures may be present after primary valve ablation in children born with PUV. The incidence of voiding dysfunction in posterior urethral obstruction has been reported to occur in 13%–38% of all patients treated, of which incontinence is the most common problem.

The main bladder anomalies causing incontinence are *detrusor overactivity, reduced compliance, and myogenic failure.* Detrusor overactivity and reduced compliance are treatable with anticholinergic pharmacotherapy, but bladder augmentation may be necessary in selected cases. Myogenic failure may be most effectively treated with clean intermittent catheterization and nocturnal bladder emptying.[38]

The evolution over the years of this severe bladder dysfunction may lead to upper tract dilatation and renal function deterioration.[29,30,38] Serial urodynamic studies, with pressure-flow analysis and evaluation of postvoiding urine residual, are necessary. Bladder activity may change over time from a hyperactive, low-compliant, and reduced-functional-volume bladder to hypocontractile, high capacity, and poor emptying behavior (decompensated bladder with myogenic failure).[41,63]

Early valve ablation, even in patients with severe bladder changes, could provide better bladder function results, with higher resolution rate of VUR and hydronephrosis. Bladder neck incision, performed simultaneously to valvulotomy or later in infancy or childhood, has been advocated to increase low-pressure bladder outlet if pharmacological treatment by alpha-1 adrenergic blockers drugs were not efficacious.[64]

VUR and hydronephrosis

The incidence of VUR in boys with PUV is high, bilateral in 37% and unilateral in 27% of patients.[65] Children born with bilateral high-grade VUR are at greater risk for CRF than those with unilateral or no VUR. Unilateral VUR may confer a protective pop-off effect in the contralateral kidney.[35]

A high rate of reflux resolution is expected after valve ablation, even in presence of vesical diverticuli, with a consistent follow-up. VUR resolution is correlated with bladder dysfunction normalization. In a recent series of Heikkila and coauthors,[65] VUR resolved spontaneously in 62%, was corrected by antireflux surgery in 21%, and required nephrectomy in 17% of boys with previous PUV. Indications for ureteral reimplantation remain undefined today, but the recent experience tends to support a less aggressive surgical approach than in the past.

Pyeloureteral dilatation persisting after treatment of an obstructing membrane is due to either vesicoureteric junction obstruction or ureteral atony. Diuretic renograms may be helpful in the differentiation between the two conditions, although temporary drainage of the upper tract may be necessary to make the diagnosis. A conservative approach, with care to bladder dysfunction treatment, is often recommended today.

Renal dysplasia

Unilateral renal dysplasia with a nonfunctioning kidney should be treated by nephroureterectomy, if at risk for blood hypertension or urinary tract infections. Bilateral renal dysplasia will go on to develop into end-stage renal disease and will require dialysis and renal transplantation.

PROGNOSTIC FACTORS IN PUV

Congenital lower urinary tract obstruction is a disease of high mortality and morbidity in pediatric age. With the widespread use of prenatal ultrasound, most children with PUV are now recognized prenatally and confirmed at birth. Several prognostic factors have been underlined to better define the long-term outcome of a baby born with PUV.

- Prenatal prognostic factors for better postnatal outcome have been presented and discussed in the section "Prenatal Diagnosis and Management." Poor prognosis is related to reduced amniotic fluid volume, presence of cortical renal cysts, and other congenital or structural anomalies of the fetus.[45]
- Ultrasound findings of reduced parenchymal thinness, increased renal echogenicity, and cystic changes in neonatal age of infancy are usually correlated with severe renal damage and dysplasia, evolving into CRF.[43]
- Urinary extravasation with or without ascites in prenatal or neonatal age, large bladder diverticula, and VURD syndrome are all factors decompressing the urinary tract and related to a better renal function outcome.[34,35]

- Delayed presentation of patients with PUV (after 2 years of life) are at higher risk of developing CRF on long-term follow-up.[66] Early vesicostomy or other urinary diversion is not confirmed to give better outcome.[67]
- Early primary valve ablation of PUV seems to lead to better outcome than urinary diversion, reducing bladder dysfunction.[62]
- Unilateral gross VUR, associated with poor-functioning ipsilateral kidney, may give a protective effect in the contralateral kidney (pop-off valve syndrome).[35]
- Bilateral high-grade VUR is at greater risk for renal insufficiency, although not always confirmed.[65]
- Severe bladder dysfunction (valve bladder syndrome) may jeopardize the upper tract and renal function at long-term follow-up.[38,41]
- Proteinuria, blood arterial hypertension, and febrile urinary tract infections do not correlate significantly with the ultimate functional outcome.[68] The nadir creatinine values of 0.8 mg/dL or higher within the first year of life are reported as the most significant prognostic factor correlated with poor renal function in the long term.[69]
- Renal transplantation can be offered to children with a history of previous PUV or congenital obstruction of the posterior urethra, with the same good results as other pediatric candidates, with preemptive urological repair of the lower urinary tract.[70]

CONCLUSIONS

Congenital obstruction of the male posterior urethra represents a spectrum of lesions, of which PUVs are the most common picture. It often remains a severe structural cause of a urinary outflow obstacle in newborn age and in infancy. It still represents one of the most significant causes of end-stage renal failure before the age of 2 years.[3,68] Prognosis of children born with PUV has improved significantly over the past two decades, but till now, a high number of patients enter CRF and progress to end-stage renal insufficiency by adolescence, with the need for a dialysis–renal transplant program.[69] A precise multidisciplinary approach may further improve the outcome of these children, providing a more pathogenetic and appropriate treatment at long-term follow-up, till adulthood.

REFERENCES

1. Parkhouse HF, Barratt TM, Dillon MJ et al. Long-term outcome of boys with posterior urethral valves. *Br J Urol* 1988; 62: 59.
2. Reinberg Y, de Castano I, Gonzalez R. Influence of initial therapy on progression of renal failure and body growth in children with posterior urethral valves. *J Urol* 1992; 148: 532.
3. Ardissino G, Daccò V, Testa S et al. Epidemiology of chronic renal failure in children: Data from the ItalKid Project. *Pediatrics* 2003; 111: 382–7.
4. Morgagni GB. *Seats and Causes of Diseases Investigated by Anatomy; in Five Books, Containing*

a Great Variety of Dissections with Remarks to which Are Added Very Accurate and Copious Indexes of the Principal Things and Names Therein Contained, 3rd edn. Millar A, Cadell T (eds). London: Johnson and Payne, 1769; 3: 540–56.

5. Langenbeck JM. Eine einfache und sichere methode des steinschnittes. 1802. In: Tolmatschen N (ed). *Ein Fall von Semilunaren Klappen der Harnrohre, und von Vergrosserter Vescicula Prostatice. Archiv Path Anat* 1870; 11; 348.

6. Velpeau AALM. Urètre et Prostate. *Traite Complet d'Anatomie Chirurgicale* 1832; 2: 247.

7. Young HH, Frontz WA, Baldwin JC. Congenital obstruction of the posterior urethra. *J Urol* 1919; 3: 289.

8. Young HH, McKay RW. Congenital valvular obstruction of the posterior urethra. *Surg Gynecol Obstet* 1929; 48: 509.

9. Macpherson RI, Leithiser RE, Gordon L et al. Posterior urethral valves: An update and review. *Radiographics* 1986; 6(5): 753–791.

10. Waterhouse K, Hamm FC. The importance of urethral valves as a cause of vesical neck obstruction in children. *J Urol* 1962; 87: 404.

11. Williams DI, Eckstein HB. Obstructive valves in the posterior urethra. *J Urol* 1965; 93: 236.

12. Gonzales ET. Posterior urethral valves and bladder neck obstruction. *Urol Clin N Am* 1978; 5: 57.

13. Glassberg KI. Current issues regarding posterior urethral valves. *Urol Clin N Am* 1985; 12: 175.

14. Dewan PA, Zappala SM, Ransley PG, Duffy PG. Endoscopic reappraisal of the morphology of congenital obstruction of the posterior urethra. *Br J Urol* 1992; 70: 439.

15. Dewan PA. Congenital obstructing posterior urethral membrane (COPUM): Further evidence for a common morphological diagnosis. *Pediatr Surg Int* 1993; 8: 45.

16. Thomas J. Etiopathogenesis and management of bladder dysfunction in patients with posterior urethral valves. *Indian J Urol* 2010 October; 26(4): 480–9. doi: 10.4103/0970-1591.74434.

17. Hendren WH. Posterior urethral valves in boys. A broad clinical spectrum. *J Urol* 1971; 106: 298.

18. Pieretti RV. The mild end of the clinical spectrum of posterior urethral valves. *J Pediatr Surg* 1993; 28: 701.

19. Colodny A. Urethral lesions in infants and children. In: Gillenwater JY, Grayhack J, Howards SS, Duckett JW (eds). *Adult and Pediatric Urology*, Chapter 53. Chicago: Year Book Medical Publishers Inc, 1987: 1782–808.

20. Livne PM, De Laune J, Gonzales ET Jr. Genetic etiology of posterior urethral valves. *J Urol* 1983; 130: 781.

21. Field PL, Stephens FD. Congenital urethral membranes causing urethral obstruction. *J Urol* 1974; 111: 250.

22. Krishnan A, De Souza A, Konijeti R, Baskin LS. The anatomy and embryology of posterior urethral valves. *J Urol* 2006; 175: 1214–20.

23. Dewan PA, Keenan RJ, Lequesne GW, Morris LL. Cobb's collar or prolapsed congenital obstructive posterior urethral membrane (COPUM). *Br J Urol* 1994; 73: 91.

24. Cobb BG, Wolf JA, Ansell JS. Congenital stricture of the proximal urethral bulb. *J Urol* 1968; 99: 629.

25. Moormann JG. Congenital bulbar urethral stenosis as a cause of disease of the urogenital junction. *Urologe* 1972; 11: 157.

26. Imaji R, Moon D, Dewan PA. Congenital posterior urethral obstruction: Variable morphological expression. *J Urol* 2001; 165: 1240.

27. Gonzales R, Reimberg Y, Burke B, Wells T, Vernier RL. Early bladder outlet obstruction in fetal lambs induces renal dysplasia and the prune-belly syndrome. *J Pediatr Surg* 1990; 25: 342.

28. Holmdahl G, Sillen U, Hansson E, Hermansson G, Hjalmas K. Bladder dysfunction in boys with posterior urethral valves before and after puberty. *J Urol* 1996; 155: 694–8.

29. Glassberg KI. The valve bladder syndrome: 20 years later. *J Urol* 2001; 166: 1406–14.

30. Mitchell ME. Persistent ureteral dilatation following valve resection. *Dial Pediatr Urol* 1982; 5: 8–11.

31. Warshaw BL, Hymes LC, Trulock TS, Woodard JR. Prognostic features in infants with obstructive uropathy due to posterior urethral valves. *J Urol* 1985; 133: 240.

32. Belloli G, Battaglino F, Mercurella A, Musi L, D'Agostino S. Evolution of upper urinary tract and renal function in patients with posterior urethral valves. *Pediatr Surg Int* 1996; 11: 339.

33. Close CE, Carr MC, Burns MW, Mitchell ME. Lower urinary tract changes after early valve ablation in neonates and infants: Is early diversion warranted? *J Urol* 1997; 157: 984.

34. Rittenberg MH, Hulbert WC, Snyder HM, Duckett JW. Protective factors in posterior urethral valves. *J Urol* 1988; 140: 993.

35. Hoover DL, Duckett JW. Posterior urethral valves, unilateral reflux and renal dysplasia: A syndrome. *J Urol* 1982; 128: 994.

36. Henneberry MO, Stephens FD. Renal hypoplasia and dysplasia in infants with posterior urethral valves. *J Urol* 1980; 123: 912.

37. Dinneen MD, Duffy PG, Barratt TM, Ransley PG. Persistent polyuria after posterior urethral valves. *Br J Urol* 1995; 75: 236.

38. Koff SA, Mutabagani KH, Jaynthi VR. The valve bladder syndrome: Pathophysiology and treatment with nocturnal bladder emptying. *J Urol* 2002; 167: 291–7.

39. Huang J, Li HJ, Wang J et al. Prenatal emotion management improves obstetric outcomes: A randomized control study. *Int J Clin Exp Med* 2015 June 15; 8(6): 9667–75.

40. Clayton DB, Brock JW 3rd. Lower urinary tract obstruction in the fetus and neonate. *Clin Perinatol* 2014 September; 41(3): 643–59.

41. De Gennaro M, Capitanucci ML, Mosiello G, Caione P, Silveri M. The changing urodynamic pattern from

infancy to adolescence in boys with posterior urethral valves. *BJU Int* 2000; 85: 1104–8.

42. Harvie S, McLeod L, Acott P et al. Abnormal antenal sonogram: An indicator of disease severity in children with posterior urethral valves. *Can Ass Radiol J* 2009; 60: 185–9.

43. Robyr R, Benachi A, Ikha-Dahmane F et al. Correlation between ultrasound and anatomical findings in fetuses with lower urinary tract obstruction in the first half of pregnancy. *Ultrasound Obstet Gynecol* 2005; 25: 478–82.

44. Glick PL, Harrison MR, Golbus MS et al. Management of the fetus with congenital hydronephrosis II: Prognostic criteria and selection for treatment. *J Pediatr Surg* 1985; 20: 376–87.

45. Ciardelli V, Rizzo N, Farina A et al. Prenatal evaluation of fetal renal function based on serum beta(2)-microglobulin assessment. *Prenat Diagn* 2001; 21(7): 586–8.

46. Quintero RA, Morales WJ, Allen MH, Bornick PW, Johnson P. Fetal hydrolaparoscopy and endoscopic cystostomy in complicated cases of lower urinary tract obstruction. *Am J Obstet Gynecol* 2000; 183: 324–30.

47. Elder JS, Duckett JW, Snyder HM. Intervention for fetal obstructive uropathy: Has it been effective? *Lancet* 1987; 2(8566): 1007.

48. Kilby MD, on behalf of the Pluto collaborative Study Group. Pluto trial protocol: Percutaneous shunting for lower urinary tract obstruction randomised controlled trial. *Br J Obst Gynaecol* 2007; 1471: 904–10.

49. Penna FJ, Bowlin P, Alyami F et al. Novel strategy for temporary decompression of the lower urinary tract in neonates using a ureteral stent. *J Urol* 2015 October; 194(4): 1086–90.

50. Bernades LS, Aksnes G, Saada J et al. Keyhole sign: How specific is it for the diagnosis of posterior urethral valves? *Ultrasound Obstet Gynecol* 2009; 34: 419–23.

51. Lal R, Bhatnager V, Mitra DK. Urethral strictures after fulguration of posterior urethral valves. *J Pediatr Surg* 1998; 33: 518–9.

52. Kyi A, Maung M, Saing H. Ablation of posterior urethral valves in the newborn using Fogarty balloon catheter: A simple method for developing countries. *J Pediatr Surg* 2001; 36: 1713–6.

53. Abraham MK. Mohan's valvotome: A new instrument. *J Urol* 1990; 144: 1196–8.

54. Whitaker RH, Sherwood T. An improved hook for destroying posterior urethral valves. *J Urol* 1986; 135: 531–3.

55. Zaontz MR, Firlit CF. Percutaneous antegrade ablation of posterior urethral valves in infants with small

caliber urethras: An alternative to urinary diversion. *J Urol* 1986; 136: 247.

56. Biewald W, Schier F. Laser treatment of posterior urethral valves in neonates. *Br J Urol* 1992; 69: 425.

57. Pagano MJ, van Batavia JP, Casale P. Laser ablation in the management of obstructive uropathy in neonates. *J Endourol* 2015 May; 29(5): 611–4.

58. Duckett Jw Jr. Cutaneous vesicostomy in childhood. The Blocksom technique. *Urol Clin N Am* 1974; 1: 485–96.

59. Krueger RP, Hardy BE, Churchill BM. Growth in boys with posterior urethral valves. Primary valve resection vs upper tract diversion. *Urol Clin N Am* 1980; 7: 265.

60. Gupta RK, Shah HS, Jadah V et al. Urethral ratio on voiding cystourethrogram: A comparative method to assess success of posterior urethral valve ablation. *J Pediatr Urol* 2010; 6(1): 32–6.

61. Bruce J, Stannard V, Small PG, Mayell MJ, Kapila L. The operative management of posterior urethral valves. *J Pediatr Surg* 1987; 22: 1081.

62. Mitchell ME, Close CE. Early primary valve ablation for posterior urethral valves. *Semin Pediatr Surg* 1996; 5: 66.

63. De Gennaro M, Capitanucci ML, Silveri M, Morini FA, Mosiello G. Detrusor hypocontractility evolution in boys with posterior urethral valves detected by pressure flow analysis. *J Urol* 2009; 165: 2248–52.

64. Kajbafzadeh AM, Payabvash S, Karimian G. The effects of bladder neck incision on urodynamic abnormalities of children with posterior urethral valves. *J Urol* 2007; 178: 2147–9.

65. Heikkila J, Rintala R, Taskinen S. Vesicoureteral reflux in conjunction with posterior urethral valves. *J Urol* 2009; 182: 1555–60.

66. Ansari MS, Singh P, Mandhani A et al. Delayed presentation in posterior urethral valve: Long-term implications and outcome. *Urology* 2008; 71(2): 230–4.

67. Godbole P, Wade A, Mushtag I, Wilcox DT. Vesicostomy vs primary ablation for posterior urethral valves: Always a difference in outcome? *J Pediatr Urol* 2007; 3: 273–5.

68. Lopez Pereira P, Espinosa L, Martinez Urrutia MT et al. Posterior urethral valves: Prognostic factors. *BJU Int* 2003; 91: 687–90.

69. Coulthard MG. Outcome of reaching end-stage renal failure in children under 2 years of age. *Arch Dis Child* 2002; 87(6): 511–7.

70. Capozza N, Collura G, Matarazzo E, Caione P. Renal transplantation and congenital anomaly of the kidney and urinary tract. *Pediatr Child Health* 2009; 19(51): 551–2.

107

Neurogenic bladder in the neonate

SALVATORE CASCIO AND MALCOLM A. LEWIS

INTRODUCTION

Neurogenic bladder in the neonate can be divided into three groups—primary, secondary, and idiopathic. *Primary neurogenic* bladder develops as a result of a lesion at any level in the central nervous system, cerebral cortex, and spinal cord, or in the peripheral nervous system. The most common causes are open or closed congenital neural tube defects (spinal dysraphism). Other forms of neurological injury (e.g., cerebral palsy) can be associated with neurogenic bladder. Outside of the spinal cord, primary neurogenic bladder can result from lesions such as sacrococcygeal teratomas. *Secondary neurogenic bladder*, also called neuropathic bladder, occurs when the bladder acts like a neurogenic bladder but is not caused by a neurological defect. Causes in a neonate include imperforate anus, prune belly syndrome, bladder exstrophy, cloacal exstrophy, and posterior urethral valves. *Idiopathic neurogenic bladder* is very rare; causes include the urofacial syndrome. Where this is not present, idiopathic neurogenic bladder is a diagnosis of exclusion once primary and secondary causes have been excluded.

The incidence of neural tube defects in Europe is heterogeneous with some regional registries showing a higher rate than others, with an overall rate across Europe of 0.49 per 1000 live births.[1] In the United States, the incidence of spina bifida has recently plateaued at approximately 0.3 per 1000 live births.[2]

The optimal management of a neurogenic bladder in the neonatal period is controversial, with no agreement among pediatric urologists and nephrologists on when clean intermittent catheterization (CIC) and anticholinergics medication should be commenced, and no consensus on the timing of renal investigations (micturating cystogram and dimercaptosuccinic acid [DMSA]), videourodynamic studies, and urological follow-up. However, general agreement exists that the key element in the urological management of these patients remains the early recognition of those bladders at risk for upper and lower urinary tract deterioration in order to start adequate medical or surgical treatment, thereby preventing renal and bladder damage and improving long-term outcome.

PRENATAL DIAGNOSIS AND COUNSELING

It is unusual to make a diagnosis of neurogenic bladder antenatally on the basis of the ultrasound (US) appearances of the renal tract. For the vast majority of patients, the diagnosis of neurogenic bladder is assumed following the finding of evidence of spinal dysraphism, open or closed, on antenatal scan. In patients with spinal dysraphism, it is virtually unknown for neurogenic bladder to present as antenatal hydronephrosis or an enlarged bladder in the absence of other congenital anomalies affecting the renal tract. The only situation where primary neurogenic bladder will present as antenatal hydronephrosis is where the child has urofacial (Ochoa) syndrome.

In cases where primary neurogenic bladder is suspected because of spinal dysraphism, it is appropriate for the urologist or nephrologist to be involved early in the counseling process. Families need to know that in cases of open spinal dysraphism, the incidence of neurogenic bladder is over 90% and what the implications of this are for the child in terms of continence, dependence, and the risk of developing renal functional impairment. The latter can occur even with optimal management of the neurogenic bladder, and it needs to be noted that, with high open spinal dysraphism lesions, accompanying renal dysplasia with the potential for renal functional impairment is more common.[3] Where a closed spinal dysraphism lesion has been detected, figures from our series of over 300 patients in Manchester, United Kingdom, show that the risk of neurogenic bladder varies from 28% in patients with isolated lesions, such as a long cord, diastem, or pure meningocele, to 66% in those with lipomyelomeningocele, to over 90% in those with sacral agenesis/dysgenesis.

The counseling process needs to provide the family with a clear outline of the problems facing the child after birth, the management options available, and the prognosis. Depending on the overall prognosis for the child, taking into account the neurological outcome based on the lesion, the availability of potential interventions and the legal requirements of the locality of the family, there are four options available. The *first* option is termination of the pregnancy. This is a common choice in some countries like the United Kingdom but rare in others. This is influenced not only by the legal framework of the locality of the family but also by their religious and ethical beliefs and those of their community. The *second* option, in cases of open spinal dysraphism, is antenatal surgical repair. This is only available in a small number of centers. As an intervention, the benefit of antenatal repair has not yet been proven. The spinal dysraphism still exists, and the antenatal surgery effectively changes an open lesion into a closed lesion. This certainly reduces the incidence of hydrocephalus and ventriculoperitoneal shunt placement with improved mental development and motor function measures at age 30 months following in utero closure.[4] However, it is unclear if prenatal closure will significantly improve bladder outcomes.[5] The process itself is far from complication-free. Preterm delivery, with secondary complications, is frequent. The *third* option is progression to term and active management of the infant after delivery. The *fourth* option, only available in cases where the combined anomalies clearly confer a very poor prognosis for the child, and where nonintervention will lead to fairly rapid death, is palliative care for the infant.

The final decision about a course of action in an individual case is dependent upon the decision of the family, influenced heavily by the legal framework of the locality and resources available. There are no "right" answers, and families have to decide which option is best for them based on the clinical information imparted to them and their own beliefs and circumstances.

In cases of neurogenic bladder secondary to other congenital anomalies of the renal tract or associated disorders, the information imparted to the family will be strongly influenced by the underlying condition. The management options will also be determined by this. The antenatal options are effectively the same as the aforementioned, though antenatal surgery is not usually an option, and antenatal drainage of a distended bladder remains an option of unproven benefit.

ANATOMY AND MICTURATION PHYSIOLOGY

The autonomic and somatic nervous systems are involved in the innervations of the bladder and sphincter; the parasympathetic component of the autonomic innervations is derived from the sacral segments of the spinal cord. These fibers emerge as preganglionic fibers within the pelvic nerve, which then joins the hypogastric nerve to form the bladders plexus. The postganglionic fibers emerge from synapses close to the bladder and urethra, where they have the overall effect of producing sustained bladder contraction. Acetylcholine is the neurotransmitter for both the preganglionic and postganglionic fibers, although there is certainly more than one principal neurotransmitter. Within the bladder, the parasympathetic cholinergic receptors are largely muscarinic (M2). Other neurotransmitters documented to be present in the bladder include the following: vasoactive intestinal peptide,

neuropeptide Y, substance P, somatostatin, calcitonin gene-related peptide, cholecystokinin, dopamine, serotonin, histamine, and tyrosine hydroxylase. The exact roles of these neurotransmitters, as well as their complex interactions, remain unclear.

The sympathetic component of the autonomic innervations arises from spinal cord segments T11–L2, with preganglionic fibers traveling to the hypogastric and inferior mesenteric ganglia, where they synapse with the noradrenergic, postganglionic fibers, which in turn travel to the bladder and urethra via the hypogastric nerve. Sympathetic input is mediated by both α and β adrenoreceptors. The α adrenoreceptors are more densely represented at the bladder base and produce contraction, while the β adrenoreceptors, which are more common in the bladder body, produce relaxation. Thus α activity promotes outlet resistance, while β activity promotes urine storage and opposes cholinergic tone.

Somatic motor innervations arise from the S2–S4 segments and pass via the pudendal nerve to the striated muscle of the external sphincter. While the external sphincter is a voluntary muscle, in infancy, external sphincter tone is mediated via spinal cord reflex. It is only as the child matures that cortical inhibitory influences develop that allow voluntary relaxation and contraction, which contribute to the development of continence.

Normal bladder sensation is relayed via pelvic and hypogastric nerves, with parasympathetic visceral afferent fibers transmitting information from pain, temperature, and stretch receptors.

In the newborn and infant, voiding occurs as a result of a spinal reflex secondary to bladder distention, which stimulates the efferent limb of the reflex arc, resulting in spontaneous detrusor contraction. Initially, as the bladder fills, the periurethral striated muscles make the external urinary sphincter contract to prevent urine loss. The act of micturition occurs with subsequent relaxation of the external sphincter, resulting in the bladder emptying at low pressure. During the first year of life, the number of voiding episodes per day remains constant at about 20, occurring both during sleep and while awake; with increased age, there is a reduction in the voiding frequency that relates to the relative increase in bladder volume and decreasing proportion of the caloric intake associated with fluid.

CLASSIFICATION

There are many classifications describing neurogenic bladder dysfunction. Most of these classifications are dependent on the site of the neurological lesions, well adapted to adult pathology but not to congenital spinal lesions. In fact, in children, there is poor correlation between the spinal level of the lesion and the clinical impact. For this reason, classification based on clinical appearance and urodynamic findings is more practical in children. The two elements determining the clinical appearance are the state of the bladder muscle and the state of the sphincter. The bladder muscle can be contractile (63%), acontractile with good compliance (20%), or acontractile with poor compliance (17%). In each of these states, the sphincter can be completely denervated (36%), partially denervated (24%), or with an intact sacral reflex arc (40%)[6] (Figure 107.1). It is the state of the sphincter that is the primary determinant of both continence and the potential for upper tract damage. A lax sphincter will be associated with urinary incontinence but safe upper tracts. A tight sphincter will be associated with urinary retention. With a tight sphincter and an acontractile bladder, there is the easy potential for continence using CIC. Where the sphincter is tight but the bladder is poorly compliant, the bladder pressures will be high, leading to obstructive uropathy. An overactive bladder will potentially both lead to urinary leakage and place the upper tracts at risk depending on how tight the sphincter is and at what pressure leakage occurs. This is where dyssynergia becomes important. If, as is commonly the case in infants with open spinal dysraphism, there is detrusor sphincter dyssynergia (DSD), then, even if the resting state of the sphincter tinge is low and leakage is readily occurring, there is a risk to the upper tracts because sphincteric spasm at the time of detrusor contractions can cause

pressures high enough to lead to obstructive uropathy. Determination of how the bladder is functioning is achieved with urodynamics. However, it needs to be appreciated that urodynamics just give a snapshot of bladder function at one moment in time. The pattern of activity seen during urodynamic testing may not be replicated throughout the day, every day. Moreover, the neurogenic bladder is not static and changes with time. Thus, urodynamic assessment cannot be used to manage the patient independently. It has to be used in combination with other investigations and full clinical assessment.

Videourodynamics

The basis for major clinical decisions in patients with neurogenic bladder rests mainly on assessment of the upper tracts with US scan and assessment of the bladder with urodynamics. It needs to be remembered that the aim in infants is to ensure the safety of the upper tracts, not provide continence. Particularly in infants, performing videourodynamics, rather than urodynamics alone, allows both functional and concurrent visual assessment of the

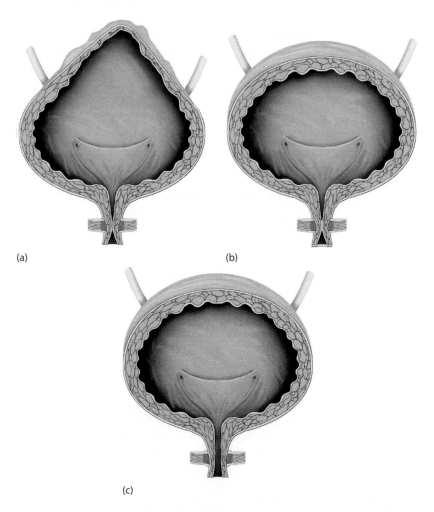

(a)

(b)

(c)

Figure 107.1 Videourodynamic findings in newborns with myelodysplasia. **(a)** Dyssynergy (37%). **(b)** Synergy (26%). **(c)** Complete denervation (36%). (From Bauer SB, Initial Management of Meningocele Children, in *Textbook of Neurogenic Bladder*, 3rd ed, pp. 633–644, Jacques Corcos, David Ginsberg, Gilles Karsenty, eds, CRC Press, Taylor & Francis Group, 2015.)

bladder, giving more information for decision making. The principles of urodynamic assessment in infants are the same as for older children and adults, but obtaining reliable and interpretable results is more difficult. Moreover, it has been well demonstrated that normal infants frequently show a picture of incomplete voiding and dyssynergic voiding on urodynamic testing.[7] Thus careful interpretation of the test, taken in conjunction with the clinical picture, the appearances on US scan, and the appearances on video images during urodynamics, is required when making decisions on urodynamic results. The mainstay of urodynamics is the measurement of detrusor pressure during a filling cycle, judging from this the bladder capacity at an acceptable pressure and the leak point pressure. The use of a rectal probe to measure abdominal pressure potentially allows the measurement of the true detrusor pressure, through subtraction of the abdominal pressure from the intravesical pressure. Sadly, getting a good rectal pressure trace can be difficult, and spontaneous rectal contractions or rectal contractions in combination with detrusor contractions are common and can give a false impression of what the true detrusor pressure is—often underestimating this. Thus, there is no substitute for carefully watching the intravesical pressure trace during a test and using this as the primary reference point. Similarly, the use of electromyography in the test will potentially give information about the background level of sphincteric activity and whether there is DSD. However, any movement makes this trace difficult to interpret, and the iron test of the risk of developing obstructive uropathy is the pressure at which leakage occurs and the intravesical volume associated with pressures over 30 cm of water. The information from concurrent videofluoroscopy is invaluable and gives a visual impression of the contour of the bladder and whether there is trabeculation of the bladder or diverticulae. The state of the bladder neck can be seen. Most importantly vesicoureteric reflux (VUR) can be identified. If VUR is present, measurements on fluoroscopy or US can be used to assess the true bladder capacity and hence compliance, which can be significantly less that the infused volume used in urodynamics with no fluoroscopy.

DIAGNOSIS AND ASSESSMENT OF NEUROGENIC BLADDER IN THE NEONATE

The initial assessment of a newborn with a neurogenic bladder begins in the first few days of life with a detailed physical examination, evaluating the presence of a palpable bladder or kidney, and a comprehensive neurological examination, looking for spontaneous movement, checking for muscle wasting and deep tendon reflexes, and testing sensation in the lower extremities and of the anus. The tone of the anal sphincter could be indicative of the type of lesion, as a patulous anus suggests a complete lower motor neuron lesion, while the presence of anal contraction to gentle scratching of the rugated perianal skin implies some intact sacral spinal cord function and reflexes.

Open neural tube defects are usually closed in the first 24–48 hours, and an indwelling Foley catheter is placed at the time of closure to ensure adequate bladder drainage and to reduce contamination of the healing wound. The catheter is left for 5–7 days, until the wound is healed and it is safe to nurse the patient on the back. Once the indwelling catheter is removed, it becomes essential to establish if the baby is able to empty the bladder. This can be achieved with a nappy alarm with assessment of voided volume (weighing the nappies) and measurement of postvoid residual with US. The constant leak of urine into the nappy with no postvoid residue would suggest a lax sphincter with a low leak point pressure, resulting in little risk to the upper tract. On the contrary, high residual (above 5 mL in the neonate) would imply a degree of sphincter spasm or dyssynergia with high leak point pressure and increased risk of upper tract deterioration. Spinal shock following myelomeningocele closure occurs in 3% of newborns, but it can last for 2–6 weeks after surgery; therefore, the initial bladder assessment might need to be repeated at the first follow-up appointment.[8] A renal and bladder US is a key element of the initial assessment. As mentioned previously, neurogenic bladder does not cause hydronephrosis and obstructive uropathy antenatally. At birth, the kidneys of neonates with neural tube defect are normal in the large majority of patients. In our database of 248 newborns with neural tube defect at the Children's University Hospital, Dublin, we have detected at birth 18 (7%) urological anomalies: 6 duplex kidney, 6 hydronephrosis, 4 horseshoe kidney, one pelvic kidney and one single kidney. Urological anomalies were found more commonly in the thoracolumbar and lumbosacral lesions with no correlation between the sensory level of the neural tube defect and the type of urological anomaly. Thus, where abnormalities are found, they are the result of concomitant renal tract anomalies or dysplasia.[3] A baseline DMSA renogram is organized after 3 months of age, while an early micturating cystourethrogram has been replaced in our institution by videourodynamics in the first 3–6 months of life (Figure 107.2).

For patients with closed lesions, there is not likely to be any early surgical intervention, so there is no need for an early indwelling catheter. Following initial clinical assessment, bladder assessment begins with the observation of the baby's voiding pattern and postmicturition volumes. These are then taken in conjunction with the renal US scan, DMSA scan, and later videourodynamics.

Management of neurogenic bladder

The initial management of a newborn with neurogenic bladder is centered on the preservation of renal function. Two different management options are available: the expectant and the proactive approach.

A relatively *expectant* approach is preferred for closed spinal defects, where the risks of neurogenic bladder are lower. In these patients, as long as initial assessment suggested they are voiding regularly, close follow-up is recommended with ultrasonography, urinary surveillance, and monitoring of bladder emptying every 3 months, together with selective

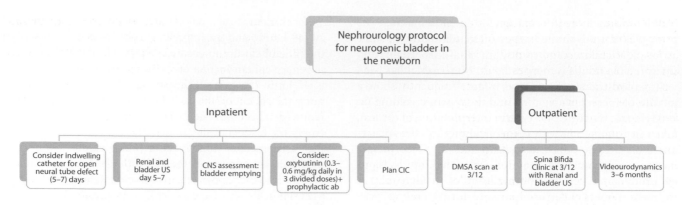

Figure 107.2 Nephrourology protocol for neurogenic bladder in the newborn.

videourodynamics according to circumstances. However, we would recommend to start in all patients daily CIC. This is neither to provide the patients with continence nor to improve bladder emptying. The CIC at this age in these patients is simply to ensure that the intervention is accepted by them, as it has been undertaken all their lives. This way, should problems become apparent during monitoring, or should the patient not develop continence in future years, the frequency of CIC can simply be increased, rather than having to go through the trauma of introducing the intervention in an older child and at a time when anxieties are raised in the family because of the child's problems.

Our preferred option for patients with open spinal defects is a *proactive* approach, as virtually all patients will have a neurogenic bladder. All the newborns are commenced, after their period of continuous catheterization, on CIC and antimuscarinic medication, to try and prevent obstructive uropathy and preserve renal function. We would also most often use prophylactic antibiotics, though there is no firm evidence base for these. The rationale for the CIC and antimuscarinic medication is based on published studies that, in the last 20 years, have shown a significant decrease in augmentation rate in patients treated proactively compared to expectantly.[9,10] In a nonrandomized prospective study, Edelstein et al.[11] found that 15% of the children treated with prophylactic intermittent catheterization had urinary tract deterioration versus nearly 80% of children followed by observation. A proactive approach is also recommended by a Dutch group, which has shown that 29 of their 65 initially "low-risk" patients later became high risk at a mean age of 3.1 years. The authors concluded that early start of CIC is essential to prevent renal damage.[12] In addition, on multivariate analysis, the late institution of CIC (after the age of 1 year) together with the presence of VUR and urinary tract infections (UTIs) has been found to be the only independent risk factor for renal cortical loss.[13]

Clean intermittent catheterization

In the management of a neurogenic bladder, CIC represents the most important modality to empty the bladder adequately and to protect the upper tract. Since its first description by Lapides in 1971, CIC has gained popularity over the years because it allows bladder emptying, avoiding any residue of urine in the bladder, thus reducing the risk of UTI and preventing the occurrence of high-pressure voiding, which is detrimental for kidney function. Even in neonates with lower motor neuron lesions, a good compliant bladder, and low leak point pressure, where CIC might be justifiably delayed, catheterization will be required at the time of toilet training to achieve continence. Our experience in patients with neurogenic bladder indicates that the early institution of CIC is better tolerated by the family and the child, becomes part of the family routine, and helps the parents to cope with their child's disease. The frequency of CIC, from twice to six times daily, will be decided on the basis of the videourodynamics (bladder capacity, activity of sphincter and detrusor, postvoid residual), fluid intake, and age of the child. Complications associated with CIC range from 0% to 40%.[14] Over a period of 16 years, approximately a quarter of boys encountered major complications following repeated catheterization, including false passages, meatal stenosis, urethral stricture, and epididymitis.[15] In young females with myelomeningocele, complications seem to be mainly difficulties in catheterization, macroscopic hematuria, and urethral polyp.[16] To prevent complications, the authors recommend early start of CIC, the use of lubricant (many modern single-use catheters are prelubricated now), and the catheterization with as large a catheter as possible that can be accepted into the urethra.

Pharmacologic treatment of neurogenic bladder overactivity

Oxybutinin hydrochloride is the only anticholinergic medication available for the treatment of neurogenic bladder in newborns and infants. It is available in liquid form, which allows easy titration according to the patient's weight; the recommended dose is 0.3–0.6 mg/ kg per day in three divided doses. It is a smooth muscle relaxant, which acts by blocking the muscarinic receptors on the detrusor muscle, which are stimulated by acetylcholine released from activated parasympathetic nerves. There are five subtypes of muscarinic receptors (M1–M5) distributed in the body. In the human detrusor muscle, M2 and M3 subtypes are found, with M2 representing two-thirds of the total number and M3 mainly responsible for normal micturition contraction.[17] The mechanism of action of oxybutinin is due to a combination of antimuscarinic receptor antagonism, direct antispasmodic effect on the smooth muscle of the bladder, as well as local anesthetic action. The latter seems to be relevant only when oxybutinin is administered intravesically.[18] An experimental study in cultured rat bladder smooth muscle cells has also shown that oxybutinin chloride is involved in bladder remodeling by decreasing smooth muscle proliferation in a dose-dependent manner, helping to prevent permanent bladder changes.[19]

The wide distribution of the muscarinic receptors in the body, brain, heart, salivary glands, and smooth muscle explains some of the common side effects encountered with its use, which include dry mouth, tachycardia, constipation, blurred vision, dizziness, headache, hallucinations, agitation, confusion, and increased postvoid residual, which is not a problem for patients on CIC.[17] Newer antimuscarinic agents are targeted to mainly M3 receptors and therefore have a lower incidence of side effects. While not available for infants, yet they are being trialed in children.

Due to its high lipophilicity, neutral charge, and relatively small molecular structure, oxybutinin easily crosses the blood–brain barrier, which has raised concerns on the association between long-term use of antimuscarinics and cognitive dysfunction. However, a recent study on a small group of patients has demonstrated no significant differences in Child Behavior Checklist scores between children with spinal dysraphism on oxybutinin from birth onward and controls at a median age of 10.6 years.[20] Moreover, a randomized double-blinded trial using long-acting oxybutynin or tolterodine in children with urgency or urge incontinence has also found that long-acting oxybutinin and tolterodine had no negative effects on short-term attention and memory.[21]

The benefit of antimuscarinics in children with detrusor hyperreflexia secondary to neurogenic conditions has been demonstrated by Franco et al.,[22] who have shown an increase in bladder capacity (maximal cystometric capacity), decrease in mean detrusor intravesical pressures, and decrease in number of patients exhibiting uninhibited detrusor contractions. The improvement was consistent across the three formulations of oxybutinin available in the market, oral, syrup, and extended release.

Botulinum toxin injections

Intravesical botulinum toxin injections have been used effectively in patients with neurogenic bladder to eradicate overactive contractions and increase functional bladder capacity. Its primary effect on the bladder is to inhibit acetylcholine release from parasympathetic nerves. The botulinum toxin is administered by intradetrusor or submucosal injection during cystoscopy. The total patient dose is divided into a number of aliquots and injected in a fan array around the bladder, avoiding the trigone.

There are two preparations of botulinum toxin available: *Botox, Allergan (onabotilinum)*, and *Dysport, Ipsen (abobotulinum)*. For Allergan, the dose administered in neurogenic bladder is 5–10 units/kg, up to a maximum of 300 units. For Dysport, the dose is 15–30 units/kg, up to a maximum of 900 units. Botulinum toxin injections can be very effective and eradicate overactivity where antimuscarinic drugs have failed. To the authors' knowledge, there are no published studies showing the efficacy of botulinum toxin in the management of neurogenic bladder in the neonatal period. A recent analysis of 10 published studies with a total of 200 patients (mean age of 9.9 years) with neurogenic bladder mostly due to myelodysplasia has clearly demonstrated that botulinum toxin increases bladder capacity, decreases the maximal detrusor pressure, increases mean continence score, and improves bladder compliance in all patients.[23] Administered correctly, there are no systemic side effects. However, the effect wears off after 6–9 months. Because general anesthesia is mandatory for botulinum toxin injection in children, alternative routes of application have been tried such as intravesical instillation or electromotive drug administration (EMDA), but initial studies require confirmation, and appropriate catheters need to be sourced.[24]

A further use for botulinum toxin is for relaxation of a tight sphincter. In cases where the sphincter is tight or severely dyssynergic, leading to obstructive uropathy, injection of botulinum toxin into the sphincter can temporarily lower the leak pressure and avoid the need for a urinary diversion.

Urinary diversion—vesicostomy

In a small selected group of patients with neurogenic bladder, in whom conservative management fails, the formation of vesicostomy should be considered. It is a simple, well-tolerated, easily reversible procedure that is highly effective in reversing upper tract dilatation. Since its first description by Duckett in 1974, numerous reports have demonstrated an improvement in the upper urinary tract dilatation in 86%–100% of patients. Indications for surgical intervention include worsening hydronephrosis, progression of renal damage, high-grade VUR, or recurrent UTIs despite maximal medical therapy. Complications are encountered in 17%–43% of patients and include peristomal dermatitis followed by bladder prolapse, stomal stenosis, bladder calculi, and recurrent UTIs.[25]

Bladder augmentation and procedures to increase outlet resistance

Other surgical procedures such as bladder augmentation, bladder outlet procedures (periurethral injection of bulking agents, autologous fascial sling, implantation of artificial sphincter), and formation of catheterizable channels for CIC (Mitrofanoff or Monti channel) are rarely required in the newborn period; therefore, their detailed discussion is beyond the scope of this chapter.

BOWEL MANAGEMENT

Spinal cord lesions affect colorectal motility, transit time, and bowel emptying, leading to constipation, fecal incontinence, or a combination of both.[26] Neurogenic bowel and bladder are closely related, and bladder symptoms correlate directly with bowel symptoms. Retained stools in the rectosigmoid can press over the bladder, impairing bladder filling, causing bladder instability, urgency, frequency, and incontinence. In addition, fecal soiling increases the risk of perineal colonization, bladder contamination, and UTI. In a neonate, bowel problems present as either constant loose stools due to complete absence of tone with a patulous anus or constipation. Constipation usually presents at around 4–6 months once solid feeds are introduced. Children with constant loose stool are at risk of excoriation of the buttocks and bleeding from the perianal skin. Barrier creams and exposing the skin to air will help. Constipation should be managed from an early age to promote cleanliness, to improve bladder dynamics, and to prevent UTIs. Early treatment with a high-fiber diet and oral laxatives (lactulose) may be sufficient in the first few years of life to soften the consistency of the stool. Glycerin and bisacodyl suppositories can be used to achieve bowel evacuation in children with an adequate rectal tone. In children with true fecal incontinence due to a deficient fecal continence mechanism and prolonged colorectal motility, mini washouts of water with either a syringe connected to a catheter or a cone-shaped tipped irrigation set can be used. A washout of 20 mL/kg tap water instilled by gravity, either daily or on alternative days, is recommended to ensure regular bowel emptying.

For children older than 3 years, different transanal irrigation systems are available in the market (Peristeen Coloplast LTD, Nene Hall, Peterborough Business Pk, Peterborough, United Kingdom; Irrimatic Pump, B. Braun Medical LTD, Thorncliffe Park, Sheffield, United Kingdom; Irrisedo Mini System, MBH-International A/S, Gydevang, 28-30, Denmark), which have been shown to be beneficial in 41%–100% of children with neurogenic fecal incontinence.[27] In older patients who fail medical therapy, an antegrade approach via the appendix to the cecum (Malone Antegrade Continence Enema [MACE] procedure) allows regular bowel emptying with improved social confidence, hygiene, and independence. Reported success rate as partial or complete fecal continence with MACE ranges from 47% to 100%,[28] with up to 80% of spina bifida patients recommending the MACE procedure to others.[29]

CONCLUSION

The management of a neonate with neurogenic bladder needs a multidisciplinary team with the urologist, renal/ bladder physician, and neurosurgeon working together. The urology nurse specialist is central to the care of the patient. CIC is the most important part of the treatment and should be started as early as possible after birth and repair of the spinal defect. The main goal of therapy is not continence but protection of the upper tracts. The secondary aim is to try and ensure that the growing child has as good a bladder capacity and compliance as possible. Each patient is individual, and therapy needs to be tailored according to the findings in each child and the family circumstances.

REFERENCES

1. McDonnell R, Delany V, O'Mahony MT, Mullaney C, Lee B, Turner MJ. Neural tube defects in the Republic of Ireland in 2009–11. *J Publ Health* 2014; 18: 1–7.
2. Lloyd JC, Wiener JS, Gargollo PC et al. Contemporary epidemiological trends in complex congenital genitourinary anomalies. *J Urol Suppl* 2013; 190: 1590.
3. Whitaker RH, Hunt GM. Incidence and distribution of renal anomalies in patients with neural tube defects. 1. *Eur Urol* 1987; 13(5): 322–3.
4. Sturm RM, Cheng EY. The management of the pediatric neurogenic bladder. *Curr Bladder Dysfunct Rep* 2016; 11: 225–33.
5. Brock JW 3rd, Carr MC, Adzick NS et al. Bladder function after fetal surgery for myelomeningocele. *Pediatrics* 2015 October; 136(4): e906–13.
6. Bauer SB. Initial management of meningocele children. In: Corcos J, Ginsberg D, Karsenty G (eds). *Textbook of Neurogenic Bladder*, 3rd edn. Boca Raton, FL: CRC Press, Taylor & Francis Group, 2015: 633–44.
7. Sillén U. Bladder function in infants. *Scand J Urol Nephrol Suppl* 2004; (215): 69–74.
8. Stoneking BJ, Borck JW, Pope JC et al. Early evolution of bladder emptying after myelomeningocele closure. *Urology* 2001; 58: 767–71.
9. Wu HY, Baskin LS, Kogan B A. Neurogenic bladder dysfunction due to myelomeningocele: Neonatal versus childhood treatment. *J Urol* 1997, 157: 2295.
10. Kaefer M, Pabby A, Kelly M et al. Improved bladder function after prophylactic treatment of the high risk neurogenic bladder in newborns with myelomeningocele. *J Urol* 1999; 162: 1068.
11. Edelstein RA, Bauer SB, Kelly MD et al. The long-term urological response of neonates with myelodysplasia treated proactively with intermittent catheterization and anticholinergic therapy. *J Urol* 1995; 154: 1500.
12. Dik P, Klijn AJ, van Gool JD et al. Early start to therapy preserves kidney function in spina bifida patients. *Eur Urol* 2006; 49: 908–13.

13. DeLair SM, Eandi J, White MJ et al. Renal cortical deterioration in children with spinal dysraphism: Analysis of risk factors. *J Spinal Cord Med* 2007; 30 Suppl 1: S30.

14. Campbell JB, Moore KN, Voaklander DC et al. Complications associated with clean intermittent catheterization in children with spina bifida. *J Urol* 2004; 171(6 Pt 1): 2420–2.

15. Lindehall B, Abrahamsson K, Hjalmas K et al. Complications of clean intermittent catheterization in boys and young males with neurogenic bladder dysfunction. *J Urol* 2004; 172(4 Pt 2): 1686–8.

16. Lindehall B, Abrahamsson K, Jodal U et al. Complications of clean intermittent catheterization in young females with myelomeningocele: 10–19 years follow up. *J Urol* 2007; 178(3 Pt 1): 1053–5.

17. Andersson KE. Antimuscarinics for treatment of overactive bladder. *Lancet Neurol* 2004 January; 3(1): 46–53.

18. Andersson KE, Chapple C, Wein A. The basis for drug treatment of the overactive bladder. *World J Urol* 2001 November; 19(5): 294–8.

19. Park JM, Bauer SB, Freeman MR et al. Oxybutynin chloride inhibits proliferation and suppresses gene expression in bladder smooth muscle cells. *J Urol* 1999 September; 162(3 Pt 2): 1110–4.

20. Veenboer PW, Huisman J, Chrzan RJ et al. Behavioral effects of long-term antimuscarinic use in patients with spinal dysraphism: A case control study. *J Urol* 2013 December; 190(6): 2228–32.

21. Giramonti KM, Kogan BA, Halpern LF. The effects of anticholinergic drugs on attention span and short-term memory skills in children. *Neurourol Urodyn* 2008; 27(4): 315–8.

22. Franco I, Horowitz M, Grady R et al. Efficacy and safety of oxybutynin in children with detrusor hyperreflexia secondary to neurogenic bladder dysfunction. *J Urol* 2005; 173: 221–5.

23. Lee B, Featherstone N, Nagappan P et al. British Association of Paediatric Urologists consensus statement on the management of the neuropathic bladder. *J Pediatr Urol* 2016; 12: 76–87.

24. Scheepe JR, Blok BF, 't Hoen LA. Applicability of botulinum toxin type A in paediatric neurogenic bladder management. *Curr Opin Urol* 2017 January; 27(1): 14–9.

25. Morrisroe SN, O'Connor RC, Nanigian DK et al. Vesicostomy revisited: The best treatment for the hostile bladder in the myelodysplastic children. *Br J Urol* 2005; 96: 397–400.

26. Krogh K, Mosdal C, Laurberg S. Gastrointestinal and segmental colonic transit times in patients with acute and chronic spinal cord lesions. *Spinal Cord* 2000; 38: 615–21.

27. Pereira PL, Salvador OP, Arcas JA. Transanal irrigation for the treatment of neuropathic bowel dysfunction. *J Pediatr Urol* 2010; 6: 134–8.

28. Gor RA, Katorski JR, Elliott SP. Medical and surgical management of neurogenic bowel. *Curr Opin Urol* 2016 July; 26(4): 369–75.

29. Imai K, Shiroyanagi Y, Kim WJ et al. Satisfaction after the Malone antegrade continence enema procedure in patients with spina bifida. *Spinal Cord* 2014; 52(1): 54e7.

FURTHER READING

De Jong TPV, Chrzan R, Klijn AJ et al. Treatment of the neurogenic bladder in spina bifida. *Ped Nephrol* 2008; 23: 889–96.

Do Ngoc C, Audry G, Forin V. Botulium toxin type A for neurogenic detrusor over activity due to spinal cord lesions in children: A retrospective study of seven cases. *J Pediatr Urol* 2009; 5: 430–6.

Karaman MI, Kaya C, Caskurlu T et al. Urodynamics findings in children with cerebral palsy. *Int J Urol* 2005; 12: 717–20.

Kiddo DA, Canning DA, Snyder HM 3rd et al. Urethral dilation as treatment for neurogenic bladder. *J Urol* 2006; 176(4 Pt 2): 1831–3.

Koff SA, Gigax MR, Jayanthi VR. Nocturnal bladder emptying: A simple technique for reversing urinary tract deterioration in children with neurogenic bladder. *J Urol* 2005; 174(4 Pt 2): 1629–31.

Lapides J, Diokno AC, Silber SJ et al. Clean, intermittent self-catheterization in the treatment of urinary tract disease. *Trans Am Assoc Genitourin Surg* 1971; 69: 142–54.

Mitrofanoff P. Cystostomie continente transappendiculaire dans le traitement des vessies neurologiques. *Chir Pediatr* 1980; 21: 297.

Nguyen MT, Pavlock CL, Zderic SA et al. Overnight catheter drainage in children with poorly compliant bladders improves post-obstructive diuresis and urinary incontinence. *J Urol* 2005; 174(4 Pt 2): 1633–6.

Wilmhurst JM, Kelly R, Borzyskowski M. Presentation and outcome of sacral agenesis: 20 years' experience. *Dev Med Child Neurol* 1999; 41: 806–12.

108

Hydrometrocolpos

DEVENDRA K. GUPTA AND SHILPA SHARMA

INTRODUCTION

Hydrometrocolpos is a condition in which the uterus and vagina are grossly distended with retained fluid other than blood, usually in the presence of distal vaginal obstruction. The diagnosis and treatment of hydrometrocolpos has now been better streamlined as the condition is being diagnosed prenatally more frequently with the use of ultrasound and fetal magnetic resonance (MR) imaging.

Hydrometrocolpos presents at the two extremes of childhood, initially during the neonatal period, when there is a high level of maternal hormones, and then at early puberty, when the patient herself begins to have production of estrogenic hormones. The distal vaginal obstruction is mostly due to imperforate hymen (in two-thirds of cases) followed by a transverse vaginal septum, and less commonly, vaginal atresia (with or without persistence of a urogenital sinus or cloaca).

Associated anomalies are common and quite often of severe nature. These include anorectal malformations and unilateral or bilateral agenesis of the kidney/s, ureters, and trigone. Uterine anomalies like didelphys may also be associated, especially in cases with common cloaca. There are often back pressure changes in the urinary tract due to the pressure effect. The vagina may be bifid in a case of common cloaca, with the terminal bowel opening directly into the intervaginal septum or even at the base of the urinary bladder. Ultrasonography, micturating cystourethrogram (MCU), dye study through a vaginostomy, panendoscopy, and MR urography would help to evaluate the complex anatomy of hydrometrocolpos associated with genitourinary anomalies.

The main treatment of hydrometrocolpos is surgical. Medical management is required to build the nutrition of the baby and make her fit for surgery. The operative procedure and timing of surgical intervention depend upon the severity of the condition, type of anomaly, and age at presentation. Early surgery is indicated in the neonatal period when a grossly distended hydrometrocolpos presents with a bulging hymen, quite often associated with complications (abdominal mass, urinary obstruction, constipation, sepsis,

dehydration). Laparotomy is indicated in patients with high vaginal obstruction and for the treatment of abdominal complications or associated anomalies.

The baby would need resuscitation and stabilization during the acute stage with antibiotics and intravenous (IV) fluids. A temporizing procedure like aspiration of the turbid infected fluid (or an abdominal tube or a flap vaginostomy) is indicated in the neonatal period to drain the infected material from the vagina. A percutaneous nephrostomy may also be needed in patients presenting with severe bilateral hydroureteronephrosis leading to urinary obstruction, uremia, and sepsis.

Hydrometrocolpos has been classified into five types on the basis of the type and level of obstruction (Figure 108.1).

I. Low hymenal obstruction
II. Midplane transverse membrane or septum
   a. Without communication
   b. With a small orifice as communication
III. High obstruction with distal vaginal atresia
   a. Without any perineal swelling
   b. With perineal swelling
IV. Vaginal atresia with persistence of the urogenital sinus
V. Vaginal atresia with cloacal anomaly

An algorithm for management of hydrometrocolpos has been suggested (Figure 108.2) [1]. Newborns presenting with complications should be managed in the intensive care unit with systemic antibiotics, IV fluids, decompression of gastrointestinal tract by nasogastric aspiration, and administration of oxygen. Fluid and electrolyte imbalance should be corrected. A Foley catheter should be inserted in the bladder for urinary drainage. In the presence of a huge distended hydrometrocolpos in a sick neonate, a preliminary drainage by puncturing the vagina under ultrasonographic guidance may be done for 24–48 hours prior to corrective surgery. Alternatively, the vaginal septum (type II anomaly) can be incised under ultrasonographic guidance safely or under vision in experienced hands.

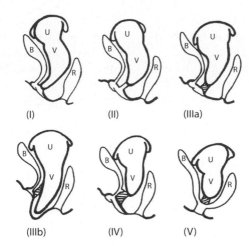

Figure 108.1 Classification. hydrometrocolpos with (I) hymenal obstruction, (II) low vaginal atresia, (IIIa) high vaginal atresia, (IIIb) high vaginal atresia with gluteal extension, (IV) urogenital sinus, and (V) common cloacal malformation.

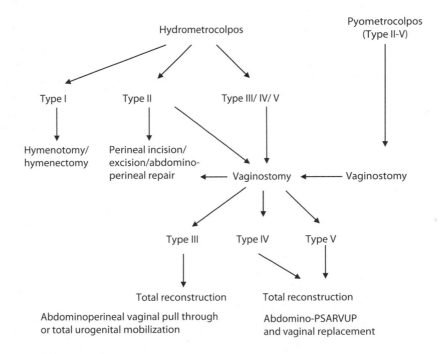

Figure 108.2 Algorithm for management of hydrometrocolpos. PSARVUP, posterior sagittal anorectal vagino-urethroplasty.

The management options depend upon the type of obstruction. Management is simple with low-level type I and II anomalies. However, patients with type III, IV, and V anomalies are usually obstructed and infected. Moreover, type IV anomaly has a valvular opening between the urethra and the vagina, allowing urine flow to the vagina during the act of micturition, and vice versa. In such cases, an attempt should be made to drain the infected material collected in the vagina by a suprapubic route (catheter or flap vaginostomy as a first-stage procedure) and allow the dilated vagina to shrink. This is followed by a definitive procedure (vaginal pull-through) later on (as a second-stage procedure). All previous attempts to drain the vagina and also simultaneously reconstruct the vaginal tract in the newborn stage carried a very high mortality, and it is thus not recommended.

DRAINAGE PROCEDURE

The advantages of an early drainage in neonates include drainage of the infected material to reduce sepsis, disconnection of the communication and retrograde flow of urine to the vagina, and allowing the inflamed vagina and uterus to shrink and occupy near-normal anatomical positions and size to allow planning of definitive surgery. In cases of common cloaca, a suprapubic cystostomy may serve to decompress the infected collection in the urogenital system. In prepubertal age, drainage allows natural passage for menstrual flow and creation of a passage for future sexual activity and fertility. The drainage procedure through the perineum may be the only definitive treatment required in types I and II.

A bulging membrane in an infant with imperforate hymen or transverse septum of the vagina may be incised without anesthesia. However, excision is preferable if the hymen is thickened or the patient is an adolescent. Hymenotomy may resolve the acute renal failure caused by hydrometrocolpos. In all cases, it is desirable to maintain the patency of the opening by the initial use of a drain followed by repeated dilatations (Figure 108.3).

In the lithotomy position, the bulging hymen becomes visible as a grayish membrane. If necessary, the abdomen may be compressed to make the hymenal bulge more prominent. A Foley catheter is inserted into the urinary bladder to decompress it as well as for the identification of the urethra during the surgery. A series of stay sutures is placed at the center of the hymen, and the vaginal fluid is aspirated and sent for microscopic examination and culture (Figure 108.4b). A circular hymenal segment is excised using a no. 11 blade (Figure 108.4c). The cut margin is oversewn and retracted with vertical mattress sutures (Figure 108.4d). The sutures are tied, exposing the vaginal cavity (Figure 108.4e). A soft Silastic catheter is inserted into the vagina. A contrast study is performed to delineate the internal anatomy. The vagina is drained for a couple of days. This procedure is simple and can be performed at the bedside or in the intensive care unit in a sick baby after assessing the depth with a needle puncture and ultrasonography. In cases of doubt, the procedure may be done in the operating room safely through the abdominal route after performing a dye study. A Hegar dilator or a finger is placed through the vaginostomy opening as a guide, to remove a disk of the septum, which may be thick. The edges are then oversewn and a drain placed. Antibiotics should be given for 5–7 days postoperatively.

A vaginostomy serves as a temporizing drainage procedure for cases with infected fluid. It may be done through the perineal route in type II after confirmation of the diagnosis with a needle aspiration. When a low transverse vaginal septum is present (between the lower one-third and

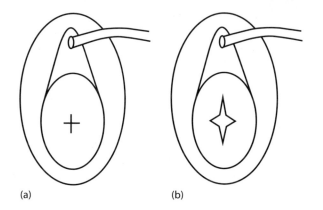

(a)   (b)

Figure 108.3 (a and b) Hymenotomy.

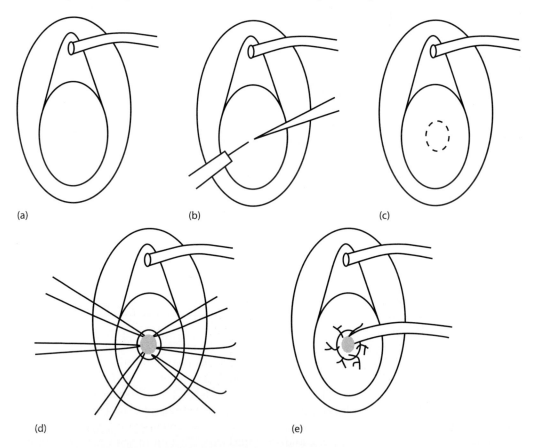

(a)   (b)   (c)

(d)   (e)

Figure 108.4 (a–e) Hymenectomy (with excision of the membrane disk).

upper two-thirds of the vagina), it presents as a bulging membrane, allowing its excision and permitting drainage by the perineal route (Figure 108.5a). In some patients, a minute vaginal orifice may be visible that may be surgically enlarged and oversewn with the placement of a catheter in the vagina for establishing drainage (Figure 108.5b).

However, even in type II anomaly, sometimes, due to secondary infection or complex anomalies, a perineal procedure may be deferred, and these babies may need suprapubic drainage by catheter or a vaginostomy. The proximal diversion stoma not only helps in decompressing the vagina but also provides a portal for detailed radiographic studies to delineate the anatomy. If the transverse septum in type II cases is more than 1 cm thick, it is wiser to perform a laparotomy and define the proper anatomy, incise the septum

precisely under direct vision, and then drain the vagina. This is performed in order to prevent injury to the urethra and rectum during the perineal dissection.

Abdominoperineal repair of type II hydrometrocolpos is as follows: A low transverse abdominal incision is made (Figure 108.6a). The hydrometrocolpos is delivered from the abdominal wound, and a purse string suture is applied on the vaginal wall. Fluid is drained out (Figure 108.6b). A Kelly forceps is then introduced through the vaginostomy opening, and the tip is advanced toward the most dependent part of the dilated vagina in the perineum (Figure 108.6c). The vaginal septum is then incised while the outer vaginal orifice is spread open by the nasal speculum and the transverse septum is pushed downward by the Kelly forceps. The septum is incised, and the Kelly forceps is pushed down and out. A Silastic catheter drains the vagina from below (Figure 108.6d). The hydrometrocolpos is also drained by an indwelling catheter from above for 5–7 days (Figure 108.6e).

For types III–V, hydrometrocolpos with atresia of the lower two-thirds of the vagina or in a case of common cloaca with hydrometrocolpos, an abdominal route is preferred for doing the vaginostomy. If the atretic lower portion of the vagina has been retracted up into the pelvis, it may be desirable to open the vagina through a laparotomy incision to avoid damage to the urethra, bladder, and rectum.

Abdominal vaginostomy may be of two types: vaginostomy with an indwelling catheter and tubed vaginostomy. The abdomen is opened with a Pfannenstiel incision. The dilated vagina is identified, and stay sutures are applied. The steps as described in Figure 108.6a–c remain the same.

1. *Vaginostomy with an indwelling catheter (Figure 108.7a–e).* Though it is easy to perform, it has certain disadvantages like infection, encrustation, and also the need to

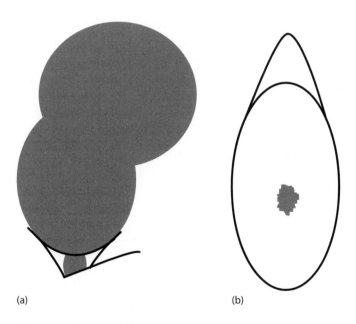

(a)   (b)

Figure 108.5 (a and b) Perineal vaginostomy.

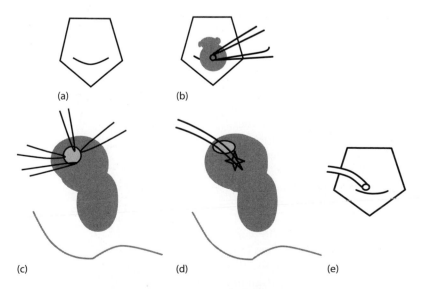

(a)   (b)

(c)   (d)   (e)

Figure 108.6 (a–e) Abdominoperineal repair (combined approach).

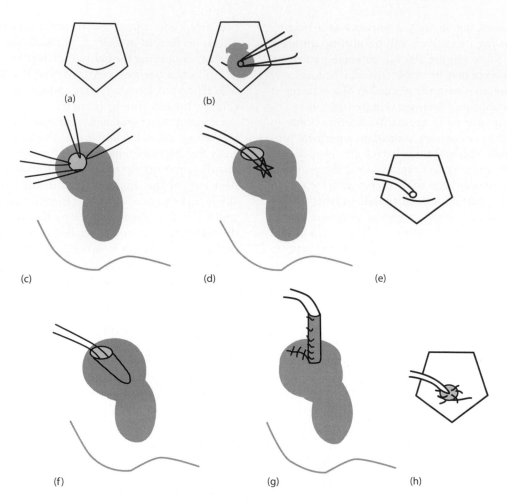

Figure 108.7 (a–e) Operative steps for abdominal vaginostomy. **(a)** Pfannesteil incision. **(b)** Stay sutures are applied on the distended vagina. **(c)** Opening in vagina is brought out and stitched to abdominal wall all around in two layers. **(d)** Malecot catheter is placed in the distended vagina. **(e)** Abdominal wound closed in layers. **(f–h)** Operative steps for tubed vaginostomy **(f)** A U-shaped flap is created with the vaginal wall. **(g)** Flap is closed in a cylindrical manner to form a tube of the vaginal wall. **(h)** Vaginal tube is brought out of the abdominal wall as a stoma. A catheter is left in for few days.

keep the tube in situ, requiring frequent changing and causing an inconvenience to the patient.

2. *Tubed vaginostomy (Figure 108.7f–h).* In this procedure, a U-shaped flap of the vagina is used to make a tube that provides drainage through the natural tract (rather than the need for a catheter) till the time of definitive surgery. The U-shaped incision is seen in Figure 108.7f. It is made into a tube, as shown in Figure 108.7g. The edge of the tube is fixed to the abdominal wall and the skin, as shown in Figure 108.7h. A tubed vaginostomy avoids the long-term use of any indwelling catheter and at the same time provides an effective drainage. This also provides easy access for performing dye studies to outline the anatomy before doing a definitive surgery.

Cases of type V hydrometrocolpos (associated with common cloaca) and a common channel more than 3 cm long require a vaginostomy and also a diverting colostomy. This is to be done keeping the good segment of the sigmoid bowel available for both vaginal replacement and bowel

pull-through in the future. Thus, a transverse colostomy is preferred (Figure 108.8).

In type IV, if the common channel of the urogenital sinus is less than 2.5 cm long, as confirmed by endoscopy

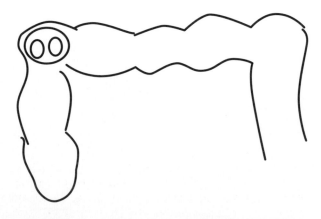

Figure 108.8 Transverse colostomy for common cloaca.

at surgery, disconnection of the fistula is done followed by total urogenital mobilization. The vagina may be exteriorized onto the perineum, while the urogenital sinus can be made to function as the main urethra. The patient is placed in lithotomy position (Figure 108.9a). Stay sutures are applied around the urogenital sinus such that the sutures lie within the line of incision (Figure 108.9b). An incision is made all around the urogenital sinus with a midline posterior incision in the sinus that extends posterolaterally in the perineum for adequate exposure and mobilization (Figure 108.9c). As the meticulous dissection continues, the urethra and the vagina become visible externally as two separate openings, and the tissues are approximated (Figure 108.9d). If the vaginal introitus is narrow, it can be widened by placing a Barrow's skin pedicle flap in its posterior wall. At times, the vagina may open into the bladder as a fistulous communication.

However, if the length of the urogenital sinus is more than 2.5 cm, then vaginal replacement would be required. The fistulous communication between the urethra and the vagina cannot be reached through the perineum. It is divided repaired with sutures, and the vagina is brought to the perineum by using the posterior sagittal route, bisecting the rectum to approach the vagina directly from behind (PSARVUP). An additional abdominal route is also required for vaginal replacement.

This is a major undertaking, and to achieve the best results, the procedure should be performed by a team of experienced surgeons preferably in a tertiary care–level center.

The common channel in type V is usually more than 3 cm, mandating a vaginal replacement. In cases with type III, IV, and V with pyometrocolpos, it may be difficult to separate it from the surrounding structures due to severe inflammation and dense adhesions. In such situations, it would be better to replace the vagina using bowel vaginoplasty. A loop of sigmoid colon or an ileum can be used for bowel vaginoplasty. An abdominoperineal approach is adopted. The abdomen is opened with a Pfannenstiel incision with extension on the left side in a hockey-stick manner (Figure 108.10a). The vaginal space is created in the perineum carefully between the

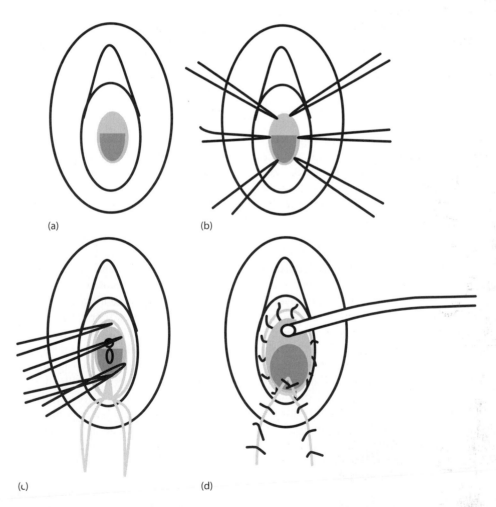

(a) (b)

(c) (d)

Figure 108.9 Total urogenital mobilization (TUM). **(a)** Diagrammatic representation of the urogenital sinus. **(b)** Stay sutures are applied all around the urogenital sinus in such a manner that an incision can be given around them. **(c)** Mobilization of the urogenital sinus is done along with a midline posterior incision or an inverted V-shaped incision (Barrow's flap). **(d)** After adequate mobilization, the urethral and vaginal openings may be visualized on the surface as two separate openings. The barrows flap if created may be used to widen the vaginal orifice.

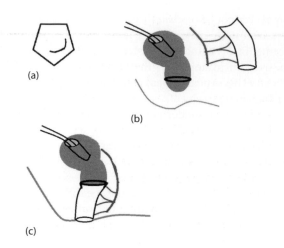

Figure 108.10 **(a–c)** Vaginal replacement with bowel segment.

rectum and the urethra and also from the abdominal side. The length of the bowel required for vaginal replacement is assessed. An adequate length of the colonic bowel segment on its mesentery with adequate blood supply is selected for the pull-through (Figure 108.10b). The upper end is anastomosed to the proximal vagina from the abdominal side, and the distal end of the bowel is anastomosed to the perineal skin at the proposed vaginal introitus, taking care not to cause any torsion to the bowel segment or traction on the blood supply (Figure 108.10c).

In cases with a narrow distal vagina or if the vagina has retracted following its repair, flaps of perineal skin may be used to contribute to the distal vaginal segment. A Barrow flap is the most commonly used procedure. An inverted-Y incision is made, with the vertical limb of the *Y* going inside the vaginal introitus for a centimeter or so in the posterior wall (Figure 108.11a). With the V-shaped perineal skin intact, blood supply is created and mobilized sufficiently. It is then advanced in the vagina and sutured to the margins of the incision edges in the introitus (Figure 108.11b).

Many surgeons prefer the use of a skin graft over a vaginal mold, a cylinder of a prosthetic patch, or a buccal mucosa graft with a mesh to form the neovagina. The results are variable, and retractions and graft contraction are not uncommon. Expertise is needed to perform such a surgery. This kind of replacement is better performed at puberty

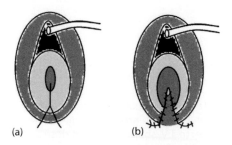

Figure 108.11 **(a** and **b)** Barrow flap vaginoplasty.

or before marriage, as it is prone to shrinkage and needs repeated dilatations.

SUMMARY

Hydrometrocolpos is a rare disorder. From a clinical point of view, there are three groups:

1. Low anomalies, usually presenting in the newborn period with a hymenal obstruction (rarely the distal vaginal obstruction) and a bulge in the perineum. The diagnosis is made on inspection and needle aspiration of the contents from the bulge under anesthesia. The contents are normally clear. A perineal incision in the bulge is curative. Though no detailed investigations are required in early infancy, the associated genitourinary anomalies should be ruled out with ultrasonography and IV pyelogram or an MR urography in due course.

2. Hydrometrocolpos with urogenital sinus anomaly. In such cases, there are two openings in the perineum instead of three: the urethra and the anus. The vagina is high up and has a tiny communication with the urinary bladder, usually at the level of the bladder neck. This communication is valvular and allows only one-way flow of urine from the urinary bladder to the vagina. A small amount of urine flows into the vagina during the act of micturition, but the vagina cannot drain it to the urethra due to the valvular effect; thus, there is slow development of hydrometrocolpos. Due to stasis of urine and the vaginal contents, the hydrometrocolpos gets infected, resulting in pyometrocolpos, and the child presents with septicemia. It is mainly the vagina that gets dilated; the uterus, not so much. The genitourinary tract is often obstructed due to the effect of pressure, and there is a bilateral hydroureteronephrosis. The patient presents in an emergency with a palpable lump in the lower abdomen, urinary obstruction, sepsis, uremia, and bilateral hydroureteronephrosis. Urgent investigations with ultrasonography, MR urography, and biochemistry are performed, and the patient is stabilized with fluids and antibiotics. The dirty fluid needs to be drained out urgently using a catheter or by fashioning a formal tube vaginostomy by the suprapubic route. Final surgery, usually after the age of 1 year or so, would require closure of the communication of the channel from the bladder and a vaginal pull-through. It is easier said than done because the vaginal walls are inflamed, thickened, and plastered to the surrounding pelvic structures, and it is not possible to mobilize them to bring them down to the perineum. Thus, it is safe to perform a vaginal replacement and bridge the gap using a segment of the colon or ileum.

3. Hydrometrocolpos with cloacal malformation. This is the most serious of all anomalies in this group. The patient has only a single opening in the perineum, into which open the urethra, the vagina, and the bowel. The

confluence is high up at the bladder neck. The vagina may be bifid with a complete or incomplete septum in between with each half of the uterus. The vagina becomes dilated so that urine can flow through the fistula. The bowel is opened with a fistulous tract either in the vaginal septum or in the bladder neck. In some cases, the whole of the colon is turned into a cesspool-like structure, called a pouch colon, having an abnormal vascular configuration. Surgery is required in the newborn period in emergencies for high-level types of anorectal abnormalities, urinary obstruction, and abdominal lump (hydrometrocolpos or pouch colon) in the form of a transverse colostomy (even ileostomy with the excision of pouch colon), closure of the fistula between the bowel and the bladder, and suprapubic tube vaginostomy to drain the vaginal contents. A urinary catheter drains the bladder well. After a year or so, the definitive surgery requires closure of the fistula between the vagina and the bladder, vaginal replacement with a segment of the bowel, a bowel pull-through with a complex reconstructive procedure by an abdomino-perineo-sacral route, called the posterior sagittal anorectal vaginourethroplasty (PSARVUP). Separation of the thick-walled vagina from the urinary bladder is tricky. A part of the vaginal wall adherent to the base of the urinary bladder can be left in situ, and the fistula can be closed to prevent damage to the urinary bladder. This should only be performed in a tertiary care–level setup by a team of experienced surgeons familiar with the anatomy and the surgical techniques.

FURTHER READING

Capito C, Belarbi N, Paye Jaouen A, Leger J, Carel JC, Oury JF, Sebag G, El-Ghoneimi A. Prenatal pelvic MRI: Additional clues for assessment of urogenital obstructive anomalies. *J Pediatr Urol* 2014; 10: 162–6.

Gupta DK, Sharma S. Hydrometrocolpos. In: Puri P, Höllwarth M, (eds). *Pediatric Surgery: Diagnosis and Management*. Berlin: Springer-Verlag, 2009: 957–66.

Gupta DK, Sharma S. Hydrometrocolpos. In: Puri P (ed). *Newborn Surgery*, 3rd edn, Chapter 101. USA: CRC Press, 2011: 940–51.

Gupta DK, Lal A. Hydrometrocolpos in the newborn. In: Gupta DK (ed).*Textbook of Neonatal Surgery*. Delhi: Modern Publishers, 2000: 518–20.

Levitt MA, Bischoff A, Peña A. Pitfalls and challenges of cloaca repair: how to reduce the need for reoperations. *J Pediatr Surg* 2011 June; 46(6) :1250–5.

Nakajima E, Ishigouoka T, Yoshida T, Sato T, Miyamoto T, Shirai M, Sengoku K. Prenatal diagnosis of congenital imperforate hymen with hydrocolpos. *J Obstet Gynaecol* 2015; 35: 311–3.

Okoro PE, Obiorah C, Enyindah CE. Experience with neonatal hydrometrocolpos in the Niger Delta area of Nigeria: Upsurge or increased recognition? *Afr J Paediatr Surg* 2016; 13: 161–5.

Speck KE, Arnold MA, Ivancic V, Teitelbaum DH. Cloaca and hydrocolpos: Laparoscopic-, cystoscopic- and colposcopic-assisted vaginostomy tube placement. *J Pediatr Surg* 2014; 49: 1867–9.

109

Disorders of sexual development

MARIA MARCELA BAILEZ

INTRODUCTION

Patients with ambiguous genitalia mostly present in the newborn period requiring a multidisciplinary team, which includes a pediatric surgeon/urologist to assign the sex of rearing as soon as possible after a thorough genetic, anatomic, functional, and socioeconomic workup.

The diagnosis of *ambiguous genitalia* is based on a meticulous perineal exam and gonadal palpation.

The feminine phenotype presents a normal-looking clitoris and no palpable gonads.

The masculine phenotype presents a normal-looking penis and two scrotal testicles.

Although exceptions to this pattern occur, e.g., a female with an inguinal hernia or a male with a mild hypospadias or an undescended testicle; if a combination of abnormal gonadal palpation and external genitalia appearance is detected, sexual ambiguity should be studied. Isolated severe defects like a perineal hypospadias or bilateral non-palpable gonads in a patient with a normal-looking phallus should also be investigated (Figures 109.1a,b and 109.2).

The Consensus Statement on Management of Intersex Disorders proposes the term *disorders of sex development* (DSDs), defined as congenital conditions in which development of chromosomal, gonadal, or anatomic sex is atypical. Occasionally, patients with previously unrecognized DSD present later in infancy or puberty. The history of DSD management shows how, in the past, the recommendations for gender assignment of infants with ambiguous genitalia have been guided by the phenotypic appearance of the genitalia. The sex of rearing was mainly decided on the basis of what was believed would facilitate the "most functional genitalia and offer the child their best opportunity to reach normality" (Hughes et al. 2006).

The assumption was that the sex assignment would later determine the child's future sexual identity. However, this simplistic approach did not always work. More recent studies have helped us to better understand what actually determines gender identity, but even now, there is a paucity of outcome data for evidence-based approaches to these rare disorders.

Contemporary management sees DSD decision making as multifaceted, involving many different factors (none to the exclusion of the others), including etiology, fertility, and most likely gender outcome. Data coming from existing studies present conflicting outcomes. New scientific acquisitions unveil the ever-evolving complexities of the neurobiological and psychosexual development regarding gender identity.

ETIOLOGY

Sex differentiation refers to the anatomic development of the internal and external genitalia as male or female dependent on the presence or absence of functioning androgens.

Genital development is constitutively female and nondependent on estrogens prenatally. In contrast, male sex differentiation is mandatorily androgen dependent and requires optimal ligand activation of the androgen receptor (AR).

Gonad development

Fifteen years have passed since the discovery of Sry as the primary "testis-determining gene" (Jager et al. 1990; Blecher and Erickson 2007) in the classic experiment of Koopman et al. showing that transgenic expression of Sry in XX mice results in testis development and male phenotype. Studies in mice are continuing to provide exciting information about differential structural changes and gene expression in normal gonad development (testis versus ovary) as well as the effect of targeted deletion of key genes involved in this process. WT1, SF1, SOX9, DHH, DMRT, SIDDT, and ARX are some of the genetic determinants of normal gonad development and gonadal dysgenesis.

Androgens

The production of androgens by fetal Leydig cells is initially gonadotropin independent. Placental human chorionic gonadotropin (HCG) is the one that ensures high

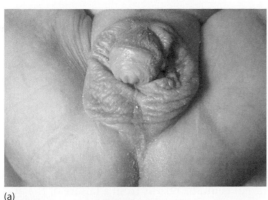

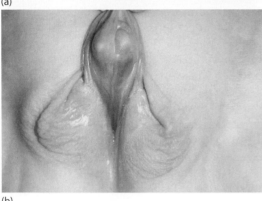

Figure 109.1 **(a)** A newborn with bilateral nonpalpable gonads but a normal-looking phallus. **(b)** Classic hyperpigmentation seen in congenital adrenal hyperplasia patients before treatment, with severe defects like a perineal hypospadias and bilateral nonpalpable gonads.

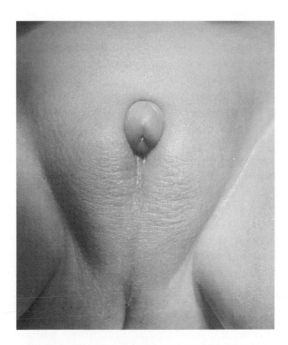

Figure 109.2 Sexual ambiguity should be studied in a patient with combined abnormal gonadal palpation and external genitalia appearance.

concentrations of androgens during the first half of gestation to stabilize Wolffian duct development and differentiation of the external genital anlage. Wolffian duct stabilization is dependent on high local concentrations of testosterone diffusing in a gradient along the duct from the adjacent ipsilateral gonad. This accounts for the asymmetric development of Wolffian ducts in some DSDs.

The androgen receptor (AR) is a transcription factor that mediates male sexual differentiation in utero and is responsible for the development and maintenance of male sexual characteristics. The AR gene is located on the X chromosome. Mutations in the AR gene may lead to diseases like androgen insensitivity syndrome (AIS). In AIS, gonadal males had a spectrum of abnormalities ranging from individuals with a female phenotype (complete AIS [CAIS]) through genital ambiguities in the partial form (partial AIS [PAIS]) to men with fertility disturbances in minimal AIS (MAIS). More than 500 mutations have now been documented in AIS.

In summary, circulating testosterone is responsible for virilization and is dependent upon 5-RD2 (transforms testosterone into dihydrotestosterone) and the presence of appropriate receptors.

Anti-Mullerian hormone

The pre-Sertoli cells secrete a glycoprotein hormone called anti-Mullerian hormone (AMH). It causes involution of the Mullerian ducts and stimulates the Leydig cells to produce testosterone. It is also responsible for the first stage of testicular descent.

The AMH receptor is different from de the. Persistent Mullerian structures in 46,XY DSD patients may be due to failure of the production of the hormone from the testes (50%) or to receptor deficiency.

Steroids

Problems in the early stages of steroid genesis can result in abnormalities of adrenal steroid synthesis, which may result in external virilization of a gonadal female-like adrenal hyperplasia (congenital adrenal hyperplasia [CAH]) or underandrogenization of the 46,XY fetus.

21-Hydroxylase is encoded by a gene on chromosome 6. Its deficiency is inherited in an autosomal recessive fashion.

Tremendous progress has been made in the past 15 years in understanding the role of mutation of factors involved in the steroid genesis process (e.g., STAR, CYP11A, HSD3B2, CYP17).

Considerably more research is needed to be able to translate this new knowledge into effective patient care and to understand the long-term outcome in specific conditions.

HISTORY

The term *intersex* was used till 2005, and subcategories included male pseudohermaphrodite, female pseudohermaphrodite, and true hermaphrodite. These terms used gender in the nomenclature and were often considered controversial or disparaging.

Therefore, revised nomenclature was proposed that incorporated genetic etiology and descriptive terminology while removing gender references.

The Lawson Wilkins Pediatric Endocrine Society (LWPES) and the European Society for Paediatric Endocrinology (ESPE) considered it timely to review the management of intersex disorders from a broad perspective, to review data on longer-term outcome, and to formulate proposals for future studies.

Advances in identification of molecular genetic causes of abnormal sex with heightened awareness of ethical issues and patient advocacy concerns necessitate a reexamination of nomenclature. Terms such as *intersex*, *pseudohermaphroditism*, *hermaphroditism*, *sex reversal*, and gender-based diagnostic labels are particularly controversial. These terms are perceived as potentially pejorative by patients and can be confusing to practitioners and parents alike. The ideal nomenclature should be sufficiently flexible to incorporate new information yet robust enough to maintain a consistent framework.

Terms should be descriptive and reflect genetic etiology when available, and accommodate the spectrum of phenotypic variation. Clinicians and scientists must value its use, and it must be understandable to patients and their families.

The Consensus Statement on Management of Intersex Disorders proposes the term *disorders of sex development* (DSDs), as defined by congenital conditions in which development of chromosomal, gonadal, or anatomic sex is atypical.

PHYSICAL EXAMINATION

External genitalia exam includes the gonadal palpation and perineal exam; both are the key to choosing the sequence of diagnostic procedures to reach an etiologic diagnosis.

The visualization of both faces of the phallus, looking for the urethral orifice, and defining its localization and aspect are important. Inguinal and perineal palpation to look for gonads is the other diagnostic key.

Each patient needs to be considered on an individual basis.

PRESENTATION

Traditionally, DSD patients were classified into three groups based on gonadal structure:

1. Presence of two well-defined ovaries with ambiguous or male external genitalia (female pseudohermaphroditism, now called overvirilized XX female). These patients have a 46,XX karyotype, and virilization of the external genitalia results from exposure to a high level of androgens in utero while they have female internal genitalia. Congenital adrenal hyperplasia (CAH) is the most common disease in this group

and accounts for 50%–80% of all the cases of ambiguity, depending on the population analyzed. The most common enzymatic defect is 21-hydroxylase deficiency. The incidence of 21-hydroxylase deficiency is 1 in 15,000–40,000 newborns. Other defects are 11-hydroxylase (hypertension) and 3-b-ol dehydrogenase or aromatase.

2. Presence of two well-defined testicles with ambiguous or female external genitalia (male pseudohermaphroditism; now called undervirilized XY male). These patients have a 46,XY karyotype, and ambiguity of the external genitalia results from a failure of the masculinization androgenic action of the male fetus. This can be due to a failure in androgenic synthesis or in the biological response. This group includes rare defects of the biosynthesis of testosterone, defect of 5-RD2 (enzyme that converts testosterone into dihydrotestosterone), and PAIS (partial defect of androgenic receptors). It is important to recognize that patients with a 46,XY karyotype and dysgenetic testicles are sometimes included in this group in the literature.

3. Presence of incomplete differentiated gonads or coexisting ovarian and testicular tissue with ambiguous or female external genitalia. This is a heterogeneous group with one common factor, which is a structural defect in gonadal differentiation with or without a chromosome alteration. Patients with mixed gonadal dysgenesis (MGD), testicular dysgenesis, and true hermaphroditism (TH, now called ovotesticular disorder of sexual development) are included in this group.

For the purpose of investigation, they are divided into the following:

1. Disorders of chromosomes (chromosomal DSD)
2. Disorders of gonad development (gonadal DSD, sex determination)
3. Disorders of sex steroid synthesis and action (phenotypic/anatomic DSD, sex differentiation)

DIAGNOSIS

According to the Consensus Statement on Management of Intersex Disorders, optimal clinical management of individuals with DSD should comprise the following: (1) gender assignment must be avoided before expert evaluation in newborns; (2) evaluation and long-term management must be performed at a center with an experienced multidisciplinary team; (3) all individuals should receive a gender assignment; (4) open communication with patients and families is essential, and participation in decision-making is encouraged; and (5) patient and family concerns should be respected and addressed in strict confidence.

The initial contact with the parents of a child with a DSD is important, because first impressions from these encounters often persist. A key point to emphasize is that the child with a DSD has the potential to become a well-adjusted, functional member of society. Although privacy needs to be respected, a DSD is not shameful. It should be explained to the parents that the best course of action may not be clear initially, but the health care team will work with the family to reach the best possible set of decisions under the circumstances. The health care team should discuss with the parents what information to share in the early stages with family members and friends. Parents need to be informed about sexual development.

A detailed personal and familiar anamnesis can give important information. Some of these pathologies recognize a sex-linked transmission (X link), and the mother will be able to transmit the defect to 50% her male children (complete or partial androgen insensitivity). Many have an autosomal recessive transmission (CAH, deficit of testosterone synthesis, deficit of 5-RD2, deficit of the lutein hormone (LH) receptor).

The finding of a neonatal death in the first days of life of male babies may be due to an unrecognized congenital adrenogenital syndrome.

Still, diagnostic algorithms are useful as guidelines to simplify the study of these complex patients.

Figure 109.3 lists the sequence of investigations used in a newborn with a suspected DSD, according to gonadal palpation.

A karyotype is mandatory, but this always requires a few days.

In the absence of palpable gonads, the first blood test are those to exclude problems that can put life at risk (blood electrolytes), commonly found in the event of salt-losing CAH. The blood sexual steroids must be determined, and among them, the level of 17-OH-progesterone, which if elevated, will make it possible to diagnose the most common cause of DSD.

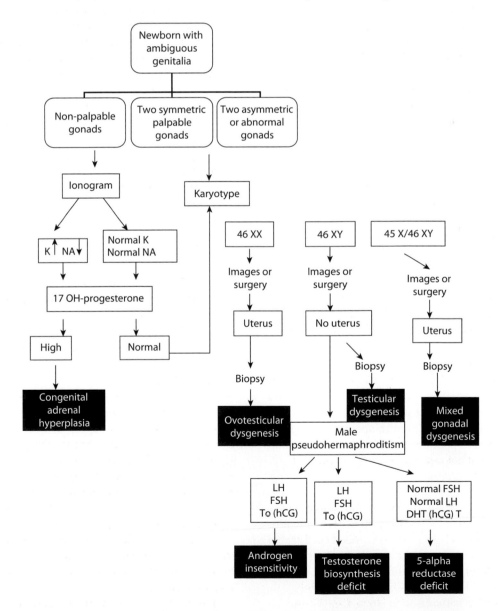

Figure 109.3 Sequence of investigations used in a newborn with a suspected disorder of sex development.

The dosage of other steroids (testosterone, dihydrotestosterone, delta-4-androstenedione, dehidroepiandrosterone [DHEA], 17-OH-pregnenolone), adrenocorticotrophine (ACTH), cortisol, and renin, will allow us to get a precise picture of the gonadal and adrenal steroidogenesis. For example, a testosterone/dehidrotestosterone (T/DHT) ratio with a value larger than 10 is suspicious for a deficit in 5-RD2 enzyme.

The most valuable stimulation tests for evaluating steroid genesis are as follows:

- HCG test for the study of testicular functionality.
- ACTH test for the study of adrenal steroid genesis.
- Low values of testosterone can be a sign of testicular dysgenesis if associated with low levels of all the other testicular steroids or of an enzyme defect of the steroid genesis path if they are associated with high levels of their precursors.
- Normal or elevated levels of T and DHT may be suggestive of a receptor resistance to androgens.
- The possibility of the ambiguous genitalia virilizing can be estimated after an HCG test or an appropriate stimulation trial with testosterone or topical DHT. This can be estimated by demonstrating the increment of the penile dimensions or indirectly by the dosage of androgen-sensitive circulating substances. Its value is reduced if the patient tissues present sensitivity for the virilizing effect of androgens.

Molecular biology techniques are more sensitive, and specific tests for assessment of the tissue sensitivity to androgens are not always available.

Histology is only required for diagnosis in patients with abnormal gonads (group 3).

Imaging tests

The primary objective of these tests is the study of the internal genitalia anatomy. The pelvic ultrasound for the demonstration of the presence of Mullerian structures is an important diagnostic element.

Genitography is very useful for the study of vaginal morphology, dimension, and relation to the urethra (Figure 109.4a,b,c). We look for the onset of the vaginal outlet in the urogenital sinus (UGS) with special attention to the proximal urethra to plan the urogenital reconstruction (see surgical treatment below).

Sex of rearing

Factors that influence gender assignment include diagnosis, genital appearance, surgical options, need for lifelong replacement therapy, potential for fertility, views of the family, and sometimes, circumstances relating to cultural practices.

More than 90% of patients with 46,XX CAH and all patients with 46,XY CAIS assigned female in infancy identify

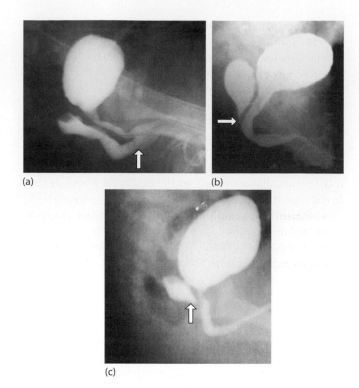

(a)   (b)

(c)

Figure 109.4 Genitography is very useful for the study of vaginal morphology, dimension, and relation to the urethra. Depending on vaginal confluence in the urogenital sinus, the vagina was classified as **(a)** low, **(b)** intermediate, or **(c)** high variant. The white arrows show the confluence of the vagina in the urogenital sinus.

as females. Evidence supports the current recommendation to raise markedly virilized 46,XX infants with CAH as female. Still, around 5% develop gender dysphoria and have more chances of homosexualism and bisexualism—1%–3% transsexuals. A consistent penile development constitutes a basic element for the male choice of rearing even if today, the criteria that must guide this choice are object of debate.

A good response in testosterone levels after HCG test and an increase in penile length after administration of testosterone in neonatal age will be useful in making the choice of male sex.

In some patients, the possibility of future virilization at puberty has to be taken into account (deficit of 5-alpha-reductase and the defect of synthesis of testosterone). Nowadays, diagnosis is easier due to the aim of molecular genetics.

Approximately 60% of 5-alpha-reductase (5-RD2)–deficient patients assigned female in infancy and virilizing at puberty (and all those assigned male) live as males. In 5-alpha-reductase and possibly 17-hydroxysteroid dehydrogenase deficiencies, for which the diagnosis is made in infancy, the combination of a male gender identity in the majority and the potential for fertility (documented in 5-RD but unknown in 17-hydroxysteroid dehydrogenase deficiencies) should be discussed when providing evidence for gender assignment.

Among patients with PAIS, androgen biosynthetic defects, and incomplete gonadal dysgenesis, there is dissatisfaction with the sex of rearing in 25% of individuals whether raised male or female.

Available data support male rearing in all patients with micropenis, taking into account equal satisfaction with assigned gender in those raised male or female without need for surgery and the potential for fertility in patients reared male.

Those making the decision on sex of rearing for those with ovotesticular DSD should consider the potential for fertility on the basis of gonadal differentiation and genital development and assuming that the genitalia are, or can be made, consistent with the chosen sex.

In the case of MGD, factors to consider include prenatal androgen exposure, testicular function at and after puberty, phallic development, and gonadal location.

MANAGEMENT

Except for gonadal biopsy or resection, no other surgery is performed in the neonatal period. Most of the reconstructive procedures, although done early, are not recommended before the first month of life.

Evolution of practice in the last years tends to postpone surgery. Sex assignment does not mean inevitable surgical intervention. Each case needs to be considered in its own terms. Preservation of tissue, particularly gonadal tissue, and maintenance of the integrity of the body as whole are aspects of care and receive higher priority.

The surgeon plays an important initial role in the interdisciplinary group that an institution is obliged to have to take care of these complex patients. He/she needs to not only take care of the best operative techniques for better functional results but also manage the proper information (after conscious discussion of the group) to be given to parents and family. The use of improper words and misinformation may result in irreversible sequelae. In our opinion, the surgeon has to be very well informed and participate actively in the preoperative workup before making contact with the family.

- **Preoperative:** A stable endocrine status, especially in CAH patients, is highly important for a well-tolerated surgical procedure and better postoperative results. The psychosocial analysis of the family is also advised. Once again, we emphasize the interaction with the clinical colleagues in charge of them. When reconstructing the UGS, a preoperative enema is indicated. Preoperative antibiotics are used according to each institution's protocols.
- **Operative:** The role of surgery consists in the following: (1) gonadal treatment, (2) feminizing genitoplasty, and (3) urethral/penile reconstruction in the undervirilized child.

Gonadal treatment

Gonadal histology is required for diagnosis in intersex patients with abnormal gonadal development like MGD and TH, recently called ovotesticular DSD. Although sex may be assigned before the biopsy is taken, histology in these patients is required for definitive diagnosis.

Gonadal biopsies must be taken along the longitudinal axis of the gonad as both ovarian and testicular tissue may be found at the polar ends of the gonad (Figure 109.5). Patients with TH may have an ovary (O) and testicle (T); bilateral ovotestes (OT); or an O and OT.

Surgical management in DSD should also consider options that will facilitate the chances of fertility. The ovarian component of ovotestes may be separated, and the testicular tissue removed, using a zoom lens, although it must be kept in mind that these gonads need to be followed closely.

If a streak gonad is recognized like in most patients with MGD, it is removed without prior biopsy together with the surrounding peritoneum and the ipsilateral gonaduct (Figure 109.6). This gonad has to be removed, avoiding previous biopsy, as it has a 25%–50% chance to develop a gonadoblastoma and or dysgerminoma and as there is the possibility of an in situ tumor at the time of the procedure. It is usually associated with an intra-abdominal or inguinal dysgenetic testicle, which is removed at the same time in patients with female sex assignment. Although there is the same risk of malignancy in the contralateral gonad (dysgenetic testicle), it may biopsied and preserved in the scrotum of patients with male sex assignment because this gonad is functional.

The highest tumor risk is found in testis-specific protein, Y-encoded (TSPY) positive gonadal dysgenesis and partial androgen insensitivity (PAIS) with intra-abdominal gonads, whereas the lowest risk (5%) is found in ovotestis and complete androgen insensitivity (CAIS).

To analyze the spectrum of gonads of the DSD patients that we treated and assess the incidence of germ cell tumors,

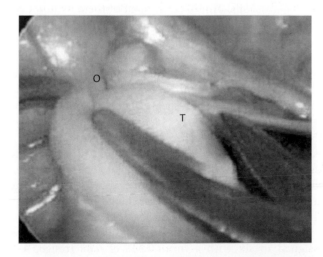

Figure 109.5 A laparoscopic view of ovotestes. This is the technique for gonadal biopsy along the longitudinal axis of the gonad. O, ovarian portion; T, testicular component.

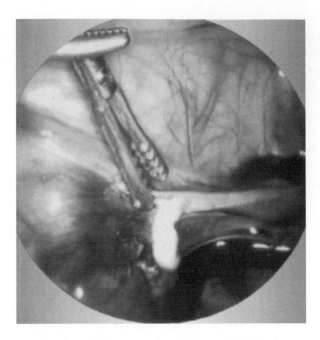

Figure 109.6 A laparoscopic view of a streak gonad. Bipolar coagulation of the gonadal pedicle. These gonads are resected en bloc with the surrounding peritoneum.

we conducted a prospective and observational study of DSD patients who underwent gonadal surgery. Age, sex assigned, scale of external masculinization (EMS), karyotype, molecular analysis, surgical approach, and pathology of the gonads were analyzed. Patients were divided into three groups: chromosomal dysgenesis (G1), 46,XX gonadal dysgenesis (G2), and 46,XY gonadal dysgenesis (G3). More than half of the gonads were intra-abdominal and were treated laparoscopically using 3 or 5 mm instruments. All streak gonads were removed, avoiding previous biopsy. We always waited for the result of biopsy before removing any gonad other than a classical streak. An inguinal approach was indicated in patients with palpable gonads. We still prefer a laparoscopic approach in most of them as it not only enables better visualization of potential Mullerian structures but also allows for treatment of a patent peritoneal sac when removing the gonads, with better cosmetic results. In total, 94 patients with a mean age of 56.42 months (range, 2–216 months) were analyzed. Forty-eight patients (19 with Turner syndrome) with a mean age of 105 months (range, 2–216 months) were included in G1. The karyotype was 45,X0/46,XY in 87.5% of them. Male sex was assigned in 19, with a mean of 7.26 EMS (range, 1–10 EMS). Histological analysis of 89 gonads was completed, identifying 52 streak gonads, 32 dysgenetic testes, and 5 ovotestes. Six germinal cell tumors (GCTs) were found in four patients. Fifteen patients with a mean age of 27.6 months (range, 2–180 months) were included in G2. Male gender was assigned to six with a mean EMS of 6.82 (range, 4–8.5 EMS). Twenty-nine gonads were analyzed: 10 ovotestes, 15 dysgenetic testes, and 4 ovaries. Bilateral gonadoblastoma was found in a 6-month-old patient with bilateral ovotestes

Mean age of the 31 patients in G3 was 69.71 months (range, 5–192 months). Five of them had an SF1 NR5A mutation, six a WT1, six a CAIS, and three a PAIS. A new mutation in the SRY (p.MET64VAL) gene was identified in two sisters. Male gender was assigned in 10 with a mean EMS of 4.52 (range, 1–10 EMS). Fifty-nine gonads were analyzed, identifying 41 dysgenetic testes, 10 streak gonads, and 8 testes, Eight GCTs were found in five patients (16%, seven in streak gonads and one in a dysgenetic testis).

We concluded that DSD patients with gonadal dysgenesis have a wide variability. The incidence of gonadoblastoma is not negligible in 46,XY, and even feasible in 46,XX. The incidence of GCT was 8.3%, 6.6%, and 16% in G1, G2, and G3, respectively. Early histological analysis and monitoring of these patients is mandatory. To our knowledge, this is the first report of bilateral gonadoblastoma in ovotestes at a very early age.

Although we used to schedule simultaneous gonadal and genitalia procedures with good results encouraged by the laparoscopically better visualization and quicker intraperitoneal access, actually we prefer to avoid resection of any gonad except a classical streak before having definitive histology and to postpone genital surgical procedures.

Sex may be assigned prior to laparoscopy in patients with 45,X0/46,XY gonadal dysgenesis. This is based on a functional and psychosocial assessment in combination with the results of karyotyping, HCG testing, and interview of the parents.

We have never found functional ovarian tissue in these patients.

TH patients do not have such a classical pattern, and definitive histology is often necessary for sex assignment. Although the most common karyotype is 46,XX and the most common gonadal combination ovary/ovotestis, each case is unique and should be treated on an individual basis. Sometimes, the macroscopic aspect of the gonad and gonaduct as well as the result of a frozen section biopsy strongly favor gonadectomy in patients with previous sex assignment. There is the advantage of a laparoscopic approach in these patients requiring secondary pelvic exploration, especially because many of them are potentially fertile.

An additional role of laparoscopy is excision of Mullerian structures and prostatic utricles and orchidopexy in patients raised as males. In patients with a symptomatic utriculus, removal is best performed laparoscopically to increase the chance of preserving continuity of the vas deferens.

An inguinal approach may be indicated in patients with palpable gonads (Figure 109.7). We still prefer a laparoscopic approach in most of them as it not only enables better visualization of potential Mullerian structures but also allows for treatment of a patent peritoneal sac when removing the gonads, with better cosmetic results. In addition, most of these patients have asymmetric gonads, with one of them being intra-abdominal. We reserve the inguinal approach for XY patients with symmetric palpable gonads, introducing the telescope through the associated hernia sac in order to rule out the presence of Mullerian structures.

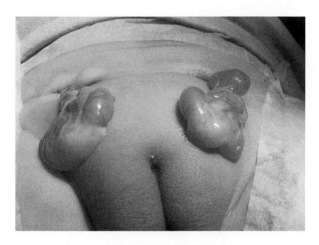

Figure 109.7 An inguinal approach for gonadectomy in a CAIS patient with palpable gonads.

Feminizing genitoplasty

Fortunately, there have been many advances in ambiguous genitalia reconstruction, with many surgeons contributing. Cosmetically, a near-normal appearance can now be achieved, but long-term functional results with newer techniques are still unknown.

Timing for this type of surgery is controversial. It is now our belief that one-stage total reconstruction can be done in most patients in the early months of life.

Nowadays, there is a strong influence of movements toward postponing any kind of surgery in the genitalia until the individual is able to decide and consent. There are even legal regulations in some countries.

Regardless of the timing or the procedure elected, the surgery must be done meticulously with a clear understanding of the anatomy and only be undertaken in centers with great experience and after all aspects of controversy have been explained in detail to the parents.

It consists in the following: (1) management of clitoral enlargement, (2) reconstruction of the UGS, and (3) labioplasty.

MANAGEMENT OF CLITORAL ENLARGEMENT

Management of clitoral enlargement remains controversial because of the ablative nature of the structure so vital to psychological body image and gender. Initial techniques consisted in total clitorectomy based on the belief that it was necessary to prevent gender dysphoria. However, new understanding that an intact clitoris plays a crucial role in the development of female sexuality has stimulated a more conservative surgical approach, but recession of the clitoris, keeping the corpora, may lead to painful erections during sexual arousal. The most used technique has been that based on Kogan's reduction clitoroplasty including removal of the corporal erectile tissue with preservation of the neurovascular bundle to the glans (Figure 109.8a,b,c). Glans reduction was accomplished by superficial excise of the epithelium of the glanular groove, avoiding a scar in the glans tissue, which is fixed to the pubis attachment.

There is evidence that innervation of the glans comes from the surrounding skin and plays an important role in sexual arousal, so in the last few years, we have been very careful in preserving most of it, trying to avoid its unnecessary sectioning. We also keep not only the dorsal pedicle but also the ventral skin and mucosal surface, and prefer not to excise the glans in any surface and but to hide it.

Recently, a nonablative and potentially reversible technique that dismembers the corporal bodies while keeping them in the labia major has been described in response to new understanding that an intact clitoris plays a crucial role in the development of female sexuality, but no long-term follow-up is available.

RECONSTRUCTION OF THE UGS

UGS abnormalities are a spectrum that goes from a labial fusion to an absent vagina depending on the location of the vaginal confluence in the UGS. Powell described four types: I, labial fusion; II, distal confluence; III, proximal confluence; and IV, absent vagina. In 1969, Hendren described different procedures required for reconstruction depending on the location of the vaginal confluence in the UGS related to the external sphincter (low when distal and high when proximal to the sphincter). This has been very helpful for reconstructive understanding, but the vagina is not always high or low and the sphincter not well seen. We have found a wide spectrum of vaginal location, from a normal position to an entrance in the bladder.

Low confluence was classically repaired by a *flap vaginoplasty* and mid to high by a *pull-through vaginoplasty*.

Even in the low type, we advocate for a very aggressive dissection of the posterior vaginal wall, separating it from the rectal wall. The vagina is then cut in the midline well back into its normal caliber, and at this point, a wide cutaneous flap can be sewn using delicate sutures. A rectal finger is very useful to facilitate vaginal exposure (Figure 109.9a,b). This maneuver of bringing the vagina out rather than skin in prevents the known complications of the Fortunoff flap (growing of hair and stenosis).

Exteriorization of the high vagina in the severely masculinized female is a surgical challenge. The vagina must be detached from the UGS and then connected to the perineum. The pull-through principle consists in placing a Fogarty balloon catheter into the vagina cystoscopically to locate it by palpation deep in the perineum later (Figure 109.10a,b). The UGS is approached like a bulbous urethra. Perineal anatomy in severe cases is like that in a normal male. The vagina is incised over the balloon and detached from its entry point in the UGS, and the anterior wall carefully dissected off the overlying urinary tract. The vaginal walls to reach the perineum may be constructed using a combination of inverted-U cutaneous flap (Fortunoff), preputial flap (Gonzalez), and redundant tissue from the UGS (Passerini flap).

The anterior sagittal transrectal approach in a prone position (ASTRA) is another way of exposure through the perineal approach.

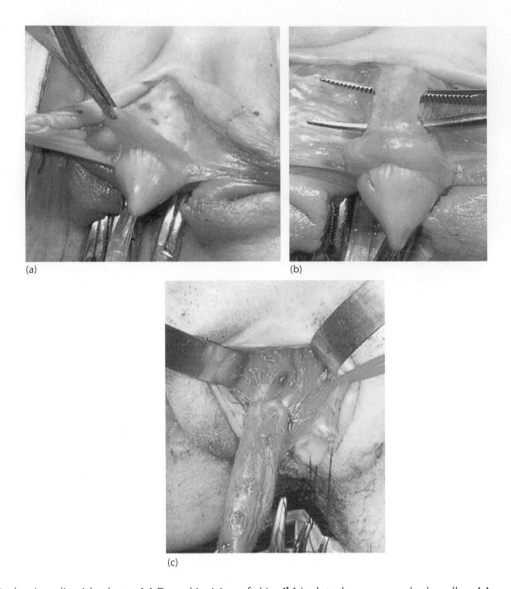

(a)

(b)

(c)

Figure 109.8 Reduction clitoridoplasty. **(a)** Dorsal incision of skin; **(b)** isolated neurovascular bundles; **(c)** corporal erectile tissue is ready to resection.

In the middle of these two points, we found what we called intermediate (IT) UGS. Although the vaginal opening is far from the UGS opening, needing an aggressive dissection to get to the vagina, there is enough proximal urethra between the bladder neck and the vaginal entrance. After Alberto Peña's (1997) description of "total urogenital mobilization" (TUM) for the treatment of cloacas, we started using this maneuver to treat intermediate UGS abnormalities. The UGS is mobilized en bloc to the perineum (Figure 109.11a,b). We used this principle but in the lithotomy position and without previous opening to prevent bleeding, and never amputate the sinus tissue until the end as it may be used to enlarge the introitus. Each patient must be individualized, and this technique can be combined with a pull-through if required, but it has simplified many of these repairs.

Richard Rink has recently described a variant that he calls partial urogenital mobilization (PUM), stopping dissection

at the level of the pubourethral ligament. Currently, regardless of the level of the confluence, he starts with PUM, allowing a unified approach to all repairs.

We always started dissection in the posterior wall of the UGS with an aggressive separation from the anterior rectal wall. If the wide portion of the vagina was reached, dissection stopped, and the UGS opened ventrally, widening to the introitus. When more dissection was required, the anterior wall of the UGS was dissected and carefully freed from the low retropubic space. Then the UGS was opened either ventrally or dorsally.

In our opinion, the best way to treat the high UGS was the combination of some of these techniques. We started by placing a balloon catheter (most of the times a Foley one using a catheter as a guide) in the vagina with a cystoscope. We mobilized the UGS in the lithotomy position without opening it (Figure 109.12a). We then turned the patient to the prone position. The perineum was incised in the midline and surrounding the anterior anus. The rectum was retracted, and only in a few patients

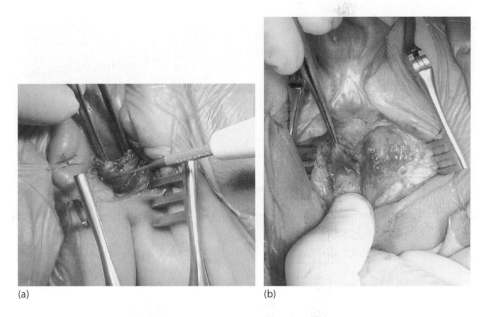

Figure 109.9 **(a)** Dissection of the posterior vaginal wall, separating it from the rectal wall before sectioning the urogenital sinus. **(b)** A rectal finger is very useful to facilitate vaginal exposure.

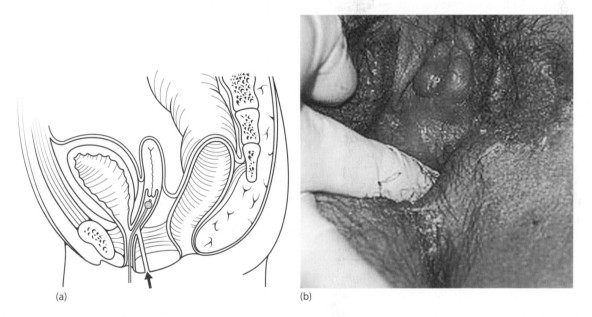

Figure 109.10 **(a)** Illustration showing the pull-through technique. The principle consists of placing a Fogarty balloon catheter into the vagina cystoscopically to locate it by palpation deep in the perineum later. **(b)** Cosmetic appearance after pull-through technique.

did the anterior wall need to be opened (Figure 109.12b). The vagina was then incised over the balloon, the Foley catheter repositioned in the proximal urethra, and the urethrovaginal fistula closed, taking care not to denervate the bladder neck (Figure 109.12c,d). The short vagina (which is usually the case in these patients) needed to be exteriorized. The transected perineal skin between the vagina and rectum was used to reconstruct the dorsal wall and the previously dissected UGS

for the ventral wall. For that purpose, it was transected ventrally and everted to reach the vagina. In this way, the proximal part of it stayed as the urethra (Figure 109.13a,b,c).

So as you can see, we combined principles (pull-through, TUM, and ASTRA) rather than using a single technique. Thus, in our experience, the technique utilized to correct UGS in CAH needs to be tailored to the individual anatomy of the patient.

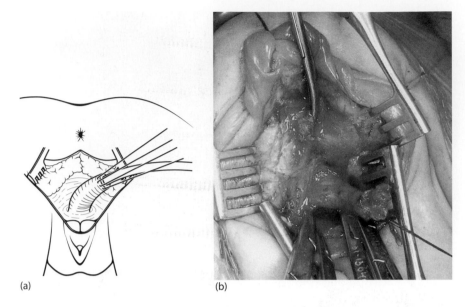

(a)   (b)

Figure 109.11 Total urogenital mobilization (TUM). The urogenital sinus is mobilized en bloc to the perineum, after it is incised in the ventral wall. **(a)** Illustration of TUM. **(b)** Operative TUM technique.

Those patients with absent vagina (type IV) should undergo vaginal replacement. Most of them are undervirilized males, and a bowel vagina (colon if possible) is preferred.

We have been doing this completely laparoscopically since 1999 (Figure 109.14).

LABIOPLASTY

Labioplasty was performed by dividing the clitoral hood skin in the midline (Byars), sewing the flaps around the clitoris and along the central mucosal strip down to the lateral vaginal walls (Figure 109.15a,b,c).

Urethral/penile reconstruction

This will be addressed in Chapter 110.

- **Postoperative:** The perineum needs to be kept dry and clean for the first week to prevent dehiscence. The urethral catheter is left depending on the technique used. We only leave it for the first postoperative day in low or intermediate UGS and for at least 3 days in high UGS.

Most of the patients only require analgesic-antipyretic and anti-inflammatory (AINES) drugs for pain treatment.

COMPLICATIONS

Techniques for vaginoplasty carry the potential for scarring at the introitus, necessitating repeated modification before sexual function.

The risks from vaginoplasty are different for high and low confluence of the urethra and vagina. The risk of urinary incontinence is decreased by recognizing the localization of the vaginal confluence for the selection of the surgical approach and avoiding unnecessary mobilization or dissection in the urethrovaginal septum.

LONG-TERM RESULTS

The pattern of surgical practice in DSD is changing with respect to the timing of surgery and the techniques used. It is essential to evaluate the effects of early versus later surgery in a holistic manner, recognizing the difficulties posed by an ever-evolving clinical practice.

Some studies suggest satisfactory outcomes from early surgery. Nevertheless, outcomes from clitoroplasty identify problems related to decreased sexual sensitivity, loss of clitoral tissue, and cosmetic issues.

Analysis of long-term outcomes is complicated by a mixture of surgical techniques.

We evaluated postoperative urinary continence in 55 patients with CAH with intermediate and high UGS who underwent a UGS mobilization maneuver. The operations we performed have not compromised urinary continence as also previously observed by others.

The outcome in undermasculinized males with a phallus depends on the degree of hypospadias and the amount of erectile tissue (Figure 109.16). Feminizing genitoplasty as opposed to masculinizing genitoplasty requires less surgery to achieve an acceptable outcome and results in fewer urologic difficulties. Long-term data regarding sexual function and quality of life among those assigned female as well as male show great variability. There are no controlled clinical trials of the efficacy of early (12 months of age) versus late (adolescence and adulthood) surgery or of the efficacy of different techniques.

Gender-role change occurs at different rates in different societies, suggesting that social factors may also be important modifiers of gender-role change.

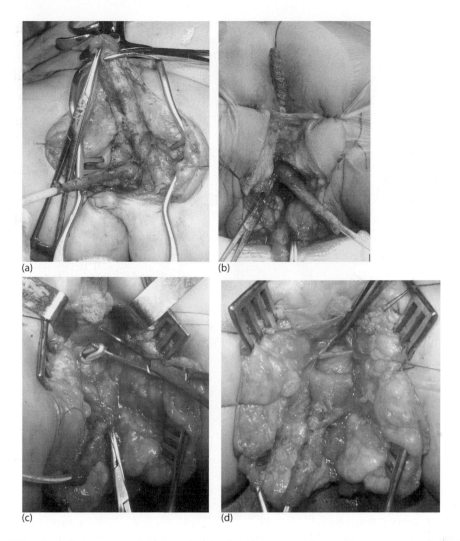

Figure 109.12 **(a)** Mobilization of the urogenital sinus in the lithotomy position without opening it. **(b)** The anterior sagittal transrectal approach. A midline sagittal incision was made through the anterior anorectal wall and provided an excellent view of the complete urethra and vagina without the need for complex preparation to gain exposure. In this patient, a previous placing of a balloon catheter in the vagina and a total urogenital mobilization were performed in the lithotomy position, and the patient was then turned to prone position. She had a very high urogenital sinus. **(c)** The vagina opened over the balloon and the Foley catheter repositioned in the proximal urethra. **(d)** The vagina is completely open.

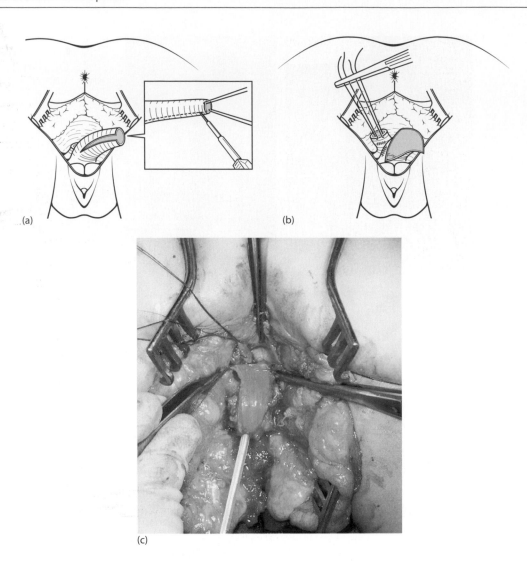

Figure 109.13 The UGS is transected dorsally (patient is in prone position) and everted to reach the anterior wall of the vagina. In this way, the proximal part of it stays as urethra.

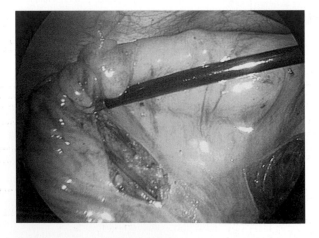

Figure 109.14 Laparoscopic aspect of an isolated piece of sigmoid colon for vaginal replacement.

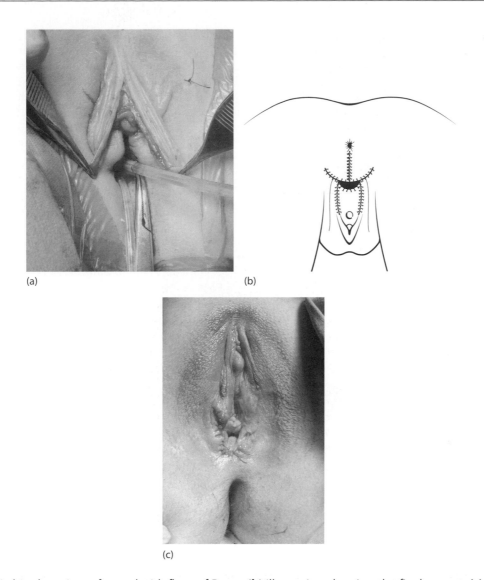

(a)   (b)

(c)

Figure 109.15 **(a)** Labioplasty is performed with flaps of Byars. **(b)** Illustration showing the final aspect. **(c)** Two weeks post-operative perineal aspect of a patient who underwent feminizing genitoplasty.

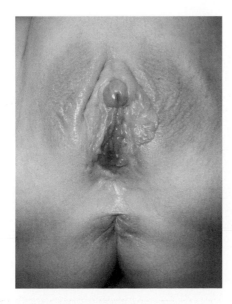

Figure 109.16 Long-term perineal aspect.

FURTHER READING

Bailez M, Dibenedetto V, Elmo G, Korman L. Laparoscopic sigmoid vaginal replacement. What we learned? *Pediatr Endosurg Innov Tech* 2004; 8(4): 295–301.

Bailez M, Fraire C. Total mobilization of the urogenital sinus for the treatment of adrenal hyperplasia. *BJU* 1998; 81: 76.

Bailez MM, Cuenca ES, Dibenedetto V. Urinary continence following repair of intermediate and high urogenital sinus (UGS) in CAH. Experience with 55 cases. *Front Pediatr* 2014 2 July. http://dx.doi.org/10.3389/fped.2014.00067

Blecher SR, Erickson RP. Genetics of sexual development: A new paradigm. *Am J Med Genet A*; 2007: 143A(24):3054–68.

Denes FT, Mendonc B, Costa E et al. Diagnostic and therapeutic laparoscopy in intersex patients. *BJU Int* 1997; 80: 176.

Dessens AB, Slijper FM, Drop SL. Gender dysphoria and gender change in chromosomal females with congenital adrenal hyperplasia. *Arch Sexual Behav* 2005; 34: 389–97.

Docimo SG, Peters C. Endourology and laparoscopy in children. In: Walsh PC, Retik AB, Vaughan CD, Wein AJ, Saunders WB (eds). *Campbells Urology*, 8th edn. Philadelphia: WB Saunders, 2002.

Gonzalez R, Fernandez E. Single-stage feminization genitoplasty. *J Urol* 1990; 143: 776–8.

Grumbach MM, Hughes IA, Conte FA. Disorders of sex differentiation. In: Larsen PR, Kronenberg HM, Melmed S, Polonsky KS (eds). *Williams Textbook of Endocrinology*, 10th edn. Heidelberg, Germany: Saunders, 2003: 842–1002.

Hendren WH, Donahoe PK. Correction of congenital abnormalities of the vagina and perineum. *J Pediatr Surg* 1980; 15: 751–63.

Hughes IA, Houk C, Ahmed SF, Lee PA, LWPES1/ESPE2 Consensus Group. Consensus statement on management of intersex disorders. *Arch Dis Child* 2006; 91(7): 554–563.

Hughes IA, Nihoul-Fékété C, Thomas B, Cohen-Kettenis PT. Consequences of the ESPE/LWPES guidelines for diagnosis and treatment of disorders of sex development. *Best Pract Res Clin Endocr Metabol* 2007; 21(3): 351–5.

Jager RJ, Anvret, M, Hall K, Scherer G. A Human XY Female with Frame Shift Mutation in the Candidate Testis-Determining Gene SRY. *Nature* 1990; 452–4.

Lee PA, Houk CP, Ahmed SF, Hughes IA; in collaboration with the participants in the International Consensus Conference on Intersex organized by the Lawson Wilkins Pediatric Endocrine Society and the European Society for Pediatric Endocrinology Department of Pediatrics, Penn State College of Medicine, Hershey. Consensus statement on management of intersex disorders. *Pediatrics* 2006;118: 488–500.

Meyer-Bahlburg HF, Gruen RS, New MI, Bell JJ, Morishima A, Shimshi M, Bueno Y, Vargas I, Baker SW. Gender change from female to male in classical congenital adrenal hyperplasia. *Horm Behav* 1996; 30(4): 319–32.

Peña A, Filmer B, Bonilla E et al. Transanorectal approach for the treatment of urogenital sinus. Preliminary report. *J Pediatr Surg* 1992; 127: 681–5.

Peña A. Total urogenital mobilization—An easier way to repair cloacas. *J Pediatr Surg* 1997; 32: 263–8.

Pippi Salle J, Braga L, Macedo N, Rosito N, Bagli D. Corporeal sparing dismembered clitoroplasty: An alternative technique for feminizing genitoplasty. *J Urol* 2007; 178(4): 1796–800.

Rossi F, De Castro R, Ceccarelli P, Domini R. Anterior sagittal transanorectal approach to the posterior urethra in the pediatric age group. *J Urol* 1998; 160(3): 1173–7.

Zucker K, Bradley SJ, Oliver G, Blake J, Fleming S, Hood J. *Horm Behav* 1996; 30: 300–18.

110

Male genital anomalies

JOHN M. HUTSON

Development of the external genitalia is a complex process in the male, which predisposes to many congenital anomalies. Understanding these anomalies requires detailed knowledge of the embryology, and particularly the central roles of androgens (in coordinating the masculinization of the anatomy) and formation of the processus vaginalis (which allows descent of the intra-abdominal fetal testis into the scrotum).

EMBRYOLOGY

Masculinization of the external genitalia occurs in normal human embryos between 8 and 12 weeks of gestation. The endodermal urethral plate canalizes and the inner genital folds fuse to create the male anterior urethra and corpus spongiosum, while the fused outer genital folds make the scrotum. The genital tubercle enlarges to form the phallus. All these processes are mediated by testosterone from the embryonic testis. An enzyme in the target tissues, 5-alpha-reductase, converts the small amount of circulating testosterone into dihydrotestosterone, which binds 5–10 times more tightly to the androgen receptor than testosterone itself, enabling androgen to act on the androgen receptors in the external genitalia. Although the genitalia appear "male" by 12 weeks of gestation, the phallus is still tiny, but it continues to grow throughout pregnancy, in response to testosterone, to reach its newborn size (3–4 cm stretched length).

Normal testicular descent is multistaged. The first phase involves enlargement of the genitoinguinal ligament (or "gubernaculum") and regression of the cranial suspensory ligament. The swollen distal gubernaculum anchors the embryonic testis near the groin during enlargement of the abdominal cavity. The hormonal regulation of this enlargement is by Leydig insulin-like hormone3 (Insl3).[1,2]

The second phase of testicular descent involves a peritoneal diverticulum (processus vaginalis) forming inside the gubernaculum, as it migrates from the external ring to the scrotum. Gubernacular migration (with elongation of the processus) to the scrotum is likely to be controlled by the genitofemoral nerve releasing calcitonin gene-related peptide, under stimulation of androgen.[3] Until migration is complete, the distal end of the gubernaculum is not anchored to the scrotum, which could predispose to perinatal (extravaginal) torsion. After migration is complete, the gubernaculum involutes and the tunica vaginalis becomes adherent inside the scrotum, preventing any further risk of extravaginal torsion.

Following testicular descent, the proximal processus vaginalis obliterates, leaving the testis within the tunica vaginalis. Failure of closure leads to inguinal hernia, hydrocele, or encysted hydrocele of the cord. In addition, failure of the fibrous tissue around the processus to disappear completely predisposes to acquired undescended testis (the "ascending" testis) later in childhood.

PENIS

The neonatal male penis is a focus of considerable parental anxiety and attention. The foreskin in a premature infant may appear relatively deficient, but by term, it protrudes beyond the glans. The inner prepuce is adherent to the glans, and the distal opening is narrow, sometimes making catheterization difficult. Phimosis or balanitis is rare in the neonatal period, although phimosis can occur secondary to neonatal cystoscopy in babies with urethral valve.

Circumcision

Neonatal circumcision is one of the commonest operations in the United States and Israel, although in other Western countries, the frequency is much lower (Dave et al. 2003).[4–6]

The procedure was known in the ancient societies of the Middle East and may have arisen as way of preventing balanitis and phimosis in an arid, sandy region. Circumcision is part of the ritual for such religions as Judaism, Christianity, and Islam, which all arose in the same geographic area.

In our own time, there is controversy over the advantages versus the risks of routine neonatal circumcision (AAP 2012).[7,8] The American Academy of Pediatrics (AAP) first issued guidelines about neonatal circumcision in 1971, concluding that there was no absolute medical indication for routine circumcision (AAP 2012). Then evidence showed a potential benefit of circumcision in preventing neonatal urinary tract infection and sexually transmitted diseases (STDs), including HIV, which led to a revision of the guidelines to balance the risks against the advantages (Bailey et al. 2007).[9] The current position of the AAP is to provide parents with an informed choice with accurate and unbiased information. Where circumcision is requested, the AAP now recommend that procedural analgesia be provided (AAP 2012).

Circumcision should prevent phimosis, paraphimosis, and balanitis, although good population studies proving this are hard to find. Learman[10] concluded that the evidence supporting circumcision was too weak to recommend routine operation. Urinary tract infection in neonatal males can be reduced by circumcision from 7/1000 to 1.9/1000,[11] but whether improved penile hygiene would have the same effect is unknown. STD rates in circumcised men are 10% lower than without circumcision, when comparing men presenting to an STD clinic in a Western country.[12] In sub-Saharan Africa, the benefits of circumcision in reducing HIV risk may be much greater,[13] although meta-analysis has not confirmed a benefit.[14,15] Circumcision is linked with a threefold reduction in penile cancer, although the low frequency of the condition does not justify routine neonatal operation. Learman[10] estimated that over 300,000 circumcisions were required to prevent one penile cancer/year. In Denmark, the incidence of penile cancer has fallen, despite no increase in circumcision, suggesting that other factors such as hygiene are important.[16]

The complications of circumcision may be extreme, including amputation or diathermy necrosis,[17] although most complications are minor (e.g., minor bleeding or infection) and uncommon (<1%)[18] (Figure 110.1). The Plastibell device and the Gomco clamp both have a low (0.2%) complication rate in neonates and are equally safe techniques.[10]

Neonatal circumcision should only be performed with adequate analgesia, using a ring penile block, local anesthetic cream, or a dorsal penile nerve block. If a Plastibell device is used, it is important to select the right size to avoid the ring slipping down the shaft and causing a form of paraphimosis.[19] The key to circumcision in the neonate is complete mobilization of the foreskin by separation from the glans with a lacrimal probe, and then inspection of the glans and urethral meatus to exclude hypospadias or other anomalies. Marking the level of the coronal groove through the base of the foreskin ensures that the skin of the shaft is not pulled up into the device.

Hypospadias

Failure of canalization of the urethral plate ± failed fusion of the inner genital folds leads to hypospadias (Greek for "hole underneath"). Secondary anomalies include deficiency of the ventral prepuce (leading to a "dorsal hood") and relative deficiency in growth of the periurethral tissues compared with dorsal structures such as the corpora cavernosa. The latter causes "chordee," or relative curvature of the penis, particularly on erection.[20]

Depending on diagnostic criteria, the incidence of hypospadias is 1/100 to 1/300.[21] Siblings or the father is affected in about 10% of patients, suggesting polygenic inheritance. Hypospadias varies widely in severity, from a minor degree of meatal ectopia on the ventral glans to severe abnormality with a perineal opening.

"Hypospadias" can be confused with more serious genital anomalies, and the most important initial aim is to exclude a serious disorder of sex development (DSD) (Figure 110.2). If hypospadias is an isolated anatomical anomaly of anterior urethral development, the rest of the external (and internal) genitalia should be normal. By contrast, patients with DSD have extensive genital abnormalities secondary to failure of all aspects of androgen-dependent development. A significant DSD can be excluded if the scrotum is completely fused

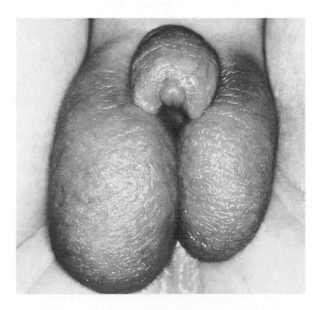

Figure 110.2 Apparent "hypospadias and bifid scrotum" in a child with a severe genital anomaly. This child needs urgent investigation for DSD.

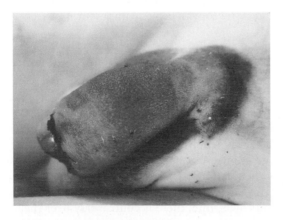

Figure 110.1 Postoperative penile hemorrhage after circumcision.

and both testes are descended. Babies with possible ambiguity need immediate referral, while those with hypospadias alone can be managed after the neonatal period.

Surgical treatment can be offered after 6 months of age, often as day surgery or overnight stay. Admission may be needed for urinary diversion, depending on severity of the anomaly and surgeon preference. A wide range of techniques are available,[22–25] which are not the main subject of this volume. Readers should consult the references for specific details.

Epispadias is a more severe and distantly related condition, which is more related to exstrophy of the bladder, which is included in Chapter 80.

Micropenis/buried penis

A small penis may be caused by inadequate hormonal stimulation during the second half of pregnancy (hypothalamic or pituitary deficiency), although in some cases, there is an anatomical deficiency. The buried penis occurs where the erectile tissue is adequate but the shaft skin is deficient.

Micropenis responds to androgen treatment, although whether postnatal hormone therapy is beneficial is controversial.[26] A number of operations have been proposed for buried penis, most of which use the foreskin.[27,28]

Penoscrotal web is a variant of buried penis where there is inadequate ventral shaft skin. This can be repaired later in infancy by Z-plasty.

Rare penile anomalies

Rare anomalies of the penis may present at birth, including urethral duplication (Figure 110.3) and megalourethra,

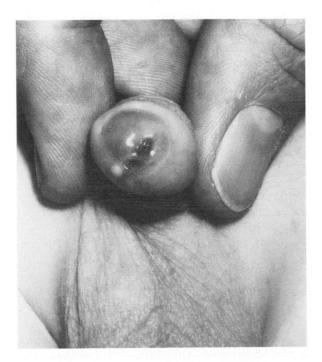

Figure 110.3 Urethral duplication in an infant.

which may be associated with prune belly syndrome.[20] Partial duplication of the caudal embryo may lead to duplication of the penis, while penile "agenesis" is usually a form of posterior ectopia, with the erectile tissue and urethra buried in the perineal body and the meatus on the anterior lip of the anal canal.[29–31] The latter anatomy is similar to the normal situation in marsupials, where the scrotum is inguinal in position and the phallus is in the perineum. Minor variants of penoscrotal transposition are common in DSD patients.[32]

Undescended testis

Any anomaly in the anatomical structures involved in testicular descent, or their hormonal regulation, will lead to congenital maldescent. Failure of the transabdominal phase causes intra-abdominal testes that are truly "cryptorchid" or hidden. Impalpable testes within the abdomen or canal are relatively uncommon (<5%–10% of patients, depending on different authors[33]).

Intra-abdominal testes are associated with hypoplasia of the ipsilateral scrotum and often with absence of the external inguinal ring. The latter is a useful clinical feature to confirm absence of any inguinoscrotal migration. When the testis is inside the canal, the external ring may be open, consistent with intermittent emergence of the canalicular gonad.

The common site for undescended testes is just outside the external ring, in the "superficial pouch," which is the name given to the tunica vaginalis when it is in the groin, superficial to the abdominal wall and deep to the superficial fascia (Scarpa).[34]

Maldescent is likely to have multiple causes, the commonest being failure of gubernacular migration for various mechanical reasons.[35] Transient deficiency of gonadal androgens related to hypothalamic or pituitary anomalies or defects in placental function also may be important.[36] A number of less common and rare causes for cryptorchidism have been proposed (Table 110.1 and Figure 110.4).

In premature infants as well as many term babies, cryptorchidism may be transitory, with further descent into the scrotum in the first 12 weeks postnatally (John Radcliffe Cryptorchidism Study Group 1992).[37] These so-called "late descenders" are at a high risk of developing acquired "ascending" testes later in childhood. The etiology of the latter is controversial, but has been proposed to be failure of the processus vaginalis to obliterate fully postnatally, leaving a fibrous remnant that prevents the normal elongation of the spermatic cord with growth.[3]

DIAGNOSIS

The aim of the physical examination is to locate the testis and determine its lowest position without undue tension. The latter corresponds with the caudal limit of the undescended tunica vaginalis.[38] In neonates, the examination may be hampered by vigorous leg movements, small size of all structures (including the testis, which is only 1–2 mL in

Table 110.1 Proposed causes of cryptorchidism in rare cases

1. Aberrant location of genitofemoral nerve (perineal testis)
2. Persistent Mullerian duct syndrome (transverse ectopia with uterus and elongated gubernaculum)
3. Prune belly syndrome (massive bladder enlargement precluding entrance into inguinal canal)
4. Posterior urethral valves (segmental mesenchymal defect)
5. Anterior abdominal wall defects (ruptured gubernaculum)
6. Connective tissue disorders (deficient gubernacular migration)
7. Neural tube defects (genitofemoral nerve anomalies)

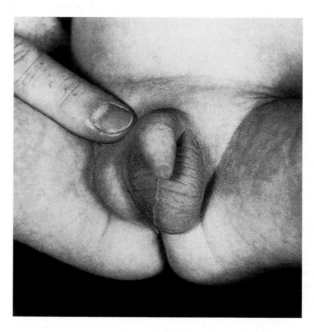

Figure 110.4 Ectopic undescended testis. In this case of perineal testis, it has been suggested that the cause is aberrant migration of the gubernaculum secondary to abnormal location of the genitofemoral nerve.

volume), and motility of the testis within the tunica vaginalis. The scrotum is hypoplastic if the testis has never reached it, and the inguinal canal is closed in intra-abdominal testes. Palpation of a triangular defect at the pubic tubercle confirms that the external ring is open and suggests that the testis is inside the canal. Conversely, hypertrophy of the contralateral testis (2–3 mL) suggests atrophy of the ipsilateral organ ("the vanishing testis").

TREATMENT

Surgical treatment of undescended testis aims to relocate the gonad into the scrotum before secondary dysfunction and degeneration occur (from high temperature). It is based on a premise, currently not proven in humans, that early placement of the testis in the scrotum will allow normal postnatal maturation of the germ cells to proceed. Careful study of testicular biopsies now suggests that the germ cells undergo transformation, from gonocytes to type A spermatogonia, within 6–12 months after birth,[3] and that this maturation is deficient or arrested in cryptorchid testes. In addition, adult dark spermatogonia are now thought to be the stem cells for subsequent spermatogenesis.

The recommended age of orchidopexy has changed over the years, reflecting accumulating knowledge about testicular function in infants. There is a current consensus that orchidopexy should be done about 6–9 months, as long as anesthetic support is adequate. Since 4%–5% of the males have undescended testes at birth, but about half of these show postnatal descent by 12 weeks, the baby should be reexamined then to confirm persisting cryptorchidism prior to referral for surgery. At this age, the operation is best performed by a trained pediatric surgeon, familiar with the handling of delicate tissues. Recent prospective trials confirm that surgery at 9 months leads to better testicular growth (measured by ultrasonography) than when operation is delayed until 3 years of age.[39]

Rare anomalies of the testis

Tumors of the testis are rare at birth, but teratomas have been reported (Figure 110.5). In a review of 68 patients with testicular tumors over 30 years, we found one newborn with a genital anomaly and a gonadoblastoma.[40] A neonatal teratoma may need to be distinguished from a hydrocele or testicular torsion. If the hydrocele is too tense to palpate a normal testis, an ultrasound examination would be useful. Most teratomas can be shelled out of the testis, thereby avoiding orchidectomy.

Exstrophy of the testis has been reported, presumably secondary to pressure necrosis of the scrotal skin from the baby's heel, and prolapse of the scrotal contents.[41] A similar defect may occur in the proximal penile urethra from probable pressure atrophy, leading to a congenital urethral fistula[42] (Figure 110.6).

Duplication of the gonadal primordium can cause polyorchidism. The presentation is of three scrotal masses, all of which feel like normal testis.[43] The differential diagnosis includes complete inguinoscrotal hernia, encysted hydrocele of the cord, and transverse testicular ectopia, where both testes are on the same side. In the latter situation, the contralateral hemiscrotum is empty. No treatment may be required, although one gonad can be removed if the vas deferens is deficient.

Transverse testicular ectopia is a rare anomaly, sometimes associated with prenatal rupture of the ipsilateral gubernaculum, allowing the testis to prolapse into the contralateral processus vaginalis. In most cases, the ectopic testis has no gubernacular attachments; the diagnosis can be confirmed on scrotal ultrasound.[44] Transverse ectopia of the testis is seen also in a rare form of DSD known as persistent Mullerian duct syndrome.[45] Transverse ectopia is treated by trans-septal scrotal orchidopexy (i.e., both testes are brought through the same inguinal canal into the scrotum, and one is placed in the contralateral hemiscrotum).

The vas deferens may be absent in the Mayer–Rokitansky–Kuster–Hauser (MRKH) syndrome type II (OMIM 601076) or in infants with cystic fibrosis. In the Rokitansky anomaly, caudal growth of the distal Wolffian duct is arrested, leading to subsequent absence of the ipsilateral vas deferens, seminal vesicle, and ureteric bud (and hence ipsilateral renal agenesis).[46] The etiology of absent vas deferens is different in cystic fibrosis, where the Wolffian ducts undergo involution/atresia in midgestation. At birth, only the head of the epididymis is palpable, and the epididymal tail and vas deferens are absent bilaterally: this finding can be used to diagnose cystic fibrosis in neonates with possible meconium ileus.[47]

Apart from DSD anomalies with separate labioscrotal folds or bifid scrotum, scrotal anomalies are rare. There are case reports of ectopic hemiscrotum and duplication, which are a local manifestation of partial twinning of the caudal embryo or compression of the perineum by the feet of the fetus.[20,48,49]

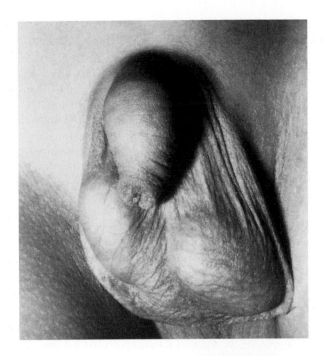

Figure 110.5 Neonate with a teratoma of the left testis.

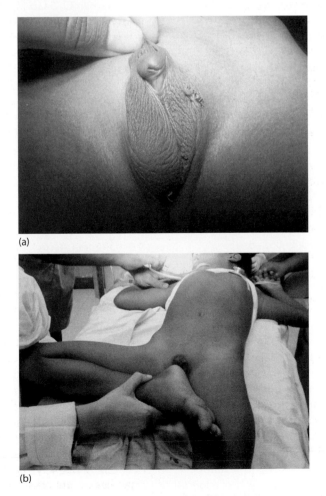

(a)

(b)

Figure 110.6 Boy with a congenital fistula of the anterior urethra caused by pressure of the heel during fetal development. **(a)** Close-up of perineum (after left scrotal orchidopexy) showing normal terminal urethral meatus on glans as well as wide-open midshaft fistula. **(b)** Folding of legs confirmed that the right heel fitted exactly over the pressure area in the anterior urethra.

REFERENCES

1. Nef S, Parada LF. Cryptorchidism in mice mutant for Insl3. *Nat Genet* 1999; 22: 295–9.
2. Zimmerman S, Stedig G, Emmen JMA, Brinkman AO, Nayernia K, Holstein AF, Engel W, Adham IM. Targeted disruption of the Insl3 gene causes bilateral cryptorchidism. *Mol Endocrinol* 1999; 13: 681–91.
3. Hutson JM, Southwell BR, Li R et al. The regulation of testicular descent and the effects of cryptorchidism. *Endocr Rev* 2013; 134: 725–52.
4. Dave S, Johnson A, Fenton K, Mercer C, Erens B, Wellings K. Male circumcision in Britain: Findings from a national probability sample survey. *Sex Transm Infect* 2003; 79(6): 499–500.
5. Merrill C, Nagamine M, Steiner C. *Circumcisions Performed in U.S. Community Hospitals 2005.* Rockville: Healthcare Cost and Utilization Project, 2008.
6. Szabo R, Short RV. How does male circumcision protect against HIV infection? *BMJ* 2000; 320: 1592–4.
7. American Academy of Pediatrics Task Force on Circumcision. Male circumcision. *Pediatrics* 2012; 130: e756–85. Technical Report.
8. Na AF, Tanny SP, Hutson JM. Circumcision: Is it worth it for 21st-century Australian boys? *J Paediatr Child Health* 2014; 51: 580–3.
9. Bailey RC, Moses S, Parker CB et al. Male circumcision for HIV prevention in young men in Kisumu, Kenya: A randomised controlled trial. *Lancet* 2007; 369: 643–56.
10. Learman LA. Neonatal circumcision: A dispassionate analysis. *Clin Obstet Gynecol* 1999; 12: 849–59.
11. Singh-Grewal D, Macdessi J, Craig J. Circumcision for the prevention of urinary tract infection in boys: A systematic review of randomised trials and observational studies. *Arch Dis Child* 2005; 90(8): 853–8.
12. Millett GA, Flores SA, Marks G et al. Circumcision status and risk of HIV and sexually transmitted infections among men who have sex with men: A meta-analysis. *JAMA* 2008; 300: 1674–84.
13. Quinn TC, Wawer MJ, Sewankambo N et al. Viral load and heterosexual transmission of human immunodeficiency virus type 1. *N Engl J Med* 2000; 342: 921–9.
14. Van Howe RS. Sexually transmitted infections and male circumcision: A systematic review and meta-analysis. *ISRN Urol* 2013; 1–42. doi: 10.1155/2013/109846.
15. Fergusson DM, Boden JM, Horwood LJ. Circumcision status and risk of sexually transmitted infection in young adult males: An analysis of a longitudinal birth cohort. *Pediatrics* 2006; 118(5): 1971–7.
16. Frisch M, Früs S, Kjear SK, Mellye M. Falling incidence of penis cancer in an uncircumcised population (Denmark 1943–90). *BMJ* 1995; 311: 1471.
17. Coskunfirat OK, Sayilkan S, Velidedeoglu H. Glans and penile skin amputation as a complication of circumcision. *Ann Plast Surg* 1999; 43: 457.
18. American Academy of Pediatrics (AAP). Circumcision policy statement. *Pediatrics* 1999; 103: 686–93.
19. Cilento BG, Holmes NM, Canning DA. Plastibell® complications revisited. *Clin Pediatr* 1999; 38: 239–42.
20. Stephens FD, Smith ED, Hutson JM. *Congenital Anomalies of the Urinary and Genital Tracts*, 2nd edn. London: Martin Dunitz, 2002.
21. Duckett JW, Baskin LS. Hypospadias. In: O'Neill JA, Grosfeld JL, Fonkalsrud EW, Coran AG, Rowe MI (eds). *Pediatric Surgery*, 5th ed. St. Louis: Mosby, 1998: 1761–81.
22. Borer JG, Retik AB. Current trends in hypospadias repair. *Urol Clin N Am* 1999; 26: 15–37.
23. Snodgrass WT. Tubularized incised plate hypospadias repair: Indications, technique and complications. *Urology* 1999; 54: 6–11.
24. Asopa HS. Newer concepts in the management of hypospadias and its complications. *Ann R Coll Surg Engl* 1998; 80: 161–8.
25. Sarhan O, Saad M, Helmy T, Hafez A. Effect of suturing technique and urethral plate characteristics on complication rate following hypospadias repair: A prospective randomized study. *J Urol* 2009; 182(2): 682–6.
26. Koff SA, Jayanthi VR. Preoperative treatment with human chorionic gonadotrophin in infancy decreases the severity of proximal hypospadias and chordee. *J Urol* 1999; 162: 1435–9.
27. Babaei A, Safarinejad MR, Farrokhi F, Iran-Pour E. Penile reconstruction: Evaluation of the most accepted techniques. *J Urol* 2010; 7(2): 71–8.
28. Donahoe PK, Keating MA. Preputial unfurling to correct the buried penis. *J Pediatr Surg* 1986; 21: 1055–7.
29. Bangroo AK, Khetri R, Tiwari S. Penile agenesis. *J Indian Assoc Pediatr Surg* 2005; 10(4): 256–7.
30. Beasley SW, Hutson JM, Howat AJ, Kelly JH. Posterior ectopia of penis mimics marsupial anatomy: Case reported in association with a primitive cloacal anomaly. *Pediatr Surg Int* 1987; 2: 127–30.
31. Gilbert J, Clark RD, Koyle MA. Penile agenesis: A fatal variation of an uncommon lesion. *J Urol* 1990; 143: 338–9.
32. Garcia RD, Banuelos A, Marin C, De Tomas E. Penoscrotal transposition. *Eur J Pediatr Surg* 1995; 5: 222–5.
33. Hutson JM, Thorup J, Beasley SW. *Descent of the testis*, 2nd edn. Springer, 2016.
34. Browne D. The diagnosis of undescended testicle. *BMJ* 1938; ii: 92–7.
35. Hutson JM, Thorup J. Evaluation and management of the infant with cryptorchidism. *Curr Opin Pediatr* 2015; 27(4): 520–4.
36. Hadziselimovic F. Letter to the editor. *J Pediatr Surg* 2013; 48: 269.

37. John Radcliffe Hospital Cryptorchidism Study Group. Cryptorchidism: A prospective study of 7500 consecutive male births, 1984-8. *Arch Dis Child* 1992; 67: 892–9.

38. Beltran-Brown F, Villegas-Alvarez F. Clinical classification for undescended testes: Experience in 1,010 orchidopexies. *J Pediatr Surg* 1988; 23: 444–7.

39. Kollin C, Hesser U, Ritzen EM, Karpe B. Testicular growth from birth to two years of age, and the effect of orchidopexy at age nine months: A randomized, controlled study. *Acta. Paediatr* 2006; 95(3): 318–24.

40. Sugita Y, Clarnette TD, Cooke-Yarborough C, Waters K, Hutson JM. Testicular and paratesticular tumours in children: 30 years' experience. *Aust NZ J Surg* 1999; 69: 505–8.

41. Heyns CF. Exstrophy of the testis. *J Urol* 1990; 144: 724–5.

42. Sharma AK, Kotharti SK, Goel D, Chaturvedi V. Congenital urethral fistula. *Pediatr Surg Int* 2000; 16: 142–3.

43. Chintamani J, Nyapathy V, Chauhan A, Krishnamurthy U. Supernumerary testis. *J Radiol Case Rep* 2009; 3(11): 29–32.

44. Chen K-C, Chu C-C, Chou T-Y. Transverse testicular ectopia: Preoperative diagnosis by ultrasonography. *Pediatr Surg Int* 2000; 16: 77–9.

45. Hutson JM, Li R, Southwell BR et al. Germ cell development in the postnatal testis: The key to prevent malignancy in cryptorchidism? *Front Endocrinol (Lausanne)* 2012; 3: 176.

46. Morcel K, Camborieux L, Guerrier D. Mayer–Rokitansky–Kuster–Hauser (MRKH) syndrome. *Orphanet J Rare Dis* 2007; 2: 13.

47. Sung V, Hutson JM. A novel way to diagnose cystic fibrosis in the neonate. *J Paediatr Child Health* 2003; 39(9): 720.

48. Hutson JM, Warne GL, Grover SR. *Disorders of Sex Development: An integrated approach to Management*. Berlin: Springer, 2012.

49. Cook WA, Stephens FD. Pathoembryology of the urinary tract. In: King LR (ed). *Urological Surgery in Neonates and Young Infants*, London: Saunders, 1988: 1–22.

111

Neonatal testicular torsion

DAVID M. BURGE AND JONATHAN DURELL

INTRODUCTION

Torsion of the neonatal testis is a well-recognized clinical entity, which accounts for about 10% of all cases of testicular torsion admitted to pediatric surgical centers.[1] A UK study estimated the incidence of neonatal testicular torsion to be 6.1 per 100,000.[2] Torsion usually occurs extravaginally, i.e., in the spermatic cord above the insertion of the tunica vaginalis (Figure 111.1), but both intravaginal and mesorchial torsion are reported.[3,4] Either testis may be involved. Bilateral torsion occurs and may be synchronous or metachronous.[5,6] Asynchronous torsion may occur in as many as 33% of cases.[7] Apparent primary infarction of the neonatal testis in the absence of torsion occurs less commonly,[8] and while it has been postulated that this represents previous torsion that has untwisted, good evidence exists to suggest that the initial event in neonatal torsion is a vascular one and that torsion may occur secondarily.[3] The neonatal testis may be prone to extravaginal torsion because of its extreme mobility within the scrotum.[9]

CLINICAL FEATURES

Neonatal torsion appears to be a condition of large term babies,[3] and it rarely, if ever, affects the preterm infant. Previously, breech delivery was suspected as being a causative factor. Recent reports, however, fail to confirm this.[3] Affected babies are usually totally asymptomatic. The typical physical features are of a hard, edematous hemiscrotum with a noticeable blue or black discoloration.

The testis feels firmly adherent to the scrotal wall and is apparently nontender. While there may be some enlargement of the hemiscrotum, this is not usually marked. These features are usually present from birth, supporting the contention that neonatal torsion is often an antenatal event. However, the clinical features are not always noted at delivery and in many cases are not detected until the second or third day of age. Occasionally, features consistent with acute torsion (sudden onset of swelling, erythema, and pain) may develop some days or weeks after delivery, and it appears that in these cases, the torsion is more likely to be intravaginal. Torsion of an undescended testis may present in this way.[3]

Diagnosis can usually be made on the clinical features alone. The differential diagnosis includes hydrocele, testicular tumor, trauma, adrenal hemorrhage, and meconium peritonitis with tracking down a patent processus. Distinction from a simple hydrocele is usually easy by transillumination. Testicular neoplasia can be excluded by the presence of bluish discoloration and scrotal edema. Torsion can only be differentiated from spontaneous infarction at surgery. Some bruising of the scrotum may occur after breech delivery,[10] but this is usually in the presence of a testis that feels normal to palpation. Intraperitoneal injury from birth trauma may result in hematocele formation, but the fluctuation of this lesion will usually distinguish it from torsion. Adrenal hemorrhage may present with features indistinguishable for torsion, but adrenal ultrasound would be diagnostic.[11] While color Doppler studies of testicular artery flow and radionuclide scanning of the scrotum might support the diagnosis, they are not required.

A clinical diagnosis of neonatal torsion is sufficient indication for scrotal exploration. While it might seem mandatory that this be conducted urgently, reports of successful testicular salvage are rare.[4,12-14] The classical clinical features seem to be due to the presence of established testicular infarction, and it can be argued that the only reason for surgery is to fix the contralateral testis. Because delayed torsion of the contralateral testis does occur and may be at the extravaginal, intravaginal, or mesorchial level, early surgery to assess the affected testis, excise it if necessary, and securely fix the contralateral testis is recommended. No specific preoperative preparation is required.

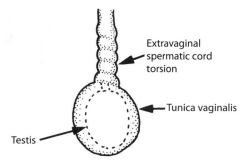

Figure 111.1 Anatomy of extravaginal torsion.

OPERATIVE TECHNIQUE

Under general anesthesia, the scrotum is incised in the midline and dissection continued into the affected hemiscrotum (Figure 111.2). Both testes are easily approached through this single incision (Figure 111.3). In most cases, established infarction will have resulted in edema and fixation of the testis to the subcutaneous tissues. It is usual, however, to find a plane of cleavage outside the tunica vaginalis, resulting in a clear demonstration of the site of torsion. In some instances, necrosis is well established, and the exact origin of the pathology cannot be identified. If, as is usually the case, the testis is clearly beyond salvage, it is wise to excise it, having transfixed the spermatic cord above the site of torsion. Retention of a necrotic testis is inadvisable as it invites sepsis, which may put the contralateral testis at risk. While there is a theoretical possibility that retention of the infarcted testis may result in some hormonal production,[9] in the majority of cases in which the affected testis is not removed, involution occurs.[3] Following excision of the affected testis, the contralateral testis is exposed through the same excision. The tunica vaginalis is opened to allow accurate inspection of the anatomy and permit effective fixation. This may be performed by placement of the testis in a subdartos pouch, as used in orchidopexy, or by suture fixation, which is now described. The tunica vaginalis is sutured to the tunica albuginea of the testis at four points, using a fine nonabsorbable monofilament material, as

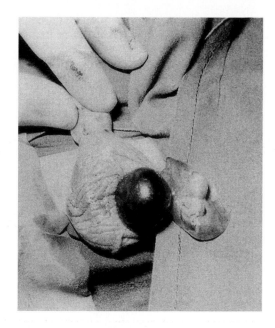

Figure 111.3 Midline exploration showing extravaginal torsion of right testis and normal left testis prior to fixation.

using an absorbable suture has been shown to have a higher rate of retorsion (88% of retorsions in the literature review used absorbable sutures),[15] thus preventing intravaginal torsion. It is wise to incorporate the scrotal septum in the two medial sutures, thus fixing the tunica vaginalis to the scrotum and preventing extravaginal torsion (Figure 111.4). Care should be taken to site these two sutures fairly deep in the wound, or else the testis will lie too superficially and skin closure will be made more difficult. The scrotal incision is then closed with a fine continuous absorbable suture. No specific postoperative care is required.

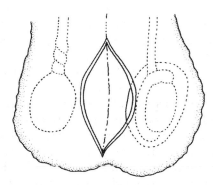

Figure 111.2 Midline scrotal incision.

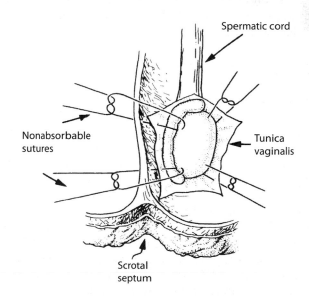

Figure 111.4 Technique of testicular fixation.

REFERENCES

1. Brereton RJ, Manley S. Acute scrotal pathology in boys. *Z Kinderchir* 1980; 29: 343–57.
2. John CM, Kooner G, Matthew DE, Ahmed S, Kenny SE. Neonatal testicular torsion—A lost cause? *Acta Paediatr* 2008; 97(4): 502.
3. Burge DM. Neonatal testicular torsion and infarction. *Br J Urol* 1987; 59: 70–3.
4. Guiney EJ, McGlinchey J. Torsion of the testis and spermatic cord in the newborn. *Surg Gynecol Obstet* 1981; 152: 273–4.
5. Gerstmann DR, Marble RD. Bilaterally enlarged testicles: An atypical presentation of intrauterine spermatic cord torsion. *Am J Dis Child* 1980; 134: 992–4.
6. Tripp BM, Homsy YL. Prenatal diagnosis of bilateral neonatal torsion: A case report. *J Urol* 1995; 153: 1990–1.
7. Baglaj M, Carachi R. Neonatal bilateral testicular torsion: A plea for emergency exploration. *J Urol* 2006; 177: 2296–9.
8. Johnston JH. The testicles and scrotum. In: Williams DI (ed). *Paediatric Urology*. London: Butterworths, 1989: 450–74.
9. Jerkins GR, Noe HN, Hollabaugh RS et al. Spermatic cord torsion in the neonate. *J Urol* 1983; 129: 121–2.
10. Dunn PM. Testicular birth trauma. *Arch Dis Child* 1975; 50: 745.
11. Liu KW, Ku KW, Cheung KL, Chan YL. Acute scrotal swelling: A sign of neonatal adrenal haemorrhage. *J Paediatr Child Health* 1994; 30: 368–9.
12. LaQuaglia MP. Bilateral neonatal torsion. *J Urol* 1987; 138: 1051–4.
13. Yerkes EB, Robertson FM, Gitlin J, Kaefer M, Cain MP, Rink RC. Management of perinatal torsion: Today, tomorrow or never? *J Urol* 2005; 174(4 Pt 2): 1579.
14. Stone KT, Kass EJ, Cacciarelli AA, Gibson DP. Management of suspected antenatal torsion: What is the best strategy. *J Urol* 1995; 153: 782–4.
15. Sells H, Moretti KL, Burfield GD. Recurrent torsion after previous testicular fixation. *ANZ J Surg* 2002; 72(1): 46–8.

PART 11

Long-term outcomes in newborn surgery

112

Long-term outcomes in newborn surgery

CHRISTIAN TOMUSCHAT, KEITH T. OLDHAM, AND CASEY M. CALKINS

INTRODUCTION

Ongoing advancements in the pre- and postoperative care of the neonate with a surgical condition have enabled the survival of an increasing number of infants with congenital malformations. For decades, surgeons have insisted on a regular self-examination of outcomes to ensure the optimal treatment of our patients. Outcome analysis traditionally relates to the rudimentary end result of an operation—utilizing variables such as mortality, operative time, specific complication rates (i.e., incidence of esophageal stricture following esophageal atresia [EA] repair), and hospital length of stay, to name a few. Recently, outcomes research has become a more complex endeavor. Measures of long-term outcomes, including "functional outcome" and "health-related quality of life," are equally important to the morbidity sustained as a result of a congenital malformation and its attendant surgical correction. The methods by which subjective assessments are expressed as a quantitative measure are therefore important for the newborn surgeon to understand. These data serve as an important adjunct to prenatal counseling, offer information about future health expectations for families, assist the surgeon in identifying potential improvements in perioperative management, and will likely be utilized by public agencies charged with implementing health policy, especially in an era of diminishing resources. Therefore, long-term outcomes are of specific import to the neonates we care for, the families we answer to, and our colleagues charged with the continued efforts to improve the surgical care of our youngest patients. This chapter will begin by focusing on the specific language and methodology of modern long-term outcomes research as a prelude to the current status of long-term outcomes assessment in newborn surgical conditions commonly treated by the pediatric surgeon.

WHAT IS AN "OUTCOME"?

In 1934, Ernest A. Codman, an orthopedic surgeon, espoused the "end result idea." In his book *The Shoulder,*

Dr. Codman introduced this "common sense notion that every hospital should follow every patient it treats long enough to determine whether or not the treatment has been successful, and to inquire 'if not, why not?'."[1] Today, this "end result idea" represents the very basis for conducting outcomes research, which examines how interventions delivered in the treatment of medical and surgical disease affect patient populations over time. It is one of many areas of investigation within the broad field of Health Services Research.[2] Although one can formally define a "health service,"[3] it seems intuitive to say that it is any organized effort to improve the health of a patient. The measurements and assessments utilized in outcomes research have changed considerably over the course of the last two decades. Regular assessment of our operative outcomes in the form of "morbidity and mortality" conferences is and continues to be an essential endeavor to ensure that we continue to improve the surgical care delivered to infants and children. It is an indispensable form of self-assessment and allows us to learn from one of the realities of human nature—error. However, assessment of individual and system failure represents only one part of how we improve the practice of pediatric surgery. Individual quality improvement depends on refining surgical technique, learning at regional and national society meetings, remaining knowledgeable by reading relevant peer-reviewed literature, and incorporating successful strategies and techniques into practice.

Assessment of patient outcomes (bad and good) helps us to understand what works and what doesn't. In this sense, an outcome can be any measure that affects the health, perceived health, physiologic function, financial status, or experience of a patient. Modern outcome measures have developed as a result of three general trends. First, traditional clinical outcomes are supplemented by measurements that take patient experience and concerns into account, especially regarding chronic illness, where the intent is typically to treat or offer palliation, rather than provide a definitive cure. Second, when making decisions regarding healthcare, patient preference is essential, and information on healthcare quality of life (QoL) or functional results of one treatment versus another may ultimately influence decision-making in this regard. Finally, healthcare policymakers remain under pressure to effectively allocate resources. Benefits and QoL perceived by patients and society as a whole may allow appropriate governmental bodies to do so with a sense of what is best for the collective good when resources may be limited. A common feature of health-related outcome measures today is the measurement of well-being from the subjective viewpoint of the individual patient (or parent—the "proxy") concerned. The three items crucial to an understanding of modern-day outcomes research are health-related quality of life (HRQoL), functional outcome, and utility (cost-effectiveness).

HEALTH-RELATED QUALITY OF LIFE

Where health and QoL clearly intersect—the concept of HRQoL assessment is born. In contrast to objective data obtained by laboratory, radiographic, or purely functional assessments, the measurement of HRQoL provides additional information about the subjective impact of a condition, or, for our purposes, the ramifications of an operation utilized to treat that condition. Transformation of qualitative assessments into quantitative data requires identification of measurable elements related to an individual's existence and assessment by way of an instrument.[4] Five general concepts define the scope of such an instrument: (1) impairment, (2) functional state, (3) health perception, (4) social opportunity, and (5) duration of life.[5] Distinct domains have been subsequently operationalized to translate these five concepts into quantifiable data. Although there is no consensus regarding a universal and inclusive set of domains, most researchers will agree that "quality of life" differs greatly from person to person. A survey respondent may weigh various domains differently, and one must decide how to assess for these differences when interpreting the results from a cohort of respondents. The seven general domains of health in most HRQoL surveys include physical functioning, social functioning, emotional functioning, cognitive functioning, pain/discomfort, vitality, and overall well-being.

Instrument standards

A HRQoL instrument is developed utilizing psychometric testing principles and, once constructed, is reviewed against standards outlined by the Scientific Advisory Committee of the Medical Outcomes Trust.[6] Evaluation criteria include appropriateness, validity, reliability, responsiveness, precision, interpretability, acceptability, and feasibility. Appropriateness is the first and most fundamental criterion to assess and asks whether the instrument measures what have been identified as the most important outcome(s) for the purposes of evaluation. Specifically, is the instrument relevant, and are the methods of evaluation and administration appropriate? Validity concerns whether an instrument measures what is intended. Face and content validity

are matters of qualitative judgment—for instance, were the patient types targeted for assessment included in the creation of the instruments' content? Construct validation refers to comparisons with other instruments, relating the scores to sociodemographic variables and comparing domain scores within the instrument itself. Reliability assesses whether or not an instrument is consistent in its measurements—both internally and over time. Responsiveness refers to the ability of an instrument to measure significant changes in health and is assessed by looking at changes in instrument scores for groups whose health is known to have changed. The precision of an instrument is measured by the range of response options and the existence of ceiling (maximum score) or floor (minimum score) effects. An instrument is likely to be acceptable to a patient or population group if it measures what they consider being important aspects of QoL. The optimal instrument is interpretable—and is able to translate a quantitative score into an external measure that has a familiar meaning. This aspect of an instrument is easily assessed when there are normative data from a representative sample of the general populous and/or patients with similar conditions for whom the instrument is intended. Finally, feasibility refers to the time and effort needed to complete the instrument, and whether such issues are prohibitive to completion of the instrument, or affect the manner in which it is completed. The United States Centers for Disease Control has established a comprehensive website that may aid the clinician when faced with the possibility of instrument evaluation or utilization (http://www.cdc.gov/hrqol/).

Unique issues in health services research for the newborn population

As the goal of adult functioning is to be self-sufficient and economically productive, adult-based measures of functioning and QoL are not likely relevant to children.[7] Furthermore, children often view health and illness as separate entities, whereas adults see these two items as part of a continuum.[8] Lack of a consensus on a theoretical framework as to the nature of HRQoL in children means that there is lack of agreement regarding the optimal domains in a pediatric HRQoL assessment tool. Even within domains, there are often variations of emphasis. For example, within the physical functioning domain, an instrument may place varied emphasis on physical symptoms, self-care, participation in physical activities, or distress caused by limitations. As a result, different instruments may yield different results depending on the age of the child, the medical or surgical condition, the emphasis of the questions within a domain, and a variety of other factors unique to pediatric healthcare.

Although adult HRQoL measures suffer from some of the same issues of validity, the common feature of most adult instruments is that they measure health from the subjective viewpoint of the individual concerned. In children, this information is not always easily obtained from the subject. Although many children are able to provide self-reports of

HRQoL if an instrument is chosen that is appropriate to his/her abilities, this assertion has not been well evaluated. Furthermore, different domains within an instrument may pose unique challenges to different age groups. Children as young as 5 years old may be able to provide accurate self-reports of pain, whereas subjective concepts such as behavior or self-esteem may not be able to be accurately assessed until 10 years of age.[9] Several self-reporting biases are also more problematic in pediatric populations. Position bias (tendency to select the first answer), acquiescent response bias (tendency to agree with questions regardless of content), failure to accurately perceive time periods, boredom with having to answer written questions, and difficulty in understanding negatively worded items make construction of pediatric outcome tools difficult. Given that self-reports suffer from such bias and many children are truly unable to fill out a self-assessment, other individuals—"proxies"—have served to provide data on the child's behalf. Parents or caregivers who have a longstanding relationship with the patient commonly complete such proxy reports. However, the choice of proxy may add further bias to the instrument. For example, fathers rate children as having fewer behavioral and psychological problems than do their mothers.[10] In another study, children aged 8–11 years with a chronic health condition reported significantly lower HRQoL than their parent proxies.[11] In one review, nearly 90% of pediatric HRQoL assessments were completed by a proxy.[12] However, most modern pediatric-specific instruments can be utilized in a self-reporting mode, and proxy assessments may apply to only the youngest of children. When possible, self-reports should always be sought over proxy-generated data.

As the development of a child is not always linear, how does one separate development from the outcome? This is one of the several questions that remain unanswered regarding the instruments currently utilized for pediatric HRQoL. Outcome measures that not only are sensitive to changes in development and health but also make allowances for different cognitive abilities of children at various ages with regard to reporting and valuing health status are required.[13] When selecting an instrument, the clinician should consider whether the concepts inherent in the tool are developmentally appropriate for age, gender, and culture. In addition, if one is interested in measuring longitudinal HRQoL in a patient cohort, selection of an instrument with items that are not overly age-related may be optimal so that children of different ages may complete the same instrument.

To get around the problematic issue of "child-friendly" tools and feasibility, some instruments have employed unique methods to entice children to complete the surveys. For example, the KINDLR instrument employs a computerized program to measure pediatric HRQoL by means of a touch-screen monitor or a mouse. It is a child-friendly (independent of reading and writing skills, in a playful format), economical, and developmentally appropriate program that is valid, reliable, and available in two languages (German and English). Other methods to entice and facilitate child participation include third-party interviewing and age-appropriate storybook formats.

Multidimensional generic measures of HRQoL

Generic quality-of-life measures are designed to assess physical, psychological, and social aspects of health without attention to a specific ailment or disability. These instruments emphasize breadth over specificity by focusing on the common elements of health that transcend all diseases. In practice, these instruments may also augment subjective and objective clinical data that focus on signs, symptoms, and effects of a specific disease.[14] The list of instruments in Table 112.1 is not, by any means, comprehensive, but serves to highlight the most common instruments available for the assessment of generic HRQoL in infants and children.

Table 112.1 HRQoL instruments

Instrument	Applicable age	Time to complete
PedsQL™	5–18 years (self) 2–18 (proxy)	<5 minutes (self or proxy)
CHIP	"CE" 6–11 years (proxy) "AE" 6–18 years (self)	20 minutes (self or proxy)
CHQ	10–18 years (self) 5–15 years (proxy)	15–30 minutes (self) 7–30 minutes (proxy)
KINDLR	4–16 years (self) 4–16 years (proxy)	10–15 minutes (self) 10 minutes (parent)
KIDSCREEN	8–18 years (self) 8 18 years (proxy)	20 minutes (52 items) 15 minutes (27 items) 5 minutes (10 items)
DISABKIDS	4–7 years (self or proxy) 8–16 (self or proxy)	20 minutes (37 items)

Note: PedsQL: Pediatric Quality of Life Inventory; CHIP: Child Health and Illness Profile; CHQ: Child Health Questionnaire.

PEDIATRIC QUALITY OF LIFE

The Pediatric Quality of Life (PedsQL™) measurement model is a modular approach to measuring HRQoL in children and adolescents who are healthy and those with acute and chronic health conditions. The model has the added ability to integrate both generic core scales and disease-specific modules into one measurement system. The PedsQL™ generic core scales include brief (23 items), practical (less than 4 minutes to complete), and flexible (designed for use with the community, school, and clinical pediatric populations). Its permutations are meant to be developmentally appropriate (different modules for ages—child self-report ages 5–7, 8–12, 13–18; parent proxy-report ages 2–4, 5–7, 8–12, 13–18). It is one of the most interpretable tools due to its widespread use. Additionally, it is translated into multiple languages including Spanish.[15] The 23-item PedsQL™ generic core scales were designed to measure the principal dimensions of health as delineated by the World Health Organization, as well as role (school) functioning. PedsQL™ condition-specific modules complement the generic core scales and are used in designated clinical populations. These are designed to provide greater measurement sensitivity for circumscribed populations (currently available for asthma, rheumatology, diabetes, cancer, and cardiac conditions, with additional modules in the development and planning stages). For the pediatric surgeon, the PedsQL™ is an attractive option as it is brief, practical, developmentally appropriate, multidimensional, reliable, valid, and responsive. It has been cited in numerous peer-reviewed publications. The instrument can measure HRQoL over time with instruments that are age appropriate and available in both patient and proxy forms.

CHILD HEALTH AND ILLNESS PROFILE

The Child Health and Illness Profile (CHIP) instruments were developed by Dr. Starfield et al.[16] at the Johns Hopkins School of Public Health. Development of the child and adolescent editions occurred over 12 years and involved more than 5000 children and adolescents from ethnically and socioeconomically diverse families. The CHIP-CE (CE = child evaluation) instruments provide a comprehensive assessment of health status that can be completed by children 6–11 years old or by their parents. It describes aspects of health that can be influenced by health systems, school health systems, and health promotion efforts. The CHIP-AE (AE = adolescent evaluation) was developed to document the state of health in adolescent age populations, identify differences in the health of subpopulations, and assess the impact of medical and surgical interventions on health.

CHILD HEALTH QUESTIONNAIRE™

Perhaps the most commonly used outcome assessment tool in contemporary health services research is the SF-36® ("short-form 36").[17] The Child Health Questionnaire (CHQ) is a by-product of the SF-36® and a more appropriate choice for use in children and adolescents. A product of the RAND-sponsored Medical Outcomes Study (MOS), the SF-36® is a 36-item general health status assessment questionnaire. It has nine separate scales, though recent work has identified two dimensions that underlie the nine subscales: physical and mental health. There are substantial reliability and validity data for the SF-36® in a wide variety of adult populations.[18] However, the 28- and 50-item CHQ short forms (which cover the same 12 concepts as the full-length CHQ) are more efficient measures than the SF-36® and are valid for use in children aged 5–18 years.[19] In the United States, normative values and benchmarks for the parent-reported versions of the CHQ are available for some specific health conditions. The youth self-report version is 87 items and was developed for use in individuals aged 10 years and older. Authorized translations and Internet-administered versions are also available.[20]

KINDLR

Initially developed in Germany, the KINDLR is a 24-item, methodologically suitable, psychometrically sound, and flexible instrument. The questionnaire can be completed by children and adolescents (aged 4–16) or by way of a parent proxy. The questionnaire is available for different age groups. The computer-assisted version (CAT-SCREEN) is a unique method of instrument administration that may be especially suitable for toddlers. Disease-specific modules exist for obesity, asthma, atopic dermatitis, cancer, and diabetes. The KINDLR has been validated and is especially effective in the assessment of psychological well-being, social relationships, physical function, and everyday life activities.[21]

KIDSCREEN

The KIDSCREEN questionnaires are a family of instruments developed and normalized for surveying HRQoL in children and adolescents aged 8–18. The questionnaires were developed simultaneously in 13 European countries with particular regard to childhood concepts of health and well-being. Three versions of the KIDSCREEN questionnaire are targeted at children, adolescents, and parents. They are available in various languages and can be applied to multiple research goals. KIDSCREEN-52 (long version) covers 10 HRQoL dimensions, KIDSCREEN-27 (short version) covers 5 HRQoL dimensions, while the KIDSCREEN-10 Index encompasses a global HRQoL measurement. In this fashion, the questionnaires measure the QoL from the child's point of view with regard to physical, mental, and social well-being (http://www.kidscreen.org).[22,23]

OTHER PEDIATRIC GENERIC INSTRUMENTS

The Infant Toddler Quality of Life Questionnaire™ (ITQOL) was developed for use in infants and toddlers from at least 2 months of age up to 5 years. The ITQOL adopts the World Health Organization's definition of health, as a state of complete physical, mental, and social well-being and not merely the absence of disease. The survey was developed following a thorough review of the infant health literature and a review of developmental guidelines used by pediatricians. The child equivalent is the aforementioned CHQ. The

Dartmouth COOP child-report charts were developed as a survey to evaluate treatment outcomes and as a tool for the detection of important health problems. It consists of six charts addressing physical fitness, emotional feelings, schoolwork, social support, family communications, and health habits.[24] The instrument was developed by a literature review and a focus group of physicians and adolescents. The tool is completed by self and is reasonably feasible in that it contains only six items. The Exeter QoL (Exqol) measure is another generic self-report HRQoL measure for children aged 6–12 years based on the authors' experience with chronically ill children. Like the KINDL CAT-SCREEN, it is computer-administered and consists of 12 gender-specific pictures—each of which is rated twice: the first in terms of "like me" and the second in terms of "as I would like to be."

Also, significant HRQoL differences exist between parents caring for children with congenital anomalies and the general population. It would be useful to improve further our understanding of the HRQoL impact of informal caregiving, separating "caregiving effects" from "family effects" and distinguishing parent–child relationships from other caregiving situations. Poley et al.[25] underline the importance of considering caregivers, also in the context of economic evaluations. It indicates that general HRQoL measures, as used in patients, may be able to detect HRQoL effects in caregivers, which facilitates the incorporation in common economic evaluations of HRQoL effects in carers. Analysts and policymakers should be aware that if HRQoL improvement is an important aim, they should register HRQoL changes not only in patients but also in their caregivers.[25]

CONDITION-SPECIFIC MEASURES OF HRQOL

Condition-specific measures aim to assess the QoL following a specific intervention or for individuals with a specific diagnosis. When condition-specific instruments are developed to assess the QoL following treatment of a specific anomaly, such measures are designed to be more sensitive to the detection of small treatment effects when compared to generic measures. In this regard, a condition-specific measure is designed to tap the domain(s) of greatest interest for the condition in question. A variety of studies have been performed with the intent of validating generic HRQoL instruments in patients with neonatal surgical disease. Furthermore, a select number of disease-specific outcome measures have been developed to assess the QoL after treatment of pediatric surgical conditions. For example, in Europe, a proxy version of EuroQOL was found to be feasible and valid in a population of children with imperforate anus.[26] Similar studies have utilized generic quality-of-life measures in children with Hirschsprung's disease,[27,28] anorectal malformations,[29] congenital diaphragmatic hernia (CDH),[30] and neurological impairment requiring gastrostomy or surgical treatment of gastroesophageal reflux,[31] to name a few. Unvalidated questionnaires have also been utilized to assess HRQoL in many conditions treated by pediatric surgeons.[32,33]

Condition-specific HRQoL measures have also been described for children with anorectal malformations and Hirschsprung's disease (HD),[34] as well as for bladder dysfunction, cancer, and inflammatory bowel disease (Table 112.2).[35–37] Very recently, the perspectives of children with EA and their parents of five HRQoL studies have been incorporated into the development of the first condition-specific HRQoL questionnaire for patients with EA.[38] However, this questionnaire needs to be validated in further studies. In summary, very few HRQoL measures, to date, have been specifically validated or developed for use in the neonatal surgical population.

FUNCTIONAL OUTCOMES

Functional outcomes can be measured in a variety of formats. It is a difficult area of health services research to define

Table 112.2 Description of disease-specific HRQoL instruments for use in pediatric age

Instrument	Disease	Applicable age (years)	Dimensions
PinQ	Bladder dysfunction	6–17	Social relation with peers, self-esteem, family and home, body image, independence, mental health, treatment
POQOLS	Cancer	3–18	Physical function and role restriction, emotional distress, reaction to current treatment
IMPACT	Inflammatory bowel disease	9–18	Bowel, body image, functional/social impairment, tests/treatments, systemic impairment
DDL	Obstructive defecation disorder	7–15	Constipation-related, emotional functioning, social functioning, treatments/interventions

Note: DDL: defecation disorder list; PinQ: QoL measure for children with bladder dysfunction; POQOLS: Pediatric Oncology QoL scale.

Table 112.3 Functional outcomes tools

Instrument	Applicable age (years)	Time to complete
FIM^SM/WeeFIMII^SM	0–18 (proxy)	15–20 minutes (18 items)
FSIIR	0–16 (proxy)	15 minutes (short)
		30 minutes (long)
PEDI™	0–7 (proxy)	45–60 minutes (237 items)

Note: FIM^SM/WeeFIMII^SM: Functional Independence Measure; FSIIR: Functional Status II; PEDI™: Pediatric Evaluation of Disability Inventory.

clearly. In one sense, these outcomes can be measured within the context of a specific disease state and the procedure that is designed to treat that disease. However, for neonatal surgery, the impact of functional outcomes may be inherently distinct from adult conditions. Take, for example, a professional football (soccer in the United States) goalie that can consistently punt the ball to the opposite penalty box. He suffers a knee injury in the prime of his career and must undergo reconstructive knee surgery. A "disease-specific" functional outcome measure following repair could be as simple as assessing his ability to kick the ball that same distance following surgery and physical rehabilitation. From the players' point of view, he is 100% functional if he can kick that same distance without any pain after treatment. However, how do we measure function in this case if he is only able to punt the same distance inconsistently? Also, what if he can punt the same distance, but suffers incredible pain in doing so—is this an issue of QoL, function, or both? Thus, the assessment of "functional outcome" is complex. However, since the sample of premier league goalies who consistently punt a soccer ball nearly the entire length of the football field is relatively small, most generic functional outcome instruments focus on the assessment of individuals with chronic health problems and their ability to "function" in everyday life. These same issues confront the newborn surgeon attempting to study functional outcomes in populations where the congenital malformations are relatively rare. Furthermore, for such measures to have a meaningful individual and societal impact, they must be measured in adult life, where independent functioning is the expectation. The ability to function is distinct from the quality of function, or life. As it relates to health services research, functional outcomes are not necessarily meant to be condition-specific but are related to any of the general domains of functional health in a survey introduced earlier: physical, social, emotional, or cognitive functioning. The following instruments are the three most common tools utilized to measure general functional outcomes in children (Table 112.3).

Functional Status II

The Functional Status II (FSIIR) can distinguish between children with and without chronic health conditions, has acceptable internal consistency and reliability, and correlates with other indicators of illness such as utilization of medical services and illness-related absenteeism.[39] The FSIIR is

a 14-item instrument administered to parents to measure their child's capacity to perform age-appropriate roles and tasks in a variety of areas such as communication, mobility, mood, energy, sleeping, and eating. Parents use a three-point categorical scale to indicate the observed frequency of specific behaviors. When impairment in child functioning is described, parents are asked to report whether each specific impairment is due to the child's illness. The total score is the sum of the scores, thus indicating the child's functional status without regard to whether or not the observed impairment is due to the child's illness. The illness score is the sum of the scores indicating the child's functional status with the deduction of points only for impairment related to the child's illness, thus often resulting in a score higher than the total score. The higher the score, the better the functional status.[40]

Pediatric Evaluation of Disability Inventory

The Pediatric Evaluation of Disability Inventory (PEDI) was developed to provide a comprehensive clinical assessment of the essential functional capabilities and performance in children between the ages of 6 months and 7 years. The PEDI was designed primarily for the functional evaluation of young children; however, it can also be used for the evaluation of older children if their functional abilities fall below that expected of a 7-year-old child. The assessment is designed to serve as a descriptive measure of the child's current functional performance, as well as a method for tracking change over time. The PEDI measures both capability and performance of functional activities in three content domains: (1) self-care, (2) mobility, and (3) social function. It has been primarily utilized in the functional evaluation following neurologic insults (i.e., traumatic brain injury or stroke).[41–43]

Functional Independence Measure

The Functional Independence Measure (FIM^SM) and its pediatric counterpart (WeeFIMII^SM) are standardized instruments initially designed to allow clinicians to document functional performance in children and adolescents with acquired or congenital disabilities.[44] These measures have been approved by the Joint Commission on Accreditation of Healthcare Organizations (JCAHO) to provide information for the ORYX initiative (a standardized initiative to allow JCAHO to measure performance standards across accredited organizations) as well as to meet accreditation standards for the Commission on Accreditation of Rehabilitation Facilities.[45]

Other assessments of functional outcome

The aforementioned scoring systems provide generic assessments of child functioning in daily life. However, a pediatric surgeon is often most interested in how a patient compares to his or her age-related peers following a specific intervention performed in the neonatal period. In this regard, disease-specific functional outcome measures have been utilized for a variety of different pediatric surgical conditions. However, "function" can be measured by various instruments and/or objective assessments pertinent to the condition in question. The literature regarding the long-term functional results of CDH illustrates this point.

The collaborative UK Extracorporeal Membrane Oxygenation (ECMO) trial concluded that a policy of ECMO support reduces the risk of death without a concomitant rise in severe disability, defined as an overall developmental quotient of <50 using the Griffiths Mental Development Scales.[46] In another study of infants with severe CDH (those that required ECMO support), survivors displayed mild neuromotor and cognitive delay in development at 24 months of age as measured by impairments in mean Bayley Mental Developmental Index and Psychomotor Developmental Index scores.[46] Both of these studies utilized cognitive functioning scores to report on the functional outcomes of infants with CDH.

Other assessments of functional outcome may be related to objective physiologic measurements. In a study of 23 adult survivors of CDH, pulmonary function tests, diffusion capacity, and a cardiopulmonary exercise test (CPET) were performed. The FEV1 and FEF25%–75% were found to be lower in CDH survivors. Despite these abnormalities, during CPET, percent predicted workload and percent predicted maximal oxygen uptake were normal in most of the patients.[47] In another study of functional respiratory outcomes of CDH patients treated in the perinatal period, 26 adolescent survivors and age- and gender-matched controls were subjected to pulmonary function testing. Significant differences were found in nearly every spirometric measurement.[48] Thus, as function relates to pulmonary mechanics in the CDH population, functional outcomes can be construed as favorable or unfavorable depending on the measure utilized.

In general, functional outcomes refer to things that are meaningful to the patient in the context of everyday living. However, for pediatric surgeons, function may be best related to how well the operation can recapitulate the "normal." In that regard, condition-specific functional outcomes are also worthy to gauge the "success" of a neonatal operation. For example, it would be helpful to the pediatric surgeon to know what percentage of patients with a Type C EA can eat any food without dysphagia in adult life. Similarly, anorectal function (fecal continence) after the period where toilet training is typically achieved is an especially significant outcome measure for patients with anorectal malformations and HD. These types of disease-specific measures are helpful for patients and their families as they consider the long-term functional issues related to the congenital malformations we are charged with treating. In the final analysis, both disease-specific and generic functional outcomes have merit in the long-term assessment of patients with neonatal surgical conditions.

COST-EFFECTIVENESS AND UTILITY MEASURES

A panel convened in 1993 by the U.S. Department of Health and Human Services suggested that standardized outcomes analyses be conducted to evaluate the cost-effectiveness of medical care.[49] One way to directly compare relative treatment effectiveness is to examine the impact of interventions on the utility gained. Cost–utility analysis fulfills this requirement.[50] In this type of analysis, health treatment effects are most commonly measured regarding quality-adjusted-life-years (QALYs) gained. Preference-based instruments allow one to compare interventions and treatment regimens for a given condition in this manner. Such analyses have become popular for examining the economic consequences of disease and the medical and surgical interventions aimed at treating such problems. A QALY takes into account both quantity and QoL generated by healthcare interventions. It is the arithmetic product of life expectancy and a measure of the quality of remaining life years. A QALY places weight on time during different health states such that a year of perfect health is worth a score of 1, whereas death receives a score of 0. Health states considered to be worse than death receive a score below zero. The strength of QALY analysis is the fact that it provides a common currency to assess the extent of benefit gained from interventions to improve the QoL. A cost–utility ratio can be calculated from a QALY assessment combined with the cost of treatment for the condition. For example, a disease that reduces the QoL by one-half will take away 0.5 QALYs over the course of 1 year. If it affects two people, it will take away 1.0 QALY (equal to 2×0.5) over a 1-year period. Medical treatment that improves the QoL by 0.2 for each of five individuals will result in a score of 1 QALY if the benefit is maintained over a 1-year period. Using this system, it is possible to express the benefits of various interventions by showing how many QALYs they produce versus the total economic cost of the intervention.[51]

Utility and cost ultimately are important components of healthcare policy formulation. Using the common metric of QALYs also allows one to introduce QoL into the direct cost comparison of programs. This approach provides a framework within which to make policy decisions that require selection between competing alternatives. Importantly, these types of analyses are potentially influential in determining the extent of funding for particular pediatric interventions.[13] The Health Utility Index (HUI), the Quality of

Table 112.4 Utility instruments

Instrument	Applicable age (years)	Time to complete
QWB	5–18 (self and proxy)	10 minutes
HUI:2	6–18 (self and proxy)	3–10 minutes
EQ-5D	5–18 (self and proxy)	1–2 minutes

Note: EQ-5D: Euro Quality of Life; HUI:2: Health Utilities Inc.; QWB: Quality of Well-Being Scale.

Well-Being Scale (QWB), and the EQ-5D are three examples of utility-based measures developed for and validated in pediatric populations (Table 112.4).

Quality of Well-Being Scale

Developed by researchers at The University of California, San Diego, the QWB assesses a patient's objective level of functioning in three areas: mobility, physical activity, and social activity.[52] An important distinction is made between "functional ability" and "functional performance"—whereby a patient is asked to report activity performed rather than what can be performed. The scoring of the instrument utilizes population-derived preference weights. Current studies are addressing the validity of the QWB-SA translated into Spanish, German, Italian, Swedish, French-Canadian, and Dutch.

Health utilities index

The HUI (HUI2, version 2; and HUI3, version 3) is a family of health status and preference-based HRQoL measures suitable for use in clinical and population studies.[53] Both HUI2 and HUI3 focus on capacity rather than performance. Each includes a health status classification system, a preference-based multiattribute utility function, data collection questionnaires, and algorithms for deriving HUI variables from questionnaire responses. The attributes of health status included in HUI were chosen on the basis of their importance to people. HUI utility scores are based on the preferences of the community. HUI2 consists of seven attributes: sensation (vision, hearing, speech), mobility, emotion, cognition, self-care, pain, and fertility.[54] Similarly, HUI3 consists of eight attributes: vision, hearing, speech, ambulation, dexterity, emotion, cognition, and pain.

EQ-5D

Established in 1987, the EuroQOL Group initially comprised a network of international, multilingual, and multidisciplinary researchers from seven centers in Finland, the Netherlands, Norway, Sweden, and the United Kingdom. Currently, the group has expanded to researchers from Canada, Denmark, Germany, Greece, Japan, New Zealand, Slovenia, Spain, the United States, and Zimbabwe. The EQ-5D is a generic measure of health status that provides a simple descriptive profile and a single index value that can be used in the clinical and economic evaluation of healthcare and in population health surveys. The EQ-5D system consists of five dimensions: mobility, self-care, usual activity, pain/discomfort, and anxiety/depression. Each dimension has three levels designated simply as no problem, some problem, or severe problem, and subjects are asked to check the level that is most descriptive of their current level of function or experience in each dimension. These five dimensions yield 243 possible distinct "health states" comprising the classification system. The classification scheme has been assigned standardized scores derived from population-based samples of respondents asked to assign values to subsets of the 243 states. A set of valuation weights has been derived from a U.S. sample.[55]

Although several measurement instruments have been developed to measure utility in children, measurement methods are seemingly fraught with inconsistencies and biases.[56] Indeed, a study of cost–utility analyses in the medical literature between 1976 and 1997 recommended the need for more consistency and clarity in reporting.[57] In response to such criticisms, the Paediatric Economic Database Evaluation Project was conceived to promote research into pediatric health economic methods. In recent years, standard methods for the conduct of economic evaluations have evolved to improve allocation decisions that are unique to the pediatric population. The database contains over 2776 citations from January 1, 1980, to December 31, 2014, and continues to be updated. Consistent with use in allocation decision-making, only full economic evaluations are accepted for inclusion.[58]

Long-term outcomes in specific neonatal surgical disease

Assessment of outcome is an important part of the practice of neonatal surgery. The current tools available to quantify the QoL, function, and cost–utility have changed dramatically over the last decade. However, this area of health research remains in its infancy where patients with neonatal surgical conditions are concerned. Unfortunately, there are a few studies in pediatric surgery that address long-term outcome. This offers an opportunity for further research, yet represents a host of difficulties. Information on long-term outcomes is difficult to obtain as studies require the meticulous collection of data over many years and are hampered by the lack of long-term follow-up (especially for those children who do well!), and attempts to corral a mobile patient population require efforts beyond the willingness or resources of most pediatric surgeons. Furthermore, relatively few clinical interventions and treatments in pediatric surgery are supported by adequately powered randomized controlled trials—which may undermine the subsequent analysis of long-term outcome. In many cases, the specific short- and long-term morbidities of each congenital malformation and its respective operative treatment have been previously addressed in the specific chapters of this text. However, we will cover some of the salient long-term standard and modern outcome measures of the most common neonatal thoracic and abdominal surgical conditions, and propose future opportunities to further our understanding of the ramifications of these malformations and the operations utilized to treat them.

LONG-TERM OUTCOMES FOR SURGERY IN THE NEWBORN PERIOD

General considerations—prematurity and low birth weight

The neonatal period is defined as the period after birth within the first 28 days of life. Indeed, no other patient demographic in medicine has achieved such a dramatic improvement in survival over the last 30 years as that of the premature neonate. Today, the survival of very low birth weight (VLBW) infants (birth weight less than 1500 gm) has increased to over 80%. Furthermore, patients weighing less than 1 kg (extremely low birth weight) have realized a survival in as many as 70%. These increases have occurred as a result of many substantive improvements in perinatal care and the expertise and methods by which that care is delivered. However, as the number of deaths from sepsis and the sequelae of group B streptococcal infection and chorioamnionitis has declined, the proportion of mortality due to congenital anomalies has increased in both the United States and the United Kingdom. The most recent national vital statistics report released by the United States Centers for Disease Control in 2014 states that the infant mortality rate of 5.96 per 1000 live births—a historical low—was 13% lower than in 2003. During the same period, the neonatal mortality rate (death rate among infants under 28 days, a subset of infant mortality) decreased 13% to 4.04 per 1000 live births, and the postneonatal mortality rate (death rate among infants 28 days through 11 months, a subset of infant mortality) declined 13% to 1.93 per 1000 live births. However, the leading cause of death in the group under 28 days of postnatal life is attributed to congenital malformations. Indeed, the yearly prevalence of congenital malformations increased from 4.0% of infants born in 1998 to 5.6% in 2007, and congenital malformations remain an important cause of neonatal morbidity and mortality among VLBW infants.[59]

In England and Wales, congenital anomalies are the second commonest cause of infant deaths overall with a rate in 2007 of 1.39 per 1000 live births; and they are the leading cause of deaths in the postneonatal (>28 days) period at 0.52 per 1000 live births.[60] For appropriately grown infants (not

suffering from intrauterine growth retardation [IUGR]) between a birth weight of 1500 and 2500 g, the mortality rate remains less than 10%. Below this weight, mortality rates incrementally increase, and survival below 500 g is uncommon. Today, the gestational age at which there is a 50% chance of survival has declined to 25 weeks.[61] Perhaps the most salient long-term outcome as it relates to prematurity and low birth weight is the incidence of impairment, disability, and handicap. According to the World Health Organization, "long-term impairment" includes any loss or abnormality of psychological, physiological, and anatomic structure or function. "Disability" is defined as any restriction of ability to perform an activity within the range considered normal for a human being. Disability reflects the consequence of impairment regarding functional performance and activity. Finally, a "handicap" is a disadvantage for a given individual resulting from an impairment or disability that limits fulfillment of the role that is normally based on age, sex, social, and cultural factors.[62] The most significant major disability affecting premature infants is cerebral palsy (CP). CP is defined as a permanent impairment of voluntary movement or posture due to damage to the developing brain. It may involve one limb (monoplegia), both lower limbs (diplegia), or all four (quadriplegia). In patients weighing less than 2 kg at birth, the incidence of CP at the age of 2 years was 8% in a geographical study of 1000 children.[63] Very and extremely low birth weight survivors are also at an increased risk for long-term visual impairment, such that approximately 5% of infants in this category are "blind." Retinopathy of prematurity is the most common cause of poor visual outcome. However, cortical blindness can occur from damage to the occipital cortex due to periventricular leukomalacia or optic atrophy as a result of hydrocephalus. Cryotherapy for retinopathy of prematurity is an effective treatment, reducing the chance of severe visual loss by 50%, and this treatment has led to an improvement in long-term visual handicaps associated with prematurity.[64] Sensorineural hearing loss (SNHL) is also a problem in survivors of premature birth. This is most frequently seen in survivors with persistent pulmonary hypertension, and high incidences are widely reported in survivors of extracorporeal life support (ECLS). In a longitudinal study of 1279 extremely premature children (gestational age ≤28 weeks; birth weight <1250 g), Robertson et al.[65] found permanent hearing loss in 3.1% and severe to profound loss in 1.9%. Among affected children, hearing loss was delayed in onset in 10% of them and was progressive in 28%. Prolonged supplemental oxygen use was the most important marker for predicting hearing loss.[65] In modern intensive care units, all infants are screened for hearing loss. Early diagnosis guides appropriate support and improves language development later in life. Whereas CP is clearly one of the most devastating long-term consequences of prematurity, cognitive impairment is a more common adverse outcome.[66] The intelligence quotient (IQ) in long-term survivors of VLBW gestations is shifted one standard deviation lower when compared to normal birth weight controls, and a significant number of these children suffer from attention deficit or hyperactivity disorders when compared with controls. However, even with an IQ in a normal range, the VLBW survivor is more likely to require special educational provisions. Also, small for gestational age infants suffer from a negative impact on school performance; 25% of such infants in 1985 were failing at school at age 10 years compared to 14% of children who had been weight appropriate for gestational age.[67] Nevertheless, small for gestational age survivors report "adequate" satisfaction with life despite the fact that these individuals are less likely to secure professional or managerial employment.[68] Finally, poor motor coordination, altered manual dexterity and balance, short attention span, and visual impairment are coexistent and together significantly impair the child's ability to function in school. The highest proportion of these adverse neurodevelopmental outcomes are seen in those treated with the highest acuity of care (i.e., ECLS).[69-71]

General considerations—psychological effects of neonatal surgery

In addition to the consequences of prematurity and low birth weight, the psychological consequences of surgery performed within the first 28 days of life should not be overlooked. Studies on the effects of hospitalization on young children show that between 6 months and 4 years of age, children will most likely demonstrate short-term emotional and behavioral problems during that admission, and later psychological disturbances were associated with repeat hospital admission, as well as those hospitalizations lasting for more than a week. Based on these observations, Dr. Loraine Ludman and colleagues at the Great Ormond Street Hospital for Children began a prospective longitudinal study to examine the psychological effects of major neonatal surgery on infants and their families. The infants studied were born at term and required major surgery within the first 28 days of life. These infants were compared to a carefully matched group of healthy newborns not requiring neonatal surgery. Interestingly, very early hospitalization and periods of separation did not differentiate between the case–control pairs at 12 months of age. However, by 3 years of age, the rate of behavioral disturbance was approximately 2.5 times greater among the patients undergoing surgery in the first 28 days of life compared to the control group (30% versus 11.5%). At that stage, the number of operative procedures that the child underwent was the strongest predictor of outcome on both verbal and nonverbal IQ measures. The two predominant factors associated with difficulty in the mother–child relationship were a lengthy first admission (more than 25 days) and/or repeat hospital admissions. In longer-term follow-up between 11 and 13 years of age, emotional and behavioral problems were more frequent in the surgical group than among the controls based on parent and teacher reports. These data suggest that surgery and repeated admissions in early childhood have long-term effects on emotional behavior adjustment. However, although a third of children were

affected by the chronic nature of their condition in their preschool years, at early adolescence, only a small proportion of those included in the dataset were regarded as having a "chronic condition." Also, the youngsters all rated themselves as "well adjusted," and there were no differences between the two groups regarding self-esteem and depression self-report scales. These data raise the need for long-term focused psychological support for children and their families who care for children with major congenital anomalies requiring surgery in the neonatal period.[72-74]

Thoracic surgery—general considerations

Some conditions diagnosed within the first 28 days of life require access to the thoracic cavity by way of thoracotomy or thoracoscopy. Neonatal thoracotomy is typically well tolerated in the short term. The recovery and return to normal physiologic function following neonatal thoracotomy is in contrast with that observed in adults—in which long-term pain and disability are more often realized in older patients. However, rapid neonatal "recovery" must be tempered by the potential for long-term chest wall growth abnormalities resulting from thoracotomy. Several types of orthopedic deformities have been described following neonatal thoracotomy, including scoliosis, rib deformities and synostosis, and shoulder deformities. Jaureguizar et al.[75] reported on 89 patients operated for EA via standard right posterolateral thoracotomy with a follow-up of 3–16 years. Of these, 32% had significant musculoskeletal deformities including "winged scapula," marked asymmetry of the thoracic cage from atrophy of the serratus anterior, rib fusion, and severe thoracic scoliosis.[75] Chetcuti et al.[76] reported on a similar experience in the study of 232 patients with esophageal congenital anomalies without preexistent congenital vertebral anomalies who underwent neonatal thoracotomy. In this series, 33% of patients later developed chest wall deformities, and 8% were reported to have scoliosis.[76] One of the purported benefits of minimally invasive access to the chest (thoracoscopy) for lung resection and repair of EA is the potential benefit of limiting this chest wall morbidity. The long-term outcome of minimally invasive access to the thorax requires assessment of this possible benefit. Because of the above concerns, many pediatric surgeons today utilize a muscle sparing thoracotomy through the auscultatory triangle while preserving the latissimus dorsi and serratus anterior musculature for infants. The long-term benefits of this type of approach also have not been reliably compared to that of a standard muscle splitting thoracotomy. Both of these newer approaches to thoracic access offer opportunities for the pediatric surgeon to assess the potential benefits of modern surgical technique to the long-term outcomes of neonatal thoracic surgery.

MALFORMATIONS OF THE TRACHEOBRONCHIAL TREE

Subglottic stenosis did not become an issue until prolonged endotracheal intubation and ventilation of neonates became commonplace in the mid-1960s. As survival of low birth weight infants increased, so did the number of patients with acquired laryngotracheal stenosis. Today, advances in the equipment utilized for neonatal endotracheal intubation, tube stabilization, and the recognition of the deleterious effects of prolonged transglottic instrumentation have decreased the incidence of laryngotracheal stenosis to less than 10%. In patients suffering significant laryngotracheal stenosis, the surgical options largely depend on the grade of stenosis realized. The functional outcomes of laryngotracheal reconstructive (LTR) surgery are clearly critical in the determination of long-term success. Studies evaluating exercise tolerance, speech, swallowing, and voice are at this point limited, owing to the relatively recent advances in the surgical correction of these disorders. Early studies of voice function after LTR surgery were entirely subjective assessments; however, recent studies in children have paired subjective observations with objective measurements.[77]

PULMONARY RESECTION

Pulmonary resection in the neonatal period may be undertaken for a congenital pulmonary airway malformation (formerly "CCAM"), pulmonary sequestration, or congenital lobar emphysema. The most significant long-term outcome facing patients undergoing neonatal pulmonary resection is that of respiratory function. Ayed and Owayed[78] reported on the safety of lung resection in the neonatal period for congenital malformations and found that none of the patients had physical limitations at a mean follow-up of 4 years. Also, Caussade et al.[79] reported normal spirometry values for vital capacity in 27 patients who underwent neonatal pulmonary lobectomy. Neonates undergoing lung resection can expect to have normal vital capacity due to the compensatory growth of the remaining lung, and most studies indicate that few children are functionally impaired by lung resection performed in the neonatal period. In addition, in patients who undergo pneumonectomy prior to the age of 5 years, ventilatory capacity is only minimally reduced when compared to that predicted for an individual with a complement of two normal lungs suggesting that "lung growth" occurs well beyond the neonatal period as a result of compensatory pulmonary hyperplasia.[80] Furthermore, no correlation could be found between age at lobectomy and future pulmonary function.[81] It appears that normal postnatal growth of lung parenchyma at the gas exchange (alveolar) level up to about 7–8 years of age contributes most of this additional reserve, as there is not regeneration of conducting airways. Whereas functional outcome studies have been limited in patients undergoing pulmonary resection in the neonatal period, reports of HRQoL are noticeably absent in this patient cohort. To date, there is no literature classifying the HRQoL of infants undergoing neonatal pulmonary resection.

MALFORMATIONS OF THE ESOPHAGUS

One of the most commonly performed operations undertaken by the pediatric surgeon in the neonatal period is the repair of EA and/or tracheoesophageal fistula. Mortality rates in patients with Waterson Risk Groups A and B EA are well below 5% overall. Today, the nature of coexisting anomalies that determine survival is best described by a newer risk stratification taking into account birth weight and the presence of cyanotic congenital heart disease.[82] Early surgical complications such as anastomotic leak, disruption, or stenosis are often associated with a favorable short-term outcome when adequately treated. In the long term, dysphagia and food impaction are the most common foregut issues facing the child with repaired EA. The motility of the esophagus is inherently abnormal to some degree in all patients despite "adequately" repaired EA.[83] Although symptoms of "choking with feeding," odynophagia, and "food impaction" are relatively common during childhood following EA repair, these problems tend to decline with age. Those who have persistent difficulties with swallowing are more likely to have or have had an esophageal stricture or significant gastroesophageal reflux. Today, radial balloon dilation of the esophagus under fluoroscopic control and medical and/or surgical control of reflux disease are useful adjuncts in the prevention of these long-term sequelae. Indeed, most adult survivors with repaired EA have minor persistent gastrointestinal symptoms such that less than 10% report dysphagia that occurs once a day, and the majority report no symptoms of gastroesophageal reflux.[84] While it is believed that persistent gastroesophageal reflux in patients undergoing EA repair contributes to dysphagia, there is little objective evidence of this. The majority of neonatal gastroesophageal reflux disease is a transient problem, can be mostly treated medically, and abates by childhood. However, a few studies report persistent gastroesophageal reflux in postoperative children after esophageal repair,[85–88] which in consequence, if untreated, can lead to esophagitis, metaplastic epithelial changes (gastric metaplasia or intestinal metaplasia), and esophageal adenocarcinoma. The metaplastic columnar mucosa, the so-called Barrett's esophagus, is found according to one study in 42% of EA patients.[87] Barrett's esophagus (BE) becomes an important risk factor for developing esophageal adenocarcinoma, and it is suggested the prevalence of BE in EA patients is higher and that it occurs at a much younger age.

Cancer in the upper gastrointestinal tract in EA patients has been described in 10 cases, of which 8 were esophageal carcinoma and 2 squamous cell carcinoma not related to the native esophagus (related to the lung and to a subcutaneous skin tube reconstruction).[89–95]

Given the high prevalence of BE, the early development of esophageal cancer, and the possible absence of symptoms in EA patients, surveillance programs seem warranted. Prospective long-term follow-up cohort studies, including endoscopic data of adult EA patients, are limited, and guidelines for follow-up are lacking.

Although adults with repaired EA may be at increased risk for developing esophageal malignancy, it is too early to tell whether or not the history of EA affects the incidence of esophageal carcinoma later in life. The concern is that esophageal dysmotility, poor esophageal clearance, and reduced lower esophageal sphincter pressure, even in the absence of symptoms, may lead to the development of Barrett's esophagus.

Several screening strategies have been suggested as a clinical screening in all patients aged 15–25 years, with endoscopy performed if any gastroesophageal reflex symptoms are present.[96] Another study suggested endoscopic surveillance at the ages of 15, 30, 40, 50, and 60 years, with intensification of this protocol if pathological observations are made: yearly in case of BE and 5-yearly in the presence of esophagitis, gastric metaplasia, severe esophageal strictures, recurrent tracheoesophageal fistula (TEF), severe GER symptoms, or the need for continuous anti-gastroesophageal reflex disease (GERD) medication.[86] Other endoscopy protocols suggest screening in all adults, from the age of 30 years for patients with significant primary surgery complications; from the age of 20 years, regardless of symptoms (5-yearly until the age of 30 years, 3-yearly until the age of 40 years, 2-yearly after 40 years of age); and screening once before adulthood with surveillance through adulthood with 5- to 10-year intervals (3-yearly in case of BE or twice a year with dysplasia).[87,88,93,97]

However, as more survivors make their way into adult and elderly life, this certainly should be a consideration for pediatric and adult surgeons caring for patients who have undergone EA repair. Follow-up should be vigilant and lifelong until the risk of malignant degeneration in these patients is better delineated.

To date, five studies have examined the HRQoL in children and adolescents after repair of EA.[33,98–101] These studies showed HRQoL experiences among children with EA and revealed that condition-specific HRQoL parameters concerned various aspects ranging from participation in play and sport, nutritional intake, social and emotional concerns, to body image issues. Several HRQoL experiences like those of stigma, isolated emotions, and impact of medical treatment are similar to those of children with other chronic health condition. As previously reported, children with EA suffer from feeding difficulties and growth retardation, particularly at early ages. Additionally, this study provides information that among EA children up to 17 years, feeding challenges and growth retardation can give rise to social and emotional strains such as being different from peers and being teased. Moreover, EA possibly affects the child's relationships and interactions with other people,[98,99] although improvement in the age group 8–13 years has been described.[100] Children with EA independent of surgical scar(s), scoliosis, or a winged scapula experienced concerns that were related to discomfort among others, to the sense of being different, or to dissatisfaction because of their appearance. Half of adults with EA had complaints of surgical scar(s), and 11% were disturbed by a disfigured or winged scapula. After esophageal replacement (mean age of patients was 34.5 years), esthetic results were the main problem, especially during adolescence. From the perspective of the pediatric surgeon, knowledge of HRQoL issues of significance to the EA children may improve the decision-making process of surgical technique and the patient–surgeon communication during the postoperative follow-up. It may permit identification of reduced HRQoL, presentation of well-directed patient and parent information, provision of relevant family support services, and, importantly, optimization of the postoperative medical management. A follow-up plan directed by the patient's needs and concerns might improve long-term health and HRQoL outcomes.

The perspectives of children with EA and their parents have been incorporated into the development of the first condition-specific HRQoL questionnaire for patients with EA.[38] According to the reported HRQoL experiences, EA interacts with various aspects of the child's life, especially among children with complex forms of EA. In addition to HRQoL issues of eating and drinking, social dimensions of relationships and interactions with other people appear to be prominent condition-specific parameters.

There are fewer problems more technically challenging for the pediatric surgeon than the patient with long-gap EA (LGEA). In the short term, the surgeon must decide on the appropriate management strategy for reconstruction of the esophageal conduit. There is a consensus among most pediatric surgeons that the conservation of the native esophagus is associated with the best postoperative results, and every effort should be made to conserve the native esophagus, as no other conduit can fully replace its function in transporting food from the oral cavity to the stomach satisfactorily. In the last 70 years, a number of innovative and sometimes controversial techniques have been introduced to reduce the distance between upper and lower esophageal segment to allow an anastomosis.[102] In 1981, Puri et al.[103] reported the observation that the spontaneous growth and hypertrophy of the esophageal segments in LGEA occur at a rate faster than overall somatic growth, in the absence of any form of mechanical stretching. The stimuli for such natural growth are the swallowing reflex and the reflux of gastric contents into the lower esophageal pouch.[104] Puri et al.[105] further noted that the maximal natural growth of the esophageal segments occurred during the first 8–12 weeks, and therefore, they suggested that the ideal time for delayed primary anastomosis (DPA) is when the infant is about 16 weeks old. A recent meta-analysis investigating long-term outcome of DPA showed that the majority of patients were able to feed normally and have normal growth and development curves after DPA.[102] However, the potential risk of Barrett's metaplasia highlights the need for continued long-term follow-up with regular endoscopic surveillance protocols as outlined above.

Although it is widely accepted that the optimal esophageal conduit is the native esophagus, some circumstances are prohibitive and surgeons use either colon, native stomach, or jejunal grafts to bridge abbreviated esophageal segments. Techniques for sequential and gradual elongation of the native esophagus such as those popularized by Foker et al.[106] and Kimura et al.[107] appear to offer favorable short-term surgical outcomes in the institutions where they are employed. These results have proven difficult to replicate, and the long-term adverse sequelae of either esophageal replacement or native esophageal lengthening remain significant. In a recent study from the Great Ormond Street Hospital, the vast majority of patients undergoing LGEA repair had long-term issues with gastroesophageal reflux.[108] A report from The Children's Hospital of Los Angeles concluded that patients with a gastric conduit had a lower overall complication rate without evidence of conduit ischemia when compared to those with a colonic interposition; however, the incidence of long-term adverse physiologic sequelae was significant. In a review of published studies for esophageal replacement in children by Arul and Parikh,[109] there was no significant difference in either early or late complications associated with the different type of conduits utilized for interposition. However, the authors did note that larger series tended to have lower complication rates than those of small series, likely reflecting the association between clinical expertise and experience and outcomes in larger surgical centers.

The short- and long-term physiologic outcome of EA and tracheoesophageal fistula could be considered favorable. However, little data exist about HRQoL in this cohort of patients. Furthermore, the long-term follow-up of patients with EA and the impact of Barrett's esophagitis and later development of adenocarcinoma is yet to be fully realized and mandates vigilant postoperative follow-up and a surveillance program that should be overseen by a practicing pediatric surgeon.

CONGENITAL DIAPHRAGMATIC HERNIA

CDH has been widely studied. The mortality rate and adverse sequelae in survivors of CDH remain significant compared to the other commonly treated newborn surgical conditions addressed by the pediatric surgeon. Historically, the long-term follow-up of patients with CDH was sporadic and uncoordinated. This likely led to an underestimation of the number and severity of problems affecting survivors of CDH repair. Data from long-term follow-up studies identify several potential morbidities involving a number of different organ systems including pulmonary, cardiac, neurologic, gastrointestinal, urogenital, and musculoskeletal systems. Today, it is recognized that these patients are best cared for in a multidisciplinary setting where coordinated follow-up care involving multiple specialties is possible.[110,111] Although this is not a widespread practice among pediatric surgeons, large pediatric centers are encouraged to develop these types of outcome clinics to coordinate follow-up and address ongoing physiologic concerns among survivors of CDH.[112] Indeed, the most remarkable accomplishment in dealing and caring for a patient with CDH is the improved survival to hospital discharge during the past decade.[113,114] However, while some authors have reported survival figures approaching 90%,[115] the current overall survival in the Unites States is 70% among 2676 live-born infants from 50 tertiary centers.[116]

The Congenital Diaphragmatic Hernia Study Group (CDHSG) is an international consortium of centers that prospectively collect and voluntarily contribute data about live-born CDH patients they manage. In total, 8279 patients were in the database as of June 2014. The vast majority are neonates (7998; 96.6%), although 281 patients were late presenters. Overall mortality decreased from >35% in 1995 to under <30% in 2013.

They reported 2014 data of more than 5000 infants (including 1127 preterm infants), compiled for over 15 years. The overall survival rate of infants in the cohort was 68.7%; term infants had a significantly higher survival rate than preterm infants: 73.1% versus 53.5%, respectively. Mortality was inversely proportional to estimated gestational age (EGA) at birth. The overall survival rate for the most premature infants, ≤28 weeks EGA, was 31.6%. Preterm infants were twice as likely as term infants to have chromosomal anomalies or cardiac defects. Whereas 86% of term infants underwent operative repair, 69% of preterm infants underwent repair. The percentage of infants who underwent operative repair decreased with decreasing gestational age.[117]

For those CDH patients who do survive to hospital discharge, long-term morbidity is a function of the severity and laterality of the defect as well as the need for extracorporeal membrane oxygenation (ECLS).[71,118,119]

Pulmonary morbidity is perhaps the most significant problem during early childhood in survivors of CDH.[120–124] Ventilatory barotrauma, bronchopulmonary dysplasia (BPD), and chronic lung disease play a larger role than previously suspected in both mortality and morbidity of those patients with CDH.[113,125] The prevalence of BPD was reported to be 41% in CDH neonates who survived until day 30. Furthermore, the severity of chronic lung disease in CDH survivors may require prolonged ventilator support and tracheostomy. CDH survivors may also suffer from recurrent respiratory tract infections in infancy and early childhood.[111,120,126] Nearly 60% of survivors require some form of medical therapy for reactive airway disease, and long-term obstructive airway disease is demonstrable in approximately 25% of patients at 5 years of follow-up.[127,128] The long-term sequelae of ventilation–perfusion mismatch may also result in significant limitations in exercise tolerance in the adolescent years.[47] Mild airway obstruction and a slightly reduced diffusion capacity for carbon monoxide are observed in most survivors of CDH.

Furthermore, pulmonary hypertension and subsequent right ventricular hypertrophy have been reported in as many as 50% of survivors of CDH treated with ECLS.[129] Nutritional morbidity and growth failure are also, unfortunately, common in patients surviving CDH. In a retrospective analysis of 121 survivors of CDH, over half of the patients were below the 25% for height and weight during the first year of life.[130] Approximately one-third of this population had issues severe enough to require a gastrostomy to provide adequate caloric intake. In two similar studies, gastrostomy tubes needed to be placed in one-third of patients in two survival cohorts due to nutritional morbidity.[70,111]

The need for ECLS and an oxygen requirement at discharge are predictive of growth failure within the first year of life. Others have reported similar trends in growth failure and nutritional morbidity.[131,132] Oral aversion, foregut dysmotility, and persistent GERD all contribute to the nutritional morbidity of CDH survivors.[123,133] Nearly 40% of babies operated on for CDH will have symptomatic GER, half of whom require antireflux surgery. The most frequently reported predictor of antireflux surgery is the need of diaphragmatic patch repair. Recurrence is more common in patients repaired with a prosthetic patch.[71,120]

Neurocognitive deficits play a significant role in the long-term functional outcome of CDH patients surviving to discharge. Bouman and colleagues reported mild to moderate development delay in more than one-third of CDH survivors followed in a multidisciplinary clinic.[134] Although the neurologic deficits in CDH survivors are the result of the critical nature of the postnatal disease process and its treatment, the contribution of ECLS on neurologic morbidity is of significant concern. The incidence of neurologic abnormalities among all neonatal survivors of ECLS ranges from 10% to 15% and includes CP, hearing loss, seizure disorder, cognitive delay, and vision impairment. However, the use of ECLS in CDH patients confers an increased risk for long-term neurocognitive impairment such that up to 70% of survivors demonstrate some type of neurocognitive deficit.[123,135–137] SNHL has also been frequently reported in CDH survivors.[111] Potential predisposing factors, including the use of ototoxic medications and prolonged mechanical ventilations with high oxygen tensions, lead to SNHL, which is found in CDH survivors treated with and without ECMO, suggesting that the use of ECMO is not the only predisposing factor for SNHL.[65,138] However, several retrospective studies found that the SNHL rate in both ECMO and non-ECMO CDH survivors is between 2.3% and 7.5%,[139–141] which approximates the SNHL rate for all neonatal intensive care unit patients.[111,142]

The orthopedic deformities associated with CDH are also of significance in that CDH survivors are prone to scoliosis and chest wall deformities. Nobuhra reported a 21% incidence of pectus deformities and a 10% incidence of mild to moderate scoliosis in long-term follow-up. These are more common among patients with an initial severe ventilatory impairment and a diaphragmatic defect requiring the need for a prosthetic patch placement.[110,112] It has been observed that these complex long-term issues appear more prevalent as newer support strategies have allowed infants with severe disease to survive.

Regarding HRQoL of CDH survivors, Peetsold et al.[101] have described a significant reduction and perception of general health in survivors of CDH compared to a reference population. Poorer functional status has also been described in CDH survivors in a recent study using the FSIIR tool.[143] These findings have been confirmed by Michel et al.,[144] who also reported a reduced QoL in children after CDH repair. They also report GER as a major marker on impact of QoL in these patients.

Furthermore, in a study from the Children's Hospital of Boston, the impact upon family was found to be profound and longstanding at a median of 8 years after surgery for a subset of CDH survivors with comorbidities and current clinical problems.[145]

ABDOMINAL CONDITIONS

General considerations

Apart from the repair of an inguinal hernia, abdominal conditions in the neonate comprise the majority of work performed by the practicing pediatric surgeon. The long-term outcome of a variety of these conditions is dependent on the method of peritoneal access. The two most significant potential adverse outcomes of laparotomy include adhesive bowel obstruction and incisional hernia. In a study from the Great Ormond Street Hospital, the authors described only four documented cases of incisional hernia in 507 pediatric laparotomies.[146] More salient to the intra-abdominal conditions of the neonate is the potential for adhesive bowel obstruction following laparotomy or laparoscopy. In a study of 649 neonates undergoing laparotomy over 10 years, 8.3% developed adhesive intestinal obstruction requiring surgical intervention.[147] In a similar study from the Netherlands of 304 neonates undergoing laparotomy, adhesive intestinal obstruction occurred in 3.3% of the cases.[148] The indication for laparotomy clearly plays a role in the incidence of postoperative adhesive bowel obstruction. In patients undergoing a Ladd's procedure, 8%–15% of patients experience one episode of postoperative adhesive bowel obstruction.[147] Techniques to prevent intestinal adhesions emphasize minimizing peritoneal trauma and separating potentially involved surfaces. Clearly one of the benefits of minimal access surgery or laparoscopic surgery is in the potential decrease in the incidence of adhesive bowel obstruction, although persuasive long-term data are yet to be realized in supporting this contention. Also, minimally invasive access to the abdominal cavity does result in a postoperative cosmetic result that is preferred by many patients, after they grow into adulthood.[149] Indeed, a noticeable scar can have physical, esthetic, and psychological consequences in children.[150] Cosmetic concerns with regard to abdominal wall scarring are likely to be more important for neonates as they grow into the teenage years. Minimizing these concerns is probably a unique benefit of minimal access neonatal surgery. Other purported benefits of minimal access laparoscopic surgery are that of a decreased inflammatory response, less postoperative pain with a subsequent reduction in the need for postoperative analgesia, and a shorter time to hospital discharge.[151–153]

Gastroschisis

The outcome of the majority of patients affected by gastroschisis is considered good in terms of growth in 75% of the cases[154,155]; the neurodevelopmental outcome seems comparable to gestational age-matched control,[155–157] and there is the possibility of reproduction and improvement in the overall QoL.[155,158] Although a minority of these infants are affected, the major impact on QoL is the occurrence of short bowel syndrome. Infants affected by short bowel syndrome can be entirely or partially dependent on total parenteral nutrition (TPN). Two-thirds can be weaned off TPN eventually, but the risk of malabsorption and nutritional deficiencies has to be considered and potentially corrected throughout their life. Some of them will remain dependent on TPN, and this anomaly still represents the largest cohort of candidates for intestinal transplantation.

On the other hand, the incidence and morbidity of intestinal adhesions leading to small bowel obstruction are estimated as 15%–27% in gastroschisis, with a mortality rate for bowel obstruction of 15%, and chronic abdominal pain is more common in these patients than in healthy peers.[155,158,159]

There is concern about the impact of adhesions among fertile women. Over 30% of women who undergo reproductive tract summary required readmission for adhesions,[160] but pregnancy is described in patients previously affected by gastroschisis, meaning that for these women, both the reproductive system and abdominal capacity can be adequate. Testicles herniated at birth in gastroschisis patients and relocated into the abdomen at first operation may descend into the scrotum spontaneously in 50% of the cases.[155,161,162] Also, the ability to participate in sports is reported as comparable to healthy peers.[155,163] The last concern is cosmesis. Indeed, 60% of patients without an umbilicus experience some psychological stress.[155,158,164] For this reason, different techniques of umbilical reconstruction are available, mainly performed by plastic surgeons at a later age or pediatric surgeons at initial repair.[155,165,166]

Omphalocele

Some long-term medical problems occur in patients with large omphaloceles. These include gastroesophageal reflux, pulmonary insufficiency, recurrent lung infections or asthma, and feeding difficulty with failure to thrive, reported in up to 60% of infants with giant omphalocele. A third of patients with omphalocele report intermittent abdominal pain persisting into young adulthood. The respiratory insufficiency associated with giant omphaloceles may be secondary to abnormal thoracic development with a narrow thorax and small lung area leading to pulmonary hypoplasia. However, a study looking at the long-term cardiopulmonary consequences of large abdominal wall defects reported normal lung volumes and oxygen consumption on long-term follow-up, although exercise tolerance was slightly reduced.[155,163] In the long-term follow-up, the most widespread concern for patients with omphalocele is cosmesis, with nearly one-half of patients expressing dissatisfaction with the lack of an umbilicus and for the large abdominal wall scar. Recent studies showed how this aspect did not affect the overall QoL, and different techniques of umbilical reconstruction have been proposed mainly by

plastic surgeons that are, usually, performed at the request of the patient.[155,163,165,166] However, this issue did not influence the QoL, which is comparable to that of healthy young adults. Parents with fetal diagnosis of omphalocele and parents of newborns with omphalocele should be informed that the high burden of surgical interventions their child will need is likely to result in good health condition in the long term, especially if there are no associated anomalies.[155,167] Patients are at risk for adhesive bowel obstruction, and a small number not treated for malrotation could develop devastating midgut volvulus with subsequent short bowel syndrome. A recent study from the Netherlands indicates that after a high level of medical intervention in early life, minor and giant omphalocele patients report similar long-term results, and the QoL in both groups is comparable to that of healthy young adults.[155,159] For the surviving patients affected by Beckwith–Wiedemann syndrome (EMG syndrome: exomphalos, macroglossia, and gigantism), a regular follow-up must be organized to make an early diagnosis of Wilms or hepatoblastoma tumor, frequently associated with this syndrome.[155,168]

Malformations of the midgut

The most profound sequelae of neonatal surgical conditions involving the midgut involve massive small bowel resection or malabsorption and altered motility. Thankfully, the outcomes of intestinal failure due to short bowel syndrome have changed dramatically over the last 30 years. The development of TPN introduced a new era in the management of children with short bowel syndrome.[169] Although the functional impairment in short bowel patients typically results from an anatomic loss or deficiency of intestinal surface area, it may also occur in the setting of a normal intestinal mucosal surface with perturbations in intestinal absorption, motility, or both. The length of the small bowel is clearly an important predictor of the development of short bowel syndrome; however, the absolute length of "viable" small intestine in the neonatal population may not be an adequate predictor of short bowel syndrome and intestinal failure. Today the consensus for the definition for short bowel syndrome is "intestinal failure as a result of surgical resection or congenital defect or disease which is associated and characterized by the inability to maintain protein-energy fluid and electrolyte or micronutrient balances on an accepted normal diet."[170] Although the amount of bowel that must be lost to produce malabsorption in short bowel syndrome is variable and depends on segments lost and whether the ileocecal valve is preserved, loss of greater than 80% of the small bowel is associated with an increased requirement for enteral nutritional support, decreased overall survival, and the need for further surgical intervention or small bowel transplantation. The neonatal surgical population at risk for developing short bowel syndrome include patients with necrotizing enterocolitis, small intestinal atresia, malrotation and midgut volvulus, and gastroschisis. The complications encountered in short bowel syndrome are varied in complexity and dependent on a variety of factors. Survival rates reported for short bowel syndrome are influenced by the variable severity of the condition, underlying disorders, and comorbidities. Potential complications are myriad and can include diarrhea and electrolyte disturbances, osteopenia, urinary oxalate stone formation, and TPN-associated liver disease. Also, the achievement of normal somatic growth is a challenge for the patient with short bowel syndrome. The most common causes of mortality following massive small intestinal resection in the neonate include liver failure and sepsis in patients requiring TPN for the majority of their nutritional support. Also, the care of the patient with short bowel syndrome entails substantial economic expense. In 1992, the annual direct cost per home for patients requiring TPN averaged approximately US$100,000.[171] A current cohort study of home parenteral nutrition patients enrolled 1251 patients between August 2011 and February 2014; of the 1251 patients, 15% (n = 188) were infants and children, with a mean age of 4.9 ± 4.9 years and with short bowel syndrome the most frequently reported TPN indication.[172] Also, the complex medical needs and potential complications of the short bowel syndrome have a clear and obvious impact on HRQoL. Although the development of home parenteral nutrition programs has provided greater independence from the hospital for these patients, the responsibility has been shifted to caretakers, which has a profound impact on the family.[173] Unfortunately, there are a few rigorous assessments of the obvious psychosocial impact of this chronic illness on both patients and their families. In adults requiring home TPN, and assessed using the SF-36, social and emotional function, as well as the QoL, were lower in patients requiring home parenteral nutrition associated with a poor QoL compared to those with short bowel syndrome, not on TPN.[174] Although it is intuitive that the QoL for both patients and their parents suffering from short bowel syndrome resulting from neonatal surgical conditions is likely to be low, about normal, the real question is whether or not subsequent surgical interventions may improve the QoL for these patients. Surgical treatment beyond the neonatal period (i.e., Bianchi procedure, longitudinal intestinal lengthening and tailoring, and the STEP procedure) may offer hope for improving the QoL for these patients.[175] Also, developing nonsurgical enteral support strategies beyond the scope of this review offers some promise.

In those patients surviving to small intestinal transplantation, relevant outcome measures include graft and patient survival. In a study from the University of Pittsburgh, the overall patient survival at 5 years following small bowel and intestinal transplantation was 56%.[176,177] At the University of Miami, the 2-year survival rate following small intestinal transplantation between 1997 and 2000 was 46%, although the current 1-year survival is approximately 85% due to improvements in surgical technique and immunosuppressive care.[178] Furthermore, combined transplantation of the intestine and the liver is associated with a 40% graft survival at 5 years,[179] although patient survival is best with isolated intestinal grafts. Both graft and patient survival will likely continue to improve with time. Also encouraging is that HRQoL is improved with intestinal transplantation in patients with short bowel syndrome. Sudan et al.[180] obtained the QoL data from 29 successful pediatric transplant patients and found that patients had comparable CHQ assessments to norms in physical function role, social limitation, general health, bodily pain, role limitations, self-esteem, health, and behavior. O'Keefe et al.[176] reported a significant improvement in overall assessment of QoL in 13 of 26 of the specific domains examined in a cohort of 46 patients after small bowel transplantation. All patients were weaned from TPN by a median of 18 days (range 1–117 days) and from tube feeding by day 69 (range 22–272 days. Their results are promising such that, with continued progress, it can potentially become an alternative to HPN for the management of permanent intestinal failure.[176]

However, the parental assessment was lower than the children in general health perception and role imitation. From a public health standpoint, the financial and emotional costs for caregivers must impact decisions regarding the allocation of medical resources. Long-term outcomes of the surgical treatment of intestinal failure including intestinal transplantation must include assessments of HRQoL, functional outcome, and utility such that families can make appropriate decisions in the neonatal period when faced with the potential for short bowel syndrome.

Malformations of the hind gut

ANORECTAL MALFORMATIONS

The QoL and functional outcomes related to anorectal malformations and their attendant surgeries must be examined with care. Perhaps one of the most notable contributions to the technical practice of pediatric surgery over the last several decades is that of the posterior sagittal approach to the repair of anorectal malformations popularized by Dr. Alberto Pena.[181] However, as advances in surgical technique have allowed us to recreate the anatomic relationships in the perineum with greater short-term "success," the functional outcomes are less clear and appear more dependent on the type of malformation encountered rather than the surgical approach.[182,183] The common relevant "functional" outcome measure is that of bowel control. We are most interested in the ability for a child to defecate normally commensurate with his or her peers. However, the implications of constipation and incontinence also have a significant impact on HRQoL.

In patients with anorectal malformations, associated anatomic malformations of the genitourinary tract, a deficient sacrum (sacral ratio <0.4), or tethered cord not only affect the surgical complexity but also impact the functional outcome and QoL. Continued evaluation after the neonatal period must address the functional sequelae of anorectal malformations. Simply put, two parameters of bowel control are particularly salient to the child with an anorectal malformation. The first is the capacity for voluntary bowel movements (VBMs). The second is the incidence of soiling or defecation between bowel movements that is uncontrolled and unwanted. The patient who can verbalize a desire to pass stool and uses the commode to pass VBMs has a significant advantage over the individual who has never had VBMs following the repair of an anorectal malformation. The latter patients are physiologically incontinent, that is, with either sensory or muscular failure (or both), and represent a specific category. In terms of soiling, Levitt and Peña[184] have categorized patients with soiling into two "grades." Grade 1 patients soil once or twice a week, where there is a spot or smear of stool in the underwear. The patient who soils every day is considered to have grade 2 soiling. Clinically, this is a straightforward and practical way to categorize patients in long-term follow-up. However, for long-term functional outcome studies, disease-specific scores to assess and quantify bowel control in these patients may be useful for academic purposes. Brandt et al.[185] have developed and validated a continence scale in children with anorectal malformations termed the Baylor Continence Scale. This disease-specific functional outcome measure is administered by recording the responses to 23 questions using a psychometric response analog scale, and the higher the score, the more significant the impact on continence. Higher scores were noted in their population of patients with anorectal malformation (ARM) compared with both enuresis and normal control groups. This type of scoring system may allow pediatric surgeons and physicians to be able to quantitate qualitative data as it relates to the postoperative function following the repair of anorectal malformations. Overall, the most salient predictor of bowel control is related to the type of anorectal malformation, bladder neck fistula, prostatic fistula, and bulbar fistula, since each one of these has a different prognosis.[183,186] Indeed, children with a perineal fistula are likely to be continent but have a higher likelihood of constipation. After anterior sagittal anorectoplasty for perineal or vestibular fistula in females, two of three patients are likely to achieve bowel control comparable to normal in the long term, and the vast majority will be socially continent.[187] Also, the majority of patients with rectal–urethral fistula achieve social continence, although for some this will require intervention with antegrade continence enema (ACE) bowel management. Approximately one-third may report VBMs and complete continence.[188] On the other hand, male patients with a rectobladder neck fistula are more likely to be incontinent of stool compared to their anatomically normal peers.[182,183]

About 50% of female patients with cloacal malformation attain fecal and urinary continence. The remaining half stay clean or dry by adjunctive measures such as bowel management by enemas or ACE channel, and continent urinary diversion or intermittent catheterization. Problems related to genital organs such as obstructed menstruations, amenorrhea, and introitus stenosis are common and often require secondary surgery. Encouragingly, most adolescent and adult patients are capable of sexual life despite often complex vaginal primary and secondary reconstructions.

Also, cloacal malformation does not preclude pregnancies, although they still are relatively rare. Pregnant patients with cloaca require special care and follow-up to guarantee uncomplicated delivery and preservation of anorectal and urinary functions. Cesarean section is recommended for cloaca patients. The self-reported QoL of cloaca patients appears to be comparable to that of female patients with less complex anorectal malformations.[189,190]

Assessment of comprehensive HRQoL in patients with ARM has been undertaken in a number of studies. The Euro QoL score has been validated in children with a history of anorectal malformation and repair.[26] In addition, disease-specific QoL questionnaires have been developed.[34,191,192] In the Brandt study from 2007, patients with anorectal malformations, in general, had a lower HRQoL score (CHQ) compared to both enuresis patients and a normal control group. Utilizing a disease-specific QoL questionnaire, Grano et al.[193] found that adults with previously repaired ARMs reported significantly lower emotional functioning and problems in the area of body image and physical symptoms when compared to those patients in the control group. In Hartman et al.'s[192] study, HRQoL is directly related to the nature and severity of the anorectal malformation. Children and adolescents with anorectal malformations reported better QoL over time. This could be attributed to coping mechanisms, utilization of a bowel management program, or more specific attention by the medical community to addressing the psychological and physiological needs of these patients in their societal context. However, approximately 13% of male ARM reported erectile dysfunction, while 50% female ARM reported sexual dysfunction not related to the QoL or type of malformation. Both ARM patients felt a need for better addressing of their sexual concerns during medical care.[194] Although psychological functioning is typically an attribute of HRQoL, specific psychological effects of anorectal malformations and their repair are also clinically relevant. A high proportion of children with previously repaired ARMs have clinically significant emotional problems based on psychiatric diagnostic interviews. Despite normal intelligence, more than half of these patients received special education or remedial teaching. In addition, problems with sustained attention were found. These findings are important for long-term care.[195] Approximately 29% of children were found to have a psychiatric disorder, with 19% having disorders severe enough to influence their daily lives.[196,197] This was significantly higher than the general child population in the United Kingdom, where the rate of a significant psychiatric disorder is 10%. Other studies have delineated similar findings.[198,199]

HIRSCHSPRUNG'S DISEASE

During the past decades, one-stage transanal endorectal pull-through (TEPT) has become one of the most commonly performed procedures for infants with Hirschsprung's disease (HD). This can be performed totally transanally or in combination with transabdominal colonic mobilization using laparotomy or laparoscopy.[200–203] The recognition of enterocolitis and its prompt treatment have decreased the short-term morbidity and mortality associated with this disorder. Early diagnosis of the disease, improvements in neonatal and anesthetic care, and surgical technical advancement have allowed for successful and prompt surgical treatment in the neonatal period. However, it has been suggested that bowel mobilization and dissection through the anus has the potential to interfere with anal sphincter integrity and rectal sensation.[200–210] For long-term outcomes, bowel function and continence again become the most salient issues. All of the operations utilized in the treatment of HD carry some risk of constipation. In most series, the severity of constipation following repair decreases with time or resolves. However, it is important to recognize and treat constipation in the postoperative period so as to prevent the long-term functional impairment of the pull-through segment. The occurrence of fecal soiling in patients who have undergone repair of HD can also affect the QoL. Indeed, the complete or partial loss of the rectal reservoir is an inevitable result of pull-through operations for HD owing to the loss or diminution of the high amplitude peristaltic contractions. The incidence of true fecal incontinence is low regardless of the operative technique utilized to address HD. However, when postoperative fecal soiling is critically assessed in childhood, the proportion of patients with some degree of fecal incontinence or soiling is approximately 50%.[27,211–214] In a cohort of 194 patients reported by Menezes and Puri, 68% ($n = 132$) of the patients had normal bowel function. Also, there was no demonstrable difference in bowel function related to the type of pull-through operation performed. They concluded that the majority of patients with HD continue to have disturbances of bowel function for many years, but most of them will attain normal continence.[215] Another study by Mills et al.[211] assessed functional outcome and HRQoL in 51 patients who had undergone surgical treatment for HD. The mean continence score as assessed by this instrument was 3.34 and categorized as "fair"; however, there was statistically significant improvement in fecal continence scores with age, confirming the previous speculation of improvement for this particular entity with time. Only 7% reported poor fecal continence in the teenage years. Good fecal continence was reported in 80% of teenagers. Utilizing the PedsQL score for HRQoL assessment, these authors found that there was no statistically significant difference between patients with HD and healthy children, either overall or by age group. Interestingly, females had noticeably higher QoL compared to their male cohorts, which also corroborates the long-held view that females with HD may fare better than their male counterparts. They state that fecal continence is a significant predictor of overall QoL in children surgically treated for HD. Although continence tends to improve with age, a number of older children still have ongoing continence problems, and they seem to be a group at risk for impaired QoL.[211] Neuvonen et al.[202] report in a cohort of 79 patients that compared with matched peers, significant impairment of fecal control prevails after TEPT in HD patients during childhood, but symptoms diminish with age. Although overall QoL appeared comparable to controls, impairment of emotional and sexual domains may be present in adulthood.[202] Another cohort of 47 patients demonstrated similar results for QoL in adults when compared to controls. However, some of them have impaired bowel function and QoL.[216]

The long-term outcomes for total colonic aganglionosis (TCA) are clearly inferior to those after surgery for classic HD.[217–220] A specific complication associated with TCA is recurrent enterocolitis, which is a long-term problem among these patients. Reports of enterocolitis post pull-through range from 2% to 55%.[217,220–222] Soiling and fecal incontinence during childhood and beyond are common in TCA patients. At least one-tird of the patients with TCA still suffer from frank fecal incontinence later in childhood or at adolescence.[217–220,223–225] Although the stooling frequency decreases over time, persistent incontinence during day- and nighttime in many of these patients has significant psychosocial implications.[217,220,225] Because of intractable incontinence or recurrent enterocolitis, some patients have opted for permanent or long-term bowel diversion. The percentage of TCA patients ending up to permanent ileostomy ranges between 5% and 18%.[217,220,224]

A significant incidence of day- or nighttime enuresis has been reported in addition to urodynamic abnormalities in children with operated HD. Urinary dysfunction was more common in patients with Swenson or Duhamel operation than in those with endorectal pull-through.[220,226]

Metabolic complications are common after repair of TCA. Growth retardation in childhood is common; it extends to adolescence and affects mainly body weight. In recent reports, severe long-term failure to thrive is, however, uncommon. Body weights and heights below the third percentile have been reported in 5%–15% of patients.[218,220,223,224]

In patients with HD, 11% of males and 53% of females report problems in the psychosexual well-being after pull-through procedures, indicating, as in patients with ARM, a need for better addressing sexual concerns during medical care.[194]

Overall, the long-term functional outcome expectancy of operated HD in terms of fecal and urinary continence is, today, relatively optimistic. Although some degree of bowel dysfunction and defect in fecal continence remain permanent in many patients, a majority of patients reaching adolescence and adulthood can maintain themselves socially continent. In some patients, however, this may require specific bowel management programs.

CONCLUSION

Today, the pediatric surgeon interested in the study of long-term outcomes must be cognizant of the tools available for outcome assessment and choose the instrument most appropriate for the patient population in question. Selection of the appropriate tool to measure an outcome is as important as the act of measuring it. Furthermore, although it is important to give emphasis to development and appropriate use of outcome instruments, it is imperative that we think of ways in which to improve the QoL or physical, cognitive, or social functioning of our patients. Interventions aimed at improving QoL may play an important adjunct in positively affecting the health of infants and children as they make the transition into adult life (i.e., counseling to teach children better coping skills, support groups, or psychological therapy). Excellent instruments already exist in the realm of generic HRQoL and functional outcomes. Choosing the appropriate instrument is dependent on knowing what the instrument is capable of measuring. National and international organizations dedicated to the surgical care of infants and children would do well to recommend specific generic or disease-specific instruments such that clinicians can utilize equalities of scale when comparing HRQoL or functional outcomes following the surgical correction of congenital or acquired disease. We owe it to our pediatric surgical patients to utilize these instruments, validate them in pediatric surgical populations, and employ strategies to ultimately improve outcomes.

REFERENCES

1. Codman EA. *The Shoulder: Rupture of the Supraspinatus Tendon and Other Lesions in or about the Subacromial Bursa.* Malabar, FL: RE Kreiger, 1934.
2. Field MJ, Tranquada RE, Feasley JC. *Health Services Research: Work Force and Educational Issues.* National Academies of Science, Institute of Medicine, Washington D.C.: National Academies Press, 1995.
3. Lieu TA, Newman TB. Issues in studying the effectiveness of health services for children. *Health Serv Res* 1998; 33: 1041–58.
4. Ware JE Jr. The status of health assessment 1994. *Ann Rev Publ Health* 1995; 16: 327–54.
5. Patrick DL, Deyo RA. Generic and disease-specific measures in assessing health status and quality of life. *Med Care* 1989; S217–32.
6. Hays RD, Anderson R, Revicki D. Psychometric considerations in evaluating health-related quality of life measures. *Qual Life Res* 1993; 2: 441–9.
7. Kozinetz CA, Warren RW, Berseth CL, Aday LA, Sachdeva R, Kirkland RT. Health status of children with special health care needs: Measurement issues and instruments. *Clin Pediatr* 1999; 38: 525–33.
8. Colver A, Jessen C. Measurement of health status and quality of life in neonatal follow-up studies. *Semin Neonatol* 2000; 5: 149–57.
9. Landgraf JM, Maunsell E, Speechley KN et al. Canadian-French, German and UK versions of the Child Health Questionnaire: Methodology and preliminary item scaling results. *Qual Life Res* 1998; 7: 433–45.
10. Drotar D. *Measuring Health-Related Quality of Life in Children and Adolescents: Implications for Research and Practice.* New York: Psychology Press, 2014.
11. Theunissen NCM, Vogels TGC, Koopman HM et al. The proxy problem: Child report versus parent report in health-related quality of life research. *Qual Life Res* 1998; 7: 387–97.
12. Bullinger M. German translation and psychometric testing of the SF-36 health survey: Preliminary results from the IQOLA project. *Soc Sci Med* 1995; 41: 1359–66.
13. Griebsch I, Coast J, Brown J. Quality-adjusted life-years lack quality in pediatric care: A critical review of published cost-utility studies in child health. *Pediatrics* 2005; 115: e600–14.
14. Higginson IJ, Carr AJ. Using quality of life measures in the clinical setting. *BMJ* 2001; 322: 1297–300.
15. Varni JW, Limbers CA, Burwinkle TM. Impaired health-related quality of life in children and adolescents with chronic conditions: A comparative analysis of 10 disease clusters and 33 disease categories/severities utilizing the PedsQL™ 4.0 Generic Core Scales. *Health Qual Life Outcomes* 2007; 5: 1.
16. Starfield B, Ensminger M, Riley A et al. Adolescent health status measurement: Development of the Child Health and Illness Profile. *Pediatrics* 1993; 91: 430–5.
17. Ware JE, Sherbourne CD. The MOS 36-item short-form health survey (SF-36). I. Conceptual framework and item selection. *Med Care* 1992; 30: 473–83.
18. McHorney CA, Ware JE, Raczek AE. The MOS 36-Item Short-Form Health Survey (SF-36): II. Psychometric and clinical tests of validity in measuring physical and mental health constructs. *Med Care* 1993; 31: 247–63.
19. Raat H, Bonsel GJ, Essink-Bot M-L, Landgraf JM, Gemke RJBJ. Reliability and validity of comprehensive health status measures in children: The Child Health Questionnaire in relation to the Health Utilities Index. *J Clin Epidemiol* 2002; 55: 67–76.
20. Raat H, Mangunkusumo RT, Landgraf JM, Kloek G, Brug J. Feasibility, reliability, and validity of adolescent health status measurement by the Child Health Questionnaire Child Form (CHQ-CF): Internet administration compared with the standard paper version. *Qual Life Res* 2007; 16: 675–85.
21. Ravens-Sieberer U, Bullinger M. Assessing health-related quality of life in chronically ill children with the German KINDL: First psychometric and content analytical results. *Qua Life Res* 1998; 7: 399–407.
22. Rankin J, Glinianaia SV, Jardine J, McConachie H, Borrill H, Embleton ND. Measuring self-reported quality of life in 8- to 11-year-old children born with gastroschisis: Is the KIDSCREEN questionnaire acceptable. *Birth Defects Res A Clin Mol Teratol* 2016; 106(4): 250–6.

23. Smits M, van Lennep M, Vrijlandt R et al. Pediatric achalasia in the Netherlands: Incidence, clinical course, and quality of life. *J Pediatr* 2016; 169: 110–5.e3.

24. Wasson JW, Kairys SW, Nelson EC, Kalishman N, Baribeau P. A short survey for assessing health and social problems of adolescents. *J Fam Pract* 1994; 38: 489–95.

25. Poley MJ, Brouwer WB, van Exel NJ, Tibboel D. Assessing health-related quality-of-life changes in informal caregivers: An evaluation in parents of children with major congenital anomalies. *Qual Life Res* 2012; 21: 849–61.

26. Stolk EA, Busschbach JJ, Vogels T. Performance of the EuroQol in children with imperforate anus. *Qual Life Res* 2000; 9: 29–38.

27. Bai Y, Chen H, Hao J, Huang Y, Wang W. Long-term outcome and quality of life after the Swenson procedure for Hirschsprung's disease. *J Pediatr Surg* 2002; 37: 639–42.

28. Fernández Ibieta M, Sánchez Morote JM, Martínez Castaño I et al. [Quality of life and long term results in Hirschsprung's disease]. *Cir Pediatr* 2014; 27: 117–24.

29. Witvliet MJ, Slaar A, Heij HA, van der Steeg AF. Qualitative analysis of studies concerning quality of life in children and adults with anorectal malformations. *J Pediatr Surg* 2013; 48: 372–9.

30. Poley MJ, Stolk EA, Tibboel D, Molenaar JC, Busschbach JJ. Short term and long term health related quality of life after congenital anorectal malformations and congenital diaphragmatic hernia. *Arch Dis Child* 2004; 89: 836–41.

31. Gatti C, di Abriola GF, Villa M et al. Esophagogastric dissociation versus fundoplication: Which is best for severely neurologically impaired children. *J Pediatr Surg* 2001; 36: 677–80.

32. Dickson A, Clarke M, Tawfik R, Thomas AG. Caregivers' perceptions following gastrostomy in severely disabled children with feeding problems. *Dev Med Child Neurol* 1997; 39: 746–51.

33. Ludman L, Spitz L. Quality of life after gastric transposition for oesophageal atresia. *J Pediatr Surg* 2003; 38: 53–7; discussion 53.

34. Hanneman MJ, Sprangers MA, De Mik EL et al. Quality of life in patients with anorectal malformation or Hirschsprung's disease: Development of a disease-specific questionnaire. *Dis Colon Rectum* 2001; 44: 1650–60.

35. Bower WF, Wong EM, Yeung CK. Development of a validated quality of life tool specific to children with bladder dysfunction. *Neurourol Urodyn* 2006; 25: 221–7.

36. Goodwin DAJ, Boggs SR, Graham-Pole J. Development and validation of the pediatric oncology quality of life scale. *Psychol Assess* 1994; 6: 321.

37. Rabbett H, Elbadri A, Thwaites R et al. Quality of life in children with Crohn's disease. *J Pediatr Gastroenterol Nutr* 1996; 23: 528–33.

38. Dellenmark-Blom M, Chaplin JE, Gatzinsky V et al. Health-related quality of life experiences among children and adolescents born with esophageal atresia: Development of a condition-specific questionnaire for pediatric patients. *J Pediatr Surg* 2015; 51(4): 563–9.

39. Lewis CC, Pantell RH, Kieckhefer GM. Assessment of children's health status. Field test of new approaches. *Med Care* 1989; 27: S54–65.

40. Stein RE, Jessop DJ. Functional status II(R). A measure of child health status. *Med Care* 1990; 28, 1041–55.

41. Andres PL, Black-Schaffer RM, Ni P, Haley SM. Computer adaptive testing: A strategy for monitoring stroke rehabilitation across settings. *Top Stroke Rehabil* 2004; 11: 33–9.

42. Haley SM, Raczek AE, Coster WJ, Dumas HM, Fragala-Pinkham MA. Assessing mobility in children using a computer adaptive testing version of the pediatric evaluation of disability inventory. *Arch Phys Med Rehabil* 2005; 86: 932–9.

43. Kothari DH, Haley SM, Gill-Body KM, Dumas HM. Measuring functional change in children with acquired brain injury (ABI): Comparison of generic and ABI-specific scales using the Pediatric Evaluation of Disability Inventory (PEDI). *Phys Ther* 2003; 83: 776–85.

44. Msall ME, DiGaudio K, Rogers BT et al. The Functional Independence Measure for Children (WeeFIM). Conceptual basis and pilot use in children with developmental disabilities. *Clin Pediatr (Phila)* 1994; 33: 421–30.

45. Slomine BS, Brintzenhofeszoc K, Salorio CF et al. A method for performance evaluation using WeeFIM data collected for the Joint Commission on Accreditation of Healthcare Organizations' ORYX initiative: The 0.5 band control chart analysis. *Arch Phys Med Rehabil* 2004; 85: 512–6.

46. The collaborative UK ECMO (Extracorporeal Membrane Oxygenation) trial: Follow-up to 1 year of age. *Pediatrics* 1998; 101: E1.

47. Peetsold MG, Vonk-Noordegraaf A, Heij HH, Gemke RJ. Pulmonary function and exercise testing in adult survivors of congenital diaphragmatic hernia. *Pediatr Pulmonol* 2007; 42: 325–31.

48. Trachsel D, Selvadurai H, Bohn D, Langer JC, Coates AL. Long-term pulmonary morbidity in survivors of congenital diaphragmatic hernia. *Pediatr Pulmonol* 2005; 39: 433–9.

49. Gold M. Panel on cost-effectiveness in health and medicine. *Med Care* 1996; 34: DS197-9.

50. Torrance GW, Feeny D. Utilities and quality-adjusted life years. *Int J Technol Assess Health Care* 1989; 5: 559–75.

51. Spilker B. *Quality of Life Assessments in Clinical Trials*. New York: Raven Press, 1990.

52. Anderson JP, Kaplan RM, Berry CC, Bush JW, Rumbaut RG. Interday reliability of function assessment for a health status measure: The Quality of Well-Being scale. *Med Care* 1989; 27: 1076–87.
53. Torrance GW, Feeny DH, Furlong WJ, Barr RD, Zhang Y, Wang Q. Multiattribute utility function for a comprehensive health status classification system: Health Utilities Index Mark 2. *Med Care* 1996; 34(7): 702–22.
54. Feeny D, Furlong W, Barr RD, Torrance GW, Rosenbaum P, Weitzman S. A comprehensive multiattribute system for classifying the health status of survivors of childhood cancer. *J Clin Oncol* 1992; 10: 923–8.
55. Johnson JA, Coons SJ, Ergo A, Szava-Kovats G. Valuation of EuroQOL (EQ-5D) health states in an adult US sample. *Pharmacoeconomics* 1998; 13: 421–33.
56. Akobundu E, Ju J, Blatt L, Mullins CD. Cost-of-illness studies: A review of current methods. *Pharmacoeconomics* 2006; 24: 869–90.
57. Neumann PJ, Stone PW, Chapman RH, Sandberg EA, Bell CM. The quality of reporting in published cost-utility analyses, 1976–1997. *Ann Intern Med* 2000; 132: 964–72.
58. Ungar WJ. Paediatric health economic evaluations: A world view. *Healthc Q* 2007; 10: 134–40, 142.
59. Adams-Chapman I, Hansen NI, Shankaran S et al. Ten-year review of major birth defects in VLBW infants. *Pediatrics* 2013; 132: 49–61.
60. Statistics OFN. Mortality Statistics, Childhood, Infant and Perinatal. Review of the National Statistician on deaths in England and Wales, 2007. Series DH3 number 40 London: Office for National Statistics 2009.
61. JM R. Perinatal mortality and morbidity: Outcome of neonatal intensive care. In: Stringer MD, Oldham KT, Mouriquand PD (eds). *Pediatric Surgery and Urology: Long Term Outcomes*. Cambridge, UK: Cambridge University Press, 2006: 39–53.
62. Bornman J. The World Health Organisation's terminology and classification: Application to severe disability. *Disabil Rehabil* 2004; 26: 182–8.
63. Pinto-Martin JA, Riolo S, Cnaan A, Holzman C, Susser MW, Paneth N. Cranial ultrasound prediction of disabling and nondisabling cerebral palsy at age two in a low birth weight population. *Pediatrics* 1995; 95: 249–54.
64. DiBiasie A. Evidence-based review of retinopathy of prematurity prevention in VLBW and ELBW infants. *Neonatal Netw* 2006; 25: 393–403.
65. Robertson CM, Howarth TM, Bork DL, Dinu IA. Permanent bilateral sensory and neural hearing loss of children after neonatal intensive care because of extreme prematurity: A thirty-year study. *Pediatrics* 2009; 123: e797–807.
66. Bhutta AT, Cleves MA, Casey PH, Cradock MM, Anand KJ. Cognitive and behavioral outcomes of school-aged children who were born preterm: A meta-analysis. *JAMA* 2002; 288: 728–37.
67. Hollo O, Rautava P, Korhonen T, Helenius H, Kero P, Sillanpää M. Academic achievement of small-for-gestational-age children at age 10 years. *Arch Pediatr Adolesc Med* 2002; 156: 179–87.
68. Strauss RS. Adult functional outcome of those born small for gestational age: Twenty-six-year follow-up of the 1970 British Birth Cohort. *JAMA* 2000; 283: 625–32.
69. Buesing KA, Kilian AK, Schaible T, Loff S, Sumargo S, Neff KW. Extracorporeal membrane oxygenation in infants with congenital diaphragmatic hernia: Follow-up MRI evaluating carotid artery reocclusion and neurologic outcome. *AJR Am J Roentgenol* 2007; 188: 1636–42.
70. Chiu PP, Sauer C, Mihailovic A et al. The price of success in the management of congenital diaphragmatic hernia: Is improved survival accompanied by an increase in long-term morbidity. *J Pediatr Surg* 2006; 41: 888–92.
71. Jaillard SM, Pierrat V, Dubois A et al. Outcome at 2 years of infants with congenital diaphragmatic hernia: A population-based study. *Ann Thorac Surg* 2003; 75: 250–6.
72. Ludman L, Lansdown R, Spitz L. Factors associated with developmental progress of full term neonates who required intensive care. *Arch Dis Child* 1989; 64: 333–7.
73. Ludman L, Spitz L, Lansdown R. Intellectual development at 3 years of age of children who underwent major neonatal surgery. *J Pediatr Surg* 1993; 28: 130–4.
74. Ludman L. Gut feelings: A psychologist's 20-year journey with paediatric surgeons. *J R Soc Med* 2003; 96: 87–91.
75. Jaureguizar E, Vazquez J, Murcia J, Diez Pardo JA. Morbid musculoskeletal sequelae of thoracotomy for tracheoesophageal fistula. *J Pediatr Surg* 1985; 20: 511–4.
76. Chetcuti P, Myers NA, Phelan PD, Beasley SW, Dickens DR. Chest wall deformity in patients with repaired esophageal atresia. *J Pediatr Surg* 1989; 24: 244–7.
77. Smith ME, Marsh JH, Cotton RT, Myer CM. Voice problems after pediatric laryngotracheal reconstruction: Videolaryngostroboscopic, acoustic, and perceptual assessment. *Int J Pediatr Otorhinolaryngol* 1993; 25: 173–81.
78. Ayed AK, Owayed A. Pulmonary resection in infants for congenital pulmonary malformation. *Chest* 2003; 124: 98–101.
79. Caussade S, Zúñiga S, García C et al. [Pediatric lung resection. A case series and evaluation of postoperative lung function]. *Arch Bronconeumol* 2001; 37: 482–8.
80. Laros CD, Westermann CJ. Dilatation, compensatory growth, or both after pneumonectomy during childhood and adolescence. A thirty-year follow-up study. *J Thorac Cardiovasc Surg* 1987; 93: 570–6.

81. Naito Y, Beres A, Lapidus-Krol E, Ratjen F, Langer JC. Does earlier lobectomy result in better long-term pulmonary function in children with congenital lung anomalies? A prospective study. *J Pediatr Surg* 2012; 47: 852–6.

82. Spitz L, Kiely EM, Morecroft JA, Drake DP. Oesophageal atresia: At-risk groups for the 1990s. *J Pediatr Surg* 1994; 29: 723–5.

83. Romeo G, Zuccarello B, Proietto F, Romeo C. Disorders of the esophageal motor activity in atresia of the esophagus. *J Pediatr Surg* 1987; 22: 120–4.

84. SW B. Esophageal atresia: Surgical aspects. In: Stringer MD, Oldham KT, Mouriquand PD (eds). *Pediatric Surgery and Urology: Long Term Outcomes*. Camridge, UK: Cambridge University Press, 2006: 192–207.

85. Deurloo JA, Ekkelkamp S, Schoorl M, Heij HA, Aronson DC. Esophageal atresia: Historical evolution of management and results in 371 patients. *Ann Thorac Surg* 2002; 73: 267–72.

86. Rintala RJ, Pakarinen MP. Long-term outcome of esophageal anastomosis. *Eur J Pediatr Surg* 2013; 23: 219–25.

87. Schneider A, Michaud L, Gottrand F. Esophageal atresia: Metaplasia, Barrett. *Dis Esophagus* 2013; 26: 425–7.

88. Sistonen SJ, Koivusalo A, Nieminen U et al. Esophageal morbidity and function in adults with repaired esophageal atresia with tracheoesophageal fistula: A population-based long-term follow-up. *Ann Surg* 2010; 251: 1167–73.

89. Adzick NS, Fisher JH, Winter HS, Sandler RH, Hendren WH. Esophageal adenocarcinoma 20 years after esophageal atresia repair. *J Pediatr Surg* 1989; 24: 741–4.

90. Alfaro L, Bermas H, Fenoglio M, Parker R, Janik JS. Are patients who have had a tracheoesophageal fistula repair during infancy at risk for esophageal adenocarcinoma during adulthood. *J Pediatr Surg* 2005; 40: 719–20.

91. Deurloo JA, van Lanschot JJ, Drillenburg P, Aronson DC. Esophageal squamous cell carcinoma 38 years after primary repair of esophageal atresia. *J Pediatr Surg* 2001; 36: 629–30.

92. Esquibies AE, Zambrano E, Ziai J et al. Pulmonary squamous cell carcinoma associated with repaired congenital tracheoesophageal fistula and esophageal atresia. *Pediatr Pulmonol* 2010; 45: 202–4.

93. Jayasekera CS, Desmond PV, Holmes JA, Kitson M, Taylor AC. Cluster of 4 cases of esophageal squamous cell cancer developing in adults with surgically corrected esophageal atresia—Time for screening to start. *J Pediatr Surg* 2012; 47: 646–51.

94. LaQuaglia MP, Gray M, Schuster SR. Esophageal atresia and ante-thoracic skin tube esophageal conduits: Squamous cell carcinoma in the conduit 44 years following surgery. *J Pediatr Surg* 1987; 22: 44–7.

95. Pultrum BB, Bijleveld CM, de Langen ZJ, Plukker JT. Development of an adenocarcinoma of the esophagus 22 years after primary repair of a congenital atresia. *J Pediatr Surg* 2005; 40: e1–4.

96. Taylor AC, Breen KJ, Auldist A et al. Gastro-esophageal reflux and related pathology in adults who were born with esophageal atresia: A long-term follow-up study. *Clin Gastroenterol Hepatol* 2007; 5: 702–6.

97. Vergouwe FW, IJsselstijn H, Wijnen RM, Bruno MJ, Spaander MC. Screening and surveillance in esophageal atresia patients: Current knowledge and future perspectives. *Eur J Pediatr Surg* 2015; 25: 345–52.

98. Dingemann C, Meyer A, Kircher G et al. Long-term health-related quality of life after complex and/or complicated esophageal atresia in adults and children registered in a German patient support group. *J Pediatr Surg* 2014; 49: 631–8.

99. Legrand C, Michaud L, Salleron J et al. Long-term outcome of children with oesophageal atresia type III. *Arch Dis Child* 2012; 97: 808–11.

100. Lepeytre C, De Lagausie P, Merrot T, Baumstarck K, Oudyi M, Dubus JC. [Medium-term outcome, follow-up, and quality of life in children treated for type III esophageal atresia]. *Arch Pediatr* 2013; 20: 1096–104.

101. Peetsold MG, Heij HA, Deurloo JA, Gemke RJ. Health-related quality of life and its determinants in children and adolescents born with oesophageal atresia. *Acta Paediatr* 2010; 99: 411–7.

102. Friedmacher F, Puri P. Delayed primary anastomosis for management of long-gap esophageal atresia: A meta-analysis of complications and long-term outcome. *Pediatr Surg Int* 2012; 28: 899–906.

103. Puri P, Blake N, O'Donnell B, Guiney EJ. Delayed primary anastomosis following spontaneous growth of esophageal segments in esophageal atresia. *J Pediatr Surg* 1981; 16: 180–3.

104. Sri Paran T, Decaluwe D, Corbally M, Puri P. Long-term results of delayed primary anastomosis for pure oesophageal atresia: A 27-year follow up. *Pediatr Surg Int* 2007; 23: 647–51.

105. Puri P, Ninan GK, Blake NS, Fitzgerald RJ, Guiney EJ, O'Donnell B. Delayed primary anastomosis for esophageal atresia: 18 months' to 11 years' follow-up. *J Pediatr Surg* 1992; 27: 1127–30.

106. Foker JE, Kendall TC, Catton K, Khan KM. A flexible approach to achieve a true primary repair for all infants with esophageal atresia. *Semin Pediatr Surg* 2005; 14: 8–15.

107. Kimura K, Nishijima E, Tsugawa C et al. Multistaged extrathoracic esophageal elongation procedure for long gap esophageal atresia: Experience with 12 patients. *J Pediatr Surg* 2001; 36: 1725–7.

108. Holland AJ, Ron O, Pierro A et al. Surgical outcomes of esophageal atresia without fistula for 24 years at a single institution. *J Pediatr Surg* 2009; 44: 1928–32.

109. Arul GS, Parikh D. Oesophageal replacement in children. *Ann R Coll Surg Engl* 2008; 90: 7–12.

110. Jancelewicz T, Vu LT, Keller RL et al. Long-term surgical outcomes in congenital diaphragmatic hernia: Observations from a single institution. *J Pediatr Surg* 2010; 45: 155–60; discussion 160.

111. Tracy S, Chen C. Multidisciplinary long-term follow-up of congenital diaphragmatic hernia: A growing trend. *Semin Fetal Neonatal Med* 2014; 19: 385–91.

112. Nobuhara KK, Lund DP, Mitchell J, Kharasch V, Wilson JM. Long-term outlook for survivors of congenital diaphragmatic hernia. *Clin Perinatol* 1996; 23: 873–87.

113. Boloker J, Bateman DA, Wung JT, Stolar CJ. Congenital diaphragmatic hernia in 120 infants treated consecutively with permissive hypercapnea/spontaneous respiration/elective repair. *J Pediatr Surg* 2002; 37: 357–66.

114. Stege G, Fenton A, Jaffray B. Nihilism in the 1990s: the true mortality of congenital diaphragmatic hernia. *Pediatrics* 2003; 112: 532–5.

115. Downard CD, Jaksic T, Garza JJ et al. Analysis of an improved survival rate for congenital diaphragmatic hernia. *J Pediatr Surg* 2003; 38: 729–32.

116. Tsao K, Lally KP. The Congenital Diaphragmatic Hernia Study Group: A voluntary international registry. *Semin Pediatr Surg* 2008; 17: 90–7.

117. Morini F, Lally PA, Lally KP, Bagolan P. The Congenital Diaphragmatic Hernia Study Group Registry. *Eur J Pediatr Surg* 2015; 25: 488–96.

118. Fisher JC, Jefferson RA, Arkovitz MS, Stolar CJ. Redefining outcomes in right congenital diaphragmatic hernia. *J Pediatr Surg* 2008; 43: 373–9.

119. Muratore CS, Kharasch V, Lund DP et al. Pulmonary morbidity in 100 survivors of congenital diaphragmatic hernia monitored in a multidisciplinary clinic. *J Pediatr Surg* 2001; 36: 133–40.

120. Bagolan P, Morini F. Long-term follow up of infants with congenital diaphragmatic hernia. *Semin Pediatr Surg* 2007; 16: 134–44.

121. Crankson SJ, Al Jadaan SA, Namshan MA, Al-Rabeeah AA, Oda O. The immediate and long-term outcomes of newborns with congenital diaphragmatic hernia. *Pediatr Surg Int* 2006; 22: 335–40.

122. Gischler SJ, van der Cammen-van Zijp MH, Mazer P et al. A prospective comparative evaluation of persistent respiratory morbidity in esophageal atresia and congenital diaphragmatic hernia survivors. *J Pediatr Surg* 2009; 44: 1683–90.

123. Peetsold MG, Heij HA, Kneepkens CM, Nagelkerke AF, Huisman J, Gemke RJ. The long-term follow-up of patients with a congenital diaphragmatic hernia: A broad spectrum of morbidity. *Pediatr Surg Int* 2009; 25: 1–17.

124. Rocha GM, Bianchi RF, Severo M et al. Congenital diaphragmatic hernia. The post-neonatal period. Part II. *Eur J Pediatr Surg* 2008; 18: 307–12.

125. Koumbourlis AC, Wung JT, Stolar CJ. Lung function in infants after repair of congenital diaphragmatic hernia. *J Pediatr Surg* 2006; 41: 1716–21.

126. Bagolan P, Casaccia G, Crescenzi F, Nahom A, Trucchi A, Giorlandino C. Impact of a current treatment protocol on outcome of high-risk congenital diaphragmatic hernia. *J Pediatr Surg* 2004; 39: 313–8; discussion 313.

127. Falconer AR, Brown RA, Helms P, Gordon I, Baron JA. Pulmonary sequelae in survivors of congenital diaphragmatic hernia. *Thorax* 1990; 45: 126–9.

128. Wischermann A, Holschneider AM, Hübner U. Long-term follow-up of children with diaphragmatic hernia. *Eur J Pediatr Surg* 1995; 5: 13–18.

129. Van Meurs KP, Robbins ST, Reed VL et al. Congenital diaphragmatic hernia: Long-term outcome in neonates treated with extracorporeal membrane oxygenation. *J Pediatr* 1993; 122: 893–9.

130. Muratore CS, Utter S, Jaksic T, Lund DP, Wilson JM. Nutritional morbidity in survivors of congenital diaphragmatic hernia. *J Pediatr Surg* 2001; 36: 1171–6.

131. Chamond C, Morineau M, Gouizi G, Bargy F, Beaudoin S. Preventive antireflux surgery in patients with congenital diaphragmatic hernia. *World J Surg* 2008; 32: 2454–8.

132. Downard CD, Wilson JM. Current therapy of infants with congenital diaphragmatic hernia. *Semin Neonatol* 2003; 8: 215–21.

133. Koivusalo AI, Pakarinen MP, Lindahl HG, Rintala RJ. The cumulative incidence of significant gastroesophageal reflux in patients with congenital diaphragmatic hernia-a systematic clinical, pH-metric, and endoscopic follow-up study. *J Pediatr Surg* 2008; 43: 279–82.

134. Bouman NH, Koot HM, Tibboel D, Hazebroek FW. Children with congenital diaphragmatic hernia are at risk for lower levels of cognitive functioning and increased emotional and behavioral problems. *Eur J Pediatr Surg* 2000; 10: 3–7.

135. Cortes RA, Keller RL, Townsend T et al. Survival of severe congenital diaphragmatic hernia has morbid consequences. *J Pediatr Surg* 2005; 40: 36–45; discussion 45.

136. Masumoto K, Nagata K, Uesugi T, Yamada T, Taguchi T. Risk factors for sensorineural hearing loss in survivors with severe congenital diaphragmatic hernia. *Eur J Pediatr* 2007; 166: 607–12.

137. van den Hout L, Sluiter I, Gischler S et al. Can we improve outcome of congenital diaphragmatic hernia. *Pediatr Surg Int* 2009; 25: 733–43.

138. Robertson CM, Tyebkhan JM, Hagler ME, Cheung PY, Peliowski A, Etches PC. Late-onset, progressive sensorineural hearing loss after severe neonatal respiratory failure. *Otol Neurotol* 2002; 23: 353–6.

139. Dennett KV, Fligor BJ, Tracy S, Wilson JM, Zurakowski D, Chen C. Sensorineural hearing loss in congenital diaphragmatic hernia survivors is associated with postnatal management and not defect size. *J Pediatr Surg* 2014; 49: 895–9.

140. Partridge EA, Bridge C, Donaher JG et al. Incidence and factors associated with sensorineural and conductive hearing loss among survivors of congenital diaphragmatic hernia. *J Pediatr Surg* 2014; 49: 890–4; discussion 894.

141. Wilson MG, Riley P, Hurteau AM, Baird R, Puligandla PS. Hearing loss in congenital diaphragmatic hernia (CDH) survivors: Is it as prevalent as we think. *J Pediatr Surg* 2013; 48: 942–5.

142. Hille ET, van Straaten HI, Verkerk PH, Dutch NICUNHSWG. Prevalence and independent risk factors for hearing loss in NICU infants. *Acta Paediatr* 2007; 96: 1155–8.

143. Chen C, Jeruss S, Chapman JS et al. Long-term functional impact of congenital diaphragmatic hernia repair on children. *J Pediatr Surg* 2007; 42: 657–65.

144. Michel F, Baumstarck K, Gosselin A et al. Health-related quality of life and its determinants in children with a congenital diaphragmatic hernia. *Orphanet J Rare Dis* 2013; 8: 89.

145. Chen C, Jeruss S, Terrin N, Tighiouart H, Wilson JM, Parsons SK. Impact on family of survivors of congenital diaphragmatic hernia repair: A pilot study. *J Pediatr Surg* 2007; 42: 1845–52.

146. Kiely EM, Spitz L. Layered versus mass closure of abdominal wounds in infants and children. *Br J Surg* 1985; 72: 739–40.

147. Wilkins BM, Spitz L. Incidence of postoperative adhesion obstruction following neonatal laparotomy. *Br J Surg* 1986; 73: 762–4.

148. Festen C. Postoperative small bowel obstruction in infants and children. *Ann Surg* 1982; 196: 580–3.

149. Haricharan RN, Aprahamian CJ, Morgan TL, Harmon CM, Georgeson KE, Barnhart DC. Smaller scars— What is the big deal: A survey of the perceived value of laparoscopic pyloromyotomy. *J Pediatr Surg* 2008; 43: 92–6; discussion 96.

150. Bayat A, McGrouther DA, Ferguson MW. Skin scarring. *BMJ* 2003; 326: 88–92.

151. Georgeson K. Minimally invasive surgery in neonates. *Semin Neonatol* 2003; 8: 243–8.

152. McHoney M, Eaton S, Pierro A. Metabolic response to surgery in infants and children. *Eur J Pediatr Surg* 2009; 19: 275–85.

153. St Peter SD, Holcomb GW, Calkins CM et al. Open versus laparoscopic pyloromyotomy for pyloric stenosis: A prospective, randomized trial. *Ann Surg* 2006; 244: 363–70.

154. Henrich K, Huemmer HP, Reingruber B, Weber PG. Gastroschisis and omphalocele: Treatments and long-term outcomes. *Pediatr Surg Int* 2008; 24: 167–73.

155. Gamba P, Midrio P. Abdominal wall defects: Prenatal diagnosis, newborn management, and long-term outcomes. *Semin Pediatr Surg* 2014; 23: 283–90.

156. Gorra AS, Needelman H, Azarow KS, Roberts HJ, Jackson BJ, Cusick RA. Long-term neurodevelopmental outcomes in children born with gastroschisis: The tiebreaker. *J Pediatr Surg* 2012; 47: 125–9.

157. Harris EL, Hart SJ, Minutillo C et al. The long-term neurodevelopmental and psychological outcomes of gastroschisis: a cohort study. *J Pediatr Surg* 2015; 51(4): 549–53.

158. Koivusalo A, Lindahl H, Rintala RJ. Morbidity and quality of life in adult patients with a congenital abdominal wall defect: A questionnaire survey. *J Pediatr Surg* 2002; 37: 1594–601.

159. van Eijck FC, Wijnen RMH, van Goor H. The incidence and morbidity of adhesions after treatment of neonates with gastroschisis and omphalocele: A 30-year review. *J Pediatr Surg* 2008; 43: 479–83.

160. Lower AM, Hawthorn RJS, O'Brien F, Buchan S, Crowe AM. The impact of adhesions on hospital readmissions over ten years after 8849 open gynaecological operations: An assessment from the Surgical and Clinical Adhesions Research Study. *Int J Obstetr Gynaecol* 2000; 107: 855–62.

161. Berger AP, Hager J. Management of neonates with large abdominal wall defects and undescended testis. *Urology* 2006; 68: 175–8.

162. Yardley IE, Bostock E, Jones MO, Turnock RR, Corbett HJ, Losty PD. Congenital abdominal wall defects and testicular maldescent—A 10-year single-center experience. *J Pediatr Surg* 2012; 47: 1118–22.

163. Zaccara A, Iacobelli BD, Calzolari A et al. Cardiopulmonary performances in young children and adolescents born with large abdominal wall defects. *J Pediatr Surg* 2003; 38: 478–81.

164. Davies BW, Stringer MD. The survivors of gastroschisis. *Arch Dis Child* 1997; 77: 158–60.

165. Dessy LA, Fallico N, Trignano E, Tarallo M, Mazzocchi M. The double opposing "Y" technique for umbilical reconstruction after omphalectomy. *Ann Ital Chir* 2011; 82: 505–10.

166. Lee Y, Lee SH, Woo KV. Umbilical reconstruction using a modified inverted CV flap with conjoint flaps. *J Plast Surg Hand Surg* 2013; 47: 334–6.

167. van Eijck FC, Hoogeveen YL, Van Weel C, Rieu PNMA, Wijnen RMH. Minor and giant omphalocele: Long-term outcomes and quality of life. *J Pediatr Surg* 2009; 44: 1355–9.

168. Calzolari E, Volpato S, Bianchi F et al. Omphalocele and gastroschisis: A collaborative study of five Italian congenital malformation registries. *Teratology* 1993; 47: 47–55.

169. JS. Intestinal failure. In: Stringer MD, Oldham KT, Mouriquand PD (eds). *Pediatric Surgery and Urology: Long-Term Outcomes*. Cambridge, UK: Cambridge University Press, 2006: 362–73.

170. O'Keefe SJ, Buchman AL, Fishbein TM, Jeejeebhoy KN, Jeppesen PB, Shaffer J. Short bowel syndrome and intestinal failure: Consensus definitions and overview. *Clin Gastroenterol Hepatol* 2006; 4: 6–10.

171. Howard L, Malone M. Current status of home parenteral nutrition in the United States. *Transplant Proc* 1996; 28: 2691–5.

172. Winkler MF, DiMaria-Ghalili RA, Guenter P et al. Characteristics of a cohort of home parenteral nutrition patients at the time of enrollment in the sustain registry. *JPEN J Parenter Enteral Nutr* 2015; 40(8): 1140–9.

173. Candusso M, Faraguna D, Sperlì D, Dodaro N. Outcome and quality of life in paediatric home parenteral nutrition. *Curr Opin Clin Nutr Metab Care* 2002; 5: 309–14.

174. Jeppesen PB, Langholz E, Mortensen PB. Quality of life in patients receiving home parenteral nutrition. *Gut* 1999; 44: 844–52.

175. Reinshagen K, Kabs C, Wirth H et al. Long-term outcome in patients with short bowel syndrome after longitudinal intestinal lengthening and tailoring. *J Pediatr Gastroenterol Nutr* 2008; 47: 573–8.

176. O'Keefe SJ, Emerling M, Koritsky D et al. Nutrition and quality of life following small intestinal transplantation. *Am J Gastroenterol* 2007; 102: 1093–100.

177. Reyes J, Mazariegos GV, Bond GM et al. Pediatric intestinal transplantation: Historical notes, principles and controversies. *Pediatr Transplant* 2002; 6: 193–207.

178. Gaynor JJ, Kato T, Selvaggi G et al. The importance of analyzing graft and patient survival by cause of failure: An example using pediatric small intestine transplant data. *Transplantation* 2006; 81: 1133–40.

179. Kato T, Selvaggi G, Gaynor J et al. Expanded use of multivisceral transplantation for small children with concurrent liver and intestinal failure. *Transplant Proc* 2006; 38: 1705–8.

180. Sudan D, Horslen S, Botha J et al. Quality of life after pediatric intestinal transplantation: The perception of pediatric recipients and their parents. *Am J Transplant* 2004; 4: 407–13.

181. Peña A, Hong A. Advances in the management of anorectal malformations. *Am J Surg* 2000; 180: 370–6.

182. Peña A. Anorectal malformations. *Semin Pediatr Surg* 1995; 4: 35–47.

183. Bischoff A, Levitt MA, Peña A. Update on the management of anorectal malformations. *Pediatr Surg Int* 2013; 29: 899–904.

184. Levitt M, Peña A. Update on pediatric faecal incontinence. *Eur J Pediatr Surg* 2009; 19: 1–9.

185. Brandt ML, Daigneau C, Graviss EA, Naik-Mathuria B, Fitch ME, Washburn KK. Validation of the Baylor Continence Scale in children with anorectal malformations. *J Pediatr Surg* 2007; 42: 1015–21; discussion 1021.

186. Holschneider A, Hutson J, Peña A et al. Preliminary report on the International Conference for the Development of Standards for the Treatment of Anorectal Malformations. *J Pediatr Surg* 2005; 40: 1521–6.

187. Kyrklund K, Pakarinen MP, Koivusalo A, Rintala RJ. Bowel functional outcomes in females with perineal or vestibular fistula treated with anterior sagittal anorectoplasty: Controlled results into adulthood. *Dis Colon Rectum* 2015; 58: 97–103.

188. Kyrklund K, Pakarinen MP, Koivusalo A, Rintala RJ. Long-term bowel functional outcomes in rectourethral fistula treated with PSARP: Controlled results after 4–29 years of follow-up: A single-institution, cross-sectional study. *J Pediatr Surg* 2014; 49: 1635–42.

189. Rintala RJ. Congenital cloaca: Long-term follow-up results with emphasis on outcomes beyond childhood. *Semin Pediatr Surg* 2016; 25: 112–6.

190. Versteegh HP, van den Hondel D, IJsselstijn H, Wijnen RM, Sloots CE, de Blaauw I. Cloacal malformation patients report similar quality of life as female patients with less complex anorectal malformations. *J Pediatr Surg* 2016; 51: 435–9.

191. Catto-Smith AG, Trajanovska M, Taylor R. *Long Term Outcome After Surgery for Anorectal Malformation*. New York: Raven Press, 2013.

192. Hartman EE, Oort FJ, Aronson DC et al. Explaining change in quality of life of children and adolescents with anorectal malformations or Hirschsprung disease. *Pediatrics* 2007; 119: e374–83.

193. Grano C, Aminoff D, Lucidi F, Violani C. Disease-specific quality of life in children and adults with anorectal malformations. *Pediatr Surg Int* 2010; 26: 151–5.

194. van den Hondel D, Sloots CE, Bolt JM, Wijnen RM, de Blaauw I, IJsselstijn H. Psychosexual well-being after childhood surgery for anorectal malformation or Hirschsprung's disease. *J Sex Med* 2015; 12: 1616–25.

195. van den Hondel D, Aarsen FK, Wijnen RM, Sloots CE, IJsselstijn H. Children with congenital colorectal malformations often require special education or remedial teaching, despite normal intelligence. *Acta Paediatr* 2016; 105: e77–84.

196. Ludman L, Spitz L, Kiely EM. Social and emotional impact of faecal incontinence after surgery for anorectal abnormalities. *Arch Dis Child* 1994; 71: 194–200.

197. Ludman L, Spitz L. Psychosocial adjustment of children treated for anorectal anomalies. *J Pediatr Surg* 1995; 30: 495–9.

198. Diseth TH, Emblem R, Solbraa IB, Vandvik IH. A psychosocial follow-up of ten adolescents with low anorectal malformation. *Acta Paediatr* 1994; 83: 216–21.

199. Diseth TH, Egeland T, Emblem R. Effects of anal invasive treatment and incontinence on mental health and psychosocial functioning of adolescents with Hirschsprung's disease and low anorectal anomalies. *J Pediatr Surg* 1998; 33: 468–75.

200. Chen Y, Nah SA, Laksmi NK et al. Transanal endorectal pull-through versus transabdominal approach for Hirschsprung's disease: A systematic review and meta-analysis. *J Pediatr Surg* 2013; 48: 642–51.

201. De La Torre L, Langer JC. Transanal endorectal pull-through for Hirschsprung disease: Technique, controversies, pearls, pitfalls, and an organized approach to the management of postoperative obstructive symptoms. *Semin Pediatr Surg* 2010; 19: 96–106.

202. Neuvonen MI, Kyrklund K, Rintala RJ, Pakarinen MP. Bowel function and quality of life after transanal endorectal pull-through for Hirschsprung disease: Controlled outcomes up to adulthood. *Ann Surg* 2016; 265(3): 622–9.

203. Stensrud KJ, Emblem R, Bjørnland K. Functional outcome after operation for Hirschsprung disease— Transanal vs transabdominal approach. *J Pediatr Surg* 2010; 45: 1640–4.

204. Kim AC, Langer JC, Pastor AC et al. Endorectal pull-through for Hirschsprung's disease—A multicenter, long-term comparison of results: Transanal vs transabdominal approach. *J Pediatr Surg* 2010; 45: 1213–20.

205. Langer JC, Durrant AC, de la Torre L et al. One-stage transanal Soave pullthrough for Hirschsprung disease: A multicenter experience with 141 children. *Ann Surg* 2003; 238: 569–76.

206. Liem NT, Hau BD, Quynh TA, Anh VTH. Early and late outcomes of primary laparoscopic endorectal colon pull-through leaving a short rectal seromuscular sleeve for Hirschsprung disease. *J Pediatr Surg* 2009; 44: 2153–5.

207. Shankar KR, Losty PD, Lamont GL et al. Transanal endorectal coloanal surgery for Hirschsprung's disease: Experience in two centers. *J Pediatr Surg* 2000; 35: 1209–13.

208. Thomson D, Allin B, Long AM, Bradnock T, Walker G, Knight M. Laparoscopic assistance for primary transanal pull-through in Hirschsprung's disease: A systematic review and meta-analysis. *BMJ open* 2015; 5(3).

209. V PMA, Thi n HHU, Hi p PMN. Transanal one-stage endorectal pull-through for Hirschsprung disease: Experiences with 51 newborn patients. *Pediatr Surg Int* 2010; 26: 589–92.

210. van de Ven TJ, Sloots CEJ, Wijnen MHWA et al. Transanal endorectal pull-through for classic segment Hirschsprung's disease: With or without laparoscopic mobilization of the rectosigmoid. *J Pediatr Surg* 2013; 48: 1914–8.

211. Mills JL, Konkin DE, Milner R, Penner JG, Langer M, Webber EM. Long-term bowel function and quality of life in children with Hirschsprung's disease. *J Pediatr Surg* 2008; 43: 899–905.

212. Minford JL, Ram A, Turnock RR et al. Comparison of functional outcomes of Duhamel and transanal endorectal coloanal anastomosis for Hirschsprung's disease. *J Pediatr Surg* 2004; 39: 161–5; discussion 161.

213. Reding R, de Ville de Goyet J, Gosseye S et al. Hirschsprung's disease: A 20-year experience. *J Pediatr Surg* 1997; 32: 1221–5.

214. Yanchar NL, Soucy P. Long-term outcome after Hirschsprung's disease: Patients' perspectives. *J Pediatr Surg* 1999; 34: 1152–60.

215. Menezes M, Corbally M, Puri P. Long-term results of bowel function after treatment for Hirschsprung's disease: A 29-year review. *Pediatr Surg Int* 2006; 22: 987–90.

216. Granström AL, Danielson J, Husberg B, Nordenskjöld A, Wester T. Adult outcomes after surgery for Hirschsprung's disease: Evaluation of bowel function and quality of life. *J Pediatr Surg* 2015; 50: 1865–9.

217. Menezes M, Pini Prato A, Jasonni V, Puri P. Long-term clinical outcome in patients with total colonic aganglionosis: A 31-year review. *J Pediatr Surg* 2008; 43: 1696–9.

218. Tsuji H, Spitz L, Kiely EM, Drake DP, Pierro A. Management and long-term follow-up of infants with total colonic aganglionosis. *J Pediatr Surg* 1999; 34, 158–61; discussion 162.

219. Wildhaber BE, Teitelbaum DH, Coran AG. Total colonic Hirschsprung's disease: A 28-year experience. *J Pediatr Surg* 2005; 40: 203–6; discussion 206.

220. Rintala RJ, Pakarinen MP. Long-term outcomes of Hirschsprung's disease. *Semin Pediatr Surg* 2012; 21: 336–43.

221. Marquez TT, Acton RD, Hess DJ, Duval S, Saltzman DA. Comprehensive review of procedures for total colonic aganglionosis. *J Pediatr Surg* 2009; 44: 257–65; discussion 265.

222. Teitelbaum DH, Coran AG. Enterocolitis. *Semin Pediatr Surg* 1998; 7: 162–9.

224. Hoehner JC, Ein SH, Shandling B, Kim PC. Long-term morbidity in total colonic aganglionosis. *J Pediatr Surg* 1998; 33: 961–5; discussion 965.

225. Ludman L, Spitz L, Tsuji H, Pierro A. Hirschsprung's disease: Functional and psychological follow up comparing total colonic and rectosigmoid aganglionosis. *Arch Dis Child* 2002; 86: 348–51.

226. Moore SW, Albertyn R, Cywes S. Clinical outcome and long-term quality of life after surgical correction of Hirschsprung's disease. *J Pediatr Surg* 1996; 31: 1496–502.

Index

Page numbers followed by f and t indicate figures and tables, respectively.